CONTENTS

W9-CFJ-669

EDITION
2

Lehne's

Pharmacotherapeutics

for Advanced Practice Nurses and Physician Assistants

Laura D. Rosenthal, DNP, ACNP, FAANP

Associate Professor, College of Nursing
University of Colorado, Anschutz Medical Campus
Denver, Colorado

Jacqueline Rosenjack Burchum, DNSc, FNP-BC, CNE

Associate Professor, College of Nursing
Department of Advanced Practice and Doctoral Studies
University of Tennessee Health Science Center
Memphis, Tennessee

ELSEVIER

Elsevier
3251 Riverport Lane
St. Louis, Missouri 63043

LEHNE'S PHARMACOTHERAPEUTICS FOR ADVANCED PRACTICE NURSES
AND PHYSICIAN ASSISTANTS, SECOND EDITION   ISBN: 978-0-323-55495-4

Previous edition copyrighted 2018.

Library of Congress Control Number: 2019940236

Executive Content Strategist: Lee Henderson
Senior Content Development Manager: Luke Held
Senior Content Development Specialist: Jennifer Wade
Publishing Services Manager: Julie Eddy
Senior Project Manager: Rachel E. McMullen
Design Direction: Renee Duenow

Printed in Canada

Last digit is the print number: 9   8   7   6   5   4

Working together
to grow libraries in
developing countries

www.elsevier.com • www.bookaid.org

*In remembrance of Victoria "Vicki" Erickson;
a nursing leader, mentor, colleague, and friend.
You are missed by many.*

LDR

*To my remarkable students.
It excites me to know that the future of nursing
is in your most capable hands.*

JRB

ACKNOWLEDGMENTS

We would like to acknowledge the support of our colleagues at Elsevier, including Lee Henderson, Executive Content Strategist; Jennifer Wade, Senior Content Development Specialist; and Rachel McMullen, Senior Project Manager. Finally, we would like to acknowledge the foundational work by Richard A. Lehne. His dedication to the Lehne Pharmacology series made this text possible.

ABOUT THE AUTHORS

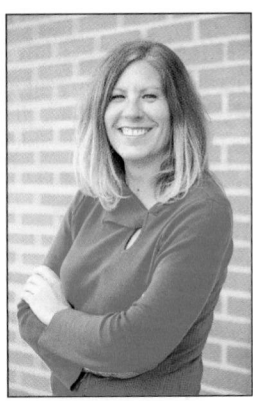

Laura D. Rosenthal, DNP, ACNP, FAANP, has been a registered nurse since graduating with her Bachelor of Science degree in Nursing from the University of Michigan in 2000. She completed her Master of Science degree in Nursing in 2006 at Case Western Reserve University in Cleveland, Ohio. She finished her nursing education at the University of Colorado, College of Nursing, graduating with her Doctor of Nursing Practice degree in 2011. Her background includes practice in acute care and inpatient medicine. While working as a nurse practitioner at the University of Colorado Hospital, she assisted in developing one of the first fellowships for advanced practice clinicians in hospital medicine.

Dr. Rosenthal serves as an associate professor at the University of Colorado, College of Nursing, where she teaches within the undergraduate and graduate programs and serves as the director of the DNP program. She received the Dean's Award for Excellence in Teaching in 2013 and the AANP State Award for Excellence in 2015.

In her spare time, Dr. Rosenthal enjoys running, skiing, and fostering retired greyhounds for Colorado Greyhound Adoption.

Jacqueline Rosenjack Burchum, DNSc, FNP-BC, CNE, has been a family nurse practitioner for over 20 years since earning her Masters of Science in Nursing degree in 1996. She completed her Doctor of Nursing Science degree in 2002. As a nurse practitioner, Dr. Burchum's work centers on addressing the needs of vulnerable populations with a special focus on immigrant and refugee populations.

Dr. Burchum currently serves as an associate professor for the University of Tennessee Health Science Center (UTHSC) College of Nursing. She is credentialed as a certified nurse educator (CNE) by the National League for Nursing. She is a three-time recipient of the UTHSC Student Government Association's Excellence in Teaching Award and a recipient of the 2014 UT Alumni Association's Outstanding Teacher Award. Dr. Burchum was also the 2016–2017 Faculty Innovation Scholar for the UTHSC Teaching and Learning Center.

Dr. Burchum has a special interest in online teaching and program quality. To this end, she serves as an on-site evaluator for the Commission on Collegiate Nursing Education (CCNE), a national agency that accredits nursing education programs. In addition, she is a Master Reviewer for Quality Matters, a program that certifies the quality of online courses.

Her favorite activities involve spending time with family. She also enjoys designing and making quilts.

CONTRIBUTOR AND REVIEWERS

CONTRIBUTOR

Courtney Quiring, BSP, BCGP
College of Pharmacy and Nutrition
University of Saskatchewan
Saskatoon, Saskatchewan, Canada
Appendix: Canadian Drug Information

REVIEWERS

Laurie M. Connors, DNP, MS
Assistant Professor
School of Nursing
Vanderbilt University
Nashville, Tennessee

Abimbola Farinde, PharmD
Professor of Health Care Administration
College of Business
Columbian Southern University
Orange Beach, Alabama

Ashley N. Fort, MS, PA-C
Assistant Professor
PA Program
LSUH Shreveport School of Allied Health Professions
Shreveport, Louisiana

James Graves, PharmD
Clinical Pharmacist
Inpatient Pharmacy
University of Missouri Columbia
Columbia, Missouri

Margaret Hammersla, BSN, MS, PhD, CRNP-A
Senior Director, DNP Program; Assistant Professor
Organizational Systems and Adult Health
University of Maryland School of Nursing
Baltimore, Maryland

Bradley R. Harrell, DNP, APRN, ACNP-BC
Assistant Professor
Loewenberg College of Nursing
The University of Memphis
Memphis, Tennessee

Robert Hawkes, MSPA, PA-C
Program Director
Master of Physician Assistant Studies
Florida Gulf Coast University
Ft. Myers, Florida

Leslie Jones Higgins, PhD, APRN, FNP-BC
Professor
Graduate Nursing Program
Belmont University School of Nursing
Nashville, Tennessee

Kathleen S. Jordan, DNP, MS, FNP-BC, ENP-BC, SANE-P
Clinical Assistant Professor
School of Nursing
The University of North Carolina at Charlotte;
Nurse Practitioner
Emergency Department
Mid-Atlantic Emergency Medicine Associates
Charlotte, North Carolina

Kathy Kemle, MS, PA-C, DFAAPA
Clinical Assistant Professor
Family Medicine
Medical Center of Central Georgia/Navicent Health
Mercer University School of Medicine
Macon, Georgia

Lisa Miklush PhD, RN, CNS
Adjunct Graduate Faculty
School of Nursing & Human Physiology
Gonzaga University
Spokane, Washington

Mary Alice Momeyer, DNP, APRN-CNP
Assistant Professor of Clinical Nursing
The Ohio State University
Columbus, Ohio

Patricia Neafsey, PhD
Professor Emeritus
School of Nursing
University of Connecticut
Storrs, Connecticut

Stephanie Neary, MPA, MMS, PA-C
Instructor, Didactic Coordinator
General Internal Medicine, PA Online Program
Yale University
New Haven, Connecticut

Teresa R. Preston, MBA, MPAS, PA-C, APWH-PA
Associate Professor, Program Director
Department of Physician Assistant Studies
Christian Brothers University
Memphis, Tennessee

James Van Rhee, MS, PA-C
Program Director, Yale Physician Assistant Online Program
Yale School of Medicine
New Haven, Connecticut

Meera K. Shah, PharmD
Clinical Pharmacist
University of Missouri, Kansas City
Kansas City, Missouri

Paula Denise Silver, BS Biology, PharmD
Medical Instructor
Medical Assisting/LPN/RN
ECPI University, School of Health Science
Newport News, Virginia

Cynthia Ann Smith, DNP, CNN-NP, FNP-BC, APRN, FNKF
Nurse Practitioner
Renal Consultants, PLLC
South Charleston, West Virginia

Jennifer K. Sofie, DNP, FNP, ANP
Associate Clinical Professor
College of Nursing
Montana State University
Bozeman, Montana

Laura Steadman, EdD, CRNP, MSN, RN
Assistant Professor
School of Nursing
The University of Alabama at Birmingham
Birmingham, Alabama;
Family Nurse Practitioner
Adult/Acute Health
Chronic Care and Foundations
Birmingham, Alabama

Mariya Tankimovich, DNP, MSN, APRN, FNP-C, CNE
Assistant Professor, FNP Track Coordinator for Clinical
Education, Simulation, and Advising
Graduate Programs
UTHealth
Houston, Texas

Daniel T. Vetrosky, PA-C, PhD, DFAAPA
Physician Assistant
Associate Professor (Ret)
Department of Physician Assistant Studies
Pat Capps Covey College of Allied Health Professions
University of South Alabama
Mobile, Alabama

Donna Warder, DNP, MS, FNP-BC, CNM
Teaching Associate
Health Systems Science
University of Illinois Chicago
College of Nursing
Chicago, Illinois

Allison White, PharmD
Pharmacist
Kansas City, Missouri

Jack A. P. Yensen, BSc (Hons), PhD, RN, MN
Instructor
DNP Program, School of Nursing
Samuel Merritt University
Oakland, California

Lisa M. Young, DNP, APRN
Assistant Professor
College of Nursing and Health Sciences
Ashland University
Mansfield, Ohio

Pharmacology and pharmacotherapeutics pervade all phases of advanced practice and relate directly to patient care and education. Despite their importance, many students—and even some teachers—are often uncomfortable with these subjects because traditional texts have stressed *memorizing* rather than *understanding*. In this text, the guiding principle is to establish further understanding of drugs and their use in patient care.

This text has two major objectives: to help you, the advanced practice student, establish a continued knowledge base in the basic science of drugs; and to show you how that knowledge can be applied in clinical practice. The methods by which these goals are achieved are described here.

LAYING FOUNDATIONS IN BASIC PRINCIPLES

To understand drugs, you need a solid foundation in basic pharmacologic principles. To help you establish that foundation, the book has major chapters on the following topics: basic principles that apply to all drugs (Chapters 4 through 7), basic principles of drug therapy across the life span (Chapters 8 through 10), basic principles of neuropharmacology (Chapter 11), and basic principles of antimicrobial therapy (Chapter 70).

REVIEWING PHYSIOLOGY AND PATHOPHYSIOLOGY

To understand the actions of a drug, it is useful to understand the biologic systems that the drug influences. Accordingly, for all major drug families, relevant physiology and pathophysiology are reviewed. In almost all cases, these reviews are presented at the beginning of each chapter rather than in a systems review at the beginning of a unit. This juxtaposition of pharmacology, physiology, and pathophysiology is designed to help you understand how these topics interrelate.

TEACHING THROUGH PROTOTYPES

Within each drug family, we can usually identify a prototype—that is, a drug that embodies characteristics shared by all members of the group. Because other family members are similar to the prototype, to know the prototype is to know the basic properties of all family members.

The benefits of teaching through prototypes can be appreciated with an example. Let's consider the nonsteroidal antiinflammatory drugs (NSAIDs), a family that includes aspirin, ibuprofen (Motrin), naproxen (Aleve), celecoxib (Celebrex), and more than 20 other drugs. Traditionally, information on these drugs is presented in a series of paragraphs describing each drug in turn. When attempting to study from such a list, you are likely to learn many drug names and little else; the important concept of similarity among family members is easily lost. In this text, the family prototype—aspirin—is discussed first and in depth. After this, the small ways in which individual NSAIDs differ from aspirin are pointed out. Not only is this approach more efficient than the traditional approach, it is also more effective, in that similarities among family members are emphasized.

USING CLINICAL REALITY TO PRIORITIZE CONTENT

This book contains two broad categories of information: pharmacology (i.e., basic science about drugs) and therapeutics (i.e., clinical use of drugs). To ensure that content is clinically relevant, we use evidence-based treatment guidelines as a basis for deciding what to stress and what to play down. Unfortunately, clinical practice is a moving target: when effective new drugs are introduced, and when clinical trials reveal new benefits or new risks of older drugs, the guidelines change—and so we have to work hard to keep this book current. Despite our best efforts, the book and clinical reality may not always agree. Some treatments discussed here will be considered inappropriate before the second edition comes out. Furthermore, in areas where controversy exists, the treatments discussed here may be considered inappropriate by some clinicians right now.

SPECIAL FEATURES

- **Summary of Key Prescribing Considerations:** This summary provides guidance for safe prescribing practices and includes information such as baseline data collection, monitoring needs, identification of high-risk patients, and evaluation for therapeutic effects.
- **Prototype Drugs:** Denoted in teal boxes; these key drugs are easy to locate.
- **Black Box Warnings:** This feature draws the reader's attention to important safety concerns related to contraindications and adverse effects.
- **Patient Education:** These boxes offer important information to provide to patients regarding their therapy.
- **Patient-Centered Care Across the Life Span:** Tables in many chapters highlight care concerns for patients throughout their lives, from infancy to older adulthood.
- **Canadian trade names** are identified by a **maple-leaf icon.**

TEACHING SUPPLEMENTS FOR INSTRUCTORS

- The Instructor Resources for the first edition are available online and include a **Test Bank,** a **PowerPoint Collection,** and an **Image Collection.**

STUDENT RESOURCES

- New online student resources include one case study per textbook section.

WAYS TO USE THIS TEXTBOOK

Thanks to its focus on essentials, this text is especially well suited to serve as the primary text for a course dedicated specifically to pharmacology and pharmacotherapeutics. In addition, the book's focused approach makes it a valuable resource for pharmacologic instruction within an integrated curriculum and for self-directed learning by students, teachers, and practitioners.

How is this focus achieved? Four primary techniques are employed: (1) teaching through prototypes, (2) using standard print for essential information and small print for secondary information, (3) limiting discussion of adverse effects and drug interactions to information that matters most, and (4) using evidence-based clinical guidelines to determine what content to stress.

Students often feel that pharmacology is one of the most difficult classes to master. Pharmacotherapeutics can be an unpopular subject because of the vast and rapidly changing area of content. We hope that this book makes the subjects of pharmacology and pharmacotherapeutics easier for you to master and more enjoyable for you to understand by allowing you to focus on the most important, umbrella concepts of pharmacology and pharmacotherapeutics as they relate to the care and safety of patients and the management of their health problems.

Laura D. Rosenthal
Jacqueline Rosenjack Burchum

CONTENTS

UNIT X Drugs for Endocrine Disorders

1

Prescriptive Authority

Our purpose in writing this book is to prepare advanced practice providers to provide safe and competent medication therapy to patients. This role requires the ability to select, prescribe, and manage medications. In this chapter we examine issues surrounding prescriptive authority and how those issues affect this fundamental aspect of comprehensive patient care.

WHAT IS PRESCRIPTIVE AUTHORITY?

Prescriptive authority is the legal right to prescribe drugs. Full prescriptive authority affords the legal right to prescribe independently and without limitation. Physicians have full prescriptive authority. For nonphysician providers, the degree of prescriptive authority varies. Some have full prescriptive authority; however, for many, prescriptive authority is restricted. Limitations are generally tied to oversight by a doctor of medicine (MD) or doctor of osteopathy (DO) as part of the provider's scope of practice.

Recall that there are two components of prescriptive authority: (1) the right to prescribe independently and (2) the right to prescribe without limitation. The provider who prescribes independently is not subject to rules requiring physician supervision or collaboration. The provider who prescribes without limitation may prescribe any drugs, including controlled drugs, with the exception of schedule I drugs, which have no current medical use.

Full practice authority is sometimes interpreted differently for advanced practice registered nurses (APRNs) and physician assistants (PAs) because supervisory requirements vary for the two professions. PAs are required to have an affiliation with a physician in order to practice and prescribe. All PAs, including those in a solo practice, must establish a relationship with physician who serves in a supervisory or collaborative role and who can be reached by telephone or other means of telecommunication. (See *PA State Laws and Regulations* available at https://www.aapa.org/download/28349 for additional information.) If the PA–physician arrangement does not limit drugs that may be prescribed and if the law allows the PA to prescribe schedule II to V drugs, the PA may enjoy a type of quasi-full prescriptive authority. Indeed, some have referred to this as full prescriptive authority; however, the issue of being affiliated to a physician still applies. Hence PAs do not have the legal right to prescribe without the PA–physician arrangement. Even for those in solo practice, there is always the possibility of dissolution of the PA–physician arrangement. In the event this occurs, the PA must affiliate with another physician or physician group to continue prescribing.

Whether APRNs possess full prescriptive authority depends on their legal right to prescribe without a supervisory or collaborative requirement. APRNs are *educated* to practice and prescribe independently without supervision; however, some state laws require that they practice in collaboration with or under the supervision of a physician. In these situations, some physicians limit the types of drugs that the APRN can prescribe. State laws may place additional restrictions with regard to controlled drugs.

Table 1.1 provides prescriptive authority status for APRNs. Table 1.2 provides prescriptive authority status for PAs. Information regarding the right to prescribe controlled drugs is available at http://www.deadiversion.usdoj.gov/drugreg/practioners.

PRESCRIPTIVE AUTHORITY REGULATIONS

Prescriptive authority is determined by state law. As a result of differences from state to state, advanced practice providers may have full prescriptive authority in some states yet face significant restrictions in other states. The stark differences particularly affect providers who serve in *locum tenens* staffing positions or who have practices in two contiguous states.

The regulation of prescriptive authority is under the jurisdiction of a health professional board. This may be the State Board of Nursing, the State Board of Medicine, or the State Board of Pharmacy, as determined by each state.

Although the federal government controls drug regulation, it has no control over prescriptive authority. However, several organizations have appealed for changes that would place scope of practice and prescriptive authority under federal regulation in an effort to expand prescriptive authority and the scope of practice of advanced practice providers. For example, National Academy of Medicine (formerly the Institute of Medicine or IOM) advocated for federal regulation in their report, *The Future of Nursing: Focus on Scope of Practice.* After noting problems with the "patchwork of state regulations," they wrote:

> *The federal government has a compelling interest in the regulatory environment for health care professions because of its responsibility to patients covered by federal programs. ... Equally important is the responsibility to all American taxpayers who fund the care provided under these programs to ensure that their tax dollars are spent efficiently. ... Scope-of-practice regulations in all states should reflect the full extent not only of nurses but of each profession's*

TABLE 1.1   Advanced Practice Registered Nurse Prescriptive Authority by State

State	Authorized to Prescribe	Scheduled Drugs	Type of Practice (Independent or Physician Collaboration Required)
AL	CNM, CNP	III–V, limited II	Collaborative
AK	CNM, CNP, CNS, CRNA	II–V	Independent
AZ	CNM, CNP	II–V	Independent
AR	CNM, CNP, CNS, CRNA	III–V	Collaborative
CA	CNM, CNP	II–V	Collaborative
CO	CNM, CNP, CNS, CRNA	II–V	Independent
CT	CNM, CNP, CRNA	II–V	Collaborative
DE	CNM, CNP, CNS, CRNA	II–V	Collaborative
FL	CNM, CNP, CRNA	III–V	Collaborative
GA	CNM, CNP, CNS, CRNA	III–V	Collaborative
HI	CNM, CNP, CNS, CRNA	II–V	Independent
ID	CNM, CNP, CNS, CRNA	II–V	Independent
IL	CNM, CNP, CNS, CRNA	III–V	Collaborative
IN	CNM, CNP, CNS	II–V (within limits)	Collaborative
IA	CNM, CNP, CNS, CRNA	II–V	Independent
KS	CNM, CNP, CNS	II–V	Collaborative
KY	CNM, CNP, CNS, CRNA	II–V	Collaborative
LA	CNM, CNP, CNS, CRNA	II–V	Collaborative
ME	CNM, CNP	II–V	Independent
MD	CNM, CNP	II–V	Independent
MA	CNM, CNP, CNS, CRNA	II–V	Collaborative: CNP, CNS, CRNA; Independent: CNM
MI	CNM, CNP, CRNA	III–V	Collaborative
MN	CNM, CNP, CNS, CRNA	II–V	Independent
MS	CNM, CNP, CRNA	II–V	Collaborative
MO	CNM, CNP, CNS, CRNA	III–V	Collaborative
MT	CNM, CNP, CNS, CRNA	II–V	Independent
NE	CNM, CNP, CRNA	II–V	Collaborative
NV	CNM, CNP, CNS	III–V	Independent
NH	CNM, CNP, CNS, CRNA	II–V	Independent
NJ	CNP, CNS, CRNA	II–V	Collaborative
NM	CNP, CNS, CRNA	II–V	Independent
NY	CNM, CNP	II–V	Independent
NC	CNM, CNP	II–V	Collaborative
ND	CNM, CNP, CNS, CRNA	II–V	Independent
OH	CNM, CNP, CNS	II–V	Collaborative
OK	CNM, CNP, CNS	III–V	Collaborative
OR	CNM, CNP, CNS, CRNA	II–V	Independent
PA	CNP	II–V	Collaborative
RI	CNP, CNS, CRNA	II–V	Independent
SC	CNM, CNP, CNS	III–V	Collaborative
SD	CNM, CNP	II–V	Independent
TN	CNM, CNP, CNS, CRNA	II–V	Collaborative
TX	CNM, CNP, CNS, CRNA	III–V	Collaborative
UT	CNM, CNP, CNS, CRNA	III–V, II if collaborative practice	Independent
VT	CNM, CNP, CNS, CRNA	II–V	Collaborative
VA	CNM, CNP, CNS	II–V	Collaborative
WA	CNM, CNP, CRNA	II–V	Independent
WV	CNM, CNP, CNS, CRNA	III–V	Collaborative
WI	CNM, CNP, CNS, CRNA	II–V	Collaborative
WY	CNM, CNP, CNS, CRNA	II–V	Independent

CNM, Certified nurse midwife; *CNP*, certified nurse practitioner; *CNS*, clinical nurse specialist; *CRNA*, certified registered nurse anesthetist.
Source: State Boards of Nursing; November 2018.

TABLE 1.2 Physician Assistants Prescriptive Authority by State

State	Scheduled Drugs	Required Physician Affiliation for Practice
AL	II–V	Supervisory
AK	II–V	Collaborative
AZ	II–V	Supervisory
AR	III–V	Supervisory
CA	II–V	Supervisory
CO	II–V	Supervisory
CT	II–V	Supervisory
DE	II–V	Supervisory
FL	II–V	Supervisory
GA	III–V	Supervisory
HI	III–V	Supervisory
ID	II–V	Supervisory
IL	II–V	Collaborative
IN	II–V	Supervisory
IA	II–V	Supervisory
KS	II–V	Supervisory
KY	No	Supervisory
LA	II–V	Supervisory
ME	II–V	Supervisory
MD	II–V	Supervisory
MA	II–V	Supervisory
MI	II–V	Participating[a]
MN	II–V	Supervisory
MS	II–V	Supervisory
MO	III–V	Supervisory
MT	III–V	Supervisory
NE	II–V	Supervisory
NV	II–V	Collaborative
NH	II–V	Supervisory
NJ	II–V	Supervisory
NM	II–V	Varies according to practice
NY	II–V	Supervisory
NC	II–V	Supervisory
ND	II–V	Supervisory
OH	II–V	Supervisory
OK	II–V	Supervisory
OR	II–V	Supervisory
PA	II–V	Supervisory
RI	II–V	Supervisory
SC	II–V	Supervisory
SD	II–V	Supervisory
TN	II–V	Supervisory
TX	III–V	Supervisory
UT	II–V	Supervisory
VT	II–V	Supervisory
VA	II–V	Supervisory
WA	II–V	Supervisory
WV	III–V	Collaborative
WI	II–V	Supervisory
WY	II–V	Supervisory

[a]Physician assistants (PAs) are required to have a PA–physician relationship that is detailed in a written practice agreement.
Source: American Medical Association. Physician assistant scope of practice; 2018. Available at: https://www.ama-assn.org/sites/ama-assn.org/files/corp/media-browser/public/arc-public/state-law-physician-assistant-scope-practice.pdf.
Drug Enforcement Agency. Mid-level practitioners—controlled substance authority by discipline within state; 2018. https://www.deadiversion.usdoj.gov/drugreg/practioners/mlp_by_state.pdf.

education and training. (http://www.nationalacademies.org/hmd/~/media/Files/Report%20Files/2010/The-Future-of-Nursing/Nursing%20Scope%20of%20Practice%202010%20Brief.pdf)

THE CASE FOR FULL PRESCRIPTIVE AUTHORITY

Advanced practice providers complete rigorous programs of study, largely in accredited programs that meet stringent national standards. Although there are differences in each program, all include common components. For example, they require extensive education focused on assessment, diagnosis, and management of health problems. Diagnostic reasoning, critical thinking, and procedural skills are evaluated in both didactic and clinical courses. National examinations validate the ability to provide safe and competent care. Licensure ensures that providers comply with standards of practice that promote public health and safety. In short, advanced practice providers are prepared to fully implement the advanced practice role in their profession.

Limited prescriptive authority creates numerous barriers to quality, affordable, and accessible patient care. For example, restrictions on the distance of the APRN or PA from the physician providing supervision or collaboration may prevent outreach to areas of greatest need. A requirement to obtain the physician's cosignature on prescriptions can increase patient waits. Despite the use of terms such as *collaborative* arrangement, these relationships create a situation in which one partner holds the power. In the event of dissolution of the arrangement, the ultimate loss is commonly assumed by the advanced practice provider rather than the physician.

In 2010, the Association of American Medical Colleges commissioned a report projecting the future of the physician workforce. The report, *The Complexities of Physician Supply and Demand: Projections from 2013 to 2025,* was released in 2015. Several of the key findings have important implications for nonphysician providers.

- By 2025, the shortage of physicians will range between 46,100 and 90,400. In primary care alone, a 12,500 to 31,100 physician shortage is anticipated. *(The lower numbers on these ranges reflect an increase in APRNs and PAs used to help offset physician shortages.)*
- As the Affordable Care Act is fully implemented, the demand for provider coverage will increase.

These findings echo the dire circumstances reported in the 2013 Department of Health and Human Services report, *Projecting the Supply and Demand for Primary Care Practitioners through 2020,* which concluded that full utilization of nurse practitioners and PAs can reduce the physician shortage.

In this scenario, in which physician demands are excessive, requiring oversight for other providers may be untenable. To adequately meet the demands for future health care needs, APRNs and PAs will need broader practice privileges than some states currently allow. This includes an imperative to afford full prescriptive authority.

PRESCRIPTIVE AUTHORITY AND RESPONSIBILITY

The possession of full prescriptive authority requires a somber responsibility. Whether you are reading this book as a student or as a practicing provider, it is essential to recognize the full obligation this requires. The safe and competent practice of prescribing and managing medications requires a sound understanding of drugs and the conditions that they are used to manage. It is our goal to help you lay that foundation. In the coming chapters, you will read about rational drug selection, writing prescriptions, and promoting positive outcomes. Then we will delve into the heart of pharmacology through a study of pharmacokinetics and pharmacodynamics as we prepare you for the study of individual drug categories.

Rational Drug Selection and Prescription Writing

RESPONSIBILITY OF PRESCRIBING

As a practitioner, you will assume great responsibility when caring for patients. The ability to prescribe medications is both a privilege and a burden. Although you may be familiar with many drugs through your previous practice as a registered nurse or other member of the health care field, giving medications and prescribing medications are two very different things. There are many different issues to consider when writing a prescription, many of which we discuss in this chapter or in the previous chapter regarding prescriptive authority.

The best way to keep your patients (and yourself) safe is to be prudent and deliberate in your decision-making process. Have a documented provider–patient relationship with the person for whom you are prescribing. Do not prescribe medications for family or friends or for yourself. Document a thorough history and physical examination in your records. Include any discussions you have with the patient regarding risk factors, side effects, or therapy options. Have a documented plan regarding drug monitoring or titration, if applicable. If you consult additional providers, note that you did so. Finally, use the references provided in the following box to assist in safely and rationally choosing one medication over another.

DRUG SELECTION

Cost

The cost of medications in the United States has risen steeply within the past 10 years. Increasing cost is related to multiple factors, including corporate competition. It is also noted that one of the reasons people do not adhere to their prescribed medication regimen is its excessive cost. Often we are so concerned with obtaining the right diagnosis and making our patient well that we overlook key pieces of information, including patient financial status. When patients cannot afford the drug you prescribe, they may not get well, even though they want to be compliant. It is of critical importance that providers ask patients if they have difficulty obtaining their medication because it is cost prohibitive.

If you find that your patient is having difficulty purchasing the prescribed medications, consider changing pharmacies or drug regimens. The cost of a drug can vary widely between pharmacies, even within the same city. Many corporations have created generic $4 lists or special prescription programs that allow patients to fill their medications for a reasonable cost. In addition, all health plans through the ACA are required to include prescription drug coverage, although these vary greatly. As a prescriber, you need to be familiar with the local resources for medication assistance and low-cost medications.

Guidelines

When in doubt, follow current guidelines for the treatment of a particular disease or symptom. Almost all medical and nursing societies have published guidelines, including the American Heart Association, the American College of Cardiology, the Infectious Diseases Society of America, and the American Diabetes Association. It is the provider's responsibility to keep abreast of new recommendations or changes in guidelines and to incorporate these into their prescribing practices. Although closely following the guidelines is desirable, we must always take into account that our patients may not fit well into these guidelines and that individualized care is always best. In these cases, it is important to document the rationale for deviating from standard of care.

Availability

Every facility and pharmacy provides drugs according to a formulary. This formulary is selected by a panel of pharmacists and providers and may be subject to following guidelines created by regulatory agencies, such as the Centers for Medicare and Medicaid Services (CMS). The formulary may also depend on regional and national drug supplies, drug costs and available rebates, and the presence of generic medications on the market.

In short, the drug you want may not be available in your facility or at a specific pharmacy. This can affect your choice in medications. Become familiar with the formulary where you are employed, and know that it can change over time. Often there are substitutes or similar medications you can order in place of what you originally intended. For example, omeprazole may be indicated for the treatment of erosive esophagitis, but the formulary contains esomeprazole instead.

Interactions

As noted throughout this text, there are very few medications that do not interact with either another medication or a food. Polypharmacy greatly increases the risk for interactions. Some of these interactions are negligible, but some can have life-threatening consequences. It is of crucial importance to ask the patient about *all* current drugs, including over-the-counter (OTC) medications and other herbal preparations. Many patients do not consider OTC or alternative pharmaceuticals as "medications" and may not mention them unless you ask specifically.

When adding a new medication to a patient regimen, check for significant interactions. There are many resources that allow checks for interactions between multiple medications or foods at one time. If there is a low-risk interaction identified, you may find it acceptable to discuss this with your patient, document the conversation, and then prescribe the medication. If there is a relative or absolute contraindication to the proposed drug combination, it is best to choose an alternative if at all possible.

Side Effects

All drugs have side effects. Some are adverse, and some may be beneficial. In addition, one patient may experience adverse effects to a medication, whereas another patient may not. It is important to note the pertinent side effects for each medication and to ask your patients about presence of symptoms after initiating, stopping, or changing a medication dose. When assessing the risk-to-benefit ratio of a medication, one must consider the severity of the side effects. If a patient started on a new antihypertensive medication has a decreased blood pressure, and therefore improvement in hypertension, but experiences fainting, a decrease in dose or a different medication should be considered.

Allergies

At times, guidelines may suggest a particular drug for a specific ailment. Unfortunately, your patient may have an allergy to that medication or class of drug. It is of critical importance to determine the type of reaction and to document in the patient's chart. Then, selection of an appropriate drug may begin.

In the case of severe allergy, such as anaphylaxis or swelling of the face, these drugs are absolutely contraindicated, but in the case of the patient who experienced vomiting or other similar reactions, the drug may be used again if necessary. The desired choice would be to use an alternate medication that is just as effective. For example, a patient with pyelonephritis who is allergic to penicillin can benefit from a fluoroquinolone instead.

Hepatic and Renal Function

Many drugs are metabolized and eliminated by the liver and kidneys. If these systems are impaired, this can lead to increased adverse effects and possible medication overdose. Frequently, drugs have special decreased doses or different dosing schedules for patients with hepatic or renal impairment. This is known as *hepatic dosing* or *renal dosing*. Despite the known safety of decreasing doses in some drugs, if there is a different option available, it is prudent to choose a different medication. For example, morphine sulfate is highly metabolized by the kidneys. For patients with renal impairment, morphine can be used to treat pain, but the better choice would be fentanyl because fentanyl does not require a dose reduction in patients with renal impairment. Although some drugs are safe to give or can be used with caution in patients with hepatic or renal dysfunction, other drugs are contraindicated in these patients and must be avoided at all costs.

Need for Monitoring

Some drugs require frequent monitoring at initiation or throughout the duration of treatment. Examples of these medications include warfarin, lithium, opioids, and immunosuppressive therapies (tacrolimus, sirolimus). When levels of these drugs are not within therapeutic range, serious patient harm can occur. If a patient does not have the ability to attend frequent laboratory appointments, cannot take their medications reliably, or is not easily reachable by phone or electronically, it may be best to try and avoid these medications if possible.

Special Populations

Populations that deserve special mention when thinking about medications include pregnant or nursing mothers, and older adults. These populations are addressed in depth in Unit III, Drug Therapy Across the Life Span. In addition, Life Span Tables are present in many of the chapters throughout the text to alert you to special considerations.

PRESCRIPTIONS

Necessities

When writing any prescription, there are key elements that must be present to compose a complete prescription. An example of a common template for a written prescription is provided in Fig. 2.1. These elements include the following:

- Prescriber name, license number, and contact information
- Prescriber U.S. Drug Enforcement Administration (DEA) number, if applicable
- Patient name and date of birth
- Patient allergies
- Name of medication
- Indication of medication (e.g., atenolol for hypertension)
- Medication strength (e.g., 25 mg, 500 mg/mL)
- Dose of medication and frequency (e.g., 12.5 mg once daily)
- Number of tablets or capsules to dispense
- Number of refills

If using an electronic medical record (EMR) to complete prescriptions, many of these elements will be mandatory for the provider, although many will already be completed by the EMR, including prescriber name and contact information. It is important to note the indication for the medication because many drugs are used for more than one purpose. This allows for the patient as well as other providers to understand your intent for prescribing this particular drug.

Types of Prescriptions
Telephone

A common and convenient way to create a new prescription or prescription refill is by telephone. A prescription can be called in to a pharmacy

---

UNIVERSITY CLINIC

Robert Smith, FNP-BC
1777 E. 17th Avenue
Las Vegas, CO 87777
Phone: 777-777-7777 Fax: 777-777-7778

Patient Name: _____ Date: _____

Allergies: _____

Medical Record#: _____ Date of Birth: _____

Medication: _____ Strength: _____ Quantity: _____

Directions for Use: 0 DAW

Indication for use: _____ Refills: _____

Prescriber Signature: _____ DEA#

License# _____ NPI # _____

Contact #/Pager # _____

Fig. 2.1 Common Example of a Written Prescription. *DEA,* U.S. Drug Enforcement Administration, *DAW,* dispense as written; *NPI,* National Provider Identifier.

Fig. 2.2 Prohibition Era Prescription for Alcohol.

by you or a specified designee. This is often done by leaving a message with the correct information. Although this is a different way of prescribing, the necessities remain the same (see earlier section "Necessities"). Certain medications cannot be prescribed or refilled by telephone. These include medications within the schedule II category. Patients must have a written prescription for these medications. The only exception to this rule is during an emergency. In this case a telephone order can be used for a limited amount of medication, but a written prescription must be presented to the pharmacy within 7 days.

Written

Providers have been writing prescriptions in the United States since the 1700s. Patients even received scripts during Prohibition in the 1920s to purchase alcohol for medicinal use (Fig. 2.2). Interestingly enough, these paper scripts did not look much different than they do nowadays. This is because the required elements for a complete prescription have not changed over the years. Although health care is making the transition to electronic prescriptions, many providers still use written scripts to prescribe medication. Written prescriptions, like telephone calls or electronic scripts, contain all the necessary elements as described earlier in this chapter. Although all the correct prompts for information may be prepopulated on your script, there are still some important points to consider. If you use a script with a different provider name or a generic script, make sure your name and contact information are printed legibly on the paper. Write all prescriptions in ink or indelible pencil. Avoid abbreviations such as U (units), MSO_4 (morphine), or QD (daily) because these can increase errors and are therefore no longer acceptable. For a list of abbreviations to avoid, see Table 2.1.

In addition, never write prescriptions on presigned scripts or presign blank scripts for other providers or staff. Although this may seem like a convenient way to ensure availability to patients at all times, it is ultimately an unsafe practice. Finally, many facilities provide tamper-resistant scripts, and some states require their use, especially in the prevention of substance misuse and abuse. A few tamper-resistant security features include Hidden Message Technology, which appears when the script is copied on a copy machine; Anti-Copy Coin Rub, which appears when rubbed with a coin; and

TABLE 2.1	**Abbreviations and Figures to Avoid**
Do *Not* Use	**Preferred**
U	Units
IU	International units
QD	Daily
QOD	Every other day
Trailing zero (X.0 mg)	Never trail (X mg)
Lack of leading zero (.X mg)	Always lead with a zero before a decimal point (0.X mg)
MS, MSO_4, $MgSO_4$	Morphine sulfate, magnesium sulfate
AS, AD, AU	Left ear, right ear, both ears
OS, OD, OU	Left eye, right eye, both eyes

distinctive security backgrounds. To learn more about these features, visit http://rxsecurityfeatures.com/.

E-Prescribing

With the advent of the EMR, many pharmacies currently have capabilities to accept electronic prescriptions. In fact, CMS provides incentives for using an EMR to prescribe medications. This program, called *Meaningful Use*, is thought to contribute to increased patient safety and improved patient outcomes.

Using an EMR allows the provider to select a specific, patient-selected pharmacy. After the correct medication information is entered, the prescription is automatically sent to the selected pharmacy. This is beneficial because there is direct transmission of information, making error less likely. In addition, the prescription can be ready for the patient when the patient leaves the facility—the patient does not need to drop off the paper script and then wait for a medication fill. Prior to the advent of Two-Factor Authentication software, limitations to e-prescribing included scheduled medications. Currently, many companies like Duo, Nexmo, and OneLogin provide an extra layer of security through use of a smartphone to verify identity at the time of prescribing. These programs are incorporated into the EMR, allowing electronic prescribing of scheduled medications directly to the pharmacy. Unfortunately, many health care organizations still do not have a functional EMR, and many pharmacies still do not have the software capabilities to process these requests. In these cases, paper prescriptions are still necessary.

Refills

There are a few things to consider when refilling a prescription. Questions you should ask yourself include the following:

- Is this a newer medication for this patient?
- Am I changing dose or frequency of the medication?
- Am I adding new medications to their regimen?
- Is the patient having undesired side effects?
- When do I expect to follow up with this patient?
- If the patient is requesting a refill by telephone, when was the last time I saw this patient? Do I need to see the patient again before refill?
- Is this a schedule II medication?

If the answer to any of these questions is "yes," consider a shorter time between refills (1 to 3 months). The exception to this question is with schedule II medications. These are not eligible for refills and must have a new prescription each renewal period. When changing or adding to current medication regimens, it is prudent to follow up with the patient by phone or in person to assess changes. This time can be used to discuss new or increased side effects, check vital signs, obtain laboratory work, or make further adjustments. When a medication, such as warfarin, requires frequent monitoring with drug levels, an even shorter refill allotment is reasonable. If the patient has been maintained on the current dose of a medication for some time and remains stable, it is likely acceptable to continue to refill that medication for a longer time period (e.g., 12 months).

ASSISTANCE

Applications for Tablets and Phones

This textbook will be paramount in your learning, but it may not be convenient to carry around in the clinical setting. Although we encourage you to use this text to the fullest extent, there are many new applications and websites available to assist providers with safe prescribing (Box 2.1). However, it must be noted that all these tools still require common sense and good judgment on the part of the prescriber. As

---

BOX 2.1 Helpful Applications and Websites for Safe Prescribing

Websites
Epocrates: http://www.epocrates.com/
LexiComp: http://online.lexi.com/action/home
Pepid: http://www.pepid.com/
Physicians' Desk Reference (PDR): http://www.pdr.net/
UptoDate: http://www.uptodate.com/contents/search

Applications for Tablets, Phones
Centers for Disease Control and Prevention Antibiotic Guidelines
Elsevier Clinical Pharmacology
Epocrates
Pepid
Prescriber's Letter

---

stated previously, one must take into account the individual patient and multiple other factors, including cost, side effects, and medication formularies. An application can assist you with the basic suggestions in dosing and duration, but ultimately there is no substitute for sound practice.

Collaboration

As reflected in this chapter, writing a prescription safely can be complicated. It is strongly encouraged that you use all available resources, including your colleagues. Developing a relationship with your pharmacist can be one of the most helpful and fruitful relationships you cultivate. Because this is their specialty, pharmacists will likely have additional information on formulary and drug interactions as well as suggestions for adequate medication dosing. In some practices, pharmacists are responsible for medication initiation and titration based on standardized protocols.

Infectious disease (ID) specialists can also be a helpful resource. Choosing an appropriate antimicrobial agent for a specific infectious process is often difficult for a new practitioner. A local ID specialist can provide guidance on resistance patterns, common local microbial flora, and correct doses, as well as on duration of treatment for specific infections.

3

Promoting Positive Outcomes of Drug Therapy

Selecting and prescribing the most appropriate drug (see Chapter 2) is just the first step in providing safe and competent medication therapy. Ensuring positive outcomes requires establishing a medication education plan, monitoring positive and negative patient responses, identifying and addressing issues of nonadherence, and managing the patient's complete medication regimen.

MEDICATION EDUCATION

Probably no other provider action influences the patient's commitment to carry out a medication plan more than medication education. This not only provides an opportunity to explain the importance of the medication but also allows the provider to dispel rumors about medications that often lead to therapy failures. Moreover, education reduces medication errors by empowering patients with accurate information and clear guidelines.

Medication Education Components

There are basic components that should be included when teaching about any new medication. These are (1) medication name, (2) purpose, (3) dosing regimen, (4) administration, (5) adverse effects, (6) any special storage needs, (7) associated laboratory testing, (8) food or drug interactions, and (9) duration of therapy. Each of these is discussed in the following sections.

Medication Name

Patients need to know the name of the medication they are taking. Unfortunately, when taking a medication history, we still have patients who refer to medications by their understood purpose (e.g., "blood pressure pill") rather than by their name. This creates a challenge for the provider who needs to select appropriate therapy. It also increases the risk for medication errors. If we teach patients the medication names, we can avoid this concern.

Patients should be encouraged to keep a list of their medications on their person at all times. Both the generic name and the brand (trade) name should be included. This can be especially important for the patient who travels and may be treated by providers unfamiliar with the patient's history. From the patient perspective, knowing the generic name empowers the patient to catch medication errors in the event that two different providers prescribe the same generic drug under different brand names.

Purpose

Patients are more likely to participate in activities when they know those activities produce positive outcomes. The same is true of taking medications. Knowing the reason the medication is prescribed propels the patient to follow through with the medication plan because the patient is aware that this action helps achieve the therapeutic goal.

Dosing

The dosing regimen, including the drug quantity and number of tablets or millimeters per dose, needs to be reviewed with the patient even though it is written on the prescription label. Doing this ensures that the patient understands how to take the medication and provides an opportunity for the patient to ask questions.

It is important to be specific when explaining the dosing regimen. For example, "four times a day" may be interpreted in various ways by different people. Can the medication be taken every 4 hours for four doses, or does it need to be spaced out evenly to every 6 hours? Does "once a day" mean that it can be taken at any time, or it is better to take the medication in the morning or evening hours? Patients need to know what to do if a dose is accidentally skipped. This is also a good time to explain why drugs should be taken exactly as prescribed.

Administration

A common patient concern is whether medication should be taken with or without food. This routine information should be provided for all drugs.

Patients also need to be informed of common administration needs that many of us take for granted. For example, suspensions should be shaken (or rolled, if shaking causes foaming) to equally disperse ingredients before administration.

Finally, some drugs require a special apparatus for administration. Inhaled drugs are a common example. Patients need to see how these are administered and should be able to repeat a demonstration before leaving with a prescription. Many manufacturers provide a "dummy" device for teaching purposes.

Adverse Effects

Some providers and other health care workers hesitate to discuss a drug's potential adverse effects. Some fear that doing so will lead to a patient's refusal to take the medications. Although that concern is understandable and the consequences may well be true, patients have a right to know of potential harms that may result from therapy. Therefore providers are ethically obligated to divulge adverse effects and other risks. That said, often the approach used in discussing these can make a difference in how patients view them.

You probably know patients who worry about taking drugs when the product labeling (i.e., package insert) lists dozens of adverse effects. Patients may not know that, for most drugs, most adverse effects occur in less than 1% to 2% of those taking the drug. Most patients are unaware that the long list of adverse effects represents all effects reported during clinical trials, regardless of whether a direct association to the drug is known. Furthermore, labeling does not mention that sometimes the incidence of adverse effects in the placebo group is similarly high. For example, in clinical trials of lovastatin, 1.8% of subjects taking 40 mg reported myalgias; however, 1.7% of subjects taking a placebo also reported myalgias.

When discussing adverse effects, focus on the adverse effects that are common and avoid undue attention on rare and unanticipated effects. If complex effects such as liver injury or pancytopenia may occur, teach patients the signs and symptoms to report. Let patients know that many adverse effects—most commonly nausea and sedation—are usually temporary and go away with continued medication use. In these discussions, it is also beneficial to emphasize benefits over risks. Patients are often willing to endure short-term adverse effects for long-term health improvement.

Storage

Storage is an important concern for some drugs. For example, some antibiotic suspensions, insulins, and rectal suppositories need to be refrigerated. Medications such as sublingual nitroglycerin and dabigatran (Pradaxa) need to be stored in their original container to prevent drug breakdown and loss of potency.

Laboratory Testing

Laboratory testing is sometimes necessary to determine whether a medication remains safe and effective. For example, liver enzymes may need to be checked periodically for drugs that can cause liver damage. Serum drug levels may need to be checked when maintaining therapeutic levels is challenging.

Patients need to know if special testing will be needed. They also need to know why the monitoring is necessary because those who understand the purpose are more likely to adhere to testing schedules. We recommend teaching what, when, where, why, and how when giving instructions (Box 3.1).

Food or Drug Interactions

Many medications interact with certain foods or other drugs (including alcohol and other recreational drugs). Patients need to know of any potential interactions and the consequence of those interactions. They also need to know if the problem with interactions can be solved by

taking substances further apart or whether they need to avoid an interacting food or drug for the duration of therapy. For example, antacids may be taken with most drugs as long as administration is separated by 2 hours; however, patients taking metronidazole must avoid alcohol for the duration of therapy.

Duration of Therapy

It is important to let the patient know if medication therapy is being prescribed for a short time (e.g., antibiotics for an acute infection) or whether ongoing long-term medication therapy is anticipated (e.g., thyroid hormone therapy for hypothyroidism). Failure to recognize the need for prolonged therapy is a common reason patients stop medications prematurely when a prescription runs out.

Written Instructions

Medication information is notoriously easy to forget, especially for patients taking numerous medications. We recommend accompanying all verbal education with written instructions. For those who are unable to read due to literacy or vision problems, video or audio instructions can be used.

The Patient Protection and Affordable Care Act of 2010, Title V, defines health literacy as "the degree to which an individual has the capacity to obtain, communicate, process, and understand basic health information and services to make appropriate health decisions." Low levels of health literacy can impair a patient's ability to understand medication instructions. Best practices in developing written patient education materials abound in the literature. Table 3.1 provides a list of those for which there is greatest consensus. An excellent resource for writing patient education materials is available at http://www.cdc.gov/healthliteracy/pdf/Simply_Put.pdf.

MONITORING

As mentioned in Chapter 2, monitoring is an important consideration in medication therapy. Ongoing monitoring of positive and negative patient responses—and acting on those responses in ways that increase benefit or decrease risk—is essential to ensure optimal outcomes.

BOX 3.1   Patient Teaching for Drug Monitoring

When testing is needed for monitoring, include the following when providing patient teaching.

What: What test is needed?

Patients like to know what test is needed. Rather than telling them that a blood test is needed, let them know the type of blood test (e.g., a test of thyroid function or cholesterol levels).

When: When is testing required?

Testing can disrupt normal routines. Patients need to know, in advance, how often testing is needed so they can make plans.

Where: Where will testing take place?

In some practices, testing takes place at locations other than the primary clinic. Patients who are unfamiliar with the area need directions to the testing site and where to go after arrival.

Why: Why is testing necessary?

Testing is often expensive and disruptive to daily lives. These barriers are common reasons that patients miss appointments. If they understand the need for testing, they are more likely to adhere to testing schedules.

How: How does the patient prepare for testing?

Some tests require special preparation. For example, many blood tests require fasting. If exercise testing is needed, patients should be told to bring comfortable shoes. It is important to let patients know of anything they need to do prior to arrival.

TABLE 3.1   Best Practices in Developing Written Patient Education Materials

Practice	Rationale
Limit content	Focus on main points. Include only the most important-to-know content.
Place important information first	People tend to remember the first things they read and may become distracted toward the end.
Write in active voice	Active voice is more direct. Passive voice is less dynamic and may be confusing.
Include adequate white space	White space does not contain text or images. White space makes the page feel less cluttered and less overwhelming.
Use meaningful illustrations	Illustrations are a useful way to break up text. Select images or drawings that have a purpose or that reinforce a point in the handout.
Avoid professional terminology	Use common terms in short, simple sentences that patients can easily understand.
Check for readability	Materials should be written at a lower education level that can be understood by most patients. Information for increasing readability is available at http://www.cdc.gov/healthliteracy/pdf/Simply_Put.pdf

TABLE 3.2   Selected Medications That Require Periodic Laboratory Monitoring

Drug or Drug Category	Laboratory Testing	Reason for Monitoring
ACEIs and ARBs	Potassium	These drugs can cause hyperkalemia.
	Serum creatinine	Renal perfusion is dependent on angiotensin in some patients; increased creatinine may require change in medication.
Amiodarone	Liver function	Hepatotoxicity is an adverse effect.
	Thyroid function	Either hypothyroidism or hyperthyroidism may occur.
	Pulmonary function and chest radiographs	Pulmonary toxicity is not uncommon; effects may be permanent.
Anticonvulsants	Serum drug levels	Determination of therapeutic dosage is needed. Some have narrow therapeutic index.
Antidiabetic drugs	Serum glucose Hemoglobin A_{1c}	Determination of glucose control is needed.
Digoxin	Digoxin level	The drugs have a narrow therapeutic index.
	Serum electrolytes if at risk	Hypokalemia, hypomagnesemia, and hypocalcemia can increase toxicity risk.
Diuretics, potassium-sparing	Serum electrolytes	Hyperkalemia can reach dangerous levels. Hypocalcemia and hypomagnesemia may occur.
Diuretics, thiazide and loop	Serum electrolytes	Hypokalemia, hypomagnesemia, and hyponatremia are common. Thiazide diuretics can cause hypercalcemia; loop diuretics can cause hypocalcemia.
Lithium	CBC	Lithium can cause leukocyte elevation.
	Lithium level	The drug has a narrow therapeutic index.
	Thyroid function	Both hypothyroidism and hyperthyroidism may occur.
	Renal function	Renal damage is a serious adverse effect.
	Serum electrolytes	Nephrogenic diabetes insipidus may occur; hyponatremia can create complications.
Methotrexate	CBC	Pancytopenia, or a decrease of any of the blood cell types, may occur.
	Liver function	Hepatotoxicity is an adverse effect.
	Renal function	Renal toxicity is an adverse effect.
NSAIDs (long-term use)	CBC	Anemia may occur, especially if there is bleeding, which may be occult.
	Serum creatinine	Prostaglandin inhibition may decrease renal perfusion, causing injury.
	Liver function	Rare but serious liver injury has occurred.
Statins	Liver function	Elevations in liver enzymes may be associated with injury.
	Creatine kinase	Creatine kinase can determine whether muscle pain is caused by injury secondary to drug use.
	Lipid panel	Lipids are checked to determine effect.
Thiazolidinediones	Liver function	These drugs are associated with a risk for hepatotoxicity.
Thyroid hormone	TSH, T_4	Monitoring is needed to optimize therapy.
Warfarin	PT/INR	Monitoring is needed to maintain therapeutic range.

ACEI, Angiotensin-converting enzyme inhibitor; *ARB,* angiotensin receptor blocker; *CBC,* complete blood count; *NSAIDs,* nonsteroidal antiinflammatory drugs; *PT/INR,* prothrombin time/international normalized ratio; *TSH,* thyroid-stimulating hormone; *T₄,* thyroxine.

There are three primary reasons for drug monitoring: (1) determining therapeutic dosage, (2) evaluating medication adequacy, and (3) identifying adverse effects. Each of these purposes is discussed in the following sections. Table 3.2 provides some common examples of drugs that require periodic laboratory monitoring.

Determining Therapeutic Dosage

Many drugs have a narrow therapeutic index (NTI) (see Chapter 4). Examples include carbamazepine, digoxin, lithium, phenytoin, and theophylline. For these drugs, the difference between an effective dose and a lethal dose is small.

To ensure safety, periodic measurement of serum drug levels is needed when drugs with an NTI are prescribed. This not only determines whether the drug is in a therapeutic range but also provides an opportunity for fine-tuning of dosage. If a drug is nearing a toxic level or a subtherapeutic level, the provider will make a dosage adjustment accordingly. How often monitoring is needed varies for each drug. In addition, patient factors such as poor liver or renal function may determine the frequency of drug level monitoring.

For some drugs with an NTI, a therapeutic dosage is determined by means other than the serum drug level. Warfarin is a drug that illustrates this method. Instead of ordering a serum warfarin level, optimal dosing is determined by measures of prothrombin time with international normalized ratio (PT/INR).

Evaluating Medication Adequacy

For some drugs, evaluation of effectiveness can be determined easily. For example, if an analgesic is given, effectiveness is determined by asking the patient to rate the pain on a scale of 0 to 10. Similarly, the adequacy of an antihypertensive medication can be evaluated by checking the patient's blood pressure. However, evaluating medication adequacy is not so simple for some conditions.

Some conditions do not cause obvious signs or symptoms. Hyperlipidemia is a common example; signs and symptoms often do not appear until after decades of accumulated damage have occurred. Other conditions may be manifested by signs and symptoms that are not easily quantifiable. A common example of this condition is hyperglycemia associated with diabetes. Some people display obvious signs and symptoms when hyperglycemic, whereas for others, the evidence is much more subtle. For conditions such as hyperlipidemia and hyperglycemia, laboratory testing offers a precisely quantifiable measure that can be used to gauge the effectiveness of medication therapy. For example, a hemoglobin A_{1c} level can be used to evaluate glucose control, and lipid panels can used to determine the effectiveness of hyperlipidemia management.

Identifying Adverse Effects

One of the most common uses of drug monitoring is that of monitoring for harm. This is a proactive undertaking to identify problems early, before they progress to the point of harm.

Many drugs are potentially dangerous. For these, monitoring depends on the type of potential injury. For example, if a drug can cause liver injury, periodic monitoring of liver enzymes (and possibly other tests of liver function) is needed. If a drug can cause bone marrow suppression, periodic monitoring of a complete blood count to assess for anemia, leukopenia, or thrombocytopenia is warranted. In addition, baseline laboratory studies are done before initiating therapy.

ADHERENCE

Medication nonadherence costs the U.S. health care system approximately $290 billion each year. It is often directly responsible for disease exacerbations, avoidable hospitalizations, transitioning to long-term (i.e., "nursing home") care, and premature deaths.

Medication adherence can be defined as the extent to which patients take their medications as prescribed by the provider and agreed to by the patient.[a] The patient who adheres to the agreed-on medication regimen takes the medication in the prescribed dose at the prescribed frequency for the length of time indicated.

In 2013, the National Community Pharmacists Association (NCPA) released *Medication Adherence in America: A National Report Card* (available at http://www.ncpa.co/adherence/AdherenceReportCard_Full.pdf with yearly progress reports at http://www.ncpanet.org/solutions/adherence-simplify-my-meds). The NCPA report identifies six nonadherent behaviors. They are, in the percentage of frequency, as follows:
- Missed a dose (57%)
- Forgot to take a dose (30%)
- Did not refill the medication in time (28%)
- Took a lower than prescribed dose (22%)
- Did not refill the medication (20%)
- Stopped taking the medication (14%)

The reasons given by patients to explain their nonadherence provide additional insight. Again, in the frequency of occurrence, they are as follows:
- Forgot to take it (42%)
- Ran out (34%)
- Was away from home (27%)
- Was trying to save money (22%)
- Didn't like the side effects (21%)
- Was too busy (17%)
- The medicine wasn't working (17%)
- Didn't believe the medicine was necessary (16%)
- Didn't like taking the medicine (12%)

[a]The addition of "agreed to by the patient" distinguishes the definition of medication adherence from medication compliance. The concept of medication compliance has fallen out of favor because it views the provider from the perspective of an authoritarian who dictates treatment rather than a provider who makes decisions that consider the patient's preferences and values.

These documents can offer valuable insight for the health care provider. Moreover, they beg the question, "What could the provider have done differently to address issues of nonadherence proactively?"

In examining these, five primary patterns emerge. These are: (1) forgetfulness, (2) lack of planning, (3) cost, (4) dissatisfaction, and (5) altered dosing. An honest and open discussion that respects both the patient and provider perspectives can be an important facilitator to promoting positive outcomes. Individualized solutions that address the specific patient's concerns are those most likely to be successful.

Forgetfulness

The most common reason cited for nonadherence was that the patient simply forgot to take the medication. Studies have demonstrated that medications are easier to remember if they are aligned with common daily activities. For example, morning medications may be taken on first arising (if they should be taken on an empty stomach) or with breakfast (if they should be taken with food). Doing this establishes habits, which are more difficult to forget.

Several memory aids are available to help patients remember to take their medications. Drug organizers are probably the most common tool used. If these are filled at the beginning of each week, the patient can tell at a glance if medications have been taken on any given day.

Numerous apps are also available for various electronic devices. These can be programmed to alarm or deliver a verbal message when it is time to take a drug. Similarly, digital assistances (e.g., Amazon's Alexa and Google Assistant) can be programmed to alert patients when it is time to take their medications.

Some patients have found that medication administration records (MARs), similar to MARs used by nurses in hospitals, can be helpful. An advantage of personalized MARs is the ability to tailor them to meet patient's vision and literacy needs.

Lack of Planning

Aligned closely with forgetfulness is the lack of planning. In this category, we include those statements aligned with failure to refill medications whether because the patient was too busy, away from home, or ran out for other reasons.

Most pharmacies offer reminder notices, either by email or automated phone calls, as part of their regular services. If being "too busy" is a concern, a pharmacy that offers a home delivery service or a mail delivery service is a viable solution.

Cost

As mentioned in Chapter 2, costs should be considered initially when selecting an appropriate drug. When possible, use of generic drugs, drugs on formulary, or drugs that are a part of a discount pharmacy program can reduce out of pocket costs. Sometimes, however, there are no adequate substitutions for a necessary but expensive drug. Fortunately, prescription assistance programs (PAPs), also called *patient assistance programs* and *pharmaceutical assistance programs*, are widely available. These offer steeply discounted drugs for those who meet eligibility requirements.

There are three sources for PAPs: pharmaceutical companies, government-run programs, and nonprofit organizations. Table 3.3 offers a program sampling. If you do not find what you need here, your likely best resource for reliable information is a local pharmacist. Warn patients to beware of discount cards that are not affiliated with known reputable organizations. Unfortunately, some criminals use applications for fake cards for illegal purposes.

Dissatisfaction

The issue of dissatisfaction as a reason for nonadherence highlights the need to identify what medications are taken and to discuss any concerns

TABLE 3.3   Patient Assistance Programs

Pharmaceutical Patient Assistance Programs

Allergan	http://www.allergan.com/responsibility/patient-resources/patient-assistance-programs
AstraZeneca	http://www.astrazeneca-us.com/medicines/help-affording-your-medicines
Boehringer Ingelheim	https://www.boehringer-ingelheim.us/our-responsibility/patient-assistance-program
Johnson & Johnson	http://www.jjpaf.org
Merck	http://www.merckhelps.com
Novartis	http://www.patientassistancenow.com
Pfizer	http://www.pfizer.com/health/financial_assistance_programs/patient_assistance_programs
Takeda	http://www.takeda.us/responsibility/patient_assistance_program.aspx

Government Programs

Medicare	https://www.medicare.gov/pharmaceutical-assistance-program
State-run programs	http://www.ncsl.org/research/health/state-pharmaceutical-assistance-programs.aspx

Nonprofit Organizations

National Council on Aging	https://www.ncoa.org/economic-security/benefits/prescriptions/lis-extrahelp
NeedyMeds	http://www.needymeds.org
Partnership for Prescription Assistance	https://www.pparx.org
RxAssist	http://www.rxassist.org
RxHope	https://www.rxhope.com/Patient/MedSearchHome.aspx
RxOutreach	https://rxoutreach.org

with the patient at each encounter. It is essential to uncover the reason for dissatisfaction (e.g., adverse effects, inconvenient dosing, or a perception that a drug is ineffective). Often the problem can be easily addressed by simple interventions. For example, taking medications with food can reduce adverse effects of nausea and gastrointestinal distress in many instances. Changing to a sustained-release drug may be all that is necessary to address problems with inconvenient dosing.

If the patient believes a drug is ineffective, it becomes important to discuss patient expectations of drug therapy and what can be realistically achieved. For some conditions (e.g., obesity), change may come slowly. For others (e.g., hypertension), the medication may cause the patient to feel worse without a perceived benefit. If the drug is truly an important one, this may be a good time to explore with the patient any consequences of not taking the drug and whether the patient is willing to assume those risks. In some instances the patient may decide to assume those risks rather than to take the medication. It is within the patient's right to do so.

Altered Dosing

It is concerning that more than 20% of patients in the NCPA report took lower than the prescribed dose. The reasons were not made clear; however, the consequence is this, because a drug must reach a therapeutic level to be effective, a subtherapeutic dose is no better than no dose at all! Furthermore, in the case of certain antimicrobial drugs, subtherapeutic levels may cause harm if the bacteria develop resistance as a result.

This finding emphasizes the necessity of not only reviewing which medications are taken at each encounter but also asking whether the medications are taken as prescribed. If dosing is altered, it is imperative to determine how and why, and then to educate the patient regarding how alterations in dosing affect outcomes.

MANAGING MEDICATION THERAPY

In addition to the medication review undertaken at each patient encounter, a more comprehensive and deliberate review is needed periodically (at least annually). This review should be approached with the intent purpose of determining whether there are better options for

medication therapy. Inherent questions that must be asked about each drug include the following:
- Is each medication accomplishing its intended purpose?
- Is each medication still necessary?
  - Has the patient's condition changed?
  - Do adverse effects or risks outweigh the benefits that some drugs provide?
  - What would happen if some medications were no longer prescribed?
- What problems does each medication create for the patient?
  - Is a medication problem amplified by other drugs the patient is taking?
  - If a medication is necessary but problematic, are drugs with fewer adverse effects available?
- If polypharmacy is an issue, are there ways to decrease the number of medications?
  - Will a combination drug simplify management?
  - Is a single drug available (and desirable) for management of two different conditions?

Ideally, these reviews should be carried out in collaboration with the patient or patient's family so that nothing is overlooked. Medication regimens can then be optimized to eliminate unnecessary drugs, add new drugs, if necessary, and ultimately improve patient satisfaction with care.

SUMMARY

We have examined four opportunities to promote positive outcomes in drug therapy. Patients need adequate drug education to take drugs correctly and to avoid complications associated with therapy. Monitoring provides a method of ensuring safe and effective therapy. Promoting adherence, by addressing common causes of nonadherence proactively, can ensure ongoing therapy without interruption. Finally, scheduled medication reviews with the intent to optimize medication regimens, based on patient experiences and needs, can help promote positive outcomes.

4

Pharmacokinetics, Pharmacodynamics, and Drug Interactions

PHARMACOKINETICS

Pharmacokinetics is the study of drug movement throughout the body.[a] There are four basic pharmacokinetic processes: absorption, distribution, metabolism, and excretion (Fig. 4.1). *Absorption* is the drug's movement from its site of administration into the blood. *Distribution* is the drug's movement from the blood to the interstitial space of tissues and from

there into cells. *Metabolism* (biotransformation) is the enzymatically mediated alteration of drug structure. *Excretion* is the movement of drugs and their metabolites out of the body. The combination of metabolism and excretion is called *elimination*. The four pharmacokinetic processes, acting in concert, determine the concentration of a drug at its sites of action.

By applying knowledge of pharmacokinetics to drug therapy, we can help maximize beneficial effects and minimize harm. Recall that the intensity of the response to a drug is directly related to the concentration of the drug at its site of action. To maximize beneficial effects, a drug must achieve concentrations that are high enough to elicit desired responses; to minimize harm, we must avoid concentrations that are too high. This balance is achieved by selecting the most appropriate route, dosage, and dosing schedule.

---

[a]Fundamental pharmacologic concepts are typically covered in undergraduate courses; however, experience has demonstrated that a refresher in the basic principles of pharmacokinetics, pharmacodynamics, and drug interactions is usually helpful. Because it is a refresher, the information in this chapter is relatively brief.

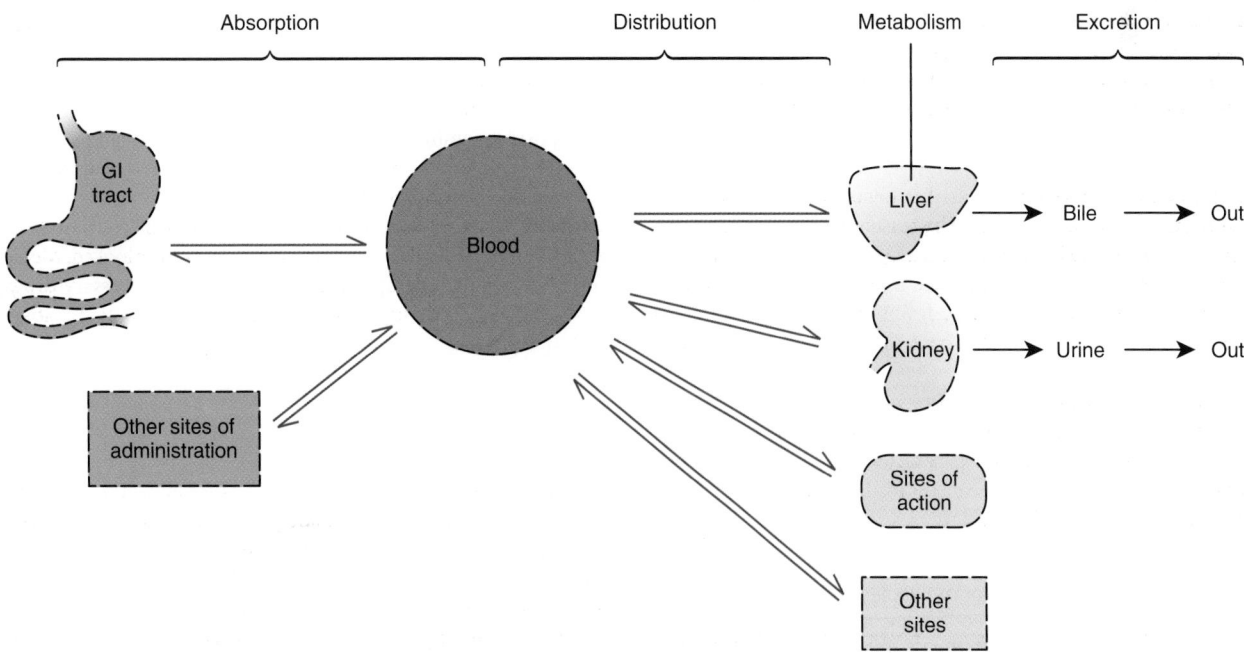

Fig. 4.1 The Four Basic Pharmacokinetic Processes. Dotted lines represent membranes that must be crossed as drugs move throughout the body. *GI,* Gastrointestinal.

PASSAGE OF DRUGS ACROSS MEMBRANES

All four phases of pharmacokinetics—absorption, distribution, metabolism, and excretion—involve drug movement. To move throughout the body, drugs must cross membranes. Drugs cross membranes as they pass from the site of administration into the bloodstream and, subsequently, as they leave the vascular system to reach the site of action. In addition, drugs must cross membranes to undergo metabolism and excretion. Accordingly, the factors that determine the passage of drugs across biologic membranes have a profound influence on all aspects of pharmacokinetics.

Biologic membranes are composed of layers of individual cells. The cells composing most membranes are very close to one another—so close, in fact, that drugs must usually pass *through* cells, rather than between them, to cross the membrane. Hence the ability of a drug to cross a biologic membrane is determined primarily by its ability to pass through single cells.

Three Ways to Cross a Cell Membrane

The three most important ways by which drugs cross cell membranes are (1) passage through channels or pores, (2) passage with the aid of a transport system, and (3) direct penetration of the membrane. Of the three, direct penetration of the membrane is most common.

Channels and Pores

Very few drugs cross membranes through channels or pores. The channels in membranes are extremely small and are specific for certain molecules. Consequently, only the smallest of compounds, such as potassium and sodium, can pass through these channels and then only if the channel is the right one.

Transport Systems

Transport systems are carriers that can move drugs from one side of the cell membrane to the other side. All transport systems are selective. Whether a transporter will carry a particular drug depends on the drug's structure.

Transport systems are an important means of drug transit. For example, certain orally administered drugs could not be absorbed unless there were transport systems to move them across the membranes that separate the lumen of the intestine from the blood. A number of drugs could not reach intracellular sites of action without a transport system to move them across the cell membrane. One transporter, known as

P-glycoprotein (PGP) or *multidrug transporter protein,* deserves special mention. PGP is a transmembrane protein that transports a wide variety of drugs *out* of cells.

Direct Penetration of the Membrane

For most drugs, movement throughout the body is dependent on the ability to penetrate membranes directly because (1) most drugs are too large to pass through channels or pores and (2) most drugs lack transport systems to help them cross all of the membranes that separate them from their sites of action, metabolism, and excretion.

A general rule in chemistry states that "like dissolves like." Membranes are composed primarily of lipids; therefore, to directly penetrate membranes, a drug must be *lipid soluble* (lipophilic).

POLAR MOLECULES AND IONS

Certain kinds of molecules are *not* lipid soluble and therefore cannot penetrate membranes. This group consists of *polar molecules* and *ions.*

Polar Molecules

Polar molecules are molecules that have no *net* charge; however, they have an uneven *distribution* of electrical charge. That is, positive and negative charges within the molecule tend to congregate separately from one another. Water is the classic example. As depicted in Fig. 4.2, the electrons (negative charges) in the water molecule spend more time in the vicinity of the oxygen atom than in the vicinity of the two hydrogen atoms. As a result, the area around the oxygen atom tends to be negatively charged, whereas the area around the hydrogen atoms tends to be positively charged. In accord with the "like dissolves like" rule, polar molecules will dissolve in *polar* solvents (such as water) but not in *nonpolar* solvents (such as lipids).

Ions

Ions are defined as molecules that have a *net electrical charge* (either positive or negative). Except for very small molecules, *ions are unable to cross membranes;* therefore they must become nonionized to cross from one side to the other. Many drugs are either weak organic acids or weak organic bases, which can exist in charged and uncharged forms. Whether a weak acid or base carries an electrical charge is determined by the pH of the surrounding medium. Acids tend to ionize in basic (alkaline) media, whereas bases tend to ionize in acidic media. Therefore drugs that are weak acids are best absorbed in an acidic environment

Fig. 4.2 Polar molecules. (A) Stippling shows the distribution of electrons within the water molecule. As indicated at the lower right, water's electrons spend more time near the oxygen atom than near the hydrogen atoms, making the area near the oxygen atom somewhat negative and the area near the hydrogen atoms more positive. (B) Gentamicin is a polar drug. The 2-OH groups of gentamicin attract electrons, thereby causing the area around these groups to be more negative than the rest of the molecule.

such as gastric acid because they remain in a nonionized form. When aspirin molecules pass from the stomach into the small intestine, where the environment is relatively alkaline, more of the molecules change to their ionized form. As a result, absorption of aspirin from the intestine is impeded.

pH Partitioning (Ion Trapping)

Because the ionization of drugs is pH dependent, when the pH of the fluid on one side of a membrane differs from the pH of the fluid on the other side, drug molecules tend to accumulate on the side where the pH most favors their ionization. Accordingly, because acidic drugs tend to ionize in basic media and because basic drugs tend to ionize in acidic media, *when there is a pH gradient between two sides of a membrane,* the following occur:
- Acidic drugs accumulate on the alkaline side.
- Basic drugs accumulate on the acidic side.

The process whereby a drug accumulates on the side of a membrane where the pH most favors its ionization is referred to as *pH partitioning or ion trapping.*

ABSORPTION

Absorption is defined as *the movement of a drug from its site of administration into the systemic circulation.* The *rate* of absorption determines how *soon* effects will begin. The *amount* of absorption helps determine how *intense* effects will be. Two other terms associated with absorption are *chemical equivalence* and *bioavailability.* Drug preparations are considered *chemically equivalent* if they contain the same amount of the identical chemical compound (drug). Preparations are considered equal in *bioavailability* if the drug they contain is absorbed at the same rate and to the same extent. It is possible for two formulations of the same drug to be chemically equivalent while differing in bioavailability. The concept of bioavailability is discussed further in Chapter 6.

Factors Affecting Drug Absorption

The rate at which a drug undergoes absorption is influenced by the physical and chemical properties of the drug and by physiologic and anatomic factors at the absorption site.

Rate of Dissolution

Before a drug can be absorbed, it must first dissolve. Hence the rate of dissolution helps determine the rate of absorption. Drugs in formulations that allow rapid dissolution have a faster onset than drugs formulated for slow dissolution.

Surface Area

The surface area available for absorption is a major determinant of the rate of absorption. When the surface area is larger, absorption is faster. For this reason, absorption of orally administered drugs is usually greater from the small intestine rather than from the stomach. (Recall that the small intestine, because of its lining of microvilli, has an extremely large surface area, whereas the surface area of the stomach is relatively small.)

Blood Flow

Drugs are absorbed most rapidly from sites where blood flow is high because blood containing a newly absorbed drug will be replaced rapidly by drug-free blood, thereby maintaining a large gradient between the concentration of drug outside the blood and the concentration of drug in the blood. The greater the concentration gradient, the more rapid absorption will be.

Lipid Solubility

As a rule, highly lipid-soluble drugs are absorbed more rapidly than drugs whose lipid solubility is low. This occurs because lipid-soluble drugs can readily cross the membranes that separate them from the blood, whereas drugs of low lipid solubility cannot.

pH Partitioning

pH partitioning can influence drug absorption. Absorption will be enhanced when the difference between the pH of plasma and the pH at the site of administration is such that drug molecules will have a greater tendency to be ionized in the plasma.

Characteristics of Commonly Used Routes of Administration

For each of the major routes of administration—oral (PO), intravenous (IV), intramuscular (IM), and subcutaneous (subQ)—the pattern of drug absorption (i.e., the rate and extent of absorption) is unique. Consequently, the route by which a drug is administered significantly affects both the onset and the intensity of effects. The distinguishing characteristics of the four major routes are summarized in Table 4.1. Additional routes of administration (e.g., topical, transdermal, inhaled) each have unique characteristics that are addressed throughout the book as we discuss specific drugs that use them.

DISTRIBUTION

Distribution is defined as *the movement of drugs from the systemic circulation to the site of drug action.* Drug distribution is determined by three major factors: blood flow to tissues, the ability of a drug to exit the vascular system, and, to a lesser extent, the ability of a drug to enter cells.

Blood Flow to Tissues

In the first phase of distribution, drugs are carried by the blood to the tissues and organs of the body. The rate at which drugs are delivered to a particular tissue is determined by blood flow to that tissue. Because most tissues are well perfused, regional blood flow is rarely a limiting factor in drug distribution.

There are two pathologic conditions—abscesses and tumors—in which low regional blood flow can affect drug therapy. An abscess has no internal blood vessels; therefore, because abscesses lack a blood supply, antibiotics cannot reach the bacteria within. Accordingly, if drug therapy is to be effective, the abscess must usually be surgically drained.

Solid tumors have a limited blood supply. Although blood flow to the outer regions of tumors is relatively high, blood flow becomes progressively lower toward the core. As a result, it may not be possible to achieve high drug levels deep inside tumors. Limited blood flow is a major reason that solid tumors are resistant to drug therapy.

Exiting the Vascular System

After a drug has been delivered to an organ or tissue by blood circulation, the next step is to exit the vasculature. Because most drugs do not produce their effects within the blood, the ability to leave the vascular system is an important determinant of drug actions. Drugs in the vascular system leave the blood at capillary beds.

Typical Capillary Beds

Most capillary beds offer no resistance to the departure of drugs because, in most tissues, drugs can leave the vasculature simply by passing through pores in the capillary wall. Because drugs pass *between* capillary cells rather

TABLE 4.1   Properties of Major Routes of Drug Administration

Route	Barriers to Absorption	Absorption Pattern	Advantages	Disadvantages
Parenteral				
Intravenous (IV)	None (absorption is bypassed)	Instantaneous	Rapid onset, and hence ideal for emergencies	Irreversible
				Expensive
			Precise control over drug levels	Inconvenient
			Permits use of large fluid volumes	Difficult to do, and hence poorly suited for self-administration
			Permits use of irritant drugs	Risk for fluid overload, infection, and embolism
				Drug must be water soluble
Intramuscular (IM)	Capillary wall (easy to pass)	Rapid with water-soluble drugs	Permits use of poorly soluble drugs	Possible discomfort
		Slow with poorly soluble drugs	Permits use of depot preparations	Inconvenient
				Potential for injury
Subcutaneous (subQ)	Same as IM	Same as IM	Same as IM	Same as IM
Enteral				
Oral (PO)	Epithelial lining of gastrointestinal tract; capillary wall	Slow and variable	Easy	Variability
			Convenient	Inactivation of some drugs by gastric acid and digestive enzymes
			Inexpensive	Possible nausea and vomiting from local irritation
			Ideal for self-medication	Patient must be conscious and cooperative.
			Potentially reversible, and hence safer than parenteral routes	

Fig. 4.3 Drug Movement at Typical Capillary Beds. In most capillary beds, "large" gaps exist between the cells that compose the capillary wall. Drugs and other molecules can pass freely into and out of the bloodstream through these gaps. As illustrated, lipid-soluble compounds can also pass directly through the cells of the capillary wall.

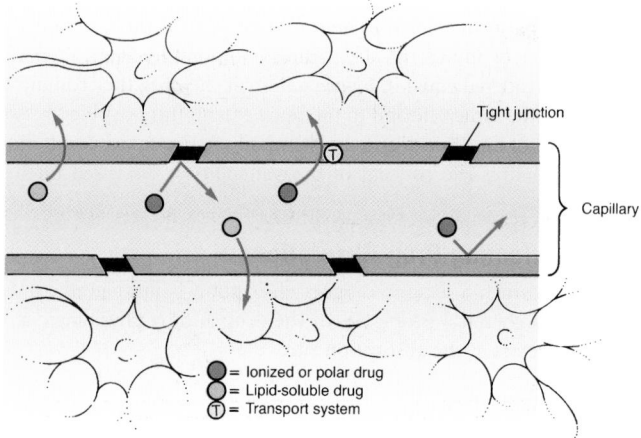

Fig. 4.4 Drug Movement Across the Blood-Brain Barrier. Tight junctions between cells that compose the walls of capillaries in the central nervous system prevent drugs from passing between cells to exit the vascular system. Consequently, to reach sites of action within the brain, a drug must pass directly through cells of the capillary wall. To do this, the drug must be lipid soluble or be able to use an existing transport system.

than *through* them, movement into the interstitial space is not impeded. The exit of drugs from a typical capillary bed is depicted in Fig. 4.3.

Blood–Brain Barrier

The term *blood–brain barrier* (BBB) refers to the unique anatomy of capillaries in the central nervous system (CNS). As shown in Fig. 4.4, there are *tight junctions* between the cells that compose the walls of most capillaries in the CNS. These junctions are so tight that they prevent drug passage. Consequently, to leave the blood and reach sites of action within the brain, a drug must be able to pass *through* cells of the capillary wall. Only drugs that are *lipid soluble* or have a *transport system* can cross the BBB to a significant degree.

Recent evidence indicates that, in addition to tight junctions, the BBB has another protective component: *PGP*. As noted earlier, PGP is a transporter that pumps a variety of drugs out of cells. In capillaries

of the CNS, PGP pumps drugs back into the blood and thereby limits their access to the brain.

The BBB is not fully developed at birth. As a result, newborns have heightened sensitivity to medicines that act on the brain. Likewise, neonates are especially vulnerable to CNS toxicity.

Placental Drug Transfer

The membranes of the placenta separate the maternal circulation from the fetal circulation (Fig. 4.5). *However, the membranes of the placenta do NOT constitute an absolute barrier to the passage of drugs.* The same factors that determine the movement of drugs across other membranes determine the movement of drugs across the placenta. Most drugs cross the placenta via simple diffusion. Lipid-soluble, nonionized compounds

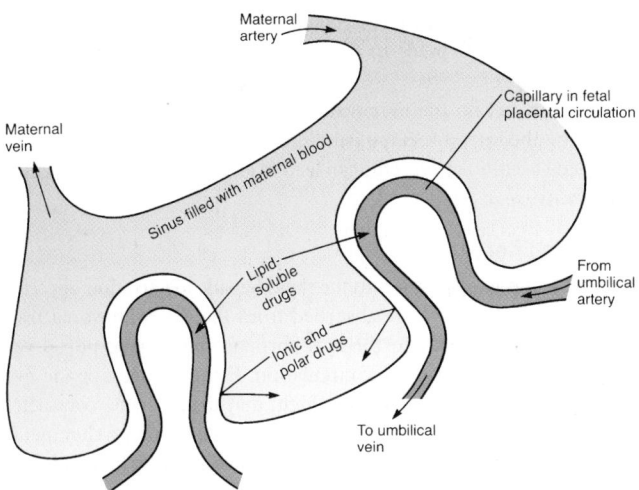

Fig. 4.5 Placental Drug Transfer. To enter the fetal circulation, drugs must cross membranes of the maternal and fetal vascular systems. Lipid-soluble drugs can readily cross these membranes and enter the fetal blood, whereas ions and polar molecules are prevented from reaching the fetal blood.

Fig. 4.6 Protein Binding of Drugs. (A) Albumin is the most prevalent protein in plasma and the most important of the proteins to which drugs bind. (B) Only unbound (free) drug molecules can leave the vascular system. Bound molecules are too large to fit through the pores in the capillary wall.

readily pass from the maternal bloodstream into the blood of the fetus. In contrast, compounds that are ionized, highly polar, or protein bound are largely excluded—as are drugs that are substrates for the PGP transporter that can pump a variety of drugs out of placental cells into the maternal blood.

Protein Binding

Drugs can form reversible bonds with various proteins in the body. Of all the proteins with which drugs can bind, *plasma albumin* is the most important. Like other proteins, albumin is a large molecule. Because of its size, albumin is too large to leave the bloodstream.

Fig. 4.6 depicts the binding of drug molecules to albumin. Note that the drug molecules are much smaller than albumin. As indicated by

the two-way arrows, binding between albumin and drugs is *reversible.* Hence drugs may be *bound* or *unbound* (free).

Even though a drug can bind albumin, only some molecules will be bound at any moment. The percentage of drug molecules that are bound is determined by the strength of the attraction between albumin and the drug. For example, the attraction between albumin and the anticoagulant warfarin is strong, causing nearly all (99%) of the warfarin molecules in plasma to be bound, leaving only 1% free. On the other hand, the attraction between the antibiotic gentamicin and albumin is relatively weak; less than 10% of the gentamicin molecules in plasma are bound, leaving more than 90% free.

An important consequence of protein binding is restriction of drug distribution. Because albumin is too large to leave the bloodstream, drug molecules that are bound to albumin cannot leave either (see Fig. 4.6B). As a result, bound molecules cannot reach their sites of action or undergo metabolism or excretion until the drug–protein bond is broken so that the drug is free to leave the circulation.

In addition to restricting drug distribution, protein binding can be a source of drug interactions. As suggested by Fig. 4.6A, each molecule of albumin has only a few sites to which drug molecules can bind. Because the number of binding sites is limited, drugs with the ability to bind albumin will compete with one another for those sites. As a result, one drug can displace another from albumin, causing the free concentration of the displaced drug to rise, thus increasing the intensity of drug responses. If plasma drug levels rise sufficiently, toxicity can result.

Entering Cells

Many drugs produce their effects by binding with receptors located on the external surface of the cell membrane; however, some drugs must enter cells to reach their sites of action, and practically all drugs must enter cells to undergo metabolism and excretion. The factors that determine the ability of a drug to cross cell membranes are the same factors that determine the passage of drugs across all other membranes, namely lipid solubility, the presence of a transport system, or both.

METABOLISM

Drug metabolism, also known as *biotransformation,* is defined as *the enzymatic alteration of drug structure.* Most drug metabolism takes place in the liver.

Hepatic Drug-Metabolizing Enzymes

Most drug metabolism that takes place in the liver is performed by the *hepatic microsomal enzyme system,* also known as the *P450 system.* The term *P450* refers to *cytochrome P450,* a key component of this enzyme system.

It is important to appreciate that cytochrome P450 is not a single molecular entity but rather a group of 12 closely related enzyme families. Three of the cytochrome P450 (CYP) families—designated CYP1, CYP2, and CYP3—metabolize drugs. The other nine families metabolize endogenous compounds (e.g., steroids, fatty acids). Each of the three P450 families that metabolize drugs is composed of multiple forms, each of which metabolizes only certain drugs. To identify the individual forms of cytochrome P450, designations such as CYP1A2, CYP2D6, and CYP3A4 are used to indicate specific members of the CYP1, CYP2, and CYP3 families, respectively.

Therapeutic Consequences of Drug Metabolism

Drug metabolism has six possible consequences of therapeutic significance:
- Accelerated renal excretion of drugs
- Drug inactivation

- Increased therapeutic action
- Activation of prodrugs
- Increased toxicity
- Decreased toxicity

Accelerated Renal Drug Excretion

The most important consequence of drug metabolism is promotion of renal drug excretion. The kidneys, which are the major organs of drug excretion, are unable to excrete drugs that are highly lipid soluble. Hence, by converting lipid-soluble drugs into more hydrophilic (water-soluble) forms, metabolic conversion can accelerate renal excretion of many agents.

Drug Inactivation

Drug metabolism can convert pharmacologically active compounds to inactive forms. This is the most common end result of drug metabolism.

Increased Therapeutic Action

Metabolism can increase the effectiveness of some drugs. For example, metabolism converts codeine into morphine. The analgesic activity of morphine is so much greater than that of codeine that formation of morphine may account for virtually all the pain relief that occurs after codeine administration.

Activation of Prodrugs

A *prodrug* is a compound that is pharmacologically inactive as administered and then undergoes conversion to its active form through metabolism. Prodrugs have several advantages; for example, a drug that cannot cross the BBB may be able to do so as a lipid-soluble prodrug that is converted to the active form in the CNS.

Increased or Decreased Toxicity

By converting drugs into inactive forms, metabolism can decrease toxicity. Conversely, metabolism can increase the potential for harm by converting relatively safe compounds into forms that are toxic. Increased toxicity is illustrated by the conversion of acetaminophen into a hepatotoxic metabolite. It is this product of metabolism, and not acetaminophen itself, that causes injury when acetaminophen is taken in overdose.

Special Considerations in Drug Metabolism

Several factors can influence the rate at which drugs are metabolized. These must be accounted for in drug therapy.

Age

The drug-metabolizing capacity of infants is limited. The liver does not develop its full capacity to metabolize drugs until approximately 1 year after birth. During the time before hepatic maturation, infants are especially sensitive to drugs, and care must be taken to avoid injury. Similarly, the ability of older adults to metabolize drugs is commonly decreased. Drug dosages may need to be reduced to prevent drug toxicity.

Induction and Inhibition of Drug-Metabolizing Enzymes

Drugs may be P450 substrates, P450 enzyme inducers, and P450 enzyme inhibitors. Drugs that are metabolized by P450 hepatic enzymes are substrates. Drugs that increase the rate of drug metabolism are inducers. Drugs that decrease the rate of drug metabolism are called *inhibitors.* Often a drug may have more than one property. For example, a drug may be both a substrate and an inducer.

Inducers act on the liver to stimulate enzyme synthesis. This process is known as *induction.* By increasing the rate of drug metabolism, the amount of active drug is decreased and plasma drug levels fall. If dosage adjustments are not made to accommodate for this, a drug may not achieve therapeutic levels.

Inhibitors act on the liver through a process known as *inhibition.* By slowing the rate of metabolism, inhibition can cause an increase in active drug accumulation. This can lead to an increase in adverse effects and toxicity.

First-Pass Effect

The term *first-pass effect* refers to the rapid hepatic inactivation of certain oral drugs. When drugs are absorbed from the gastrointestinal tract, they are carried directly to the liver through the hepatic portal vein before they enter the systemic circulation. If the capacity of the liver to metabolize a drug is extremely high, that drug can be completely inactivated on its first pass through the liver. As a result, no therapeutic effects can occur. To circumvent the first-pass effect, a drug that undergoes rapid hepatic metabolism is often administered parenterally. This permits the drug to temporarily bypass the liver, thereby allowing it to reach therapeutic levels in the systemic circulation before being metabolized.

Nutritional Status

Hepatic drug-metabolizing enzymes require a number of cofactors to function. In the malnourished patient, these cofactors may be deficient, causing drug metabolism to be compromised.

Competition Between Drugs

When two drugs are metabolized by the same metabolic pathway, they may compete with each other for metabolism and may thereby decrease the rate at which one or both agents are metabolized. If metabolism is depressed enough, a drug can accumulate to dangerous levels.

Enterohepatic Recirculation

As noted earlier and depicted in Fig. 4.7, enterohepatic recirculation is a repeating cycle in which a drug is transported from the liver into the duodenum (through the bile duct) and then back to the liver (through the portal blood). However, it is important to note that only certain drugs are affected. Specifically, the process is limited to drugs that have undergone *glucuronidation,* a process that converts lipid-soluble drugs to water-soluble drugs by binding them to glucuronic acid. After glucuronidation, these drugs can enter the bile and then pass to the duodenum. In the intestine, some drugs can be hydrolyzed by intestinal β-glucuronidase, an enzyme that breaks the bond between the original drug and the glucuronide moiety, thereby releasing the free drug. Because the free drug is more lipid soluble than the glucuronidated form, the free drug can undergo reabsorption across the intestinal wall, followed by transport back to the liver, where the cycle can start again. Because of enterohepatic recycling, drugs can remain in the body much longer than they otherwise would.

EXCRETION

Drug excretion is defined as *the removal of drugs from the body.* Drugs and their metabolites can exit the body in urine, bile, sweat, saliva, breast milk, and expired air. The most important organ for drug excretion is the kidney.

Renal Drug Excretion

The kidneys account for the majority of drug excretion. When the kidneys are healthy, they serve to limit the duration of action of many drugs. Conversely, if renal failure occurs, both the duration and intensity of drug responses may increase.

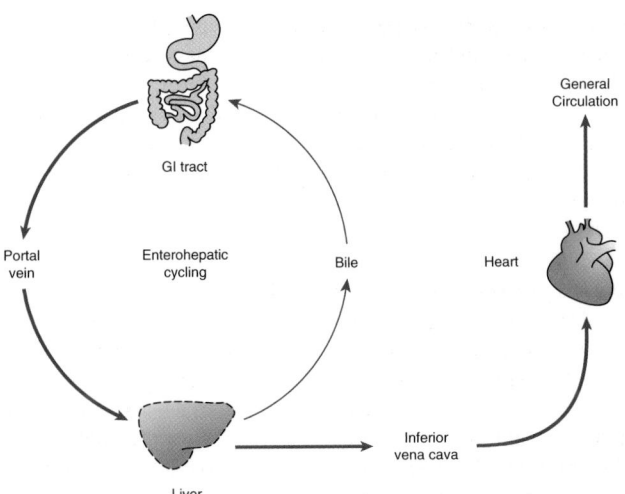

Fig. 4.7 Movement of Drugs After Gastrointestinal *(GI)* Absorption. All drugs absorbed from sites along the GI tract—stomach, small intestine, and large intestine (but not the oral mucosa or distal rectum)—must go through the liver, through the portal vein, on their way to the heart and then the general circulation. For some drugs, passage is uneventful. Others undergo extensive hepatic metabolism, and still others undergo *enterohepatic recirculation,* a repeating cycle in which a drug moves from the liver into the duodenum (through the bile duct) and then back to the liver (through the portal blood). As discussed in the text under *Enterohepatic Recirculation,* the process is limited to drugs that have first undergone hepatic glucuronidation.

Steps in Renal Drug Excretion

Urinary excretion is the net result of three processes: (1) glomerular filtration, (2) passive tubular reabsorption, and (3) active tubular secretion.

Glomerular filtration. Renal excretion begins at the glomerulus of the kidney tubule. As blood flows through the glomerular capillaries, fluids and small molecules—including drugs—are forced through the pores of the capillary wall. This process, called *glomerular filtration,* moves drugs from the blood into the tubular urine. Blood cells and large molecules (e.g., proteins) are too big to pass through the capillary pores and therefore do not undergo filtration. Because large molecules are not filtered, drugs bound to albumin remain in the blood.

Passive tubular reabsorption. As depicted in Fig. 4.8, the vessels that deliver blood to the glomerulus return to proximity with the renal tubule at a point distal to the glomerulus. At this distal site, drug concentrations in the blood are lower than drug concentrations in the tubule. This concentration gradient acts as a driving force to move drugs from the lumen of the tubule back into the blood. Because lipid-soluble drugs can readily cross the membranes that compose the tubular and vascular walls, *drugs that are lipid soluble undergo passive reabsorption from the tubule back into the blood.* In contrast, drugs that are not lipid soluble (ions and polar compounds) remain in the urine to be excreted.

Active tubular secretion. There are active transport systems in the kidney tubules that pump drugs from the blood to the tubular urine. These pumps have a relatively high capacity and play a significant role in excreting certain compounds.

Factors That Modify Renal Drug Excretion

Renal drug excretion varies from patient to patient. Conditions such as chronic renal disease may cause profound alterations. Three other important factors to consider are pH-dependent ionization, competition for active tubular transport, and patient age.

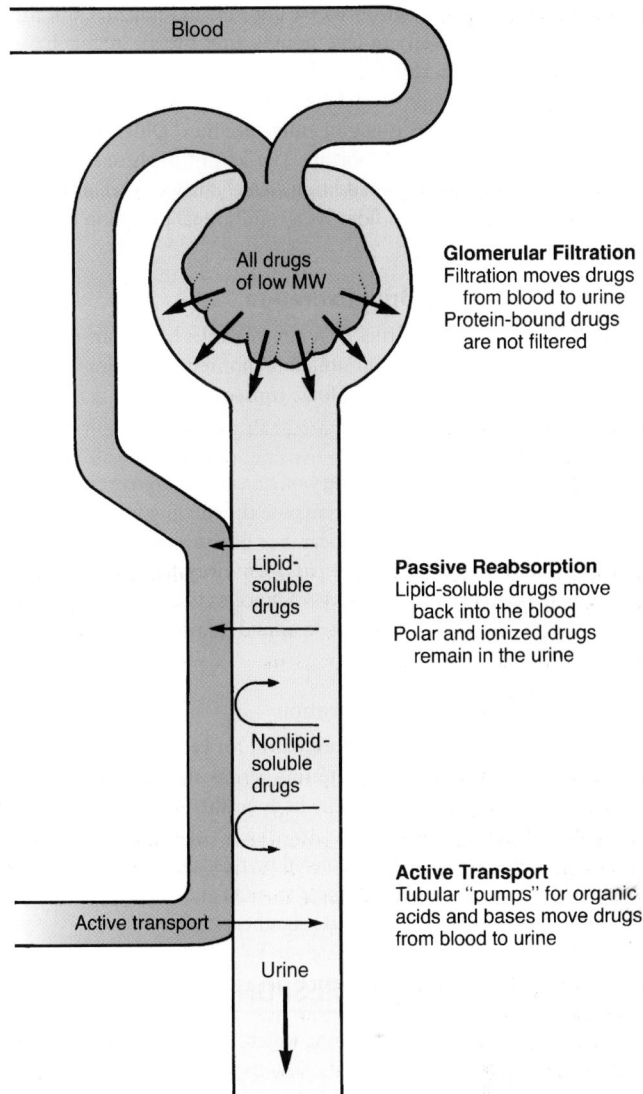

Fig. 4.8 Renal Drug Excretion. *MW,* Molecular weight.

pH-dependent ionization. The phenomenon of pH-dependent ionization can be used to accelerate renal excretion of drugs. Recall that passive tubular reabsorption is limited to lipid-soluble compounds. Because ions are not lipid soluble, drugs that are ionized at the pH of tubular urine will remain in the tubule and be excreted. Consequently, by manipulating urinary pH in such a way as to promote the ionization of a drug, we can decrease passive reabsorption back into the blood and can thereby hasten the drug's elimination. This principle has been used to promote the excretion of poisons and medications that have been taken in toxic doses.

Competition for active tubular transport. Competition between drugs for active tubular transport can delay renal excretion, thereby prolonging effects. The active transport systems of the renal tubules can be envisioned as motor-driven revolving doors that carry drugs from the plasma into the renal tubules. These "revolving doors" can carry only a limited number of drug molecules per unit of time. Accordingly, if there are too many molecules present, some must wait their turn. Because of competition, if we administer two drugs at the same time and if both drugs use the same transport system, excretion of each will be delayed by the presence of the other.

Age. The kidneys of newborns are not fully developed. Until their kidneys reach full capacity (a few months after birth), infants have a limited capacity to excrete drugs. This must be accounted for when medicating an infant.

In older adults, renal function often declines. Older adults have smaller kidneys and fewer nephrons. The loss of nephrons results in decreased blood filtration. In addition, vessel changes such as atherosclerosis reduce renal blood flow. As a result, renal excretion of drugs is decreased.

Nonrenal Routes of Drug Excretion

In most cases, excretion of drugs by nonrenal routes has minimal clinical significance. However, in certain situations, nonrenal excretion can have important therapeutic and toxicologic consequences.

Breast Milk

Some drugs taken by breast-feeding women can undergo excretion into milk. As a result, breastfeeding can expose the nursing infant to drugs. The factors that influence the appearance of drugs in breast milk are the same factors that determine the passage of drugs across membranes. Accordingly, lipid-soluble drugs have ready access to breast milk, whereas drugs that are polar, ionized, or protein bound cannot enter in significant amounts.

Other Nonrenal Routes of Excretion

The *bile* is an important route of excretion for certain drugs. Because bile is secreted into the small intestine, drugs that do not undergo enterohepatic recirculation leave the body in the feces.

The *lungs* are the major route by which volatile anesthetics are excreted. Alcohol is partially eliminated by this route.

Small amounts of drugs can appear in *sweat* and *saliva*. These routes have little therapeutic or toxicologic significance.

TIME COURSE OF DRUG RESPONSES

It is possible to regulate the time at which drug responses start, the time they are most intense, and the time they cease. Because the four pharmacokinetic processes—absorption, distribution, metabolism, and excretion—determine how much drug will be at its sites of action at any given time, these processes are the major determinants of the time course over which drug responses take place.

Plasma Drug Levels

In most cases the time course of drug action bears a direct relationship to the concentration of a drug in the blood. Hence, before discussing the time course per se, we need to review several important concepts related to plasma drug levels.

Clinical Significance of Plasma Drug Levels

Providers frequently monitor plasma drug levels in efforts to regulate drug responses. When measurements indicate that drug levels are inappropriate, these levels can be adjusted up or down by changing dosage size, dosage timing, or both.

The practice of regulating plasma drug levels to control drug responses should seem a bit odd, given that (1) drug responses are related to drug concentrations at sites of action and (2) the site of action of most drugs is not in the blood. More often than not, it is a practical impossibility to measure drug concentrations at sites of action. Experience has shown that, for most drugs, *there is a direct correlation between therapeutic and toxic responses and the amount of drug present in plasma.* Therefore, although we cannot usually measure drug concentrations at sites of action, we *can* determine plasma drug concentrations that, in turn, are

highly predictive of therapeutic and toxic responses. Accordingly, the dosing objective is commonly spoken of in terms of achieving a specific plasma level of a drug.

Two Plasma Drug Levels Defined

Two plasma drug levels are of special importance: (1) the minimum effective concentration (MEC) and (2) the toxic concentration. These levels are depicted in Fig. 4.9.

Minimum effective concentration. The MEC is defined as *the plasma drug level less than which therapeutic effects will not occur.* Hence, to be of benefit, a drug must be present in concentrations at or greater than the MEC.

Toxic concentration. Toxicity occurs when plasma drug levels climb too high. The plasma level at which toxic effects begin is termed the *toxic concentration.* Doses must be kept small enough so that the toxic concentration is not reached.

Therapeutic Range

As indicated in Fig. 4.9, there is a range of plasma drug levels, falling between the MEC and the toxic concentration, which is termed the *therapeutic range.* When plasma levels are within the therapeutic range, there is enough drug present to produce therapeutic responses but not so much that toxicity results. *The objective of drug dosing is to maintain plasma drug levels within the therapeutic range.*

The width of the therapeutic range is a major determinant of the ease with which a drug can be used safely. Drugs that have a narrow therapeutic range are difficult to administer safely. Conversely, drugs that have a wide therapeutic range can be administered safely with relative ease. The principle is the same as that of the therapeutic index discussed in Chapter 3. The therapeutic range is quantified, or measured, by the therapeutic index.

Understanding the concept of therapeutic range can facilitate patient care. Because drugs with a narrow therapeutic range are more dangerous than drugs with a wide therapeutic range, patients taking drugs with a narrow therapeutic range are the most likely to require intervention for drug-related complications. The provider who is aware of this fact can focus additional attention on monitoring these patients for signs and symptoms of toxicity.

Single-Dose Time Course

Fig. 4.9 shows how plasma drug levels change over time after a single dose of an oral medication. Drug levels rise as the medicine undergoes

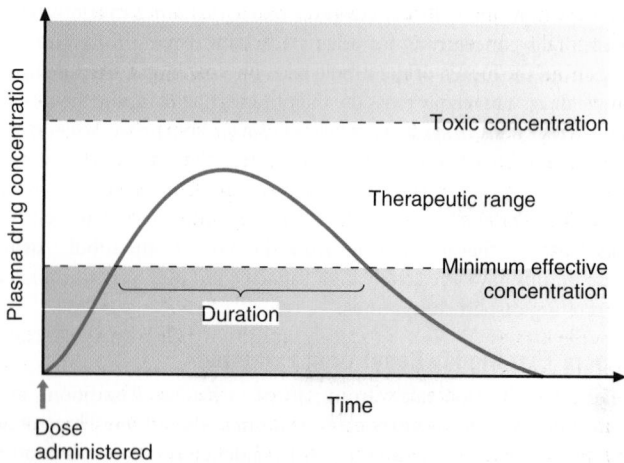

Fig. 4.9 Single-Dose Time Course.

absorption. Drug levels then decline as metabolism and excretion eliminate the drug from the body.

Because responses cannot occur until plasma drug levels have reached the MEC, there is a latent period between drug administration and onset of effects. The extent of this delay is determined by the rate of absorption.

The duration of effects is determined largely by the combination of metabolism and excretion. As long as drug levels remain greater than the MEC, therapeutic responses will be maintained; when levels fall to less than the MEC, benefits will cease. Because metabolism and excretion are the processes most responsible for causing plasma drug levels to fall, these processes are the primary determinants of how long drug effects will persist.

Drug Half-Life

Before proceeding to the topic of multiple dosing, we need to discuss the concept of half-life. When a patient ceases drug use, the combination of metabolism and excretion will cause the amount of drug in the body to decline. The half-life of a drug is an index of just how rapidly that decline occurs for most drugs. The concept of half-life does not apply to the elimination of all drugs. A few agents, most notably ethanol (alcohol), leave the body at a *constant rate*, regardless of how much is present. The implications of this kind of decline for ethanol are discussed in Chapter 32.

Drug half-life is defined as *the time required for the amount of drug in the body to decrease by 50%*. A few drugs have half-lives that are extremely short—on the order of minutes or less. In contrast, the half-lives of some drugs exceed 1 week.

Note that, in our definition of half-life, a *percentage*—not a specific *amount*—of drug is lost during one half-life. That is, the half-life does not specify, for example, that 2 g or 18 mg will leave the body in a given time. Rather, the half-life tells us that, no matter what the amount of drug in the body may be, half (50%) will leave during a specified period of time (the half-life). The actual amount of drug that is lost during one half-life depends on just how much drug is present: the more drug in the body, the larger the amount lost during one half-life.

The concept of half-life is best understood through an example. Morphine provides a good illustration. The half-life of morphine is approximately 3 hours. By definition, this means that body stores of morphine will decrease by 50% every 3 hours—regardless of how much morphine is in the body. If there are 50 mg of morphine in the body, 25 mg (50% of 50 mg) will be lost in 3 hours; if there are only 2 mg of morphine in the body, only 1 mg (50% of 2 mg) will be lost in 3 hours. Note that, in both cases, morphine levels drop by 50% during an interval of one half-life. However, the actual *amount* lost is larger when total body stores of the drug are higher.

The half-life of a drug determines the dosing interval (i.e., how much time separates each dose). For drugs with a short half-life, the dosing interval must be correspondingly short. If a long dosing interval is used, drug levels will fall to less than the MEC between doses, and therapeutic effects will be lost. Conversely, if a drug has a long half-life, a long time can separate doses without loss of benefits.

Drug Levels Produced With Repeated Doses

Multiple dosing leads to drug accumulation. When a patient takes a single dose of a drug, plasma levels simply go up and then come back down. In contrast, when a patient takes repeated doses of a drug, the process is more complex and results in drug accumulation. The factors that determine the rate and extent of accumulation are considered next.

Plateau Drug Levels

Administering repeated doses will cause a drug to build up in the body until a *plateau* (steady level) has been achieved. What causes drug levels to reach plateau? If a second dose of a drug is administered before all of the prior dose has been eliminated, total body stores of that drug will be higher after the second dose than after the initial dose. As succeeding doses are administered, drug levels will climb even higher. The drug will continue to accumulate until a state has been achieved in which the amount of drug eliminated between doses equals the amount administered. *When the amount of drug eliminated between doses equals the dose administered, average drug levels will remain constant and plateau will have been reached* (Fig. 4.10).

Time to Plateau

When a drug is administered repeatedly in the same dose, *plateau will be reached in approximately four half-lives*. For the hypothetical agent illustrated in Fig. 4.10, total body stores approached their peak near the beginning of day 5, or approximately 4 full days after treatment began. Because the half-life of this drug is 1 day, reaching plateau in 4 days is equivalent to reaching plateau in four half-lives.

As long as dosage remains constant, the time required to reach plateau is independent of dosage size. Put another way, the time required to reach plateau when giving repeated large doses of a particular drug is identical to the time required to reach plateau when giving repeated small doses of that drug. Referring to the drug in Fig. 4.10, just as it took four half-lives (4 days) to reach plateau when a dose of 2 g was administered daily, it would also take four half-lives to reach plateau if a dose of 4 g were administered daily. It is true that the *height* of the plateau would be greater if a 4-g dose were given, but the time required to reach plateau would not be altered by the increase in dosage. To confirm this statement, substitute a dose of 4 g in the previous exercise and see when plateau is reached.

Techniques for Reducing Fluctuations in Drug Levels

As illustrated in Fig. 4.10, when a drug is administered repeatedly, its level will fluctuate between doses. The highest level is referred to as the *peak concentration*, and the lowest level is referred to as the *trough concentration*. The acceptable height of the peaks and troughs will depend on the drug's therapeutic range: the peaks must be kept less than the toxic concentration, and the troughs must be kept greater than the MEC. If there is not much difference between the toxic concentration and the MEC, then fluctuations must be kept to a minimum.

Three techniques can be used to reduce fluctuations in drug levels. One technique is to *administer drugs by continuous infusion*. With this

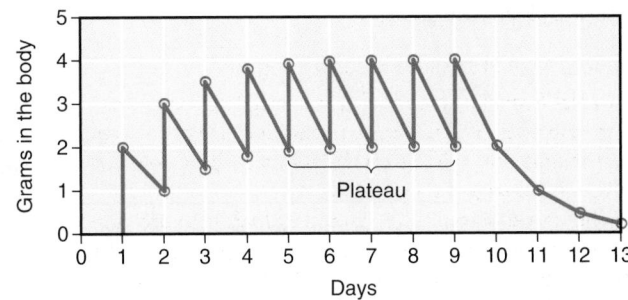

Fig. 4.10 Drug Accumulation With Repeated Administration. The drug has a half-life of 1 day. The dosing schedule is 2 g given once a day on days 1 through 9. Note that plateau is reached at about the beginning of day 5 (i.e., after four half-lives). Note also that, when administration is discontinued, it takes approximately 4 days (four half-lives) for most (94%) of the drug to leave the body.

procedure, plasma levels can be kept nearly constant. Another is to *administer a depot preparation,* which releases the drug slowly and steadily. The third is to *reduce both the size of each dose and the dosing interval* (keeping the total daily dose constant). For example, rather than giving the drug from Fig. 4.10 in 2-g doses once every 24 hours, we could give this drug in 1-g doses every 12 hours. With this altered dosing schedule, the total daily dose would remain unchanged, as would total body stores at plateau. However, instead of fluctuating over a range of 2 g between doses, levels would fluctuate over a range of 1 g.

Loading Doses Versus Maintenance Doses

As discussed previously, if we administer a drug in repeated doses of *equal size,* an interval equivalent to approximately four half-lives is required to achieve plateau. When plateau must be achieved more quickly, a large initial dose can be administered. This large initial dose is called a *loading dose.* After high drug levels have been established with a loading dose, plateau can be maintained by giving smaller doses. These smaller doses are referred to as *maintenance doses.*

The claim that use of a loading dose will shorten the time to plateau may appear to contradict an earlier statement, which said that the time to plateau is not affected by dosage size. However, there is no contradiction. For any *specified dosage,* it will always take about four half-lives to reach plateau. When a loading dose is administered followed by maintenance doses, the plateau is not reached *for the loading dose.* Rather, we have simply used the loading dose to rapidly produce a drug level equivalent to the plateau level for a smaller dose. To achieve plateau level for the loading dose, it would be necessary to either administer repeated doses equivalent to the loading dose for a period of four half-lives or administer a dose even larger than the original loading dose.

Decline From Plateau

When drug administration is discontinued, most (94%) of the drug in the body will be eliminated over an interval equal to approximately four half-lives. The time required for drugs to leave the body is important when toxicity develops. If a drug has a short half-life, body stores will decline rapidly, thereby making management of overdose less difficult. However, when an overdose of a drug with a long half-life occurs, toxic levels of the drug will remain in the body for a long time. Additional management may be needed in these instances.

▌PHARMACODYNAMICS

Pharmacodynamics is the study of the biochemical and physiologic effects of drugs on the body and the molecular mechanisms by which those effects are produced. To participate rationally in achieving the therapeutic objective, an understanding of pharmacodynamics is essential.

DOSE–RESPONSE RELATIONSHIPS

The dose–response relationship (i.e., the relationship between the size of an administered dose and the intensity of the response produced) is a fundamental concern in therapeutics. Dose–response relationships determine the minimal amount of drug needed to elicit a response, the maximal response a drug can elicit, and how much to increase the dosage to produce the desired increase in response.

Basic Features of the Dose–Response Relationship

The basic characteristics of dose–response relationships are illustrated in Fig. 4.11. Part A shows dose–response data plotted on *linear* coordinates. Part B shows the same data plotted on *semilogarithmic* coordinates (i.e., the scale on which dosage is plotted is logarithmic rather than linear). The most obvious and important characteristic revealed by these curves is that the dose–response relationship is *graded.* That is, as the dosage increases, the response becomes progressively larger. Because drug responses are graded, therapeutic effects can be adjusted to fit the needs of each patient by raising or lowering the dosage until a response of the desired intensity is achieved.

As indicated in Fig. 4.11, the dose–response relationship can be viewed as having three phases. Phase 1 (see Fig. 4.11B) occurs at low

Fig. 4.11 Basic Components of the Dose-Response Curve. (A) A dose–response curve with dose plotted on a linear scale. (B) The same dose–response relationship shown in A but with the dose plotted on a logarithmic scale. Note the three phases of the dose–response curve: *Phase 1,* The curve is relatively flat; doses are too low to elicit a significant response. *Phase 2,* The curve climbs upward as bigger doses elicit correspondingly bigger responses. *Phase 3,* The curve levels off; bigger doses are unable to elicit a further increase in response. (Phase 1 is not indicated in A because very low doses cannot be shown on a linear scale.)

doses. The curve is flat during this phase because doses are too low to elicit a measurable response. During phase 2, an increase in dose elicits a corresponding increase in the response. This is the phase during which the dose–response relationship is graded. As the dose goes higher, eventually a point is reached where an increase in dose is unable to elicit a further increase in response. At this point, the curve flattens out into phase 3.

Maximal Efficacy and Relative Potency

Dose–response curves reveal two characteristic properties of drugs: *maximal efficacy* and *relative potency*. Curves that reflect these properties are shown in Fig. 4.12.

Maximal Efficacy

Maximal efficacy is defined as *the largest effect that a drug can produce*. Maximal efficacy is indicated by the *height* of the dose–response curve.

The concept of maximal efficacy is illustrated by the dose–response curves for meperidine (Demerol) and pentazocine (Talwin), two morphine-like pain relievers (see Fig. 4.12A). As you can see, the curve for pentazocine levels off at a maximal height less than that of the curve for meperidine. This tells us that the maximal degree of pain relief we can achieve with pentazocine is smaller than the maximal degree of pain relief we can achieve with meperidine. Put another way, no matter how much pentazocine we administer, we can never produce the degree of pain relief that we can with meperidine. Accordingly, we would say that meperidine has greater maximal efficacy than pentazocine.

Despite what intuition might tell us, a drug with very high maximal efficacy is not always more desirable than a drug with lower efficacy. Recall that we want to match the intensity of the response to the patient's needs. This may be difficult to do with a drug that produces extremely intense responses. For example, certain diuretics (e.g., furosemide) have such high maximal efficacy that they can cause dehydration. If we want to mobilize only a modest volume of water, a diuretic with lower maximal efficacy (e.g., hydrochlorothiazide) would be preferred. Similarly, in a patient with a mild headache, we would not select a powerful analgesic (e.g., morphine) for relief. Rather, we would select an analgesic with lower maximal efficacy, such as aspirin.

Relative Potency

The term *potency* refers to the amount of drug we must give to elicit an effect. Potency is indicated by the relative position of the dose-response curve along the *x* (dose) axis.

The concept of potency is illustrated by the curves in Fig. 4.12B. These curves plot doses for two analgesics—morphine and meperidine—versus the degree of pain relief achieved. As you can see, for any particular degree of pain relief, the required dose of meperidine is larger than the required dose of morphine. Because morphine produces pain relief at lower doses than meperidine, we would say that morphine is more potent than meperidine. That is, a potent drug is one that produces its effects at low doses.

Potency is rarely an important characteristic of a drug. The only consequence of having greater potency is that a drug with greater potency can be given in smaller doses.

It is important to note that the potency of a drug implies nothing about its maximal efficacy! Potency and efficacy are completely independent qualities. Drug A can be more effective than drug B even though drug B may be more potent. In addition, drugs A and B can be equally effective even though one may be more potent. As shown in Fig. 4.12B, although meperidine happens to be less potent than morphine, the maximal degree of pain relief that we can achieve with these drugs is identical.

A final comment on the word *potency* is in order. In everyday parlance, people tend to use the word *potent* to express the pharmacologic concept of effectiveness. That is, when most people say, "This drug is very potent," what they mean is, "This drug produces powerful effects." They do not mean, "This drug produces its effects at low doses." In pharmacology, we use the words *potent* and *potency* with the specific and appropriate terminology.

DRUG–RECEPTOR INTERACTIONS

Introduction to Drug Receptors

Drugs produce their effects by interacting with other chemicals. Receptors are the special chemical sites in the body that most drugs interact with to produce effects.

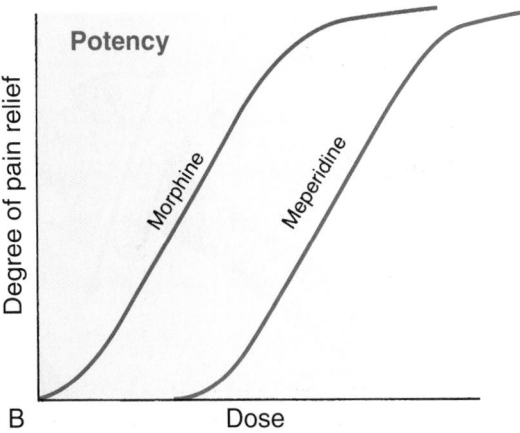

Fig. 4.12 Dose–Response Curves Demonstrating Efficacy and Potency. (A) Efficacy, or maximal efficacy, is an index of the maximal response a drug can produce. The efficacy of a drug is indicated by the height of its dose–response curve. In this example, meperidine has greater efficacy than pentazocine. Efficacy is an important quality in a drug. (B) Potency is an index of how much drug must be administered to elicit a desired response. In this example, achieving pain relief with meperidine requires higher doses than with morphine. We would say that morphine is more potent than meperidine. Note that, if administered in sufficiently high doses, meperidine can produce just as much pain relief as morphine. Potency is usually not an important quality in a drug.

We can define a receptor as *any functional macromolecule in a cell to which a drug binds to produce its effects*. However, although the formal definition of a receptor encompasses all functional macromolecules, the term *receptor* is generally reserved for the body's own receptors for hormones, neurotransmitters, and other regulatory molecules. The other macromolecules to which drugs bind, such as enzymes and ribosomes, can be thought of simply as target molecules rather than as true receptors.

Binding of a drug to its receptor is usually *reversible*. Receptors are activated by interaction with other molecules (Fig. 4.13). Under physiologic conditions, endogenous compounds (neurotransmitters, hormones, other regulatory molecules) are the molecules that bind to receptors to produce a response. When a drug is the molecule that binds to a receptor, all that it can do is mimic or block the actions of endogenous regulatory molecules. By doing so, the drug will either increase or decrease the rate of the physiologic activity normally controlled by that receptor.

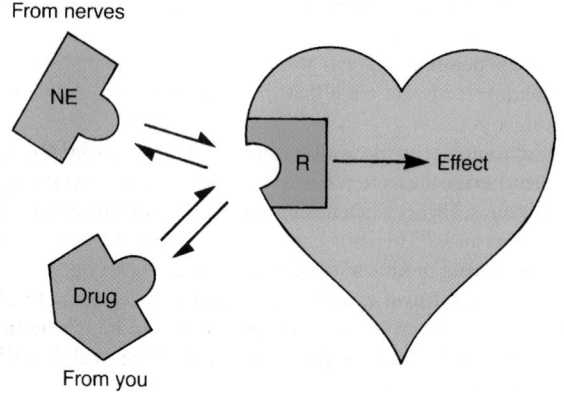

Fig. 4.13 Interaction of Drugs With Receptors for Norepinephrine. Under physiologic conditions, cardiac output can be increased by the binding of norepinephrine *(NE)* to receptors *(R)* on the heart. Norepinephrine is supplied to these receptors by nerves. These same receptors can be acted on by drugs, which can either mimic the actions of endogenous NE (and thereby increase cardiac output) or block the actions of endogenous NE (and thereby reduce cardiac output).

Because drug action is limited to mimicking or blocking the body's own regulatory molecules, drugs cannot give cells new functions. In other words, drugs cannot make the body do anything that it is not already capable of doing.[b]

Receptors and Selectivity of Drug Action

Selectivity, the ability to elicit only the response for which a drug is given, is a highly desirable characteristic of a drug. The more selective a drug is, the fewer side effects it will produce. Selective drug action is possible in large part because drugs act through specific receptors. There are receptors for each neurotransmitter (e.g., norepinephrine [NE], acetylcholine, dopamine); there are receptors for each hormone (e.g., progesterone, insulin, thyrotropin); and there are receptors for all of the other molecules the body uses to regulate physiologic processes (e.g., histamine, prostaglandins, leukotrienes). As a rule, each type of receptor participates in the regulation of just a few processes (Fig. 4.14). If a drug interacts with only one type of receptor, and if that receptor type regulates just a few processes, then the effects of the drug will be limited. Conversely, if a drug interacts with several different receptor types, then that drug is likely to elicit a wide variety of responses.

How can a drug interact with one receptor type and not with others? In some important ways, a receptor is analogous to a lock and a drug is analogous to a key for that lock: just as only keys with the proper profile can fit a particular lock, only those drugs with the proper size, shape, and physical properties can bind to a particular receptor (Fig. 4.15).

Theories of Drug-Receptor Interaction

In the discussion that follows, we consider two theories of drug–receptor interaction: (1) the simple occupancy theory and (2) the modified occupancy theory. These theories help explain dose–response relationships and the ability of drugs to mimic or block the actions of endogenous regulatory molecules.

---

[b]The only exception to this rule is gene therapy. By inserting genes into cells, we actually can make them do something they were previously incapable of doing.

Fig. 4.14 The Four Primary Receptor Families. *1,* Cell membrane–embedded enzyme. *2,* Ligand-gated ion channel. *3,* G protein–coupled receptor system (*G,* G protein). *4,* Transcription factor. (See text for details.)

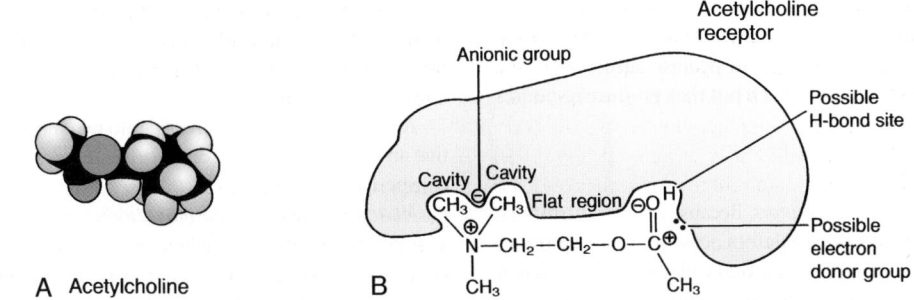

Fig. 4.15 Interaction of Acetylcholine With Its Receptor. (A) Three-dimensional model of the acetylcholine molecule. (B) Binding of acetylcholine to its receptor. Note how the shape of acetylcholine closely matches the shape of the receptor. Note also how the positive charges on acetylcholine align with the negative sites on the receptor.

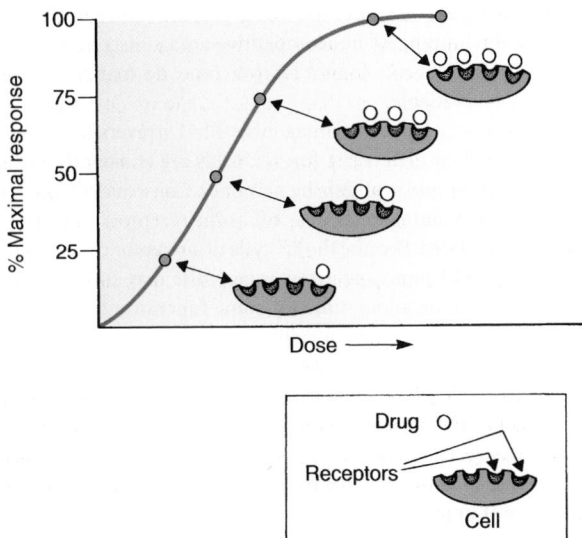

Fig. 4.16 Model of Simple Occupancy Theory. The simple occupancy theory states that the intensity of response to a drug is proportional to the number of receptors occupied; maximal response is reached with 100% receptor occupancy. Because the hypothetical cell in this figure has only four receptors, maximal response is achieved when all four receptors are occupied. (*Note:* Real cells have thousands of receptors.)

Simple Occupancy Theory

The simple occupancy theory of drug–receptor interaction states that (1) the intensity of the response to a drug is proportional to the number of receptors occupied by that drug and (2) a maximal response will occur when *all* available receptors have been occupied. This relationship between receptor occupancy and the intensity of the response is depicted in Fig. 4.16.

Although certain aspects of dose–response relationships can be explained by the simple occupancy theory, other important phenomena cannot. Specifically, there is nothing in this theory to explain why one drug should be more potent than another. In addition, this theory cannot explain how one drug can have higher maximal efficacy than another. That is, according to this theory, two drugs acting at the same receptor should produce the same maximal effect, provided that their dosages were high enough to produce 100% receptor occupancy. However, we have already seen this is not true. As illustrated in Fig. 4.12A, there is a dose of pentazocine greater than which no further increase in response can be elicited. Presumably, all receptors are occupied when

the dose-response curve levels off. However, at 100% receptor occupancy, the response elicited by pentazocine is less than that elicited by meperidine. Simple occupancy theory cannot account for this difference.

Modified Occupancy Theory

The modified occupancy theory of drug–receptor interaction explains certain observations that cannot be accounted for with the simple occupancy theory. The modified theory ascribes two qualities to drugs: *affinity* and *intrinsic activity*. The term *affinity* refers to the strength of the attraction between a drug and its receptor. *Intrinsic activity* refers to the ability of a drug to activate the receptor after binding. *Affinity and intrinsic activity are independent properties.*

Affinity. As noted, the term *affinity* refers to the strength of the attraction between a drug and its receptor. Drugs with high affinity are strongly attracted to their receptors. Conversely, drugs with low affinity are weakly attracted.

The affinity of a drug for its receptor is reflected in its *potency*. Because they are strongly attracted to their receptors, drugs with high affinity can bind to their receptors when present in low concentrations. Because they bind to receptors at low concentrations, drugs with high affinity are effective in low doses. That is, *drugs with high affinity are very potent*. Conversely, drugs with low affinity must be present in high concentrations to bind to their receptors. Accordingly, these drugs are less potent.

Intrinsic activity. The term *intrinsic activity* refers to the ability of a drug to activate a receptor upon binding. Drugs with high intrinsic activity cause intense receptor activation. Conversely, drugs with low intrinsic activity cause only slight activation.

The intrinsic activity of a drug is reflected in its *maximal efficacy*. Drugs with high intrinsic activity have high maximal efficacy. That is, by causing intense receptor activation, they are able to cause intense responses. Conversely, if intrinsic activity is low, maximal efficacy will be low as well.

It should be noted that, under the modified occupancy theory, the intensity of the response to a drug is still related to the number of receptors occupied. The wrinkle added by the modified theory is that intensity is also related to the ability of the drug to activate receptors after binding has occurred. Under the modified theory, two drugs can occupy the same number of receptors but produce effects of different intensity; the drug with greater intrinsic activity will produce the more intense response.

Agonists, Antagonists, and Partial Agonists

As previously noted, when drugs bind to receptors, they can do one of two things: they can either *mimic* the action of endogenous regulatory molecules or they can *block* the action of endogenous regulatory molecules. Drugs that mimic the body's own regulatory molecules are called *agonists*. Drugs that block the actions of endogenous regulators are called *antagonists*. Like agonists, *partial agonists* also mimic the actions of endogenous regulatory molecules, but they produce responses of intermediate intensity.

Agonists

Agonists are molecules that activate receptors. Because neurotransmitters, hormones, and other endogenous regulators activate the receptors to which they bind, all of these compounds are considered agonists. When drugs act as agonists, they simply bind to receptors and mimic the actions of the body's own regulatory molecules. For example, dobutamine is a drug that mimics the action of NE at receptors on the heart, thereby causing heart rate and force of contraction to increase.

In terms of the modified occupancy theory, an agonist is a drug that has both *affinity* and *high intrinsic activity*. Affinity allows the agonist to bind to receptors, whereas intrinsic activity allows the bound agonist to activate or turn on receptor function.

Antagonists

Antagonists produce their effects by preventing receptor activation by endogenous regulatory molecules and drugs. Antagonists have virtually no effects of their own on receptor function.

In terms of the modified occupancy theory, an antagonist is a drug with affinity for a receptor but with no intrinsic activity. Affinity allows the antagonist to bind to receptors, but lack of intrinsic activity prevents the bound antagonist from causing receptor activation.

Although antagonists do not cause receptor activation, they most certainly *do* produce pharmacologic effects. Antagonists produce their effects by *preventing the activation of receptors* by endogenous regulatory molecules. For example, antihistamines are histamine receptor antagonists that suppress allergy symptoms by binding to receptors for histamine, thereby preventing activation of these receptors by histamine released in response to allergens.

It is important to note that the response to an antagonist is determined by how much *agonist* is present. Because antagonists act by preventing receptor activation, *if there is no agonist present, administration of an antagonist will have no observable effect*; the drug will bind to its receptors, but nothing will happen. On the other hand, if receptors are undergoing

activation by agonists, administration of an antagonist will shut the process down, resulting in an observable response. An example is the use of the opioid antagonist naloxone, which is used to block opioid receptors in the event of an opioid overdose.

Antagonists can be subdivided into two major classes: (1) noncompetitive antagonists and (2) competitive antagonists. Most antagonists are competitive.

Noncompetitive (insurmountable) antagonists. Noncompetitive antagonists bind *irreversibly* to receptors. The effect of irreversible binding is equivalent to reducing the total number of receptors available for activation by an agonist. Because the intensity of the response to an agonist is proportional to the total number of receptors occupied and because noncompetitive antagonists decrease the number of receptors available for activation, noncompetitive antagonists *reduce the maximal response* that an agonist can elicit. If sufficient antagonist is present, agonist effects will be blocked completely. Dose–response curves illustrating inhibition by a noncompetitive antagonist are shown in Fig. 4.17A.

Because the binding of noncompetitive antagonists is irreversible, inhibition by these agents cannot be overcome, no matter how much agonist may be available.

Although noncompetitive antagonists bind irreversibly, this does not mean that their effects last forever. Cells are constantly breaking down old receptors and synthesizing new ones. Consequently, the effects of noncompetitive antagonists wear off as the receptors to which they are bound are replaced. Because the life cycle of a receptor can be relatively short, the effects of noncompetitive antagonists may subside in a few days. Still, this can be a long time for some functions; therefore these agents are rarely used therapeutically.

Competitive (surmountable) antagonists. Competitive antagonists bind *reversibly* to receptors. As their name implies, competitive antagonists produce receptor blockade by competing with agonists for receptor binding. If an agonist and a competitive antagonist have equal affinity for a particular receptor, then the receptor will be occupied by whichever agent—agonist or antagonist—is present in the highest concentration. If there are more antagonist molecules present than agonist molecules, antagonist molecules will occupy the receptors and receptor activation will be blocked. Conversely, if agonist molecules outnumber the antagonists, receptors will be occupied mainly by the agonist and little inhibition will occur.

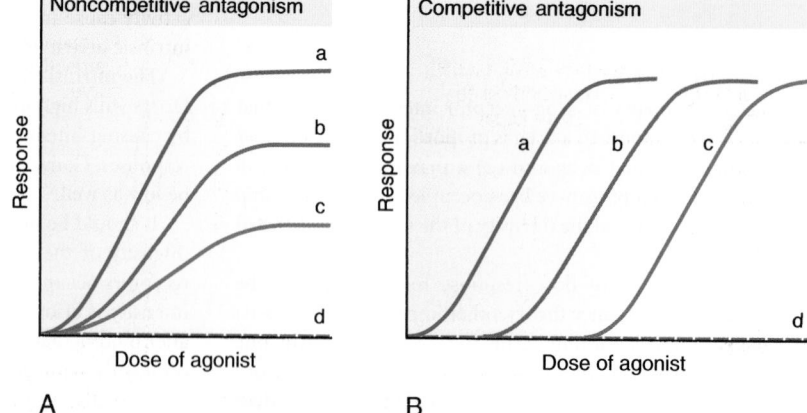

a = Agonist alone
b = Agonist + antagonist (low dose)
c = Agonist + antagonist (higher dose)
d = Antagonist alone

Fig. 4.17 Dose–Response Curves in the Presence of Competitive and Noncompetitive Antagonists. (A) Effect of a noncompetitive antagonist on the dose–response curve of an agonist. Note that noncompetitive antagonists decrease the maximal response achievable with an agonist. (B) Effect of a competitive antagonist on the dose–response curve of an agonist. Note that the maximal response achievable with the agonist is not reduced. Competitive antagonists simply increase the amount of agonist required to produce any given intensity of response.

Because competitive antagonists bind reversibly to receptors, the inhibition they cause is *surmountable.* In the presence of sufficiently high amounts of agonist, agonist molecules will occupy all receptors and inhibition will be completely overcome. The dose–response curves shown in Fig. 4.17B illustrate the process of overcoming the effects of a competitive antagonist with large doses of an agonist.

Partial Agonists

A partial agonist is an agonist that has only moderate intrinsic activity. As a result, *the maximal effect that a partial agonist can produce is lower than that of a full agonist.* Pentazocine is an example of a partial agonist. As the curves in Fig. 4.12A indicate, the degree of pain relief that can be achieved with pentazocine is much lower than the relief that can be achieved with meperidine (a full agonist).

Partial agonists are interesting in that they can act as *antagonists* as well as *agonists.* For this reason, they are sometimes referred to as agonists-antagonists. For example, when pentazocine is administered by itself, it occupies opioid receptors and produces moderate relief of pain. In this situation, the drug is acting as an agonist. However, if a patient is already taking meperidine (a full agonist at opioid receptors) and is then given a large dose of pentazocine, pentazocine will occupy the opioid receptors and prevent their activation by meperidine. As a result, rather than experiencing the high degree of pain relief that meperidine can produce, the patient will experience only the limited relief that pentazocine can produce. In this situation, pentazocine is acting as both an agonist (producing moderate pain relief) and an antagonist (blocking the higher degree of relief that could have been achieved with meperidine by itself).

Regulation of Receptor Sensitivity

Receptors are dynamic components of the cell. In response to continuous activation or continuous inhibition, the number of receptors on the cell surface can change, as can their sensitivity to agonist molecules. For example, when the receptors of a cell are continually exposed to an *agonist,* the cell usually becomes less responsive. When this occurs, the cell is said to be *desensitized* or *refractory* or to have undergone *downregulation.* Several mechanisms may be responsible, including destruction of receptors by the cell and modification of receptors such that they respond less fully. Continuous exposure to antagonists has the opposite effect, causing the cell to become *hypersensitive* (also referred to as *supersensitive*). One mechanism that can cause hypersensitivity is synthesis of more receptors.

DRUG RESPONSES THAT DO NOT INVOLVE RECEPTORS

Although the effects of most drugs result from drug–receptor interactions, some drugs do not act through receptors. Rather, they act through simple physical or chemical interactions with other small molecules.

Common examples of these drugs include antacids, antiseptics, saline laxatives, and chelating agents. Antacids neutralize gastric acidity by direct chemical interaction with stomach acid. The antiseptic action of ethyl alcohol results from precipitating bacterial proteins. Magnesium sulfate, a powerful laxative, acts by retaining water in the intestinal lumen through an osmotic effect. Dimercaprol, a chelating agent, prevents toxicity from heavy metals (e.g., arsenic, mercury) by forming complexes with these compounds. All of these pharmacologic effects are the result of simple physical or chemical interactions and not interactions with cellular receptors.

INTERPATIENT VARIABILITY IN DRUG RESPONSES

The dose required to produce a therapeutic response can vary substantially from patient to patient because people differ from one another. In this section we consider interpatient variation as a general issue. The specific kinds of differences that underlie variability in drug responses are discussed in Chapter 6.

To promote the therapeutic objective, you must be alert to interpatient variation in drug responses. Because of interpatient variation, it is not possible to predict exactly how an individual patient will respond to medication. The provider who appreciates the reality of interpatient variability will be better prepared to anticipate, evaluate, and respond appropriately to each patient's therapeutic needs.

Fig. 4.18 illustrates an example of interpatient variability in response to a drug. Fig. 4.18A represents incremental increases in the milligram dose of drug to elevated gastric pH coupled with the number of patients who had a therapeutic response (pH of 5) at each dose. In Fig. 4.18B, these results are plotted on a *frequency distribution curve.* We can see

Dose of Drug (mg)	Number of Subjects Responding at Each Dose
100	2
120	6
140	17
160	25
180	25
200	17
220	6
240	2

A

B

Fig. 4.18 Interpatient Variation in Drug Responses. (A) Data from tests of a hypothetical acid suppressant in 100 patients. The goal of the study is to determine the dosage required by each patient to elevate gastric pH to 5. Note the wide variability in doses needed to produce the target response for the 100 subjects. (B) Frequency distribution curve for the data in A. The dose at the middle of the curve is termed the ED_{50}—the dose that will produce a predefined intensity of response in 50% of the population.

from the curve that a wide range of doses is required to produce the desired response in all subjects. For some subjects, a dose of only 100 mg was sufficient to produce the target response. For other subjects, the therapeutic end point was not achieved until the dose totaled 240 mg.

ED_{50}

The dose at the middle of the frequency distribution curve is termed the ED_{50} (see Fig. 4.18B). (ED_{50} is an abbreviation for *average effective dose.*) The ED_{50} is defined as *the dose that is required to produce a defined therapeutic response in 50% of the population.* In the case of the drug in our example, the ED_{50} was 170 mg—the dose needed to elevate gastric pH to a value of 5 in 50% of the 100 people tested.

The ED_{50} can be considered a standard dose and, as such, is frequently the dose selected for initial treatment. After evaluating a patient's response to this standard dose, we can then adjust subsequent doses up or down to meet the patient's needs.

Clinical Implications of Interpatient Variability

Interpatient variation has four important clinical consequences. As a provider you should be aware of these implications:

- The initial dose of a drug is necessarily an approximation. Subsequent doses may need to be fine-tuned based on the patient's response.
- When given an ED_{50}, some patients will be undertreated, whereas others will have received more drug than they need. Accordingly, when therapy is initiated with a dose equivalent to the ED_{50}, it is especially important to evaluate the response. Patients who fail to respond may need an increase in dosage. Conversely, patients who show signs of toxicity will need a dosage reduction.
- Because drug responses are not completely predictable, you must monitor the patient's response for both positive effects and adverse effects to determine whether too much or too little medication has been administered. In other words, dosage should be adjusted on

the basis of the patient's response and not just on the basis of clinical guidelines.

THERAPEUTIC INDEX

The therapeutic index is a measure of a drug's safety. The therapeutic index is defined as *the ratio of a drug's LD_{50} to its ED_{50}.* (The LD_{50}, or average lethal dose, is the dose that is lethal to 50% of the subjects treated.) A large (or high or wide) therapeutic index indicates that a drug is relatively safe. Conversely, a small (or low or narrow) therapeutic index indicates that a drug is relatively unsafe.

The concept of therapeutic index is illustrated by the frequency distribution curves in Fig. 4.19. Part A of the figure shows curves for therapeutic and lethal responses to drug X. Part B shows equivalent curves for drug Y. As you can see in Fig. 4.19A, the LD_{50} (100 mg) for drug X is much larger than the average therapeutic dose (10 mg). Because this drug's lethal dose is much larger than its therapeutic dose, common sense tells us that the drug should be relatively safe. The safety of this drug is reflected in its high therapeutic index, which is 10. In contrast, drug Y is unsafe. As shown in Fig. 4.19B, the LD_{50} for drug Y (20 mg) is only twice the average therapeutic dose (10 mg). Hence, for drug Y, a dose only twice the ED_{50} could be lethal to 50% of those treated. Clearly, drug Y is not safe. This lack of safety is reflected in its low therapeutic index.

The curves for drug Y illustrate a phenomenon that is even more important than the therapeutic index. As you can see, there is *overlap* between the curve for therapeutic effects and the curve for lethal effects. This overlap tells us that the high doses needed to produce therapeutic effects in some people may be large enough to cause death in others. The message here is that, if a drug is to be truly safe, the highest dose required to produce therapeutic effects must be substantially lower than the lowest dose required to produce death.

Fig. 4.19 Therapeutic Index. (A) Frequency distribution curves indicating the average effective dose *(ED_{50})* and average lethal dose *(LD_{50})* for drug X. Because its LD_{50} is much greater than its ED_{50}, drug X is relatively safe. (B) Frequency distribution curves indicating the ED_{50} and LD_{50} for drug Y. Because its LD_{50} is very close to its ED_{50}, drug Y is not very safe. Also note the overlap between the effective-dose curve and the lethal-dose curve.

DRUG INTERACTIONS

A drug interaction occurs when another substance alters a drug's efficacy, effects, or safety. These are usually the result of interactions with other drugs, food, or supplements.

DRUG–DRUG INTERACTIONS

Drug–drug interactions can occur whenever a patient takes two or more drugs. Some interactions are both intended and desired, as when we combine drugs to treat hypertension. In contrast, some interactions are both unintended and undesired.

Consequences of Drug–Drug Interactions

When two drugs interact, there are three possible outcomes: (1) one drug may intensify the effects of the other, (2) one drug may reduce the effects of the other, or (3) the combination may produce a new response not seen with either drug alone.

Intensification of Effects

When one drug intensifies, or potentiates, the effects of the other, this type of interaction is often termed *potentiative*. Potentiative interactions may be beneficial or detrimental.

Increased therapeutic effects. The interaction between sulbactam and ampicillin represents a beneficial potentiative interaction. When administered alone, ampicillin undergoes rapid inactivation by bacterial enzymes. Sulbactam inhibits those enzymes and thereby prolongs and intensifies ampicillin's therapeutic effects.

Increased adverse effects. The interaction between aspirin and warfarin represents a potentially detrimental potentiative interaction. Both aspirin and warfarin suppress formation of blood clots; aspirin does this through antiplatelet activity, and warfarin does this through anticoagulant activity. As a result, if aspirin and warfarin are taken concurrently, the risk for bleeding is significantly increased.

Reduction of Effects

Interactions that result in reduced drug effects are often termed *inhibitory*. As with potentiative interactions, inhibitory interactions can be beneficial or detrimental. Inhibitory interactions that reduce toxicity are beneficial. Conversely, inhibitory interactions that reduce therapeutic effects are detrimental.

Reduced therapeutic effects. The interaction between propranolol and albuterol represents a detrimental inhibitory interaction. Albuterol is taken by people with asthma to dilate the bronchi. Propranolol, a drug for cardiovascular disorders, can act in the lung to block the effects of albuterol. Hence, if propranolol and albuterol are taken together, propranolol can reduce albuterol's therapeutic effects.

Reduced adverse effects. The use of naloxone to treat morphine overdose is an excellent example of a beneficial inhibitory interaction. When administered in excessive dosage, morphine can produce coma, profound respiratory depression, and eventual death. Naloxone blocks morphine's actions and can completely reverse all symptoms of toxicity.

Creation of a Unique Response

Rarely, the combination of two drugs produces a new response not seen with either agent alone. To illustrate, let's consider the combination of alcohol with disulfiram (Antabuse)], a drug used to treat alcohol use disorder. When alcohol and disulfiram are combined, a host of unpleasant and dangerous responses can result; however, these effects do not occur when disulfiram or alcohol is used alone.

Basic Mechanisms of Drug–Drug Interactions

Drugs can interact through four basic mechanisms: (1) direct chemical or physical interaction, (2) pharmacokinetic interaction, (3) pharmacodynamic interaction, and (4) combined toxicity.

Direct Chemical or Physical Interactions

Some drugs, because of their physical or chemical properties, can undergo direct interaction with other drugs. Direct physical and chemical interactions usually render both drugs inactive.

Direct interactions occur most commonly when drugs are combined in IV solutions. Frequently, the interaction produces a precipitate; however, direct drug interactions may not always leave visible evidence. Hence you cannot rely on simple inspection to reveal all direct interactions. Because drugs can interact in solution, *it is essential to consider and verify drug incompatibilities when ordering medications.*

The same kinds of interactions that can take place when drugs are mixed together in an IV solution can also occur when incompatible drugs are taken by other routes. However, because drugs are diluted in body water after administration, and because dilution decreases chemical interactions, significant interactions within the patient are much less likely than in IV solutions.

Pharmacokinetic Interactions

Drug interactions can affect all four of the basic pharmacokinetic processes. That is, when two drugs are taken together, one may alter the absorption, distribution, metabolism, or excretion of the other.

Altered absorption. Drug absorption may be enhanced or reduced by drug interactions. There are several mechanisms by which one drug can alter the absorption of another.

- By elevating gastric pH, antacids can decrease the ionization of basic drugs in the stomach, increasing the ability of basic drugs to cross membranes and be absorbed. Antacids have the opposite effect on acidic drugs.
- Laxatives can reduce absorption of other oral drugs by accelerating their passage through the intestine.
- Drugs that depress peristalsis (e.g., morphine, atropine) prolong drug transit time in the intestine, thereby increasing the time for absorption.
- Drugs that induce vomiting can decrease absorption of oral drugs.
- Orally administered adsorbent drugs that do not undergo absorption (e.g., cholestyramine) can adsorb other drugs onto themselves, thereby preventing absorption of the other drugs into the blood.
- Drugs that reduce regional blood flow can reduce absorption of other drugs from that region. For example, when epinephrine is injected together with a local anesthetic, the epinephrine causes local vasoconstriction, thereby reducing regional blood flow and delaying absorption of the anesthetic.

Altered distribution. There are two principal mechanisms by which one drug can alter the distribution of another: (1) competition for protein binding and (2) alteration of extracellular pH.

Competition for protein binding. When two drugs bind to the same site on plasma albumin, coadministration of those drugs produces competition for binding. As a result, binding of one or both agents is reduced, causing plasma levels of free drug to rise. In theory, the increase in free drug can intensify effects. However, because the newly freed drug usually undergoes rapid elimination, the increase in plasma levels of free drug is rarely sustained or significant unless the patient has liver problems that interfere with drug metabolism or has renal problems that interfere with drug excretion.

Alteration of extracellular pH. A drug with the ability to change extracellular pH can alter the distribution of other drugs. For example, if a drug were to increase extracellular pH, that drug would increase the ionization of acidic drugs in extracellular fluids (i.e., plasma and interstitial fluid). As a result, acidic drugs would be drawn from within cells (where the pH was less than that of the extracellular fluid) into the extracellular space. Hence the alteration in pH would change drug distribution.

The ability of drugs to alter pH and thereby alter the distribution of other drugs can be put to practical use in the management of poisoning. For example, symptoms of aspirin toxicity can be reduced with sodium bicarbonate, a drug that elevates extracellular pH. By increasing the pH outside cells, bicarbonate causes aspirin to move from intracellular sites into the interstitial fluid and plasma, thereby minimizing injury to cells.

Altered metabolism. Altered metabolism is one of the most important—and most complex—mechanisms by which drugs interact. Some drugs *increase* the metabolism of other drugs, and some drugs *decrease* the metabolism of other drugs. Drugs that increase the metabolism of other drugs do so by inducing synthesis of hepatic drug-metabolizing enzymes. Drugs that decrease the metabolism of other drugs do so by inhibiting those enzymes.

As discussed earlier in this chapter, the majority of drug metabolism is catalyzed by the cytochrome P450 enzymes, which are composed of a large number of isoenzyme families (CYP1, CYP2, and CYP3) that are further divided into specific forms. Five isoenzyme forms are responsible for the metabolism of most drugs: CYP1A2, CYP2C9, CYP2C19, CYP2D6, and CYP3A4. Table 4.2 lists major drugs that are metabolized by each isoenzyme and indicates drugs that can inhibit or induce those isoenzymes.

Induction of CYP enzymes. In our discussion of metabolism earlier in the chapter, you learned about induction of CYP enzymes.

When it is essential that an inducing agent is taken with another medicine, dosage of the other medicine may need adjustment. For example, if a woman taking oral contraceptives were to begin taking phenobarbital, induction of drug metabolism by phenobarbital would accelerate metabolism of the contraceptive, thereby lowering its level. If drug metabolism were increased enough, protection against pregnancy would be lost. To maintain contraceptive efficacy, dosage of the contraceptive should be increased. Conversely, when a patient *discontinues* an inducing agent, dosages of other drugs may need to be *lowered*. If dosage is not reduced, drug levels may climb dangerously high as rates of hepatic metabolism decline to their baseline (noninduced) values.

Inhibition of CYP enzymes. If drug A inhibits the metabolism of drug B, then levels of drug B will rise. The result may be beneficial or harmful. The interactions of cobicistat (a strong CYP3A4 inhibitor) and atazanavir (an expensive drug used to treat HIV infection) provide an interesting case in point. Because cobicistat inhibits CYP3A (the CYP isoenzyme that metabolizes atazanavir), if cobicistat is combined with atazanavir, the plasma level of atazanavir will rise. In this instance, inhibition of CYP3A4 allows us to achieve therapeutic drug levels at lower doses, thereby greatly reducing the cost of treatment.

Although inhibition of drug metabolism can be beneficial, as a rule inhibition has undesirable results. That is, in most cases, when an inhibitor increases the level of another drug, the outcome is toxicity. Accordingly, when a patient is taking an inhibitor along with his or her other medicines, you should be alert for possible adverse effects. Unfortunately, because the number of possible interactions of this type is large, keeping track is a challenge. The safest practice is to check for drug interactions in one of the reliable software applications that are widely available.

Altered renal excretion. Drugs can alter all three phases of renal excretion: filtration, reabsorption, and active secretion. By doing so, one drug can alter the renal excretion of another. Glomerular filtration can be decreased by drugs that reduce cardiac output: a reduction in cardiac output decreases renal perfusion, which decreases drug filtration

at the glomerulus, which in turn decreases the rate of drug excretion. By altering urinary pH, one drug can alter the ionization of another and thereby increase or decrease the extent to which that drug undergoes passive tubular reabsorption. Finally, competition between two drugs for active tubular secretion can decrease the renal excretion of both agents.

Interactions that involve P-glycoprotein. As discussed earlier in this chapter, PGP is a transmembrane protein that transports a wide variety of drugs *out* of cells, including cells of the intestinal epithelium, placenta, BBB, liver, and kidney tubules. Like P450 isoenzymes, PGP is subject to induction and inhibition by drugs. In fact (and curiously), most of the drugs that induce or inhibit P450 have the same effect on PGP. Drugs that *induce* PGP can have the following effects on other drugs:

- *Reduced absorption*—by increasing drug export from cells of the intestinal epithelium into the intestinal lumen
- *Reduced fetal drug exposure*—by increasing drug export from placental cells into the maternal blood
- *Reduced brain drug exposure*—by increasing drug export from cells of brain capillaries into the blood
- *Increased drug elimination*—by increasing drug export from liver into the bile and from renal tubular cells into the urine
  Drugs that inhibit PGP will have opposite effects.

Pharmacodynamic Interactions

By influencing pharmacodynamic processes, one drug can alter the effects of another. Pharmacodynamic interactions are of two basic types: (1) interactions in which the interacting drugs act at the *same* site and (2) interactions in which the interacting drugs act at *separate* sites. Pharmacodynamic interactions may be potentiative or inhibitory and can be of great clinical significance.

Interactions at the same receptor. Interactions that occur at the same receptor are almost always *inhibitory*. Inhibition occurs when an antagonist drug blocks access of an agonist drug to its receptor. There are many agonist–antagonist interactions of clinical importance. Some reduce therapeutic effects and are therefore undesirable. Others reduce toxicity and are of obvious benefit. The interaction between naloxone and morphine noted earlier in this chapter is an example of a beneficial inhibitory interaction: by blocking access of morphine to its receptors, naloxone can reverse all symptoms of morphine overdose.

Interactions resulting from actions at separate sites. Even though two drugs have different mechanisms of action and act at separate sites, if both drugs influence the same physiologic process, then one drug can alter responses produced by the other. Interactions resulting from effects produced at different sites may be potentiative or inhibitory.

The interaction between morphine and diazepam (Valium) illustrates a potentiative interaction resulting from concurrent use of drugs that act at separate sites. Morphine and diazepam are CNS depressants, but these drugs do not share the same mechanism of action. Hence, when these agents are administered together, the ability of each to depress CNS function reinforces the depressant effects of the other. This potentiative interaction can result in profound CNS depression.

The interaction between two diuretics—hydrochlorothiazide and spironolactone—illustrates how the effects of a drug acting at one site can counteract the effects of a second drug acting at a different site. Hydrochlorothiazide acts on the distal convoluted tubule of the nephron to increase excretion of potassium. Acting at a different site in the kidney, spironolactone works to decrease renal excretion of potassium. Consequently, when these two drugs are administered together, the potassium-sparing effects of spironolactone tend to balance the potassium-wasting effects of hydrochlorothiazide, leaving renal excretion of potassium at approximately the same level it would have been had no drugs been given at all.

TABLE 4.2 Drugs That Are Important Substrates, Inhibitors, or Inducers of Specific CYP Isoenzymes

CYP	Substrates	Inhibitors	Inhibitors	Inducers
CYP1A2	*CNS drugs:* amitriptyline, clomipramine, clozapine, desipramine, duloxetine, fluvoxamine, haloperidol, imipramine, methadone, ramelteon, rasagiline, ropinirole, tacrine *Others:* theophylline, tizanidine, warfarin	Acyclovir Ciprofloxacin Ethinyl estradiol Fluvoxamine Isoniazid Norfloxacin Oral contraceptives Zafirlukast Zileuton		Carbamazepine Phenobarbital Phenytoin Primidone Rifampin Ritonavir Tobacco St. John's wort
CYP2C9	Diazepam, phenytoin, ramelteon, voriconazole, warfarin	Amiodarone Azole antifungals Efavirenz Fenofibrate Fluorouracil Fluoxetine	Fluvastatin Fluvoxamine Gemfibrozil Isoniazid Leflunomide Zafirlukast	Aprepitant Carbamazepine Phenobarbital Phenytoin Primidone Rifampin Rifapentine Ritonavir St. John's wort
CYP2C19	Citalopram, clopidogrel, methadone, phenytoin, thioridazine, voriconazole	Chloramphenicol Cimetidine Esomeprazole Etravirine Felbamate Fluconazole Fluoxetine	Fluvoxamine Isoniazid Ketoconazole Lansoprazole Modafinil Omeprazole Ticlopidine Voriconazole	Carbamazepine Phenobarbital Phenytoin St. John's wort Tipranavir/ritonavir
CYP2D6	*CNS drugs:* amitriptyline, atomoxetine, clozapine, desipramine, donepezil, doxepin, duloxetine, fentanyl, haloperidol, iloperidone, imipramine, meperidine, nortriptyline, tetrabenazine, thioridazine, tramadol, trazodone *Antidysrhythmic drugs:* flecainide, mexiletine, propafenone *β blocker:* metoprolol Opioids: codeine, dextromethorphan, hydrocodone	Amiodarone Cimetidine Darifenacin Darunavir/ritonavir Duloxetine Fluoxetine Methadone	Paroxetine Propranolol Quinidine Ritonavir Sertraline Tipranavir/ritonavir	Not an inducible enzyme
CYP3A4	*Antibacterials/antifungals:* clarithromycin, erythromycin, ketoconazole, itraconazole, rifabutin, telithromycin, voriconazole *Anticancer drugs:* busulfan, dasatinib, doxorubicin, erlotinib, etoposide, ixabepilone, lapatinib, paclitaxel, pazopanib, romidepsin, sunitinib, tamoxifen, vinblastine, vincristine *Calcium channel blockers:* amlodipine, felodipine, isradipine, nifedipine, nimodipine, nisoldipine, verapamil *Drugs for HIV infection:* amprenavir, atazanavir, darunavir, etravirine, indinavir, maraviroc, nelfinavir, ritonavir, saquinavir, tipranavir *Drugs for erectile dysfunction:* sildenafil, tadalafil, vardenafil *Drugs for urge incontinence:* darifenacin, fesoterodine, solifenacin, tolterodine *Immunosuppressants:* cyclosporine, everolimus, sirolimus, tacrolimus *Opioids:* alfentanil, alfuzosin, fentanyl, methadone, oxycodone *Sedative-Hypnotics:* alprazolam, eszopiclone, midazolam, ramelteon, triazolam *Statins:* atorvastatin, lovastatin, simvastatin *Antidysrhythmics drugs:* disopyramide, dronedarone, lidocaine, quinidine *Others:* aprepitant, bosentan, cinacalcet, cisapride, colchicine, conivaptan, dihydroergotamine, dronabinol, eplerenone, ergotamine, estrogens, ethosuximide, fluticasone, guanfacine, iloperidone, ondansetron, oral contraceptives, pimozide, ranolazine, rivaroxaban, saxagliptin, sertraline, silodosin, tiagabine, tolvaptan, trazodone, warfarin	Amiodarone Amprenavir Aprepitant Atazanavir Azole antifungals Chloramphenicol Cimetidine Clarithromycin Cobicistat Conivaptan Cyclosporine Darunavir/ritonavir Delavirdine Diltiazem Dronedarone Erythromycin Fluvoxamine Fosamprenavir Grapefruit juice	Indinavir Isoniazid Methylprednisolone Nefazodone Nelfinavir Nicardipine Nifedipine Norfloxacin Pazopanib Prednisone Protease inhibitors Quinine Quinupristin/ dalfopristin Ritonavir Saquinavir Telithromycin Tipranavir/ritonavir Verapamil	Amprenavir Aprepitant Bosentan Carbamazepine Dexamethasone Efavirenz Ethosuximide Etravirine Garlic supplements Nevirapine Oxcarbazepine Phenobarbital Phenytoin Primidone Rifabutin Rifampin Rifapentine Ritonavir St. John's wort

This list is not comprehensive.
CNS, Central nervous system; *HIV,* human immunodeficiency virus.

Combined Toxicity

If drug A and drug B are both toxic to the same organ, then taking them together will cause more injury than if they were not combined. For example, when we treat tuberculosis with isoniazid and rifampin, both of which are hepatotoxic, the potential to cause liver injury is greater than it would be if we used just one of the drugs. As a rule, drugs with overlapping toxicity are not used together. Unfortunately, when treating tuberculosis, the combination is essential.

Clinical Significance of Drug–Drug Interactions

Clearly, drug interactions have the potential to affect the outcome of therapy. As a result of drug–drug interactions, the intensity of responses may be increased or reduced. Interactions that increase therapeutic effects or reduce toxicity are desirable. Conversely, interactions that reduce therapeutic effects or increase toxicity are detrimental.

Interactions are especially important for drugs that have a narrow therapeutic range. For these agents, an interaction that produces a modest increase in drug levels can cause toxicity. Conversely, an interaction that produces a modest decrease in drug levels can cause therapeutic failure.

Although a large number of important interactions have been documented, many more are yet to be identified. Therefore if a patient develops unusual symptoms, it is wise to suspect that a drug interaction may be the cause—especially because yet another drug might be given to control the new symptoms.

Minimizing Adverse Drug–Drug Interactions

We can minimize adverse interactions in several ways. The most obvious is to minimize the number of drugs a patient receives. A second and equally important way to avoid detrimental interactions is to take a thorough drug history. A history that identifies all drugs the patient is taking, including illicit and over-the-counter preparations, allows the provider to adjust the regimen accordingly. Additional measures for reducing adverse interactions include adjusting the dosage when an inducer of metabolism is added to or deleted from the regimen, adjusting the timing of administration to minimize interference with absorption, monitoring for early signs of toxicity when combinations of toxic agents cannot be avoided, and being especially vigilant when the patient is taking a drug with a narrow therapeutic range.

DRUG–FOOD INTERACTIONS

Coadministration with food can significantly alter the efficacy and safety of some drugs. The primary mechanisms are by decreased or increased absorption and altered metabolism.

Decreased Absorption

Food frequently decreases the *rate* of drug absorption and occasionally decreases the *extent* of absorption. Reducing the rate of absorption merely delays the onset of effects; peak effects are not lowered. In contrast, reducing the extent of absorption reduces the intensity of peak responses.

The interaction between calcium-containing foods and tetracycline antibiotics is a classic example of food reducing drug absorption. Tetracyclines bind with calcium to form an insoluble and nonabsorbable complex. Hence, if tetracyclines are administered with milk products or calcium supplements, absorption is reduced and antibacterial effects may be lost.

High-fiber foods can reduce absorption of some drugs. For example, absorption of digoxin (Lanoxin), used for cardiac disorders, is reduced significantly by wheat bran, rolled oats, and sunflower seeds. This reduced absorption can result in therapeutic failure.

Increased Absorption

With some drugs, food increases the extent of absorption. When this occurs, peak effects are heightened. For example, a high-calorie meal more than doubles the absorption of saquinavir (Invirase), a drug for HIV infection. If saquinavir is taken without food, absorption may be insufficient for antiviral activity.

Effects of Food on Drug Metabolism: The Grapefruit Juice Effect

Grapefruit juice can inhibit the metabolism of certain drugs, thereby raising their blood levels. Four compounds have been identified as the responsible agents: two furanocoumarins (*bergapten* and *6′,7′-dihydroxybergamottin*) and two flavonoids (*naringin* and *naringenin*). This effect is *not* seen with orange juice; however, other citrus fruits related to grapefruit–Seville oranges, pomelos, and tangelos–contain furanocoumarins. Drug interactions with these fruits have not been adequately tested. Until more is known, these should be treated with the same caution as grapefruit juice.

Grapefruit juice raises drug levels mainly by inhibiting CYP3A4 metabolism. CYP3A4 is an isoenzyme of cytochrome P450 found in the liver and the intestinal wall. Inhibition of the *intestinal* isoenzyme is much greater than inhibition of the liver isoenzyme. By inhibiting CYP3A4, grapefruit juice decreases the intestinal metabolism of many drugs (Table 4.3) and thereby increases the amount available for absorption. As a result, blood levels of these drugs rise, causing peak effects to be more intense. Because inhibition of CYP3A4 in the liver is minimal, grapefruit juice does not usually affect metabolism of drugs after they have been absorbed. Importantly, grapefruit juice has little or no effect on drugs administered intravenously. Why? Because, with IV administration, intestinal metabolism is not involved. Inhibition of CYP3A4 is dose dependent; the more grapefruit juice the patient drinks, the greater the inhibition.

Inhibition of CYP3A4 persists after grapefruit juice is consumed, so the problem cannot be easily resolved by scheduling medication hours after drinking the juice. In fact, when grapefruit juice is consumed on a regular basis, inhibition can persist up to 3 days after the last drink.

The effects of grapefruit juice vary considerably among patients because levels of CYP3A4 show great individual variation. In patients with very little CYP3A4, inhibition by grapefruit juice may be sufficient to stop metabolism completely. As a result, large increases in drug levels may occur. Conversely, in patients with an abundance of CYP3A4, metabolism may continue more or less normally, despite inhibition by grapefruit juice.

The effects of grapefruit juice also vary considerably among CYP3A4 substrates. In one study, coadministration of grapefruit juice produced a 406% increase in blood levels of the calcium channel blocker felodipine (Plendil). For some other drugs metabolized by these isoenzymes, the effects are negligible.

The clinical consequences of inhibition may be good or bad. As indicated in Table 4.3, by elevating levels of certain drugs, grapefruit juice can increase the risk for serious toxicity. On the other hand, by increasing levels of two drugs—saquinavir and cyclosporine—grapefruit juice can intensify therapeutic effects to promote positive outcomes.

What should providers do if the drugs they are prescribing can be affected by grapefruit juice? Unless a predictable effect is known or desirable, prudence dictates advising patients to avoid grapefruit juice entirely.

Effects of Food on Drug Toxicity

Drug–food interactions sometimes increase toxicity. The most dramatic example is the interaction between monoamine oxidase (MAO) inhibitors

TABLE 4.3   Some Drugs Whose Levels Can Be Increased by Grapefruit Juice

Drug	Indications	Potential Consequences of Increased Drug Levels
Dihydropyridine CCBs: felodipine, nifedipine, nimodipine, nisoldipine	Hypertension; angina pectoris	Toxicity: flushing, headache, tachycardia, hypotension
Nondihydropyridine CCBs: verapamil	Hypertension; angina pectoris	Toxicity: bradycardia, AV heart block, hypotension, constipation
Statins: atorvastatin, lovastatin, simvastatin (minimal effect on fluvastatin, pravastatin, or rosuvastatin)	Cholesterol reduction	Toxicity: headache, GI disturbances, liver and muscle toxicity
Amiodarone	Cardiac dysrhythmias	Toxicity
Caffeine	Prevents sleepiness	Toxicity: restlessness, insomnia, convulsions, tachycardia
Carbamazepine	Seizures; bipolar disorder	Toxicity: ataxia, drowsiness, nausea, vomiting, tremor
Buspirone	Anxiety	Drowsiness, dysphoria
Triazolam	Anxiety; insomnia	Increased sedation
Midazolam	Induction of anesthesia; conscious sedation	Increased sedation
Saquinavir	HIV infection	Increased therapeutic effect
Cyclosporine	Prevents rejection of organ transplants	Increased therapeutic effects; if levels rise too high, renal and hepatic toxicity will occur
Sirolimus and tacrolimus	Prevent rejection of organ transplants	Toxicity
SSRIs: fluoxetine, fluvoxamine, sertraline	Depression	Toxicity: serotonin syndrome
Pimozide	Tourette syndrome	Toxicity: QT prolongation resulting in a life-threatening ventricular dysrhythmia
Praziquantel	Schistosomiasis	Toxicity
Dextromethorphan	Cough	Toxicity
Sildenafil	Erectile dysfunction	Toxicity

AV, Atrioventricular; *CCBs,* calcium channel blockers; *GI,* gastrointestinal; *HIV,* human immunodeficiency virus; *SSRIs,* selective serotonin reuptake inhibitors.

and foods rich in tyramine (e.g., aged cheeses, yeast extracts, Chianti wine). If an MAO inhibitor is combined with these foods, blood pressure can rise to a life-threatening level. To avoid disaster, patients taking MAO inhibitors must be warned about the consequences of consuming tyramine-rich foods and must be given a list of foods to strictly avoid (see Chapter 26). Other drug–food combinations that can increase toxicity include the following:

- Theophylline (an asthma medicine) plus caffeine, which can result in excessive CNS excitation
- Potassium-sparing diuretics (e.g., spironolactone) plus salt substitutes, which can result in dangerously high potassium levels
- Aluminum-containing antacids (e.g., Maalox) plus citrus beverages (e.g., orange juice), which can result in excessive absorption of aluminum

Effects of Food on Drug Action

Although most drug–food interactions concern drug absorption or drug metabolism, food may also (rarely) have a direct effect on drug action. For example, foods rich in vitamin K (e.g., broccoli, Brussels sprouts, cabbage) can reduce the effects of warfarin, an anticoagulant. This occurs because warfarin inhibits vitamin K–dependent clotting factors. Accordingly, when vitamin K is more abundant, warfarin is less able to inhibit the clotting factors and therapeutic effects decline.

Timing of Drug Administration With Respect to Meals

Prescribing the administration of drugs at the appropriate time with respect to meals is an important part of drug therapy. As discussed, the absorption of some drugs can be significantly decreased by food, and hence these drugs should be prescribed to be administered on an empty stomach (i.e., at least 1 hour before or 2 hours after a meal). Conversely, the absorption of other drugs can be increased by food, and hence these drugs should be prescribed to be administered with meals.

Many drugs cause stomach upset when taken without food. If food does not significantly reduce their absorption, then these drugs should be administered with meals. However, if food does reduce their absorption, then we have a difficult choice: we can administer them with food and thereby reduce stomach upset but also reduce absorption, or we can administer them without food and thereby improve absorption but also increase stomach upset. Unfortunately, the correct choice is not obvious. The best solution, when possible, may be to select an alternative drug that does not upset the stomach.

DRUG–SUPPLEMENT INTERACTIONS

Dietary supplements (herbal medicines and other nonconventional remedies) create the potential for frequent and significant interactions with conventional drugs. Of greatest concern are interactions that reduce beneficial responses to conventional drugs and interactions that increase toxicity. These interactions occur through the same pharmacokinetic and pharmacodynamic mechanisms by which conventional drugs interact with each other. Unfortunately, reliable information about dietary supplements is largely lacking, including information on interactions with conventional agents. Interactions that *have* been well documented are discussed as appropriate throughout this text.

5

Adverse Drug Reactions and Medication Errors

In this chapter we discuss two related issues of drug safety: (1) adverse drug reactions (ADRs), also known as *adverse drug events*; and (2) medication errors, a major cause of ADRs. We begin with ADRs and then discuss medication errors.

ADVERSE DRUG REACTIONS

An *ADR*, as defined by the World Health Organization, is "any noxious, unintended, and undesired effect that occurs at normal drug doses." Adverse reactions can range in intensity from mildly annoying to life threatening. Among the milder reactions are drowsiness, nausea, itching, and rash. Severe reactions include potentially fatal conditions such as neutropenia, hepatocellular injury, cardiac dysrhythmias, anaphylaxis, and hemorrhage.

Scope of the Problem

A 2018 statistical brief by the Agency for Healthcare Research and Quality highlighted a decrease in the occurrence of ADRs for inpatients. These are believed to be the result of intensive efforts to implement system-wide changes to decrease ADRs. For outpatients, however, ADRs have increased. In 2014, more than 1,110,000 outpatients were admitted to hospitals because of ADRs. This represented an increase of 100,000 compared with the year 2010. Box 5.1 lists the most common causes of these ADRs. Many of these incidences were preventable, but fortunately, when drugs are carefully prescribed and when patients are well educated on proper use, many ADRs can be avoided or minimized.

Definitions

Side Effect

A *side effect* is formally defined as a nearly unavoidable secondary drug effect produced at therapeutic doses. Common examples include drowsiness caused by traditional antihistamines and gastric irritation caused by aspirin. Side effects are generally predictable, and their intensity is dose dependent. Some side effects develop soon after drug use starts, whereas others may not appear until a drug has been taken for weeks or months.

Toxicity

The formal definition of *toxicity* is the degree of detrimental physiologic effects caused by excessive drug dosing. Examples include profound respiratory depression from an overdose of morphine and severe hypoglycemia from an overdose of insulin. Although the formal definition of toxicity includes only those severe reactions that occur when dosage is excessive, in everyday language the term *toxicity* has come to mean any severe ADR, regardless of the dose that caused it. For example, when administered in therapeutic doses, many anticancer drugs cause neutropenia, thereby putting the patient at high risk for infection. This neutropenia may be called "toxicity" even though it was produced when dosage was therapeutic.

Allergic Reaction

An allergic reaction is an immune response. For an allergic reaction to occur, there must be prior sensitization of the immune system. After the immune system has been sensitized to a drug, reexposure to that drug can trigger an allergic response. The intensity of allergic reactions can range from mild itching to severe rash to anaphylaxis. Estimates suggest that less than 10% of ADRs are of the allergic type.

The intensity of an allergic reaction is determined primarily by the degree of sensitization of the immune system, not by drug dosage. Put another way, *the intensity of allergic reactions is largely independent of dosage.* As a result, a dose that elicits a very strong reaction in one allergic patient may elicit a very mild reaction in another. Furthermore, because a patient's sensitivity to a drug can change over time, a dose that elicits a mild reaction early in treatment may produce an intense reaction later on.

Very few medications cause severe allergic reactions. In fact, most serious reactions are caused by just one drug family—the *penicillins.* Other drugs noted for causing allergic reactions include the nonsteroidal antiinflammatory drugs (e.g., aspirin) and the sulfonamide group of compounds, which includes certain diuretics, antibiotics, and oral hypoglycemic agents.

Idiosyncratic Effect

An idiosyncratic effect is defined as *an uncommon drug response resulting from a genetic predisposition.* An example of an idiosyncratic effect occurs in people with glucose-6-phosphate dehydrogenase (G6PD) deficiency. G6PD deficiency is an X-linked inherited condition that occurs primarily in people with African and Mediterranean ancestry. When people with G6PD deficiency take drugs such as sulfonamides or aspirin, they develop varying degrees of red blood cell hemolysis, which may become life threatening.

Paradoxical Effect

A paradoxical effect is the opposite of the intended drug response. A common example is the excitement that may occur when some children take first-generation antihistamines (available over-the-counter as a sleep aid). Similarly, older adults may experience paradoxical excitement when they are given benzodiazepines for sedation.

Iatrogenic Disease

An iatrogenic disease is a disease that occurs as the result of medical care or treatment. The term *iatrogenic disease* is also used to denote a disease produced by drugs.

Iatrogenic diseases are nearly identical to naturally occurring diseases. For example, patients taking certain antipsychotic drugs may develop

BOX 5.1   Ranking of Drugs Requiring Hospitalization for Adverse Drug Reactions

Antibiotics/anti-infectives (21.6%)
Systemic agents[a] (13.5%)
Hormones (13.3%)
Analgesics (13.1%)
Hematologic agents (10%)
Psychotropic drugs (8.1%)
Cardiovascular drugs (6.6%)
Water, mineral, and uric acid metabolism drugs (4.9%)
Sedatives or hypnotics (3.6%)
Anticonvulsants and anti-Parkinson drugs (2.5%)
Central nervous system (CNS) depressants and anesthetics (1.9%)
Smooth muscle and respiratory drugs (1.3%)
CNS drugs not previously identified (1%)
Autonomic nervous system drugs (0.7%)
Gastrointestinal drugs (0.4%)
Eye, skin, and mucous membrane drugs (0.3%)
Vaccines (0.1%)
Drug not identified (14.4%)

[a]Anticancer drugs, antiallergy and antiemetic drugs, and other systemic agents.
Adapted from an Agency for Healthcare Research and Quality 2014 examination of hospital admissions in 28 states. See https://www.hcup-us.ahrq.gov/reports/statbriefs/sb234-Adverse-Drug-Events.pdf.

a syndrome with symptoms that closely resemble those of Parkinson disease.

Physical Dependence

Physical dependence is a state in which the body has adapted to drug exposure in such a way that an abstinence syndrome will result if drug use is discontinued. Physical dependence develops during long-term use of certain drugs, such as opioids, alcohol, barbiturates, and amphetamines. The precise nature of the abstinence syndrome is determined by the drug involved.

Although physical dependence is usually associated with opioids, these are not the only dependence-inducing drugs. A variety of other centrally acting drugs (e.g., ethanol, barbiturates, amphetamines) can promote dependence. Furthermore, some drugs that work outside the central nervous system can cause physical dependence of a sort. Because a variety of drugs can cause physical dependence of one type or another, and because withdrawal reactions have the potential for harm, *patients should be warned against abrupt discontinuation of any medication without first consulting a health professional.*

Carcinogenic Effect

The term *carcinogenic effect* refers to the ability of certain medications and environmental chemicals to cause cancers. Fortunately, only a few therapeutic agents are carcinogenic. Ironically, several of the drugs used to *treat* cancer are among those with the greatest carcinogenic potential.

Evaluating drugs for the ability to cause cancer is extremely difficult. Evidence of neoplastic disease may not appear until 20 or more years after initial exposure to a cancer-causing compound.

Teratogenic Effect

A *teratogenic effect* is a drug-induced birth defect. Medicines and other chemicals capable of causing birth defects are called *teratogens.* Teratogenesis is discussed in Chapter 8.

Organ-Specific Toxicity

Many drugs are toxic to specific organs. Common examples include injury to the kidneys caused by amphotericin B (an antifungal drug), injury to the heart caused by doxorubicin (an anticancer drug), injury to the lungs caused by amiodarone (an antidysrhythmic drug), and injury to the inner ear caused by aminoglycoside antibiotics (e.g., gentamicin). Patients using these drugs should be monitored for signs of developing injury. In addition, patients should be educated about these signs and advised to seek medical attention if they appear.

Two types of organ-specific toxicity deserve special comment. These are (1) injury to the liver and (2) altered cardiac function, as evidenced by a prolonged QT interval on the electrocardiogram. Both are discussed next.

Hepatotoxic Drugs

As some drugs undergo metabolism by the liver, they are converted to toxic products that can injure liver cells. These drugs are called *hepatotoxic drugs.*

In the United States, drugs are the leading cause of acute liver failure, a rare condition that can rapidly prove fatal. Fortunately, liver failure from using known hepatotoxic drugs is rare, with an incidence of less than 1 in 50,000. (Drugs that cause liver failure more often than this are removed from the market—unless they are indicated for a life-threatening illness.) More than 50 drugs are known to be hepatotoxic. Some examples are listed in Table 5.1.

Combining a hepatotoxic drug with certain other drugs may increase the risk of liver damage. Acetaminophen (Tylenol) is a hepatotoxic drug that can damage the liver when taken in excessive doses. When taken in therapeutic doses, acetaminophen does not usually create a risk for liver injury; however, if the drug is taken with just two or three alcoholic beverages, severe liver injury can result.

QT Interval Drugs

The term *QT interval drugs*—or simply *QT drugs*—refers to the ability of some medications to prolong the QT interval on the electrocardiogram, thereby creating a risk for serious dysrhythmias. The QT interval is a measure of the time required for the ventricles to repolarize after each contraction. When the QT interval is prolonged (more than 470 ms for postpubertal males or more than 480 ms for postpubertal females), patients can develop a dysrhythmia known as *torsades de pointes,* which can progress to potentially fatal ventricular fibrillation.

More than 100 drugs are known to cause QT prolongation, torsades de pointes, or both. As shown in Table 5.2, QT drugs are found in many drug families. Several QT drugs have been withdrawn from the market because of deaths linked to their use, and the use of another QT drug—cisapride (Propulsid)—is now restricted. To reduce the risks from QT drugs, the US Food and Drug Administration (FDA) now requires that all new drugs be tested for the ability to cause QT prolongation.

Identifying Adverse Drug Reactions

It can be very difficult to determine whether a specific drug is responsible for an observed adverse event because other factors—especially the underlying illness and other drugs being taken—could be the actual cause. To help determine whether a particular drug is responsible, the following questions should be considered:
- Did symptoms appear shortly after the drug was first used?
- Did symptoms abate when the drug was discontinued?
- Did symptoms reappear when the drug was reinstituted?
- Is the illness itself sufficient to explain the event?
- Are other drugs in the regimen sufficient to explain the event?

If the answers reveal a temporal relationship between the presence of the drug and the adverse event, and if the event cannot be explained

TABLE 5.1 Some Hepatotoxic Drugs

Statins and Other Lipid-Lowering Drugs
Atorvastatin (Lipitor)
Fenofibrate (TriCor, Trilipix, Lipidil EZ)
Fluvastatin (Lescol)
Gemfibrozil (Lopid)
Lovastatin (Mevacor)
Niacin (Niaspan, others)
Pitavastatin (Livalo)
Pravastatin (Pravachol)
Rosuvastatin (Crestor)
Simvastatin (Zocor)

Oral Antidiabetic Drugs
Acarbose (Precose, Glucobay)
Pioglitazone (Actos)
Rosiglitazone (Avandia)

Antiseizure Drugs
Carbamazepine (Tegretol)
Felbamate (Felbatol)
Phenytoin (Dilantin)
Valproic acid (Depakene, others)

Antifungal Drugs
Fluconazole (Diflucan)
Griseofulvin (Grifulvin V, Gris-PEG)
Itraconazole (Sporanox)
Ketoconazole (Nizoral)
Terbinafine (Lamisil)

Antigout Drugs
Allopurinol (Zyloprim)
Febuxostat (Uloric)

Antidepressant/Antipsychotic Drugs
Bupropion (Wellbutrin, Zyban)
Duloxetine (Cymbalta)
Nefazodone
Trazodone
Tricyclic antidepressants

Antimicrobial Drugs
Amoxicillin–clavulanic acid (Augmentin)
Erythromycin
Minocycline (Minocin)
Nitrofurantoin (Macrodantin, Macrobid)
Penicillin
Trimethoprim-sulfamethoxazole (Septra, Bactrim)

Drugs for Tuberculosis
Isoniazid
Pyrazinamide
Rifampin (Rifadin)

Immunosuppressants
Azathioprine (Imuran)
Leflunomide (Arava)
Methotrexate (Rheumatrex)

Antiretroviral Drugs
Nevirapine (Viramune)
Ritonavir (Norvir)

Other Drugs
Acetaminophen (Tylenol), but only when combined with alcohol or taken in excessive dose
Amiodarone (Cordarone)
Baclofen (Lioresal, Gablofen)
Celecoxib (Celebrex)
Diclofenac (Voltaren)
Labetalol (Trandate)
Lisinopril (Prinivil, Zestril)
Losartan (Cozaar)
Methyldopa (Aldomet)
Omeprazole (Prilosec)
Procainamide
Tamoxifen (Nolvadex)
Testosterone
Zileuton (Zyflo)

by the illness itself or by other drugs in the regimen, then there is a high probability that the drug under suspicion is indeed the culprit. Unfortunately, this process is limited. It can only identify adverse effects that occur while the drug is being used; it cannot identify adverse events that develop years after drug withdrawal. Nor can it identify effects that develop slowly over the course of prolonged drug use.

Adverse Reactions to New Drugs

Preclinical and clinical trials of new drugs cannot detect all of the ADRs that a drug may be able to cause. In fact, about 50% of all new drugs have serious ADRs that are not revealed during phase 1 and phase 3 trials.

Because newly released drugs may have as yet unreported adverse effects, you should be alert for unusual responses when prescribing new drugs. If the patient develops new symptoms, it is wise to suspect that the drug may be responsible—even if the symptoms are not described in the literature. It is a good practice to initially check postmarket drug evaluations at www.fda.gov/Drugs/GuidanceComplianceRegulatoryInformation/

Surveillance/ucm204091.htm to determine whether serious problems have been reported. If the drug is especially new, however, you may be the first provider to have observed the effect. If you suspect a drug of causing a previously unknown adverse effect, you should report the effect to MedWatch, the FDA Medical Products Reporting Program. You can file your report online at www.fda.gov/medwatch. Because voluntary reporting by health care professionals is an important mechanism for bringing ADRs to light, you should report all suspected ADRs, even if absolute proof of the drug's complicity has not been established.

Ways to Minimize Adverse Drug Reactions

The responsibility for reducing ADRs lies with everyone associated with drug production and use. The pharmaceutical industry must strive to produce the safest medicines possible; the provider must select the least harmful medicine for a particular patient and provide clear instructions for its use; the nurse must evaluate patients for ADRs and educate patients in ways to avoid or minimize harm; and patients and their

TABLE 5.2 Drugs That Prolong the QT Interval, Induce Torsades De Pointes, or Both

Cardiovascular: Antidysrhythmics
Amiodarone (Cordarone)
Disopyramide (Norpace)
Dofetilide (Tikosyn)
Dronedarone (Multaq)
Flecainide (Tambocor)
Ibutilide (Corvert)
Mexiletine (Mexitil)
Procainamide (Procan, Pronestyl)
Quinidine
Sotalol (Betapace)

Cardiovascular: ACE Inhibitors/Calcium Channel Blockers
Bepridil (Vascor)
Isradipine (DynaCirc)
Moexipril
Nicardipine (Cardene)

Antibiotics
Azithromycin (Zithromax)
Clarithromycin (Biaxin)
Erythromycin
Gemifloxacin (Factive)
Levofloxacin (Levaquin)
Moxifloxacin (Avelox)
Ofloxacin (Floxin)
Telithromycin

Antifungal Drugs
Fluconazole (Diflucan)
Voriconazole (Vfend)

Antidepressants
Amitriptyline (Elavil)
Citalopram (Celexa)
Desipramine (Norpramin)
Doxepin (Sinequan)
Escitalopram (Lexapro)
Fluoxetine (Prozac)
Imipramine (Tofranil)
Mirtazapine (Remeron)
Protriptyline (Pamelor, Aventyl)
Sertraline (Zoloft)
Trimipramine (Surmontil)
Venlafaxine (Effexor)

Antipsychotics
Chlorpromazine (Thorazine)
Clozapine (Clozaril)
Haloperidol (Haldol)
Iloperidone (Fanapt)
Paliperidone (Invega)
Pimozide (Orap)
Quetiapine (Seroquel)
Risperidone (Risperdal)
Thioridazine (Mellaril)
Ziprasidone (Geodon)

Antiemetics/Antinausea Drugs
Dolasetron (Anzemet)
Domperidone (Motilium) ♣
Droperidol (Inapsine)
Granisetron (Kytril)
Ondansetron (Zofran)

Anticancer Drugs
Arsenic trioxide (Trisenox)
Eribulin (Halaven)
Lapatinib (Tykerb)
Nilotinib (Tasigna)
Sunitinib (Sutent)
Tamoxifen (Nolvadex)
Vandetanib (Caprelsa)
Vorinostat (Zolinza)

Drugs for Attention-Deficit/Hyperactivity Disorder
Amphetamine/dextroamphetamine (Adderall)
Atomoxetine (Strattera)
Dexmethylphenidate (Focalin)
Dextroamphetamine (Dexedrine)
Methylphenidate (Ritalin, Concerta)

Nasal Decongestants
Phenylephrine (Neo-Synephrine, Sudafed PE)
Pseudoephedrine (Sudafed)

Other Drugs
Alfuzosin (Uroxatral)
Amantadine (Symmetrel)
Chloroquine (Aralen)
Cisapride (Propulsid)[a]
Cocaine
Felbamate (Felbatol)
Fingolimod (Gilenya)
Foscarnet (Foscavir)
Fosphenytoin (Cerebyx)
Galantamine (Razadyne)
Halofantrine (Halfan)
Indapamide (Lozol)
Lithium (Lithobid, Eskalith)
Methadone (Dolophine)
Midodrine (ProAmatine)
Octreotide (Sandostatin)
Pasireotide (Signifor)
Pentamidine (Pentam, Nebupent)
Phentermine (Fastin)
Ranolazine (Ranexa)
Ritodrine (Yutopar)
Salmeterol (Serevent)
Saquinavir (Invirase)
Solifenacin (Vesicare)
Tacrolimus (Prograf)
Terbutaline
Tizanidine (Zanaflex)
Tolterodine (Detrol)
Vardenafil (Levitra)

[a]Restricted availability.

families must take medication only as directed, watch for signs that an ADR may be developing, and seek medical attention if one appears.

When patients are using drugs that are toxic to specific organs, function of the target organ should be monitored. The liver, kidneys, and bone marrow are important sites of drug toxicity. For drugs that are toxic to the liver, the patient should be monitored for signs and symptoms of liver damage (jaundice, dark urine, light-colored stools, nausea, vomiting, malaise, abdominal discomfort, loss of appetite), and periodic tests of liver function (e.g., *aspartate aminotransferase* [AST] and *alanine aminotransferase* [ALT]) should be performed. For drugs that are toxic to the kidneys, the patient should undergo routine urinalysis and measurement of serum creatinine or creatinine clearance. For drugs that are toxic to bone marrow, periodic complete blood cell counts are required.

Individualizing therapy can reduce adverse effects. When choosing a drug for a patient, the provider must balance the drug's risks and benefits. Drugs that are likely to harm a specific patient should be avoided unless the benefit of the drug exceeds the risk for injury.

Special Alerts and Management Guidelines

To decrease harm associated with drugs that cause serious adverse effects, the FDA requires special alerts and management guidelines. These may take the form of a *Medication Guide* for patients, a *boxed warning* to alert providers, or a *Risk Evaluation and Mitigation Strategy* (REMS), which can involve patients, providers, and pharmacists.

Medication Guides

Medication Guides, commonly called MedGuides, are FDA-approved documents created to educate patients about how to minimize harm from potentially dangerous drugs. In addition, a MedGuide is required when the FDA has determined that (1) patient adherence to directions for drug use is essential for efficacy or (2) patients need to know about potentially serious effects when deciding to use a drug.

All MedGuides use a standard format that provides information under the following main headings:
- What is the most important information I should know about *(name of drug)*?
- What is *(name of drug)*? Include a description of the drug and its indications.
- Who should not take *(name of drug)*?
- How should I take *(name of drug)*? Include importance of adherence to dosing instructions, special instructions about administration, what to do in case of overdose, and what to do if a dose is missed.
- What should I avoid while taking *(name of drug)*? Include activities (e.g., driving, sunbathing), other drugs, foods, pregnancy, and breastfeeding.
- What are the possible or reasonably likely side effects of *(name of drug)*?
- General information about the safe and effective use of prescription drugs.

Additional headings may be added by the manufacturer as appropriate, with the approval of the FDA. MedGuides for all drug products that require one are available online at https://www.accessdata.fda.gov/scripts/cder/daf/index.cfm?event=medguide.page. The MedGuide should be provided whenever a prescription is filled, and even when drug samples are handed out.

Boxed Warnings

The *boxed warning*, also known as a *black box warning*, is the strongest safety warning a drug can carry and still remain on the market. Text for the warning is presented inside a box with a heavy black border. The FDA requires a boxed warning on drugs with serious or life-threatening risks. The purpose of the warning is to alert providers to (1) potentially severe side effects (e.g., life-threatening dysrhythmias, suicidality, major fetal harm) as well as (2) ways to prevent or reduce harm (e.g., avoiding a teratogenic drug during pregnancy). The boxed warning provides a *concise summary* of the adverse effects of concern. A boxed warning must appear prominently on the package insert, on the product label, and even in magazine advertising. Drugs that have a boxed warning must also have a MedGuide. An example of a drug with a boxed warning is promethazine (Phenergan). Promethazine is contraindicated in patients less than 2-years-old because it can cause respiratory depression. Additionally, when administered by injection, there is a risk for severe tissue injury and necrosis.

Risk Evaluation and Mitigation Strategies

A REMS is simply a plan to minimize drug-induced harm. For most drugs that have a REMS, a MedGuide is all that is needed. For a few drugs, however, the REMS may have additional components. For example, the REMS for the antiacne drug isotretinoin has provisions that pertain to the patient, provider, and pharmacist. This program, known as iPledge, is needed because isotretinoin can cause serious birth defects. The iPledge program was designed to ensure that patients who are pregnant, or may become pregnant, will not have access to the drug. Details of the iPledge program are presented in Chapter 87. All REMS that have received FDA approval can be found online at https://www.accessdata.fda.gov/scripts/cder/rems/index.cfm.

MEDICATION ERRORS

Medication errors are a major cause of morbidity and mortality. According to the National Academy of Medicine (formerly the Institute of Medicine [IOM]), every year medication errors injure at least 1.5 million Americans and kill an estimated 7000. The financial costs are staggering: among hospitalized patients alone, treatment of drug-related injuries costs at least $3.5 billion per year.

What Is a Medication Error?

The National Coordinating Council for Medication Error Reporting and Prevention (NCC MERP) defines a medication error as "any preventable event that may cause or lead to inappropriate medication use or patient harm, while the medication is in the control of the healthcare professional, patient, or consumer. Such events may be related to professional practice, healthcare products, procedures, and systems, including prescribing; order communication; product labeling, packaging and nomenclature; compounding; dispensing; distribution; administration; education; monitoring; and use." Note that, by this definition, medication errors can be made by many people—beginning with workers in the pharmaceutical industry, followed by people in the health care delivery system, and ending with patients and their family members. In this chapter, we focus on medication errors attributed to health care providers. These typically fall into one of the following categories:

Prescribing Practices
- Inappropriate drug selection
- Error in drug dosage
- Lack of clear instructions
- Illegible writing

Oversight
- Failure to keep an up-to-date medication list
- Failure to continue or discontinue medications
- Absence of medication reconciliation

Communication

- Inadequate or unclear instructions
- Failure to verify drugs that sound alike
- Inadequate patient education

Ways to Reduce Medication Errors

Organizations throughout many countries are working to design and implement measures to reduce medication errors. Changes having the most dramatic effect have been those that focused on the National Academy of Medicine recommendations to (1) help and encourage patients and their families to be active, informed members of the health care team, and (2) give health care providers the tools and information needed to prescribe, dispense, and administer drugs as safely as possible. Foremost among these recommendations are requiring electronic prescribing, making drug reference material available electronically, and regulating abbreviations.

Implementation of technology to reduce errors has had remarkable success, as well. For example, replacing handwritten medication orders with a computerized order entry system has reduced medication errors by 50%. Using barcode systems that match the patient's armband bar code to a drug barcode has decreased medication errors in some institutions by as much as 85%.

Targeted interventions to address provider-related errors can be employed to decrease medication errors by health care providers. These are provided in Table 5.3.

TABLE 5.3 Provider-Related Medication Errors and Interventions

Errors	Interventions
Prescribing Practices	
Inappropriate drug selection	Verify that the drug selected is the drug intended. (See Table 5.4 for a list of drugs that look or sound like other drugs.)
	Drug information changes frequently; make sure that drug references are authoritative and up to date.
	Verify allergies when ordering new medications. Display allergies prominently in the patient record.
	Check for interactions of new medications against all currently prescribed medications, over-the-counter medications, herbal remedies, nutritional supplements, and recreational drugs that the patient is taking. Authoritative drug interaction application software is recommended.
	Verify that patients can afford the medication; otherwise, this increases the likelihood of errors due to taking subtherapeutic doses, if filled at all.
	Consider individualized patient factors (e.g., age, pregnancy, comorbidities) when selecting the most appropriate drug.
	Consider whether drug therapy is necessary; use nonpharmacologic interventions when practical to do so.
Error in drug dosage	Verify unit of measure (e.g., milligram vs. microgram).
	Verify height and weight and verify unit of measure (e.g., kilograms vs. pounds) for dosage calculations.
	Verify decimal placement; follow the ISMP recommendations in Table 5.5.
Lack of clear labeling instructions	Incorporate ISMP-recommended substitutions for any error-prone abbreviations. (See Table 5.5.)
	Write precise and detailed instructions. Avoid "Take as directed" and similar nonspecific labeling.
	Request large font labeling for patients who have difficulty reading small print.
Illegible writing	Use print instead of cursive writing.
	Check spelling, placement of decimals, and clarity of numerals.
	Convert to computerized provider order entry at earliest possibility.
Oversight	
Failure to keep an up-to-date medication list	When taking a medication history, assess not only how a medication is prescribed to be taken but also how the patient actually takes it in order to identify discrepancies and why they occur.
	Include dates when drugs are stopped, started, or altered, as well as the reasons for these changes.
Failure to continue/discontinue medications	Update patient medications at every visit and compare this list with prior lists to identify drugs that should have been continued or that should be discontinued or weaned.
	Avoid polypharmacy when possible; determine whether all drugs prescribed are necessary and if new drugs are truly needed.
Absence of medication reconciliation	Medication reconciliation should occur any time there is a transfer of patients to another provider or to another facility (see Box 5.2).
	Develop interprofessional relationships to facilitate communication regarding reconciliation needs.
Communication	
Inadequate or unclear instructions	Reserve verbal orders for emergency situations.
	When verbal orders are required, have the nurse repeat them to ensure that they are understood and are what you intended.
Inadequate patient education	Develop strong collaborative partnerships with patients (or their caretakers) and consider their perspectives and preferences when making treatment decisions.
	Verify patient understanding of teaching by repeating instructions or demonstrating procedures.
	Provide handouts to reinforce teaching. These should be written at the 5th grade level or, at most, the 8th grade level.

ISMP, Institute for Safe Medical Practices.

Incorporating *medication reconciliation* (Box 5.2) has resulted in decreasing medication errors by 70% and reducing ADRs by 15%.

Words that look alike or sound alike are a common source of medication errors (Table 5.4). The Institute for Safe Medical Practices (ISMP) recommends interventions for look-alike drugs (e.g., including brand and generic names when writing prescriptions), but these recommendations do not address sound-alike drugs. When it is necessary to give a verbal order, as in an emergency situation, asking for a verbalization of the order adds an extra layer of safety.

Many medication errors result from using error-prone abbreviations, symbols, and dose designations. To address this concern, the ISMP and the FDA together compiled a list of error-prone abbreviations, symbols, and dose designations (Table 5.5) and have recommended against their use. This list includes eight entries (presented at the top of Table 5.5) that have been *banned* by The Joint Commission (TJC). These banned abbreviations can no longer be used by hospitals and other organizations that require TJC accreditation. The full list is available online at www.ismp.org/tools/errorproneabbreviations.pdf.

A wealth of information is available on reducing medication errors. See Table 5.6 for some good places to start.

How to Report a Medication Error

You can report a medication error through the Medication Error Reporting (MER) Program, a nationwide system run by the ISMP. All reporting is confidential and can be done by phone or through the Internet. Details on submitting a report are available at www.ismp.org/orderForms/reporterrortoISMP.asp. The MER Program encourages participation by all health care providers, including pharmacists, nurses, physicians, and students. The objective is not to establish blame, but instead to improve patient safety by increasing our knowledge of medication errors. All information gathered by the MER Program is forwarded to the FDA, the ISMP, and the product manufacturer.

TABLE 5.4 Examples of Drugs With Names That Sound Alike or Look Alike

Amicar	*Omacor*
Anaspaz	*Antispas*
Celebrex	*Cerebyx*
Clinoril	*Clozaril*
Cycloserine	Cyclosporine
Depo-Estradiol	*Depo-Testadiol*
Dioval	*Diovan*
Estratab	*Estratest*
Etidronate	Etretinate
Flomax	*Volmax*
Lamisil	*Lamictal*
Levoxine	*Levoxyl*
Lithobid	*Lithostat*
Lodine	Iodine
Naprelan	*Naprosyn*
Nasarel	*Nizoral*
Neoral	*Neosar*
Nicoderm	*Nitroderm*
Sarafem	*Serophene*
Serentil	*Seroquel*
Tamiflu	*Theraflu*
Tramadol	*Toradol*

Trade names are italicized; generic names are not.

BOX 5.2   Medication Reconciliation

What Is Medication Reconciliation and When Is It Done?
Medication reconciliation is the process of comparing a list of all medications that a patient is currently taking with a list of new medications that are about to be provided. Reconciliation is conducted whenever a patient undergoes a *transition in care* in which new medications may be ordered or existing orders may be changed. Transitions in care include hospital admission, hospital discharge, moving to a different level of care within a hospital, transfer to another facility, or discharge home.

How Is Medication Reconciliation Conducted?
There are five steps:
Step 1. Create a list of current medications. For each drug, include the name, indication, route, dosage size, and dosing interval. For patients entering a hospital, the list would consist of all medications being taken at home, including vitamins, herbal products, and prescription and nonprescription drugs.
Step 2. Create a list of all medications to be prescribed in the new setting.
Step 3. Compare the medications on both lists.
Step 4. Adjust medications based on the comparison. For example, the provider would discontinue drugs that are duplicates or inappropriate and would avoid drugs that can interact adversely.
Step 5. When the next transition in care occurs, provide the updated, reconciled list to the patient and the new provider. By consulting the list, the new provider will be less likely to omit a prescribed medication or commit a dosing error and will be less likely to prescribe a new medication that might duplicate or negate

the effects of a current medication or interact with a current medication to cause a serious adverse event.

Every time a new transition in care occurs, reconciliation should be conducted again.

Does Medication Reconciliation Reduce Medication Errors?
Definitely. Approximately 60% of medication errors occur when patients undergo a transition in care. Medication reconciliation can eliminate most of these errors.

Should Medication Reconciliation Be Conducted at Discharge?
When patients leave a facility, they should receive a single, clear, comprehensive list of *all* medications they will be taking after discharge. The list should include any medications ordered at the time of discharge, as well as any other medications the patient will be taking, including over-the-counter drugs, vitamins, and herbal products and other nutritional supplements. In addition, the list should include all prescription medications that the patient had been taking at home but had been temporarily discontinued during the episode of care. The discharge list should *not* include drugs that had been used during the episode of care but are no longer needed. The patient and, with the patient's permission, the next provider of care should receive the discharge list so that the new provider will be able to continue the reconciliation process.

TABLE 5.5   Abbreviations, Symbols, and Dose Designations That Can Promote Medication Errors

Abbreviations, Symbols, or Dose Designations	Intended Meaning	Potential Misinterpretation	Preferred Alternative
Abbreviations and Notations for Which the Alternative *Must* Be Used (TJC Mandated)			
U or u	Unit	Misread as 0 or 4 (e.g., 4U seen as 40; 4u seen as 44); mistaken to mean "cc" so dose given in volume instead of units (e.g., 4u mistaken to mean 4 cc)	Write "unit"
IU	International unit	Misread as IV (intravenous) or "10"	Write "international unit"
q.d./Q.D.	Every day	Misread as q.i.d. (4 times a day)	Write "daily"
q.o.d./Q.O.D.	Every other day	Misread as q.d. (daily) or q.i.d. (4 times a day)	Write "every other day"
MS or MSO_4	Morphine sulfate	Mistaken as magnesium sulfate	Write "morphine sulfate"
$MgSO_4$	Magnesium sulfate	Mistaken as morphine sulfate	Write "magnesium sulfate"
Trailing zero after final decimal point (e.g., 1.0 mg)	1 mg	Mistaken as 10 mg if the decimal point is missed	Never write a zero by itself after a decimal point
Leading decimal point not preceded by a zero (e.g., .5 mg)	0.5 mg	Mistaken as 5 mg if the decimal point is missed	Write "0" before a leading decimal point
Some Abbreviations and Notations for Which the Alternative Is *Recommended* (But Not Yet TJC Mandated)			
µg	Microgram	Mistaken as "mg"	Write "mcg"
cc	Cubic centimeters	Mistaken as "u" (units)	Write "mL"
IN	Intranasal	Mistaken as "IM" or "IV"	Write "intranasal" or "NAS"
H.S.; hs	Half-strength; at bedtime	Mistaken as opposite of what was intended	Write "half-strength" or "at bedtime"
qhs	At bedtime	Mistaken as qhr (every hour)	Write "at bedtime"
q1d	Daily	Mistaken as q.i.d. (4 times daily)	Write "daily"
q6PM, etc.	Nightly at 6 PM	Mistaken as every 6 hours	Write "nightly at 6 PM"
T.I.W.	3 times a week	Mistaken as 3 times a day or twice weekly	Write "3 times weekly"
SC, SQ, sub q	Subcutaneous	SC mistaken as "SL" (sublingual); SQ mistaken as "5 every"; the "q" in "sub q" mistaken as "every" (e.g., a heparin dose ordered "sub q 2 hours before surgery" mistaken as "every 2 hours before surgery")	Write "subQ," "sub-Q," "subcut," or "subcutaneously"; write "every"
D/C	Discharge or discontinue	Premature discontinuation of medications if D/C (intended to mean "discharge") has been interpreted as "discontinued" when followed by a list of discharge medications	Write "discharge" or "discontinue"
AD, AS, AU	Right ear, left ear, each ear	Mistaken as OD, OS, OU (right eye, left eye, each eye)	Write "right ear," "left ear," or "each ear"
OD, OS, OU	Right eye, left eye, each eye	Mistaken as AD, AS, AU (right ear, left ear, each ear)	Write "right eye," "left eye," or "each eye"
Per os	By mouth, orally	The "os" can be mistaken as "left eye" (OS = oculus sinister)	Write "PO," "by mouth," or "orally"
> or <	Greater than or less than	Mistaken for the opposite	Write "greater than" or "less than"
AZT	Zidovudine (Retrovir)	Mistaken as azathioprine or aztreonam	Write complete drug name
CPZ	Prochlorperazine (Compazine)	Mistaken as chlorpromazine	Write complete drug name
ARA A	Vidarabine	Mistaken as cytarabine (ARAC)	Write complete drug name
HCT	Hydrocortisone	Mistaken as hydrochlorothiazide	Write complete drug name
HCTZ	Hydrochlorothiazide	Mistaken as hydrocortisone	Write complete drug name

TJC, The Joint Commission.
Adapted from a list compiled by the Institute for Safe Medication Practices. The official TJC list is available at http://www.jointcommission.org/assets/1/18/dnu_list.pdf. The complete ISMP list is available at www.ismp.org/tools/errorproneabbreviations.pdf.

TABLE 5.6 Resources on Decreasing Medication Errors

Resource	Location
Agency for Healthcare Research and Quality's Patient Safety Network	https://psnet.ahrq.gov
Institute for Safe Medication Practices	www.ismp.org
Institute for Healthcare Improvement	http://www.ihi.org/topics/adesmedicationreconciliation/Pages/default.aspx
Medication Reconciliation Information and Tools	
National Coordinating Council for Medication Error Reporting and Prevention	www.nccmerp.org
Institute of Medicine: Preventing Medication Errors	https://www.nap.edu/catalog/11623/preventing-medication-errors
US Food and Drug Administration: Medication Errors Related to Drugs	www.fda.gov/Drugs/DrugSafety/MedicationErrors/default.htm

Individual Variation in Drug Responses

6

In this chapter, we discuss the major factors that can cause one patient to respond to drugs differently than another. With this information, you will be better prepared to reduce individual variation in drug responses, thereby maximizing the benefits of treatment and reducing the potential for harm.

BODY WEIGHT AND COMPOSITION

The intensity of the response to a drug is determined in large part by the concentration of the drug at its sites of action—the higher the concentration, the more intense the response. Thus body size can be a significant determinant of drug effects. If we give the same dose to a small person and a large person, the drug will achieve a higher concentration in the small person and therefore will produce more intense effects. The potential consequences are that we will produce toxicity in the smaller person and undertreat the larger person. To compensate for this potential source of individual variation, the size of the patient should be considered when prescribing drug dosage. This is especially important for pediatric patients.

Adjustments in dosage are typically based on body surface area because surface area determinations account not only for the patient's weight but also for the patient's relative amount of body adiposity. Because percentage of body fat can change drug distribution, and because altered distribution can change the concentration of a drug at its sites of action, dosage adjustments based on body surface area provide a more precise means of controlling drug responses compared to adjustments based on weight alone.

AGE

Drug sensitivity varies with age. Infants and older adults are especially sensitive to drugs. In the very young patient, heightened drug sensitivity is the result of organ immaturity. In older adults, heightened sensitivity results largely from decline in organ function. Other factors that affect sensitivity in older adults are the presence of multiple comorbidities and treatment with multiple drugs. The clinical challenge created by heightened drug sensitivity in very young or in older adult patients is the subject of Chapters 9 and 10.

PATHOPHYSIOLOGY

Physiologic alterations can modify drug responses. Four pathologic conditions, in particular, may have a profound effect: (1) kidney disease, (2) liver disease, (3) acid-base imbalance, and (4) altered electrolyte status.

Kidney Disease

Kidney disease can reduce drug excretion, causing drugs to accumulate in the body. If dosage is not lowered, drugs may accumulate to toxic levels. Accordingly, if a patient is taking a drug that is eliminated by the kidneys, and if renal function declines, dosage must be decreased.

Liver Disease

Like kidney disease, liver disease can cause drugs to accumulate. This occurs because the liver is the major site of drug metabolism. Therefore if liver function declines, the rate of metabolism will decline, causing drug levels to climb. Accordingly, to prevent accumulation to toxic levels, the dosage of drugs eliminated through hepatic metabolism must be reduced or discontinued if liver disease develops.

Acid–Base Imbalance

By altering pH partitioning (see Chapter 4), changes in acid–base status can alter the absorption, distribution, metabolism, and excretion of drugs. Because of pH partitioning, if there is a difference in pH on two sides of a membrane, a drug will accumulate on the side where the pH most favors its ionization. Because acidic drugs ionize in alkaline media, acidic drugs will accumulate on the alkaline side of the membrane. Conversely, basic drugs will accumulate on the acidic side.

Altered Electrolyte Status

Electrolytes (e.g., potassium, sodium, calcium, magnesium, phosphorus) have important roles in cell physiology. Consequently, when electrolyte levels become disturbed, multiple cellular processes can be disrupted. Excitable tissues (nerves and muscles) are especially sensitive to alterations in electrolyte status. Given that disturbances in electrolyte balance can have widespread effects on cell physiology, we might expect that electrolyte imbalances would cause profound and widespread effects on responses to drugs. However, this does not seem to be the case; examples in which electrolyte changes have a significant effect on drug responses are rare. An exception is digoxin in the presence of hypokalemia. When potassium levels are low, the ability of digoxin to induce dysrhythmias is greatly increased. Accordingly, all patients receiving digoxin must undergo regular measurement of serum potassium to ensure that levels remain within a safe range.

TOLERANCE

Tolerance is a *decreased responsiveness to a drug as a result of repeated drug administration*. Patients who are tolerant to a drug require higher doses to produce effects equivalent to those that could be achieved with lower doses before tolerance developed. There are three categories of drug tolerance: (1) pharmacodynamic tolerance, (2) metabolic tolerance, and (3) tachyphylaxis.

Pharmacodynamic Tolerance

The term *pharmacodynamic tolerance* refers to the familiar type of tolerance associated with long-term administration of drugs such as morphine and heroin. Pharmacodynamic tolerance is the result of adaptive processes that occur in response to chronic receptor occupation. Because increased drug levels are required to produce an effective response, the minimum effective concentration (MEC) of a drug becomes abnormally high.

Metabolic Tolerance

Metabolic tolerance is defined as tolerance resulting from accelerated drug metabolism. This form of tolerance is brought about by the ability of certain drugs (e.g., barbiturates) to induce the synthesis of hepatic drug-metabolizing enzymes, thereby causing rates of drug metabolism to increase. Because of increased metabolism, dosage must be increased to maintain therapeutic drug levels. Unlike pharmacodynamic tolerance, which causes the MEC to increase, metabolic tolerance does not affect the MEC.

Tachyphylaxis

Tachyphylaxis is a reduction in drug responsiveness brought on by repeated dosing over a short time. This is unlike pharmacodynamic tolerance and metabolic tolerance, which take days or longer to develop. Transdermal nitroglycerin provides a good example of tachyphylaxis. When nitroglycerin is administered using a transdermal patch, effects are lost in less than 24 hours if the patch is left in place around the clock. As discussed in Chapter 44, the loss of effect results from depletion of a cofactor required for nitroglycerin to act. When nitroglycerin is administered on an intermittent schedule, rather than continuously, the cofactor can be replenished between doses, and no loss of effect occurs.

PLACEBO EFFECT

A *placebo* is devoid of intrinsic pharmacologic activity; therefore any response that a patient may have to a placebo is based solely on the patient's psychological reaction to the idea of taking a medication and not to any direct physiologic or biochemical action of the placebo itself. The primary use of the placebo is as a control preparation during clinical trials.

In pharmacology, the *placebo effect* is defined as the component of a drug response that is caused by psychological factors and not by the biochemical or physiologic properties of the drug. It is widely believed that with practically all medications, some fraction of the total response results from a placebo effect. Although placebo effects are determined by psychological factors and not physiologic responses to the inactive placebo, the presence of a placebo response does not imply that a patient's original pathology was imaginary.

Not all placebo responses are beneficial. If a patient believes that a medication is going to be effective, then placebo responses are likely to help promote recovery. Conversely, if a patient is convinced that a particular medication is ineffective or perhaps even harmful, then placebo effects are likely to detract from his or her progress.

Because the placebo effect depends on the patient's attitude toward medicine, fostering a positive attitude may help promote beneficial effects. In this regard, it is desirable that all members of the health care team present the patient with an optimistic (but realistic) assessment of the effects that therapy is likely to produce.

VARIABILITY IN ABSORPTION

Both the rate and extent of drug absorption can vary among patients. As a result, both the timing and intensity of responses can be changed.

Bioavailability

The term *bioavailability* refers to the amount of an active drug that reaches the systemic circulation from its site of administration. Different formulations of the same drug can vary in bioavailability. Factors such as tablet disintegration time, enteric coatings, and sustained-release formulations can alter bioavailability and can thereby make drug responses variable.

Differences in bioavailability occur primarily with oral preparations rather than parenteral preparations. Fortunately, even with oral agents, when differences in bioavailability do exist between preparations, those differences are usually so small that they lack clinical significance.

Differences in bioavailability are of greatest concern for drugs with a narrow therapeutic range, because with these agents, a relatively small change in drug level can produce a significant change in response: a small decline in drug level may cause therapeutic failure, whereas a small increase in drug level may cause toxicity. Under these conditions, differences in bioavailability could have a significant effect.

Individual Causes of Variable Absorption

Individual variations that affect the speed and degree of drug absorption affect bioavailability and can thereby lead to variations in drug responses. Alterations in gastric pH can affect absorption through the pH partitioning effect. For drugs that undergo absorption in the intestine, absorption will be delayed when gastric emptying time is prolonged. Diarrhea can reduce absorption by accelerating the transport of drugs through the intestine. Conversely, constipation may enhance the absorption of some drugs by prolonging the time available for absorption.

GENETICS AND PHARMACOGENOMICS

A patient's unique genetic makeup can lead to drug responses that are qualitatively and quantitatively different from those of the population at large. Adverse effects and therapeutic effects may be increased or reduced. Idiosyncratic responses to drugs may also occur. This topic is explored extensively in Chapter 7.

GENDER- AND RACE-RELATED VARIATIONS

Gender- and race-related differences in drug responses are, ultimately, genetically based. However, a general discussion is warranted.

Gender

Men and women can respond differently to the same drug. A drug may be more effective in men than in women, or vice versa. Likewise, adverse effects may be more intense in men than in women, or vice versa. Unfortunately, for most drugs, we do not have adequate knowledge about gender-related differences because before 1997, when the FDA pressured drug companies to include women in trials of new drugs, essentially all drug research was done in men. Since that time, research has demonstrated that significant gender-related differences really do exist. Here are four examples:

- When used to treat heart failure, digoxin may *increase* mortality in women while having no effect on mortality in men.
- Alcohol is metabolized more slowly by women than by men. As a result, a woman who drinks the same amount as a man (on a weight-adjusted basis) will become more intoxicated.

- Certain opioid analgesics (e.g., pentazocine, nalbuphine) are much more effective in women than in men. As a result, pain relief can be achieved at lower doses in women.
- Quinidine causes greater QT interval prolongation in women than in men. As a result, women given the drug are more likely to develop torsades de pointes, a potentially fatal cardiac dysrhythmia.

Although there is still a lack of adequate data related to drug effects in women, information generated by these drug trials, coupled with current and future trials, will permit drug therapy in women to be more rational than is possible today. In the meantime, clinicians must keep in mind that the information currently available may fail to accurately predict responses in female patients. Accordingly, clinicians should remain alert for treatment failures and unexpected adverse effects.

Race

In 2005, BiDil, a fixed-dose combination of two vasodilators (isosorbidide dinitrate [ISDN] and hydralazine), became the first drug product approved by the FDA for treatment of a single racial group. Approval was based on results of the African American Heart Failure Trial (A-HeFT), which demonstrated that, in self-described black patients, adding ISDN plus hydralazine to standard therapy of heart failure reduced 1 year mortality by 43%—a very impressive and welcome result. The approval was controversial; however, because populations other than self-described black patients were excluded from clinical trials. Hence, there is no evidence that BiDil will not work just as well (and possibly even better) among some other group.

The greatest concern surrounding race-based therapy has to do with genetic variability. We know there is great diversity within and among racial groups; therefore, a "one fits all" approach based on race is unwise. Still, we can use known associations to guide choices. For example, differences in metabolism between people with East Asian and European heritage are common. The provider can use this knowledge to guide initial dosing (with adjustment, as indicated based on response) if genetic testing is not feasible or warranted.

COMORBIDITIES AND DRUG INTERACTIONS

Individuals often have two or more medical conditions or disease processes. When this occurs, drugs taken to manage one condition may complicate management of the other condition. As an example, if a person who has both asthma and hypertension is prescribed a nonselective β-adrenergic antagonist (β blocker) to control blood pressure, this may worsen the patient's asthma symptoms if the dose is sufficient to cause airway constriction. This illustrates the necessity for the provider to consider the whole patient, not only the disease being treated, when selecting drug therapy.

Because patients with comorbidities often take multiple medications, there is the increased likelihood of drug interactions. Drug interactions can be an important source of variability. The mechanisms by which one drug can alter the effects of another and the clinical consequences of drug interactions are discussed at length in Chapter 4.

7

Genetic and Genomic Considerations in Pharmacotherapeutics

Scientists completed sequencing of the human genome in 2003. Since that time, patients have benefited from great advances in the science and technology of genomics. Before we discuss pharmacogenomics in more depth, it is helpful to differentiate between genetics and genomics. The study of genetics has existed since the time of Gregor Mendel and his pea pods in the 1800s. Genetics is the examination of passing genetic traits from one generation to another through human genes. The examination of the effects of genes (through creation of specific proteins) also falls under the study of genetics. As we have found, patients with the same genes may experience different diseases or different expression of disease traits.

The National Human Genome Research Institute defines the *genome* as all of a person's genes. Going further, the study of the genome, as well as how genes interact with each other and the environment, is referred to as *genomics*. Genomics often involves investigation into diseases, such as asthma, heart disease, and cancer, as these conditions are often the result of complex interactions between a person's genome and their personal environment. The study of human genomics encompasses many areas of science, including epigenomics, proteomics, microbiomics, and of course, pharmacogenomics.

Besides the definitions discussed previously, how does genomics *really* differ from genetics? As we have found, patients with the same genes may experience different diseases or different expression of disease traits. This phenomenon is due to the variances in where a person lives, what they eat, how much they sleep, how much the work and what they do for work, and, as you can imagine, many other factors. Genomics takes into account a person's environment and lifestyle.

PHARMACOGENOMICS

The National Institutes of Health define pharmacogenomics as the study of how genes affect a person's response to drugs. The purpose of pharmacogenomics is to combine the sciences of genomics and pharmacology to provide individualized, targeted, safe drug therapies to patients. Some may include pharmacogenomics within the practice of *Personalized Medicine* or *Precision Medicine*, but truly, pharmacogenomics falls under the category of precision medicine. Although the two terms are often used interchangeably, *precision medicine* refers to a more general approach to finding effective strategies for treatment of similar groups of patients with specific genetic, lifestyle, and environmental factors. The name *precision medicine* developed from the ideas of *personalized medicine*. The reason *personalized medicine* has fallen out of favor is that while providers are treating patients on an individual basis, scientists are not developing novel treatments for every individual on the planet.

Although pharmacogenomics is a relatively young science, it has produced significant clinically relevant information—information that can be used to enhance therapeutic effects and reduce harm. A patient's unique genetic makeup can lead to drug responses that are qualitatively and quantitatively different from those of the population at large. Adverse

effects and therapeutic effects may be increased or reduced. Idiosyncratic responses to drugs may also occur. Discovery of genetic variants between individuals allows prescribers to select a more appropriate medication for a patient.

The US Food and Drug Administration (FDA) lists adverse drug reactions as the fourth leading cause of death in the United States, noting more than 100,000 deaths and 2 million serious adverse drug events each year. As a result, the FDA has more than 150 medications that have pharmacogenomic biomarkers included in the drug package insert (Fig. 7.1). Of these medications, 38 are required to include pharmacogenetics information on their package inserts. Genetic testing is now done routinely for some drugs. In fact, for a few drugs, such as maraviroc (Selzentry) and trastuzumab (Herceptin), the FDA now requires genetic testing before use, and for a few other drugs, including warfarin (Coumadin) and carbamazepine (Tegretol), genetic testing is recommended but not required.

Genomics Education and Competencies

Key organizations in health care voiced the need for additional education in the field of genomics and pharmacogenomics to improve patient outcomes. In their 2015 publication, *Improving Genetics Education in Graduate and Continuing Health Professional Education*, the National Academy of Medicine (NAM), formerly the Institute of Medicine (IOM), stated genomics education should be provided for all health professionals. Providers should possess knowledge in patient education, genetic testing and interpretation, and management of appropriate drug therapies. In September 2011, the American Nurses Association (ANA) published *Essential Genetic and Genomic Competencies for Nurses with Graduate Degrees*. This document discussed 38 competencies for nurses in the areas of risk assessment and interpretation, genetic education, clinical management, as well as ethical, legal, and social implications.

Other strong proponents of genomics education and application include the National Institutes of Nursing Research (NINR) and American Association of Physician Assistants (AAPA). The Society of PAs in Genetics and Genomics (SPAGG) is a significant interest group affiliated with AAPA. Resources for further information surrounding genetics and genomics are located in Table 7.1.

APPLICATION OF PHARMACOGENOMICS

In the discussion that follows, we look at ways in which genetic variations can influence an individual's responses to drugs, and then indicate how pharmacogenomic tests may be used to guide treatment (Table 7.2). Specifically in pharmacogenomics, we perform testing for gene characteristics related to drug responses. These gene characteristics are also known as *biomarkers*. The technical definition of a *biomarker* is a measurable substance that, when present in an organism, indicates the presence of a specific phenomenon. In simple terms, a biomarker tells practitioners about the existence of genetic variation. Not only are

Warfarin Package Insert Section 12.5 Pharmacogenomics

CYP2C9 and VKORC1 Polymorphisms

The *S*-enantiomer of warfarin is mainly metabolized to 7-hydroxywarfarin by CYP2C9, a polymorphic enzyme. The variant alleles, CYP2C9*2 and CYP2C9*3, result in decreased *in vitro* CYP2C9 enzymatic 7-hydroxylation of S-warfarin. The frequencies of these alleles in Caucasians are approximately 11% and 7% for CYP2C9*2 and CYP2C9*3, respectively.

Other CYP2C9 alleles associated with reduced enzymatic activity occur at lower frequencies, including *5, *6, and *11 alleles in populations of African ancestry and *5, *9, and *11 alleles in Caucasians.

Warfarin reduces the regeneration of vitamin K from vitamin K epoxide in the vitamin K cycle through inhibition of VKOR, a multiprotein enzyme complex. Certain single nucleotide polymorphisms in the VKORC1 gene (e.g., −1639G>A) have been associated with variable warfarin dose requirements. VKORC1 and CYP2C9 gene variants generally explain the largest proportion of known variability in warfarin dose requirements.

Fig. 7.1 Warfarin Package

TABLE 7.1   Pharmacogenomic and Genetic Resources for Health Care Providers

Organization	Resource	Website
Clinical Pharmacogenetics Implementation Consortium (CPIC)	Guidelines to assist providers in using genetic testing to optimize drug therapy	https://epicpgx.org
US Food and Drug Administration (FDA)	*Table of Pharmacogenomic Biomarkers in Drug Labeling*	http://www.fda.gov/drugs/scienceresearch/researchareas/pharmacogenetics/ucm083378.htm
Genetics/Genomics Competency Center (G2C2)	Genetics and genomics resource-specific search engine	https://genomicseducation.net/
Genetics in Primary Care Institute (GPCI)	Multiple resources for application into primary practice	https://www.aap.org/en-us/advocacy-and-policy/aap-health-initiatives/Pages/Genetics-in-Primary-Care-Institute.aspx
Personalized Medicine Coalition	Variety of resources including tables that link drugs, biomarkers, and indications	http://www.personalizedmedicinecoalition.org/Education/Therapies
Pharmacogenomics Knowledgebase (PharmGKB)	A wealth of information including a listing of drugs having labels with genetic information approved by the FDA and Health Canada	https://www.pharmgkb.org/

biomarkers used to diagnose certain disease processes; they can also be used in pharmacogenomics to determine reaction to drug treatment. As discussed previously, there are many drugs that mention biomarkers in their labels.

Genetic Variants That Alter Drug Metabolism

The most common mechanism by which genetic variants modify drug responses is by altering drug metabolism. These gene-based changes can either accelerate or slow the metabolism of many drugs. The usual consequence is either a reduction in benefits or an increase in toxicity.

For drugs that have a high therapeutic index (TI), altered rates of metabolism may have little effect on the clinical outcome. However, if the TI is low or narrow, then relatively small increases in drug levels can lead to toxicity, and relatively small decreases in drug levels can lead to therapeutic failure. In these cases, altered rates of metabolism can be significant.

The following examples show how a genetically determined variation in drug metabolism can *reduce the benefits of therapy.*

- Variants in the gene that codes for cytochrome P450-2D6 (CYP2D6) can greatly reduce the benefits of tamoxifen (Soltamox), a drug used to prevent breast cancer recurrence. To work, tamoxifen must first be converted to its active form—endoxifen—by CYP2D6. Women with an inherited deficiency in the CYP2D6 gene cannot activate the drug well, so they get minimal benefit from treatment. In one study, the cancer recurrence rate in those poor

metabolizers was 9.5 times higher than in good metabolizers. Between 8% and 10% of women of European ancestry and up to 40% of Asian descent have gene variants that prevent them from metabolizing tamoxifen to endoxifen. At this time, the FDA neither requires nor recommends testing for variants in the CYP2D6 gene. However, given these numbers, testing is very reasonable and a test kit is available.

- Variants of the gene that codes for CYP2C19 can greatly reduce the benefits of clopidogrel (Plavix), a drug that prevents platelet aggregation. Like tamoxifen, clopidogrel is a prodrug that must undergo conversion to an active form. With clopidogrel, the conversion is catalyzed by CYP2C19. Unfortunately, about 25% of patients produce a variant form of the enzyme—CYP2C19*2. As a result, these people experience a weak antiplatelet response, which places them at increased risk for stroke, myocardial infarction, and other events. People with this genetic variation should use a different antiplatelet drug.

- Among Americans of European heritage, about 52% metabolize isoniazid (a drug for tuberculosis) slowly, and 48% metabolize it rapidly. Owing to genetic differences, people of this ancestry may produce two different forms of N-acetyltransferase-2, the enzyme that metabolizes isoniazid. If dosage is not adjusted for these differences, the rapid metabolizers may experience treatment failure and the slow metabolizers may experience toxicity.

- About 1 in 14 people of European heritage have a form of CYP2D6 that is unable to convert codeine into morphine, the active form of codeine. As a result, codeine cannot relieve pain in these people.

TABLE 7.2   Examples of How Genetic Variations Can Affect Drug Responses

Genetic Variation	Drug Affected	Effect of the Genetic Variation	Explanation	FDA Stand on Genetic Testing
Variants That Alter Drug Metabolism				
CYP2D6 variants	Tamoxifen (Nolvadex)	Reduced therapeutic effect	Women with inadequate CYP2D6 activity cannot convert tamoxifen to its active form; therefore the drug cannot adequately protect them from breast cancer	No recommendation
CYP2C19 variants	Clopidogrel (Plavix)	Reduced therapeutic effect	Patients with inadequate CYP2C19 activity cannot convert clopidogrel to its active form; therefore the drug cannot protect them against cardiovascular events	Recommended
CYP2C9 variants	Warfarin (Coumadin)	Increased toxicity	In patients with abnormal CYP2C9, warfarin may accumulate to a level that causes bleeding	Recommended
TMPT variants	Thiopurines (e.g., thioguanine, mercaptopurine)	Increased toxicity	In patients with reduced TPMT activity, thiopurines can accumulate to levels that cause severe bone marrow toxicity	Recommended
Variants That Alter Drug Targets on Normal Cells				
ADRB1 variants	Metoprolol and other β blockers	Increased therapeutic effect	β_1 receptors produced by ADRB1 variant genes respond more intensely to β agonists, causing enhanced effects of blockade by β antagonists	No recommendation
VKORC1 variants	Warfarin (Coumadin)	Increased drug sensitivity	Variant VKORC1 is readily inhibited by warfarin, allowing anticoagulation with a reduced warfarin dosage	Recommended
Variants That Alter Drug Targets on Cancer Cells or Viruses				
HER2 overexpression	Trastuzumab (Herceptin)	Increased therapeutic effect	Trastuzumab only acts against breast cancers that overexpress HER2	Required
EGFR expression	Cetuximab (Erbitux)	Increased therapeutic effect	Cetuximab only works against colorectal cancers that express EGFR	Required
CCR5 tropism	Maraviroc (Selzentry)	Increased therapeutic effect	Maraviroc only acts against HIV strains that express CCR5	Required
Variants That Alter Immune Responses to Drugs				
HLA-B*1502	Carbamazepine (Tegretol)	Increased toxicity	The HLA-B*1502 variant increases the risk for life-threatening skin reaction in patients taking carbamazepine	Recommended for patients of Asian descent
HLA-B*5701	Abacavir (Ziagen)	Increased toxicity	The HLA-B*5701 variant increases the risk for fatal hypersensitivity reactions in patients taking abacavir	Recommended

ADRB1, β1-adrenergic receptor; *CCR5*, chemokine receptor 5; *CYP2C9*, 2C9 isozyme of cytochrome P450 (CYP); *CYP2C19*, 2C19 isozyme of cytochrome P450 (CYP); *CYP2D6*, 2D6 isozyme of cytochrome P450 (CYP); *EGFR*, epidermal growth factor receptor; *FDA*, US Food and Drug Administration; *HER2*, human epidermal growth factor receptor type 2; *HLA-B*1502*, human leukocyte antigen B*1502; *HLA-B*5701*, human leukocyte antigen B*5701; *TPMT*, thiopurine methyltransferase; *VKORC1*, vitamin K epoxide reductase complex 1.

The following examples show how a genetically determined variation in drug metabolism can *increase drug toxicity*.

- Variants in the gene that codes for CYP2C9 can increase the risk for toxicity from warfarin (Coumadin), an anticoagulant with a narrow TI. Bleeding occurs because (1) warfarin is inactivated by CYP2C9 and (2) patients with altered CYP2C9 genes produce a form of the enzyme that metabolizes warfarin slowly, allowing it to accumulate to dangerous levels. To reduce bleeding risk, the FDA now recommends that patients be tested for variants of the CYP2C9 gene. It should be noted, however, that in this case outcomes using expensive genetic tests are no better than outcomes using cheaper traditional tests, which directly measure the effect of warfarin on coagulation.
- Variants in the gene that codes for thiopurine methyltransferase (TPMT) can reduce TPMT activity and can thereby delay the metabolic inactivation of two thiopurine anticancer drugs: *thioguanine* (generic only) and *mercaptopurine* (Purinethol). As a result, in patients with inherited TPMT deficiency, standard doses of thiopurine or mercaptopurine can accumulate to high levels, posing a risk for potentially fatal bone marrow damage. To reduce risk, the FDA recommends testing for TPMT variants before using either drug. Patients who are found to be TPMT deficient should be given these drugs in reduced dosages.
- In the United States, about 1% of the population produces a form of *dihydropyrimidine dehydrogenase* that does a poor job of metabolizing *fluorouracil*, a drug used to treat cancer. Several people with this inherited difference, while receiving standard doses of fluorouracil, have died from central nervous system injury because of accumulation of the drug to toxic levels.

Genetic Variants That Alter Drug Targets

Genetic variations can alter the structure of drug receptors and other target molecules and can thereby influence drug responses. These variants have been documented in normal cells and in cancer cells and viruses.

Genetic variants that affect drug targets on *normal cells* are illustrated by the following two examples:

- Variants in the genes that code for the *β_1-adrenergic receptor* (ADRB1) produce receptors that are hyperresponsive to activation, which can be a mixed blessing. The bad news is that, in people with hypertension, activation of these receptors may produce an exaggerated *increase* in blood pressure. The good news is that in people with hypertension, blockade of these receptors will therefore produce an exaggerated decrease in blood pressure. Population studies indicate that variant ADRB1 receptors occur more often in people of European ancestry than in people of African ancestry, which may explain why β blockers work better, on average, against hypertension in people with light skin than in people with dark skin.
- The anticoagulant, warfarin works by inhibiting *vitamin K epoxide reductase complex 1* (VKORC1). Variant genes that code for VKORC1 produce a form of the enzyme that can be easily inhibited, and hence anticoagulation can be achieved with low warfarin doses. If normal doses are given, anticoagulation will be excessive, and bleeding could result. To reduce risk, the FDA recommends testing for variants in the VKORC1 gene before warfarin is used.

Genetic variants that affect drug targets on *cancer cells and viruses* are illustrated by these three examples. Many of these targets are the focus of immunologic therapy, further discussed with a quickly emerging class of drugs, the biologics, in Chapter 83.

- *Trastuzumab* (Herceptin), used for breast cancer, only works against tumors that overexpress human epidermal growth factor receptor type 2 (HER2). The HER2 protein, which serves as a receptor for hormones that stimulate tumor growth, is overexpressed in about 25% of breast cancer patients. Overexpression of HER2 is associated with a poor prognosis but also predicts a better response to trastuzumab. Accordingly, the FDA requires a positive test result for HER2 overexpression before trastuzumab is used.
- *Cetuximab* (Erbitux), used mainly for metastatic colorectal cancer, only works against tumors that express the epidermal growth factor receptor (EGFR). All other tumors are unresponsive. Accordingly, the FDA requires evidence of EGFR expression if the drug is to be used.
- *Maraviroc* (Selzentry), a drug for HIV infection, works by binding with a viral surface protein known as chemokine receptor 5 (CCR5), which certain strains of HIV require for entry into immune cells. HIV strains that use CCR5 are known as being *CCR5 tropic*. If maraviroc is to be of benefit, patients must be infected with one of these strains. Therefore, before maraviroc is used, the FDA requires that testing be done to confirm that the infecting strain is indeed CCR5 tropic.

Genetic Variants That Alter Immune Responses to Drugs

Genetic variants that affect the immune system can increase the risk for severe hypersensitivity reactions to certain drugs. Two examples are as follows:

- Carbamazepine (Tegretol), used for epilepsy and bipolar disorder, can cause life-threatening skin reactions in some patients—specifically patients of Asian ancestry who carry genes that code for an unusual *human leukocyte antigen* (HLA) known as *HLA-B*1502*. Although the mechanism underlying toxicity is unclear, a good guess is that interactions between HLA-B*1502 molecules and carbamazepine (or a metabolite) may trigger a cellular immune response. To reduce risk, the FDA recommends that patients of Asian descent be screened for the HLA-B*1502 gene before carbamazepine is used. If the test is positive, carbamazepine should be avoided.
- Abacavir (Ziagen), used for HIV infection, can cause potentially fatal hypersensitivity reactions in patients who have a variant gene that codes for HLA-B*5701. Accordingly, the FDA recommends screening for the variant gene before using this drug. If the test is positive, abacavir should be avoided.

Genetic and Pharmacogenomic Testing

To perform complete testing, providers must have access to a facility approved to complete accurate laboratory analysis of genetic biomarkers. Blood, saliva, urine, amniotic fluid, tissue, or hair may be used, depending on the test requirements. Due to the explosive increase in research and technology, there are now more than 70,000 genetic testing products on the market in the United States. About 10 new products enter the market on a daily basis. Many tests are now available in a panel, allowing assessment for multiple biomarkers with one sample.

The ability of the public to access genetic testing is increasing. In 2018, the FDA approved the first direct-to-consumer genetic test kit for assessment of breast cancer risk. The test kit, provided by *23andMe*, tests for three of the BRCA1 and BRCA2 gene mutations through a saliva sample provided by the consumer. Although this is a step forward in the increasing the availability of genetic testing, the FDA cautions patients and providers about using this test as a definitive guide for treatment. One of the reasons is that the BRCA1 and BRCA2 genes have more than 1000 mutations, and this test only diagnoses 3 "founder" mutations.

Shortly after the approval of the *23andMe* BRCA test kit, the FDA also approved *23andMe* to provide another direct-to-consumer test, the *23andMe Personal Genome Service Pharmacogenetic Report*, that provides information about genetic variants that may affect drug metabolism.

BARRIERS TO PHARMACOGENOMIC APPLICATION IN PRACTICE

Lack of Education

Because pharmacogenomics is a relatively new and rapidly developing science, many health care providers do not possess the knowledge or comfort to order or interpret testing. In addition, patient education must be incorporated into treatment. How can we educate patients if we do not have the information ourselves? Although there are pockets of valuable resources available on the internet, provider education remains lacking within graduate programs of study.

Financial Cost for Testing

Many insurance plans do not cover genetic testing as a preventive option. As precision medicine becomes more prominent, more insurance companies are beginning to pay for all or part of certain tests, especially if recommended by a provider. Costs for genetic tests can vary from $100 to $2000, depending on the intricacy of the test or test panel.

IMPLICATIONS AND ETHICS

Patients need to know the full implications of testing before undergoing evaluation. Providers must obtain informed consent and educate the patient on the reason for testing, the potential results, and options for treatment based on the results. Providers should also inform patients that they may not have the results of their test for weeks or more. Results of genetic testing must remain confidential, as with any other piece of medical information shared between the provider and patient.

The fear of discrimination from employers, insurance companies, or providers is real. In 2008, the Genetic Information Nondiscrimination Act (GINA) was passed. This provides patient protection from discrimination from employers and insurance providers based on genetic information. Although these laws exist, patients are still at risk for discrimination. GINA does not apply to patients receiving care in the military, through the Veteran's Administration, Indian Health Services, or for life or long-term care insurance.

GUIDELINES

Few clinical guidelines exist in the area of pharmacogenomics, as it remains a newer science. Currently, the Clinical Pharmacogenetics Implementation Consortium (CPIC) provides the largest amount of guidelines for clinical practice. As of 2018, CPIC published 35 guidelines on individual medications, including codeine, warfarin, clopidogrel, allopurinol, and others. Each guideline contains commonly tested variants and their effects on specific drugs, and therapy recommendations based on gene variation.

The Royal Dutch Association for the Advancement of Pharmacy-Pharmacogenetics Working Group (DPWG) and the Canadian Pharmacogenomics Network for Drug Safety (CPNDS) have also published a number of clinical practice recommendations regarding the use of drug therapy in patients with genetic variation. These guidelines are compiled through PharmGKB and located on their website (see Table 7.1).

Clinical practice societies are examining guidelines for their use in specialty practice. As of 2018, the American Psychiatric Association Task Force for Novel Biomarkers and Treatments feels there is a lack of evidence on which to base clinical guidelines. The National Comprehensive Cancer Network (NCCN) publishes multiple guidelines on the treatment of specific malignancies with pharmacologic therapy based on the genetic variant of the cancer. The American Society of Nephrology (ASN) published their article, *Clinical Pharmacogenomics: Applications in Nephrology*, in October 2018. This article contained a clinical guidance summary for commonly used drugs within the practice of nephrology.

In the future, pharmacogenomic analysis of each patient may allow us to engage in revolutionary personalized medicine that addresses the individual patient's genotype. For the present, however, although many advances have been made in pharmacogenomics knowledge, the science is still relatively new (as science goes). Nevertheless, the rapid expanse of knowledge in this area is astonishing.

8

Drug Therapy During Pregnancy and Breastfeeding

This chapter addresses drug therapy in women who are pregnant or breastfeeding. The clinical challenge is to provide effective treatment for the patient while avoiding harm to the fetus or nursing infant. Unfortunately, meeting this challenge is confounded by a shortage of reliable data on drug toxicity during pregnancy or breastfeeding.

DRUG THERAPY DURING PREGNANCY: BASIC CONSIDERATIONS

Drug use during pregnancy is common: about two-thirds of pregnant patients take at least one medication, and the majority take more. Some drugs are used to treat pregnancy-related conditions, such as nausea, constipation, and preeclampsia. Some are used to treat chronic disorders, such as hypertension, diabetes, and epilepsy. Still others are used for the management of invasive conditions, such as infectious diseases or cancer. In addition to taking these therapeutic agents, pregnant patients may use drugs of abuse, such as alcohol, cocaine, and heroin.

Drug therapy in pregnancy presents a vexing dilemma. In pregnant patients, as in all other patients, the benefits of treatment must balance the risks. Of course, when drugs are used during pregnancy, risks apply to the fetus as well. Unfortunately, most drugs have not been tested during pregnancy. As a result, the risks for most drugs are unknown—hence the dilemma: the provider is obliged to balance risks versus benefits, without always knowing what the risks really are.

Despite the imposing challenge of balancing risks versus benefits, drug therapy during pregnancy cannot and should not be avoided. Because the health of the fetus depends on the health of the mother, conditions that threaten the mother's health must be addressed. Chronic asthma is a good example. Uncontrolled maternal asthma is far more dangerous to the fetus than the drugs used to treat it. The incidence of stillbirth is doubled among pregnant patients who do not take medications for asthma control.

One of the greatest challenges in identifying drug effects on a developing fetus has been the lack of clinical trials, which, by their nature, would put the developing fetus at risk. Current research often focuses on comparing histories of women who have had children with and without congenital anomalies. An early example was the National Birth Defects Prevention Study (http://www.nbdps.org), which examined births from 1997 to 2011. More recently, the Birth Defects Study to Evaluate Pregnancy Exposures (http://www.cdc.gov/ncbddd/birthdefects/bd-steps.html) began collecting data on children born in January 2014 and beyond. Additionally, there are several pregnancy registries in which a woman who needs to take a drug while pregnant can enroll. This allows researchers to monitor pregnancy outcomes associated with a drug. The US Food and Drug Administration (FDA) provides a list of pregnancy exposure registries at http://www.fda.gov/ScienceResearch/SpecialTopics/WomensHealthResearch/ucm134848.htm. Although some studies are devoted to a single drug and its effect on pregnancy and the fetus, many study multiple drugs.

Physiologic Changes During Pregnancy

Pregnancy brings on physiologic changes that can alter drug disposition. Changes in the kidney, liver, and gastrointestinal (GI) tract are of particular interest. Because of these changes, a compensatory change in dosage may be needed.

By the third trimester, renal blood flow is doubled, causing a large increase in the glomerular filtration rate. As a result, there is accelerated clearance of drugs that are eliminated by glomerular filtration. Elimination of lithium, for example, is increased by 100%. To compensate for accelerated excretion, dosage must be increased.

For some drugs, hepatic metabolism increases during pregnancy. Three antiseizure drugs—phenytoin, carbamazepine, and valproic acid—provide examples.

Tone and motility of the bowel decrease in pregnancy, causing intestinal transit time to increase. Because of prolonged transit, there is more time for drugs to be absorbed. In theory, this could increase levels of drugs whose absorption is normally poor. Similarly, there is more time for the reabsorption of drugs that undergo enterohepatic recirculation, possibly resulting in a prolongation of drug effects. In both cases, a reduction in dosage might be needed.

Placental Drug Transfer

The factors that determine drug passage across the membranes of the placenta are the same factors that determine drug passage across all other membranes. Accordingly, drugs that are lipid soluble cross the placenta easily, whereas drugs that are ionized, highly polar, or protein bound cross with difficulty. Nonetheless, for practical purposes, the provider should assume that *any drug taken during pregnancy will reach the fetus.*

Adverse Reactions During Pregnancy

Not only are pregnant patients subject to the same adverse effects as nonpregnant patients, but they may also suffer effects unique to pregnancy. For example, when heparin (an anticoagulant) is taken by pregnant patients, it can cause osteoporosis, which in turn can cause compression fractures of the spine. The use of prostaglandins (e.g., misoprostol), which stimulate uterine contraction, can cause abortion. Conversely, the use of aspirin near term can suppress contractions in labor. In addition, aspirin increases the risk for serious bleeding.

Drugs taken during pregnancy can adversely affect the patient as well as the fetus. Regular use of dependence-producing drugs (e.g., heroin, barbiturates, alcohol) during pregnancy can result in the birth of a drug-dependent infant. If the newborn's dependence is not supported with drugs, a withdrawal syndrome will ensue. Symptoms include shrill crying, vomiting, and extreme irritability. The neonate should be weaned from dependence by giving progressively smaller doses of the drug on which he or she is dependent. Additionally, certain pain relievers used during delivery can depress respiration in the neonate. The infant must be closely monitored until respiration is normal.

The drug effect of greatest concern is teratogenesis. This is the production of congenital anomalies (also known as birth defects) in the fetus.

DRUG THERAPY DURING PREGNANCY: TERATOGENESIS AND OTHER RISKS

The term *teratogenesis* is derived from *teras,* the Greek word for monster. Translated literally, teratogenesis means *to produce a monster.* Consistent with this derivation, we usually think of congenital anomalies in terms of gross malformations, such as cleft palate, clubfoot, and hydrocephalus.

Incidence and Causes of Congenital Anomalies

The incidence of *major* structural abnormalities (e.g., abnormalities that are life threatening or require surgical correction) is between 1% and 3%. Half of these are obvious and are reported at birth. The other half involve internal organs (e.g., heart, liver, GI tract) and are not discovered until later in life or at autopsy. The incidence of minor structural abnormalities is unknown, as is the incidence of functional abnormalities (e.g., growth delay, intellectual disabilities).

Congenital anomalies have multiple causes, including genetic predisposition, environmental chemicals, and drugs. Genetic factors account for about 25% of all congenital anomalies. Of the genetically based anomalies, Down syndrome is the most common. Less than 1% of all congenital anomalies are caused by drugs. For most congenital anomalies, the cause is unknown.

Teratogenesis and Stage of Development

Fetal sensitivity to teratogens changes during development; thus the effect of a teratogen is highly dependent on when the drug is given. As shown in Fig. 8.1, development occurs in three major stages: the *preimplantation/presomite period* (conception through week 2), the *embryonic period* (weeks 3 through 8), and the *fetal period* (week 9 through term). During the preimplantation/presomite period, teratogens act in an all-or-nothing fashion. That is, if the dose is sufficiently high, the result is death of the conceptus. Conversely, if the dose is sublethal, the conceptus is likely to recover fully.

Gross malformations are produced by exposure to teratogens during the *embryonic period* (roughly the first trimester). This is the time when the basic shape of internal organs and other structures is being established. Because the fetus is especially vulnerable during the embryonic period, pregnant patients must take special care to avoid teratogen exposure during this time.

Teratogen exposure during the *fetal period* (i.e., the second and third trimesters) usually disrupts *function* rather than gross anatomy. Of the developmental processes that occur in the fetal period, growth and development of the brain are especially important. Disruption of brain development can result in learning deficits and behavioral abnormalities.

Identification of Teratogens

For the following reasons, human teratogens are extremely difficult to identify:

- The incidence of congenital anomalies is generally low.
- Animal tests may not be applicable to humans.
- Prolonged drug exposure may be required.
- Teratogenic effects may be delayed.
- Behavioral effects are difficult to document.
- Controlled experiments cannot be done in humans.

As a result, only a few drugs are considered *proven* teratogens. Drugs whose teratogenicity has been documented (or at least is highly suspected) are listed in Table 8.1. However, it is important to note that *lack of proof of teratogenicity does not mean that a drug is safe*—it only means that the available data are insufficient to make a definitive judgment. Conversely, *proof of teratogenicity does not mean that every exposure will result in a congenital anomaly.* In fact, with most teratogens, the risk for malformation after exposure is only about 10%.

To prove that a drug is a teratogen, three criteria must be met:

- The drug must cause a characteristic set of malformations.
- The drug must act only during a specific window of vulnerability (e.g., weeks 4 through 7 of gestation).
- The incidence of malformations should increase with increasing dosage and duration of exposure.

Obviously, we cannot do experiments on humans to determine whether a drug meets these criteria. The best we can do is systematically collect and analyze data on drugs taken during pregnancy in the hope that useful information on teratogenicity will be revealed.

Studies in animals may be of limited value, in part because teratogenicity may be species specific. That is, drugs that are teratogens in laboratory animals may be safe in humans. Conversely, and more important, drugs that fail to cause anomalies in animals may later prove teratogenic in humans. The most notorious example is thalidomide. In studies with pregnant animals, thalidomide was harmless; however, when pregnant patients took thalidomide, about 30% had babies with severe malformations. The take-home message is this: *lack of teratogenicity in animals is not proof of safety in humans.* Accordingly, we cannot assume that a new drug is safe for use in human pregnancy just because it has met FDA requirements based on tests done in pregnant animals.

Some teratogens act quickly, whereas others require prolonged exposure. Thalidomide represents a fast-acting teratogen: a single dose can cause malformation. In contrast, alcohol (ethanol) must be taken repeatedly in high doses if gross malformation is to result. (Lower doses of alcohol may produce subtle anomalies.) Because a single exposure to a rapid-acting teratogen can produce obvious malformation, they are easier to identify than slow-acting teratogens.

Teratogens that produce delayed effects are among the hardest to identify. The best example is diethylstilbestrol, an estrogenic substance that causes vaginal cancer in female offspring 18 years or so after they were born.

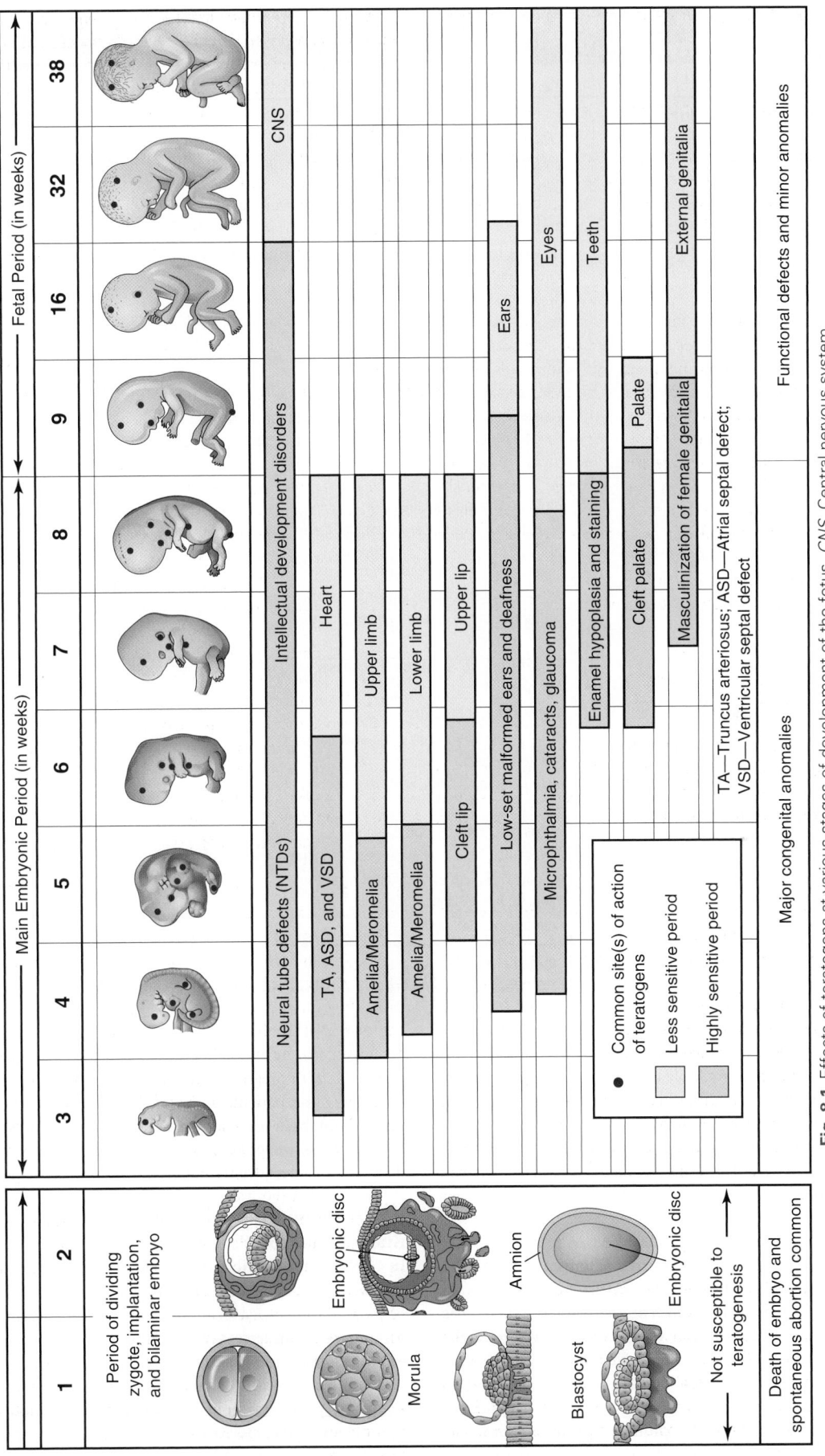

Fig. 8.1 Effects of teratogens at various stages of development of the fetus. *CNS,* Central nervous system. (From Moore K, Persaud TVN, Torchia M. *The Developing Human: Clinically Oriented Embryology.* 9th ed. Philadelphia: Elsevier; 2012, with permission.)

TABLE 8.1 Drugs That Should Be Avoided During Pregnancy Because of Proven or Strongly Suspected Teratogenicity

Drug	Teratogenic Effect
Anticancer/Immunosuppressant Drugs	
Cyclophosphamide	CNS malformation, secondary cancer
Methotrexate	CNS and limb malformations
Thalidomide	Shortened limbs, internal organ defects
Antiseizure Drugs	
Carbamazepine	Neural tube defects, craniofacial defects, malformations of the heart, hypospadias
Phenytoin	Growth delay, CNS defects
Topiramate	Growth delay, cleft lip with cleft palate
Valproic acid	Neural tube defects, craniofacial defects, malformations of the heart and extremities, and hypospadias
Sex Hormones	
Androgens (e.g., danazol)	Masculinization of the female fetus
Diethylstilbestrol	Vaginal carcinoma in female offspring
Estrogens	Congenital defects of female reproductive organs
Antimicrobial Drugs	
Tetracycline	Tooth and bone anomalies
Trimethoprim-sulfamethoxazole	Neural tube defects, cardiovascular malformations, cleft palate, clubfoot, and urinary tract abnormalities
Other Drugs	
Alcohol	Fetal alcohol syndrome, stillbirth, spontaneous abortion, low birth weight, intellectual disabilities
5-α-reductase inhibitors (e.g., dutasteride, finasteride)	Malformations of external genitalia in males
Angiotensin-converting enzyme inhibitors	Renal failure, renal tubular dysgenesis, skull hypoplasia (from exposure during the second and third trimesters)
Antithyroid drugs (propylthiouracil, methimazole)	Goiter and hypothyroidism
HMG CoA reductase inhibitors (atorvastatin, simvastatin)	Facial malformations and CNS anomalies, including holoprosencephaly (single-lobed brain) and neural tube defects
Isotretinoin and other vitamin A derivatives (etretinate, megadoses of vitamin A)	Multiple defects (CNS, craniofacial, cardiovascular, others)
Lithium	Epstein anomaly (cardiac defects)
Nicotine replacement products	Orofacial clefts, intrauterine growth restriction, CNS defects
NSAIDs	Premature closure of the ductus arteriosus
Oral hypoglycemic drugs (e.g., tolbutamide)	Neonatal hypoglycemia
Warfarin	Skeletal and CNS defects

The absence of a drug from this table does not mean that the drug is not a teratogen.
CNS, Central nervous system; *HMG CoA*, 3-hydroxy-3methylglutaryl coenzyme A; *NSAIDs*, nonsteroidal antiinflammatory drugs.

Teratogens that affect behavior may be nearly impossible to identify. Behavioral changes are often delayed and therefore may not become apparent until the child goes to school. By this time, it may be difficult to establish a correlation between drug use during pregnancy and the behavioral deficit. Furthermore, if the deficit is subtle, it may not even be recognized.

Although we have been discussing the effect of teratogens, it is important to note that drug-related effects are not limited to the distortions of gross anatomy caused by teratogens. Drugs may also include neurobehavioral and metabolic anomalies. For example, benzodiazepines taken late in pregnancy may cause hypoglycemia and respiratory complications along with a hypotonic state that is commonly called *floppy infant syndrome*. The aminoglycoside streptomycin provides another example. Although the teratogen risk of aminoglycosides is low, children born to women taking streptomycin have been born with congenital deafness. Some drugs taken by pregnant women may be dangerous (e.g., the anticoagulant warfarin has been associated with fetal hemorrhage) or life threatening (e.g., misoprostol, a drug taken to protect the stomach of people taking nonsteroidal antiinflammatory drugs) can cause a spontaneous abortion.

US Food and Drug Administration Pregnancy Risk Categories

In 1979, the FDA established a system for classifying drugs according to their probable risks to the fetus. According to this system, *drugs can be put into one of five risk categories: A, B, C, D, and X* (Table 8.2). Although this rating system is helpful, it is far from ideal. For example, some drugs that were placed in Category B—to indicate animal reproduction studies—do not indicate risk, and may not have undergone an adequate type or number of studies to adequately determine risk. Because of problems and confusion with the rating system, the FDA decided to phase it out over a period that will end in 2020. Nevertheless, because

TABLE 8.2 US Food and Drug Administration Pregnancy Risk Categories

Category	Category Description
A	*Remote risk for fetal harm:* Controlled studies in women have been done and have failed to demonstrate a risk for fetal harm during the first trimester, and there is no evidence of risk in later trimesters
B	*Slightly more risk than A:* Animal studies show no fetal risk, but controlled studies have not been done in women. *or* Animal studies do show a risk for fetal harm, but controlled studies in women have failed to demonstrate a risk during the first trimester, and there is no evidence of risk in later trimesters
C	*Greater risk than B:* Animal studies show a risk for fetal harm, but no controlled studies have been done in women. *or* No studies have been done in women or animals
D	*Proven risk for fetal harm:* Studies in women show proof of fetal damage, but the potential benefits of use during pregnancy may be acceptable despite the risks (e.g., treatment of life-threatening disease for which safer drugs are ineffective). A statement on risk will appear in the WARNINGS section of drug labeling
X	*Proven risk for fetal harm:* Studies in women or animals show definite risk for fetal abnormality. *or* Adverse reaction reports indicate evidence of fetal risk. The risks clearly outweigh any possible benefit. A statement on risk will appear in the CONTRAINDICATIONS section of drug labeling

Pregnancy Risk Categories became obsolete in 2020.

these categories are frequently referenced in recent pre-2020 literature, it is wise for the provider to have some familiarity with these categories.

US Food and Drug Administration Pregnancy and Lactation Labeling Rule

In December 2014, the FDA issued the Pregnancy and Lactation Labeling Rule (PLLR) providing new guidance for labeling.

The PLLR requires three sections for labeling: (1) pregnancy, (2) lactation, and (3) females and males of reproductive potential. These are further divided into subsections containing specified content (Table 8.3). The full report is available at http://www.fda.gov/downloads/drugs/guidancecomplianceregulatoryinformation/guidances/ucm450636.pdf.

Minimizing Drug Risk During Pregnancy

A first step in decreasing drug risk during pregnancy is to develop a comprehensive list of current drugs used. It is crucial to include not only prescription drugs but also over-the-counter and nutritional supplements, as well as recreational drug use, at every visit. A drug as common as vitamin A is dangerous when taken in excess. Vitamin A can cause craniofacial anomalies and central nervous system, cardiac, and thymus abnormalities.

If pregnancy status is unknown and a high-risk drug is recommended for management of a condition, a pregnancy test should be performed before prescribing. As noted, some disease states (e.g., epilepsy, asthma, diabetes) pose a greater risk to fetal health than the drugs used for treatment. However, even with these disorders, in which drug therapy reduces the risk for disease-induced fetal harm, we must still take steps to minimize harm from drugs. Accordingly, drugs that pose a high risk for danger to the developing embryo or fetus should be discontinued, and safer alternatives substituted.

Sometimes the use of a high-risk drug is unavoidable. Some anticancer drugs, for example, are highly toxic to the developing fetus, yet cannot be ethically withheld from the pregnant patient. If a patient elects to use such drugs, termination of pregnancy should be considered. Reducing the risk for dangerous drug effects also applies to female patients who

are *not* pregnant because approximately 50% of pregnancies are unintended. Accordingly, if a patient of reproductive age is taking a teratogenic medication, she should be educated about the teratogenic risk as well as the necessity of using at least one reliable form of birth control.

Responding to Teratogen Exposure

When a pregnant patient has been exposed to a known teratogen, the first step is to determine exactly when the drug was taken and exactly when the pregnancy began. If drug exposure was not during the period of organogenesis (i.e., weeks 3 through 8), the patient should be reassured that the risk of drug-induced malformation is minimal.

What should be done if the exposure *did* occur during organogenesis? First, a reference (such as FDA-approved prescribing information for the drug) should be consulted to determine the type of malformation expected. Next, at least two ultrasound scans should be done to assess the extent of injury. If the malformation is severe, termination of pregnancy should be considered. If the malformation is minor (e.g., cleft palate), it may be correctable by surgery, either shortly after birth or later in childhood.

DRUG THERAPY DURING BREASTFEEDING

Drugs taken by lactating patients can be excreted in breast milk. Although nearly all drugs can enter breast milk, the extent of entry varies greatly. The factors that determine entry into breast milk are the same factors that determine passage of drugs across membranes. Accordingly, drugs that are lipid soluble enter breast milk readily, whereas drugs that are ionized, highly polar, or protein bound tend to be excluded. If drug concentrations in milk are high enough, a pharmacologic effect can occur in the infant, raising the possibility of harm.

To address concerns about drug risks for breastfed infants and children, the US National Library of Medicine created the LactMed database. (See https://toxnet.nlm.nih.gov/newtoxnet/lactmed.htm) LactMed is a comprehensive searchable site that provides the most current information on prescription and nonprescription drugs and

TABLE 8.3   FDA Pregnancy and Lactation Labeling Rule Requirements

Sections	Subsections	Headings and/or Content
Pregnancy	Pregnancy Exposure Registry *(This subsection is omitted if there are no known pregnancy exposure registries for the drug.)*	*If a pregnancy exposure registry exists, the following sentence will be included.* "There is a pregnancy exposure registry that monitors pregnancy outcomes in women exposed to (name of drug) during pregnancy." *The statement is followed by registry enrollment information*
	Risk Summary *(This subsection is required.)*	*Risk summaries are statements that summarize outcomes for the following content relative to drug dosage, length of time drug was taken, and weeks of gestation when the drug was taken as well as known pharmacologic mechanisms of action.* Human data Animal data Pharmacology
	Clinical Considerations *(This subsection is omitted if none of the headings is applicable.)*	*Information is provided for the following five headings.* Disease-associated maternal and/or embryo/fetal risk Dose adjustments during pregnancy and the postpartum period Maternal adverse reactions Fetal/neonatal adverse reactions Labor or delivery *(Any heading that is not applicable is omitted.)*
	Data *(This subsection is omitted if none of the headings is applicable.)*	*This section describes research that served as a source of data for Risk Summaries. The following categories are included.* a. Human data b. Animal data *(Any heading that is not applicable is omitted.)*
Lactation	Risk Summary *(This subsection is required.)*	*Risk summaries are statements that summarize outcomes for the following content.* Presence of drug in human milk Effects of drug on the breastfed child Effects of drug on milk production/excretion Risk and benefit statement
	Clinical Considerations *(This subsection is omitted if none of the headings is applicable.)*	*Information is provided for the following headings.* Minimizing exposure Monitoring for adverse reactions *(Any heading that is not applicable is omitted.)*
	Data *(This subsection is omitted if none of the headings is applicable.)*	*This section expands on the Risk Summary and Clinical Considerations subsections. There are no defined headings.*
Females and males of reproductive potential	*(There is no defined subsection for this section.)*	*The following headings are included to address the need for pregnancy testing or contraception and adverse effects associated with preimplantation loss or adverse effects on fertility.* a. Pregnancy testing b. Contraception c. Infertility *(Any heading that is not applicable is omitted.)*

Adapted from U.S. Department of Health and Human Services, Food and Drug Administration. (2015, June). Appendix A: Organization and Format for Pregnancy, Lactation, and Females and Males of Reproductive Potential Subsections. *Pregnancy, Lactation, and Reproductive Potential: Labeling for Human Prescription Drug and Biological Products—Content and Format.* Available at http://www.fda.gov/downloads/drugs/guidancecomplianceregulatoryinformation/guidances/ucm450636.pdf.

their effects on breastfed infants and children. Unfortunately, relatively little systematic research has been done on many drugs. As a result, although a few drugs are known to be hazardous (Table 8.4), the possible danger posed by many others remains undetermined.

Fortunately, most drugs detected in milk are in concentrations that are too low to cause harm. Still, prudence is in order: if the nursing patient can avoid drugs that may pose a risk, she should. Moreover, when these drugs *must* be used, steps should be taken to minimize risk. These include the following:

- Dosing immediately *after* breastfeeding (to minimize drug concentrations in milk at the next feeding)
- Avoiding drugs that have a long half-life
- Avoiding sustained-release formulations
- Choosing drugs that tend to be excluded from milk
- Choosing drugs that are least likely to affect the infant (Table 8.5)
- Avoiding drugs that are known to be hazardous (see Table 8.4)
- Using the lowest effective dosage for the shortest possible time
- Abandoning plans to breastfeed if a necessary drug is known to be harmful to the child

TABLE 8.4   Drugs That Are Contraindicated During Breastfeeding

Controlled Substances
Amphetamine
Cocaine
Heroin
Marijuana
Phencyclidine

Anticancer Agents/Immunosuppressants
Cyclophosphamide
Cyclosporine
Doxorubicin
Methotrexate

Others
Atenolol
Bromocriptine
Ergotamine
Lithium
Nicotine
Radioactive compounds (temporary cessation)

TABLE 8.5   Drugs of Choice for Breastfeeding Patients

Drug Category	Drugs and Drug Groups of Choice	Comments
Analgesic drugs	Acetaminophen, ibuprofen, flurbiprofen, ketorolac, mefenamic acid, sumatriptan, morphine	Sumatriptan may be given for migraine. Morphine may be given for severe pain
Anticoagulant drugs	Warfarin, acenocoumarol ♣, heparin (unfractionated)	Among breastfed infants whose mothers were taking warfarin, the drug was undetectable in plasma, and bleeding time was not affected. The large molecular size of unfractionated heparin decreases the amount excreted in breast milk. Furthermore, it is not bioavailable from the GI tract, so heparin in breast milk is not systemically absorbed
Antidepressant drugs	Sertraline, paroxetine, TCAs	Fluoxetine (Prozac) may be given if other SSRIs are ineffective; however, caution is needed because levels are higher in breast milk than levels of other SSRIs. Infant risk with TCAs cannot be ruled out; however, no significant adverse effects have been reported
Antiepileptic drugs	Carbamazepine, phenytoin, valproic acid	The estimated level of exposure to these drugs in infants is less than 10% of the therapeutic dose standardized by weight
Antihistamines (histamine-1 blockers)	Loratadine, fexofenadine	First-generation antihistamines are associated with irritability or sedation and may decrease milk supply
Antimicrobial drugs	Penicillins, cephalosporins, aminoglycosides, macrolides	Avoid chloramphenicol and tetracycline
β-adrenergic antagonists	Labetalol, metoprolol, propranolol	Angiotensin-converting enzyme inhibitors and calcium channel–blocking agents are also considered safe
Endocrine drugs	Propylthiouracil, insulin, levothyroxine	The estimated level of exposure to propylthiouracil in breastfeeding infants is less than 1% of the therapeutic dose standardized by weight; thyroid function of the infant is not affected
Glucocorticoids	Prednisolone and prednisone	The amount of prednisolone the infant would ingest in breast milk is less than 0.1% of the therapeutic dose standardized by weight

This list is not exhaustive. Cases of overdoses of these drugs must be assessed on an individual basis.
GI, Gastrointestinal; *SSRI*, selective serotonin reuptake inhibitor; *TCA*, tricyclic antidepressant.

9

Drug Therapy in Pediatric Patients

Young patients respond differently to drugs than do the rest of the population. Most differences are *quantitative*. Specifically, younger patients are more sensitive to drugs than adult patients, and they show greater individual variation. Drug sensitivity in the very young results largely from *organ system immaturity*. Because of heightened drug sensitivity, they are at increased risk for adverse drug reactions. In this chapter we discuss the physiologic factors that underlie heightened drug sensitivity in pediatric patients and ways to promote safe and effective drug use.

Pediatrics covers all patients up to age 16 years. Because of ongoing growth and development, pediatric patients in different age groups present different therapeutic challenges. Traditionally, the pediatric population is subdivided into six groups:

- Premature infants (less than 36 weeks gestational age)
- Full-term infants (36 to 40 weeks gestational age)
- Neonates (first 4 postnatal weeks)
- Infants (postnatal weeks 5 to 52)
- Children (1 to 12 years)
- Adolescents (12 to 16 years)

Not surprisingly, as young patients grow older, they become more like adults physiologically, and hence more like adults with regard to drug therapy. Conversely, the very young—those younger than 1 year, and especially those younger than 1 month—are very different from adults. If drug therapy in these patients is to be safe and effective, we must account for these differences.

Managing pediatric drug therapy is made even more difficult by insufficient drug information. To address this deficit, the US Food and Drug Administration (FDA) Safety and Innovation Act of 2012 permanently reauthorized two laws previously enacted by Congress to promote drug research in children: the Best Pharmaceuticals for Children Act (BPCA) and the Pediatric Research Equity Act (PREA). Additionally, in 2012, the National Academies of Medicine (formerly the Institutes of Medicine [IOM]), published a synopsis of findings from previous research conducted under the BPCA and PREA. This report is available at http://nationalacademies.org/hmd/reports/2012/safe-and-effective-medicines-for-children.aspx.

As more studies are done, the gaps in our knowledge will shrink. In the meantime, we must still treat children with drugs—even though we lack the information needed to prescribe rationally. Similar to drug therapy during pregnancy, providers must try to balance benefits and risks, without precisely knowing what the benefits and risks really are.

PHARMACOKINETICS: NEONATES AND INFANTS

Pharmacokinetic factors determine the concentration of a drug at its sites of action and hence determine the intensity and duration of responses. If drug levels are elevated, responses will be more intense. If drug elimination is delayed, responses will be prolonged. Because the organ systems that regulate drug levels are not fully developed in very young patients, they are at risk for both drug effects that are unusually intense *and* prolonged. By accounting for pharmacokinetic differences in the very young, we can increase the chances that drug therapy will be both effective and safe.

Fig. 9.1 illustrates how drug levels differ between infants and adults after administration of doses adjusted for body weight. When a drug is administered *intravenously*, levels decline more slowly in the infant than in the adult. As a result, drug levels in the infant remain above the minimum effective concentration (MEC) longer than in the adult, thereby causing effects to be prolonged. When a drug is administered *subcutaneously*, not only do levels in the infant remain above the MEC *longer* than in the adult, but these levels also rise *higher*, causing effects to be more intense as well as prolonged. From these illustrations, it is clear that adjustment of dosage for infants on the basis of body size alone is not sufficient to achieve safe results.

If small body size is not the major reason for heightened drug sensitivity in infants, what is? The increased sensitivity of infants is due largely to the immature state of five pharmacokinetic processes: (1) drug absorption, (2) protein binding of drugs, (3) exclusion of drugs from the central nervous system (CNS) by the blood-brain barrier, (4) hepatic drug metabolism, and (5) renal drug excretion.

Absorption
Oral Administration

Gastrointestinal physiology in the infant is very different from that in the adult. As a result, drug absorption may be enhanced or impeded, depending on the physicochemical properties of the drug involved.

Gastric emptying time is both prolonged and irregular in early infancy, and then gradually reaches adult values by 6 to 8 months. For drugs that are absorbed primarily from the stomach, delayed gastric emptying enhances absorption. On the other hand, for drugs that are absorbed primarily from the intestine, absorption is delayed. Because gastric emptying time is irregular, the precise effect on absorption is not predictable.

Gastric acidity is very low 24 hours after birth and does not reach adult values for 2 years. Because of low acidity, absorption of acid-labile drugs is increased.

Intramuscular Administration

Drug absorption after intramuscular injection in the *neonate* is *slow* and *erratic*. Delayed absorption is due in part to low blood flow through muscle during the first days of postnatal life. By early *infancy*, absorption of intramuscular drugs becomes more *rapid* than in neonates and adults.

Transdermal Absorption

Drug absorption through the skin is more rapid and complete in infants than in older children and adults. The stratum corneum of the infant's

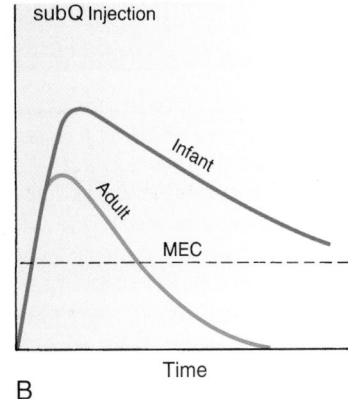

Fig. 9.1 Comparison of Plasma Drug Levels in Adults and Infants. (A) Plasma drug levels after intravenous injection. Dosage was adjusted for body weight. Note that plasma levels remain above the minimum effective concentration *(MEC)* much longer in the infant. (B) Plasma drug levels after subcutaneous injection. Dosage was adjusted for body weight. Note that both the maximal drug level and the duration of action are greater in the infant.

skin is very thin, and blood flow to the skin is greater in infants than in older patients. Because of this enhanced absorption, infants are at increased risk for toxicity from topical drugs.

Distribution
Protein Binding
Binding of drugs to albumin and other plasma proteins is limited in the infant because (1) the amount of serum albumin is relatively low, and (2) endogenous compounds (e.g., fatty acids, bilirubin) compete with drugs for available binding sites. Consequently, drugs that ordinarily undergo extensive protein binding in adults undergo much less binding in infants. As a result, the concentration of *free* levels of such drugs is relatively high in the infant, thereby intensifying the effects. To ensure that the effects are not too intense, dosages in infants should be reduced. Protein-binding capacity reaches adult values within 10 to 12 months.

Blood–Brain Barrier
The blood–brain barrier is not fully developed at birth. As a result, drugs and other chemicals have relatively easy access to the CNS, making the infant especially sensitive to drugs that affect CNS function. Accordingly, all medicines employed for their CNS effects (e.g., morphine, phenobarbital) should be given in reduced dosage. Dosage also should be reduced for drugs used for actions *outside* the CNS if those drugs are capable of producing CNS toxicity as a side effect.

Hepatic Metabolism
The drug-metabolizing capacity of newborns is low. As a result, neonates are especially sensitive to drugs that are eliminated primarily by hepatic metabolism. When these drugs are used, dosages must be reduced. The capacity of the liver to metabolize many drugs increases rapidly about 1 month after birth and approaches adult levels a few months later. Complete maturation of the liver develops by 1 year.

Renal Excretion
Renal drug excretion is significantly reduced at birth. Renal blood flow, glomerular filtration, and active tubular secretion are all low during infancy. Because the drug-excreting capacity of infants is limited, drugs that are eliminated primarily by renal excretion must be given in reduced dosage or at longer dosing intervals, or both. Adult levels of renal function are achieved by 1 year.

PHARMACOKINETICS: CHILDREN 1 YEAR AND OLDER
By age 1 year, most pharmacokinetic parameters in children are similar to those in adults. Therefore drug sensitivity in children older than 1 year is more like that of adults than that of the very young. Although pharmacokinetically similar to adults, children do differ in one important way: they metabolize drugs *faster* than adults. Drug-metabolizing capacity is markedly elevated until age 2 years and then gradually declines. A further sharp decline takes place at puberty, when adult values are reached. Because of enhanced drug metabolism in children, an increase in dosage or a reduction in dosing interval may be needed for drugs that are eliminated by hepatic metabolism.

ADVERSE DRUG REACTIONS
Like adults, pediatric patients are subject to adverse reactions when drug levels rise too high. In addition, pediatric patients are vulnerable to unique adverse effects related to organ system immaturity and to ongoing growth and development. Among these age-related effects are growth suppression (caused by glucocorticoids), discoloration of developing teeth (caused by tetracyclines), and kernicterus (caused by sulfonamides). Table 9.1 presents a list of drugs that can cause unique adverse effects in pediatric patients of various ages. These drugs should be avoided in patients whose age puts them at risk.

DOSAGE DETERMINATION
Because of the pharmacokinetic factors discussed previously, dosage selection for pediatric patients can be challenging. Selecting a dosage is especially difficult in the very young because pharmacokinetic factors are undergoing rapid change.

Pediatric doses have been established for a few drugs, but not for most. For drugs that do not have an established pediatric dose, dosage can be extrapolated from adult doses. The method of conversion employed most commonly is based on body surface area (BSA):

$$\text{Child's BSA} \times \text{adult dosage} \div 1.73\,\text{m}^2 = \text{pediatric dosage}$$

Please note that initial pediatric doses—whether based on established pediatric doses or extrapolated from adult doses—are at best an

TABLE 9.1   Adverse Drug Reactions Unique to Pediatric Patients

Drug	Adverse Effect
Androgens	Premature puberty in males; reduced adult height from premature epiphyseal closure
Aspirin and other salicylates	Severe intoxication from acute overdose (acidosis, hyperthermia, respiratory depression); Reye syndrome in children with chickenpox or influenza
Chloramphenicol	Gray syndrome (neonates and infants)
Fluoroquinolones	Tendon rupture
Glucocorticoids	Growth suppression with prolonged use
Hexachlorophene	Central nervous system toxicity (infants)
Nalidixic acid	Cartilage erosion
Phenothiazines	Sudden infant death syndrome
Promethazine	Pronounced respiratory depression in children younger than 2 years
Sulfonamides	Kernicterus (neonates)
Tetracyclines	Staining of developing teeth

TABLE 9.2   Strategies to Promote Medication Adherence in Children

Strategies for Providers

Prescribe drugs that can be taken once daily or less often, when possible.

Consider drug costs and insurance coverage when choosing medications; discuss options with the caregiver.

Use drug information sheets to reinforce verbal instructions.

Give caregivers age-appropriate and condition-specific reading or coloring books to teach children

Strategies for Caregivers

Suggest medication reminders to avoid missed doses, such as pillboxes, calendars, computer alert systems.

Recommend a reward system to prompt the child to take medication, such as stickers.

Provide pleasant-tasting medication when possible. If the medication is unpalatable, consider the following:

- Suggest keeping it refrigerated, even if not required for storage.
- Administer with food to mask taste, unless contraindicated.
- Have the child suck on a frozen treat to decrease taste sensation before administration.
- Offer a treat to "get the taste out" immediately after taking the medication.
- Praise the child for taking the medication well.

Strategies for Older Children and Adolescents

Simplify medication regimens, when possible.

Treat the patient with respect and develop trust.

Teach and reinforce necessary skills (e.g., inhaler administration, insulin injection) to improve confidence.

Provide developmentally appropriate information, games, software, and videos to reinforce teaching.

Proactively address adverse effects when possible and collaborate with the patient on preferred methods to manage them when they occur.

Set up networks to connect the child or adolescent with others managing similar illnesses and medication regimens.

Employ an interprofessional team approach for support and encouragement

approximation. Subsequent doses must be adjusted on the basis of clinical outcome and plasma drug concentrations. These adjustments are especially important in neonates and younger infants. If dosage adjustments are to be optimal, it is essential that we monitor the patient for therapeutic and adverse responses as a component of optimizing dosage.

PROMOTING ADHERENCE

Achieving accurate and timely dosing requires informed participation of the child's caregiver and, to the extent possible, active involvement of the child as well. Effective education is critical. The following issues should be addressed:

- Dosage size and timing
- Route and technique of administration
- Duration of treatment
- Drug storage
- The nature and time course of desired responses
- The nature and time course of adverse responses

Written instructions should be provided to reinforce verbal instructions. For techniques of administration that are difficult, a demonstration should be made, after which the child's caregivers should repeat the procedure to ensure they understand. With young children, spills and spitting out are common causes of inaccurate dosing; parents should be taught to estimate the amount of drug lost and to readminister that amount, being careful not to overcompensate. When more than one person is helping medicate a child, all participants should be warned against multiple dosing. Multiple dosing can be avoided by maintaining a drug administration chart. With some disorders—especially infections—symptoms may resolve before the prescribed course of treatment has been completed. Parents should be instructed to complete the full course nonetheless. Additional strategies to promote adherence are presented in Table 9.2.

10

Drug Therapy in Geriatric Patients

Drug use among older adults (those 65 years and older) is disproportionately high. While older adults constitute only 12.8% of the US population, they consume 33% of the nation's prescribed drugs. The reasons for this intensive use of drugs include increased severity of illness, multiple pathologies, and excessive prescribing.

Drug therapy in older adults represents a special therapeutic challenge. As a rule, older patients are more sensitive to drugs and they show wider individual variation. In addition, older adults experience more adverse drug reactions (ADRs) and drug–drug interactions. The principal factors underlying these complications are (1) altered pharmacokinetics (secondary to organ system degeneration), (2) multiple and severe illnesses, (3) multidrug therapy, and (4) poor adherence. To help ensure that drug therapy is as safe and effective as possible, *individualization of treatment is essential: each patient must be monitored for desired and adverse responses, and the regimen must be adjusted accordingly.* Because older adults often suffer from incurable chronic illnesses, the usual objective is to reduce symptoms and improve quality of life.

PHARMACOKINETIC CHANGES IN OLDER ADULTS

The aging process can affect all phases of pharmacokinetics. From early adulthood on, there is a gradual, progressive decline in organ function. This decline can alter the absorption, distribution, metabolism, and excretion of drugs. As a rule, these pharmacokinetic changes increase drug sensitivity (largely from reduced hepatic and renal drug elimination). However, it should be noted that the extent of change varies greatly among patients: pharmacokinetic changes may be minimal in patients who have remained physically fit, whereas they may be dramatic in patients who have aged less fortunately. Accordingly, you should keep in mind that age-related changes in pharmacokinetics are not only a potential source of increased sensitivity to drugs but also a potential source of increased variability. The physiologic changes that underlie alterations in pharmacokinetics are summarized in Table 10.1.

Absorption

Altered gastrointestinal absorption is not a major factor in drug sensitivity in older adults. As a rule, the *percentage* of an oral dose that becomes absorbed does not usually change with age. However, the *rate* of absorption may be slowed (because of delayed gastric emptying and reduced splanchnic blood flow). As a result, drug responses may be somewhat delayed. Gastric acidity is reduced in older adults and may alter the absorption of certain drugs. For example, some drug formulations require high acidity to dissolve, and hence their absorption may be reduced.

Distribution

Four major factors can alter drug distribution in older adults: (1) increased percentage of body fat, (2) decreased percentage of lean body mass, (3) decreased total body water, and (4) reduced concentration of serum albumin. The increase in body fat seen in older adults provides a storage depot for *lipid-soluble* drugs (e.g., propranolol). As a result, plasma levels of these drugs are reduced, causing a reduction in responses. Because of the decline in lean body mass and total body water, *water-soluble* drugs (e.g., ethanol) become distributed in a smaller volume than in younger adults. As a result, the concentration of these drugs is increased, causing effects to be more intense. Although albumin levels are only slightly reduced in healthy older adults, these levels can be significantly reduced in older adults who are malnourished. Because of reduced albumin levels, sites for protein binding of drugs decrease, causing levels of free drug to rise. Accordingly, drug effects may be more intense.

Metabolism

Rates of hepatic drug metabolism tend to decline with age. The principal reasons are reduced hepatic blood flow, reduced liver mass, and decreased activity of some hepatic enzymes. Because liver function is diminished, the half-lives of certain drugs may be increased, thereby prolonging responses. Responses to oral drugs that ordinarily undergo extensive first-pass metabolism may be enhanced because fewer drugs are inactivated before entering the systemic circulation. However, it is important to note that the degree of decline in drug metabolism varies greatly among individuals. As a result, we cannot predict whether drug responses will be significantly reduced in any particular patient.

Excretion

Renal function, and hence renal drug excretion, undergoes progressive decline beginning in early adulthood. *Drug accumulation secondary to reduced renal excretion is the most important cause of ADRs in older adults.* The decline in renal function is the result of reductions in renal blood flow, glomerular filtration rate, active tubular secretion, and number of nephrons. Renal pathology can further compromise kidney function. The degree of decline in renal function varies greatly among individuals. Accordingly, when patients are taking drugs that are eliminated primarily by the kidneys, renal function should be assessed. In older adults, the proper index of renal function is *creatinine clearance,* not *serum creatinine levels.* Creatinine levels do not adequately reflect kidney function in older adults because the source of serum creatinine—lean muscle mass—declines in parallel with the decline in kidney function. Accordingly, creatinine levels may be normal even though renal function is greatly reduced. Although most medication adjustments for renal problems use creatinine clearance, for a few medications the estimated glomerular filtration rate (eGFR) is used. The National Kidney Foundation offers online calculators to determine the creatinine clearance at https://www.kidney.org/professionals/KDOQI/gfr_calculatorCoc and the eGFR at https://www.kidney.org/professionals/kdoqi/gfr_calculator.

TABLE 10.1   Physiologic Changes That Can Affect Pharmacokinetics in Older Adults

Absorption of Drugs
Increased gastric pH
Decreased absorptive surface area
Decreased splanchnic blood flow
Decreased gastrointestinal motility
Delayed gastric emptying

Distribution of Drugs
Increased body fat
Decreased lean body mass
Decreased total body water
Decreased serum albumin
Decreased cardiac output

Metabolism of Drugs
Decreased hepatic blood flow
Decreased hepatic mass
Decreased activity of hepatic enzymes

Excretion of Drugs
Decreased renal blood flow
Decreased glomerular filtration rate
Decreased tubular secretion
Decreased number of nephrons

PHARMACODYNAMIC CHANGES IN OLDER ADULTS

Alterations in receptor properties may underlie altered sensitivity to some drugs. However, information on such pharmacodynamic changes is limited. In support of the possibility of altered pharmacodynamics is the observation that beta-adrenergic blocking agents (drugs used primarily for cardiac disorders) are *less* effective in older adults than in younger adults, even when present in the same concentrations. Possible explanations for this observation include (1) a reduction in the number of beta receptors and (2) a reduction in the affinity of beta receptors for beta-receptor blocking agents. Other drugs (warfarin, certain central nervous system depressants) produce effects that are more intense in older adults, suggesting a possible increase in receptor number, receptor affinity, or both. Unfortunately, our knowledge of pharmacodynamic changes in older adults is restricted to a few families of drugs.

ADVERSE DRUG REACTIONS AND DRUG INTERACTIONS

ADRs are seven times more common in older adults than in younger adults, accounting for about 16% of hospital admissions among older individuals and 50% of all medication-related deaths. Most of these reactions are dose related, not idiosyncratic. Symptoms in older adults are often nonspecific (e.g., dizziness, cognitive impairment), making identification of ADRs difficult. Furthermore, older adults may be less comfortable revealing alcohol or recreational drug use because of generational taboos in some segments of society. This can confound efforts to identify the source of a new ADR-related symptom.

Perhaps surprisingly, the increase in ADRs seen in older adults is often not the direct result of aging. Rather, multiple factors predispose older patients to ADRs, the most important of which follow:
- Drug accumulation secondary to reduced renal function
- Polypharmacy (treatment with multiple drugs)

BOX 10.1   Measures to Reduce Adverse Drug Reactions in Older Adults

- Take a thorough drug history, including over-the-counter medications, herbal remedies, and dietary supplements
- Account for the pharmacokinetic and pharmacodynamic changes that occur with aging
- Initiate therapy with low doses and titrating upward gradually ("start low and go slow")
- Monitor clinical responses and plasma drug levels to provide a rational basis for dosage adjustment
- Employ the simplest medication regimen possible
- Monitor for drug–drug interactions and iatrogenic illness
- Periodically review the need for continued drug therapy, and discontinue medications as appropriate
- Encourage the patient to dispose of old medications
- Take steps to promote adherence
- Avoid drugs included in *Beers Criteria for Potentially Inappropriate Medication Use in Older Adults* (the Beers list) unless benefits outweigh risks.

- Greater severity of illness
- Presence of comorbidities
- Use of drugs that have a low therapeutic index (e.g., digoxin, a drug for heart failure)
- Increased individual variation secondary to altered pharmacokinetics
- Inadequate supervision of long-term therapy
- Poor patient adherence

Most ADRs in older adults are avoidable. Measures that can reduce their incidence are presented in Box 10.1.

Synthesizing information on disparate drugs that can cause harm has presented a challenge. A few lists have emerged over the years, but perhaps the most well known are the Beers List and START/STOPP criteria. Both identify drugs that are potentially inappropriate. As with all drug decisions, the provider must weigh benefits and risks. The patient's individual history must also be taken into account. For example, often patients are started on these medications well before they reach age 65. If the drugs are meeting the patient's needs and not causing problems, it would be illogical to stop them or reduce their dosage based on age alone.

The *Beers List* identifies drugs with a high likelihood of causing adverse effects in older adults. Accordingly, drugs on this list should generally be avoided in adults older than 65 years except when the benefits are significantly greater than the risks. A partial listing of these drugs appears in Table 10.2. The full list, updated in 2019, is available online at https://onlinelibrary.wiley.com/doi/pdf/10.1111/jgs.15767.

STOPP stands for Screening Tool of Older People's potentially inappropriate Prescriptions. Like the Beers List, STOPP criteria also identify drugs that may be dangerous if prescribed for older adults. It has an advantage of also considering the economic costs of drug therapy. Additionally, when combined with the Screening Tool to Alert doctors to Right Treatment (START), the set can be used to promote the selection of appropriate treatment in addition to the avoidance of inappropriate treatment. The article detailing START/STOPP criteria is available at https://academic.oup.com/ageing/article/44/2/213/2812233.

PROMOTING ADHERENCE

Between 26% and 59% of older adult patients fail to take their medicines as prescribed. Some patients never fill their prescriptions, some fail to refill their prescriptions, and some don't follow the prescribed dosing schedule. Nonadherence can result in therapeutic failure (from

TABLE 10.2 Some Drugs to Generally Avoid in Older Adults

Drugs	Reason for Concern	Alternative Treatments
Analgesics Indomethacin (Indocin) Ketorolac (Toradol) Chronic use of non---COX-2 selective NSAIDs (e.g., ibuprofen, aspirin >325 mg/day)	Risk of GI bleeding and acute renal failure. Indomethacin is more prone to affect the CNS than other NSAIDs.	Mild pain: acetaminophen, codeine, COX-2–selective inhibitors if no heart failure risk, *short-term* use of *low-dose* NSAIDs
Meperidine (Demerol)	Not effective at usual doses, risk for neurotoxicity, confusion, delirium	Moderate to severe pain: morphine, oxycodone, hydrocodone
Tricyclic Antidepressants, First Generation Amitriptyline Clomipramine (Anafranil) Doxepin (>6 mg/day) Imipramine (Tofranil)	Anticholinergic effects (constipation, urinary retention, blurred vision), risk for cognitive impairment, delirium, syncope	SSRIs with shorter half-life, (e.g., paroxetine, sertraline, fluvoxamine), SNRIs, or other antidepressants
Antihistamines, First Generation Chlorpheniramine (Chlor-Trimeton, Teldrin, Chlor-Tripolon ♦) Diphenhydramine (Benadryl) Hydroxyzine (Vistaril, Atarax ♦) Promethazine (Phenergan)	Anticholinergic effects (constipation, urinary retention, blurred vision), sedation, orthostatic hypotension	Second-generation antihistamines, such as cetirizine (Zyrtec), fexofenadine (Allegra), or loratadine (Claritin)
Antihypertensives, α-Adrenergic Blocking Agents α₁ blockers (e.g., doxazosin [Cardura], prazosin [Minipress], terazosin [Hytrin])	High risk for orthostatic hypotension and falls; less dangerous drugs are available	Thiazide diuretic, ACE inhibitor, beta-adrenergic blocker, calcium channel blocker
Sedative-Hypnotics Barbiturates (e.g., butalbital [component of Fiorinal], phenobarbital, secobarbital [Seconal])	Physical dependence; compared with other hypnotics, higher risk for falls, confusion, cognitive impairment	Short-term zolpidem (Ambien), zaleplon (Sonata), or eszopiclone (Lunesta) Low-dose ramelteon (Rozerem) or low-dose doxepin Nonpharmacologic interventions (e.g., cognitive behavioral therapy)
Benzodiazepines, both short acting (e.g., alprazolam [Xanax], lorazepam [Ativan]) and long acting (e.g., chlordiazepoxide [Librium], diazepam [Valium])	Sedation, cognitive impairment, risk for falls, delirium risk	Low-dose ramelteon (Rozerem) or low-dose doxepin Nonpharmacologic interventions (e.g., cognitive behavioral therapy)
Drugs for Urge Incontinence Oxybutynin (Ditropan) Tolterodine (Detrol)	Anticholinergic effects, urinary retention, confusion, hallucinations, sedation	Behavioral therapy (e.g., bladder retraining, urge suppression)
Muscle Relaxants Carisoprodol (Soma) Cyclobenzaprine Metaxalone (Skelaxin) Methocarbamol (Robaxin)	Anticholinergic effects, sedation, cognitive impairment; may not be effective at tolerable dosage	Antispasmodics, such as baclofen (Lioresal) Nonpharmacologic interventions (e.g., exercises, proper body mechanics)
Proton Pump Inhibitors (chronic use exceeding 8 weeks) Esomeprazole (Nexium) Lansoprazole (Prevacid) Omeprazole (Prilosec)	Increased risk for *Clostridium difficile* infection, decreased bone integrity, and fractures	Histamine-2 receptor antagonists (e.g., famotidine (Pepcid), ranitidine (Zantac)) Nonpharmacologic interventions (e.g., deleting foods that increase gastric acidity, such as high-fat foods, and deleting substances that lower esophageal sphincter pressure such as alcohol)

ACE, Angiotensin-converting enzyme; *CNS*, central nervous system; *COX-2*, cyclooxygenase-2; *GI*, gastrointestinal; *NSAIDs*, nonsteroidal antiinflammatory drugs; *SNRI*, serotonin/norepinephrine reuptake inhibitor; *SSRI*, selective serotonin reuptake inhibitor.
Adapted from American Geriatrics Society 2019 updated Beers criteria for potentially inappropriate medication use in older adults. *J Am Geriatr Soc.* 2019; 674–694. (*Note:* The original document lists many drugs in addition to those in this table.)

underdosing or erratic dosing) or toxicity (from overdosing). Of the two possibilities, underdosing with resulting therapeutic failure is by far (90%) the more common. Problems arising from nonadherence account for up to 10% of all hospital admissions, and their management may cost more than $100 billion a year.

Multiple factors underlie nonadherence to the prescribed regimen (Box 10.2). Among these are forgetfulness; failure to comprehend instructions (because of intellectual, visual, or auditory impairment); inability to pay for medications; and use of complex regimens (several drugs taken several times a day). All of these factors can contribute to *unintentional* nonadherence. However, in most cases (about 75%), nonadherence among older adults is *intentional*. The principal reason given for intentional nonadherence is the patient's conviction that the drug was simply not needed in the dosage prescribed. Unpleasant side effects and expense also contribute to intentional nonadherence.

Several measures can promote adherence, including the following:

- Simplifying the regimen so that the number of drugs and doses per day is as small as possible
- Explaining the treatment plan using clear, concise, verbal and written instructions
- Choosing an appropriate dosage form (e.g., a liquid formulation if the patient has difficulty swallowing)
- Requesting that the pharmacist label drug containers using a large print size and provide containers that are easy to open by patients with impaired dexterity (e.g., those with arthritis)
- Suggesting the use of a calendar, diary, or pill counter to record drug administration
- Asking the patient if he or she has access to a pharmacy and can afford the medication
- Enlisting the aid of a friend, relative, or visiting health care professional
- Monitoring for therapeutic responses, adverse reactions, and plasma drug levels

However, it must be noted that the benefits of these measures will be restricted primarily to patients whose nonadherence is *unintentional*. Unfortunately, these measures are generally inapplicable to the patient whose nonadherence is *intentional*. For these patients, intensive education may help.

CONSIDERATIONS FOR END-OF-LIFE CARE

End-of-life care poses a set of different concerns regarding the choice of drugs to best meet the needs of older patients. Priority treatment varies as goals shift from disease prevention and management to the provision of comfort measures. Drugs that were once considered important in care (e.g., drugs for cholesterol management) may no longer be relevant and can be discontinued. Drugs that were once considered inappropriate due to patient age (e.g., sedatives) may need to become a predominant feature of care. Table 10.3 explores medication considerations and choices for concerns that patients sometimes encounter near the end of life. Additional information is available at https://www.cancer.gov/about-cancer/advanced-cancer/caregivers/planning/last-days-hp-pdq#section/_7. The National Academy of Medicine's report *Dying in America: Improving Quality and Honoring Individual Preferences Near the End of Life* addresses multiple concerns of dying patients and their families, and is available at http://www.nap.edu/read/18748/chapter/1.

BOX 10.2 Factors That Increase Risk for Poor Adherence in Older Adults

- Multiple chronic disorders
- Multiple prescription medications
- Multiple doses per day for each medication
- Drug packaging that is difficult to open
- Multiple prescribers
- Changes in the regimen (addition of drugs, changes in dosage size or timing)
- Cognitive or physical impairment (reduction in memory, hearing, visual acuity, color discrimination, or manual dexterity)
- Living alone
- Recent discharge from hospital
- Low literacy
- Inability to pay for drugs
- Personal conviction that a drug is unnecessary or the dosage too high
- Presence of side effects

TABLE 10.3 Pharmacological Considerations for End-of-Life Care

Problems	Considerations	Drug Choice
Constipation	Constipation may be opioid-induced; an order for opioids should be accompanied by an order to treat constipation. Stimulants typically cause some degree of abdominal cramping. Drugs specifically formulated for opioid-induced constipation (i.e., methylnaltrexone) are very expensive and may not be warranted if other interventions are effective. Increased fiber may cause constipation if there is insufficient fluid intake	First-line choices are osmotic laxatives (e.g., lactulose, polyethylene glycol). Stimulants with stool softener (e.g., senna with docusate) are second-line choices if abdominal cramping is a concern; otherwise, they may be given as a first-line choice. For those who cannot swallow, bisacodyl rectal suppositories or enemas can provide relief. Methylnaltrexone may be used for refractory opioid-induced constipation
Delirium	Delirium may be a manifestation of pain. Delirium may be a manifestation of opioid-induced neurotoxicity. Benzodiazepines may cause a paradoxical agitation but may be helpful if delirium is related to alcohol withdrawal or as an *adjunct* to antipsychotics. Underlying causes (constipation, urinary retention, infection) should be treated, if identified	Treat with antipsychotics such as haloperidol or olanzapine. Benzodiazepines such as midazolam may be helpful short term to supplement antipsychotics for acute episodes of delirium. Consider adding analgesics (or evaluate adequacy of currently prescribed analgesics). For patients taking opioids (e.g., morphine), changing to a different opioid (e.g., fentanyl) has been helpful.

TABLE 10.3   Pharmacological Considerations for End-of-Life Care—cont'd

Problems	Considerations	Drug Choice
Dyspnea	Dyspnea may or may not be associated with hypoxemia. Management should consider severity of associated manifestations (e.g., profound fatigue exacerbated by respiratory effort). Bronchodilators may increase anxiety which can further worsen sensation of shortness of breath	Oxygen therapy is indicated if hypoxemia is present. Opioids are a first-line drug choice. Glucocorticoids are often helpful, if not contraindicated. Consider bronchodilators only if dyspnea is associated with bronchospasm
Fatigue	Dexamphetamine has only short-term benefit due to tolerance; one study showed that benefit did not extend past 8 days	Methylphenidate has demonstrated improvement in some studies
Nausea and vomiting	Management should be tailored to the underlying cause	Chemotherapy or radiation-induced N/V: 5-HT3 receptor antagonists (e.g., ondansetron) or neurokinin1 receptor antagonist (e.g., aprepitant) or glucocorticoid (e.g., dexamethasone). Metoclopramide is recommended first line for N/V due to gastroparesis, liver failure and unknown causes. Haloperidol, a dopamine receptor antagonist, is often effective in relieving N/V of unknown causes and is first line for N/V due to bowel obstruction and renal failure. Glucocorticoids may be helpful in treating N/V secondary to brain tumors and bowel obstructions. For N/V of unknown cause, metoclopramide may be supplemented with 5HT3-receptor antagonists or dopamine receptor antagonists
Pain	Pain associated with conditions such as cancer is often intractable. Concerns about addiction are generally irrelevant at this stage of life, so highly addictive drugs may be employed. Opioids undergo hepatic metabolism and most undergo renal excretion. As organ failure occurs, opioids may accumulate to toxic levels. TCAs have adverse effects and drug–drug interactions that create complications when used for neuropathic pain	Fentanyl is the drug of choice for severe pain in patients with renal and/or hepatic dysfunction. Methadone is a drug of choice for patients with renal dysfunction but without hepatic dysfunction. Schedule medication around the clock rather than prn. Gabapentin or pregabalin are recommended for management of neuropathic pain. SSRIs and SNRIs also may be helpful
Respiratory secretions "Death Rattle"	Accumulation of secretions in the airway occurs as the patient nears death (within 2 weeks or less) and ineffective cough progresses to loss of cough reflex and pooling of secretions. Suctioning may be inadequate to relieve this problem. Expert opinion is divided regarding whether treatment is warranted. Many believe that the death rattle does not cause patient distress, but it can be upsetting to families	If drug therapy is desired, anticholinergics are often effective in decreasing secretions. Glycopyrrolate is the anticholinergic of choice due to decreased CNS adverse effects. Some studies have indicated that hyoscyamine is a good choice for this purpose

CNS, Central nervous system; *N/V,* nausea and vomiting; *SNRI,* serotonin-norepinephrine reuptake inhibitor; *SSRI,* selective serotonin reuptake inhibitor; *TCA,* tricyclic antidepressants.

11

Basic Principles of Neuropharmacology

Neuropharmacology can be defined as the study of drugs that alter processes controlled by the nervous system. Neuropharmacologic drugs produce effects equivalent to those produced by the excitation or suppression of neuronal activity. Neuropharmacologic agents can be divided into two broad categories: (1) peripheral nervous system (PNS) drugs and (2) central nervous system (CNS) drugs.

The neuropharmacologic drugs constitute a large and important family of therapeutic agents. These drugs are used to treat conditions ranging from depression to epilepsy to hypertension to asthma. The clinical significance of these agents is reflected in the fact that more than 25% of this text is dedicated to them.

Because the nervous system participates in the regulation of practically all bodily processes, practically all bodily processes can be influenced by drugs that alter neuronal regulation. By mimicking or blocking neuronal regulation, neuropharmacologic drugs can modify such diverse processes as skeletal muscle contraction, cardiac output, vascular tone, respiration, gastrointestinal function, uterine motility, glandular secretion, and functions unique to the CNS, such as ideation, mood, and perception of pain. Given the broad spectrum of processes that neuropharmacologic drugs can alter, and given the potential benefits to be gained by manipulating those processes, it is no surprise that neuropharmacologic drugs have widespread clinical applications.

We begin our study of neuropharmacology by discussing PNS drugs (Chapters 12 through 17), after which we discuss CNS drugs (Chapters 18 through 22). The principal rationale for this order of presentation is that our understanding of PNS pharmacology is much clearer than our understanding of CNS pharmacology because the PNS is less complex than the CNS, and more accessible to experimentation. By placing our initial focus on the PNS, we can establish a firm knowledge base in neuropharmacology before proceeding to the less definitive and vastly more complex realm of CNS pharmacology.

HOW NEURONS REGULATE PHYSIOLOGIC PROCESSES

As a rule, if we want to understand the effects of a drug on a particular physiologic process, we must first understand the process itself. Accordingly, if we wish to understand the effects of drugs on neuronal regulation of bodily function, we must first understand how neurons regulate bodily function when drugs are absent.

Fig. 11.1 illustrates the basic process by which neurons elicit responses from other cells. The figure depicts two cells: a neuron and a postsynaptic cell. The postsynaptic cell might be another neuron, a muscle cell, or a cell within a secretory gland. As indicated, there are two basic steps—*axonal conduction* and *synaptic transmission*—in the process by which the neuron influences the behavior of the postsynaptic cell. Axonal conduction is simply the process of conducting an action potential down the axon of the neuron. Synaptic transmission is the process by which information is carried across the gap between the neuron and the postsynaptic cell. As shown in the figure, synaptic transmission requires the release of neurotransmitter molecules from the axon terminal followed by binding of these molecules to receptors on the postsynaptic cell. As a result of transmitter–receptor binding, a series of events is initiated in the postsynaptic cell, leading to a change in its behavior. The precise nature of the change depends on the identity of the neurotransmitter and the type of cell involved. If the postsynaptic cell is another neuron, it may increase or decrease its firing rate; if the cell is part of a muscle, it may contract or relax; and if the cell is glandular, it may increase or decrease secretion.

BASIC MECHANISMS BY WHICH NEUROPHARMACOLOGIC AGENTS ACT

Sites of Action: Axons Versus Synapses

To influence a process under neuronal control, a drug can alter one of two basic neuronal activities: axonal conduction or synaptic transmission. *Most neuropharmacologic agents act by altering synaptic transmission.* Only a few alter axonal conduction. This is to our advantage because drugs that alter synaptic transmission can produce effects that are much more *selective* than those produced by drugs that alter axonal conduction.

Axonal Conduction

Drugs that act by altering axonal conduction are not very selective. Recall that the process of conducting an impulse along an axon is essentially the same in all neurons. As a consequence, a drug that alters axonal conduction will affect conduction in all nerves to which it has access. Such a drug cannot produce selective effects.

Local anesthetics are drugs that work by decreasing axonal conduction. Because these agents produce nonselective inhibition of axonal conduction, they suppress transmission in any nerve they reach. Hence, although local anesthetics are certainly valuable, their indications are limited.

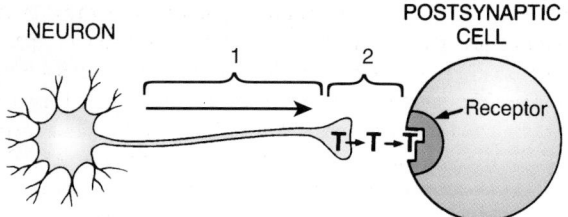

Fig. 11.1 How Neurons Regulate Other Cells. There are two basic steps in the process by which neurons elicit responses from other cells: (1) axonal conduction and (2) synaptic transmission. T, Neurotransmitter.

Synaptic Transmission

In contrast to drugs that alter axonal conduction, drugs that alter synaptic transmission can produce effects that are highly selective. This selectivity can occur because synapses, unlike axons, differ from one another. Synapses at different sites employ different transmitters. In addition, for most transmitters, the body employs more than one type of receptor. Hence, by using a drug that selectively influences a specific type of neurotransmitter or receptor, we can alter one neuronally regulated process while leaving most others unchanged. Because of their relative selectivity, drugs that alter synaptic transmission have many uses.

Receptors

The ability of a neuron to influence the behavior of another cell depends, ultimately, on the ability of that neuron to alter receptor activity on the target cell. As discussed, neurons alter receptor activity by releasing transmitter molecules, which diffuse across the synaptic gap and bind to receptors on the postsynaptic cell. If the target cell lacked receptors for the transmitter that a neuron released, that neuron would be unable to affect the target cell.

The effects of neuropharmacologic drugs, like those of neurons, depend on altering receptor activity. That is, no matter what its precise mechanism of action, a neuropharmacologic drug ultimately works by influencing receptor activity on target cells. This concept is central to understanding the actions of neuropharmacologic drugs. In fact, this concept is so critical to our understanding of neuropharmacologic agents that I will repeat it: *the effect of a drug on a neuronally regulated process is dependent on the ability of that drug to directly or indirectly influence receptor activity on target cells.*

Steps in Synaptic Transmission

To understand how drugs alter receptor activity, we must first understand the steps by which synaptic transmission takes place because it is by modifying these steps that neuropharmacologic drugs influence receptor function. The steps in synaptic transmission are shown in Fig. 11.2.

Step 1: Transmitter Synthesis

For synaptic transmission to take place, molecules of transmitter must be present in the nerve terminal. Hence, we can look on transmitter synthesis as the first step in transmission. In the figure, the letters Q, R, and S represent the precursor molecules from which the transmitter (T) is made.

Step 2: Transmitter Storage

After transmitter is synthesized, it must be stored until the time of its release. Transmitter storage takes place within vesicles—tiny packets

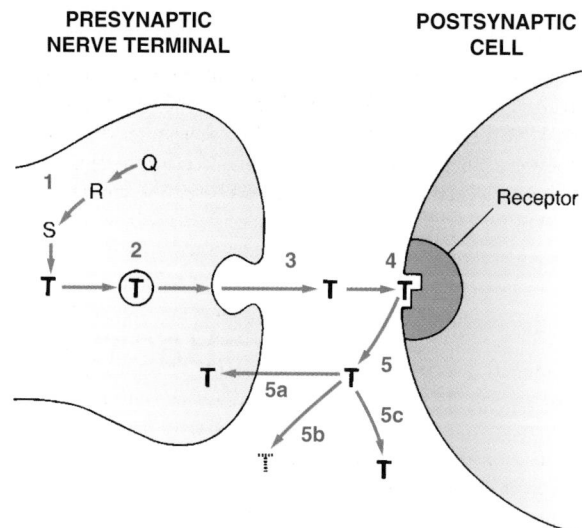

Fig. 11.2 Steps in Synaptic Transmission. *Step 1,* Synthesis of transmitter *(T)* from precursor molecules *(Q, R,* and *S). Step 2,* Storage of transmitter in vesicles. *Step 3,* Release of transmitter: in response to an action potential, vesicles fuse with the terminal membrane and discharge their contents into the synaptic gap. *Step 4,* Action at receptor: transmitter binds (reversibly) to its receptor on the postsynaptic cell, causing a response in that cell. *Step 5,* Termination of transmission: transmitter dissociates from its receptor and is then removed from the synaptic gap by *(a)* reuptake into the nerve terminal, *(b)* enzymatic degradation, or *(c)* diffusion away from the gap.

present in the axon terminal. Each nerve terminal contains a large number of transmitter-filled vesicles.

Step 3: Transmitter Release

Release of transmitter is triggered by the arrival of an action potential at the axon terminal. The action potential initiates a process in which vesicles undergo fusion with the terminal membrane, causing release of their contents into the synaptic gap. Each action potential causes only a small fraction of all vesicles present in the axon terminal to discharge their contents.

Step 4: Receptor Binding

After release, transmitter molecules diffuse across the synaptic gap and then undergo *reversible* binding to receptors on the postsynaptic cell. This binding initiates a cascade of events that result in altered behavior of the postsynaptic cell.

Step 5: Termination of Transmission

Transmission is terminated by dissociation of transmitter from its receptors, followed by removal of a free transmitter from the synaptic gap. Transmitter can be removed from the synaptic gap by three processes: (1) reuptake, (2) enzymatic degradation, and (3) diffusion. In those synapses where transmission is terminated by reuptake, axon terminals contain "pumps" that transport transmitter molecules back into the neuron from which they were released (Step 5a in Fig. 11.2). After reuptake, molecules of transmitter may be degraded, or they may be packaged in vesicles for reuse. In synapses where transmitter is cleared by enzymatic degradation (Step 5b), the synapse contains large quantities of transmitter-inactivating enzymes. Although simple diffusion away from the synaptic gap (Step 5c) is a potential means of terminating transmitter action, this process is very slow and generally of little significance.

Effects of Drugs on the Steps of Synaptic Transmission

As emphatically noted, all neuropharmacologic agents (except local anesthetics) produce their effects by directly or indirectly altering receptor activity. We also noted that the way in which drugs alter receptor activity is by interfering with synaptic transmission. Because synaptic transmission has multiple steps, the process offers several potential targets for drugs. In this section, we examine the specific ways in which drugs can alter the steps of synaptic transmission.

Before discussing specific mechanisms by which drugs can alter receptor activity, we need to understand what drugs can do to receptors in general terms. From the broadest perspective, when a drug influences receptor function, that drug can do just one of two things: it can enhance receptor activation, or it can reduce receptor activation. What do we mean by *receptor activation*? For our purposes, we can define *activation* as an effect on receptor function equivalent to that produced by the natural neurotransmitter at a particular synapse. Hence a drug whose effects mimic the effects of a natural transmitter would be said to *increase* receptor activation. Conversely, a drug whose effects were equivalent to reducing the amount of natural transmitter available for receptor binding would be said to *decrease* receptor activation.

Please note that activation of a receptor does not necessarily mean that a physiologic process will go faster; receptor activation can also make a process go slower. For example, the heart rate will decline when the endogenous neurotransmitter acetylcholine activates cholinergic receptors on the heart; therefore, a drug that mimics acetylcholine at receptors on the heart will cause the heart to beat more slowly.

Having defined receptor activation, we are ready to discuss the mechanisms by which drugs, acting on specific steps of synaptic transmission, can increase or decrease receptor activity (Table 11.1). As we consider these mechanisms one by one, their logical associations should become apparent.

Transmitter Synthesis

There are three different effects that drugs are known to have on transmitter synthesis. They can (1) increase transmitter synthesis, (2) decrease transmitter synthesis, or (3) cause the synthesis of transmitter molecules that are more effective than the natural transmitter itself.

A drug that increases transmitter synthesis will cause receptor activation to increase. The process is this: as a result of increased transmitter synthesis, storage vesicles will contain transmitter in abnormally high amounts. Hence, when an action potential reaches the axon terminal, more transmitter will be released, and therefore more transmitter will be available to receptors on the postsynaptic cell, causing activation of those receptors to increase. Conversely, a drug that decreases transmitter synthesis will cause the transmitter content of vesicles to decline, resulting in reduced transmitter release and decreased receptor activation.

Some drugs can cause neurons to synthesize transmitter molecules whose structure is different from that of normal transmitter molecules. For example, by acting as substrates for enzymes in the axon terminal, drugs can be converted into "super" transmitters (molecules whose ability to activate receptors is greater than that of the naturally occurring transmitter at a particular site). Release of these supertransmitters will cause receptor activation to increase.

Transmitter Storage

Drugs that interfere with transmitter storage will cause receptor activation to decrease. This occurs because disruption of storage depletes vesicles of their transmitter content, thereby decreasing the amount of transmitter available for release.

Transmitter Release

Drugs can either *promote* or *inhibit* transmitter release. Drugs that promote release will increase receptor activation. Conversely, drugs that inhibit release will reduce receptor activation. The amphetamines represent drugs that act by promoting transmitter release. Botulinum toxin, in contrast, acts by inhibiting transmitter release.

Receptor Binding

Many drugs act directly at receptors. These agents can (1) bind to receptors and cause activation, (2) bind to receptors and thereby block receptor activation by other agents, or (3) bind to receptor components and thereby enhance receptor activation by the natural transmitter at the site.

In the terminology introduced in Chapter 4, drugs that directly activate receptors are called *agonists*, whereas drugs that prevent receptor activation are called *antagonists*. The direct-acting receptor agonists and antagonists constitute the largest and most important groups of neuropharmacologic drugs. (There is no single name or category for drugs that bind to receptors to enhance natural transmitter effects.)

Examples of drugs that act directly at receptors are numerous. Drugs that bind to receptors and cause *activation* include morphine (used for its effects on the CNS), epinephrine (used mainly for its effects on the cardiovascular system), and insulin (used for its effects in diabetes). Drugs that bind to and block receptors to *prevent* their activation include naloxone (used to treat overdose with opioid drugs), antihistamines (used to treat allergic disorders), and metoprolol (used to treat hypertension, angina pectoris, and cardiac dysrhythmias). Benzodiazepines are excellent examples of drugs that bind to receptors and thereby enhance the actions of a natural transmitter. Drugs in this family, which includes diazepam (Valium) and related agents, are used to treat anxiety, seizure disorders, and muscle spasms.

Termination of Transmitter Action

Drugs can interfere with the termination of transmitter action by two mechanisms: (1) blockade of transmitter reuptake and (2) inhibition of transmitter degradation. Drugs that act by either mechanism will increase transmitter availability, thereby causing receptor activation to increase.

TABLE 11.1	**Effects of Drugs on Synaptic Transmission and the Resulting Effect on Receptor Activation**	
Step of Synaptic Transmission	**Drug Action**	**Effect on Receptor Activation**[a]
1. Synthesis of transmitter	Increased synthesis of T	Increase
	Decreased synthesis of T	Decrease
	Synthesis of "super" T	Increase
2. Storage of transmitter	Reduced storage of T	Decrease
3. Release of transmitter	Promotion of T release	Increase
	Inhibition of T release	Decrease
4. Binding to receptor	Direct receptor activation	Increase
	Enhanced response to T	Increase
	Blockade of T binding	Decrease
5. Termination of transmission	Blockade of T reuptake	Increase
	Inhibition of T breakdown	Increase

[a]Receptor activation is defined as producing an effect equivalent to that produced by the natural transmitter that acts on a particular receptor.

T, Transmitter.

MULTIPLE RECEPTOR TYPES AND SELECTIVITY OF DRUG ACTION

As we discussed in Chapter 4, selectivity is one of the most desirable qualities a drug can have. A selective drug can alter a specific disease process while leaving other physiologic processes largely unaffected.

Many neuropharmacologic agents display a high degree of selectivity. This selectivity is possible because the nervous system works through multiple types of receptors to regulate processes under its control. The relationship between multiple receptor types and selective drug action is illustrated by Mort and Merv, whose unique physiologies are depicted in Fig. 11.3. Let's begin with Mort. Mort can perform four functions: he can pump blood, digest food, shake hands, and empty his bladder. All four functions are under neuronal control, and in all cases, that control is exerted by activation of the same type of receptor (designated *A*).

As long as Mort remains healthy, having only one type of receptor to regulate his various functions is no problem. Selective *physiologic* regulation can be achieved simply by sending impulses down the appropriate nerves. When there is a need to increase cardiac output, impulses are sent down the nerve to his heart; when digestion is needed, impulses are sent down the nerve to his stomach; and so forth.

Although having only one receptor type is no disadvantage when all is well, if Mort gets sick, having only one receptor type creates a therapeutic challenge. Let's assume he develops heart disease and we need to provide a drug that will help increase cardiac output. To stimulate cardiac function, we need to administer a drug that will activate receptors on his heart. Unfortunately, because the receptors on his heart are the same as the receptors on his other organs, a drug that stimulates cardiac function will stimulate his other organs, too. Consequently, any attempt to improve cardiac output with drugs will necessarily be accompanied by side effects. These will range from silly (compulsive handshaking) to embarrassing (enuresis) to hazardous (gastric ulcers). Please note that these undesirable effects are the direct result of Mort having a nervous system that works through just one type of receptor to regulate all organs. That is, the presence of only one receptor type has made selective drug action impossible.

Now let's consider Merv. Although Merv appears to be Mort's twin, Merv differs in one important way: whereas all functions in Mort are regulated through just one type of receptor, Merv employs different receptors to control each of his four functions. Because of this simple but important difference, the selective drug action that was impossible with Mort can be achieved easily with Merv. We can, for example, selectively enhance cardiac function in Merv without risking the side effects to which Mort was predisposed. This can be done simply by administering an agonist agent that binds selectively to receptors on the heart (type A receptors). If this medication is sufficiently selective for type A receptors, it will not interact with receptor types B, C, or D. Hence, function in structures regulated by those receptors will be unaffected. Note that our ability to produce selective drug action in Merv is made possible because his nervous system works through different types of receptors to regulate function in his various organs. The message from this example is clear: *the more types of receptors we have to work with, the greater our chances of producing selective drug effects.*

AN APPROACH TO LEARNING ABOUT PERIPHERAL NERVOUS SYSTEM DRUGS

To understand any particular PNS drug, you need three types of information: (1) the type (or types) of receptor through which the drug acts; (2) the normal response to activation of those receptors; and (3) what the drug in question does to receptor function (i.e., does it increase or decrease receptor activation?). Armed with these three types of information, you can predict the major effects of any PNS drug. (Information about PNS function is reviewed in Chapter 12.)

An example will illustrate this process. Let's consider the drug named *isoproterenol*. The first information we need is the identity of the receptors at which isoproterenol acts. Isoproterenol acts at two types of receptors, named β_1- and β_2-adrenergic receptors. Next, we need to know the normal responses to activation of these receptors. The most prominent responses to activation of β_1 receptors are *increased heart rate* and *increased force of cardiac contraction*. The primary responses to activation of β_2 receptors are *bronchial dilation* and *elevation of blood glucose levels*. Finally, we need to know whether isoproterenol increases or decreases

Mort   **Merv**

Fig. 11.3 Multiple Drug Receptors and Selective Drug Action. All of the **Mort** organs are regulated through activation of type A receptors. Drugs that affect type A receptors on one organ will affect type A receptors on all other organs. Hence, selective drug action is impossible. **Merv** has four types of receptors (*A, B, C,* and *D*) to regulate his four organs. A drug that acts at one type of receptor will not affect the others. Hence, selective drug action is possible.

the activation of β_1 and β_2 receptors. At both types of receptor, isoproterenol causes *activation*. Armed with these three primary pieces of information about isoproterenol, we can now predict the principal effects of this drug. By *activating* β_1 and β_2 receptors, isoproterenol can elicit three major responses: (1) increased cardiac output (by increasing heart rate and force of contraction), (2) dilation of the bronchi, and (3) elevation of blood glucose.

From this example, you can see how easy it is to predict the effects of a PNS drug. Accordingly, I strongly encourage you to take the approach suggested when studying these agents. That is, for each PNS drug, you should learn (1) the identity of the receptors at which that drug acts, (2) the normal responses to activation of those receptors, and (3) whether the drug increases or decreases receptor activation.

12

Physiology of the Peripheral Nervous System

To understand peripheral nervous system (PNS) drugs, it is necessary to first understand the PNS. The purpose of this chapter is to help you develop that understanding.

Because the ultimate goal of this book concerns pharmacology—and not physiology—the discussion is limited to those aspects of PNS physiology that have a direct bearing on the ability to understand drugs.

DIVISIONS OF THE NERVOUS SYSTEM

The nervous system has two main divisions, the *central nervous system* (CNS) and the *peripheral nervous system*. The PNS has two major subdivisions: (1) the *somatic motor system*, and (2) the *autonomic nervous system*. The autonomic nervous system is further subdivided into the *parasympathetic nervous system* and the *sympathetic nervous system*. The somatic motor system controls voluntary movement of muscles. The two subdivisions of the autonomic nervous system regulate many involuntary processes.

The autonomic nervous system is the principal focus of this chapter. The somatic motor system is also considered, but discussion is brief.

OVERVIEW OF AUTONOMIC NERVOUS SYSTEM FUNCTIONS

The autonomic nervous system has three principal functions: (1) regulation of the *heart*, (2) regulation of *secretory glands* (salivary, gastric, sweat, and bronchial glands), and (3) regulation of *smooth muscles* (muscles of the bronchi, blood vessels, urogenital system, and gastrointestinal [GI] tract). These regulatory activities are shared between the sympathetic and parasympathetic divisions of the autonomic nervous system.

Functions of the Parasympathetic Nervous System

The parasympathetic nervous system performs seven regulatory functions that have particular relevance to drugs. Specifically, stimulation of appropriate parasympathetic nerves causes the following:
- Slowing of heart rate
- Increased gastric secretion
- Emptying of the bladder
- Emptying of the bowel
- Focusing the eye for near vision
- Constricting the pupil
- Contracting bronchial smooth muscle

Just how the parasympathetic nervous system elicits these responses is discussed later in the section "Functions of Cholinergic Receptor Subtypes."

From the previous discussion we can see that the parasympathetic nervous system is concerned primarily with what might be called the "housekeeping" chores of the body (digestion of food and excretion of wastes). In addition, the system helps control vision by constricting the pupil and conserves energy by reducing cardiac work.

Therapeutic agents that alter parasympathetic nervous system function are used primarily for their effects on the GI tract, bladder, and eye. Occasionally, these drugs are also used for effects on the heart and lungs.

A variety of poisons act by mimicking or blocking effects of parasympathetic stimulation. Among these are insecticides, nerve gases, and toxic compounds found in certain mushrooms and plants.

Functions of the Sympathetic Nervous System

The sympathetic nervous system has three main functions:
- Regulating the cardiovascular system
- Regulating body temperature
- Implementing the acute stress response (commonly called a "fight-or-flight" reaction)

The sympathetic nervous system exerts multiple influences on the heart and blood vessels. Stimulation of sympathetic nerves to the heart increases cardiac output. Stimulation of sympathetic nerves to arterioles and veins causes vasoconstriction. Release of epinephrine from the adrenal medulla results in vasoconstriction in most vascular beds and vasodilation in certain others. By influencing the heart and blood vessels, the sympathetic nervous system can achieve three homeostatic objectives:
- Maintenance of blood flow to the brain
- Redistribution of blood flow during exercise
- Compensation for loss of blood, primarily by causing vasoconstriction

The sympathetic nervous system helps regulate body temperature in three ways: (1) By regulating blood flow to the skin, sympathetic nerves can increase or decrease heat loss. By dilating surface vessels, sympathetic nerves increase blood flow to the skin and thereby accelerate heat loss. Conversely, constricting cutaneous vessels conserves heat. (2) Sympathetic nerves to sweat glands promote the secretion of sweat, thereby helping the body cool. (3) By inducing piloerection (erection of hair), sympathetic nerves can promote heat conservation.

When we are faced with an acute stress-inducing situation, the sympathetic nervous system orchestrates the fight-or-flight response, which consists of the following:
- Increasing heart rate and blood pressure
- Shunting blood away from the skin and viscera and into skeletal muscles
- Dilating the bronchi to improve oxygenation
- Dilating the pupils (perhaps to enhance visual acuity)
- Mobilizing stored energy, thereby providing glucose for the brain and fatty acids for muscles

Many therapeutic agents produce their effects by altering functions under sympathetic control. These drugs are used primarily for effects on the heart, blood vessels, and lungs. Agents that alter cardiovascular function are used to treat hypertension, heart failure, angina pectoris, and other disorders. Drugs affecting the lungs are used primarily for asthma.

AUTONOMIC NERVOUS SYSTEM REGULATION OF PHYSIOLOGIC PROCESSES

To understand how drugs influence processes under autonomic control, we must first understand how the autonomic nervous system itself regulates those activities. The basic mechanisms by which the autonomic nervous system regulates physiologic processes are discussed in the following sections.

Patterns of Innervation and Control

Most structures under autonomic control are innervated by sympathetic nerves and parasympathetic nerves. The relative influence of sympathetic and parasympathetic nerves depends on the organ under consideration.

In many organs that receive dual innervation, the influence of sympathetic nerves *opposes* that of parasympathetic nerves. For example, in the heart, *sympathetic* nerves *increase* the heart rate, whereas *parasympathetic* nerves *slow* the heart rate.

In some organs that receive nerves from both divisions of the autonomic nervous system, the effects of sympathetic and parasympathetic nerves are *complementary* rather than opposite. For example, in the male reproductive system, erection is regulated by parasympathetic nerves, whereas ejaculation is controlled by sympathetic nerves. If attempts at reproduction are to succeed, cooperative interaction of both systems is needed.

A few structures under autonomic control receive innervation from only one division. The principal example is blood vessels, which are innervated exclusively by sympathetic nerves.

In summary, there are three basic patterns of autonomic innervation and regulation:
- Innervation by *both* divisions of the autonomic nervous system in which the effects of the two divisions are *opposed*
- Innervation by *both* divisions of the autonomic nervous system in which the effects of the two divisions are *complementary*
- Innervation and regulation by *only one* division of the autonomic nervous system

Feedback Regulation

Feedback regulation is a process that allows a system to adjust itself by responding to incoming information. Practically all physiologic processes are regulated at least in part by feedback control.

Fig. 12.1 depicts a feedback loop typical of those used by the autonomic nervous system. The main elements of this loop are (1) a *sensor*, (2) an *effector*, and (3) *neurons* connecting the sensor to the

effector. The purpose of the sensor is to monitor the status of a physiologic process. Information picked up by the sensor is sent to the CNS (spinal cord and brain), where it is integrated with other relevant information. Signals (instructions for change) are then sent from the CNS along nerves of the autonomic system to the effector. In response to these instructions, the effector makes appropriate adjustments in the process. The entire procedure is called a *reflex*.

Baroreceptor Reflex

From a pharmacologic perspective, the most important feedback loop of the autonomic nervous system is one that helps regulate blood pressure. This system is referred to as the *baroreceptor reflex*. (Baroreceptors are receptors that sense blood pressure.) This reflex is important to us because it frequently opposes our attempts to modify blood pressure with drugs.

Feedback (reflex) control of blood pressure is achieved as follows: (1) Baroreceptors located in the carotid sinus and aortic arch monitor changes in blood pressure and send this information to the brain. (2) In response, the brain sends impulses along nerves of the autonomic nervous system, instructing the heart and blood vessels to behave in a way that restores blood pressure to normal. Accordingly, when blood pressure *falls*, the baroreceptor reflex causes vasoconstriction and increases cardiac output. Both actions help bring blood pressure back up. Conversely, when the blood pressure *rises* too high, the baroreceptor reflex causes vasodilation and reduces cardiac output, thereby causing the blood pressure to drop. The baroreceptor reflex is discussed in greater detail in Chapter 36.

Autonomic Tone

Autonomic tone is the steady, day-to-day influence exerted by the autonomic nervous system on a particular organ or organ system. Autonomic tone provides a basal level of control over which reflex regulation is superimposed.

When an organ is innervated by both divisions of the autonomic nervous system, one division—either sympathetic or parasympathetic—provides most of the basal control, thereby obviating conflicting instruction. Recall that, when an organ receives nerves from both divisions of the autonomic nervous system, those nerves frequently exert opposing influences. If both divisions were to send impulses simultaneously, the resultant conflicting instructions would be counterproductive (like running heating and air conditioning simultaneously). By having only one division of the autonomic nervous system provide the basal control to an organ, conflicting signals are avoided.

The branch of the autonomic nervous system that controls organ function most of the time is said to provide the *predominant tone* to that organ. *In most organs, the parasympathetic nervous system provides the predominant tone.* The vascular system, which is regulated almost exclusively by the *sympathetic* nervous system, is the principal exception.

ANATOMIC CONSIDERATIONS

Although a great deal about the anatomy of the PNS is known, very little of this information contributes to an understanding of PNS drugs. The few details that *do* pertain to pharmacology are shown in Fig. 12.2.

Parasympathetic Nervous System

Pharmacologically relevant aspects of parasympathetic anatomy are shown in Fig. 12.2. Note that there are *two* neurons in the pathway leading from the spinal cord to organs innervated by parasympathetic nerves. The junction (synapse) between these two neurons occurs within a structure called a *ganglion*. (A ganglion is simply a mass of nerve cell

Fig. 12.1 Feedback Loop of the Autonomic Nervous System.

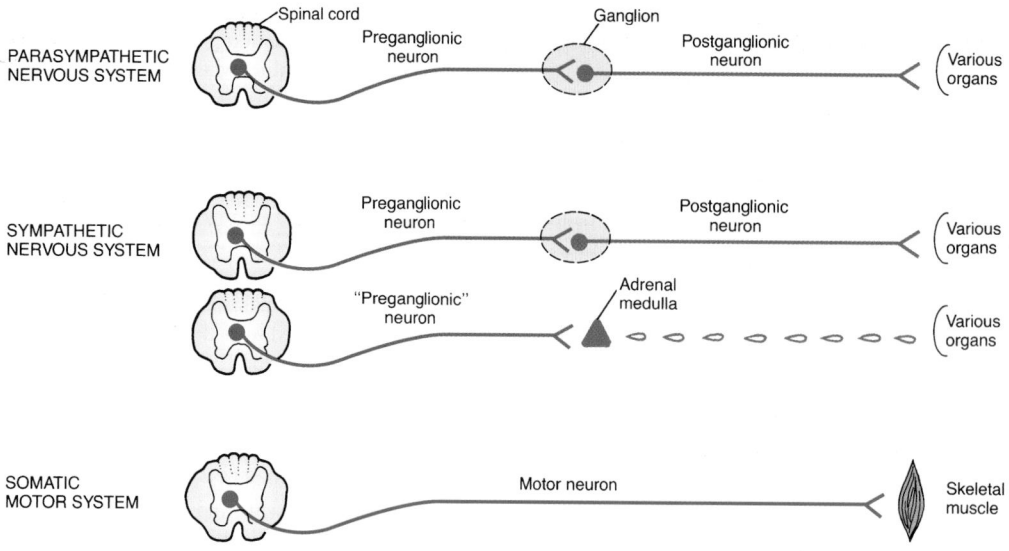

Fig. 12.2 The Basic Anatomy of the Parasympathetic and Sympathetic Nervous Systems and the Somatic Motor System.

bodies.) The neurons that go from the spinal cord to the parasympathetic ganglia are called *preganglionic neurons*, whereas the neurons that go from the ganglia to effector organs are called *postganglionic neurons*. The anatomy of the parasympathetic nervous system offers two general sites at which drugs can act: (1) the synapses between preganglionic neurons and postganglionic neurons, and (2) the junctions between postganglionic neurons and their effector organs.

Sympathetic Nervous System

Pharmacologically relevant aspects of sympathetic nervous system anatomy are illustrated in Fig. 12.2. As you can see, these features are nearly identical to those of the parasympathetic nervous system. Like the parasympathetic nervous system, the sympathetic nervous system employs two neurons in the pathways leading from the spinal cord to organs under its control. As with the parasympathetic nervous system, the junctions between those neurons are located in *ganglia*. Neurons leading from the spinal cord to the sympathetic ganglia are termed *preganglionic neurons*, and neurons leading from ganglia to effector organs are termed *postganglionic neurons*.

The *medulla of the adrenal gland* is a feature of the sympathetic nervous system that requires comment. Although not a neuron per se, the adrenal medulla can be looked on as the functional equivalent of a postganglionic neuron of the sympathetic nervous system. (The adrenal medulla influences the body by releasing epinephrine into the bloodstream, which then produces effects much like those that occur in response to the stimulation of postganglionic sympathetic nerves.) Because the adrenal medulla is similar in function to a postganglionic neuron, the nerve leading from the spinal cord to the adrenal gland is commonly referred to as a preganglionic neuron, even though there is no ganglion in this pathway.

As with the parasympathetic nervous system, drugs that affect the sympathetic nervous system have two general sites of action: (1) the synapses between preganglionic and postganglionic neurons (including the adrenal medulla), and (2) the junctions between postganglionic neurons and their effector organs.

Somatic Motor System

Pharmacologically relevant anatomy of the somatic motor system is depicted in Fig. 12.2. Note that there is *only one* neuron in the pathway from the spinal cord to the muscles innervated by somatic motor nerves. Because this pathway contains only one neuron, peripherally acting drugs that affect somatic motor system function have only one site of action: the *neuromuscular junction* (i.e., the junction between the somatic motor nerve and the muscle).

TRANSMITTERS OF THE PERIPHERAL NERVOUS SYSTEM

The PNS employs three neurotransmitters: *acetylcholine, norepinephrine,* and *epinephrine.* Any given junction in the PNS uses only one of these transmitter substances. A fourth compound—*dopamine*—may also serve as a PNS transmitter, but this role has not been demonstrated conclusively.

To understand PNS pharmacology, it is necessary to know the identity of the transmitter employed at each of the junctions of the PNS. This information is shown in Fig. 12.3. As indicated, acetylcholine (ACh) is the transmitter employed at most junctions of the PNS. ACh is the transmitter released by (1) all preganglionic neurons of the parasympathetic nervous system, (2) all preganglionic neurons of the sympathetic nervous system, (3) all postganglionic neurons of the parasympathetic nervous system, (4) all motor neurons to skeletal muscles, and (5) most postganglionic neurons of the sympathetic nervous system that go to sweat glands.

Norepinephrine is the transmitter released by practically all postganglionic neurons of the sympathetic nervous system. The only exceptions are the postganglionic sympathetic neurons that go to sweat glands, which employ ACh as their transmitter.

Epinephrine is the major transmitter released by the adrenal medulla. (The adrenal medulla also releases some norepinephrine.)

RECEPTORS OF THE PERIPHERAL NERVOUS SYSTEM

The PNS works through several different types of receptors. Understanding these receptors is central to understanding PNS pharmacology. All effort that you invest in learning about these receptors now will be rewarded as we discuss PNS drugs in later chapters. Much of what follows is based on the information in Fig. 12.3.

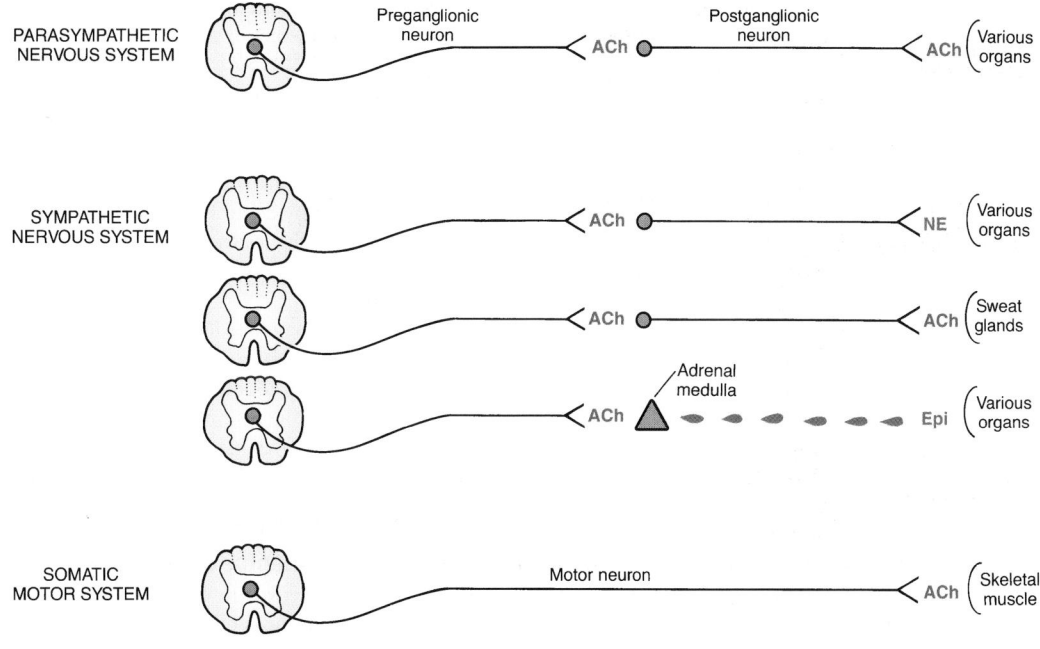

ACh = acetylcholine, NE = norepinephrine, Epi = epinephrine

Fig. 12.3 Transmitters Employed at Specific Junctions of the Peripheral Nervous System. (1) *All preganglionic neurons of the parasympathetic and sympathetic nervous systems release acetylcholine as their transmitter.* (2) *All postganglionic neurons of the parasympathetic nervous system release acetylcholine as their transmitter.* (3) *Most postganglionic neurons of the sympathetic nervous system release norepinephrine as their transmitter.* (4) *Postganglionic neurons of the sympathetic nervous system that innervate sweat glands release acetylcholine as their transmitter.* (5) *Epinephrine is the principal transmitter released by the adrenal medulla.* (6) *All motor neurons to skeletal muscles release acetylcholine as their transmitter.*

Primary Receptor Types: Cholinergic Receptors and Adrenergic Receptors

There are two basic categories of receptors associated with the PNS: *cholinergic receptors* and *adrenergic receptors*. Cholinergic receptors are defined as receptors that mediate responses to ACh. These receptors mediate responses at all junctions where ACh is the transmitter. Adrenergic receptors are defined as receptors that mediate responses to epinephrine (adrenaline) and norepinephrine. These receptors mediate responses at all junctions where norepinephrine or epinephrine is the transmitter.

Subtypes of Cholinergic and Adrenergic Receptors

Not all cholinergic receptors are the same; likewise, not all adrenergic receptors are the same. For each of these two major receptor classes there are receptor subtypes. There are three major subtypes of cholinergic receptors, referred to as nicotinic$_N$, nicotinic$_M$, and muscarinic.[a] There are four major subtypes of adrenergic receptors, referred to as α_1, α_2, β_1, and β_2.

---

[a]Evidence indicates that muscarinic receptors, like nicotinic receptors, come in subtypes. Five have been identified. Of these, only three—designated M_1, M_2, and M_3—have clearly identified functions. At this time, practically all drugs that affect muscarinic receptors are nonselective. Accordingly, because our understanding of these receptors is limited, and because drugs that can selectively alter their function are few, we will not discuss muscarinic receptor subtypes further in this chapter. However, we will discuss them in Chapter 14, in the context of drugs for overactive bladder.

In addition to the four major subtypes of adrenergic receptors, there is another adrenergic receptor type, referred to as the *dopamine* receptor. Although dopamine receptors are classified as adrenergic, these receptors do not respond to epinephrine or norepinephrine. Rather, they respond only to dopamine, a neurotransmitter found primarily in the CNS.

EXPLORING THE CONCEPT OF RECEPTOR SUBTYPES

The concept of receptor subtypes is important and potentially confusing. In this section we discuss what a receptor subtype is and why receptor subtypes matter.

What Is a Receptor Subtype?

Receptors that respond to the same transmitter but nonetheless are different from one another are called *receptor subtypes*. For example, peripheral receptors that respond to ACh can be found (1) in ganglia of the autonomic nervous system, (2) at neuromuscular junctions, and (3) on organs regulated by the parasympathetic nervous system. However, even though all of these receptors can be activated by ACh, there is clear evidence that the receptors at these three sites are, in fact, different from one another. Hence, although all of these receptors belong to the same major receptor category (cholinergic), they are sufficiently different as to constitute distinct receptor subtypes.

How Do We Know That Receptor Subtypes Exist?

Historically, our knowledge of receptor subtypes came from observing responses to drugs. In fact, were it not for drugs, receptor subtypes might never have been discovered.

Table 12.1 illustrates the types of drug responses that led to the realization that receptor subtypes exist. These data summarize the results of an experiment designed to study the effects of a natural transmitter (ACh) and a series of drugs (nicotine, muscarine, d-tubocurarine, and atropine) on two tissues: skeletal muscle and ciliary muscle. (The ciliary muscle is the muscle responsible for focusing the eye for near vision.) Although skeletal muscle and ciliary muscle both contract in response to ACh, these tissues differ in their responses to drugs. In the discussion that follows, we examine the selective responses of these tissues to drugs and see how those responses reveal the existence of receptor subtypes.

At synapses on skeletal muscle and ciliary muscle, ACh is the transmitter employed by neurons to elicit contraction. Because both types of muscle respond to ACh, it is safe to conclude that both muscles have receptors for this substance. Because ACh is the natural transmitter for these receptors, we would classify them as *cholinergic*.

What do the effects of nicotine on skeletal muscle and ciliary muscle suggest? There are four possible conclusions: (1) Because skeletal muscle contracts in response to nicotine, we can conclude that skeletal muscle has receptors at which nicotine can act. (2) Because ciliary muscle does *not* respond to nicotine, we can tentatively conclude that ciliary muscle does not have receptors for nicotine. (3) Because nicotine mimics the effects of ACh on skeletal muscle, we can conclude that nicotine may act at the same skeletal muscle receptors where ACh acts. (4) Because both skeletal and ciliary muscle have receptors for ACh, and because nicotine appears to act only at the ACh receptors on skeletal muscle, we can tentatively conclude that the ACh receptors on skeletal muscle are different from the ACh receptors on ciliary muscle.

What do the responses to muscarine suggest? The conclusions that can be drawn are exactly parallel to those drawn for nicotine. They are that (1) ciliary muscle has receptors that respond to muscarine, (2) skeletal muscle may not have receptors for muscarine, (3) muscarine may be acting at the same receptors on ciliary muscle where ACh acts, and (4) the receptors for ACh on ciliary muscle may be different from the receptors for ACh on skeletal muscle.

The responses of skeletal muscle and ciliary muscle to nicotine and muscarine suggest but do not prove that the cholinergic receptors on these two tissues are different. However, the responses of these two tissues to d-*tubocurarine* and *atropine*, both of which are receptor *blocking agents,* eliminate any doubts as to the presence of cholinergic receptor subtypes. When both types of muscle are pretreated with d-tubocurarine and then exposed to ACh, the response to ACh is blocked in skeletal muscle but not in ciliary muscle. Tubocurarine pretreatment does not reduce the ability of ACh to stimulate ciliary muscle. Conversely, pretreatment with atropine selectively blocks the response to ACh in ciliary muscle—but atropine does nothing to prevent ACh from stimulating receptors on skeletal muscle. Because tubocurarine can selectively block cholinergic receptors in skeletal muscle (whereas atropine can selectively

block cholinergic receptors in ciliary muscle), we can conclude with certainty that the receptors for ACh in these two types of muscle must be different.

The data just discussed illustrate the essential role of drugs in revealing the presence of receptor subtypes. If ACh were the only probe that we had, all that we would have been able to observe is that both skeletal muscle and ciliary muscle can respond to this agent. This simple observation would provide no basis for suspecting that the receptors for ACh in these two tissues were different. It is only through the use of selectively acting drugs that the presence of receptor subtypes was initially revealed.

Today, the technology for identifying receptors and their subtypes is extremely sophisticated—not that studies like the one just discussed are no longer of value. In addition to performing traditional drug-based studies, scientists are now cloning receptors using DNA hybridization technology. As you can imagine, this allows us to understand receptors in ways that were unthinkable in the past.

How Can Drugs Be More Selective Than Natural Transmitters at Receptor Subtypes?

Drugs achieve their selectivity for receptor subtypes by having structures that are different from those of natural transmitters. The relationship between structure and receptor selectivity is illustrated in Fig. 12.4. Drawings are used to represent drugs (nicotine and muscarine), receptor subtypes (nicotinic and muscarinic), and ACh (the natural transmitter at nicotinic and muscarinic receptors). From the structures shown, we can easily imagine how ACh is able to interact with both kinds of receptor subtypes, whereas nicotine and muscarine can interact only with the receptor subtypes whose structure is complementary to their own. By synthesizing chemicals that are structurally related to natural transmitters, pharmaceutical chemists have been able to produce drugs that are more selective for specific receptor subtypes than are the natural transmitters that act at those sites.

Why Do Receptor Subtypes Exist and Why Do They Matter?

The physiologic benefits of having multiple receptor subtypes for the same transmitter are not immediately obvious. In fact, as noted previously, were it not for drugs, we probably wouldn't know that receptor subtypes existed at all. Although receptor subtypes are of uncertain physiologic relevance, from the viewpoint of therapeutics, they are invaluable.

Nicotinic cholinergic receptor

Muscarinic cholinergic receptor

Acetylcholine

Nicotine

Muscarine

Fig. 12.4 Drug Structure and Receptor Selectivity. The relationship between structure and receptor selectivity is shown. The structure of acetylcholine allows this transmitter to interact with both receptor subtypes. In contrast, because of their unique structures, nicotine and muscarine are selective for the cholinergic receptor subtypes whose structure complements their own.

TABLE 12.1	Responses of Skeletal Muscle and Ciliary Muscle to a Series of Drugs	
	RESPONSE	
Drug	**Skeletal Muscle**	**Ciliary Muscle**
Acetylcholine	Contraction	Contraction
Nicotine	Contraction	No response
Muscarine	No response	Contraction
Acetylcholine		
After d-tubocurarine	No response	Contraction
After atropine	Contraction	No response

The presence of receptor subtypes makes possible a dramatic increase in drug selectivity. For example, thanks to the existence of subtypes of cholinergic receptors (and the development of drugs selective for those receptor subtypes), it is possible to influence the activity of certain cholinergic receptors (e.g., receptors of the neuromuscular junction) without altering the activity of all other cholinergic receptors (e.g., the cholinergic receptors found in all autonomic ganglia and all target organs of the parasympathetic nervous system). Were it not for the existence of receptor subtypes, a drug that acted on cholinergic receptors at one site would alter the activity of cholinergic receptors at all other sites. Clearly, the existence of receptor subtypes for a particular transmitter makes drug actions possible, which are much more selective than could be achieved if all of the receptors for that transmitter were the same. (Recall our discussion of Mort and Merv in Chapter 11.)

LOCATIONS OF RECEPTOR SUBTYPES

Because many of the drugs discussed in later chapters are selective for specific receptor subtypes, knowledge of the sites at which specific receptor subtypes are located will help us predict which organs a drug will affect. Accordingly, in laying our foundation for studying PNS drugs, it is important to learn the sites at which the subtypes of adrenergic and cholinergic receptors are located. This information is shown in Fig. 12.5. You will find it helpful to master the content of this figure before proceeding. (In the interest of minimizing confusion, subtypes of adrenergic receptors in Fig. 12.5 are listed simply as α and β rather than as α_1, α_2, β_1, and β_2. The locations of all four subtypes of adrenergic receptors are discussed in the section that follows.)

FUNCTIONS OF CHOLINERGIC AND ADRENERGIC RECEPTOR SUBTYPES

Knowledge of receptor function is essential for understanding PNS drugs. By knowing the receptors at which a drug acts, and by knowing what those receptors do, we can predict the major effects of any PNS drug.

Tables 12.2 and 12.3 show the pharmacologically relevant functions of PNS receptors. Table 12.2 summarizes responses elicited by the activation of *cholinergic* receptor subtypes. Table 12.3 summarizes responses to the activation of *adrenergic* receptor subtypes. You should master Table 12.2 before studying cholinergic drugs (Chapters 13 and 14.) You should master Table 12.3 before studying adrenergic drugs (Chapters 15 to 17.) If you master these tables in preparation for learning about PNS drugs, you will find the process of learning the pharmacology relatively simple. Conversely, if you attempt to study the pharmacology without first mastering the appropriate table, you are likely to meet with frustration.

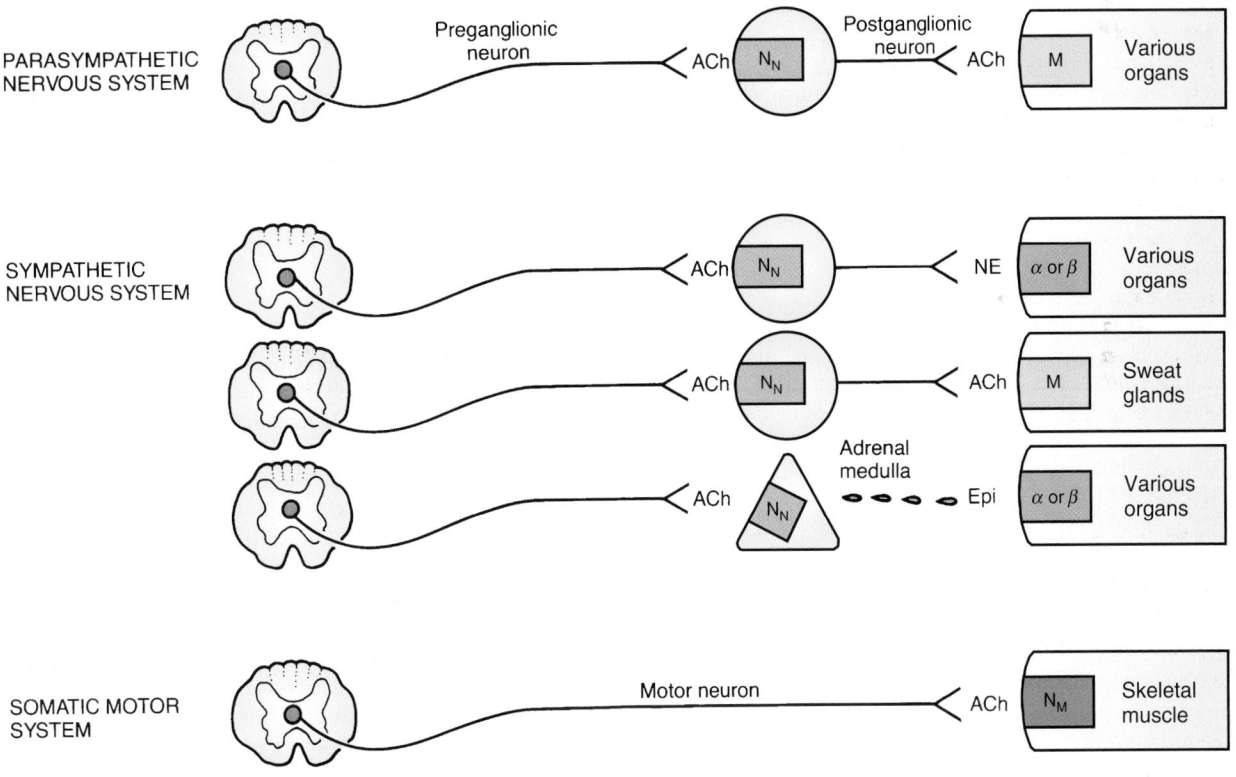

Cholinergic receptor subtypes: N_N = nicotinic$_N$, N_M = nicotinic$_M$, and M = muscarinic.
Adrenergic receptor subtypes: α = alpha and β = beta.

Fig. 12.5 Locations of Cholinergic and Adrenergic Receptor Subtypes. (1) *Nicotinic$_N$* receptors are located on the *cell bodies of all postganglionic neurons* of the *parasympathetic* and *sympathetic* nervous systems. Nicotinic$_N$ receptors are also located on cells of the *adrenal medulla*. (2) *Nicotinic$_M$* receptors are located on *skeletal muscle*. (3) *Muscarinic* receptors are located on *all organs* regulated by the *parasympathetic* nervous system (i.e., organs innervated by postganglionic parasympathetic nerves). *Muscarinic* receptors are also located on *sweat glands*. (4) *Adrenergic* receptors—α, β, or both—are located on *all organs* (except sweat glands) regulated by the *sympathetic* nervous system (i.e., organs innervated by postganglionic sympathetic nerves). *Adrenergic* receptors are also located on organs regulated by epinephrine released from the *adrenal medulla*. *ACh*, Acetylcholine.

TABLE 12.2 Functions of Peripheral Cholinergic Receptor Subtypes

Receptor Subtype	Location	Response to Receptor Activation
Nicotinic$_N$	All autonomic nervous system ganglia and the adrenal medulla	Stimulation of parasympathetic and sympathetic postganglionic nerves and release of epinephrine from the adrenal medulla
Nicotinic$_M$	Neuromuscular junction	Contraction of skeletal muscle
Muscarinic	All parasympathetic target organs:	
	Eye	Contraction of the ciliary muscle focuses the lens for near vision
		Contraction of the iris sphincter muscle causes miosis (decreased pupil diameter)
	Heart	Decreased rate
	Lung	Constriction of bronchi
		Promotion of secretions
	Bladder	Contraction of detrusor increases bladder pressure
		Relaxation of trigone and sphincter allows urine to leave the bladder
		Coordinated contraction of detrusor and relaxation of trigone and sphincter causes voiding of the bladder
	Gastrointestinal tract	Salivation
		Increased gastric secretions
		Increased intestinal tone and motility
		Defecation
	Sweat glands[a]	Generalized sweating
	Sex organs	Erection
	Blood vessels[b]	Vasodilation

[a]Although sweating is due primarily to stimulation of muscarinic receptors by acetylcholine, the nerves that supply acetylcholine to sweat glands belong to the sympathetic nervous system rather than the parasympathetic nervous system.
[b]Cholinergic receptors on blood vessels are not associated with the nervous system.

Functions of Cholinergic Receptor Subtypes

Table 12.2 shows the pharmacologically relevant responses to activation of the three major subtypes of cholinergic receptors: nicotinic$_N$, nicotinic$_M$, and muscarinic.

Responses to cholinergic receptor activation can be grouped into three major categories based on the subtype of receptor involved:

- Activation of *nicotinic$_N$* (neuronal) receptors promotes *ganglionic transmission* at all ganglia of the sympathetic and parasympathetic nervous systems. In addition, activation of nicotinic$_N$ receptors promotes *release of epinephrine from the adrenal medulla.*
- Activation of *nicotinic$_M$* (muscle) receptors causes *contraction of skeletal muscle.*
- Activation of *muscarinic* receptors, which are located on target organs of the parasympathetic nervous system, elicits an appropriate response from the organ involved. Specifically, muscarinic activation causes

TABLE 12.3 Functions of Peripheral Adrenergic Receptor Subtypes

Receptor Subtype	Location	Response to Receptor Activation
α_1	Eye	Contraction of the radial muscle of the iris causes mydriasis (increased pupil size)
	Arterioles	Constriction
	Skin	
	Viscera	
	Mucous membranes	
	Veins	Constriction
	Sex organs, male	Ejaculation
	Prostatic capsule	Contraction
	Bladder	Contraction of trigone and sphincter
α_2	Presynaptic nerve terminals[a]	Inhibition of transmitter release
β_1	Heart	Increased rate
		Increased force of contraction
		Increased atrioventricular conduction velocity
	Kidney	Release of renin
β_2	Arterioles	Dilation
	Heart	
	Lung	
	Skeletal muscle	
	Bronchi	Dilation
	Uterus	Relaxation
	Liver	Glycogenolysis
	Skeletal muscle	Enhanced contraction, glycogenolysis
Dopamine	Kidney	Dilation of kidney vasculature

(1) increased glandular secretions (from pulmonary, gastric, intestinal, and sweat glands), (2) contraction of smooth muscle in the bronchi and GI tract, (3) slowing of the heart rate, (4) contraction of the sphincter muscle of the iris, resulting in miosis (reduction in pupillary diameter), (5) contraction of the ciliary muscle of the eye, causing the lens to focus for near vision, (6) dilation of blood vessels, and (7) voiding of the urinary bladder (by causing contraction of the detrusor muscle [which forms the bladder wall] and relaxation of the trigone and sphincter muscles [which block the bladder neck when contracted]).

Muscarinic cholinergic receptors on blood vessels require additional comment. These receptors are not associated with the nervous system in any way. That is, no autonomic nerves terminate at vascular muscarinic receptors. It is not at all clear as to how, or even if, these receptors are activated physiologically. However, regardless of their physiologic relevance, the cholinergic receptors on blood vessels do have *pharmacologic* significance because drugs that are able to activate these receptors cause vasodilation, which in turn causes blood pressure to fall.

Functions of Adrenergic Receptor Subtypes

Adrenergic receptor subtypes and their functions are shown in Table 12.3.

α_1 Receptors

α_1 receptors are located in the eyes, blood vessels, male sex organs, prostatic capsule, and bladder (trigone and sphincter).

Ocular α_1 receptors are present on the radial muscle of the iris. Activation of these receptors leads to *mydriasis* (dilation of the pupil).

α_1 receptors are present on veins and on arterioles in many capillary beds. Activation of α_1 receptors in blood vessels produces *vasoconstriction*.

Activation of α_1 receptors in the sexual apparatus of males causes *ejaculation*. Activation of α_1 receptors in smooth muscle of the bladder (trigone and sphincter) and prostatic capsule causes *contraction*.

α_2 Receptors

α_2 receptors of the PNS are located on nerve terminals (see Table 12.3) and not on the organs innervated by the autonomic nervous system. Because α_2 receptors are located on nerve terminals, these receptors are referred to as *presynaptic* or *prejunctional*. The function of these receptors is to *regulate transmitter release*. As depicted in Table 12.3, norepinephrine can bind to α_2 receptors located on the same neuron from which the norepinephrine was released. The consequence of this norepinephrine–receptor interaction is suppression of further norepinephrine release. Hence, presynaptic α_2 receptors can help reduce transmitter release when too much transmitter has accumulated in the synaptic gap. Drug effects resulting from activation of *peripheral* α_2 receptors are of minimal clinical significance.

α_2 receptors are also present in the CNS. In contrast to peripheral α_2 receptors, central α_2 receptors are therapeutically relevant. We will consider these receptors in later chapters.

β_1 Receptors

β_1 receptors are located in the heart and the kidney. Cardiac β_1 receptors have great therapeutic significance. Activation of these receptors *increases heart rate, force of contraction*, and *velocity of impulse conduction through the atrioventricular node*.

Activation of β_1 receptors in the kidney causes *release of renin* into the blood. Because renin promotes synthesis of angiotensin, a powerful vasoconstrictor, activation of renal β_1 receptors is a means by which the nervous system helps elevate blood pressure. (The role of renin in the regulation of blood pressure is discussed in depth in Chapter 38.)

β_2 Receptors

β_2 receptors mediate several important processes. Activation of β_2 receptors in the lung leads to *bronchial dilation*. Activation of β_2 receptors in the uterus causes *relaxation of uterine smooth muscle*. Activation of β_2 receptors in arterioles of the heart, lungs, and skeletal muscles causes *vasodilation* (an effect opposite to that of α_1 activation). Activation of β_2 receptors in the liver and skeletal muscle promotes *glycogenolysis* (breakdown of glycogen into glucose), thereby increasing blood levels of glucose. In addition, activation of β_2 receptors in skeletal muscle enhances *contraction*.

Dopamine Receptors

In the periphery, the only dopamine receptors of clinical significance are located in the vasculature of the kidney. Activation of these receptors *dilates renal blood vessels*, enhancing renal perfusion.

In the CNS, receptors for dopamine are of great therapeutic significance. The functions of these receptors are discussed in Chapters 19 and 26.

RECEPTOR SPECIFICITY OF THE ADRENERGIC TRANSMITTERS

The receptor specificity of adrenergic transmitters is more complex than the receptor specificity of ACh. Whereas ACh can activate all three subtypes of cholinergic receptors, not every adrenergic transmitter (epinephrine, norepinephrine, dopamine) can interact with each of the five subtypes of adrenergic receptors.

Receptor specificity of adrenergic transmitters is as follows: (1) *epinephrine* can activate all α and β receptors, but not dopamine receptors, (2) *norepinephrine* can activate α_1, α_2, and β_1 receptors, but not β_2 or dopamine receptors, and (3) *dopamine* can activate α_1, β_1, and dopamine receptors. (Note that dopamine itself is the only transmitter capable of activating dopamine receptors.) Receptor specificity of the adrenergic transmitters is shown in Table 12.4.

Knowing that epinephrine is the only transmitter that acts at β_2 receptors can serve as an aid to remembering the functions of this receptor subtype. Recall that epinephrine is released from the adrenal medulla—not from neurons—and that the function of epinephrine is to prepare the body for fight or flight. Accordingly, because epinephrine is the only transmitter that activates β_2 receptors, and because epinephrine is released only in preparation for fight or flight, times of fight or flight will be the only occasions on which β_2 receptors will undergo significant physiologic activation. As it turns out, the physiologic changes elicited by β_2 activation are precisely those needed for success in the fight-or-flight response. Specifically, activation of β_2 receptors will (1) dilate blood vessels in the heart, lungs, and skeletal muscles, thereby increasing blood flow to these organs, (2) dilate the bronchi, thereby increasing oxygenation, (3) increase glycogenolysis, thereby increasing available energy, and (4) relax uterine smooth muscle, thereby preventing delivery (a process that would be inconvenient for a pregnant woman preparing to fight or flee). Accordingly, if you think of the physiologic requirements for success during fight or flight, you will have a good picture of the responses that β_2 activation can cause.

TRANSMITTER LIFE CYCLES

In this section we consider the life cycles of ACh, norepinephrine, and epinephrine. Because a number of drugs produce their effects by interfering with specific phases of the transmitters' life cycles, knowledge of these cycles helps us understand drug actions.

Life Cycle of Acetylcholine

The life cycle of ACh is depicted in Fig. 12.6. The cycle begins with synthesis of ACh from two precursors: choline and acetylcoenzyme A. After synthesis, ACh is stored in vesicles and later released in response to an action potential. After release, ACh binds to receptors (nicotinic$_N$,

TABLE 12.4 Receptor Specificity of Adrenergic Transmitters

Transmitter	α_1	α_2	β_1	β_2	Dopamine
Epinephrine	←			→	
Norepinephrine	←		→		
Dopamine	↔		↔		↔

Arrows indicate the range of receptors that the transmitters can activate.

nicotinic$_M$, or muscarinic) located on the postjunctional cell. Upon dissociating from its receptors, ACh is destroyed almost instantaneously by *acetylcholinesterase* (AChE), an enzyme present in abundance on the surface of the postjunctional cell. AChE degrades ACh into two inactive products: acetate and choline. Uptake of choline into the cholinergic nerve terminal completes the life cycle of ACh. Note that an inactive substance (choline), and not the active transmitter (ACh), is taken back up for reuse.

Therapeutic and toxic agents can interfere with the ACh life cycle at several points. Botulinum toxin inhibits ACh release. A number of medicines and poisons act at cholinergic receptors to mimic or block the actions of ACh. Several therapeutic and toxic agents act by inhibiting AChE, thereby causing ACh to accumulate in the junctional gap.

Life Cycle of Norepinephrine

The life cycle of norepinephrine is depicted in Fig. 12.7. As indicated, the cycle begins with synthesis of norepinephrine from a series of precursors. The final step of synthesis takes place within vesicles, where norepinephrine is then stored before release. After release, norepinephrine binds to adrenergic receptors. Norepinephrine can interact with *postsynaptic* α_1 and β_1 receptors (but not with β_2 receptors) and with *presynaptic* α_2 receptors. Transmission is terminated by *reuptake* of norepinephrine back into the nerve terminal. (Note that the termination process for norepinephrine differs from that for ACh, whose effects are terminated by enzymatic degradation rather than reuptake.) After reuptake, norepinephrine can undergo one of two fates: (1) uptake into

Fig. 12.6 Life Cycle of Acetylcholine. Transmission is terminated by enzymatic degradation of acetylcholine *(ACh)* and not by the uptake of intact ACh back into the nerve terminal. *Acetyl CoA*, Acetylcoenzyme A; *AChE*, acetylcholinesterase.

Fig. 12.7 Life Cycle of Norepinephrine. Note that transmission mediated by norepinephrine *(NE)* is terminated by the reuptake of NE into the nerve terminal and not by enzymatic degradation. Be aware that although postsynaptic cells may have α_1, β_1, and β_2 receptors, NE can only activate postsynaptic α_1 and β_1 receptors; physiologic activation of β_2 receptors is done by epinephrine. *DA*, Dopamine; *MAO*, monoamine oxidase.

vesicles for reuse, or (2) inactivation by monoamine oxidase (MAO), an enzyme found in the nerve terminal.

Practically every step in the life cycle of norepinephrine can be altered by therapeutic agents. We have drugs that alter the synthesis, storage, and release of norepinephrine; we have drugs that act at adrenergic receptors to mimic or block the effects of norepinephrine; we have drugs, such as cocaine and tricyclic antidepressants, that inhibit the reuptake of norepinephrine (and thereby intensify transmission); and we have drugs that inhibit the breakdown of norepinephrine by MAO, causing an increase in the amount of transmitter available for release.

Life Cycle of Epinephrine

The life cycle of epinephrine is much like that of norepinephrine—although there are significant differences. The cycle begins with synthesis of epinephrine within chromaffin cells of the adrenal medulla. These cells produce epinephrine by first making norepinephrine, which is then converted enzymatically to epinephrine. (Because sympathetic neurons lack the enzyme needed to convert norepinephrine to epinephrine, epinephrine is not produced in sympathetic nerves.) After synthesis, epinephrine is stored in vesicles to await release. When released, epinephrine travels through the bloodstream to target organs throughout the body, where it can activate α_1, α_2, β_1, and β_2 receptors. Termination of epinephrine actions is accomplished primarily by hepatic metabolism, and not by uptake into nerves.

13

Muscarinic Agonists and Cholinesterase Inhibitors

INTRODUCTION TO CHOLINERGIC DRUGS

Cholinergic drugs are agents that influence the activity of cholinergic receptors. Most of these drugs act directly at cholinergic receptors, where they either mimic or block the actions of acetylcholine. The remainder—the cholinesterase inhibitors—activate cholinergic receptors indirectly by preventing the breakdown of acetylcholine.

The cholinergic drugs have both therapeutic and toxicologic significance. Therapeutic applications are limited but valuable. The toxicology of cholinergic drugs is extensive, encompassing such agents as nicotine, insecticides, and compounds designed for chemical warfare.

There are six categories of cholinergic drugs. These categories are muscarinic agonists, muscarinic antagonists, cholinesterase inhibitors, ganglionic stimulating agents, ganglionic blocking agents, and neuromuscular blocking agents. The muscarinic antagonists, ganglionic blocking agents, and neuromuscular blocking agents (commonly referred to as anticholinergic agents) are discussed in Chapter 14.

The *muscarinic agonists* selectively mimic the effects of acetylcholine at muscarinic receptors. The *cholinesterase inhibitors* prevent the breakdown of acetylcholine by acetylcholinesterase. As a result, more acetylcholine remains available to activate cholinergic receptors.

Ganglionic stimulating agents selectively mimic the effects of acetylcholine at nicotinic$_N$ (neuronal) receptors of autonomic ganglia. These drugs have little therapeutic value beyond the use of nicotine in smoking cessation programs (see Chapter 34). *Ganglionic blocking agents*, represented by mecamylamine, selectively block ganglionic nicotinic$_N$ receptors. *Neuromuscular blocking agents*, represented by *d*-tubocurarine and succinylcholine, selectively block the effects of acetylcholine at nicotinic$_M$ (muscle) receptors at the neuromuscular junction (NMJ). Ganglionic and neuromuscular blocking agents are used in specialty settings and are beyond the scope of this text.

Table 13.1 is your key to understanding the cholinergic drugs. It lists the three major subtypes of cholinergic receptors (muscarinic, nicotinic$_N$, and nicotinic$_M$) and indicates the following for each receptor type: (1) location, (2) responses to activation, (3) drugs that produce activation (agonists), and (4) drugs that prevent activation (antagonists). This information, along with the detailed information on cholinergic receptor function summarized in Table 12.2 in Chapter 12, provides the information you need to predict the actions of cholinergic drugs.

An example will demonstrate the combined value of Tables 13.1 and 12.2. Let's consider bethanechol. As shown in Table 13.1, bethanechol is a selective *agonist* at *muscarinic* cholinergic receptors. Referring to Table 12.2, we see that activation of muscarinic receptors can produce the following: ocular effects (miosis and ciliary muscle contraction), slowing of heart rate, bronchial constriction, urination,

glandular secretion, stimulation of the gastrointestinal (GI) tract, and vasodilation. Because bethanechol *activates* muscarinic receptors, the drug is capable of eliciting all of these responses. Therefore, by knowing which receptors bethanechol activates (from Table 13.1), and by knowing what those receptors do (from Table 12.2), you can predict the kinds of responses you might expect bethanechol to produce.

Next we will examine the muscarinic agonists, cholinesterase inhibitors, and muscarinic antagonists. The muscarinic agonists and antagonists produce their effects through *direct* interaction with muscarinic receptors. The muscarinic agonists cause receptor activation; the antagonists produce receptor blockade. Like the muscarinic agonists, another group of drugs—the cholinesterase inhibitors—can also cause receptor activation, but they do so by an *indirect* mechanism.

MUSCARINIC AGONISTS

The muscarinic agonists bind to muscarinic receptors and thereby cause receptor activation. Because nearly all muscarinic receptors are associated with the parasympathetic nervous system, responses to muscarinic agonists closely resemble those produced by stimulation of parasympathetic nerves. Accordingly, muscarinic agonists are also known as *parasympathomimetic agents*.

Bethanechol

Bethanechol (Urecholine, Duvoid ✦) embodies the properties that typify all muscarinic agonists and will serve as our prototype for the group.

Mechanism of Action

Bethanechol is a direct-acting muscarinic agonist. The drug binds reversibly to muscarinic cholinergic receptors to cause activation. At therapeutic doses, bethanechol acts selectively at muscarinic receptors, having little or no effect on nicotinic receptors, either in ganglia or in skeletal muscle.

Pharmacologic Effects

Bethanechol can elicit all of the responses typical of muscarinic receptor activation. Accordingly, we can readily predict the effects of bethanechol by knowing the information on muscarinic responses summarized in Table 12.2.

The principal structures affected by muscarinic activation are the *heart, exocrine glands, smooth muscles,* and *eyes*. Muscarinic agonists act on the heart to cause bradycardia (decreased heart rate) and on exocrine glands to increase sweating, salivation, bronchial secretions, and secretion of gastric acid. In smooth muscles of the lungs and GI tract, muscarinic agonists promote contraction. The result is constriction of the bronchi and increased tone and motility of GI smooth muscle. In the bladder, muscarinic activation causes *contraction* of the detrusor muscle and *relaxation* of the trigone and sphincter; the result is bladder emptying. In vascular smooth muscle, these drugs cause relaxation; the resultant vasodilation can produce hypotension. Activation of muscarinic receptors in the eyes has two effects: (1) miosis (pupillary constriction) and (2) contraction of the ciliary muscle, resulting in accommodation for near vision. (The ciliary muscle, which is attached to the lens, focuses the eyes for near vision by altering lens curvature.)

Pharmacokinetics. Bethanechol is available for oral administration. Effects begin in 30 to 60 minutes and persist for about 1 hour. Because bethanechol is a quaternary ammonium compound that always carries a positive charge, the drug crosses membranes poorly. As a result, only a small fraction of each dose is absorbed. Additional information on pharmacokinetics of bethanechol and other muscarinic agonists is provided in Table 13.2.

Preparations, dosage, and administration. Preparation and dosing of bethanechol and other muscarinic agonists is provided in Table 13.3.

Therapeutic Uses

Although bethanechol can produce a broad spectrum of pharmacologic effects, the drug is approved only for urinary retention.

Urinary retention. Bethanechol relieves urinary retention by activating muscarinic receptors of the urinary tract. Muscarinic activation relaxes the trigone and sphincter muscles and increases voiding pressure by contracting the detrusor muscle, which composes the bladder wall. It is approved to treat urinary retention in postoperative and postpartum patients and to treat retention secondary to neurogenic atony of the bladder. The drug should not be used to treat urinary retention caused by physical obstruction of the urinary tract because increased pressure in the tract in the presence of blockage could cause injury.

Gastrointestinal uses. Bethanechol has been used off-label to treat *gastroesophageal reflux*. Benefits may result from increased esophageal motility and increased pressure in the lower esophageal sphincter.

Bethanechol can help treat disorders associated with GI paralysis. Benefits derive from increased tone and motility of GI smooth muscle. Specific applications are *adynamic ileus*, *gastric atony*, and *postoperative abdominal distention*. Bethanechol should not be given if physical obstruction of the GI tract is present, because in the presence of blockage, increased propulsive contractions might result in damage to the intestinal wall.

TABLE 13.1 Cholinergic Drugs and Their Receptors

	RECEPTOR SUBTYPE		
	Muscarinic	Nicotinic$_N$	Nicotinic$_M$
Receptor Location	Sweat glands Blood vessels All organs regulated by the parasympathetic nervous system	All ganglia of the autonomic nervous system	Neuromuscular junctions
Effects of Receptor Activation	Many, including: ↓ Heart rate ↑ Gland secretion Smooth muscle contraction	Promotes ganglionic transmission	Skeletal muscle contraction
Receptor Agonists	Bethanechol	Nicotine	(Nicotine[a])
Indirect-Acting Cholinomimetics	Cholinesterase inhibitors: physostigmine, neostigmine, and other cholinesterase inhibitors can activate *all* cholinergic receptors (by causing accumulation of acetylcholine at cholinergic junctions)		

[a]The doses of nicotine needed to activate nicotinic$_M$ receptors of the neuromuscular junctions are much higher than the doses needed to activate nicotinic$_N$ receptors in autonomic ganglia.

TABLE 13.3 Preparation and Dosage of Muscarinic Agonists

Drug Class or Drug	Preparation	Dosage
Muscarinic Agonists		
Bethanechol (Urecholine, Duvoid ♦)	Tablets: 5, 10, 25, and 50 mg	10–50 mg 3–4 times a day
Cevimeline (Evoxac)	Capsules: 30 mg	30 mg 3 times a day
Pilocarpine ophthalmic (Isopto Carpine, Diocarpine ♦, Pilopine HS)	Solution: 1% in 15 mL, 2% in 15 mL, and 4% in 15 mL Gel: 4%	Solution: 1–2 drops to affected eye up to 6 times a day Gel: apply a 0.5-inch ribbon onto the lower conjunctival sac at bedtime
Pilocarpine systemic (Salagen)	Tablets: 5 mg, 7.5 mg	Sjögren syndrome: 5 mg 4 times a day Postradiotherapy for cancer: 5 mg 3 times a day initially; may be titrated upward to 10 mg 3 times a day

TABLE 13.2 Pharmacokinetics of Muscarinic Agonists

Drug	Peak	Protein Binding	Metabolism	Half-Life	Elimination
Bethanechol (Urecholine, Duvoid ♦)	1–1.5 h	UK	UK	2 h	UK
Cevimeline (Evoxac)	1.5–2 h	<20%	Hepatic (CYP2D6, CYP3A3, & CYP3A4)	4–6 h	Urine, 84% Feces
Pilocarpine (Isopto Carpine, Diocarpine ♦, Pilopine HS, Salagen)	Ophthalmic: 0.5–1 h	UK	Hepatic	1–1.5 h	Urine

h, Hour(s); *UK*, unknown.

PATIENT-CENTERED CARE ACROSS THE LIFE SPAN

Muscarinic Agonists

Life Stage	Patient Care Concerns
Children	Safety and effectiveness in children has not been established for bethanechol and cevimeline.
Pregnant women	It is unknown whether bethanechol or cevimeline cause fetal harm. Reproduction studies in animals suggest that cevimeline may decrease implantation.
Breastfeeding women	It is unknown whether bethanechol or cevimeline are excreted in breast milk. As a cautionary measure, manufacturers recommend that nursing be discontinued while taking these drugs.
Older adults	Because older patients may have decreased cardiac, hepatic, or renal function, care must be taken to evaluate risks on an individual basis.

Adverse Effects

In theory, bethanechol can produce the full range of muscarinic responses as side effects. However, with oral dosing, side effects are relatively rare.

Cardiovascular system. Bethanechol can cause *hypotension* (secondary to vasodilation) and *bradycardia*. Accordingly, the drug is contraindicated for patients with low blood pressure or low cardiac output.

Gastrointestinal system. At usual therapeutic doses, bethanechol can cause *excessive salivation, increased secretion of gastric acid, abdominal cramps*, and *diarrhea*. Higher doses can cause involuntary defecation. Bethanechol is contraindicated in patients with gastric ulcers because stimulation of acid secretion could intensify gastric erosion, causing bleeding and possibly perforation. The drug is also contraindicated for patients with *intestinal obstruction* and for those recovering from recent *surgery of the bowel*. In both cases, the ability of bethanechol to increase the tone and motility of intestinal smooth muscle could result in rupture of the bowel wall.

Urinary tract. Because of its ability to contract the bladder detrusor and thereby *increase pressure within the urinary tract*, bethanechol can be hazardous to patients with urinary tract obstruction or weakness of the bladder wall. In both groups, elevation of pressure within the urinary tract could rupture the bladder. Accordingly, bethanechol is contraindicated for patients with either disorder.

Exacerbation of asthma. By activating muscarinic receptors in the lungs, bethanechol can cause bronchoconstriction. Accordingly, the drug is contraindicated for patients with latent or active asthma. Of course, it stands to reason that muscarinic agonists may also complicate other respiratory disorders.

Dysrhythmias in patients with hyperthyroidism. Bethanechol is contraindicated for people with hyperthyroidism. *If given to patients with this condition, bethanechol may increase heart rate to the point of initiating a dysrhythmia. (Note that increased heart rate is opposite to the effect that muscarinic agonists have in most patients.)* The mechanism of dysrhythmia induction is explained here.

When patients with hyperthyroidism are given bethanechol, their initial cardiovascular responses are like those of anyone else: bradycardia and hypotension. In reaction to hypotension, the baroreceptor reflex attempts to return blood pressure to normal. Part of this reflex involves the release of norepinephrine from sympathetic nerves that regulate heart rate. In patients who do not have hyperthyroidism, norepinephrine release serves to increase cardiac output and thus helps restore blood pressure. However, in patients, norepinephrine can induce cardiac

dysrhythmias. The reason for this unusual response is that, in patients with hyperthyroidism, the heart is exquisitely sensitive to the effects of norepinephrine, and hence relatively small amounts can cause stimulation sufficient to elicit a dysrhythmia.

SUMMARY OF KEY PRESCRIBING CONSIDERATIONS

Bethanechol

Therapeutic Goal: Treatment of nonobstructive urinary retention.

Baseline Data: Vital signs, urination trends (times and amounts)

Monitoring: Intake and output. Observe for signs of excessive muscarinic response (abnormal salivation, sweating, urinary urgency, bradycardia, and hypotension).

Identifying High-Risk Patients: Bethanechol is *contraindicated* for patients with peptic ulcer disease, urinary tract obstruction, intestinal obstruction, coronary insufficiency, hypotension, asthma, and hyperthyroidism.

Evaluating Therapeutic Effects: Absence of bladder distension or suprapubic discomfort. Adequate urinary output.

Minimizing Adverse Effects: Taking on an empty stomach can help reduce nausea and vomiting. Treat excessive muscarinic stimulation with atropine and supportive measures.

Other Muscarinic Agonists

Cevimeline

Actions and uses. Cevimeline (Evoxac) is a derivative of acetylcholine with actions much like those of bethanechol. The drug is indicated for relief of xerostomia (dry mouth) in patients with Sjögren syndrome, an autoimmune disorder. Xerostomia, left untreated, can lead to multiple complications, including periodontal disease, dental caries, altered taste, oral ulcers and candidiasis, and difficulty eating and speaking. Cevimeline relieves dry mouth by activating muscarinic receptors on residual healthy tissue in salivary glands, thereby promoting salivation. Because it stimulates salivation, cevimeline may also benefit patients with xerostomia induced by radiation therapy for head and neck cancer, although the drug is not approved for this use. Cevimeline has also been used to manage keratoconjunctivitis sicca (inflammation of the cornea and conjunctiva) and dry eye. It increases tear production, which can help relieve discomfort associated with these conditions.

Adverse effects. Adverse effects result from activating muscarinic receptors and hence are similar to those of bethanechol. The most common effects are excessive sweating, nausea, rhinitis, and diarrhea. There is also an increased incidence of urinary tract infections (UTIs). To compensate for fluid loss caused by sweating and diarrhea, patients should increase fluid intake. Like bethanechol, cevimeline promotes miosis (constriction of the pupil) and may also cause blurred vision. Both actions can make driving dangerous, especially at night.

Activation of cardiac muscarinic receptors can reduce heart rate and slow cardiac conduction. Accordingly, cevimeline should be used with caution in patients with a history of heart disease.

Because muscarinic activation increases airway resistance, cevimeline is contraindicated for patients with uncontrolled asthma and should be used with caution in patients with controlled asthma, chronic bronchitis, or chronic obstructive pulmonary disease (COPD). Cevimeline is also contraindicated for people with both narrow-angle glaucoma and iritis.

Drug interactions. Cevimeline can intensify cardiac depression caused by β blockers because both drugs decrease heart rate and cardiac conduction.

Beneficial effects of cevimeline can be antagonized by drugs that block muscarinic receptors. Among these are atropine, tricyclic antidepressants (e.g., imipramine), antihistamines (e.g., diphenhydramine), and phenothiazine antipsychotics (e.g., chlorpromazine).

Pilocarpine

Pilocarpine is a muscarinic agonist used mainly for topical therapy of glaucoma, an ophthalmic disorder characterized by elevated intraocular pressure (IOP) with subsequent injury to the optic nerve. The basic pharmacology of pilocarpine and its use in glaucoma are discussed in Chapter 87.

In addition to its use in glaucoma, oral pilocarpine is approved for treatment of dry mouth resulting from Sjögren syndrome or from salivary gland damage caused by radiation therapy of head and neck cancer. For these applications, pilocarpine is available under the trade name Salagen. It may also be given to manage dry mouth secondary to head and neck cancer. At lower doses, the principal adverse effect is sweating. However, if dosage is excessive, pilocarpine can produce the full spectrum of muscarinic effects.

Toxicology of Muscarinic Agonists
Sources of Muscarinic Poisoning

Muscarinic poisoning can result from overdose with two kinds of medications: (1) direct-acting muscarinic agonists (e.g., bethanechol, pilocarpine) and (2) indirect-acting cholinomimetics (e.g., cholinesterase inhibitors; discussed later). Muscarinic poisoning can also occur following ingestion of certain mushrooms (e.g., *Inocybe* and *Clitocybe* spp.).

Symptoms

Manifestations of muscarinic poisoning result from excessive activation of muscarinic receptors. Prominent symptoms are (1) respiratory (bronchospasm and excessive bronchial secretions), (2) cardiovascular (bradycardia and hypotension), (3) GI (profuse salivation, nausea and vomiting, abdominal pain, diarrhea, and fecal incontinence), (4) genitourinary (excessive urination and urinary incontinence), (5) integumentary (diaphoresis), and (5) visual (lacrimation and miosis). Severe poisoning can produce cardiovascular collapse. (Mnemonics for muscarinic poisoning are presented in Box 13.1.)

Treatment

Management is direct and specific: administer *atropine* (a selective muscarinic blocking agent) and provide supportive therapy. By blocking access of muscarinic agonists to their receptors, atropine can reverse most signs of toxicity.

PROTOTYPE DRUGS

Cholinergic Agents

Muscarinic Agonists
    Bethanechol (Urecholine, Duvoid)
Cholinesterase Inhibitors
    Pyridostigmine (Mestinon, Regonol)
Muscarinic Antagonist
    Atropine (AtroPen, others)

PATIENT EDUCATION

Muscarinic Agonists and Cholinesterase Inhibitors

Advise patients to take these drugs 1 h before meals or 2 h after meals to decrease incidence of nausea and vomiting.

Inform patients about manifestations of muscarinic excess and advise them to seek medical treatment if they occur.

BOX 13.1   Muscarinic (Cholinergic) Toxicity

Muscarinic (cholinergic) toxicity can be caused by either muscarinic agonists or cholinesterase inhibitors. Some common mnemonics can help you to identify this potentially dangerous condition.

Mnemonic 1: Dumbels
Diaphoresis/**D**iarrhea
Urination
Miosis
Bradycardia/**B**ronchospasm/**B**ronchorrhea
Emesis
Lacrimation
Salivation

Mnemonic 2: Sludge and the Killer Bs
Salivation
Lacrimation
Urination
Diaphoresis/**D**iarrhea
Gastrointestinal cramping
Emesis
Bradycardia
Bronchospasm
Bronchorrhea

CHOLINESTERASE INHIBITORS

Cholinesterase inhibitors are drugs that prevent the degradation of acetylcholine by acetylcholinesterase (also known simply as *cholinesterase*). Cholinesterase inhibitors are also known as *anticholinesterase* drugs. By preventing the breakdown of acetylcholine, cholinesterase inhibitors increase the amount of acetylcholine available to activate receptors, thus enhancing cholinergic action. Because cholinesterase inhibitors do not bind directly with cholinergic receptors, they are viewed as indirect-acting cholinergic agonists. Use of cholinesterase inhibitors results in transmission at all cholinergic junctions (muscarinic, ganglionic, and neuromuscular), so these drugs can elicit a broad spectrum of responses. Because they lack selectivity, cholinesterase inhibitors are limited to only a few therapeutic applications: treatment of myasthenia gravis (MG), glaucoma, Alzheimer disease, Parkinson disease dementia, and poisoning by muscarinic antagonists. In specialty areas, they are used to reverse competitive (nondepolarizing) neuromuscular blockade. Applications of individual agents are shown in Table 13.4.

There are two basic categories of cholinesterase inhibitors: (1) *reversible inhibitors* and (2) *irreversible inhibitors*. The reversible inhibitors produce effects of moderate duration, and the irreversible inhibitors produce effects of long duration.

Reversible Cholinesterase Inhibitors
Pyridostigmine

Pyridostigmine (Mestinon, Regonol) typifies the reversible cholinesterase inhibitors and will serve as our prototype for the group. Pyridostigmine is the drug of choice for management of MG. It is also approved for reversal of nondepolarizing muscle relaxants.

Pyridostigmine contains a quaternary nitrogen atom and hence always carries a positive charge. Because of this charge, pyridostigmine cannot readily cross membranes, including those of the GI tract, blood–brain barrier, and placenta. Consequently, pyridostigmine is absorbed poorly after oral administration and has minimal effects on the brain and fetus.

Mechanism of action. Pyridostigmine and the other reversible cholinesterase inhibitors act as substrates for cholinesterase. As indicated in Fig. 13.1, the normal function of cholinesterase is to break down acetylcholine into choline and acetic acid. (This process is called a *hydrolysis reaction* because of the water molecule involved.) The overall reaction between acetylcholine and cholinesterase is extremely fast. As a result, one molecule of cholinesterase can break down a huge amount of acetylcholine in a very short time.

The reaction between pyridostigmine and cholinesterase is much like the reaction between acetylcholine and cholinesterase. The only difference is that cholinesterase splits pyridostigmine more slowly than it splits acetylcholine. Hence, after pyridostigmine becomes bound to cholinesterase, the drug remains in place for a relatively long time. Because cholinesterase remains bound until it finally succeeds in degrading pyridostigmine, less cholinesterase is available to catalyze the breakdown of acetylcholine. As a result, more acetylcholine is available to activate cholinergic receptors.

Pharmacologic effects. By decreasing breakdown of acetylcholine, pyridostigmine and the other cholinesterase inhibitors make more acetylcholine available, and this can intensify transmission at virtually all junctions where acetylcholine is the transmitter. In sufficient doses, cholinesterase inhibitors can produce skeletal muscle stimulation, ganglionic stimulation, activation of peripheral muscarinic receptors, and activation of cholinergic receptors in the central nervous system (CNS). However, when used *therapeutically*, cholinesterase inhibitors usually affect only muscarinic receptors on organs and nicotinic receptors of the NMJ. Ganglionic transmission and CNS function are usually unaltered.

Muscarinic responses. Muscarinic effects of the cholinesterase inhibitors are identical to those of the direct-acting muscarinic agonists. By preventing breakdown of acetylcholine, cholinesterase inhibitors can cause bradycardia, bronchial constriction, urinary urgency, increased glandular secretions, increased tone and motility of GI smooth muscle, miosis, and focusing of the lens for near vision.

Neuromuscular effects. The effects of cholinesterase inhibitors on skeletal muscle are dose dependent. At *therapeutic* doses, these drugs *increase* force of contraction. In contrast, *toxic* doses *reduce* force of contraction. Contractile force is reduced because excessive amounts of

---

🔲 PATIENT-CENTERED CARE ACROSS THE LIFE SPAN

Cholinesterase Inhibitors

Life Stage	Considerations or Concerns
Children	Safety has not been established. As with all patients, benefits must be considered relative to risks.
Pregnant Women	When given for myasthenia gravis, cholinesterase inhibitors may be necessary during pregnancy and during labor. Neonatal myasthenia gravis has occurred, but this effect is transient.
Breast-feeding Women	It is unknown whether cholinesterase inhibitors are excreted in sufficient amounts in breast milk to cause harm to nursing infants. Of note, women with myasthenia gravis may have difficulty breast-feeding due to fatigue.
Older Adults	Older adults are the greatest recipients of cholinesterase inhibitors prescribed for dementia associated with Alzheimer Disease. Doses may need lowered if renal function is decreased.

TABLE 13.4 Clinical Applications of Cholinesterase Inhibitors

Generic Name (Trade Name)	Routes	Myasthenia Gravis		Glaucoma	Reversal of Competitive Neuromuscular Blockade	Antidote to Poisoning by Muscarinic Antagonists	Alzheimer Disease
		Diagnosis	Treatment				
Reversible Inhibitors							
Neostigmine (Prostigmin)	PO, IM, IV, subQ		✓		✓		
Pyridostigmine (Mestinon)	PO		✓				
Edrophonium (Enlon)	IM, IV	✓			✓		
Physostigmine (generic)	IM, IV					✓	
Donepezil (Aricept)[a]	PO						✓
Galantamine (Razadyne)	PO						✓
Rivastigmine (Exelon)[a]	PO, Transdermal						✓
Irreversible Inhibitor							
Echothiophate (Phospholine Iodide)	Topical			✓			

[a]Also used for Parkinson disease dementia.
IM, Intramuscular; *IV,* intravenous; *PO,* oral; *subQ,* subcutaneous.

Fig. 13.1 Hydrolysis of Acetylcholine by Cholinesterase.

TABLE 13.5 Pharmacokinetics: Cholinesterase Inhibitors

Drug	Peak	Protein Binding	Metabolism	Half-Life	Elimination
Neostigmine (Prostigmin)	1–2 h	15%–25%	Hepatic	0.5–1.5 h	Urine
Physostigmine	UK	UK	Hydrolysis by cholinesterases	1–2 h	Urine
Pyridostigmine (Mestinon Regonol, Mestinon-SR ♣)	1–2 h	None	Hydrolysis by cholinesterases	1–2 h	Urine

h, Hour(s); *UK*, unknown.

TABLE 13.6 Preparation and Dosage of Cholinesterase Inhibitors

Drug Class or Drug	Preparation	Dosage
Cholinesterase Inhibitors		
Neostigmine (Prostigmin ♣)	Prostigmin ♣: 0.5-mg/mL solution available in 1-mL and 10-mL vials Generic: 0.5 mg/mL and 1 mg/mL, both in 10-mL vials	Reversal of effects of nondepolarizing neuromuscular blocking agents after surgery: 0.03 mg/kg to 0.07 mg/kg over 1 minute. Myasthenia gravis treatment, approved in Canada (highly individualized): 0.5 mg IM or subQ initially with additional dosing based on patient response. Typical dosing is 15–375 mg/day in divided doses.
Physostigmine	1 mg/mL in 2-mL vials	Reversal of anticholinergic toxicity: adults—0.5–2 mg IM or IV Children: 0.02 mg/kg Dose may be repeated every 10–30 min as needed
Pyridostigmine (Mestinon Regonol, Mestinon-SR ♣)	Syrup: 60 mg/5 mL Tablet IR: 60 mg Tablet ER: 180 mg	Myasthenia gravis treatment (highly individualized) IR: 60–1,500 mg/day Typical dosing 600 mg/day divided into 5 doses ER: 180–540 mg once or twice a day (It may be necessary to use both IR and ER dosing to sustain effects)

ER, Extended release; *IM*, intramuscular; *IR*, immediate release; *IV*, intravenous; *subQ*, subcutaneous.

acetylcholine at the NMJ keep the motor end plate in a state of constant depolarization, causing depolarizing neuromuscular blockade.

Central nervous system effects. Effects on the CNS vary with drug concentration. *Therapeutic* levels can produce mild *stimulation*, whereas *toxic* levels *depress* the CNS, including the areas that regulate respiration. However, keep in mind that for CNS effects to occur, the inhibitor must first penetrate the blood–brain barrier, which some cholinesterase inhibitors can do only when present in very high concentrations.

Pharmacokinetics. Pharmacokinetics of pyridostigmine and other cholinesterase inhibitors is provided in Table 13.5.

Preparation and dosage. Preparation and dosage of pyridostigmine and other cholinesterase inhibitors are provided in Table 13.6.

Therapeutic uses. MG is a major indication for pyridostigmine and several other reversible cholinesterase inhibitors. Treatment of MG is discussed separately.

Adverse effects

Excessive muscarinic stimulation. Accumulation of acetylcholine at muscarinic receptors can result in excessive salivation, increased gastric secretions, increased tone and motility of the GI tract, urinary urgency, bradycardia, sweating, miosis, and spasm of accommodation (focusing of the lens for near vision). If necessary, these responses can be suppressed with atropine.

Neuromuscular blockade. If administered in toxic doses, cholinesterase inhibitors can cause accumulation of acetylcholine in amounts sufficient to produce depolarizing neuromuscular blockade. Paralysis of the respiratory muscles can be fatal.

Precautions and contraindications. Most of the precautions and contraindications regarding the cholinesterase inhibitors are the same as those for the direct-acting muscarinic agonists. These include obstruction of the GI tract, obstruction of the urinary tract, peptic ulcer disease, asthma, coronary insufficiency, and hyperthyroidism.

Drug interactions. The effects of cholinesterase inhibitors at muscarinic receptors are opposite to those of atropine (and all other muscarinic antagonists). Consequently, cholinesterase inhibitors can be used to overcome excessive muscarinic blockade caused by atropine. Conversely, atropine can be used to reduce excessive muscarinic stimulation caused by cholinesterase inhibitors.

Other Reversible Cholinesterase Inhibitors

Neostigmine. Neostigmine (Bloxiverz, Prostigmin ♣) has pharmacologic effects much like those of other cholinesterase inhibitors. Because neostigmine carries a positive charge, the drug is poorly absorbed after oral administration; hence oral formulations have been discontinued in the United States, although they remain available in some other countries. After it is absorbed, neostigmine can reach sites of action at the NMJ and peripheral muscarinic receptors but it cannot cross the blood-brain barrier to affect the CNS.

Neostigmine is widely available as a generic drug. Formulations marketed as branded drugs are not used interchangably. Prostigmin is approved in Canada for management of MG. Bloxiverz is used to reverse the actions of nondepolarizing neuromuscular blockade after surgery; however, this use is beyond the scope of this book.

Physostigmine. The basic pharmacology of physostigmine is essentially the same as that of neostigmine. In contrast to neostigmine, physostigmine is *not* a quaternary ammonium compound and hence does *not* carry a charge. Because physostigmine is uncharged, physostigmine readily crosses membranes, whereas neostigmine does not. As a result of this important difference, although their pharmacology is the same, their uses are very different.

Because physostigmine can cross the blood–brain barrier, it is the drug of choice for treating *poisoning by atropine and other drugs that cause muscarinic blockade*, including antihistamines and phenothiazine antipsychotics—but *not* tricyclic antidepressants, owing to a risk for causing seizures and cardiotoxicity. Physostigmine counteracts

SUMMARY OF KEY PRESCRIBING CONSIDERATIONS

Pyridostigmine

Therapeutic Goal: Treatment of myasthenia gravis

Baseline Data: Heart rate, blood pressure, ECG. Determine the extent of neuromuscular dysfunction by assessing muscle strength, fatigue, ptosis, and ability to swallow.

Monitoring: Heart rate, blood pressure. Recheck ECG if bradycardic or for patient reports of palpitations, chest pain, shortness of breath. Additionally, monitor and record (1) times of drug administration; (2) times at which fatigue occurs; (3) state of muscle strength, ptosis, and ability to swallow; and (4) signs of excessive muscarinic stimulation. Titrate dose based on these observations.

Monitor for *myasthenic crisis* (extreme muscle weakness, paralysis of respiratory muscles), which can occur when cholinesterase inhibitor dosing is insufficient. Manage with respiratory support and increased dosage. (Be certain to distinguish myasthenic crisis from cholinergic crisis. This is done by observing for signs of excessive muscarinic stimulation, which will accompany cholinergic crisis but not myasthenic crisis.)

Identifying High-Risk Patients: Cholinesterase inhibitors are *contraindicated* for patients with mechanical obstruction of the intestine or urinary tract. Exercise *caution* in patients with peptic ulcer disease, bradycardia, asthma, or hyperthyroidism. For patients with decreased renal function, start with low-dose therapy.

Evaluating Therapeutic Effects: Assess for increased strength and muscle control.

Minimizing Adverse Effects: For minor effects, common nursing measures (e.g., adequate lighting to address decreased night vision due to miosis and more frequent linen changes to address discomfort due to sweating) are adequate. Cholinergic crisis can result from cholinesterase inhibitor overdose. Manifestations are skeletal muscle paralysis (from depolarizing neuromuscular blockade) and signs of excessive muscarinic stimulation (e.g., excessive salivation, sweating, bradycardia, urinary incontinence). Manage with mechanical ventilation and atropine.

antimuscarinic poisoning by causing acetylcholine to build up at muscarinic junctions. The accumulated acetylcholine competes with the muscarinic blocker for receptor binding and thereby reverses receptor blockade.

Edrophonium. Edrophonium (Enlon, Tensilon ♣) has pharmacologic effects much like those of pyridostigmine. It is noteworthy for its very brief duration of action. Edrophonium is also unique in that it is indicated for diagnosis, but not treatment, of MG. In current practice, though, edrophonium is not commonly used for this purpose because better and more accurate testing is now available.

Drugs for Alzheimer disease. Three cholinesterase inhibitors—donepezil (Aricept), galantamine (Razadyne), and rivastigmine (Exelon)—are approved for management of Alzheimer disease, and one of them—rivastigmine—is also approved for dementia of Parkinson disease. With all three, benefits derive from inhibiting cholinesterase in the CNS. The pharmacology of these drugs is discussed in Chapter 20.

Irreversible Cholinesterase Inhibitors

The irreversible cholinesterase inhibitors have only one indication: treatment of *glaucoma*. For that indication, only one drug—echothiophate (Phospholine Iodide)—is available. The use of echothiophate for glaucoma is discussed in Chapter 87.

The limited indications for irreversible cholinesterase inhibitors is in large part because these agents are highly toxic. During World War II, huge quantities of irreversible cholinesterase inhibitors were produced for possible use as *nerve agents* but were never deployed. Today, there is concern that these agents might be employed as weapons of terrorism.

Basic Pharmacology

All irreversible cholinesterase inhibitors contain an atom of *phosphorus*. Because of this phosphorus atom, the irreversible inhibitors are known as *organophosphate* cholinesterase inhibitors.

Almost all irreversible cholinesterase inhibitors are *highly lipid soluble*. As a result, these drugs are readily absorbed from all routes of administration. They can even be absorbed directly through the skin. Easy absorption, coupled with high toxicity, is what makes these drugs good insecticides—and gives them potential as agents of chemical warfare. After they are absorbed, the organophosphate inhibitors have ready access to all tissues and organs, including the CNS.

Mechanism of action. The irreversible cholinesterase inhibitors bind to the active center of cholinesterase, preventing the enzyme from hydrolyzing acetylcholine. Although these drugs can be split from cholinesterase, the splitting reaction is *extremely* slow. Hence, under normal conditions, their binding to cholinesterase can be considered irreversible. Because binding is irreversible, effects persist until new molecules of cholinesterase can be synthesized.

Although we normally consider the bond between irreversible inhibitors and cholinesterase permanent, this bond can, in fact, be broken. To break the bond and reverse the inhibition of cholinesterase, we must administer *pralidoxime*, a cholinesterase reactivator.

Pharmacologic effects. The irreversible cholinesterase inhibitors produce essentially the same spectrum of effects as the reversible inhibitors. The principal difference is that responses to irreversible inhibitors last a long time, whereas responses to reversible inhibitors are brief.

Toxicology of Cholinesterase Inhibitors
Sources of Poisoning

Poisoning by organophosphate cholinesterase inhibitors is a common occurrence. Cholinesterase inhibitors are employed primarily as *insecticides*. Agricultural workers have been poisoned by accidental ingestion of organophosphate insecticides and by absorption of these lipid-soluble compounds through the skin. In addition, because organophosphate insecticides are readily available to the public, poisoning may occur accidentally or from attempted homicide or suicide. As mentioned previously, exposure could also occur if these drugs were used as instruments of warfare or terrorism.

Symptoms

Toxic doses of irreversible cholinesterase inhibitors produce excessive muscarinic, nicotinic, and CNS effects. This condition, known as a *cholinergic crisis*, is characterized by *excessive muscarinic stimulation* and *depolarizing neuromuscular blockade*. Overstimulation of muscarinic receptors results in profuse secretions from salivary and bronchial glands, involuntary urination and defecation, laryngospasm, and bronchoconstriction. Prominent nicotinic effects reflect nicotinic activity at NMJs, resulting in muscle weakness, fasciculations, cramps, and twitching. Neuromuscular blockade can result in paralysis, followed by death from apnea. CNS effects may range from anxiety and confusion to delirium. Convulsions of CNS origin precede paralysis and apnea.

Treatment

Pharmacologic treatment involves giving *atropine* to reduce muscarinic stimulation, giving *pralidoxime* to reverse inhibition of cholinesterase (primarily at the NMJ), and giving a benzodiazepine such as *diazepam* to suppress convulsions. Respiratory depression from cholinesterase inhibitors cannot be managed with drugs. Rather, treatment consists of mechanical ventilation with oxygen.

Pralidoxime. Pralidoxime is a specific antidote to poisoning by the irreversible (organophosphate) cholinesterase inhibitors; the drug is *not* effective against poisoning by reversible cholinesterase inhibitors. In poisoning by irreversible inhibitors, benefits derive from causing the inhibitor to dissociate from the active center of cholinesterase. Reversal is most effective at the NMJ. Pralidoxime is much less effective at reversing cholinesterase inhibition at muscarinic and ganglionic sites. Furthermore, because pralidoxime is a quaternary ammonium compound, it cannot cross the blood–brain barrier and therefore cannot reverse cholinesterase inhibition in the CNS. To be effective, pralidoxime must be administered soon after organophosphate poisoning has occurred.

Use of Cholinesterase Inhibitors in Practice: Myasthenia Gravis
Pathophysiology

MG is a neuromuscular disorder characterized by fluctuating muscle weakness and a predisposition to rapid fatigue. Common symptoms include ptosis (drooping eyelids), difficulty swallowing, and weakness of skeletal muscles. Patients with severe MG may have difficulty breathing owing to weakness of the muscles of respiration.

Symptoms of MG result from an autoimmune process in which the patient's immune system produces antibodies that attack nicotinic$_M$ receptors on skeletal muscle. As a result, the number of functional receptors at the NMJ is reduced by 70% to 90%, causing muscle weakness.

Treatment with Cholinesterase Inhibitors

Beneficial effects. Reversible cholinesterase inhibitors (e.g., pyridostigmine) are the mainstay of therapy. By preventing acetylcholine inactivation, anticholinesterase agents can intensify the effects of acetylcholine released from motor neurons, increasing muscle strength. Cholinesterase inhibitors do not cure MG. Rather, they only produce symptomatic relief, so patients usually need therapy lifelong.

When working with patients with MG, keep in mind that muscle strength may be insufficient to permit swallowing. Accordingly, you should assess the ability to swallow before prescribing oral medications. If the patient is unable to swallow water, parenteral medication must be substituted for oral medication.

Side effects. Because cholinesterase inhibitors can inhibit acetylcholinesterase at any location, these drugs will cause acetylcholine to accumulate at muscarinic junctions as well as at NMJs. If muscarinic responses are excessive, atropine may be given to suppress them. However, atropine should not be employed *routinely* because the drug can mask the early signs (e.g., excessive salivation) of overdose with anticholinesterase agents.

Dosage adjustment. In the treatment of MG, establishing an optimal dosage for cholinesterase inhibitors can be a challenge. Dose determination is accomplished by administering a small initial dose followed by additional small doses until an optimal level of muscle function has been achieved. Important signs of improvement include increased ease of swallowing and increased ability to raise the eyelids. You can help establish a correct dosage by having the patient or family keep records of (1) times of drug administration, (2) times at which fatigue occurs, (3) the state of muscle strength before and after drug administration, and (4) signs of excessive muscarinic stimulation.

To maintain optimal responses, patients must occasionally modify the dose themselves. To do this, they must be taught to recognize signs of undermedication (ptosis, difficulty in swallowing) and signs of overmedication (excessive salivation and other muscarinic responses). Patients may also need to modify a dose in anticipation of exertion. For example, they may find it necessary to take supplementary medication 30 to 60 minutes before activities such as eating or shopping.

It is important to recognize that lack of clinical improvement with pyridostigmine may indicate either an underdose or overdose. It is important to monitor for signs of toxicity before increasing the dose.

Myasthenic Crisis and Cholinergic Crisis

Myasthenic crisis. Patients who are inadequately medicated may experience myasthenic crisis, a state characterized by extreme muscle weakness caused by insufficient acetylcholine at the NMJ. Left untreated, myasthenic crisis can result in death from paralysis of the muscles of respiration. A cholinesterase inhibitor (e.g., neostigmine) is used to relieve the crisis.

Cholinergic crisis. As noted previously, overdose with a cholinesterase inhibitor can produce cholinergic crisis. Like myasthenic crisis, cholinergic crisis is characterized by extreme muscle weakness or frank paralysis. In addition, cholinergic crisis is accompanied by signs of excessive muscarinic stimulation. Treatment consists of respiratory support plus atropine. The offending cholinesterase inhibitor should be withheld until muscle strength has returned.

Distinguishing myasthenic crisis from cholinergic crisis. Because myasthenic crisis and cholinergic crisis share similar symptoms (muscle weakness or paralysis) but are treated very differently, it is essential to distinguish between them. A history of medication use or signs of excessive muscarinic stimulation are usually sufficient to permit a differential diagnosis. If these clues are inadequate, the provider may elect to administer a challenging dose of *edrophonium,* an ultrashort-acting cholinesterase inhibitor. If edrophonium-induced elevation of acetylcholine levels alleviates symptoms, the crisis is myasthenic. Conversely, if edrophonium intensifies symptoms, the crisis is cholinergic. Because the symptoms of cholinergic crisis will be made even worse by edrophonium and could be life-threatening, atropine and oxygen should be immediately available whenever edrophonium is used for this test. For this reason, and because cholinergic crisis is relatively rare for patients with MG, the use of edrophonium for this purpose is controversial.

PATIENT EDUCATION
Cholinesterase Inhibitors for Myasthenia Gravis

- It may be helpful to take this drug before engaging in activities that create difficulty. Depending on the patient's condition, this challenging activities may range from eating to carrying out activities of daily living to more strenuous tasks.
- If a dose is missed, patients should, not take an extra dose the next time it is scheduled. Stress the importance of not taking more drug more than prescribed because high doses can cause serious complications.
- Have the patient report difficulty breathing, drooling, vomiting, diarrhea, excessive sweating, or the new onset of other problems.
- Because of the possibility of experiencing either myasthenic crisis or cholinergic crisis, patients with MG should keep a list of medications and dosages with them at all times. They should also be encouraged to wear a Medic Alert bracelet or some other form of identification to inform emergency medical personnel of their condition in the event that they become unable to communicate.

14

Muscarinic Antagonists

INTRODUCTION TO ANTICHOLINERGIC DRUGS

Anticholinergic drugs are agents that block the activity of cholinergic receptors. These drugs act directly at cholinergic receptors, where they block the actions of acetylcholine.

There are three categories of anticholinergic drugs. These categories are muscarinic antagonists, ganglionic blocking agents, and neuromuscular blocking agents. Of the three, muscarinic antagonists are the most commonly used. Although muscarinic antagonist is the more specific term, these are more often called simply anticholinergic drugs.

The *muscarinic antagonists*, represented by atropine, selectively block the effects of acetylcholine (and other muscarinic agonists) at muscarinic receptors. *Ganglionic blocking agents* selectively block ganglionic nicotinic$_N$ receptors. *Neuromuscular blocking agents* selectively block the effects of acetylcholine at nicotinic$_M$ (muscle) receptors at the neuromuscular junction (NMJ). Ganglionic and neuromuscular blocking agents are used in specialty settings and are beyond the scope of this text.

We recommend the same approach to learning muscarinic antagonists as we advised for the muscarinic agonists (Chapter 13). Table 14.1 is your key to understanding the anticholinergic drugs. It lists the three major subtypes of cholinergic receptors (muscarinic, nicotinic$_N$, and nicotinic$_M$) and indicates for each receptor type the (1) location, (2) responses to activation, (3) drugs that prevent activation (antagonists). This information, along with the detailed information on cholinergic receptor function summarized in Table 12.2 in Chapter 12, provides the information you need to predict the actions of anticholinergic drugs.

MUSCARINIC ANTAGONISTS (ANTICHOLINERGIC DRUGS)

Muscarinic antagonists competitively block the actions of acetylcholine at muscarinic receptors. Because most muscarinic receptors are located on structures innervated by parasympathetic nerves, the muscarinic antagonists are also known as *parasympatholytic drugs*. Additional names for these agents are *antimuscarinic drugs, muscarinic blockers,* and *anticholinergic drugs.*

The term *anticholinergic* can be a source of confusion and requires comment. This term is unfortunate in that it implies blockade at *all* cholinergic receptors. However, as normally used, the term *anticholinergic* only denotes blockade of *muscarinic* receptors. Therefore, when a drug is characterized as being anticholinergic, you can take this to mean that it produces selective *muscarinic* blockade—and not blockade of all cholinergic receptors. In this chapter, the terms *muscarinic antagonist* and *anticholinergic agent* are used interchangeably.

PATIENT-CENTERED CARE ACROSS THE LIFE SPAN

Anticholinergic Drugs

Life Stage	Patient Care Concerns
Children	Anticholinergics have a prominent role in the management of respiratory conditions in childhood. Administration by inhalation decreases systemic effects. There is no contraindication to systemic use due to age, but due to numerous adverse effects, benefits should be weighed against risk.
Pregnant women	Oxybutynin is relatively safe when taken during pregnancy; however, due to a lack of sufficient animal studies and clinical trials, the full risk of most of these drugs is unknown. Caution is recommended with a strong consideration of whether benefits derived are worth potential risks.
Breastfeeding women	Anticholinergics may inhibit lactation in some women, resulting in decreased production of breast milk. Due to a lack of studies, full risks of breastfeeding are unknown. If decisions to breastfeed are made, monitor the infant to identify possible anticholinergic effects.
Older adults	Anticholinergic drugs have been designated as potentially inappropriate for use in geriatric patients. They can cause confusion, blurred vision, tachycardia, urinary retention, and constipation. Many of these complicate preexisting conditions (e.g., urinary retention secondary to benign prostatic hyperplasia) and increase the risk for other conditions (e.g., narrow-angle glaucoma risk secondary to pupil dilation and heat-related illness secondary to hyperthermia and impaired sweating mechanisms).

PROTOTYPE DRUGS

Anticholinergic Agents

Muscarinic Antagonist
Atropine (AtroPen, others)

TABLE 14.1 Anticholinergic Drugs and Their Receptors

	RECEPTOR SUBTYPE		
	Muscarinic	**Nicotinic$_N$**	**Nicotinic$_M$**
Receptor Location	Sweat glands Blood vessels All organs regulated by the parasympathetic nervous system	All ganglia of the autonomic nervous system	Neuromuscular junctions
Effects of Receptor Activation	Many, including: ↓ Heart rate ↑ Gland secretion Smooth muscle contraction	Promotes ganglionic transmission	Skeletal muscle contraction
Receptor Antagonists	Atropine	Mecamylamine	d-Tubocurarine, succinylcholine

TABLE 14.2 Relationship Between Dose and Responses to Atropine

Dose of Atropine	Response Produced
Low dose ↓ High dose	Salivary glands—decreased secretion Sweat glands—decreased secretion Bronchial glands—decreased secretion Heart—increased rate Eyes—mydriasis, blurred vision Urinary tract—interference with voiding Intestines—decreased tone and motility Lungs—dilation of bronchi[a] Stomach—decreased acid secretion[a]

[a]Doses of atropine that are high enough to dilate the bronchi or decrease gastric acid secretion will also affect all other structures under muscarinic control. As a result, atropine and most other muscarinic antagonists are not very desirable for treating peptic ulcer disease or asthma.

Atropine

Atropine (AtroPen, others) is the best-known muscarinic antagonist and will serve as our prototype for the group. The actions of all other muscarinic blockers are much like those of this drug.

Atropine is found naturally in a variety of plants, including *Atropa belladonna* (deadly nightshade) and *Datura stramonium* (also known as Jimson weed, stinkweed, and devil's apple). Because of its presence in *A. belladonna*, atropine is referred to as a *belladonna alkaloid*.

Mechanism of Action

Atropine produces its effects through competitive blockade at muscarinic receptors. Like all other receptor antagonists, atropine has no direct effects of its own. Rather, all responses to atropine result from *preventing receptor activation* by endogenous acetylcholine (or by drugs that act as muscarinic agonists).

At therapeutic doses, atropine produces selective blockade of muscarinic cholinergic receptors. However, if the dose is sufficiently high, the drug will produce some blockade of nicotinic receptors, too.

It is important to note that not all muscarinic receptors are equally sensitive to blockade by atropine and most other anticholinergic drugs: at some sites, muscarinic receptors can be blocked with relatively low doses; whereas at other sites, much higher doses are needed. Table 14.2 indicates the sequence in which specific muscarinic receptors are blocked as the dose of atropine is increased.

Pharmacologic Effects

Because atropine acts by causing muscarinic receptor blockade, its effects are opposite to those caused by muscarinic activation. Accordingly, we can readily predict the effects of atropine by knowing the normal responses to muscarinic receptor activation (see Table 12.2) and by knowing that atropine will reverse those responses. Like the muscarinic agonists, the muscarinic antagonists exert their influence primarily on the *heart*, *exocrine glands*, *smooth muscles*, and *eyes*.

Heart. Atropine *increases heart rate*. Because activation of cardiac muscarinic receptors decreases heart rate, blockade of these receptors will cause heart rate to increase.

Exocrine glands. Atropine *decreases secretion* from salivary glands, bronchial glands, sweat glands, and the acid-secreting cells of the stomach. Note that these effects are opposite to those of muscarinic agonists, which increase secretion from exocrine glands.

Smooth muscle. By preventing activation of muscarinic receptors on smooth muscle, atropine causes *relaxation of the bronchi*, *decreased tone of the urinary bladder detrusor*, and *decreased tone and motility of the GI tract*. In the absence of an exogenous muscarinic agonist (e.g., bethanechol), muscarinic blockade has no effect on vascular smooth muscle tone because there is no parasympathetic innervation to muscarinic receptors in blood vessels.

Eyes. Blockade of muscarinic receptors on the iris sphincter causes *mydriasis* (dilation of the pupil). Blockade of muscarinic receptors on the ciliary muscle produces *cycloplegia* (relaxation of the ciliary muscle), thereby focusing the lens for far vision.

Central nervous system. At therapeutic doses, atropine can cause mild *CNS excitation*. Toxic doses can cause *hallucinations* and *delirium*, which can resemble psychosis. Extremely high doses can result in coma, respiratory arrest, and death.

Pharmacokinetics

Atropine may be administered topically (to the eye), and parenterally (IM, IV, and subQ routes). The drug is rapidly absorbed after administration and distributes to all tissues, including the CNS. Peak effect occurs in 30 minutes to an hour. Atropine has a half-life of approximately 3 hours but may be as long as 10 to 17 hours in older patients. Elimination is by a combination of hepatic metabolism and urinary excretion.

Therapeutic Uses

Except for ophthalmic formulations, atropine is used short term (typically one dose or repeated dosing within a short period of time). It is approved for use prior to surgery, as an antidote to anticholinesterase poisoning, and for treatment of sinus bradycardia and atrioventricular (AV) block. It may be used off-label to treat other conditions; these are discussed next.

Preanesthetic medication. The cardiac effects of atropine can help during surgery. Procedures that stimulate baroreceptors of the carotid body can initiate reflex slowing of the heart, resulting in profound bradycardia. Because this reflex is mediated by muscarinic receptors on the heart, pretreatment with atropine can prevent a dangerous reduction in heart rate.

Certain anesthetics irritate the respiratory tract and thereby stimulate secretion from salivary, nasal, pharyngeal, and bronchial glands. If these secretions are sufficiently profuse, they can interfere with respiration. By blocking muscarinic receptors on secretory glands, atropine can help prevent excessive secretions. Fortunately, modern anesthetics are much less irritating. The availability of these new anesthetics has greatly reduced the use of atropine for this purpose during anesthesia.

Disorders of the eyes. By blocking muscarinic receptors in the eyes, atropine can cause mydriasis and paralysis of the ciliary muscle. Both actions can be of help during eye examinations and ocular surgery. The ophthalmic uses of atropine and other muscarinic antagonists are discussed in Chapter 87.

Bradycardia. Atropine can accelerate heart rate in certain patients with bradycardia. Heart rate is increased because blockade of cardiac muscarinic receptors reverses parasympathetic slowing of the heart.

Intestinal hypertonicity and hypermotility. By blocking muscarinic receptors in the intestine, atropine can decrease both the tone and motility of intestinal smooth muscle. This can be beneficial in conditions characterized by excessive intestinal motility, such as mild dysentery and diverticulitis. When taken for these disorders, atropine can reduce both the frequency of bowel movements and associated abdominal cramps.

Peptic ulcer disease. Because it can suppress secretion of gastric acid, atropine has been used to treat peptic ulcer disease. Unfortunately, when administered in doses that are strong enough to block the muscarinic receptors that regulate secretion of gastric acid, atropine also blocks most other muscarinic receptors (see Table 14.2). Therefore, the use of atropine in treatment of ulcers is associated with a broad range of antimuscarinic side effects (dry mouth, blurred vision, urinary retention, constipation, and so on). Because of these side effects, atropine is reserved for rare cases in which symptoms cannot be relieved with preferred medications (e.g., antibiotics, histamine-2 receptor antagonists, proton pump inhibitors).

Asthma. By blocking bronchial muscarinic receptors, atropine can promote bronchial dilation, thereby improving respiration in patients with asthma. Unfortunately, in addition to dilating the bronchi, atropine also causes drying and thickening of bronchial secretions—effects that can be harmful to patients with asthma. Furthermore, when given in the doses needed to dilate the bronchi, atropine causes a variety of antimuscarinic side effects (see Table 14.2). Because of the potential for harm, and because superior medicines are available, atropine is rarely used for asthma.

Biliary colic. Biliary colic is characterized by intense abdominal pain brought on by passage of a gallstone through the bile duct. In some cases, atropine may be combined with analgesics such as morphine to relax biliary tract smooth muscle, thereby helping alleviate discomfort.

Muscarinic agonist poisoning. As mentioned in Chapter 13, atropine is a specific antidote to poisoning by agents that activate muscarinic receptors. By blocking muscarinic receptors, atropine can reverse all signs of muscarinic poisoning. An atropine autoinjector (Atropen) is approved for use in people exposed to the irreversible cholinesterase inhibitor nerve agents or insecticides discussed previously (Box 14.1).

Adverse Effects

Most adverse effects of atropine and other anticholinergic drugs are the direct result of muscarinic receptor blockade. Accordingly, these effects can be predicted from your knowledge of muscarinic receptor function.

Xerostomia. Blockade of muscarinic receptors on salivary glands can inhibit salivation, thereby causing dry mouth. Not only is this uncomfortable; it also can impede swallowing and can promote tooth decay, gum problems, and oral infections. Patients should be informed that dryness can be alleviated by sipping fluids, chewing sugar-free gum, and using salivary stimulants (citrus-flavored or tart sugarless candies, maltose lozenges). If these do not provide adequate relief, oral moisturizers (saliva substitutes) such as Biotene dry mouth spray and

---

BOX 14.1 AtroPen for Cholinesterase Inhibitor Poisoning

The AtroPen is a prefilled autoinjector indicated for intramuscular treatment of poisoning with an organophosphate cholinesterase inhibitor (nerve agent or insecticide). Four strengths are available: 0.25 and 0.5 mg (for children weighing <40 pounds), 1 mg (for children 40–90 pounds), and 2 mg (for adults and children >90 pounds). The AtroPen should be used immediately on exposure or if exposure is strongly suspected. Injections are administered into the lateral thigh, directly through clothing, if necessary.

Dosing is determined by symptom severity and weight. Dose by weight is as follows:

- <6.8 kg (<15 lb): administer 0.25 mg/dose
- 6.8–18 kg (15–40 lb): administer 0.5 mg/dose
- 18–41 kg (40–90 lb): administer 1 mg/dose
- >41 kg (>90 lb): administer 2 mg/dose

Multiple doses are often required. If symptoms are severe, three weight-based doses should be administered rapidly. If symptoms are mild, one dose should be given; if severe symptoms develop afterward, additional doses can be given up to a maximum of three doses.

XyliMelts are available over-the-counter. Owing to increased risk for tooth decay, patients should avoid sugary gum and hard candy.

Blurred vision and photophobia. The blockade of muscarinic receptors on the ciliary muscle and the sphincter of the iris can paralyze these muscles. Paralysis of the ciliary muscle focuses the eye for far vision, causing nearby objects to appear blurred. Patients should be forewarned about this effect and advised to avoid hazardous activities if vision is impaired.

In addition, paralysis of the iris sphincter prevents constriction of the pupil, thereby rendering the eye unable to adapt to bright light. Patients should be advised to wear dark glasses if photophobia is a problem. Room lighting for hospitalized patients should be kept low.

Elevation of intraocular pressure. Paralysis of the iris sphincter can raise IOP by a mechanism discussed in Chapter 87. Because they can increase IOP, anticholinergic drugs are contraindicated for patients with glaucoma, a disease characterized by abnormally high IOP. In addition, these drugs should be used with caution in patients who may not have glaucoma per se but for whom a predisposition to glaucoma may be present.

Urinary retention. Blockade of muscarinic receptors in the urinary tract reduces pressure within the bladder and increases the tone of the urinary sphincter and trigone. These effects can produce urinary hesitancy or urinary retention. In the event of severe urinary retention, catheterization or treatment with a muscarinic agonist (e.g., bethanechol) may be required. Patients should be advised that urinary retention can be minimized by voiding just before taking their medication.

Constipation. Muscarinic blockade decreases the tone and motility of intestinal smooth muscle. The resultant delay in transit through the intestine can produce constipation. Patients should be informed that constipation can be minimized by increasing dietary fiber, fluids, and physical activity. A laxative may be needed if constipation is severe. Because of their ability to decrease smooth muscle tone, muscarinic antagonists are contraindicated for patients with intestinal atony, a condition in which intestinal tone is already low.

Anhidrosis. Blockade of muscarinic receptors on sweat glands can produce anhidrosis (a deficiency or absence of sweat). Because sweating is necessary for cooling, people who cannot sweat are at risk for hyperthermia. Patients should be warned of this possibility and advised to avoid activities that might lead to overheating (e.g., exercising on a hot day).

Tachycardia. Blockade of cardiac muscarinic receptors eliminates parasympathetic influence on the heart. By removing the "braking" influence of parasympathetic nerves, anticholinergic agents can cause tachycardia. Exercise caution in patients with preexisting tachycardia.

Asthma. In patients with asthma, antimuscarinic drugs can cause thickening and drying of bronchial secretions and can thereby cause bronchial plugging. Consequently, although muscarinic antagonists can be used to treat asthma, they can also do harm.

Drug Interactions

Several drugs that are not classified as muscarinic antagonists can nonetheless produce significant muscarinic blockade. Among these are antihistamines, phenothiazine antipsychotics, and tricyclic antidepressants. Because of their prominent anticholinergic actions, these drugs can greatly enhance the antimuscarinic effects of atropine and related agents. Accordingly, it is wise to avoid combined use of atropine with other drugs that can cause muscarinic blockade.

 ## SUMMARY OF KEY PRESCRIBING CONSIDERATIONS

Atropine

Therapeutic Goal: Treatment of bradycardia or atrioventricular block, antidote to anticholinesterase poisoning, or as a preanesthetic medication.
Baseline Data: Heart rate, blood pressure, ECG.
Monitoring: Heart rate, blood pressure. Recheck ECG for patient reports of palpitations or chest pain.
Identifying High-Risk Patients: Exercise caution with patients with non-bradycardic dysrhythmias, especially tachydysrhythmias, and in patients with myocardial ischemia. May precipitate acute glaucoma. May precipitate a myasthenic crisis in patients with MG. Can cause urinary retention, especially in patients with benign prostatic hyperplasia.
Evaluating Therapeutic Effects: Depending on purpose of administration, restoration of normal sinus rhythm, prevention of anesthetic or surgical associated complications, reversal of anticholinesterase poisoning.
Minimizing Adverse Effects: Treat dry mouth with fluids, saliva stimulants (sour or tart candies, sugar-free chewing gum), and oral moisturizers. Manage photophobia with reduced lighting or sunglasses. Void prior to taking medication to decrease incidence of urinary retention. Be prepared for catheter insertion, if necessary.

Other Muscarinic Antagonists
Scopolamine

Scopolamine is an anticholinergic drug with actions much like those of atropine, but with two exceptions. First, whereas therapeutic doses of atropine produce mild CNS excitation, therapeutic doses of scopolamine produce sedation. And second, scopolamine suppresses emesis and motion sickness, whereas atropine does not. Principal uses for scopolamine are motion sickness (see Chapter 66), production of cycloplegia and mydriasis for ophthalmic procedures (see Chapter 87), and production of preanesthetic sedation and obstetric amnesia.

Ipratropium Bromide

Ipratropium (Atrovent) is an anticholinergic drug used to treat asthma, COPD, and rhinitis caused by allergies or the common cold. The drug is administered by inhalation for asthma and COPD and by nasal spray for rhinitis. Systemic absorption is minimal for both formulations. As a result, therapy is not associated with typical antimuscarinic side effects (dry mouth, blurred vision, urinary hesitancy, constipation, and so forth). Ipratropium is discussed fully in Chapter 62.

Dicyclomine

Dicyclomine (Bentyl, Bentylol) is indicated for irritable bowel syndrome (spastic colon, mucous colitis). It is also used for functional bowel disorders such as diarrhea and hypermotility.

Antisecretory Anticholinergics

Muscarinic blockers can be used to suppress gastric acid secretion in patients with peptic ulcer disease. However, because superior antiulcer drugs are available, and because anticholinergic agents produce significant side effects, most of these drugs have been withdrawn. Today, only four agents—glycopyrrolate (Robinul, Cuvposa), mepenzolate (Cantil), methscopolamine (Pamine), and propantheline (generic)—remain on the market. Glycopyrrolate oral solution (Cuvposa) is also approved for reducing severe drooling in children with chronic severe neurologic disorders. The drug is also approved for reducing salivation caused by anesthesia. Although it was originally approved as an adjunct in treatment of peptic ulcer disease, it is no longer indicated for this purpose.

Mydriatic Cycloplegics

Five muscarinic antagonists—atropine, homatropine, scopolamine, cyclopentolate, and tropicamide—are employed to produce mydriasis and cycloplegia in ophthalmic procedures. These applications are discussed in Chapter 87.

Centrally Acting Anticholinergics

Several anticholinergic drugs, including benztropine (Cogentin) and trihexyphenidyl, are used to treat Parkinson disease and drug-induced parkinsonism. Benefits derive from blockade of muscarinic receptors in the CNS. The centrally acting anticholinergics and their use in Parkinson disease are discussed in Chapter 19.

Use of Muscarinic Antagonists in Practice: Overactive Bladder
Pathophysiology

Overactive bladder (OAB)—also known as *urgency incontinence*—is a disorder with four major symptoms: urinary urgency (a sudden, compelling desire to urinate), urinary frequency (voiding 8 or more times in 24 hours), nocturia (waking 2 or more times to void), and urge incontinence (involuntary urine leakage associated with a strong urge to void). In most cases, urge incontinence results from *involuntary contractions of the bladder detrusor* (the smooth muscle component of the bladder wall). These contractions are often referred to as detrusor instability or detrusor overactivity. Urge incontinence should not be confused with *stress incontinence,* defined as involuntary urine leakage caused by activities (e.g., exertion, sneezing, coughing, laughter) that increase pressure within the abdominal cavity, or *overflow incontinence,* which is the involuntary leakage of urine from an overly distended bladder.

OAB is a common disorder, affecting up to one-third of Americans. The condition can develop at any age but is most prevalent in older populations. Among people ages 40 to 44 years, symptoms are reported by 3% of men and 9% of women. In comparison, among those 75 years and older, symptoms are reported by 42% of men and 31% of women. Because urine leakage, the most disturbing symptom, is both unpredictable and potentially embarrassing, many people with OAB curtail travel, social activities, and even work.

Treatment

OAB has two primary modes of treatment: *behavioral therapy* and *drug therapy* (Fig. 14.1). Behavioral therapy, which is at least as effective as drug therapy and lacks side effects, should be tried first. Behavioral interventions include scheduled voiding, timing fluid intake, doing Kegel

Diagnosis & Treatment Algorithm: American Urological Association (AUA)/Society of Urodynamics, Female Pelvic Medicine & Urogenital Reconstruction (SUFU) Guideline on Non-Neurogenic Overactive Bladder in Adults

Fig. 14.1 Algorithm for Management of Overactive Bladder. *OAB,* Overactive bladder. (From the American Urologic Association. Available at: https://www.auanet.org/Documents/education/clinical-guidance/OAB-Algorithm.pdf.)

exercises (to strengthen pelvic floor muscles), and avoiding caffeine, a diuretic that may also increase detrusor activity. As a rule, drugs should be reserved for patients who don't respond adequately to behavioral measures. If behavioral therapy and drugs are inadequate, a provider may offer specialized treatments (e.g., sacral neuromodulation, peripheral tibial nerve stimulation).

When drug therapy *is* indicated, *anticholinergic agents* (e.g., oxybutynin, tolterodine) are indicated. These drugs block muscarinic receptors on the bladder detrusor and thereby inhibit bladder contractions and the urge to void.

Unfortunately, drugs that block muscarinic receptors in the bladder can also block muscarinic receptors elsewhere and cause the typical anticholinergic side effects previously described. Anticholinergic side effects can be reduced in at least three ways: (1) using long-acting formulations, (2) using drugs that don't cross the blood–brain barrier, and (3) using drugs that are selective for muscarinic receptors in the bladder. Long-acting formulations (e.g., extended-release [ER] capsules,

transdermal patches) reduce side effects by providing a steady but relatively low level of drug, thereby avoiding the high peak levels that can cause intense side effects. Drugs that can't cross the blood–brain barrier are unable to cause CNS effects.

What about drugs that are selective for muscarinic receptors in the bladder? To answer this question, we must first discuss muscarinic receptor subtypes. As noted in Chapter 12, there are five known muscarinic receptor subtypes. However, only three—designated M_1, M_2, and M_3—have clearly identified functions. Locations of these receptor subtypes, and responses to their activation and blockade, are shown in Table 14.3. As indicated, M_3 receptors are the most widely distributed, being found in salivary glands, the bladder detrusor, GI smooth muscle, and the eyes. M_2 receptors are found only in the heart and M_1 receptors are found in salivary glands and the CNS. At each location, responses to receptor activation are the same as we discussed in Chapter 12— although, in that chapter, we didn't identify the receptors by subtype; rather, we called all of them *muscarinic*.

TABLE 14.3 Muscarinic Receptor Subtypes

Muscarinic Subtype	Location	Response to Activation	Impact of Blockade
M$_1$	Salivary glands	Salivation	Dry mouth
	CNS	Enhanced cognition	Confusion, hallucinations
M$_2$	Heart	Bradycardia	Tachycardia
M$_3$	Salivary glands	Salivation	Dry mouth
	Bladder: detrusor	Contraction (increased pressure)	Relaxation (decreased pressure)
	GI smooth muscle	Increased tone and motility	Decreased tone and motility (constipation)
	Eyes: iris sphincter	Contraction (miosis)	Relaxation (mydriasis)
	Eyes: ciliary muscle	Contraction (accommodation)	Relaxation (blurred vision)
	Eyes: lacrimal gland	Tearing	Dry eyes

CNS, Central nervous system; *GI*, gastrointestinal.

TABLE 14.4 Preparation and Dosage of Anticholinergic Drugs for Overactive Bladder

Generic and Trade Names	Formulation	DOSAGE Initial	Maximum
Highly M$_3$ Selective			
Darifenacin			
Enablex	ER tablets	7.5 mg once daily	15 mg once daily
Primarily M$_3$ Selective			
Oxybutynin			
(generic only)	Syrup	5 mg 2–3 times/day	5 mg 4 times/day
(generic only)	IR tablets	5 mg 2–3 times/day	5 mg 4 times/day
Ditropan XL	ER tablets	5 mg once daily	30 mg once daily[a]
Oxytrol	Transdermal patch	1 patch twice weekly (delivers 3 mg/day)	1 patch twice weekly
Gelnique	Topical gel	3%: 3 pumps once daily	100 mg once daily
		10%: one 100-mg/1-g gel packet once daily	
Solifenacin			
VESIcare	Tablets	5 mg once daily	10 mg once daily
Nonselective			
Fesoterodine			
Toviaz	ER tablets	4 mg once daily	8 mg once daily
Tolterodine			
Detrol	IR tablets	1–2 mg twice daily	2 mg twice daily
Detrol LA	ER capsules	2–4 mg once daily	4 mg once daily
Trospium			
(generic only in United States) Trosec ♦	Tablets	20 mg twice daily[b]	20 mg twice daily
Sanctura XR ♦	ER capsules	60 mg once daily	60 mg once daily[b]

[a]Titrate dose upward as needed and tolerated.
[b]For patients with severe renal impairment, decrease dosage to 20 mg once daily at bedtime.
ER, Extended release; *IR*, immediate release.

With this background, we can consider how receptor selectivity might decrease anticholinergic side effects of drugs for OAB. To be beneficial, an anticholinergic agent must block muscarinic receptors in the bladder detrusor. That is, it must block the M$_3$ receptor subtype. Because M$_3$ receptors are also found in GI smooth muscle, the eyes, and salivary glands, an M$_3$-selective blocker will still have some unwanted anticholinergic effects—namely, constipation (from reducing bowel motility), blurred vision and photophobia (from preventing contraction of the ciliary muscle and iris sphincter), dry eyes (from blocking tear production), and *some* degree of dry mouth (from blocking salivary gland M$_3$ receptors, while sparing salivary M$_1$ receptors). What an M$_3$-selective blocker will *not* do is cause tachycardia (because muscarinic receptors in the heart are the M$_2$ type) or impairment of CNS function (because muscarinic receptors in the brain are primarily the M$_1$ type).

Specific Anticholinergic Drugs for Overactive Bladder

In the United States, six anticholinergic drugs are approved specifically for OAB (Table 14.4). All six work by M$_3$-muscarinic receptor blockade, although most block M_1 and M_2 receptors as well. With all of these drugs, we want sufficient M_3 blockade to reduce symptoms of OAB, but not so much as to cause urinary retention. You should be aware that responses to these agents are relatively modest and, for many patients, only slightly better than a placebo. None of the anticholinergics used for OAB are clearly superior to the others. However, if one anticholinergic fails to reduce symptoms, success may occur with a different anticholinergic approved for OAB.

Of note, in 2012, the FDA approved mirabegron (Myrbetriq), a β_3 agonist, for management of OAB. It has not demonstrated increased efficacy compared to anticholinergics, and it may be cost-prohibitive for many patients; however, it remains an alternative for patients who should not take anticholinergics or for whom anticholinergic side effects are intolerable. It may also be added to an anticholinergic regimen as an OAB management option (β agonists are discussed in Chapter 15).

Oxybutynin. Oxybutynin (Ditropan XL, Gelnique, Oxytrol) is an anticholinergic agent that acts primarily at M_3 muscarinic receptors. The drug is approved only for OAB. Benefits derive from blocking M_3 receptors on the bladder detrusor.

Oxybutynin is available in five formulations. Two are short acting (syrup and immediate-release [IR] tablets), and three are long acting (transdermal patch, topical gel, and ER tablets). The short-acting formulations have a short half-life (2 to 3 hours), and hence multiple daily doses are required. Another disadvantage of the IR formulation is that side effects are more intense. For these reasons, most patients prefer long-acting formulations of the drug. Dosing of oxybutynin and other drugs for OAB is provided in Table 14.4. Pharmacokinetics of anticholinergic drugs for OAB are provided in Table 14.5.

Anticholinergic side effects are common. The incidence of dry mouth is very high, in part because of muscarinic blockade by oxybutynin itself, and in part because of blockade by N-desethyloxybutynin. Other common side effects include constipation, tachycardia, urinary hesitancy, urinary retention, mydriasis, blurred vision, and dry eyes. In the CNS, cholinergic blockade can result in confusion, hallucinations, insomnia, and nervousness. In postmarketing reports of CNS effects, hallucinations and agitation were prominent among reports involving pediatric patients, whereas hallucinations, confusion, and sedation were prominent among reports involving older-adult patients. The combined use of oxybutynin

with other anticholinergic agents (e.g., antihistamines, tricyclic antidepressants, phenothiazine antipsychotics) can intensify all anticholinergic side effects.

Drugs that inhibit or induce CYP3A4 may alter oxybutynin blood levels and may thereby either increase toxicity (inhibitors of CYP3A4) or reduce effectiveness (inducers of CYP3A4).

Darifenacin. Of the anticholinergic agents used for OAB, darifenacin (Enablex) displays the greatest degree of M_3 selectivity. As a result, the drug can reduce OAB symptoms while having no effect on M_1 receptors in the brain or M_2 receptors in the heart. However, darifenacin does block M_3 receptors outside the bladder, so it can still cause dry mouth, constipation, and other M_3-related effects.

Clinical benefits are similar to those of oxybutynin and tolterodine. On average, treatment reduces episodes of urge incontinence from 15/week down to 7/week (using 7.5 mg/day) and from 17/week down to 6/week (using 15 mg/day).

Darifenacin is relatively well tolerated. The most common side effect is dry mouth. Constipation is also common. Other adverse effects include dyspepsia, gastritis, and headache. Darifenacin has little or no effect on memory, reaction time, word recognition, or cognition. The drug does not increase heart rate.

Levels of darifenacin can be raised significantly by strong inhibitors of CYP3A4. Among these are azole antifungal drugs (e.g., ketoconazole, itraconazole), certain protease inhibitors used for HIV/AIDS (e.g., ritonavir, nelfinavir), and clarithromycin (a macrolide antibiotic). If darifenacin is combined with any of these, its dosage must be kept low.

In patients with moderate liver impairment and in those taking powerful inhibitors of CYP3A4, doses should be kept low. In patients with severe liver impairment, darifenacin should be avoided.

Solifenacin. Solifenacin (VESIcare) is very similar to darifenacin, although it's not quite as M_3 selective. In clinical trials, the drug reduced episodes of urge incontinence from 18/week down to 8/week (using 5 mg/day) and from 20/week down to 8/week (using 10 mg/day).

The most common adverse effects are dry mouth, constipation, and blurred vision. Dyspepsia, urinary retention, headache, and nasal dryness occur infrequently. Rarely, solifenacin has caused potentially fatal angioedema of the face, lips, tongue, and larynx. At high doses (10 to 30 mg/day), solifenacin can prolong the QT interval, thereby posing a

TABLE 14.5 Pharmacokinetics: Anticholinergic Drugs for Overactive Bladder

Drug	Peak	Protein Binding	Metabolism	Half-Life	Elimination
Darifenacin (Enablex)	7 h	98%	Hepatic (CYP3A4 & CYP2D6)	13–19 h	Urine, 60% Feces, 40%
Oxybutynin (Ditropan XL, Gelnique, Oxytrol)	IR: 1 h ER: 4–6 h Transdermal: 24–48 h	More than 99%	Hepatic (CYP3A4)	IR: 2–3 h ER: 13 h Transdermal: 64 h	Urine
Solifenacin (VESIcare)	3–8 h	98%	Hepatic (N-oxidation, 4 R-hydroxylation, CYP3A4)	45–68 h	Urine, 69% Feces
Fesoterodine (Toviaz)	5 h	50%	Hepatic (CYP2D6, CYP3A4, nonspecific esterases)	7 h	Urine, 70% Feces
Tolterodine (Detrol, Detrol LA)	IR: 1–2 h ER: 2–6 h	96%	Hepatic (CYP2D6, CYP3A4)	IR: 2–10 h[a] ER: 7–18 h[a]	Urine, 77%, feces
Trospium (Trosec, Sanctura XR) (generic in United States)	5–6 h	48%–85%	Esterase hydrolysis and conjugation	IR: 20 h ER: 35 h	Feces 85%, Urine

[a]Longer half-life characteristic of poor metabolizers.
IR, Immediate release; *ER*, extended release; *h*, hour(s).

risk for a fatal dysrhythmia. Accordingly, caution is needed in patients with a history of QT prolongation and in those taking other QT-prolonging drugs. As with darifenacin, levels of solifenacin can be increased by strong inhibitors of CYP3A4 (e.g., ketoconazole, ritonavir, clarithromycin).

Solifenacin should be swallowed intact with liquid. Dosing may be done with or without food. For patients with moderate hepatic impairment or severe renal impairment, and for those taking a powerful CYP3A4 inhibitor, dosage should not exceed 5 mg/day. For patients with severe hepatic impairment, solifenacin should be not be used.

Tolterodine. Tolterodine (Detrol, Detrol LA) is a nonselective muscarinic antagonist approved only for OAB. Like oxybutynin, tolterodine is available in short- and long-acting formulations. Anticholinergic side effects are less intense with the long-acting form.

Anticholinergic side effects with tolterodine affect fewer patients compared with other anticholinergics prescribed for OAB. For example, dry mouth occurs in 35% of patients taking IR tolterodine versus 70% with IR oxybutynin. At a dose of 2 mg twice daily, the most common side effects are dry mouth, constipation, and dry eyes. Effects on the CNS—somnolence, vertigo, dizziness—occur infrequently. The incidence of both tachycardia and urinary retention is less than 1%. Anticholinergic effects can be intensified by concurrent use of other drugs with anticholinergic actions (e.g., antihistamines, tricyclic antidepressants, phenothiazine antipsychotics). Drugs that inhibit CYP3A4 (e.g., erythromycin, ketoconazole) can raise levels of tolterodine and can thereby intensify beneficial and adverse effects.

In addition to its anticholinergic effects, tolterodine can prolong the QT interval and can thereby promote serious cardiac dysrhythmias. Because of this risk, dosage should not exceed 4 mg/day.

Fesoterodine. Fesoterodine (Toviaz) is a nonselective muscarinic antagonist very similar to tolterodine. Both fesoterodine and tolterodine are used only for OAB, and at a dosage of 4 mg/day, both are equally effective. Furthermore, both agents undergo conversion to the same active metabolite—5-hydroxymethyl tolterodine—which is later inactivated by CYP3A4 and CYP2D6. In patients taking a strong inhibitor of CYP3A4 (e.g., ketoconazole, clarithromycin), beneficial and adverse effects are increased. Conversely, in patients taking a strong inducer of CYP3A4 (e.g., rifampin, carbamazepine), beneficial and adverse effects are reduced. As with tolterodine, the most common side effect is dry mouth. Another common side effect is constipation. Less common side effects include dizziness, fatigue, and blurred vision. Unlike tolterodine, fesoterodine has not been associated with QT prolongation and hence probably does not pose a risk for dysrhythmia.

Trospium. Trospium (Sanctura XR, Trosec ✦) is a nonselective muscarinic blocker indicated only for OAB. Compared with other drugs for OAB, trospium is notable for its low bioavailability, lack of CNS effects, and lack of metabolism-related interactions with other drugs.

Trospium IR tablets (Trosec) reduce episodes of urge incontinence from 27/week down to 12/week (compared with 30/week down to 16/week with placebo). Reductions in urinary frequency are minimal.

Trospium is generally well tolerated. The most common side effects are dry mouth and constipation. Rarely, the drug causes dry eyes and urinary retention. Trospium is a quaternary ammonium compound. Owing to its positive charge, trospium cannot cross the blood–brain barrier and hence is devoid of CNS effects.

Few studies of drug interactions have been done. However, because trospium is eliminated by the kidneys, we can assume it may compete with other drugs that undergo renal tubular excretion. Among these are vancomycin (an antibiotic), metformin (used for diabetes), and digoxin and procainamide (both used for cardiac disorders). Because trospium is not metabolized by CYP enzymes, the drug is unlikely to influence the hepatic metabolism of other agents.

PATIENT EDUCATION
Muscarinic Antagonists

- Teach patients that dry mouth can be relieved by sipping fluids, chewing sugar-free gum, treating the mouth with a saliva substitute, and using an alcohol-free mouthwash. Owing to increased risk for tooth decay, advise patients to avoid sugared gum, hard candy, and cough drops.
- Because these drugs can cause blurred vision, advise patients to avoid hazardous activities if vision is impaired. Recommend wearing sunglasses to decrease discomfort due to glare and excessive light related to pupil dilation. Indoors, lights may need to be turned down.
- Advise patients that urinary retention can be minimized by voiding just before taking anticholinergic medication.
- Counsel patients that constipation can be reduced by increasing dietary fiber and fluids and can be treated with a laxative if severe. Reinforce the need for adequate fluids if fiber supplements are taken to avoid worsening constipation.
- Caution patients to avoid vigorous exercise in warm environments to prevent hyperthermia. Heat-related illness is a particular concern in older patients taking anticholinergic drugs.

Toxicology of Muscarinic Antagonists
Sources of Antimuscarinic Poisoning

Sources of poisoning include natural products (e.g., *A. belladonna, D. stramonium*) and selective antimuscarinic drugs (e.g., atropine, scopolamine). Drugs with pronounced antimuscarinic properties (e.g., antihistamines, phenothiazines, tricyclic antidepressants) can also cause toxicity.

Symptoms

Symptoms of antimuscarinic poisoning, which are the direct result of excessive muscarinic blockade, include dry mouth, blurred vision, photophobia secondary to mydriasis, hyperthermia, CNS effects (hallucinations, delirium), and skin that is hot, dry, and flushed. Death results from respiratory depression secondary to blockade of cholinergic receptors in the brain. (See Box 14.2 for a mnemonic to help you remember antimuscarinic poisoning.)

Treatment

Treatment consists of (1) minimizing intestinal absorption of the antimuscarinic agent and (2) administering an antidote. Minimizing absorption is accomplished by administering activated charcoal, which will adsorb the poison within the intestine, thereby preventing its absorption into the blood.

The most effective antidote to antimuscarinic poisoning is *physostigmine*, an inhibitor of acetylcholinesterase. By inhibiting cholinesterase, physostigmine causes acetylcholine to accumulate at all cholinergic

---

BOX 14.2 Antimuscarinic (Anticholinergic) Toxicity

A mnemonic is commonly used to remember the signs and symptoms of antimuscarinic (anticholinergic) toxicity.

Hot as a hare (hyperthermia)
Dry as a bone (dry eyes, dry mouth, dry skin)
Red as a beet (flushed face)
Blind as a bat (mydriasis)
Mad as a hatter (delirium)

junctions. As acetylcholine builds up, it competes with the antimuscarinic agent for receptor binding, thereby reversing excessive muscarinic blockade.

Warning

It is important to differentiate between antimuscarinic poisoning, which often resembles psychosis (hallucinations, delirium), and an actual psychotic episode. We need to make the differential diagnosis because some antipsychotic drugs have antimuscarinic properties of their own and hence will intensify symptoms if given to a victim of antimuscarinic poisoning. Fortunately, because a true psychotic episode is not ordinarily associated with signs of excessive muscarinic blockade (dry mouth, hyperthermia, dry skin, and so forth), differentiation is not usually difficult.

📄 SUMMARY OF KEY PRESCRIBING CONSIDERATIONS

Atropine and Other Muscarinic Antagonists

Assessment
Therapeutic Goal
Atropine has many applications, including treatment of bradycardia, biliary colic, intestinal hypertonicity and hypermotility, and muscarinic agonist poisoning.

Identifying High-Risk Patients
Atropine and other muscarinic antagonists are *contraindicated* for patients with glaucoma, intestinal atony, urinary tract obstruction, and tachycardia. Use with *caution* in patients with asthma.

Administration Considerations
Dry mouth from muscarinic blockade may interfere with swallowing. Advise patients to moisten the mouth by sipping water before oral administration.

Ongoing Monitoring and Interventions
Minimizing Adverse Effects
Xerostomia
Decreased salivation can dry the mouth. Common interventions such as sipping fluids frequently, chewing gum, and sucking on hard candies will usually alleviate symptoms. Saliva substitutes are available for severe cases.

Blurred Vision
Paralysis of the ciliary muscle may reduce visual acuity. Patients should not participate in activities such as driving where good vision is necessary.

Photophobia
Muscarinic blockade prevents the pupil from constricting in response to bright light. Keep room lighting low to reduce visual discomfort. Sunglasses are often required.

Urinary Retention
Muscarinic blockade in the urinary tract can cause urinary hesitancy or retention. If urinary retention is severe, catheterization or treatment with bethanechol (a muscarinic agonist) may be required. Keep in mind, however, that a muscarinic agonist will also counteract positive effects of anticholinergics.

Constipation
Reduced tone and motility of the gut may cause constipation. Increasing fluids, fiber, and activity will be helpful.

Hyperthermia
Suppression of sweating may result in hyperthermia.

Tachycardia
Blockade of cardiac muscarinic receptors can accelerate heart rate. Monitor pulse and report significant increases.

Minimizing Adverse Interactions
Antihistamines, tricyclic antidepressants, and *phenothiazines* have prominent antimuscarinic actions. Combining these agents with atropine and other anticholinergic drugs can cause excessive muscarinic blockade.

Management of Acute Toxicity
Symptoms
Overdose produces dry mouth, blurred vision, photophobia, hyperthermia, hallucinations, and delirium; the skin becomes hot, dry, and flushed. Differentiate muscarinic antagonist poisoning from psychosis!

Treatment
Treatment centers on limiting absorption of ingested poison (e.g., by giving activated charcoal to adsorb the drug) and administering physostigmine, an inhibitor of acetylcholinesterase.

15

Adrenergic Agonists

Adrenergic agonists produce their effects by activating adrenergic receptors. Because the sympathetic nervous system acts through these same receptors, responses to adrenergic agonists and responses to stimulation of the sympathetic nervous system are very similar. Because of this similarity, adrenergic agonists are often referred to as *sympathomimetics*. They have a broad spectrum of indications, ranging from heart failure to asthma to preterm labor.

Learning about adrenergic agonists can be a challenge. To facilitate the process, our approach to these drugs has four stages. We begin with the general mechanisms by which drugs can activate adrenergic receptors. Next, we establish an overview of the major adrenergic agonists, focusing on their receptor specificity and chemical classification. Then we address the adrenergic receptors themselves; for each receptor type—α_1, α_2, β_1, β_2, and dopamine—we discuss the beneficial and harmful effects that can result from receptor activation. Finally, we integrate all of this information by discussing the characteristic properties of representative sympathomimetic drugs.

This chapter is intended only as an *introduction* to the adrenergic agonists. Our objective is to discuss the basic properties of the sympathomimetic drugs and to establish an overview of their applications and adverse effects. In later chapters, we will discuss the clinical applications of these agents in greater depth.

MECHANISMS OF ADRENERGIC RECEPTOR ACTIVATION

Drugs can activate adrenergic receptors by four basic mechanisms: (1) direct receptor binding, (2) promotion of norepinephrine (NE) release, (3) blockade of NE reuptake, and (4) inhibition of NE inactivation. Note that only the first mechanism is *direct*. With the other three mechanisms, receptor activation occurs by an *indirect* process. Examples of drugs that act by these four mechanisms are presented in Table 15.1.

Direct Receptor Binding

Direct interaction with receptors is the most common mechanism by which drugs activate peripheral adrenergic receptors. The direct-acting receptor stimulants produce their effects by binding to adrenergic receptors and mimicking the actions of natural transmitters (NE, epinephrine, dopamine). All of the drugs discussed in this chapter activate receptors directly.

Promotion of Norepinephrine Release

By acting on terminals of sympathetic nerves to cause NE release, drugs can bring about indirect activation of adrenergic receptors. Agents that act by this mechanism include amphetamines and ephedrine. (Ephedrine can also activate adrenergic receptors directly.)

Inhibition of Norepinephrine Reuptake

Recall that reuptake of NE into terminals of sympathetic nerves is the major mechanism for terminating adrenergic transmission. By blocking NE reuptake, drugs can cause NE to accumulate within the synaptic gap and can thereby increase receptor activation. Agents that act by this mechanism include cocaine and the tricyclic antidepressants.

Inhibition of Norepinephrine Inactivation

As discussed in Chapter 12, some of the NE in terminals of adrenergic neurons is subject to inactivation by monoamine oxidase (MAO). Hence drugs that inhibit MAO can increase the amount of NE available for release and enhance receptor activation. (In addition to being present in sympathetic nerves, MAO is present in the liver and the intestinal wall. The significance of MAO at these other sites is considered later.)

In this chapter, which focuses on *peripherally* acting sympathomimetics, nearly all of the drugs discussed act exclusively by *direct* receptor activation. The only exception is *ephedrine,* a drug that works by a combination of direct receptor activation and the promotion of NE release.

Most of the indirect-acting adrenergic agonists are used for their ability to activate adrenergic receptors in the central nervous system (CNS)—not for their effects in the periphery. The indirect-acting sympathomimetics (e.g., amphetamine, cocaine) are mentioned here to emphasize that, although these agents are employed for effects on the brain, they can and will cause activation of adrenergic receptors in the periphery. Peripheral activation is responsible for certain toxicities of these drugs (e.g., cardiac dysrhythmias, hypertension).

OVERVIEW OF THE ADRENERGIC AGONISTS

Chemical Classification: Catecholamines Versus Noncatecholamines

The adrenergic agonists fall into two major chemical classes: catecholamines and noncatecholamines, which differ in three important respects: (1) availability for oral use, (2) duration of action, and (3) ability to act in the CNS. Accordingly, if we know to which category a particular adrenergic agonist belongs, we will know three of its prominent features.

Catecholamines

The catecholamines are so named because they contain a *catechol* group and an *amine* group. A catechol group is simply a benzene ring that has hydroxyl groups on two adjacent carbons. The amine component

TABLE 15.1   Mechanisms of Adrenergic Receptor Activation

Mechanism of Stimulation	Examples
Direct Mechanism	
Receptor activation through direct binding	Dopamine
	Epinephrine
	Isoproterenol
	Ephedrine[a]
Indirect Mechanisms	
Promotion of NE release	Amphetamine
	Ephedrine[a]
Inhibition of NE reuptake	Cocaine
	Tricyclic antidepressants
Inhibition of MAO	MAO inhibitors

[a]Ephedrine is a mixed-acting drug that activates receptors directly and by promoting release of norepinephrine.
MAO, Monoamine oxidase; *NE,* norepinephrine.

of the catecholamines is *ethylamine.* Structural formulas for each of the major catecholamines—epinephrine, NE, isoproterenol, dopamine, and dobutamine—are shown in Fig. 15.1. Because of their chemistry, all catecholamines have three properties in common: (1) they cannot be used orally, (2) they have a brief duration of action, and (3) they cannot cross the blood–brain barrier.

The actions of two enzymes—*monoamine oxidase* and *catechol-O-methyltransferase* (COMT)—explain why the catecholamines have short half-lives and cannot be used orally. MAO and COMT are located in the liver and intestinal wall. Both enzymes are very active and quickly destroy catecholamines administered by any route. Because these enzymes are located in the liver and intestinal wall, catecholamines that are administered orally become inactivated before they can reach the systemic circulation. Hence catecholamines are ineffective if given by mouth. Because of rapid inactivation by MAO and COMT, three catecholamines—NE, dopamine, and dobutamine—are effective only if administered by continuous infusion. Administration by other parenteral routes (e.g., subcutaneously, intramuscularly) will not yield adequate blood levels, owing to rapid hepatic inactivation.

Catecholamines are polar molecules, so they cannot cross the blood–brain barrier. (Recall from Chapter 4 that polar compounds penetrate membranes poorly.) The polar nature of the catecholamines is due to the hydroxyl groups on the catechol portion of the molecule. Because they cannot cross the blood-brain barrier, catecholamines have minimal effects on the CNS.

Be aware that catecholamine-containing solutions, which are colorless when first prepared, turn pink or brown over time. This pigmentation is caused by oxidation of the catecholamine molecule. *Catecholamine solutions should be discarded as soon as discoloration develops.* The only exception is dobutamine, which can be used up to 24 hours after the solution was made, even if discoloration appears.

Noncatecholamines

The noncatecholamines have ethylamine in their structure (see Fig. 15.1), but do not contain the catechol moiety that characterizes the catecholamines. Here we discuss three noncatecholamines: ephedrine, albuterol, and phenylephrine.

The noncatecholamines differ from the catecholamines in three important respects. First, because they lack a catechol group,

noncatecholamines are not substrates for COMT and are metabolized slowly by MAO. As a result, the half-lives of noncatecholamines are much longer than those of catecholamines. Second, because they do not undergo rapid degradation by MAO and COMT, noncatecholamines can be given orally, whereas catecholamines cannot. Third, noncatecholamines are considerably less polar than catecholamines and hence are more able to cross the blood–brain barrier.

Receptor Specificity

To understand the actions of individual adrenergic agonists, we need to know their receptor specificity. Variability in receptor specificity among the adrenergic agonists can be illustrated with three drugs: albuterol, isoproterenol, and epinephrine. Albuterol is highly selective, acting at β_2 receptors only. Isoproterenol is less selective, acting at β_1 receptors and β_2 receptors. Epinephrine is even less selective, acting at all four adrenergic receptor subtypes: α_1, α_2, β_1, and β_2.

The receptor specificities of the major adrenergic agonists are shown in Table 15.2. In the upper part of the table, receptor specificity is presented in tabular form. In the lower part, the same information is presented schematically. By learning this content, you will be well on your way to understanding the pharmacology of the sympathomimetic drugs.

Note that the concept of receptor specificity is relative, not absolute. The ability of a drug to selectively activate certain receptors to the exclusion of others depends on the dose: at low doses, selectivity is maximal; as the dose increases, selectivity declines. For example, when albuterol is administered in low to moderate doses, the drug is highly selective for β_2-adrenergic receptors. However, if the dose is high, albuterol will activate β_1 receptors as well. The information on receptor specificity in Table 15.2 refers to usual therapeutic doses. So-called selective agents will activate additional adrenergic receptors if the dose is abnormally high.

THERAPEUTIC APPLICATIONS AND ADVERSE EFFECTS OF ADRENERGIC RECEPTOR ACTIVATION

In this section we discuss the responses—both therapeutic and adverse—that can be elicited with sympathomimetic drugs. Because many adrenergic agonists activate more than one type of receptor (see Table 15.2), it could be quite confusing if we were to talk about the effects of the sympathomimetics while employing specific drugs as examples. Consequently, rather than attempting to structure this presentation around representative drugs, we discuss the actions of the adrenergic agonists one receptor at a time. Our discussion begins with α_1 receptors, and then moves to α_2 receptors, β_1 receptors, β_2 receptors, and finally dopamine receptors. For each receptor type, we discuss both the therapeutic and adverse responses that can result from receptor activation.

To understand the effects of any specific adrenergic agonist, all you need are two types of information: (1) the identity of the receptors at which the drug acts, and (2) the effects produced by activating those receptors. Combining this information will reveal a profile of drug action. This is the same approach to understanding neuropharmacologic agents that we discussed in Chapter 11.

Before you continue, it may be helpful to review Table 12.3 in Chapter 12. We are about to discuss the clinical consequences of adrenergic receptor activation, and Table 12.3 shows the responses to activation of those receptors.

Clinical Consequences of α_1 Activation

In this section we discuss the therapeutic and adverse effects that can result from activation of α_1-adrenergic receptors. As shown in

Fig. 15.1 Structures of Representative Catecholamines and Noncatecholamines. *Catecholamines:* All of the catecholamines share the same basic chemical formula. Because of their biochemical properties, the catecholamines cannot be used orally, cannot cross the blood–brain barrier, and have short half-lives (owing to rapid inactivation by monoamine oxidase [MAO] and catechol-*O*-methyltransferase [COMT]). *Noncatechol-amines:* Although structurally similar to catecholamines, noncatecholamines differ from catecholamines in three important ways: they can be used orally; they can cross the blood–brain barrier; and, because they are not rapidly metabolized by MAO or COMT, they have much longer half-lives.

Table 15.2, drugs capable of activating α_1 receptors include epinephrine, NE, phenylephrine, ephedrine, and dopamine.

Therapeutic Applications of α_1 Activation

Activation of α_1 receptors elicits two responses that can be of therapeutic use: (1) *vasoconstriction* (in blood vessels of the skin, viscera, and mucous membranes), and (2) *mydriasis*. Of the two, vasoconstriction is the one for which α_1 agonists are used most often. Using these drugs for mydriasis is rare.

Hemostasis. Hemostasis is defined as the arrest of bleeding, which α_1 agonists support through vasoconstriction. α_1 agonists are given to stop bleeding primarily in the skin and mucous membranes. Epinephrine, applied topically, is the α_1 agonist used most for this purpose.

Nasal decongestion. Nasal congestion results from dilation and engorgement of blood vessels in the nasal mucosa. Drugs can relieve congestion by causing α_1-mediated vasoconstriction. Specific α_1-activating agents employed as nasal decongestants include phenylephrine (administered topically) and pseudoephedrine (administered orally).

TABLE 15.2   Receptor Specificity of Representative Adrenergic Agonists

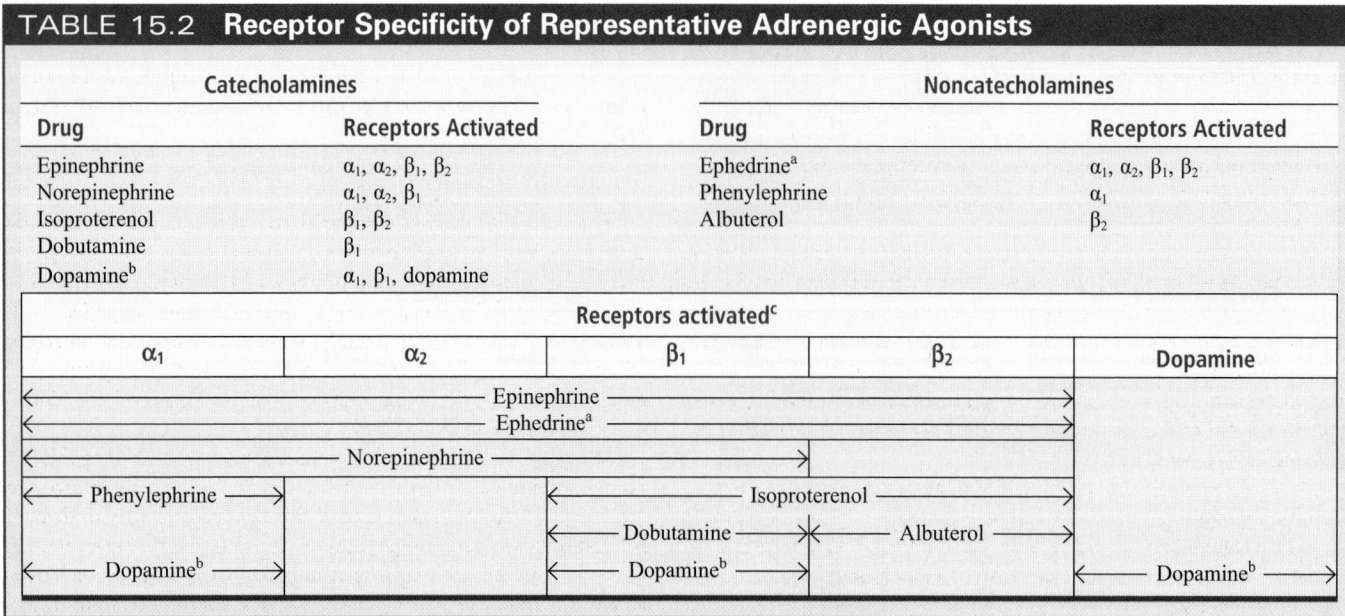

Catecholamines		Noncatecholamines	
Drug	**Receptors Activated**	**Drug**	**Receptors Activated**
Epinephrine	$\alpha_1, \alpha_2, \beta_1, \beta_2$	Ephedrine[a]	$\alpha_1, \alpha_2, \beta_1, \beta_2$
Norepinephrine	$\alpha_1, \alpha_2, \beta_1$	Phenylephrine	α_1
Isoproterenol	β_1, β_2	Albuterol	β_2
Dobutamine	β_1		
Dopamine[b]	$\alpha_1, \beta_1,$ dopamine		

[a]Ephedrine is a mixed-acting agent that causes NE release and activates α and β receptors directly.
[b]Receptor activation by dopamine is dose dependent.
[c]This chart presents in graphic form the same information on receptor specificity given above. *Arrows* indicate the range of receptors that the drugs can activate (at usual therapeutic doses).
α, Alpha; β, beta; *NE*, norepinephrine.

Adjunct to local anesthesia. α_1 agonists are frequently combined with local anesthetics to delay systemic absorption. The mechanism is α_1-mediated vasoconstriction, which reduces blood flow to the site of anesthetic administration. Why delay anesthetic absorption? Because keeping the drug at the local site of action prolongs anesthesia, allows a reduction in the anesthetic dose, and reduces the systemic effects that a local anesthetic might produce. The drug used most frequently to delay anesthetic absorption is epinephrine.

Elevation of blood pressure. Because of their ability to cause vasoconstriction, α_1 agonists can elevate blood pressure in hypotensive patients. However, α_1 agonists are not the primary therapy for hypotension. Rather, they are reserved for situations in which fluid replacement and other measures either are contraindicated or have failed to restore blood pressure to a satisfactory level.

Mydriasis. Activation of α_1 receptors on the radial muscle of the iris causes mydriasis (dilation of the pupil), which can facilitate eye examinations and ocular surgery. Note that producing mydriasis is the only clinical use of α_1 activation that is not based on vasoconstriction.

Adverse Effects of α_1 Activation

All adverse effects caused by α_1 activation result directly or indirectly from vasoconstriction.

Hypertension. α_1 agonists can produce hypertension by causing widespread vasoconstriction. Severe hypertension is most likely with parenteral dosing. Accordingly, when α_1 agonists are given intravenously, the patient's cardiac rhythm must be monitored continuously, and other indicators of cardiovascular status and perfusion (e.g., blood pressure, peripheral pulses, urine output) should be assessed frequently.

Necrosis. If the intravenous (IV) solution containing an α_1 agonist extravasates, seepage of the drug into the surrounding tissues may result in necrosis. The cause is lack of blood flow to the affected area secondary to intense local vasoconstriction. If extravasation occurs, the area should be infiltrated with an α_1-blocking agent (e.g., phentolamine), which

will counteract α_1-mediated vasoconstriction and thereby help minimize injury.

Bradycardia. α_1 agonists can cause reflex slowing of the heart. This occurs when: α_1-mediated vasoconstriction elevates blood pressure, which triggers the baroreceptor reflex, causing the heart rate to decline. In patients with marginal cardiac reserve, the decrease in cardiac output may compromise tissue perfusion.

Clinical Consequences of α_2 Activation

α_2 receptors in the periphery are located *presynaptically,* and their activation inhibits NE release. Several adrenergic agonists (e.g., epinephrine, NE) are capable of causing α_2 activation. However, their ability to activate α_2 receptors in the periphery has little clinical significance because there are no therapeutic applications related to activation of peripheral α_2 receptors. Furthermore, activation of these receptors rarely causes significant adverse effects.

In contrast to α_2 receptors in the *periphery,* α_2 receptors in the *CNS* are of great clinical significance. By activating central α_2 receptors, we can produce two useful effects: (1) *reduction* of sympathetic outflow to the heart and blood vessels, and (2) relief of severe pain. The central α_2 agonists used for effects on the heart and blood vessels, and the agents used to relieve pain, are discussed in Chapters 17 and 24, respectively.

Clinical Consequences of β_1 Activation

All of the clinically relevant responses to activation of β_1 receptors result from activating β_1 receptors in the *heart;* activation of renal β_1 receptors is not associated with either beneficial or adverse effects. As indicated in Table 15.2, β_1 receptors can be activated by epinephrine, NE, isoproterenol, dopamine, dobutamine, and ephedrine.

Therapeutic Applications of β_1 Activation

Heart failure. Heart failure is characterized by a reduction in the force of myocardial contraction, resulting in insufficient cardiac output.

Because activation of β_1 receptors in the heart has a positive inotropic effect (i.e., increases the force of contraction), drugs that activate these receptors can improve cardiac performance.

Shock. Shock is characterized by profound hypotension and greatly reduced tissue perfusion. The primary goal of treatment is to maintain blood flow to vital organs. By increasing heart rate and force of contraction, β_1 stimulants can increase cardiac output and thereby improve tissue perfusion.

Atrioventricular heart block. Atrioventricular (AV) heart block is a condition in which impulse conduction from the atria to the ventricles is either impeded or blocked entirely. As a consequence, the ventricles are no longer driven at an appropriate rate. Because activation of cardiac β_1 receptors can enhance impulse conduction through the AV node, β_1 stimulants can help overcome AV block. However, it should be noted that drugs are only a temporary form of treatment. For long-term management, a pacemaker is implanted.

Cardiac arrest. By activating cardiac β_1 receptors, drugs have a role in initiating contraction in asystole or pulseless ventricular rhythms. However, it should be noted that drugs are not the preferred treatment. Initial management focuses on cardiopulmonary resuscitation, external pacing, or defibrillation (whichever is applicable), and identification and treatment of the underlying cause (e.g., hypoxia, severe acidosis, drug overdose). When a β_1 agonist *is* indicated, epinephrine, administered intravenously, is the preferred drug. If IV access is not possible, epinephrine can be administered endotracheally or by intraosseous infusion.

Adverse Effects of β_1 Activation

All of the adverse effects of β_1 activation result from activating β_1 receptors in the heart. Activating renal β_1 receptors is not associated with untoward effects.

Altered heart rate or rhythm. Overstimulation of cardiac β_1 receptors can produce *tachycardia* and *dysrhythmias*.

Angina pectoris. In some patients, drugs that activate β_1 receptors can precipitate an attack of angina pectoris, a condition characterized by substernal pain in the region of the heart. Anginal pain occurs when cardiac oxygen supply is insufficient to meet cardiac oxygen needs. The most common cause of angina is coronary atherosclerosis (accumulation of lipids and other substances in coronary arteries). Because β_1 agonists increase cardiac oxygen demand (by increasing heart rate and force of contraction), patients with compromised coronary circulation are at risk for an anginal attack.

Clinical Consequences of β_2 Activation

Applications of β_2 activation are limited to the *lungs* and the *uterus*. Drugs used for their β_2-activating ability include epinephrine, isoproterenol, and albuterol.

Therapeutic Applications of β_2 Activation

Asthma. Asthma is a chronic condition characterized by inflammation and bronchoconstriction occurring in response to a variety of stimuli. During a severe attack, the airflow reduction can be life threatening. Because drugs that activate β_2 receptors in the lungs promote bronchodilation, these drugs can help relieve or prevent asthma attacks.

For therapy of asthma, adrenergic agonists that are *selective for β_2 receptors* (e.g., albuterol) are preferred to less selective agents (e.g., isoproterenol). This is especially true for patients who also suffer from *angina pectoris* or *tachycardia* because drugs that activate β_1 receptors can aggravate these cardiac disorders.

Most β_2 agonists used to treat asthma are administered by *inhalation.* This route is desirable in that it helps minimize adverse systemic effects. However, it should be noted that inhalation does not guarantee safety: serious systemic toxicity can result from overdosing with inhaled

sympathomimetics, so patients must be warned against inhaling too much drug.

Delay of preterm labor. Activation of β_2 receptors in the uterus relaxes uterine smooth muscle. This action can be employed to delay preterm labor.

Adverse Effects of β_2 Activation

Hyperglycemia. The most important adverse response to β_2 activation is hyperglycemia. The mechanism is activation of β_2 receptors in the liver and skeletal muscles, which promotes breakdown of glycogen into glucose. As a rule, β_2 agonists cause hyperglycemia only in patients with *diabetes;* in patients with normal pancreatic function, insulin release will maintain blood glucose at an appropriate level. If hyperglycemia develops in the patient with diabetes, medications used for glucose control will need to be adjusted.

Tremor. Tremor is the most common side effect of β_2 agonists. It occurs because activation of β_2 receptors in skeletal muscle enhances contraction. This effect can be confounding for patients with diabetes because tremor is a common symptom of hypoglycemia; however, when due to β_2 activation, it may be accompanied by hyperglycemia. Fortunately, the tremor generally fades over time and can be minimized by initiating therapy at low doses.

Clinical Consequences of Dopamine Receptor Activation

Activation of peripheral dopamine receptors causes dilation of the renal vasculature. This effect is employed in the treatment of *shock:* by dilating renal blood vessels, we can improve renal perfusion and can thereby reduce the risk for renal failure. *Dopamine* is the only drug available that can activate dopamine receptors. It should be noted that, when dopamine is given to treat shock, the drug also enhances cardiac performance because it activates β_1 receptors in the heart.

Multiple Receptor Activation: Treatment of Anaphylactic Shock
Pathophysiology of Anaphylaxis

Anaphylaxis can be triggered by a variety of substances, including bee venom, wasp venom, latex rubber, certain foods (e.g., peanuts, shellfish), and certain drugs (e.g., penicillins).

Anaphylactic shock is a manifestation of severe allergy. The reaction is characterized by *hypotension* (from widespread vasodilation), *bronchoconstriction,* and *edema of the glottis.* Although histamine contributes to these responses, symptoms are due largely to the release of other mediators (e.g., leukotrienes). For this reason, antihistamines are not especially useful against anaphylaxis.

Treatment. Epinephrine, injected intramuscularly or intravenously, is the treatment of choice for anaphylactic shock. Benefits derive from activating three types of adrenergic receptors: α_1, β_1, and β_2. By activating these receptors, epinephrine can reverse the most severe manifestations of the anaphylactic reaction. Activation of β_1 receptors increases cardiac output, helping to elevate blood pressure. Blood pressure is also increased because epinephrine promotes α_1-mediated vasoconstriction. In addition to increasing blood pressure, vasoconstriction helps suppress glottal edema. By activating β_2 receptors, epinephrine can counteract bronchoconstriction.

Individuals who are prone to severe allergic responses should carry an epinephrine autoinjector (EpiPen, EpiPen Jr., Auvi-Q, Adrenaclick, Allerject, generic) at all times. Because the mechanism of administration varies among products, it is important to review the specific auto-injector instructions on the product's package insert with the patient and to verify that the patient can use the auto-injector prior to discharge.

PATIENT EDUCATION
Epinephrine Auto-Injectors

- Fill your prescription immediately and replace it if it expires.
- Keep your epinephrine auto-injector with you at all times and inform friends and family of its location in the event of an emergency.
- Use the auto-injector immediately if exposure to an allergen causes you to have difficulty breathing, makes you feel lightheaded like you may pass out, or if you feel a tightening in your throat. Do not wait to see if symptoms will worsen.
- After using the auto-injector, call for ambulance transport to the local emergency department. They will need to monitor your condition. Additional epinephrine or other treatment may be necessary. (Be sure to take your auto-injector with you to the emergency department. Personnel there will want to know of prior treatment and dispose of it for you.)

PROPERTIES OF REPRESENTATIVE ADRENERGIC AGONISTS

Our aim in this section is to establish an overview of the adrenergic agonists. The information is presented in the form of "drug digests," which highlight characteristic features of representative sympathomimetic agents. Some of these drugs are used in specialty areas; however, the choices of representative drugs will increase the understanding of adrenergic receptor activation. This knowledge will be helpful for later chapters.

As noted, there are two keys to understanding individual adrenergic agonists: (1) knowledge of the receptors that the drug can activate, and (2) knowledge of the therapeutic and adverse effects that receptor activation can elicit. By integrating these two types of information, you can easily predict the spectrum of effects that a particular drug can produce.

Unfortunately, knowing the effects that a drug is *capable* of producing does not always indicate how that drug is *actually used* in a clinical setting. Safer alternatives are often available. For example, NE can activate α_1 receptors and can therefore produce mydriasis, but safer drugs are available for this purpose. Similarly, although isoproterenol is capable of producing uterine relaxation through β_2 activation, it is no longer used for this purpose because safer drugs are available. Because receptor specificity is not always a predictor of the therapeutic applications of a particular adrenergic agonist, for each of the drugs discussed next, approved clinical applications are indicated.

Epinephrine

- *Receptor specificity:* α_1, α_2, β_1, β_2
- *Chemical classification:* catecholamine

Epinephrine (Adrenalin, others) was among the first adrenergic agonists employed clinically and can be considered the prototype of the sympathomimetic drugs. Because of its prototypic status, epinephrine is discussed in detail.

Therapeutic Uses

Epinephrine can activate all four subtypes of adrenergic receptors. As a consequence, the drug can produce a broad spectrum of beneficial sympathomimetic effects:
- Because it can cause α_1-mediated vasoconstriction, epinephrine is used to (1) delay absorption of local anesthetics, (2) control superficial bleeding, and (3) elevate blood pressure.
- Because it can activate β_1 receptors, epinephrine may be used to (1) overcome AV heart block and (2) restore cardiac function in patients

PATIENT-CENTERED CARE ACROSS THE LIFE SPAN
Adrenergic Agonists

Life Stage	Considerations or Concerns
Children	These drugs are commonly used in emergency situations. There are no contraindications for children.
Pregnant Women	No known fetal abnormalities are associated with Dobutamine. With epinephrine, norepinephrine, and dopamine, vasoconstriction in the uterus may decrease oxygenation to the fetus. Albuterol is associated with rare congenital anomalies. Albuterol also may decrease uterine contractility. In any case, when used for emergencies in which the woman's life is at risk, treatment should not be withheld.
Breast-feeding Women	Manufacturers recommend caution if the patient is breast-feeding because adequate studies are not available. Breast-feeding infants should be monitored for adrenergic effects.
Older Adults	Older adult patients may be more disposed to the adverse effects of these drugs (e.g., blood pressure elevation, tachycardia, shakiness). Adrenergic agonists may also contribute to urinary retention. For life-threatening emergencies requiring use of these drugs, benefits are greater than risks.

PROTOTYPE DRUGS
Adrenergic Agonists

Epinephrine

in cardiac arrest experiencing ventricular fibrillation, pulseless ventricular tachycardia, pulseless electrical activity, or asystole.
- Activation of β_2 receptors in the lung promotes bronchodilation, which can be useful in patients with asthma (although epinephrine is not the drug of choice for this purpose).
- Because it can activate a combination of α and β receptors, epinephrine is the treatment of choice for anaphylactic shock.

Pharmacokinetics

Epinephrine may be administered topically or by injection. The drug cannot be given orally because epinephrine and other catecholamines undergo destruction by MAO and COMT before reaching the systemic circulation. After subcutaneous injection, absorption is slow owing to epinephrine-induced local vasoconstriction. Absorption is more rapid after intramuscular injection and is immediate with IV administration.

Epinephrine has a short half-life because of two processes: enzymatic inactivation and uptake into adrenergic nerves. The enzymes that inactivate epinephrine and other catecholamines are MAO and COMT.

Additional information on the pharmacokinetics of epinephrine and other adrenergic agonists is provided in Table 15.3.

Adverse Effects

Because it can activate the four major adrenergic receptor subtypes, epinephrine can produce multiple adverse effects.

TABLE 15.3 Pharmacokinetics: Adrenergic Agonists (Intravenous Administration Except Where Indicated)

Drug	Onset of Action	Metabolism	Half-Life	Duration	Elimination
Epinephrine[a]	Immediate	MAO and COMT	<5 min	UK	Urine
Norepinephrine	Immediate	MAO and COMT	UK	1–2 min	Urine
Isoproterenol	Immediate	COMT	2.5–5 min	10–15 min	Urine
Dopamine	<5 min	MAO and COMT	2 min	<10 min	Urine
Dobutamine	1–2 min	COMT	2 min	UK	Urine
Phenylephrine[b]	Immediate	Hepatic (oxidative deamination)	5 min	15–20 min	Urine
Albuterol[c]	10–30 min	Hepatic	3.8–5 h	2–6 h	Urine, feces
Ephedrine	Immediate	UK	3–6 h depending on urinary pH (half-life increases as pH increases)	UK	Urine

[a]Also available for oral inhalation and nasal administration.
[b]Also available for topical, nasal, and ophthalmic administration.
[c]Administration by inhalation.
COMT, Catechol-o-methyltransferase; *h,* hour; *MAO,* monoamine oxidase; *min,* minutes.

Hypertensive crisis. Vasoconstriction secondary to excessive α_1 activation can produce a dramatic increase in blood pressure. Cerebral hemorrhage can occur. Because of the potential for severe hypertension, patients receiving *parenteral* epinephrine must undergo continuous cardiovascular monitoring with frequent assessment of vital signs.

Dysrhythmias. Excessive activation of β_1 receptors in the heart can produce dysrhythmias. Because of their sensitivity to catecholamines, hyperthyroid patients are at high risk for epinephrine-induced dysrhythmias.

Angina pectoris. By activating β_1 receptors in the heart, epinephrine can increase cardiac work and oxygen demand. If the increase in oxygen demand is significant, an anginal attack may ensue. Provocation of angina is especially likely in patients with coronary atherosclerosis.

Post-extravasation necrosis. If an IV solution containing epinephrine extravasates, the ensuing localized vasoconstriction may result in necrosis. Because of this possibility, the IV site should be monitored closely. If extravasation occurs, injury can be minimized by local injection of phentolamine, an α-adrenergic antagonist.

Hyperglycemia. In patients with diabetes, epinephrine can cause hyperglycemia. How? By causing breakdown of glycogen secondary to activation of β_2 receptors in the liver and in skeletal muscle. If hyperglycemia develops, dosage adjustments will need to be made for medications used to manage diabetes.

Drug Interactions

Monoamine oxidase inhibitors. As their name implies, MAO inhibitors suppress the activity of MAO. These drugs are used primarily to treat depression (see Chapter 27). Because MAO is one of the enzymes that inactivate epinephrine and other catecholamines, inhibition of MAO will prolong and intensify epinephrine's effects. In most situations, patients receiving an MAO inhibitor should not receive epinephrine.

Tricyclic antidepressants. Tricyclic antidepressants block the uptake of catecholamines into adrenergic neurons. Because neuronal uptake is one mechanism by which the actions of NE and other catecholamines are terminated, blocking uptake can intensify and prolong epinephrine's effects. Accordingly, patients receiving a tricyclic antidepressant may require a lower dose of epinephrine.

General anesthetics. Several inhalation anesthetics render the myocardium hypersensitive to activation by β_1 agonists. When the heart is in this hypersensitive state, exposure to epinephrine and other β_1 agonists can cause tachydysrhythmias.

α-Adrenergic blocking agents. Drugs that block α-adrenergic receptors can prevent α-adrenergic receptor activation by epinephrine. α blockers (e.g., phentolamine) can be used to treat toxicity (e.g., hypertension, local vasoconstriction) caused by excessive epinephrine-induced α activation.

β-Adrenergic blocking agents. Drugs that block β-adrenergic receptors can prevent β-adrenergic receptor activation by epinephrine. β-blocking agents (e.g., metoprolol) can reduce adverse effects (e.g., dysrhythmias, anginal pain) caused by epinephrine and other β_1 agonists.

Norepinephrine

- *Receptor specificity:* α_1, α_2, β_1
- *Chemical classification:* catecholamine

Norepinephrine (Levophed) is similar to epinephrine in several respects. With regard to receptor specificity, NE differs from epinephrine only in that NE does not activate β_2 receptors. Accordingly, NE can elicit all of the responses that epinephrine can, except those that are β_2 mediated. Because NE is a catecholamine, the drug is subject to rapid inactivation by MAO and COMT, and hence cannot be given orally. Adverse effects are nearly identical to those of epinephrine: tachydysrhythmias, angina, hypertension, and local necrosis on extravasation. In contrast to epinephrine, NE does not promote hyperglycemia, a response that is β_2 mediated. As with epinephrine, responses to NE can be modified by MAO inhibitors, tricyclic antidepressants, general anesthetics, and adrenergic blocking agents.

Despite its similarity to epinephrine, NE has limited clinical applications. The only recognized indications are hypotensive states and cardiac arrest.

Isoproterenol

- *Receptor specificity:* β_1 and β_2
- *Chemical classification:* catecholamine

Isoproterenol (Isuprel) differs significantly from NE and epinephrine in that isoproterenol acts only at β-adrenergic receptors. Isoproterenol was the first β-selective agent employed clinically.

Therapeutic Uses

By activating β_1 receptors in the heart, isoproterenol can benefit patients with cardiovascular disorders. Specifically, it is used to manage AV heart block, to improve outcomes in cardiac arrest, and to increase cardiac output during shock.

Adverse Effects

Because isoproterenol does not activate α-adrenergic receptors, it produces fewer adverse effects than NE or epinephrine. The major undesired responses, caused by activating β_1 receptors in the heart, are *tachydysrhythmias* and *angina pectoris*. In patients with diabetes, isoproterenol can cause *hyperglycemia* by promoting β_2-mediated glycogenolysis.

Drug Interactions

The major drug interactions of isoproterenol are nearly identical to those of epinephrine. Effects are enhanced by MAO inhibitors and tricyclic antidepressants and reduced by β-adrenergic blocking agents. Like epinephrine, isoproterenol can cause dysrhythmias in patients receiving certain inhalation anesthetics.

Dopamine

- *Receptor specificity:* dopamine, β_1, and, at high doses, α_1
- *Chemical classification:* catecholamine

Receptor Specificity

Dopamine has *dose-dependent* receptor specificity. When administered in low therapeutic doses, dopamine acts on dopamine receptors only. At moderate therapeutic doses, dopamine activates β_1 receptors in addition to dopamine receptors. And at very high doses, dopamine activates α_1 receptors along with β_1 and dopamine receptors.

Therapeutic Uses

The major indication for dopamine is shock. Benefits derive from effects on the heart and renal blood vessels. By activating β_1 receptors in the heart, dopamine can increase cardiac output, improving tissue perfusion. By activating dopamine receptors in the kidney, dopamine can dilate renal blood vessels, improving renal perfusion; however, studies indicate that it is not effective in preventing acute renal failure. Moreover, at very high doses that activate α_1 receptors, vasoconstriction may decrease renal perfusion, overriding the effects of dopamine activation. Therefore monitoring urine output is an essential component of care for patients on this drug.

Dopamine is also indicated for the treatment of heart failure. Heart failure is characterized by reduced tissue perfusion secondary to reduced cardiac output. Dopamine can help alleviate symptoms by activating β_1 receptors on the heart, which increases myocardial contractility and thereby increases cardiac output.

Adverse Effects

The most common adverse effects of dopamine—*tachycardia, dysrhythmias,* and *anginal pain*—result from activation of β_1 receptors in the heart. Because of its cardiac actions, dopamine is contraindicated for patients with tachydysrhythmias or ventricular fibrillation. Because high concentrations of dopamine cause α_1 activation, extravasation may result in *necrosis* from localized vasoconstriction. Tissue injury can be minimized by local infiltration of phentolamine, an α-adrenergic antagonist.

Drug Interactions

MAO inhibitors can intensify the effects of dopamine on the heart and blood vessels. If a patient is receiving an MAO inhibitor, the dosage of dopamine must be reduced by at least 90%. Tricyclic antidepressants can also intensify dopamine's actions, but not to the extent seen with MAO inhibitors. Certain general anesthetics can sensitize the myocardium to stimulation by dopamine and other catecholamines, thereby increasing the risk for dysrhythmias. Diuretics can complement the beneficial effects of dopamine on the kidney.

Dobutamine

- *Receptor specificity:* β_1
- *Chemical classification:* catecholamine

Action and Uses

At therapeutic doses, dobutamine causes selective activation of β_1-adrenergic receptors. The only indication for the drug is heart failure.

Adverse Effects

The major adverse effect is tachycardia. Blood pressure and the electrocardiogram should be monitored closely.

Drug Interactions

Effects of dobutamine on the heart and blood vessels are intensified greatly by MAO inhibitors. Accordingly, in patients receiving an MAO inhibitor, dobutamine dosage must be reduced at least 90%. Concurrent use of tricyclic antidepressants may cause a moderate increase in the cardiovascular effects. Certain general anesthetics can sensitize the myocardium to stimulation by dobutamine, thereby increasing the risk for dysrhythmias.

Phenylephrine

- *Receptor specificity:* α_1
- *Chemical classification:* noncatecholamine

Phenylephrine (Neo-Synephrine, others) is a selective α_1 agonist. The drug can be administered locally to reduce nasal congestion and parenterally to elevate blood pressure. In addition, phenylephrine eye drops can be used to dilate the pupil. Also, phenylephrine can be coadministered with local anesthetics to delay anesthetic absorption.

Albuterol

- *Receptor specificity:* β_2
- *Chemical classification:* noncatecholamine

Therapeutic Uses

Albuterol (Proventil, Ventolin, VoSpire, others) is a drug of choice in the treatment of asthma. It can reduce airway resistance in asthma by causing β_2-mediated bronchodilation. Because albuterol is relatively selective for β_2 receptors, it produces much less activation of cardiac β_1 receptors than does isoproterenol. As a result, albuterol and other β_2-selective agents have replaced isoproterenol for the therapy of asthma. However, remember that receptor selectivity is only relative: if administered in large doses, albuterol will lose selectivity and will activate β_1 receptors as well as β_2 receptors. Accordingly, patients should be warned not to exceed recommended doses because doing so may cause undesired cardiac stimulation. Preparations and dosages for asthma are presented in Chapter 62.

Adverse Effects

Adverse effects are minimal at therapeutic doses. *Tremor* is most common. If dosage is excessive, albuterol can cause *tachycardia* by activating β_1 receptors in the heart.

Ephedrine

- *Receptor specificity:* α_1, α_2, β_1, β_2
- *Chemical classification:* noncatecholamine

Ephedrine is referred to as a mixed-acting drug because it activates adrenergic receptors by direct and indirect mechanisms. Direct activation results from the binding of the drug to α and β receptors. Indirect activation results from the release of NE from adrenergic neurons.

Owing to the development of more selective adrenergic agonists, uses for ephedrine are limited. By promoting β2-mediated bronchodilation, ephedrine can benefit patients with asthma. By activating a combination of α and β receptors, ephedrine can improve hemodynamic status in patients with shock. It may also be used to manage anesthesia-induced hypotension.

Because ephedrine activates the same receptors as epinephrine, both drugs share the same adverse effects: hypertension, dysrhythmias, angina, and hyperglycemia. In addition, because ephedrine can cross the blood-brain barrier, it can act in the CNS to cause insomnia.

All of the drugs presented here are also discussed in chapters that address specific applications (Table 15.4).

TABLE 15.4 Discussion of Adrenergic Agonists in Other Chapters

Drug Class	Discussion Topic	Chapter
α₁ agonists	Nasal congestion	63
	Ophthalmology	87
α₂ agonists	Hypertension	41
	Ophthalmology	87
β₁ agonists	Heart failure	42
β₂ agonists	Asthma	62
Amphetamines	Attention-deficit/hyperactivity disorder	31
	Substance use disorder	35
	Appetite suppression	68

16

Adrenergic Antagonists

Adrenergic antagonists cause direct blockade of adrenergic receptors. With one exception, all of the adrenergic antagonists produce *reversible* (competitive) blockade.

Unlike many adrenergic agonists, which act at both α- *and* β-adrenergic receptors, most adrenergic antagonists are more selective. As a result, the adrenergic antagonists can be neatly divided into two major groups (Table 16.1): (1) *α-adrenergic blocking agents* (drugs that produce selective blockade of α-adrenergic receptors); and (2) *β-adrenergic blocking agents* (drugs that produce selective blockade of β receptors).[a]

Our approach to the adrenergic antagonists mirrors the approach we took with the adrenergic agonists. We begin by discussing the therapeutic and adverse effects that can result from α- and β-adrenergic blockade, after which we discuss the individual drugs that produce receptor blockade.

It is much easier to understand responses to the adrenergic drugs if you first understand the responses to the activation of adrenergic receptors. If you have not yet mastered Table 12.3 in Chapter 12, you should do so now (or be prepared to consult the table as we proceed).

α-ADRENERGIC ANTAGONISTS

Therapeutic and Adverse Responses to α Blockade

In this section we discuss the beneficial and adverse responses that can result from the blockade of α-adrenergic receptors. Then, properties of individual α-blocking agents are discussed.

Therapeutic Applications of α Blockade

Most clinically useful responses to α-adrenergic antagonists result from blockade of α_1 receptors on blood vessels. Blockade of α_1 receptors in the bladder and prostate can help those with benign prostatic hyperplasia (BPH). Blockade of α_1 receptors in the eyes and blockade of α_2 receptors have no recognized therapeutic applications.

Essential hypertension. Hypertension can be treated with a variety of drugs, including the α-adrenergic antagonists. α antagonists lower blood pressure by causing vasodilation which results from blocking α_1 receptors on arterioles and veins. Dilation of arterioles reduces arterial pressure directly. Dilation of veins lowers arterial pressure by an indirect process: in response to venous dilation, return of blood to the heart decreases, thereby decreasing cardiac output, which in turn reduces arterial pressure. The role of α-adrenergic blockers in essential hypertension is discussed further in Chapter 41.

Reversal of toxicity from α_1 agonists. Overdose with an α-adrenergic agonist (e.g., epinephrine) can produce *hypertension* secondary to

excessive activation of α_1 receptors on blood vessels. When this occurs, blood pressure can be lowered by reversing the vasoconstriction with an α-blocking agent.

If an intravenous (IV) line containing an α agonist extravasates, necrosis can occur secondary to intense local vasoconstriction. By infiltrating the region with phentolamine (an α-adrenergic antagonist), we can block the vasoconstriction and thereby prevent injury.

Benign prostatic hyperplasia. BPH results from a proliferation of cells in the prostate gland. Symptoms include dysuria, increased frequency of daytime urination, nocturia, urinary hesitancy, urinary urgency, a sensation of incomplete voiding, and a reduction in the size and force of the urinary stream. All of these symptoms can be improved with drugs that block α_1 receptors. Benefits derive from reduced contraction of smooth muscle in the prostatic capsule and the bladder neck (trigone and sphincter). BPH and its treatment are discussed in Chapter 53.

Pheochromocytoma. A pheochromocytoma is a catecholamine-secreting tumor derived from cells of the sympathetic nervous system. These tumors are usually located in the adrenal medulla. If secretion of catecholamines (epinephrine, norepinephrine) is sufficiently great, persistent hypertension can result. The principal cause of hypertension is the activation of α_1 receptors on blood vessels, although the activation of β_1 receptors on the heart can also contribute. The preferred treatment is surgical removal of the tumor, but α-adrenergic blockers also may be employed.

α-blocking agents have two roles in managing pheochromocytoma. First, in patients with inoperable tumors, α blockers are given long term to suppress hypertension. Second, when surgery is indicated, α blockers are administered preoperatively to reduce the risk for acute hypertension during the procedure. This is necessary because manipulation of the tumor can cause massive catecholamine release.

Raynaud disease. Raynaud disease is a peripheral vascular disorder characterized by vasospasm in the toes and fingers. Prominent symptoms are local sensations of pain and cold. α blockers can suppress symptoms by preventing α-mediated vasoconstriction. However, it should be noted that although α blockers can relieve symptoms of Raynaud disease, they are generally ineffective against other peripheral vascular disorders that involve inappropriate vasoconstriction.

Adverse Effects of α Blockade

The most significant adverse effects of the α-adrenergic antagonists result from the blockade of α_1 receptors. Detrimental effects associated with α_2 blockade are minor.

Orthostatic hypotension. Orthostatic (postural) hypotension is the most serious adverse response to α-adrenergic blockade. This hypotension can reduce blood flow to the brain, causing dizziness, lightheadedness, and even syncope.

The cause of orthostatic hypotension is blockade of α receptors on *veins,* which reduces muscle tone in the venous wall. Because of reduced venous tone, blood tends to pool in veins when the

---

[a]Only two adrenergic antagonists—carvedilol and labetalol—act on both alpha *and* beta receptors.

TABLE 16.1 Receptor Specificity of Adrenergic Antagonists

Category	Drugs	Receptors Blocked
α-Adrenergic Blocking Agents		
Nonselective agents	Phenoxybenzamine	α_1, α_2
	Phentolamine	α_1, α_2
α_1-selective agents	Alfuzosin	α_1
	Doxazosin	α_1
	Prazosin	α_1
	Silodosin	α_1
	Tamsulosin	α_1
	Terazosin	α_1
β-Adrenergic Blocking Agents		
Nonselective agents	Carteolol	β_1, β_2
	Nadolol	β_1, β_2
	Pindolol	β_1, β_2
	Propranolol	β_1, β_2
	Sotalol	β_1, β_2
	Timolol	β_1, β_2
	Carvedilol	$\beta_1, \beta_2, \alpha_1$
	Labetalol	$\beta_1, \beta_2, \alpha_1$
β_1-selective agents	Acebutolol	β_1
	Atenolol	β_1
	Betaxolol	β_1
	Bisoprolol	β_1
	Esmolol	β_1
	Metoprolol	β_1
	Nebivolol	β_1

patient stands. As a result, return of blood to the heart is reduced, which decreases cardiac output, which in turn causes blood pressure to fall.

Patients should be informed about symptoms of orthostatic hypotension (e.g., lightheadedness or dizziness on standing) and be advised to sit or lie down if these occur. In addition, patients should be informed that orthostatic hypotension can be minimized by avoiding abrupt transitions from a supine or sitting position to an erect posture.

Reflex tachycardia. α-adrenergic antagonists can increase heart rate by triggering the baroreceptor reflex. This occurs because: (1) blockade of vascular α_1 receptors causes vasodilation; (2) vasodilation reduces blood pressure; and (3) baroreceptors sense the reduction in blood pressure and, in an attempt to restore normal pressure, initiate a reflex increase in heart rate via the autonomic nervous system. If necessary, reflex tachycardia can be suppressed with a β-adrenergic blocking agent.

Nasal congestion. α blockade can dilate the blood vessels of the nasal mucosa, producing nasal congestion.

Inhibition of ejaculation. Because activation of α_1 receptors is required for ejaculation (see Table 12.3), blockade of these receptors can cause sexual dysfunction. This form of dysfunction is reversible and resolves when the α blocker is withdrawn. If a patient deems the adverse sexual effects of α blockade unacceptable, a change in medication will be required. Because males may be reluctant to discuss such concerns, a tactful interview may be needed to discern whether drug-induced sexual dysfunction is discouraging adherence to the medication regimen.

Sodium retention and increased blood volume. By reducing blood pressure, α blockers can promote renal retention of sodium and water, thereby causing blood volume to increase. The steps in this process are as follows: (1) by reducing blood pressure, α_1 blockers decrease renal blood flow; (2) in response to reduced renal perfusion, the kidney excretes less sodium and water; and (3) the resultant retention of sodium and water increases blood volume. As a result, blood pressure is elevated, blood flow to the kidney is increased, and, as far as the kidney is concerned, all is well. Unfortunately, when α blockers are used to treat hypertension (which they often are), this compensatory elevation in blood pressure can negate beneficial effects. To prevent the kidney from "neutralizing" hypotensive actions, α-blocking agents are usually combined with a diuretic when used in patients with hypertension.

Adverse Effects of α_2 Blockade

The most significant adverse effect associated with an α_2 blockade is potentiation of the reflex tachycardia that can occur in response to the blockade of α_1 receptors. This effect occurs because peripheral α_2 receptors are located presynaptically and activation of these receptors inhibits norepinephrine release. Hence, if α_2 receptors are blocked, the release of norepinephrine will increase. Because the reflex tachycardia caused by the α_1 blockade is ultimately the result of increased firing of the sympathetic nerves to the heart, and because the α_2 blockade will cause each nerve impulse to release a greater amount of norepinephrine, the α_2 blockade will potentiate reflex tachycardia initiated by the blockade of α_1 receptors. Accordingly, drugs such as phentolamine, which block α_2 as well as α_1 receptors, cause greater reflex tachycardia than do drugs that block α_1 receptors only.

⊕ PATIENT-CENTERED CARE ACROSS THE LIFE SPAN

α-Adrenergic Antagonists

Life Stage	Patient Care Concerns
Children	α-blockers are not approved for use in children with the exceptions of OraVerse (the agent approved for reversal of local anesthesia following dental surgery) and phentolamine for the prevention of tissue damage that can occur with extravasation of intravenous vasopressors. Phenoxybenzamine has used off-label for treatment of hypertension due to pheochromocytoma in children.
Pregnant women	Alfuzosin, silodosin, and tamsulosin are not known to cause problems when taken during pregnancy; however, it is important to note that these three drugs are only approved for treatment of benign prostatic hyperplasia. The remaining α-adrenergic blockers have either caused concerns in animal studies or have been inadequately studied in pregnant women.
Breast-feeding women	Manufacturers of phenoxybenzamine and phentolamine recommend that women taking this drug not breastfeed due to inadequate studies and potential risks. Labeling for the remaining drugs in this class recommend exercising caution.
Older adults	Older adults are especially vulnerable to the first-dose effects of α blockers. α blockers are also associated with worsening of urinary incontinence in women and increases of syncope in both genders. Beers criteria specifically identifies the peripheral α_1 blockers doxazosin, prazosin, and terazosin as potentially inappropriate for older adults due to the high incidence of orthostatic hypotension. Commonly prescribed drugs, such as diuretics and central nervous system depressants, can cause additive adverse effects when given with α blockers.

Adrenergic Antagonists

α Adrenergic Antagonists
Prazosin (Minipress)

First-Generation β Blockers
Propranolol (Inderal LA, InnoPran XL)

Second-Generation β Blockers
Metoprolol (Lopressor, Toprol XL)

Properties of Individual α Blockers

Eight α-adrenergic antagonists are employed clinically. Because the α blockers often cause postural hypotension, therapeutic uses are limited.

As indicated in Table 16.1, the α-adrenergic blocking agents can be subdivided into two major groups. One group, represented by *prazosin*, contains drugs that produce *selective α₁ blockade.* The second group, represented by *phentolamine*, consists of *nonselective α blockers,* which block α_1 and α_2 receptors.

Prazosin

Actions and uses. Prazosin (Minipress), our prototype, is a competitive antagonist that produces selective blockade of α_1-adrenergic receptors. The results are dilation of arterioles and veins and relaxation of smooth muscle in the bladder neck (trigone and sphincter) and prostatic capsule. Prazosin is approved only for hypertension, but it can also benefit men with BPH.

Pharmacokinetics. Pharmacokinetics of prazosin and the remaining α-blockers is available in Table 16.2. Preparations and dosages are provided in Table 16.3.

Adverse effects. Blockade of α_1 receptors can cause *orthostatic hypotension, reflex tachycardia,* and *nasal congestion.* The most serious of these is hypotension. Patients should be educated about the symptoms of orthostatic hypotension and be advised to sit or lie down if they occur. Also, patients should be informed that orthostatic hypotension can be minimized by moving slowly when changing from a supine or sitting position to an upright position.

About 1% of patients lose consciousness 30 to 60 minutes after receiving their initial prazosin dose. This "first-dose" effect is the result of severe postural hypotension. To minimize the first-dose effect, the initial dose should be small (no more than 1 mg). Subsequent doses can be gradually increased with little risk for fainting. Patients who are starting treatment should be forewarned about the first-dose effect and advised to avoid driving and other hazardous activities for 12 to 24 hours. Administering the initial dose immediately before going to bed eliminates the risk for a first-dose effect.

Terazosin

Actions and uses. Like prazosin, terazosin is a selective, competitive antagonist at α_1-adrenergic receptors. The drug is approved for hypertension and BPH.

Adverse effects. Like other α-blocking agents, terazosin can cause orthostatic hypotension, reflex tachycardia, and nasal congestion. In addition, terazosin is associated with a high incidence (16%) of headache. As with prazosin, the first dose can cause profound hypotension. To minimize this first-dose effect, the initial dose should be administered at bedtime.

Doxazosin

Actions and uses. Doxazosin (Cardura, Cardura XL) is a selective, competitive inhibitor of α_1-adrenergic receptors. Immediate release forms of this drug are indicated for hypertension and BPH. Extended release doxazosin (Cardura XL) is approved for management of BPH only.

Adverse effects. Like prazosin and terazosin, doxazosin can cause orthostatic hypotension, reflex tachycardia, and nasal congestion. As with prazosin and terazosin, the first dose can cause profound hypotension, which can be minimized by giving the initial dose at bedtime.

Tamsulosin

Actions and uses. Tamsulosin (Flomax) is an α_1-adrenergic antagonist that causes "selective" blockade of α_1 receptors on the smooth muscle of the bladder neck (trigone and sphincter), prostatic capsule, and prostatic urethra; blockade of vascular α_1 receptors is weak. The drug is approved only for BPH. It is not useful for hypertension. In men with BPH, tamsulosin increases the urine flow rate and

TABLE 16.2 α-Adrenergic Antagonists: Pharmacokinetic Properties

Drugs	Route	Peak	Half-Life	Metabolism[a]	Excretion
Nonselective Agents					
Phenoxybenzamine	PO, IV	PO: 4–6 h	PO: unknown IV: 24	Hepatic	Urine (primary), Bile
Phentolamine	IM, IV, Local infiltration	IM: 30–45 min IV: 1–2 min	IM: unknown IV: 20 min	Hepatic	Urine
α₁-Selective Agents					
Alfuzosin	PO	8 h	10 h[b]	Hepatic	Feces
Doxazosin	PO	2–3 h	22 h[c]	Hepatic	Bile
Prazosin	PO	1–3 h	2–3 h	Hepatic	Bile
Silodosin	PO	3–6 h	13–24 h[c]	Hepatic	Feces (primary), Urine
Tamsulosin	PO	4–5 h (with food) 6–7 h (without food)	9–15 h[c]	Hepatic	Urine (primary), Feces
Terazosin	PO	1–2 h	9–12 h[c]	Hepatic	Bile (primary), Urine

[a]Primary mechanism of metabolism.
[b]80%–90% protein-bound.
[c]Greater than 90% protein-bound.
IN, Intramuscular; *IV,* intravenous; *PO,* per os (by mouth).

TABLE 16.3 α-Adrenergic Antagonists: Preparations and Dosage

Drug Name	Preparations	Dosage
Nonselective Agents		
Phenoxybenzamine (Dibenzyline)	Tablets: 10 mg	10 mg twice daily up to 20–40 mg 2–3 times daily
Phentolamine (OraVerse)	Sol: 5 mg/2 mL (concentrated) OraVerse: 0.4 mg/1.7 mL (Use of OraVerse is limited to reversal of anesthetic following dental surgery.)	Infiltration post IV extravasation: 5–10 mg diluted in 10 mL saline. To prevent hypertension during surgical excision of a pheochromocytoma: 5 mg (IM or IV) given 1–2 h before surgery.
α₁-Selective Agents		
Alfuzosin (ER) (Uroxatral)	Tablet: 10 mg	10 mg/day
Doxazosin (IR) (Cardura)	Tablets: 1, 2, 4, 8 mg	1–8 mg/day max: 16 mg/day
Doxazosin (ER) (Cardura XL)	Tablets: 4, 8 mg	4–8 mg/day
Prazosin (Minipress)	Tablets: 1, 2, 5 mg	1–2 mg 2–3 times daily up to 20 mg twice daily
Silodosin	Capsules: 4, 8 mg	8 mg/day
Tamsulosin (Flomax)	Capsules: 0.4 mg	0.4 mg/day
Terazosin (Hytrin)	Tablets: 1, 2, 5, 10 mg Capsules: 1, 2, 5, 10 mg	1–5 mg/day for hypertension 10 mg/day for BPH max: 20 mg

BPH, Benign prostatic hyperplasia; *ER,* extended release; *IM,* intramuscular; *IR,* immediate release; *IV,* intravenous; *max,* maximum dose; *NIOSH,* National Institute for Occupational Safety and Health; *Sol,* solution.

decreases the residual urine volume. Maximum benefits develop within 2 weeks.

Adverse effects. The most common adverse effects are headache and dizziness. Between 8% and 18% of patients experience abnormal ejaculation (ejaculation failure, ejaculation decrease, retrograde ejaculation). In addition, the drug is associated with increased incidence of rhinitis.

Drug interactions. Combined use with cimetidine increases tamsulosin serum levels, which may cause toxicity. Combined use with hypotensive drugs—including phosphodiesterase type 5 (PDE-5) inhibitors such as sildenafil (Viagra)—may cause a significant reduction in blood pressure.

Alfuzosin

Actions and uses. Like tamsulosin, alfuzosin (Uroxatral, Xatral ♣) is an α₁ blocker with selectivity for α₁ receptors in the prostate and urinary tract. At recommended doses, the blockade of α₁ receptors on blood vessels is weak. Therefore, alfuzosin is indicated only for BPH.

Adverse effects. Alfuzosin is generally well tolerated. The most common adverse effect is dizziness. Syncope and clinically significant hypotension are rare. Unlike tamsulosin, alfuzosin does not interfere with ejaculation.

Doses four times greater than recommended can prolong the QT interval and might thereby pose a risk for ventricular dysrhythmias. In patients with moderate to severe hepatic impairment, alfuzosin levels increase three- to fourfold, thus increasing the likelihood of ventricular rhythm disturbances. The drug is contraindicated for these patients.

Drug interactions. Levels of alfuzosin are markedly raised by powerful inhibitors of CYP3A4. Among these are erythromycin, clarithromycin, itraconazole, ketoconazole, nefazodone, and the HIV protease inhibitors, such as ritonavir. Concurrent use of alfuzosin with these drugs is contraindicated.

Although alfuzosin does not lower blood pressure much, combining it with other hypotensive agents could produce a more dramatic reduction. Accordingly, such combinations should be used with caution. Drugs of concern include organic nitrates, antihypertensive agents, and the PDE-5 inhibitors used for sexual dysfunction (e.g., sildenafil [Viagra]).

Silodosin

Actions and uses. Silodosin (Rapaflo) is an α-adrenergic antagonist that selectively blocks α₁ receptors in the prostate, bladder, and urethra. Blockade of vascular α receptors is weak. The drug is indicated only for BPH.

Adverse effects. Silodosin is generally well tolerated. However, like tamsulosin, silodosin can greatly reduce or eliminate release of semen during orgasm. This effect reverses when the drug is discontinued. Although blockade of vascular α receptors is usually minimal, silodosin can produce dizziness, lightheadedness, and nasal congestion.

Phentolamine

Actions and uses. Like prazosin, phentolamine (OraVerse, Rogitine ♣) is a competitive adrenergic antagonist. However, in contrast to prazosin, phentolamine blocks α₂ receptors as well as α₁ receptors. Phentolamine has three approved applications: (1) diagnosis and treatment of pheochromocytoma; (2) prevention of tissue necrosis after extravasation of drugs that produce α₁-mediated vasoconstriction (e.g., norepinephrine); and (3) reversal of soft tissue anesthesia. (Local anesthetics are often combined with epinephrine, which prolongs anesthetic action by causing α₁-mediated vasoconstriction. Phentolamine blocks epinephrine-mediated vasoconstriction and thereby increases local blood flow, which increases the rate of anesthetic removal.)

Adverse effects. Like prazosin, phentolamine can produce the typical adverse effects associated with α-adrenergic blockade: orthostatic hypotension, reflex tachycardia, nasal congestion, and inhibition of ejaculation. Because it blocks α₂ receptors, phentolamine produces greater reflex tachycardia than prazosin. If reflex tachycardia is especially severe, the heart rate can be reduced with a β blocker. Because tachycardia can aggravate angina pectoris and myocardial infarction (MI), phentolamine is contraindicated for patients with either disorder.

Overdose can produce profound hypotension. If necessary, blood pressure can be elevated with norepinephrine. Epinephrine should not be used because the drug can cause blood pressure to drop even further. In the presence of α₁ blockade, the ability of epinephrine to promote vasodilation (through the activation of vascular β₂ receptors) may outweigh the ability of epinephrine to cause vasoconstriction (through the activation of vascular α₁ receptors). Further lowering of blood pressure is not a significant problem with norepinephrine because norepinephrine does not activate β₂ receptors.

Phenoxybenzamine

Actions and uses. Phenoxybenzamine (Dibenzyline) is an old drug that, like phentolamine, blocks α₁ and α₂ receptors. However, unlike all of the other α-adrenergic antagonists, phenoxybenzamine is a noncompetitive receptor antagonist. Hence receptor blockade is not reversible. As a result, the effects of phenoxybenzamine are long lasting. (Responses to a single dose can persist for several days.) Effects subside as newly synthesized receptors replace the ones that have been irreversibly blocked. Phenoxybenzamine is approved only for pheochromocytoma.

Adverse effects. Like the other α-adrenergic antagonists, phenoxybenzamine can produce orthostatic hypotension, reflex tachycardia, nasal congestion, and inhibition of ejaculation. Reflex tachycardia is greater than that caused by prazosin and about equal to that caused by phentolamine.

If dosage is excessive, phenoxybenzamine, like phentolamine, will cause profound hypotension. Furthermore, because hypotension is the result of irreversible α₁ blockade, it cannot be corrected with an α₁ agonist. To restore blood pressure, patients must be given IV fluids, which elevate blood pressure by increasing blood volume.

PATIENT EDUCATION
α1-Adrenergic Antagonists

Forewarn patients about first-dose hypotension. Advise them to sit or lie down if dizziness or lightheadedness occurs on standing. Teach patients to move slowly when changing from a supine or sitting position to an upright posture. Urge them to avoid driving and other hazardous activities for 12–24 h after the initial dose. Reinforce the importance of taking the initial dose at bedtime to minimize the first-dose effect.

Outpatients need to be taught how to monitor heart rate and blood pressure. Instruct them to hold the drug and notify the provider if sustained bradycardia or hypotension develop.

SUMMARY OF KEY PRESCRIBING CONSIDERATIONS
α1-Adrenergic Antagonists

Therapeutic Goal: Manage hypertension (doxazosin, prazosin, terazosin) and reduce symptoms of BPH (doxazosin, terazosin, alfuzosin, silodosin, tamsulosin)

Baseline Data: Hypertension: Assess heart rate, blood pressure, ECG (if indicated by patient age and status), and general cardiovascular status; BPH: Determine the degree of nocturia, daytime frequency, hesitance, intermittency, terminal dribbling, urgency, impairment of size and force of urinary stream, dysuria, and sensation of incomplete voiding.

Monitoring: Heart rate, blood pressure, evaluation for adverse effects (with symptom-targeted assessment if indicated)

Identifying High-Risk Patients: The only contraindication is hypersensitivity to these drugs.

Evaluating Therapeutic Effects: Hypertension: Normalization of blood pressure; BPH: Improvement from baseline symptoms

Minimizing Adverse Effects: α₁ blockade can cause postural hypotension. Effects may be minimized by instructing patient to sit or lie down if these occur. Patients need to move slowly when changing from a supine or sitting position to an upright posture. The first dose (and, for some, the first few doses) may cause severe orthostatic hypotension. This can be minimized by prescribing the first doses to be taken at bedtime.

BPH, Benign prostatic hyperplasia; *ECG*, electrocardiogram.

β-ADRENERGIC ANTAGONISTS

Therapeutic and Adverse Responses to β Blockade

In this section we consider the beneficial and adverse responses that can result from blockade of β-adrenergic receptors. Then we examine the properties of individual β blockers.

Therapeutic Applications of β Blockade

Practically all of the therapeutic effects of the β-adrenergic antagonists result from the blockade of β₁ receptors in the heart. The major consequences of blocking these receptors are (1) reduced heart rate; (2) reduced force of contraction; and (3) reduced velocity of impulse conduction through the atrioventricular (AV) node. Because of these effects, β blockers are useful in a variety of cardiovascular disorders.

Angina pectoris. Angina pectoris occurs when oxygen supplied to the heart through coronary circulation is insufficient to meet cardiac oxygen demand. Anginal attacks can be precipitated by exertion, intense emotion, and other factors. β-adrenergic blockers are a mainstay of antianginal therapy. By blocking β₁ receptors in the heart, these drugs decrease cardiac workload. This reduces oxygen demand, bringing it back into balance with oxygen supply and thereby preventing ischemia and pain.

Hypertension. For years, β blockers were considered drugs of choice for hypertension. However, more recent data indicate that they are less beneficial than previously believed.

The exact mechanism by which β blockers reduce blood pressure is not known. Older proposed mechanisms include the reduction of cardiac output through blockade of β₁ receptors in the heart and suppression of renin release through the blockade of β₁ receptors in the kidney (see Chapter 38 for a discussion of the role of renin in blood pressure control). More recently, we have learned that, with long-term use, β blockers reduce peripheral vascular resistance, which could account for much of their antihypertensive effects.

Cardiac dysrhythmias. β-adrenergic blocking agents are especially useful for treating dysrhythmias that involve excessive electrical activity in the sinus node and atria. By blocking cardiac β₁ receptors, these drugs can (1) decrease the rate of sinus nodal discharge; and (2) suppress conduction of atrial impulses through the AV node, thereby preventing the ventricles from being driven at an excessive rate.

Myocardial infarction. As you know, an MI is a region of myocardial necrosis caused by localized interruption of blood flow to the heart wall. Treatment with a β blocker can reduce pain, infarct size, mortality, and the risk for reinfarction. To be effective, therapy with a β blocker must begin soon after an MI has occurred and should be continued for several years.

Reduction of perioperative mortality. β blockers may decrease the risk for mortality associated with noncardiac surgery in high-risk patients. In the DECREASE-IV trial, pretreatment with bisoprolol reduced the incidence of perioperative MI and death. However, for treatment to be both safe and effective, dosing should begin *early* (several days to weeks before surgery) and *doses should be low initially and then titrated up* (to achieve a resting heart rate of 60 to 80 beats/min). In addition, treatment should continue for 1 month after surgery. As shown in an earlier trial, known as POISE, if the β blocker is started *late* (just before surgery), and if the doses are *large*, such treatment can actually *increase* the risk for perioperative mortality.

Heart failure. β blockers are now considered standard therapy for heart failure. This application is relatively new and may come as a surprise to some readers because, until recently, heart failure was considered an absolute *contraindication* to β blockers. At this time, only three β blockers—carvedilol, bisoprolol, and metoprolol—have been shown effective for heart failure.

Hyperthyroidism. Hyperthyroidism is associated with an increase in the sensitivity of the heart to catecholamines (e.g., norepinephrine, epinephrine). As a result, normal levels of sympathetic activity to the heart can generate tachydysrhythmias and angina pectoris. The blockade of cardiac β₁ receptors suppresses these responses.

Migraine prophylaxis. When taken prophylactically, β-adrenergic blocking agents can reduce the frequency and intensity of migraine attacks. However, although β blockers are effective as prophylaxis, these drugs are not able to abort a migraine headache after it has begun. The mechanism by which β blockers prevent migraine is not known.

Performance anxiety. Public speakers and other performers sometimes experience performance anxiety ("stage fright"). Prominent symptoms are tachycardia, tremors, and sweating brought on by generalized discharge of the sympathetic nervous system. Some of you may experience similar symptoms when taking tests. β blockers help prevent performance anxiety—including test anxiety—by preventing β_1-mediated tachycardia.

Pheochromocytoma. As discussed earlier in the chapter, a pheochromocytoma secretes large amounts of catecholamines, which can cause excessive stimulation of the heart resulting in life-threatening hypertension. Cardiac stimulation can be prevented by a β_1 blockade.

Glaucoma. β blockers are important drugs for treating glaucoma, a condition characterized by elevated intraocular pressure with subsequent injury to the optic nerve. The group of β blockers used in glaucoma is different from the group of β blockers discussed here. Glaucoma treatment is discussed in Chapter 87.

Adverse Effects of β Blockade

Although therapeutic responses to β blockers are due almost entirely to the blockade of β_1 receptors, adverse effects involve both β_1 and β_2 blockade. Consequently, the nonselective β-adrenergic blocking agents (drugs that block both β_1 and β_2 receptors) produce a broader spectrum of adverse effects than do the "cardioselective" β-adrenergic antagonists (drugs that block only β_1 receptors at therapeutic doses).

All of the adverse effects of β_1 blockade are the result of blocking β_1 receptors in the heart. Blockade of renal β_1 receptors is not a concern.

Bradycardia. Blockade of cardiac β_1 receptors can produce bradycardia. If necessary, the heart rate can be increased using a β-adrenergic agonist, such as isoproterenol, and atropine (a muscarinic antagonist). Isoproterenol competes with the β blocker for cardiac β_1 receptors, thereby promoting cardiac stimulation. By blocking muscarinic receptors on the heart, atropine prevents slowing of the heart by the parasympathetic nervous system.

Reduced cardiac output. β_1 blockade can reduce cardiac output by decreasing the heart rate and the force of myocardial contraction. Because they can decrease cardiac output, *β blockers must be used with great caution in patients with heart failure or reduced cardiac reserve.* In both cases, any further decrease in cardiac output could result in insufficient tissue perfusion.

Precipitation of heart failure. In some patients, suppression of cardiac function with a β blocker can be so great as to cause heart failure. Patients should be informed about the early signs of heart failure (e.g., shortness of breath, night coughs, swelling of the extremities) and instructed to notify the prescriber if these occur. It is notable that, although β blockers can precipitate heart failure, they are also used to *treat* heart failure.

Atrioventricular heart block. AV heart block is defined as a delay in the conduction of electrical impulses through the AV node. In its most severe form, AV block prevents *all* atrial impulses from reaching the ventricles. Because the blockade of cardiac β_1 receptors can suppress AV conduction, the production of AV block is a potential complication of β-blocker therapy. These drugs are contraindicated for patients with preexisting AV block.

Rebound cardiac excitation. Long-term use of β blockers can sensitize the heart to catecholamines. As a result, if a β blocker is withdrawn *abruptly,* anginal pain or ventricular dysrhythmias may

develop. This phenomenon of increased cardiac activity in response to abrupt cessation of β-blocker therapy is referred to as *rebound excitation.* The risk for rebound excitation can be minimized by withdrawing these drugs gradually (e.g., by tapering the dosage over a period of 1 to 2 weeks). If rebound excitation occurs, dosing should be temporarily resumed. Patients should be warned against abrupt cessation of treatment. Also, they should be advised to carry an adequate supply of their β blocker when traveling.

Adverse effects of β_2 blockade

Bronchoconstriction. Blockade of β_2 receptors in the lungs can cause constriction of the bronchi. (Recall that activation of these receptors promotes bronchodilation.) For most people, the degree of bronchoconstriction is insignificant. However, when bronchial β_2 receptors are blocked in patients with asthma, the resulting increase in airway resistance can be life threatening. Accordingly, *drugs that block β_2 receptors are contraindicated for people with asthma.* If these individuals must use a β blocker, they should use an agent that is β_1 selective (e.g., metoprolol).

Hypoglycemia from inhibition of glycogenolysis. Epinephrine, acting at β_2 receptors in skeletal muscle and the liver, can stimulate glycogenolysis (breakdown of glycogen into glucose). β_2 blockade will inhibit this process, posing a risk for hypoglycemia in susceptible individuals. Although suppression of β_2-mediated glycogenolysis is inconsequential for most people, interference with this process can be detrimental to patients with *diabetes mellitus.* These people are especially dependent on β_2-mediated glycogenolysis as a way to overcome insulin-induced hypoglycemia. If the patient with diabetes requires a β blocker, a β_1-selective agent is preferable.

Adverse effects in neonates from β_1 and β_2 blockade. The use of β blockers during pregnancy can have residual effects on the newborn infant. Specifically, because β blockers can remain in the circulation for several days after birth, neonates may be at risk for bradycardia (from β_1 blockade), respiratory distress (from β_2 blockade), and hypoglycemia (from β_2 blockade). Accordingly, for 3 to 5 days after birth, newborns should be closely monitored for these effects. Adverse neonatal effects have been observed with at least one β blocker (betaxolol) and may be a risk with others as well.

Properties of Individual β Blockers

The β-adrenergic antagonists can be subdivided into three groups:

- *First-generation (nonselective) β blockers* (e.g., propranolol), which block β_1 and β_2 receptors
- *Second-generation (cardioselective) β blockers* (e.g., metoprolol), which produce selective blockade of β_1 receptors (at usual doses)
- *Third-generation (vasodilating) β blockers* (e.g., carvedilol), which act on blood vessels to cause dilation, but may produce nonselective or cardioselective β blockade

Our discussion of the individual β blockers focuses on two prototypes: propranolol and metoprolol.

Propranolol

Propranolol (Inderal LA, InnoPran XL), our prototype of the first-generation β blockers, produces a *nonselective* β blockade. That is, this drug blocks both β_1- and β_2-adrenergic receptors. Propranolol was the first β blocker to receive widespread clinical use and remains one of our most important β-blocking agents.

Pharmacologic effects. By blocking *cardiac* β_1 receptors, propranolol can *reduce the heart rate, decrease the force of ventricular contraction, and suppress impulse conduction through the AV node.* The net effect is a reduction in cardiac output.

By blocking *renal* β_1 receptors, propranolol can *suppress the secretion of renin.*

By blocking β_2 receptors, propranolol can produce three major effects: (1) *bronchoconstriction* (through β_2 blockade in the lungs); (2) *vasoconstriction* (through β_2 blockade on certain blood vessels); and (3) *reduced glycogenolysis* (through β_2 blockade in skeletal muscle and liver).

Pharmacokinetics. Propranolol is *highly lipid soluble*. Because of its ability to cross membranes, propranolol is widely distributed to all tissues and organs, including the central nervous system (CNS). Additional information on pharmacokinetics of propranolol and other β blockers is provided in Table 16.4.

Therapeutic uses. Practically all of the applications of propranolol are based on the blockade of β_1 receptors in the heart. The most important indications are *hypertension, angina pectoris, cardiac dysrhythmias,* and *myocardial infarction.* The role of propranolol and other β blockers in these disorders is discussed in Chapters 41, 43, 45, and 91. Additional indications include the prevention of migraine headache and the management of performance anxiety.

Adverse effects. The most serious adverse effects result from the blockade of β_1 receptors in the heart and the blockade of β_2 receptors in the lungs.

Bradycardia. β_1 blockade in the heart can cause bradycardia. If necessary, the heart rate can be increased by administering atropine and isoproterenol.

Atrioventricular heart block. By slowing conduction of impulses through the AV node, propranolol can cause AV heart block. The drug is contraindicated for patients with preexisting AV block (if the block is greater than first degree).

Heart failure. In patients with heart disease, suppression of myocardial contractility by propranolol can result in heart failure. Patients should be informed about the early signs of heart failure (shortness of breath on mild exertion or when lying supine, night coughs, swelling of the extremities, weight gain from fluid retention) and be instructed to notify the prescriber if these occur. Propranolol is generally contraindicated for patients with preexisting heart failure (although other β blockers are used to *treat* heart failure).

Rebound cardiac excitation. Abrupt withdrawal of propranolol can cause rebound excitation of the heart, resulting in tachycardia and ventricular dysrhythmias. This problem is especially dangerous for patients with preexisting cardiac ischemia. To avoid rebound excitation, propranolol should be withdrawn slowly by giving progressively smaller doses over 1 to 2 weeks. Patients should be warned against abrupt cessation of treatment. In addition, they should be advised to carry an adequate supply of propranolol when traveling.

Bronchoconstriction. The blockade of β_2 receptors in the lungs can cause bronchoconstriction. As a rule, increased airway resistance is hazardous only to patients with asthma and other obstructive pulmonary disorders.

Inhibition of glycogenolysis. The blockade of β_2 receptors in skeletal muscle and the liver can inhibit glycogenolysis. This effect can be dangerous for people with diabetes, as discussed previously in this chapter.

Central nervous system effects. Because of its lipid solubility, propranolol can readily cross the blood–brain barrier and hence has ready access sites in the CNS. However, although propranolol is reputed to cause a variety of CNS reactions—depression, insomnia, nightmares, and hallucinations—these reactions are, in fact, very rare. Because of the possible risk for depression, prudence dictates avoiding propranolol in patients who already have this disorder.

Effects in neonates. Propranolol crosses the placental barrier. Using propranolol and potentially, some other β blockers (except labetalol) during pregnancy may put the neonate at risk for bradycardia, respiratory distress, and hypoglycemia. Neonates should be closely monitored for these effects. The American College of Obstetricians and Gynecologists recommend labetalol as one of three drugs of first choice for the

TABLE 16.4 β-Adrenergic Antagonists: Pharmacokinetics and Pharmacologic Properties

Generic Name	ISA	Lipid Solubility	Peak	Half-Life (Adults)	Metabolism	Excretion
First Generation: Nonselective β Blockers						
Nadolol	0	Low	3–4 h	20–24 h	Not Metabolized	Urine (unchanged drug)
Pindolol	+++	Moderate	1 h	3–4 h	Hepatic	Urine
Propranolol	0	High	1–4 h	3–5 h	Hepatic	Urine
Sotalol	0	High	2.5–4 h	12 h	None	Urine (unchanged drug)
Timolol	0	Low	1–2 h	4 h	Hepatic	Urine
Second Generation: Cardioselective β Blockers						
Acebutolol	+	Moderate	2–4 h	Drug: 3–4 h Metabolite: 8–13 h		Feces (primary), Urine
Atenolol	0	Low	2–4 h	6–9 h	Hepatic	Feces (primary), Urine
Betaxolol	0	Low	1.5–6 h	14–22 h	Hepatic	Urine
Bisoprolol	0	Moderate	2–4 h	9–12 h	Hepatic	Urine
Esmolol	0	Low	1–2 min	Drug: 9 min Metabolite: 3–4 h	Red cell esterases	Urine
Metoprolol	0	High	IV: 20 min PO: 1–2 h	3–7 h	Hepatic	Urine
Third Generation: β Blockers With Vasodilating Actions						
Carvedilol	0	Moderate	1–2 h	5–11 h	Hepatic	Feces (primary), Urine
Labetalol	0	Low	IV: 5–15 min PO: 2–4 min	6–8 h	Hepatic	Urine (primary), Feces
Nebivolol	0	High	1.5–4 h	12–19 h	Hepatic	Urine (primary), Feces

ISA, Intrinsic sympathomimetic activity (partial agonist activity); *IV,* intravenous; *PO,* per os (by mouth).

management of hypertension in pregnant women. (The others are methyldopa, a centrally-acting α_2 agonist, and nifedipine, a calcium channel blocker.)

Precautions, warnings, and contraindications

Severe allergy. Propranolol should be avoided in patients with a history of severe allergic reactions (anaphylaxis). Recall that epinephrine, the drug of choice for anaphylaxis, relieves symptoms in large part by activating β_1 receptors in the heart and β_2 receptors in the lungs. If these receptors are blocked by propranolol, the ability of epinephrine to help will be impaired.

Diabetes Mellitus. Propranolol can be detrimental to patients with diabetes mellitus in two ways. First, by blocking β_2 receptors in muscle and liver, propranolol can suppress glycogenolysis, thereby eliminating an important mechanism for correcting insulin-induced hypoglycemia. Second, by blocking β_1 receptors, propranolol can suppress tachycardia, tremors, and perspiration, which normally serve as an early warning signal that blood glucose levels are falling too low. By "masking" symptoms of hypoglycemia, propranolol can delay awareness of hypoglycemia, thereby compromising the patient's ability to correct the problem in a timely fashion. Patients with diabetes who take propranolol should be warned that these common symptoms may no longer be a reliable indicator of hypoglycemia. In addition, they should be taught to recognize alternative symptoms (e.g., hunger, fatigue, poor concentration) that blood glucose is falling perilously low.

Cardiac, respiratory, and psychiatric disorders. Propranolol can exacerbate *heart failure, AV heart block, sinus bradycardia, asthma,* and *bronchospasm.* Accordingly, the drug is contraindicated for patients with these disorders. In addition, propranolol should be used with caution in patients with a history of *depression.*

Drug interactions. Calcium channel blockers. The cardiac effects of two calcium channel blockers—verapamil and diltiazem—are identical to those of propranolol: reduction of heart rate, suppression of AV conduction, and suppression of myocardial contractility. When propranolol is combined with either of these drugs, excessive cardiosuppression may result.

Insulin. As discussed previously, propranolol can impede early recognition of insulin-induced hypoglycemia. In addition, propranolol can block glycogenolysis, the body's mechanism for correcting hypoglycemia.

General dosing considerations. Establishing an effective propranolol dosage is difficult for two reasons: (1) patients vary widely in their requirements for propranolol; and (2) there is a poor correlation between blood levels of propranolol and therapeutic responses. The explanation for these observations is that responses to propranolol are dependent on the activity of the sympathetic nervous system. If sympathetic activity is high, then the dose needed to reduce receptor activation will be high. Conversely, if sympathetic activity is low, then low doses will usually be sufficient to produce receptor blockade. Because sympathetic activity varies among patients, propranolol requirements also vary. Accordingly, the dosage must be adjusted by monitoring the patient's response rather than relying on dosing information in a drug reference. Typical dosing for propranolol and other β blockers is provided in Table 16.6.

Metoprolol

Metoprolol (Lopressor, Toprol XL), our prototype of the second-generation β blockers, produces the selective blockade of β_1 receptors in the heart. At usual therapeutic doses, the drug does not cause β_2 blockade. However, selectivity for β_1 receptors is not absolute: at higher doses, metoprolol and the other cardioselective agents will block β_2 receptors as well. Because their effects on β_2 receptors are normally minimal, cardioselective agents are not likely to cause

bronchoconstriction or hypoglycemia. Accordingly, these drugs are preferred to the nonselective β blockers for patients with asthma or diabetes.

Pharmacologic effects. By blocking cardiac β_1 receptors, metoprolol has the same impact on the heart as propranolol: it reduces heart rate, force of contraction, and conduction velocity through the AV node. Also, like propranolol, metoprolol reduces the secretion of renin by the kidney. In contrast to propranolol, metoprolol does not block bronchial β_2 receptors at usual doses and therefore does not increase airway resistance.

Pharmacokinetics. Metoprolol is very lipid soluble and, like propranolol, is widely distributed. See Table 16.4 for additional information on pharmacokinetics.

Therapeutic uses. The primary indication for metoprolol is *hypertension.* The drug is also approved for *angina pectoris, heart failure,* and *myocardial infarction.*

Adverse effects. Major adverse effects involve the heart. Like propranolol, metoprolol can cause *bradycardia, reduced cardiac output, AV heart block,* and *rebound cardiac excitation after abrupt withdrawal.* Also, even though metoprolol is approved for *treating* heart failure, it can *cause* heart failure if used incautiously. In contrast to propranolol, metoprolol causes minimal bronchoconstriction and does not interfere with β_2-mediated glycogenolysis.

Precautions, warnings, and contraindications. Like propranolol, metoprolol is contraindicated for patients with *sinus bradycardia* and *AV block greater than first degree.* In addition, it should be used with great care in patients with *heart failure.* Because metoprolol produces only minimal blockade of β_2 receptors, the drug is safer than propranolol for patients with asthma or a history of severe allergic reactions. In addition, because metoprolol does not suppress β_2-mediated glycogenolysis, it can be used more safely than propranolol by patients with diabetes. However, please note that metoprolol, like propranolol, will mask common signs and symptoms of hypoglycemia, thereby depriving the patient with diabetes of an early indication that hypoglycemia is developing.

Other β-Adrenergic Blockers

In the United States, 16 β blockers are approved for cardiovascular disorders (hypertension, angina pectoris, cardiac dysrhythmias, MI). Principal differences among these drugs concern receptor specificity, pharmacokinetics, indications, side effects, intrinsic sympathomimetic activity (ISA), and the ability to cause vasodilation.

In addition to the agents used for cardiovascular disorders, there is a group of β blockers used for glaucoma (see Chapter 87).

Receptor specificity. With regard to receptor specificity, β blockers fall into two groups: nonselective agents and cardioselective agents. The nonselective agents block β_1 *and* β_2 receptors, whereas the cardioselective agents block β_1 receptors only when prescribed at usual doses. Because of their limited side effects, the cardioselective agents are preferred for patients with asthma or diabetes. Two β blockers—*labetalol* and *carvedilol*—differ from all the others in that they block α-adrenergic receptors in addition to β receptors. The receptor specificity of individual β blockers is indicated in Table 16.1.

Pharmacokinetics. Pharmacokinetic properties of the β blockers are shown in Table 16.4. The relative lipid solubility of these agents is of particular importance. The drugs with high solubility (e.g., propranolol, metoprolol) have two prominent features: (1) they penetrate the blood-brain barrier with ease; and (2) they are eliminated primarily by hepatic metabolism. Conversely, the drugs with low lipid solubility (e.g., nadolol, atenolol) penetrate the blood-brain barrier poorly and are eliminated primarily by renal excretion.

PATIENT-CENTERED CARE ACROSS THE LIFE SPAN

Adrenergic Antagonists

Life Stage	Patient Care Concerns
Children	These drugs are commonly used in children. Typical monitoring for adverse effects is needed.
Pregnant women	Some β blockers have been associated with decreased intrauterine growth. They may cause decreased heart rate in both the fetus and neonate. Neonates born to women taking β blockers may experience hypoglycemia. Risks must be compared to benefits, which include that untreated dysrhythmias and hypertension also create risks for the fetus and neonate. Acebutolol, labetalol, pindolol, and sotalol are considered safest when taken during pregnancy and, of these, labetalol is a drug of first choice for the management of hypertension in pregnant patients.
Breastfeeding women	β-blockers may enter breast milk in varying amounts; those that are more lipid soluble can cross into breast milk in greater quantities. Betaxolol is more extensively excreted into breast milk than other β blockers. When a β blocker is necessary, it may be better to prescribe an alternate β-blocking agent when prescribing to breastfeeding mothers. There are no contraindications to breastfeeding; however, caution and close monitoring of breastfed infants is recommended.
Older adults	β-blockers are commonly prescribed for older adults. As with most drugs for this age group, attention should be paid to hepatic and renal function; if function is decreased, impaired metabolism and elimination by these pathways may result in increased drug levels.

BLACK BOX WARNING

Sotalol (Betapace, Betapace AF)

When starting or restarting sotalol, patients should be in a facility that can provide continuous electrocardiogram monitoring and cardiopulmonary resuscitation for a minimum of 3 days to minimize problems associated with induced arrhythmia.

Creatinine clearance should be established before initiating this drug.

Betapace cannot be substituted for Betapace AF when treating atrial fibrillation.

Therapeutic uses. Principal indications for the β-adrenergic blockers are *hypertension, angina pectoris,* and *cardiac dysrhythmias.* Other uses include prophylaxis of *migraine headache,* treatment of *myocardial infarction,* symptom suppression in individuals with *situational anxiety* (e.g., stage fright), and treatment of *heart failure* (see Chapter 42). Approved and off-label uses of the β blockers are shown in Table 16.5. Preparations and dosages are presented in Table 16.6.

Esmolol and *sotalol* differ from the other β blockers in that they are not used for hypertension. Because of its very short half-life (15 minutes), *esmolol* is clearly unsuited for treating hypertension, which

requires the maintenance of blood levels throughout the day, every day, for an indefinite time. The only approved indication for esmolol is emergency IV therapy of *supraventricular tachycardia. Sotalol* is approved for *ventricular dysrhythmias* and for the maintenance of normal sinus rhythm in patients who previously experienced symptomatic atrial fibrillation or atrial flutter. Esmolol and sotalol are discussed in Chapter 43.

Adverse effects. By blocking β_1 receptors in the heart, all of the β blockers can cause *bradycardia, AV heart block,* and, rarely, *heart failure.* By blocking β_2 receptors in the lung, the nonselective agents can cause significant *bronchoconstriction* in patients with asthma or chronic obstructive pulmonary disease. In addition, by blocking β_2 receptors in the liver and skeletal muscle, the *nonselective* agents can *inhibit glycogenolysis,* compromising the ability of patients with diabetes to compensate for insulin-induced hypoglycemia. Because of their ability to block α-adrenergic receptors, *carvedilol* and *labetalol* can cause *postural hypotension.*

Although *CNS effects* (insomnia, depression) can occur with all β blockers, these effects are rare and are most likely with the more lipid-soluble agents. Abrupt discontinuation of any β blocker can produce *rebound cardiac excitation.* Accordingly, all β blockers should be withdrawn slowly (by tapering the dosage over 1 to 2 weeks).

Intrinsic sympathomimetic activity (partial agonist activity). The term *intrinsic sympathomimetic activity* refers to the ability of certain β blockers—especially *pindolol*—to act as *partial agonists* at β-adrenergic receptors. (A partial agonist is a drug that, when bound to a receptor, produces a limited degree of receptor activation while preventing strong agonists from binding to that receptor to cause full activation.)

In contrast to other β blockers, agents with ISA have very little effect on the resting heart rate and cardiac output. When patients are at rest, stimulation of the heart by the sympathetic nervous system is low. If an ordinary β blocker is given, it will block sympathetic stimulation, causing the heart rate and cardiac output to decline. However, if a β blocker has ISA, its own ability to cause limited receptor activation will compensate for blocking receptor activation by the sympathetic nervous system, and, consequently, resting heart rate and cardiac output are not reduced. A comparison of ISA activity among β blockers is included in Table 16.4.

Because of their ability to provide a low level of cardiac stimulation, β blockers with ISA are preferred to other β blockers for use in patients with bradycardia. Conversely, these agents should not be given to patients with MI because their ability to cause even limited cardiac stimulation can be detrimental.

Vasodilation. The third-generation β blockers—*carvedilol, labetalol,* and *nebivolol*—can dilate blood vessels. Two mechanisms are employed: carvedilol and labetalol block vascular α_1 receptors; nebivolol promotes synthesis and the release of nitric oxide from the vascular epithelium. The exact clinical benefit of vasodilation by these drugs has not been clarified.

All of the drugs presented in this chapter are also discussed in chapters that address specific applications (Table 16.7).

BLACK BOX WARNING:

Atenolol, Metoprolol, Nadolol, Timolol

Abrupt discontinuation may cause exacerbation of angina and increases the risk for myocardial infarction.

TABLE 16.5　β-Adrenergic Blocking Agents: Summary of Therapeutic Uses

	Hypertension	Angina Pectoris	Myocardial Infarction or Prophylaxis	Cardiac Dysrhythmia/Rate Control	Heart Failure	Glaucoma	Migraine Prophylaxis	Hyperthyroidism/Thyrotoxicosis	Performance Anxiety	Tremor or Movement Disorder
First Generation: Nonselective β Blockers										
Carteolol	A					A				
Nadolol	A	A		O			O	O		
Pindolol	A	O[a]		O						
Propranolol	A	A	A	A			A	O	O	O
Sotalol			A	A						
Timolol	A	A	A	O		A	A			
Second Generation: Cardioselective β Blockers										
Acebutolol	A	O		A						
Atenolol	A	A	A	O				O		
Betaxolol	A	O		O		A				
Bisoprolol	A	O		O	O					
Esmolol				A				O		
Metoprolol	A	A	A	O	A		O	O		
Third Generation: β Blockers With Vasodilating Actions										
Carvedilol	A	O		O						
Labetalol	A									
Nebivolol	A								O	O

[a]Approved for use in Canada but not in the United States.
A, U.S. Food and Drug Administration–approved use; O, off-label use.

TABLE 16.6   β-Adrenergic Antagonists: Preparations and Dosage[a]

Drug Name	Preparations	Typical Dosage Range[b]
First Generation: Nonselective β Blockers		
Nadolol (Corgard)	Tablets: 20, 40, 80 mg	40–80 mg/day; max 240 mg/day
Pindolol (Visken)	Tablets: 5, 10, 15 mg	10–40 mg/day; max 60 mg/day
Propranolol (IR)	Tablets: 10, 20, 40, 60, 80 mg	Tablets: 60–120 mg twice daily
(generic only)	IV sol: 1 mg/mL	IV sol: highly individualizing; typically begins at 1–3 mg
Propranolol (ER) (Inderal LA, InnoPran XL)	Capsules: 60, 80, 120, 160 mg	80–120 mg/day; max 120 mg/day
Sotalol (Betapace, Betapace AF, Sorine)	Tablets: 80, 120, 160, 240 mg	Tablets: 80–120 mg twice daily; max 160 mg twice daily
	IV sol: 150 mg/10 mL	IV sol: 112.5 mg twice daily; max 300 mg/day
Timolol (Blocadren)	Tablets: 5, 10, 20 mg	10–20 mg twice daily; max 60 mg/day
Second Generation: Cardioselective β Blockers		
Acebutolol (Sectral)	Tablets: 100, 200, 400 mg	400–800 mg/day; max 1200 mg/day
Atenolol (Tenormin)	Tablets: 25, 50, 100 mg	25–50 mg/day; max 100 mg/day
Betaxolol (Kerlone)	Tablets: 10, 20 mg	PO: 10–20 mg/day; max 20 mg
Bisoprolol (Zebeta)	Tablets: 5, 10 mg	5–10 mg/day
Esmolol (Brevibloc)	Sol: 100 mg/10 mL; 200 mg/200 mL NaCl; 2500 mg/250 mL NaCl	Individualized
Metoprolol Tartrate (IR) (Lopressor, Betaloc)	Tablets: 25, 37.5, 50, 75, 100 mg	PO: 50–100 mg/day; max 200 mg/day
	IV sol: 1 mt/mL in 5 mL, 5 mg/5 mL in 5 mL	IV: 1.25–5 mg 2–4 times daily
Metoprolol Succinate (ER) (Toprol XL, Betaloc CR)	Tablets: 25, 50, 100, 200 mg	100 mg/day; max 400 mg/day
Third Generation: β Blockers With Vasodilating Actions		
Carvedilol (IR) (Coreg)	Tablets: 3.125, 6.25, 12.5. 25 mg	6.5–25 mg twice daily; max 25 mg twice daily
Carvedilol (ER) (Coreg CR)	Capsules: 10, 20, 40, 80 mg	20–40 mg/day; max 80 mg/day
Labetalol (Trandate)	Tablets: 100, 200, 300 mg	100–300 mg twice daily
	IV sol: 5 mg/mL in 4, 20, 40 mL	
Nebivolol (Bystolic)	Tablets: 2.5, 5, 10, 20 mg	5–20 mg/day; max 40 mg/day

[a]Ophthalmic preparations are covered in Chapter 87.
[b]Dosage may vary depending on treatment purpose.
ER, Extended release; *IR*, immediate release; *IV*, intravenous; *max*, maximum dosage; *PO*, per os (by mouth); *sol*, solution.

TABLE 16.7   Discussion of Adrenergic Antagonists in Other Chapters

Drug Class	Discussion Topic	Chapter
α-Adrenergic Blocking Agents		
Nonselective agents	Vasodilators	40
α₁-selective agents	Vasodilators	40
	Hypertension	41
	Benign prostatic hypertrophy	53
β-Adrenergic Blocking Agents		
Nonselective agents	Migraine headache	25
	Hypertension	41
	Dysrhythmias	43
	Angina	45
	Glaucoma	87
β₁-selective agents	Migraine headache	25
	Hypertension	41
	Heart failure	42
	Dysrhythmias	43
	Angina	45
	Myocardial infarction	91

PATIENT EDUCATION
β Blockers

β₁ blockade can mask early signs and symptoms of hypoglycemia by preventing common tachycardia, tremors, and perspiration. Warn patients with diabetes that tachycardia, tremors, and perspiration cannot be relied on as indicators of impending hypoglycemia, and teach them to recognize other indicators (e.g., hunger, fatigue, poor concentration) that blood glucose is falling dangerously low.

Inform patients about early signs of heart failure (shortness of breath, night coughs, swelling of the extremities), and instruct them to notify the provider if these occur.

Warn patients against abruptly discontinuing β blockers because this may cause tachycardia and other dysrhythmias. Advise patients, when traveling, to carry an adequate supply of medication plus a copy of their prescription.

SUMMARY OF KEY PRESCRIBING CONSIDERATIONS

β-*Adrenergic Antagonists*

Therapeutic Goal: Principal indications are hypertension, angina pectoris, heart failure, and cardiac dysrhythmias. Indications for individual agents are shown in Table 16.5.

Baseline Data: Heart rate, blood pressure (supine, sitting, and standing depending on patient status), ECG (if indicated by patient age and status), and general cardiovascular status

Monitoring: Heart rate, blood pressure, evaluation for adverse effects (with symptom-focused assessment if indicated). Advise patients to record the incidence, circumstances, and severity of any symptoms that may indicate inadequate control of symptoms for which the drug is given (e.g., angina) or a new onset of adverse effects.

Identifying High-Risk Patients: β blockers are contraindicated for patients with sinus bradycardia or AV heart block greater than first degree and must be used with great caution in patients with heart failure. Use with caution (especially the nonselective agents) in patients with asthma, bronchospasm, diabetes, or a history of severe allergic reactions. Use all β blockers with caution in patients with a history of depression and in patients taking calcium channel blockers.

Evaluating Therapeutic Effects: Evaluate for improvement of indication for which the drug was prescribed.

Minimizing Adverse Effects:

- β_1 blockade can reduce heart rate; decrease dosage if bradycardia is sustained.
- β_1 blockade can decrease AV conduction; carefully weigh benefits versus risks if first degree AV block develops and discontinue β blockers for patients who develop AV block greater than first degree.

- Suppression of myocardial contractility can cause heart failure; development of signs or symptoms of heart failure (e.g., shortness of breath, orthopnea, and peripheral edema) may require medication adjustment or discontinuation.
- Abrupt withdrawal of β blockers can cause tachycardia and ventricular dysrhythmias; taper off gradually when discontinuing this drug.
- By blocking α-adrenergic receptors, *carvedilol* and *labetalol* can cause postural hypotension; these effects may be minimized by having patients move slowly when changing from a supine or sitting position to an upright posture and by having them sit or lie down if they feel lightheaded.
- β_2 blockade can cause substantial airway constriction in patients with asthma; cardioselective drugs should be preferentially prescribed for patients with asthma and other respiratory problems.
- β_1 blockade can mask early signs and symptoms of hypoglycemia by preventing common tachycardia, tremors, and perspiration; patients will need to rely on indicators such as hunger and poor concentration to identify hypoglycemia. It may be necessary to monitor fingerstick glucose more closely until recognition is well established.
- β_2 blockade can prevent glycogenolysis—an emergency means of increasing blood glucose. Patients may need to reduce their insulin dosage. Cardioselective β blockers are preferred to nonselective agents in patients with diabetes.
- Maternal use of betaxolol during pregnancy may cause bradycardia, respiratory distress, and hypoglycemia in the infant; Accordingly, for 3–5 days after birth, newborns should be closely monitored for these effects. (β blockers other than betaxolol may pose a similar risk.)
- Rarely, β blockers cause depression, insomnia, and nightmares; switching to a β blocker with low lipid solubility may help (see Table 16.4).

AV, Atrioventricular; *ECG*, electrocardiogram.

17

Indirect-Acting Antiadrenergic Agents

The indirect-acting antiadrenergic agents are drugs that prevent the activation of peripheral adrenergic receptors by mechanisms that do not involve direct interaction with peripheral receptors. These drugs, the *centrally acting α_2 agonists,* act within the central nervous system (CNS) to reduce the outflow of impulses along sympathetic neurons.[a] The pharmacologic effects of the indirect-acting adrenergic blocking agents are very similar to those of drugs that block adrenergic receptors directly. Their primary use is for hypertension.

CENTRALLY ACTING α_2 AGONISTS

The mechanism by which an adrenergic agonist acts as an antiadrenergic agent requires an understanding of presynaptic and postsynaptic receptors. α_2 receptors in the CNS are located on *presynaptic* nerve terminals. As norepinephrine (NE) accumulates in the synapse, it activates α_2 receptors. This activation signals that adequate NE is available (Fig. 17.1). As a result, synthesis of NE is decreased. The decrease of available NE results in vasodilation, which in turn decreases blood pressure.

Why are we discussing centrally acting drugs in a unit on peripheral nervous system pharmacology? Because the effects of these drugs are ultimately the result of decreased activation of α- and β-adrenergic receptors in the periphery. That is, by inhibiting the firing of sympathetic neurons, the centrally acting agents decrease the release of NE from sympathetic nerves and thereby decrease activation of peripheral adrenergic receptors. Therefore, although these drugs act within the CNS Because of this action, their effects are like those of the direct-acting adrenergic receptor blockers even though they act within the CNS.

PROTOTYPE

Centrally Acting α_2 Agonists

Clonidine

Clonidine

Clonidine (Catapres, Catapres-TTS, Duraclon, Kapvay, Dixarit ♦) is a centrally acting α_2 agonist with three approved indications: *hypertension, severe pain,* and *attention-deficit/hyperactivity disorder (ADHD).* The use for hypertension is discussed here. The use against pain is discussed in Chapter 24. The use in ADHD management is discussed in Chapter 31.

[a]A second class of indirect-acting adrenergic blocking agents, the adrenergic neuron-blocking agents, represented by reserpine, is no longer available in the United States.

PATIENT EDUCATION

Clonidine

Advise the patient to take the major portion of the daily dose at bedtime to minimize daytime sedation. For transdermal clonidine, instruct the patient to apply transdermal patches to hairless, intact skin on the upper arm or torso, and to apply a new patch every 7 days. Additionally, because patches contain metal, they must be removed prior to magnetic resonance imaging (MRI).

Have the patient record their blood pressure daily and call the clinic if hypotension develops. Warn patients against abruptly discontinuing this drug because this may cause tachycardia and other dysrhythmias. Advise patients, when traveling, to carry an adequate supply of medication plus a copy of their prescription.

Inform patients about possible CNS depression. Warn them to avoid hazardous activities if alertness is reduced.

Dry mouth can be significant. Inform patients that discomfort can be reduced by chewing sugarless chewing gum, sucking hard candy, and taking frequent sips of fluids.

Inform patients about the potential for rebound hypertension. Advise them to refill their prescription promptly so that they do not run out of medication and warn them not to discontinue clonidine without consulting the prescriber.

Mechanism of Antihypertensive Action

Clonidine is an α_2-adrenergic agonist that causes selective activation of α_2 receptors in the CNS—specifically, in brainstem areas associated with autonomic regulation of the cardiovascular system. By activating central α_2 receptors, clonidine reduces sympathetic outflow to blood vessels and to the heart (see Fig. 17.1).

Pharmacologic Effects

The most significant effects of clonidine concern the heart and vascular system. By suppressing the firing of sympathetic nerves to the heart, clonidine can cause *bradycardia* and *a decrease in cardiac output.* By suppressing the sympathetic regulation of blood vessels, the drug promotes *vasodilation.* The net result of cardiac suppression and vasodilation is *decreased blood pressure.* Blood pressure is reduced in both supine and standing subjects. Because the hypotensive effects of clonidine are not posture dependent, orthostatic hypotension is minimal.

Pharmacokinetics

Clonidine is very lipid soluble. As a result, the drug is readily absorbed after oral dosing and is widely distributed throughout the body, including the CNS. Hypotensive responses begin 30 to 60 minutes after administration. Additional pharmacokinetic information for Clonidine and other centrally acting α_2 agonists is provided in Table 17.1.

Therapeutic Uses

As mentioned earlier, clonidine has three *approved* applications: treatment of hypertension (its main use), relief of severe cancer-related pain, and management of ADHD. It has been used off-label for treating pain, managing opioid and methadone withdrawal, facilitating smoking cessation, treating conduct disorder and oppositional defiant disorder in children, and treating Tourette syndrome—a CNS disease characterized by uncontrollable tics and verbal outbursts that are frequently obscene.

Adverse Effects

Drowsiness. CNS depression is common. About 35% of patients experience drowsiness; an additional 8% experience outright sedation. These responses become less intense with continued drug use. Patients in their early weeks of treatment should be advised to avoid hazardous activities if alertness is impaired.

Xerostomia. Xerostomia is common, occurring in about 40% of patients. The reaction usually diminishes over the first 2 to 4 weeks of therapy. Although not dangerous, xerostomia can be annoying enough to discourage drug use.

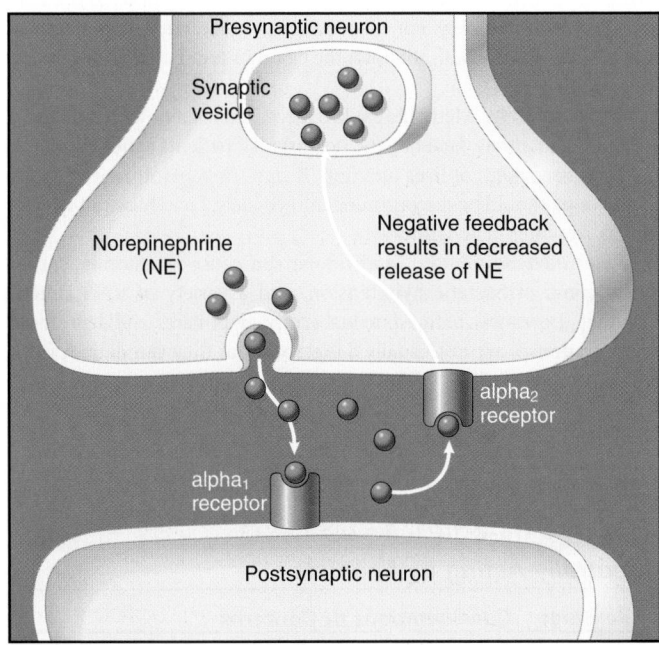

Fig. 17.1 Mechanism of Centrally Acting α_2 Agonist Action. The α_2 agonist activates receptors on presynaptic nerve terminals in the CNS. Receptor activation signals that there is sufficient norepinephrine in the synapse, so release of norepinephrine from the presynaptic neuron decreases. As a result of decreased norepinephrine in the synapse, there is decreased activation of α_1 receptors on the post-synaptic neuron. This inhibits firing of sympathetic neurons, resulting in decreased activation of peripheral adrenergic receptors. *CNS,* Central nervous system.

Rebound hypertension. Rebound hypertension is characterized by a large increase in blood pressure occurring in response to abrupt clonidine withdrawal. This rare but serious reaction is caused by overactivity of the sympathetic nervous system and can be accompanied by nervousness, tachycardia, and sweating. Left untreated, the reaction may persist for a week or more. If blood pressure climbs dangerously high, it should be lowered with a combination of α- and β-adrenergic blocking agents. Rebound effects can be avoided by withdrawing clonidine slowly (over 2 to 4 days).

Use in pregnancy. Clonidine is embryotoxic in animals. Because of the possibility of fetal harm, clonidine is not recommended for pregnant women. Pregnancy should be ruled out before clonidine is prescribed.

Abuse. People who abuse cocaine, opioids (e.g., morphine, heroin), and other drugs frequently abuse clonidine as well. At high doses, clonidine can cause subjective effects—euphoria, sedation, hallucinations—which some individuals find desirable. In addition, clonidine can intensify the subjective effects of some abused drugs, including benzodiazepines, cocaine, and opioids.

Other adverse effects. Clonidine can cause a variety of adverse effects, including constipation, impotence, gynecomastia, and adverse CNS effects (e.g., vivid dreams, nightmares, anxiety, depression). Localized skin reactions are common with transdermal clonidine patches.

Preparations, Dosage, and Administration

Clonidine is available in oral and transdermal formulations and as a solution for epidural administration. Branded products have specific uses. The drug is sold as as Catapres (tablet) and Catpres-TTS (patch) for treatment of hypertension. Duraclon is an epidural injection for pain. Kapvay is an extended-release tablet used for management of ADHD. Information on dosages and administration is provided in Table 17.2.

Guanfacine

The pharmacology of guanfacine (Intuniv) is very similar to that of clonidine. Like clonidine, guanfacine is indicated for hypertension. In addition, guanfacine is used for ADHD. (See Chapter 31.) Benefits in hypertension derive from activating brainstem α_2-adrenergic receptors, an action that reduces sympathetic outflow to the heart and blood vessels. The result is a reduction in cardiac output and blood pressure. Guanfacine has the same major adverse effects as clonidine: sedation and dry mouth. In addition, it can cause rebound hypertension after abrupt withdrawal.

Methyldopa and Methyldopate

Methyldopa is an oral antihypertensive agent that lowers blood pressure by acting at sites within the CNS. Two side effects—hemolytic anemia and hepatic necrosis—can be severe. Methyldopate, an intravenous agent, is nearly identical to methyldopa in structure and pharmacologic effects. In the discussion below, the term *methyldopa* is used in reference to both methyldopate and methyldopa.

TABLE 17.1	Pharmacokinetics: Centrally Acting α_2 Agonists				
Drug Class	**Peak**	**Protein Binding**	**Metabolism**	**Half-Life**	**Elimination**
Clonidine (Catapres, Catapres-TTS-1, Catapres-TTS-2, Catapres-TTS-3, Kapvay, Dixarit ✦)	IR: 1–3 h ER: 7–8 h	20%–40%	Hepatic (enterohepatic recirculation occurs)	12–16 h (20 h with transdermal route)	Urine
Guanfacine [Intuniv]	2–6 h	70%	Hepatic (CYP3A4)	17 h	Urine
Methyldopa (generic)	3–6 h	10%–15%	Intestinal and hepatic	1.5–2 h	Urine

ER, Extended release; *IR,* immediate release; *TTS,* transdermal therapeutic system.

TABLE 17.2   Preparation, Dosage, and Administration of Centrally Acting α_2 Agonists

Drug	Preparation	Dosage	Prescribing Considerations
Clonidine (Catapres, Catapres-TTS-1, Catapres-TTS-2, Catapres-TTS-3, Kapvay, Dixarit ✦)	Tablets IR: 0.1 mg, 0.2 mg, 0.3 mg Tablets ER: 0.1 mg, 0.2 mg Transdermal patch: 2.5-mg patch delivers 0.1 mg/24 h 5-mg patch delivers 0.2 mg/24 h 7.5-mg patch delivers 0.3 mg/24 h	IR: 0.1 mg twice a day; typical maintenance dose 0.1–0.8 mg/d in divided doses ER: 0.1–0.4 mg/d Patches: 1 every 7 days	When immediate-release (twice-daily) dosing is used, scheduling most of the daily dose at bedtime can minimize daytime sedation. Patches should be applied to hairless, intact skin on the upper arm or torso
Guanfacine (Intuniv)	Tablets: 1 mg, 2 mg	Usual dose: 1 mg/d	Prescribe IR tablets to be taken at bedtime to minimize daytime sedation. Advise not to take with grapefruit juice
Methyldopa	Tablets: 250 mg, 500 mg	Initial dose: 250 mg 2–3 times a day Maintenance dose: 0.5–2 g in 2–4 divided doses	If dosage is increased, scheduling the increase at bedtime can decrease daytime drowsiness

ER, Extended release; *IR,* immediate release.

Mechanism of Action

Methyldopa works much like clonidine. Like clonidine, methyldopa inhibits sympathetic outflow from the CNS by causing α_2 activation in the brain. However, methyldopa differs from clonidine in that methyldopa itself is not an α_2 agonist. Thus before it can act, methyldopa must first be taken up into brainstem neurons, where it is converted to methylnorepinephrine, a compound that *is* an effective α_2 agonist. Release of methylnorepinephrine results in α_2 activation.

Pharmacologic Effects

The most prominent response to methyldopa is a drop in blood pressure. The principal mechanism is vasodilation, not cardiosuppression. Vasodilation occurs because of reduced sympathetic stimulation of blood vessels. At usual therapeutic doses, methyldopa does not decrease heart rate or cardiac output. The hemodynamic effects of methyldopa are very much like those of clonidine: both drugs lower blood pressure in supine and standing subjects, and both produce relatively little orthostatic hypotension.

Therapeutic Use

The only indication for methyldopa is *hypertension*. Studies regarding methyldopa use in pregnant patients have shown improved outcomes without fetal harm, so the American College of Obstetricians and Gynecologists has designated methyldopa as one of three preferred drugs for the management of hypertension during pregnancy. (The other preferred drugs are labetalol, a β blocker, and nifedipine, a calcium channel blocker.)

Adverse Effects

Positive Coombs test and hemolytic anemia. Approximately 10% to 20% of patients who take methyldopa chronically will have a positive Coombs test. A Coombs test should be performed before treatment and 6 to 12 months later. Blood counts (hematocrit, hemoglobin, or red cell count) should also be obtained before treatment and periodically thereafter. If the test turns positive, it usually occurs between 6 and 12 months of treatment. Of the patients who have a positive Coombs test, about 5% develop hemolytic anemia. Coombs-positive patients who

do not develop hemolytic anemia may continue methyldopa treatment. However, if hemolytic anemia does develop, methyldopa should be withdrawn immediately. For most patients, hemolytic anemia quickly resolves after withdrawal, although the Coombs test may remain positive for months.

Hepatotoxicity. Methyldopa has been associated with hepatitis, jaundice, and, rarely, fatal hepatic necrosis. All patients should undergo periodic assessment of liver function. If signs of hepatotoxicity appear, methyldopa should be discontinued immediately. Liver function usually normalizes after drug withdrawal.

Other adverse effects. Methyldopa can cause xerostomia, sexual dysfunction, orthostatic hypotension, and a variety of CNS effects, including drowsiness, reduced mental acuity, nightmares, and depression. These responses are not usually dangerous, but they can detract from adherence.

🔲 PATIENT-CENTERED CARE ACROSS THE LIFE SPAN

Centrally-Acting α_2 Agonists

Life Stage	Considerations or Concerns
Children	Centrally acting agonists are approved for use in children 6 years and older, although clonidine has been used in children as young as 5 years (for conduct/oppositional defiance disorders).
Pregnant women	Because clonidine has caused embryotoxicity in some animal reproduction studies, it should not be prescribed for women who are pregnant. Animal studies have not demonstrated adverse events for guanfacine and methyldopa (noninjectable) except when administered at toxic levels. Methyldopa is designated a drug of choice for pregnant women.
Breastfeeding women	Clonidine is excreted in relatively large amounts in breast milk. Breastfeeding is not recommended for women taking clonidine, especially if large doses are required, and should be avoided altogether in women breastfeeding premature infants.
Older adults	The Beers Criteria recommend avoidance of centrally acting α blockers in patients 65 years and older.

---

[b]The Coombs test detects the presence of antibodies directed against the patient's own red blood cells. These antibodies can cause hemolysis (i.e., red blood cell lysis).

SUMMARY OF KEY PRESCRIBING CONSIDERATIONS

Central α₂ Agonists

Therapeutic Goal: Reduce blood pressure in patients with hypertension.[a]

Baseline Data: Assess heart rate, blood pressure, and general cardiovascular status. For methyldopa, obtain a baseline CBC and liver enzymes.

Monitoring: Assess heart rate, blood pressure, and cardiovascular status at each visit. For methyldopa, check CBC (or, at least, hematocrit and hemoglobin then a CBC if low), Coombs test, and liver enzymes if signs or symptoms of anemia or liver problems develop or 6–12 weeks into treatment, and then periodically.

Identifying High-Risk Patients: Use with caution in patients with bradycardia (clonidine and guanfacine). Dosing adjustments may be needed for patients who take CNS depressants. Clonidine should not be given to patients who are pregnant. Methyldopa should not be given to patients with active liver disease or a history of methyldopa-induced liver dysfunction.

Evaluating Therapeutic Effects: Blood pressure (or other reasons for taking) effectively controlled.

Minimizing Adverse Effects:

- CNS depression increases the risk of accidents; safety precautions should be initiated for patients at risk of falls.
- Severe hypertension occurs rarely after abrupt clonidine withdrawal; manage with a combination of α- and β-adrenergic blockers. To prevent rebound hypertension, withdraw clonidine slowly over 2–4 days.
- People who abuse cocaine, opioids, and other drugs frequently abuse clonidine as well; be alert for signs of clonidine abuse (e.g., questionable or frequent requests for a prescription).
- Methyldopa can cause hemolytic anemia; if this occurs, withdraw methyldopa immediately. Hemolytic anemia usually resolves quickly.
- Methyldopa can cause hepatitis, jaundice, and fatal hepatic necrosis. If liver dysfunction develops, discontinue methyldopa immediately. In most cases, liver function returns to previous status quickly.

[a]For clonidine and guanfacine, the goal may be the management of symptoms of ADHD. For clonidine, the goal may be to decrease pain.
ADHD, Attention deficit/hyperactivity disorder; *CBC*, complete blood count; *CNS*, central nervous system.

18

Introduction to Central Nervous System Pharmacology

Central nervous system (CNS) drugs are agents that act on the brain and spinal cord. Medical applications include relief of pain, suppression of seizures, production of anesthesia, and treatment of mental health conditions. CNS drugs are sometimes abused for their stimulant, depressant, euphoriant, and other "mind-altering" abilities.

Despite the widespread use of CNS drugs, knowledge of these agents is limited. Much of our ignorance stems from the anatomic and neurochemical complexity of the brain and spinal cord. (There are more than 50 billion neurons in the cerebral hemispheres alone.) We are a long way from fully understanding both the CNS and the drugs used to affect it.

TRANSMITTERS OF THE CENTRAL NERVOUS SYSTEM

In contrast to the peripheral nervous system, in which only three compounds—acetylcholine, norepinephrine, and epinephrine—serve as neurotransmitters, the CNS contains at least 21 compounds that serve as neurotransmitters (Box 18.1). Furthermore, there are numerous sites within the CNS for which no transmitter has been identified, so it is clear that additional compounds, yet to be discovered, also mediate central neurotransmission.

None of the compounds believed to be CNS neurotransmitters has actually been *proved* to serve this function. The reason for uncertainty lies with the technical difficulties involved in CNS research. However, although absolute proof may be lacking, the evidence supporting a neurotransmitter role for several compounds (e.g., dopamine, norepinephrine, enkephalins) is completely convincing.

Although much is known about the actions of CNS transmitters at various sites in the brain and spinal cord, it is not usually possible to precisely relate these known actions to behavioral or psychologic processes. For example, we know the locations of specific CNS sites at which norepinephrine appears to act as a transmitter, and we know the effect of norepinephrine at most of these sites (suppression of neuronal excitability), but we do not know the precise relationship between suppression of neuronal excitability at each of these sites and the effect of that suppression on the overt function of the organism. This example shows the state of our knowledge of CNS transmitter function: we have a great deal of detailed information about the biochemistry and electrophysiology of CNS transmitters, but we are as yet unable to assemble those details into a completely meaningful picture.

THE BLOOD–BRAIN BARRIER

The blood–brain barrier impedes the entry of drugs into the brain. Passage across the barrier is limited to lipid-soluble agents and to drugs that cross by way of specific transport systems. Protein-bound drugs and highly ionized drugs cannot cross.

From a therapeutic perspective, the blood–brain barrier presents an advantage and a disadvantage. The barrier protects the brain from injury by potentially toxic substances, but it can also be a significant obstacle to entry of therapeutic agents.

The blood–brain barrier is not fully developed at birth. Accordingly, infants are much more sensitive to CNS drugs than are older children and adults.

HOW CENTRAL NERVOUS SYSTEM DRUGS PRODUCE THERAPEUTIC EFFECTS

Although much is known about the biochemical and electrophysiologic effects of CNS drugs, in most cases we cannot state with certainty the relationship between these effects and production of beneficial responses. To fully understand how a drug alters symptoms, we must understand, at a biochemical and physiologic levels, the pathophysiology of the disorder being treated. In the case of most CNS disorders, our knowledge is limited: we do not fully understand the brain in either health or disease. Therefore we must exercise caution when attempting to assign a precise mechanism for a drug's therapeutic effects.

Although we cannot state with certainty how CNS drugs act, we do have sufficient data to permit formulation of plausible hypotheses. Consequently, as we study CNS drugs, proposed mechanisms of action are presented. Keep in mind, however, that these mechanisms are tentative, representing our best scientifically-informed guesses based on available data. As we learn more, it is almost certain that these concepts will be modified if not discarded.

ADAPTATION OF THE CENTRAL NERVOUS SYSTEM TO PROLONGED DRUG EXPOSURE

When CNS drugs are taken long term, their effects may differ from those produced during initial use. These altered effects are the result of adaptive changes that occur in the brain in response to prolonged drug exposure. The brain's ability to adapt to drugs can produce alterations in therapeutic effects and side effects. Adaptive changes are often beneficial, although they can also be detrimental.

Increased Therapeutic Effects

Certain drugs used in psychiatry—antipsychotics and antidepressants—must be taken for several weeks and up to 2 months before full therapeutic effects develop. Beneficial responses may be delayed because they result from adaptive changes, not from direct effects of drugs on synaptic

BOX 18.1 Neurotransmitters of the Central Nervous System

Monoamines
Dopamine
Epinephrine
Norepinephrine
Serotonin

Amino Acids
Aspartate
Gamma-aminobutyric acid
Glutamate
Glycine

Purines
Adenosine
Adenosine monophosphate
Adenosine triphosphate

Opioid Peptides
Dynorphins
Endorphins
Enkephalins

Nonopioid Peptides
Neurotensin
Oxytocin
Somatostatin
Substance P
Vasopressin

Others
Acetylcholine
Histamine

function. Hence full therapeutic effects are not seen until the CNS has had time to modify in response to prolonged drug exposure.

Decreased Side Effects

When CNS drugs are taken long term, the intensity of side effects may decrease. For example, phenobarbital (an antiseizure drug) produces sedation during the initial phase of therapy; however, with continued treatment, sedation declines while full protection from seizures is retained. Adaptations within the brain are believed to underlie this phenomenon.

Tolerance and Physical Dependence

Tolerance and physical dependence are special manifestations of CNS adaptation. *Tolerance* is a decreased response that occurs with prolonged drug use. *Physical dependence* is a state in which abrupt discontinuation of drug use will precipitate a withdrawal syndrome. The kinds of adaptive changes that underlie tolerance and dependence are such that, after they have taken place, continued drug use is required for the brain to function "normally." If drug use is stopped, the drug-adapted brain can no longer function properly, and a withdrawal syndrome ensues. The withdrawal reaction continues until the adaptive changes have had time to revert, restoring the CNS to its pretreatment state.

DEVELOPMENT OF NEW PSYCHOTHERAPEUTIC DRUGS

Because of deficiencies in our knowledge of the neurochemical and physiologic changes that underlie mental disease, it is impossible to take a rational approach to the development of truly new (nonderivative) psychotherapeutic agents. History bears this out: virtually all of the major advances in psychopharmacology have been serendipitous.

In addition to our relative ignorance of the neurochemical and physiologic correlates of mental illness, two other factors contribute to the difficulty in generating truly new psychotherapeutic agents. First, in contrast to many other diseases, we lack adequate animal models of mental illness. Accordingly, animal research is not likely to reveal new types of psychotherapeutic agents. Second, mentally healthy individuals cannot be used as subjects to assess potential psychotherapeutic agents because most psychotherapeutic drugs either have no effect on healthy individuals or produce paradoxical effects.

After a new drug has been found, variations on that agent can be developed systematically: (1) structural analogs of the new agent are synthesized; (2) these analogs are run through biochemical and physiologic screening tests to determine whether they possess activity similar to that of the parent compound; and (3) after serious toxicity has been ruled out, promising agents are tested in humans for possible psychotherapeutic activity. Using this procedure, it is possible to develop drugs that have fewer side effects than the original drug and perhaps even superior therapeutic effects. However, although this procedure may produce small advances, it is not likely to yield a major therapeutic breakthrough.

APPROACHING THE STUDY OF CENTRAL NERVOUS SYSTEM DRUGS

Because our understanding of the CNS is less complete than our understanding of the peripheral nervous system, our approach to studying CNS drugs differs from the approach we took with peripheral nervous system agents. When we studied the pharmacology of the peripheral nervous system, we emphasized the importance of understanding transmitters and their receptors before embarking on a study of drugs. Because our knowledge of CNS transmitters is insufficient to allow this approach, rather than making a detailed examination of CNS transmitters before we study CNS drugs, we will discuss drugs and transmitters concurrently.

19

Drugs for Parkinson Disease

Parkinson disease (PD) is a slowly progressive neurodegenerative disorder that afflicts more than 1 million Americans, making it second only to Alzheimer disease as the most common degenerative disease of neurons. Cardinal symptoms are resting tremor, rigidity, postural instability, and slowed movement. In addition to these motor symptoms, most patients also experience nonmotor symptoms such as depression, fatigue, and sleep disturbances, as well as autonomic disturbances such as constipation, urinary retention, incontinence, and dysphasia. Psychosis and dementia can also occur with PD. Years before functional impairment develops, patients may experience early symptoms of PD, including loss of smell, excessive salivation, clumsiness of the hands, worsening of handwriting, bothersome tremor, slower gait, and reduced voice volume. Symptoms first appear in middle age and progress relentlessly. The underlying cause of motor symptoms is loss of dopaminergic neurons in the substantia nigra. Although there is no cure for motor symptoms, drug therapy can maintain functional mobility for years and can thereby substantially prolong quality of life and life expectancy.

THE PATHOPHYSIOLOGY UNDERLYING MOTOR SYMPTOMS

Motor symptoms result from damage to the *extrapyramidal system*, a complex neuronal network that helps regulate movement. When extrapyramidal function is disrupted, *dyskinesias* (disorders of movement) result. The dyskinesias that characterize PD are tremor at rest, rigidity, postural instability, and bradykinesia (slowed movement). In severe PD, bradykinesia may progress to *akinesia*, the complete absence of movement.

In people with PD, neurotransmission is disrupted primarily in the brain's *striatum*. A simplified model of striatal neurotransmission is depicted in Fig. 19.1A. As indicated, proper function of the striatum requires a balance between two neurotransmitters: *dopamine* and *acetylcholine*. Dopamine is an *inhibitory* transmitter; acetylcholine is an *excitatory* transmitter. The neurons that release dopamine inhibit neurons that release γ-aminobutyric acid (GABA), transmitter that contributes to motor control. In contrast, the neurons that release acetylcholine excite the neurons that release GABA. Movement is normal when the inhibitory influence of dopamine and the excitatory influence of acetylcholine are in balance. In PD, there is an imbalance between dopamine and acetylcholine in the striatum (see Fig. 19.1B). As noted, the imbalance results from *degeneration of the neurons in the substantia nigra that supply dopamine to the striatum*. In the absence of dopamine, the excitatory influence of acetylcholine goes unopposed, causing excessive stimulation of the neurons that release GABA. Overactivity of these GABAergic neurons contributes to the motor symptoms that characterize PD. That said, between 70% and 80% of these neurons must be lost before PD becomes clinically recognizable. Because this loss takes place over 5 to 20 years, neuronal degeneration begins long before overt motor symptoms appear.

No one knows for sure what causes degeneration of dopaminergic neurons. However, some evidence strongly implicates α-*synuclein*—a potentially toxic protein synthesized by dopaminergic neurons. Under normal conditions, α-synuclein is rapidly degraded. As a result, it does not accumulate and no harm occurs. Degradation of α-synuclein requires two other proteins: *parkin* and *ubiquitin*. (Parkin is an enzyme that catalyzes the binding of α-synuclein to ubiquitin. When bound to ubiquitin, α-synuclein can be degraded.) If any of these proteins—α-synuclein, parkin, or ubiquitin—is defective, degradation of α-synuclein cannot take place. When this occurs, α-synuclein accumulates inside the cell, forming neurotoxic fibrils. At autopsy, these fibrils are visible as *Lewy bodies*, which are characteristic of PD pathology. Failure to degrade α-synuclein appears to result from two causes: genetic vulnerability and toxins in the environment. Defective genes coding for all three proteins have been found in families with inherited forms of PD. In people with PD that is not inherited, environmental toxins may explain the inability to degrade α-synuclein.

As discussed in Chapter 26, movement disorders similar to those of PD can occur as side effects of antipsychotic drugs. These dyskinesias, which are referred to as *extrapyramidal side effects*, result from blockade of dopamine receptors in the striatum. This drug-induced parkinsonism can be managed with some of the drugs used to treat PD.

OVERVIEW OF MOTOR SYMPTOM MANAGEMENT

Therapeutic Goal

The ideal treatment would reverse neuronal degeneration or at least prevent further degeneration and control symptoms. Unfortunately the ideal treatment does not exist: we have no drugs that can prevent neuronal damage or reverse damage that has already occurred. Drugs can only provide symptomatic relief; they do not cure PD. Furthermore, there is no convincing proof that any current drug can delay disease progression. Hence the goal of pharmacologic therapy is simply to improve the patient's ability to carry out activities of daily living. Drug selection and dosage are determined by the extent to which PD interferes with work, walking, dressing, eating, bathing, and other activities. Drugs benefit the patient primarily by improving bradykinesia, gait disturbance, and postural instability. Tremor and rigidity, although disturbing, are less disabling.

Drugs Employed

Given the neurochemical basis of parkinsonism—too little striatal dopamine and too much acetylcholine—the approach to treatment is obvious: give drugs that can restore the functional balance between dopamine and acetylcholine. To accomplish this, two types of drugs are used: (1) *dopaminergic agents* (i.e., drugs that directly or indirectly activate dopamine receptors) and (2) *anticholinergic agents* (i.e., drugs that block receptors for acetylcholine). Of the

127

Fig. 19.1 A Model of Neurotransmission in the Healthy Striatum and Parkinsonian Striatum. (A) In the healthy striatum, dopamine *(DA)* released from neurons originating in the substantia nigra *inhibits* the firing of neurons in the striatum that release γ-aminobutyric acid *(GABA)*. Conversely, neurons located within the striatum, which release acetylcholine *(ACh)*, *excite* the GABAergic neurons. Therefore, under normal conditions, the inhibitory actions of DA are balanced by the excitatory actions of ACh, and controlled movement results. (B) In Parkinson disease, the neurons that supply DA to the striatum degenerate. In the absence of sufficient DA, the excitatory effects of ACh go unopposed, and disturbed movement results.

two groups, dopaminergic agents are by far the more widely employed.

As shown in Table 19.1, dopaminergic drugs act by several mechanisms: levodopa is converted to dopamine, which activates dopamine receptors directly; inhibitors of monoamine oxidase-B (MAO-B) prevent dopamine breakdown; amantadine promotes dopamine release (and may also block dopamine reuptake); and the inhibitors of catechol-O-methyltransferase (COMT) enhance the effects of levodopa by blocking its degradation.

In contrast to the dopaminergic drugs, which act by multiple mechanisms to increase dopamine activity, all of the anticholinergic agents share the same mechanism: blockade of muscarinic receptors in the striatum to decrease acetylcholine activity.

Clinical Guidelines

Management of PD is generally under the guidance of a neurologist or providers working collaboratively in a neurology practice. Because these patients often have co-morbidities or are followed elsewhere for management of primary care needs, it is important for all providers involved in care to have a familiarity with the drugs used to manage PD.

The most current (2018) set of guidelines for the management of motor symptoms is provided by the International Parkinson and Movement Disorder Society. These are available at https://www.movement disorders.org/MDS-Files1/Resources/PDFs/TreatmentsforMotor SymptomsofPD-2018.pdf

The recommendations that follow are based on these guidelines.

Drug Selection
Initial Treatment

For patients with mild symptoms, treatment can begin with an MAO-B inhibitor. MAO-B inhibitors confer mild symptomatic benefit.

For patients with more severe symptoms, treatment should begin with either levodopa (combined with carbidopa) or a dopamine agonist. Levodopa is more effective than the dopamine agonists, but long-term use carries a higher risk for disabling dyskinesias. Hence the choice must be tailored to the patient: if improving motor function is the primary objective, then levodopa is preferred. However, if drug-induced dyskinesias are a primary concern, then a dopamine agonist would be preferred.

Management of Motor Fluctuations

Long-term treatment with levodopa or dopamine agonists is associated with two types of motor fluctuations: *"off"* times (loss of symptom relief) and *drug-induced dyskinesias* (involuntary movements). Off times can be reduced with three types of drugs: dopamine agonists, COMT inhibitors, and MAO-B inhibitors. Evidence of efficacy is strongest for entacapone (a COMT inhibitor) and rasagiline (an MAO-B inhibitor). The only drug recommended for dyskinesias is amantadine.

Neuroprotection

To date there is no definitive proof that any drug can protect dopaminergic neurons from progressive degeneration. However, although no drug has yet been proved to provide neuroprotective effects for people with PD, studies suggest that some drugs are promising. For example, MAO-B inhibitors have provided neuroprotective effects in animal

TABLE 19.1 Dopaminergic Agents for Parkinson Disease

Drug	Mechanism of Action	Therapeutic Role
Dopamine Replacement		
Levodopa/carbidopa Levodopa/carbidopa/entacapone	Levodopa undergoes conversion to DA in the brain and then activates DA receptors (carbidopa blocks destruction of levodopa in the periphery)	First-line drug, or supplement to a dopamine agonist
Dopamine Agonists **Nonergot Derivatives** • Apomorphine • Pramipexole • Ropinirole • Rotigotine **Ergot Derivatives** • Bromocriptine • Cabergoline	Directly activate DA receptors	Pramipexole and ropinirole are first-line drugs, or supplements to levodopa. Apomorphine—a subQ nonergot agent—is reserved for rescue therapy during "off" times. Ergot derivatives are generally avoided.
Comt Inhibitors Entacapone Tolcapone	Inhibit breakdown of levodopa by COMT	Adjunct to levodopa to decrease "wearing off"; entacapone is more effective and safer than tolcapone
MAO-B Inhibitors Rasagiline Selegiline	Inhibit breakdown of DA by MAO-B	Used in newly diagnosed patients and for managing "off" times during levodopa therapy
Dopamine Releaser Amantadine	Promotes release of DA from remaining DA neurons; may also block DA reuptake	May help reduce levodopa-induced dyskinesias

COMT, Catechol-*O*-methyltransferase; *DA,* dopamine; *MAO-B,* type B monoamine oxidase.

studies. Similarly, dopamine agonists have demonstrated neuroprotective effects in laboratory studies. For both drug categories, however, clinical studies in humans have been inconclusive. A growing body of research with levodopa supports a likely role for neuroprotection; however, because some studies demonstrate toxic effects in patients with PD, the risks may outweigh the benefits when the drug is given for this purpose.

PHARMACOLOGY OF THE DRUGS USED FOR MOTOR SYMPTOMS

Levodopa

Levodopa was introduced in the 1960s and has been a cornerstone of PD treatment ever since. Unfortunately, although the drug is highly effective, beneficial effects diminish over time.

Use in Parkinson Disease

Beneficial effects. Levodopa is the most effective drug for PD. At the beginning of treatment, about 75% of patients experience a 50% reduction in symptom severity. Levodopa is so effective, in fact, that a diagnosis of PD should be questioned if the patient fails to respond.

Full therapeutic responses may take several months to develop. Consequently, although the effects of levodopa can be significant, patients should not expect immediate improvement. Rather, they should be informed that beneficial effects are likely to increase steadily over the first few months.

In contrast to the dramatic improvements seen during initial therapy, long-term therapy with levodopa has been disappointing. Although symptoms may be well controlled during the first 2 years of treatment, by the end of year 5, the ability to function may deteriorate to pretreatment levels. This probably reflects disease progression and not the development of tolerance to levodopa.

Acute loss of effect. Acute loss of effect occurs in two patterns: gradual loss and abrupt loss. Gradual loss—"wearing off"—develops near the end of the dosing interval and simply indicates that drug levels have declined to a subtherapeutic value. Wearing off can be minimized in three ways: (1) shortening the dosing interval, (2) giving a drug that prolongs levodopa's plasma half-life (e.g., entacapone), and (3) giving a direct-acting dopamine agonist.

Abrupt loss of effect, often referred to as the "on-off" phenomenon, can occur at any time during the dosing interval—even while drug levels are high. Off times may last from minutes to hours. Over the course of treatment, off periods are likely to increase in both intensity and frequency. Drugs that can help reduce off times are listed in Table 19.2. As discussed later, avoiding high-protein meals may also help.

Mechanism of Action

Levodopa reduces symptoms by increasing dopamine synthesis in the striatum (Fig. 19.2). Levodopa enters the brain through an active transport system that carries it across the blood–brain barrier. When in the brain, the drug undergoes uptake into the remaining dopaminergic nerve terminals that remain in the striatum. After uptake, levodopa, which has no direct effects of its own, is converted to dopamine, its active form. As dopamine, levodopa helps restore a proper balance between dopamine and acetylcholine.

Conversion of levodopa to dopamine is depicted in Fig. 19.3. As indicated, the enzyme that catalyzes the reaction is called a *decarboxylase* (because it removes a carboxyl group from levodopa). The activity of decarboxylases is enhanced by *pyridoxine* (vitamin B_6).

Why is PD treated with levodopa and not with dopamine itself? There are two reasons. First, dopamine cannot cross the blood–brain barrier (see Fig. 19.2). As noted, levodopa crosses the barrier by means of an active transport system, a system that does not transport dopamine.

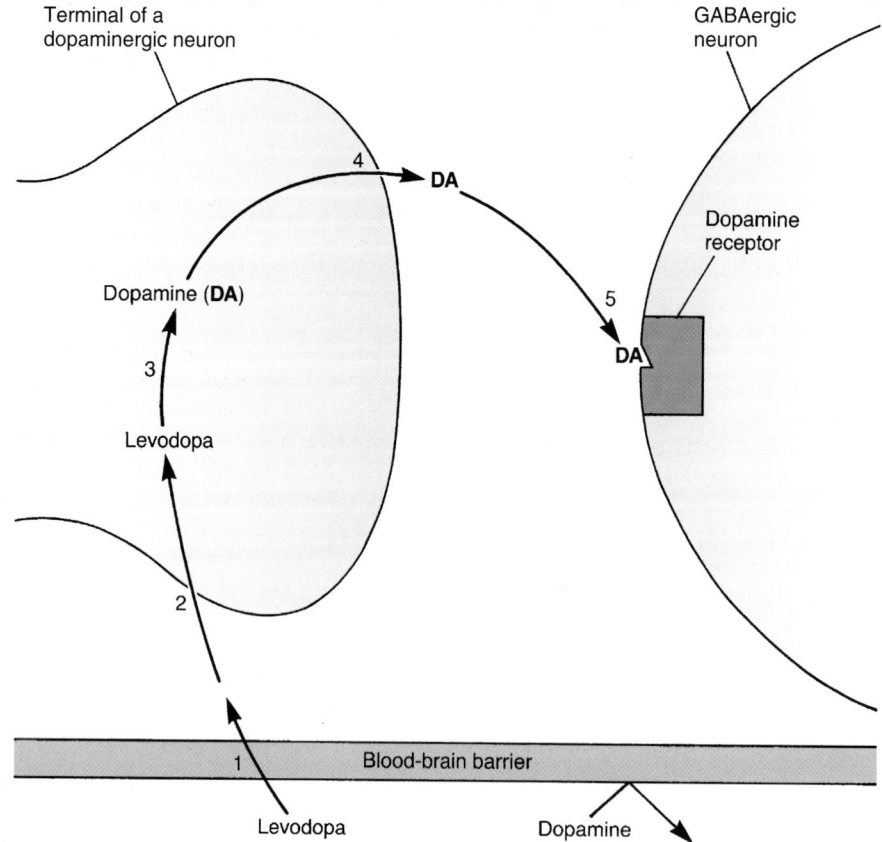

Fig. 19.2 Steps Leading to Alteration of Central Nervous System Function by Levodopa. To produce its beneficial effects in Parkinson disease (PD), levodopa must be *(1)* transported across the blood-brain barrier; *(2)* taken up by dopaminergic nerve terminals in the striatum; *(3)* converted into dopamine; *(4)* released into the synaptic space; and *(5)* bound to dopamine receptors on striatal GABAergic neurons, causing them to fire at a slower rate. Note that dopamine itself is unable to cross the blood–brain barrier and hence cannot be used to treat PD.

TABLE 19.2 **Drugs for Motor Complications of Levodopa Therapy**	
Drug	**Drug Class**
Drugs for Off Times	
Definitely Effective	
Entacapone	COMT inhibitor
Rasagiline	MAO-B inhibitor
Probably Effective	
Rotigotine	DA agonist
Pramipexole	DA agonist
Ropinirole	DA agonist
Tolcapone	COMT inhibitor
Possibly Effective	
Apomorphine	DA agonist
Cabergoline	DA agonist
Selegiline	MAO-B inhibitor
Drug for Levodopa-Induced Dyskinesias	
Amantadine	DA-releasing agent

COMT, Catechol-*O*-methyltransferase; *DA*, dopamine; *MAO-B*, type B monoamine oxidase

Fig. 19.3 Conversion of Levodopa to Dopamine. Decarboxylases present in the brain, liver, and intestine convert levodopa into dopamine. Pyridoxine (vitamin B6) accelerates the reaction.

Second, dopamine has such a short half-life in the blood that it would be impractical to use even if it could cross the blood–brain barrier.

Pharmacokinetics

Levodopa is administered orally and undergoes rapid absorption from the small intestine. Food delays absorption by slowing gastric emptying. Furthermore, because neutral amino acids compete with levodopa for intestinal absorption (and for transport across the blood-brain barrier as well), high-protein foods will reduce therapeutic effects.

Only a small fraction of each dose reaches the brain. Most is metabolized in the periphery, primarily by *decarboxylase enzymes* and to a lesser extent by COMT. Peripheral decarboxylases convert levodopa into dopamine, an active metabolite. In contrast, COMT converts levodopa into an inactive metabolite. Like the enzymes that decarboxylate levodopa within the brain, peripheral decarboxylases work faster in the presence of pyridoxine. Because of peripheral metabolism, less than 2% of each dose enters the brain if levodopa is given alone. For this reason, levodopa is now available only in combination preparations with either carbidopa or carbidopa and entacapone. These additional agents decrease the amount of decarboxylation in the periphery so that more of the drug can enter the central nervous system (CNS). This is discussed in greater detail later in the chapter. A summary of pharmacokinetics for levodopa combinations and other drugs in this chapter is provided in Table 19.3.

Adverse Effects

Most side effects of levodopa are dose dependent. Older adult patients, who are the primary users of levodopa, are especially sensitive to adverse effects.

Nausea and vomiting. Most patients experience nausea and vomiting early in treatment. The cause is activation of dopamine receptors in the chemoreceptor trigger zone (CTZ) of the medulla. Nausea and vomiting can be reduced by administering levodopa in low initial doses and with meals. (Food delays levodopa absorption, causing a decrease in peak plasma drug levels and a corresponding decrease in stimulation of the CTZ.) However, because administration with food can reduce therapeutic effects by decreasing levodopa absorption, administration with meals should be avoided if possible. Giving additional carbidopa can help reduce nausea and vomiting. Why carbidopa helps is unknown, but studies show that peripheral decarboxylase is saturated by carbidopa at approximately 70 to 100 mg a day. Patients receiving less than this amount of carbidopa are more likely to experience nausea and vomiting.

Dyskinesias. Ironically, levodopa, which is given to *alleviate* movement disorders, actually *causes* movement disorders in many patients. About 80% develop involuntary movements within the first year. Some dyskinesias are just annoying (e.g., head bobbing, tics, grimacing), whereas others can be disabling (e.g., ballismus, a rapid involuntary jerking or flinging of proximal muscle groups, or choreoathetosis, a slow involuntary writhing movement). These dyskinesias develop just before or soon after optimal levodopa dosage has been achieved. Dyskinesias can be managed in three ways: drug therapy, surgery, or electrical stimulation. First, the dosage of levodopa can be reduced. However, dosage reduction may allow PD symptoms to reemerge. Second, amantadine (discussed later) can be given, which can reduce dyskinesias in some patients. If these measures fail, surgery and electrical stimulation remain as options.

Cardiovascular effects. Postural hypotension is common early in treatment. The underlying mechanism is unknown. Hypotension can be reduced by increasing intake of salt and water. An α-adrenergic agonist can help too.

Conversion of levodopa to dopamine in the periphery can produce excessive activation of β_1 receptors in the heart. *Dysrhythmias* can result, especially in patients with heart disease.

Psychosis. Psychosis develops in about 20% of patients. Prominent symptoms are visual hallucinations, vivid dreams or nightmares, and paranoid ideation (fears of personal endangerment, sense of persecution, feelings of being followed or spied on). Activation of dopamine receptors is thought to be involved. Symptoms can be reduced by lowering the levodopa dosage, but this will reduce beneficial effects as well.

Treatment of levodopa-induced psychosis with first-generation antipsychotics is problematic. Yes, these agents can decrease psychologic symptoms; however, they will also *intensify* symptoms of PD because they block receptors for dopamine in the striatum. In fact, when first-generation antipsychotic agents are used for schizophrenia, the biggest problem is parkinsonian side effects, referred to as extrapyramidal symptoms (EPS).

Two second-generation antipsychotics—*clozapine* and *quetiapine*—have been used successfully to manage levodopa-induced psychosis. Unlike the first-generation antipsychotic drugs, clozapine and quetiapine cause little or no blockade of dopamine receptors in the striatum, so they do not cause EPSs. In patients taking levodopa, these drugs can reduce psychotic symptoms without intensifying symptoms of PD. Clozapine and quetiapine are discussed in Chapter 26.

Central nervous system effects. Levodopa may cause several CNS effects. These range from anxiety and agitation to memory and cognitive impairment. Insomnia and nightmares are common. Some patients experience problems with impulse control, resulting in behavioral changes associated with promiscuity, gambling, binge eating, or alcohol abuse.

Other adverse effects. Levodopa may *darken sweat and urine;* patients should be informed about this is a harmless effect. Some studies suggest that levodopa can *activate malignant melanoma;* however, others have failed to support this finding. Until more is known it is important to perform a careful skin assessment of patients who are taking levodopa.

TABLE 19.3   Pharmacokinetics of Drugs for Parkinson Disease

Drug Name	Peak	Protein Binding	Metabolism	Half-Life	Elimination
Levodopa Combinations					
Levodopa/carbidopa (Sinemet, Rytary, Duopa, Duodopa 🍁)[a]	IR: 0.5 h ER: 2 h Intestinal suspension: 2.5 h Intestinal gel: UK	10%–30%	COMT Decarboxylation[b]	IR: 0.75–1.5 h ER: 1.5–2 h	Urine
Levodopa/carbidopa/entacapone (Stalevo)[a]	1–2 h	10%–30%	COMT Decarboxylation[b]	1–3 h	Urine
Dopamine Agonists: Ergot Derivatives					
Bromocriptine (Parlodel)	Parlodel 0.5–4.5 h	90%–96%	Hepatic (CYP3A)	5–6 h	Feces 82% Urine
Cabergoline (Dostinex 🍁, generic in the United States)	2–3 h	40%–42%	Hepatic (hydrolysis, minimal CYP450)	60–70 h	Feces 60% Urine
Dopamine Agonists: Nonergot Derivatives					
Pramipexole (Mirapex, Mirapex ER)	IR: 2 h ER: 6 h	15%	Minimal	8.5 h (up to 12 h in older adults)	Urine (almost all as unchanged drug)
Ropinirole (Requip, Requip XL)	IR: 1–2 h ER: 6–10 h	40%	Hepatic (CYP1A2)	6 h	Urine
Rotigotine (Neupro)	15–18 h typically (range 4–27 h)	90%	Extensive via multiple mechanism including multiple CYP450 isoenzymes	5–7 h (after removal of patch)	Urine (71%) Feces
Apomorphine (Apokyn, Movapo)	10 min to 1 h	50%	Hepatic (but not CYP450)	40 min	UK
Comt Inhibitors					
Entacapone (Comtan)	1 h	98%	Isomerization and glucuronidation	2.5–3 h	Feces (90%) Urine
Tolcapone (Tasmar)	2 h	99.9%	Hepatic via glucuronidation	2–3 h	Urine (60%) Feces
MAO-B Inhibitors					
Selegiline (Eldepryl, Emsam, Zelapar)	<1 h	85%–90%	Hepatic (CYP2B6, CYP2C9, CYP3A with CYP2A6 having a minimal role)	10 h	Urine
Rasagiline (Azilect)	1 h	88%–94%	Hepatic (CYP1A2)	3 h	Urine (62%) Feces
Antiviral Agent					
Amantadine (Gocovri, Osmolex ER)	IR: 2–4 h ER: 7.5–12 h	67%	Minimal	10–22 h	Urine (80%–90% unchanged)
Centrally Acting Anticholinergic Drugs					
Benztropine (Cogentin, Kynesia)	7 h	UK	Hepatic	UK	UK
Trihexyphenidyl (generic)	1.3 h	UK	Hydroxylation	33 h	Urine, Bile

[a]For levodopa combination drugs, pharmacokinetics for the levodopa component are provided.
[b]Decarboxylation inhibited by carbidopa.
COMT, Catechol-*O*-methyltransferase; *ER*, extended release; *GI*, gastrointestinal; *h*, Hour(s); *IR*, immediate release; *MAO*, monoamine oxidase; *min*, Minutes; *UK*, unknown.

Drug Interactions

Interactions between levodopa and other drugs can (1) increase the beneficial effects of levodopa, (2) decrease the beneficial effects of levodopa, and (3) increase toxicity from levodopa. Major interactions are shown in Table 19.4. Several important interactions are discussed later in this chapter.

First-generation antipsychotic drugs. All of the first-generation antipsychotic drugs (e.g., chlorpromazine, haloperidol) block receptors for dopamine in the striatum. As a result, they can decrease the therapeutic effects of levodopa. Accordingly, concurrent use of levodopa and these drugs should be avoided. As discussed previously, two second-generation agents—clozapine and quetiapine—do not block dopamine receptors in the striatum, so they can be used safely in patients with PD.

Monoamine oxidase inhibitors. Levodopa can cause a hypertensive crisis if it is administered to an individual taking a *nonselective* inhibitor

TABLE 19.4   Major Drug Interactions of Levodopa

Drug Category	Drug	Mechanism of Interaction
Drugs that *increase* beneficial effects of levodopa	Carbidopa	Inhibits peripheral decarboxylation of levodopa
	Entacapone, tolcapone	Inhibit destruction of levodopa by COMT in the intestine and peripheral tissues
	Rotigotine, apomorphine, bromocriptine, cabergoline, pramipexole, ropinirole	Stimulate dopamine receptors directly; add to the effects of dopamine derived from levodopa
	Amantadine	Promotes release of dopamine
	Anticholinergic drugs	Block cholinergic receptors in the CNS; help restore balance between dopamine and ACh
Drugs that *decrease* beneficial effects of levodopa	Antipsychotic drugs[a]	Block dopamine receptors in the striatum
Drugs that *increase* levodopa toxicity	MAO inhibitors (especially *nonselective* MAO inhibitors)	Inhibit MAO; increase risk for severe levodopa-induced hypertension

[a]First-generation antipsychotic agents block dopamine receptors in the striatum and can thereby nullify the therapeutic effects of levodopa. Two second-generation antipsychotics—clozapine (Clozaril) and quetiapine (Seroquel)—do not block dopamine receptors in the striatum and thus do not nullify the therapeutic effects of levodopa.
ACh, Acetylcholine; *CNS*, central nervous system; *COMT*, catechol-*O*-methyltransferase; *MAO*, monoamine oxidase

of MAO. The mechanism is as follows: (1) Levodopa elevates neuronal stores of dopamine and norepinephrine (NE) by promoting the synthesis of both transmitters. (2) Because intraneuronal MAO serves to inactivate dopamine and NE, inhibition of MAO allows elevated neuronal stores of these transmitters to grow even larger. (3) Because both dopamine and NE promote vasoconstriction, release of these agents in supranormal amounts can lead to massive vasoconstriction, thereby causing blood pressure to rise dangerously high. To avoid hypertensive crisis, nonselective MAO inhibitors should be withdrawn at least 2 weeks before giving levodopa.

Anticholinergic drugs. As discussed previously, excessive stimulation of cholinergic receptors contributes to the dyskinesias of PD. Therefore, by blocking these receptors, anticholinergic agents can enhance responses to levodopa.

Pyridoxine. You may read advice indicating that the intake of pyridoxine (vitamin B₆) should be limited. It is true that pyridoxine accelerates the decarboxylation of levodopa at the periphery; however, because levodopa is now always combined with carbidopa, a drug that suppresses decarboxylase activity, this potential interaction is no longer a clinical concern.

Food Interactions

High-protein meals can reduce therapeutic responses to levodopa. Neutral amino acids compete with levodopa for absorption from the intestine and for transport across the blood-brain barrier. Therefore a high-protein meal can significantly reduce both the amount of levodopa absorbed and the amount transported into the brain. It has been suggested that a high-protein meal could trigger an abrupt loss of effect (i.e., an off episode). Accordingly, patients should be advised to spread their protein consumption evenly throughout the day.

High-fat foods can decrease absorption, delaying peak effects by several hours. High-fat foods should be avoided. Patients should take these drugs, if tolerated, on an empty stomach.

Preparations

At one time levodopa was available as a single drug. However, such single-drug preparations have been withdrawn from the market. Levodopa is now available only in combination preparations, either levodopa/carbidopa or levodopa/carbidopa/entacapone. A summary of preparations that include levodopa and other drugs for PD is provided in Table 19.5.

Levodopa/carbidopa and levodopa/carbidopa/entacapone. The combination of levodopa plus carbidopa is our most effective therapy

for PD. Levodopa plus carbidopa is available under three trade names: *Rytary*, *Sinemet*, and *Duopa*.

Mechanism of action. Carbidopa has no therapeutic effects of its own; however, it inhibits the decarboxylation of levodopa in the intestine and peripheral tissues, making more levodopa available to the CNS. Carbidopa does not prevent the conversion of levodopa to dopamine by decarboxylases in the brain because carbidopa is unable to cross the blood-brain barrier.

The effect of carbidopa is shown schematically in Fig. 19.4, which compares the fate of levodopa in the presence and absence of carbidopa. As mentioned previously, in the absence of carbidopa, about 98% of levodopa is lost in the periphery, leaving only 2% available to the brain. Why is levodopa lost? Primarily because decarboxylases in the gastrointestinal (GI) tract and peripheral tissues convert it to dopamine, which cannot cross the blood-brain barrier. When these decarboxylases are inhibited by carbidopa, only 90% of levodopa is lost in the periphery, leaving 10% for actions in the brain.

Advantages of carbidopa. The combination of levodopa plus carbidopa is superior to levodopa alone in three ways:
- By increasing the fraction of levodopa available for actions in the CNS, carbidopa allows the dosage of levodopa to be reduced by about 75%. As illustrated in Fig. 19.4, to provide 10 mg of dopamine to the brain, we must administer 500 mg of levodopa if carbidopa is absent but only 100 mg if carbidopa is present.
- By reducing the production of dopamine at the periphery, carbidopa reduces cardiovascular responses to levodopa as well as nausea and vomiting.
- By causing direct inhibition of decarboxylase, carbidopa eliminates concerns about decreasing the effects of levodopa by taking a vitamin preparation that contains pyridoxine.

Disadvantages of carbidopa. Carbidopa has no adverse effects of its own. Accordingly, any adverse responses from carbidopa/levodopa are the result of potentiating the effects of levodopa. When levodopa is combined with carbidopa, abnormal movements and psychiatric disturbances can occur sooner and can be more intense than with levodopa alone.

Carbidopa as a single drug. Carbidopa without levodopa, sold as Lodosyn, is available by special request. When carbidopa is added to levodopa/carbidopa, carbidopa can reduce levodopa-induced nausea and vomiting. It also allows smaller doses of levodopa to be used while promoting a faster response.

TABLE 19.5   Preparation, Dosage, and Administration of Drugs for Parkinson Disease

Drug Name	Preparation	Daily Dosage	Administration Considerations
Levodopa Combinations			
Levodopa/carbidopa (Sinemet, Rytary, Duopa, Duodopa ♣)	Sinemet (IR): 10 mg carbidopa/100 mg levodopa; 25 mg carbidopa/100 mg levodopa; 25 mg carbidopa/250 mg levodopa Sinemet CR: 25 mg carbidopa/100 mg levodopa; 50 mg carbidopa/200 mg levodopa Rytary: carbidopa 23.75 mg/levodopa 95 mg; carbidopa 36.25 mg/levodopa 145 mg; carbidopa 48.75 mg/levodopa 195 mg; carbidopa 61.25 mg/levodopa 245 mg Duopa enteral suspension: carbidopa 4.63 mg/levodopa 20 mg/mL Duodopa ♣ intestinal gel: carbidopa 5 mg/levodopa 20 mg/1 mL	Dosage is highly individualized. Typical dosage is 1 tablet daily or every other day initially and then gradually increased up to a maximum of 8 tablets a day, regardless of strength, administered in divided doses. Duopa and Duodopa are both highly individualized to the patient with dosage adjustments sometimes made on a daily basis.	Food (especially if high fat or high protein) reduces absorption delaying peak by up to 2.5–3 h. Duopa enteral suspension and Duodopa intestinal gel are administered via PEG-J tube infusion.
Levodopa/carbidopa/ entacapone (Stalevo)	Stalevo 50: carbidopa 12.5 mg/levodopa 50 mg/entacapone 200 mg Stalevo 75: carbidopa 18.75 mg/levodopa 75 mg/entacapone 200 mg Stalevo 100: carbidopa 25 mg/levodopa 100 mg/entacapone 200 mg Stalevo 125: carbidopa 31.25 mg/levodopa 125 mg/entacapone 200 mg Stalevo 150: carbidopa 37.5 mg/levodopa 150 mg/entacapone 200 mg Stalevo 200: carbidopa 50 mg/levodopa 200 mg/entacapone 200 mg	Dosage is highly individualized. Typical dosage is 1 tablet of any strength at each dosing interval up to a maximum daily limit of 8 tablets of Stalevo 50 to Stalevo 150 or 6 tablets of Stalevo 200. Dosing intervals are determined by patient response.	Foods that are high in fat may delay absorption. Although this combination may be taken with food, taking habitually on an empty stomach can prevent inadvertent interactions.
Dopamine Agonists: Ergot Derivatives			
Bromocriptine (Parlodel)	Parlodel: 2.5 tablet (scored) Parlodel: 5-mg capsule	Initial: 1.25 mg bid. Gradually increase dosage to achieve desired response or until side effects become intolerable. Maintenance: 30–100 mg/day.	Advise patients to take with food or meals to decrease GI symptoms. Taper dose gradually.
Cabergoline (Dostinex ♣, generic in U.S.)	0.5-mg tablet	Initial: 1 mg/day. Increase using 0.5–1 mg at 1–2 weeks intervals. Maintenance: 2–3 mg/day.	Advise patients to take with food or meals to decrease GI symptoms.
Dopamine Agonists: Nonergot Derivatives			
Pramipexole (Mirapex, Mirapex ER)	IR tablets: 0.125, 0.25, 0.5, 0.75, 1, and 1.5 mg ER tablets: 0.375, 0.75, 1.5, 2.25, 3, and 4.5 mg	IR tablets: 0.125 mg 3 tid initially, and then increased over 7 weeks to a maximum of 1.5 mg tid. ER tablets: 0.375 mg qd initially, then gradually increased to a maximum of 4.5 mg/daily. Reduced dosage for significant renal impairment.	Advise patients that taking with food decreases GI upset. Reduce dosage for significant renal impairment. Taper dose gradually.
Ropinirole (Requip, Requip XL)	IR tablets: 0.25, 0.5, 1, 2, 3, 4, and 5 mg ER tablets: 2, 4, 6, 8, and 12 mg	IR tablets: 0.25 mg tid initially. Can increase over several months to a maximum of 8 mg tid. ER tablets: 2 mg/day initially. Can increase over several months to a maximum of 24 mg/day.	Advise patient that taking with food decreases GI upset. Taper dose gradually.

TABLE 19.5 Preparation, Dosage, and Administration of Drugs for Parkinson Disease—cont'd

Drug Name	Preparation	Daily Dosage	Administration Considerations
Rotigotine (Neupro)	24-h transdermal patch: 1, 2, 3, 4, 6, or 8 mg	Early-stage PD: Usual starting dose is one 2-mg patch q24h. Increase by 2 mg/week until lowest effective dose is attained or until maximal dose of 6 mg/24 h is reached. Advanced-stage PD: Usual starting dose is one 4-mg patch q24h. Increased by 2 mg weekly up to a maximum of 8 mg/24 h. If it becomes necessary to discontinue treatment, withdrawal should be done at the same rate of 2 mg/week.	Advise patient that rotating sites with each application will decrease skin reactions. Allow at least a 2-week lapse before applying the patch to a site used previously. Taper dose gradually.
Apomorphine (Apokyn, Movapo)	10 mg/mL in 3-mL cartridges to be used with a multidose injector pen (provided)	2–6 mg (0.2–0.6 mL) subQ for each "off" episode. Maximum: 5 doses/day	Package labeling states that all patients should take an antiemetic (e.g., trimethobenzamide, 300 mg tid), starting 3 days before the first apomorphine dose.

Comt Inhibitors

Drug Name	Preparation	Daily Dosage	Administration Considerations
Entacapone (Comtan)	200 mg tablets	Initial: 200 mg. Can increase to a maximum of 8 doses (1600 mg) a day.	Advise patient to take with each dose of levodopa/carbidopa.
Tolcapone (Tasmar)	100-mg tablets	100 mg tid. Increase to 200 mg tid if needed.	The first dose should be taken in the morning along with levodopa/carbidopa. The next two doses are taken 6 and 12 h later.

MAO-B Inhibitors

Drug Name	Preparation	Daily Dosage	Administration Considerations
Selegiline (Eldepryl, Emsam, Zelapar)	Capsule: (Eldepryl, generic): 5 mg; Tablet (generic): 5 mg; Dispersible tablet (Zelapar): 1.25 mg (A 24-h patch marketed as Emsam is available, but this is not approved for management of PD.)	5 mg taken with breakfast and lunch, for a total of 10 mg/day. This dosage produces complete inhibition of MAO-B, and hence larger doses are unnecessary. Orally disintegrating tablets: 1.25 mg/day for 6 weeks. Can increase to a maximal dose of 2.5 mg/day if needed.	Bioavailability increased 3–4 times when taken with food. Dispersible tablet should be place on top of tongue and allowed to dissolve. Advise the patient to wait at least 5 min before drinking or eating.
Rasagiline (Azilect)	0.5- and 1-mg tablets	Monotherapy: usual dosage is 1 mg/day or 0.5 mg/day for mild hepatic impairment. Adjunctive therapy with levodopa: 0.5 mg/day initially. Increase to 1 mg/day if needed.	The drug should be decreased by half in mild hepatic impairment. Patients with moderate to severe hepatic impairment should not use this drug.

Antiviral Agent

Drug Name	Preparation	Daily Dosage	Administration Considerations
Amantadine (Gocovri, Osmolex ER)	Tablet: 100 mg; Capsules: 100 mg; Syrup: 10 mg/mL	100 mg twice daily initially. May increase to 400 mg/day in divided doses. Dosage for patients taking high doses of other drugs for PD: 100 mg/day initially. May increase to 200 mg/day in divided doses.	Advise patient that taking with food decreases GI upset.

Centrally Acting Anticholinergic Drugs

Drug Name	Preparation	Daily Dosage	Administration Considerations
Benztropine (Cogentin, Kynesia)	Tablet: 0.5, 1, and 2 mg; Solution for injection: 1 mg/mL in 2-mL vials	Initial: 0.5–1 mg at bedtime. May increase by 0.5 mg every 5–6 days to a maximal dose of 6 mg/day.	IM injection is preferable because, for PD, IV injection does not provide an advantage.
Trihexyphenidyl (generic)	Tablet: 2 mg, 5 mg; Elixir: 0.4/mL	Initial: 1 mg once a day. May increase by 2 mg every 3–5 days to a maximal dose of 15 mg/day.	May be taken with or without food.

CR, Controlled release; ER, extended release; GI, gastrointestinal; IR, immediate release; MAO, monoamine oxidase; PEG, percutaneous endoscopic gastrostomy; PD, Parkinson disease, subQ, subcutaneous

Fig. 19.4 Fate of Levodopa in the Presence and Absence of Carbidopa. In the absence of carbidopa, 98% of an administered dose of levodopa is metabolized in intestinal and peripheral tissues—either by decarboxylases or catechol-*O*-methyltransferase (COMT)—leaving only 2% for actions in the brain. Therefore to deliver 10 mg of levodopa to the brain, the dose of levodopa must be large (500 mg). By inhibiting intestinal and peripheral decarboxylases, carbidopa increases the percentage of levodopa available to the brain. Thus the dose needed to deliver 10 mg is greatly reduced (to 100 mg in this example). Since carbidopa cannot cross the blood-brain barrier, it does not suppress conversion of levodopa to dopamine in the brain. Furthermore, since carbidopa reduces peripheral production of dopamine (from 140 mg to 50 mg in this example), peripheral toxicity (nausea, cardiovascular effects) is greatly reduced. *GI,* Gastrointestinal.

📄 SUMMARY OF KEY PRESCRIBING CONSIDERATIONS

Levodopa Combinations

Therapeutic Goal: To maintain or improve the patient's ability to carry out activities of daily living.

Baseline Data: Heart rate and blood pressure and general cardiovascular (especially if apomorphine or cabergoline are being considered) and neurologic assessment. In particular, motor symptoms—bradykinesia, akinesia, postural instability, tremor, rigidity—should be assessed as well as the extent to which these interfere with activities of daily living (e.g., ability to work, dress, bathe, walk). Because some studies suggest that levodopa can activate malignant melanoma, a careful skin assessment should also be performed.

Monitoring: Orthostatic vital signs must be assessed at each clinic visit. If the patient reports palpitations or if dysrhythmias are suspected, an electrocardiogram (ECG) or monitoring may be indicated. Motor function must be evaluated and compared with baseline.

Identifying High-Risk Patients: Caution must be exercised in dealing with patients who have cardiac disease or psychiatric disorders and in those taking selective monoamine oxidase-B (MAO-B) inhibitors.

Evaluating Therapeutic Effects: Patients should be evaluated for improvements in activities of daily living and for reductions in bradykinesia, postural instability, tremor, and rigidity.

Minimizing Adverse Effects

* Nausea and vomiting—Medications are best taken with a nonfat, nonprotein snack (e.g., fruit) if nausea/vomiting is a problem.
* Dyskinesias—A reduction in dosage may be needed. Amantadine may help with dyskinesias.
* Orthostatic hypotension—Patients should be advised to change from supine or sitting to standing slowly. Fall precautions must be implemented if a patient is hospitalized.

Psychosis—Clozapine or quetiapine may be beneficial.

* Acute loss of effect—Off times can be reduced by combining levodopa/carbidopa with a dopamine agonist (e.g., pramipexole), a catechol-*O*-methyltransferase inhibitor (e.g., entacapone), or a MAO-B inhibitor (e.g., rasagiline).

Dopamine Agonists

Dopamine agonists are first-line drugs for PD. Beneficial effects result from direct activation of dopamine receptors in the striatum. For patients with mild or moderate symptoms, dopamine agonists are the drugs of first choice. Although dopamine agonists are less effective than levodopa, they still have advantages. Specifically, in contrast to levodopa, they are not dependent on enzymatic conversion to become active, are not converted to potentially toxic metabolites, and do not compete with dietary proteins for uptake from the intestine or transport across the blood-brain barrier. In addition, when used long term, dopamine agonists have a lower incidence of response failures and are less likely to cause disabling dyskinesias. However, dopamine agonists do cause serious side effects—especially hallucinations, daytime sleepiness, and postural hypotension. As a result, these drugs are usually reserved for younger patients, who tolerate their side effects better than do the older patients.

The dopamine agonists fall into two groups: derivatives of ergot (an alkaloid found in plants) and nonergot derivatives. The nonergot derivatives—*pramipexole, ropinirole, rotigotine,* and *apomorphine*—are highly selective for dopamine receptors. In contrast, the ergot derivatives—*bromocriptine* and *cabergoline*—are less selective. In addition to activating dopamine receptors, these drugs cause mild *blockage* of serotonergic and α-adrenergic receptors. Because of their selectivity, the nonergot derivatives cause fewer side effects than the ergot derivatives and hence are preferred.

PROTOTYPE DRUGS

Drugs for Parkinson Disease

Dopaminergic Drugs
- Levodopa (increases dopamine [DA] synthesis)
- Carbidopa (blocks levodopa destruction)
- Pramipexole (DA receptor agonist)
- Entacapone (inhibits COMT)
- Selegiline (inhibits MAO-B)
- Amantadine (promotes DA release)

Centrally Acting Anticholinergic Drugs
- Benztropine

Nonergot Derivatives: Pramipexole, Ropinirole, Rotigotine, and Apomorphine

Pramipexole

Actions and uses. Pramipexole (Mirapex) is a nonergot dopamine receptor agonist. The drug is used alone in early-stage PD and is combined with levodopa in advanced-stage PD. Pramipexole binds selectively to dopamine-2 (D_2) and dopamine-3 (D_3) receptors. Binding to D_2 receptors underlies therapeutic effects. The significance of D_3 binding is unknown. When used as monotherapy in early PD, pramipexole can produce significant improvement in motor performance. When combined with levodopa in advanced PD, the drug can reduce fluctuations in motor control and may permit a reduction in levodopa dosage. In both cases, maximal benefits take several weeks to develop. Compared with levodopa, pramipexole is less effective at controlling the motor symptoms of PD, but it is also less likely to cause motor fluctuations.

In addition to its use in PD, pramipexole is approved for patients with moderate to severe *restless legs syndrome* (RLS), a sensorimotor disorder characterized by unpleasant leg sensations that create an urge to move the legs in an effort to ease discomfort. Symptoms are usually more intense in the evening and often disrupt sleep. People with severe RLS experience sleep loss, daytime exhaustion, and diminished quality of life.

Adverse effects and interactions. Pramipexole can produce a variety of adverse effects, primarily by activating dopamine receptors. The most common effects seen when pramipexole is used *alone* are nausea, dizziness, daytime somnolence, insomnia, constipation, weakness, and hallucinations. When the drug is *combined with levodopa*, about 50% of patients experience orthostatic hypotension and dyskinesias, which are not seen when the drug is used by itself. In addition, the incidence of hallucinations nearly doubles.

A few patients have reported *sleep attacks* (overwhelming and irresistible sleepiness that comes on without warning). Sleep attacks should not be equated with the normal sleepiness that occurs with dopaminergic agents.

Pramipexole has been associated with *impulse control disorders*, including compulsive gambling, shopping, binge eating, and hypersexuality. These behaviors are dose related, begin about 9 months after starting pramipexole, and reverse when the drug is discontinued. Risk factors include younger adulthood, a family or personal history of alcohol abuse, and a personality trait called novelty seeking, characterized by impulsivity, a quick temper, and a low threshold for boredom. Before prescribing pramipexole, providers should screen patients for compulsive behaviors.

Cimetidine (a drug for peptic ulcer disease) can inhibit the renal excretion of pramipexole, thereby increasing its blood level.

Ropinirole

Actions and uses. Ropinirole (Requip), a nonergot dopamine agonist, is similar to pramipexole with respect to receptor specificity, mechanism of action, indications, and adverse effects. Like pramipexole, ropinirole is highly selective for D_2 and D_3 receptors, and both drugs share the same indications: PD and RLS. In patients with early PD, ropinirole can be used as monotherapy and in patients with advanced PD, it is used as an adjunct to levodopa.

Adverse effects. Some adverse effects are more common than those with pramipexole. When ropinirole is used alone, the most common effects are nausea, dizziness, somnolence, and hallucinations. Rarely, sleep attacks occur. When ropinirole is combined with levodopa, the most important side effects are dyskinesias, hallucinations, and postural hypotension. Note that these occur less frequently than when pramipexole is combined with levodopa. Like pramipexole, ropinirole can promote compulsive gambling, shopping, and eating as well as hypersexuality.

Rotigotine

Actions and uses. Rotigotine (Neupro) is a nonergot dopamine agonist that is specific for selected dopamine receptors. Although the exact mechanism of action is unknown, it is believed that rotigotine improves dopamine transmission by activating postsynaptic dopamine receptors in the substantia nigra. Rotigotine is approved for the management of PD from its early to advanced stages. It is also approved for the management of moderate to severe primary RLS.

Adverse effects. The most common adverse effects are associated with the CNS and neuromuscular systems. These include a variety of sleep disorders, dizziness, headache, dose-related hallucinations, and dose-related dyskinesia. Orthostatic hypotension and peripheral edema may occur. Nausea and vomiting are common, especially when beginning the drug. Some patients develop skin reactions at the site of application, and hyperhidrosis (excessive perspiration) may occur.

Apomorphine

Actions and use. Apomorphine (Apokyn, Movapo) is a nonergot dopamine agonist approved for the acute treatment of hypomobility during off episodes in patients with advanced PD. Unlike other dopamine agonists, the drug is not given by mouth. Also unlike other dopamine agonists, apomorphine is not indicated for routine PD management. Instead, apomorphine is reserved for the rescue treatment of hypomobility during off episodes in patients with advanced PD.

When tested in patients experiencing at least 2 hours of off time a day, apomorphine produced a 62% improvement in PD rating scores compared with no improvement in patients receiving placebo. Benefits were sustained during 4 weeks of use. Apomorphine is a derivative of morphine but is devoid of typical opioid effects (e.g., analgesia, euphoria, respiratory depression).

Adverse effects. The most common adverse effects are injection-site reactions, hallucinations, yawning, drowsiness, dyskinesias, rhinorrhea, and nausea and vomiting. During clinical trials, there was a 4% incidence of serious cardiovascular events: angina, myocardial infarction, cardiac arrest, or sudden death. Postural hypotension and fainting occurred in 2% of patients. Similar to other dopamine agonists, apomorphine poses a risk for daytime sleep attacks. In addition, apomorphine can promote hypersexuality and enhanced erections (the drug is used in Europe to treat erectile dysfunction). Rarely, apomorphine causes priapism (sustained, painful erection), possibly requiring surgical intervention.

Combined use with an antiemetic. To prevent nausea and vomiting during clinical trials, nearly all patients were treated with an antiemetic, starting 3 days before the first dose of apomorphine. The antiemetic chosen was trimethobenzamide (Tigan, others). Two classes of antiemetics cannot be used: serotonin receptor antagonists (e.g., ondansetron [Zofran]) and dopamine receptor antagonists (e.g., prochlorperazine [Compazine]). Serotonin receptor antagonists will increase the risk for orthostatic (postural) hypotension while having no effect on the nausea, and dopamine receptor antagonists will decrease the effectiveness of apomorphine and most other drugs for PD. About half the trial participants discontinued the antiemetic at some point but continued taking apomorphine.

PATIENT EDUCATION
Dopamine Agonists

Patients should be informed that nausea and vomiting can be reduced by taking oral dopamine agonists with food and told to notify their provider if the nausea and vomiting persist or become severe. Patients taking apomorphine may be pretreated with trimethobenzamide (Tigan), an antiemetic.

Patients should be informed about symptoms of orthostatic hypotension (dizziness, lightheadedness on standing) and advised to sit or lie down if these occur. They should also be told to move slowly when sitting up or standing up.

The potential for movement disorders (tremor, dystonic movements, twitching) should be explained; if these occur, patients should notify their provider.

Forewarn patients that dopamine agonists can cause hallucinations, especially in older adults, and instruct them to notify you if these develop.

Patients should also be aware that pramipexole, ropinirole, rotigotine, and apomorphine can cause sleep attacks. If a sleep attack occurs, patients should avoid potentially hazardous activities (e.g., driving) until these attacks have been adequately managed.

Patients of childbearing age should know that ropinirole may harm the developing fetus and advised to use effective birth control.

Ergot Derivatives: Bromocriptine and Cabergoline

Two ergot derivatives—bromocriptine and cabergoline—are used to manage PD. Bromocriptine is approved for PD; cabergoline is not. These drugs are poorly tolerated, so their use is limited. The side-effect profile of the ergot derivatives differs from that of the nonergot agents because, in addition to activating dopamine receptors, the ergot drugs cause mild blockade of serotonergic and α-adrenergic receptors.

Bromocriptine. Bromocriptine (Parlodel), a derivative of ergot, is a direct-acting dopamine agonist. Beneficial effects derive from activating dopamine receptors in the striatum. Responses are equivalent to those seen with pramipexole and ropinirole. Bromocriptine is used alone in early PD and in combination with levodopa in advanced PD. When combined with levodopa, bromocriptine can prolong therapeutic responses and reduce motor fluctuations. In addition, because bromocriptine allows the dosage of levodopa to be reduced, the incidence of levodopa-induced dyskinesias may be reduced.

Adverse effects are dose dependent and are seen in 30% to 50% of patients. Nausea is most common. The most common dose-limiting effects are psychological reactions (confusion, nightmares, agitation, hallucinations, paranoid delusions). These occur in about 30% of patients and are most likely when the dosage is high. Like levodopa, bromocriptine can cause dyskinesias and postural hypotension. Rarely, bromocriptine causes retroperitoneal fibrosis, pulmonary infiltrates, a Raynaud-like phenomenon, and erythromelalgia (vasodilation in the feet and sometimes hands, resulting in swelling, redness, warmth, and burning pain). In addition, the ergot derivatives have been associated with valvular heart disease. The probable cause is the activation of serotonin receptors on heart valves.

Cabergoline. Cabergoline, a drug approved for treatment of hyperprolactinemic disorders, is used occasionally in PD, although it is not approved by the U.S. Food and Drug Administration (FDA) for this disorder. According to the AAN guidelines, the drug is "possibly effective" for improving off times during levodopa therapy; however, the supporting evidence is weak. Consequently cabergoline is rarely used unless other management attempts have failed. Common side effects are headaches, dizziness, nausea, and weakness. A more concerning adverse effect is the development of cardiac valve regurgitation and the subsequent development of heart failure. Pulmonary and pericardial fibrosis have also occurred.

Catechol-*O*-Methyltransferase Inhibitors

Two COMT inhibitors are available: entacapone and tolcapone. With both drugs, benefits derive from inhibiting metabolism of levodopa in the periphery; these drugs have no direct therapeutic effects of their own. Entacapone is safer and more effective than tolcapone and hence is preferred.

Entacapone

Actions and use. Entacapone (Comtan) is a selective, reversible inhibitor of COMT indicated only for use with levodopa. Like carbidopa, entacapone inhibits the metabolism of levodopa in the intestine and peripheral tissues. However, the drugs inhibit different enzymes: carbidopa inhibits decarboxylases, whereas entacapone inhibits COMT. By inhibiting COMT, entacapone prolongs the plasma half-life of levodopa and thereby prolongs the time that levodopa is available to the brain. In addition, entacapone increases levodopa availability by a second mechanism: By inhibiting COMT, entacapone decreases the production of levodopa metabolites that compete with levodopa for transport across the blood-brain barrier. In clinical trials, entacapone increased the half-life of levodopa by 50% to 75% and thereby caused levodopa blood levels to be more stable and sustained. As a result, entacapone is especially beneficial for patients who experience a wearing off of the effects of levodopa/carbidopa. Entacapone may also permit a reduction in levodopa dosage.

Adverse effects. Most adverse effects result from increasing levodopa levels, although some are caused by entacapone itself. By increasing levodopa levels, entacapone can cause dyskinesias, orthostatic hypotension, nausea, hallucinations, sleep disturbances, and impulse control disorders (see Pramipexole). These can be managed by decreasing the dosage of levodopa. Entacapone should not be stopped abruptly, however. Doing so can result in a significant worsening of symptoms.

SUMMARY OF KEY PRESCRIBING CONSIDERATIONS

Dopamine Agonists

Therapeutic Goal: To maintain or improve the patient's ability to carry out activities of daily living.

Baseline Data: Heart rate and blood pressure and general cardiovascular assessment (especially if apomorphine or cabergoline are being considered) and neurologic assessment. In particular, assess motor symptoms—bradykinesia, akinesia, postural instability, tremor, rigidity—and the extent to which these interfere with activities of daily living (e.g., ability to work, dress, bathe, walk).

Monitoring: Assess orthostatic vital signs at each visit. Evaluate motor function and compare to baseline.

Identifying High-Risk Patients: Use all dopamine agonists with caution in older-adult patients and in those with psychiatric disorders. Use pramipexole with caution in patients with kidney dysfunction. Avoid ropinirole during pregnancy. Use pramipexole and ropinirole with caution in patients prone to compulsive behavior.

Evaluating Therapeutic Effects: Evaluate for improvements in activities of daily living and for reductions in bradykinesia, postural instability, tremor, and rigidity.

Minimizing Adverse Effects:
- Multiple adverse effects—To minimize adverse effects, dosage should be low initially and then gradually increased.
- Nausea, vomiting, orthostatic hypotension—Nausea and vomiting and orthostatic hypotension are addressed through teaching. (See the box "Patient Education: Dopamine Agonists.") Avoid serotonin receptor antagonists and dopamine receptor antagonists for the management of nausea and vomiting because the former can worsen orthostatic (postural) hypotension and the later can decrease the effectiveness of drugs prescribed for PD.
- Dyskinesias, hallucinations, sleep attacks—For complications such as dyskinesias, hallucinations, or sleep attacks, medication adjustments may be necessary.
- Fetal injury—If pregnancy occurs and will be continued, switching to a dopamine agonist other than ropinirole is advised.
- Impulse-control disorders—Pramipexole and ropinirole may induce compulsive, self-rewarding behaviors, including compulsive gambling, eating, and shopping as well as hypersexuality. Before prescribing these drugs, providers should screen patients for a history of compulsive behaviors.

Entacapone itself is responsible for fewer adverse effects. The most common are vomiting, diarrhea, constipation, and yellow-orange discoloration of the urine.

Drug interactions. Because it inhibits COMT, entacapone can, in theory, increase levels of drugs metabolized by COMT. In addition to levodopa, these include methyldopa (an antihypertensive agent), dobutamine (an adrenergic agonist), and isoproterenol (a β-adrenergic agonist). If entacapone is combined with these drugs, a reduction in their dosages may be needed.

Tolcapone

Actions and use. Tolcapone (Tasmar) is a COMT inhibitor used only in conjunction with levodopa—and only if safer agents are ineffective or inappropriate. As with entacapone, benefits derive from inhibiting levodopa metabolism in the periphery, which prolongs levodopa availability. When given to patients taking levodopa, tolcapone improves motor function and may allow a reduction in levodopa dosage. For many patients, the drug reduces the wearing-off effect that can occur with levodopa, thereby extending the effects of levodopa by as much as 2.9 hours a day. Unfortunately, although tolcapone is effective, it is

also potentially dangerous: deaths from liver failure have occurred. Because it carries a serious risk, tolcapone should be reserved for patients who cannot be treated, or treated adequately, with safer drugs. When tolcapone is used, treatment should be limited to 3 weeks in the absence of a beneficial response.

Adverse effects

Liver failure. Tolcapone can cause severe hepatocellular injury, which is sometimes fatal. Because of this risk, a black box warning is mandated by the FDA. Before treatment, patients should be fully apprised of the risks. They should also be informed about signs of emergent liver dysfunction (persistent nausea, fatigue, lethargy, anorexia, jaundice, dark urine) and instructed to report these immediately. Patients with preexisting liver dysfunction should not take the drug. If liver injury is diagnosed, tolcapone should be discontinued and never used again.

BLACK BOX WARNING

Tolcapone (Tasmar)

Tolcapone increases the risk for hepatotoxicity. Liver injury and liver failure may be fatal. Close monitoring is required. Tolcapone should be discontinued if clinical signs or symptoms of liver injury occur or if aspartate aminotransferase (AST) or alanine aminotransferase (ALT) elevation is twice the upper range of normal.

Laboratory monitoring of liver enzymes is required. Tests for serum ALT and AST should be conducted before treatment and then throughout treatment as follows: every 2 weeks for the first year, every 4 weeks for the next 6 months, and every 8 weeks thereafter. If ALT or AST levels exceed the upper limit of normal, tolcapone should be discontinued. Monitoring may not prevent liver injury, but early detection and immediate drug withdrawal can minimize harm.

Other adverse effects. By increasing the availability of levodopa, tolcapone can intensify levodopa-related effects, especially dyskinesias, orthostatic hypotension, nausea, hallucinations, sleep disturbances, and impulse control disorders (see the section on "Pramipexole"); a reduction in levodopa dosage may be required. Tolcapone itself can cause diarrhea, hematuria, and yellow-orange discoloration of the urine. Abrupt withdrawal of tolcapone can produce symptoms that resemble those of neuroleptic malignant syndrome (fever, muscular rigidity, altered consciousness). In rats, large doses have caused renal tubular necrosis and tumors of the kidneys and uterus.

Levodopa/Carbidopa/Entacapone

Levodopa, carbidopa, and entacapone are now available in fixed-dose combinations sold as Stalevo. As discussed earlier, both carbidopa and entacapone inhibit the enzymatic degradation of levodopa and thereby enhance therapeutic effects. The triple combination is more convenient than taking levodopa/carbidopa and entacapone separately, and it also costs a little less. Unfortunately Stalevo is available only in immediate-release tablets and only in specific strengths (see Table 19.4).

Patients who need more flexibility in their regimen cannot be treated with Stalevo, nor can patients who require a sustained-release formulation.

Monoamine Oxidase-B Inhibitors

The MAO-B inhibitors—selegiline and rasagiline—are considered first-line drugs for PD even though benefits are modest. When combined with levodopa, they can reduce the wearing-off effect.

Selegiline

Selegiline (Eldepryl, Emsam, Zelapar), also known as *deprenyl*, was the first MAO inhibitor approved for PD. The drug may be used alone or

BLACK BOX WARNING
Selegiline (Eldepryl, Emsam, Zelapar)

Antidepressants are associated with an increased risk for suicide in patients younger than 24 years. Selegiline, an antidepressant as well as a drug for PD, is included in this warning.

Selegiline carries an increased risk for hypertensive crisis in younger patients and is contraindicated for children younger than 12 years.

in combination with levodopa. In either case, improvement of motor function is modest. There is some evidence suggesting that selegiline may delay neurodegeneration and hence may delay disease progression. However, conclusive proof of neuroprotection is lacking. Nonetheless, current guidelines suggest trying selegiline in newly diagnosed patients just in case the drug *does* confer some protection.

Actions and use. Selegiline causes *selective, irreversible* inhibition of MAO-B, the enzyme that inactivates dopamine in the striatum. Because selegiline causes irreversible inhibition of MAO-B, effects persist until more MAO-B can be synthesized.

Another form of MAO, known as monoamine oxidase-A (MAO-A), inactivates NE and serotonin. As discussed in Chapter 27, nonselective inhibitors of MAO (i.e., drugs that inhibit MAO-A *and* MAO-B) are used to treat depression—and pose a risk for hypertensive crisis as a side effect. Because selegiline is a selective inhibitor of MAO-B, the drug is not an antidepressant and, *at recommended doses,* poses little or no risk for hypertensive crisis.

Selegiline appears to benefit patients with PD in two ways. First, when used as an adjunct to levodopa, selegiline can suppress the destruction of dopamine derived from levodopa. The mechanism is inhibition of MAO-B. By helping preserve dopamine, selegiline can prolong the effects of levodopa and can thereby decrease fluctuations in motor control. Unfortunately these benefits decline dramatically within 12 to 24 months.

In addition to preserving dopamine, there is some hope that selegiline may delay the progression of PD. When used early in the disease, selegiline can delay the need for levodopa. This may reflect a delay in the progression of the disease, or it may simply reflect direct symptomatic relief from selegiline itself.

Adverse effects. When selegiline is used alone, the principal adverse effect is insomnia, presumably because selegiline is metabolized to l-amphetamine and l-methamphetamine, resulting in CNS excitation. (These metabolites, which do not appear to have therapeutic effects, can be harmful.) Insomnia can be minimized by administering the last daily dose no later than noon. Other adverse effects include orthostatic hypotension, dizziness, and GI symptoms. Patients taking selegiline oral disintegrating tablets (ODTs) may experience irritation of the buccal mucosa.

Hypertensive crisis. Although selegiline is selective for MAO-B, high doses can inhibit MAO-A, which creates a risk for hypertensive crisis, especially in younger patients. As discussed in Chapter 27, when a patient is taking a MAO inhibitor, hypertensive crisis can be triggered by taking certain drugs, including sympathomimetics, and by ingesting foods that contain tyramine. Tyramine is especially high in foods that are aged, cured, or fermented (Box 19.1). Accordingly, patients should be instructed to avoid these foods and drugs, both while taking selegiline and for 2 weeks after stopping it.

Drug interactions

Levodopa. When used with levodopa, selegiline can intensify adverse responses to levodopa-derived dopamine. These reactions—orthostatic hypotension, dyskinesias, and psychologic disturbances

(hallucinations, confusion)—can be reduced by decreasing the dosage of levodopa.

Meperidine. Like the nonselective MAO inhibitors, selegiline can cause a dangerous interaction with meperidine (Demerol). Symptoms include stupor, rigidity, agitation, and hyperthermia. The combination should be avoided.

Selective serotonin reuptake inhibitors. Selegiline should not be combined with selective serotonin reuptake inhibitors (SSRIs) such as fluoxetine (Prozac). The combination of an MAO-B inhibitor plus an SSRI can cause fatal serotonin syndrome. Accordingly, SSRIs should be withdrawn at least 5 weeks before giving selegiline.

Rasagiline

Actions and use. Rasagiline (Azilect) is another MAO-B inhibitor for PD. Like selegiline, rasagiline is a selective, irreversible inhibitor of MAO-B. Benefits derive from preserving dopamine in the brain. The drug is approved for initial monotherapy of PD and for combined use with levodopa. Rasagiline is similar to selegiline in most regards. As with selegiline, benefits are modest. The drugs differ primarily in that rasagiline is not converted to amphetamine or methamphetamine.

Adverse effects. When used as monotherapy, rasagiline is generally well tolerated. The most common side effects are headache, arthralgia, dyspepsia, depression, and flu-like symptoms. Unlike selegiline, rasagiline does not cause insomnia.

When rasagiline is combined with levodopa, side effects increase. The most common additional reactions are dyskinesias, accidental injury, nausea, orthostatic hypotension, constipation, weight loss, and hallucinations. Like selegiline, rasagiline may pose a risk for hypertensive crisis (owing to inhibition of MAO-A, especially at higher doses); hence patients should be instructed to avoid tyramine-containing foods and certain drugs, including sympathomimetic agents.

Rasagiline may increase the risk for malignant melanoma. Periodic monitoring of the skin is recommended.

Drug and food interactions. Rasagiline has the potential to interact adversely with multiple drugs. Drugs that should be used with caution include the following:

- *Levodopa.* Like selegiline, rasagiline can intensify adverse responses to levodopa-derived dopamine. If the patient develops dopaminergic side effects, including dyskinesias or hallucinations, a reduction in the dosage of levodopa, not rasagiline, should be considered.
- *CYP1A2 inhibitors,* Blood levels of rasagiline can be raised by ciprofloxacin and other drugs that inhibit CYP1A2, the hepatic enzyme that inactivates rasagiline. For patients taking these drugs, the daily dosage should be reduced.

Drugs and foods that are contraindicated include the following:

- *MAO inhibitors.* Combining rasagiline with another MAO inhibitor increases the risk for hypertensive crisis. At least 2 weeks should separate use of these drugs.
- *Sympathomimetics.* These drugs (e.g., amphetamines, ephedrine, phenylephrine, pseudoephedrine) increase the risk for hypertensive crisis and must be avoided.

- *Tyramine-containing foods.* These agents increase the risk for hypertensive crisis and must be avoided.
- *Antidepressants.* Combining rasagiline with mirtazapine, SSRIs, serotonin-norepinephrine reuptake inhibitors, and tricyclic antidepressants may pose a risk for hyperpyrexia and death. These drugs should be discontinued at least 2 weeks before starting rasagiline. Fluoxetine (an SSRI) should be discontinued at least 5 weeks before starting rasagiline.
- *Analgesics.* Combining rasagiline with meperidine, methadone, or tramadol may pose a risk for serious reactions, including coma, respiratory depression, convulsions, hypertension, hypotension, and even death. At least 2 weeks should separate use of these drugs.
- *Dextromethorphan.* Combining rasagiline with dextromethorphan may pose a risk for brief episodes of psychosis and bizarre behavior.
- *Cyclobenzaprine.* This drug is structurally related to the tricyclic antidepressants, so it should be avoided.

An Antiviral Agent
Amantadine
Actions and uses. Amantadine (Gocovri, Osmolex ER) was developed as an antiviral agent and was later found to be effective in PD. Possible mechanisms include the inhibition of dopamine uptake, stimulation of dopamine release, blockade of cholinergic receptors, antagonism of *N*-methyl-D-aspartate (NMDA) receptors, and blockade of glutamate receptors. Responses develop rapidly—often within 2 to 3 days—but are much less profound than with levodopa or the dopamine agonists. Furthermore, responses may begin to diminish within 3 to 6 months. Accordingly, amantadine is not considered a first-line agent. However, the drug may be helpful for managing dyskinesias caused by levodopa. If effects diminish, they can be restored by increasing the dosage or by discontinuing treatment for several weeks.

Adverse effects. Amantadine can cause adverse CNS effects (confusion, lightheadedness, anxiety) and peripheral effects that are thought to result from muscarinic blockade (blurred vision, urinary retention, dry mouth, constipation). All of these are generally mild when amantadine is used alone. However, if amantadine is combined with an anticholinergic agent, both the CNS and peripheral responses will be intensified.

Patients taking amantadine for 1 month or longer often develop livedo reticularis, a condition characterized by mottled discoloration of the skin. Livedo reticularis is benign and gradually subsides after amantadine withdrawal.

Centrally Acting Anticholinergic Drugs
Anticholinergic drugs have been used in PD since 1867, making them the oldest medicines for this disease. These drugs alleviate symptoms by blocking muscarinic receptors in the striatum, thereby improving the balance between dopamine and acetylcholine. Anticholinergic drugs can reduce tremor and possibly rigidity, but not bradykinesia. These drugs are less effective than levodopa or the dopamine agonists but are better tolerated. Today, anticholinergics are used as second-line therapy for tremor. They are most appropriate for younger patients with mild symptoms. Anticholinergics are generally avoided in older patients, who are intolerant of CNS side effects (sedation, confusion, delusions, and hallucinations).

Although the anticholinergic drugs used today are somewhat selective for cholinergic receptors in the CNS, they can also block cholinergic receptors in the periphery. As a result, they can cause dry mouth, blurred vision, photophobia, urinary retention, constipation, and tachycardia. These effects are usually dose limiting. Blockade of cholinergic receptors in the eye may precipitate or aggravate glaucoma. Accordingly, intraocular

pressure should be measured periodically. Peripheral anticholinergic effects are discussed in Chapter 14.

The anticholinergic agents used most often are benztropine (Cogentin, Kynesia) and trihexyphenidyl, formerly available as Artane. Providers need to be aware that if anticholinergic drugs are discontinued abruptly, symptoms of PD may be intensified.

PATIENT-CENTERED CARE ACROSS THE LIFE SPAN
Drugs for Parkinson Disease

Life Stage	Considerations or Concerns
Children	Juvenile Parkinson disease (PD) in patients younger than 18 years is extremely rare; therefore many drugs for PD have not been tested in children. Only amantadine, benztropine, and bromocriptine have approval for pediatric populations. Selegiline is contraindicated in children younger than 12 years.
Pregnant women	Bromocriptine and cabergoline are not associated with adverse outcomes; however, the manufacturer recommends stopping them after pregnancy is determined. Animal reproduction studies for the remaining drugs have demonstrated a possibility for fetal harm. For ropinirole, in particular, animal studies have demonstrated teratogenic effects and embryonic loss. Of note, it is rare for a woman of childbearing age to develop PD.
Breastfeeding women	Bromocriptine and cabergoline interfere with lactation. Anticholinergics such as benztropine can suppress lactation. Breastfeeding is not recommended in this chapter for women taking other drugs.
Older adults	The average age at PD diagnosis is 62 years; therefore most prescriptions are written for older adults. Adverse effects tend to be more common and more serious in these patients. Beers criteria designate anticholinergic drugs (e.g., benztropine and trihexyphenidyl) as potentially inappropriate for use in geriatric patients.

NONMOTOR SYMPTOMS AND THEIR MANAGEMENT

In addition to experiencing characteristic motor symptoms, about 90% of patients with PD develop nonmotor symptoms, notably autonomic disturbances, sleep disturbances, depression, dementia, and psychosis. Management is addressed in two evidence-based AAN guidelines: *Practice Parameter: Evaluation and Treatment of Depression, Psychosis, and Dementia in Parkinson Disease* and *Practice Parameter: Treatment of Nonmotor Symptoms of Parkinson Disease.*

Autonomic Symptoms
Disruption of autonomic function can produce a variety of symptoms, including constipation, urinary incontinence, drooling, orthostatic hypotension, cold intolerance, and erectile dysfunction. The intensity of these symptoms increases in parallel with the intensity of motor symptoms. Erectile function can be managed with sildenafil (Viagra) and other inhibitors of type 5 phosphodiesterase (see Chapter 53). Orthostatic hypotension can be improved by increasing one's intake of salt and fluid and possibly by taking fludrocortisone, a mineralocorticoid. Urinary incontinence may improve with oxybutynin and other peripherally acting anticholinergic drugs (see Chapter 14). Constipation can be

managed by getting regular exercise and maintaining adequate intake of fluid and fiber. Polyethylene glycol (an osmotic laxative) or a stool softener (e.g., docusate) may also be tried (see Chapter 65).

Sleep Disturbances

PD is associated with excessive daytime sleepiness (EDS), periodic limb movements of sleep (PLMS), and insomnia (which may include either difficulty falling asleep or difficulty staying asleep). EDS may respond to modafinil (Provigil, Alertec ♣), a nonamphetamine CNS stimulant (see Chapter 31). For PLMS, levodopa/carbidopa should be considered; the nonergot dopamine agonists—pramipexole and ropinirole—may also help. Insomnia may be improved by levodopa/carbidopa and melatonin (see Chapter 29). Levodopa/carbidopa helps by reducing motor symptoms that can impair sleep. Melatonin helps by making people feel they are sleeping better, even though objective measures of sleep quality may not improve.

Depression

About 50% of PD patients develop depression, partly in reaction to having a debilitating disease and partly due to the disease process itself. According to the AAN guidelines, only one drug—amitriptyline—has been proved effective in these patients. Unfortunately amitriptyline, a tricyclic antidepressant, has anticholinergic effects that can exacerbate dementia as well as antiadrenergic effects that can exacerbate orthostatic hypotension. Data for other antidepressants, including SSRIs and bupropion, are insufficient to prove or disprove efficacy in PD.

Dementia

Dementia occurs in 40% of PD patients. The AAN guidelines recommend considering treatment with two drugs: donepezil and rivastigmine. Both drugs are cholinesterase inhibitors developed for Alzheimer disease (see Chapter 20). In patients with PD, these drugs can produce a modest improvement in cognitive function without causing significant worsening of motor symptoms, even though these drugs increase availability of acetylcholine at central synapses.

Psychosis

In patients with PD, psychosis is usually caused by the drugs taken to control motor symptoms. Most of these drugs—levodopa, dopamine agonists, amantadine, and anticholinergic drugs—can cause hallucinations. Therefore, if psychosis develops, dopamine agonists, amantadine, and anticholinergic drugs should be withdrawn, and the dosage of levodopa should be reduced to the lowest effective amount. If antipsychotic medication is needed, first-generation antipsychotics should be avoided because these drugs block receptors for dopamine and hence can intensify motor symptoms. Accordingly, the AAN guidelines recommend considering two second-generation antipsychotics: clozapine and quetiapine. Because clozapine can cause agranulocytosis, many clinicians prefer quetiapine. The guidelines recommend against the routine use of olanzapine, another second-generation agent. The antipsychotic drugs are discussed in Chapter 26.

20

Drugs for Alzheimer Disease

Alzheimer disease (AD) is a devastating illness characterized by progressive memory loss, impaired thinking, neuropsychiatric symptoms (e.g., hallucinations, delusions), and the inability to perform routine tasks of daily living. More than 5.5 million Americans have AD. It is the sixth leading cause of death, with an annual cost of about $277 billion. Major pathologic findings are cerebral atrophy, degeneration of cholinergic neurons, and the presence of neuritic plaques and neurofibrillary tangles—all of which begin to develop years before clinical symptoms appear. This neuronal damage is irreversible, so AD cannot be cured. Drugs in current use do little to relieve symptoms or prevent neuronal loss. Furthermore, for many patients there is no significant delay in the progression of AD or in cognitive decline.

PATHOPHYSIOLOGY OF ALZHEIMER DISEASE

The underlying cause of AD is still unknown. Scientists have discovered important pieces of the AD puzzle but still do not know how they fit together. It may well be that AD results from a combination of factors rather than from a single cause.

Degeneration of Neurons

Neuronal degeneration occurs in the hippocampus early in AD, followed later by degeneration of neurons in the cerebral cortex and subsequent decline in cerebral volume. The hippocampus serves an important role in memory. The cerebral cortex is central to speech, perception, reasoning, and other higher functions. As hippocampal neurons degenerate, short-term memory begins to fail. As cortical neurons degenerate, patients begin having difficulty with language. With advancing cortical degeneration, more severe symptoms appear. These include complete loss of speech, loss of bladder and bowel control, and complete inability for self-care. AD eventually destroys enough brain function to cause death.

Reduced Cholinergic Transmission

In patients with advanced AD, levels of acetylcholine are 90% below normal. Loss of acetylcholine is significant for two reasons. First, acetylcholine is an important transmitter in the hippocampus and cerebral cortex—the regions where neuronal degeneration occurs. Second, acetylcholine is critical to forming memories, and its decline has been linked to memory loss. However, cholinergic transmission is essentially normal in patients with mild AD. Hence, loss of cholinergic function cannot explain the cognitive deficits that occur early in the disease process.

β-Amyloid and Neuritic Plaques

Neuritic plaques, which form outside of neurons, are a hallmark of AD. These spherical bodies are composed of a central core of β-amyloid (a protein fragment) surrounded by neuron remnants. Neuritic plaques are seen mainly in the hippocampus and cerebral cortex.

In patients with AD, β-amyloid is present in high levels and may contribute to neuronal injury. Accumulation of β-amyloid begins early in the disease process, perhaps 10 to 20 years before the first symptoms of AD appear. Because of the central role that beta-amyloid appears to play in AD, treatments directed against β-amyloid are in development.

Neurofibrillary Tangles and Tau

Like neuritic plaques, neurofibrillary tangles are a prominent feature of AD. These tangles, which form inside of neurons, result when the orderly arrangement of microtubules becomes disrupted (Fig. 20.1). The underlying cause is production of an abnormal form of tau, a protein that, in healthy neurons, forms cross-bridges between microtubules and thereby keeps their configuration stable. In patients with AD, tau twists into paired helical filaments that form tangles.

Apolipoprotein E4

Apolipoprotein E (apoE), long known for its role in cholesterol transport, may also contribute to AD. ApoE has three forms, named apoE2, apoE3, and apoE4. Only one form—apoE4—is associated with AD. Genetic research has shown that individuals with one or two copies of the gene that codes for apoE4 are at increased risk for AD; however, many people with AD do not have the gene for apoE4.

Endoplasmic Reticulum–Associated Binding Protein

The discovery of endoplasmic reticulum–associated binding protein (ERAB) adds another piece to the AD puzzle. ERAB is present in high concentration in the brains of patients with AD. These high concentrations of ERAB enhance the neurotoxic effects of β-amyloid.

Homocysteine

Elevated plasma levels of homocysteine are associated with an increased risk for AD. Fortunately, the risk can be easily reduced: levels of homocysteine can be lowered by eating foods rich in folic acid and vitamins B_6 and B_{12}, or by taking dietary supplements that contain these compounds.

RISK FACTORS AND SYMPTOMS

Risk Factors

The major known risk factor for AD is advancing age. In 90% of patients, the age of onset is 65 years or older. After age 65 years, the risk for acquiring AD increases exponentially, doubling every 10 years until age 85 to 90 years, after which the risk for getting AD levels off or declines. The only other known risk factor is a family history of AD. Being female *may* be a risk factor. However, the higher incidence of AD in women may occur simply because women generally live longer than men. Other possible risk factors include head injury, low educational level, production of apoE4, high levels of homocysteine, low levels of folic acid, estrogen/

Normal

A

Alzheimer's disease

B

Fig. 20.1 Histologic Changes in Alzheimer Disease. (A) Healthy neuron. (B) Neuron affected by Alzheimer disease, showing characteristic intracellular neurofibrillary tangles. Note also extracellular neuritic plaques.

progestin therapy, sedentary lifestyle, smoking, and chronic exposure to second hand smoke.

Symptoms

The symptoms of AD progress relentlessly from mild to moderate to severe (Table 20.1). Symptoms typically begin after age 65 years but may appear in people as young as 40 years. Early in the disease, patients begin to experience memory loss and confusion. They may be disoriented and get lost in familiar surroundings. Judgment becomes impaired, and personality may change. As the disease progresses, patients have increasing difficulty with self-care. Between 70% and 90% eventually develop behavior problems (wandering, pacing, agitation, screaming). Symptoms may intensify in the evening, a phenomenon known as "*sundowning.*" In the final stages of AD, the patient is unable to recognize close family members or to communicate in any way. All sense of identity is lost, and the individual is completely dependent on others for survival. The time from onset of symptoms to death may be 20 years or longer, but it is usually 4 to 8 years. Although there is no clearly effective therapy for *core symptoms,* other symptoms (e.g., incontinence, depression) can be treated.

PROTOTYPE DRUGS

Alzheimer Disease

Cholinesterase Inhibitors
Donepezil (Aricept)

N-methyl-D-aspartate (NMDA) receptor antagonists
Memantine (Namenda, Namenda XR, Ebixa)

TABLE 20.1	Symptoms of Alzheimer Disease
Mild symptoms	Confusion and memory loss
	Disorientation; getting lost in familiar surroundings
	Problems with routine tasks
	Changes in personality and judgment
Moderate symptoms	Difficulty with activities of daily living, such as feeding and bathing
	Anxiety, suspiciousness, agitation
	Sleep disturbances
	Wandering, pacing
	Difficulty recognizing family and friends
Severe symptoms	Loss of speech
	Loss of appetite; weight loss
	Loss of bladder and bowel control
	Total dependence on caregiver

DRUGS FOR COGNITIVE IMPAIRMENT

Ideally, the goal of AD treatment is to improve symptoms and to reverse cognitive decline (Fig. 20.2). Unfortunately, available drugs cannot do this. At best, drugs currently in use may slow loss of memory and cognition and prolong independent function. However, for many patients, even these modest goals are elusive.

Four drugs are approved for treating AD dementia. Three of the drugs—donepezil, galantamine, and rivastigmine—are cholinesterase inhibitors. The fourth drug—memantine—blocks neuronal receptors for *N*-methyl-D-aspartate (NMDA). Treatment of dementia with these drugs can yield improvement that is statistically significant but clinically marginal. As one expert put it, the benefits of these drugs are equivalent to losing half a pound after taking a weight loss drug for 6 months. Given the modest benefits of these drugs, evidence-based clinical guidelines in the U.S. do not recommend that all patients receive drug therapy; this decision is left to the patient, family, and prescriber. No single drug is more effective than the others, so selection should be based on tolerability, ease of use, and cost. Research has not established an optimal treatment duration. Severity indications for drug choice are shown in Table 20.2.

Cholinesterase Inhibitors

The cholinesterase inhibitors were the first drugs approved by the U.S. Food and Drug Administration (FDA) to treat AD. Three cholinesterase inhibitors are available.

Group Properties

Mechanism of action. Cholinesterase inhibitors prevent the breakdown of acetylcholine by acetylcholinesterase (AChE) and thereby increase the availability of acetylcholine at cholinergic synapses. In patients with AD, the result is enhanced transmission by central cholinergic neurons that have not yet been destroyed. Cholinesterase inhibitors do not cure AD, and they do not stop disease progression—although they may slow progression by a few months.

Therapeutic effect. All cholinesterase inhibitors are approved for patients with *mild to moderate* symptoms, and one agent—donepezil—is also approved for those with *severe* symptoms. Unfortunately, treatment only benefits 1 in 12 patients. Among those who do benefit, improvements are seen in quality of life and cognitive functions (e.g., memory, thought, reasoning). However, these improvements are modest and short lasting. There is no convincing evidence of marked improvement

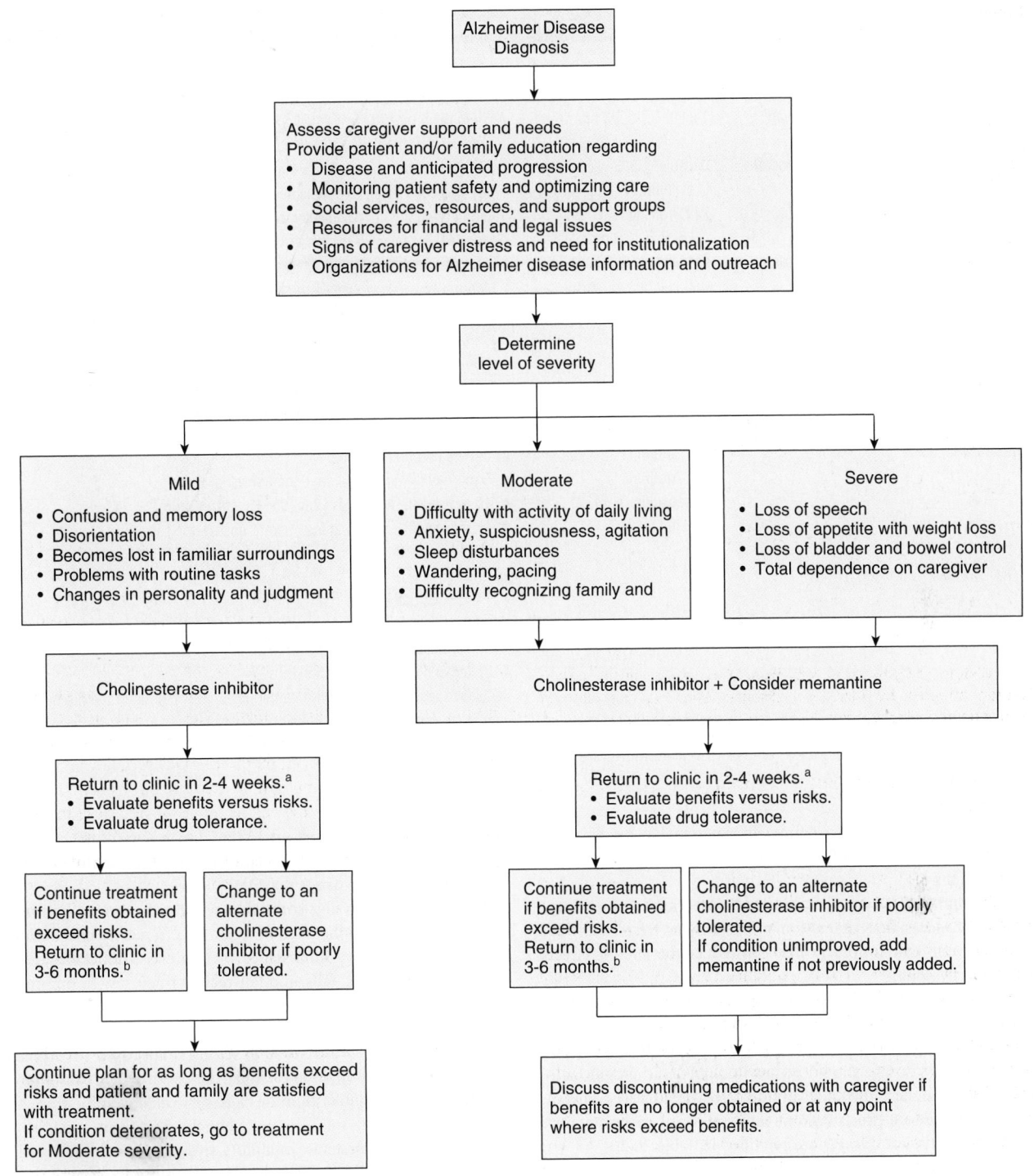

Fig. 20.2 Algorithm for Treating Alzheimer Disease. (American Family Physician available online at http://www.aafp.org/afp/2011/0615/p1403.pdf.)

or significant delay of disease progression. Nonetheless, although improvements are not universal, dramatic, or long lasting, and although side effects are common, the benefits may still be worth the risks for some patients.

Adverse effects. By elevating acetylcholine in the periphery, all cholinesterase inhibitors can cause typical cholinergic side effects. Gastrointestinal (GI) effects—*nausea, vomiting, dyspepsia, diarrhea*—occur often. *Dizziness* and *headache* are also common. The elevation of acetylcholine at synapses in the lungs can cause *bronchoconstriction.* Accordingly, cholinesterase inhibitors should be used with caution in patients with asthma or chronic obstructive pulmonary disease (COPD).

Cardiovascular effects, although uncommon, are a serious concern. Increased activation of cholinergic receptors in the heart can cause symptomatic bradycardia, leading to fainting, falls, fall-related fractures,

TABLE 20.2 Preparations and Dosages of Drugs for Cognitive Impairment

Drug	Indication (AD Severity)	Preparations	Dosing Schedule
Donepezil (Aricept)	Mild to severe	Tablet: 5, 10, 23 mg	*Mild to moderate AD:* 5 mg daily. After 4–6 weeks, may increase to 10 mg daily *Severe AD:* 10 mg daily. After 3 months, may increase to 23 mg daily
Rivastigmine (Exelon)	Mild to moderate	Capsule: 1.5, 3, 4.5, 6 mg Oral solution: 2 mg/mL 24-h transdermal patch: 4.6, 9.5, 13.3 mg	*Mild to moderate AD:* Oral: 1.5 mg twice daily. May increase weekly by 3 mg/day (1.5 each meal) to a maximum of 6 mg twice daily Patch: 4.6-mg patch daily. May increase to a higher dose, if needed *Severe AD:* Initially 4.6-mg patch titrated up to a maximum of 13.3 mg daily
Galantamine (Razadyne, Razadyne ER)	Mild to moderate	IR tablet: 4, 8, 12 mg Oral solution: 4 mg/mL ER tablet: 8, 16, 24 mg	IR tablets and oral solution: 4 mg twice daily × 4 weeks; may increase dosage by 4 mg twice daily every 4 weeks. Maintenance: 8–12 mg twice daily Extended-release capsules: 8 mg once daily × 4 weeks; may increase to 16 mg daily × 4 weeks and then to 24 mg twice daily Maintenance: 16–24 mg daily For patients with moderate hepatic or renal impairment, maximal dose is 16 mg/day. Avoid in patients with severe impairment
Memantine (Namenda, Namenda XR, Ebixa)	Moderate to severe	IR tablet: 5, 10 mg Oral solution: 2 mg/mL, 10 mg/5 mL ER capsules: 7, 14, 21, 28 mg	Increase gradually using the following schedules for IR and ER formulations. IR tablets and oral solution: • 5 mg/day (5 mg once a day), for 1 week or more • 10 mg/day (5 mg twice a day), for 1 week or more • 15 mg/day (5 and 10 mg in separate doses), for 1 week or more • 20 mg/day (10 mg twice a day), for maintenance ER capsules: • 7 mg once daily for 1 week or more • 14 mg once daily for 1 week or more • 21 mg once daily for 1 week or more • 21 mg once daily for maintenance Reduce dosage in patients with moderate renal impairment and discontinue in patients with severe renal impairment

AD, Alzheimer disease; *ER,* extended release; *IR,* immediate release; *NMDA, N*-methyl-D-aspartate.

and pacemaker placement. If a patient is experiencing bradycardia, fainting, or falls, drug withdrawal may be indicated, especially if cognitive benefits are lacking.

Drug interactions. Drugs that block cholinergic receptors (e.g., anticholinergic agents, first-generation antihistamines, tricyclic antidepressants, conventional antipsychotics) can reduce therapeutic effects and should be avoided.

Dosage and duration of treatment. Dosage should be carefully titrated, and treatment should continue as long as clinically indicated. The highest doses produce the greatest benefits—but also the most intense side effects. Accordingly, dosage should be low initially and then gradually increased to the highest tolerable amount. Treatment can continue indefinitely or until side effects become intolerable or benefits are lost. Preparations and typical dosages are provided in Table 20.2.

Properties of Individual Cholinesterase Inhibitors

These drugs have not been directly compared with one another for efficacy. However, they appear to offer equivalent benefits. Accordingly, selection among them is based on side effects, ease of dosing, and cost.

Donepezil. Donepezil (Aricept) is indicated for mild, moderate, or severe AD. The drug causes reversible inhibition of AChE—but is more selective for the form of AChE found in the brain than that found in the periphery. Like other cholinesterase inhibitors, donepezil does not affect the underlying disease process.

Donepezil is well absorbed after oral administration and undergoes metabolism by hepatic CYP2D6 and CYP3A4 isoenzymes. Elimination is mainly in the urine and partly in the bile. Donepezil is highly protein bound and has a prolonged plasma half-life (about 60 hours). According

to FDA labeling, it takes about 15 days for donepezil to achieve steady state. See Table 20.3 for a summary of pharmacokinetic properties for donepezil and other drugs for AD.

Although donepezil is somewhat selective for brain cholinesterase, it can still cause peripheral cholinergic effects; nausea and diarrhea are most common. Like other drugs in this class, donepezil can cause bradycardia, fainting, falls, and fall-related fractures. To minimize side effects, patients are stabilized on the initial dosage for 1 to 3 months before an increase in dosage.

Rivastigmine. Rivastigmine (Exelon) is approved for AD and for dementia of Parkinson disease. Unlike donepezil, which causes reversible inhibition of AChE, rivastigmine causes irreversible inhibition. As with other cholinesterase inhibitors, the benefits in AD are modest.

Like other cholinesterase inhibitors, rivastigmine can cause peripheral cholinergic side effects. These occur with more frequency compared with the other two drugs. With oral dosing, the most common cholinergic effects are nausea, vomiting, diarrhea, abdominal pain, tremors, and anorexia. Weight loss (7% of initial weight) occurs in 18% of male to 26% of female patients. By enhancing cholinergic transmission, rivastigmine can intensify symptoms in patients with peptic ulcer disease, bradycardia, sick sinus syndrome, urinary obstruction, and lung disease; caution is advised. Like other drugs in this class, rivastigmine can cause bradycardia, fainting, falls, and fall-related fractures. Blood levels are lower with transdermal dosing than with oral dosing, and hence the intensity of side effects is lower as well. Rivastigmine has no significant drug interactions, probably because it does not interact with hepatic drug-metabolizing enzymes. (In contrast to other cholinesterase inhibitors, rivastigmine is converted to inactive metabolites by AChE.)

TABLE 20.3 Drugs for Alzheimer Disease: Pharmacokinetic Properties

Drugs	Route	Peak	Half-Life	Metabolism	Excretion
Donepezil (Aricept)	PO	3 h (8 h for 23 mg film-coated tablet)	70 h	Hepatic (CYP2D6, CYP3A4 and glucuronidation)	Urine (primary), bile
Rivastigmine (Exelon)	PO, transdermal	PO: 1 h Transdermal: >8 h	1.5 h	AChE in the brain	Urine (primary), feces
Galantamine (Razadyne, Razadyne ER Reminyl ER)	PO	IR tablet without food: 1 h IR tablet with food: 2.5 h ER tablet: 5 h	7 h	Hepatic (predominantly CYP2D6 and CYP3A4)	Urine
Memantine (Namenda, Namenda XR, Ebixa)	PO	3–7 h	60–80 h	Hepatic (primarily non-CYP450)	Urine

AChE, Acetylcholinesterases; *ER*, extended release; *IR*, immediate release; *PO*, per os.

Galantamine. Galantamine (Razadyne, Razadyne ER Reminyl ER) is a reversible cholinesterase inhibitor indicated for mild to moderate AD. The drug is prepared by extraction from daffodil bulbs. In clinical trials, galantamine improved cognitive function, behavioral symptoms, quality of life, and the ability to perform activities of daily living. However, as with other cholinesterase inhibitors, benefits were modest and short lasting.

The most common adverse effects are nausea, vomiting, diarrhea, anorexia, and weight loss. Nausea and other GI complaints are greater than with donepezil but less than with oral rivastigmine. By increasing cholinergic stimulation in the heart, galantamine can cause bradycardia, fainting, falls, and fall-related fractures. Like other cholinesterase inhibitors, galantamine can cause bronchoconstriction and hence must be used with caution in patients with asthma or COPD. Drugs that block cholinergic receptors (e.g., anticholinergics, first-generation antihistamines, tricyclic antidepressants, conventional antipsychotics) can reduce therapeutic effects and should be avoided.

N-Methyl-D-Aspartate Receptor Antagonist
Memantine

Memantine (Namenda, Namenda XR, Ebixa) is a first-in-class NMDA receptor antagonist. Unlike the cholinesterase inhibitors, which can be used for mild AD, memantine is indicated only for *moderate or severe* AD. Although memantine helps treat symptoms of AD, there is no evidence that it modifies the underlying disease process.

Therapeutic effects. In patients with moderate to severe AD, memantine appears to confer modest benefits. For many patients, the drug can slow the decline in function, and in some cases it may actually cause symptoms to improve. In one study, patients taking memantine for 28 weeks scored higher on tests of cognitive function and day-to-day function than did those taking placebo, suggesting that memantine slowed functional decline. In another study that compared treatment with memantine plus donepezil (a cholinesterase inhibitor) with donepezil alone, after 24 weeks, those taking the combination showed less decline in cognitive and day-to-day function than those taking donepezil alone. This suggests that either (1) the two agents confer independent benefits or (2) they act synergistically to enhance each other's effects.

Mechanism of action. Memantine modulates the effects of glutamate (the major excitatory transmitter in the central nervous system) at NMDA receptors, which are believed to play a critical role in learning and memory. The NMDA receptor—a transmembrane protein with a central channel—regulates calcium entry into neurons. The binding of glutamate to the receptor promotes calcium influx.

Under healthy conditions, an action potential releases a burst of glutamate into the synaptic space. Glutamate then binds with the NMDA

SUMMARY OF KEY PRESCRIBING CONSIDERATIONS
Cholinesterase Inhibitors

Therapeutic Goal: Improved cognition and function for patients with Alzheimer disease by increasing availability of acetylcholine at cholinergic synapses.

Baseline Data: Assess cognitive and functional neurological status. Assess for evidence of gastrointestinal problems. Check baseline weight and basic respiratory and cardiovascular status.

Monitoring: At each visit, assess orientation, cognition, and functional status. Check weight and examine for changes in respiratory, cardiovascular, or gastrointestinal status compared to baseline. If significant adverse effects occur, consider the degree of drug benefit achieved when determining whether to continue therapy.

Identifying High-Risk Patients: Cholinesterase inhibitors should be prescribed cautiously for patients with a history of respiratory or peptic ulcer disease. Exercise caution when prescribing for patients with bradycardia or first-degree heart block; benefits may not be worth the risks. Avoid prescribing to patients with higher degrees of heart block.

Evaluating Therapeutic Effects: Evaluate for improvement of cognitive and functional status.

Minimizing Adverse Effects:
- Most adverse effects (e.g., nausea, diarrhea, insomnia) are dose related and can be decreased by starting with lower doses and increasing gradually. These symptoms usually abate in 2–3 weeks.
- Falls are more likely to occur as a result of bradycardia and other cardiac changes. Initiate fall precautions if hospitalized and teach patient and family how to prevent falls at home.
- To prevent weight loss, encourage nutritional supplements (e.g., Boost) and snacks between meals. Schedule an appointment with a registered dietician.

PATIENT EDUCATION
Cholinesterase Inhibitors

- Explain that this drug is prescribed to improve thinking and function in patients with Alzheimer disease. It does not work on everyone.
- Explain that lightheadedness may occur and that this increases the risk for falls. If these symptoms occur, sit or lie down until it passes. It may help to move slowly when changing to a standing position because sudden movement may increase dizziness.
- Encourage patient and family to insure adequate intake with supplemental meals and snacks to maintain optimal weight.
- Have the patient keep a list of new symptoms and problems so that these can be discussed at each patient encounter.

Normal physiology

A   Resting state   Activated state   Return to resting state

Pathophysiology

B   Activated state   Persistent activated state

KEY

NMDA receptor

△ Glutamate

● Magnesium

○ Calcium

∨ Memantine

Effect of memantine

C   Blockade of further calcium entry   Return to normal resting state   Normal activation

Fig. 20.3 Memantine Mechanism of Action. (A) *Normal physiology.* In the resting postsynaptic neuron, magnesium occupies the *N*-methyl-D-aspartate *(NMDA)* receptor channel, blocking calcium entry. Binding of glutamate to the receptor displaces magnesium, which allows calcium to enter. When glutamate dissociates from the receptor, magnesium returns to the channel and blocks further calcium inflow. The brief period of calcium entry constitutes a "signal" in the learning and memory process. (B) *Pathophysiology.* Slow but steady leakage of glutamate from the presynaptic neuron keeps the NMDA receptor in a constantly activated state. This allows excessive calcium influx, which can impair memory and learning and can eventually cause neuronal death. (C) *Effect of memantine.* Memantine blocks calcium entry when extracellular glutamate is low and thereby stops further calcium entry, which allows intracellular calcium levels to normalize. When a burst of glutamate is released in response to an action potential, the resulting high level of glutamate is able to displace memantine, causing a brief period of calcium entry. Not shown: When glutamate diffuses away, memantine reblocks the channel and thereby stops further calcium entry, despite continuing low levels of glutamate in the synapse.

receptor and displaces magnesium from the receptor channel, permitting calcium entry (Fig. 20.3A). Glutamate then quickly dissociates from the receptor, permitting magnesium to reblock the channel, and thereby prevents further calcium influx. The brief period of calcium entry constitutes a "signal" in the learning and memory process.

Under pathologic conditions, there is slow but steady leakage of glutamate from the presynaptic neuron and surrounding glia. As a result, the channel in the NMDA receptor is kept open, allowing excessive influx of calcium (see Fig. 20.3B). High intracellular calcium has two

effects: (1) impaired learning and memory (because the "noise" created by excessive calcium overpowers the "signal" created when calcium enters in response to glutamate released by a nerve impulse) and (2) neurodegeneration (because too much intracellular calcium is toxic).

How does memantine help? It blocks calcium influx when extracellular glutamate is low but permits calcium influx when extracellular glutamate is high. As shown in Fig. 20.3C, when the glutamate level is low, memantine is able to occupy the NMDA receptor channel and thereby block the steady entry of calcium. As a result, the level of intracellular calcium is able to normalize. Then, when a burst of glutamate is released in response to an action potential, the resulting high level of extracellular glutamate is able to displace memantine, causing a brief period of calcium entry. Because intracellular calcium is now low, normal signaling can occur. When glutamate diffuses away from the receptor, memantine reblocks the channel and thereby stops further calcium entry, despite continuing low levels of glutamate in the synapse.

Adverse effects. Memantine is well tolerated. The most common side effects are dizziness, headache, and confusion—and these occur in only 5% to 7% of those taking the drug. Other less common effects include diarrhea or constipation. In clinical trials, the incidence of all these effects was about the same as in patients taking placebo. Rarely, skin reactions, such as erythema multiforme and Stevens–Johnson syndrome, and cardiovascular events, such as bradycardia, hypertension, and angina, have occurred. Dosage adjustment is required for patients with renal impairment having creatinine clearance of less than 30 mL/min. Canadian labeling also recommends avoiding memantine in patients with severe hepatic impairment as a precaution due to inadequate studies and in patients with corneal conditions as these have worsened during treatment.

Drug interactions. In theory, combining memantine with another NMDA antagonist, such as amantadine or ketamine, could have an undesirable additive effect. Accordingly, such combinations should be used with caution.

Sodium bicarbonate and other drugs that alkalinize the urine can greatly decrease the renal excretion of memantine. Accumulation of the drug to toxic levels might result.

 ## SUMMARY OF KEY PRESCRIBING CONSIDERATIONS

Memantine

Therapeutic Goal: Slow cognitive and functional decline of patients with moderate to severe Alzheimer disease.

Baseline Data: Cognitive and functional neurological status. Rule out corneal conditions and hepatic conditions.

Monitoring: At each visit, assess cognition, and functional status. Canadian labeling recommends scheduling ophthalmic exams while taking this drug.

Identifying High-Risk Patients: Use caution with prescribing to patients with a history of cardiovascular disease, hepatic or renal impairment, or ophthalmic disease.

Evaluating Therapeutic Effects: Evaluate for improvement of cognitive and functional status.

Minimizing Adverse Effects:
- Dizziness can increase the risk for falls. Institute fall risks if hospitalized.
- Advise patients to take acetaminophen or an nonsteroidal antiinflammatory for headaches.

PATIENT EDUCATION
Memantine

- Explain that this drug is prescribed to improve thinking and function in patients with Alzheimer disease. It does not work on everyone.
- Explain that dizziness may occur and, if it does, sit or lie down until it passes. It may help to move slowly when changing to a standing position because sudden movement may increase dizziness.
- Have the patient notify you if they have changes in vision, develop a rash, or have chest pain or other new symptoms.

Drugs for Neuropsychiatric Symptoms

Neuropsychiatric symptoms (e.g., agitation, aggression, delusions, hallucinations) occur in more than 80% of people with AD. Although multiple drug classes—antipsychotics, cholinesterase inhibitors, mood stabilizers, antidepressants, anxiolytics, NMDA receptor antagonists—have been tried as treatment, very few are effective, and even then the benefits are limited. There *is* convincing evidence that neuropsychiatric symptoms can be reduced with two atypical antipsychotics: *risperidone* (Risperdal) and *olanzapine* (Zyprexa). However, benefits are modest, and these drugs slightly *increase* mortality, mainly from cardiovascular events and infection. Cholinesterase inhibitors may offer modest help. There is little or no evidence for a benefit from conventional antipsychotics (e.g., haloperidol, chlorpromazine), mood stabilizers (valproate, carbamazepine, lithium), antidepressants, or memantine.

Can We Prevent Alzheimer Disease or Delay Cognitive Decline?

Despite extensive research to find ways to prevent AD or to delay the cognitive decline associated with this condition, a 2017 systematic review by the Agency of Healthcare Research and Quality (see https://effectivehealthcare.ahrq.gov/topics/cognitive-decline/research-2017) found we have very little good evidence supporting the association of any *modifiable* factor—diet, exercise, social interaction, economic status, nutritional supplements, medications, environmental toxins—with reduced risk for AD. However, this discouraging conclusion does not mean that all available interventions have been proved not to work. Rather, it means that the evidence is too meager or the findings are contradictory to prove that some interventions *might* work.

21

Drugs for Seizure Disorders

In this chapter, we focus on drugs for seizure disorders. Epilepsy is a common condition associated with seizure disorders, so we begin with a short discussion of this condition.

The term *epilepsy* refers to a group of chronic neurologic disorders characterized by recurrent seizures, brought on by excessive excitability of neurons in the brain. Symptoms can range from brief periods of unconsciousness to violent convulsions. Patients may also experience problems with learning, memory, and mood, which can be just as troubling as their seizures.

In the United States, about 3.4 million people have epilepsy, according to the Centers for Disease Control and Prevention. The incidence is highest in the very young and in older adults. The total direct and indirect costs of epilepsy are estimated at $15.5 billion a year.

The terms *seizure* and *convulsion* are not synonymous. *Seizure* is a general term that applies to all types of epileptic events. In contrast, *convulsion* has a more limited meaning, applying only to abnormal motor phenomena, for example, the jerking movements that occur during a tonic-clonic attack. Accordingly, although all convulsions may be called seizures, it is not correct to call all seizures convulsions. Absence seizures, for example, manifest as brief periods of unconsciousness, which may or may not be accompanied by involuntary movements. Because not all seizures involve convulsions, we will refer to the agents used to treat seizures as *antiseizure drugs*, rather than anticonvulsants.

GENERATION OF SEIZURES

Seizures are initiated by synchronous, high-frequency discharge from a group of hyperexcitable neurons, called a *focus*. A focus may result from several causes, including congenital defects, hypoxia at birth, head trauma, brain infection, stroke, cancer, and genetic disorders. Seizures occur when discharge from a focus spreads to other brain areas, thereby recruiting normal neurons to discharge abnormally. The overt manifestations of any particular seizure disorder depend on the location of the seizure focus and the neuronal connections to that focus. The connections to the focus determine the brain areas to which seizure activity can spread.

TYPES OF SEIZURES

Seizure can be divided into two broad categories: *partial (focal) seizures* and *generalized seizures*. In partial seizures, seizure activity undergoes a very limited spread to adjacent cortical areas beyond the focus. In generalized seizures, focal seizure activity is conducted widely throughout both hemispheres. As a rule, partial seizures and generalized seizures are treated with different drugs; however, there are some exceptions (Table 21.1).

Partial Seizures

Partial seizures fall into three groups: simple partial seizures, complex partial seizures, and partial seizures that evolve into secondarily generalized seizures.

Simple Partial Seizures

These seizures manifest with discrete symptoms that are determined by the brain region involved. Hence the patient may experience discrete motor symptoms (e.g., twitching thumb), sensory symptoms (e.g., local numbness; auditory, visual, or olfactory hallucinations), autonomic symptoms (e.g., nausea, flushing, salivation, urinary incontinence), or psychoillusory symptoms (e.g., feelings of unreality, fear, or depression). Simple partial seizures are distinguished from complex partial seizures in that there is *no loss of consciousness*. These seizures persist for 20 to 60 seconds.

Complex Partial Seizures

These seizures are characterized by *impaired consciousness* and lack of responsiveness. At seizure onset, the patient becomes motionless and stares with a fixed gaze. This state is followed by a period of *automatism*, in which the patient performs repetitive, purposeless movements, such as lip smacking or hand wringing. Seizures last 45 to 90 seconds.

Secondarily Generalized Seizures

These seizures begin as simple or complex partial seizures and then evolve into generalized tonic-clonic seizures. Consciousness is lost. These seizures last 1 to 2 minutes.

Generalized Seizures

Generalized seizures may be convulsive or nonconvulsive. As a rule, they produce immediate loss of consciousness. The major generalized seizures are discussed briefly in the sections that follow.

Tonic-Clonic Seizures

In tonic-clonic seizures (formerly known as grand mal seizures), neuronal discharge spreads throughout both hemispheres of the cerebral cortex. These seizures manifest as major convulsions, characterized by a period of muscle rigidity (tonic phase) followed by synchronous muscle jerks (clonic phase). Tonic-clonic seizures often cause urination but not defecation. Convulsions may be preceded by a loud cry, caused by forceful expiration of air across the vocal cords. Tonic-clonic seizures are accompanied by marked impairment of consciousness and are followed by a period of central nervous system (CNS) depression, referred to as the *postictal state*. The seizure itself typically lasts 90 seconds or less.

Absence Seizures (Petit Mal)

Absence seizures are characterized by loss of consciousness for a brief time (10 to 30 seconds). Seizures usually involve mild, symmetrical motor activity (e.g., eye blinking) but may occur with no motor activity at all. The patient may experience hundreds of absence attacks a day. Absence seizures occur primarily in children and usually cease during the early teen years.

TABLE 21.1   Drugs for Specific Types of Seizures

Seizure Type	Traditional Antiseizure Drugs	Newer Antiseizure Drugs
Partial		
Simple partial, complex partial, and secondarily generalized	Carbamazepine Fosphenytoin Phenobarbital Phenytoin Primidone Valproic acid	Brivaracetam Ezogabine Felbamate Gabapentin Lacosamide Lamotrigine Levetiracetam Oxcarbazepine Pregabalin Tiagabine Topiramate Vigabatrin Zonisamide
Primary Generalized		
Tonic-clonic	Carbamazepine Fosphenytoin Phenobarbital Phenytoin Primidone Valproic acid	Lamotrigine Levetiracetam Topiramate
Absence	Ethosuximide Valproic acid	Lamotrigine
Myoclonic	Valproic acid	Lamotrigine Levetiracetam Topiramate

Atonic Seizures

These seizures are characterized by sudden loss of muscle tone. If seizure activity is limited to the muscles of the neck, "head drop" occurs. However, if the muscles of the limbs and trunk are involved, a "drop attack" can occur, causing the patient to suddenly collapse. Atonic seizures occur mainly in children.

Myoclonic Seizures

These seizures consist of sudden muscle contraction that lasts for just 1 second. Seizure activity may be limited to one limb (focal myoclonus), or it may involve the entire body (massive myoclonus).

Status Epilepticus

Status epilepticus (SE) is defined as a seizure that persists for 15 to 30 minutes or longer or a series of recurrent seizures during which the patient does not regain consciousness. There are several types of SE, including generalized convulsive SE, absence SE, and myoclonic SE.

Febrile Seizures

Fever-associated seizures are common among children aged 6 months to 5 years. Febrile seizures typically manifest as generalized tonic-clonic convulsions of short duration. Children who experience these seizures are *not* at high risk for developing epilepsy later in life.

Mixed Seizures: Lennox-Gastaut Syndrome

Lennox-Gastaut syndrome is a severe form of epilepsy that usually develops during the preschool years. The syndrome is characterized by developmental delay and a mixture of partial and generalized seizures. Seizure types include partial, atonic, tonic, generalized tonic-clonic, and atypical absence. In children with Lennox-Gastaut syndrome, seizures can be very difficult to manage.

HOW ANTISEIZURE DRUGS WORK

We have long known that antiseizure drugs can (1) suppress discharge of neurons within a seizure focus and (2) suppress propagation of seizure activity from the focus to other areas of the brain. However, until recently, we did not know how these effects were achieved. It now appears that nearly all antiseizure drugs act through five basic mechanisms: suppression of sodium influx, suppression of calcium influx, promotion of potassium efflux, blockade of receptors for glutamate, and potentiation or increase of gamma-aminobutyric acid (GABA). Categorization of antiseizure drugs by mechanism of action, when known, is displayed in Box 21.1.

Suppression of Sodium Influx

Before discussing antiseizure drug actions, we need to review sodium channel physiology. Neuronal action potentials are propagated by influx of sodium through sodium channels, which are gated pores in the cell membrane that control sodium entry. For sodium influx to occur, the channel must be in an *activated state*. Immediately after sodium entry, the channel goes into an *inactivated state*, during which further sodium entry is prevented. Under normal circumstances, the inactive channel very quickly returns to the activated state, thereby permitting more sodium entry and propagation of another action potential.

Several antiseizure drugs, including phenytoin, carbamazepine, and lamotrigine, reversibly bind to sodium channels while they are in the inactivated state and thereby prolong channel inactivation. By delaying return to the active state, these drugs decrease the ability of neurons to fire at high frequency. As a result, seizures that depend on high-frequency discharge are suppressed.

Suppression of Calcium Influx

In axon terminals, influx of calcium through voltage-gated calcium channels promotes transmitter release. Hence drugs that block these calcium channels can suppress transmission. Ethosuximide acts by this mechanism.

Promotion of Potassium Efflux

During an action potential, influx of sodium causes neurons to depolarize, and then efflux of potassium causes neurons to repolarize. One antiseizure drug—ezogabine (retigabine)—acts on voltage-gated potassium channels to facilitate potassium efflux. This action is believed to underlie the drug's ability to slow repetitive neuronal firing and thereby provide seizure control.

Antagonism of Glutamate

Glutamic acid (glutamate) is the primary excitatory transmitter in the CNS. The compound works through two receptors: (1) *N*-methyl-D-aspartate (NMDA) receptors and (2) alpha-amino-3-hydroxy-5-methyl-4-isoxazole propionic acid (AMPA) receptors. Perampanel is an AMPA glutamate receptor antagonist. Two other drugs—felbamate and topiramate—block the actions of glutamate at NMDA receptors and thereby suppress neuronal excitation.

Potentiation of Gamma-Aminobutyric Acid

Several antiseizure drugs potentiate the actions of GABA, an inhibitory neurotransmitter that is widely distributed throughout the brain. By augmenting the inhibitory influence of GABA, these drugs decrease

BOX 21.1 Categorization of Antiseizure Drugs by Mechanism of Action

Drugs That Affect Sodium Influx
Phenytoin
Lamotrigine
Carbamazepine
Eslicarbazepine
Oxcarbazepine
Lacosamide
Rufinamide
Zonisamide
Topiramate[a]

Drugs That Affect Calcium Influx
Ethosuximide

Drugs That Affect Potassium Efflux
Ezogabine

Drugs That Affect GABA Activity
Benzodiazepines (e.g., diazepam)
Barbiturates (e.g., phenobarbital)
Gabapentin
Tiagabine
Vigabatrin
Valproic acid

Drugs That Affect Glutamate Receptors
Perampanel
Felbamate
Topiramate[a]

Drugs With Uncertain Mechanisms of Action
Pregabalin
Levetiracetam
Brivaracetam

[a]Drug possesses more than one mechanism of action

neuronal excitability and thereby suppress seizure activity. Drugs increase the influence of GABA by several mechanisms. Benzodiazepines and barbiturates enhance the effects of GABA by mechanisms that involve direct binding to GABA receptors. Gabapentin promotes GABA release. Tiagabine inhibits GABA reuptake, and vigabatrin inhibits the enzyme that degrades GABA and thereby increases GABA availability.

BASIC THERAPEUTIC CONSIDERATIONS

Therapeutic Goal and Treatment Options

The goal in treating epilepsy is to reduce seizures to an extent that enables the patient to live a normal or nearly normal life. Ideally, treatment should eliminate seizures entirely. However, this may not be possible without causing intolerable side effects. Therefore we must balance the desire for complete seizure control against the acceptability of side effects.

Epilepsy may be treated with drugs or with nondrug therapies. As noted, drugs can benefit 60% to 70% of patients. This means that, of the 3.4 million Americans with epilepsy, over a million people *cannot* be treated successfully with drugs. For these people, nondrug therapy may well help. Three options exist: neurosurgery, vagus nerve stimulation, and the ketogenic diet. Of the three, neurosurgery has the best success rate, but vagus nerve stimulation is used most widely.

Diagnosis and Drug Selection

Control of seizures requires proper drug selection. As indicated in Table 21.1, many antiseizure drugs are selective for specific seizure disorders. Phenytoin, for example, is useful for treating tonic-clonic and partial seizures but not absence seizures. Conversely, ethosuximide is active against absence seizures but not against tonic-clonic or partial seizures. Only one drug—valproic acid—appears effective against practically all forms of epilepsy. Because most antiseizure drugs are selective for certain seizure disorders, effective treatment requires a proper match between the drug and the seizure. To make this match, the seizure type must be accurately diagnosed.

Making a diagnosis requires physical, neurologic, and laboratory evaluations along with a thorough history. The history should determine the age at which seizures began, the frequency and duration of seizure events, precipitating factors, and times when seizures occur. Physical and neurologic evaluations may reveal signs of head injury or other disorders that could underlie seizure activity, although in many patients the physical and neurologic evaluations may be normal. An electroencephalogram is essential for diagnosis. Other diagnostic tests that may be employed include computed tomography, positron emission tomography, and magnetic resonance imaging.

Pharmacologic management with antiseizure drugs is highly individualized. Very often, patients must try several drugs before a regimen that is both effective and well tolerated can be established. Initial treatment should be done with just one antiseizure drug. If this drug fails, it should be discontinued and a different antiseizure drug should be tried. If this second drug fails, two options are open: (1) treatment with a third antiseizure drug alone or (2) treatment with a combination of antiseizure drugs.

Drug Evaluation

After an antiseizure drug has been selected, a trial period is needed to determine its effectiveness. During this time there is no guarantee that seizures will be controlled. Until seizure control is certain, the patient should be warned not to participate in driving and other activities that could be hazardous should a seizure occur.

Maintenance of a seizure frequency chart is important. The chart should be kept by the patient or a family member and should contain a complete record of all seizure events. This record can be used to help guide the provider in optimizing pharmacologic management.

During the process of drug evaluation, adjustments in dosage are often needed. No drug should be considered ineffective until it has been tested in sufficiently high dosages and for a reasonable time. Knowledge of plasma drug levels can be a valuable tool for establishing dosage and evaluating the effectiveness of a specific drug.

Monitoring Plasma Drug Levels

Safe and effective levels have been firmly established for most antiseizure drugs (Table 21.2). Monitoring these levels can help guide dosage adjustments.

Monitoring plasma drug levels is especially helpful when treating major convulsive disorders (e.g., tonic-clonic seizures). Because these seizures can be dangerous, and because delay of therapy may allow the condition to worsen, rapid control of seizures is desirable. However, because these seizures occur infrequently, a long time may be needed to establish control if clinical outcome is relied on as the only means of determining an effective dosage. By adjusting initial doses on the basis of plasma drug levels (rather than on the basis of seizure control), we can readily achieve drug levels that are likely to be effective, thereby increasing our chances of establishing control quickly.

TABLE 21.2 Preparations and Dosage of Antiseizure Drugs

Drug	Preparations	DAILY MAINTENANCE DOSAGE[a] Adults (mg)	Children (mg/kg)	Target Serum Level (μg/mL)
Traditional Antiseizure Drugs				
Carbamazepine (Tegretol, Tegretol-XR, Carbatrol, Equetro, Epitol, Carnexiv)	IR tablets: 200 mg Chewable tablets: 100 mg ER tablets: 100, 200, 400 mg ER capsules: 100, 200, 300 mg Oral suspension: 20 mg/mL IV: 200 mg/20 mL (10 mg/mL)	800–1200	10–35	4–12
Ethosuximide (Zarontin)	Capsules: 250 mg Syrup: 250 mg/5 mL	750	20	40–100[b]
Phenobarbital (Phenobarb)	Tablets: 15 mg, 16.2 mg, 30 mg, 32.4 mg, 60 mg, 64.8 mg, 97.2 mg, 100 mg Elixir: 20 mg/5 mL Oral solution: 20 mg/5 mL Solution for injection: 65 mg/mL, 130 mg/mL	50–120	3–8	15–45
Phenytoin (Dilantin-125, Dilantin Infatab, Phenytek [ER capsules], Dilantin [ER capsules])	Chewable tablets: 50 mg Capsules: 30, 100, 200, 300 mg Oral suspension: 125 mg/5 mL Solution for injection: 50 mg/mL	300–600	4–8	10–20
Fosphenytoin (Cerebyx)	Solution for injection: 100 mg PE/2 mL, 500 mg	4–6 mg PE/kg/day	ND	10–20 as phenytoin
Primidone (Mysoline)	Tablets: 50 mg, 250 mg	500–750	10–25	5–12[c]
Valproic acid (Depakene, Depakote, Depakote Sprinkles, Epival, Depakote ER)	Capsules: 250 mg Syrup: 250 mg/5 mL Tablets ER: 125, 250, 500 mg Capsules "Sprinkles" containing enteric-coated granules: 125 mg	500–3000	15–60	50–100
Newer Antiseizure Drugs				
Brivaracetam (Briviact, Brivlera)	Tablets: 10 mg, 25 mg, 50 mg, 75 mg, 100 mg Oral solution: 10 mg/mL Solution for injection: 50 mg/5 mL	100–200 100–200[d]	1–5	ND
Eslicarbazepine (Aptiom)	Tablets: 400 mg, 600 mg, 800 mg	800–1600	N/A	ND
Ezogabine (Potiga)	Tablets: 50 mg, 200 mg, 300 mg, 400 mg	600–1200	ND	ND
Felbamate (Felbatol)	Tablets: 400 mg, 600 mg Oral suspension: 600 mg/5 mL	1200–3600	15–45	ND
Gabapentin (Neurontin)	Tablets: 600 mg, 800 mg Capsule: 100 mg, 300 mg, 400 mg, 600 mg, 800 mg Oral solution: 250 mg/5 mL	1200–3600	25–50	12–20
Lacosamide (Vimpat)	Tablets: 50 mg, 100 mg, 150 mg, 200 mg Oral solution: 10 mg/mL IV solution: 200 mg/20 mL	200–400	ND	ND
Lamotrigine (Lamictal, Lamictal ODT, Lamictal XR)	Tablets: 25 mg, 100 mg, 150 mg, 200 mg Chewable tablets: 5 mg, 25 mg ODT: 25 mg, 50 mg, 100 mg, 200 mg ER tablet: 25 mg, 50 mg, 100 mg, 200 mg, 250 mg, 300 mg	400–600[e,f]	5[e,f]	3–14
Levetiracetam (Keppra, Keppra XR)	IR tablet: 250 mg, 500 mg, 750 mg, 1000 mg ER tablets: 500 mg, 750 mg ODT: 250 mg, 500 mg, 750 mg, 1000 mg Oral solution: 100 mg/mL IV solution: 500 mg/5 mL, 500 mg/100 mL, 1 gm/100 mL, 1.5 gm/100 mL	2000–3000	40–100	10–40
Oxcarbazepine (Trileptal Oxtellar XR)	IR tablets: 150 mg, 300 mg, 600 mg ER tablets: 150 mg, 300 mg, 600 mg Oral suspension: 300 mg/5 mL	900–2400 1200–2400	30–46 20–29 kg: 900 mg/day; 29.1–39 kg: 1200 mg/day; >39 kg: 1800 mg/day	3–40

Continued

TABLE 21.2　Preparations and Dosage of Antiseizure Drugs—cont'd

Drug	Preparations	DAILY MAINTENANCE DOSAGE[a]		Target Serum Level (µg/mL)
		Adults (mg)	Children (mg/kg)	
Perampanel (Fycompa)	Tablets: 2 mg, 4 mg, 6 mg, 8 mg, 10 mg, 12 mg	8–12	N/A	ND
Pregabalin (Lyrica)	Capsule: 25 mg, 50 mg, 75 mg, 100 mg, 150 mg, 200 mg, 225 mg, 300 mg Oral solution: 20 mg/mL	150–600	ND	ND
Rufinamide (Banzel)	Tablets: 200 mg, 400 mg Oral suspension: 40 mg/mL	3200	45	ND
Tiagabine (Gabitril)	Tablets: 2 mg, 4 mg, 12 mg, 16 mg	16–32	0.4[f]	ND
Topiramate (Topamax, Trokendi XR, Qudexy XR)	Tablets: 25 mg, 50 mg, 100 mg, 200 mg Sprinkle capsule: 15 mg, 25 mg ER sprinkle capsule: 25 mg, 50 mg, 100 mg, 150 mg, 200 mg ER capsule: 25 mg, 50 mg, 100 mg, 200 mg	100–400	3–9	5–25
Vigabatrin (Sabril)	Tablets: 500 mg Solution: 500 mg	3000–6000	50–150	ND
Zonisamide (Zonegran)	Capsules: 25 mg, 50 mg, 100 mg	200–400	4–12	10–40

[a]Dosing for AEDs is highly individualized. These represent averages, which may be subtherapeutic for some patients but toxic for others.
[b]Monitoring the clinical response rather than plasma drug levels is the preferred method for ethosuximide dosage determination.
[c]Target serum level is 5 to 12 mcg/mL for primidone itself, and 15 to 40 mcg/mL for phenobarbital derived from primidone.
[d]According to product labeling "Briviact injection should be administered intravenously to adult patients at the same dosage and same frequency as Briviact tablets and oral solution."
[e]Dosage must be decreased in patients taking valproic acid.
[f]Dosage must be increased in patients taking drugs that induce hepatic drug-metabolizing enzymes.
AED, Antiepileptic drug; *CR*, controlled release; *ER*, extended release; *IR*, immediate release; *IV*, intravenous; *ND*, not determined; *ODT*, orally disintegrating tablet; *XR*, extended release; *PE*, phenytoin equivalent.

Measurements of plasma drug levels are less important for determining effective dosages for absence seizures. Because absence seizures occur very frequently (up to several hundred a day), observation of the patient is the best means for establishing an effective dosage: if seizures stop, dosage is sufficient; if seizures continue, it is likely that more drug is needed.

In addition to serving as a guide for dosage adjustment, knowledge of plasma drug levels can serve as an aid to (1) monitoring patient adherence, (2) determining the cause of lost seizure control, and (3) identifying causes of toxicity, especially in patients taking more than one drug.

Promoting Patient Adherence

Epilepsy is a chronic condition that requires regular and continuous therapy. As a result, seizure control is highly dependent on patient adherence. In fact, it is estimated that nonadherence accounts for about 50% of all treatment failures. Accordingly, promoting adherence should be a priority for all members of the health care team. Measures that can help include the following:

- Educating patients and families about the chronic nature of epilepsy and the importance of adhering to the prescribed regimen
- Monitoring plasma drug levels to encourage and evaluate adherence
- Deepening patient and family involvement by having them maintain a seizure frequency chart

Withdrawing Antiseizure Drugs

Some forms of epilepsy undergo spontaneous remission, and hence discontinuing treatment may eventually be appropriate. Unfortunately, there are no firm guidelines to indicate the most appropriate time to withdraw antiseizure drugs. However, after the decision to discontinue treatment has been made, agreement does exist on how drug withdrawal should be accomplished. The most important rule is that *antiseizure drugs be withdrawn slowly* (over a period of 6 weeks to several months).

Failure to gradually reduce dosage is a frequent cause of SE. If the patient is taking two drugs to control seizures, they should be withdrawn sequentially, not simultaneously.

Suicide Risk With Antiseizure Drugs

In 2008, the U.S. Food and Drug Administration (FDA) warned that all antiseizure drugs can increase suicidal thoughts and behavior. However, data gathered since 2008 suggest that the risk may be lower than previously believed and may apply only to certain antiseizure drugs.

Since the FDA issued its warning, other large studies have been conducted to clarify the relationship between antiseizure drugs and suicidality. Unfortunately, these studies have yielded conflicting results. Nonetheless, they do suggest three things. First, only some antiseizure drugs—especially topiramate and lamotrigine—are likely to increase suicidality, not all antiseizure drugs as warned by the FDA. Second, the risk for suicidal behavior may be related more to the illness than the medication: by analyzing data on 5,130,795 patients, researchers in the United Kingdom found that antiseizure drugs produced a small increase in suicidal behavior in patients with *depression* but did *not* increase suicidal behavior in patients with *epilepsy* or *bipolar disorder*. And third, even if these drugs do promote suicidality, antiseizure drug-related suicide attempts and completed suicides are very rare.

Given the uncertainty regarding antiseizure drugs and suicidality, what should the clinician do? Because epilepsy itself carries a risk for suicide, and because patients with epilepsy often have depression or anxiety (which increases the risk for suicide), prudence dictates screening all patients for suicide risk, regardless of whether these drugs increase that risk. In addition, after treatment begins, all patients should be monitored for increased anxiety, agitation, mania, and hostility—signs that may indicate the emergence or worsening of depression—and an increased risk for suicidal thoughts or behavior. Patients, families, and caregivers should be alerted to these signs and advised to report them immediately. Finally, two antiseizure drugs—topiramate and lamotrigine—should be used with special caution, given their significant association with suicidality.

Contraception and Pregnancy Concerns

For women of childbearing age who are not pregnant, it is essential to consider interactions of antiseizure drugs with oral contraceptives. Eight antiseizure drugs decrease the effectiveness of oral contraceptives: carbamazepine, eslicarbazepine, lamotrigine, oxcarbazepine, phenytoin, phenobarbital, rufinamide, and topiramate. If it is necessary to prescribe any of these drugs, it is important to advise the patient of the risks and the need for additional contraceptives if pregnancy is not desired.

There is a risk of congenital anomalies with antiseizure drugs; however, it is important that pregnant women with seizures take these drugs. Two important reasons for this are: (1) risk to a fetus from uncontrolled seizures is greater than the risk from antiseizure drugs, and (2) more than 90% of women who take antiseizure drugs while pregnant have normal pregnancies and their infants are born without problems.

The following guidelines can help decrease fetal risk.

- Avoid valproic acid unless it is absolutely necessary and then only if no other drug is effective.
- The lowest effective dosage should be determined and maintained.
- Use just one drug whenever possible.
- To reduce the risk for neural tube defects that can occur with antiseizure drugs, pregnant patients should take supplemental folic acid before conception and throughout pregnancy. (The American Academy of Neurology and the American Epilepsy Society recommend the same 0.4 mg/daily dosage currently recommended for all pregnant women.)
- Maternal and fetal or infant bleeding risks are also a concern. Because phenytoin, phenobarbital, carbamazepine, and primidone can decrease synthesis of vitamin K–dependent clotting factors, some experts advocate administering vitamin K to the mother for 1 month before delivery and during delivery. (The American Academy of Neurology does not recommend this practice because there is insufficient evidence to support a benefit.)

To increase data on pregnancy outcomes, pregnant women taking antiseizure drugs are encouraged to enroll in the North American Antiepileptic Drug Pregnancy Registry at www.aedpregnancyregistry.org. As information is collected, outcomes and new recommendations will be disseminated to guide decision making.

CLASSIFICATION OF ANTISEIZURE DRUGS

The antiseizure drugs can be grouped into two major categories: *traditional antiseizure drugs* and *newer antiseizure drugs*. The traditional group has seven major members. The group of newer antiseizure drugs has 14 members. As shown in Table 21.3, both groups have their advantages and disadvantages. For example, clinical experience with the older antiseizure drugs is more extensive than with the newer ones, and the older drugs cost less. Both facts make the older drugs attractive. However, the older antiseizure drugs also have drawbacks, including troublesome side effects and complex drug interactions. Of importance, drugs in both groups appear equally effective—although few direct comparisons have been made. Neither group is clearly superior. Hence when selecting an antiseizure drug, drugs in both groups should be considered.

TRADITIONAL ANTISEIZURE DRUGS

The traditional antiseizure drugs have been in use for decades. Because of this extensive clinical experience, the efficacy and therapeutic niche of the traditional antiseizure drugs are well established. As a result, these drugs are prescribed more widely than the newer antiseizure drugs.

TABLE 21.3 Comparison of Traditional and Newer Antiseizure Drugs

Area of Comparison	ANTISEIZURE DRUG GROUP	
	Traditional Antiseizure Drugs[a]	Newer Antiseizure Drugs[b]
Efficacy	Well established	Equally good (probably), but less well established
Clinical experience	Extensive	Less extensive
Therapeutic niche	Well established	Evolving
Tolerability	Less well tolerated	Better tolerated (usually)
Pharmacokinetics	Often complex	Less complex
Drug interactions	Extensive, owing to induction of drug-metabolizing enzymes	Limited, owing to little or no induction of drug-metabolizing enzymes
Safety in pregnancy	Less safe	Safer
Cost	Less expensive	More expensive

[a]Carbamazepine, ethosuximide, phenobarbital, fosphenytoin, phenytoin, primidone, and valproic acid.
[b]Ezogabine, felbamate, gabapentin, lacosamide, lamotrigine, levetiracetam, oxcarbazepine, pregabalin, rufinamide, tiagabine, topiramate, vigabatrin, and zonisamide.

Although familiarity makes the traditional antiseizure drugs appealing, these drugs do have drawbacks. In general, they are less well tolerated than the newer antiseizure drugs, and they pose a greater risk to the developing fetus. Furthermore, owing to effects on drug-metabolizing enzymes (either induction or inhibition), they have complex interactions with other drugs, including other antiseizure drugs.

In the discussion that follows, we focus first on the major traditional antiseizure drugs. They are phenytoin, fosphenytoin, carbamazepine, valproic acid, ethosuximide, phenobarbital, and primidone.

PROTOTYPE DRUGS

Drugs for Seizure Disorders

Traditional Agents
Phenytoin

Newer Agents
Oxcarbazepine

Phenytoin

Phenytoin (Dilantin, Phenytek) is our most widely used antiseizure drug, despite having tricky kinetics and troublesome side effects. The drug is active against partial seizures as well as primary generalized tonic-clonic seizures. Phenytoin is of historical importance in that it was the first drug to suppress seizures without depressing the entire CNS. Consequently, phenytoin heralded the development of selective medications that could treat epilepsy while leaving most CNS functions undiminished.

Mechanism of Action

At the concentrations achieved clinically, phenytoin causes selective inhibition of sodium channels. Specifically, the drug slows recovery of sodium channels from the inactive state back to the active state. As a result, entry of sodium into neurons is inhibited, and hence action potentials are suppressed. Blockade of sodium entry is limited to neurons that are hyperactive. As a result, the drug suppresses activity of seizure-generating neurons while leaving healthy neurons unaffected.

Pharmacokinetics

The pharmacokinetic properties of phenytoin and other drugs is provided in Table 21.4. It is important to discuss some pharmacokinetic properties of phenytoin in greater depth, however, because phenytoin has unusual pharmacokinetics that must be accounted for in therapy. Because of saturation kinetics, small changes in dosage can produce disproportionately large changes in serum drug levels. As a result, a dosage that is both effective and safe is difficult to establish.

The capacity of the liver to metabolize phenytoin is limited. Doses of phenytoin needed to produce therapeutic effects are only slightly smaller than the doses needed to saturate the hepatic enzymes that metabolize phenytoin. Consequently, if phenytoin is administered in doses only slightly greater than those needed for therapeutic effects, the liver's capacity to metabolize the drug will be overwhelmed, causing plasma levels of phenytoin to rise dramatically. This unusual relationship between dosage and plasma levels is illustrated in Fig. 21.1A. As you can see, after plasma levels have reached the therapeutic range, small changes in dosage produce large changes in plasma levels. As a result, small increases in dosage can cause toxicity, and small decreases can cause therapeutic failure. This relationship makes it difficult to establish and maintain a dosage that is both safe and effective. For this reason, serum drug levels and trough levels are often used, along with assessments of seizure control, to determine dosage.

The relationship between dosage and plasma levels that exists for most drugs is detailed in Fig. 21.1B. As indicated, this relationship is *linear*, in contrast to the nonlinear relationship that exists for phenytoin. Accordingly, for most drugs, if the patient is taking doses that produce plasma levels that are within the therapeutic range, small deviations from that dosage produce only small deviations in plasma drug levels. Because of this relationship, with most drugs it is relatively easy to maintain plasma levels that are safe and effective.

Because of saturation kinetics, the half-life of phenytoin varies with dosage. At low doses, the half-life is relatively short—about 8 hours. However, at higher doses, the half-life becomes prolonged—in some cases up to 60 hours. At higher doses, there is more drug present than the liver can process. As a result, metabolism is delayed, causing the half-life to increase.

Therapeutic Uses

Phenytoin can be used to treat all major forms of epilepsy except absence seizures. The drug is especially effective against tonic-clonic seizures,

and phenytoin is a drug of choice for treating these seizures in adults and older children. (Carbamazepine is preferred to phenytoin for treating tonic-clonic seizures in young children.) Although phenytoin can be used to treat simple and complex partial seizures, the drug is less effective against these seizures than against tonic-clonic seizures. Phenytoin can be administered by intravenous (IV) injection to treat generalized convulsive SE, but other drugs are preferred.

Phenytoin is active against certain types of dysrhythmias and was used for management of dysrhythmias in the past. Because newer and better agents are now available, phenytoin has fallen out of favor for this purpose.

Dosage Considerations

Dosing is highly individualized. Plasma drug levels are often monitored as an aid to establishing dosage. *The dosing objective is to produce levels between 10 and 20 µg/mL.* Levels below 10 µg/mL are too low to control seizures; levels above 20 µg/mL produce toxicity. Because phenytoin has a relatively narrow therapeutic range (between 10 and 20 µg/mL), and because of the nonlinear relationship between phenytoin dosage and phenytoin plasma levels, after a safe and effective dosage has been established, the patient should adhere to it rigidly. For a summary of preparations and typical dosages of phenytoin and other antiseizure drugs, see Table 21.2.

When treatment is discontinued, dosage should be reduced gradually. Abrupt withdrawal may precipitate seizures.

Adverse Effects

Effects on the central nervous system. Although phenytoin acts on the CNS in a relatively selective fashion to suppress seizures, the drug can still cause CNS side effects—especially when dosage is excessive. At therapeutic levels (10 to 20 µg/mL), sedation and other CNS effects are mild. At plasma levels above 20 µg/mL, toxicity can occur. Nystagmus (continuous back-and-forth movements of the eyes) is relatively common. Other manifestations of excessive dosage include sedation, ataxia (staggering gait), diplopia (double vision), and cognitive impairment.

Gingival hyperplasia. Gingival hyperplasia (excessive growth of gum tissue) is characterized by swelling, tenderness, and bleeding of the gums. In extreme cases, patients require gingivectomy (surgical removal of excess gum tissue). Gingival hyperplasia is seen in about 20% of patients who take phenytoin. Can risk be reduced? Possibly. Risk may be minimized by good oral hygiene, including dental flossing and gum massage. Patients should be taught these techniques and encouraged to practice them. Supplemental folic acid is often recommended for this adverse effect based on studies that demonstrated that supplemental

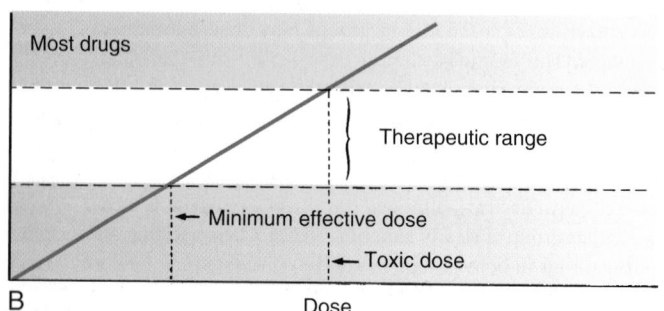

Fig. 21.1 Relationship Between Dose and Plasma Level for Phenytoin Compared With Most Other Drugs. (A) Within the therapeutic range, small increments in phenytoin dosage produce sharp increases in plasma drug levels. This relationship makes it difficult to maintain plasma phenytoin levels within the therapeutic range. (B) Within the therapeutic range, small increments in dosage of most drugs produce small increases in drug levels. With this relationship, moderate fluctuations in dosage are unlikely to result in either toxicity or therapeutic failure.

TABLE 21.4 Pharmacokinetics of Antiseizure Drugs[a]

Drug Name	Route	Peak	Half-Life[b]	Metabolism	Induces Hepatic Drug Metabolism	Excretion
Briviact	PO, IV	0.25–3 h	9 h	CYP2C19 and other non-P450	No	Urine
Carbamazepine	PO, IV	Suspension: 1.5 h IR: 4–5 hr ER: 3–26 h	Variable due to auto-induction. Initially 25–65 h; after stabilization, 8–14 h (children) to 12–17 h (adults)	CYP3A4 (induces its own metabolism)	Yes	Urine (primary), feces
Ethosuximide	PO	1–7 h	Children: 30 h; Adults: 50–60 h	CYP3A4, CYP2E1	No	Urine
Phenobarbital	PO, IM, IV	PO: 1.4 h IV: 15 min	Children: 110 h (range 60–180 h) Adults: 79 h (range 53–118 h)	CYP2C9 (primary), CYP2C19, CYP2E1	Yes	Urine (primary), feces
Phenytoin	PO, IV	IR: 1.5–3 h ER: 4–12 h	7–42 h	CYP2C9, CYP2C19	Yes	Urine
Fosphenytoin	IM, IV	IV: 15 min IM: 30 min	Conversion to phenytoin: 15 min	Initial conversion to phenytoin: probably phosphatases	Yes	Following conversion to phenytoin: urine
Primidone	PO	0.5–9 h	5–16 h	Hepatic via oxidation	Yes	Urine
Valproic acid	PO, IV	IR: 4 h ER: 4–17 h	9–19 h	Hepatic via glucuronide conjugation and mitochondrial beta-oxidation	No	Urine
Eslicarbazepine	PO	1–4 h	13–20 h	Hydrolysis	Yes	Urine
Ezogabine	PO	0.5–2 h	7–11 h	Glucuronidation, acetylation	No	Urine (primary), feces
Felbamate	PO	2–6 h	20–23 h	CYP3A4	Yes	Urine
Gabapentin	PO	2–4 h	Children: 4.7 h Adults: 5–7 h	Not metabolized	No	Urine
Lacosamide	PO, IV	1–4 h	13 h	CYP3A4, CYP2C9, CYP2C19	No	Urine
Lamotrigine	PO	IR: 1–4 h ER: 4–11 h	25–33 h as monotherapy	Hepatic via glucuronidation (primary), renal	No	Urine
Levetiracetam	PO, IV	Solution: 1 h IR: 1 h ER: 4 h	Children: 7.2–9.3 h (MHD) Adults: 9–11 h (MHD)	Hydrolysis by enzymes in the blood	No	Urine
Oxcarbazepine	PO	IR: 3–4 h (MHD) ER: 7 h	Children: 4.8–9 h Adults: 9–11 h	Hepatic cytosolic enzymes MHD, then glucuronide conjugation	Yes[c]	Urine
Perampanel	PO	2–2.5 h Food delays by 1–2 h	105 h	CYP3A4/5, (primary), CYP1A2, CYP2B6	Yes (weak)	Feces (primary), urine
Pregabalin	PO	1.5 h Food delays by 1.5 h	6.3 h	Negligible	No	Urine
Rufinamide	PO	4–6 h	6–10 h	carboxylesterase-mediated hydrolysis		Urine
Tiagabine	PO	45 min	Children 2–10 h Adults 7–9 h	CYP3A4 (major)	No	Feces (primary), urine
Topiramate	PO	IR: 1–4.3 h ER: 20–24 h	Children: 12–13 h Adults: 19–23 h	Minimal via hydroxylation, hydrolysis, glucuronidation	No	Urine
Vigabatrin	PO	1 h Food delays by1 h	Children: 5.5–9.5 h Adults: 10.5 h	Negligible	Yes	Urine
Zonisamide	PO	2–6 h	63 h (range 50–68)	CYP3A4	No	Urine

[a]Peaks and half-lives are often highly variable and depended on multiple individual factors.

[b]Half-lives are based on monotherapy. Administration of other drugs can significantly alter timing. Those with prolonged half-lives may take many days or even weeks to reach a steady state.

[c]Oxcarbazepine does not induce enzymes that metabolize antiseizure drugs, but does induce enzymes that metabolize other drugs.

ER, Extended release; *IR*, immediate release; *MHD*, 10-monohydroxy metabolite (the active metabolite); *PE*, phenytoin equivalent; *PO*, by mouth.

folic acid (0.5 mg/day) reduces gingival overgrowth. However, other research did not demonstrate this benefit. A subsequent Cochrane review established that only 15 of the studies met inclusion criteria and even those had issues with methodological quality. Their conclusion: Current evidence is insufficient to support the use of folic acid to prevent gingival hyperplasia so additional randomized control trials are needed.

Dermatologic effects. Between 2% and 5% of patients develop a morbilliform (measles-like) rash. Rarely, morbilliform rash progresses to much more severe reactions: *Stevens-Johnson syndrome* (SJS) or *toxic epidermal necrolysis* (TEN). Product labeling warns that the risk for developing SJS or TEN is strongly associated with a genetic mutation known as *human leukocyte antigen (HLA)-B*1502,* which occurs almost exclusively in people of Asian descent. For this reason, phenytoin should not be prescribed for patients known to have this mutation.

Drug Reaction with Eosinophilia and Systemic Symptoms (DRESS). Rarely, patients can experience signs and symptoms of hypersensitivity with systemic involvement. This potentially fatal reaction, also associated with HLA-B*1502, is characterized by skin eruptions, lymphadenopathy, fever, and multi-organ involvement (most commonly hepatic, renal, pulmonary, and hematologic system). Discontinuation of the drug is required.

Effects in pregnancy. Phenytoin is a teratogen. It can cause cleft palate, heart malformations, and *fetal hydantoin syndrome,* characterized by growth deficiency, motor or mental deficiency, microcephaly, craniofacial distortion, positional deformities of the limbs, hypoplasia of the nails and fingers, and impaired neurodevelopment. Because of these effects, phenytoin should be used during pregnancy only if safer alternatives are not effective and if the benefits of seizure control are deemed to outweigh the risk to the fetus.

Phenytoin can decrease synthesis of vitamin K–dependent clotting factors and can thereby increase the risk for *bleeding tendencies in newborns.*

Cardiovascular effects. When phenytoin is administered by IV injection (to treat SE), cardiac dysrhythmias and hypotension may result. These dangerous responses can be minimized by injecting phenytoin no faster than 50 mg/min.

 BLACK BOX WARNING

Phenytoin (Dilantin, Phenytek) and Fosphenytoin (Cerebyx)

> When administered intravenously at rates exceeding 50 mg/min in adults, or at the slower rate of either 1 to 3 mg/kg/min *or* 50 mg/min in children, phenytoin can cause severe hypotension and cardiac dysrhythmias. Cardiac monitoring should be in place before administration.

Other adverse effects. Hirsutism (overgrowth of hair in unusual places) can be a disturbing response, especially in young women. Interference with vitamin D metabolism may cause rickets and osteomalacia (softening of the bones). Interference with vitamin K metabolism can lower prothrombin levels, thereby causing bleeding tendencies in newborns. Very rarely, liver damage may occur, probably because of drug allergy. Oral preparations may cause gastric discomfort.

Significant Drug Interactions

Phenytoin interacts with a large number of drugs. The more important interactions are discussed here.

Induction of hepatic drug-metabolizing enzymes. Phenytoin stimulates synthesis of hepatic drug-metabolizing enzymes CYP2C8, CYP2C9, CYP3A4, and, to a lesser degree, CYP2B6. As a result, phenytoin can decrease the effects of other drugs, including *oral contraceptives,*

warfarin (an anticoagulant), and *glucocorticoids* (antiinflammatory and immunosuppressive drugs). Because avoiding pregnancy is desirable while taking antiseizure medications, and because phenytoin can decrease the effectiveness of oral contraceptives, the provider may need to increase the contraceptive dosage, or a switch to an alternative form of contraception may need to be made.

Drugs that increase plasma levels of phenytoin. Because the therapeutic range of phenytoin is narrow, slight increases in phenytoin levels can cause toxicity. Consequently, caution must be exercised when phenytoin is used with drugs that can increase its level. Drugs known to elevate phenytoin levels include *diazepam* (an antianxiety agent and antiseizure drug), *isoniazid* (a drug for tuberculosis), *cimetidine* (a drug for gastric ulcers), and *alcohol* (when taken acutely). These agents increase phenytoin levels by reducing the rate at which phenytoin is metabolized. *Valproic acid* (an antiseizure drug) elevates levels of free phenytoin by displacing phenytoin from binding sites on plasma proteins.

Drugs that decrease plasma levels of phenytoin. *Carbamazepine, phenobarbital,* and *alcohol* (when used chronically) can accelerate the metabolism of phenytoin, thereby decreasing its level. Breakthrough seizures can result.

Central nervous system depressants. The depressant effects of *alcohol, barbiturates,* and *other CNS depressants* will add with those of phenytoin. Advise patients to avoid alcohol and all other drugs with CNS-depressant actions.

Enteral tube feedings. Tube feedings decrease phenytoin absorption and can lead to subtherapeutic serum levels. Manufacturer labeling recommends against administering the drug with feedings. For patients receiving continuous tube feedings, hold the feeding for 1 to 2 hours before and after phenytoin administration.

Fosphenytoin
Mechanism of Action

Fosphenytoin (Cerebyx) is a prodrug that is converted to phenytoin when metabolized. It is recommended as a substitute for oral phenytoin when the oral route is contraindicated.

Therapeutic Use

Because fosphenytoin is converted to phenytoin, the therapeutic uses are the same as those of phenytoin. It is active against both generalized tonic-clonic seizures and partial seizures.

Dosage Considerations

Fosphenytoin has a unique dosing system. Although 150 mg of fosphenytoin will hydrolyze to 100 mg of phenytoin, rather than use standard milligram dosing, fosphenytoin is dosed in phenytoin equivalents (PE). Using this alternative, fosphenytoin 1 mg PE equals phenytoin 1 mg.

Unlike phenytoin, the IV formulation of fosphenytoin is compatible with standard IV solutions. When the drug is administered intramuscularly (IM), the full dose may need to be divided into two to four separate injections.

Adverse Effects

Adverse effects of fosphenytoin are the same as those of phenytoin, with one notable exception. During IV infusion, temporary paresthesias and itching, especially in the groin area, may occur. This infusion-related reaction will resolve when the infusion rate is decreased or within 10 minutes after completion of the infusion.

Carbamazepine

Carbamazepine (Tegretol, Tegretol-XR, Tegretol CR ♦, Carbatrol, Epitol, Equetro) is a cornerstone of epilepsy therapy. The drug is active against partial seizures and tonic-clonic seizures but not absence seizures.

Mechanism of Action

Carbamazepine suppresses high-frequency neuronal discharge in and around seizure foci. The mechanism appears to be the same as that of phenytoin: delayed recovery of sodium channels from their inactivated state.

Pharmacokinetics

Carbamazepine is unusual in that its half-life decreases as therapy progresses. During the initial phase of treatment, the half-life is about 40 hours. With continued treatment, the half-life decreases to about 15 hours because carbamazepine, like phenytoin and phenobarbital, induces hepatic drug-metabolizing enzymes. By increasing its own metabolism, carbamazepine causes its own half-life to decline. See Table 21.4 for other pharmacokinetic properties.

Therapeutic Uses

Carbamazepine is effective against tonic-clonic, simple partial, and complex partial seizures. Because the drug causes fewer adverse effects than phenytoin and phenobarbital, it is often preferred to these agents. Many prescribers consider carbamazepine the drug of first choice for partial seizures. Carbamazepine is not effective against absence, myoclonic, or atonic seizures.

Carbamazepine can provide symptomatic control in patients with bipolar disorder (manic-depressive illness) and is often effective in patients who are refractory to lithium. The role of carbamazepine in bipolar disorder is discussed in Chapter 28.

Carbamazepine can reduce neuralgia associated with the trigeminal and glossopharyngeal nerves. It should be noted that, although carbamazepine can reduce pain in these specific neuralgias, it is not generally effective as an analgesic and is not indicated for other kinds of pain.

Dosage Considerations

Administering the largest portion of the daily carbamazepine dose at bedtime can help reduce adverse CNS effects. To minimize side effects, dosage is low initially and then increased gradually (every 1 to 3 weeks) until seizure control is achieved.

Adverse Effects

In contrast to phenytoin and phenobarbital, carbamazepine has minimal effects on cognitive function. This is a primary reason for selecting carbamazepine over other antiseizure drugs.

Carbamazepine can cause a variety of *neurologic effects,* including visual disturbances (nystagmus, blurred vision, diplopia), ataxia, vertigo, unsteadiness, and headache. These reactions are common during the first weeks of treatment, affecting 35% to 50% of patients. Fortunately, tolerance usually develops with continued use. These effects can be minimized by initiating therapy at low doses and giving the largest portion of the daily dose at bedtime.

Carbamazepine-induced bone marrow suppression can cause *leukopenia, anemia,* and *thrombocytopenia.* However, serious reactions are rare. Thrombocytopenia and anemia, which have an incidence of 5%, respond to drug discontinuation. Leukopenia, which has an incidence of 10%, is usually transient and subsides even with continued drug use. Accordingly, carbamazepine should not be withdrawn unless the white blood cell count drops below 3000/mm³.

Fatal *aplastic anemia* has occurred during carbamazepine therapy. This reaction is extremely rare, having an incidence of 1 in 200,000.

To monitor for serious hematologic effects, complete blood counts should be performed before treatment and periodically thereafter. Patients with preexisting hematologic abnormalities should not use this drug. Patients should be informed about manifestations of hematologic abnormalities (fever, sore throat, pallor, weakness, infection, easy bruising, petechiae) and instructed to notify the prescriber if these occur.

Carbamazepine is teratogenic. In humans, the drug is associated with a 2.6-fold increase in the risk for spina bifida, a neural tube defect. Because it can harm the fetus, carbamazepine should be used only if the benefits of seizure control are deemed to outweigh risks to the fetus.

Carbamazepine can inhibit renal excretion of water, apparently by promoting secretion of antidiuretic hormone. The resulting water retention can reduce the osmolarity of blood and other body fluids, thereby posing a threat to patients with heart failure. Hyponatremia is a particular concern and appears to be dose-dependent. Periodic monitoring of serum sodium levels is recommended, especially in older patients who are at greater risk for hyponatremia when taking this drug.

Carbamazepine has been associated with several dermatologic effects, including morbilliform rash (10% incidence), photosensitivity reactions, SJS, and TEN. Mild reactions can often be treated with prednisone (an antiinflammatory agent) or an antihistamine. Severe reactions—SJS and TEN—necessitate drug withdrawal. With skin eruptions, it is important to be alert for signs and symptoms of DRESS. As discussed earlier, this rare condition, severe dermatologic reactions are accompanied by systemic symptoms (e.g., fever, generalized lympadenopathy) and multi-organ involvement.

▶▶ BLACK BOX WARNING

Carbamazepine (Carbatrol, Epitol, Equetro, Tegretol)

Carbamazepine may cause serious skin reactions such as SJS and TEN. Fatalities may occur. The risk for a reaction is strongly associated with the HLA-B*1502 variant of the HLA-B gene that is found predominantly in people of Asian ancestry.

Aplastic anemia and agranulocytosis occurred in patients taking carbamazepine. Incidence is rare (±2 to 6 patients for each 1 million taking the drug).

A major risk factor for SJS TEN, and DRESS is HLA-B*1502, a genetic variation seen primarily in people of Asian descent. Among people with the variant gene, about 5% develop SJS or TEN with carbamazepine. Accordingly, to reduce the risk for severe reactions, the FDA recommends that, before receiving carbamazepine, patients of Asian descent be tested for HLA-B*1502. Of note, this was the first time that the FDA recommended genetic screening for a major drug. As discussed previously, the presence of HLA-B*1502 *may* also increase the risk for SJS and TEN in patients taking phenytoin. Accordingly, phenytoin should not be used as an alternative to carbamazepine in patients with the mutation.

Hepatic and renal failure have occurred with carbamazepine. Although this is uncommon, monitoring of hepatic and renal function is recommended. Drug reaction with eosinophilia and systemic symptoms (DRESS) may occur 2 to 6 weeks following initiation of therapy.

Significant Drug and Food Interactions

Carbamazepine induces hepatic drug-metabolizing enzymes and hence can increase the rate at which it and other drugs are inactivated. Accelerated inactivation of *oral contraceptives* and *warfarin* is of particular concern.

Both phenytoin and phenobarbital induce hepatic drug metabolism. Thus if either drug is taken with carbamazepine, induction of metabolism is likely to be greater than with carbamazepine alone. Accordingly, phenytoin and phenobarbital can further accelerate the metabolism of carbamazepine, thereby decreasing its effects.

As discussed in Chapter 4, grapefruit juice can inhibit the metabolism of many drugs, thereby causing their plasma levels to rise. Grapefruit juice can increase peak and trough levels of carbamazepine by 40%. Advise patients to avoid grapefruit juice.

Valproic Acid

Valproic acid (Depakene, Depakote, Depakote ER, Depakote Sprinkles, Depacon, Epival) is an important antiseizure drug used widely to treat all major seizure types. In addition to its use in epilepsy, valproic acid is used for bipolar disorder and migraine headache.

Nomenclature

Valproic acid is available in three closely related chemical forms: (1) valproic acid; (2) the sodium salt of valproic acid, known as *valproate*; and (3) *divalproex sodium,* a combination of valproic acid plus its sodium salt. All three forms have identical antiseizure actions. In this chapter, the term *valproic acid* is used in reference to all three.

Mechanism of Action

The exact mechanism of valproic acid is unknown. Though several mechanisms have been suggested, most experts now believe it may augment the inhibitory influence of GABA or increase GABA concentration in the brain.

Therapeutic Uses

Valproic acid is considered a first-line drug for all partial and generalized seizures. As mentioned previously, this drug also is indicated for management of bipolar disorder (see Chapter 28) and migraine headache prophylaxis (see Chapter 25).

Dosage Considerations

Therapeutic responses are often seen at plasma levels of 50 to 100 µg/mL. However, the correlation between plasma levels and therapeutic effects is not very narrow.

Adverse Effects

Valproic acid is generally well tolerated and causes minimal sedation and cognitive impairment. Gastrointestinal effects are most common. Hepatotoxicity and pancreatitis are rare but serious.

▶▶ BLACK BOX WARNING

Valproate and Valproic Acid (Depacon, Depakene, Depakote, Stavzor)

Fatal hepatic failure has occurred; young children and patients with mitochondrial disease are at increased risk.

Fatal and rapidly progressing pancreatitis has occurred. Common symptoms include nausea, vomiting, anorexia, and abdominal pain.

Valproate is highly teratogenic. Neonates who survive may have major congenital malformations and decreased mental capacity.

Valproic acid can cause common but transient nausea, vomiting, and indigestion. These effects are most intense with formulations that are not enteric coated. Gastrointestinal reactions can be minimized by administering valproic acid with food and by using an enteric-coated product.

Rarely, valproic acid has been associated with fatal liver failure. Most deaths have occurred within the first few months of therapy. The overall incidence of fatal hepatotoxicity is about 1 in 40,000. However, in high-risk patients—children younger than 2 years receiving multidrug therapy—the incidence is much higher: 1 in 500. To minimize the risk for fatal liver injury, the following guidelines have been established:

- Don't use valproic acid in conjunction with other drugs in children younger than 2 years.
- Don't use valproic acid in patients with preexisting liver dysfunction.

- Evaluate liver function at baseline and periodically thereafter. (Unfortunately, monitoring liver function may fail to provide advance warning of severe hepatotoxicity. Fatal liver failure can develop so rapidly that it is not preceded by an abnormal test result.)
- Inform patients about signs and symptoms of liver injury (reduced appetite, malaise, nausea, abdominal pain, jaundice) and instruct them to notify the prescriber if these develop.
- Use valproic acid in the lowest effective dosage.

Life-threatening pancreatitis may develop in children and adults. Some cases have been hemorrhagic, progressing rapidly from initial symptoms to death. Pancreatitis can develop soon after starting therapy or after years of drug use. Patients should be informed about signs of pancreatitis (abdominal pain, nausea, vomiting, anorexia) and instructed to obtain immediate evaluation if these develop. If pancreatitis is diagnosed, valproic acid should be withdrawn, and alternative medication should be substituted as indicated.

Valproic acid is *highly teratogenic,* especially when taken during the first trimester. The risk for a major congenital malformation is 4 times higher than with other antiseizure drugs. Neural tube defects (e.g., spina bifida) are the greatest concern. The risk is 1 in 20 among women taking valproic acid, versus 1 in 1000 among women in the general population. In addition to neural tube defects, valproic acid can cause five other major congenital malformations: atrial septal defect, cleft palate, hypospadias, polydactyly, and craniosynostosis.

Exposure to valproic acid in utero can *impair cognitive function.* Children exposed to valproic acid had IQ scores that were significantly lower than those of children exposed to other antiseizure drugs (carbamazepine, phenytoin, or lamotrigine). These deficits persist for at least 4.5 years, and perhaps longer. Research also indicates an increased risk for autism.

Other adverse effects of valproic acid include rash, weight gain, hair loss, tremor, and blood dyscrasias (leukopenia, thrombocytopenia, red blood cell aplasia). Significant CNS effects are uncommon.

Significant Drug Interactions

Valproic acid decreases the rate at which phenobarbital is metabolized. Blood levels of phenobarbital may rise by 40%, resulting in significant CNS depression. When the combination is used, levels of phenobarbital should be monitored, and if they rise too high, phenobarbital dosage should be reduced.

Valproic acid can displace phenytoin from binding sites on plasma proteins. The resultant increase in free phenytoin may lead to phenytoin toxicity. Phenytoin levels and clinical status should be monitored.

Combining valproic acid with topiramate poses a risk for hyperammonemia, which may occur with or without encephalopathy. Symptoms include vomiting, lethargy, altered level of consciousness, and altered cognitive function. If these symptoms develop, hyperammonemic encephalopathy should be suspected, and blood ammonia should be measured. As a rule, symptoms abate after removal of either drug.

Two carbapenem antibiotics—meropenem and imipenem/cilastatin—can reduce plasma levels of valproic acid. Breakthrough seizures have occurred. Of note, increasing the dosage of valproic acid may be insufficient to overcome this effect. Accordingly, meropenem and imipenem/cilastatin should be avoided in patients taking valproic acid.

Ethosuximide
Mechanism of Action

Ethosuximide suppresses neurons in the thalamus that are responsible for generating absence seizures. The specific mechanism is inhibition of low-threshold calcium currents, known as T currents. Ethosuximide does not block sodium channels and does not enhance GABA-mediated neuronal inhibition.

PATIENT-CENTERED CARE ACROSS THE LIFE SPAN

Antiseizure Drugs

Life Stage	Considerations or Concerns
Children	FDA approved antiseizure drugs are approved for children, with the exception of eslicarbazepine. Children younger than 2 years who take valproate are at higher risk for hepatotoxicity, which can be fatal. Although approved for pediatric use, prescribing information for many antiseizure drugs mentions that inadequate studies have been done in younger children.
Pregnant women	Valproate can cause severe physical malformations and markedly decreased cognitive function in children born to women taking the drug and should only be prescribed as a drug of last resort. Canadian labeling additionally prohibits the prescribing of vigabatrin to pregnant women. Human fetal harm has also been documented for carbamazepine, lamotrigine, phenytoin, phenobarbital, and topiramate. For the remaining drugs, fetal harm has been documented in animal studies but not in humans. The lack of documented harm in humans often reflects a lack of studies rather than positive outcomes. Because phenytoin, phenobarbital, carbamazepine, and primidone can decrease synthesis of vitamin K–dependent clotting factors, some experts advocate administering vitamin K to the mother for 1 month before delivery and during delivery.
Breastfeeding women	Manufacturers advise carefully weighing the benefits of breastfeeding over the risks for adverse effects in the infant. Valproic acid and phenytoin are often selected preferentially because they are highly protein bound. Of note, for women taking vigabatrin, Canadian labeling contraindicates breastfeeding.
Older adults	Beers Criteria list carbamazepine, oxcarbazepine, and phenobarbital among the drugs deemed possibly inappropriate for adults 65 years and older. Additionally, the Pharmacy Quality Alliance identifies phenobarbital as a high-risk medication for patients 56 years and older. Because elderly patients are at increased risk for adverse events (e.g., falls because of sedation), cautious prescribing of all antiseizure drugs, often at lower initial doses, is advisable.

Therapeutic Use

Ethosuximide (Zarontin) is the drug of choice for absence seizures, the only indication it has. Absence seizures are eliminated in 60% of patients, and, in newly diagnosed patients, practical control is achieved in 80% to 90% of cases.

Dosage Considerations

Ethosuximide has a long half-life. This allows dosing to be done just once a day; however, dosing twice a day is better tolerated.

Because absence seizures occur many times each day, monitoring the clinical response rather than plasma drug levels is the preferred method for dosage determination. Dosage should be increased until seizures have been controlled or until adverse effects become too great. Trough levels are commonly used to help guide dosing.

Adverse Effects

Ethosuximide is generally devoid of significant adverse effects and interactions. During initial treatment, it may cause drowsiness, dizziness, and lethargy. These diminish with continued use. Nausea and vomiting may occur and can be reduced by administering the drug with food. Rare but serious reactions include systemic lupus erythematosus, leukopenia, aplastic anemia, and SJS.

Phenobarbital

Phenobarbital, one of our oldest antiseizure drugs, is effective and inexpensive, and it can be administered just once a day. Unfortunately, certain side effects—lethargy, depression, learning impairment—can be significant. Hence although phenobarbital was used widely in the past, it has largely been replaced by newer drugs that are equally effective but better tolerated.

Phenobarbital belongs to the barbiturate family. However, in contrast to most barbiturates, which produce generalized depression of the CNS, phenobarbital can suppress seizures at doses that produce only moderate disruption of CNS function. Because it does not cause significant sedation at doses typically used to reduce seizures, phenobarbital is classified as an *anticonvulsant barbiturate* (to distinguish it from most other barbiturates, which are employed primarily as sedatives).

The U.S. Drug Enforcement Agency (DEA) has classified phenobarbital under Schedule IV of the Controlled Substances Act. Phenobarbital can cause physical dependence; however, at the doses employed to treat epilepsy, significant dependence is unlikely.

The basic pharmacology of the barbiturates is discussed in Chapter 29. Discussion here is limited to the use of phenobarbital for seizures.

Mechanism of Action

Phenobarbital suppresses seizures by potentiating the effects of GABA. Specifically, the drug binds to GABA receptors, causing the receptors to respond more intensely to GABA itself.

Therapeutic Uses

Phenobarbital is effective against partial seizures and generalized tonic-clonic seizures but not absence seizures. IV phenobarbital can be used for generalized convulsive SE, but other antiseizure drugs are preferred. Like other barbiturates, phenobarbital can be used for sedation and to promote sleep at night. These applications are discussed in Chapter 29.

Dosage Considerations

Phenobarbital has a long half-life—about 4 days. In addition to permitting once-daily dosing, the long half-life has another consequence: 2 to 3 weeks are required for plasma levels to reach plateau. To address this concern, loading doses are often given to increase serum levels. Loading doses are higher than typical doses. For example, doses that are twice normal can be given for the first 4 days.

Adverse Effects

Drowsiness is the most common CNS effect. During the initial phase of therapy, sedation develops in practically all patients. With continued treatment, tolerance to sedation develops. Some children and older patients experience paradoxical responses: instead of becoming sedated, they may become irritable and hyperactive. Cognitive deficits may occur in children. Depression may occur in adults. Older adult patients may experience agitation and confusion.

Phenobarbital and other barbiturates can increase the risk for acute intermittent porphyria. Accordingly, barbiturates are absolutely contraindicated for patients with a personal or family history of this disorder.

Phenobarbital can cause respiratory depression. It should not be prescribed for patients with significant respiratory compromise.

Like phenytoin, phenobarbital can interfere with the metabolism of vitamins D and K. Disruption of vitamin D metabolism can cause rickets and osteomalacia. Patients should be advised to eat foods high in vitamins D, K, and calcium. Supplementation may be indicated for some patients.

Toxicity

When taken in moderately excessive doses, phenobarbital causes nystagmus and ataxia. Severe overdose produces generalized CNS depression; death results from depression of respiration. Barbiturate toxicity and its treatment are discussed in Chapter 29.

Significant Drug Interactions

Phenobarbital induces hepatic drug-metabolizing enzymes CYP1A2, CYP2A6, CYP2C8, CYP2C9, CYP3A4, and, to a lesser degree CYP2B6. As a result, it can accelerate the metabolism of drugs that are substrates for these enzymes, causing a loss of therapeutic effects. This is of particular concern with oral contraceptives and warfarin.

Because phenobarbital is a CNS depressant, it can intensify CNS depression caused by other drugs (e.g., alcohol, benzodiazepines, opioids). Severe respiratory depression and coma can result. Patients should be warned against combining phenobarbital with other drugs that have CNS-depressant actions.

Valproic acid is an antiseizure drug that has been used in combination with phenobarbital. By competing with phenobarbital for drug-metabolizing enzymes, valproic acid can increase plasma levels of phenobarbital by approximately 40%. Hence when this combination is used, the dosage of phenobarbital must be reduced.

Drug Withdrawal

When phenobarbital is withdrawn, dosage should be reduced gradually because abrupt withdrawal can precipitate SE. Patients should be warned of this danger and instructed not to discontinue phenobarbital too quickly.

Primidone
Mechanism of Action

Primidone (Mysoline) is nearly identical in structure to phenobarbital. As a result, the pharmacology of both agents is very similar.

Therapeutic Uses

Primidone is effective against tonic-clonic, simple partial, and complex partial seizures. The drug is not active against absence seizures.

As a rule, primidone is employed in combination with another antiseizure drug, usually phenytoin or carbamazepine. Primidone is never taken together with phenobarbital because phenobarbital is an active metabolite of primidone, so concurrent use would be irrational.

Dosage Considerations

Therapeutic plasma levels range from 5 to 12 µg/mL. Levels above 15 µg/mL are considered toxic.

Adverse Effects

Sedation, ataxia, and dizziness are common during initial treatment but diminish with continued drug use. Like phenobarbital, primidone can cause confusion in older adults and paradoxical hyperexcitability in children. A sense of acute intoxication can occur shortly after dosing. As with phenobarbital, primidone is absolutely contraindicated for patients with acute intermittent porphyria. Serious adverse reactions

(acute psychosis, leukopenia, thrombocytopenia, systemic lupus erythematosus) can occur but are rare.

Significant Drug Interactions

Drug interactions for primidone are similar to those for phenobarbital. Primidone can induce hepatic drug-metabolizing enzymes and can thereby reduce the effects of oral contraceptives, warfarin, and other drugs. In addition, primidone can intensify responses to other CNS depressants.

PATIENT EDUCATION
Antiseizure Drugs

Explain that finding the optimal dose takes time and that the medication regimen may require tweaking over the next several appointments.

To promote adherence, educate patients about the importance of taking antiseizure drugs exactly as prescribed. Inform them that, after a safe and effective dosage has been established, small deviations in dosage can lead to toxicity or to loss of seizure control.

Inform patients about the dangers of abrupt drug withdrawal and instruct them never to discontinue drug use without consulting the prescriber. Advise patients who are planning a trip to carry extra medication to ensure an uninterrupted supply in the event they become stranded where medication is unavailable. Explain the need to obtain refills on time so that they do not run out of drugs.

Teach the patient (or a family member) to maintain a seizure frequency chart, indicating the date, time, and nature of all seizure events. They should bring this with them to all clinic appointments.

If the drug requires periodic measurement of drug levels or other laboratory studies, explain the purpose and the importance of keeping those appointments.

Advise patients to avoid potentially hazardous activities (e.g., driving, operating dangerous machinery) until seizure control is achieved. It may be necessary to explain laws concerning this risk. Also, because seizures may recur after they are largely under control, advise patients to carry some form of identification (e.g., Medic Alert bracelet) to aid in diagnosis and treatment if a seizure occurs.

Forewarn patients about CNS depression that can occur as a drug side effect. Advise them to avoid driving and other hazardous activities if CNS depression is significant. To prevent additive CNS depressant effects, warn patients against using alcohol and other CNS depressants.

To reduce the risk for neural tube defects, advise women to take folic acid supplements before and throughout pregnancy.

Educate patients, families, and caregivers about signs that may precede suicidal behavior (e.g., increased anxiety, agitation, mania, or hostility) and advise them to report these immediately.

NEWER ANTISEIZURE DRUGS

The group of newer antiseizure drugs has 15 members. Although most newer antiseizure drugs have not been compared directly with the traditional antiseizure drugs (or with each other, for that matter), all of these drugs appear equally effective.

The newer antiseizure drugs have properties that make them more appealing than the traditional antiseizure drugs. As a group, they are better tolerated than the traditional antiseizure drugs and may pose a smaller risk to the developing fetus. Furthermore, only one—oxcarbazepine—induces drug-metabolizing enzymes to a significant degree, and hence interactions with other drugs, including other antiseizure drugs, are relatively minor.

The subject of approved indications for the newer antiseizure drugs requires comment. When these drugs were introduced, FDA-approved indications were limited to *adjunctive* therapy of certain seizure disorders. None of these drugs was approved for *monotherapy* because clinical trials were limited to patients who were refractory to traditional antiseizure drugs. When the trials were conducted, rather than switching patients from a traditional antiseizure drug to the experimental antiseizure drug, the experimental antiseizure drug was *added* to the existing regimen. Hence when the trials were completed, all we knew for sure was that the new antiseizure drugs were effective when used together with older antiseizure drugs. We had no data on use of the newer antiseizure drug alone. As a result, the FDA had no option but to approve the new drug for adjunctive therapy. Since being released, seven of the newer antiseizure drugs have received FDA approval for monotherapy. These are eslicarbazepine, felbamate, lacosamide, lamotrigine, oxcarbazepine, topiramate, and vigabatrin.

To help prescribers be more comfortable with the newer antiseizure drugs, two organizations—the American Academy of Neurology (AAN) and American Epilepsy Society (AES)—convened a panel to evaluate the efficacy and tolerability of these drugs. For some of the newer antiseizure drugs, the AAN/AES panel recommended uses not yet approved by the FDA. These recommendations, along with FDA-approved indications, are discussed in the sections that follow.

Oxcarbazepine

Oxcarbazepine (Oxtellar XR, Trileptal) will serve as our prototype for the newer antiseizure drugs. It is a derivative of carbamazepine; therefore they share some of the same features.

Mechanism of Action

Antiseizure effects result from blockade of voltage-sensitive sodium channels in neuronal membranes, an action that stabilizes hyperexcitable neurons and thereby suppresses seizure spread. The drug does not affect neuronal GABA receptors.

Therapeutic Uses

Oxcarbazepine is indicated for both monotherapy and adjunctive therapy for management of partial seizures. It is approved for use in both adults and children. As monotherapy, it is approved for children aged 4 years and older; as adjunctive therapy, it may be prescribed for children as young as 2 years. Of note, in Canada, this drug is only approved for children aged 6 years and older.

Adverse Effects

Central nervous system effects. The most common adverse effects are dizziness, drowsiness, double vision, nystagmus, headache, nausea, vomiting, and ataxia. Patients should avoid driving and other hazardous activities, unless the degree of drowsiness is low.

Hyponatremia. Clinically significant *hyponatremia* (sodium concentration below 125 mmol/L) develops in 2.5% of patients. Signs include nausea, drowsiness, headache, and confusion. If oxcarbazepine is combined with other drugs that can decrease sodium levels (especially diuretics), monitoring of sodium levels may be needed.

Dermatologic effects. Like carbamazepine, oxcarbazepine can cause *serious skin reactions,* including SJS and TEN. There is 30% cross-sensitivity among patients with hypersensitivity to carbamazepine. Accordingly, patients with a history of severe reactions to either drug should probably not use the other.

Hematologic effects. Oxcarbazepine does not usually cause the severe hematologic abnormalities seen with carbamazepine; however, they have occurred rarely. Accordingly, routine monitoring of blood counts is not usually required, unless the patient is at risk, though some experts suggest periodic monitoring. In either case, patients should be assessed for evidence of blood dyscrasias (e.g., pallor, fatigue, weakness, exercise intolerance, fever, infection, easy bleeding or bruising, petechiae), and a complete blood count (CBC) should be ordered for confirmation as needed.

Hypersensitivity effects. Oxcarbazepine has been associated with serious *multiorgan hypersensitivity reactions.* Although manifestations vary, patients typically present with fever and rash, associated with one or more of the following: lymphadenopathy, hematologic abnormalities, pruritus, hepatitis, nephritis, hepatorenal syndrome, oliguria, arthralgia, or asthenia. If this reaction is suspected, oxcarbazepine should be discontinued.

Other adverse effects. Long-term use of oxcarbazepine may cause decreased bone mineral density. This can result in osteopenia and osteoporosis with an increased risk for fractures.

Significant Drug Interactions

Phenytoin. Oxcarbazepine's interaction with phenytoin has multiple implications. Oxcarbazepine inhibits the enzymes that metabolize phenytoin, thus raising phenytoin levels. Conversely, phenytoin may decrease serum concentrations of oxcarbazepine. When this combination is used, phenytoin toxicity and subtherapeutic levels of oxcarbazepine can result. Phenytoin and oxcarbazepine levels should be monitored and dosages adjusted accordingly.

Perampanel, phenobarbital, and valproic acid. Perampanel can increase serum levels of oxcarbazepine. Valproic acid can decrease levels of oxcarbazepine. Phenobarbital can decrease serum levels of oxcarbazepine's active metabolite. If these drugs are given together, oxcarbazepine levels will need to be monitored and dosages adjusted accordingly.

Eslicarbazepine. Oxcarbazepine can increase serum levels of eslicarbazepine. This combination is not recommended.

Oral contraceptives. Oxcarbazepine induces enzymes that metabolize both estrogens and progestins, which are ingredients in *oral contraceptives*. Accordingly, women who are at risk of becoming pregnant should employ an alternative birth control method.

Sodium-depleting drugs. Sodium-depleting drugs can increase the risk of hyponatremia. Oxcarbazepine should be used with caution in patients taking *diuretics* and other drugs that can lower sodium levels.

Alcohol. Alcohol can intensify CNS depression caused by oxcarbazepine. It should be avoided.

Lamotrigine
Mechanism of Action

Lamotrigine (Lamictal) has a broad spectrum of antiseizure activity. Benefits derive mainly from blocking sodium channels and partly from blocking calcium channels. Both actions decrease release of glutamate, an excitatory neurotransmitter.

Therapeutic Uses

Lamotrigine (Lamictal) has a broad spectrum of antiseizure activity. The drug is FDA approved for (1) adjunctive therapy of partial seizures in adults and children older than 2 years, (2) adjunctive therapy of generalized seizures associated with Lennox-Gastaut syndrome in adults and children older than 2 years, (3) adjunctive therapy of primary generalized tonic-clonic seizures in adults and children older than 2 years, and (4) monotherapy of partial seizures in patients at least 16 years old who are converting from another antiseizure drug. In addition, the AAN/AES guidelines recommend using lamotrigine for absence seizures. Lamotrigine is also FDA approved for long-term maintenance therapy of bipolar disorder (see Chapter 28).

Adverse Effects

Common side effects include dizziness, diplopia (double vision), blurred vision, nausea, vomiting, and headache. Of much greater concern, patients may develop life-threatening rashes, including SJS and TEN and DRESS. Deaths have occurred. The incidence of severe rash is about 0.8% in patients younger than 16 years and 0.3% in adults. Concurrent use of valproic acid increases this risk. If a rash develops, lamotrigine should be withdrawn immediately.

Blood dyscrasias may occur. Hypersensitivity and immune system reactions have occurred. Very rarely, patients experience aseptic meningitis (inflammation of the meninges in the absence of bacterial infection). Patients who develop symptoms of meningitis—headache, fever, stiff neck, nausea, vomiting, rash, sensitivity to light—should undergo immediate evaluation to determine the cause. Treatable causes should be managed as indicated. If no clear cause other than lamotrigine is identified, discontinuation of lamotrigine should be considered.

Risk for suicide may be greater than with most other antiseizure drugs. Screen patients for suicidality before starting treatment and monitor for suicidality during the treatment course.

Significant Drug Interactions

The half-life of lamotrigine is dramatically affected by drugs that induce or inhibit hepatic drug-metabolizing enzymes. Enzyme inducers (e.g., carbamazepine, phenytoin, phenobarbital) decrease the half-life of lamotrigine to 10 hours, whereas valproate (an enzyme inhibitor) increases the half-life to about 60 hours. Lamotrigine itself is not an inducer or inhibitor of drug metabolism.

Estrogens can lower lamotrigine levels, whereas lamotrigine may lower progestin levels. This can create unique concerns for the provider caring for a woman of childbearing age who wants to take oral contraceptives.

Gabapentin
Mechanism of Action

Gabapentin (Neurontin) is an analog of GABA but does not directly affect GABA receptors. Its precise mechanism of action is unknown, but it may enhance GABA release, thereby increasing GABA-mediated inhibition of neuronal firing.

Therapeutic Uses

Gabapentin has a broad spectrum of antiseizure activity. However, its only FDA-approved use in epilepsy is adjunctive therapy of partial seizures (with or without secondary generalization). The AAN/AES guidelines also recommend the drug for monotherapy of partial seizures. Gabapentin also has approval for treating postherpetic neuralgia. Interestingly, more than 80% of prescriptions are written for off-label uses, including diabetic neuropathy, prophylaxis of migraine, treatment of fibromyalgia, restless leg syndrome, alcohol withdrawal, chronic cough, and hiccups. However, benefits in these disorders are modest, at best. Gabapentin does not appear effective in bipolar disorder.

Two forms of gabapentin are *not currently indicated* for management of epilepsy and, therefore should not be confused with the form of gabapentin known as Neurontin. These are gabapentin ER (Gralise), which is approved for management of postherpetic neuralgia; and gabapentin enacarbil (Horizant), a prodrug form of gabapentin approved for treatment of moderate to severe restless legs syndrome. Owing to differences in pharmacokinetics, these forms of gabapentin are *not interchangeable with each other or with Neurontin.*

Dosage Considerations

Absorption of gabapentin is not affected by food. However, as the dosage gets larger, the percentage absorbed gets smaller. This occurs because, at high doses, the intestinal transport system for uptake of the drug becomes saturated.

Adverse Reactions

Gabapentin is very well tolerated. The most common side effects are somnolence, dizziness, ataxia, fatigue, nystagmus, and peripheral edema. These are usually mild to moderate and often diminish with continued drug use. Patients should avoid driving and other hazardous activities until they are confident they are not impaired.

Significant Drug Interactions

Unlike most antiseizure drugs, gabapentin is devoid of significant interactions. It does not induce or inhibit drug-metabolizing enzymes and does not affect the metabolism of other drugs. As a result, gabapentin is well suited for combined use with other antiseizure drugs.

Pregabalin
Mechanism of Action

Pregabalin (Lyrica), an analog of GABA, is much like gabapentin; however, although pregabalin is an analog of GABA, the drug does not bind with GABA receptors or with benzodiazepine receptors, and hence does not work by mimicking or enhancing the inhibitory actions of GABA. Although the precise mechanism of action has not been established, we do know that pregabalin can bind with calcium channels on nerve terminals, and can thereby inhibit calcium influx, which in turn can inhibit release of several neurotransmitters, including glutamate, norepinephrine, and substance P. Reduced transmitter release may underlie seizure control and relief of neuropathic pain.

Therapeutic Uses

Like gabapentin, pregabalin is used for seizures and neuropathic pain. Pregabalin has four approved indications: neuropathic pain associated with diabetic neuropathy, postherpetic neuralgia, adjunctive therapy of partial seizures, and fibromyalgia.

Adverse Effects

Pregabalin can cause a variety of adverse effects. The most common are dizziness and somnolence, which often persist as long as the drug is being taken. Blurred vision may develop during early therapy but resolves with continued drug use. About 8% of patients experience significant weight gain (7% or more of body weight in just a few months). Other adverse effects include difficulty thinking, headache, peripheral edema, and dry mouth.

Postmarketing reports indicate a risk for hypersensitivity reactions, including life-threatening angioedema, characterized by swelling of the face, tongue, lip, gums, throat, and larynx. Patients should discontinue pregabalin immediately at the first sign of angioedema or any other hypersensitivity reaction (blisters, hives, rash, dyspnea, wheezing).

In clinical trials, three patients developed rhabdomyolysis (muscle breakdown). However, it is not clear that pregabalin was the cause. Nonetheless, patients should be instructed to report signs of muscle injury (pain, tenderness, weakness). If rhabdomyolysis is diagnosed, or even suspected, pregabalin should be withdrawn.

Abuse Potential and Physical Dependence

In contrast to most other antiseizure agents, pregabalin is regulated under the Controlled Substances Act. In clinical trials, 4% to 12% of patients reported euphoria as a side effect. When given to recreational users of sedative-hypnotic drugs, pregabalin produced subjective effects perceived as similar to those of diazepam (Valium). On the basis of these data, the DEA has classified pregabalin under Schedule V of the Controlled Substances Act.

Abrupt discontinuation can cause insomnia, nausea, headache, diarrhea, and other symptoms that suggest physical dependence. To avoid withdrawal symptoms, pregabalin should be discontinued slowly, over 1 week or more.

Reproductive Risks for Women and Men

Pregabalin has demonstrated adverse effects on reproduction and fetal development in *both male and female* animals. When given to pregnant female rats and rabbits, pregabalin caused fetal growth delay, fetal death, structural abnormalities (e.g., skeletal and visceral malformation), and impaired function of the nervous system and reproductive system.

When given to male rats before and during mating with untreated females, pregabalin decreased sperm counts and motility, decreased fertility, reduced fetal weight, and caused fetal abnormalities. Although data on human reproduction are lacking, men using the drug should be informed about the possibility of decreased fertility and male-mediated teratogenicity. Men taking pregabalin should wear a condom when having sex with women who may become pregnant.

Significant Drug Interactions

Alcohol, opioids, benzodiazepines, and other CNS depressants may intensify the depressant effects of pregabalin. Accordingly, such combinations should be avoided.

Extensive studies have failed to show pharmacokinetic interactions with any other drugs. Pregabalin does not inhibit cytochrome P450 isoenzymes. Whether it can induce these isoenzymes is unknown. Pregabalin does not interact with oral contraceptives and does not alter the kinetics of any antiseizure drugs studied (carbamazepine, lamotrigine, phenobarbital, phenytoin, topiramate, valproic acid, and tiagabine).

Levetiracetam
Mechanism of Action

Levetiracetam (Keppra) is a unique agent that is chemically and pharmacologically different from all other antiseizure drugs. How levetiracetam acts is unknown; however, we know that it does not bind to receptors for GABA or any other known neurotransmitter.

Therapeutic Uses

In the United States levetiracetam is approved for adjunctive therapy of (1) myoclonic seizures in adults and adolescents 12 years and older, (2) partial-onset seizures in adults and children 4 years and older, and (3) primary generalized tonic-clonic seizures in adults and children 6 years and older. Unlabeled uses include migraine, bipolar disorder, and new-onset pediatric epilepsy. In Europe, the drug is approved for monotherapy of partial seizures, for which it is highly effective.

Adverse Effects

In 2017, Health Canada reported a possible link between levetiracetam and renal injury. Other than this potential exception, adverse effects are generally mild to moderate. The most common are drowsiness and asthenia (lack of strength, weakness). Neuropsychiatric symptoms (agitation, anxiety, depression, psychosis, hallucinations, depersonalization) occur in less than 1% of patients. In contrast to other antiseizure drugs, levetiracetam does not impair speech, concentration, or other cognitive functions.

Unlike most other antiseizure drugs, levetiracetam does not interact with other drugs. It does not alter plasma concentrations of oral contraceptives, warfarin, digoxin, or other antiseizure drugs. These benefits are primarily attributable to the fact that levetiracetam is not metabolized by P450 isoenzymes.

Topiramate
Mechanism of Action

Topiramate (Topamax) is another broad-spectrum antiseizure agent. Seizure reduction occurs by four mechanisms: (1) potentiation of GABA-mediated inhibition, (2) blockade of voltage-dependent sodium channels, (3) blockade of calcium channels, and (4) blockade of receptors for glutamate, an excitatory neurotransmitter.

Therapeutic Uses

The drug is FDA approved for (1) adjunctive treatment of adults and children 2 years and older with partial seizures, primary generalized tonic-clonic seizures, and seizures associated with Lennox-Gastaut syndrome; (2) monotherapy of adults and children 10 years and older with partial seizures or primary generalized tonic-clonic seizures; and (3) prophylaxis of migraine in adults (see Chapter 25). Unlabeled uses include bipolar disorder, cluster headaches, neuropathic pain (including the pain of diabetic neuropathy), infantile spasms, essential tremor, binge-eating disorder, bulimia nervosa, and weight loss. Studies also show promise for management of alcohol and cocaine dependence.

Adverse Effects

Although topiramate is generally well tolerated, it can cause multiple adverse effects. Common effects include somnolence, dizziness, ataxia, nervousness, diplopia, nausea, anorexia, and weight loss. Cognitive effects (confusion, memory difficulties, altered thinking, reduced concentration, difficulty finding words) can occur, but the incidence is low at recommended dosages. Kidney stones and paresthesias occur rarely.

Topiramate can cause metabolic acidosis. The drug inhibits carbonic anhydrase and thereby increases renal excretion of bicarbonate, which causes plasma pH to fall. Hyperventilation is the most characteristic symptom. Mild to moderate metabolic acidosis develops in 30% of adult patients, but severe acidosis is rare. Risk factors include renal disease, severe respiratory disorders, diarrhea, and a ketogenic diet. Prolonged metabolic acidosis can lead to kidney stones, fractures, and growth delay. Serum bicarbonate should be measured at baseline and periodically thereafter. Advise patients to inform the prescriber if they experience hyperventilation and other symptoms (fatigue, anorexia). If metabolic acidosis is diagnosed, topiramate should be given in reduced dosage or discontinued. If discontinuation is needed, be aware that rebound effects can occur if stopped abruptly; tapering off is recommended if possible.

Topiramate can cause hypohidrosis (reduced sweating), thereby posing a risk for hyperthermia. Significant hyperthermia is usually associated with vigorous activity and an elevated environmental temperature.

There have been case reports of angle-closure glaucoma. Left untreated, this rapidly leads to blindness. Patients should be informed about symptoms of glaucoma (ocular pain, unusual redness, sudden worsening or blurring of vision) and instructed to seek immediate attention if these develop. Fortunately, topiramate-induced glaucoma is rare.

Topiramate should be used only if the benefits of maternal seizure control are deemed to outweigh the risk to the fetus. Women using topiramate should use an effective form of birth control or should switch to a safer antiseizure drug if pregnancy is intended.

Risk for suicide may be greater than with most other antiseizure drugs. Screen patients for suicidality before starting treatment and monitor for suicidality during the treatment course.

Significant Drug Interactions

Phenytoin and carbamazepine can decrease levels of topiramate by about 45%. Topiramate may increase levels of phenytoin. As mentioned previously, there is an increased risk for hyperammonemia (with or without encephalopathy) when topiramate is combined with valproic acid.

Tiagabine
Mechanism of Action

Tiagabine (Gabitril) blocks reuptake of GABA by neurons and glia. As a result, the inhibitory influence of GABA is intensified, and seizures are suppressed.

Therapeutic Uses

Tiagabine (Gabitril) is FDA approved only for adjunctive therapy of partial seizures in patients at least 12 years old. Off-label uses include management of generalized anxiety disorder, multiple sclerosis, neuropathic pain, posttraumatic stress disorder, psychosis, and spasticity. Recent studies show promise for use of tiagabine in migraine prophylaxis as well as management of bipolar disorder and insomnia. However, owing to a risk for seizures (see *Adverse Effects*), such off-label use is discouraged.

Adverse Effects

Tiagabine is generally well tolerated. Common adverse effects are dizziness, somnolence, asthenia, nausea, nervousness, and tremor. Like most other antiseizure drugs, tiagabine can cause dose-related cognitive effects (e.g., confusion, abnormal thinking, trouble concentrating).

Tiagabine has caused seizures in some patients—but only in those using the drug off-label (i.e., those using the drug for a condition other than epilepsy). A few patients have developed SE, which can be life threatening. In most cases, seizures occurred soon after starting tiagabine or after increasing the dosage. Because of seizure risk, off-label use of tiagabine usually should be avoided. Why are people without epilepsy at risk? Possibly because they are not taking antiseizure drugs. Remember, tiagabine is approved only for adjunctive use with other antiseizure drugs. It may be that these drugs protect against tiagabine-induced seizures. Because people without epilepsy take tiagabine by itself, they are not protected from seizure development.

Significant Drug Interactions

Tiagabine does not alter the metabolism or serum concentrations of other antiseizure drugs. However, levels of tiagabine can be decreased by phenytoin, phenobarbital, and carbamazepine—all of which induce drug-metabolizing enzymes.

Zonisamide
Mechanism of Action

Zonisamide (Zonegran) belongs to the same chemical family as the sulfonamide antibiotics but lacks antimicrobial activity. In animal models, zonisamide suppresses focal seizure activity and spread. The underlying mechanism appears to be blockade of neuronal sodium channels and calcium channels.

Therapeutic Uses

Zonisamide is approved only for adjunctive therapy of partial seizures in adults. This drug is sometimes used off-label for management of bipolar disorder, migraine prophylaxis, and Parkinson disease.

Adverse Effects

The most common adverse effects are drowsiness, dizziness, anorexia, headache, and nausea. Metabolic acidosis is also common. Like most other antiseizure drugs, zonisamide can impair speech, concentration, and other cognitive processes. Because the drug can reduce alertness and impair cognition, patients should avoid driving and other hazardous activities until they know how the drug affects them.

Zonisamide can have severe psychiatric effects. During clinical trials, 2.2% of patients either discontinued treatment or were hospitalized because of severe depression; 1.1% attempted suicide.

Zonisamide can trigger hypersensitivity reactions, including some that are potentially fatal (e.g., SJS, TEN, fulminant hepatic necrosis). Patients who develop a rash should be followed closely because rash can evolve into a more serious event. If severe hypersensitivity develops, zonisamide should be withdrawn immediately. Fortunately, serious reactions and fatalities are rare.

Zonisamide has adverse effects on the kidneys. In clinical trials, about 4% of patients developed nephrolithiasis (kidney stones). The risk can be reduced by drinking 6 to 8 glasses of water a day (to maintain hydration and urine flow). Patients should be informed about signs of kidney stones (sudden back pain, abdominal pain, painful urination, bloody or dark urine) and instructed to report them immediately. In addition to nephrolithiasis, zonisamide can impair glomerular filtration. Because of its effects on the kidney, zonisamide should be used with caution in patients with kidney disease.

Like topiramate, zonisamide inhibits carbonic anhydrase and can thereby cause metabolic acidosis. The condition develops in up to 90% of children and 43% of adults, usually early in treatment. Risk is increased by renal disease, respiratory disease, diarrhea, and following a ketogenic diet. Metabolic acidosis can delay growth in children, and, over time, can lead to kidney stones and fractures in all patients. Advise patients to report hyperventilation and other signs of metabolic acidosis (e.g., fatigue, anorexia). Determine plasma bicarbonate at baseline and periodically thereafter. If metabolic acidosis is diagnosed, zonisamide should be discontinued or given in reduced dosage.

Rarely, zonisamide causes hypohidrosis (decreased sweating) and hyperthermia. Pediatric patients may be at special risk. In warm weather, hypohidrosis may lead to heat stroke and subsequent hospitalization. Patients should be monitored closely for reduced sweating and increased body temperature.

Drug and Food Interactions

Levels of zonisamide can be affected by agents that induce or inhibit CYP3A4. Inducers of CYP3A4—including St. John's wort (an herbal supplement used for depression) and several antiseizure drugs (e.g., phenytoin, phenobarbital, carbamazepine)—can accelerate the metabolism of zonisamide and can thereby reduce the drug's half-life (to as little as 27 hours). Conversely, inhibitors of CYP3A4—including grapefruit juice, azole antifungal agents (e.g., ketoconazole), and several protease inhibitors (e.g., ritonavir)—can slow the metabolism of zonisamide and thereby prolong and intensify its effects.

Felbamate
Mechanism of Action

Felbamate (Felbatol) increases seizure threshold and suppresses seizure spread. The underlying mechanism is unknown. Unlike some antiseizure drugs, such as phenobarbital and benzodiazepines, felbamate does not interact with GABA receptors and does not enhance the inhibitory actions of GABA.

Therapeutic Uses

Felbamate is an effective antiseizure drug with a broad spectrum of antiseizure activity. It is approved for (1) adjunctive or monotherapy in adults with partial seizures (with or without generalization) and (2) adjunctive therapy in children with Lennox-Gastaut syndrome. However, because adverse effects can be severe, use of the drug is very limited.

Adverse Effects

Felbamate can cause aplastic anemia. Because of the high risk associated with this danger, felbamate has a black box warning for this concern.

Felbamate can also cause liver damage. Because of the risk for liver failure, felbamate should not be used by patients with preexisting liver dysfunction. In addition, patients taking the drug should be monitored for indications of liver injury.

The most common adverse effects are GI disturbances (anorexia, nausea, vomiting) and CNS effects (insomnia, somnolence, dizziness, headache, diplopia). These occur more frequently when felbamate is combined with other drugs.

BLACK BOX WARNING
Felbamate (Felbatol)

> Felbamate has been associated with an increased risk for aplastic anemia. Associated fatality rates have been estimated at 20% to 30%; however, rates up to 70% have been attributed to this drug.
>
> Felbamate may cause acute liver failure. Though uncommon, 67% of reported cases were either fatal or required liver transplants.

Significant Drug Interactions

Felbamate can alter plasma levels of other antiseizure drugs, and vice versa. Felbamate increases levels of phenytoin and valproic acid. Levels of felbamate are increased by valproic acid and reduced by phenytoin and carbamazepine. Increased levels of phenytoin and valproic acid (and possibly felbamate) could lead to toxicity; reduced levels of felbamate could lead to therapeutic failure. Therefore to keep levels of these drugs within the therapeutic range, drug levels should be monitored and dosages adjusted accordingly.

Lacosamide
Mechanism of Action

Benefits of lacosamide (Vimpat) appear to derive from slow inactivation of sodium channels. This results in stabilization of hyperexcitable neuronal membranes and subsequent inhibition of repetitive firing.

Therapeutic Uses

Lacosamide is indicated for add-on therapy of partial-onset seizures in patients 17 years and older. Monotherapy was added as an indication in 2015 labeling updates. In patients with refractory partial-onset seizures, adding lacosamide to the regimen reduced seizure frequency by 50% or more in roughly 40% of those treated. Compared with other drugs for partial-onset seizures, lacosamide has two advantages. First, it has few drug interactions. Second, it can be administered IV as well as orally.

Adverse Effects

Lacosamide is generally well tolerated. The most common adverse effects are dizziness, headache, diplopia, and nasopharyngitis. Other effects include vomiting, fatigue, incoordination, blurred vision, tremor, somnolence, and cognitive changes (e.g., impaired memory, confusion, attention disruption). Lacosamide can prolong the PR interval, so it should be used with caution in patients with cardiac conduction problems and in those taking other drugs that prolong the PR interval. About 1% of patients experience euphoria. As a result, lacosamide is classified as a Schedule V drug under the Controlled Substances Act. Like other antiseizure drugs, lacosamide carries a small risk for suicidal thoughts or behavior.

Significant Drug Interactions

Lacosamide has few drug interactions. In clinical trials, it had little effect on plasma levels of other antiseizure drugs; however, carbamazepine, fosphenytoin, phenytoin, and phenobarbital may decrease the serum concentration of lacosamide. As noted, lacosamide should be used with caution in patients taking other drugs that can prolong the PR interval (e.g., β-blockers, calcium channel blockers).

Rufinamide
Mechanism of Action

Rufinamide (Banzel) has actions similar to some other antiseizure drugs (e.g., phenytoin, carbamazepine) in that rufinamide appears to suppress seizure activity by prolonging the inactive state of neuronal sodium channels.

Therapeutic Uses

Rufinamide is approved as add-on therapy for seizures associated with Lennox-Gastaut syndrome, a severe form of childhood epilepsy. In clinical trials, the drug reduced seizure frequency and severity.

Adverse Effects

Adverse effects differ somewhat between children and adults. In children, the most common adverse effects are somnolence, vomiting, and headache. In adults, the most common effects are dizziness, fatigue, nausea, and somnolence. Rufinamide can reduce the QT interval on the electrocardiogram, so it should not be used by patients with familial short QT syndrome. Like all other antiseizure drugs, rufinamide may increase suicidal thoughts and behavior.

Significant Drug Interactions

Four antiseizure drugs—carbamazepine, phenobarbital, phenytoin, and primidone—can significantly reduce levels of rufinamide. Because rufinamide is not metabolized by P450 isoenzymes, induction of cytochrome P450 cannot be the mechanism. One antiseizure drug—valproic acid—can increase rufinamide levels by up to 70%. Rufinamide causes mild induction of CYP3A4 and can thereby reduce levels of ethinyl estradiol and norethindrone, common components of oral contraceptives. An alternative form of contraception may be needed. Because rufinamide shortens the QT interval, other drugs that shorten the interval (e.g., digoxin) should be used with caution.

Vigabatrin
Mechanism of Action

Benefits of Vigabatrin (Sabril) derive from inhibiting GABA transaminase, the enzyme that inactivates GABA in the CNS. By preventing GABA inactivation, vigabatrin increases GABA availability, and thereby enhances GABA-mediated inhibition of neuronal activity.

Therapeutic Uses

Vigabatrin has two indications: (1) add-on therapy of complex partial seizures in adults who are refractory to other drugs and (2) monotherapy of infantile spasms in children ages 6 months to 2 years. Vigabatrin is the first drug approved in the United States for infantile spasms, a severe seizure disorder that occurs in children during the first year of life.

Adverse Effect

Vigabatrin can cause irreversible damage to the retina, usually manifesting as progressive narrowing of the visual field. Severe damage can produce tunnel vision. Some degree of visual field reduction occurs in 30% or more of patients. Some patients experience retinal damage within days to weeks of treatment onset, whereas others may use the drug for months to years before damage occurs.

BLACK BOX WARNING
Vigabatrin (Sabril)

> Vigabatrin can cause permanent loss of peripheral vision. Vision should be tested at baseline, then at 4 weeks, and then every 3 months as long as therapy continues.

To reduce the extent of damage, vision should be tested at baseline and every 3 months thereafter. If vision loss is detected, vigabatrin should be discontinued. Stopping will not reverse damage that has already occurred but may limit development of further damage. Unfortunately, even with periodic testing, some patients will develop severe vision loss.

Owing to the risk for vision loss, vigabatrin is available only through a restricted use program, known as SHARE (Support, Help, and Resources for Epilepsy). The goal is to monitor for vision damage and discontinue the drug as soon as possible when damage is detected. SHARE requires registration by prescribers, pharmacists, adult patients, and parents/guardians of young patients. In addition, the program requires that adult and pediatric patients undergo regular vision testing.

In clinical trials, the most common adverse effects in adults (who received vigabatrin plus other antiseizure drugs) were headache, somnolence, fatigue, dizziness, convulsions, increased weight with edema, and depression. Anemia has occurred. Like other antiseizure drugs, vigabatrin can promote suicidal thoughts and behavior. Among children, the most common adverse effects were somnolence, bronchitis, and otitis media.

Significant Drug Interactions

The risk for retinal damage is increased by combining vigabatrin with other drugs that can directly damage the retina (e.g., hydroxychloroquine) or with drugs that can promote glaucoma (e.g., glucocorticoids, tricyclic antidepressants). Vigabatrin can reduce levels of phenytoin (by inducing CYP2C9, the 2C9 isoenzyme of cytochrome P450) and can increase levels of clonazepam (by a mechanism that is unknown).

Ezogabine
Mechanism of Action

Ezogabine (generic) activates voltage-gated potassium channels in the neuronal membrane, and thereby facilitates potassium efflux. As a result, repetitive neuronal firing and related seizure activity are reduced.

Therapeutic Uses

Ezogabine is a first-in-class potassium channel opener. The drug is approved for adjunctive treatment of partial-onset seizures. Because of its abuse potential, ezogabine is a Schedule V controlled substance.

Adverse Effects

Previously, adverse effects due to ezogabine were thought to be minimal. Fortunately, subjects enrolled in clinical trials continued in extension trials post-marketing. As a result of these post-marketing trials, researchers discovered that prolonged use of ezogabine can lead to retinal abnormalities. Moreover, of those taking the drug for 4 years, approximately a third of patients demonstrated retinal changes on eye examinations and some of those had associated vision loss. As a result of this finding, ezogabine is recommend for use only for those in whom other antiseizure drugs do not work and in whom benefits exceed the risk of vision loss.

 BLACK BOX WARNING
Ezogabine (Generic)

Ezogabine may cause retinal abnormalities and potential vision loss.

Another concerning adverse effect is urinary retention. This occurs because, in addition to activating voltage-gated potassium channels in the neuronal membrane, ezogabine also activates potassium channels in the bladder epithelium and thereby promotes urinary retention, a unique side effect among the antiseizure drugs. Because of its effects on the bladder, ezogabine should be used with caution (if at all) in patients with preexisting voiding difficulty.

The most common adverse reactions are somnolence, dizziness, fatigue, confusion, vertigo, tremor, incoordination, double vision, memory impairment, and reduced strength. In addition, ezogabine can cause hallucinations and other symptoms of psychosis. Like all other antiseizure drugs, ezogabine may increase the risk for suicidal thinking or behavior.

Long-term use of ezogabine can also cause blue, gray-blue, and brown skin discoloration. This occurs most commonly in the nailbed and perioral area; however, it may become generalized. The drug can impart a red-orange color to urine. This effect is dose related and doesn't occur in most patients. When it does, it is harmless and unrelated to urinary retention.

In contrast to many antiseizure drugs, ezogabine has few interactions with other drugs. Both carbamazepine and phenytoin can decrease plasma concentrations of the drug, so higher doses of ezogabine may be needed when adding either drug to the medication regimen.

Eslicarbazepine
Mechanism of Action

The mechanism of action of eslicarbazepine (Aptiom) appears to be related to blockade of sodium channels. It is a prodrug that is metabolized to its active eslicarbazepine metabolite on first-pass metabolism.

Therapeutic Uses

Eslicarbazepine is approved for management of partial seizures. It may be used as either monotherapy or as an adjunct to ongoing therapy.

Adverse Effects

Most of eslicarbazepine's adverse effects are related to actions on the CNS. These include dizziness and sedation. More than 10% of patients have developed headache and diplopia. Less common adverse effects include blood dyscrasias, hepatic impairment, and an increased risk for SJS and TEN. Hyponatremia may also occur.

Significant Drug Interactions

Eslicarbazepine is a CYP2C19 inhibitor and a CYP3A4 inducer. This is the mechanism behind many of the interactions with this drug.

When prescribed with phenytoin, eslicarbazepine can increase phenytoin levels and phenytoin can decrease eslicarbazepine levels. Carbamazepine and phenobarbital can also decrease levels of eslicarbazepine.

Other significant interactions may occur with statins, hormonal contraceptives, and warfarin. Eslicarbazepine can lower levels of all these drugs. Dosage adjustments may be required, and alternate forms of birth control may need to be considered.

Perampanel
Mechanism of Action

The antiseizure effects of perampanel (Fycompa) are the result of AMPA glutamate antagonism. It blocks AMPA glutamate receptors on post-synaptic neurons.

Therapeutic Uses

Perampanel is approved for adjunctive therapy for treatment of both tonic-clonic seizures and partial seizures. It is not approved for use in children under 12 years of age.

Adverse Effects

Perampanel has been associated with serious psychiatric reactions. These include anger, aggression, hostility, violence, and even homicidal ideation. This atypical anger and aggression may occur in as many as 20% of patients taking the drug.

 BLACK BOX WARNING
Perampanel (Fycompa)

Perampanel has been associated with serious psychiatric reactions. These include anger, aggression, hostility, violence, and even homicidal ideation.

Other than hostility, the most common adverse effects are dizziness, drowsiness, fatigue, and headache. Nausea, vomiting, abdominal discomfort, and weight gain may also occur.

Significant Drug Interactions

Perampanel can decrease the effectiveness of hormonal contraceptives, particularly progestins. It can enhance the effect of CNS depressants, thus increasing risks related to sedation and, if significant, respiratory drive.

Phenytoin, carbamazepine, and oxcarbazepine can decrease perampanel levels by 50% or more through hepatic enzyme induction. Care must be undertaken to adjust for this when making adjustments in therapy.

Brivaracetam

Approved in 2016, brivaracetam (Briviact, Brivlera ♣) is the latest drug to receive FDA approval.

Mechanism of Action

The exact mechanism of action is unknown. Brivaracetam is known to have a selective affinity for a synaptic vesicle protein located in the brain and it is hypothesized that this may be a contributing factor.

Therapeutic Uses

Brivaracetam is approved for management of partial onset seizures in patients age 4 years and older, with brivaracetam injection restricted to patients age 16 years and older. It may be used as either monotherapy or adjunctive therapy.

Adverse Effects

Brivaracetam shares the same general adverse reactions as other antiseizure drugs (i.e., CNS depression, suicidal risk, and other mental health concerns). It may also cause neutrophil count to decrease and may cause serious hypersensitivity reactions. It should be used cautiously in patients with hepatic or renal impairment and is contraindicated for end-stage renal failure.

Significant Drug Interactions

Because brivaracetam is a CYP2C19 substrate, strong CYP2C19 inducers may reduce serum levels while CYP2C19 inhibitors may increase serum levels of the drug. As with all antiseizure drugs, other CNS depressants will have an additive effect.

MANAGEMENT OF GENERALIZED CONVULSIVE STATUS EPILEPTICUS

Convulsive SE is defined variably as either a prolonged tonic-clonic seizure lasting at least 5 minutes, a series of tonic-clonic seizures occurring without recovery of consciousness between seizures, or repeated seizures lasting 30 minutes or longer. Tachycardia, elevation of blood pressure, and hyperthermia are typical. Metabolic sequelae include hypoglycemia and acidosis. If SE persists for more than 20 minutes, it can cause permanent neurologic injury (cognitive impairment, memory loss, worsening of the underlying seizure disorder) and even death. Generalized convulsive SE is a medical emergency that requires immediate treatment. Management of SE is discussed in Chapter 92.

SPECIAL INTEREST TOPIC
Cannabidiol for Seizures

For decades there has been anecdotal reports of improved seizure control using marijuana. Unfortunately, randomized controlled trials (RCTs) were few and those yielded conflicting findings. Recommendations for and against use of marijuana for seizure control were hotly debated.

In 2018, the FDA approved cannabidiol (Epidiolex) for the management of seizures associated with Lennox-Gastaut syndrome (LGS) or Dravet syndrome (DS) in children age 2 years and older. LGS and DS are rare and severe forms of epilepsy that can be difficult to manage. In clinical trials with patients with LGS, there were 42% fewer seizures for those taking 20 mg/day compared to 37% fewer in those taking 10 mg/day. (At both dosages, those taking placebos had a decrease of 17%.) Clinical trials with patients with DS demonstrated a 44% decrease in seizures (22% with placebo). As with other medications, off-label use is anticipated.

Cannabidiol (CBD) is a product of the cannabis sativa plant. Unlike delta-9-tetrahydrocannabinol (THC), CBD is devoid of psychoactive effects. Still, the U.S. Drug Enforcement Agency (DEA) has designated CBD as a Schedule V drug. It is important that patients be instructed that highly controlled medical-grade CBD is different from that sold elsewhere. They cannot be used interchangeably.

Compared to other drugs for seizures, CBD has a relatively mild adverse effect profile. The most common adverse effects are alterations in sleep (both somnolence and insomnia), decreased appetite, diarrhea, fatigue, malaise, and decreased strength. Hepatic enzyme elevations have occurred so hepatic function should be tested before starting CBD and monitored periodically.

Full prescribing information is available at https://www.accessdata.fda.gov/drugsatfda_docs/label/2018/210365lbl.pdf.

SUMMARY OF KEY PRESCRIBING CONSIDERATIONS
Drugs for Seizure Disorders

Therapeutic Goal
To minimize or eliminate seizure events

Baseline Data
Pregnancy test. For all antiseizure drugs, assess seizure frequency and type and conduct a depression screening.

Additional Baseline Data Are Needed for the Following Drugs
Brivaracetam: CBC with differential, liver function, renal function
Carbamazepine: CBC with differential, liver function, renal function. Screen for HLA-B*1502 allele variant for patients of Asian ancestry
Eslicarbazepine: CBC with differential, liver function, serum sodium
Ethosuximide: CBC with differential

Felbamate: CBC with differential, liver function
Gabapentin: Renal function
Lacosamide: ECG, check for history of drug abuse and assess potential for dependency
Lamotrigine: CBC with differential
Oxcarbazepine: CBC with differential, serum sodium
Phenobarbital: CBC with differential, liver function, renal function. Check for history of drug abuse and assess potential for dependency
Phenytoin: Screen for HLA-B*1502 allele variant for patients of Asian ancestry (increased risk for SJS/TEN)
Rufinamide: ECG
Tiagabine: Liver function
Valproic Acid: Liver function

SUMMARY OF KEY PRESCRIBING CONSIDERATIONS—cont'd

Vigabatrin: Hematocrit and hemoglobin (if abnormal, obtain CBC), visual acuity and dilated ophthalmologic exam

Zonisamide: CBC with differential, liver function, renal function, metabolic panel, serum bicarbonate

Monitoring

For all antiseizure drugs, ongoing monitoring includes evaluating frequency and type of seizures, degree of CNS change, and depression, suicidality, or behavior change.

Additional Monitoring Is Needed for the Following Drugs as Clinically Indicated

Brivaracetam: CBC with differential, liver function, renal function

Carbamazepine: CBC with differential, liver function, renal function, serum iron. Assess for rash as a precursor to SJS or TEN. Assess signs and symptoms of blood abnormalities (e.g., pallor and fatigue associated with anemia, easy bruising and petechiae associated with thrombocytopenia, or symptoms of infection associated with leukopenia)

Eslicarbazepine: CBC with differential for signs of blood abnormalities, liver function, serum sodium for signs of hyponatremia. Assess for rash because this can progress to SJS or TEN

Ethosuximide: Trough concentrations to guide dosage. Assess for rash and other skin reactions

Felbamate: CBC with differential, liver function

Gabapentin: Renal function

Lacosamide: ECG after patient is on maintenance or if there are signs or symptoms suggestive of atrioventricular block or other cardiac rhythm disturbances

Lamotrigine: CBC with differential. Assess for rash because this may progress to SJS or TEN. Ask about suicide and depression; risk is higher for this drug

Oxcarbazepine: Serum sodium, CBC with differential for evidence of blood abnormalities (e.g., pallor, fatigue, weakness, exercise intolerance, fever, infection, easy bleeding or bruising, petechiae). Assess for rash because this may progress to SJS or TEN

Phenobarbital: CBC with differential, liver function, renal function. Serum drug levels at maintenance and when clinically indicated

Phenytoin: Obtain serum drug level and trough concentrations for dosage considerations. Assess for rash because this may progress to SJS or TEN. Assess for gingival hyperplasia

Rufinamide: ECG if history or physical examination positive for palpitations or other indications of cardiac rhythm changes

Tiagabine: Liver function

Valproic Acid: Liver function. Assess for signs and symptoms of pancreatitis

Vigabatrin: CBC if signs and symptoms of anemia develop. Dilated ophthalmologic exam every 3 months. Assess for fluid retention

Zonisamide: CBC with differential, liver function, renal function, metabolic panel, serum bicarbonate

Identifying High-Risk Patients

Depression is a concern for all antiseizure drugs. Pregnancy is a concern; however, when antiseizure drugs are necessary, benefits exceed risks.

High-Risk Patients for Specific Drugs Are

Brivaracetam: Cautious use recommended for patients with hepatic and renal impairment. Contraindicated for patients in end-stage renal failure

Carbamazepine: Contraindicated for patients with a history of bone marrow depression or preexisting hematologic abnormalities. There is an increased risk for SJS or TEN in patients with the variant HLA-B*1502 allele

Eslicarbazepine: Not recommended for patients with impaired liver function

Felbamate: Contraindicated for patients with anemia and hepatic impairment

Gabapentin: Caution and dosage adjustment is recommended for patients with renal impairment. The risk for psychological and physical dependence is increased in patients with a history of drug abuse

Lacosamide: Not recommended for patients with cardiac conduction disorders or patients who are taking drugs that can prolong the PR interval. The risk for abuse and dependency may be increased in patients with a history of abuse or dependency with other drugs

Oxcarbazepine: May worsen preexisting osteopenia and osteoporosis

Phenobarbital: Contraindicated in patients with a personal or family history of porphyria and in patients with marked anemia, or liver impairment. It should not be prescribed to patients with significant respiratory disease

Phenytoin: IV phenytoin is contraindicated for patients with bradycardia or atrioventricular block. Oral phenytoin may potentially worsen these conditions

Rufinamide: Contraindication for patients with a family history of short QT syndrome

Tiagabine: Not recommended for patients with hepatic impairment

Valproic Acid: Contraindicated for patients with significant hepatic dysfunction and in children younger than 3 years who are taking other antiseizure drugs. For pregnant women, valproic acid should be the drug of last resort, and only if use is essential

Vigabatrin: Caution prescribing to patients with anemia or vision loss

Zonisamide: Contraindicated for patients with conditions that contribute to a tendency toward metabolic acidosis. It should not be prescribed to patients with sulfa allergies

Evaluating Therapeutic Effects: Teach the patient (or a family member) to maintain a seizure frequency chart, indicating the date, time, and nature of all seizure events. This record can be used to evaluate treatment, make dosage adjustments, and alter drug selections.

Minimizing Adverse Effects
Central Nervous System Depression

Signs of CNS depression (sedation, drowsiness, lethargy) are most prominent during the initial phase of treatment and decline with continued drug use. Until this effect declines, patients should avoid driving and other hazardous activities. Until then, to minimize adverse CNS effects, use low initial doses and give the largest portion of the daily dose at bedtime.

Withdrawal Seizures

Abrupt discontinuation of antiseizure drugs can lead to status epilepticus. Consequently, medication should be withdrawn slowly (over 6 weeks to several months). Patients will need to take precautions not to run out of medications. Alerting patients of the need for follow-up visits prior to time for medication refills may be helpful.

Usage in Pregnancy

In most cases, the risk from uncontrolled seizures exceeds the risk from medication, and hence women with major seizure disorders should continue to take antiseizure drugs during pregnancy. However, the lowest effective dosage should be employed, and, if possible, only one drug should be used. Valproic acid should be avoided unless no other drugs are effective because this drug is highly teratogenic and can decrease the IQ of children exposed to it in utero. To reduce the risk for neural tube defects, pregnant patients taking any AED should be prescribed at least 0.04 mg of folic acid daily. Ideally, this should be started prior to becoming pregnant.

Suicidal Thoughts and Behavior

Screen for depression and suicidality before starting treatment and assess for these at clinic appoints. Involve families or significant others in care if antiseizure drugs are required for patient with depression for whom suicide is a risk factor and assess for these concerns at every clinical encounter.

22

Drugs for Muscle Spasm and Spasticity

In this chapter we consider two groups of drugs that cause skeletal muscle relaxation. One group is used for localized muscle spasm. The other is used for spasticity. As a rule, the drugs used to treat spasticity do not relieve acute muscle spasm, and the drugs used to treat acute muscle spasm do not relieve spasticity; therefore the two groups are not interchangeable. Ten muscle relaxants are currently approved for these purposes (Table 22.1). With the exception of one direct-acting muscle relaxer, these drugs produce their effects through actions in the central nervous system (CNS).

DRUGS FOR SPASTICITY

The term *spasticity* refers to a group of movement disorders of CNS origin. These disorders are characterized by heightened muscle tone, spasm, and loss of dexterity. The most common causes are multiple sclerosis and cerebral palsy. Other causes include traumatic spinal cord lesions and stroke. Spasticity is managed with a combination of drugs and physical therapy.

Four drugs—baclofen, diazepam, dantrolene, and tizanidine—can relieve spasticity. Baclofen, diazepam, and tizanidine act in the CNS. In contrast, dantrolene acts directly on skeletal muscle. Diazepam (Diastat, Valium) is a member of the benzodiazepine family. Although diazepam is the only benzodiazepine labeled for treating spasticity, other benzodiazepines have been used off-label for this purpose. The basic pharmacology of the benzodiazepines is discussed in Chapter 29.

PROTOTYPE DRUGS

Muscle Spasm

Centrally Acting Muscle Relaxer for Spasticity
Baclofen (Lioresal, Gablofen)

Centrally Acting Muscle Relaxer for Localized Muscle Spasm
Cyclobenzaprine (Amrix, Fexmid)

Direct Acting Muscle Relaxer
Dantrolene (Dantrium)

Baclofen

Baclofen (Lioresal, Gablofen) will serve as our prototype for centrally acting drugs that relieve spasticity. Baclofen is helpful in relieving spasm related to multiple sclerosis and some spinal cord injuries. It is not approved for management of spasticity related to cerebral palsy, stroke, Parkinson disease, or Huntington chorea.

Mechanism of Action

Baclofen acts within the spinal cord to suppress hyperactive reflexes involved in regulation of muscle movement. The precise mechanism of reflex attenuation is unknown. Because baclofen is a structural analog of the inhibitory neurotransmitter γ-aminobutyric acid (GABA), it may act by mimicking the actions of GABA on spinal neurons. Baclofen has no direct effects on skeletal muscle.

Therapeutic Use

As mentioned earlier, baclofen can reduce spasticity associated with multiple sclerosis and spinal cord injury. The drug decreases flexor and extensor spasms and suppresses resistance to passive movement. These actions reduce the discomfort of spasticity and allow increased performance. Because baclofen has no direct muscle relaxant action, it does not decrease muscle strength. For this reason, baclofen is preferred to dantrolene, a direct-acting muscle relaxer, when spasticity is associated with significant muscle weakness.

Preparations, Dosages, and Pharmacokinetics

Preparations and dosages of baclofen and other drugs in this chapter are provided in Table 22.1. Pharmacokinetics of these drugs are provided in Table 22.2.

Adverse Effects

The most common side effects involve the CNS and gastrointestinal tract. Approximately 10% of patients taking baclofen develop hypotension. Serious adverse effects are rare.

Central nervous system effects. Baclofen is a CNS depressant and hence frequently causes *drowsiness, dizziness, weakness,* and *fatigue.* These responses are most intense during the early phase of therapy and diminish with continued drug use. CNS depression can be minimized with doses that are small initially and then gradually increased. Patients should be cautioned to avoid alcohol and other CNS depressants because baclofen will potentiate the depressant actions of these drugs.

Overdose can produce *coma* and *respiratory depression.* Because there is no antidote to baclofen overdose, treatment for overdose is supportive and should be started immediately.

Withdrawal. Although baclofen does not appear to cause physical dependence, abrupt discontinuation has been associated with adverse reactions. Abrupt withdrawal of *oral* baclofen can cause visual hallucinations, paranoid ideation, and seizures. Accordingly, withdrawal should be done slowly (over 1 to 2 weeks). (Although not typically ordered by advanced practice registered nurses and physician assistants, it is interesting to note that a black box warning alerts providers against abrupt withdrawal of *intrathecal* baclofen. Potential reactions include high fever, altered mental status, exaggerated rebound spasticity, and muscle rigidity that, in rare cases, has advanced to rhabdomyolysis, multiple organ system failure, and death.)

Other adverse effects. Baclofen causes nausea, vomiting, constipation, and urinary retention in approximately 8%–10% of patients. Hypotension may also occur. Patients should be warned about these possible reactions.

TABLE 22.1   Drugs for Muscle Spasm and Spasticity

Drug Name	Preparation	Indication	Usual Adult Oral Maintenance Dosage	Common Adverse Effects	Considerations
Centrally Acting Muscle Relaxants					
Baclofen (Lioresal, Gablofen)	Tablet: 10 mg, 20 mg Suspension: 1 mg/mL, 5 mg/mL Cream: 1%, 2% Intrathecal Solution[a]: 50 µg/mL (0.05 mg/mL), 10 mg/5 mL, 10,000 µg/20 mL (10 mg/20 mL), 20,000 µg/20 mL, 40,000 µg/20 mL (40 mg/20 mL)	Spasticity due to spinal cord injury or CNS condition.	15–20 mg 3 or 4 times/day	CNS depression, dizziness, headache, nausea, vomiting, constipation, urinary retention	Abrupt withdrawal can cause seizures and hallucinations. Taper slowly over at least 1–2 weeks.
Carisoprodol (Soma)	Tablets: 250 mg, 350 mg	Musculoskeletal pain and muscle spasms	250–350 mg 3 or 4 times/day	CNS depression, dizziness, headaches, euphoria.	Controlled substance (schedule IV) Avoid in patients with porphyria.
Chlorzoxazone (Lorzone)	Tablets: 375 mg, 500 mg, 750 mg	Musculoskeletal pain and muscle spasms	500–750 mg 3 or 4 times/day	CNS depression, dizziness	Paradoxical CNS stimulation may occur. May color urine orange to purple-red. Rare hepatotoxicity can be fatal.
Cyclobenzaprine (Amrix, Fexmid)	IR tablets: 5 mg, 7.5 mg, 10 mg ER capsule: 15 mg, 30 mg Suspension: 1 mg/mL Cream: 5%, 20 mg/g	Musculoskeletal pain and muscle spasms	IR (tablets or solution): 5 mg 3 times daily initially then increase up to 10 mg 3 times daily ER: 15 or 30 mg once daily	CNS depression, dizziness, anticholinergic effects (dry mouth, blurred vision, photophobia, urinary retention, constipation)	Recommended for short-term use not to exceed 2–3 weeks. Administration with food increases bioavailability.[b] Contraindicated for patients taking MAO inhibitors. May cause serotonin syndrome in patients taking SSRIs and related antidepressants
Diazepam (Diastat, Valium)	Tablets: 2 mg, 5 mg, 10 mg Oral solution: 1 mg/mL Oral concentrate: 5 mg/mL Rectal gel: 2.5 mg, 10 mg, 20 mg Injection solution: 5 mg/mL Auto-injector: 10 mg/2 mL	Spasticity due to spinal cord injury or CNS condition Musculoskeletal pain and muscle spasms. Muscle spasms associated with localized musculoskeletal pain, inflammation, or trauma.	2–10 mg 3 or 4 times/ day	CNS depression, hypotension	Controlled substance (C-IV) May cause paradoxical CNS stimulation and/or antegrade amnesia.
Metaxalone (Skelaxin)	Tablets: 400 mg, 800 mg	Musculoskeletal pain and muscle spasms	800 mg 3 or 4 times/ day	CNS depression, dizziness, headache	Administration with food increases bioavailability.[b] May cause liver damage. May cause serotonin syndrome in patients taking serotonergic drugs (e.g., SSRIs and related antidepressants).
Methocarbamol (Robaxin)	Tablets: 500 mg, 750 mg Injection solution: 1000 mg/10 mL	Musculoskeletal pain and muscle spasms	1000 mg 4 times/day	CNS depression, amnesia, headache, hypotension, bradycardia, nausea	Have patient stay in a lying position for 10–15 min after IV administration. Less sedation than most. May color urine green to brown-black.
Orphenadrine (Norflex)	ER tablet: 100 mg Injection solution: 30 mg/ mL	Musculoskeletal pain and muscle spasms	100 mg twice a day	CNS depression, headache, euphoria, palpitations, tachycardia, anticholinergic effects (dry mouth, blurred vision, photophobia, urinary retention, constipation)	May worsen cardiac conditions such as heart failure

TABLE 22.1   Drugs for Muscle Spasm and Spasticity—cont'd

Drug Name	Preparation	Indication	Usual Adult Oral Maintenance Dosage	Common Adverse Effects	Considerations
Tizanidine (Zanaflex)	Tablet: 2 mg, 4 mg Capsule: 2 mg, 4 mg, 6 mg	Spasticity due to spinal cord injury or CNS condition.	Initially 2 mg every 6–8 h, then may increase to 8 mg every 6–8 h	CNS depression, dizziness, hypotension, weakness, bradycardia, dry mouth.	Administration with food increases bioavailability.[b] May cause liver damage. More sedation than most. Hallucinations and psychosis may occur.
Direct-Acting Muscle Relaxants					
Dantrolene (Dantrium, Revonto, Ryanodex)	Capsule: 25 mg, 50 mg, 100 mg IV solution: 20 mg, 250 mg	Spasticity due to spinal cord injury or CNS condition.	Initial adult dosage is 25 mg once daily for 1 week then increase gradually up to 100 mg 3 times/day	Muscle weakness, drowsiness, dysphagia, hoarseness, nausea, erectile dysfunction, diarrhea. Flushing with IV administration.	Hepatic toxicity can be life-threatening. If some degree of spasticity is required for maintenance of posture and mobility, negative effects associated with loss of function may exceed any positive benefit.

[a]Gablofen is dosed in micrograms; Lioresal is dosed in milligrams.
[b]Increases in bioavailability can increase adverse effects. To stabilize dosing, administer consistently either with or without food.
CNS, Central nervous system; *ER*, extended release; *IR*, immediate release; *MAO*, monoamine oxidase.

TABLE 22.2   Pharmacokinetics: Drugs for Muscle Spasm and Spasticity

Drug	Peak	Protein Binding	Metabolism	Half-Life	Elimination
CENTRALLY ACTING MUSCLE RELAXANTS					
Baclofen (Lioresal, Gablofen)	1 h	30%	Hepatic	3–5 h	Urine (70%) Feces
Carisoprodol (Soma)	1.5–2 h	70%	Hepatic via CYP2C19	2 h	Urine
Chlorzoxazone (Lorzone)	1–2 h	UK	Hepatic via glucuronidation	1 h	Urine
Cyclobenzaprine (Amrix, Fexmid)	IR: 4 h ER: 7–8 h	UK	Hepatic via CYP3A4, CYP1A2, CYP2D6	8–37 h (Up to 188 h with hepatic impairment)	Urine
Diazepam (Diastat, Valium)	0.25–2.5 h[a]	95%–98%	Hepatic via CYP3A4, CYP2C19	44–48 h Active metabolite: up to 100 h and greater	Urine
Metaxalone (Skelaxin)	3 h	UK	Hepatic primarily via CYP1A2, CYP2D6, CYP2E1, CYP3A4 additionally via CYP2C8, CPY2C9, CYP2C19	6–14 h	Urine
Methocarbamol (Robaxin)	1–2 h	45%–50%	Hepatic	1–2 h	Urine
Orphenadrine (Norflex)	2–4 h	20%	Hepatic	14–16 h	Urine
Tizanidine (Zanaflex)	1–4 h[a]	30%	Hepatic via CYP1A2	2.5 h	Urine (60%) Feces
Direct-Acting Muscle Relaxants					
Dantrolene (Dantrium, Revonto, Ryanodex)	Oral: UK IV: 1 h	UK[b]	Hepatic	4–11 h (mean: 8.7 h)	Feces (45%–50%) Urine

[a]Later peak times reflect drug taken with food
[b]Product labeling states "significant binding"
ER, Extended release; *IR*, immediate release; *UK*, unknown.

PATIENT EDUCATION
Baclofen

Tell patients about possible depressant effects such as drowsiness, lightheadedness, and fatigue, and warn them to avoid hazardous activities such as driving. Caution patients to avoid other central nervous system depressants because these drugs will intensify the depressant effects of baclofen. Baclofen frequently causes hypotension, nausea, constipation, and urinary retention. Patients should be warned about these possible reactions and provided with interventions to manage these conditions. It is also important to warn patients that abrupt discontinuation may cause psychiatric symptoms such as visual hallucinations, paranoia, and seizures.

Contraindications and Interactions
Alcohol and Other Central Nervous System Depressants

Baclofen can cause additive CNS depression when given with CNS depressant agents such as alcohol, opioids, or benzodiazepines. Any centrally acting muscle relaxant in combination with a CNS depressant can cause severe respiratory depression.

Urinary Retention

Baclofen can cause acute urinary retention. Patients with a history of benign prostatic hypertrophy and those taking drugs that can cause urinary retention (e.g., anticholinergics) should be monitored closely for this complication.

Psychiatric Conditions

Baclofen may exacerbate psychotic conditions and confusion. Patients with a history of schizophrenia or other psychiatric illnesses may require close observation to determine progression of symptoms.

PATIENT EDUCATION
Centrally Acting Skeletal Muscle Relaxants

Inform patients about possible depressant effects such as drowsiness, lightheadedness, and fatigue. Advise them to avoid driving and other hazardous activities if significant impairment occurs. If they must be taken by older patients, it is essential to explain about the increased risk of falls. Teach patients and family members home safety measures to decrease fall risk such as ensuring adequate lighting and avoiding scatter rugs. Let patients know that central nervous system (CNS) depressant effects are worsened by intake of other CNS depressants, including alcohol and first-generation antihistamines. Warn patients against abrupt discontinuation to avoid withdrawal reactions.

Diazepam

Diazepam (Diastat, Valium) is a member of the benzodiazepine family. Although diazepam is the only benzodiazepine labeled for treating spasticity, other benzodiazepines have been used off-label. The basic pharmacology of the benzodiazepines is discussed in Chapter 29.

Mechanism of Action

Like baclofen, diazepam acts in the CNS to suppress spasticity. Beneficial effects appear to result from mimicking the actions of GABA at receptors in the spinal cord and brain. Diazepam does not affect skeletal muscle directly. Because diazepam has no direct effects on muscle strength, the drug is preferred to dantrolene when muscle strength is marginal.

Adverse Effects

Sedation is common when treating spasticity. To minimize sedation, initial doses should be low. Other adverse effects are discussed in Chapter 29.

Dantrolene

Dantrolene (Dantrium) will serve as our prototype for direct-acting drugs that relieve spasticity.

Mechanism of Action

Unlike baclofen, which acts within the CNS, dantrolene (Dantrium) acts directly on skeletal muscle. The drug relieves spasm by suppressing release of calcium from the sarcoplasmic reticulum; therefore the muscle is less able to contract. Fortunately, therapeutic doses have only minimal effects on contraction of smooth muscle and cardiac muscle.

PATIENT EDUCATION
Dantrolene

Inform patients about possible depressant effects (drowsiness, dizziness, lightheadedness, fatigue), and advise them to avoid driving and other hazardous activities if significant impairment occurs. Inform patients about signs of liver dysfunction (e.g., jaundice, abdominal pain, malaise), and instruct them to seek medical attention if these develop. Warn patients to avoid central nervous system depressants (e.g., alcohol, benzodiazepines, opioids, antihistamines) because these drugs will intensify depressant effects of dantrolene.

Therapeutic Uses

Spasticity. Dantrolene can relieve spasticity associated with multiple sclerosis, cerebral palsy, and spinal cord injury. It is also used to manage muscle contraction and rigidity associated with malignant hyperthermia.

Unfortunately, because dantrolene suppresses spasticity by causing a generalized reduction in the ability of skeletal muscle to contract, treatment may be associated with a significant reduction in strength. As a result, overall function may be reduced rather than improved. Accordingly, care must be taken to ensure that the benefits of therapy (reduced spasticity) outweigh the harm (reduced strength). If beneficial effects do not develop within 45 days, dantrolene should be discontinued.

Adverse Effects

Hepatic toxicity. Dose-related liver damage is the most serious adverse effect. The incidence is 1 in 1000. Deaths have occurred. Hepatotoxicity is most common in women older than 35 years. By contrast, liver injury is rare in children younger than 10 years. To reduce the risk for liver damage, liver function tests (LFTs) should be performed at baseline and periodically thereafter. If LFTs indicate liver injury, dantrolene should be withdrawn. Because of the potential for liver damage, dantrolene should be administered in the lowest effective dosage and for the shortest time necessary.

Other adverse effects. Muscle weakness, drowsiness, and diarrhea are the most common side effects. Muscle weakness is a direct extension of dantrolene's pharmacologic action. Other adverse effects may include dysphagia and hoarseness, nausea and vomiting, and erectile dysfunction. Almost a third of patients receiving intravenous (IV) dantrolene will experience flushing.

⏵⏵ BLACK BOX WARNING
Dantrolene

Fatal hepatotoxicity has occurred, especially at higher doses, even with short-term therapy. The lowest effective dose should be used. Because patients may be asymptomatic, baseline liver function tests should be obtained followed by frequent monitoring of these levels throughout therapy.

SUMMARY OF KEY PRESCRIBING CONSIDERATIONS

Direct-Acting Muscle Relaxants

The prescribing implications summarized here apply only to the use of dantrolene for spasticity.

Therapeutic Goal: Management of spasticity

Baseline Data: Motor function, including spasm, rigidity, range of motion, dexterity, and associated pain. Liver function tests.

Monitoring: Motor function, including reduction in rigidity, spasm, and pain and for improvements in dexterity and range of motion. Liver function tests. (Discontinue dantrolene if liver impairment develops.)

Identifying High-Risk Patients: Contraindicated with hepatic disease (e.g., cirrhosis or hepatitis)

Evaluating Therapeutic Effects: Demonstrates improvement in function and quality of life

Minimizing Adverse Effects:

Central Nervous System Depression

Dantrolene is a central nervous system depressant. Depressant effects such as drowsiness, lightheadedness, and fatigue pose a danger if patients engage in hazardous activities. Initiate fall precautions if hospitalized.

Muscle Weakness

Dantrolene can decrease muscle strength. Evaluate muscle function to ensure that benefits of therapy (decreased spasticity) are not outweighed by reductions in strength. Patients may need additional help with ambulation and other activities initially

DRUGS FOR LOCALIZED MUSCLE SPASM

Muscle spasm is defined as involuntary contraction of a muscle or muscle group. Muscle spasm is often painful and reduces the ability to function. Spasm can result from a variety of causes, including epilepsy, hypocalcemia, acute and chronic pain syndromes, and localized muscle injury. Discussion here is limited to spasm resulting from acute musculoskeletal injury.

Treatment of acute muscle spasm involves physical measures and drug therapy. Examples of these measures include physical therapy, specific exercises, whirlpool baths, and heat application. Although application of cold compresses is commonly used initially following a musculoskeletal injury, its purpose is to relieve pain and reduce swelling, not to relieve muscle spasm. Current evidence does not support cold treatments for management of muscle spasm.

For drug therapy, two groups of medicines are used: (1) analgesics such as acetaminophen or nonsteroidal antiinflammatory drugs (NSAIDs); and (2) centrally acting muscle relaxants. The analgesics are discussed in Chapter 57. The centrally acting muscle relaxants used to relieve muscle spasm are carisoprodol, chlorzoxazone, cyclobenzaprine, diazepam, metaxalone, methocarbamol, and orphenadrine. Cyclobenzaprine (Amrix, Fexmid) will serve as our prototype for drugs used to treat local muscle spasm.

CYCLOBENZAPRINE

Mechanism of Action

Cyclobenzaprine is a centrally acting skeletal muscle relaxant. Its activity takes place primarily in the brain stem and results in a reduction of tonic motor activity.

Therapeutic Use

Cyclobenzaprine is used for relief of muscle spasm and associated pain. It is considered the most efficacious of the drugs used for this purpose; therefore it is typically the drug of first choice for acute muscle spasm. It is ineffective as a treatment for spasticity.

Adverse Effects

Central Nervous System Effects

Cyclobenzaprine is a CNS depressant, so drowsiness, dizziness, and fatigue are common. As with baclofen, these responses are most intense during the early phase of therapy and diminish with continued drug use.

Anticholinergic Effects

Cyclobenzaprine is structurally similar to tricyclic antidepressants (see Chapter 27). This similarity explains the presence of anticholinergic effects. Common anticholinergic adverse effects include dry mouth, blurred vision, photophobia, urinary retention, and constipation.

Cardiac Rhythm Disturbances

Cyclobenzaprine can cause cardiac rhythm disturbances similar to those of tricyclic antidepressants. These include a wide variety of dysrhythmias including sinus tachycardia and significant conduction delays.

Contraindications and Interactions

Antidepressants

Cyclobenzaprine use is contraindicated for patients taking monoamine oxidase (MAO) inhibitors. For patients previously undergoing therapy with MAO inhibitors, at least 2 weeks must have passed after discontinuing the drug before starting cyclobenzaprine. Failure to do so has led to potentially fatal serotonin syndrome manifested by high fever, seizures, and rhabdomyolysis.

Serotonin syndrome may also occur if cyclobenzaprine is given with selective serotonin reuptake inhibitors (SSRIs), serotonin and norepinephrine reuptake inhibitors (SNRIs), and tricyclic antidepressants. Symptoms may range from mild agitation and tremor to the high fevers and seizures that can occur with MAO inhibitors (Box 22.1).

Alcohol and Other Central Nervous System Depressants

Cyclobenzaprine will cause additive CNS depression when given with other CNS depressants such as alcohol. Patients must be advised to avoid these combinations.

Other Centrally Acting Muscle Relaxants

We have discussed our prototype drugs—baclofen, dantrolene, and cyclobenzaprine—in detail. All centrally acting muscle relaxers have

---

BOX 22.1 Manifestations of Serotonin Syndrome

System	Manifestation
Central Nervous System	Agitation, restlessness, confusion, hallucinations, headache, unconsciousness
Autonomic Nervous System	Hyperthermia, diaphoresis, blood pressure elevation, tachycardia, pupil dilation
Neuromuscular System	Tremor, hyperreflexia, ataxia, muscle twitching, muscle rigidity, seizures
Gastrointestinal System	Nausea, vomiting, diarrhea

LIFE SPAN CONSIDERATIONS: DRUGS FOR MUSCLE SPASM AND SPASTICITY

Life Stage	Considerations or Concerns
Children	Chlorzoxazone, orphenadrine, and tizanidine are not approved for use in children.
Pregnant women	Cyclobenzaprine is considered relatively safe for pregnant women. Diazepam is a teratogen. Diazepam is associated with low birth weights, prematurity, hypoglycemia, and respiratory depression. Neonatal withdrawal syndrome has been observed with benzodiazepines (e.g., alprazolam, diazepam, lorazepam) and baclofen. Animal reproduction studies have yielded adverse events for baclofen, carisoprodol, tizanidine, and dantrolene. There are insufficient animal studies conducted for chlorzoxazone, methocarbamol, and orphenadrine. Human trials are lacking. Animal studies did not identify any adverse events for metaxalone.
Breast-feeding women	These drugs can cause adverse effects in infants. Breastfeeding is not recommended.
Older adults	At the dosage required to have adequate effect, these drugs may cause sedation and cognitive impairment, thus creating a fall risk. Carisoprodol, chlorzoxazone, cyclobenzaprine, metaxalone, methocarbamol, and orphenadrine are listed in Beers Criteria as potentially inappropriate for older adults. Cyclobenzaprine and orphenadrine have more anticholinergic effects (e.g., blurred vision, constipation, urinary retention, elevated heart rate) that may create additional problems for older adult patients. Long-acting benzodiazepines such as diazepam are particularly troublesome because older adult patients tend to have a slower metabolism. Elimination may be delayed, and active drug may accumulate.

similar pharmacologic properties, so we will consider the remaining (nonprototype) agents as a group.

Mechanism of Action

For most centrally acting muscle relaxants, the mechanism of spasm relief is unclear. In laboratory animals, high doses can depress spinal motor reflexes. However, these doses are much higher than those used in humans. Hence many investigators believe that relaxation of spasm results primarily from the *sedative properties* of these drugs and not from specific actions exerted on CNS pathways that control muscle tone.

The drugs for spasticity—diazepam and tizanidine—are thought to relieve spasm by enhancing presynaptic inhibition of motor neurons in the CNS. Diazepam promotes presynaptic inhibition by enhancing the effects of GABA, an inhibitory neurotransmitter. Tizanidine promotes inhibition by acting as an agonist at presynaptic α_2 receptors.

Therapeutic Use

Tizanidine is indicated for treating spasticity and has been used off-label to treat acute back pain. Carisoprodol, chlorzoxazone, metaxalone, methocarbamol, and orphenadrine are used to relieve localized muscle spasm. Diazepam is approved for treatment of both spasticity and muscle spasm.

Adverse Effects
Central Nervous System Depression
All centrally acting muscle relaxants can cause CNS depression. Depressant effects may include drowsiness, lightheadedness, and fatigue. These may be dangerous if the patient must engage in hazardous activities (e.g., truck-driving or construction). If necessary for treatment of older adults, fall precautions should be instituted. Patients should be advised to avoid alcohol and all other CNS depressants.

Hepatic Toxicity
Tizanidine (Zanaflex) and *metaxalone* (Skelaxin) can cause liver damage. Liver function should be assessed before starting treatment and periodically thereafter. If liver injury develops, these drugs should be discontinued. If the patient has preexisting liver disease, these drugs should be avoided.

Chlorzoxazone (Lorzone) can cause hepatitis and potentially fatal hepatic necrosis. Because of this potential for harm and because other drugs are more effective, the risk of harm generally exceeds the drug's benefits.

Physical Dependence
Chronic, high-dose therapy can cause physical dependence, manifesting as a potentially life-threatening abstinence syndrome if these drugs are abruptly withdrawn. Accordingly, withdrawal should be done slowly. Two of the muscle relaxants, diazepam and carisprodol, are schedule IV controlled drugs.

Other Adverse Effects
Cyclobenzaprine and orphenadrine have significant anticholinergic (atropine-like) properties and hence may cause dry mouth, blurred vision, photophobia, urinary retention, and constipation.

Methocarbamol may turn urine brown, black, or dark green. Chlorzoxazone may color urine orange to purple-red. This appears to be dose related. The effect is harmless.

Tizanidine can cause dry mouth, hypotension, hallucinations, and psychotic symptoms.

Tizanidine is similar to clonidine and can cause hypotension. When discontinuing this drug, it may be necessary to taper dosage to avoid rebound hypertension.

Carisoprodol can be hazardous to patients predisposed to intermittent porphyria. It is contraindicated for patients with this condition.

▤ SUMMARY OF KEY PRESCRIBING CONSIDERATIONS

Centrally Acting Skeletal Muscle Relaxants

Except where noted, the nursing implications summarized here apply to all centrally acting muscle relaxants used to treat muscle spasm.

Therapeutic Goal: To relieve muscle spasm/spasticity

Baseline Data:

All drugs: Degree of spasm, functional ability, pain, premedication central nervous system (CNS) status.

Chlorozoxazone: Liver function

Diazepam: Complete blood count (CBC), liver function, renal function

Metaxalone: CBC, liver function, renal function

Tizanidine: Blood pressure, liver function, renal function.

Monitoring:

All drugs: Compare degree of spasm, functional ability, CNS status, and pain to premedication level.

Baclofen: Seizure activity and EEG in patients who have epilepsy (needed because loss of seizure control has been reported)

Carisoprodol, diazepam, orphenadrine: Evidence of drug misuse or abuse (Carisoprodol and diazepam are controlled drugs. Orphenadrine is known to cause euphoria so there is a potential for abuse.)

Chlorozoxazone: Liver function tests. Assess for signs and symptoms of hepatotoxicity (e.g., jaundice, anorexia, nausea, fatigue, dark urine).

Cyclobenzaprine: Assess for signs/ symptoms serotonin syndrome if taking SSRI, SNRI, or other serotonergic drugs. ECG, if indicated.

Diazepam: Liver function, renal function. Assess for signs and symptoms of hepatotoxicity or decreased renal function.

Metaxalone: CBC, liver function, renal function. Assess for signs and symptoms of anemia, hepatotoxicity, or decreased renal function.

Tizanidine: Heart rate, blood pressure. Liver function, renal function. Assess for signs and symptoms of hepatotoxicity or decreased renal function.

Identifying High-Risk Patients:

All drugs: Patients having CNS depression or taking CNS depressants may have an additive effect.

Carisoprodol, diazepam: Patients with a history of drug abuse may be more likely to misuse or abuse these drugs.

Chlorzoxazone: Patients with liver disease should not take chlorzoxazone.

Cyclobenzaprine: Patients taking serotonergic drugs (e.g., selective serotonin reuptake inhibitors, serotonin and norepinephrine reuptake inhibitors) are at risk for serotonin syndrome if cyclobenzaprine is prescribed. Cyclobenzaprine is contraindicated in patients taking a monoamine oxidase (MAO) inhibitor; at least 14 days without an MAO inhibitor should elapse prior to initiating therapy with cyclobenzaprine. Use caution prescribing for patients with cardiac rhythm disturbances.

Diazepam: Diazepam is contraindicated for patients with both narrow-angle and open-angle glaucoma, severe respiratory or liver impairment, sleep apnea, and myasthenia gravis.

Metaxalone: Patients with impaired hepatic function, renal function, or history of anemias (especially if drug induced or hemolytic) should not take this drug. Increases risk for serotonin syndrome in patients taking serotonergic drugs.

Methocarbamol: Not recommended for patients with seizure disorders or renal impairment but not contraindicated. Hepatic impairment may cause toxic serum levels.

Orphenadrine: Contraindicated for patients with glaucoma, myasthenia gravis, gastrointestinal obstruction, and urinary bladder outlet obstruction. Cautious use is recommended for patients with coronary insufficiency, heart failure, cardiac decompensation.

Tizanidine: Prescribe cautiously for patients with hepatic disease.

Evaluating Therapeutic Effects: Improved function, decreased pain

Minimizing Adverse Effects:

Withdrawal Reactions

Central muscle relaxants can cause physical dependence. To avoid an abstinence syndrome, withdraw gradually.

23

Local Anesthetics

Local anesthetics are drugs that suppress pain by blocking impulse conduction along axons. Conduction is blocked only in neurons located near the site of administration. The great advantage of local anesthesia, compared with inhalation anesthesia, is that pain can be suppressed without causing generalized depression of the entire nervous system. Local anesthetics carry much less risk than do general anesthetics.

We begin the chapter by considering the pharmacology of the local anesthetics as a group. After that, we discuss three prototypic agents: procaine, lidocaine, and cocaine. We conclude by discussing specific routes of anesthetic administration.

BASIC PHARMACOLOGY OF THE LOCAL ANESTHETICS

Classification

There are two major groups of local anesthetics: *esters* and *amides*. The ester-type anesthetics, represented by *procaine* (Novocain), contain an ester linkage in their structure. In contrast, the amide-type agents, represented by *lidocaine* (Xylocaine), contain an amide linkage. The ester-type agents and amide-type agents differ in two important ways: (1) method of inactivation and (2) promotion of allergic responses. Contrasts between the esters and amides are shown in Table 23.1.

Mechanism of Action

Local anesthetics stop axonal conduction by *blocking sodium channels* in the axonal membrane. Recall that propagation of an action potential requires movement of sodium ions from outside the axon to the inside. This influx takes place through specialized sodium channels. By blocking axonal sodium channels, local anesthetics prevent sodium entry and thereby block conduction.

Selectivity of Anesthetic Effects

Local anesthetics are nonselective modifiers of neuronal function. That is, they will block action potentials in all neurons to which they have access. The only way to achieve selectivity is by delivering the anesthetic to a limited area.

Although local anesthetics can block traffic in all neurons, blockade develops more rapidly in some neurons than in others. Specifically, small, nonmyelinated neurons are blocked more rapidly than large, myelinated neurons. Because of this differential sensitivity, some

sensations are blocked sooner than others. Specifically, perception of pain is lost first, followed in order by perception of cold, warmth, touch, and deep pressure.

The effects of local anesthetics are not limited to sensory neurons: these drugs also block conduction in motor neurons.

PATIENT EDUCATION
Self-Inflicted Injury

Because anesthetics eliminate pain and because pain can be a warning sign of complications, patients recovering from anesthesia must be protected from inadvertent harm until the anesthetic wears off. Caution the patient against activities that might result in unintentional harm.

Time Course of Local Anesthesia

Ideally, local anesthesia would begin promptly and would persist no longer (or shorter) than needed. Unfortunately, although onset of anesthesia is usually rapid (Tables 23.2 and 23.3), duration of anesthesia is often less than ideal. In some cases, anesthesia persists longer than needed. In others, repeated administration is required to maintain anesthesia of sufficient duration.

Onset of local anesthesia is determined largely by the molecular properties of the anesthetic. Before anesthesia can occur, the anesthetic must diffuse from its site of administration to its sites of action within the axon membrane. Anesthesia is delayed until this movement has occurred. The ability of an anesthetic to penetrate the axon membrane is determined by three properties: *molecular size, lipid solubility,* and *degree of ionization at tissue pH.* Anesthetics of small size, high lipid solubility, and low ionization cross the axon membrane rapidly. In contrast, anesthetics of large size, low lipid solubility, and high ionization cross slowly. Obviously, anesthetics that penetrate the axon most rapidly have the fastest onset.

Termination of local anesthesia occurs as molecules of anesthetic diffuse out of neurons and are carried away in the blood. The same factors that determine onset of anesthesia (molecular size, lipid solubility, degree of ionization) also help determine duration. In addition, *regional blood flow* is an important determinant of how long anesthesia will last. In areas where blood flow is high, anesthetic is carried away quickly and effects terminate with relative haste. In regions where blood flow is low, anesthesia is more prolonged.

Use With Vasoconstrictors

Local anesthetics are frequently administered in combination with a vasoconstrictor, usually *epinephrine*. The vasoconstrictor decreases local blood flow and thereby delays systemic absorption of the anesthetic. Delaying absorption has two benefits: It *prolongs anesthesia* and *reduces the risk for toxicity*. Because absorption is slowed, less anesthetic is used and a more favorable balance is established between the rate of entry of anesthetic into circulation and the rate of its conversion into inactive metabolites.

It should be noted that absorption of the vasoconstrictor itself can result in systemic toxicity (e.g., palpitations, tachycardia, nervousness, hypertension). If adrenergic stimulation from absorption of epinephrine is excessive, symptoms can be controlled with α- and β-adrenergic antagonists.

Pharmacokinetics
Absorption and Distribution

Although administered for local effects, local anesthetics do get absorbed into the blood and become distributed to all parts of the body. The rate of absorption is determined largely by blood flow to the site of administration.

Metabolism

The process by which a local anesthetic is metabolized depends on the class—ester or amide—to which it belongs. *Ester-type* local anesthetics are metabolized in the blood by enzymes known as *esterases*. In contrast, *amide-type* anesthetics are metabolized by enzymes in the *liver*. For both types of anesthetic, metabolism results in inactivation.

The balance between rate of absorption and rate of metabolism is clinically significant. If a local anesthetic is absorbed more slowly than it is metabolized, its level in blood will remain low and systemic reactions will be minimal. Conversely, if absorption outpaces metabolism, plasma drug levels will rise and the risk for systemic toxicity will increase.

Adverse Effects

Adverse effects can occur locally or distant from the site of administration. Local effects are less common.

Central Nervous System

When absorbed in sufficient amounts, local anesthetics cause central nervous system (CNS) excitation followed by depression. During the excitation phase, *seizures* may occur. If needed, excessive excitation can be managed with an intravenous benzodiazepine (diazepam or midazolam). Depressant effects range from *drowsiness* to *unconsciousness* to *coma*. Death can occur secondary to *depression of respiration*. If respiratory depression is prominent, mechanical ventilation with oxygen is indicated.

Cardiovascular System

When absorbed in sufficient amounts, local anesthetics can affect the heart and blood vessels. In the heart, these drugs suppress excitability in the myocardium and conducting system and thereby can cause *bradycardia, heart block, reduced contractile force,* and *even cardiac arrest.* In blood vessels, anesthetics relax vascular smooth muscle; the resultant vasodilation can cause *hypotension.*

TABLE 23.3   Injectable Local Anesthetics: Trade Names and Time Course of Action

Chemical Class	Generic Name	Trade Name	Onset (min)	Duration (h)
Amides	Lidocaine[b]	Xylocaine	<2	0.5–1
	Bupivacaine	Marcaine	5	2–4
	Mepivacaine	Carbocaine	3–5	0.75–1.5
	Prilocaine	Citanest	<2	≥1
	Ropivacaine	Naropin	10–30[c]	0.5–6[c]
Esters[d]	Procaine	Novocain	2–5	0.25–1
	Chloroprocaine	Nesacaine	6–12	0.5
	Tetracaine[b]	Pontocaine	≤15	2–3

(Header spanning Onset and Duration columns: TIME COURSE OF ACTION[a])

[a]Values are for *infiltration* anesthesia in the absence of epinephrine (epinephrine prolongs duration twofold to threefold).
[b]Also administered topically.
[c]Values are for epidural administration (without epinephrine).
[d]Because of the risk for allergic reactions, the ester anesthetics are rarely administered by injection.

TABLE 23.1   Contrasts Between Ester and Amide Local Anesthetics

Property	Ester-Type Anesthetics	Amide-Type Anesthetics
Characteristic chemistry	Ester bond	Amide bond
Representative agent	Procaine	Lidocaine
Incidence of allergic reactions	Low	Very low
Method of metabolism	Plasma esterases	Hepatic enzymes

TABLE 23.2   Topical Local Anesthetics: Trade Names, Indications, and Time Course of Action

Chemical Class	Generic Name	Trade Name	Skin	Mucous Membranes	Peak Effect (min)	Duration (min)
Amides	Dibucaine	Nupercainal	✓		<5	15–45
	Lidocaine[b]	Xylocaine, Lidoderm, others	✓	✓	2–5	15–45
Esters	Benzocaine	Many names	✓	✓	<5	15–45
	Cocaine	Generic only	✓	✓	1–5	30–60
	Tetracaine[b]	None[c]	✓	✓	3–8	30–60
Others	Dyclonine	Sucrets (spray)		✓	<10	<60
	Pramoxine	Tronolane, others	✓		3–5	—

(Header spanning Skin/Mucous Membranes columns: INDICATIONS; header spanning Peak Effect/Duration columns: TIME COURSE OF ACTION[a])

[a]Based primarily on application to mucous membranes.
[b]Also administered by injection.
[c]For application to the skin, tetracaine is available only in combination products, such as Cetacaine.

Allergic Reactions

An array of hypersensitivity reactions, ranging from *allergic dermatitis* to *anaphylaxis,* can be triggered by local anesthetics. These reactions, which are relatively uncommon, are much more likely with the *ester-type* anesthetics (e.g., procaine) than with the amides. Patients allergic to one ester-type anesthetic are likely to be allergic to all other ester-type agents. Fortunately, cross-hypersensitivity between the esters and amides has not been observed. Therefore the amides can be used when allergies contraindicate use of ester-type anesthetics. Because they are unlikely to cause hypersensitivity reactions, the amide-type anesthetics have largely replaced the ester-type agents when administration by injection is required.

Methemoglobinemia

Topical *benzocaine* can cause methemoglobinemia, a blood disorder in which hemoglobin is modified such that it cannot release oxygen to tissues. If enough hemoglobin is converted to methemoglobin, death can result. Methemoglobinemia has been associated with benzocaine liquids, sprays, and gels. Most cases were in children younger than 2 years treated with benzocaine gel for teething pain. Because of this risk, topical benzocaine should not be used in children younger than 2 years without the advice of a health care professional and should be used with caution in older children and adults when applied to mucous membranes of the mouth.

PROPERTIES OF INDIVIDUAL LOCAL ANESTHETICS

Procaine

Procaine (Novocain) is the prototype of the ester-type local anesthetics. The drug is not effective topically and must be given by injection. Administration in combination with epinephrine delays absorption. Although procaine is readily absorbed, systemic toxicity is rare because plasma esterases rapidly convert the drug to inactive, nontoxic products. Being an ester-type anesthetic, procaine poses a greater risk for allergic reactions than do the amide-type anesthetics. Individuals allergic to procaine should be considered allergic to all other ester-type anesthetics but not to the amides.

PROTOTYPE DRUGS

Local Anesthetics

Ester-Type Local Anesthetics
Procaine

Amide-Type Local Anesthetics
Lidocaine

Preparations and Dosage

Drug	Forms	Usual Adult Doses
Procaine (Novocain)	Injection 0.25%–2%	Inject small volumes subcutaneously until the entire area is anesthetized. Maximal dose of 1000 mg 1% strength
Lidocaine (Xylocaine)	Injection 0.5%–5%	Inject small volumes subcutaneously until the entire area is anesthetized (about 1-3 minutes). Maximal dose of 300 mL 1% strength
Cocaine oronasolaryngeal	Solution 4% and 10%	1 mg/kg topically once. Alt: 1–2 mL of solution per nostril once. Maximal dose of 3 mg/kg or 200 mg.

Lidocaine

Lidocaine, introduced in 1948, is the prototype of the amide-type agents. Currently one of the most widely used local anesthetics, lidocaine can be administered topically and by injection. Anesthesia with lidocaine is more rapid, more intense, and more prolonged than an equal dose of procaine. Effects can be extended by coadministration of epinephrine. Allergic reactions are rare, and individuals allergic to ester-type anesthetics are not cross-allergic to lidocaine. If plasma levels of lidocaine climb too high, CNS and cardiovascular toxicity can result. Inactivation is by hepatic metabolism.

In addition to its use in local anesthesia, lidocaine is used to treat dysrhythmias (see Chapter 92 on drugs for acute care). Control of dysrhythmias results from suppression of cardiac excitability secondary to blockade of cardiac sodium channels.

Cocaine

Cocaine was our first local anesthetic. It is an ester-type anesthetic. Administered topically, the drug is used for anesthesia of the ear, nose, and throat. Anesthesia develops rapidly and persists for approximately 1 hour. Unlike other local anesthetics, cocaine causes intense vasoconstriction (by blocking norepinephrine uptake at sympathetic nerve terminals on blood vessels) which is especially useful for the treatment of expistaxis. Accordingly, the drug should not be given in combination with epinephrine or any other vasoconstrictor. In addition to causing local anesthesia, cocaine has pronounced effects on the sympathetic and CNSs. These sympathetic and CNS effects are due largely to blocking the reuptake of norepinephrine by adrenergic neurons.

Central Nervous System Effects

Cocaine produces generalized CNS stimulation. Moderate doses cause euphoria, talkativeness, reduced fatigue, and increased sociability and alertness. Excessive doses can cause seizures. Excitation is followed by CNS depression. Respiratory arrest and death can result.

Although cocaine does not seem to cause substantial physical dependence, psychological dependence can be profound. The drug is subject to widespread abuse and is classified under schedule II of the Controlled Substances Act. Cocaine abuse is discussed in Chapter 35.

Cardiovascular Effects

Cocaine stimulates the heart and causes vasoconstriction. These effects result from (1) central stimulation of the sympathetic nervous system and (2) blockade of norepinephrine uptake in the periphery. Stimulation of the heart can produce *tachycardia* and potentially fatal *dysrhythmias.* Vasoconstriction can cause *hypertension.* Cocaine presents an especially serious risk to individuals with cardiovascular disease (e.g., hypertension, dysrhythmias, angina pectoris).

Other Local Anesthetics

In addition to the drugs discussed previously, several other local anesthetics are available. These agents differ with respect to indications, route of administration, mode of elimination, duration of action, and toxicity.

The local anesthetics can be grouped according to route of administration: topical versus injection. (Very few agents are administered by both routes, primarily because the drugs that are suitable for topical application are usually too toxic for parenteral use.) Table 23.2 lists the topically administered local anesthetics, trade names, and their time course of action. Table 23.3 presents equivalent information for the injectable agents.

CLINICAL USE OF LOCAL ANESTHETICS

Local anesthetics may be administered *topically* (for surface anesthesia) and *by injection* (for infiltration anesthesia, nerve block anesthesia, intravenous regional anesthesia, epidural anesthesia, and spinal anesthesia). The uses and hazards of these anesthesia techniques are discussed next.

Topical Administration

Surface anesthesia is accomplished by applying the anesthetic directly to the skin or a mucous membrane. The agents used most commonly are *lidocaine, tetracaine,* and *cocaine.*

Therapeutic Uses

Local anesthetics are applied to the *skin* to relieve pain, itching, and soreness of various causes, including infection, thermal burns, sunburn, diaper rash, wounds, bruises, abrasions, plant poisoning, and insect bites. Application may also be made to *mucous membranes* of the nose, mouth, pharynx, larynx, trachea, bronchi, vagina, and urethra. In addition, local anesthetics may be used to relieve discomfort associated with hemorrhoids, anal fissures, and pruritus ani.

Systemic Toxicity

Topical anesthetics applied to the skin can be absorbed in amounts sufficient to produce serious or even life-threatening effects. Cardiac toxicity can result in bradycardia, heart block, or cardiac arrest. CNS toxicity can result in seizures, respiratory depression, and coma. Obviously, the risk for toxicity increases with the amount absorbed, which is determined primarily by (1) the amount applied, (2) skin condition, and (3) skin temperature. Accordingly, to minimize the amount absorbed, and thereby minimize risk, patients should do the following:

- Apply the smallest amount needed.
- Avoid application to large areas.
- Avoid application to broken or irritated skin.
- Avoid strenuous exercise, wrapping the site, and heating the site, all of which can accelerate absorption by increasing skin temperature.

Administration by Injection

Injection of local anesthetics carries significant risk and requires special skills. Injections are usually performed by an anesthesiologist. Because severe systemic reactions may occur, equipment for resuscitation should be immediately available. In addition, an intravenous line should be in place to permit rapid treatment of toxicity. Inadvertent injection into an artery or vein can cause severe toxicity. To ensure the needle is not in a blood vessel, it should be aspirated before injection. After administration, the patient should be monitored for cardiovascular status, respiratory function, and state of consciousness. To reduce the risk for toxicity, local anesthetics should be administered in the lowest effective dose.

Infiltration Anesthesia

Infiltration anesthesia is achieved by injecting a local anesthetic directly into the immediate area of surgery or manipulation. Anesthesia can be prolonged by combining the anesthetic with epinephrine. The agents used most frequently for infiltration anesthesia are lidocaine and bupivacaine.

Nerve Block Anesthesia

Nerve block anesthesia is achieved by injecting a local anesthetic into or near nerves that supply the surgical field but at a site distant from the field itself. This technique has the advantage of producing anesthesia with doses that are smaller than those needed for infiltration anesthesia. Drug selection is based on required duration of anesthesia. For shorter procedures, lidocaine or mepivacaine might be used. For longer procedures, bupivacaine would be appropriate.

 SUMMARY OF KEY PRESCRIBING CONSIDERATIONS

Local Anesthetics

Therapeutic Goal: Reduction of discomfort associated with local disorders of the skin and mucous membranes.

Identifying High-Risk Patients: *Ester-type* local anesthetics are *contraindicated* for patients with a history of serious allergic reactions to these drugs. Avoid topical *benzocaine* in children younger than the age of 2 years.

Minimizing Adverse Effects: Absorption into the general circulation can cause systemic toxicity. Effects on the heart (bradycardia, atrioventricular [AV] heart block, cardiac arrest) and central nervous system (excitation, possibly including seizures, followed by depression) are of greatest concern. Monitor blood pressure, pulse rate, respiratory rate, and state of consciousness. Have facilities for cardiopulmonary resuscitation available.

The risk of systemic toxicity is determined by the extent of absorption. To minimize absorption, apply topical anesthetics to the smallest surface area needed and, when possible, avoid application to injured skin.

24

Opioid Analgesics, Opioid Antagonists, and Nonopioid Centrally Acting Analgesics

Analgesics are drugs that relieve pain without causing loss of consciousness. In this chapter, we focus mainly on the opioid analgesics, the most effective pain relievers available. The opioid family, whose name derives from *opium,* includes such widely used agents as morphine, fentanyl, codeine, and oxycodone (OxyContin).

OPIOID ANALGESICS

Introduction to the Opioids

Terminology

An *opioid* is any drug, natural or synthetic, that has actions similar to those of morphine. The term *opiate* is more specific and applies only to compounds present in opium (e.g., morphine, codeine).

Endogenous Opioid Peptides

The body has three families of peptides—*enkephalins, endorphins,* and *dynorphins*—that have opioid-like properties. Endogenous opioid peptides are found in the central nervous system (CNS) and in peripheral tissues. Although we know that endogenous opioid peptides serve as neurotransmitters, neurohormones, and neuromodulators, their precise physiologic role is not fully understood.

Opioid Receptors

There are three main classes of opioid receptors, designated μ, κ, and δ. From a pharmacologic perspective, μ receptors are the most important because opioid analgesics act primarily by activating μ receptors, although they also produce weak activation of κ receptors. As a rule, opioid analgesics do not interact with δ receptors. In contrast to opioid analgesics, endogenous opioid peptides act through all three opioid receptors, including δ receptors. Important responses to activation of μ and κ receptors are shown in Table 24.1.

μ receptors. Responses to activation of μ receptors include analgesia, respiratory depression, euphoria, and sedation. In addition, μ activation is related to physical dependence.

A study in genetically engineered mice underscores the importance of μ receptors in drug action. In this study, researchers studied mice that lacked the gene for μ receptors. When these mice were given morphine, the drug had no effect. It did not produce analgesia or physical dependence, and it did not reinforce social behaviors that are thought to indicate subjective effects. Hence, at least in mice, μ receptors appear both necessary and sufficient to mediate the major actions of opioid drugs.

κ receptors. As with μ receptors, activation of κ receptors can produce analgesia and sedation. In addition, κ activation may underlie psychotomimetic effects seen with certain opioids.

Classification of Drugs That Act at Opioid Receptors

Drugs that act at opioid receptors are classified on the basis of how they affect receptor function. At each type of receptor, a drug can act in one of three ways: as an *agonist, partial agonist,* or *antagonist.* Based on these actions, drugs that bind opioid receptors fall into three major groups: (1) pure opioid agonists, (2) agonist-antagonist opioids, and (3) pure opioid antagonists. The actions of drugs in these groups at μ and κ receptors are shown in Table 24.2.

Pure opioid agonists. The pure opioid agonists activate μ receptors and κ receptors. By doing so, the pure agonists can produce analgesia, euphoria, sedation, respiratory depression, physical dependence, constipation, and other effects. The pure agonists can be subdivided into two groups: *strong opioid agonists* and *moderate to strong opioid agonists.* Morphine is the prototype of the strong agonists. Codeine is the prototype of the moderate to strong agonists.

Agonist-antagonist opioids. Four agonist-antagonist opioids are currently available: pentazocine, nalbuphine, butorphanol, and buprenorphine. The actions of these drugs at μ and κ receptors are shown in Table 24.2. When administered alone, the agonist-antagonist opioids produce analgesia. However, if given to a patient who is taking a pure opioid agonist, these drugs can *antagonize* analgesia caused by the pure agonist. Pentazocine is the prototype of the agonist-antagonists.

Pure opioid antagonists. The pure opioid antagonists act as antagonists at μ and κ receptors. These drugs do not produce analgesia or any of the other effects caused by opioid agonists. Their principal use is reversal of respiratory and CNS depression caused by overdose with opioid agonists. In addition, one of these drugs—methylnaltrexone—is used to treat opioid-induced constipation. Naloxone (Narcan) is the prototype of the pure opioid antagonists.

PROTOTYPE DRUGS

Opioid Analgesics and Antagonists

Pure Opioid Agonists
Morphine

Agonist-Antagonist Opioids
Pentazocine

Pure Opioid Antagonists
Naloxone

BASIC PHARMACOLOGY OF THE OPIOIDS

Morphine

Morphine is the prototype of the strong opioid analgesics and remains the standard by which newer opioids are measured. Morphine has multiple pharmacologic effects, including analgesia, sedation, euphoria, respiratory depression, cough suppression, and suppression of bowel motility.

TABLE 24.1   Important Responses to Activation of μ and κ Receptors

Response	RECEPTOR TYPE	
	μ	κ
Analgesia	✓	✓
Respiratory depression	✓	
Sedation	✓	✓
Euphoria	✓	
Physical dependence	✓	
Decreased gastrointestinal motility	✓	✓

TABLE 24.2   Drug Actions at μ and κ Receptors

Drugs	RECEPTOR TYPE	
	μ	κ
Pure Opioid Agonists		
Morphine, codeine, meperidine, and others	Agonist	Agonist
Agonist-Antagonist Opioids		
Pentazocine, nalbuphine, butorphanol	Antagonist	Agonist
Buprenorphine	Partial agonist	Antagonist
Pure Opioid Antagonists		
Naloxone, naltrexone, others	Antagonist	Antagonist

Overview of Pharmacologic Actions

Morphine has multiple pharmacologic actions. In addition to relieving pain, the drug causes drowsiness and mental clouding, reduces anxiety, and creates a sense of well-being. Through actions in the CNS and periphery, morphine can cause respiratory depression, constipation, urinary retention, orthostatic hypotension, emesis, miosis, cough suppression, and biliary colic. With prolonged use, the drug produces tolerance and physical dependence.

Therapeutic Use: Relief of Pain

The principal indication for morphine is relief of moderate to severe pain. The drug can relieve postoperative pain, pain of labor and delivery, and chronic pain caused by cancer and other conditions.

The drug is more effective against constant, dull pain than against sharp, intermittent pain. However, sharp pain can even be relieved by large doses. The ability of morphine to cause mental clouding, sedation, euphoria, and anxiety reduction can contribute to relief of pain.

The use of morphine and other opioids to relieve pain is discussed further in this chapter and in Chapter 86. Additional information regarding morphine and other opiates are located in Tables 24.3 through 24.6.

Adverse Effects

Respiratory depression. Respiratory depression is the most serious adverse effect. At equianalgesic doses, all of the pure opioid agonists depress respiration to the same extent. Death after an overdose is almost always from respiratory arrest. Opioids depress respiration primarily through activation of μ receptors, although activation of κ receptors also contributes.

The time course of respiratory depression begins up to 90 minutes after PO ingestion. With prolonged use of opioids, tolerance develops

TABLE 24.3   Interactions of Opioid Agonists Drugs With Other Drugs

Interacting Drugs	Outcome of the Interaction
Adverse Interactions	
CNS depressants	Increased respiratory depression and sedation
Barbiturates	
Benzodiazepines	
Alcohol	
General anesthetics	
Antihistamines	
Phenothiazines	
Agonist-antagonist opioids	Precipitation of a withdrawal reaction
Anticholinergic drugs	Increased constipation and urinary retention
Atropinelike drugs	
Antihistamines	
Phenothiazines	
Tricyclic antidepressants	
Hypotensive agents	Increased hypotension
Monoamine oxidase inhibitors	Hyperpyrexic coma
Beneficial Interactions	
Amphetamines	Increased analgesia and decreased sedation
Antiemetics	Suppression of nausea and vomiting
Naloxone	Suppression of symptoms of opioid overdose
Dextromethorphan	Increased analgesia; possible reduction in tolerance

CNS, Central nervous system.

TABLE 24.4   Morphine Preparations

Formulation	Available Doses
IR tablets	15, 30 mg
ER tablets (Arymo ER, Morphabond ER, MS Contin)	15, 30, 60, 100, 200 mg
ER capsules (Twice-daily dosing) (Kadian)	10, 20, 30, 50, 60, 80, 100 mg
ER capsules (Daily dosing)	30, 45, 60, 75, 90, 120 mg
Suppository	5, 10, 20, 30 mg
Oral solution (MSIR)	10 mg/5 mL, 20 mg/5 mL, 100 mg/5 mL
Solution for injection	Various

ER, Extended release; *IR,* instant release.

to respiratory depression. Certain patients, including the very young, older adults, and those with respiratory disease (e.g., asthma, emphysema), are especially sensitive to respiratory depression and hence must be monitored closely. Outpatients should be informed about the risk for respiratory depression and instructed to notify the prescriber if respiratory distress occurs.

PATIENT EDUCATION

Respiratory Depression

Respiratory depression is increased by concurrent use of other drugs with CNS-depressant actions (e.g., alcohol, barbiturates, benzodiazepines). Accordingly, these drugs should be avoided. Outpatients should be warned against use of alcohol and all other CNS depressants.

TABLE 24.5 Clinical Pharmacology and Pharmacokinetics of Pure Opioid Agonists

Drug and Route[a]	Equianalgesic Dose (mg)[b]	TIME COURSE OF ANALGESIC EFFECTS			Metabolism	Excretion
		Onset (min)	Peak (min)	Duration (h)		
Codeine					Hepatic CYP450: 2D6	Renal
PO	200	30–45	60–120	4–6		
Fentanyl					Hepatic CYP450: 3A4	Renal
Transdermal	—	Delayed	24–72	72		
Transmucosal[c]	—	10–15	20	1–2		
Nasal spray	—	10–15	15–20	1–2		
Hydrocodone					Hepatic CYP450: 3A4, 2B6, 2D6	Renal
PO	30	10–30	30–60	4–6		
Hydromorphone					Hepatic	Renal, gastrointestinal (bile)
PO (IR)	7.5	30	90–120	4		
PO (ER)	7.5	—	360–480	18–24		
Levorphanol					Hepatic	Renal
PO	4	10–60	90–120	6–8		
Meperidine						
PO	300	15	60–90	2–4		
Methadone					Hepatic CYP450: 2B6, 3A4	Gastrointestinal (feces), renal
PO	20	30–60	90–120	4–6[d]		
Morphine					Hepatic, gastrointestinal	Gastrointestinal (feces) renal
PO (IR)	30	—	60–120	4–5		
PO (ER)	30	—	420	8–12		
Oxycodone					Hepatic CYP450: 3A4, 2D6	Renal
PO (IR)	20	15–30	60	3–4		
PO (CR)	20	—	120–180	Up to 12		
Oxymorphone					Hepatic	Gastrointestinal (feces), renal
PO (IR)	10	—	—	4–6		
PO (ER)	10	—	—	Up to 12		
Rectal	10	15–30	120	3–6		
Tapentadol					Hepatic CYP450: 2C9/19	Renal
PO	100	45–60	90–120	4–8		

[a]IM administration should be avoided whenever possible.
[b]Dose in milligrams that produces a degree of analgesia equivalent to that produced by a 10-mg IM dose of morphine.
[c]Data are for the Actiq lozenge on a stick.
[d]With repeated doses, methadone's duration of action may increase up to 48 hours.
CR, Controlled release; *ER,* extended release; *IM,* intramuscular; *IR,* immediate release; *PO,* by mouth.

TABLE 24.6 Fentanyl Preparations

Formulations	Available Doses	Usual Initial Dose	Indications
Buccal Tablets (Fentora)	100, 200, 400, 600, 800 mcg	100 mcg x1, may repeat after 30 min	Breakthrough cancer pain in opioid tolerant patients
Intranasal (Lazanda)	100, 300, 400 mcg per actuation	100 mcg intranasally x1	
Lozenge on a Stick (Actiq)	200, 400, 600, 800, 1200, 1600 mcg	200 mcg orally x1, may repeat after 30 min	
Sublingual Spray (Subsys)	100, 200, 400, 600, 800 mcg per actuation	100 mcg SL x1, may repeat after 30 min	
Sublingual Tablets (Abstral)	100, 200, 300, 400, 600, 800 mcg	100 mcg SL x1, may repeat after 30 min	
Transdermal Patch (Duragesic)	12, 25, 37.5, 50, 62.5, 75, 87.5, 100 mcg/h	Individualize dose based on current opioid intake	Severe, chronic pain
Transdermal Iontophoretic System			

SL, Sublingual.

Pronounced respiratory depression can be reversed with naloxone (Narcan), an opioid antagonist. However, dosing must be carefully titrated because excessive doses will completely block the analgesic effects of morphine, causing pain to return.

Constipation. Opioids promote constipation through actions in the CNS and gastrointestinal (GI) tract. Specifically, by activating μ receptors in the gut, these drugs can suppress propulsive intestinal contractions,

▶ BLACK BOX WARNING

Opioids

Opioid medications can cause respiratory arrest in both opioid-naïve and opioid-tolerant patients. Monitor for respiratory depression, especially during new-onset therapy or after escalation of dose.

intensify nonpropulsive contractions, increase the tone of the anal sphincter, and inhibit secretion of fluids into the intestinal lumen. As a result, constipation can develop after a few days of opioid use. Potential complications of constipation include fecal impaction, bowel perforation, rectal tearing, and hemorrhoids.

Opioid-induced constipation can be managed with a combination of pharmacologic and nonpharmacologic measures. The goal is to produce a soft, formed stool every 1 to 2 days. Principal nondrug measures are physical activity and increased intake of fiber and fluids (for prevention) and enemas (for treatment). Most patients also require *prophylactic drugs*: a stimulant laxative, such as senna, is given to counteract reduced bowel motility, plus polyethylene glycol (an osmotic laxative) can provide additional benefit. If these prophylactic drugs prove inadequate, the patient may need *rescue therapy* with a strong osmotic laxative, such as lactulose or sodium phosphate. As a last resort, patients may be given *methylnaltrexone* (Relistor), an oral drug that blocks μ receptors in the intestine. As discussed later in the chapter, methylnaltrexone cannot cross the blood-brain barrier and hence does not reverse opioid-induced analgesia.

Orthostatic hypotension. Opioid agonists lower blood pressure by blunting the baroreceptor reflex and by dilating peripheral arterioles and veins. Peripheral vasodilation results primarily from morphine-induced release of histamine.

PATIENT EDUCATION

Hypotension

Hypotension is mild in the recumbent patient but can be significant when the patient stands up. Patients should be informed about symptoms of hypotension (lightheadedness, dizziness) and instructed to sit or lie down if they occur. Also, patients should be informed that hypotension can be minimized by moving slowly when changing from a supine or seated position to an upright position. Patients should be warned against walking if hypotension is substantial. Hospitalized patients may require ambulatory assistance. Hypotensive drugs can exacerbate opioid-induced hypotension.

Urinary retention. Morphine can cause urinary hesitancy and urinary retention. Three mechanisms are involved. First, morphine increases tone in the bladder sphincter. Second, morphine increases tone in the detrusor muscle, thereby elevating pressure within the bladder, causing a sense of urinary urgency. Third, in addition to its direct effects on the urinary tract, morphine may interfere with voiding by suppressing awareness of bladder stimuli. To reduce discomfort, patients should be encouraged to void every 4 hours. Urinary hesitancy or retention is especially likely in patients with benign prostatic hypertrophy. Drugs with anticholinergic properties (e.g., tricyclic antidepressants, antihistamines) can exacerbate the problem.

Emesis. Morphine promotes nausea and vomiting through direct stimulation of the chemoreceptor trigger zone of the medulla. Emetic reactions are greatest with the initial dose and then diminish with subsequent doses. Nausea and vomiting are uncommon in recumbent patients but occur in 15% to 40% of ambulatory patients, suggesting a vestibular component. Nausea and vomiting can be reduced by pretreatment with an antiemetic (e.g., prochlorperazine) and by having the patient remain still.

Sedation. When administered to relieve pain, morphine is likely to cause drowsiness and some mental clouding. Although these effects can complement analgesic actions, they can also be detrimental. Outpatients should be warned about CNS depression and advised to avoid hazardous activities (e.g., driving) if sedation is significant. Sedation

can be minimized by taking smaller doses more often or using opioids that have short half-lives.

Neurotoxicity. Opioid-induced neurotoxicity can cause delirium, agitation, myoclonus, hyperalgesia, and other symptoms. Primary risk factors are renal impairment, preexisting cognitive impairment, and prolonged, high-dose opioid use. Management consists of hydration and dose reduction. For patients who must take opioids long term, opioid rotation (periodically switching from one opioid to another) may reduce neurotoxicity development.

Tolerance and physical dependence. With continuous use, morphine can cause tolerance and physical dependence. These phenomena, which are generally inseparable, reflect cellular adaptations that occur in response to prolonged opioid exposure. For definitions and further discussion of tolerance and physical dependence, please refer to Chapter 32.

Drug Interactions

The major interactions between morphine and other drugs are shown in Table 24.3. Some interactions are adverse, and some are beneficial.

Toxicity

Clinical manifestations. Opioid overdose produces a classic triad of signs: *coma, respiratory depression,* and *pinpoint pupils.* Coma is profound, and the patient cannot be aroused. Respiratory rate may be as low as 2 to 4 breaths/minute. Although the pupils are constricted initially, they may dilate as hypoxia sets in (secondary to respiratory depression). Hypoxia may cause blood pressure to fall. Prolonged hypoxia may result in shock. When death occurs, respiratory arrest is almost always the immediate cause.

Treatment. Treatment consists primarily of *ventilatory support* and giving an *opioid antagonist.* Naloxone (Narcan) is the traditional antagonist of choice. The pharmacology of the opioid antagonists is discussed later.

Other Strong Opioid Agonists

In an effort to produce a strong analgesic with a low potential for respiratory depression and abuse, pharmaceutical scientists have created many new opioid analgesics. However, none of the newer pure opioid agonists can be considered truly superior to morphine; these drugs are essentially equal to morphine with respect to analgesic action, abuse liability, and the ability to cause respiratory depression. Also, to varying degrees, they all cause sedation, euphoria, constipation, urinary retention, cough suppression, hypotension, and miosis. However, despite their similarities to morphine, the newer drugs do have unique qualities. Hence one agent may be more desirable than another in a particular

TABLE 24.7 Hydromorphone, Oxymorphone, and Levorphanol Preparations

Drug	Preparations
Hydromorphone (Dilaudid, Exalgo, Jurnista)	IR tablets: 2, 4, 8 mg ER tablets: 8, 12, 16, 32 mg Oral liquid: 1 mg/mL Rectal suppositories: 3 mg Solution for injection varies
Oxymorphone (Opana)	IR tablets: 5, 10 mg ER tablets: 5, 7.5, 10, 15, 20, 30, 40 mg
Levorphanol	IR tablets: 2 mg

ER, Extended release; *IR,* instant release.

clinical setting. With all of the newer pure opioid agonists, toxicity can be reversed with an opioid antagonist (e.g., naloxone). Important differences between morphine and the newer strong opioid analgesics are discussed later. Tables 24.4 and Table 24.7 show dosages, routes, and time courses for morphine and the newer agents.

Fentanyl

Fentanyl (Duragesic, Abstral, Actiq, Fentora, Lazanda, Subsys) is a strong opioid analgesic with a high milligram potency (about 100 times that of morphine). Eight formulations are available for administration by four different routes: parenteral, transdermal, transmucosal, and intranasal (see Table 24.6). Depending on the route, fentanyl may be used for surgical analgesia, chronic pain control, and control of breakthrough pain in patients taking other opioids. All preparations are regulated under schedule II of the Controlled Substances Act.

Fentanyl, regardless of route, has the same adverse effects as other opioids: respiratory depression, sedation, constipation, urinary retention, and nausea. Of these, respiratory depression is the greatest concern. Signs of toxicity can be reversed with an opioid antagonist (e.g., naloxone).

Fentanyl is metabolized by CYP3A4 (the 3A4 isoenzyme of cytochrome P450), and hence fentanyl levels can be increased by CYP3A4 inhibitors (e.g., ritonavir, ketoconazole). Patients taking these inhibitors should be closely monitored for severe respiratory depression and other signs of toxicity.

Transdermal system. The fentanyl transdermal system (Duragesic) consists of a fentanyl-containing patch that is applied to the skin of the upper torso. The drug is slowly released from the patch and absorbed through the skin, reaching effective levels in 24 hours. Levels remain steady for another 48 hours, after which the patch should be replaced. If a new patch is not applied, effects will nonetheless persist for several hours, owing to continued absorption of residual fentanyl remaining in the skin.

Transdermal fentanyl is indicated only for persistent severe pain in patients who are already opioid tolerant. Use in nontolerant patients can cause fatal respiratory depression. The patch should not be used in children younger than 2 years or in anyone younger than 18 years who weighs less than 110 pounds. Also, the patch should not be used for postoperative pain, intermittent pain, or pain that responds to a less powerful analgesic.

Like other strong opioids, fentanyl overdose poses a risk for fatal respiratory depression. If respiratory depression develops, it may persist for hours after patch removal, due to continued absorption of fentanyl from the skin.

All transmucosal products are approved only for breakthrough cancer pain in patients at least 18 years old who are already taking opioids around-the-clock and have developed some degree of tolerance, defined as needing, for 1 week or longer, at least: 60 mg of oral morphine a day, or 30 mg of oral oxycodone a day, or 25 mg of oral oxymorphone a day, or 8 mg of oral hydromorphone a day, or 25 mcg of fentanyl per hour, or an equianalgesic dose of another opioid. Transmucosal fentanyl must not be used for acute pain, postoperative pain, headache, or athletic injuries. Furthermore, it is essential to appreciate that the dose of fentanyl in these formulations is sufficient to kill nontolerant individuals—especially children. Accordingly, these products must be stored in a secure, child-resistant location.

Because of differences in bioavailability, *transmucosal fentanyl products are not interchangeable on a microgram-for-microgram basis*. For example, a 100-mcg buccal tablet produces about the same fentanyl blood level as does a 200-mcg lozenge. Accordingly, if a patient switches from one transmucosal product to another, dosage of the new product must be titrated to determine a strength that is safe and effective.

 BLACK BOX WARNING

Fentanyl

Products containing fentanyl can cause fatal respiratory depression. Many of these products are only available through restricted distribution programs secondary to misuse and abuse.

Methadone

Methadone (Diskets, Dolophine, Methadose) has pharmacologic properties very similar to those of morphine. The drug is effective orally and has a long duration of action. Repeated dosing can result in accumulation. Because of methadone's long half-life and potential to cause QTc prolongation, consultation with a pain specialist is recommended when starting or titrating methadone in any patient. Methadone is used to relieve pain and to treat opioid addiction. Use of methadone for pain control has risen dramatically. The use of methadone in drug-abuse treatment programs is discussed in Chapter 35.

Because methadone can cause QT prolongation, all patients should receive an electrocardiogram (ECG) before treatment, 30 days later, and annually thereafter. If the QT interval exceeds 500 ms, stopping methadone or reducing the dosage should be considered.

PATIENT EDUCATION

Methadone Toxicity

To reduce risk for methadone toxicity, patients should be warned against taking more methadone than was prescribed and should be cautioned to avoid other CNS depressants, such as benzodiazepines, alcohol, and other opioids.

BLACK BOX WARNING

Methadone

Methadone prolongs the QT interval and hence may pose a risk for potentially fatal dysrhythmia. Torsades de pointes has developed in patients taking 65 to 400 mg/day. To reduce risk, methadone should be used with great caution—if at all—in patients with existing QT prolongation or a family history of long QT syndrome and in those taking other QT-prolonging drugs. In addition, methadone causes severe respiratory depression that can be potentially fatal.

Hydromorphone, Oxymorphone, and Levorphanol

Basic pharmacology. All three drugs are strong opioid agonists with pharmacologic actions like those of morphine, and all three are indicated for moderate to severe pain. Dosages and time courses are shown in Table 24.5. Formulations are available in Table 24.7. Adverse effects include respiratory depression, sedation, cough suppression, constipation, urinary retention, nausea, and vomiting. Of note, hydromorphone may cause less nausea than morphine. Toxicity can be reversed with an opioid antagonist (e.g., naloxone). All three drugs are schedule II agents.

BLACK BOX WARNING

Hydromorphone and Oxymorphone

Hydromorphone and oxymorphone have high abuse potential and can cause fatal respiratory depression, especially when used in combination with other sedating agents such as alcohol. Long-acting forms of oxymorphone should be prescribed only by a provider with additional education regarding chronic pain.

Moderate to Strong Opioid Agonists

The moderate to strong opioid agonists are similar to morphine in most respects. Like morphine, these drugs produce analgesia, sedation, and euphoria. In addition, they can cause respiratory depression, constipation, urinary retention, cough suppression, and miosis. Differences between the moderate to strong opioids and morphine are primarily quantitative: the moderate to strong opioids produce less analgesia and respiratory depression than morphine and have a somewhat lower potential for abuse. As with morphine, toxicity from the moderate to strong agonists can be reversed with naloxone.

Codeine

Codeine is indicated for relief of mild to moderate pain. The drug is usually administered by mouth. Side effects are dose limiting. As a result, although taking codeine can produce significant pain relief, the degree of pain relief that can be achieved *safely* is quite low—much lower than with morphine. When taken in its usual analgesic dose (30 mg), codeine produces about as much pain relief as 325 mg of aspirin or 325 mg of acetaminophen.

For analgesic use, codeine is formulated alone and in combination with nonopioid analgesics (either aspirin or acetaminophen). Because codeine and nonopioid analgesics relieve pain by different mechanisms, the combinations can produce greater pain relief than either agent alone. Codeine alone is classified under schedule II of the Controlled Substances Act. The combination preparations are classified under schedule III. Although codeine is classified along with morphine in schedule II, the abuse liability of codeine appears to be significantly lower.

Codeine is an extremely effective cough suppressant and is widely used for this action. The antitussive dose (10 mg) is lower than analgesic doses. Codeine is formulated in combination with various agents to suppress cough. These mixtures are classified under schedule V.

> ### ▶ BLACK BOX WARNING
> #### *Codeine*
>
> In the liver, about 10% of each dose of codeine undergoes conversion to *morphine,* the active form of codeine. The enzyme responsible is CYP2D6 (the *2D6* isoenzyme of cytochrome P450). Among ultrarapid metabolizers, which carry multiple copies of the *CYP2D6* gene, codeine is unusually effective and has led to death in some children. Severe toxicity can also develop in breastfed infants whose mothers are taking codeine. The cause is high levels of morphine in breast milk, due to ultrarapid codeine metabolism.

Oxycodone

Oxycodone (OxyContin, Roxicodone) has analgesic actions equivalent to those of codeine. Administration is oral. Oxycodone is available by itself or in combination with adjuvant drugs. All formulations are classified under schedule II.

> ### ▶ BLACK BOX WARNING
> #### *Oxycodone*
>
> Like oxymorphone and hydromorphone, oxycodone has a high potential for abuse and can cause fatal respiratory depression. Long-acting forms of oxycodone should be prescribed only by providers with additional education regarding chronic pain.

Hydrocodone

Hydrocodone has analgesic actions equivalent to those of codeine. The drug is taken orally to relieve pain and to suppress cough. The usual instant release (IR) dosage is 5 mg (see Table 24.8). Extended-release (ER) products (Zohydro ER, Hysingla ER) contain only hydrocodone and are taken every 12 to 24 hours. IR hydrocodone is combined with acetaminophen or ibuprofen. For cough suppression, the drug is combined with antihistamines and nasal decongestants. All of these products are currently classified under schedule II. Trade names for combination products containing hydrocodone include *Vicodin, Vicoprofen,* and *Lortab.*

> ### ▶ BLACK BOX WARNING
> #### *Hydrocodone*
>
> All forms of hydrocodone contain a black box warning. Products that contain acetaminophen (Vicodin) are associated with hepatotoxicity. The extended-release forms of hydrocodone can cause fatal respiratory depression and should only be prescribed by providers with additional education regarding chronic pain.

Tapentadol

Actions and uses. Tapentadol (Nucynta) is indicated for oral therapy of moderate to severe pain—acute or chronic—in patients aged 18 years and older. Analgesic effects are equivalent to those of oxycodone. Like other opioids, tapentadol can cause CNS depression and respiratory depression and has a significant potential for abuse. However, the drug differs from other opioids in two important ways. First, in addition to

TABLE 24.8 Moderate to Strong Opioid Agonists-Preparations and Dosages		
Drug	**Preparations**	**Usual Adult Analgesic Dose**
Codeine	Tablets: 15, 30, 60 mg Oral solution: 30 mg/5 mL	15–60 mg every 3 to 6 h Maximum 120 mg in 24 h
Oxycodone (Oxaydo, OxyContin, Roxicodone, Xtampza ER)	IR tablets: 5, 7.5, 15, 30 mg ER tablets: 10, 15, 20, 30, 40, 60, 80 mg ER capsules: 9, 13.5, 18, 27, 36 mg	Opiate-naïve patients: 5–10 mg IR every 4–6 h Opiate-tolerant patients: 10 mg ER every 12 h
Hydrocodone (Hysingla ER, Zohydro ER, Norco)	IR tablets (hydrocodone with acetaminophen): 5/325, 7.5/325, 10/325 mg ER tablets: 20, 30, 40, 60, 80, 100, 120 mg ER capsules: 10, 15, 20, 30, 40, 50 mg	Acute pain: 5/325 mg IR every 4–6 h Severe, chronic pain: 20 mg ER every 24 h
Tapentadol (Nucynta, Nucynta ER)	IR tablets: 50, 75, 100 mg ER tablets: 50, 100, 150, 200, 250 mg	Acute pain: 50–100 mg IR every 4–6 h Severe, chronic pain: 50 mg ER every 12 h

ER, Extended release; *IR,* instant release.

TABLE 24.9 Clinical Pharmacology of Opioid Agonist-Antagonists

Drug and Route	Equianalgesic Dose (mg)[a]	TIME COURSE OF ANALGESIC EFFECTS		
		Onset (min)	Peak (min)	Duration (h)
Buprenorphine				
IM	0.3	15	60	Up to 6
IV	0.3	Under 15	Under 60	Up to 6
Butorphanol				
IM	2–3	10	30–60	3–4
IV	2–3	2–3	30–60	3–4
Intranasal	2–3	Within 15	60–120	4–5
Nalbuphine				
IM	10	Within 15	60	3–6
IV	10	2–3	30	3–6
SubQ	10	Within 15	60	3–6
Pentazocine				
PO	—	15–30	60–90	3[b]
IM	30	15–20	30–60	4–6[b]
IV	30	2–3	15–30	4–6[b]
SubQ	30	15–20	30–60	4–6[b]

[a]Dose in milligrams that produces a degree of analgesia equivalent to that produced by a 10-mg IM dose of morphine.
[b]Duration may increase greatly in patients with liver disease.
IM, Intramuscular; *IV,* intravenous; *PO,* by mouth; *subQ,* subcutaneous.

activating μ opioid receptors, tapentadol blocks reuptake of norepinephrine, similar to tramadol, discussed later. Second, tapentadol causes less constipation than traditional opioids.

Agonist-Antagonist Opioids

Compared with pure opioid agonists, the agonist-antagonists have a low potential for abuse, produce less respiratory depression, and generally have less powerful analgesic effects. If given to a patient who is physically dependent on a pure opioid agonist, these drugs can precipitate withdrawal. The clinical pharmacology of the agonist-antagonists is shown in Table 24.9.

Pentazocine

Actions and uses. Pentazocine (Talwin) was the first agonist-antagonist opioid available and can be considered the prototype for the group. The drug is indicated for mild to moderate pain. Pentazocine is much less effective than morphine against severe pain.

Pentazocine acts as an *agonist* at κ receptors and as an *antagonist* at μ receptors. By activating κ receptors, the drug produces analgesia, sedation, and respiratory depression. However, unlike the respiratory depression caused by morphine, *respiratory depression caused by pentazocine is limited:* beyond a certain dose, no further depression occurs. Because it lacks agonist actions at μ receptors, pentazocine produces little or no euphoria. In fact, at supratherapeutic doses, pentazocine produces unpleasant reactions (anxiety, strange thoughts, nightmares, hallucinations). These psychotomimetic effects may result from activation of κ receptors. Because of its subjective effects, pentazocine has a low potential for abuse and is classified between schedule II and schedule IV depending on the state regulations.

If administered to a patient who is physically dependent on a pure opioid agonist, pentazocine can precipitate withdrawal. Recall that μ receptors mediate physical dependence on pure opioid agonists and that pentazocine acts as an antagonist at these receptors. By blocking access of the pure agonist to μ receptors, pentazocine will prevent receptor

TABLE 24.10 Formulations of Agonist-Antagonist Opioids

Drug	Formulation
Buprenorphine[a]	
Buccal strip [Belbuca]	75, 150, 300, 450, 600, 750, 900 mcg
Transdermal patch [Butrans]	5, 7.5, 10, 15, 20 mcg/h
Solution for injection [Buprenex]	300 mcg /mL
Butorphanol	
Nasal Spray	1 mg per actuation
Solution for injection	1 mg/2 mL, 2 mg/2 mL
Pentazocine	
Pentazocine/naloxone tablets	50 mg/0.5 mg
Solution for injection (Talwin)	30 mg/mL

[a]Formulations for treating opioid dependence are located in Chapter 35.

activation, thereby triggering withdrawal. Accordingly, *pentazocine and other drugs that block μ receptors should never be administered to a person who is physically dependent on a pure opioid agonist.* If a pentazocinelike agent is to be used, the pure opioid agonist must be withdrawn first.

Physical dependence can occur with pentazocine, but symptoms of withdrawal are generally mild (e.g., cramps, fever, anxiety, restlessness). Treatment is rarely required. As with pure opioid agonists, toxicity from pentazocine can be reversed with naloxone. Pentazocine is available in combination with naloxone for oral therapy Table 24.10.

Buprenorphine

Basic pharmacology. Buprenorphine (Butrans) differs significantly from other opioid agonist-antagonists. The drug is a partial agonist at μ receptors and an antagonist at κ receptors. Analgesic effects are like those of morphine, but significant tolerance has not been observed. Although buprenorphine can depress respiration, severe respiratory depression has not been reported. Like pentazocine, buprenorphine can precipitate a withdrawal reaction in persons physically dependent on a pure opioid agonist. Physical dependence on buprenorphine develops, but symptoms of abstinence are delayed: Peak responses may not occur until 2 weeks after the final dose was taken. Although pretreatment with naloxone can prevent toxicity from buprenorphine, naloxone cannot readily reverse toxicity that has already developed. (Buprenorphine binds very tightly to its receptors and hence cannot be readily displaced by naloxone.) Buprenorphine is classified as a schedule III substance. In addition to its use for analgesia, buprenorphine is used to treat opioid addiction (see Chapter 35).

Buprenorphine prolongs the QT interval, posing a risk for potentially fatal dysrhythmias. Accordingly, the drug should not be used by patients with long QT syndrome or a family history of long QT syndrome, or by patients using QT-prolonging drugs (e.g., quinidine, amiodarone).

The risk for adverse effects may be increased by coexisting conditions, including psychosis, alcoholism, adrenocortical insufficiency, and severe liver or renal impairment.

OPIOID ANTAGONISTS

Opioid antagonists are drugs that block the effects of opioid agonists. Principal uses are treatment of opioid overdose, relief of opioid-induced constipation, reversal of postoperative opioid effects (e.g., respiratory depression, ileus), and management of opioid addiction. Four pure antagonists are available and three are discussed here: naloxone (Narcan), methylnaltrexone (Relistor), and naltrexone (ReVia, Vivitrol).

Naloxone
Mechanism of Action
Naloxone (Narcan) is a structural analog of morphine that acts as a competitive antagonist at opioid receptors, thereby blocking opioid actions. Naloxone can reverse most effects of the opioid agonists, including respiratory depression, coma, and analgesia.

Pharmacologic Effects
When administered in the absence of opioids, naloxone has no significant effects. If administered before giving an opioid, naloxone will block opioid actions. If administered to a patient who is already receiving opioids, naloxone will reverse analgesia, sedation, euphoria, and respiratory depression. If administered to an individual who is physically dependent on opioids, naloxone will precipitate an immediate withdrawal reaction.

Pharmacokinetics
Naloxone was traditionally restricted for use in the inpatient setting. Now with new legislation, naloxone is available for use by patients and families in the outpatient setting to help prevent opioid-related deaths from accidental overdose. After intramuscular (IM) or subcutaneous (subQ) injection, effects begin within 2 to 5 minutes and persist for several hours. Elimination is by hepatic metabolism. The half-life is approximately 2 hours. Naloxone cannot be used orally because of rapid first-pass inactivation.

Therapeutic Uses
Reversal of opioid overdose. Naloxone is the drug of choice for treating overdose with a pure opioid agonist. The drug reverses respiratory depression, coma, and other signs of opioid toxicity. Naloxone can also reverse toxicity from agonist-antagonist opioids (e.g., pentazocine,

nalbuphine). However, the doses required may be higher than those needed to reverse poisoning by pure agonists.

Dosage must be carefully titrated when treating toxicity in opioid addicts because the degree of physical dependence in these individuals is usually high and hence an excessive dose of naloxone can transport the patient from a state of poisoning to one of acute withdrawal. Accordingly, treatment should be initiated with a series of small doses rather than one large dose. Because the half-life of naloxone is shorter than that of most opioids, repeated dosing is required until the crisis has passed. If the patient received a dose of naloxone by a friend or family member for a suspected overdose, the patient should be transported by emergency providers to the nearest emergency department for further evaluation.

In some cases of accidental poisoning, there may be uncertainty as to whether unconsciousness is due to opioid overdose or to overdose with a general CNS depressant (e.g., barbiturate, alcohol, benzodiazepine). When uncertainty exists, naloxone is nonetheless indicated. If the cause of poisoning is a barbiturate or another general CNS depressant, naloxone will be of no benefit—but neither will it cause any harm.

Other Opioid Antagonists
Methylnaltrexone, Naloxegol, and Naldemedine
Actions and therapeutic use. Methylnaltrexone (Relistor), naloxegol (Movantik), and naldemedine (Symproic) are selective μ opioid antagonists indicated for opioid-induced constipation in patients with chronic pain who are taking opioids continuously and who have not responded to standard laxative therapy. Benefits derive from blocking μ opioid receptors in the GI tract. These drugs work in the periphery and hence do not block opioid receptors in the CNS. Accordingly, the drugs do not decrease analgesia and cannot precipitate opioid withdrawal.

Pharmacokinetics. Methylnaltrexone is rapidly absorbed after subQ injection, reaching peak plasma levels within 30 minutes. Naloxegol and naldemedine can be taken orally on a daily basis and have a slightly longer half-life (6 to 11 hours) than methylnaltrexone. Methylnaltrexone undergoes minimal metabolism and is excreted in the urine (50%) and feces (50%), primarily as unchanged drug. The terminal half-life is 8 hours. Naloxegol is metabolized in the liver and largely excreted in the feces (68%). Naldemedine is metabolized in the urine and excreted renally and in the feces.

Adverse effects, precautions, and drug interactions. Methylnaltrexone, naloxegol, and naldemedine are generally well tolerated. The most common adverse effects are *abdominal pain, flatulence, nausea, dizziness,* and *diarrhea.* In the event of severe or persistent diarrhea, these drugs should be discontinued. In patients with known or suspected mechanical GI obstruction, all three drugs should be avoided. No significant drug interactions have been reported with methylnaltrexone. Naloxegol and naldemedine should be used with caution in patients taking CYP3A4 inhibitors.

Naltrexone
Naltrexone (ReVia, Vivitrol), given PO or IM, is a pure opioid antagonist used for opioid and alcohol abuse. In opioid abuse, the goal is to prevent euphoria if the abuser should take an opioid. Because naltrexone can precipitate a withdrawal reaction in persons who are physically dependent on opioids, candidates for treatment must be rendered opioid free before naltrexone is started. Although naltrexone can block opioid-induced euphoria, the drug does not prevent craving for opioids. As a result, many addicts fail to comply with treatment. Therapy with naltrexone has been considerably less successful than with methadone, a drug that eliminates craving for opioids while blocking euphoria. Use of naltrexone for alcohol dependence and opioid addiction is discussed in Chapters 34 and 35, respectively.

When dosage is excessive, naltrexone can cause hepatocellular injury. Accordingly, the drug is contraindicated for patients with acute hepatitis or liver failure. Warn patients about the possibility of liver injury and advise them to discontinue the drug if signs of hepatitis develop.

IM administration can cause injection-site reactions, which are sometimes severe. Moderate reactions include pain, tenderness, induration, swelling, erythema, bruising, and pruritus. Severe reactions—cellulitis, hematoma, abscess, necrosis—can cause significant scarring and may require surgical intervention.

Naltrexone is available in two formulations: (1) 50-mg tablets, for oral dosing; and (2) an ER suspension (380 mg/vial), marketed as Vivitrol, for IM dosing. For oral therapy, a typical dosing schedule consists of 100 mg on Monday and Wednesday and 150 mg on Friday. Alternatively, the drug can be administered daily in 50-mg doses. For IM dosing, the usual regimen is 380 mg once a month.

Morphine and naltrexone (embeda). In 2010, the US Food and Drug Administration (FDA) approved Embeda, a fixed-dose combination of morphine and naltrexone. The product is designed to discourage morphine abuse. Embeda capsules are filled with tiny pellets that have an outer layer of ER morphine and an inner core of naltrexone. When the capsules are swallowed intact, only the morphine is absorbed. However, if the pellets are crushed, the naltrexone will be absorbed too, thereby blunting the effects of the morphine. As a result, potential abusers cannot get a quick high by crushing the pellets to release all of the morphine at once. However, abusers can still get high by simply taking a large dose. Embeda capsules are more expensive than other ER morphine products and should be prescribed only when abuse appears likely.

Alcohol can accelerate release of morphine from Embeda pellets. As a result, the entire dose can be absorbed quickly—rather than over 24 hours—thereby causing a potentially fatal spike in morphine blood levels. Accordingly, patients should be warned against alcohol consumption.

Embeda capsules are available in six morphine/naltrexone strengths: 20 mg/0.8 mg, 30 mg/1.2 mg, 50 mg/2 mg, 60 mg/2.4 mg, 80 mg/3.2 mg, and 100 mg/4 mg. Dosing is done once or twice daily. Patients can swallow Embeda capsules whole, or they can open the capsules and sprinkle the pellets on applesauce, which must be ingested without chewing.

NONOPIOID CENTRALLY ACTING ANALGESIC—TRAMADOL

Tramadol (Ultram, Ultram ER, Ryzolt, Rybix ODT) is a moderately strong analgesic with a low potential for dependence, abuse, or respiratory depression. The drug relieves pain through a combination of opioid and nonopioid mechanisms.

Tramadol (Ultram) relieves pain by mechanisms largely or completely unrelated to opioid receptors. This drug causes little or no respiratory depression, physical dependence, or abuse.

Mechanism of Action

Tramadol is an analog of codeine that relieves pain in part through weak agonist activity at μ opioid receptors. However, it seems to work primarily by blocking uptake of norepinephrine and serotonin, thereby activating monoaminergic spinal inhibition of pain. Naloxone, an opioid antagonist, only partially blocks tramadol's effects.

Therapeutic Use

Tramadol is approved for moderate to moderately severe pain. The drug is less effective than morphine and no more effective than codeine combined with aspirin or acetaminophen. Analgesia begins 1 hour after oral dosing, is maximum at 2 hours, and continues for 6 hours.

Pharmacokinetics

Tramadol is administered by mouth and reaches peak plasma levels in 2 hours. Elimination is by hepatic metabolism and renal excretion. The half-life is 5 to 6 hours.

Adverse Effects

Tramadol has been used by millions of patients, and serious adverse effects have been rare. Respiratory depression is minimum at recommended doses. The most common side effects are sedation, dizziness, headache, dry mouth, and constipation. Seizures have been reported in more than 280 patients, and hence the drug should be avoided in patients with epilepsy and other neurologic disorders. Severe allergic reactions occur rarely. Although generally very safe, tramadol can be fatal in overdose, especially when combined with another CNS depressant.

Drug Interactions

Tramadol can intensify responses to CNS depressants (e.g., alcohol, benzodiazepines) and therefore should not be combined with these drugs.

By inhibiting uptake of norepinephrine, tramadol can precipitate a hypertensive crisis if combined with a monoamine oxidase inhibitor (MAOI). Accordingly, the combination is absolutely contraindicated.

By inhibiting uptake of serotonin, tramadol can cause serotonin syndrome in patients taking drugs that enhance serotonergic transmission. Among these are selective serotonin reuptake inhibitors (SSRIs), serotonin and norepinephrine reuptake inhibitors, tricyclic antidepressants, MAOIs, and triptans. If these drugs must be combined with tramadol, the patient should be monitored carefully, especially during initial therapy and times of dosage escalation.

Abuse Liability

Abuse liability is very low, and hence tramadol is classified as schedule IV under the Controlled Substances Act. There have been reports of abuse, dependence, withdrawal, and intentional overdose, presumably for subjective effects. Consequently, tramadol should not be given to patients with a history of drug abuse, and the recommended dosage should not be exceeded.

PRESCRIBING OPIOIDS FOR CHRONIC, NONCANCER PAIN DURING A NATIONAL OPIOID CRISIS

The Opioid Epidemic

A radical change in the way providers managed pain occurred in the 1990s. It was determined that health care teams were doing a poor job of managing pain. At that time, pain became "what the patient said it was." Pain was treated as the "5th vital sign." Patient feedback regarding pain management was linked to performance and reimbursement. This request for more aggressive pain management led to an increase in opioid prescriptions.

The amount of prescription opioids has risen steeply in the 2000s. Efforts to improve pain management led to a 10-fold increase in opioid prescriptions, accompanied by a substantial increase in abuse, serious injuries, and deaths. In 2016, there were more than 63,000 overdose deaths in the United States (about 115 deaths per day). Over 65% of these deaths involved an opioid medication.

In 2017, the office of Health and Human Services (HHS) declared a national public health emergency to address the opioid crisis in the United States. In addition to the declaration, HHS provided a strategy for management of the crisis. The top five priorities are as follows:

- Improving access to treatment and recovery services
- Promoting use of overdose-reversing drugs
- Strengthening our understanding of the epidemic through better public health surveillance
- Providing support for cutting-edge research on pain and addiction
- Advancing better practices for pain management

Efforts to Decrease Opioid Abuse and Misuse

Prior to the announcement of the opioid crisis in 2017, pharmaceutical companies and the FDA attempted to do their part in decreasing opioid abuse and misuse through strengthening warning labels and through creation and approval of drugs especially designed to deter misuse.

Drug Reformulations

The first opiate product to undergo reformulation, in 2010, was OxyContin. Reformulation occurred because abusers could crush the OxyContin tablets and then "snort" the resulting powder, or dissolve the powder in water and inject it intravenously. The reformulated tablets are much harder to crush into a powder, and if exposed to water or alcohol, the tablets form a thick gel, rather than a solution that can be drawn into a syringe and injected.

After the reformulation of OxyContin, multiple other companies followed suit. Currently, the FDA approves seven drugs for labeling describing abuse-deterrent properties. These drugs are shown in Table 24.11.

Risk Evaluation and Mitigation Strategy to Reduce Opioid-Related Morbidity, Mortality, and Abuse

In 2018, the FDA updated the Risk Evaluation and Mitigation Strategy (REMS) to include IR opioids, ER opioids, and long-acting prescription opioids.

The central component is education for prescribers (e.g., physicians, nurse practitioners, physician assistants) and patients. In addition, education must now be available for all health-care providers involved in caring for the patient experiencing pain, including nurses and pharmacists. Training for prescribers focuses on patient selection, balancing the risks and benefits of opioids, monitoring treatment, and recognizing opioid misuse, abuse, and addiction. In addition, prescribers are taught how to counsel patients on the safe use of opioids and are given written instructions for their patients. When patients have a prescription filled, the pharmacy provides a medication guide. Newer education for the entire health-care team includes fundamentals of acute and chronic pain management, monitoring patients receiving opioids, and use of appropriate clinical oversight.

Changes in Legislation

Between the years 2016 and 2018, more than 30 states passed legislation regarding the prescription of opioid therapy. The majority of these laws limit the number of opioids prescribed at one time, especially with first-time prescriptions. Many of these laws also specify other prescribing requirements, including providing patient education, checking prescription drug monitoring websites, and obtaining additional education on safe prescribing. Information on your state may be found at http://www.ncsl.org/research/health/prescribing-policies-states-confront-opioid-overdose-epidemic.aspx.

Prescribing Guidelines

In patients with chronic pain of nonmalignant origin, opioids can reduce discomfort, improve mood, and enhance function. In addition, patients still have a right to effective treatment. Hence there is a need to balance patients' rights with prescribers' concerns. To assist in decreasing the amount of undue harm from opiate therapy, a number of guidelines were created to assist providers in balancing adequate pain control with safe prescribing.

Before the creation of the Centers for Disease Control and Prevention (CDC) pain guidelines in 2016 (Box 24.1), the American Academy of Pain Medicine and the American Pain Society issued guidelines for using opioids in patients with chronic noncancer pain. Provisions include the following:

- Using opioids only after nonopioid analgesics or more conservative methods have failed
- Discussing the benefits and risks of long-term opioids with the patient
- When possible, using only one prescriber and one pharmacy
- Ensuring comprehensive follow-up to assess efficacy and side effects of treatment and to monitor for signs of opioid abuse
- Stopping opioids after an attempt at opioid rotation has produced inadequate benefit
- Fully documenting the entire process

In 2018, the Society of Hospital Medicine issued a consensus statement on the treatment of pain in hospitalized patients: "Society of Hospital Medicine Recommendation on Improving the Safety of Opioid Use for Acute Noncancer Pain in Hospitalized Adults Outside of Intensive Care, Palliative Care, and End-of Life Care." This consensus statement can be found at https://www.journalofhospitalmedicine.com/jhospmed/article/161929/hospital-medicine/safe-opioid-prescribing-acute-noncancer-pain-hospitalized.

Safe Opiate Prescribing Considerations
Pain Assessment

Assessment is an essential component of pain management. Pain and current functional status should be evaluated at every patient appointment. Assessment should include documentation of where the pain is located, what type of pain is present (e.g., dull, sharp, stabbing), how the pain changes with time, what makes the pain better, what makes it worse, and how much the pain impairs the patient's ability to function. In addition, you should assess for psychological factors that can reduce pain threshold (anxiety, depression, fear, anger).

TABLE 24.11 Opioids With FDA-Approved Labeling Describing Abuse-Deterrent Properties

Drug[a]	Abuse-Deterrent Properties
OxyContin	Formulated with inactive ingredients that resist crushing, breaking, or dissolving
Embeda	Contains naltrexone, an opioid antagonist
Hysingla ER	Formulated with inactive ingredients that resist crushing, breaking, or dissolving
MorphaBond ER	Retains extended release properties, even when manipulated
Xtampza ER	Formulated with inactive ingredients that resist crushing, breaking, or dissolving
Arymo ER	Formulated with inactive ingredients that resist crushing, breaking, or dissolving
RoxyBond	Formulated with inactive ingredients that resist crushing, breaking, or dissolving

[a]Currently, there are no generic drugs available with abuse-deterrent properties.

ER, Extended release.

BOX 24.1   CDC Guidelines for Safe Opiate Prescribing

Determining When to Initiate or Continue Opioids for Chronic Pain

1. Nonpharmacologic therapy and nonopioid pharmacologic therapy are preferred for chronic pain. Clinicians should consider opioid therapy only if expected benefits for both pain and function are anticipated to outweigh risks to the patient. If opioids are used, they should be combined with nonpharmacologic therapy and nonopioid pharmacologic therapy, as appropriate.

2. Before starting opioid therapy for chronic pain, clinicians should establish treatment goals with all patients, including realistic goals for pain and function, and should consider how therapy will be discontinued if benefits do not outweigh risks. Clinicians should continue opioid therapy only if there is clinically meaningful improvement in pain and function that outweighs risks to patient safety.

3. Before starting and periodically during opioid therapy, clinicians should discuss with patients known risks and realistic benefits of opioid therapy and patient and clinician responsibilities for managing therapy.

Opioid Selection, Dosage, Duration, Follow-Up, and Discontinuation

4. When starting opioid therapy for chronic pain, clinicians should prescribe immediate-release opioids instead of extended-release/long-acting (ER/A) opioids.

5. When opioids are started, clinicians should prescribe the lowest effective dosage. Clinicians should use caution when prescribing opioids at any dosage, should carefully reassess evidence of individual benefits and risks when increasing dosage to ≥50 morphine milligram equivalents (MME)/day, and should avoid increasing dosage to ≥90 MME/day or carefully justify a decision to titrate dosage to ≥90 MME/day.

6. Long-term opioid use often begins with treatment of acute pain. When opioids are used for acute pain, clinicians should prescribe the lowest effective dose of immediate-release opioids and should prescribe no greater quantity than needed for the expected duration of pain severe enough to require opioids. Three days or less will often be sufficient; more than seven days will rarely be needed.

7. Clinicians should evaluate benefits and harms with patients within 1 to 4 weeks of starting opioid therapy for chronic pain or of dose escalation.

Clinicians should evaluate benefits and harms of continued therapy with patients every 3 months or more frequently. If benefits do not outweigh harms of continued opioid therapy, clinicians should optimize other therapies and work with patients to taper opioids to lower dosages or to taper and discontinue opioids.

Assessing Risk and Addressing Harms of Opioid Use

8. Before starting and periodically during continuation of opioid therapy, clinicians should evaluate risk factors for opioid-related harms. Clinicians should incorporate into the management plan strategies to mitigate risk, including considering offering naloxone when factors that increase risk for opioid overdose, such as history of overdose, history of substance use disorder, higher opioid dosages (≥50 MME/day), or concurrent benzodiazepine use, are present.

9. Clinicians should review the patient's history of controlled substance prescriptions using state prescription drug monitoring program (PDMP) data to determine whether the patient is receiving opioid dosages or dangerous combinations that put him or her at high risk for overdose. Clinicians should review PDMP data when starting opioid therapy for chronic pain and periodically during opioid therapy for chronic pain, ranging from every prescription to every 3 months.

10. When prescribing opioids for chronic pain, clinicians should use urine drug testing before starting opioid therapy and consider urine drug testing at least annually to assess for prescribed medications as well as other controlled prescription drugs and illicit drugs.

11. Clinicians should avoid prescribing opioid pain medication and benzodiazepines concurrently whenever possible.

12. Clinicians should offer or arrange evidence-based treatment (usually medication-assisted treatment with buprenorphine or methadone in combination with behavioral therapies) for patients with opioid use disorder.

All recommendations are category A (apply to all patients outside of active cancer treatment, palliative care, and end-of-life care) except recommendation 10 (designated category B, with individual decision making required); see full guideline for evidence ratings.

From Dowell D, Haegerich TM, Chou R. CDC recommendations for prescribing opioids for chronic pain—United States, 2016. *MMWR Recomm Rep.* 2016;65(1):1–49.

Patient Education

It is crucial that the patient understand the risks and benefits of using opioids to treat chronic, noncancer pain. The provider should discuss goals of care regarding pain and function. Treatment goals set by the patient and provider should be realistic. These goals should be revisited at each patient appointment. If the risks begin to outweigh the benefits of opioid therapy, a new plan should be developed.

Initiating Therapy

Nonpharmacologic therapy and nonopioid therapy should be used to treat chronic pain before starting opioid therapy. If these modalities are not successful in improving patient pain and function, opioid therapy can be considered. Although research is lacking regarding the safest way to initiate opiate therapy in the patient with chronic pain, there is evidence to suggest that starting patients on ER or long-acting medications before starting with IR medications may lead to increases in medication overdose. Therefore current recommendations suggest initiating therapy with IR medications first. In addition, use of nonopioid, adjuvant medications should continue to maximize pain control and patient function. The CDC has included a checklist for providers

initiating opioid therapy. This can be found at http://stacks.cdc.gov/view/cdc/38025.

Assessing Risk

Prior to initiation of opioid therapy, the first step is to identify patients at risk for abuse by using a screening tool, such as *NIDA-Modified ASSIST*, available at www.drugabuse.gov/nidamed/screening/nmassist.pdf.

The second step is to become familiar with the state prescription drug monitoring program (PDMP). This database contains information regarding all scheduled medications prescribed to a patient, including who prescribed them and the amount prescribed. Providers should carefully review the patient's history with controlled substances and check the PDMP at initiation of opioid therapy and periodically during the course of treatment. Evaluation of the database allows providers to assess for medication combinations that may promote dangerous side effects.

Finally, the provider should consider obtaining a urine drug test for controlled substances, including illicit drugs, before initiation of therapy and at least annually after that. Patients taking multiple medications, including those like benzodiazepines, other opiates, or heroin, may be at increased risk for fatal overdose. Providers that receive unexpected results can use this opportunity to educate the patient or change the patient's treatment plan.

Dosage Determination

Providers should start with the lowest effective dosage for the patient. "Standard" doses cannot be relied on as appropriate for all patients. For example, if a "standard" 10-mg dose of morphine were employed for all adults, only 70% would receive adequate relief; the other 30% would be undertreated. Not all patients have the same tolerance for pain, and hence some need larger doses than others for the same disorder. Some conditions hurt more than others. Older-adult patients metabolize opioids slowly and therefore require lower doses than younger adults. Because the blood–brain barrier of newborns is poorly developed, these patients are especially sensitive to opioids; therefore they generally require smaller doses (on a milligram-per-kilogram basis) than do older infants and young children.

To minimize physical dependence and abuse, opioid analgesics should be administered in the lowest effective dosages for the shortest time needed. Be aware, however, that larger doses are needed for patients who have more intense pain and for those who have developed tolerance. As pain diminishes, opioid dosage should be reduced. As soon as possible, the patient should be switched to a nonopioid analgesic, such as aspirin or acetaminophen.

Avoiding a Withdrawal Reaction

When opioids are administered in high doses for 20 days or more, clinically significant physical dependence may develop. Under these conditions, abrupt withdrawal will precipitate an abstinence syndrome. To minimize symptoms of abstinence, opioids should be withdrawn slowly, tapering the dosage over 3 days. If the degree of dependence is especially high, as can occur in opioid addicts, dosage should be tapered over 7 to 10 days.

Cancer-Related Pain

Treating chronic pain of cancer differs substantially from treating acute pain of other disorders. When treating cancer pain, the objective is to maximize comfort. Psychological and physical dependence are minimal concerns. Patients should be given as much medication as needed to relieve pain. In the words of one pain specialist, "No patient should wish for death because of the physician's reluctance to use adequate amounts of opioids." With proper therapy, cancer pain can be effectively managed in about 90% of patients. Cancer pain is discussed fully in Chapter 86.

PATIENT-CENTERED CARE ACROSS THE LIFE SPAN

Opioid Analgesics

Life Stage	Patient Care Concerns
Infants	Regular use of opioids during pregnancy can cause physical dependence in the fetus, resulting in withdrawal after delivery.
Children	Adequately assess pain with a standardized pain scale. Aspirin, as an adjuvant to opioids, should be avoided because of risk for Reye syndrome. There remains lack of research regarding best practice in treatment of chronic noncancer pain in children.
Pregnant women	Taking opioids in early pregnancy can increase the risk for congenital heart defects, spina bifida, and gastroschisis.
Breastfeeding women	Limited data suggest small amounts of opioids are excreted in breast milk. This can result in infant drowsiness.
Older adults	Persistent pain is often undertreated in the frail older-adult population. The American Geriatrics Association recommends that providers consider treating moderate to severe uncontrolled pain with opiates after a trial of acetaminophen.

25

Drugs for Headache

Headache is a common symptom that can be triggered by a variety of stimuli, including stress, fatigue, acute illness, and sensitivity to alcohol. Some people experience severe, recurrent, debilitating headaches that are frequently unresponsive to aspirin-like drugs. For these individuals, medical attention is merited. In this chapter, we focus on severe forms of headache—specifically, migraine, cluster, and tension-type headaches.

When attempting to treat headache, we must differentiate between headaches that have an identifiable underlying cause (e.g., severe hypertension; hyperthyroidism; tumors; infection; disorders of the eyes, ears, nose, sinuses, and throat) and headaches that have no identifiable cause (e.g., migraine and cluster headaches). If there is a clear cause, it should be treated directly (Table 25.1).

As we consider drugs for headache, keep three basic principles in mind. First, antiheadache drugs may be used in two ways: to abort an ongoing attack or to prevent an attack from occurring. Second, not all patients with a particular type of headache respond to the same drugs. Hence therapy must be individualized. Third, several of the drugs employed to treat severe headaches (e.g., ergotamine, opioids) can cause physical dependence. Accordingly, every effort should be made to keep dependence from developing. If dependence does develop, a withdrawal procedure is needed.

MIGRAINE HEADACHE

Characteristics, Pathophysiology, and Overview of Treatment

Characteristics

Migraine headache is characterized by throbbing head pain of moderate to severe intensity that may be unilateral (60%) or bilateral (40%). Most patients also experience nausea and vomiting, along with neck pain and sensitivity to light and sound. Physical activity intensifies the pain. During a prolonged attack, patients develop *hyperalgesia* (augmented responses to painful stimuli) and *allodynia* (painful responses to normally innocuous stimuli). Migraines usually develop in the morning after arising. Pain increases gradually and lasts 4 to 72 hours (median duration, 24 hours). On average, attacks occur 1.5 times a month. Precipitating factors include anxiety, fatigue, stress, menstruation, alcohol, weather changes, and tyramine-containing foods.

Migraine has two primary forms: migraine *with aura* and migraine *without aura*. In migraine with aura, the headache is preceded by visual symptoms (flashes of light, a blank area in the field of vision, zigzag patterns). Of the two forms, migraine without aura is more common, affecting about 70% of people with migraine.

Migraine afflicts 36 million people in the United States and more than 10% of the population worldwide. The headaches are more common and more severe in females, with a lifetime incidence of 43%, compared with 18% in males. About 65% of people with migraine are women in their late teens, 20s, or 30s. With some women, migraine attacks are worse during menstruation but subside during pregnancy and cease after menopause, indicating a hormonal component to the attacks. A family history of the disease is typical.

Pathophysiology

Migraine headache is a *neurovascular* disorder that involves *dilation* and *inflammation* of intracranial blood vessels. Headache generation begins with neural events that trigger vasodilation. Vasodilation then leads to pain, which leads to further neural activation, thereby amplifying pain-generating signals. Neurons of the trigeminal vascular system, which innervate intracranial blood vessels, are key components.

The exact cause of migraine pain is not completely understood—although vasodilation and inflammation are clearly involved. Available data suggest that two compounds—*calcitonin gene–related peptide* (CGRP) and *serotonin* (5-hydroxytryptamine [5-HT])—play important roles. The role of CGRP is to *promote migraine,* and the role of 5-HT is to *suppress* migraine. Data that implicate CGRP as a cause of migraine include the following:

- Plasma levels of CGRP rise during a migraine attack.
- Stimulation of neurons of the trigeminal vascular system promotes release of CGRP, which in turn promotes vasodilation and release of inflammatory neuropeptides.
- Dosing with sumatriptan—a drug that relieves migraine—lowers elevated levels of CGRP.
- Sumatriptan can suppress the release of CGRP from cultured trigeminal neurons.
Data that support a protective role for 5-HT include the following:
- Plasma levels of 5-HT drop by 50% during a migraine attack.
- Depletion of 5-HT with reserpine can precipitate an attack in migraine-prone individuals.
- Administration of 5-HT or sumatriptan—both of which activate 5-HT receptors—can abort an ongoing attack.

Overview of Treatment

Drugs for migraine are employed in two ways: to abort an ongoing attack and to prevent attacks from occurring. Drugs used to abort an attack fall into two groups: nonspecific analgesics (aspirin-like drugs and opioid analgesics) and migraine-specific drugs (serotonin$_{1B/1D}$ receptor agonists [triptans] and ergot alkaloids). Drugs employed for prophylaxis include β blockers (e.g., propranolol), tricyclic antidepressants (e.g., amitriptyline), CGRP receptor antagonists, and antiepileptic drugs (e.g., divalproex).

Abortive Therapy

The objective of abortive therapy is to eliminate headache pain and suppress associated nausea and vomiting. Treatment should commence at the earliest sign of an attack. Because migraine causes gastrointestinal (GI) disturbances (nausea, vomiting, and gastric stasis), oral therapy may be ineffective after an attack has begun. Hence, for treatment of

TABLE 25.1   Treatment of Headache

Migraine Treatment	Cluster Headache Treatment

Select treatment based on severity and functional impairment	Determine acute treatment
	   Oxygen
	   Sumatriptan

Mild	Determine prophylactic treatment

Aspirin or aspirin combinations
Triptans
	Verapamil
	   Corticosteroids
	   Lithium

Moderate	Patient education and lifestyle modifications
DHE	
Ergotamine	
NSAID combination products	
Severe	
Metoclopramide	
Triptans	
Ergotamine or DHE	
NSAIDs (Ketorolac)	
Prophylaxis	
β blockers	
Tricyclic antidepressants	
Antiepileptics	
Consider hormonally related migraine in females	
CGRP receptor antagonists	
NSAIDs	
Triptans	
Prophylaxis with estrogen	
Patient education and lifestyle modifications	

CGRP, Calcitonin gene–related peptide; DHE, dihydroergotamine; NSAID, nonsteroidal antiinflammatory drug.
Adapted from Diagnosis and treatment of headache. *ICHI Health Care Guideline.* 11th ed. https://www.icsi.org/guideline/headache/. January 2013.

TABLE 25.2   Migraine Headache: Drugs for Abortive Therapy

Nonspecific Analgesics	Usual Dosage
NSAIDs and NSAID Combinations	
Aspirin, naproxen, diclofenac	Per specific drug instructions
Acetaminophen + aspirin + caffeine (Excedrin Migraine)	2 caplets (250 mg/250 mg/65 mg) once at onset
Opioid Analgesics	
Butorphanol nasal spray	1 spray (1 mg) in one nostril; may repeat in 60 min See Table 25.3
Migraine-Specific	**Drugs**
Selective Serotonin$_{1B/1D}$ Receptor Agonists (Triptans)	
Almotriptan (Axert)	
Eletriptan (Relpax)	
Frovatriptan (Frova)	
Naratriptan (Amerge)	
Rizatriptan (Maxalt)	
Sumatriptan (Imitrex, Sumavel DosePro, Onzetra Xsail)	
Zolmitriptan (Zomig)	
Ergot Alkaloids	
Dihydroergotamine intranasal spray (Migranal)	1 spray (0.5 mg) each nostril and repeat in 15 min
Ergotamine sublingual (Ergomar)	1 tablet (2 mg) under tongue at onset; may administer 1 additional tablet at 30-min intervals ×2.
Ergotamine + caffeine (Cafergot, Migergot)	1–2 tablets (1 mg/100 mg) at onset; may administer 1 additional tablet at 30-min intervals ×4.

NSAIDs, Nonsteroidal inflammatory drugs.

an established attack, a drug that can be administered by injection, nasal spray, or rectal suppository may be best. As noted, two types of drugs are used: nonspecific analgesics and migraine-specific agents. Representative drugs are listed in Table 25.2.

Drug selection depends on the intensity of the attack. For mild to moderate symptoms, an NSAID (e.g., aspirin, naproxen) may be sufficient. For moderate to severe symptoms, patients should take a *migraine-specific drug,* such as a serotonin$_{1B/1D}$ agonist, or—less frequently used—an ergot alkaloid (ergotamine or dihydroergotamine). If these agents fail to relieve pain, an *opioid analgesic* (e.g., butorphanol) may be needed. Note that opioids should be reserved for treatment in patients with migraines resistant to all other treatments.

The use of abortive medications (both nonspecific and migraine specific) should be limited to 1 or 2 days a week. More frequent use can lead to *medication overuse headache* (MOH), also known as drug-induced headache or drug-rebound headache (see section on MOH).

Antiemetics are important adjuncts to migraine therapy. By reducing nausea and vomiting, these drugs can (1) make the patient more comfortable, and (2) permit therapy with oral antimigraine drugs. Two antiemetics—*metoclopramide* (Reglan) and *prochlorperazine* (formerly available as *Compazine*)—are used most often.

Analgesics

NSAIDs. Aspirin, naproxen, diclofenac, and other aspirin-like analgesics can provide adequate relief of mild to moderate migraine attacks. In fact, when combined with metoclopramide (to enhance absorption), aspirin may work as well as sumatriptan, a highly effective antimigraine drug. Moreover, the combination of aspirin plus metoclopramide costs less than sumatriptan and causes fewer adverse effects.

Acetaminophen. Acetaminophen should be used only in combination with other drugs, not alone. One effective combination, marketed as *Excedrin Migraine,* consists of acetaminophen, aspirin, and caffeine.

Opioid analgesics. Opioid analgesics are reserved for severe migraine that has not responded to first-line medications. This is because of the potential for abuse as well as MOH. The recommended agent is *butorphanol nasal spray.*

Serotonin$_{1B/1D}$ Receptor Agonists (Triptans)

The serotonin$_{1B/1D}$ receptor agonists, also known as *triptans*, are first-line drugs for terminating a migraine attack. These agents relieve pain by constricting intracranial blood vessels and suppressing release of inflammatory neuropeptides. All are well tolerated. Rarely, they cause symptomatic coronary vasospasm. Table 25.3 presents the clinical pharmacology of the triptans.

Sumatriptan. Sumatriptan (Imitrex, Sumavel DosePro) was the first triptan available and will serve as our prototype for the group. The drug can be administered by mouth, nasal inhalation, or subcutaneous (subQ) injection.

TABLE 25.3   Clinical Pharmacology of the Triptans

Generic Name (Trade Name)	Route	Onset (min)	Duration	Half-Life (h)	Dosage	SSRIs, SNRIs, Triptans, Ergots	MAOIs	CYP3A4 Inhibitors	Comments
						CONTRAINDICATED DRUGS			
Sumatriptan									
(Imitrex)	Oral	30–60	Short	2.5	25, 50, or 100 mg; may repeat in 2 h (max. 200 mg/24 h)	✓	✓		First triptan available and best understood. Available in three fast-acting formulations: nasal spray, an inhaled nasal powder, an autoinjector for subQ dosing (using a needle), and a needle-free device for subQ dosing (Sumavel DosePro).
(Imitrex)	Nasal spray	15–20			5 or 20 mg; may repeat in 2 h (max. 40 mg/24 h)				
(Imitrex)	SubQ, with needle	10-15			6 mg; may repeat in 1 h (max. 12 mg/24 h)				
Onzetra Xsail	Nasal powder	15			1 capsule (11 mg) in each nostril				
(Sumavel DosePro)	SubQ, needle-free	10			6 mg; may repeat in 1 h (max. 12 mg/24 h)				
Almotriptan (Axert)	Oral	30–120	Short	3–4	6.25 or 12.5 mg; may repeat in 2 h (max. 25 mg/24 h)	✓			Incidence of chest Discomfort (pain, tightness, pressure) is lower than with other triptans. Decrease dosage if combined with a CYP3A4 inhibitor.
Eletriptan (Relpax)	Oral	60	Short	4	20 or 40 mg; may repeat in 2 h (max. 40 mg/24 h)	✓		✓	Bioavailability increased by high-fat meal. Good balance between fast onset and long duration
Frovatriptan (Frova)	Oral	120–180	Long	26	2.5 mg; may repeat in 2 h	✓			Slowest onset, longest half-life, and lowest rate of headache recurrence. Decrease dose if combined with propranolol
Naratriptan (Amerge)	Oral	60–180	Intermediate	6	1 or 2.5 mg; may repeat in 4 h (max. 5 mg/24 h)	✓			Slower onset and longer duration than most triptans
Rizatriptan (Maxalt, Maxalt MLT)	Oral	30–120	Short	2–3	5 or 10 mg; may repeat in 2 h (max. 30 mg/24 h)	✓	✓		May be the most consistently effective triptan. Decrease dose if combined with propranolol. Available in melt-in-the-mouth wafers (Maxalt MLT) that can be taken without water
Zolmitriptan (Zomig, Zomig ZMT)	Oral	45	Short	3	2.5 or 5 mg; may repeat in 2 h (max. 10 mg/24 h)	✓	✓		Available in a fast-acting nasal spray, and in melt-in-the-mouth wafers (Zomig ZMT) that can be taken without water
(Zomig)	Nasal spray	15			5 mg; may repeat in 2 h (max. 10 mg/24 h)				
(Zecuity)	Transdermal	60	Short	3.1	6.5 mg patch; may repeat in 4 h (max. two patches in 24 h.)	✓	✓		Newest form of sumatriptan approved for transdermal use in 2013. Requires use of a metal transdermal system that cannot get wet

CYP3A4, The 3A4 isozyme of cytochrome P450; *MAOI*, monoamine oxidase inhibitor; *SNRI*, serotonin and norepinephrine reuptake inhibitor; *SSRI*, selective serotonin reuptake inhibitor; *subQ*, subcutaneous.

Sumatriptan is also available in a fixed-dose combination with naproxen under the trade name Treximet.

Mechanism of action. Sumatriptan, an analog of 5-HT, causes selective activation of $5\text{-}HT_{1B}$ and $5\text{-}HT_{1D}$ receptors ($5\text{-}HT_{1B/1D}$ receptors). The drug has no affinity for $5\text{-}HT_2$ or $5\text{-}HT_3$ receptors, nor does it bind to adrenergic, dopaminergic, muscarinic, or histaminergic receptors. Binding to $5\text{-}HT_{1B/1D}$ receptors on intracranial blood vessels causes vasoconstriction. Binding to $5\text{-}HT_{1B/1D}$ receptors on sensory nerves of the trigeminal vascular system suppresses the release of CGRP, a compound that promotes release of inflammatory neuropeptides. As a result, sumatriptan reduces release of inflammatory neuropeptides and thereby diminishes perivascular inflammation. Both actions—vasoconstriction and decreased perivascular inflammation—help relieve migraine pain.

Therapeutic use. Sumatriptan is taken to abort an ongoing migraine attack. The drug relieves headache and associated symptoms (nausea, neck pain, photophobia, phonophobia). In clinical trials, sumatriptan gave complete relief to most patients. Beneficial effects begin about 15 minutes after subQ or intranasal dosing and 30 to 60 minutes after oral dosing. Complete relief occurs in 40% to 60% of patients 2 hours after subQ dosing, in 30% to 60% of patients 2 hours after intranasal dosing, in 18% of patients 2 hours after transdermal dosing, and in 50% to 60% of patients 4 hours after oral dosing. Unfortunately, headache returns in about 40% of patients within 24 hours. In comparison, the 24-hour recurrence rate with dihydroergotamine is only 14%. In patients who respond to subQ sumatriptan, subsequent administration of oral sumatriptan can delay recurrence but does not prevent it. In addition to migraine, sumatriptan is approved for cluster headaches.

Pharmacokinetics. With oral or intranasal dosing, bioavailability is low (about 15%). The transdermal system has even lower bioavailability (about 6%), whereas with subQ dosing, bioavailability is high (97%). As a result, oral and intranasal doses are considerably higher than subQ and transdermal doses. Sumatriptan undergoes extensive hepatic metabolism, primarily by monoamine oxidase (MAO), followed by excretion in the urine. The half-life is short—about 2.5 hours.

Adverse effects. Sumatriptan is generally well tolerated. Most side effects are transient and mild. The most common side effect, affecting up to 25% of patients, is a bad taste in the mouth after administration. Coronary vasospasm is the biggest concern.

Chest symptoms. About 50% of patients experience unpleasant chest symptoms, usually described as "heavy arms" or "chest pressure" rather than pain. These symptoms are transient and *not* related to ischemic heart disease. Possible causes are pulmonary vasoconstriction, esophageal spasm, intercostal muscle spasm, and bronchoconstriction. Patients should be forewarned of these symptoms and reassured that they are not dangerous.

Coronary vasospasm. Very rarely, sumatriptan and other triptans can cause angina secondary to coronary vasospasm. Electrocardiographic changes have been observed in patients with coronary artery disease (CAD) or Prinzmetal (vasospastic) angina. To reduce the risk for angina, avoid sumatriptan in patients with risk factors for CAD until CAD has been ruled out. These patients include postmenopausal women, men older than 40 years, smokers, and patients with hypertension, hypercholesterolemia, diabetes, or a family history of CAD. Owing to the risk for coronary vasospasm, sumatriptan is contraindicated for patients with a history of ischemic heart disease, myocardial infarction (MI), uncontrolled hypertension, or other heart disease.

Teratogenesis. *Sumatriptan should be avoided during pregnancy.* When given daily to pregnant rabbits, the drug was embryolethal at blood levels only three times higher than those achieved with a 6-mg subQ injection in humans (a typical dose). Accordingly, unless the prescriber directs otherwise, women should be instructed to avoid the drug if they are pregnant or think they might be, if they are trying to become pregnant, or if they are not using an adequate form of contraception.

Drug interactions

Ergot alkaloids and other triptans. Sumatriptan, other triptans, and ergot alkaloids (e.g., ergotamine, dihydroergotamine) all cause vasoconstriction. Accordingly, if one triptan is combined with another or with an ergot alkaloid, excessive and prolonged vasospasm could result. Therefore sumatriptan should not be used within 24 hours of an ergot derivative or another triptan.

Monoamine oxidase inhibitors. Monoamine oxidase inhibitors (MAOIs) can suppress hepatic degradation of sumatriptan, causing its plasma level to rise. Toxicity can result. Accordingly, sumatriptan should not be combined with an MAOI and should not be used within 2 weeks of stopping an MAOI.

Selective serotonin reuptake inhibitors and serotonin/norepinephrine reuptake inhibitors. As discussed in Chapter 27, the selective serotonin reuptake inhibitors (SSRIs) (e.g., fluoxetine [Prozac]) and serotonin/norepinephrine reuptake inhibitors (SNRIs) (e.g., duloxetine [Cymbalta]) indirectly activate serotonin receptors in the brain (by increasing the availability of serotonin at brain synapses). If receptor activation is excessive, serotonin syndrome can occur. Signs and symptoms include altered mental status (agitation, confusion, disorientation, anxiety, hallucinations, poor concentration) as well as incoordination, myoclonus, hyperreflexia, excessive sweating, tremor, and fever. Deaths have occurred. Because the triptans *directly* activate serotonin receptors, and the SSRIs and SNRIs *indirectly* activate serotonin receptors, you can see how combining these drugs could lead to excessive receptor activation. Accordingly, these combinations should not be used.

📄 SUMMARY OF KEY PRESCRIBING CONSIDERATIONS

Triptans

Therapeutic Goal: Termination of migraine headache

Baseline Data: Assess for possible underlying causes of headache, including severe hypertension, hyperthyroidism, tumors, or infection.

Monitoring: No laboratory monitoring necessary with this drug class.

Identifying High-Risk Patients: All triptans are contraindicated for patients with ischemic heart disease, prior MI, or uncontrolled hypertension.

Evaluating Therapeutic Effects: Determine the size and frequency of doses used and the extent to which therapy has reduced the intensity and duration of attacks.

Minimizing Adverse Effects: Sumatriptan can cause birth defects in laboratory animals, and must not be used during pregnancy. Interactions with ergot alkaloids, SSRIs, SNRIs, MAOIs should be considered.

PROTOTYPE DRUGS

Drugs for Migraine Headache

Nonsteroidal Antiinflammatory Drugs
Aspirin

Selective Serotonin Receptor Agonists
Sumatriptan

Ergot Alkaloids
Ergotamine

Ergot Alkaloids

Ergotamine

Mechanism of antimigraine action. Ergotamine has complex actions, and the precise mechanism by which it aborts migraine is unknown. Ergotamine can alter transmission at serotonergic, dopaminergic, and α-adrenergic junctions. Current evidence suggests that antimigraine effects are related to agonist activity at subtypes of serotonin receptors, specifically 5-HT$_{1B}$ and 5-HT$_{1D}$ receptors. Additional evidence indicates that ergotamine can block inflammation associated with the trigeminal vascular system, perhaps by suppressing release of CGRP. Relief also may be related to vascular effects. In cranial arteries, ergotamine acts directly to promote constriction and to reduce the amplitude of pulsations. In addition, the drug can affect blood flow by depressing the vasomotor center.

Therapeutic uses. Ergotamine is used as a second-line drug for stopping an ongoing migraine attack in patients who have not responded to a triptan. Owing to the risk for dependence (see later), ergotamine should not be taken daily on a long-term basis.

Pharmacokinetics. Administration may be oral, sublingual, or rectal. Bioavailability with oral and sublingual administration is low. Bioavailability with rectal administration is higher. Although the half-life of ergotamine is only 2 hours, pharmacologic effects can still be observed 24 hours after dosing. Ergotamine undergoes metabolism by CYP3A4, followed by excretion in the bile.

Adverse effects. Ergotamine is well tolerated at the usual therapeutic doses. The drug can stimulate the chemoreceptor trigger zone, causing *nausea and vomiting* in about 10% of patients, thereby augmenting nausea and vomiting caused by the migraine itself. Concurrent treatment with metoclopramide or prochlorperazine can help reduce these responses. Other common side effects include *weakness in the legs, myalgia, numbness and tingling in the fingers and toes, angina-like pain,* and *tachycardia or bradycardia.*

Overdose. Acute or chronic overdose can cause serious toxicity referred to as *ergotism.* In addition to the adverse effects seen at therapeutic doses, overdose can cause ischemia secondary to constriction of peripheral arteries and arterioles: the extremities become cold, pale, and numb; muscle pain develops; and gangrene may eventually result. Patients should be informed about these responses and instructed to seek immediate medical attention if they develop. The risk for ergotism is highest in patients with sepsis, peripheral vascular disease, and renal or hepatic impairment.

Drug interactions

Triptans. Ergotamine should not be combined with triptans (e.g., sumatriptan, zolmitriptan) because a prolonged vasospastic reaction could occur. To avoid this problem, dosing with ergotamine and serotonin agonists should be separated by at least 24 hours.

Physical dependence. Regular daily use of ergotamine, even in moderate doses, can cause physical dependence. The withdrawal syndrome is characterized by headache, nausea, vomiting, and restlessness. That is, withdrawal resembles a migraine attack. Patients who experience these symptoms are likely to resume taking the drug, thereby perpetuating the cycle of dependence. Hospitalization may be required to break the cycle. To avoid dependence, the dosage and duration of treatment must be restricted (see dosing guidelines later).

Contraindications. Ergotamine is contraindicated for patients with hepatic or renal impairment, sepsis (gangrene has resulted), CAD, peripheral vascular disease, and uncontrolled hypertension, and for those taking potent inhibitors of CYP3A4. In addition, the drug should not be taken during pregnancy because it can promote uterine contractions and hence might cause fetal harm or abortion. Women of childbearing age should be warned to avoid pregnancy while using this drug.

Dihydroergotamine

Therapeutic uses. Parenteral dihydroergotamine (D.H.E. 45, Migranal)—given by the intramuscular (IM), intravenous (IV), or subQ route—is a second-line drug for terminating a migraine attack. The drug also may be given by intranasal spray. Intranasal dihydroergotamine is less effective than intranasal sumatriptan but is associated with a lower rate of migraine recurrence.

Pharmacologic effects. The actions of dihydroergotamine are similar to those of ergotamine. Like ergotamine, dihydroergotamine alters transmission at serotonergic, dopaminergic, and α-adrenergic junctions. In contrast to ergotamine, dihydroergotamine causes little nausea and vomiting, no physical dependence, and minimal peripheral vasoconstriction (when used alone). However, diarrhea is prominent.

Pharmacokinetics. Dihydroergotamine may be administered parenterally or by nasal spray—but not by mouth (owing to extensive first-pass metabolism). In the liver, the drug is metabolized by CYP3A4. An active metabolite (8′-hydroxydihydroergotamine) contributes to therapeutic effects. The half-life of dihydroergotamine plus the active metabolite is about 21 hours.

 BLACK BOX WARNING:
Ergotamine and Dihydroergotamine

Potent inhibitors of CYP3A4 can raise ergotamine to dangerous levels, posing a risk for intense vasospasm. Cerebral and/or peripheral ischemia can result. Accordingly, concurrent use with CYP3A4 inhibitors is contraindicated.

SUMMARY OF KEY PRESCRIBING CONSIDERATIONS

Ergot Alkaloids

Therapeutic Goal: Termination of migraine or cluster headache.
Baseline Data: Assess for possible underlying causes of headaches including severe hypertension, hyperthyroidism, tumors, or infection.
Monitoring: No laboratory monitoring is necessary with this medication class.
Identifying High-Risk Patients: Ergot alkaloids are contraindicated in patients with hepatic or renal impairment, CAD, and PVD.
Evaluating Therapeutic Effects: Determine the size and frequency of doses used and the extent to which therapy has reduced the intensity and duration of attacks.
Adverse Effects: Toxicity (ergotism) can result from acute or chronic overdose. Signs include muscle pain, paresthesia, and cold extremities.

Preventive Therapy

In 2015, the American Academy of Neurology and the American Headache Society published new guidelines on the pharmacologic treatment for the prevention of migraines, the *Evidence-Based Guideline Update: Pharmacologic Treatment for Episodic Migraine Prevention in Adults.* Prophylactic therapy can reduce the frequency, intensity, and duration of migraine attacks and can improve responses to abortive drugs. Preventive treatment is indicated for patients who have frequent attacks (three or more a month), attacks that are especially severe, or attacks that do not respond adequately to abortive agents. Preferred drugs for prophylaxis include propranolol, divalproex, and amitriptyline. All three are effective and well tolerated, and with all three, the benefits take 4 to 6 weeks to develop. Major preventive agents are listed in Table 25.4.

β Blockers

β blockers are first-line drugs for migraine prevention. Of the available β blockers, *propranolol* is used most often, although *metoprolol* is now deemed to be just as effective. Treatment can reduce the number and intensity of attacks in 70% of patients. Benefits take a few weeks to develop. In addition to propranolol and metoprolol, three other β blockers—*timolol, atenolol,* and *nadolol*—can help prevent migraine

TABLE 25.4 Migraine Headache: Drugs for Preventive Therapy

Drugs	Usual Daily Dosage (mg)
β-Adrenergic Blocking Agents	
Propranolol (Inderal)	80–240
Metoprolol (Lopressor)	50–200
Antiepileptic Drugs	
Divalproex (Depakote ER)	500–1000
Topiramate (Topamax)	Initiate with 25 nightly for 1 week. Advance to 25 twice daily for additional week Third week increase to 25 a.m. and 50 p.m. Final dosing 50 PO twice daily
Tricyclic Antidepressants	
Amitriptyline (Elavil)	25–150 at bedtime
Estrogens (for Menstrually Associated Migraine)	
Estrogen gel	1.5 × 7 days starting 2 days before the expected attack
Estrogen patch (Alora, Climara, Vivelle-Dot)	0.01 daily × 7 days starting 2 days before the expected attack
Calcitonin Gene-Related Peptide Receptor Antagonist	
Erenumab (Aimovig)	70–140 SubQ every month

PO, Per os (by mouth); *subQ,* subcutaneous.

attacks. In contrast, β blockers that possess intrinsic sympathomimetic activity (e.g., acebutolol, pindolol) are *not* effective. The basic pharmacology of the β blockers is discussed in Chapter 16.

Antiepileptic Drugs

Several drugs that were developed for epilepsy can reduce migraine attacks. Proof of efficacy is strongest for divalproex (Depakote ER) and topiramate (Topamax). Gabapentin (Neurontin) and tiagabine (Gabitril) appear promising, although extensive proof of efficacy is lacking.

Divalproex. Divalproex (Depakote ER), employed first for epilepsy and later for bipolar disorder (manic-depressive illness), is now approved for prophylaxis of migraine too. The drug is a form of valproic acid (see Chapter 21). Divalproex reduces the incidence of attacks by 50% or more in 30% to 50% of patients. However, when attacks do occur, their intensity and duration are not diminished. In patients with migraine, the most common side effect is nausea. Other side effects include fatigue, weight gain, tremor, bone loss, and reversible hair loss.

▶▶ BLACK BOX WARNING

Divalproex

> Potentially fatal pancreatitis and hepatitis can occur. In addition, divalproex can cause neural tube defects in the developing fetus, and hence is contraindicated during pregnancy.

Topiramate. Topiramate (Topamax), originally developed for epilepsy, was approved for migraine prophylaxis in 2004. Benefits take several weeks to develop and appear equal to those of β blockers, tricyclic antidepressants, or divalproex. However, topiramate costs much more than these drugs. In clinical trials, topiramate reduced migraine frequency by at least 50% in 83% of adolescents and about 50% of adults. The drug also reduced the need for rescue medication. Unfortunately, side

effects are common, especially paresthesias, fatigue, and cognitive dysfunction (psychomotor slowing, word-finding difficulty, and impairment of concentration and memory). Other side effects include metabolic acidosis and moderate weight loss (owing to anorexia, nausea, and diarrhea). To minimize side effects, dosage should be low initially and then gradually increased. The basic pharmacology of topiramate is discussed in Chapter 21.

Tricyclic Antidepressants

Tricyclic antidepressants can prevent migraine and tension-type headaches in some patients. The underlying mechanism has not been established but may involve inhibiting reuptake of serotonin, making more of the transmitter available for action. The tricyclic agent used most often is *amitriptyline* (Elavil). Because amitriptyline is effective in patients who are not depressed, it would seem that benefits do not depend on elevation of mood. Like other tricyclic antidepressants, amitriptyline can cause hypotension and anticholinergic effects (dry mouth, constipation, urinary retention, blurred vision, tachycardia). Excessive doses can cause dysrhythmias. The basic pharmacology of amitriptyline is discussed in Chapter 27.

Estrogens and Triptans for Menstrually Associated Migraine

Menstrually associated migraine is defined as migraine that routinely occurs within 2 days of the onset of menses. An important trigger is the decline in estrogen levels that precedes menstruation. For many women, menstrually associated migraine can be prevented by taking estrogen supplements, which compensate for the premenstrual estrogen drop. Topical preparations—estrogen gel and estrogen patches (e.g., Divigel, Climara)—work well.

Perimenstrual triptans can also help. For example, frovatriptan, naratriptan, and zolmitriptan can reduce the frequency, intensity, and duration of menstrually associated migraine. Dosing is done for 6 days each month, beginning 2 days before the expected onset of menses.

In addition, naproxen sodium at a dosage of 550 mg twice daily, given 6 days before to 7 days after menses, has demonstrated effectiveness in the prevention of migraine.

Other Drugs for Prophylaxis

Erenumab: a calcitonin gene-related peptide receptor antagonist. In 2018, the FDA approved a new human immunoglobulin G2 monoclonal antibody, erenumab (Aimovig), for the prevention of migraine headache. This antibody binds to, and antagonizes the function of, the CGRP receptors, and is thought to play an important role in the development of migraine headache, as mentioned above under pathophysiology. Monoclonal antibodies are discussed in further detail in Chapter 84.

Pharmacokinetics. Bioavailability after subcutaneous injection is about 82%. In low concentrations, erenumab undergoes elimination mainly through binding to the receptor target. At higher concentrations, it is degraded through a nonspecific proteolytic pathway. Because the drug is administered once monthly, the half-life is long—about 28 days. Erenumab appears safe to use in patients with renal and hepatic impairment.

Adverse effects. Erenumab is a subcutaneous injection, and the most common adverse effect is injection site reaction. Constipation and muscle cramping were also reported in the study population. As with other monoclonal antibodies, there exists the risk of antibody formation to the treatment. In patients receiving 70 mg and 140 mg once monthly, the incidence of anti-erenumab antibody formation was 6.2% and 2.6%, respectively.

Botulinum toxin. Injections of botulinum toxin A (Botox) are approved for the prevention of headaches in adults with chronic migraine (defined as having 15 or more headache days per month), but not for patients with less frequent headaches. Treatment consists of 31 injections, made into muscles of the scalp, neck, and upper back. The treatment is expensive, and the benefits are modest: on average, patients experience about two fewer headache days a month.

BLACK BOX WARNING
Botulinum Toxin

> Botulinum toxin can spread from the site of injection and produce muscle weakness, difficulty with respiration, and swallowing difficulties that can be life threatening.

CLUSTER HEADACHES

Characteristics

Cluster headaches occur in a series or "cluster" of attacks. Each attack lasts 15 minutes to 2 hours and is characterized by severe, throbbing, unilateral pain in the orbital-temporal area (i.e., near the eye). A typical cluster consists of one or two such attacks every day for 2 to 3 months. An attack-free interval of months to years separates each cluster. Along with headache, patients usually experience lacrimation, conjunctival redness, nasal congestion, rhinorrhea, ptosis (drooping eyelid), and miosis (constriction of the pupil)—all on the same side as the headache. Although related to migraine, cluster headaches differ in several ways: (1) they are not preceded by an aura, (2) they do not cause nausea and vomiting, (3) they can be more debilitating, (4) they are less common and occur mostly in males (5:1 ratio), (5) they are not associated with a family history of attacks, and (6) management is different.

Drug Therapy
Prophylaxis

Primary therapy is directed at prophylaxis. The American Headache Society produced guideleines in 2016 regarding treatment of cluster headache. These can be located at https://onlinelibrary.wiley.com/doi/epdf/10.1111/head.12866. Agents deemed probably effective by the American Headache Society include glucocorticoids (prednisone and dexamethasone), verapamil, and lithium. Suboccipital steroid injections are the only established effective treatment in the prophylaxis of cluster headache. Verapamil is a first-line agent for preventing chronic cluster headache. This drug is effective, easy to use, and safe. Lithium is considered a second-line drug for prophylaxis. The drug is effective but can cause multiple adverse effects, and dosing is difficult. To ensure therapeutic effects and to minimize toxicity, blood levels of lithium must be monitored; the target range is 0.4 to 0.8 mEq/L. With all of these drugs, prophylactic therapy should be limited to the cluster cycle and then discontinued when the current cycle is over. Drugs for prophylaxis are listed in Table 25.5.

Treatment

If an attack occurs despite preventive therapy, it can be aborted with sumatriptan or oxygen. Sumatriptan (6 mg subQ) is the treatment of choice for cluster headaches. Inhaling 100% oxygen (7 to 10 L/min for 15 to 20 minutes) is also highly effective and has virtually no adverse effects. In the past, ergot preparations (e.g., intravenous dihydroergotamine, sublingual ergotamine) were commonly used. However, their use today is limited because modern trials are small in population and lack evidence that these drugs work any better at relieving cluster headaches than placebo.

TABLE 25.5 Drugs Used for Prophylaxis of Cluster Headache

Drug[a]	Usual Daily Dosage (mg)
Calcium Channel Blockers	
Verapamil (Calan, others)	240–420
Neurostabilizers	
Divalproex (Depakote)	500–1500
Lithium (Lithobid)	600–1200[b]
Topiramate (Topamax)	50–200
Nonsteroidal Antiinflammatory Drugs	
Indomethacin	100–150
Naproxen	1000–1500
Glucocorticoids	
Dexamethasone	8
Prednisone	40–80
Ergot Alkaloids	
Ergotamine	1.2

[a]None of the drugs listed is approved by the FDA for cluster headache prophylaxis.
[b]Dosage is adjusted on the basis of serum lithium levels.

MEDICATION OVERUSE HEADACHE

MOH is a chronic headache that develops in response to frequent use of headache medicines and that resolves days to weeks after the overused drug is withdrawn. The stage for MOH is set when headache drugs are taken too often, especially if the dosage is high. Discontinuing the medication brings on the MOH, which causes the patient to resume taking medicine—setting up a repeating cycle of MOH, followed by medication use and discontinuation, followed by another MOH, and so on. One reason the cycle gets established is that patients do not realize that the drugs they are taking to *treat* headache can, if taken too often, become the *cause* of headache. Failing to recognize MOH for what it is, patients take more and more medicine to make their headaches go away, but only succeed in making MOH worse.

Almost all of the medicines used for abortive headache therapy can cause MOH: analgesics (aspirin-like drugs, opioids), triptans, ergotamine (but not dihydroergotamine), and caffeine.

The treatment for MOH is to stop taking all headache medicines. Unfortunately, when medication is withdrawn, headaches increase for a while. Their duration and intensity depend on the drug that was overused. With triptans, withdrawal headaches are relatively mild and often resolve in a few days. In contrast, with analgesics or ergots, withdrawal headaches are more intense and may persist for 2 weeks or more.

Several measures can *decrease the risk* for developing MOH. The most important is to limit the use of abortive medicines. If possible, patients should take these drugs no more than 2 or 3 times a week—and doses should be no higher than actually needed. Alternating headache medicines may help, too, because this would limit exposure to any one drug. If headaches begin to occur more than two or three times a month, prophylactic therapy should be tried. Implementing nondrug measures—stress reduction, avoidance of triggers, getting sufficient sleep, relaxation techniques, and biofeedback—can reduce the need for headache medicines and decrease exposure to drugs that cause MOH.

26

Antipsychotic Agents and Their Use in Schizophrenia

Antipsychotic agents are a chemically diverse group of compounds used for a broad spectrum of psychotic disorders. Specific indications include schizophrenia, delusional disorders, bipolar disorder, depressive psychoses, and drug-induced psychoses. As a rule, antipsychotics should not be used to treat dementia-related psychosis in older adults, owing to a risk for increased mortality.

Since their introduction in the early 1950s, the antipsychotic agents have catalyzed revolutionary change in the management of psychotic illnesses. Before these drugs were available, psychoses were largely untreatable and patients were fated to a life of institutionalization. With the advent of antipsychotic medications, many patients with schizophrenia and other severe psychotic disorders have been able to leave psychiatric hospitals and return to the community. Others have been spared hospitalization entirely. For those who must be institutionalized, antipsychotic drugs have at least reduced suffering.

The antipsychotic drugs fall into two major groups: (1) *first-generation antipsychotics* (FGAs), also known as *conventional antipsychotics*; and (2) *second-generation antipsychotics* (SGAs), also known as *atypical antipsychotics*. Both groups are equally effective. All of the FGAs produce a strong blockade of dopamine in the central nervous system (CNS). As a result, they all can cause serious movement disorders, known as *extrapyramidal symptoms* (EPSs). The SGAs produce a moderate blockade of receptors for dopamine and a much stronger blockade of receptors for serotonin. Because dopamine receptor blockade is only moderate, the risk for EPSs is lower than with the FGAs. However, although the SGAs carry a reduced risk for EPSs, they carry a significant risk of *metabolic effects*—weight gain, diabetes, and dyslipidemia—that can cause cardiovascular events and early death.

SCHIZOPHRENIA: CLINICAL PRESENTATION AND ETIOLOGY

Clinical Presentation

Schizophrenia is a chronic psychotic illness characterized by disordered thinking and a reduced ability to comprehend reality. Symptoms usually emerge during adolescence or early adulthood. In the United States about 2.2 million people are affected.

Three Types of Symptoms

Symptoms of schizophrenia can be divided into three groups: positive symptoms, negative symptoms, and cognitive symptoms. Positive and negative symptoms are shown in Table 26.1.

PROTOTYPE DRUGS

Antipsychotic Agents

Traditional (First Generation) Antipsychotics
Chlorpromazine (a low-potency agent)
Haloperidol (a high-potency agent)

Atypical (Second Generation) Antipsychotic
Clozapine

Positive symptoms and negative symptoms. Positive symptoms can be viewed as an exaggeration or distortion of normal function, whereas negative symptoms can be viewed as a loss or diminution of normal function. Positive symptoms include hallucinations, delusions, agitation, tension, and paranoia. Negative symptoms include lack of motivation, poverty of speech, blunted affect, poor self-care, and social withdrawal. Positive and negative symptoms respond equally to FGAs and SGAs.

Cognitive symptoms. Cognitive symptoms include disordered thinking, reduced ability to focus attention, and prominent learning and memory difficulties. Subtle changes may appear years before symptoms become florid, when thinking and speech may be completely incomprehensible to others. Cognitive symptoms may respond equally to FGAs and SGAs.

Acute Episodes

During an acute schizophrenic episode, delusions (fixed false beliefs) and hallucinations are frequently prominent. Delusions are typically religious, grandiose, or persecutory. Auditory hallucinations, which are more common than visual hallucinations, may consist of voices arguing or commenting on one's behavior. The patient may feel controlled by external influences. Disordered thinking and loose association may render rational conversation impossible. Affect may be blunted or labile. Misperception of reality may result in hostility and lack of cooperation. Impaired self-care skills may leave the patient disheveled and dirty. Patterns of sleeping and eating are usually disrupted.

Residual Symptoms

After florid symptoms (e.g., hallucinations, delusions) of an acute episode remit, less vivid symptoms may remain. These include suspiciousness, poor anxiety management, and diminished judgment, insight, motivation, and capacity for self-care. As a result, patients frequently find it difficult

TABLE 26.1   Positive and Negative Symptoms of Schizophrenia

Positive symptoms	Hallucinations
	Delusions
	Disordered thinking
	Disorganized speech
	Combativeness
	Agitation
	Paranoia
Negative symptoms	Social withdrawal
	Emotional withdrawal
	Lack of motivation
	Poverty of speech
	Blunted affect
	Poor insight
	Poor judgment
	Poor self-care

to establish close relationships, maintain employment, and function independently in society. Suspiciousness and poor anxiety management contribute to social withdrawal. The inability to appreciate the need for continued drug therapy may cause nonadherence, resulting in relapse and perhaps hospital readmission.

Long-Term Course

The long-term course of schizophrenia is characterized by episodic acute exacerbations separated by intervals of partial remission. As the years pass, some patients experience progressive decline in mental status and social functioning. However, many others stabilize, or even improve. Maintenance therapy with antipsychotic drugs reduces the risk for acute relapse but may fail to prevent long-term deterioration.

Etiology

Although there is strong evidence that schizophrenia has a biologic basis, the exact etiology is unknown. Genetic, perinatal, neurodevelopmental, and neuroanatomic factors may all be involved. Possible primary defects include excessive activation of CNS receptors for dopamine and insufficient activation of CNS receptors for glutamate. Although psychosocial stressors can precipitate acute exacerbations in susceptible patients, they are not considered causative.

FIRST-GENERATION (CONVENTIONAL) ANTIPSYCHOTICS

The FGAs have been in use for decades, and their pharmacology is well understood. Accordingly, it seems appropriate to begin with these drugs, even though their use has greatly declined. Because the pharmacology of the FGAs and SGAs is very similar, when you understand the FGAs, you will know a great deal about the SGAs as well.

Group Properties

In this section we discuss pharmacologic properties shared by all FGAs. Much of our attention focuses on adverse effects. Of these, extrapyramidal side effects are of particular concern. Because of these neurologic side effects, the FGAs are also known as *neuroleptics*.

Classification

The FGAs can be classified by potency or chemical structure. From a clinical viewpoint, classification by potency is more helpful.

Classification by potency. FGAs can be classified as *low potency, medium potency,* or *high potency* (Table 26.2). The low-potency drugs, represented by chlorpromazine, and the high-potency drugs, represented by haloperidol, are of particular interest.

It is important to note that, although the FGAs differ from one another in potency, they all have the same ability to relieve symptoms of psychosis. Recall that the term *potency* refers only to the size of the dose needed to elicit a given response; potency implies nothing about the maximal effect a drug can produce. Hence when we say that haloperidol is more potent than chlorpromazine, we only mean that the dose of haloperidol required to relieve psychotic symptoms is smaller than the required dose of chlorpromazine. We do not mean that haloperidol can produce greater effects. When administered in therapeutically equivalent doses, both drugs elicit an equivalent antipsychotic response.

If low-potency and high-potency neuroleptics are equally effective, why distinguish between them? The answer is that, although these agents produce identical *antipsychotic* effects, they differ significantly in *side effects*. Hence by knowing the potency category to which a particular neuroleptic belongs, we can better predict its undesired responses. This knowledge is useful in drug selection and providing patient care and education.

Chemical classification. The FGAs fall into four major chemical categories (Table 26.3). One of these categories, the phenothiazines, has three subgroups. Drugs in all groups are equivalent with respect to antipsychotic actions, and hence chemical classification is not emphasized in this chapter.

Two chemical categories—*phenothiazines* and *butyrophenones*—deserve attention. The phenothiazines were the first modern antipsychotic agents. Chlorpromazine, our prototype of the low-potency neuroleptics, belongs to this family. The butyrophenones stand out because they are the family to which haloperidol belongs. Haloperidol is the prototype of the high-potency FGAs.

Mechanism of Action

The FGAs block a variety of receptors within and outside the CNS. To varying degrees, they block receptors for dopamine, acetylcholine, histamine, and norepinephrine. There is little question that blockade at these receptors is responsible for the major *adverse effects* of the antipsychotics. However, because the etiology of psychotic illness is unclear, the relationship of receptor blockade to *therapeutic effects* can only be guessed. The current dominant theory suggests that FGA drugs suppress symptoms of psychosis by blocking dopamine$_2$ (D$_2$) receptors in the mesolimbic area of the brain. In support of this theory is the observation that all of the FGAs produce a D$_2$ receptor blockade. Furthermore, there is a close correlation between the clinical potency of these drugs and their potency as D$_2$ receptor antagonists.

Therapeutic Use: Schizophrenia

Schizophrenia is the primary indication for antipsychotic drugs. These agents effectively suppress symptoms during acute psychotic episodes and, when taken chronically, can greatly reduce the risk for relapse. Initial effects may be seen in 1 to 2 days, but substantial improvement usually takes 2 to 4 weeks, and full effects may not develop for several months. Positive symptoms may respond somewhat better than negative symptoms or cognitive dysfunction. All of the FGA agents are equally effective, although individual patients may respond better to one FGA than to another. Consequently, selection among these drugs is based primarily on their side effect profiles, rather than on therapeutic effects. It must be noted that antipsychotic drugs do not alter the underlying pathology of schizophrenia. Hence treatment is not curative—it offers only symptomatic relief. The management of schizophrenia is discussed later in the chapter.

TABLE 26.2 Antipsychotic Drugs: Relative Potency and Incidence of Selected Side Effects

INCIDENCE OF SIDE EFFECTS

Drug	Trade Name	Equivalent Oral Dose (mg)[a]	Extrapyramidal Effects[b]	Sedation	Orthostatic Hypotension	Anticholinergic Effects	Metabolic Effects: Weight Gain, Diabetes Risk, Dyslipidemia	Significant QT Prolongation	Prolactin Elevation	Metabolized by CYP3A4
First-Generation (Conventional) Antipsychotics										
Low Potency										
Chlorpromazine	generic only	100	Moderate	High	High	Moderate	Moderate	Yes	Low	—
Thioridazine	generic only	100	Low	High	High	High	Moderate	Yes	Low	—
Medium Potency										
Loxapine	Loxitane	13	Moderate	Moderate	Low	Low	Low	No	Moderate	—
Perphenazine	generic only	8	Moderate	Moderate	Low	Low	—	No	Low	—
High Potency										
Fluphenazine	generic only	1	Very high	Low	Low	Low	—	No	Moderate	—
Haloperidol	Haldol	2	Very high	Low	Low	Low	Moderate	Yes	Moderate	—
Pimozide	Orap	1	High	Moderate	Low	Moderate	—	Yes	Moderate	—
Thiothixene	Navane	2	High	Low	Moderate	Low	Moderate	No	Moderate	—
Trifluoperazine	generic only	2	High	Low	Low	Low	—	No	Moderate	—
Second-Generation (Atypical) Antipsychotics										
Aripiprazole	Abilify	2	Very low	Low	Low	None	None/low	No	Low	Yes
Asenapine	Saphris	4	Moderate	Moderate	Moderate	Low	Low	Yes	Low	Slightly
Brexpiprazole	Rexulti	2	Very low	Very low	Low	None	Low	No	Low	Yes
Cariprazine	Vraylar	1.5	Very low	Moderate	Low	Low	Moderate	No	No	Yes
Clozapine	Clozaril, FazaClo, Versacloz	75	Very low	High	Moderate	High	High	No	Low	Yes
Iloperidone	Fanapt	4	Very low	Moderate	Moderate	Moderate	Moderate	Yes	Low	Yes
Lurasidone	Latuda	10	Moderate	Moderate	Low	None	None/low	No	Low	Yes
Olanzapine	Zyprexa	3	Low	Moderate	Moderate	Moderate	High	No	Low	No
Paliperidone	Invega	2	Moderate	Low	Low	None	Moderate	Yes	High	Slightly
Quetiapine	Seroquel	95	Very low	Moderate	Moderate	None	Moderate/high	Yes	Low	Yes
Risperidone	Risperdal	1	Moderate	Low	Low	None	Moderate	No	High	No
Ziprasidone	Geodon, Zeldox	20	Low	Moderate	Moderate	None	None/low	Yes	Low	Yes

[a]Doses listed are the therapeutic equivalent of 100 mg of oral chlorpromazine.
[b]Incidence here refers to *early* extrapyramidal reactions (acute dystonia, parkinsonism, akathisia). The incidence of *late* reactions (tardive dyskinesia) is the same for all traditional antipsychotics.

TABLE 26.3 Antipsychotic Drugs: Preparations and Dosages

Chemical Group and Generic Name	Trade Name	Availability	Usual Total Daily Dose for Schizophrenia (mg)[a]
Phenothiazine: Aliphatic			
Chlorpromazine	generic only	10-, 25-, 50-, 100-, 200-mg tablets	200–1000
Phenothiazine: Piperidine			
Thioridazine	generic only	10-, 25-, 50-, 100-mg tablets 100-mg/mL solution	200–800
Phenothiazine: Piperazine			
Fluphenazine	generic only	1-, 2.5-, 5-, 10-mg tablets 2.5-mg/mL elixir 5-mg/mL oral concentrate	5–20
Perphenazine	generic only	2-, 4-, 8-, 16-mg tablets	12–64
Trifluoperazine	generic only	1-, 2-, 5-, 10-mg tablets	15–40
Thioxanthene			
Thiothixene	generic only	1-, 2-, 5-, 10-mg capsules	15–50
Butyrophenone			
Haloperidol	Haldol	0.5-, 1-, 2-, 5-, 10-, 20-mg tablets	6–40
Dibenzoxazepine			
Loxapine	Loxitane	5-, 10-, 25-, 50-mg capsules	30–100
Aripiprazole	Abilify	2-, 5-, 10-, 15-, 20-, 30-mg tablets 1-mg/mL oral solution 10-, 15-mg orally disintegrating tablets	10–30
Asenapine	Saphris	2.5-, 5-, 10-mg sublingual tablets	5–10
Brexpiprazole	Rexulti	0.25-, 0.5-, 1-, 2-, 3-, 4-mg tablets	2–3
Cariprazine	Vraylar	1.5-, 3-, 4.5-, 6-mg capsules	1.5–6
Clozapine	Clozaril, FazaClo, Versacloz	12.5-, 25-, 50-, 100-, 200-mg tablets 50-mg/mL oral suspension 12.5-, 25-, 100-, 150-, 200-mg orally disintegrating tablets	150–600
Iloperidone	Fanapt	1-, 2-, 4-, 6-, 8-, 10-, 12-mg tablets	12–24
Lurasidone	Latuda	20-, 40-, 60-, 80-, 120-mg tablets	40–160
Olanzapine	Zyprexa	2.5-, 5-, 7.5-, 10-, 15-, 20-mg tablets 5-, 10-, 15-, 20-mg orally disintegrating tablets	5–20
Paliperidone	Invega	1.5-, 3-, 6-, 9-mg extended release tablets	3–12
Quetiapine	Seroquel	25-, 50-, 100-, 200-, 300-, 400-mg immediate release tablets 50-, 150-, 200-, 300-, 400- mg extended-release tablets	300–800
Risperidone	Risperdal	0.25-, 0.5-, 1-, 2-, 3-, 4-mg film-coated tablets 1-mg/mL oral solution 0.5-, 1-, 2-, 3-, 4-mg orally disintegrating tablets	2–8
Ziprasidone	Geodon, Zeldox	20-, 40-, 60-, 80-mg capsules	20–160

[a]Higher doses may be given for acute symptom management or in patients with refractory symptoms.

Adverse Effects

The antipsychotic drugs block several kinds of receptors and produce an array of side effects, including a variety of undesired effects. However, these drugs are generally very safe; death from overdose is practically unheard of. Among the many side effects FGAs can produce, the most troubling are the extrapyramidal reactions—especially tardive dyskinesia (TD).

Extrapyramidal symptoms. EPSs are movement disorders resulting from effects of antipsychotic drugs on the extrapyramidal motor system. The extrapyramidal system is the same neuronal network whose malfunction is responsible for the movement disorders of Parkinson disease (PD). Although the exact cause of EPSs is unclear, blockade of D_2 receptors is strongly suspected.

Four types of EPS occur. They differ with respect to time of onset and management. Three of these reactions—acute dystonia, parkinsonism, and akathisia—occur early in therapy and can be managed with a variety of drugs. The fourth reaction—TD—occurs late in therapy and has no satisfactory treatment. Characteristics of EPSs are shown in Table 26.4.

TABLE 26.4 Extrapyramidal Side Effects of Antipsychotic Drugs

Type of Reaction	Time of Onset	Features	Management
Early Reactions			
Acute dystonia	A few hours to 5 days	Spasm of muscles of tongue, face, neck, and back; opisthotonus	Anticholinergic drugs (e.g., benztropine) IM or IV
Parkinsonism	5–30 days	Bradykinesia, mask-like facies, tremor, rigidity, shuffling gait, drooling, cogwheeling, stooped posture	Anticholinergics (e.g., benztropine, diphenhydramine), amantadine, or both. For severe symptoms, switch to a second-generation antipsychotic.
Akathisia	5–60 days	Compulsive, restless movement; symptoms of anxiety, agitation	Reduce dosage or switch to a low-potency antipsychotic. Treat with a benzodiazepine, β blocker, or anticholinergic drug
Late Reaction			
Tardive dyskinesia	Months to years	Oral-facial dyskinesias, choreoathetoid movements	Best approach is prevention; no reliable treatment. Discontinue all anticholinergic drugs. Give benzodiazepines. Reduce antipsychotic dosage. For severe TD, switch to a second-generation antipsychotic

IM, Intramuscular; *IV*, intravenous; *TD*, tardive dyskinesia.

The *early* reactions occur *less frequently* with *low-potency* agents (e.g., chlorpromazine) than with high-potency agents (e.g., haloperidol). In contrast, the risk for TD is equal with all FGAs.

For many patients, EPSs are uncomfortable, disturbing, and sometimes dangerous. Some manifestations of EPSs, such as TD, are irreversible. It is crucial to monitor patients treated with antipsychotic medications for evidence of EPSs.

Acute dystonia. Acute dystonia can be both disturbing and dangerous. The reaction develops within the first few days of therapy and frequently within hours of the first dose. Typically, the patient develops severe spasm of the muscles of the tongue, face, neck, or back. Oculogyric crisis (involuntary upward deviation of the eyes) and opisthotonus (tetanic spasm of the back muscles causing the trunk to arch forward while the head and lower limbs are thrust backward) may also occur. Severe cramping can cause joint dislocation. Laryngeal dystonia can impair respiration.

Intense dystonia is a crisis that requires rapid intervention. Initial treatment consists of an anticholinergic medication (e.g., benztropine, diphenhydramine) administered by the intramuscular (IM) or intravenous (IV) route. As a rule, symptoms resolve within 5 minutes of IV dosing and within 15 to 20 minutes of IM dosing.

It is important to differentiate between acute dystonia and psychotic hysteria. Misdiagnosis of acute dystonia as hysteria could result in giving bigger antipsychotic doses, thereby causing the acute dystonia to become even worse.

Parkinsonism. Antipsychotic-induced parkinsonism is characterized by bradykinesia, mask-like facies, drooling, tremor, rigidity, shuffling gait, cogwheeling, and stooped posture. Symptoms develop within the first month of therapy and are indistinguishable from those of idiopathic PD.

Neuroleptics cause parkinsonism by blocking dopamine receptors in the striatum. Because idiopathic PD is also due to reduced activation of striatal dopamine receptors (see Chapter 19), it is no wonder that PD and neuroleptic-induced parkinsonism share the same symptoms.

Neuroleptic-induced parkinsonism is treated with some of the drugs used for idiopathic PD. Specifically, centrally acting *anticholinergic drugs* (e.g., benztropine, diphenhydramine) and *amantadine* (Symmetrel) may be employed. Levodopa and direct dopamine agonists (e.g., bromocriptine) should be avoided because these drugs activate dopamine receptors

and might thereby counteract the beneficial effects of antipsychotic treatment.

Use of antiparkinsonism drugs should not continue indefinitely. Antipsychotic-induced parkinsonism tends to resolve spontaneously, usually within months of its onset. Accordingly, antiparkinsonism drugs should be withdrawn after a few months to determine whether they are still needed.

If parkinsonism is severe, switching to an SGA is likely to help. As discussed later, the risk for parkinsonism with SGAs is much lower than with FGAs.

Akathisia. Akathisia is characterized by pacing and squirming brought on by an uncontrollable need to be in motion. This profound sense of restlessness can be very disturbing. The syndrome usually develops within the first 2 months of treatment. Like other early EPSs, akathisia occurs most frequently with high-potency FGAs.

Three types of drugs have been used to suppress symptoms: *β blockers, benzodiazepines,* and *anticholinergic drugs.* Although these drugs can help, reducing antipsychotic dosage or switching to a low-potency FGA may be more effective.

It is important to differentiate between akathisia and exacerbation of psychosis. If akathisia were to be confused with anxiety or psychotic agitation, it is likely that antipsychotic dosage would be increased, thereby making akathisia more intense.

Tardive dyskinesia. TD, the most troubling EPS, develops in about 5.5% of patients during long-term therapy with FGAs. The risk is related to the duration of treatment and the dosage size. For many patients, symptoms are irreversible.

TD is characterized by involuntary choreoathetoid (twisting, writhing, worm-like) movements of the tongue and face. Patients may also present with lip-smacking movements, and their tongues may flick out in a "fly catching" motion. One of the earliest manifestations of TD is slow, worm-like movement of the tongue. Involuntary movements that involve the tongue and mouth can interfere with chewing, swallowing, and speaking. Eating difficulties can result in malnutrition and weight loss. Over time, TD produces involuntary movements of the limbs, toes, fingers, and trunk. For some patients, symptoms decline after a dosage reduction or drug withdrawal. For others, TD is irreversible.

The cause of TD is complex and not completely understood. One theory suggests that symptoms result from excessive *activation* of dopamine receptors. It is postulated that, in response to chronic receptor blockade, dopamine receptors of the extrapyramidal system undergo a functional change such that their sensitivity to activation is increased. Stimulation of these "supersensitive" receptors produces an imbalance in favor of dopamine and thereby produces abnormal movement. In support of this theory is the observation that symptoms of TD can be reduced (temporarily) by *increasing* antipsychotic dosage, which increases dopamine receptor blockade. (Because symptoms eventually return even though antipsychotic dosage is kept high, dosage elevation cannot be used to treat TD.)

Until recently, there were no pharmaceutical options for the management of TD. In 2017, the U.S. Food and Drug Administration approved valbenazine (Ingrezza) for the treatment of TD in adults. Shortly following valbenazine approval, deutetrabenazine (Austedo) was approved for TD as well as chorea associated with Huntington disease. Both drugs are vesicular monoamine transporter 2 (VMAT2) inhibitors.

The VMAT2 transporters recycle dopamine and return it back to presynaptic vesicles, thus getting dopamine ready for re-release into the synaptic space and protecting it from degradation by monoamine oxidase. Although the true mechanism of action of VMAT2 inhibitors is not fully understood, it is thought that by blocking these transporters, dopamine is not stored in the vesicles, leaving it to be broken down by monoamine oxidase. Said more simply, there is now less dopamine available to interact with overly sensitive dopamine receptors.

In clinical trials, both drugs significantly reduced abnormal, involuntary movements associated with TD. Although a reduction in TD severity was achieved, these drugs are not curative and produce their own side effects.

Valbenazine and deutetrabenazine both cause QT prolongation and somnolence. They should be avoided in patients taking other QT prolonging drugs or those with known QT prolongation. In addition, VMAT2 inhibitors should be used with caution in patients taking monoamine oxidase inhibitors or drugs that inhibit the CYP2D6 pathway.

In addition to these new drugs, measures that may be tried to manage TD include gradually withdrawing anticholinergic drugs, giving benzodiazepines, and reducing the dosage of the offending FGA. For patients with severe TD, switching to an SGA may help because SGAs are less likely to promote TD.

Although newer treatments are available, prevention remains the best approach. Antipsychotic drugs should be used in the lowest effective dosage for the shortest time required. After 12 months, the need for continued therapy should be assessed. If drug use must continue, a neurologic evaluation should be done at least every 3 months to detect early signs of TD. For patients with chronic schizophrenia, dosage should be tapered periodically (at least annually) to determine the need for continued treatment.

Other adverse effects

Neuroleptic malignant syndrome. Neuroleptic malignant syndrome (NMS) is a rare but serious reaction that carries a 4% risk for mortality—down from 30% in the past, thanks to early diagnosis and intervention. Primary symptoms are "lead pipe" rigidity, sudden high fever (temperature may exceed 41°C), sweating, and autonomic instability, manifested as dysrhythmias and fluctuations in blood pressure. The patient's level of consciousness may rise and fall, they may appear confused or mute, and seizures or coma may develop. Death can result from respiratory failure, cardiovascular collapse, dysrhythmias, and other causes. NMS is more likely with high-potency FGAs than with low-potency FGAs.

Treatment consists of supportive measures, drug therapy, and immediate withdrawal of antipsychotic medication. Hyperthermia should be controlled with cooling blankets and antipyretics (e.g., aspirin, acetaminophen). Hydration should be maintained with fluids. Benzodiazepines may relieve anxiety and help reduce blood pressure and

tachycardia. Two drugs—*dantrolene* and *bromocriptine*—may be especially helpful. Dantrolene is a direct-acting muscle relaxant (see Chapter 22). In patients with NMS, this drug reduces rigidity and hyperthermia. Bromocriptine is a dopamine receptor agonist (see Chapter 19) that may relieve CNS toxicity.

Resumption of antipsychotic therapy carries a small risk for NMS recurrence. The risk can be minimized by (1) waiting at least 2 weeks before resuming antipsychotic treatment; (2) using the lowest effective dosage; and (3) avoiding high-potency agents. If a second episode occurs, switching to an SGA may help.

Anticholinergic effects. First-generation agents produce varying degrees of muscarinic cholinergic blockade (see Table 26.2) and can elicit the full spectrum of anticholinergic responses (dry mouth, blurred vision, photophobia, urinary hesitancy, constipation, tachycardia). Patients should be informed about these responses and taught how to minimize danger and discomfort. As indicated in Table 26.2, anticholinergic effects are more likely with low-potency FGAs than with high-potency FGAs. Anticholinergic effects and their management are discussed in detail in Chapter 14.

Orthostatic hypotension. Antipsychotic drugs promote orthostatic hypotension by blocking α_1-adrenergic receptors on blood vessels. α-adrenergic blockade prevents compensatory vasoconstriction when the patient stands, thereby causing blood pressure to fall. Hypotension is more likely with low-potency FGAs than with the high-potency FGAs (see Table 26.2). Tolerance to hypotension develops in 2 to 3 months.

PATIENT EDUCATION
First Generation Antipsychotics

Patients should be informed about signs of hypotension (lightheadedness, dizziness) and advised to sit or lie down if these occur. In addition, patients should be informed that hypotension can be minimized by moving slowly when assuming an erect posture. Patients should be warned against participating in hazardous activities (e.g., driving) until sedative effects diminish.

Sedation. Sedation is common during the early days of treatment but subsides within a week or so. Neuroleptic-induced sedation is thought to result from the blockade of histamine-1 (H_1) receptors in the CNS. Daytime sedation can be minimized by giving the entire daily dose at bedtime.

Neuroendocrine effects. Antipsychotics increase levels of circulating *prolactin* by blocking the inhibitory action of dopamine on prolactin release. Elevation of prolactin levels promotes *gynecomastia* (breast growth) and *galactorrhea* in up to 57% of women. Up to 97% of women experience menstrual irregularities. Gynecomastia and galactorrhea can also occur in males. Because prolactin can promote growth of prolactin-dependent carcinoma of the breast, neuroleptics should be avoided in patients with this form of cancer. (It should be noted that, although FGAs can promote the growth of cancers that already exist, there is no evidence that FGAs actually *cause* cancer.)

Seizures. First-generation agents can reduce seizure threshold, thereby increasing the risk for seizure activity. The risk for seizures is greatest in patients with seizure disorders. These patients should be monitored, and, if loss of seizure control occurs, the dosage of their antiseizure medication must be increased.

Sexual dysfunction. First-generation agents can cause sexual dysfunction in women and men. In women, these drugs can suppress libido and impair the ability to achieve orgasm. In men, FGAs can suppress libido and cause erectile and ejaculatory dysfunction; the incidence is 25% to 60%. Drug-induced sexual dysfunction can make treatment unacceptable to sexually active patients, thereby leading to poor adherence. A reduction in dosage or switching to a high-potency FGA may reduce adverse sexual effects. Patients should be counseled about possible sexual dysfunction and encouraged to report any problems.

Agranulocytosis. Agranulocytosis is a rare but serious reaction. Among the FGAs, the risk is highest with chlorpromazine and certain other phenothiazines. Because agranulocytosis severely compromises the ability to fight infection, a white blood cell (WBC) count should be done whenever signs of infection (e.g., fever, sore throat) appear. If agranulocytosis is diagnosed, the neuroleptic should be withdrawn. Agranulocytosis will then reverse.

Severe dysrhythmias. Four FGAs—*chlorpromazine, haloperidol, thioridazine,* and *pimozide*—pose a risk for fatal cardiac dysrhythmias. The mechanism is prolongation of the QT interval, an index of cardiac function that can be measured with an electrocardiogram (ECG). Drugs that prolong the QT interval increase the risk for torsades de pointes, a dysrhythmia than can progress to fatal ventricular fibrillation. To reduce the risk for dysrhythmias, patients should undergo an ECG and serum potassium determination before treatment and periodically thereafter. In addition, they should avoid other drugs that cause QT prolongation, as well as drugs that can increase levels of these four FGAs.

▶ BLACK BOX WARNING
Antipsychotic Drugs

When used off-label to treat older adult patients with dementia-related psychosis, all antipsychotics (FGAs and SGAs) approximately double the rate of mortality. Most deaths result from heart-related events (e.g., heart failure, sudden death) or from infection (mainly pneumonia). Because antipsychotics are not approved for treating dementia-related psychosis, and because doing so increases the risk for death, such use is not recommended.

Signs of withdrawal and extrapyramidal symptoms in neonates. Neonates exposed to antipsychotic drugs (first or second generation) during the third trimester of pregnancy may experience EPSs and signs of withdrawal. Symptoms include tremor, agitation, sleepiness, difficulty feeding, severe breathing difficulty, and altered muscle tone (increased or decreased). Fortunately, the risk appears low. Neonates who present with EPSs or signs of withdrawal should be monitored. Some will recover within hours or days, but others may require prolonged hospitalization. Despite the risk to the infant, women who become pregnant should not discontinue their medication without consulting the prescriber.

PATIENT EDUCATION
Sun Exposure and Dermatitis

Patients should be warned against excessive exposure to sunlight and advised to apply a sunscreen and wear protective clothing. Handling antipsychotics can cause contact dermatitis in patients and health care workers. Dermatitis can be prevented by avoiding direct contact with these drugs.

Physical and Psychological Dependence

Development of physical and psychological dependence is rare. Patients should be reassured that addiction and dependence are not likely.

Although physical dependence is minimal, abrupt withdrawal of FGAs *can* precipitate a mild abstinence syndrome. Symptoms, which are related to chronic cholinergic blockade, include restlessness, insomnia, headache, gastric distress, and sweating. The syndrome can be avoided by withdrawing FGAs gradually.

Drug Interactions

Anticholinergic drugs. Drugs with anticholinergic properties will intensify anticholinergic responses to neuroleptics. Patients should be advised to avoid all drugs with anticholinergic actions, including antihistamines and certain over-the-counter sleep aids.

Central nervous system depressants. Neuroleptics can intensify CNS depression caused by other drugs. Patients should be warned against using alcohol and all other drugs with CNS-depressant actions (e.g., antihistamines, benzodiazepines, barbiturates).

Levodopa and direct dopamine receptor agonists. Levodopa (a drug for PD) may counteract the antipsychotic effects of neuroleptics. Conversely, neuroleptics may counteract the therapeutic effects of levodopa. These interactions occur because levodopa and neuroleptics have opposing effects on receptors for dopamine: levodopa activates dopamine receptors, whereas neuroleptics cause receptor blockade. Like levodopa, the direct dopamine receptor agonists (e.g., bromocriptine) activate dopamine receptors and hence have interactions with neuroleptics identical to those of levodopa.

Toxicity

FGAs are very safe; death by overdose is extremely rare. With chlorpromazine, for example, the therapeutic index is about 200; that is, the lethal dose is 200 times the therapeutic dose.

Overdose produces hypotension, CNS depression, and extrapyramidal reactions. Extrapyramidal reactions can be treated with antiparkinsonism drugs. Hypotension can be treated with IV fluids plus an α-adrenergic agonist (e.g., phenylephrine). There is no specific antidote to CNS depression. Excess drug should be removed from the stomach by gastric lavage. Emetics cannot be used because their effects would be blocked by the antiemetic action of the neuroleptic.

Properties of Individual Agents

All of the FGAs are equally effective at alleviating symptoms of schizophrenia, although individual patients may respond better to one FGA than to another. Differences among these agents relate primarily to side effects (see Table 26.2). Because the high-potency agents produce fewer side effects than the low-potency agents, high-potency agents are used more often.

High-Potency Agents

Compared with the low-potency FGAs, the high-potency FGAs cause more early EPSs but cause less sedation, orthostatic hypotension, and anticholinergic effects. Because they cause fewer side effects, high-potency agents are generally preferred for initial therapy.

Haloperidol

Actions and uses. Haloperidol (Haldol), a member of the *butyrophenone* family, is the prototype of the high-potency FGAs. Principal indications are schizophrenia and acute psychosis. The drug also can be used to control severe behavior problems in children (e.g., combative, explosive hyperexcitability unrelated to any immediate provocation), but only as a last resort. Haloperidol is used more than other FGAs.

Adverse effects. As indicated in Table 26.2, early extrapyramidal reactions (acute dystonia, parkinsonism, akathisia) occur frequently, whereas sedation, hypotension, and anticholinergic effects are uncommon. Note that the incidence of these reactions is opposite to that seen with the low-potency agents. However, the incidence of TD is the same as with all other FGAs. Neuroendocrine effects—galactorrhea, gynecomastia, menstrual irregularities—are seen occasionally. NMS, photosensitivity, convulsions, and impotence are rare.

Haloperidol can prolong the QT interval and hence may pose a risk for *serious dysrhythmias,* especially when given by the IV route or in high doses. The drug should be used with caution in patients with dysrhythmia risk factors, including long QT syndrome, hypokalemia or hyperkalemia, or a history of dysrhythmias, heart attack, or severe heart failure. Combined use with other QT-prolonging drugs (e.g., amiodarone, erythromycin, quinidine) should be avoided.

 ## SUMMARY OF KEY PRESCRIBING CONSIDERATIONS

First-Generation (Conventional) Antipsychotics

Therapeutic Goal: Treatment of schizophrenia: (1) suppression of acute episodes; (2) prevention of acute exacerbations; and (3) maintenance of the highest possible level of functioning.

Baseline Data: Complete blood count (CBC), electrolytes, hepatic function, cardiac function.

Monitoring: Patients with history of dysrhythmias should be monitored carefully for palpitations, QT prolongation, or electrolyte imbalances.

Identifying High-Risk Patients: First-generation antipsychotics are contraindicated in patients who are comatose or severely depressed, or in patients with Parkinson disease. All FGAs increase the risk of mortality when used to treat dementia-related psychosis in older adult patients.

Evaluating Therapeutic Effects: Improvement in psychotic symptoms, including suppression of hallucinations, delusions, agitation, and tension. Improvement in self-care, social skills and patterns of sleeping and eating.

Minimizing Adverse Effects: Avoid use with QT prolonging drugs. Have patients report symptoms of TD immediately (muscle spasm of tongue, face, neck, or back; restless movement; tremor; rigidity).

SECOND-GENERATION (ATYPICAL) ANTIPSYCHOTICS

The SGAs, also known as *atypical antipsychotics*, quickly took over 90% of the market, owing to the perception of superior efficacy and greater safety. However, neither initial perception has held up. Thanks to two large, government-sponsored studies, one in the United States and the other in Great Britain, we now know that in most cases, SGAs and FGAs are equally effective. As for major side effects, the SGAs *are* less likely to cause EPSs, including TD. However, three SGA's, clozapinem quetiapine, and olanzapine carry an even greater risk of their own, namely, serious metabolic effects—weight gain, diabetes, and dyslipidemia—that can lead to cardiovascular events and premature death. Furthermore, like the FGAs, the SGAs can cause sedation and orthostatic hypotension and can increase the risk for death when used to treat dementia-related psychosis in older adults. Finally, even though SGAs have no clear clinical advantage over FGAs, the SGAs cost 10 to 20 times as much.

In addition to their use in schizophrenia, all of the SGAs are approved for bipolar disorder (see Chapter 28).

Clozapine

Clozapine (Clozaril, FazaClo, Versacloz) was the first SGA and will serve as our prototype for the group—even though other SGAs are now used more widely. This drug is our most effective agent for schizophrenia, the only indication it has.

 ## BLACK BOX WARNING

Clozapine

Clozapine can cause life-threatening agranulocytosis. Its use should be reserved for patients who have not responded to safer alternatives.

Mechanism of Action

Antipsychotic effects result from blockade of receptors for dopamine and serotonin (5-hydroxytryptamine [5-HT]). Like the FGAs, clozapine blocks D_2 dopamine receptors, but its affinity for these receptors is relatively low. In contrast, the drug produces strong blockade of 5-HT_2 serotonin receptors. The combined blockade of D_2 receptors and 5-HT_2 receptors is thought to underlie therapeutic effects. Low affinity for D_2 receptors may explain why SGAs cause fewer EPSs than do the FGAs. In addition to blocking receptors for dopamine and serotonin, clozapine blocks receptors for norepinephrine (α_1), histamine, and acetylcholine.

Therapeutic Use

Schizophrenia. Clozapine is approved for relieving general symptoms of schizophrenia and for reducing suicidal behavior in patients with schizophrenia or schizoaffective disorder who are at chronic suicide risk. The drug is highly effective and often works when all other antipsychotics have failed. Like the FGAs, clozapine improves positive, negative, and cognitive symptoms of schizophrenia. Because the incidence of EPSs with clozapine is low, the drug is well suited for patients who have experienced severe EPSs with an FGA.

Adverse Effects and Interactions

Common adverse effects include sedation and weight gain (from blocking H_1 receptors); orthostatic hypotension (from blocking α-adrenergic receptors); and dry mouth, blurred vision, urinary retention, constipation, and tachycardia (from blocking muscarinic cholinergic receptors). Neuroendocrine effects (galactorrhea, gynecomastia, amenorrhea) and interference with sexual function are minimal. Compared with the FGAs, clozapine carries a low risk for extrapyramidal effects, including TD.

Agranulocytosis. Clozapine produces agranulocytosis in 1% to 2% of patients. The overall risk for death is about 1 in 5000. The usual cause is gram-negative septicemia. Agranulocytosis typically occurs during the first 6 months of treatment, and the onset is usually gradual. Why agranulocytosis occurs is unknown.

Because of the risk for fatal agranulocytosis, providers are required to enroll in the Clozapine REMS program prior to prescribing clozapine. Monitoring of the WBC count *and* absolute neutrophil count (ANC) is mandatory. Before starting clozapine, both the total WBC count and ANC must be in the normal range (i.e., WBC count of 3500/mm³ or greater and ANC of 2000/mm³ or greater). During treatment, the WBC count and ANC must be monitored weekly for the first 6 months, then every 2 weeks for an additional 6 months. Additional testing may be completed when considering the possibility of neutropenia, when adding other antipsychotics, or when clinically indicated. If the total WBC count falls below 3000/mm³ or if the ANC falls below 1500/mm³, treatment should be interrupted. When subsequent *daily* monitoring indicates that counts have risen above these values, clozapine can be resumed. If the total WBC count falls below 2000/mm³ or if the ANC falls below 1000/mm³, clozapine should be permanently discontinued. Blood counts should be monitored for 4 weeks after drug withdrawal.

Patients should be informed about the risk for agranulocytosis and told that clozapine will not be dispensed if the blood tests have not been done. Also, patients should be informed about early signs of infection (fever, sore throat, fatigue, mucous membrane ulceration) and instructed to report these immediately.

Metabolic effects: weight gain, diabetes, and dyslipidemia. Clozapine and the other SGAs can cause a group of closely linked metabolic effects—obesity, diabetes, and dyslipidemia—all of which increase the risk for cardiovascular events. As indicated in Table 26.2, risk is highest with clozapine and olanzapine and lowest with aripiprazole, lurasidone, and ziprasidone.

Weight gain is the metabolic effect of greatest concern because it seems to underlie development of diabetes and dyslipidemia. Antipsychotic drugs promote weight gain through the blockade of H1 receptors in the brain; they also cause a decrease in body temperature, which decreases energy expenditure. Among patients taking clozapine, weight gain can be significant. Patients should be informed about the possibility. Body mass index should be measured at baseline, at every visit for 6 months, and every 3 months thereafter. In addition, waist circumference should be measured at baseline and annually thereafter. If significant weight gain occurs, it can be managed with a combination of lifestyle measures and *metformin,* an oral drug used for diabetes. In one study, metformin was more effective than lifestyle measures, and the combination of metformin plus lifestyle measures was more effective than either intervention alone.

Clozapine and all other SGAs can cause *new-onset diabetes.* Patients taking these drugs have developed typical diabetes symptoms, including hyperglycemia, polyuria, polydipsia, polyphagia, and dehydration. In extreme cases, hyperglycemia has led to ketoacidosis, hyperosmolar coma, and even death. Because of diabetes risk, fasting blood sugar should be measured before starting clozapine, then 12 weeks later, and annually thereafter. Patients with documented diabetes at treatment onset should be monitored for worsening of glucose control. All patients should be informed about symptoms of diabetes and instructed to report them. If diabetes develops, it can be managed with insulin or an oral antidiabetic drug, such as metformin. Discontinuing clozapine is also an option. However, if the drug has produced control of psychotic symptoms, continuing clozapine and treating the diabetes would seem preferable.

Dyslipidemia associated with clozapine and other SGAs can manifest as increased total cholesterol, low-density lipoprotein (LDL) cholesterol, and triglycerides, along with decreased high-density lipoprotein (HDL) cholesterol. This lipid profile increases the risk for atherosclerosis and coronary heart disease. To monitor the effects on lipids, a fasting lipid profile should be obtained at baseline and every 6 months thereafter. A fasting lipid profile should be obtained more frequently for patients on high-risk medications, including clozapine and olanzapine.

Seizures. Generalized tonic-clonic convulsions occur in 3% of patients. The risk for seizures is dose related. Patients should be warned not to drive or to participate in other potentially hazardous activities if a seizure has occurred. Patients with a history of seizure disorders should use the drug with great caution.

Extrapyramidal symptoms. Although the risk for EPSs with SGAs is relatively low, it is not zero. Hence, like the FGAs, clozapine and other SGAs can cause parkinsonism, acute dystonia, akathisia, and TD.

BLACK BOX WARNING
Clozapine

Very rarely, clozapine has been associated with myocarditis (inflammation of the heart muscle), which can be fatal. If a patient develops signs and symptoms (e.g., unexplained fatigue, dyspnea, tachypnea, chest pain, palpitations), clozapine should be withheld until myocarditis has been ruled out. If myocarditis is diagnosed, clozapine should not be used again.

Orthostatic hypotension. Clozapine can cause orthostatic hypotension, sometimes with fainting. Rarely, collapse is severe and accompanied by respiratory or cardiac arrest, or both. Hypotension is most likely during initial dosage titration, especially if dosage escalation is rapid.

Effects in older adult patients with dementia. Like the FGAs, the SGAs approximately double the rate of mortality when used off-label to treat dementia-related psychosis in older adults. Accordingly, because SGAs are not approved for this use, and because they pose a risk to these patients, it is clear that SGAs should not be prescribed for this condition.

Drug Interactions

Because it can cause agranulocytosis, clozapine is contraindicated for patients taking other drugs that can suppress bone marrow function, including many anticancer drugs.

Drugs that induce cytochrome P450 isoenzymes (e.g., phenytoin, rifampin) can lower clozapine levels, and drugs that inhibit P450 isoenzymes (e.g., ketoconazole, erythromycin) can raise clozapine levels. These inducers and inhibitors should be used with caution.

 SUMMARY OF KEY PRESCRIBING CONSIDERATIONS
Second-Generation (Atypical) Antipsychotics

Therapeutic Goal: Treatment of schizophrenia: (1) suppression of acute episodes; (2) prevention of acute exacerbations; and (3) maintenance of the highest possible level of functioning.

Baseline Data: Patient weight, baseline glucose levels, fasting lipid levels, CBC, electrolytes, hepatic function, cardiac function.

Monitoring: Regular CBC in patients taking clozapine is mandatory to assess for agranulocytosis. Patients with a history of dysrhythmias should be monitored carefully for palpitations, QT prolongation, or electrolyte imbalances.

Identifying High-Risk Patients: Use with caution in patients with diabetes. Mortality risk is increased when used to treat dementia-related psychosis in older adult patients.

Evaluating Therapeutic Effects: Improvement in psychotic symptoms, including suppression of hallucinations, delusions, agitation, and tension. Improvement in self-care, social skills and patterns of sleeping and eating.

Minimizing Adverse Effects: Avoid use with QT prolonging drugs. Have patients report weight gain or an increase in blood glucose (in patients who monitor at home).

DEPOT ANTIPSYCHOTIC PREPARATIONS

Depot antipsychotics are long-acting, injectable formulations used for long-term maintenance therapy of schizophrenia. The objective is to prevent relapse and maintain the highest possible level of functioning. As a rule, the rate of relapse is lower with depot therapy than with oral therapy. Depot preparations are valuable for all patients who need long-term treatment—not just for patients who have difficulty with adherence. There is no evidence that depot preparations pose an increased risk for side effects, including NMS and TD. In fact, because depot therapy permits a reduction in the total drug burden (the dose per unit time is lower than with oral therapy), the risk for TD is actually reduced.

Eight depot preparations are currently available: *haloperidol decanoate* (Haldol Decanoate), *fluphenazine decanoate* (generic only), *risperidone microspheres* (Risperdal Consta), *paliperidone palmitate* (Invega Sustenna, Invega Trinza), *aripiprazole* (Abilify Maintena, Aristada), and *olanzapine pamoate* (Zyprexa Relprevv). After the injection, the active drug is slowly absorbed into the blood. Because of this slow, steady absorption, plasma levels remain relatively constant between doses. The dosing interval is 2 to 4 weeks. Typical maintenance dosages are shown in Table 26.5.

TABLE 26.5   Depot Antipsychotic Preparations

Generic Name (Trade Name)	Availability	Route	Typical Maintenance Dosage
Haloperidol decanoate (Haldol Decanoate)	50 mg/mL and 100 mg/mL	IM	50–200 mg every 4 weeks
Fluphenazine decanoate (generic only)	25 mg/mL	IM, subQ	12.5–50 mg every 2 weeks
Risperidone microspheres (Risperdal Consta)	12.5-, 25-, 37.5-, 50-mg microspheres in 2-mL diluent	IM	25–50 mg every 2 weeks
Paliperidone palmitate (Invega Sustenna)	39-, 78-, 117-, 156-, 234-mg prefilled syringes	IM	117 mg every 4 weeks
(Invega Trinza)	273-, 410-, 546-, or 819-mg prefilled syringes		273–819 mg every 12 weeks to be started after stable on Sustenna
Olanzapine pamoate (Zyprexa Relprevv)	150-mg/mL injection	IM	210–300 mg every 2 weeks or 405 mg every 4 weeks
Aripiprazole (Abilify Maintena)	300-mg/1.5 mL, 400-mg/1.5 mL single-use vials 300-, 400-mg single-use prefilled syringe	IM	400 mg every 4 weeks
Aripiprazole lauroxil (Aristada)	441-, 662-, 882-, 1064-mg single-use prefilled syringe	IM	441 mg every 4 weeks or 882 mg every 6 weeks

IM, Intramuscular; *subQ*, subcutaneous.

MANAGEMENT OF SCHIZOPHRENIA

Drug Therapy

Drug therapy of schizophrenia has three major objectives: (1) suppression of acute episodes; (2) prevention of acute exacerbations; and (3) maintenance of the highest possible level of functioning.

Drug Selection

Like all other drugs, antipsychotics should be selected on the basis of effectiveness, tolerability, and cost. Currently, SGAs are prescribed 10 times more often than FGAs, but that may change. When the SGAs were introduced, available data suggested they were more effective than FGAs and safer. However, we now know otherwise. A comparative effectiveness review compared FGAs with SGAs in the treatment of schizophrenia in adults. In 113 studies, clozapine was more effective than chlorpromazine in treating the core illness of schizophrenia. Yet when looking at functional outcomes, quality of life, and adverse events, there was no difference between the FGAs and SGAs. Regarding serious side effects, SGAs were initially thought to be safer than FGAs because SGAs pose a lower risk for EPSs. However, over time, it became clear that some SGAs posed a serious risk of their own: potentially fatal

metabolic effects. Hence rather than being *free* of serious side effects, the SGAs simply substituted a new serious effect for the old one. As for cost, FGAs are much cheaper. In summary, here's what we know:

- Most FGAs and SGAs are equally effective, except for clozapine, which is more effective than the rest.
- Whereas FGAs pose a greater risk for EPSs, SGAs pose a significant risk for metabolic effects, which may be more detrimental than EPSs.
- FGAs cost much less than SGAs.

Given this information, which drug should we choose? That's still hard to answer. With regard to efficacy and safety, no single agent is clearly superior to the others. So, we're back to our initial selection criteria: efficacy, safety, and cost. For a patient who is treatment resistant, a trial with clozapine might be reasonable. For a patient with a history of diabetes or dyslipidemia, an FGA might be a good choice, as might aripiprazole or ziprasidone—two SGAs with a low risk for metabolic effects. If there's no clinical reason to select an SGA over an FGA, cost considerations would suggest choosing an FGA.

Dosing

Dosing with antipsychotics is highly individualized. Older adult patients require relatively small doses—typically 30% to 50% of those for younger patients. Poorly responsive patients may need larger doses. However, very large doses should generally be avoided because huge doses are probably no more effective than moderate doses and will increase the risk for side effects.

Dosage size and timing are likely to change over the course of therapy. During the initial phase, antipsychotics should be administered in divided daily doses. After an effective dosage has been determined, the entire daily dose can often be given at bedtime. Because antipsychotics cause sedation, bedtime dosing helps promote sleep while decreasing daytime drowsiness. Doses used early in therapy to gain rapid control of behavior are often very high. For long-term therapy, the dosage should be reduced to the lowest effective amount.

Routes

Oral. Oral dosing is preferred for most patients. Antipsychotics are available in tablets, capsules, and liquids for oral use.

The liquid formulations require special handling. These preparations are concentrated and must be diluted before use. Dilution may be performed with a variety of fluids, including milk, fruit juices, and carbonated beverages. Some oral liquids are light sensitive and must be stored in amber or opaque containers. Liquid formulations of *phenothiazines* can cause contact dermatitis; nurses and patients should take care to avoid skin contact with these preparations.

A new oral formulation of aripiprazole, Abilify MYCITE, consists of a conventional aripiprazole tablet containing a sensor. When the tablet is ingested, it transmits a signal to a transdermal patch worn by the patient. This patch, in turn, sends data regarding date and time of ingestion to a database, including a smartphone application. This allows providers to monitor dose adherence. The phone app notifies the patient when the patch should be changed (about once weekly).

Sublingual. One SGA—asenapine (Saphris)—is administered as a sublingual tablet designed to be absorbed through the oral mucosa (to avoid first-pass hepatic metabolism). This route has the additional advantage of preventing "cheeking" because doing so will simply cause the drug to be absorbed as intended.

Intramuscular. IM injection is generally reserved for patients with severe, acute schizophrenia and for long-term maintenance. Depot preparations are given every 2 to 4 weeks (see Table 26.5).

Inhaled. Loxapine (Adasuve) is a formula used for the acute treatment of agitation associated with schizophrenia. Adasuve is available as a 10-mg inhaled powder. Only one inhalation is recommended in a 24-hour period.

Initial Therapy

With adequate dosing, symptoms begin to resolve within 1 to 2 days. However, significant improvement takes 1 to 2 weeks, and a full response may not be seen for several months.

Some symptoms resolve sooner than others. During the first week, the goal is to reduce agitation, hostility, anxiety, and tension and to normalize patterns of sleeping and eating. Over the next 6 to 8 weeks, symptoms should continue to steadily improve. The goals over this interval are increased socialization and improved self-care, mood, and formal thought processes. Of the patients who have not responded within 6 weeks, 50% are likely to respond by the end of 12 weeks.

Maintenance Therapy

Schizophrenia is a chronic disorder that usually requires prolonged treatment. The purpose of long-term therapy is to reduce the recurrence of acute florid episodes and to maintain the highest possible level of functioning. Unfortunately, although long-term treatment can be very effective, it also carries a risk for adverse effects, especially TD.

After control of an acute episode, antipsychotic therapy should continue indefinitely. Withdrawal of medication is associated with relapse. Accordingly, patients must be convinced to continue therapy even though they may be symptom free and consider themselves "cured."

When long-term therapy is conducted, dosage should be adjusted with care. To reduce the risk for TD and other adverse effects, a minimal effective dosage should be established. Annual attempts should be made to lower the dosage.

Long-acting (depot) antipsychotics are especially well suited for prolonged treatment. Depot therapy has three major advantages over oral therapy: (1) the relapse rate may be lower; (2) drug levels are more stable between doses; and (3) the total dose per unit time is lower, thereby reducing the risk for adverse effects, including TD. In the United States, only a small number of patients receive depot therapy. The low rate is due in large part to the widely held (but unfounded) perception that depot therapy is for patients who suffer recurrent relapse because of persistent nonadherence with oral therapy.

Promoting Adherence

Poor adherence is a common cause of therapeutic failure and underlies a significant proportion of hospital readmissions. Adherence can be difficult to achieve because treatment is prolonged and because patients may fail to appreciate the need for therapy, or they may be unwilling or unable to take medicine as prescribed. In addition, side effects can discourage adherence. Adherence can be enhanced in the following ways:

- Encouraging family members to oversee medication management
- Establishing a good therapeutic relationship with the patient and family
- Using an IM depot preparation (e.g., fluphenazine decanoate, haloperidol decanoate) for long-term therapy

PATIENT EDUCATION
Importance of Following Dosage Instructions

Provide patients with written and verbal instructions on dosage size and timing, and encourage them to take their medicine exactly as prescribed. Inform patients and their families that antipsychotics must be taken on a regular schedule to be effective and hence should not be used as needed. Educate patients about the side effects of treatment and teach them how to minimize undesired responses. Assure patients that antipsychotic drugs do not cause addiction.

Nondrug Therapy

Although drugs can be of great benefit in schizophrenia, medication alone does not constitute optimal treatment. The acutely ill patient needs care, support, and protection; a period of hospitalization may be essential. Counseling can offer the patient and family insight into the nature of schizophrenia and can facilitate adjustment and rehabilitation. Although conventional psychotherapy is of little value in reducing symptoms of schizophrenia, establishing a good therapeutic relationship can help promote adherence and can help the prescriber evaluate the patient, which in turn can facilitate dosage adjustment and drug selection. Behavioral therapy can help reduce stress. Vocational training in a sheltered environment offers the hope of productivity and some measure of independence. Ideally, the patient will be provided with a comprehensive therapeutic program to complement the benefits of medication. Unfortunately, ideal situations don't always exist, leaving many patients to rely on drugs as their sole treatment modality.

27

Antidepressants

Our principal focus in this chapter is drugs used to treat major depression. We begin by discussing depression itself and the basic approach to treatment. After that, we discuss the antidepressant drugs and therapies.

MAJOR DEPRESSION: CLINICAL FEATURES, PATHOGENESIS, AND TREATMENT OVERVIEW

Depression is the most common psychiatric disorder. In the United States, about 15 million adults are affected per year. The incidence in women is twice that in men. The risk for suicide among depressed people is high. Unfortunately, depression is underdiagnosed and undertreated: only 35% of depressed individuals had seen a mental health provider. This is especially sad in that treatment can help many people: about 30% of those given antidepressants achieve full remission; an additional 20% to 30% achieve at least a 50% reduction in symptom severity.

Clinical Features

The principal symptoms of major depression are depressed mood and loss of pleasure or interest in all or nearly all of one's usual activities and pastimes. Associated symptoms include insomnia (or sometimes hypersomnia); anorexia and weight loss (or sometimes hyperphagia and weight gain); mental slowing and loss of concentration; feelings of guilt, worthlessness, and helplessness; thoughts of death and suicide; and overt suicidal behavior. For a diagnosis to be made, symptoms must be present most of the day, nearly every day, for at least 2 weeks.

It is important to distinguish between major depression and normal grief or sadness. Whereas major depression is an illness, grief or sadness is not. Rather, grief and sadness are appropriate reactions to a major life stressor (e.g., death of a loved one, loss of a job). In most cases, grief and sadness resolve spontaneously over several weeks and do not require medical intervention. However, if symptoms are unusually intense, and if they fail to resolve within an appropriate time, a major depressive episode may have been superimposed. If this occurs, treatment is indicated.

Pathogenesis

The etiology of major depression is complex and incompletely understood. For some individuals, depression seems to descend "out of the blue"; otherwise healthy people—unexpectedly and without apparent cause—find themselves feeling profoundly depressed. For many others, depressive episodes are brought on by stressful life events, such as bereavement, loss of a job, or childbirth. Because depression does not occur in everyone, it would appear that some people are more vulnerable than others. Factors that may contribute to vulnerability include genetic heritage, a difficult childhood, and chronic low self-esteem.

Clinical observations made in the 1960s led to the formulation of the monoamine-deficiency hypothesis of depression, which asserts that depression is caused by a functional deficiency of monoamine neurotransmitters (norepinephrine [NE], serotonin, or both). Findings that support the hypothesis include (1) induction of depression with reserpine, a drug that depletes monoamines from the brain; (2) induction of depression with inhibitors of tyrosine hydroxylase, an enzyme needed for monoamine transmitter synthesis; and (3) relief of depression with drugs that intensify monoamine-mediated neurotransmission. Although these observations lend support to the monoamine-deficiency hypothesis, it is clear that the hypothesis is too simplistic. However, despite its shortcomings, the monoamine-deficiency hypothesis does provide a useful conceptual framework for understanding antidepressant drugs.

Treatment Overview

Depression can be treated with three major modalities: (1) pharmacotherapy, (2) depression-specific psychotherapy (e.g., cognitive behavioral therapy or interpersonal psychotherapy), and (3) somatic therapies, such as electroconvulsive therapy and transcranial magnetic stimulation. For patients with mild to moderate depression, drug therapy and psychotherapy can be equally effective. For those with more severe depression, a combination of drug therapy and psychotherapy is better than either intervention alone. Electroconvulsive therapy can be used when a rapid response is needed or when drugs and psychotherapy have not worked. For all patients, aerobic exercise and resistance training can improve mood.

PROTOTYPE DRUGS

Antidepressants

Selective Serotonin Reuptake Inhibitor
Fluoxetine

Serotonin-Norepinephrine Reuptake Inhibitor
Venlafaxine

Tricyclic Antidepressant
Imipramine

Monoamine Oxidase Inhibitor
Phenelzine

Atypical Antidepressant
Bupropion

DRUGS USED FOR DEPRESSION

Drugs are the primary therapy for major depression. However, benefits are limited mainly to patients with severe depression. In patients with mild to moderate depression, antidepressants have little or no beneficial effect.

Available antidepressants are listed in Table 27.1. As indicated, these drugs fall into five major classes: selective serotonin reuptake inhibitors (SSRIs), serotonin-norepinephrine reuptake inhibitors (SNRIs), tricyclic antidepressants (TCAs), monoamine oxidase inhibitors (MAOIs), and atypical antidepressants. All of these classes are equally effective, as are the individual drugs within each class. Hence differences among these drugs relate mainly to side effects and drug interactions.

Basic Considerations

In this section, we consider basic issues that apply to all antidepressant drugs. The information on suicide risk is especially important.

Time Course of Response

With all antidepressants, symptoms resolve slowly. Initial responses develop in 1 to 3 weeks. Maximal responses may not be seen until 12 weeks. Because therapeutic effects are delayed, antidepressants cannot be used PRN. Furthermore, a therapeutic trial should not be considered a failure until a drug has been taken for at least 1 month without success.

Drug Selection

Because all antidepressants have nearly equal efficacy, selection among them is based largely on tolerability and safety. Additional considerations are drug interactions, patient preference, and cost. The usual drugs of first choice are the SSRIs, SNRIs, bupropion, and mirtazapine. Older antidepressants—TCAs and MAOIs—have more adverse effects and are less well tolerated than the first-line agents, and hence are generally reserved for patients who have not responded to the first-line drugs.

In some cases, the side effects of a drug, when matched to the right patient, can actually be beneficial. Here are some examples:

- For a patient with fatigue, choose a drug that causes central nervous system (CNS) stimulation (e.g., fluoxetine, bupropion).

TABLE 27.1 Antidepressant Classes and Adult Dosages

Generic Name	Trade Name	Availability	Initial Dose[a,b] (mg/day)	Maintenance Dose[a] (mg/day)
Selective Serotonin Reuptake Inhibitors (SSRIs)				
Citalopram	Celexa	10-mg/5-mL oral solution 10-, 20-, 40-mg tablets	20	20–40
Escitalopram	Lexapro, Cipralex ♦	5-mg/5-mL oral solution 5-, 10-, 20-mg tablets	10	10–20
Fluoxetine	Prozac, Sarafem	20-mg/5-mL oral solution 10-, 20-, 60-mg tablets 90-mg delayed-release tablets 10-, 20-, 40-mg capsules	20	20–80
Fluvoxamine[c]	Luvox CR	25-, 50-, 100-mg tablets 100-, 150-mg controlled-release capsules	50	100–300
Paroxetine	Paxil, Pexeva	10-mg/5-mL oral solution 7.5-mg capsules 10-, 20-, 30-, 40-mg tablets 12.5-, 25-, 37.5-mg controlled-release tablets	12.5–20	20–50
Sertraline	Zoloft	20-mg/mL oral solution 25-, 50-, 100-mg tablets	50	50–200
Vortioxetine	Trintellix	5-, 10-, 20-mg tablets	10	10–20
Serotonin-Norepinephrine Reuptake Inhibitors (SNRIs)				
Desvenlafaxine	Pristiq	25-, 50-, 100-mg extended-release tablets	50	50–100
Duloxetine	Cymbalta	20-, 30-, 60-mg delayed-release tablets	40–60	60–120
Levomilnacipran	Fetzima	20-, 40-, 80-, 120-mg capsules	20 mg	40–120
Venlafaxine	Effexor XR	25-, 37.5-, 50-, 75-, 100-mg tablets 37.5-, 75-, 150-, 225-mg extended-release tablets 37.5-, 75-, 150-mg extended-release capsules	37.5–75	75–375
Tricyclic Antidepressants (TCAs)				
Amitriptyline	Generic only	10-, 25-, 50-, 75-, 100-, 125-, 150-mg tablets	25–50	100–300
Clomipramine[c]	Anafranil	25-, 50-, 75-mg tablets	25	100–250
Desipramine	Norpramin	10-, 25-, 50-, 75-, 100-, 150-mg tablets	25–50	100–300
Doxepin	Sinequan[d]	10-mg/mL oral solution 10-, 25-, 50-, 75-, 100-, 150-mg tablets	50	75–300
Imipramine	Tofranil	10-, 25-, 50-mg tablets 75-, 100-, 125-, 150-mg capsules	25–50	100–200
Maprotiline	Generic only	25-, 50-, 75-mg tablets	75	100–225
Nortriptyline	Pamelor	10-mg/5-mL oral solution 10-, 25-, 50-, 75-mg tablets	75–100	50–150
Protriptyline	Vivactil	5-, 10-mg tablets	15–40	20–60
Trimipramine	Surmontil	10-mg tablets	75–100	75–200

Continued

TABLE 27.1 Antidepressant Classes and Adult Dosages—cont'd

Generic Name	Trade Name	Availability	Initial Dose[a,b] (mg/day)	Maintenance Dose[a] (mg/day)
Monoamine Oxidase Inhibitors (MAOIs)				
Isocarboxazid	Marplan	10-mg tablets	10–20	30–60
Phenelzine	Nardil	15-mg tablets	45	60–90
Selegiline (transdermal)	Emsam	6-, 9-, 12-mg/24 h transdermal patches	6	6–12
Tranylcypromine	Parnate	10-mg tablets	10–30	30–60
Atypical Antidepressants				
Amoxapine	Generic only	25-, 50-, 100-, 150-mg tablets	100	200–400
Bupropion	Wellbutrin, others	75-, 100-mg tablets; 100-, 150-, 200-, 300-mg sustained-release tablets	200	300–450
Mirtazapine	Remeron	7.5-, 15-, 30-, 45-mg tablets; 15-, 30-, 45-mg orally disintegrating tablets	15	15–45
Nefazodone	Generic only	50-, 100-, 150-, 200-, 250-mg tablets	200	300–600
Trazodone	Generic only	50-, 100-, 150-, 300-mg tablets	150	150–600
Trazodone ER	Oleptro	150-, 300-mg extended-release tablets	150	150–375
Vilazodone	Viibryd	10-, 20-, 40-mg tablets	10	40

[a]Doses listed are total daily doses. Depending on the drug and the patient, the total dose may be given in a single dose or in divided doses.
[b]Initial doses are employed for 4 to 8 weeks, the time required for most symptoms to respond. Dosage is gradually increased as required.
[c]Fluvoxamine and clomipramine are not approved for major depression.
[d]Doxepin is also available in a low-dose formulation, sold as Silenor, for treating insomnia.

- For a patient with insomnia, choose a drug that causes substantial sedation (e.g., mirtazapine).
- For a patient with sexual dysfunction, choose bupropion, a drug that enhances libido.
- For a patient with chronic pain, choose duloxetine or a TCA, drugs that can relieve chronic pain.

Managing Treatment

After a drug has been selected for initial treatment, it should be used for 4 to 8 weeks to assess efficacy. As a rule, dosage should be low initially (to reduce side effects) and then gradually increased (see Table 27.1). If the initial drug is not effective, we have four major options:

- Increase the dosage.
- Switch to another drug in the same class.
- Switch to another drug in a different class.
- Add a second drug, such as an atypical antidepressant.

After symptoms are in remission, treatment should continue for at least 4 to 9 months to prevent relapse. To this end, patients should be encouraged to take their drugs, even if they are symptom free and hence feel that continued dosing is unnecessary. When antidepressant therapy is discontinued, dosage should be gradually tapered over several weeks because abrupt withdrawal can trigger withdrawal symptoms.

▶▶ BLACK BOX WARNING

Suicide Risk With Antidepressant Drugs

Patients with depression often think about or attempt suicide. During treatment with antidepressants, especially early on, the risk for suicide may actually increase. Concerns about antidepressant-induced suicide apply mainly to children, adolescents, and adults younger than 25 years.

To reduce the risk for suicide, patients taking antidepressant drugs should be observed closely for suicidality, worsening mood, and unusual changes in behavior. Close observation is especially important during the first few months of therapy and whenever antidepressant dosage is changed (either increased or decreased). Ideally, the patient or caregiver should meet with the prescriber at least weekly during the first 4 weeks of treatment, then biweekly for the next 4 weeks, then once 1 month later, and periodically thereafter. Phone contact may be appropriate between visits. In addition, family members or caregivers should monitor the patient daily, being alert for symptoms of decline (e.g., anxiety, agitation, panic attacks, insomnia, irritability, hostility, impulsivity, hypomania, and, of course, emergence of suicidality). If these symptoms are severe or develop abruptly, the patient should see his or her prescriber immediately.

Because antidepressant drugs can be used to commit suicide, prescriptions should be written for the smallest number of doses consistent with good patient management. What should be done if suicidal thoughts emerge during drug therapy, or if depression is persistently worse while taking drugs? One option is to switch to another antidepressant. However, as noted, the risk for suicidality appears equal with all antidepressants. Another option is to stop antidepressants entirely. However, this option is probably unwise because the long-term risk for suicide from untreated depression is much greater than the long-term risk associated with antidepressant drugs. If the risk for suicide appears high, temporary hospitalization may be the best protection.

Selective Serotonin Reuptake Inhibitors

The SSRIs were introduced in 1987 and have since become our most commonly prescribed antidepressants. These drugs are indicated for major depression as well as several other psychological disorders (Table 27.2). Characteristic side effects are nausea, agitation and insomnia, and sexual dysfunction (especially anorgasmia). Like all other antidepressants, SSRIs may increase the risk for suicide. Compared with the TCAs and MAOIs, SSRIs are equally effective, better tolerated, and much safer. Death by overdose is extremely rare.

TABLE 27.2 Therapeutic Uses of Selective Serotonin Reuptake Inhibitors and Serotonin-Norepinephrine Reuptake Inhibitors

Drug	THERAPEUTIC USE[a]								
	Major Depression	OCD	Panic Disorder	Social Phobia	GAD	PTSD	PMDD	Bulimia Nervosa	Chronic Pain Disorders[b]
Citalopram (Celexa)	A	U	U	U	U	U	U		
Escitalopram (Lexapro)	A	U	U		A	U			
Fluoxetine (Prozac)	A	A	A	U	U	U	A	A	
Fluvoxamine (Luvox CR)	U	A	U	A	U	U	U	U	
Paroxetine (Paxil)	A	A	A	A	A	A	A		
Sertraline (Zoloft)	A	A	A	A	U	A	A		
Vortioxetine (Trintellix)	A				U				
Desvenlafaxine (Pristiq)	A		U	U	U				U
Duloxetine (Cymbalta)	A				A				A
Levomilnacipran (Fetzima)	A				U				U
Venlafaxine (Effexor)	A		A	A	A				U

[a]A, Approved use; U, unlabeled use.
[b]Chronic musculoskeletal pain, neuropathic pain, or fibromyalgia.
GAD, Generalized anxiety disorder; OCD, obsessive-compulsive disorder; PMDD, premenstrual dysphoric disorder; PTSD, posttraumatic stress disorder.

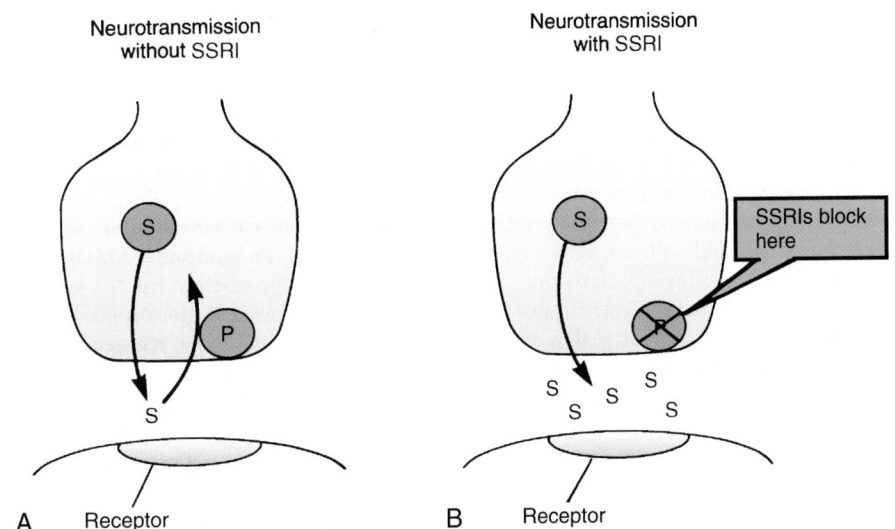

Fig. 27.1 Mechanism of Action of Selective Serotonin Reuptake Inhibitors. (A) Under drug-free conditions, the actions of serotonin are terminated by active uptake of the transmitter back into the nerve terminals from which it was released. (B) By inhibiting the reuptake pump for serotonin, the selective serotonin reuptake inhibitors *(SSRIs)* cause the transmitter to accumulate in the synaptic space, thereby intensifying transmission. *P*, Reuptake pump; *S*, serotonin.

Fluoxetine

Fluoxetine (Prozac, Prozac Weekly), the first SSRI available, will serve as our prototype for the group. At one time, this drug was the most widely prescribed antidepressant in the world.

Mechanism of action. The mechanism of action of fluoxetine and the other SSRIs is depicted in Fig. 27.1. As shown, SSRIs selectively block neuronal reuptake of serotonin (5-hydroxytryptamine [5-HT]), a monoamine neurotransmitter. As a result of reuptake blockade, the concentration of 5-HT in the synapse increases, causing increased activation of postsynaptic 5-HT receptors. This mechanism is consistent with the theory that depression stems from a deficiency in monoamine-mediated transmission—and hence should be relieved by drugs that can intensify monoamine effects.

It is important to appreciate that blockade of 5-HT reuptake, by itself, cannot fully account for therapeutic effects. Clinical responses to SSRIs (relief of depressive symptoms) and the biochemical effect of the SSRIs (blockade of 5-HT reuptake) do not occur in the same time frame. That is, whereas SSRIs block 5-HT reuptake within hours of dosing, relief of depression takes several weeks to fully develop. This delay suggests that therapeutic effects are the result of adaptive cellular changes that take place in response to prolonged reuptake blockade. Fluoxetine and the other SSRIs do not block reuptake of dopamine or NE. In contrast to the TCAs (as discussed later), fluoxetine does not block cholinergic, histaminergic, or α_1-adrenergic receptors. Furthermore, fluoxetine produces CNS excitation rather than sedation.

Therapeutic uses. Fluoxetine is used primarily for major depression. In addition, the drug is approved for bipolar disorder (see Chapter 28), obsessive-compulsive disorder (see Chapter 30), panic disorder (see Chapter 30), bulimia nervosa, and premenstrual dysphoric disorder (see Chapter 51).

Pharmacokinetics. Fluoxetine is well absorbed after oral administration, even in the presence of food. The drug is widely distributed and highly bound to plasma proteins. Fluoxetine undergoes extensive hepatic metabolism, primarily by CYP2D6 (the 2D6 isoenzyme of cytochrome P450). The major metabolite—norfluoxetine—is active, and later undergoes metabolic inactivation, followed by excretion in the urine. The half-life of fluoxetine is 2 days, and the half-life of norfluoxetine is 7 days. Because the effective half-life is prolonged, about 4 weeks are required to produce steady-state plasma drug levels—and about 4 weeks are required for washout after dosing stops.

Adverse effects. Fluoxetine is safer and better tolerated than TCAs and MAOIs. Death from overdose with fluoxetine alone has not been reported. In contrast to TCAs, fluoxetine does not block receptors for histamine, NE, or acetylcholine, and hence does not cause sedation, orthostatic hypotension, anticholinergic effects, or cardiotoxicity. The most common side effects are sexual dysfunction, nausea, headache, and manifestations of CNS stimulation, including nervousness, insomnia, and anxiety. Weight gain can also occur.

Sexual dysfunction. Fluoxetine causes sexual problems (impotence, delayed or absent orgasm, delayed or absent ejaculation, decreased sexual interest) in nearly 70% of men and women. The underlying mechanism is unknown.

Sexual dysfunction can be managed in several ways. In some cases, reducing the dosage or taking "drug holidays" (e.g., discontinuing medication on Fridays and Saturdays) can help. Although this approach can be helpful in some patients, close provider management is required. Another solution is to add a drug that can overcome the problem. Among these are yohimbine, buspirone (BuSpar), and three atypical antidepressants: bupropion (Wellbutrin, others), nefazodone, and mirtazapine (Remeron). Drugs such as sildenafil (Viagra) can also help. In men, these drugs improve erectile dysfunction as well as arousal, ejaculation, orgasm, and overall satisfaction; in women, they can improve delayed orgasm. If all of these measures fail, the patient can try a different antidepressant. Agents that cause the least sexual dysfunction are the same three atypical antidepressants just mentioned.

Sexual problems often go unreported, either because patients are uncomfortable discussing them or because patients don't realize their medicine is the cause. Accordingly, patients should be informed about the high probability of sexual dysfunction and told to report any problems so that they can be addressed.

Weight gain. Like many other antidepressants, fluoxetine and other SSRIs cause weight gain. When these drugs were first introduced, we thought they caused weight loss. During the first few weeks of therapy, patients lose weight, perhaps because of drug-induced nausea and vomiting. However, with long-term treatment, the lost weight is regained. Furthermore, about one-third of patients continue gaining weight. Although the reason is unknown, a good possibility is decreased sensitivity of 5-HT receptors that regulate appetite.

Serotonin syndrome. By increasing serotonergic transmission in the brainstem and spinal cord, fluoxetine and other SSRIs can cause serotonin syndrome. This syndrome usually begins 2 to 72 hours after treatment onset. Signs and symptoms include altered mental status (agitation, confusion, disorientation, anxiety, hallucinations, poor concentration) as well as incoordination, myoclonus, hyperreflexia, excessive sweating, tremor, and fever. Deaths have occurred. The syndrome resolves spontaneously after discontinuing the drug. The risk for serotonin syndrome is increased by concurrent use of MAOIs and other drugs (see the "Drug Interactions" section).

PATIENT EDUCATION
Withdrawal Syndrome

Abrupt discontinuation of selective serotonin reuptake inhibitors can cause a withdrawal syndrome. Symptoms include dizziness, headache, nausea, sensory disturbances, tremor, anxiety, and dysphoria. These begin within days to weeks of the last dose and then persist for 1 to 3 weeks. Resumption of drug use will make symptoms subside. The withdrawal syndrome can be minimized by tapering the dosage slowly.

Neonatal effects from use in pregnancy. The use of fluoxetine and other SSRIs late in pregnancy poses a small risk for two adverse effects in the newborn: (1) neonatal abstinence syndrome (NAS) and (2) persistent pulmonary hypertension of the newborn (PPHN). NAS is characterized by irritability, abnormal crying, tremor, respiratory distress, and possibly seizures. The syndrome can be managed with supportive care and generally abates within a few days. PPHN, which compromises tissue oxygenation, carries a significant risk for death and, among survivors, a risk for cognitive delay, hearing loss, and neurologic abnormalities. Treatment measures include providing ventilatory support, giving oxygen and nitric oxide (to dilate pulmonary blood vessels), and giving intravenous (IV) sodium bicarbonate (to maintain alkalosis) and dopamine or dobutamine (to increase cardiac output and thereby maintain pulmonary perfusion). Infants exposed to SSRIs late in gestation should be monitored closely for NAS and PPHN.

Teratogenesis. The risk for birth defects when taking fluoxetine and other SSRIs appears to be very low. Two SSRIs—paroxetine and fluoxetine—may cause septal heart defects. But even with these agents, the absolute risk is very low.

Drug interactions

Monoamine oxidase inhibitors and other drugs that increase the risk for serotonin syndrome. MAOIs increase 5-HT availability and hence greatly increase the risk for serotonin syndrome. Accordingly, use of MAOIs with SSRIs is contraindicated. Because MAOIs cause irreversible inhibition of monoamine oxidase their effects persist long after dosing stops. Therefore MAOIs should be withdrawn at least 14 days before starting an SSRI. Because fluoxetine and its active metabolite have long half-lives, at least 5 weeks should elapse between stopping fluoxetine and starting an MAOI. For other SSRIs, at least 2 weeks should elapse between treatment cessation and starting an MAOI.

Other drugs that increase the risk for serotonin syndrome include the serotonergic drugs listed in Table 27.3—drugs that inhibit CYP2D6 (and thereby raise fluoxetine levels), tramadol (an analgesic), and linezolid (an antibiotic that inhibits MAO).

Tricyclic antidepressants and lithium. Fluoxetine can elevate plasma levels of TCAs and lithium. Exercise caution if fluoxetine is combined with these agents.

Antiplatelet drugs and anticoagulants. Antiplatelet drugs (e.g., aspirin, nonsteroidal antiinflammatory drugs [NSAIDs], and anticoagulants (e.g., warfarin) increase the risk for gastrointestinal (GI) bleeding. Exercise caution if fluoxetine is combined with these drugs.

The risk for bleeding with warfarin is compounded by a pharmacokinetic interaction. Because fluoxetine is highly bound to plasma proteins, it can displace other highly bound drugs. Displacement of warfarin is of particular concern. Monitor responses to warfarin closely.

Other Selective Serotonin Reuptake Inhibitors

In addition to fluoxetine, five other SSRIs are available: citalopram (Celexa), escitalopram (Lexapro, Cipralex ♦), fluvoxamine (Luvox CR), paroxetine (Paxil, Pexeva), and sertraline (Zoloft). All five are similar

TABLE 27.3   Drugs That Promote the Activation of Serotonin Receptors

Drug	Mechanism
Selective Serotonin Reuptake Inhibitors (SSRIs)	
Citalopram (Celexa)	Block 5-HT reuptake and thereby
Escitalopram (Lexapro, Cipralex ♦)	increase 5-HT in the synapse
Fluoxetine (Prozac)	
Fluvoxamine (Luvox CR)	
Paroxetine (Paxil)	
Sertraline (Zoloft)	
Vortioxetine (Trintellix)	
Serotonin/Norepinephrine Reuptake Inhibitors (SNRIs)	
Desvenlafaxine (Pristiq)	Same as SSRIs
Duloxetine (Cymbalta)	
Venlafaxine (Effexor XR)	
Levomilnacipran (Fetzima)	
Tricyclic Antidepressants (TCAs)	
Amitriptyline	Same as SSRIs
Clomipramine (Anafranil)	
Desipramine (Norpramin)	
Doxepin (Sinequan)	
Imipramine (Tofranil)	
Trimipramine (Surmontil)	
Monoamine Oxidase Inhibitors (MAOIs)	
Isocarboxazid (Marplan)	Inhibit neuronal breakdown of 5-HT
Phenelzine (Nardil)	by MAO and thereby increase
Selegiline (Emsam)	stores of 5-HT available for release
Atypical Antidepressants	
Mirtazapine (Remeron)	Promotes release of 5-HT
Nefazodone	Same as SSRIs
Trazodone (Oleptro)	Same as SSRIs
Analgesics	
Meperidine (Demerol)	Same as SSRIs and MAOIs
Methadone (Dolophine)	Same as SSRIs and MAOIs
Tramadol (Ultram)	Same as SSRIs
Triptan Antimigraine Drugs	
Almotriptan (Axert)	Cause direct activation of serotonin
Eletriptan (Relpax)	receptors
Frovatriptan (Frova)	
Rizatriptan (Maxalt)	
Sumatriptan (Imitrex)	
Zolmitriptan (Zomig)	
Others	
St. John's wort	Same as SSRIs *and* MAOIs
Linezolid (Zyvox)	Same as MAOIs

5-HT, 5-hydroxytryptamine (serotonin); *MAO*, monoamine oxidase.

principal differences among the SSRIs relate to duration of action. Patients who experience intolerable adverse effects with one SSRI may find a different SSRI more acceptable. As with fluoxetine, withdrawal should be done slowly. In contrast to the TCAs, the SSRIs do not cause hypotension or anticholinergic effects and, with the exception of fluvoxamine, do not cause sedation. When taken in overdose, these drugs do not cause cardiotoxicity. Therapeutic uses for individual SSRIs are shown in Table 27.2.

PATIENT-CENTERED CARE ACROSS THE LIFE SPAN

Antidepressants

Life Stage	Patient Care Concerns
Children/ adolescents	Antidepressants may increase the risk for suicide, especially during the early phase of treatment.
Pregnant women	Use of SSRIs late in pregnancy may promote PPHN. Paroxetine and Fluoxetine may cause septal heart defects. Use of SSRIs in late pregnancy poses a small risk for NAS, charactized by abnormal crying, irritability, tremor, and possible seizures.
Breastfeeding women	Antidepressants are generally safe in breastfeeding women. Sertraline has been shown to be especially safe.
Older adults	Treatment with SSRIs or SNRIs is generally safe, providing less medication interaction and smaller side-effect profiles.

NAS, Neonatal abstinence syndrome; *PPHN,* persistent pulmonary hypertension of the newborn; *SNRI,* serotonin-norepinephrine reuptake inhibitor; *SSRI,* selective serotonin reuptake inhibitor.

Serotonin-Norepinephrine Reuptake Inhibitors

Four drugs—venlafaxine, desvenlafaxine, duloxetine, and levomilnacipran—block neuronal reuptake of serotonin and NE, with minimal effects on other transmitters or receptors. Pharmacologic effects are similar to those of the SSRIs, although the SSRIs may be better tolerated. The SNRIs are indicated for major depression as well as other disorders (see Table 27.2).

Venlafaxine

Venlafaxine (Effexor XR), the first SNRI available, is approved for major depression, generalized anxiety disorder, social anxiety disorder, and panic disorder. The drug produces powerful blockade of NE and 5-HT reuptake and weak blockade of dopamine reuptake. The relationship of these actions to therapeutic effects is uncertain. Venlafaxine does not block cholinergic, histaminergic, or α_1-adrenergic receptors. Despite impressions that venlafaxine may be superior to SSRIs, when compared directly in clinical trials, the drugs were about equally effective—and SSRIs are probably safer.

Venlafaxine is well absorbed after oral administration, in both the presence and absence of food. In the liver, much of each dose is converted to desvenlafaxine, an active metabolite. The half-life is 5 hours for the parent drug and 11 hours for the active metabolite.

Venlafaxine can cause a variety of adverse effects. The most common is nausea (37% to 58%), followed by headache, anorexia, nervousness, sweating, somnolence, and insomnia. Dose-dependent weight loss may occur secondary to anorexia. Venlafaxine can also cause dose-related sustained diastolic hypertension; blood pressure should be monitored. Sexual dysfunction may occur too. Some patients experience sustained mydriasis, which can increase the risk for eye injury in those with elevated intraocular pressure or glaucoma. Like the SSRIs, venlafaxine

to fluoxetine. Antidepressant effects equal those of TCAs. Characteristic side effects are nausea, insomnia, headache, nervousness, weight gain, sexual dysfunction, hyponatremia, GI bleeding, and NAS and PPHN (in infants who were exposed to these drugs late in gestation). Serotonin syndrome is a potential complication with all SSRIs, especially if these agents are combined with MAOIs or other serotonergic drugs. The can cause hyponatremia, especially in older adult patients taking diuretics. Like all other antidepressants, venlafaxine may increase the risk for suicide, especially in children and young adults.

The combined use of venlafaxine with MAOIs and other serotonergic drugs (see Table 27.3) increases the risk for serotonin syndrome, a potentially fatal reaction. If the clinical situation demands, venlafaxine may be cautiously combined with an SSRI or another SNRI. However, combined use with an MAOI is contraindicated. Accordingly, MAOIs should be withdrawn at least 14 days before starting venlafaxine. When switching from venlafaxine to an MAOI, venlafaxine should be discontinued 7 days before starting the MAOI.

As with the SSRIs, the use of venlafaxine late in pregnancy can result in a neonatal withdrawal syndrome, characterized by irritability, abnormal crying, tremor, respiratory distress, and possibly seizures. Symptoms, which can be managed with supportive care, generally abate within a few days.

Abrupt discontinuation can cause an intense withdrawal syndrome. Symptoms include anxiety, agitation, tremors, headache, vertigo, nausea, tachycardia, and tinnitus. Worsening of pretreatment symptoms may also occur. Withdrawal symptoms can be minimized by tapering the dosage over 2 to 4 weeks. Warn patients not to stop venlafaxine abruptly.

SUMMARY OF KEY PRESCRIBING CONSIDERATIONS

Selective Serotonin Reuptake Inhibitors and Serotonin/Norepinephrine Reuptake Inhibitors

Therapeutic Goal: Alleviation of symptoms of major depression. In addition, some drugs may relieve symptoms of obsessive-compulsive disorder, panic disorder, social phobia, generalized anxiety disorder, and chronic pain.

Baseline Data: Serum sodium should be checked in older adults and patients on diuretic therapy.

Monitoring: Serum sodium should be monitored in older adults and patients on diuretic therapy.

Identifying High-Risk Patients: Selective serotonin reuptake inhibitors and serotonin/norepinephrine reuptake inhibitors are contraindicated for patients taking monoamine oxidase inhibitors and should be used with caution in patients taking other serotonergic drugs.

Evaluating Therapeutic Effects: Assess patients for improvement in symptoms, especially depressed mood and loss of interest or pleasure in usual activities.

Minimizing Adverse Effects: Educate patients that abrupt cessation of these drugs is not recommended. Patients should also report thoughts of suicide or self-harm immediately.

Tricyclic Antidepressants

The first TCA—imipramine—was introduced to psychiatry in the late 1950s. Since then, the ability of TCAs to relieve depressive symptoms has been firmly established. For decades, TCAs were drugs of first choice for depression. However, owing to the development of safer alternatives, especially the SSRIs, the use of TCAs has greatly declined. The most common adverse effects are sedation, orthostatic hypotension, and anticholinergic effects. The most dangerous effect is cardiac toxicity. When taken in overdose, TCAs can readily prove lethal. Like all other antidepressants, TCAs may increase the risk for suicide. Because all of the TCAs have similar properties, we will discuss these drugs as a group rather than focusing on a representative prototype.

Chemistry

The structure of imipramine, a representative TCA, is very similar to the structure of the phenothiazine antipsychotics. Because of this

similarity, TCAs and phenothiazines have several actions in common. Specifically, both groups produce varying degrees of sedation, orthostatic hypotension, and anticholinergic effects.

Mechanism of Action

The TCAs block neuronal reuptake of two monoamine transmitters: NE and 5-HT. As a result, TCAs increase the concentration of these transmitters at CNS synapses and thereby intensify their effects. As indicated in Table 27.4, some TCAs block reuptake of NE and 5-HT, whereas others only block reuptake of NE. As with the SSRIs, biochemical effects (blockade of transmitter reuptake) occur within hours, whereas therapeutic effects (relief of depression) develop over several weeks. This delay suggests that antidepressant effects are due to adaptive changes brought on by prolonged reuptake blockade, and not to reuptake blockade directly.

Pharmacokinetics

The half-lives of TCAs are long and variable. Because their half-lives are long, TCAs can usually be administered in a single daily dose. Because their half-lives are variable, TCAs require individualization of dosage.

Therapeutic Uses

Depression. TCAs are effective agents for major depression. These drugs can elevate mood, increase activity and alertness, decrease morbid preoccupation, improve appetite, and normalize sleep patterns. Despite their efficacy, TCAs are generally considered second-line drugs, owing to the development of safer and better-tolerated alternatives.

Fibromyalgia syndrome. Fibromyalgia syndrome is a chronic disorder characterized by diffuse musculoskeletal pain, profound fatigue, disturbed sleep, and cognitive dysfunction. TCAs are the most effective drugs available for reducing symptoms.

Other uses. TCAs can benefit patients with neuropathic pain (see Chapter 86), chronic insomnia (see Chapter 29), attention-deficit/hyperactivity disorder (see Chapter 31), and panic disorder or obsessive-compulsive disorder (see Chapter 30).

Adverse Effects

The most common adverse effects are orthostatic hypotension, sedation, and anticholinergic effects. The most serious adverse effect is cardiotoxicity. These effects occur because, in addition to blocking reuptake of NE and 5-HT, TCAs cause direct blockade of receptors for histamine, acetylcholine, and NE. Adverse effects of individual agents are shown in Table 27.4.

Orthostatic hypotension. Orthostatic hypotension is the most serious of the common adverse responses to TCAs. Hypotension is due in large part to blockade of α_1-adrenergic receptors on blood vessels.

PATIENT EDUCATION
Orthostatic Hypotension

Patients should be informed that they can minimize orthostatic hypotension by moving slowly when assuming an upright posture. In addition, patients should be instructed to sit or lie down if symptoms (dizziness, lightheadedness) occur.

Anticholinergic effects. The TCAs block muscarinic cholinergic receptors and can thereby cause an array of anticholinergic effects (dry mouth, blurred vision, photophobia, constipation, urinary hesitancy, and tachycardia). Patients should be informed about possible anticholinergic responses and instructed in ways to minimize discomfort. A detailed discussion of anticholinergic effects and their management is presented in Chapter 14.

TABLE 27.4 Antidepressants: Adverse Effects and Impact on Neurotransmitters

	Transmitters Affected	Agitation/ Insomnia[a]	Anticholinergic Activity	Sedation	Hypotension	Seizure Risk	Cardiac Toxicity	Weight Gain	Sexual Dysfunction	Other Side Effects
Selective Serotonin Reuptake Inhibitors (SSRIs)										
Citalopram	5-HT	++	0/+		0	0/+	0	+	+++	GI bleeding, hyponatremia, NAS and PPHN in newborns. Citalopram may cause dysrhythmias.[c]
Escitalopram	5-HT	++	0/+	0/+	0	0/+	0	+	+++	
Fluoxetine	5-HT	++	0	b	0	0/+	0/+	+	+++	
Fluvoxamine	5-HT	++	0/+	0/+	0	0/+	0	+	+++	
Paroxetine	5-HT	++	0/+	b	0	0/+	0	+	+++	
Sertraline	5-HT	++	0	b	0	0/+	0	0	+++	
Vortioxetine	5-HT3, 5-HT1A	++	0/+	b	0	0/+	0	0	++	
Serotonin-Norepinephrine Reuptake Inhibitors (SNRIs)										
Desvenlafaxine	NE, 5-HT	++	0	0	0	0/+	0/+	0	++	
Duloxetine	NE, 5-HT	++	0	0	0/+	0/+	0/+	0/+	+	Hepatotoxicity
Venlafaxine	NE, 5-HT	++	0	0	0	0/+	0/+	0	+++	
Levomilnacipran	NE, 5-HT	++	0	0	0	d	0/+	0	++	Hyponatremia
Tricyclic Antidepressants (TCAs)										
Amitriptyline	NE, 5-HT	0/+	++++	+++	++	++	+++	+++	++	
Clomipramine	NE, 5-HT	+	++	++	++	++	++++	++	++	
Doxepin	NE, 5-HT	0/+	++	+++	++	++	+++	+++	++	
Imipramine	NE, 5-HT	+	++	++	++	++	+++	++	++	
Trimipramine	NE, 5-HT	0/+	+++	+++	++	++	+++	++	++	
Desipramine	NE	+	+	b	+	+	++	+	++	
Maprotiline	NE	+	++	++	+	++	++	++	++	
Nortriptyline	NE	+	+	+	+	+	++	+	++	
Protriptyline	NE	++	++	b	+	+	+++	+	++	
Monoamine Oxidase Inhibitors (MAOIs)										
Isocarboxazid	NE, 5-HT, DA	++	0	+	+	0	0	+	++	Hypertensive crisis from tyramine in food[e]
Phenelzine	NE, 5-HT, DA	++	0	++	+	0	0	++	++	
Selegiline	NE, 5-HT, DA	++	0	0	0/+	0	0	0	+	
Tranylcypromine	NE, 5-HT, DA	++	0	b	+	0	0	+	++	
Atypical Antidepressants										
Amoxapine	NE, ↓DA	0/+	+	+	+	++	++	+	++	Parkinsonism
Bupropion	DA	++	0/+	b	0	+++	0	0	f	Seizures
Mirtazapine	NE, 5-HT	0/+	0/+	++++	0/+	0	0	++++	0	
Nefazodone	5-HT	0/+	0/+	++	0	0	0/+	0/+	0/+	
Trazodone	5-HT	0/+	0/+	++++	+	0	0/+	+	+	Priapism
Vilazodone	5-HT	++	0	++	0	0	0	0	++	Bleeding, hyponatremia

[a]All of the antidepressants increase synaptic activity of the transmitters indicated—with the exception of amoxapine, which increases activity of NE but blocks receptors for DA. The TCAs, SSRIs, SNRIs, amoxapine, bupropion, nefazodone, and trazodone decrease transmitter reuptake; vilazodone blocks transmitter reuptake and directly activates 5-HT receptors; MAOIs block transmitter breakdown; and mirtazapine promotes transmitter release.

[b]Produces moderate stimulation, not sedation.

[c]NAS, Neonatal abstinence syndrome; PPHN, persistent pulmonary hypertension of the newborn.

[d]Levomilnacipran was not tested in patients with seizure disorders.

[e]Hypertensive crisis is not a risk with low-dose (6 mg/day) transdermal selegiline, and possibly not with higher doses.

[f]Bupropion may increase sexual desire.

DA, Dopamine; 5-HT, 5-hydroxytryptamine (serotonin); NE, norepinephrine.

Diaphoresis. Despite their anticholinergic properties, TCAs often cause diaphoresis. The mechanism of this paradoxical effect is unknown.

Sedation. Sedation is a common response to TCAs. The cause is blockade of histamine receptors in the CNS. Patients should be advised to avoid hazardous activities if sedation is prominent.

Cardiac toxicity. Tricyclics can adversely affect cardiac function. However, in the absence of an overdose or preexisting cardiac impairment, serious effects are rare. The TCAs affect the heart by (1) decreasing vagal influence on the heart (secondary to muscarinic blockade) and (2) acting directly on the bundle of His to slow conduction. Both effects increase the risk of dysrhythmias. To minimize risk, all patients should undergo ECG evaluation before treatment and periodically thereafter. Risk for cardiac toxicity may be higher with desipramine than with other TCAs.

Seizures. TCAs lower seizure threshold and thereby increase seizure risk. Exercise caution in patients with seizure disorders.

BLACK BOX WARNING

Suicide Risk With Tricyclic Antidepressants

Tricyclic antidepressants and all other antidepressants may increase the risk for suicide in depressed patients, especially during the early phase of treatment. The risk for antidepressant-induced suicide is greatest among children, adolescents, and young adults.

Drug Interactions

Monoamine oxidase inhibitors. The combination of a TCA with an MAOI can lead to severe hypertension, owing to excessive adrenergic stimulation of the heart and blood vessels. Excessive adrenergic stimulation occurs because (1) inhibition of MAO causes accumulation of NE in adrenergic neurons and (2) blockade of NE reuptake by the tricyclics decreases NE inactivation. Because of the potential for hypertensive crisis, combined therapy with TCAs and MAOIs is generally avoided.

Direct-acting sympathomimetic drugs. Tricyclics potentiate responses to direct-acting sympathomimetics (i.e., drugs such as epinephrine and dopamine that produce their effects by direct interaction with adrenergic receptors). Because TCAs block uptake of these agents into adrenergic nerve terminals, they prolong the presence of these agents in the synaptic space.

Indirect-acting sympathomimetic drugs. TCAs decrease responses to indirect-acting sympathomimetics (i.e., drugs such as ephedrine and amphetamine that promote release of transmitter from adrenergic nerves). TCAs block the uptake of these agents into adrenergic nerves, thereby preventing them from reaching their site of action within the nerve terminal.

Anticholinergic agents. Because TCAs have anticholinergic actions of their own, they will intensify the effects of other anticholinergic medications. Consequently, patients receiving TCAs should be advised to avoid all other drugs with anticholinergic properties, including antihistamines and certain over-the-counter sleep aids.

Central nervous system depressants. CNS depression caused by TCAs will add with CNS depression caused by other drugs. Accordingly, patients should be warned against taking all other CNS depressants, including alcohol, antihistamines, opioids, and barbiturates.

Toxicity

Overdose with a TCA can be life threatening. The lethal dose is only eight times the average therapeutic dose. To minimize the risk for death by suicide, consider prescribing smaller amounts with increased follow-up appointments in acutely depressed patients.

Clinical Manifestations

Symptoms result primarily from anticholinergic and cardiotoxic actions. The combination of cholinergic blockade and direct cardiotoxicity can produce dysrhythmias, including tachycardia, intraventricular blocks, complete atrioventricular block, ventricular tachycardia, and ventricular fibrillation. Responses to peripheral muscarinic blockade include hyperthermia, flushing, dry mouth, and dilation of the pupils. CNS symptoms are prominent. Early responses are confusion, agitation, and hallucinations. Seizures and coma may follow.

Treatment

Absorption of ingested drug can be reduced with gastric lavage followed by administration of activated charcoal. IV administration of sodium bicarbonate is recommended to control dysrhythmias caused by cardiac toxicity. Dysrhythmias should not be treated with procainamide or quinidine, because these drugs cause cardiac depression.

Drug selection

Selection among TCAs is based on side effects. For example, if the patient is experiencing insomnia, a drug with prominent sedative properties (e.g., doxepin) might be selected. Conversely, if daytime sedation is undesirable, a less sedating agent (e.g., desipramine) might be preferred. Older adult patients with glaucoma or constipation and males with benign prostatic hypertrophy can be especially sensitive to anticholinergic effects. Hence, for these patients, a drug with weak anticholinergic properties (e.g., nortriptyline) would be appropriate.

SUMMARY OF KEY PRESCRIBING CONSIDERATIONS

Tricyclic Antidepressants

Therapeutic Goal: Alleviation of symptoms of major depression.
Baseline Data: ECG should be checked, especially in patients with known dysrhythmias or patients older than 40 years of age.
Monitoring: Periodic ECG should be completed.
Identifying High-Risk Patients: Tricyclic antidepressants (TCAs) are generally contraindicated in patients taking monoamine oxidase inhibitors. Also use with caution in patients with urinary retention, cardiac disorders, and liver or kidney dysfunction.
Evaluating Therapeutic Effects: Assess patients for improvement in symptoms, especially depressed mood and loss of interest or pleasure in usual activities.
Minimizing Adverse Effects: Educate patients regarding orthostatic hypotension and anticholinergic effects, including dry mouth, blurred vision, constipation, and urinary hesitancy.

Monoamine Oxidase Inhibitors

The MAOIs are second- or third-choice antidepressants for most patients. Although these drugs are as effective as the SSRIs and TCAs, they are more hazardous. The greatest concern is hypertensive crisis, which can be triggered by eating foods rich in tyramine. At this time, MAOIs are drugs of choice only for atypical depression. Three MAOIs (isocarboxazid [Marplan], phenelzine [Nardil], and tranylcypromine [Parnate]) are administered orally, and one (selegiline [Emsam]) is administered by transdermal patch.

Oral Monoamine Oxidase Inhibitors

Mechanism of action. Before discussing the MAOIs, we need to discuss MAO itself. MAO is an enzyme found in the liver, the intestinal wall, and terminals of monoamine-containing neurons. The function of MAO in neurons is to convert monoamine neurotransmitters—NE, 5-HT, and dopamine—into inactive products. In the liver and intestine,

MAO serves to inactivate tyramine and other biogenic amines in food. In addition, these enzymes inactivate biogenic amines administered as drugs.

The body has two forms of MAO, named MAO-A and MAO-B. In the brain, MAO-A inactivates NE and 5-HT, whereas MAO-B inactivates dopamine. In the intestine and liver, MAO-A acts on dietary tyramine and other compounds. All of the MAOIs used for depression are nonselective. That is, at therapeutic doses, they inhibit both MAO-A and MAO-B. One agent—selegiline (used for depression and Parkinson disease)—is selective for MAO-B at the low doses used for Parkinson disease but is nonselective at the higher doses used for depression.

Antidepressant effects of the MAOIs result from inhibiting MAO-A in nerve terminals (Fig. 27.2). By inhibiting intraneuronal MAO-A, these drugs increase the amount of NE and 5-HT available for release, and thereby intensify transmission at noradrenergic and serotonergic junctions.

Note that antidepressant effects of the MAOIs cannot be fully explained by MAO inhibition alone. The biochemical action of MAOIs (inhibition of MAO) takes place rapidly, whereas the clinical response to MAOIs (relief of depression) develops slowly. In the interval between initial inhibition of MAO and relief of depression, secondary neurochemical events must be taking place. These secondary events, which have not been identified, are ultimately responsible for the beneficial response to treatment.

The MAOIs can act on MAO in two ways: reversibly and irreversibly. All of the MAOIs in current use cause irreversible inhibition. Because recovery from irreversible inhibition requires synthesis of new MAO molecules, effects of the irreversible inhibitors persist for about 2 weeks after drug withdrawal. In contrast, recovery from reversible inhibition is more rapid, occurring in 3 to 5 days.

Therapeutic uses

Depression. MAOIs are equal to SSRIs and TCAs for relieving depression. However, because MAOIs can be hazardous, they are generally reserved for patients who have not responded to SSRIs, TCAs, and other safer drugs. Nonetheless, there is one group of patients—those with atypical depression—for whom MAOIs are the treatment of choice. As

with other antidepressants, beneficial effects do not reach their peak for several weeks.

Adverse effects

Central nervous system stimulation. MAOIs cause direct CNS stimulation (in addition to exerting antidepressant effects). Excessive stimulation can produce anxiety, insomnia, agitation, hypomania, and even mania.

Orthostatic hypotension. Despite their ability to increase the NE content of peripheral sympathetic neurons, the MAOIs reduce blood pressure when administered in usual therapeutic doses. Patients should be informed about signs of hypotension (dizziness, lightheadedness) and advised to sit or lie down if these occur. Also, they should be informed that hypotension can be minimized by moving slowly when assuming an erect posture.

MAOIs reduce blood pressure through actions in the CNS. The following sequence has been proposed: (1) Inhibition of MAO increases the NE content of neurons within the vasomotor center. (2) When NE is released, it binds to postsynaptic α receptors on neurons within the vasomotor center, thereby decreasing the firing rate of sympathetic nerves that control vascular tone. (3) This reduction in sympathetic activity results in vasodilation, causing blood pressure to fall.

Hypertensive crisis from dietary tyramine. Although the MAOIs normally produce hypotension, they can be the cause of severe hypertension if the patient eats food that is rich in tyramine, a substance that promotes the release of NE from sympathetic neurons. Hypertensive crisis is characterized by severe headache, tachycardia, hypertension, nausea, vomiting, confusion, and profuse sweating—possibly leading to stroke and death.

Before considering the mechanism by which hypertensive crisis is produced, let's consider the effect of dietary tyramine under drug-free conditions. In the absence of MAO inhibition, dietary tyramine is not a threat. Much of the tyramine in food is metabolized by MAO in the intestinal wall. Furthermore, as shown in Fig. 27.3A, any dietary tyramine that gets through the intestinal wall intact will then pass directly to the liver through the hepatic portal circulation. When in the liver, tyramine is immediately inactivated by MAO there. Hence, as long as intestinal

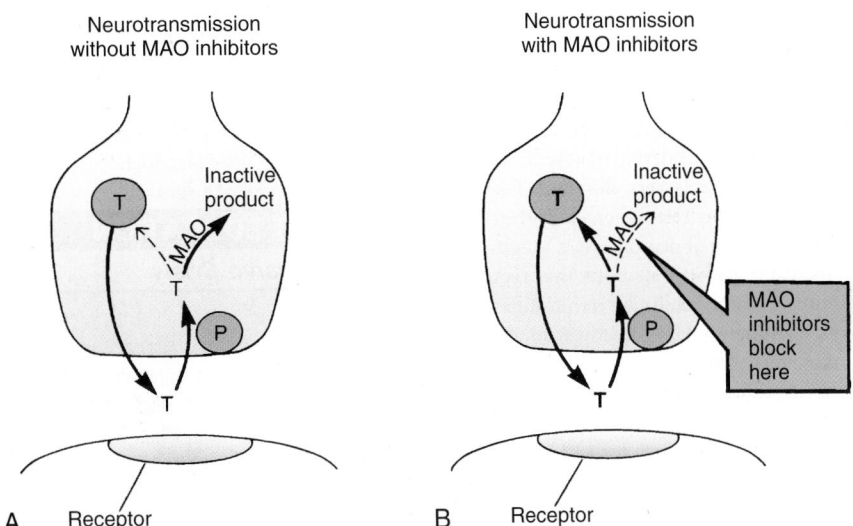

Fig. 27.2 Mechanism of Action of Monoamine Oxidase Inhibitors. (A) Under drug-free conditions, much of the norepinephrine or serotonin that undergoes reuptake into nerve terminals becomes inactivated by monoamine oxidase *(MAO)*. Inactivation helps maintain an appropriate concentration of transmitter within the terminal. (B) monoamine oxidase inhibitors prevent inactivation of norepinephrine and serotonin, thereby increasing the amount of transmitter available for release. Release of supranormal amounts of transmitter intensifies transmission. *P*, Reuptake pump; *T*, transmitter [norepinephrine or serotonin].

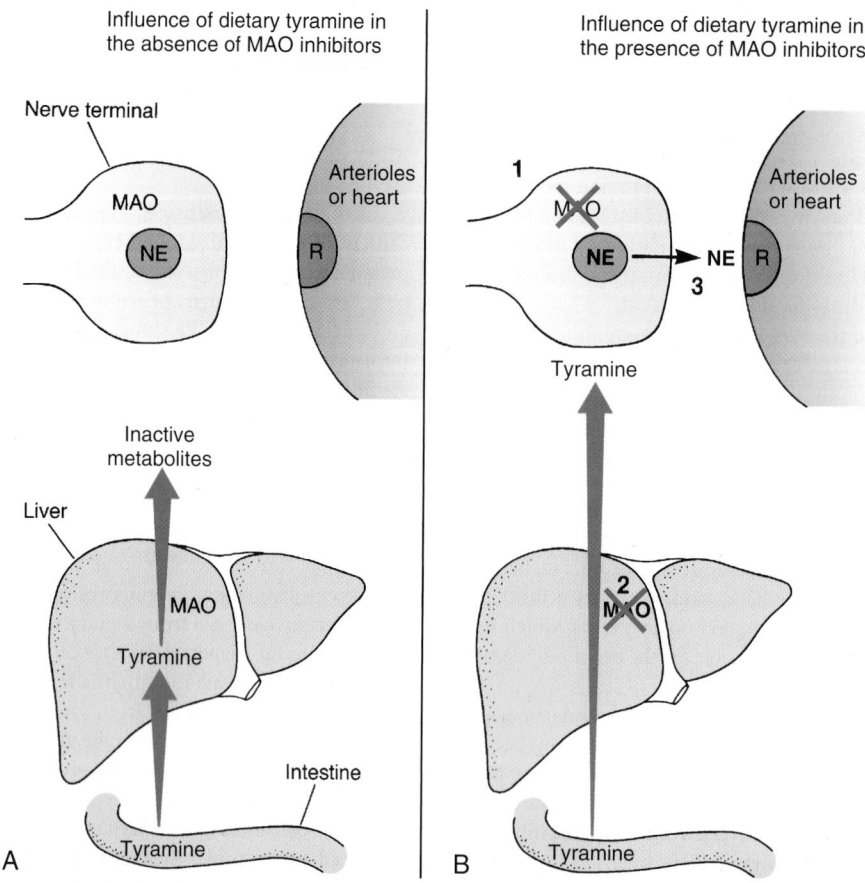

Fig. 27.3 Interaction Between Dietary Tyramine and Monoamine Oxidase Inhibitors. (A) In the absence of monoamine oxidase inhibitors *(MAOIs)*, much of ingested tyramine is inactivated by monoamine oxidase (MAO) in the intestinal wall (not shown in the figure). Any dietary tyramine that is not metabolized in the intestinal wall is transported directly to the liver, where it undergoes immediate inactivation by hepatic MAO. No tyramine reaches the general circulation. (B) Three events occur in the presence of MAOIs: (1) Inhibition of neuronal MAO raises levels of norepinephrine in sympathetic nerve terminals. (2) Inhibition of intestinal and hepatic MAO allows dietary tyramine to pass through the intestinal wall and liver to enter the systemic circulation intact. (3) On reaching peripheral sympathetic nerve terminals, tyramine promotes the release of accumulated norepinephrine stores, thereby causing massive vasoconstriction and excessive stimulation of the heart. *NE,* Norepinephrine; *R,* receptor for norepinephrine.

and hepatic MAO is functioning, dietary tyramine is prevented from reaching the general circulation and therefore is devoid of adverse effects.

In the presence of MAOIs, the picture is very different: Dietary tyramine can produce a life-threatening hypertensive crisis. Three steps are involved (see Fig. 27.3B). First, inhibition of neuronal MAO augments NE levels within the terminals of sympathetic neurons that regulate cardiac function and vascular tone. Second, inhibition of intestinal and hepatic MAO allows dietary tyramine to pass directly through the intestinal wall and liver and then enter the systemic circulation intact. Third, on reaching peripheral sympathetic nerves, tyramine stimulates the release of the accumulated NE, thereby causing massive vasoconstriction and intense stimulation of the heart. Hypertensive crisis results. To reduce the risk for tyramine-induced hypertensive crisis, the following precautions must be taken:

- MAOIs must not be dispensed to patients considered incapable of rigid adherence to dietary restrictions.
- Before an MAOI is dispensed, the patient must be fully informed about the hazard of ingesting tyramine-rich foods.
- The patient must be given a detailed list of foods and beverages to avoid.

- The patient should be instructed to avoid all drugs not specifically approved by the prescriber.

PATIENT EDUCATION

Hypertensive Crisis

Patients should be informed about the symptoms of hypertensive crisis (headache, tachycardia, palpitations, nausea, vomiting, sweating) and instructed to seek immediate medical attention if these develop.

In addition to tyramine, several other dietary constituents (e.g., caffeine, phenylethylamine) can precipitate hypertension in patients taking MAOIs. Foods that contain these compounds are listed in Table 27.5. Patients should be instructed to avoid them.

Drug interactions. The MAOIs can interact with many drugs to cause potentially harmful results. Accordingly, patients should be instructed to avoid all medications—prescription drugs and over-the-counter drugs—that have not been specifically approved by the prescriber.

TABLE 27.5   Foods That Can Interact With Monoamine Oxidase Inhibitors

Foods That Contain Tyramine

Category	Foods With High Tyramine Content	Foods With Little or No Tyramine
Vegetables	Avocados, especially if overripe; fermented bean curd; fermented soybean; soybean paste	Most vegetables
Fruits	Figs, especially if overripe; bananas, in large amounts	Most fruits
Meats	Meats that are fermented, smoked, or otherwise aged; spoiled meats; liver, unless very fresh	Meats that are known to be fresh (exercise caution in restaurants; meat may not be fresh)
Sausages	Fermented varieties: bologna, pepperoni, salami, others	Nonfermented varieties
Fish	Dried or cured fish; fish that is fermented, smoked, or otherwise aged; spoiled fish	Fish that is known to be fresh; vacuum-packed fish, if eaten promptly or refrigerated only briefly after opening
Milk, milk products	Practically all cheeses	Milk, yogurt, cottage cheese, cream cheese
Foods with yeast	Yeast extract (e.g., Marmite, Bovril)	Baked goods that contain yeast
Beer, wine	Some imported beers, Chianti wine	Major domestic brands of beer, most wines
Other foods	Protein dietary supplements; soups (may contain protein extract); shrimp paste; soy sauce	

Foods That Contain Nontyramine Vasopressors

Food	Comments
Chocolate	Contains phenylethylamine, a pressor agent; large amounts can cause a reaction
Fava beans	Contain dopamine, a pressor agent; reactions are most likely with overripe beans
Ginseng	Headache, tremulousness, and manic-like reactions have occurred
Caffeinated beverages	Caffeine is a weak pressor agent; large amounts may cause a reaction

Indirect-acting sympathomimetic agents. Indirect-acting sympathomimetics (e.g., ephedrine, amphetamine) are drugs that promote the release of NE from sympathetic nerves. In patients taking MAOIs, these drugs can produce hypertensive crisis. The mechanism is the same as that described for tyramine. Patients should be instructed to avoid all sympathomimetic drugs, including ephedrine, methylphenidate, amphetamines, and cocaine. Sympathomimetic agents may be present in cold remedies, nasal decongestants, and asthma medications; all of these should be avoided unless approved by the prescriber.

Interactions secondary to inhibition of hepatic monoamine oxidase. Inhibition of MAO in the liver can decrease the metabolism of several drugs, including epinephrine, NE, and dopamine. These drugs must be used with caution because their effects will be more intense and prolonged.

Tricyclic antidepressants. The combination of a TCA with an MAOI may produce hypertensive episodes or hypertensive crisis. As a result, this combination of antidepressants is not employed routinely. However, although potentially dangerous, the combination can benefit certain patients. If concurrent use is employed, caution must be exercised.

Serotonergic drugs. Combining MAOIs with SSRIs and other serotonergic drugs (see Table 27.3) poses a risk for serotonin syndrome. Accordingly, these combinations should be avoided.

Antihypertensive drugs. Combined use of MAOIs and antihypertensive agents may result in excessive lowering of blood pressure.

Transdermal Monoamine Oxidase Inhibitors: Selegiline

Transdermal selegiline (Emsam) is the first and only transdermal treatment for major depression. Selegiline inhibits MAO-A as well as MAO-B. Like other MAOIs, selegiline should be reserved for patients who have not responded to preferred antidepressant drugs.

The pharmacology of transdermal selegiline is much like that of the oral MAOIs but with one important difference: the risk for hypertensive crisis from dietary tyramine is much lower than with oral dosing. With transdermal dosing, selegiline enters the systemic circulation without first passing through the GI tract. As a result, it can achieve therapeutic levels in the CNS while preserving activity of MAO-A in the intestinal wall and liver. Therefore dietary tyramine will be destroyed before it can promote NE release in the periphery. Clinical trials have shown that restricting dietary tyramine is unnecessary with low-dose selegiline (6 mg/24 hours). However, owing to a lack of data, tyramine restriction is recommended at higher selegiline doses. Furthermore, with all doses of selegiline, sympathomimetic drugs (e.g., phenylephrine, ephedrine, pseudoephedrine, amphetamines) are still able to promote NE release and hence must be avoided, just as with oral MAOIs.

Two drugs—carbamazepine (Tegretol) and oxcarbazepine (Trileptal)—can significantly raise levels of selegiline. Accordingly, these drugs are contraindicated.

The most common adverse reaction is localized rash, which develops in about one-third of patients. Rash can be managed with topical glucocorticoids.

SUMMARY OF KEY PRESCRIBING CONSIDERATIONS

Monoamine Oxidase Inhibitors

Therapeutic Goal: Alleviation of symptoms of major depression, especially atypical depression.

Baseline Data: Baseline blood pressure should be obtained.

Monitoring: Blood pressures can be obtained periodically.

Identifying High-Risk Patients: Monoamine oxidase inhibitors are contraindicated in patients taking SSRIs, patients with heart failure, severe renal impairment, hypertension, and cardiovascular disease. Also use with caution in patients taking serotonergic drugs.

Evaluating Therapeutic Effects: Assess patients for improvement in symptoms, especially depressed mood and loss of interest or pleasure in usual activities.

Minimizing Adverse Effects: Educate patients on foods containing tyramine and to report signs of hypertensive crisis (nausea, vomiting, profuse sweating, severe headache) immediately.

Atypical Antidepressants

Bupropion

Actions and uses. Bupropion (Wellbutrin, Forfivo XL, Aplenzin) is a unique antidepressant similar in structure to amphetamine. Like amphetamine, bupropion has stimulant actions and suppresses appetite. Antidepressant effects begin in 1 to 3 weeks. The mechanism by which depression is relieved is unclear but may be related to blockade of dopamine or NE reuptake. The drug does not affect serotonergic, cholinergic, or histaminergic transmission, and does not inhibit MAO. In contrast to SSRIs, bupropion does not cause weight gain or sexual dysfunction. In fact, it appears to increase sexual desire and pleasure, so bupropion has been used to counteract sexual dysfunction in patients taking SSRIs and heighten sexual interest in women with hypoactive sexual desire disorder. Because of its efficacy and side-effect profile, bupropion is a good alternative to SSRIs for patients who cannot tolerate SSRIs. Bupropion has two antidepressant indications: (1) major depressive disorder and (2) prevention of seasonal affective disorder (SAD). In addition to its use in depression, bupropion, marketed as Zyban and Buproban, is approved as an aid to quit smoking (see Chapter 34). Unlabeled uses include relief of neuropathic pain, treatment of depressive episodes in bipolar disorder, and management of attention-deficit/hyperactivity disorder.

Pharmacokinetics. Bupropion is administered orally. With the immediate-release tablets, plasma levels peak about 2 hours after dosing. Bioavailability is low: in animals, only 5% to 20% of each dose reaches the systemic circulation. Bupropion undergoes extensive hepatic metabolism, primarily by CYP2B6. The elimination half-life ranges from 8 to 24 hours.

Adverse effects. Bupropion is generally well tolerated but can cause seizures. The most common adverse effects are agitation, headache, dry mouth, constipation, weight loss, GI upset, dizziness, tremor, insomnia, blurred vision, and tachycardia. In addition, bupropion carries a small risk for causing psychotic symptoms, including hallucinations and delusions. Accordingly, the drug should not be used in patients with psychotic disorders. Like other antidepressants, bupropion may increase the risk for suicide in children, adolescents, and young adults. In contrast to many other antidepressants, bupropion does not cause adverse sexual effects.

Seizures are the side effect of greatest concern. At doses greater than 450 mg/day, bupropion produces seizures in about 0.4% of patients. Seizure risk can be reduced by avoiding the following:

- Doses above 450 mg/day
- Rapid dosage titration (as discussed later)
- Bupropion in patients with seizure risk factors, such as head trauma, preexisting seizure disorder, CNS tumor, and use of other drugs that lower seizure threshold
- Bupropion in patients with anorexia nervosa or bulimia, which seem to increase seizure risk
- Drugs that inhibit CYP2B6, which can elevate bupropion levels

Drug interactions. As noted, drugs that inhibit CYP2B6 (e.g., sertraline, fluoxetine, paroxetine) can elevate bupropion levels, thereby increasing the risk for seizures. Combined use with these drugs should be avoided.

MAOIs can increase the risk for bupropion toxicity. Accordingly, patients should discontinue MAOIs at least 2 weeks before starting bupropion.

Mirtazapine

Mirtazapine (Remeron) is the first representative of a new class of antidepressants. Benefits appear to result from increased release of 5-HT and NE. The mechanism is blockade of presynaptic α_2-adrenergic receptors that serve to inhibit release. In addition to promoting transmitter release, mirtazapine is a powerful blocker of two serotonin receptor subtypes: 5-HT$_2$ and 5-HT$_3$. The contribution of this effect is unclear. Mirtazapine blocks histamine receptors and thus promotes sedation and weight gain. Antidepressant effects equal those of SSRIs and may develop faster.

Mirtazapine is well absorbed after oral dosing and reaches peak plasma levels in 2 hours. The drug undergoes extensive hepatic metabolism followed by excretion in the urine (75%) and feces (25%). The elimination half-life is 20 to 40 hours.

Mirtazapine is generally well tolerated. Somnolence is the most prominent adverse effect, occurring in 54% of patients. Weight gain, increased appetite, and elevated cholesterol are also common. Sexual dysfunction is minimal. Reversible agranulocytosis was reported in early trials but was not confirmed in later clinical experience. Blockade of muscarinic receptors is moderate, and hence anticholinergic effects are mild. Mirtazapine-induced somnolence can be exacerbated by alcohol, benzodiazepines, and other CNS depressants. Accordingly, these agents should be avoided. Mirtazapine should not be combined with MAOIs.

PERIPARTUM DEPRESSION

Most women (about 80%) experience depressive symptoms after giving birth. For most, the symptoms are mild and transient, reflecting a condition sometimes called the "baby blues." For others, symptoms are severe and persistent, reflecting true postpartum depression, a condition that merits rapid medical attention.

An estimated 60% to 70% of women experience depression postpartum, and in 50% of these depression begins before delivery—hence the term peripartum depression. Symptoms include tearfulness, sadness, nervousness, irritability, and anxiety, along with difficulty eating and sleeping. The new mother may feel overwhelmed, vulnerable, weak, and alone. She may cry for no clear reason. Her self-esteem and self-confidence may decline, and she may feel unqualified to care for her baby. Fortunately, all of these symptoms pass quickly: they develop a few days after delivery and are gone by day 10. Because these symptoms are so common, they're considered a normal postpartum event. Treatment is neither necessary nor recommended.

True peripartum depression is different. The condition is much less common than the "baby blues" but much more serious. Left untreated, peripartum depression lasts for months and is likely to become worse as time passes. The condition is detrimental to the mother, and it can adversely affect the child, preventing secure attachment and impairing cognitive, emotional, and behavioral development. Immediate intervention is indicated.

True peripartum depression is an episode of major depression that starts in the weeks before or just after giving birth. Otherwise, the diagnostic criteria are the same as for all other episodes of major depression. According to the *Diagnostic and Statistical Manual of Mental Disorders, Fifth Edition* (DSM-5), for a depressive episode to qualify as having peripartum onset, symptoms must begin within 4 weeks of delivery. However, most clinicians who study the disorder use a different criterion: to them, depression is considered postpartum if it begins within 3 months of delivery—not just within 4 weeks.

Who is likely to suffer peripartum depression? Sometimes the condition occurs in first-time mothers, and sometimes it doesn't strike until a second, third, or fourth child is born. Among first-time mothers, the incidence is between 8% and 15% (about 1 in 8). For women with a history of the disorder, the risk increases to 33% (1 in 3). In addition to a prior history of the disorder, risk factors include a history of depression unrelated to childbirth, history of premenstrual dysphoric disorder (i.e., severe premenstrual syndrome), and major stress related to family, work, or residence (e.g., death of a loved one, loss of a job, moving away from a familiar town or city).

The underlying cause of peripartum depression is unknown, but several factors are thought to contribute. Heading the list is the sharp drop in estrogen and progesterone levels that occurs after delivery. (Levels of these hormones increase 10-fold during pregnancy and return to baseline after the placenta is expelled.) However, because hormone levels fall in all women, but only some get peripartum depression, other factors—physical, emotional, and social—must be involved. The birthing process may leave women feeling weak and fatigued. Caring for a baby, who needs round-the-clock attention and feeding, exacerbates tiredness and exhaustion. Emotional and social factors may also play a role. Feelings of loss are common: women experience loss of freedom, loss of control, and even loss of identity. Stress increases substantially, owing to increased workload and responsibilities, coupled with feelings of self-doubt and inadequacy, and compounded by a self-imposed (albeit highly unrealistic) expectation to be a "perfect" parent. Stress can be made even worse by financial insecurity and inadequate support from one's partner, family, and friends. Thyroid insufficiency may also contribute: levels of thyroid hormone often decline after delivery, causing symptoms that can mimic depression. Accordingly, thyroid levels should be checked and, if indicated, replacement therapy should be implemented.

Screening for peripartum depression should be contemplated in all women, although evidence is lacking regarding universal screening. Women with multiple risk factors should be strongly considered. Screening can be accomplished with a quick test: the Edinburgh Postnatal Depression Scale.

Treatment of peripartum depression is much like treatment of major depression unrelated to pregnancy. The goals are to normalize mood and to optimize maternal and social functioning. The principal treatment modalities are psychotherapy and antidepressant drugs, both of which can be effective. In addition, the woman should be encouraged to nurture herself in the following ways:

- Reduce isolation (by going out for at least a short time each day).
- Ensure adequate rest (by doing only what's really needed and letting the rest go).
- Spend time alone with her partner.

Other beneficial measures include joining a support group for new mothers and recruiting family members and friends to assist with household and baby-related chores.

Although antidepressants are clearly appropriate, there are few published data to guide selection. In one study of women with postpartum depression, fluoxetine (Prozac), an SSRI, was compared with psychotherapy. Both treatments were equally effective, and both were superior to placebo. Efficacy has also been demonstrated for sertraline (Zoloft), venlafaxine (Effexor), and certain TCAs. For initial therapy, an SSRI is an attractive choice because these drugs are effective and well tolerated and present little risk for toxicity if taken in overdose. However, if a woman has responded to an antidepressant from a different class in the past, that drug should be tried first. To minimize side effects, dosage should be low initially (50% of the usual starting dosage) and then gradually increased. To reduce the risk for relapse, treatment should continue for at least 6 months after symptoms have resolved. Unfortunately, even then the relapse rate is high: between 50% and 85% of patients experience at least one more depressive episode. With each succeeding episode, the risk for another recurrence increases. Accordingly, long-term prophylactic therapy should be considered.

Which antidepressants can be taken safely while breastfeeding? All of these drugs can be detected in breast milk—but levels of some are lower (safer) than levels of others. Sertraline, for example, appears safe. Studies show that drug activity in breastfed infants is extremely low, and no adverse reactions have been observed. The TCAs (e.g., nortriptyline, desipramine) also appear safe: levels are too low for detection in breastfed infants, and follow-up studies have found no developmental deficits. In contrast to sertraline and the TCAs, fluoxetine appears unsafe: the drug and its metabolites reach therapeutic levels in breastfed infants; potential consequences include colic and impaired weight gain. Infants of breastfeeding mothers on antidepressants should be monitored closely for these side effects.

28

Drugs for Bipolar Disorder

Bipolar disorder (BPD), formerly known as *manic-depressive illness*, afflicts an estimated 4.4% of the adult population—more than 6.7 million Americans. The mainstays of therapy are lithium and divalproex sodium (valproate), drugs that can stabilize mood. Many patients also receive an antipsychotic agent, and some may require an antidepressant. BPD is a chronic condition that requires lifelong treatment.

CHARACTERISTICS OF BIPOLAR DISORDER

BPD is a severe biologic illness characterized by recurrent fluctuations in mood. Typically patients experience alternating episodes in which mood is abnormally elevated or abnormally depressed, separated by periods in which mood is relatively normal. Symptoms usually begin in adolescence or early adulthood but can occur before adolescence or as late as the fifth decade of life. In the absence of treatment, episodes of mania or depression generally persist for several months. As time passes, manic and depressive episodes tend to recur more frequently. Although the precise etiology of BPD is unknown, it is clear that symptoms are caused by altered brain physiology, not by a character flaw or an unstable personality.

Types of Mood Episodes Seen in Bipolar Disorder

Patients with BPD may experience four types of mood episodes: pure manic, hypomanic, major depressive, and mixed.

Pure Manic Episode (Euphoric Mania)

Manic episodes are characterized by persistently heightened, expansive, or irritable mood—typically associated with hyperactivity, excessive enthusiasm, pressured speech, and flight of ideas. Manic individuals display overactivity at work and at play and have a reduced need for sleep. Mania produces excessive sociability and talkativeness. Extreme self-confidence, grandiose ideas, and delusions of self-importance are common. Manic individuals often indulge in high-risk activities (e.g., questionable business deals, reckless driving, gambling, sexual indiscretions), giving no forethought to the consequences. In severe cases, symptoms may resemble those of paranoid schizophrenia (hallucinations, delusions, bizarre behavior).

Hypomanic Episode (Hypomania)

Hypomania can be viewed as a mild form of mania. As in mania, mood is persistently elevated, expansive, or irritable. However, symptoms are not severe enough to cause marked impairment in social or occupational functioning or to require hospitalization. Psychotic symptoms are absent.

Major Depressive Episode (Depression)

A major depressive episode is characterized by depressed mood and loss of pleasure or interest in all or nearly all of one's usual activities and pastimes. Associated symptoms include disruption of sleeping and eating patterns; difficulty concentrating; feelings of guilt, worthlessness, and helplessness; and thoughts of death and suicide.

The characteristics of major depression are discussed further in Chapter 27.

Mixed Episode

In a true mixed episode, patients experience symptoms of mania and depression simultaneously. Patients may be agitated and irritable (as in mania) but may also feel worthless and depressed. The combination of high energy and depression puts them at significant risk for suicide.

Patterns of Mood Episodes

Among people with BPD, mood episodes can occur in a variety of patterns. Contrary to popular belief, not all patients alternate repeatedly between mania and depression. Some experience repeated episodes of mania, and some experience repeated episodes of depression (with an occasional episode of mania). Mood may be normal between episodes of mania and depression, or it may be slightly elevated (hypomania) or slightly depressed (dysphoria).

Mood episodes can vary greatly with respect to how often they occur and how long they last. A single episode may last for days, weeks, months, or more than a year. In the absence of treatment, episodes of mania or hypomania typically last a few months, whereas episodes of major depression typically last at least 6 months. On average, people with BPD experience only four episodes during the first 10 years of their illness. However, some people cycle much more rapidly, experiencing many episodes every year.

On the basis of mood episode type and frequency, BPD can be subdivided into two major categories:
- *Bipolar I disorder*—patients experience manic or mixed episodes and usually depressive episodes too.
- *Bipolar II disorder*—patients experience hypomanic or depressive episodes but not manic or mixed episodes.

Etiology

Theories regarding the etiology of BPD continue to evolve. In the past there was general agreement that BPD was due primarily to an imbalance in neurotransmitters. Today researchers suspect that the real cause may be disruption of neuronal growth and survival. First, neuroimaging studies have shown an association between prolonged mood disorders and atrophy of specific brain regions—especially the subgenual prefrontal cortex, an area involved in emotionality. Second, mood-stabilizing drugs can prevent or reverse neuronal atrophy in patients with BPD, apparently by influencing signaling pathways that regulate neuronal growth and survival.

PROTOTYPE DRUGS

Mood-Stabilizing Drugs for Bipolar Disorder

Lithium
Carbamazepine
Valproic acid

TREATMENT OF BIPOLAR DISORDER

Types of Drugs Employed

BPD is treated with three major groups of drugs: mood stabilizers, antipsychotics, and antidepressants. In addition, benzodiazepines are frequently used for sedation.

Mood Stabilizers

Mood stabilizers are drugs that (1) relieve symptoms during manic and depressive episodes, (2) prevent the recurrence of manic and depressive episodes, and (3) do not worsen symptoms of mania or depression or accelerate the rate of cycling. The principal mood stabilizers are *lithium* and two drugs originally developed for epilepsy: *divalproex sodium* (valproate) and *carbamazepine*. These drugs are the mainstays of treatment. The pharmacology of lithium and the antiepileptic drugs is discussed later.

Antipsychotics

In patients with BPD, antipsychotic drugs are given to help control symptoms during severe manic episodes, even if psychotic symptoms are absent. Although antipsychotics can be used alone, they are usually employed in combination with a mood stabilizer. For reasons discussed later, the second-generation antipsychotics (e.g., olanzapine, risperidone) are generally preferred to the first-generation agents (e.g., haloperidol).

Antidepressants

Antidepressants may be needed during a depressive episode. However, in patients with BPD, antidepressants are almost always combined with a mood stabilizer because of the long-held belief that, when used alone, antidepressants may elevate mood so much that a hypomanic or manic episode will result. However, data indicate that the risk for inducing mania may be much lower than previously thought. Nonetheless, the current guidelines suggest continuing the traditional practice of using an antidepressant only if a mood stabilizer is being used as well.

Although antidepressants have been studied extensively in patients with major depression, research is still lacking in patients with BPD. At this time there are insufficient data on which to base drug selection. Even so, experts do have their preferences. Among clinicians with extensive experience in BPD, the following are considered antidepressants of choice: *bupropion* (Wellbutrin), *venlafaxine* (Effexor XR), and the selective serotonin reuptake inhibitors (SSRIs) such as fluoxetine (Prozac) and sertraline (Zoloft). One thing we do know is that the use of tricyclic antidepressants (TCAs) appears to promote more incidents of mania; therefore TCAs are not recommended in the treatment of BPD. The pharmacology of these drugs is discussed in Chapter 27.

Drug Selection

Acute Therapy: Manic Episodes

Two mood stabilizers—lithium and valproate—are preferred drugs for the acute management of manic episodes in combination with a second-generation (atypical) antipsychotic medication. Lithium is the drug of choice. If the patient does not respond adequately to lithium or valproate alone, the drugs may be used together. Responses to mood stabilizers develop slowly, taking 2 or more weeks to become maximal.

Seven second-generation antipsychotic medications are approved for the management of acute manic or mixed episodes occurring in bipolar depression. These medications are often used for the short-term management of severe mania as adjunctive therapy to the mood stabilizers. Table 28.1 lists common dosages.

If needed for episodes of severe mania, a benzodiazepine may be added to the regimen for the acute management of symptoms (e.g., insomnia, anxiety, agitation). For patients with hypoactive mania, an

antipsychotic may be employed as monotherapy; olanzapine or risperidone would be a good choice.

Acute Therapy: Depressive Episodes

Depressive episodes may be treated with a mood stabilizer, an atypical antipsychotic, or a mood stabilizer or antipsychotic *plus* an antidepressant but rarely with an antidepressant alone (because hypomania or mania might result). If depression is mild, monotherapy with a mood stabilizer

TABLE 28.1 Adult Oral Dosages for Atypical Antipsychotics Used in Bipolar Disorder	
Drug	**Dosage**
Aripiprazole (Abilify)	*Acute mania:* Start with 15 mg once daily and increase to 30 mg once daily if needed. Do not exceed 30 mg qd.
Asenapine (Saphris)	*Acute mania/mixed episode:* Start with 10 mg qd and increase to 20 mg qd if needed.
Cariprazine (Vraylar)	*Acute mania:* Start with 1.5 mg once daily and increase by 1.5 mg daily to a daily dose of 3–6 mg.
Olanzapine (Zyprexa)	*Acute mania:* Start with 10–15 mg once daily. Increase in increments of 5-mg/day as indicated. The effective range is 5–20 mg once daily. *Maintenance therapy:* The effective range is 5–20 mg once daily.
Olanzapine/ fluoxetine (Symbyax)	*Depressive episodes:* Start with 6 mg olanzapine/25 mg fluoxetine once daily in the evening. The effective range for antidepressant effects is olanzapine 6–12 mg and fluoxetine 25–50 mg.
Quetiapine (Seroquel)	*Acute mania (with normal liver function):* Give in two divided doses as follows: 100 mg on day 1, 200 mg on day 2, 300 mg on day 3, and 400 mg on day 4. If needed, increase to 600 mg on day 5 and 800 mg on day 6. *Acute mania (with liver impairment):* Give 25 mg on day 1, then increase by 25–50 mg/day until symptoms are controlled or side effects are intolerable, whichever comes first. *Depressive episodes:* Give once-daily doses at bedtime as follows: 50 mg on day 1, 100 mg on day 2, 200 mg on day 3, and 300 mg on day 4; if needed, increase to 400 mg on day 5, and 600 mg on day 8.
Risperidone, short-acting (Risperdal)	*Acute mania:* Start with 2–3 mg once daily; increase to a maximum of 6 mg once daily if needed.
Risperidone, long-acting (Risperdal Consta)	*Maintenance therapy:* Start with 25 mg intramuscularly (IM) every 2 weeks. After at least 4 weeks, dosage may be increased to 37.5 mg IM every 2 weeks. After at least 4 more weeks, increased again to 50 mg IM every 2 weeks.
Ziprasidone (Geodon)	*Acute mania:* On day 1, give 80 mg (in two divided doses with food). On day 2, increase to 60 or 80 mg bid. Based on tolerability and efficacy, adjust dosage within the range of 40–80 mg bid. *Maintenance therapy:* The effective range is 15–30 mg qd.

(lithium or valproate) may be sufficient. If the mood stabilizer is inadequate, an antidepressant or antipsychotic can be added. Benefits may be limited with the addition of an antidepressant. Preferred antidepressants are bupropion, venlafaxine, or an SSRI. There is even a combination drug that consists of an atypical antipsychotic and an SSRI specifically designed for this purpose (see Table 28.1).

Long-Term Preventive Treatment

The purpose of long-term therapy is to prevent recurrence of both mania and depression. As a rule, one or more mood stabilizers are employed. Drug selection is based on what worked acutely. For example, if the patient responded to acute therapy with lithium alone, then lithium alone should be tried long term. Other long-term options include valproate alone and valproate plus lithium. More recently antipsychotic agents have been employed for long-term maintenance, either as monotherapy or in combination with a mood stabilizer.

Promoting Adherence

Poor patient adherence can frustrate attempts to treat a manic episode. Patients may resist treatment because they fail to see anything wrong with their thinking or behavior. Furthermore, the experience is not necessarily unpleasant. In fact, individuals going through a manic episode may well enjoy it. Therefore, to ensure adherence, short-term hospitalization may be required. To achieve this, collaboration with the patient's family may be needed. Because hospitalization per se will not guarantee success, lithium administration should be directly observed to ensure that each dose is actually taken.

PATIENT EDUCATION

Adherence to Long-Term Therapy

After an acute manic episode has been controlled, long-term prophylactic therapy is indicated, making adherence an ongoing issue. To promote adherence, the patient and family should be educated about the nature of bipolar disorder and the importance of taking medications as prescribed. Family members can help ensure adherence by overseeing medication use and urging the patient to visit his or her prescriber or a psychiatric clinic if a pattern of nonadherence develops.

MOOD-STABILIZING DRUGS

As noted, mood stabilizers are drugs that can relieve an acute manic or depressive episode and prevent symptoms from recurring—all without aggravating mania or depression and without accelerating cycling. The agents used most often are lithium, valproate, and carbamazepine.

Lithium

Lithium (Lithobid, Carbolith ♣) can stabilize mood in patients with BPD. Its beneficial effects were first described in 1949 by John Cade, an Australian psychiatrist. Because of concerns about toxicity, lithium was not approved for use in the United States until 1970. Lithium has a low therapeutic index. As a result, toxicity can occur at blood levels only slightly greater than therapeutic levels. Accordingly, the monitoring of lithium levels is mandatory.

Chemistry

Lithium is a simple inorganic ion that carries a single positive charge. In the periodic table of elements, lithium is in the same group as potassium and sodium. Not surprisingly, lithium has properties in common with both elements. Lithium is found naturally in animal tissues but has no known physiologic function.

Therapeutic Uses

Bipolar disorder. Lithium is a drug of choice for controlling acute manic episodes in patients with BPD and for long-term prophylaxis against the recurrence of mania or depression. In manic patients, lithium reduces euphoria, hyperactivity, and other symptoms but does not cause sedation. Antimanic effects begin 5 to 7 days after treatment onset, but full benefits may not develop for 2 to 3 weeks. Lithium is considered the drug of choice for all patients experiencing an acute manic episode regardless of clinical presentation.

Mechanism of Action

Although lithium has been studied extensively, the precise mechanism by which it stabilizes mood is unknown. In the past, research focused on three aspects of brain neurochemistry: (1) altered distribution of certain ions (calcium, sodium, magnesium) that are critical to neuronal function; (2) altered synthesis and release of norepinephrine, serotonin, and dopamine; and (3) effects on second messengers (e.g., cyclic adenosine monophosphate, phosphatidylinositol), which mediate intracellular responses to neurotransmitters. Unfortunately this research has failed to provide a definitive explanation of how lithium works. Current neurochemical research suggests that lithium may work by (1) altering glutamate uptake and release, (2) blocking the binding of serotonin to its receptors, or (3) inhibiting glycogen synthase kinase-3 β.

There has been growing interest in the neurotrophic and neuroprotective actions of lithium. As noted earlier, there is evidence that symptoms of BPD may result from neuronal atrophy in certain brain areas. In animal studies, "therapeutic" doses of lithium doubled the level of neurotrophic Bcl-2 proteins. In addition, lithium has been shown to facilitate the regeneration of damaged optic nerves. In patients with BPD taking lithium long term, the volume of the subgenual prefrontal cortex is greater than that in untreated patients. Furthermore, lithium can increase total gray matter in regions known to atrophy in BPD, including the prefrontal cortex, hippocampus, and caudate nucleus. All of these studies suggest that the benefits of lithium may result at least in part from an ability to protect against neuronal atrophy or promote neuronal growth.

Pharmacokinetics

Absorption and distribution. Lithium is well absorbed after oral administration. The drug distributes evenly to all tissues and body fluids.

Excretion. Lithium has a short half-life owing to its rapid renal excretion. Because of its short half-life (and high toxicity), the drug must be administered in divided daily doses. Large single daily doses cannot be used, even when a slow-release preparation is prescribed. Because lithium is excreted by the kidneys, it must be employed with great care in patients with renal impairment.

Renal excretion of lithium is affected by blood levels of sodium. Specifically, lithium excretion is *reduced* when levels of sodium are *low*, because the kidney processes lithium and sodium in the same way. Hence, when the kidney senses that sodium levels are inadequate, it retains lithium in an attempt to compensate. Because of this relationship, lithium can accumulate to toxic levels in the presence of low sodium. Accordingly, it is important that sodium levels remain normal. Patients should be instructed to maintain normal sodium intake. Because diuretics promote sodium loss, these agents must be employed with caution. Also, sodium loss secondary to diarrhea can be sufficient to cause lithium accumulation. The patient should be told about this possibility.

Dehydration will cause lithium retention by the kidneys, posing the risk for accumulation to dangerous levels. Potential causes of dehydration include hot weather and diarrhea. Patients should be counseled to maintain adequate hydration.

Monitoring plasma lithium levels. Measurement of plasma lithium levels is an essential component of treatment. *Lithium levels must be kept below 1.5 mEq/L; levels greater than this can produce significant toxicity.* Lithum levels should range from 0.4 to 1 mEq/L. Generally levels should be between 0.6 and 0.8 mEq/L. Levels of 0.8 to 1 mEq/L may be more effective but carry a greater risk of adverse effects. Blood for lithium determinations should be drawn in the morning, 12 hours after the evening dose. During maintenance therapy, lithium levels should be measured every 3 to 6 months.

Adverse Effects

The adverse effects of lithium can be divided into two categories (1) effects that occur at therapeutic lithium levels and (2) effects that occur at excessive lithium levels. Certain toxicities are closely correlated with the concentration of lithium in blood. As indicated in Table 28.2, mild responses (e.g., fine hand tremor, gastrointestinal [GI] upset, thirst, muscle weakness) can develop at lithium levels that are still within the therapeutic range (i.e., less than 1.5 mEq/L). When plasma levels exceed 1.5 mEq/L, more serious toxicities appear. At drug levels higher than 2.5 mEq/L, death can occur. In the following discussion, effects produced at therapeutic levels are considered individually. Effects produced at excessive lithium levels are considered as a group.

⏩ BLACK BOX WARNING

Lithium Toxicity

> Lithium toxicity is closely related to serum lithium levels and can occur at doses close to therapeutic levels. Facilities for prompt and accurate serum lithium determinations should be available before initiating therapy.

Adverse effects that occur at therapeutic levels of lithium

Early adverse effects. Several responses occur early in treatment and then usually subside. *GI effects* (e.g., nausea, diarrhea, abdominal bloating, anorexia) are common but transient. About 30% of patients experience *transient fatigue, muscle weakness, headache, confusion,* and *memory impairment. Polyuria* and *thirst* occur in 30% to 50% of patients and may persist.

Tremor. Patients may develop a fine hand tremor, especially in the fingers, that can interfere with writing and other motor skills. Lithium-induced tremor can be augmented by stress, fatigue, and certain drugs

TABLE 28.2   Toxicities Associated With Excessive Plasma Levels of Lithium

Plasma Lithium Level (mEq/L)	Signs of Toxicity
Less than 1.5	Nausea, vomiting, diarrhea, thirst, polyuria, lethargy, slurred speech, muscle weakness, fine hand tremor
1.5–2	Persistent GI upset, coarse hand tremor, confusion, hyperirritability of muscles, ECG changes, sedation, incoordination
2–2.5	Ataxia, giddiness, high output of dilute urine, serious ECG changes, fasciculations, tinnitus, blurred vision, clonic movements, seizures, stupor, severe hypotension, coma, death (usually secondary to pulmonary complications)
More than 2.5	Symptoms may progress rapidly to generalized convulsions, oliguria, and death

ECG, Electrocardiographic; *GI,* gastrointestinal.

(antidepressants, antipsychotics, caffeine). Tremor can be reduced with a beta blocker (e.g., propranolol) and by measures that reduce peak levels of lithium (i.e., dosage reduction, use of divided doses, or use of a sustained-release formulation).

Polyuria. Polyuria occurs in 50% to 70% of patients taking lithium chronically. In some patients, daily urine output may exceed 3 L. Lithium promotes polyuria by antagonizing the effects of antidiuretic hormone. To maintain adequate hydration, patients should be instructed to drink 8 to 12 glasses of fluids daily. Polyuria, nocturia, and excessive thirst can discourage patients from adhering to the regimen.

Lithium-induced polyuria can be reduced with *amiloride* (Midamor), a potassium-sparing diuretic. Amiloride appears to help by reducing the entry of lithium into epithelial cells of the renal tubule. Polyuria can also be reduced with a thiazide diuretic. However, because thiazides can lower levels of sodium (see Chapter 37) and would thereby increase lithium retention, amiloride is preferred.

Renal toxicity. Chronic lithium use has been associated with degenerative changes in the kidney. The risk for renal injury can be reduced by keeping the dosage low and, when possible, avoiding long-term lithium therapy. Kidney function should be assessed before treatment and once a year thereafter.

Goiter and hypothyroidism. Lithium can reduce the incorporation of iodine into thyroid hormone and can inhibit thyroid hormone secretion. With long-term use, the drug can cause *goiter* (enlargement of the thyroid gland). Although usually benign, lithium-induced goiter is sometimes associated with *hypothyroidism.* Treatment with thyroid hormone (levothyroxine) or withdrawal of lithium will reverse both goiter and hypothyroidism. Levels of thyroid hormones—triiodothyronine (T_3) and thyroxine (T_4)—and levels of thyroid-stimulating hormone (TSH) should be measured before giving lithium and annually thereafter.

Teratogenesis. Lithium may or may not be a teratogen. In older studies, lithium appeared to have significant teratogenic effects: drug use during the first trimester of pregnancy was associated with an 11% incidence of birth defects (usually malformations of the heart). However, in more recent studies, lithium showed little or no teratogenic potential. Nonetheless, to minimize any potential fetal risk, *lithium should be avoided during the first trimester of pregnancy.* Unless the benefits of therapy clearly outweigh the risks, it should be avoided during the remainder of pregnancy as well. Women of childbearing age should be counseled to avoid pregnancy while taking lithium. Also, pregnancy should be ruled out before initiating lithium therapy.

Use in lactation. Lithium readily enters breast milk and can achieve concentrations that might harm the nursing infant. Consequently breastfeeding during lithium therapy should be discouraged.

Lithium toxicity. Patients should be informed about early signs of toxicity and instructed to interrupt lithium dosing if these appear. In adherent patients, the most common cause of lithium accumulation is sodium depletion.

To keep lithium levels within the therapeutic range, plasma drug levels should be monitored routinely. Levels should be measured every 2 to 3 days at the beginning of treatment and every 3 to 6 months during maintenance therapy.

Treatment of acute overdose is primarily supportive; there is no specific antidote. The severely intoxicated patient should be hospitalized. Hemodialysis is an effective means of lithium removal and should be considered whenever drug levels exceed 2.5 mEq/L.

Drug Interactions

Diuretics. Diuretics promote sodium loss and can thereby increase the risk for lithium toxicity. Toxicity can occur because renal excretion of lithium is reduced in the presence of low sodium, causing lithium levels to rise.

TABLE 28.3   Lithium Preparations

Formulation	Lithium Content[a]	Trade Name	Usual Adult Dose
Capsules	4.06 mEq lithium (150 mg Li₂CO₃)	Generic only	300 mg PO three or four times daily
	8.12 mEq lithium (300 mg Li₂CO₃)	Carbolith	300 mg PO three or four times daily
	16.24 mEq lithium (600 mg Li₂CO₃)	Generic only	600 mg PO twice daily
Oral solution	Lithium citrate 8 mEq/5 mL (300 mg Li₂CO₃)	Generic only	300 mg PO three or four times daily
Immediate-release tablets	8.12 mEq lithium (300 and 450 mg Li₂CO₃)	Generic only	300 mg PO three or four times daily
Slow-release tablets	8.12 mEq lithium (300 and 450 mg Li₂CO₃)	Lithobid	600 mg PO twice daily

[a]Lithium content is expressed in two ways: milliequivalents (mEq) of lithium ion and milligrams (mg) of lithium carbonate.
PO, Given by mouth.

Nonsteroidal antiinflammatory drugs. Nonsteroidal antiinflammatory drugs (NSAIDs) can increase lithium levels by as much as 60%. By suppressing prostaglandin synthesis in the kidney, NSAIDs can increase renal reabsorption of lithium (and also sodium), causing lithium levels to rise. NSAIDs known to increase lithium levels include ibuprofen (Motrin, others), naproxen (Naprosyn), piroxicam (Feldene), indomethacin (Indocin), and celecoxib (Celebrex). Interestingly, aspirin (the prototype NSAID) and sulindac (Clinoril) do *not* increase lithium levels. Accordingly, if a mild analgesic is needed, aspirin or sulindac would be a good choice.

Anticholinergic drugs. Anticholinergics can cause urinary hesitancy. Coupled with lithium-induced polyuria, this can result in considerable discomfort. Accordingly, patients should avoid drugs with prominent anticholinergic actions (e.g., antihistamines, phenothiazine antipsychotics, TCAs).

Dosage and Administration

Dosing. Lithium dosing is highly individualized. Dosage adjustments are based on plasma drug levels and clinical response (Table 28.3).

Plasma levels should be kept within the therapeutic range. Lithium levels should remain between 0.4 and 1 mEq/L. (Levels of 0.6 to 0.8 mEq/L are effective for most patients.) To avoid serious toxicity, *lithium levels should not exceed 1.5 mEq/L.*

Knowledge of plasma drug levels is not the only guide to lithium dosing; the clinical response is at least as important. Accordingly, when lithium dosage is being evaluated, we must not forget to look at the patient. Laboratory tests are all well and good, but they are not a substitute for clinical assessment. For example, if blood levels of lithium appear proper but clinical evaluation indicates toxicity, there is no question as to what should be done: reduce the dosage, despite the apparent acceptability of the dosage as reflected by plasma lithium levels.

 ### BLACK BOX WARNING

Life-Threatening Adverse Reactions to Lithium

Lithium is associated with hepatotoxicity and pancreatitis, including fatalities, usually during the first 6 months of treatment. Children younger than 2 years and patients with mitochondrial disorders are at higher risk.

Lithium is linked to increased fetal risk, particularly neural tube defects, other major malformations, and decreased IQ.

Antiepileptic Drugs

Three antiepileptic drugs—divalproex sodium, carbamazepine, and lamotrigine—can suppress mania and depression and can stabilize mood in patients with BPD (Table 28.4). The efficacy of these agents is firmly established. In fact, one drug, divalproex sodium, is so effective that it has replaced lithium as the drug of choice for many patients. The basic

SUMMARY OF KEY PRESCRIBING CONSIDERATIONS

Lithium

Therapeutic Goal: Control of acute manic episodes in patients with bipolar disorder (BPD) and prophylaxis against recurrent mania and depression in patients with BPD.

Baseline Data: Complete blood count, electrolytes, hepatic function, cardiac function, and thyroid function.

Monitoring: Lithium levels should be measured every 2–3 days during initial therapy and every 3–6 months during maintenance.

Identifying High-Risk Patients: Lithium should be avoided during the first trimester of pregnancy and used with caution during the remainder of pregnancy. Monitor use closely in patients with renal disease and patients on concurrent diuretic therapy.

Evaluating Therapeutic Effects: Evaluate the patient for abatement of manic symptoms and mood stabilization.

Minimizing Adverse Effects: Educate patients on signs of toxicity, including nausea, vomiting, tremor, confusion, blurred vision, and tinnitus.

pharmacology of the antiepileptic drugs and their use in seizure disorders is discussed in Chapter 21. Discussion here focuses on their use in BPD.

Divalproex Sodium (Valproate)

Divalproex sodium[a] (Depakote, Epival), or simply valproate, was the first antiseizure agent approved for BPD. Valproate can control symptoms in acute manic episodes and can help prevent relapse into mania. However, the drug is less effective at the treatment and prevention of depressive episodes. As with lithium, benefits appear to result at least in part from neurotrophic and neuroprotective effects. In patients with BPD, valproate compares favorably with lithium. Both drugs are highly effective; moreover, valproate works faster and has a higher therapeutic index and a more desirable side-effect profile. However, lithium *is* superior in two important respects. First, lithium is better at reducing the risk for suicide. And second, lithium is more effective at preventing relapses. Nonetheless, because of its rapid onset, safety, and overall efficacy, valproate has become a first-line treatment for BPD.

Although valproate has a higher therapeutic index than lithium and is generally better tolerated, it *can* cause serious toxicity. Of greatest concern are rare cases of thrombocytopenia, pancreatitis, and liver failure, all of which require immediate drug withdrawal. In addition, valproate is a teratogen and hence should not be used during pregnancy.

---

[a]As discussed in Chapter 21, divalproex sodium (Depakote) is a mixture of valproic acid (Depakene, Depacon) and its sodium salt (sodium valproate). Only divalproex sodium is approved for BPD, although all three preparations have identical actions.

TABLE 28.4 Antiepileptic Drugs Used in Bipolar Disorder

Drug	Trade Name(s)	Availability	Usual Initial Dose	Usual Maintenance Dose/Day
Divalproex sodium	Depakote Depakote ER	125-, 250-, 500-mg DR tablets 125-mg DR capsules 250-, 500-mg ER tablets	250 mg PO three times daily or 500 mg PO at every bedtime	1000–2500 mg
Carbamazepine	Equetro	100-, 200-, 300-mg ER tablets	200 mg PO twice daily	Gradually increase to max dose of 1600 mg
Lamotrigine	Lamictal Lamictal XR	25-, 100-, 150-, 200-mg tablets 25-, 50-, 100-, 200-mg orally dissolving tablets 25-, 50-, 100-, 200-, 250-, 300-mg ER tablets 2-, 5-, 25-mg chewable tablets	25–50 mg PO daily	Gradually increase to 200 mg

DR, Delayed-release; *ER*, extended-release; *PO*, given by mouth; *XR*, extended-release

GI disturbances (nausea, vomiting, diarrhea, dyspepsia, indigestion) are common. Despite causing GI distress, valproate frequently causes weight gain, a serious and chronic complication of treatment.

 BLACK BOX WARNING

Hepatotoxicity and Pancreatitis With Divalproex

Serious or fatal hepatic failure has occurred with use of Depakote ER. In addition, life-threatening pancreatitis has been reported.

Depakote is also linked to increased fetal risk, particularly neural tube defects, other major malformations, and decreased IQ.

Carbamazepine

Carbamazepine (Tegretol, Equetro) is approved for the treatment and prevention of manic episodes in patients with BPD. Like valproate, carbamazepine appears less effective in the treatment and prevention of depression. The target trough plasma level is 4 to 12 μg/mL. Neurologic side effects (visual disturbances, ataxia, vertigo, unsteadiness, headache) are common early in treatment but generally resolve despite continued drug use. Hematologic effects (leukopenia, anemia, thrombocytopenia, aplastic anemia) are relatively uncommon but can be severe. Accordingly, CBCs, including platelets, should be obtained at baseline and periodically thereafter. Carbamazepine induces cytochrome P450 isoenzymes and can thereby accelerate its own metabolism and the metabolism of other drugs (e.g., oral contraceptives, warfarin, valproate, TCAs). To maintain efficacy, dosages of carbamazepine and these other drugs should be increased as needed.

Drug products containing carbamazepine are available under four trade names: *Carbatrol, Equetro, Epitol,* and *Tegretol.* Carbamazepine formulations with any of these names can be used for BPD. However, only one product—Equetro—is actually *approved* for BPD.

 BLACK BOX WARNING

Serious Adverse Reactions to Carbamazepine

Serious and sometimes fatal dermatologic reactions—including toxic epidermal necrolysis and Stevens-Johnson syndrome—have been reported during treatment with carbamazepine.

Aplastic anemia and agranulocytosis have also been reported in association with the use of carbamazepine.

Lamotrigine

Lamotrigine (Lamictal) is indicated for long-term maintenance therapy of BPD. The goal is to prevent affective relapses into mania or depression.

Lamotrigine may be used alone or in combination with other mood-stabilizing agents. Side effects include headache, dizziness, double vision, and, rarely, life-threatening rashes (Stevens-Johnson syndrome, toxic epidermal necrolysis).

 BLACK BOX WARNING

Serious Adverse Reactions to Lamotrigine

Serious and sometimes fatal dermatologic reactions, including toxic epidermal necrolysis and Stevens-Johnson syndrome, have been reported during treatment with lamotrigine.

ANTIPSYCHOTIC DRUGS

In patients with BPD, antipsychotic drugs are used *acutely* to control symptoms during manic episodes, and *long term* to help stabilize mood. These drugs benefit patients with or without psychotic symptoms. Although antipsychotics can be used alone, they are usually employed in combination with a mood stabilizer, typically lithium or valproate.

As discussed in Chapter 26, the antipsychotic drugs fall into two major groups: first-generation antipsychotics (conventional antipsychotics) and second-generation antipsychotics (atypical antipsychotics). Compared with the conventional agents, the atypical agents carry a lower risk for extrapyramidal side effects, including tardive dyskinesia. Accordingly, the atypical agents are preferred for BPD.

Eight atypical antipsychotics—*olanzapine* (Zyprexa), *quetiapine* (Seroquel), *risperidone* (Risperdal), *aripiprazole* (Abilify), *lurasidone* (Latuda), *cariprazine* (Vraylar), *asenapine* (Saphris), and *ziprasidone* (Geodon)—are approved for BPD. (Another one—*clozapine* (Clozaril)—although highly effective in BPD, is not used owing to a risk for agranulocytosis.) All of these drugs are effective against acute mania when used alone or combined with lithium or valproate. Currently only three atypical agents—aripiprazole, olanzapine, and ziprasidone—are approved for long-term use to prevent the recurrence of mood episodes. Dosages for patients with BPD are shown in Table 28.1.

The pharmacology of the antipsychotics is presented in Chapter 26.

BLACK BOX WARNING

Increased Mortality in Older Adults

Elderly patients with dementia-related psychosis treated with antipsychotic drugs are at an increased risk for death.

29

Sedative-Hypnotic Drugs

The sedative-hypnotics are drugs that depress the function of the central nervous system (CNS). CNS depression is more generalized with some of these drugs than with others. The sedative-hypnotics are used primarily for two common disorders: anxiety and insomnia. Agents given to relieve anxiety are known as *antianxiety agents* or *anxiolytics*. Agents given to promote sleep are known as *hypnotics*. The distinction between antianxiety effects and hypnotic effects is often a matter of dosage: typically sedative-hypnotics relieve anxiety in low doses and induce sleep in higher doses. Hence a single drug may be considered both an antianxiety agent and a hypnotic agent, depending on the reason for its use and the dosage employed.

There are four major groups of sedative-hypnotics: barbiturates (e.g., secobarbital), benzodiazepines (e.g., diazepam), benzodiazepine-like drugs (e.g., zolpidem), and new agents with unique mechanisms of action (suvorexant, ramelteon). The barbiturates were introduced in the early 1900s, the benzodiazepines in the 1950s, and the benzodiazepine-like drugs in the 1990s. Although barbiturates were widely used as sedative-hypnotics in the past, they are rarely used for this purpose today, having been replaced by the newer drugs.

Before the benzodiazepines became available, anxiety and insomnia were treated with barbiturates and other *general CNS depressants*—drugs with multiple undesirable qualities. First, these drugs are powerful respiratory depressants that can readily prove fatal in overdose. As a result, they are commonly used drugs for suicide. Second, because they produce subjective effects that many individuals find desirable, most general CNS depressants have a high potential for abuse. Third, with prolonged use, most of these drugs produce significant tolerance and physical dependence. And fourth, barbiturates and some other CNS depressants induce the synthesis of hepatic drug-metabolizing enzymes and can thereby decrease responses to other drugs. Because the benzodiazepines are just as effective as the general CNS depressants but do not share their undesirable properties, the benzodiazepines are clearly preferred to the general CNS depressants for treating anxiety and insomnia.

This chapter begins by discussing the basic pharmacology of the sedative-hypnotics and ends by discussing their use in insomnia. Use of these drugs for anxiety disorders is addressed in Chapter 30.

BENZODIAZEPINES

Benzodiazepines, along with the newer benzodiazepine receptor agonists, are drugs of first choice for anxiety and insomnia. In addition, these drugs are used to induce general anesthesia and to manage seizure disorders, muscle spasm, and withdrawal from alcohol.

Benzodiazepines were introduced in the late 1950s and remain important today. Perhaps the most familiar member of the family is diazepam (Valium). The most frequently prescribed members are lorazepam (Ativan) and alprazolam (Xanax, Xanax XR, Niravam).

Although triazolam is our prototype for the benzodiazepines, because all drugs in this category produce nearly identical effects, these can be considered as a group.

Overview of Pharmacologic Effects

Practically all responses to benzodiazepines result from actions in the CNS. Benzodiazepines have few direct actions outside the CNS. All of the benzodiazepines produce a similar spectrum of responses. However, because of pharmacokinetic differences, individual benzodiazepines may differ in clinical applications.

Central Nervous System

All of the beneficial effects of benzodiazepines as well as most of their adverse effects result from depressant actions in the CNS. With increasing dosage, effects progress from sedation to hypnosis to stupor.

Benzodiazepines depress neuronal function at multiple sites in the CNS. They *reduce anxiety* through effects on the limbic system, a neuronal network associated with emotionality. They *promote sleep* through effects on cortical areas and on the sleep–wakefulness "clock." They *induce muscle relaxation* through effects on supraspinal motor areas, including the cerebellum. Two important side effects—*confusion* and *antero-grade amnesia*—result from effects on the hippocampus and cerebral cortex.

Cardiovascular System

When taken *orally*, benzodiazepines have almost no effect on the heart and blood vessels. In contrast, when administered *intravenously*, even in therapeutic doses, benzodiazepines can produce profound hypotension and cardiac arrest.

Respiratory System

In contrast to the barbiturates, the benzodiazepines are weak respiratory depressants. When taken alone in therapeutic doses, benzodiazepines produce little or no depression of respiration; with toxic doses, respiratory depression is moderate at most. With oral therapy, clinically significant respiratory depression occurs only when benzodiazepines are combined with other CNS depressants (e.g., opioids, barbiturates, alcohol).

Although benzodiazepines generally have minimal effects on respiration, they can be a problem for patients with respiratory disorders. In patients with chronic obstructive pulmonary disease (COPD), benzodiazepines may worsen hypoventilation and hypoxemia. In patients with obstructive sleep apnea (OSA), benzodiazepines may exacerbate apneic episodes. In patients who snore, benzodiazepines may convert partial airway obstruction into OSA.

Molecular Mechanism of Action

Benzodiazepines *potentiate the actions of γ-aminobutyric acid* (GABA), an inhibitory neurotransmitter found throughout the CNS. These drugs enhance the actions of GABA by binding to specific receptors in a supramolecular structure known as the GABA receptor–chloride channel complex. Note that benzodiazepines do not act as direct GABA agonists; they simply intensify the effects of GABA.

Because benzodiazepines act by amplifying the actions of endogenous GABA rather than by directly mimicking GABA, there is a limit to how much CNS depression benzodiazepines can produce. This explains why benzodiazepines are so much safer than the barbiturates—drugs that can directly mimic GABA. Because benzodiazepines simply potentiate the inhibitory effects of endogenous GABA and because the amount of GABA in the CNS is finite, there is a built-in limit to the depth of CNS depression the benzodiazepines can produce. In contrast, because the barbiturates are direct-acting CNS depressants, maximal effects are limited only by the amount of barbiturate administered.

Pharmacokinetics

Absorption and Distribution

Most benzodiazepines are well absorbed after oral administration. Because of their high lipid solubility, benzodiazepines readily cross the blood–brain barrier to reach sites in the CNS.

Metabolism

Most benzodiazepines undergo extensive metabolic alterations. With few exceptions, the *metabolites are pharmacologically active*. As a result, responses produced by administering a particular benzodiazepine often persist long after the parent drug has disappeared. Hence there may be a poor correlation between the plasma half-life of the parent drug and duration of pharmacologic effects. Flurazepam, for example, whose plasma half-life is only 2 to 3 hours, is converted into an active metabolite with a half-life of 50 hours. Hence giving flurazepam produces long-lasting effects, even though flurazepam itself is gone from the plasma in 8 to 12 hours (about four half-lives).

In patients with liver disease, metabolism of benzodiazepines may be reduced, thereby prolonging excretion and intensifying responses. Because certain benzodiazepines (oxazepam, temazepam, and lorazepam) undergo very little metabolic alteration, they may be preferred for patients with hepatic impairment.

Time Course of Action

Benzodiazepines differ significantly from one another with respect to time course. Specifically, they differ in onset and duration of action and in their tendency to accumulate with repeated dosing.

Because all benzodiazepines have essentially equivalent pharmacologic actions, selection among them is based largely on differences in time course. For example, if a patient needs medication to accelerate falling asleep, a benzodiazepine with a rapid onset (e.g., triazolam) would be indicated. However, if medication is needed to prevent waking later in the night, a benzodiazepine with a slower onset (e.g., estazolam) would be preferred. For treatment of anxiety, a drug with an intermediate duration is desirable. For treatment of any benzodiazepine-responsive condition in older adults, a drug such as lorazepam, which is not likely to accumulate with repeated dosing, is generally preferred.

Therapeutic Uses

The benzodiazepines have three principal indications: (1) anxiety, (2) insomnia, and (3) seizure disorders. In addition, they are used as preoperative medications and to treat muscle spasm and withdrawal from alcohol. Although all benzodiazepines share the same pharmacologic properties and therefore might be equally effective for all applications, not every benzodiazepine is actually employed for all potential uses. The principal factors that determine the actual applications of a particular benzodiazepine are (1) the pharmacokinetic properties of the drug itself and (2) the research and marketing decisions of pharmaceutical companies. Specific applications of individual benzodiazepines are shown in Table 29.1.

Anxiety

Benzodiazepines are drugs of first choice for acute anxiety. Although all benzodiazepines have anxiolytic actions, only six are marketed for this indication (see Table 29.1). Anxiolytic effects result from depressing neurotransmission in the limbic system and cortical areas. Use of benzodiazepines to treat anxiety disorders is discussed in Chapter 30.

Insomnia

Benzodiazepines are also used in the treatment of insomnia. These drugs decrease latency time to falling asleep, reduce awakenings, and increase total sleeping time. The role of benzodiazepines in managing insomnia is discussed in depth later.

TABLE 29.1 Applications of the Benzodiazepines

	APPROVED APPLICATIONS						
Generic Name (Trade Name)	GAD	Insomnia	Seizures	Muscle Spasm, Spasticity	Alcohol Withdrawal	Anesthesia Induction or Preanesthetic	Anxiety
Alprazolam (Xanax, Xanax XR, Niravam)	✓						✓
Chlordiazepoxide (Librium)	✓				✓		✓
Clonazepam (Klonopin, Rivotril🍁)			✓				✓
Clorazepate (Tranxene-T)	✓		✓		✓		
Diazepam (Valium, Diastat AcuDial)	✓		✓	✓	✓	✓	
Estazolam (generic only)		✓					
Flurazepam (generic only)		✓					
Lorazepam (Ativan)	✓	✓	✓				
Midazolam (Versed)						✓[a]	
Oxazepam (generic only)	✓				✓		
Temazepam (Restoril)		✓					
Triazolam (Halcion)		✓					

[a]Midazolam, in conjunction with an opioid analgesic, is also used to produce *conscious sedation*, a semiconscious state suitable for minor surgeries and endoscopic procedures.
GAD, Generalized anxiety disorder.

Seizure Disorders

Four benzodiazepines—diazepam, clonazepam, lorazepam, and clorazepate—are employed for seizure disorders. Antiseizure applications are discussed in Chapter 21.

Muscle Spasm

One benzodiazepine—diazepam—is used to relieve muscle spasm and spasticity (see Chapter 22). Effects on muscle tone are secondary to actions in the CNS. Diazepam cannot relieve spasm without causing sedation.

Alcohol Withdrawal

Diazepam and other benzodiazepines may be administered to ease withdrawal from alcohol (see Chapter 33). Benefits derive from cross-dependence with alcohol, which enables benzodiazepines to suppress symptoms brought on by alcohol abstinence.

Adverse Effects

Benzodiazepines are generally well tolerated, and serious adverse reactions are rare. In contrast to barbiturates and other general CNS depressants, benzodiazepines are remarkably safe.

Central Nervous System Depression

When taken to promote sleep, benzodiazepines cause drowsiness, lightheadedness, incoordination, and difficulty concentrating. When these effects occur at bedtime, they are generally inconsequential. However, if sedation and other manifestations of CNS depression persist beyond waking, interference with daytime activities can result.

Anterograde Amnesia

Benzodiazepines can cause anterograde amnesia (impaired recall of events that take place after dosing). Anterograde amnesia has been especially troublesome with *triazolam* (Halcion). If patients complain of forgetfulness, the possibility of drug-induced amnesia should be evaluated.

Sleep Driving and Other Complex Sleep-Related Behaviors

Patients taking benzodiazepines in sleep-inducing doses may carry out complex behaviors and then have no memory of their actions. Reported behaviors include sleep driving, preparing and eating meals, and making phone calls. Although these events can occur with normal doses, they are more likely when doses are excessive and when benzodiazepines are combined with alcohol and other CNS depressants. Because of the potential for harm, benzodiazepines should be withdrawn if sleep driving is reported. To minimize withdrawal symptoms, dosing should be tapered slowly rather than discontinued abruptly.

Paradoxical Effects

When employed to treat anxiety, benzodiazepines sometimes cause paradoxical responses, including insomnia, excitation, euphoria, heightened anxiety, and rage. If these occur, the benzodiazepine should be withdrawn.

Respiratory Depression

Benzodiazepines are weak respiratory depressants. Death from overdose with oral benzodiazepines alone has never been documented. Hence, in contrast to the barbiturates, benzodiazepines present little risk as vehicles for suicide. It must be emphasized, however, that although respiratory depression with *oral* therapy is rare, benzodiazepines can cause severe respiratory depression when administered *intravenously*. In addition, substantial respiratory depression can result from combining oral benzodiazepines with other CNS depressants (e.g., alcohol, barbiturates, opioids).

Abuse

Benzodiazepines have a lower abuse potential than barbiturates and most other general CNS depressants. The behavior pattern that constitutes "addiction" is uncommon among people who take benzodiazepines for therapeutic purposes. When asked about their drug use, individuals who regularly abuse drugs rarely express a preference for benzodiazepines over barbiturates. Because their potential for abuse is low, the benzodiazepines are classified under Schedule IV of the Controlled Substances Act. This contrasts with the barbiturates, most of which are classified under Schedule III.

Use in Pregnancy and Lactation

Benzodiazepines are highly lipid soluble and can readily cross the placental barrier. Use of benzodiazepines during the first trimester of pregnancy is associated with an increased risk for congenital malformations such as cleft lip, inguinal hernia, and cardiac anomalies. Use near term can cause CNS depression in the neonate. Women of childbearing age should be warned about the potential for fetal harm and instructed to discontinue benzodiazepines if pregnancy occurs.

Benzodiazepines enter breast milk with ease and may accumulate to toxic levels in the breastfed infant. Accordingly, these drugs should be avoided by nursing mothers.

Drug Interactions

Benzodiazepines undergo very few important interactions with other drugs. Unlike barbiturates, benzodiazepines do not induce hepatic drug-metabolizing enzymes. Hence benzodiazepines do not accelerate the metabolism of other drugs.

Central Nervous System Depressants

The CNS-depressant actions of benzodiazepines add to those of other CNS depressants (e.g., alcohol, barbiturates, opioids). Hence, although benzodiazepines are very safe when used alone, they can be extremely hazardous in combination with other depressants. Combined overdose with a benzodiazepine plus another CNS depressant can cause profound respiratory depression, coma, and death. Patients should be warned against the use of alcohol and all other CNS depressants.

Tolerance and Physical Dependence
Tolerance

With prolonged use of benzodiazepines, tolerance develops to some effects but not to others. No tolerance develops to anxiolytic effects, and tolerance to hypnotic effects is generally low. In contrast, significant tolerance develops to antiseizure effects. Patients tolerant to barbiturates, alcohol, and other general CNS depressants show some cross-tolerance to benzodiazepines.

Physical Dependence

Benzodiazepines can cause physical dependence, but the incidence of *substantial* dependence is low. When benzodiazepines are discontinued after short-term use at therapeutic doses, the resulting withdrawal syndrome is generally mild and often goes unrecognized. Symptoms include anxiety, insomnia, sweating, tremors, and dizziness. Withdrawal from long-term, high-dose therapy can cause more serious reactions such as panic, paranoia, delirium, hypertension, muscle twitches, and seizures. Symptoms of withdrawal are usually more intense with benzodiazepines that have a short duration of action. With one agent—*alprazolam* (Xanax, Xanax XR, Niravam)—dependence may be a greater problem than with other benzodiazepines. Because the benzodiazepine withdrawal syndrome can resemble an anxiety disorder, it is important to differentiate withdrawal symptoms from the return of the original symptoms of anxiety.

The intensity of withdrawal symptoms can be minimized by discontinuing treatment gradually. Doses should be slowly tapered over several weeks or months. Substituting a benzodiazepine with a long half-life for one with a short half-life is also helpful. Patients should be warned against abrupt cessation of treatment. After discontinuation of treatment, patients should be monitored for 3 weeks for indications of withdrawal or recurrence of original symptoms.

 ## SUMMARY OF KEY PRESCRIBING CONSIDERATIONS

Benzodiazepines

Therapeutic Goal: Benzodiazepines, among other uses, are employed to promote sleep.

Baseline Data: Determine the nature of the sleep disturbance (frequent awakenings, early morning awakening, prolonged latency).

Monitoring: No routine monitoring required.

Identifying High-Risk Patients: Benzodiazepines are contraindicated in pregnancy and should be used with extreme caution in patients who experience sleep apnea. Consider use in patients with a history of substance abuse.

Evaluating Therapeutic Effects: Insomnia is usually self-limiting. Consequently drug therapy is usually short term.

Minimizing Adverse Effects: Warn patients against abrupt discontinuation of treatment.

PROTOTYPE DRUGS

Sedative-Hypnotic Drugs

Benzodiazepine
Triazolam

Benzodiazepine-Like Drugs
Zolpidem
Zaleplon

Barbiturate
Secobarbital

Melatonin Receptor Agonist
Ramelteon

Orexin Receptor Agonist
Suvorexant

BENZODIAZEPINE-LIKE DRUGS

Three benzodiazepine-like drugs are available: zolpidem, zaleplon, and eszopiclone. All three are preferred agents for insomnia. They are not indicated for anxiety. These drugs are structurally different from benzodiazepines, but nonetheless share the same mechanism of action: they all act as *agonists at the benzodiazepine receptor site* on the GABA receptor–chloride channel complex. Like the benzodiazepines, these drugs have a low potential for tolerance, dependence, and abuse and are classified as Schedule IV substances.

Zolpidem

Zolpidem (Ambien, Ambien CR, Edluar, Intermezzo, Zolpimist), our most widely used hypnotic, is approved only for the short-term management of insomnia. However, although approval is limited to short-term use, many patients have taken the drug long term with no apparent tolerance or increase in adverse effects. All zolpidem formulations have a rapid onset and hence can help people who have difficulty falling asleep. In addition, the extended-release formulation—Ambien CR—can help people who have difficulty maintaining sleep.

Although structurally unrelated to the benzodiazepines, zolpidem binds to the benzodiazepine receptor site on the GABA receptor–chloride channel complex and shares some properties of the benzodiazepines. Like the benzodiazepines, zolpidem can reduce sleep latency and awakenings and prolong sleep duration. The drug does not significantly reduce time in rapid eye movement (REM) sleep and causes little or no rebound insomnia when therapy is discontinued. In contrast to the benzodiazepines, zolpidem lacks anxiolytic, muscle relaxant, and anticonvulsant actions because zolpidem does not bind with all benzodiazepine receptors. Rather, binding is limited to the benzodiazepine-1 subtype of benzodiazepine receptors. The pharmacokinetics of zolpidem is displayed in Table 29.2.

Zolpidem has a side-effect profile like that of the benzodiazepines. *Daytime drowsiness and dizziness* are most common, and these occur in only 1% to 2% of patients. Like the benzodiazepines, zolpidem has been associated with *sleep driving* and other complex *sleep-related behaviors*. At therapeutic doses, zolpidem causes little or no respiratory depression. Safety in pregnancy has not been established. According to the U.S. Food and Drug Administration (FDA), zolpidem may pose a small risk for anaphylaxis and angioedema.

Short-term treatment is not associated with significant tolerance or physical dependence. Withdrawal symptoms are minimal or absent. Similarly, the abuse liability of zolpidem is low. Accordingly, the drug is classified under Schedule IV of the Controlled Substances Act.

TABLE 29.2 Pharmacokinetic Properties of Sedative-Hypnotic Drugs

Drug	Route	Peak[a] (h)	Half-Life[a] (h)	Metabolism	Excretion
Benzodiazepine-Like Drugs					
Eszopiclone (Lunesta)	PO	1–2	6	Hepatic	Renal
Zaleplon (Sonata)	PO	1	1	Hepatic	Renal
Zolpidem (Ambien)	PO, SL	2	2.5	Hepatic	Gastrointestinal (bile, feces), renal
Melatonin Receptor Agonist					
Ramelteon (Rozarem)	PO	1	2–5	Hepatic	Renal
Orexin Receptor Antagonist					
Suvorexant (Belsomra)	PO	2	12	Hepatic	Gastrointestinal (feces) renal

[a]With oral administration.

Like other sedative-hypnotics, zolpidem can intensify the effects of other CNS depressants. Patients should be warned against combining zolpidem with alcohol and all other drugs that depress CNS function.

Zaleplon

Zaleplon (Sonata) is the first representative of a new class of hypnotics, the pyrazolopyrimidines. The drug is approved only for the short-term management of insomnia, but prolonged use does not appear to cause tolerance. Like zolpidem, zaleplon binds to the benzodiazepine-1 receptor site on the GABA receptor–chloride channel complex, enhancing the depressant actions of endogenous GABA. In contrast to zolpidem, zaleplon has a very rapid onset and short duration of action and hence is good for helping patients fall asleep but not for maintaining sleep.

Zaleplon is well tolerated. The most common side effects are headache, nausea, drowsiness, dizziness, myalgia, and abdominal pain. Like the benzodiazepines, zaleplon has been associated with rare cases of sleep driving and other complex sleep-related behaviors. Respiratory depression has not been observed. Physical dependence is minimal, the only sign being mild rebound insomnia the first night after drug withdrawal. Next-day sedation and hangover have not been reported. Like the benzodiazepines, zaleplon has a low potential for abuse and hence is classified as a Schedule IV drug.

Eszopiclone

Eszopiclone (Lunesta), like zaleplon and zolpidem, binds selectively with the benzodiazepine-1 receptor on the GABA receptor–chloride channel complex and thereby enhances the depressant actions of endogenous GABA.

Eszopiclone is approved for treating insomnia, with no limitation on how long it can be used. This contrasts with zaleplon and zolpidem, which are approved for short-term use only. Does this mean that eszopiclone is safer than the other two drugs, or is it less likely to promote tolerance? Not necessarily. It only means that the manufacturer of eszopiclone conducted a prolonged (6-month) study whereas the manufacturers of the other two drugs did not. In that prolonged study, eszopiclone reduced sleep latency and nighttime awakening, increased total sleep time and sleep quality, had no significant effect on sleep architecture, and showed no indication of tolerance.

Eszopiclone is generally well tolerated. The most common adverse effect is a bitter aftertaste, reported by 17% of patients dosed with 2 mg and 34% of those dosed with 3 mg. Other common effects are headache, somnolence, dizziness, and dry mouth. Rebound insomnia may occur on the first night after discontinuing the drug. Like the benzodiazepines and the other benzodiazepine-like drugs, eszopiclone has been associated with cases of sleep driving and other complex sleep-related behaviors. Rarely, eszopiclone may cause anaphylaxis or angioedema. Eszopiclone has a low potential for abuse and hence is classified as a Schedule IV drug.

SUMMARY OF KEY PRESCRIBING CONSIDERATIONS

Benzodiazepine-Like Drugs

Therapeutic Goal: Assist patients in both falling asleep and staying asleep.
Baseline Data: Determine the nature of the sleep disturbance (frequent awakenings, early morning awakening, prolonged latency).
Monitoring: No routine monitoring required.
Identifying High-Risk Patients: Safety in pregnancy has not been established.
Evaluating Therapeutic Effects: Insomnia is usually self-limiting; consequently drug therapy is usually short term.
Minimizing Adverse Effects: Educate patients regarding the possibility of sleep driving and other complex sleep-related behaviors.

RAMELTEON: A MELATONIN AGONIST

Ramelteon (Rozerem) is a relatively new hypnotic with a unique mechanism of action: activation of receptors for melatonin. The drug is approved for treating chronic insomnia characterized by difficulty with sleep onset but not with sleep maintenance. Long-term use is permitted. Of the major drugs for insomnia, ramelteon is the only one not regulated as a controlled substance.

Therapeutic Use

Ramelteon has a rapid onset (about 30 minutes) and short duration of action and hence is good for inducing sleep but not maintaining it. There are no significant residual effects on the day after dosing, nor is there any rebound insomnia when treatment is stopped after 35 consecutive nights of use. In approving the drug, the FDA put no limit on how long it may be used.

Mechanism of Action

Ramelteon activates receptors for melatonin—specifically the MT_1 and MT_2 subtypes, which are key mediators of the normal sleep–wake cycle. Sleep promotion derives primarily from activating MT_1 receptors. (Under physiologic conditions, activation of MT_1 receptors by endogenous melatonin induces sleepiness.) Ramelteon does not activate MT_3 receptors, which help regulate numerous systems unrelated to sleep. Selectivity for MT_1 and MT_2 receptors explains why ramelteon is superior to melatonin itself for treating insomnia. Ramelteon does not bind with the GABA receptor–chloride channel complex or with receptors for neuropeptides, benzodiazepines, dopamine, serotonin, norepinephrine, acetylcholine, or opioids.

Adverse Effects

Ramelteon is very well tolerated. In clinical trials, the incidence of adverse effects was nearly identical to that of placebo. The most common side effects are somnolence, dizziness, and fatigue. According to the FDA, ramelteon may share the ability of benzodiazepines to cause sleep driving and other complex sleep-related behaviors. Very rarely, patients have reported hallucinations, agitation, and mania.

Ramelteon can increase levels of prolactin and reduce levels of testosterone. As a result, the drug has the potential to cause amenorrhea, galactorrhea, reduced libido, and fertility problems. If these occur, the prescriber should be consulted.

Postmarketing reports indicate a small risk for severe allergic reactions. Rarely, patients have experienced angioedema of the tongue, glottis, or larynx. Some patients also experienced dyspnea and throat constriction, suggestive of anaphylaxis. Patients who experience these symptoms should discontinue ramelteon and never use it again.

Drug Interactions

Fluvoxamine (Luvox), a strong inhibitor of CYP1A2, can increase levels of ramelteon more than 50-fold. Accordingly, the combination should be avoided. Weaker inhibitors of CYP1A2 should be used with caution. Alcohol can intensify sedation and hence should also be avoided.

Precautions

Ramelteon should be used with caution by patients with moderate hepatic impairment and should be avoided by those with severe hepatic impairment. Because ramelteon promotes sedation, patients should be advised to avoid dangerous activities such as driving or operating heavy machinery.

Use in Pregnancy and Breastfeeding

Effects during human pregnancy have not been studied. Until more is known, prudence dictates avoiding the drug during pregnancy (or at least using it with caution). Ramelteon is not recommended for use by nursing mothers.

SUVOREXANT: AN OREXIN ANTAGONIST

Suvorexant (Belsomra) is a sedative that selectively blocks receptors for orexin, a neurotransmitter in the brain that promotes wakefulness. The drug is approved for treating chronic insomnia characterized by difficulty with sleep onset and/or sleep maintenance. Similar to the benzodiazepine-like drugs, suvorexant is regulated as a Schedule IV substance.

Adverse Effects

The most common side effects are somnolence, headache, dizziness, diarrhea, dry mouth, and cough. Hallucinations, sleep paralysis, and vivid, disturbing perceptions have been reported by some patients.

Physical Dependence and Abuse

Suvorexant is classified by the US Drug Enforcement Administration (DEA) as a Schedule IV medication. An abuse study conducted with suvorexant revealed that patients had similar subjective ratings of "drug liking" as that of zolpidem, also a Schedule IV drug. Patients with a history of drug abuse or addiction may be at an increased risk for the abuse of suvorexant.

Drug Interactions

Use with strong inhibitors of CYP3A (ketoconazole, clarithromycin, others) can increase the effects of suvorexant; therefore such use is not recommended. Suvorexant can also increase digoxin levels; therefore close monitoring is indicated.

Precautions

Suvorexant should be used with caution by patients with compromised respiratory function, such as severe COPD or obstructive sleep apnea (OSA). Because suvorexant promotes sedation, its use is contraindicated in patients with narcolepsy.

Use in Pregnancy and Breastfeeding

Adequate human studies on the effects of suvorexant in pregnant women are lacking. Administration to pregnant rats resulted in decreased fetal body weight with increased doses. Whether suvorexant is expressed in breast milk remains unknown. When this medication is used during pregnancy, the benefits should clearly outweigh the risks.

BARBITURATES

The barbiturates have been available for more than 100 years. These drugs cause relatively nonselective depression of CNS function and are the prototypes of the general CNS depressants. Because they depress multiple aspects of CNS function, barbiturates can be used for daytime sedation, induction of sleep, suppression of seizures, and general anesthesia. Barbiturates cause tolerance and dependence, have a high abuse potential, and are subject to multiple drug interactions. Moreover, barbiturates are powerful respiratory depressants that can be fatal in overdose. Because of these undesirable properties, barbiturates are now used much less than in the past, having been replaced by newer and safer drugs—primarily the benzodiazepines and benzodiazepine-like drugs (e.g., zolpidem). However, although their use has declined greatly, barbiturates still have important applications in seizure control and anesthesia. Moreover, barbiturates are valuable from an instructional point of view: by understanding these prototypic agents, we gain an understanding of the general CNS depressants as a group along with an appreciation of why barbiturates are no longer used for anxiety and insomnia.

Classification

Duration of action influences the clinical applications of barbiturates. The ultra-short-acting agents (e.g., methohexital) are used for induction of anesthesia. The short- to intermediate-acting agents (e.g., secobarbital) are used as sedatives and hypnotics. The long-acting agents (e.g., phenobarbital) are used primarily as antiseizure drugs.

Mechanism of Action

Like benzodiazepines, barbiturates bind to the GABA receptor–chloride channel complex. By doing so, these drugs can (1) enhance the inhibitory actions of GABA and (2) directly mimic the actions of GABA.

Because barbiturates can directly mimic GABA, there is no ceiling to the degree of CNS depression they can produce. Hence, in contrast to the benzodiazepines, these drugs can readily cause death by overdose. Although barbiturates can cause general depression of the CNS, they show some selectivity for depressing the reticular activating system (RAS), a neuronal network that helps regulate the sleep–wake cycle. By depressing the RAS, barbiturates produce sedation and sleep.

Pharmacologic Effects
Central Nervous System Depression

Most effects of barbiturates—both therapeutic and adverse—result from generalized depression of CNS function. With increasing dosage, responses progress from sedation to sleep to general anesthesia.

Most barbiturates can be considered nonselective CNS depressants. The main exception is phenobarbital, a drug used to control seizures. Seizure control is achieved at doses that have minimal effects on other aspects of CNS function.

Cardiovascular Effects

At hypnotic doses, barbiturates produce modest reductions in blood pressure and heart rate. In contrast, toxic doses can cause profound hypotension and shock. At high doses, barbiturates depress the myocardium and vascular smooth muscle along with all other electrically excitable tissues.

Induction of Hepatic Drug-Metabolizing Enzymes

Barbiturates stimulate the synthesis of hepatic microsomal enzymes, the principal drug-metabolizing enzymes of the liver. As a result, barbiturates can accelerate their own metabolism and the metabolism of many other drugs by promoting the synthesis of porphyrin. Porphyrin is then converted into heme, which in turn is incorporated into cytochrome P450, a key component of the hepatic drug-metabolizing system.

Tolerance and Physical Dependence
Tolerance

When barbiturates are taken regularly, tolerance develops to many but not all of their CNS effects. Specifically, tolerance develops to sedative and hypnotic effects and to other effects that underlie barbiturate abuse. However, even with chronic use, very little tolerance develops to toxic effects.

In the tolerant user, doses must be increased to produce the same intensity of response that could formerly be achieved with smaller doses. Hence individuals who take barbiturates for prolonged periods—be it for therapy or recreation—require steadily increasing doses to achieve the effects they desire.

It is important to note that very little tolerance develops to respiratory depression. Because tolerance to respiratory depression is minimum and tolerance does develop to therapeutic effects, the lethal (respiratory-depressant) dose with continued treatment remains relatively constant whereas the therapeutic dose climbs higher and higher (Fig. 29.1). As

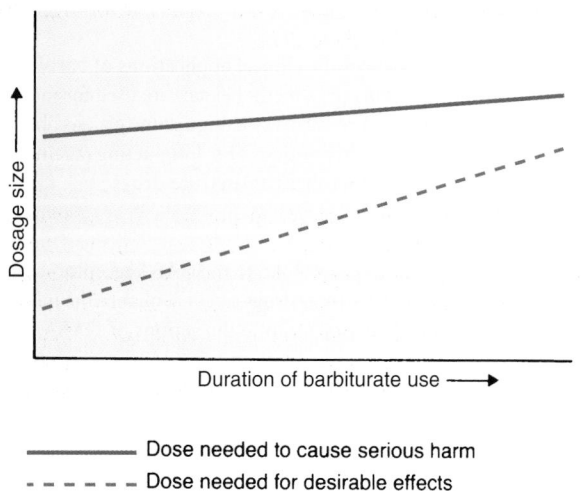

Fig. 29.1 Development of Tolerance to the Toxic and Subjective Effects of Barbiturates. With prolonged barbiturate use, tolerance develops. However, less tolerance develops to toxic effects than to desired effects. Consequently, as duration of use increases, the difference between the dose producing desirable effects and the dose producing toxicity becomes progressively smaller, thereby increasing the risk for serious harm.

tolerance to therapeutic effects increases, the therapeutic dose grows steadily closer to the lethal dose—a situation that is clearly hazardous.

As a rule, tolerance to one general CNS depressant bestows tolerance to all other general CNS depressants. Hence there is cross-tolerance among barbiturates, alcohol, benzodiazepines, general anesthetics, and certain other agents. Tolerance to barbiturates and the other general CNS depressants does not produce significant cross-tolerance with opioids (e.g., morphine).

Physical Dependence

Prolonged use of barbiturates results in physical dependence, a state in which continued use is required to avoid an abstinence syndrome. Physical dependence results from adaptive neurochemical changes that occur in response to chronic drug exposure.

Individuals who are physically dependent on barbiturates exhibit cross-dependence with other general CNS depressants. Because of cross-dependence, a person physically dependent on barbiturates can prevent withdrawal symptoms by taking any other general CNS depressant (e.g., alcohol, benzodiazepines). As a rule, cross-dependence exists among all of the general CNS depressants. However, there is no significant cross-dependence with opioids.

The general CNS-depressant abstinence syndrome can be severe. Abrupt withdrawal from general CNS depressants is more dangerous than withdrawal from opioids. Although withdrawal from opioids is certainly unpleasant, the risk for serious injury is low. In contrast, the abstinence syndrome associated with general CNS depressants can be fatal.

Withdrawal from general CNS depressants can be dangerous. Early reactions include weakness, restlessness, insomnia, hyperthermia, orthostatic hypotension, confusion, and disorientation. By the third day, seizures may develop. Approximately 75% of patients experience psychotic delirium (a state similar to alcoholic delirium tremens). In extreme cases, these symptoms may be followed by exhaustion, cardiovascular collapse, and death. The entire abstinence syndrome evolves over approximately 8 days. Symptom intensity can be greatly reduced by withdrawing barbiturates and other general CNS depressants slowly.

A long-acting barbiturate (e.g., phenobarbital) may be administered to facilitate the withdrawal process. Because of cross-dependence, phenobarbital can substitute for other CNS depressants and can thereby suppress symptoms of withdrawal. Because phenobarbital is eliminated from the body slowly, treatment permits a gradual transition from a drug-dependent state to a drug-free state. When phenobarbital is given to aid withdrawal, its dosage should be reduced gradually over 10 days to 3 weeks.

Therapeutic Uses
Seizure Disorders

Phenobarbital is used for seizure disorders (see Chapter 21). This drug suppresses seizures at doses that are essentially nonsedative.

Insomnia

By depressing the CNS, barbiturates can promote sleep. However, because they can cause multiple undesired effects, barbiturates have been replaced by benzodiazepines and related drugs as treatments of choice for insomnia.

Adverse Effects
Respiratory Depression

Barbiturates reduce ventilation by two mechanisms: (1) depression of brain stem neurogenic respiratory drive and (2) depression of chemoreceptive mechanisms that control respiratory drive. Doses only three times greater than those needed to induce sleep can cause complete suppression of the neurogenic respiratory drive. With severe overdose, barbiturates can cause apnea and death.

For most patients, the degree of respiratory depression produced at therapeutic doses is not significant. However, in older adult patients and those with respiratory disease, therapeutic doses can compromise respiration substantially. Combining a barbiturate with another CNS depressant intensifies respiratory depression.

Abuse

Barbiturates produce subjective effects that many individuals find desirable. As a result, they are popular drugs of abuse. The barbiturates most prone to abuse are those in the short- to intermediate-acting group (e.g., secobarbital). Individual barbiturates within the group are classified under Schedule III of the Controlled Substances Act, reflecting their high potential for abuse. Although barbiturates are frequently abused in nonmedical settings, they are rarely abused during medical use.

MANAGEMENT OF INSOMNIA

Insomnia can be defined as an inability to sleep well. Some people have difficulty falling asleep, some have difficulty maintaining sleep, some are troubled by early-morning awakening, and some have sleep that is not refreshing. Insomnia is transient for some people and chronic for others. In any given year, about 30% of Americans experience intermittent insomnia and about 10% experience chronic insomnia.

Therapy With Hypnotic Drugs

Hypnotics should be used only when insomnia cannot be managed by other means. Hence, before resorting to drugs, nondrug measures should be implemented, and any pathology that may underlie inadequate sleep should be treated.

Drug therapy of transient insomnia should be short term (just 2 to 3 weeks). The patient should be reassessed on a regular basis to determine whether drug therapy is still needed.

Escalation of dosage should be avoided. A need for increased dosage suggests the development of tolerance. If hypnotic effects are lost in the course of treatment, it is preferable to interrupt therapy rather than to elevate dosage. Interruption will allow tolerance to decline, thereby restoring responsiveness to treatment.

In certain patients, hypnotics must be employed with special caution. Patients who snore heavily and those with respiratory disorders have reduced respiratory reserve, which can be further compromised by the respiratory depressant actions of hypnotics. Hypnotic agents are generally contraindicated for use during pregnancy; these drugs have the potential to cause fetal harm, and their use is rarely an absolute necessity.

Patients taking hypnotics should be forewarned that residual CNS depression may persist the next day. Although CNS depression may not be pronounced, it may still compromise intellectual or physical performance.

When hypnotics are employed, care must be taken to prevent *drug-dependency insomnia*, a condition that can lead to the inappropriate prolongation of therapy. Drug-dependency insomnia is a particular problem with older hypnotics (e.g., barbiturates) and develops as follows:
1. Insomnia motivates treatment with hypnotics.
2. With continuous drug use, low-level physical dependence develops.
3. Upon cessation of treatment, a mild withdrawal syndrome occurs and disrupts sleep.
4. Failing to recognize that the inability to sleep is a manifestation of drug withdrawal, the patient becomes convinced that insomnia has returned and resumes drug use.
5. Continued drug use leads to heightened physical dependence, making it even more difficult to withdraw medication without producing another episode of drug-dependency insomnia.

To minimize drug-dependency insomnia, hypnotics should be employed judiciously. That is, they should be used in the lowest effective dosage for the shortest time required. Common dosages of major drugs for insomnia are located in Table 29.3.

OTHER HYPNOTICS

Antidepressants

Trazodone

Trazodone (Oleptro) is an atypical antidepressant with strong sedative actions. The drug can decrease sleep latency and prolong sleep duration; it does not cause tolerance or physical dependence. Trazodone is especially useful for treating insomnia resulting from use of antidepressants that cause significant CNS stimulation (e.g., fluoxetine [Prozac], bupropion [Wellbutrin]). Principal adverse effects are daytime grogginess and postural hypotension. (Hypotension results from alpha-adrenergic blockade.)

Doxepin

Doxepin is an old tricyclic antidepressant (TCA) with strong sedative actions. In 2010, the FDA approved a new low-dose formulation for treating patients who have trouble staying asleep. The new formulation (3- and 6-mg tablets) is sold as Silenor. In clinical trials of adults with chronic insomnia, Doxepin (Silenor) increased total sleep time and maintained the effect for more than 12 weeks. These benefits probably derive from blockage of the receptors for histamine.

In the low doses used for sleep maintenance, doxepin is well tolerated. The most common adverse effects are sedation, nausea, and upper respiratory infection. In the high doses used for depression, doxepin can cause hypotension, dysrhythmias, and anticholinergic effects (e.g., dry mouth, constipation, urinary retention, blurred vision). Owing to the risk for anticholinergic effects, doxepin is contraindicated for patients

TABLE 29.3 Major Drugs for Insomnia

Drug	TIME COURSE		USE IN INSOMNIA		BEDTIME DOSAGE (mg)	
	Onset (min)	Duration	DFA	DMS	Younger Adult	Older Adult
Benzodiazepines						
Triazolam [Halcion]	15–30	Short	✓		0.125–0.25	0.125
Flurazepam[a] (generic only)	30–60	Long	✓	✓	15–30	15
Estazolam (generic only)	15–60	Intermediate		✓	1–2	0.5–1
Quazepam[a] (Doral)	20–45	Long	✓	✓	15	7.5
Temazepam (Restoril)	45–60	Intermediate		✓	15–30	7.5–15
Benzodiazepine-Like Drugs						
Eszopiclone (Lunesta)	30	Intermediate	✓	✓	2–3	1–2
Zolpidem						
Extended-release tablets (Ambien CR)	30	Intermediate	✓	✓	12.5	6.25
Immediate-release tablets (Ambien)	30	Short	✓		10	5
Sublingual (Intermezzo)	30	Short	✓	✓	1.75 for females and 3.5 for males	1.75
Sublingual (Edluar)	30	Short	✓		10	5
Oral spray (Zolpimist)	30	Short	✓		5–10	5
Zaleplon (Sonata)	15–30	Ultrashort	✓		5–10	5
Melatonin Receptor Agonist						
Ramelteon (Rozerem)	30	Short	✓		8	8
Orexin Receptor Antagonist						
Suvorexant (Belsomra)	30	Intermediate	✓	✓	10	10

[a]Because of its long duration of action, this drug is not generally recommended.
DFA, Difficulty falling asleep; *DMS,* difficulty maintaining sleep.

with untreated narrow-angle glaucoma or severe urinary retention. In addition, doxepin is contraindicated for patients who have taken a monoamine oxidase inhibitor within the previous 2 weeks. Unlike the benzodiazepines and benzodiazepine-like drugs, doxepin has little or no potential for abuse and hence is not regulated under the Controlled Substances Act. Accordingly, the drug may be especially appropriate when drug abuse is a concern.

Antihistamines

Two antihistamines—diphenhydramine (Nytol, Sominex, others) and doxylamine (Unisom)—are FDA-approved for use as "sleep aids" and can be purchased without a prescription. These drugs are less effective than benzodiazepines and benzodiazepine-like drugs and tolerance develops quickly (in 1 to 2 weeks). Daytime drowsiness and anticholinergic effects (e.g., dry mouth, blurred vision, urinary hesitancy, constipation) are common.

Melatonin

Of the alternative medicines employed to promote sleep, only one—melatonin—appears to be moderately effective. Melatonin is a hormone that helps regulate the circadian clock, the timekeeping mechanism that controls the sleep–wake cycle. The principal uses of melatonin include the treatment of insomnia and jet lag. Of note, melatonin is the only hormone that can be purchased without a prescription. The compound is available in health-food stores, vitamin shops, and even airport newsstands.

Melatonin is produced by the pineal gland, a structure located at the base of the brain. Secretion is suppressed by environmental light and stimulated by darkness. Normally, secretion is low during the day, begins to rise around 9 p.m., reaches a peak between 2 a.m. and 4 a.m., and returns to baseline by morning. Signals that control secretion travel along a multineuron pathway that connects the retina to the pineal gland.

Several trials indicate that melatonin promotes sleep. For example, doses of 0.3 to 1 mg taken 1 to 2 hours before bedtime can hasten sleep onset and the time to REM sleep without reducing total time in REM sleep. Melatonin may also ease symptoms of jet lag by resetting the circadian clock to the new time zone. Of all treatments for jet lag, melatonin is the most widely studied. To date, there have been 11 double-blind, placebo-controlled trials. In eight of these trials, melatonin produced significant benefit. Of the three negative studies, two were too small to permit firm conclusions and one involved subjects whose baseline circadian rhythm may have been inappropriate for evaluation.

When used short term in low doses (e.g., less than 2 mg), melatonin has no observable adverse effects. However, short-term use of large doses can cause hangover, headache, nightmares, hypothermia, and transient depression. In one case, reversible psychosis occurred with a huge daytime dose. Possible adverse effects of long-term use are unknown.

30

Management of Anxiety Disorders

Anxiety is an uncomfortable state that has both psychological and physical components. The psychological component can be characterized with terms such as *fear, apprehension, dread,* and *uneasiness.* The physical component manifests as tachycardia, palpitations, trembling, dry mouth, sweating, weakness, fatigue, and shortness of breath.

Anxiety is a nearly universal experience that often serves an adaptive function. When anxiety is moderate and situationally appropriate, therapy may not be needed, or even desirable. In contrast, when anxiety is persistent and disabling, intervention is clearly indicated.

Anxiety disorders are among the most common psychiatric illnesses. In the United States about 25% of people develop pathologic anxiety at some time in their lives. As a rule, the incidence is higher in women than in men.

In this chapter, we focus on five of the more common anxiety disorders: generalized anxiety disorder (GAD), panic disorder (PD), obsessive-compulsive disorder (OCD), social anxiety disorder (SAD), and posttraumatic stress disorder (PTSD). Although each type is distinct, they all have one element in common: an unhealthy level of anxiety. In addition, with all anxiety disorders, depression is frequently comorbid.

Fortunately, anxiety disorders often respond well to treatment—either psychotherapy, drug therapy, or both. For most patients, a combination of psychotherapy and drug therapy is more effective than either modality alone.

As indicated in Table 30.1, two classes of drugs are used most: *serotonergic reuptake inhibitors (SRIs)* which encompass both selective serotonin reuptake inhibitors (SSRIs) and serotonin-norepinephrine reuptake inhibitors (SNRIs), and *benzodiazepines.* Benzodiazepines are used primarily for two conditions: GAD and PD. In contrast, the SRIs are now used for *all* anxiety disorders. It should be noted that although SRIs were developed as antidepressants, they can be very effective against anxiety—whether or not depression is present.

GENERALIZED ANXIETY DISORDER

Characteristics

GAD is a chronic condition characterized by uncontrollable worrying. Of all anxiety disorders, GAD is the least likely to remit. Most patients with GAD also have another psychiatric disorder, usually depression. GAD should not be confused with *situational anxiety,* which is a normal response to a stressful situation; symptoms may be intense, but they are temporary.

The hallmark of GAD is unrealistic or excessive anxiety about several events or activities (e.g., work or school performance) that lasts 6 months or longer. Other psychological manifestations include vigilance, tension, apprehension, poor concentration, and difficulty falling or staying asleep. Somatic manifestations include trembling, muscle tension, restlessness, and signs of autonomic hyperactivity, such as palpitations, tachycardia, sweating, and cold clammy hands.

PROTOTYPE DRUGS

Drugs for Anxiety Disorders

Serotonergic Reuptake Inhibitors (SRIs)
Paroxetine (selective serotonin reuptake inhibitor [SSRI])
Venlafaxine (serotonin-norepinephrine reuptake inhibitor [SNRI])

Nonbenzodiazepine-Nonbarbiturate
Buspirone

Benzodiazepine
Diazepam

Treatment

GAD can be managed with nondrug therapy and with drugs. Nondrug approaches include supportive therapy, cognitive behavioral therapy (CBT), biofeedback, and relaxation training. These can help relieve symptoms and improve coping skills in anxiety-provoking situations. When symptoms are mild, nondrug therapy may be all that is needed. However, if symptoms are intensely uncomfortable or disabling, drugs are indicated. Current U.S. Food and Drug Administration (FDA)–approved first-line choices include SRIs (including both SSRIs and SNRIs) and buspirone. Second-line choices include the benzodiazepines. With the benzodiazepines, onset of relief is rapid. In contrast, with buspirone and the antidepressants, onset is delayed. Accordingly, benzodiazepines can be utilized for immediate stabilization, especially when anxiety is severe. However, for long-term management, buspirone and the antidepressants are preferred. Because GAD is a chronic disorder, initial drug therapy should be prolonged, lasting at least 12 months and possibly longer. Unfortunately, even after extended treatment, drug withdrawal frequently results in relapse. Hence, for many patients, drug therapy must continue indefinitely.

Serotonergic Reuptake Inhibitors

Both SSRIs and SNRIs are considered first-line treatment for GAD. At this time, only four antidepressants—venlafaxine (Effexor XR), duloxetine (Cymbalta), paroxetine (Paxil), and escitalopram (Lexapro, Cipralex♣)—are approved for GAD. Venlafaxine and duloxetine are SNRIs; paroxetine and escitalopram are SSRIs. All four drugs are especially well suited for patients who have depression in addition to GAD. However, they are also effective even when depression is absent. Anxiolytic effects develop slowly: initial responses can be seen in a week, but optimal responses require several more weeks to develop. Because relief is delayed, the antidepressants cannot be used on an as-needed basis (PRN). Compared with benzodiazepines, the antidepressants do a better job of decreasing cognitive and psychic symptoms of anxiety, but are not as good at decreasing somatic symptoms. In contrast to the

TABLE 30.1   First-Line Drugs for Anxiety Disorders

Anxiety Disorder	Benzodiazepines	SSRIs	SNRIs/ Others
Generalized anxiety disorder	Alprazolam Chlordiazepoxide Clorazepate Diazepam Lorazepam Oxazepam	Escitalopram Paroxetine	Buspirone Duloxetine Venlafaxine
Panic disorder	Alprazolam Clonazepam	Fluoxetine Paroxetine Sertraline	Venlafaxine
Obsessive-compulsive disorder		Citalopram Escitalopram Fluoxetine Fluvoxamine Paroxetine Sertraline	
Social anxiety disorder		Fluvoxamine Paroxetine Sertraline	Venlafaxine
Posttraumatic stress disorder		Fluoxetine Paroxetine Sertraline	Venlafaxine

SSRIs, Selective serotonin reuptake inhibitors.

benzodiazepines, antidepressants have no potential for abuse. However, abrupt discontinuation *can* produce withdrawal symptoms.

Venlafaxine, an SNRI, was the first antidepressant approved for GAD. The drug has been proved effective for both short-term and long-term use. The most common side effect is nausea, which develops in 37% of patients. Fortunately, nausea subsides despite continued treatment. Other common reactions include headache, anorexia, nervousness, sweating, daytime somnolence, and insomnia. In addition, venlafaxine can cause hypertension, although this is unlikely at the doses used in GAD. Combining venlafaxine with a monoamine oxidase inhibitor (MAOI) can result in serious toxicity and hence must be avoided.

Paroxetine and *escitalopram* are the only SSRIs approved for GAD. These drugs are as effective as the benzodiazepines but not as well tolerated. The basic pharmacology of venlafaxine, paroxetine, escitalopram, and duloxetine is discussed in Chapter 27.

Buspirone

Actions and therapeutic use. Buspirone (BuSpar) is an anxiolytic drug that differs significantly from the benzodiazepines. Most notably, buspirone is *not* a central nervous system (CNS) depressant. For treatment of anxiety, buspirone is as effective as the benzodiazepines and has two distinct advantages: it has no abuse potential and does not intensify the effects of CNS depressants (benzodiazepines, alcohol, and barbiturates). Its major disadvantage is that anxiolytic effects develop *slowly:* initial responses take a week to appear, and several more weeks must pass before responses peak. Because therapeutic effects are delayed, buspirone is not suitable for PRN use or for patients who need immediate relief. Buspirone has no abuse potential and thus may be especially appropriate for patients known to abuse alcohol or other drugs.

Because it lacks depressant properties, buspirone is an attractive alternative to benzodiazepines in patients who require long-term therapy but cannot tolerate benzodiazepine-induced sedation and psychomotor slowing. Buspirone is labeled only for *short-term* treatment of anxiety.

However, the drug has been taken for as long as a year with no reduction in benefit. Buspirone does not display cross-dependence with benzodiazepines. Hence when patients are switched from a benzodiazepine to buspirone, the benzodiazepine must be tapered slowly. Furthermore, because the effects of buspirone are delayed, buspirone should be initiated 2 to 4 weeks before beginning benzodiazepine withdrawal. The mechanism by which buspirone relieves anxiety has not been established. The drug binds with high affinity to receptors for serotonin and with lower affinity to receptors for dopamine. Buspirone does not bind to receptors for γ-aminobutyric acid (GABA) or benzodiazepines.

Adverse effects. Buspirone is generally well tolerated. The most common reactions are *dizziness, nausea, headache, nervousness, sedation, lightheadedness,* and *excitement.* Furthermore, it poses little or no risk for suicide; extremely high doses (375 mg/day) have been given to healthy volunteers with only moderate adverse effects (nausea, vomiting, dizziness, drowsiness, miosis).

Drug and food interactions. Levels of buspirone can be greatly increased (5- to 13-fold) by *erythromycin* and *ketoconazole.* Levels can also be increased by *grapefruit juice.* Elevated levels may cause drowsiness and subjective effects (dysphoria, feeling "spacey"). Buspirone does not enhance the depressant effects of alcohol, barbiturates, and other general CNS depressants.

Tolerance, dependence, and abuse. Buspirone has been used for up to a year without evidence of tolerance, physical dependence, or psychological dependence. No withdrawal symptoms have been observed on termination. There is no cross-tolerance or cross-dependence between buspirone and the sedative-hypnotics (e.g., benzodiazepines, barbiturates). Buspirone appears to have no potential for abuse and hence is not regulated under the Controlled Substances Act.

Benzodiazepines

Benzodiazepines are first-choice drugs for acute anxiety. Benefits derive from enhancing responses to GABA, an inhibitory neurotransmitter. Onset of benefits is immediate, and the margin of safety is high. Principal side effects are sedation and psychomotor slowing. Patients should be warned about these effects and informed that they will subside in 7 to 10 days. Although they are considered first choice drugs for acute anxiety, their use must be carefully considered. Because of their abuse potential, benzodiazepines should be used with caution in patients known to abuse alcohol or other psychoactive substances.

Long-term use of benzodiazepines carries a risk for physical dependence. Withdrawal symptoms include panic, paranoia, and delirium. These can be especially troubling for patients with GAD. Furthermore, they can be confused with a return of pretreatment symptoms. Accordingly, clinicians must differentiate between a withdrawal reaction and relapse. To minimize withdrawal symptoms, benzodiazepines should be tapered gradually—over a period of several months. If relapse occurs, treatment should resume.

Of the 13 benzodiazepines available, 6 are approved for anxiety. The agents prescribed most often are alprazolam (Xanax, Xanax XR, Niravam) and lorazepam (Ativan). However, there is no proof that any one benzodiazepine is clearly superior to the others. Hence, selection among them is largely a matter of prescriber preference. Dosages for anxiety are shown in Table 30.2.

PANIC DISORDER

Characteristics

PD is characterized by recurrent, intensely uncomfortable episodes known as *panic attacks.* A panic attack is an abrupt surge of intense fear or intense discomfort during which four or more of the following are present:

TABLE 30.2   Medications Approved for Anxiety Disorders

Generic Name	Trade Name	Indication	DOSAGE Initial	DOSAGE Usual Range (mg/day)
Alprazolam	Xanax, Niravam	GAD	0.25–0.5 mg 3 times/day	0.5–4
	Xanax XR		0.5–1 mg once/day	4
Buspirone	Generic only	GAD	7.5 mg 2 times/day	30–60
Chlordiazepoxide	Librium	GAD	—	15–100
Citalopram	Celexa	OCD	20 mg once/day	40
Clorazepate	Tranxene-T	GAD	—	15–60
Diazepam	Valium	GAD	—	4–40
Duloxetine	Cymbalta	GAD	30–60 mg once/day	30–60
Escitalopram	Lexapro	GAD	10 mg once/day	20
		OCD	10 mg once/day	20
Fluoxetine	Prozac	PD	10 mg once/day	20
		OCD	20 mg once/day	80
Fluvoxamine	Luvox	OCD	50 mg once/day	300
Lorazepam	Ativan	GAD	0.5–1 mg 3 times/day	2–6
Oxazepam	Generic only	GAD	—	30–120
Paroxetine	Paxil	GAD	20 mg once/day	20–50
		PD	10 mg once/day	20–40
		OCD	20 mg once/day	60
		SAD	20 mg once/day	20–40
Sertraline	Zoloft	PD	25 mg once/day	50–200
		OCD	50 mg once/day	200
Venlafaxine	Effexor XR	GAD	37.5 mg once/day	75–225

GAD, Generalized anxiety disorder; *OCD*, obsessive-compulsive disorder; *PD*, panic disorder; *SAD*, social anxiety disorder.

- Palpitations, pounding heart, racing heartbeat
- Sweating
- Trembling or shaking
- Sensation of shortness of breath or smothering
- Feeling of choking
- Chest pain or discomfort
- Nausea or abdominal distress
- Feeling dizzy, unsteady, lightheaded, or faint
- Chills or heat sensations
- Paresthesias (numbness or tingling sensations)
- Derealization (feelings of unreality) or depersonalization (feeling detached from oneself)
- Fear of losing control or going crazy
- Fear of dying

Panic symptoms reach a peak in a few minutes and then dissipate within 30 minutes. Many patients go to an emergency department because they think they are having a heart attack. Some patients experience panic attacks daily; others have only one or two per month. PD is a common condition that affects 1.6% of Americans at some time in their lives. The incidence in women is 2 to 3 times the incidence in men. Onset of PD usually occurs in the late teens or early 20s.

The underlying cause of PD is unknown. However, malfunction of the brain's "alarm system" is suspected. This malfunction may result from abnormalities in noradrenergic systems, serotonergic systems, or benzodiazepine receptors. Genetic vulnerability also may play a role.

Treatment

Between 70% and 90% of patients with PD respond well to treatment. Two modalities may be employed: drug therapy and CBT. Combining drug therapy with CBT is more effective than either modality alone. As a rule, patients experience rapid and significant improvement. Drug therapy helps suppress panic attacks, whereas CBT helps patients become more comfortable with situations and places they've been avoiding. Additional benefit can be derived from avoiding caffeine and sympathomimetics (which can trigger panic attacks), avoiding sleep deprivation (which can predispose to panic attacks), and doing regular aerobic exercise (which can reduce anxiety).

Drug therapy should continue at least 6 to 9 months. Stopping sooner is associated with a high rate of relapse.

Antidepressants

PD responds well to all four classes of antidepressants: SSRIs, SNRIs, tricyclic antidepressants (TCAs), and MAOIs. With all classes, full benefits take 6 to 12 weeks to develop. Owing to better tolerability, SSRIs are generally preferred. The basic pharmacology of the antidepressants is discussed in Chapter 27.

Selective serotonin reuptake inhibitors. The SSRIs are first-line drugs for PD. At this time, only three SSRIs—fluoxetine (Prozac), paroxetine (Paxil), and sertraline (Zoloft)—are approved for this condition. However, the other SSRIs appear just as effective. The SSRIs decrease anticipatory anxiety, avoidance behavior, and the frequency and intensity of attacks. Furthermore, SSRIs decrease panic attacks regardless of whether the patient is actually depressed. However, if the patient does have coexisting depression, antidepressants will benefit the depression and PD simultaneously. Common side effects include nausea, headache, insomnia, weight gain, and sexual dysfunction. In addition, SSRIs can *increase* anxiety early in treatment.

OBSESSIVE-COMPULSIVE DISORDER

Characteristics

OCD is a potentially disabling condition characterized by persistent obsessions and compulsions that cause marked distress, consume at least 1 hour a day, and significantly interfere with daily living. An *obsession* is defined as a recurrent, persistent thought, impulse, or mental image that is unwanted and distressing and comes involuntarily to mind despite attempts to ignore or suppress it. Common obsessions include fear of contamination (e.g., acquiring a disease by touching another person), aggressive impulses (e.g., harming a family member), a need for orderliness or symmetry (e.g., personal bathroom items must be arranged in a precise way), and repeated doubts (e.g., did I unplug the iron?). A *compulsion* is a ritualized behavior or mental act that the patient is driven to perform in response to his or her obsessions. In the patient's mind, carrying out the compulsion is essential to prevent some horrible event from occurring (e.g., death of a loved one). If performing the compulsion is suppressed or postponed, the patient experiences increased anxiety. Common compulsions include hand washing, mental counting, arranging objects symmetrically, and hoarding. Patients usually understand that their compulsive behavior is excessive and senseless but nonetheless are unable to stop.

Treatment

Patients with OCD respond to drugs and to behavioral therapy. Optimal treatment consists of both. As a last resort, patients with severe, resistant OCD can be treated with deep brain stimulation.

Behavioral therapy is probably more important in OCD than in any other psychiatric disorder. In the technique employed, patients are exposed to sources of their fears while being encouraged to refrain from acting out their compulsive rituals. When no dire consequences come to pass, despite the absence of "protective" rituals, patients are able to gradually give up their compulsive behavior. Although this form of therapy causes great anxiety, the success rate is high.

Five drugs are approved to treat OCD: four SSRIs and one TCA (clomipramine). All five enhance serotonergic transmission. The SSRIs are better tolerated than clomipramine and hence are preferred.

Selective Serotonin Reuptake Inhibitors

The SSRIs are first-line drugs for OCD. Only four SSRIs—fluoxetine (Prozac), fluvoxamine (Luvox), sertraline (Zoloft), and paroxetine (Paxil)—are approved for OCD. However, the remaining two—citalopram (Celexa) and escitalopram (Lexapro, Cipralex✚)—are also effective. All six reduce symptoms by enhancing serotonergic transmission. They all are equally effective, although individual patients may respond better to one than to another. With all six, beneficial effects develop slowly, taking several months to become maximal. Common side effects include nausea, headache, insomnia, and sexual dysfunction. Weight gain can also occur. Despite this array of side effects, SSRIs are safer than clomipramine and better tolerated.

Therapy of an initial episode should continue for at least 1 year, after which discontinuation can be tried. Withdrawal should be done slowly, reducing the dosage by 25% every 1 to 2 months. Unfortunately, relapse is common; estimates range from 23% to as high as 90%. If relapse continues to occur after three or four attempts at withdrawal, lifelong treatment may be indicated.

SOCIAL ANXIETY DISORDER

Characteristics

SAD is characterized by an intense, irrational fear of situations in which one might be scrutinized by others, or might do something that is embarrassing or humiliating. Exposure to the feared situation almost always elicits anxiety. As a result, the person avoids the situation or, if it can't be avoided, endures it with intense anxiety (manifestations include blushing, stuttering, sweating, palpitations, dry throat, and muscle tension and twitches).

SAD has two principal forms: generalized and performance only. In the generalized form, the person fears nearly all social and performance situations. In the performance-only form, fear is limited to speaking or performing in public.

SAD can be very debilitating. In younger people, it can delay social development, inhibit participation in social activities, impair acquisition of friends, and make dating difficult or even impossible. It can also preclude pursuit of higher education. In older people, it can severely limit social and occupational options.

SAD is one of the most common psychiatric disorders, and *the* most common anxiety disorder. In the United States, 13% to 14% of the population is affected at some time in their lives. The disorder typically begins during the teenage years and, left untreated, is likely to continue lifelong.

Treatment

SAD can be treated with psychotherapy, drug therapy, or both. Studies indicate that psychotherapy—both cognitive and behavioral—can be as effective as drugs. However, a combination of psychotherapy *plus* drugs is likely to be more effective than either modality alone.

The SSRIs are considered first-line drugs for most patients. These drugs are especially well suited for patients who fear multiple situations and are obliged to face those situations on a regular basis. Only two SSRIs—paroxetine (Paxil) and sertraline (Zoloft)—are approved for SAD, but available data indicate that the other SSRIs are effective also. Initial effects take about 4 weeks to develop; optimal effects are seen in 8 to 12 weeks. Patients should be informed that benefits will be delayed.

Benzodiazepines (e.g., clonazepam [Klonopin, Rivotril✚], alprazolam [Xanax]) are an option for some patients. These drugs are well tolerated and their benefits are immediate, unlike those of the SSRIs. As a result, benzodiazepines can provide rapid relief and can be used PRN. Accordingly, these drugs are well suited for people whose fear is limited to performance situations and who must face those situations only occasionally. The usual dosage is 1 to 3 mg/day for clonazepam and 1 to 4 mg/day for alprazolam.

Propranolol (Inderal) and other β blockers can benefit patients with performance anxiety. When taken 1 to 2 hours before a scheduled performance, beta blockers can reduce symptoms caused by autonomic hyperactivity (e.g., tremors, sweating, tachycardia, palpitations). Doses are relatively small—only 10 to 80 mg for propranolol.

POSTTRAUMATIC STRESS DISORDER

Characteristics

PTSD develops after a *traumatic event* that elicited an immediate reaction of *fear, helplessness,* or *horror.* PTSD has three core symptoms: *reexperiencing* the event, *avoiding reminders* of the event (coupled with generalized emotional numbing), and a persistent state of *hyperarousal.* A traumatic event is one that involves a threat of injury or death or a threat to one's physical integrity. Many events meet this criterion. Among these are physical or sexual assault, rape, torture, combat, industrial explosions, serious accidents, natural disasters, being taken hostage, displacement as a refugee, and terrorist attacks. It should be noted that PTSD can affect persons who were only *witnesses* to a traumatic event—not just those who were directly involved.

The epidemiology of PTSD is revealing. In the United States, more than 8 million Americans have PTSD in any given year, making PTSD the fourth most common psychiatric disorder. PTSD develops in 4% of men at some time in their lives, and in 10% to 14% of women. Traumatic events that involve interpersonal violence (e.g., assault, rape, torture) are more likely to cause PTSD than are traumatic events that do not (e.g., car accidents, natural disasters). For example, among rape victims, the incidence of PTSD is 45.9% for women and 65% for men. In contrast, among natural disaster survivors, the incidence is 5.4% for women and 3.7% for men. Combat carries a high risk for PTSD: the disorder develops in up to 40% of soldiers who go to war.

Treatment

PTSD can be treated with psychotherapy and with drugs, as described in a recent evidence-based guideline—*VA/DoD Clinical Practice Guideline for the Management of Post-Traumatic Stress*—released by the Department of Veterans Affairs and Department of Defense in 2010. Two basic types of psychotherapy are recommended: *trauma-focused therapy* and *stress inoculation training*. Trauma-focused therapy uses a variety of cognitive behavioral techniques, including a very effective one known as *exposure therapy*, in which patients repeatedly reimagine traumatic events as a way to make those events lose their power. Stress inoculation training helps patients identify cues that can trigger fear and anxiety and then teaches them techniques to cope with those disturbing reactions.

Regarding drugs, evidence of efficacy is strongest for three SSRIs (fluoxetine, paroxetine, and sertraline) and one SNRI (venlafaxine). Of these four drugs, only two—paroxetine (Paxil) and sertraline (Zoloft)—are approved by the FDA for PTSD. If none of the first-line drugs is effective, the guidelines suggest several alternatives: mirtazapine, a TCA (amitriptyline or imipramine), or an MAOI (phenelzine). Current evidence does *not* support the use of monotherapy with bupropion, buspirone, trazodone, or a benzodiazepine.

31

Central Nervous System Stimulants and Attention-Deficit/Hyperactivity Disorder

CENTRAL NERVOUS SYSTEM STIMULANTS

Central nervous system (CNS) stimulants increase the activity of CNS neurons. Most stimulants act by enhancing neuronal excitation. A few act by suppressing neuronal inhibition. In sufficient doses, all stimulants can cause seizures.

Clinical applications of the CNS stimulants are limited. Currently these drugs have two principal indications: attention-deficit/hyperactivity disorder (ADHD) and narcolepsy.

Please note that CNS stimulants are not the same as antidepressants. The antidepressants act selectively to elevate mood and hence can relieve depression without affecting other CNS functions. In contrast, CNS stimulants cannot elevate mood without producing generalized excitation. Accordingly, the role of stimulants in treating depression is minor.

Our principal focus is on *amphetamines*, *methylphenidate* (Ritalin, others), and *methylxanthines* (e.g., caffeine). These are by far the most widely used stimulant drugs.

Amphetamines

The amphetamine family consists of amphetamine, dextroamphetamine, methamphetamine, and lisdexamfetamine. All are powerful CNS stimulants. In addition to their CNS actions, amphetamines have significant peripheral actions—actions that can cause cardiac stimulation and vasoconstriction. The amphetamines have a high potential for abuse.

PROTOTYPE DRUGS

Central Nervous System Stimulants

Amphetamine
Amphetamine sulfate

Amphetamine-Like Drug
Methylphenidate

Methylxanthine
Caffeine

Drugs for Attention-Deficit/Hyperactivity Disorder
CNS Stimulants
Methylphenidate

Nonstimulants
Atomoxetine

Amphetamine

The term *amphetamine* refers not to a single compound but rather to a 50:50 mixture of dextroamphetamine and levoamphetamine.

Lisdexamfetamine

Lisdexamfetamine (Vyvanse) is a prodrug composed of dextroamphetamine covalently linked to L-lysine. After oral dosing, the drug undergoes rapid hydrolysis by enzymes in the intestine and liver to yield lysine and free dextroamphetamine, the active form of the drug. If lisdexamfetamine is inhaled or injected, hydrolysis will not take place, and hence the drug is not effective by these routes. Accordingly, it may have a lower abuse potential than other forms of amphetamine.

Methamphetamine

Methamphetamine is simply dextroamphetamine with an additional methyl group.

Mechanism of action. The amphetamines act primarily by causing release of norepinephrine (NE) and dopamine (DA) and partly by inhibiting reuptake of both transmitters. These actions take place in the CNS and in peripheral nerves. Most pharmacologic effects result from release of NE.

Pharmacologic effects

Central nervous system. The amphetamines have prominent effects on mood and arousal. At usual doses, they increase wakefulness and alertness, reduce fatigue, elevate mood, and augment self-confidence and initiative. Euphoria, talkativeness, and increased motor activity are likely. Task performance that had been reduced by fatigue or boredom improves.

Amphetamines can stimulate respiration and suppress appetite and perception of pain. Stimulation of the medullary respiratory center increases respiration. Effects on the hypothalamic feeding center depress appetite. By a mechanism that is not understood, amphetamines can enhance the analgesic effects of morphine and other opioids.

Cardiovascular system. Cardiovascular effects occur secondary to release of NE from sympathetic neurons. NE acts in the heart to increase heart rate, atrioventricular conduction, and force of contraction. Excessive cardiac stimulation can cause dysrhythmias. In blood vessels, NE promotes constriction. Excessive vasoconstriction can cause hypertension.

Tolerance. With regular amphetamine use, tolerance develops to elevation of mood, suppression of appetite, and stimulation of the heart and blood vessels. In highly tolerant users, doses up to 1000 mg given intravenously every few *hours* may be required to maintain *euphoric* effects. This compares with *daily* doses of 5 to 30 mg for nontolerant individuals.

Physical dependence. Chronic amphetamine use produces physical dependence. If amphetamines are abruptly withdrawn from a dependent person, an abstinence syndrome will ensue. Symptoms include exhaustion, depression, prolonged sleep, excessive eating, and a craving for more amphetamine. Sleep patterns may take months to normalize.

Abuse. Because amphetamines can produce euphoria (extreme mood elevation), they have a high potential for abuse. Psychological dependence can occur. (Users familiar with CNS stimulants find the psychological effects of amphetamines nearly identical to those of cocaine.) Because of their abuse potential, all amphetamines, including lisdexamfetamine, are classified under Schedule II of the Controlled Substances Act and must be dispensed accordingly. Whenever amphetamines are used therapeutically, their potential for abuse must be weighed against their potential benefits.

Adverse effects

Central nervous system stimulation. Stimulation of the CNS can cause insomnia and restlessness. These effects can occur at therapeutic doses.

Weight loss. By suppressing appetite, amphetamines can cause weight loss.

Cardiovascular effects. At recommended doses, stimulants produce a small increase in heart rate and blood pressure. For most patients, these increases lack clinical significance. However, for patients with preexisting cardiovascular disease, stimulants may cause dysrhythmias, anginal pain, or hypertension. Accordingly, amphetamines must be employed with extreme caution in these people. Any patient who develops cardiovascular symptoms while using a stimulant should be evaluated immediately.

Do amphetamines increase the risk for *sudden death*? Probably not. Sudden death in children on these medications is very rare, and evidence is conflicting regarding risk for sudden death. Should children *routinely* receive an electrocardiogram (ECG) before using these drugs? Probably not—despite a 2008 statement from the American Heart Association (AHA) saying it would be reasonable to consider obtaining an ECG in children being evaluated for stimulant therapy of ADHD. The AHA developed this statement because 14 children, 5 with heart defects, died suddenly while using Adderall, a mixture of amphetamine and dextroamphetamine. However, given that millions of children have used the drug, the death rate is no greater than would be expected for a group this size, whether or not Adderall was being used. The bottom line? First, there are conflicting data showing that stimulants increase the risk for sudden death, even in children with heart disease. Second, there are no data showing that limiting the use of stimulants in children with heart defects will protect them from sudden death. And third, there are no data showing that screening for heart disease with an ECG before starting stimulants will be of benefit. Therefore it would seem that *routine* ECGs are unnecessary before starting a child on stimulant therapy, especially if there is no evidence of heart disease. However, if there *is* evidence of heart disease, or evidence of hereditary cardiovascular defects, an ECG might be appropriate.

Psychosis. Excessive amphetamine use produces a state of paranoid psychosis, characterized by hallucinations and paranoid delusions. Amphetamine-induced psychosis looks very much like schizophrenia. Symptoms are thought to result from release of DA. Consistent with this hypothesis is the observation that symptoms can be alleviated with a DA receptor blocking agent (e.g., haloperidol). After amphetamine withdrawal, psychosis usually resolves spontaneously within a week.

In some individuals, amphetamines can unmask latent schizophrenia. For these people, symptoms of psychosis do not clear spontaneously, and hence psychiatric care is indicated.

Therapeutic uses

Attention-deficit/hyperactivity disorder. The role of amphetamines in ADHD is discussed later.

Narcolepsy. Narcolepsy is a disorder characterized by daytime somnolence and uncontrollable attacks of sleep. By stimulating the CNS, amphetamines can promote arousal and thereby alleviate symptoms.

BLACK BOX WARNING
Amphetamine Abuse

> Amphetamines have a high potential for abuse and dependence. In patients who use amphetamines chronically, withdrawal may occur if use of these medications is suddenly stopped.

Methylphenidate and Dexmethylphenidate

Methylphenidate and dexmethylphenidate are nearly identical in structure and pharmacologic actions. Furthermore, the pharmacology of both drugs is nearly identical to that of the amphetamines.

Methylphenidate

Although methylphenidate (Ritalin, Metadate, Methylin, Concerta, Daytrana, Biphentin ✤) is structurally dissimilar from the amphetamines, the pharmacologic actions of these drugs are essentially the same. Consequently, methylphenidate can be considered an amphetamine in all but structure and name. Methylphenidate and amphetamine share the same mechanism of action (promotion of NE and DA release, and inhibition of NE and DA reuptake), adverse effects (insomnia, reduced appetite, emotional lability), and abuse liability (Schedule II). Like amphetamine, methylphenidate is not a single compound, but rather a 50:50 mixture of dextro and levo isomers. Methylphenidate has two indications: ADHD and narcolepsy.

BLACK BOX WARNING
Methylphenidate Abuse

> Chronic abuse of methylphenidate can lead to marked tolerance and psychological dependence with varying degrees of abnormal behavior and possible frank psychotic episodes.

Dexmethylphenidate

Dexmethylphenidate (Focalin, Focalin XR), a drug for ADHD, is simply the dextro isomer of methylphenidate. As noted, the dextro isomer accounts for most of the pharmacologic activity of methylphenidate, a 50:50 mixture of dextro and levo isomers. Accordingly, the pharmacology of dexmethylphenidate is nearly identical to that of methylphenidate. The only difference is that the dosage of dexmethylphenidate is one-half the dosage of methylphenidate.

Methylxanthines

The methylxanthines are methylated derivatives of xanthine, hence the family name. These compounds consist of a xanthine nucleus with one or more methyl groups attached. Caffeine, the most familiar member of the family, will serve as our prototype.

Caffeine

Caffeine is consumed worldwide for its stimulant effects. In the United States, per capita consumption is about 200 mg/day, mostly in the form of coffee. Although clinical applications of caffeine are few, caffeine remains of interest because of its widespread ingestion for nonmedical purposes.

Mechanism of action. Several mechanisms of action have been proposed. These include (1) reversible blockade of adenosine receptors, (2) enhancement of calcium permeability in the sarcoplasmic reticulum, and (3) inhibition of cyclic nucleotide phosphodiesterase, resulting in accumulation of cyclic adenosine monophosphate (cyclic AMP). Blockade of adenosine receptors appears responsible for most effects.

PATIENT-CENTERED CARE ACROSS THE LIFE SPAN

Stimulants

Life Stage	Patient Care Concerns
Infants	Caffeine citrate (Cafcit) is used for neonatal apnea. Other central nervous system stimulants should be avoided in this population.
Children	The stimulant class of drugs for treatment of attention-deficit/hyperactivity disorder (ADHD) has been proved safe and effective for this population. Atomoxetine, a nonstimulant for ADHD, may cause suicidal thinking in children and adolescents.
Pregnant women	Caffeine may pose a small risk for birth defects, although human data are lacking. Adverse fetal effects have been demonstrated in animal studies.
Breastfeeding women	Stimulants, such as methylphenidate, do not have any reported side effects in the breastfeeding infant. There are limited to no data on the nonstimulants and the effects on breastfeeding infants.
Older adults	Most studies focus on patients older than 65 years because stimulants are often used for treatment of apathy, depression, and fatigue in the older adult population. Stimulants should be avoided in patients with cardiac disease or glaucoma. Consider a lower starting dose and monitor heart rate, blood pressure, and weight.

Therapeutic uses

Neonatal apnea. Premature infants may experience prolonged apnea (lasting 15 seconds or more) along with bradycardia. Hypoxemia and neurologic damage may result. Caffeine and other methylxanthines can reduce the number and duration of apnea episodes and can promote a more regular pattern of breathing.

Promoting wakefulness. Caffeine is used commonly to aid in staying awake. The drug is marketed in various over-the-counter (OTC) preparations (Maximum Strength NoDoz, Vivarin, others) for this purpose. Of course, individuals desiring increased alertness can get just as much caffeine by drinking coffee or some other caffeine-containing beverage.

Miscellaneous Central Nervous System Stimulants
Modafinil

Therapeutic use. Modafinil (Provigil, Alertec ♣), a unique non-amphetamine stimulant, is approved for promoting wakefulness in patients with excessive sleepiness associated with three disorders: narcolepsy, shift-work sleep disorder (SWSD), and obstructive sleep apnea–hypopnea syndrome (OSAHS). However, although the drug has only three approved uses, most prescriptions (95%) are written for off-label uses, including fatigue, depression, ADHD, jet lag, and sleepiness caused by medications. Investigational uses include ADHD and fatigue associated with multiple sclerosis. The military studied the drug for use in sustaining alertness in helicopter pilots and found it superior to placebo.

In clinical trials, modafinil has been moderately effective. In patients with narcolepsy, modafinil increased wakefulness, but only to about 50% of the level seen in normal people. In contrast, methylphenidate and dextroamphetamine increase wakefulness to about 70% of normal. In patients with SWSD and OSAHS, benefits are about the same as those seen in narcolepsy.

Mechanism of action. The drug seems to influence hypothalamic areas involved in maintaining the normal sleep–wakefulness cycle. Also,

there is evidence that modafinil inhibits the activity of sleep-promoting neurons (in the ventrolateral preoptic nucleus) by blocking reuptake of NE.

Pharmacokinetics. Modafinil is rapidly absorbed from the gastro-intestinal (GI) tract. Plasma levels peak in 2 to 4 hours. Food decreases the rate of absorption but not the extent. Elimination is by hepatic metabolism followed by renal excretion. The half-life is about 15 hours.

Adverse effects. Modafinil is generally well tolerated. The most common adverse effects are headache, nausea, nervousness, diarrhea, and rhinitis. Modafinil does not disrupt nighttime sleep. In clinical trials, only 5% of patients dropped out because of undesired effects. Initially, the drug was believed devoid of cardiovascular effects. However, we now know it can increase heart rate and blood pressure, apparently by altering autonomic function. Subjective effects—euphoria; altered perception, thinking, and feeling—are like those of other CNS stimulants. However, modafinil has less abuse potential and hence is regulated as a Schedule IV substance. Physical dependence and withdrawal have not been reported. Modafinil is embryotoxic in laboratory animals and hence should be avoided during pregnancy.

Postmarketing reports link modafinil to rare cases of serious skin reactions, including Stevens-Johnson syndrome, erythema multiforme, and toxic epidermal necrolysis. Patients should be informed about signs of these reactions—swelling or rash, especially in the presence of fever or changes in the oral mucosa—and instructed to discontinue the drug if they develop.

Drug interactions. Modafinil inhibits some forms of cytochrome P450 (CYP) and induces others. Induction of CYP3A4 (the 3A4 iso-enzyme of P450) may accelerate the metabolism of oral contraceptives, cyclosporine, and certain other drugs, thereby causing their levels to decline. Caution is advised.

ATTENTION-DEFICIT/HYPERACTIVITY DISORDER

Our discussion of ADHD has two parts. We begin by addressing basic concepts in ADHD—specifically, signs and symptoms, etiology, and treatment strategy. After that, we discuss the pharmacology of the drugs used for treatment (Table 31.1).

Basic Considerations
Attention-Deficit/Hyperactivity Disorder in Children

ADHD is the most common neuropsychiatric disorder of childhood, affecting 5% to 11% of school-aged children. The incidence in boys is two to three times the incidence in girls. Symptoms begin between ages 3 and 7 years, usually persist into the teens, and often persist on into adulthood. Most (60% to 70%) children respond well to stimulant drugs. Methylphenidate (Ritalin, Concerta, others) is the agent employed most.

Signs and symptoms. ADHD is characterized by *inattention*, *hyperactivity*, and *impulsivity*. Affected children are fidgety, unable to concentrate on schoolwork, and unable to wait their turn; switch excessively from one activity to another; call out excessively in class; and never complete tasks. To make a diagnosis, symptoms must appear before age 7 years and be present for at least 6 months. Because other disorders—especially anxiety and depression—may cause similar symptoms, diagnosis must be done carefully.

ADHD can be subclassified as predominantly inattentive type, predominantly hyperactive-impulsive type, or combined type, depending on symptom profile.

Etiology. Although various theories have been proposed, the underlying pathophysiology of ADHD is only partially understood. Neuroimaging studies indicate structural and functional abnormalities in multiple brain areas, including the frontal cortex, basal ganglia, brainstem,

TABLE 31.1 Major Drugs for Attention-Deficit/Hyperactivity Disorder

Drug	Trade Name	Availability	Duration (h)	Dosing Schedule	Usual Pediatric Maintenance Dosage
Stimulants					
Methylphenidate					
Immediate release	Ritalin, Methylin	5-, 10-, 20-mg tablets 2.5-, 5-, 10-mg chewables 5- and 10-mg/mL solution	3–5	2 or 3 times daily	10 mg at 8:00 AM and noon, and 5 mg at 4:00 PM
Sustained release	Ritalin-SR, Metadate ER, Quillivant XR	20-mg tablets 25-mg/5-mL oral suspension	6–8	Once or twice daily	20 or 40 mg in AM plus 20 mg in the early PM if needed
24-hour	Concerta	18-, 27-, 36-, 54-mg tablets. Osmotic-Release Oral System (OROS)	10–12	Once daily	36 mg in the AM
	Metadate CD	10-, 20-, 30-, 40-, 50-, 60-mg capsules containing IR and DR beads	8–12	Once daily	30 mg in the AM
	Ritalin LA	10-, 20-, 30-, 40-mg ER capsules	8–12	Once daily	30 mg in the AM
	Daytrana	10-, 15-, 20-, 30-mg/9-h transdermal patches	10–12	Once daily	One 15- or 20-mg patch, applied in the AM and removed 9 h later
Dexmethylphenidate					
Immediate release	Focalin	2.5-, 5-, 10-mg tablets	4–5	Twice daily	10 mg in the AM plus 10 mg in the early PM
Sustained release	Focalin XR	5-, 10-, 15-, 20-, 30-, 35-, 40-mg capsules	12	Once daily	10 mg in the AM
Dextroamphetamine					
Immediate release	Dexedrine, ProCentra	5-, 10-mg tablets 5-mg/mL solution	4–6	Once or twice daily	5 mg in the AM
Sustained release	Dexedrine Spansule	5-, 10-, 15-mg capsules	6–10	Once or twice daily	10 mg at 8:00 AM
Amphetamine Mixture					
Immediate release	Adderall	5-, 7.5-, 10-, 12.5-, 15-, 20-, 30-mg tablets	4–6	Twice daily	5 mg in the AM and 4–6 h later
Sustained release	Adderall XR	5-, 10-, 15-, 20-, 25-, 30-mg capsules	10–12	Once daily	20 mg in the AM
Lisdexamfetamine					
Sustained release	Vyvanse	20-, 30-, 40-, 50-, 60-, 70-mg capsules	13	Once daily	30 mg in the AM
Nonstimulants					
Atomoxetine	Strattera	10-, 18-, 25-, 40-, 60-, 80-, 100-mg capsules	24	Once or twice daily	80 mg in the AM *or* 40 mg in the AM and early PM
Guanfacine	Intuniv	1-, 2-, 3-, 4-mg ER tablets	24	Once daily	1–4 mg in the AM
Clonidine	Kapvay	0.1-, 0.2-mg ER tablets	24	Twice daily	0.1–0.2 mg in the AM and PM

DR, Delayed release; *ER*, extended release; *IR*, immediate release.

and cerebellum—regions involved with regulating attention, impulsive behavior, and motor activity. Several theories implicate dysregulation in neuronal pathways that employ NE, DA, and serotonin as transmitters. These theories would be consistent with the effects of atomoxetine (which blocks NE reuptake), imipramine (which blocks NE and serotonin uptake), and stimulant drugs (which promote release of NE and DA and, to some degree, block their uptake). Genetic factors play a significant role.

Management overview. Multiple strategies may be employed to manage ADHD. In addition to drugs, which are considered first-line treatment, the management program can include family therapy, parent training, and cognitive therapy for the child. Guidelines issued by the American Academy of Pediatrics emphasize the importance of a comprehensive treatment program, involving collaboration among clinicians, families, and educators. For long-term gains, a combination of cognitive therapy and stimulant drugs appears most effective. Of the drugs employed for ADHD, stimulants are most effective and hence are considered agents of choice. The nonstimulants (e.g., atomoxetine, guanfacine, clonidine) are less effective than stimulants and hence are considered second-choice drugs.

Attention-Deficit/Hyperactivity Disorder in Adults

In about 30% to 60% of cases, childhood ADHD persists into adulthood. In the United States, about 8 million adults are afflicted, although an estimated 90% are undiagnosed and untreated. Symptoms include poor concentration, stress intolerance, antisocial behavior, outbursts of anger, and inability to maintain a routine. Also, adults with ADHD experience more job loss, divorce, and driving accidents. As in childhood ADHD, therapy with a stimulant drug is the foundation of treatment. Methylphenidate is prescribed most often. About 33% of adults fail to respond to stimulants or cannot tolerate their side effects. For these patients, a trial with a nonstimulant may help. Combining behavioral therapy with drug therapy may be more effective than drug therapy alone.

Drugs Used for Attention-Deficit/Hyperactivity Disorder

Central Nervous System Stimulants

Stimulant drugs are the mainstay of ADHD therapy. Drugs with proven efficacy include *methylphenidate* (Ritalin, Concerta, others), *dexmethylphenidate* (Focalin), *dextroamphetamine-amphetamine mixture* (Adderall), and *lisdexamfetamine* (Vyvanse). There are no data to support use of one stimulant over another. If one stimulant is ineffective, another should be tried before considering a second-line agent.

The response to stimulants can be dramatic. These drugs can increase attention span and goal-oriented behavior while decreasing impulsiveness, distractibility, hyperactivity, and restlessness. Tests of cognitive function (memory, reading, arithmetic) often improve significantly. Unfortunately, although benefits can be dramatic initially, in children they diminish after 2 to 3 years, as reported in a 2009 paper: *MTA at 8 Years: Prospective Follow-up of Children Treated for Combined-Type ADHD in a Multisite Study.* Nonetheless, stimulant therapy can still buy time to teach children behavioral strategies to help them combat inattention and hyperactivity over the long term.

Although reduction of impulsiveness and hyperactivity with a stimulant may seem paradoxical, it isn't. Stimulants don't suppress rowdy behavior directly. Rather, they improve attention and focus. Impulsiveness and hyperactivity decline because the child is now able to concentrate on the task at hand. It should be noted that stimulants do not create *positive* behavior; they only reduce *negative* behavior. Accordingly, stimulants cannot give a child good study skills and other appropriate behaviors. Rather, these must be learned when the disruptive behavior is no longer an impediment.

Principal adverse effects of the stimulants are *insomnia* and *growth suppression.* Insomnia results from CNS stimulation and can be minimized by reducing the size of the afternoon dose and taking it no later than 4:00 PM. Growth suppression occurs secondary to appetite suppression. Growth reduction can be minimized by administering stimulants during or after meals (which reduces the impact of appetite suppression). In addition, some clinicians recommend taking "drug holidays" on weekends and in the summer (which creates an opportunity for growth to catch up). However, other clinicians argue against this strategy because depriving children of medication during these unstructured times can be hard on them. When stimulants are discontinued, a rebound increase in growth will take place; as a result, adult height may not be affected. Other adverse effects include *headache* and *abdominal pain,* which have an incidence of 10%; and *lethargy* and *listlessness,* which can occur when dosage is excessive.

Nonstimulants

Several nonstimulants are used for ADHD, although only three of them—atomoxetine, guanfacine, and clonidine—are approved by the U.S. Food and Drug Administration (FDA) for this use. The nonstimulants are less effective than the stimulants and hence are considered second-choice drugs. For treatment of ADHD, the nonstimulants may be employed as monotherapy, or as add-on therapy with a stimulant. Unlike the stimulants, the nonstimulants are not regulated as controlled substances.

Atomoxetine, a norepinephrine uptake inhibitor

Description and therapeutic effects. Atomoxetine (Strattera) is a unique drug approved for ADHD in children and adults. It was the first *nonstimulant* approved for ADHD, and one of only three drugs approved for ADHD in adults (the others are amphetamine-dextroamphetamine mixture (Adderall XR) and lisdexamfetamine (Vyvanse). In contrast to the CNS stimulants, atomoxetine has no potential for abuse and hence is not regulated as a controlled substance. As a result, prescriptions can be refilled over the phone, making atomoxetine more convenient than the stimulants. Like the long-acting stimulants, atomoxetine can be administered just once a day.

In clinical trials comparing atomoxetine with placebo in children or adults with ADHD, atomoxetine was clearly superior at reducing symptoms. It should be noted that responses develop slowly: the initial response takes a few days to develop, and the maximal response is seen in 1 to 3 weeks. This contrasts with the CNS stimulants, where the effects are near maximal with the first dose.

Mechanism of action. Atomoxetine is a *selective inhibitor of NE reuptake* and hence causes NE to accumulate at synapses. Although the precise relationship between this neurochemical action and symptom relief is unknown, it would appear that *adaptive changes* that occur after uptake blockade underlie benefits. Uptake blockade occurs immediately, whereas full therapeutic effects are not seen for at least a week—suggesting that after uptake blockade occurs, additional processes must take place before benefits can be seen.

Pharmacokinetics. Atomoxetine is rapidly and completely absorbed after oral administration. Plasma levels peak in 1 to 3 hours, depending on whether the drug was taken without or with food. Atomoxetine is metabolized in the liver, primarily by CYP2D6 (the 2D6 isoenzyme of cytochrome P450). For most patients, the half-life is 5 hours. However, for 5% to 10% of patients, the half-life is much longer: 24 hours. These patients have an atypical form of CYP2D6, which metabolizes atomoxetine slowly. Dosage should be reduced in these people.

Adverse effects. Like the CNS stimulants, atomoxetine is generally well tolerated. In clinical trials, the most common effects were GI reactions (dyspepsia, nausea, and vomiting), reduced appetite, dizziness, somnolence, mood swings, and trouble sleeping. Sexual dysfunction and urinary retention were seen in adults. Severe allergic reactions, including angioneurotic edema, occurred rarely. If allergy develops, patients should discontinue the drug and contact their prescriber immediately.

Atomoxetine may cause *suicidal thinking* in children and adolescents but not in adults. Fortunately, the incidence is relatively low: about 4 cases per 1000 patients. Risk is greatest during the first few months of treatment. Young patients should be monitored closely for suicidal thinking and behavior and for signs of clinical worsening (e.g., agitation, irritability).

Appetite suppression may result in *weight loss and growth delay.* Among children who took atomoxetine for 18 months or longer, mean height and weight percentiles declined. Because experience with the drug is limited, we don't know if expected adult height will be affected. Nor do we know if "drug holidays" would have an effect on growth.

Atomoxetine poses a small risk for *severe liver injury* that may progress to outright liver failure, resulting in death or the need for a liver transplantation. Patients should be informed about signs of liver injury—jaundice, dark urine, abdominal tenderness, unexplained flu-like symptoms—and instructed to report these immediately. In the event of jaundice or laboratory evidence of liver injury, atomoxetine should be discontinued.

Atomoxetine *may raise or lower blood pressure.* During clinical trials, some patients experienced a small increase in blood pressure and heart rate. Accordingly, atomoxetine should be used with caution by patients with hypertension or tachycardia. During postmarketing surveillance, some patients experienced *hypotension and syncope* (fainting). Patients should be informed of this possibility and advised to sit or lie down if they feel faint.

Drug interactions. *Inhibitors of CYP2D6* can increase levels of atomoxetine and hence must be used with caution. Common examples include paroxetine (Paxil), fluoxetine (Prozac), and quinidine.

Role in attention-deficit/hyperactivity disorder therapy. Atomoxetine is recommended for treatment of ADHD in cases in which there may be concern for stimulant abuse or there exists a strong aversion to treatment with stimulant medications. Because CNS stimulants are more effective and have a long record of safety and efficacy, it would seem prudent to reserve atomoxetine for patients who are unresponsive to or intolerant of the stimulants. In the absence of a compelling reason, patients doing well on the stimulants should not switch.

α_2-adrenergic agonists. Two α_2-adrenergic agonists—guanfacine and clonidine—are approved for ADHD. Both drugs appear less effective than CNS stimulants. Principal side effects are sedation, hypotension, and fatigue. Unlike the CNS stimulants, guanfacine and clonidine are not controlled substances and do not cause anorexia or insomnia. The basic pharmacology of these drugs is discussed in Chapter 17.

32

Substance Use Disorders I:
Basic Considerations

Mind-altering drugs have intrigued human beings since the dawn of civilization. Throughout history, people have taken drugs to elevate mood, release inhibitions, distort perceptions, induce hallucinations, and modify thinking. Many of those who take mind-altering drugs restrict use to socially approved patterns. However, many others self-administer drugs to excess. Excessive drug use is our focus in this chapter and the three that follow.

Substance abuse extracts a huge toll on the individual and on society. Tobacco alone kills approximately 480,000 Americans each year. Alcohol and illicit drugs kill another 100,000. In addition to putting people at risk for death, drug abuse puts them at risk for long-term illness and impairs their ability to fulfill role obligations at home, school, and work. The economic burden of drug abuse is staggering: the combined direct and indirect costs from abusing nicotine, alcohol, and illicit substances are estimated at more than $700 *billion* each year.

Substance abuse confronts clinicians in a variety of ways, making knowledge of abuse a necessity. Important areas in which expertise on substance use may be applied include (1) diagnosis and treatment of acute toxicity, (2) diagnosis and treatment of secondary medical complications of drug abuse, (3) the facilitation of drug withdrawal, and (4) education and counseling to maintain long-term abstinence.

Our discussion of substance abuse occurs in two stages. In this chapter, we discuss basic concepts in drug abuse. In Chapters 33, 34, and 35, we focus on the pharmacology of specific abused agents and methods of treatment.

DEFINITIONS

Drug Abuse

Drug abuse can be defined as *using a drug in a fashion inconsistent with medical or social norms.* Traditionally, the term also implies drug use that is harmful to the individual or society. As we shall see, although we can give abuse a general definition, deciding whether a particular instance of drug use constitutes "abuse" is often difficult.

Whether or not drug use is considered abuse depends, in part, on the purpose for which a drug is taken. Not everyone who takes large doses of psychoactive agents has a disorder. For example, we do not consider it abuse to take large doses of opioids long term to relieve pain caused by cancer. However, we do consider it abusive for an otherwise healthy individual to take those same opioids in the same doses to produce euphoria.

Abuse can have different degrees of severity. For example, some people use heroin only occasionally, whereas others use it habitually and compulsively. Although both patterns of drug use are socially condemned and therefore constitute abuse, there is an obvious quantitative difference between taking heroin once or twice and taking it routinely and compulsively.

Note that, by the previous definition, substance abuse is culturally defined. Because abuse is culturally defined and because societies differ from one another and are changeable, there can be wide variations in what is labeled abuse. What is defined as abuse can vary from one culture to another. For example, in many societies, moderate consumption of alcohol is not usually considered abuse. In contrast, any ingestion of alcohol may be considered abuse in some Muslim societies. Furthermore, what is defined as abuse can vary from one time to another within the same culture. For example, when a few Americans first experimented with lysergic acid diethylamide (LSD) and other psychedelic drugs, these agents were legal and their use was not generally disapproved. However, when use of psychedelics became widespread, our societal posture changed, and legislation was passed to make the manufacture, sale, and use of these drugs illegal.

As we can see, distinguishing between culturally acceptable drug use and drug use that is abuse is more in the realm of social science than pharmacology. Accordingly, because this is a pharmacology text and not a sociology text, we will not attempt to define just what patterns of drug use do or do not constitute abuse. Instead, we will focus on the pharmacologic properties of abused drugs. Fortunately, we can identify the drugs that tend to be misused and discuss their pharmacology.

Substance Use Disorder

According to the American Psychiatric Association (APA), substance use disorder (SUD) is defined as a *cluster of cognitive, behavioral, and physiological symptoms indicating that the individual continues using the substance despite significant substance-related problems.* Please note that this definition does not equate SUD solely with physical dependence. As discussed elsewhere in this chapter, although physical dependence can contribute to addictive behavior, it is neither necessary nor sufficient for addiction to occur.

Other Definitions

Tolerance results from regular drug use and can be defined as a state in which a particular dose elicits a smaller response than it did with initial use. As tolerance increases, higher and higher doses are needed to elicit desired effects.

Cross-tolerance is a state in which tolerance to one drug confers tolerance to another. Cross-tolerance generally develops among drugs

255

within a particular class and not between drugs in different classes. For example, tolerance to one opioid (e.g., heroin) confers cross-tolerance to other opioids (e.g., morphine) but not to central nervous system (CNS) depressants, psychostimulants, psychedelics, or nicotine.

Psychological dependence can be defined as an intense subjective need for a particular psychoactive drug.

Physical dependence can be defined as a state in which an abstinence syndrome will occur if drug use is discontinued. Physical dependence is the result of neuroadaptive processes that take place in response to prolonged drug exposure.

Cross-dependence refers to the ability of one drug to support physical dependence on another drug. When cross-dependence exists between drug A and drug B, taking drug A will prevent withdrawal in a patient physically dependent on drug B, and vice versa. As with cross-tolerance, cross-dependence generally exists among drugs in the same pharmacologic family but not between drugs in different families.

A *withdrawal syndrome* is a constellation of signs and symptoms that occurs in physically dependent individuals when they discontinue drug use. Quite often, the symptoms seen during withdrawal are opposite to effects the drug produced before it was withdrawn. For example, discontinuation of a CNS depressant can cause CNS excitation.

DIAGNOSTIC CRITERIA FOR SUBSTANCE USE DISORDER

SUD is best defined as *continued use of a substance despite significant substance-related problems*. There exists a change in brain circuitry that persists despite detoxification from a particular substance. Diagnosis of substance abuse disorder is based on behaviors related to continued use of a substance.

Tolerance and withdrawal are among the criteria established by the APA for having an SUD. However, please note that tolerance and withdrawal, by themselves, are neither necessary nor sufficient for a SUD to exist. Put another way, the pattern of drug use that constitutes a SUD can exist in persons who are not physically dependent on drugs and who have not developed tolerance. This distinction is extremely important. *Being physically dependent on a drug is not the same as having a substance use disorder.* Many people are physically dependent but do not meet the criteria for a diagnosed disorder. These people are not considered to have SUD because they do not demonstrate the behavior pattern that constitutes substance dependence. For example, individuals with terminal cancer are often physically dependent on opioids. However, because their lives are not disrupted by their medication (quite the contrary), their drug use does not meet the criteria for a SUD. Similarly, some degree of physical dependence occurs in all patients who take phenobarbital to control seizure disorders. However, despite their physical dependence, patients with seizure do not carry out addictive behavior and therefore do not have a SUD.

Having stressed that physical dependence and SUD are different from each other, we must note that the two states are not entirely unrelated. As discussed in the sections that follow, although physical dependence is not the same as SUD, physical dependence often contributes to addictive behavior.

FACTORS THAT CONTRIBUTE TO SUBSTANCE USE DISORDER

SUD is the end result of a progressive involvement with drugs. Taking psychoactive drugs is usually initiated out of curiosity. From this initial involvement, an individual can progress to occasional use. Occasional use may evolve into compulsive use. Factors that play a role in the progression from experimental use to compulsive use are discussed next.

Reinforcing Properties of Drugs

Reinforcement by drugs can occur in two ways. First, drugs can give the individual an experience that is pleasurable. For example, cocaine produces a state of euphoria. Second, drugs can reduce the intensity of unpleasant experiences. For example, drugs can reduce anxiety and stress.

The reinforcing properties of drugs can be clearly demonstrated in experiments with animals. In the laboratory, animals will self-administer most of the drugs that are abused by humans (e.g., opioids, barbiturates, alcohol, cocaine, amphetamines, phencyclidine, nicotine, caffeine). When these drugs are made freely available, animals develop patterns of drug use that are similar to those of humans. Animals will self-administer these drugs (except for nicotine and caffeine) in preference to eating, drinking, and sex. When permitted, their preference for a substance will lead to death due to lack of food and fluid. These observations strongly suggest that preexisting psychopathology is not necessary for drug abuse to develop. Rather, these studies suggest that drug abuse results, in large part, from the reinforcing properties of drugs themselves.

Physical Dependence

As defined earlier in this chapter, *physical dependence* is a state in which a withdrawal syndrome will occur if drug use is discontinued. The degree of physical dependence is determined largely by dosage and duration of drug use. Physical dependence is greatest in people who take large doses for a long time. The more physically dependent a person is, the more intense the withdrawal syndrome. Substantial physical dependence develops to opioids (e.g., morphine, heroin) and other CNS depressants (e.g., barbiturates, alcohol). Physical dependence tends to be less prominent with other abused drugs (e.g., psychostimulants, psychedelics, marijuana).

Physical dependence can contribute to compulsive drug use. After dependence has developed, the desire to avoid withdrawal becomes a motivator for continued dosing. Furthermore, if the drug is administered after the onset of withdrawal, its ability to alleviate the discomfort of withdrawal can reinforce its desirability. However, please note, that although physical dependence plays a role in the abuse of drugs, physical dependence should not be viewed as the primary cause of addictive behavior. Rather, physical dependence is just one of several factors that can contribute to the development and continuation of compulsive use.

Psychological Dependence

Psychological dependence is defined as *an intense subjective need for a drug*. Individuals who are psychologically dependent feel strongly that their sense of well-being is dependent on continued drug use; a sense of "craving" is felt when the drug is unavailable. There is no question that psychological dependence can be a major factor in addictive behavior. For example, it is psychological dependence—and not physical dependence—that plays the principal role in causing renewed use of opioids by addicts who had previously gone through withdrawal.

Social Factors

Social factors can play an important role in the development of SUDs. The desire for social status and approval is a common reason for initiating drug use. In addition, because initial drug experiences are frequently unpleasant, the desire for social approval can be one of the most compelling reasons for repeating drug use after the initial exposure. For example, most people do not especially enjoy their first cigarette; were it not for peer pressure, many would quit before they smoked enough for it to become pleasurable. Similarly, initial use of heroin, with its associated nausea and vomiting, is often deemed unpleasant; peer pressure is a common reason for continuing heroin use long enough to develop tolerance to these undesirable effects.

Drug Availability

Drug availability is clearly a factor in the development and maintenance of abuse. Abuse can flourish only in environments where drugs can be readily obtained. In contrast, where procurement is difficult, abuse is minimal. The ready availability of drugs in hospitals and clinics is a major reason for the high rate of addiction among pharmacists, nurses, and physicians.

Vulnerability of the Individual

Some individuals are more prone to becoming drug abusers than others. By way of illustration, let us consider three individuals from the same social setting who have equal access to the same psychoactive drug. The first person experiments with the drug briefly and never uses it again. The second person progresses from experimentation to occasional use. The third goes on to take the drug compulsively. Because social factors, drug availability, and the properties of the drug itself are the same for all three people, these factors cannot explain the three different patterns of drug use. Therefore we must conclude that the differences must lie in the people: one individual was not prone to drug abuse, one had only moderate tendencies toward abuse, and the third was highly vulnerable to becoming an abuser.

Several psychological factors have been associated with tendencies toward drug abuse. Drug abusers are frequently individuals who are impulsive, have a low tolerance for frustration, and are rebellious against social norms. Other psychological factors that seem to predispose individuals to abusing drugs include depressive disorders, anxiety disorders, and antisocial personality. It is also clear that individuals who abuse one type of drug are likely to abuse other drugs.

There is speculation that some instances of drug abuse may actually represent self-medication to relieve emotional discomfort. For example, some people may use alcohol and other depressants to control severe anxiety. Although their drug use may appear excessive, it may be no more than they need to neutralize intolerable feelings.

Genetics also contributes to drug abuse. For example, vulnerability to alcoholism may result from an inherited predisposition.

NEUROBIOLOGY OF SUBSTANCE USE DISORDERS

Repeated use of a drug contributes to the transition from voluntary drug use to compulsive use by causing molecular changes in the brain. Each time the drug is taken, it causes changes that promote further drug use. With repeated drug exposure, these changes are reinforced, making drug use increasingly more difficult to control.

Molecular changes occur in the *reward circuit*—a system that normally serves to reinforce behaviors essential for survival, such as eating and reproductive activities. Neurons of the reward circuit originate in the ventral tegmental area of the midbrain and project to the nucleus accumbens. Their major transmitter is *dopamine.* Under normal circumstances, biologically critical behavior, such as sexual intercourse, activates the circuit. The resultant release of dopamine rewards and reinforces the behavior. Like natural positive stimuli, addictive drugs can also activate the circuit and thereby cause dopamine release. In fact, drugs are so effective at activating the circuit that the amount of dopamine released may be 2 to 10 times the amount released by natural stimuli. Ultimately, whether the system is activated by use of drugs or by behavior essential for survival, the outcome is the same: a tendency to repeat the behavior that turned the system on. With repeated activation over time, the system undergoes synaptic remodeling, thereby consolidating changes in brain function. This neural remodeling persists after drug use has ceased.

An important aspect of drug-induced remodeling is a phenomenon known as *downregulation,* which serves to *reduce* the response to drugs. Because drugs release abnormally large amounts of dopamine, the reward circuit is put in a state of excessive activation. In response, the brain (1) produces less dopamine and (2) reduces the number of dopamine receptors. As a result, responses to drugs are reduced. Unfortunately, the ability of natural stimuli to activate the circuit is reduced as well. In the absence of pleasurable feelings from natural stimuli, the abuser is left feeling flat, lifeless, and depressed. The good news is that, when drug use stops, neural remodeling tends to gradually reverse.

PRINCIPLES OF SUBSTANCE USE DISORDER TREATMENT

SUD is a treatable disease of the brain. With therapy, between 40% and 60% of addicts can reduce drug use. The first science-based guide on addiction therapy—*Principles of Drug Addiction Treatment*—was published by the National Institute on Drug Abuse in 1999 and later revised in 2009 and 2012. The guide centers on 13 principles of effective treatment, shown in Box 32.1.

Ideally, the goal of treatment is *complete cessation* of drug use. However, total abstinence is not the only outcome that can be considered successful. Treatment that changes drug use from compulsive to moderate will permit increased productivity, better health, and a decrease in socially unacceptable behavior. Clearly, this outcome is beneficial both to the individual and to society—even though some degree of drug use continues. However, it must be noted that in the treatment of some forms of abuse, nothing short of total abstinence can be considered a true success. Experience has shown that abusers of *cigarettes, alcohol,* and *opioids* are rarely capable of sustained moderation. Hence, for many of these individuals, abstinence must be complete if there is to be any hope of avoiding a return to compulsive use.

Recovery from addiction is a prolonged process that typically requires multiple treatment episodes because addiction is a *chronic, relapsing* illness. As such, periods of treatment-induced abstinence will very likely be followed by relapse. This does not mean that treatment has failed. Rather, it simply means that at least one more treatment episode is needed. Eventually, many patients achieve stable, long-term abstinence, along with a more productive and rewarding life.

Because addiction is a complex illness that affects all aspects of life, the treatment program must be comprehensive and multifaceted. In addition to addressing drug use itself, the program should address any related medical, psychological, social, vocational, and legal problems. Obviously, treatment must be tailored to the individual; no single approach works for all people. Multiple techniques are used. Techniques with proven success include (1) group and individual therapy directed at resolving emotional problems that underlie drug use, (2) substituting alternative rewards for the rewards of drug use, and (3) use of pharmacologic agents to modify the effects of abused drugs. The most effective treatment programs incorporate two or more of these methods. When possible, a specialist in addiction medicine or substance use should be involved in the patient's care.

CONTROLLED SUBSTANCES ACT

The *Comprehensive Drug Abuse Prevention and Control Act of 1970,* known informally as the *Controlled Substances Act* (CSA), is the principal federal legislation addressing drug abuse. One objective of the CSA is to reduce the chances that drugs originating from legitimate sources will be diverted to abusers. To accomplish this goal, the CSA sets forth regulations for the handling of controlled substances by manufacturers,

---

BOX 32.1 Principles of Drug Addiction Treatment

1. **Addiction is a complex but treatable disease that affects brain function and behavior.** Drugs of abuse alter brain structure and function, resulting in changes that may persist long after drug use has stopped. These persistent changes may explain why former abusers are at the risk for relapse after prolonged abstinence.

2. **No single treatment is appropriate for everyone.** It is critical to match treatment settings, interventions, and services to each patient's problems and needs.

3. **Treatment must be readily available.** Treatment applicants can be lost if treatment is not immediately available or readily accessible. As with other chronic diseases, the earlier treatment is offered in the disease process, the greater the likelihood of positive outcomes.

4. **Effective treatment must attend to multiple needs of the individual, not solely drug use.** In addition to addressing drug use, treatment must address the individual's medical, psychological, social, vocational, and legal problems.

5. **Remaining in treatment for an adequate time is critical.** Treatment duration is based on individual need. Most patients require at least 3 months of treatment to significantly reduce or stop drug use. Additional treatment can produce further progress. As with other chronic illnesses, relapses can occur, signaling a need for treatment to be reinstated or adjusted. Programs should include strategies to prevent patients from leaving prematurely.

6. **Individual and/or group counseling and other behavioral therapies are the most common forms of drug abuse treatment.** In therapy, patients address motivation, build skills to resist drug use, replace drug-using activities with constructive and rewarding activities, and improve problem-solving abilities. Behavioral therapy also addresses incentives for abstinence and facilitates interpersonal relationships. Ongoing group therapy and other peer support programs can help to maintain abstinence.

7. **Medication can be an important element of treatment, especially when combined with counseling and other behavioral therapies.** Methadone, buprenorphine, and naltrexone can help persons addicted to opioids. Nicotine replacement therapy (e.g., patches, gum), bupropion, and varenicline can help persons addicted to nicotine. Disulfiram, naltrexone, topiramate, and acamprosate can help persons addicted to alcohol.

8. **Because needs of the individual can change, the plan for treatment and services must be reassessed continually and modified as indicated.** At different times during treatment, a patient may develop a need for medications, medical services, family therapy, parenting instruction, vocational rehabilitation, and social and legal services.

9. **Many drug-addicted individuals also have other mental disorders, which must be addressed.** Because drug addiction often cooccurs with other mental illnesses, patients presenting with one condition should be assessed for other conditions and treated as indicated.

10. **Medically assisted detoxification is only the first stage of addiction treatment and, by itself, does little to change long-term drug use.** Medical detoxification manages the acute physical symptoms of withdrawal—and can serve as a precursor to effective long-term treatment.

11. **Treatment need not be voluntary to be effective.** Sanctions or enticements coming from the family, employer, or criminal justice system can significantly increase treatment entry, retention, and success.

12. **Drug use during treatment must be monitored continuously because relapses during treatment do occur.** Knowing that drug use is being monitored (e.g., through urinalysis) can help the patient to withstand urges to use drugs. Monitoring also can provide early evidence of drug use, thereby allowing timely adjustment of the treatment program.

13. Treatment programs should provide assessment for HIV/AIDS, hepatitis B and C, tuberculosis, and other infectious diseases, along with counseling to help patients modify behaviors that place them or others at risk.

HIV/AIDS, Human immunodeficiency virus/acquired immunodeficiency syndrome.
Adapted from National Institute on Drug Abuse. *Principles of drug addiction treatment: a research-based guide.* 3rd ed. (Publication No. 12-4180). Bethesda, MD: National Institutes of Health; 2012.

---

distributors, pharmacists, nurses, and physicians. Enforcement of the CSA is the responsibility of the *Drug Enforcement Agency* (DEA), an arm of the U.S. Department of Justice.

Record Keeping

To keep track of controlled substances that originate from legitimate sources, a written record must be made of all transactions involving these agents. Every time a controlled substance is purchased or dispensed, the transfer must be recorded. Providers, pharmacists, and hospitals must keep an inventory of all controlled substances in stock. This inventory must be reported to the DEA every 2 years. Although not specifically obliged to do so by the CSA, many hospitals use medication-dispensing machines that count the controlled substances dispensed during each shift.

Drug Enforcement Agency Schedules

Each drug preparation regulated under the CSA has been assigned to one of five categories: schedule I, II, III, IV, or V. Drugs in schedule I have a high potential for abuse and no approved medical use in the United States. In contrast, drugs in schedules II through V all have approved applications. Assignment to schedules II through V is based on abuse potential and potential for causing physical or psychological dependence. Of the drugs that have medical applications, those in schedule II have the highest potential for abuse and dependence. Drugs

in the remaining schedules have decreasing abuse and dependence liabilities. Table 32.1 lists the primary drugs that come under the five DEA schedules.

Scheduling of drugs under the CSA undergoes periodic reevaluation. With increased understanding of the abuse and dependence liabilities of a drug, the DEA or individual states may choose to reassign it to a different schedule.

Prescriptions

The CSA places restrictions on prescribing drugs in schedules II through V. (Drugs in schedule I have no approved uses and hence are not prescribed.) Only prescribers registered with the DEA are authorized to prescribe controlled drugs. Regulations on prescribing controlled substances are summarized next.

Schedule II

All prescriptions for schedule II drugs must be typed or filled out in ink or indelible pencil and signed by the prescriber. Alternatively, prescribers may submit prescriptions using an electronic prescribing procedure. Oral prescriptions may be called in but only in emergencies, and a written prescription must follow within 72 hours. Prescriptions for schedule II drugs cannot be refilled. However, a DEA rule allows a prescriber to write multiple prescriptions on the same day—for the same patient and same drug.

TABLE 32.1	**Drug Enforcement Agency Classification of Controlled Substances**			
Schedule I Drugs	**Schedule II Drugs**	**Schedule III Drugs**	**Schedule IV Drugs**	**Schedule V Drugs**
Opioids	Opioids	Opioids	Opioids	Opioids
Acetylmethadol	Alfentanil	Buprenorphine	Butorphanol	Diphenoxylate plus atropine
Heroin	Codeine	Paregoric	Pentazocine	Pregabalin
Normethadone	Fentanyl	Cannabinoids	Stimulants	
Many others	Hydrocodone	Dronabinol (THC)	Diethylpropion	
Psychedelics	Hydromorphone	Stimulants	Fenfluramine	
Bufotenin	Levorphanol	Benzphetamine	Mazindol	
Diethyltryptamine	Meperidine	Phendimetrazine	Pemoline	
Dimethyltryptamine	Methadone	Barbiturates	Phentermine	
Ibogaine	Morphine	Aprobarbital	Barbiturates	
d-Lysergic acid diethylamide (LSD)	Opium tincture	Butabarbital	Methohexital	
Mescaline	Oxycodone	Talbutal	Phenobarbital	
3,4-Methylenedioxy-methamphetamine (MDMA)	Oxymorphone	Thiamylal	Benzodiazepines	
	Remifentanil	Thiopental	Alprazolam	
Psilocin	Sufentanil	Miscellaneous Depressants	Chlordiazepoxide	
Psilocybin	Psychostimulants	Methyprylon	Clonazepam	
Cannabis Derivatives	Amphetamine	Anabolic Steroids	Clorazepate	
Marijuana	Cocaine	Fluoxymesterone	Diazepam	
Others	Dextroamphetamine	Methyltestosterone	Estazolam	
Gamma-hydroxybutyrate	Methamphetamine	Nandrolone	Flurazepam	
Methaqualone	Methylphenidate	Oxandrolone	Lorazepam	
	Phenmetrazine	Stanozolol	Midazolam	
	Barbiturates	Testosterone	Oxazepam	
	Amobarbital	Many others	Prazepam	
	Pentobarbital	Others	Quazepam	
	Secobarbital	Ketamine	Temazepam	
	Miscellaneous Depressants		Triazolam	
	Glutethimide		Benzodiazepine-like Drugs	
			Zaleplon	
			Zolpidem	
			Miscellaneous Depressants	
			Chloral hydrate	
			Dichloralphenazone	
			Ethchlorvynol	
			Ethinamate	
			Meprobamate	
			Paraldehyde	

Schedules III and IV

Prescriptions for drugs in schedules III and IV may be oral, written, or electronic. If authorized by the prescriber, these prescriptions may be refilled up to 5 times. Refills must be made within 6 months of the original order. If additional medication is needed beyond the amount provided for in the original prescription, a new prescription must be written.

Schedule V

The same regulations for prescribing drugs in schedules III and IV apply to drugs in schedule V. In addition, schedule V drugs may be dispensed without a prescription provided the following conditions are met: (1) the drug is dispensed by a pharmacist; (2) the amount dispensed is very limited; (3) the recipient is at least 18 years old; (4) the pharmacist writes and initials a record indicating the date, the name and amount of the drug, and the name and address of the recipient; and (5) state and local laws do not prohibit dispensing schedule V drugs without a prescription.

Labeling

When drugs in schedules II, III, and IV are dispensed, their containers must bear this label: *Caution—Federal law prohibits the transfer of this drug to any person other than the patient for whom it was prescribed.*

State Laws

All states have their own laws regulating drugs of abuse. In many cases, state laws are more stringent than federal laws. As a rule, whenever there is a difference between state and federal laws, the more restrictive of the two takes precedence.

33

Substance Use Disorders II: Alcohol

Alcohol (ethyl alcohol, ethanol) is the most commonly used and abused psychoactive agent in the United States. Although alcohol does have some therapeutic applications, the drug is of interest primarily for its nonmedical use. When consumed in moderation, alcohol prolongs life and reduces the risk for dementia and cardiovascular disorders. Conversely, when consumed in excess, alcohol diminishes life in both quality and quantity.

In approaching our study of alcohol, we begin by discussing the basic pharmacology of alcohol, and then we discuss alcohol use disorder (AUD) and the drugs used for treatment.

BASIC PHARMACOLOGY OF ALCOHOL
Central Nervous System Effects
Acute Effects

Alcohol has two acute effects on the brain: (1) general depression of central nervous system (CNS) function and (2) activation of the reward circuit.

For many years, we believed that alcohol simply dissolved into the neuronal membrane, thereby disrupting the ordered arrangement of membrane phospholipids. However, we currently know that alcohol interacts with specific proteins—certain receptors, ion channels, and enzymes—that regulate neuronal excitability. Three target proteins are of particular importance, namely (1) receptors for γ-aminobutyric acid (GABA), (2) receptors for glutamate, and (3) the 5-HT$_3$ subset of receptors for serotonin (5-hydroxytryptamine [5-HT]). The *depressant* effects of alcohol result from binding with receptors for GABA (the principal inhibitory transmitter in the CNS) and receptors for glutamate (a major excitatory transmitter in the CNS). When alcohol binds with GABA receptors, it enhances GABA-mediated inhibition, causing widespread depression of CNS activity. When alcohol binds with glutamate receptors, it blocks glutamate-mediated excitation and thereby reduces overall CNS activity. The *rewarding* effects of alcohol result from binding with 5-HT$_3$ receptors in the brain's reward circuit. When these receptors are activated, they promote release of dopamine, the major transmitter of the reward system. When alcohol binds with these receptors, it enhances serotonin-mediated release of dopamine and intensifies the reward process.

The depressant effects of alcohol are dose dependent. When dosage is low, higher brain centers (cortical areas) are primarily affected. As dosage increases, more primitive brain areas (e.g., medulla) become depressed. With depression of cortical function, thought processes and learned behaviors are altered, inhibitions are released, and self-restraint is replaced by increased sociability and expansiveness. Cortical depression also impairs motor function. As CNS depression deepens, reflexes diminish greatly and consciousness becomes impaired. At very high doses, alcohol produces a state of general anesthesia. (Alcohol cannot be used for anesthesia because the doses required are close to lethal.)

Chronic Effects

When consumed chronically and in excess, alcohol can produce severe neurologic and psychiatric disorders. Injury to the CNS is caused by the direct actions of alcohol and by the nutritional deficiencies often seen in chronic heavy drinkers.

Two neuropsychiatric syndromes are common in alcoholics: *Wernicke encephalopathy* and *Korsakoff psychosis*. Both disorders are caused by thiamin deficiency, which results from poor diet and alcohol-induced suppression of thiamin absorption. Wernicke encephalopathy is characterized by confusion, nystagmus, and abnormal ocular movements. This syndrome is readily reversible with thiamin. Korsakoff psychosis is characterized by polyneuropathy, inability to convert short-term memory into long-term memory, and confabulation (unconscious filling of gaps in memory with fabricated facts and experiences). Korsakoff psychosis is not reversible.

Perhaps the most dramatic effect of long-term excessive alcohol consumption is enlargement of the cerebral ventricles, presumably in response to atrophy of the cerebrum itself. These gross anatomic changes are associated with impairment of memory and intellectual function. With cessation of drinking, ventricular enlargement and cognitive deficits partially reverse but only in some individuals.

Impact on Cognitive Function

Low to moderate alcohol consumption helps preserve cognitive function in older people and may protect against development of dementia. Although drinking alcohol in general may sound like a sufficient way to protect ourselves from developing dementia, the findings have been isolated to red wine only. Resveratrol, a natural molecule found in red wine, is thought to be responsible for neuroprotection.

Effect on Sleep

Although alcohol is commonly used as a sleep aid, it actually disrupts sleep. Drinking can alter sleep cycles, decrease total sleeping time, and reduce the quality of sleep. In addition, alcohol can intensify snoring and exacerbate obstructive sleep apnea.

Other Pharmacologic Effects
Cardiovascular System

When alcohol is consumed acutely and in moderate doses, cardiovascular effects are minor. The most prominent effect is *dilation of cutaneous blood vessels,* causing increased blood flow to the skin. By doing so, alcohol imparts a sensation of warmth—but at the same time promotes loss of heat.

Although the cardiovascular effects of moderate alcohol consumption are unremarkable, chronic and excessive consumption is clearly harmful. Abuse of alcohol results in *direct damage to the myocardium,* thereby increasing the risk for heart failure. Some investigators believe that alcohol may be a major cause of cardiomyopathy in the Western world.

In addition to damaging the heart, alcohol produces a dose-dependent *elevation of blood pressure.* The cause is vasoconstriction in vascular beds of skeletal muscle brought on by increased activity of the sympathetic nervous system. Estimates suggest that heavy drinking may be responsible for 10% of all cases of hypertension.

Not all of the cardiovascular effects of alcohol are deleterious: there is clear evidence that people who drink *moderately* (two drinks a day or less for men, one drink a day or less for women) experience less ischemic stroke, coronary artery disease (CAD), myocardial infarction (MI), and heart failure than do abstainers. However, it is important to note that *heavy* drinking (five or more drinks per day) *increases* the risk for heart disease and stroke. Moderate drinking protects against heart disease primarily by raising levels of high-density lipoprotein (HDL) cholesterol. As discussed in Chapter 44, HDL cholesterol protects against CAD, whereas low-density lipoprotein (LDL) cholesterol promotes CAD. Of all the agents that can raise HDL cholesterol, alcohol is one of the most effective known. In addition to raising HDL cholesterol, alcohol may confer protection through four other mechanisms: decreasing platelet aggregation, decreasing levels of fibrinogen (the precursor of fibrin, which reinforces clots), increasing levels of tissue plasminogen activator (a clot-dissolving enzyme), and suppressing the inflammatory component of atherosclerosis. The degree of cardiovascular protection is nearly equal for beer, wine, and distilled spirits. That is, protection is determined primarily by the *amount* of alcohol consumed—not by the particular beverage the alcohol is in. In addition, the *pattern* of drinking matters: protection is greater for people who drink moderately 3 or 4 days a week than for people who drink just 1 or 2 days a week. Finally, cardioprotection is greatest for those with an *un*healthy lifestyle: among people who exercise, eat fruits and vegetables, and do not smoke, alcohol has little or no effect on the incidence of coronary events; conversely, among people who lack these behaviors, moderate alcohol intake is associated with a 50% reduction in coronary risk.

Glucose Metabolism

Alcohol has several effects on glucose metabolism that may decrease the risk for type 2 diabetes. For example, alcohol raises levels of adiponectin, a compound that enhances insulin sensitivity. In addition, alcohol suppresses gluconeogenesis, blunts the postprandial rise in blood glucose, and lowers fasting levels of both glucose and insulin.

Bone Health

Alcohol increases bone mineral density, probably by increasing levels of sex hormones.

Respiration

Like all other CNS depressants, alcohol depresses respiration. Respiratory depression from moderate drinking is negligible. However, when consumed in excess, alcohol can cause death by respiratory arrest. The respiratory depressant effects of alcohol are potentiated by other CNS depressants (e.g., benzodiazepines, opioids, barbiturates).

Liver

Alcohol-induced liver damage can progress from fatty liver to hepatitis to cirrhosis, depending on the amount consumed. Acute drinking causes reversible accumulation of fat and protein in the liver. With more chronic drinking, nonviral *hepatitis* develops in approximately 90% of heavy users. In 8% to 20% of patients with chronic AUD, hepatitis evolves into cirrhosis—a condition characterized by proliferation of fibrous tissue and destruction of liver parenchymal cells. Although various factors other than alcohol can cause cirrhosis, alcohol abuse is unquestionably the major cause of *fatal* cirrhosis.

Stomach

Excessive use of alcohol can cause *erosive gastritis*. Approximately one-third of patients with AUD have this disorder. Two mechanisms are involved.

First, alcohol stimulates secretion of gastric acid. Second, when present in high concentrations, alcohol can injure the gastric mucosa directly.

Kidney

Alcohol is a diuretic. It promotes urine formation by inhibiting the release of antidiuretic hormone (ADH) from the pituitary. Because ADH acts on the kidney to promote water reabsorption, thereby decreasing urine formation, a reduction in circulating ADH will increase urine production.

Pancreas

Approximately 35% of cases of acute pancreatitis can be attributed to alcohol, making alcohol the second most common cause of the disorder. Flare-ups typically occur after a bout of heavy drinking. Only 5% of alcoholics develop pancreatitis and then only after years of overindulgence.

Sexual Function

Alcohol has both psychological and physiologic effects related to human sexual behavior. Although alcohol is not exactly an aphrodisiac, its ability to release inhibitions has been known to motivate sexual activity. Ironically, the physiologic effects of alcohol may frustrate attempts at consummating the activity that alcohol inspired: Objective measurements in males and females show that alcohol significantly decreases our physiologic capacity for sexual responsiveness. In males, long-term use of alcohol may induce *feminization*. Symptoms include testicular atrophy, impotence, sterility, and breast enlargement.

Cancer

Alcohol—even in moderate amounts—is associated with an increased risk for several common cancers. Among these are cancers of the breast, liver, rectum, and aerodigestive tract, which includes the lips, tongue, mouth, nose, throat, vocal cords, and portions of the esophagus and trachea. According to a 2016 study, alcohol is linked to seven cancers. The fraction attributable to alcohol is highest for aerodigestive tract cancers. Data suggest that, regarding cancer risk, no amount of alcohol can be considered safe—although risk is lowest with moderate drinking (two drinks or less a day for men and one drink or less a day for women).

Pregnancy

Effects of alcohol on the developing fetus are dose dependent. Risk for fetal injury is greatest with heavy drinking and much lower with light drinking. Is there some low level of drinking that is *completely* safe? We do not know.

Fetal alcohol exposure can cause structural and functional abnormalities, ranging from mild neurobehavioral deficits to facial malformation and developmental delay. The term *fetal alcohol spectrum disorder* (FASD) is used in reference to the *full range* of outcomes—from mild to severe—that drinking during pregnancy can cause. In contrast, the term *fetal alcohol syndrome* (FAS) is reserved for the most severe cases of FASD, characterized by craniofacial malformations, growth restriction (including microcephaly), and neurodevelopmental abnormalities, manifesting during childhood as cognitive and social dysfunction. In addition to causing FASD and FAS, heavy drinking during pregnancy can result in stillbirth, spontaneous abortion, and giving birth to an alcohol-dependent infant.

Is *light* drinking safe during pregnancy? The data are unclear. Two studies published in 2010 suggest that light drinking may carry little risk. One study, conducted in the United Kingdom, found no clinically relevant behavioral or cognitive problems in 5-year-olds whose mothers consumed one to two drinks a week during pregnancy. The other study, conducted in Australia, found no link between *low to moderate* alcohol consumption during pregnancy and alcohol-related birth defects (ARBDs), although the same study did show that *heavy* drinking was associated with a fourfold increased risk for an ARBD. These results are consistent with other recent studies, which have failed to show a relationship between occasional or light drinking during pregnancy and abnormalities in newborns or older children. However, because all of these studies were observational, rather than randomized controlled trials, the negative results might be explained by confounding factors, especially educational level, income, or access to prenatal care. Furthermore, because the follow-up time for these studies was relatively short (only 5 years), the long-term effects of light drinking remain unknown.

If there *is* some amount of alcohol that is safe during pregnancy, that amount is very low. Accordingly, despite the studies noted previously, the American College of Obstetricians and Gynecologists (ACOG) and the American Academy of Pediatrics continue to maintain the long-held position that no amount of alcohol can be considered safe during pregnancy. Therefore in the interests of fetal health, all women should be advised to avoid alcohol *entirely* while pregnant or trying to conceive. Having said that, it is important to appreciate that a few drinks early in pregnancy are not likely to harm the fetus. Consequently, if a woman consumed a little alcohol before realizing she was pregnant, she should be reassured that the risk to the fetus—if any—is extremely low.

Lactation

The concentration of alcohol in breast milk parallels the concentration in blood. Recent data indicate that drinking while breastfeeding can adversely affect the infant's feeding and behavior.

Impact on Longevity

The effects of alcohol on life span depend on the amount consumed. *Heavy* drinkers have a higher mortality rate than the population at large. Causes of death include cirrhosis, respiratory disease, cancer, and fatal accidents. The risk for mortality associated with alcohol abuse increases markedly in individuals who consume six or more drinks a day.

Interestingly, people who consume *moderate* amounts of alcohol live *longer* than those who abstain—and combining regular exercise with moderate drinking prolongs life even more. Compared with nondrinkers, moderate drinkers have a 30% lower mortality rate, a 50% lower incidence of MI, and a 59% lower incidence of heart failure. According to a study by the American Medical Association, if all Americans were to give up drinking, deaths from heart disease would *increase* by 81,000 a year. Hence, for people who already *are* moderate drinkers, continued moderate drinking would seem beneficial. Conversely, despite the apparent benefits of drinking—and the apparent health disadvantage of abstinence—no one is recommending that abstainers take up drinking. Furthermore, when the risks of alcohol outweigh any possible benefits—such as in pregnancy—then alcohol consumption should be avoided entirely.

Pharmacokinetics
Absorption
Alcohol is absorbed from the stomach and small intestine. Approximately 20% of ingested alcohol is absorbed from the stomach. Gastric absorption is relatively slow and is delayed even further by the presence of food. Absorption from the small intestine is rapid and largely independent of food; approximately 80% of ingested alcohol is absorbed from this site. Because most alcohol is absorbed from the small intestine, gastric emptying time is a major determinant of individual variation in alcohol absorption.

Distribution
Because alcohol is both nonionic and water soluble, it distributes well to all tissues and body fluids. The drug crosses the blood–brain barrier with ease, allowing alcohol in the brain to equilibrate rapidly with alcohol in the blood. Alcohol also crosses the placenta and hence can affect the developing fetus.

Distribution in body water partly explains why women are more sensitive to alcohol than men. As a rule, women have a lower percentage of body water than do men. Hence, when a woman drinks, the alcohol is diluted in a smaller volume of water, causing the concentration of alcohol in tissues and fluids to be relatively high, which causes the effects of alcohol to be more intense.

Metabolism

Alcohol is metabolized in both the liver and stomach. The liver is the primary site. The process begins with conversion of alcohol to acetaldehyde, a reaction catalyzed by *alcohol dehydrogenase*. This reaction is slow and puts a limit on the rate at which alcohol can be inactivated. When formed, acetaldehyde undergoes *rapid* conversion by aldehyde dehydrogenase to acetic acid. Through a series of reactions, acetic acid is then used to synthesize cholesterol, fatty acids, and other compounds.

The kinetics of alcohol metabolism differ from those of most other drugs. With most drugs, as plasma drug levels rise, the amount of drug metabolized per unit time also increases. This is not true for alcohol: as the alcohol content of blood increases, there is almost no change in the speed of alcohol breakdown. That is, alcohol is metabolized at a relatively *constant rate*—regardless of how much alcohol is present. The average rate at which individuals can metabolize alcohol is approximately *15 mL (0.5 oz) per hour.*

Because alcohol is metabolized at a slow and constant rate, there is a limit to how much alcohol one can consume without having the drug accumulate. For practical purposes, that limit is approximately *one drink per hour.* Consumption of more than one drink per hour—be that drink beer, wine, straight whiskey, or a cocktail—will result in alcohol accumulation. One drink is defined as 5 ounces of wine, 12 ounces of beer, or 1.5 ounces of liquor.

When used on a regular basis, alcohol induces hepatic drug-metabolizing enzymes, thereby increasing the rate of its own metabolism and that of other drugs. As a result, individuals who consume alcohol routinely in high amounts can metabolize the drug faster than people who drink occasionally and moderately.

Males and females differ with respect to activity of alcohol dehydrogenase in the stomach. Specifically, women have lower activity than men. As a result, gastric metabolism of alcohol is significantly less in women. This difference partly explains why women achieve higher blood alcohol levels than men after consuming the same number of drinks.

Tolerance

Chronic consumption of alcohol produces tolerance. As a result, to alter consciousness, people who drink on a regular basis require larger amounts of alcohol than people who drink occasionally. Tolerance to alcohol confers cross-tolerance to general anesthetics, barbiturates, and other general CNS depressants. However, no cross-tolerance develops to opioids. Tolerance subsides within a few weeks after drinking cessation.

Although tolerance develops to many of the effects of alcohol, *very little tolerance develops to respiratory depression.* Consequently, the lethal dose of alcohol for chronic, heavy drinkers is not much bigger than the lethal dose for nondrinkers. Alcoholics may tolerate blood alcohol levels as high as 0.4% (five times the amount defined by law as intoxicating) with no marked reduction in consciousness. However, if blood levels rise only slightly above this level, death may ensue.

Physical Dependence

Chronic use of alcohol produces physical dependence. If alcohol is withdrawn abruptly, an abstinence syndrome will result. The intensity of the abstinence syndrome is proportional to the degree of physical dependence. Individuals who are physically dependent on alcohol show cross-dependence with other general CNS depressants (e.g., barbiturates, chloral hydrate, benzodiazepines) but not with opioids.

Drug Interactions
Central Nervous System Depressants
The CNS effects of alcohol are additive with those of other CNS depressants (e.g., barbiturates, benzodiazepines, opioids). Consumption of alcohol with other CNS depressants intensifies the psychological and physiologic manifestations of CNS depression and greatly increases the risk for death from respiratory depression.

Nonsteroidal Antiinflammatory Drugs
Like alcohol, aspirin, ibuprofen, and other nonsteroidal antiinflammatory drugs (NSAIDs) can injure the gastrointestinal (GI) mucosa. The combined effects of alcohol and NSAIDs can result in significant gastric bleeding.

Acetaminophen
The combination of acetaminophen (Tylenol, others) with alcohol poses a risk for potentially fatal liver injury. The interaction between alcohol and acetaminophen is discussed further in Chapter 57.

Disulfiram
The combination of alcohol with disulfiram (Antabuse) can cause a variety of adverse effects, some of which are dangerous. These effects, and the use of disulfiram to maintain abstinence, are discussed later.

Antihypertensive Drugs
Because alcohol raises blood pressure, it tends to counteract the effects of antihypertensive medications. However, elevation of blood pressure is significant only when alcohol dosage is high. Conversely, when the dosage is low, alcohol may actually help: among hypertensive men, light to moderate alcohol consumption is associated with reduced risk for both cardiovascular mortality and all-cause mortality.

Acute Overdose
Acute overdose produces vomiting, coma, pronounced hypotension, and respiratory depression. The combination of vomiting and unconsciousness can result in aspiration, which in turn can result in pulmonary obstruction and pneumonia. Alcohol-induced hypotension results from a direct effect on peripheral blood vessels and cannot be corrected with vasoconstrictors (e.g., epinephrine). Hypotension can lead to renal failure (secondary to compromised renal blood flow) and cardiovascular shock, a common cause of alcohol-related death. Although death can also result from respiratory depression, this is not the usual cause.

Because symptoms of acute alcohol poisoning can mimic symptoms of other pathologies (e.g., diabetic coma, skull fracture), a definitive diagnosis may not be possible without measuring alcohol in the blood, urine, or expired air. The smell of "alcohol" on the breath is not a reliable means of diagnosis because the breath odors we associate with alcohol are due to impurities in alcoholic beverages—and not to alcohol itself. Hence these odors may or may not be present.

Alcohol poisoning is treated like poisoning with all other general CNS depressants. Details of management are discussed in Chapter 29. Alcohol can be removed from the body by gastric lavage and dialysis. Stimulants (e.g., caffeine) should not be given.

Precautions and Contraindications
Alcohol can injure the GI mucosa and should not be consumed by persons with *peptic ulcer disease*. Alcohol is harmful to the liver and should not be used by individuals with *liver disease*. Alcohol should be avoided during *pregnancy* owing to the risk for FASD (including FAS), stillbirth, spontaneous abortion, and neurodevelopmental abnormalities.

Alcohol must be used with caution by patients with *epilepsy*. During alcohol use, the CNS is depressed. When alcohol consumption ceases, the CNS undergoes rebound excitation; seizures can result.

Alcohol causes a dose-related increase in the risk for *breast cancer*. All women—and especially those at high risk—should minimize alcohol consumption. Alcohol also increases the risk for cancer of the liver, rectum, and aerodigestive tract.

ALCOHOL USE DISORDER

Alcohol use disorder is a chronic, relapsing disorder characterized by impaired control over drinking, preoccupation with alcohol consumption, use of alcohol despite awareness of adverse consequences, and distortions in thinking, especially as evidenced by denial of a drinking problem. The development and manifestations of AUD are influenced by genetic, psychosocial, and environmental factors. The disease is progressive and often fatal. In the United States, approximately 6% of the adult population are diagnosed with AUD.

AUD is defined as a problematic pattern of alcohol use leading to clinically significant impairment or distress occurring within a 12-month period. Manifestations of AUD can include recurrent alcohol use in situations in which it is physically hazardous; recurrent use resulting in a failure to fulfill major role obligations at work, school, or home; and spending a great deal of time in activities necessary to obtain alcohol, use alcohol, or recover from alcohol.

PATIENT-CENTERED CARE ACROSS THE LIFE SPAN

Alcohol

Life Stage	Patient Care Concerns
Infants	See later entry, "Breastfeeding women"
Children/adolescents	Adolescents are more sensitive to alcohol-induced memory impairment than adults but less sensitive to the motor effects of alcohol. Alcohol exposure during adolescence affects brain functioning during adulthood.
Pregnant women	Use of alcohol while pregnant can cause structural and functional abnormalities in the fetus. These abnormalities are termed *fetal alcohol spectrum disorder* (FASD). It is recommended that pregnant women abstain from alcohol.
Breastfeeding women	The concentration of alcohol in breast milk parallels the concentration in blood. Breastfeeding while consuming alcohol can affect infant behavior.
Older adults	Aging lowers the body's tolerance for alcohol. Many older adults may not metabolize alcohol as efficiently as younger adults. Many older adults take medications that interact with alcohol.

In the United States, misuse of alcohol is responsible for 6 million nonfatal injuries each year and 85,000 deaths. Causes of death range from liver disease to automobile wrecks. Fully 50% of all fatal highway crashes are alcohol related. Among teens, alcohol-related crashes are the leading cause of death. Alcohol also causes industrial accidents and is responsible for 40% of industrial fatalities.

TABLE 33.1   Screening Instrument: The Alcohol Use Disorders Identification Test

	0	1	2	3	4	Score
How often do you have a drink containing alcohol?	Never	Monthly or less	2–4 times a month	2–3 times a week	4 or more times a week	
How many drinks containing alcohol do you have on a typical day when you are drinking?	1 or 2	3 or 4	5 or 6	7–9	10 or more	
How often do you have 5 or more drinks on one occasion?	Never	Less than monthly	Monthly	Weekly	Daily or almost daily	
How often during the last year have you found that you were not able to stop drinking once you had started?	Never	Less than monthly	Monthly	Weekly	Daily or almost daily	
How often during the last year have you failed to do what was normally expected of you because of drinking?	Never	Less than monthly	Monthly	Weekly	Daily or almost daily	
How often during the last year have you needed a first drink in the morning to get yourself going after a heavy drinking session?	Never	Less than monthly	Monthly	Weekly	Daily or almost daily	
How often during the last year have you had a feeling of guilt or remorse after drinking?	Never	Less than monthly	Monthly	Weekly	Daily or almost daily	
How often during the last year have you been unable to remember what happened the night before because of your drinking?	Never	Less than monthly	Monthly	Weekly	Daily or almost daily	
Have you or someone else been injured because of your drinking?	No		Yes, but not in the last year		Yes, during the last year	
Has a relative, friend, doctor, or other health care worker been concerned about your drinking or suggested you cut down?	No		Yes, but not in the last year		Yes, during the last year	
Total score						

Instructions to patient: Circle the option that best describes your answer to each question.
Scoring: Record the score (0, 1, 2, 3, or 4) for each response in the blank box at the end of each line, and then add up the total score. The maximum possible is 40. A total score of 8 or more (for men up to age 60 years), or 4 or more (for women, adolescents, and men older than 60 years) is considered a positive screen. For patients with totals near the cutoff points, clinicians may wish to examine individual responses to questions and clarify them during the clinical examination.
Reprinted with permission from the World Health Organization. To reflect standard drink sizes in the United States, the number of drinks in question 3 was changed from 6 to 5.

Alcohol abuse is a major public health problem, and its consequences are numerous. Alcoholism produces psychological derangements, including anxiety, depression, and suicidal ideation. Malnutrition, secondary to inadequate diet and malabsorption, is common. Poor work performance and disruption of family life reflect the social deterioration suffered by alcoholics. Alcohol abuse during pregnancy can result in FASD (including FAS), stillbirth, and spontaneous abortion. Lastly, chronic alcohol abuse is harmful to the body; consequences include liver disease, cardiomyopathy, and brain damage—not to mention injury and death from accidents.

In 2016 the National Institute on Alcohol Abuse and Alcoholism (NIAAA) updated its document—*Helping Patients Who Drink Too Much: A Clinician's Guide*—that contains clear, concise information on screening, counseling, and treatment of AUDs. By following this guide, clinicians can help reduce morbidity and mortality among people who drink more than is safe, defined as more than four drinks in a day (or 14/week) for men or more than three drinks in a day (or 7/week) for women. Helping patients involves four simple steps:

- Ask about alcohol use.
- Assess for AUDs, using the Alcohol Use Disorders Identification Test (AUDIT).
- Advise and assist (brief intervention).
- At follow-up: continue support.

This process is founded in part on two lines of evidence. First, we can identify people who misuse alcohol with an easily administered questionnaire, such as AUDIT (Table 33.1). Second, for many people, alcohol consumption can be reduced through brief interventions, such as offering feedback and advice about drinking and about setting goals. Long-term follow-up studies have shown that these simple interventions can decrease hospitalization and lower mortality rates. The guide is available at www.niaaa.nih.gov/guide.

To help individuals who drink too much, the NIAAA created an interactive website, located at rethinkingdrinking.niaaa.nih.gov. Content includes tools to identify and manage problem drinking, plus a calculator for determining the alcohol content of various beverages.

DRUGS FOR ALCOHOL USE DISORDER

In the United States, approximately 1 million people with AUD seek treatment every year. Although the success rate is discouraging—nearly 50% relapse during the first few months—treatment should nonetheless be tried. The objective is to modify drinking patterns (i.e., to reduce or completely eliminate alcohol consumption). Drugs can help in two ways. First, they can facilitate withdrawal. Second, they can help maintain abstinence after withdrawal has been accomplished.

Drugs Used to Facilitate Withdrawal

Management of withdrawal depends on the degree of dependence. When dependence is mild, withdrawal can be accomplished on an outpatient basis without drugs. However, when dependence is great, withdrawal carries a risk for death. Accordingly, hospitalization and drug therapy are indicated. The goals of management are to minimize symptoms of withdrawal, prevent seizures and delirium tremens, and facilitate

TABLE 33.2 Drugs Used to Treat the Symptoms of Alcohol Withdrawal

Drug	Benefit During Withdrawal
Benzodiazepines	
Chlordiazepoxide	Decrease withdrawal symptoms; stabilize vital signs; prevent seizures and delirium tremens
Clorazepate	
Diazepam	
Lorazepam	
Oxazepam	
β-Adrenergic Blockers	
Atenolol	Improve vital signs; decrease craving; decrease autonomic component of withdrawal symptoms
Propranolol	
Central α₂-Adrenergic Agonist	
Clonidine	Decreases autonomic component of withdrawal symptoms
Antiepileptic Drug	
Carbamazepine	Decreases withdrawal symptoms; prevents seizures

transition to a program for maintaining abstinence. In theory, any drug that has cross-dependence with alcohol (i.e., any of the general CNS depressants) should be effective. However, in actual practice, benzodiazepines are the drugs of choice. The benefits of benzodiazepines and other drugs used during withdrawal are shown in Table 33.2.

Benzodiazepines

Of the drugs used to facilitate alcohol withdrawal, benzodiazepines are the most effective. Furthermore, they are safe for use in both the inpatient and outpatient settings. In patients with severe alcohol dependence, benzodiazepines can stabilize vital signs, reduce symptom intensity, and decrease the risk for seizures and delirium tremens. Although all benzodiazepines are effective, agents with longer half-lives are generally preferred because they provide the greatest protection against seizures and breakthrough symptoms. The benzodiazepines used most often are chlordiazepoxide (generic only), clorazepate (Tranxene), oxazepam (generic only), and lorazepam (Ativan). Traditionally, benzodiazepines have been administered around-the-clock on a fixed schedule. However, PRN administration (in response to symptoms) can be just as effective.

Adjuncts to Benzodiazepines

Combining a benzodiazepine with another drug may improve withdrawal outcome. Agents that have been tried include carbamazepine (an antiepileptic drug), clonidine (an α₂-adrenergic agonist), and atenolol and propranolol (β-adrenergic blockers). Carbamazepine may reduce withdrawal symptoms and the risk for seizures. Clonidine and the β-blockers reduce the autonomic component of withdrawal symptoms. In addition, the β-blockers may improve vital signs and decrease craving. However, it should be stressed that these drugs are not very effective as monotherapy. Hence they should be viewed only as adjuncts to benzodiazepines—not as substitutes.

Drugs Used to Maintain Abstinence

After detoxification has been accomplished, the goal is to prevent—or at least minimize—future drinking. The ideal goal is complete abstinence. However, if drinking must resume, keeping it to a minimum is still beneficial because doing so will reduce alcohol-related morbidity.

In trials of drugs used to maintain abstinence, several parameters are used to measure efficacy. These include the following:

- Proportion of patients who maintain complete abstinence
- Days to relapse
- Number of drinking days
- Number of drinks per drinking day

In the United States, only three drugs—naltrexone, acamprosate, and disulfiram—are approved for maintaining abstinence. Naltrexone blocks the pleasurable effects of alcohol and decreases craving. Acamprosate reduces some of the unpleasant feelings (e.g., tension, dysphoria, anxiety) brought on by alcohol abstinence. Disulfiram works by causing an unpleasant reaction if alcohol is consumed. Of the three drugs, naltrexone appears most effective. However, even with this agent, benefits are modest.

Owing to the risk for relapse, prolonged treatment is needed. The minimal duration is 3 months. However, continuing for a year or more is not unreasonable. If the first drug fails, clinicians often try a different one.

Naltrexone

Naltrexone (Vivitrol) is a pure opioid antagonist that decreases craving for alcohol and blocks alcohol's reinforcing (pleasurable) effects. Patients with AUD report that naltrexone decreases their "high." Although the mechanism underlying these effects is uncertain, one possibility is blockade of dopamine release secondary to blockade of opioid receptors. Naltrexone is generally well tolerated. Nausea is the most common adverse effect, followed by headache, anxiety, and sedation. Because naltrexone is an opioid antagonist, the drug will precipitate withdrawal if given to a patient who is opioid dependent. Conversely, if a patient taking naltrexone needs emergency treatment with an opioid analgesic, high doses of the opioid will be required.

Naltrexone was approved for AUD on the basis of randomized clinical trials that combined extensive counseling along with the drug. In these trials, naltrexone cut the relapse rate by 50%. Compared with patients taking placebo, those taking naltrexone reported less craving for alcohol, fewer days drinking, fewer drinks per occasion, and reduced severity of alcohol-related problems. In contrast to the original trials, a more recent trial, conducted by the U.S. Department of Veterans Affairs, failed to show any benefit of naltrexone in maintaining abstinence. Why did naltrexone work in the original trials but not in the more recent one? The most likely reason is that the subjects in the two trials were very different: the alcoholic veterans suffered from long-term alcoholism, had little or no social support, and received minimal counseling during the trial, whereas subjects in the earlier studies were younger, had good support systems, and received extensive counseling along with naltrexone. Hence the new study does not prove that naltrexone does not work. Rather, it proves only that naltrexone does not work for all individuals and does not work in the absence of adequate counseling. The basic pharmacology of naltrexone is discussed in Chapter 24.

Acamprosate

Therapeutic use. Acamprosate is approved for maintaining abstinence in patients with alcohol dependence after detoxification. Benefits derive from reducing unpleasant feelings (e.g., tension, dysphoria, anxiety) brought on by abstinence. This effect contrasts with the effects of disulfiram (which makes drinking unpleasant) and naltrexone (which blocks the pleasant feelings that alcohol can cause). Acamprosate should be used only as part of a comprehensive management program that includes psychosocial support.

In clinical trials, acamprosate was moderately effective. Compared with patients taking placebo, those taking acamprosate abstained from their first drink longer, had greater rates of complete abstinence, and were abstinent for more total days. Benefits may be related to the degree of alcohol dependence: the greater the dependence, the more likely that

TABLE 33.3   Preparations, Dosage, Mechanism of Action, Pharmacokinetics, Adverse Effects, and Administration

Drug	Preparations	Mechanism of Action	Pharmacokinetics	Adverse Effects	Usual Adult Dosage and Administration
Naltrexone (generic)	50-mg tablets	Possible blockade of dopamine release secondary to blockade of opioid receptors	Half-life: 13–14 h (active metabolite) Metabolism: Hepatic Excretion: Urine	Can precipitate withdrawal in opioid dependent patients	50 mg PO daily
Naltrexone (Vivitrol)	Solution for IM injection	Possible blockade of dopamine release secondary to blockade of opioid receptors	Half-life: 5–10 days Metabolism: Hepatic Excretion: Urine	Can precipitate withdrawal in opioid dependent patients	380 mg IM every 4 weeks
Acamprosate (generic)	333-mg delayed-release tablets	Possible restoration of balance between inhibitory (GABA) and excitatory (glutamate) neurotransmitters	Half-life: 20–33 h Unmetabolized Excretion: Urine	Diarrhea	666 mg PO three times daily, taken with meals
Disulfiram (Antabuse)	250- and 500-mg tablets	Disruption of alcohol metabolism through irreversible inhibition of aldehyde dehydrogenase	Half-life: 60–120 h Metabolism: Hepatic Excretion: Urine	Acetaldehyde syndrome	Initial dosage 500 mg PO daily for 1–2 weeks Maintenance dose 125–500 mg PO daily

GABA, γ-Aminobutyric acid; *IM*, intramuscular; *PO*, oral administration.

acamprosate will help. Among patients who lack psychosocial support, little or no benefit is seen.

Disulfiram Aversion Therapy

Therapeutic effects. Disulfiram (Antabuse) helps individuals with AUD avoid drinking by causing unpleasant effects if alcohol is ingested. Disulfiram has no applications outside the treatment of AUD.

Although disulfiram has been used for decades, its efficacy is only moderate. Due to low rates of patient adherence, it is no longer recommended as a first-line treatment agent. In clinical trials, there is emerging evidence that the drug may be only slightly better than placebo at maintaining long-term abstinence; however, long-term studies have not been completed. Disulfiram does decrease the frequency of drinking after relapse has occurred—presumably because of the unpleasant reaction that the patient is now familiar with. Supervised administration of disulfiram may be more effective than when patients self-administer the drug.

Pharmacologic effects. The constellation of effects caused by alcohol plus disulfiram is referred to as the *acetaldehyde syndrome,* a potentially dangerous event. In its "mild" form, the syndrome manifests as nausea, copious vomiting, flushing, palpitations, headache, sweating, thirst, chest pain, weakness, blurred vision, and hypotension; blood pressure may ultimately decline to shock levels. This reaction, which may last from 30 minutes to several hours, can be brought on by consuming as little as 7 mL of alcohol.

In its most severe manifestation, the acetaldehyde syndrome is life threatening. Possible reactions include marked respiratory depression, cardiovascular collapse, cardiac dysrhythmias, MI, acute congestive heart failure, convulsions, and death. Clearly, the acetaldehyde syndrome is not simply unpleasant; this syndrome can be extremely hazardous and must be avoided.

In the absence of alcohol, disulfiram rarely causes significant effects. Drowsiness and skin eruptions may occur during initial use, but they diminish with time.

Patient selection. Owing to the severity of the acetaldehyde syndrome, candidates must be carefully chosen. Alcoholics who lack the determination to stop drinking should not receive disulfiram. In other words, disulfiram must not be administered to individuals who are likely to attempt drinking while undergoing treatment.

 ## BLACK BOX WARNING
Disulfiram

Disulfiram should never be administered to a patient experiencing alcohol intoxication because this may cause a potentially fatal reaction.

Preparations, dosage, and administration. See Table 33.3 for preparations, dosage, and administration.

SUMMARY OF KEY PRESCRIBING CONSIDERATIONS
Drugs to Maintain Abstinence

Therapeutic Goal: Maintaining alcohol abstinence

Identifying High-Risk Patients: Disulfiram is contraindicated for patients suspected of being incapable of abstinence from alcohol; for patients with myocardial disease, coronary occlusion, or psychosis; and for patients who have recently received alcohol, metronidazole, or alcohol-containing medications (e.g., cough syrups).

Measures to Enhance Therapeutic Effects: Warn patients to avoid all forms of alcohol, including alcohol in vinegar, sauces, and cough syrups and alcohol applied to the skin in aftershave lotions and colognes.

Minimizing Adverse Effects: The first dose of disulfiram should not be administered until at least 12 h after the last alcoholic drink consumed. When stopping disulfiram, the effects can last up to 2 weeks after the last dose.

34

Substance Use Disorders III: Nicotine and Smoking

Cigarette smoking remains the greatest single cause of preventable illness and premature death. In the United States, smoking kills more than 480,000 adults each year—approximately one of every five deaths. Around the world, tobacco kills more than 6 million people each year. On average, male smokers die 13.2 years prematurely, and female smokers die 14.5 years prematurely. According to the Centers for Disease Control and Prevention, most deaths result from lung cancer (127,000), heart disease (99,300), and chronic airway obstruction (100,600). Not only do cigarettes kill people who smoke, but also every year, through secondhand smoke, cigarettes kill approximately 41,000 nonsmoking Americans and approximately 600,000 nonsmokers worldwide. The direct medical costs of smoking exceed $170 billion a year. Indirect costs, including lost time from work and disability, add up to an additional $156 billion. In the United States, the prevalence of smoking among adults fell steadily from 1965 (42%) through the 1980s and 1990s but decreased only slightly between 2004 (20.9%) and 2015 (15.1%).

Although tobacco smoke contains many dangerous compounds, nicotine is of greatest concern. Other hazardous components in tobacco smoke include carbon monoxide, hydrogen cyanide, ammonia, nitrosamines, and tar. Tar is composed of various polycyclic hydrocarbons, some of which are proven carcinogens.

Until recently, cigarettes had avoided virtually all federal regulation. However, strong regulations are currently in place. Under the *Family Smoking Prevention and Tobacco Control Act*, the U.S. Food and Drug Administration (FDA) currently has the authority to:

- Strengthen advertising restrictions, including the prohibition on marketing to youth
- Require revised and more prominent warning labels
- Require disclosure of all ingredients in tobacco products and restrict harmful additives
- Monitor nicotine yields and mandate gradual nicotine reduction to nonaddictive levels

BASIC PHARMACOLOGY OF NICOTINE

Mechanism of Action

The effects of nicotine result from actions at nicotinic receptors. Whether these receptors are activated or inhibited depends on nicotine dosage. *Low* doses *activate* nicotinic receptors; *high* doses *block* them. The amount of nicotine received from cigarettes is relatively low. Accordingly, cigarette smoking causes receptor *activation*.

Nicotine can activate nicotinic receptors at several locations. Most effects result from activating nicotinic receptors in autonomic ganglia and the adrenal medulla. In addition, nicotine can activate nicotinic receptors in the carotid body, aortic arch, and central nervous system (CNS). As discussed later, actions in the CNS mimic those of cocaine and other highly addictive substances. When present at the levels produced by smoking, nicotine has no significant effect on nicotinic receptors of the neuromuscular junction.

Pharmacokinetics

Absorption of nicotine depends on whether the delivery system is a cigarette, a cigar, or smokeless tobacco. Nicotine in cigarette smoke is absorbed primarily from the lungs. When cigarette smoke is inhaled, between 90% and 98% of nicotine in the lungs enters the blood. Unlike nicotine in cigarette smoke, nicotine in cigar smoke is absorbed primarily from the mouth, as is nicotine in smokeless tobacco.

Nicotine can cross membranes easily and is widely distributed throughout the body. When inhaled in cigarette smoke, nicotine reaches the brain in just 10 seconds.

Nicotine is rapidly metabolized to inactive products. Nicotine and its metabolites are excreted by the kidney. The drug's half-life is 1 to 2 hours.

Pharmacologic Effects

The pharmacologic effects discussed in this section are associated with *low* doses of nicotine. These are the effects caused by smoking cigarettes. Responses to *high* doses are discussed later under "Acute Poisoning."

Cardiovascular Effects

The cardiovascular effects of nicotine result primarily from activating nicotinic receptors in *sympathetic ganglia* and the *adrenal medulla*. Activation of these receptors promotes release of norepinephrine from sympathetic nerves and release of epinephrine (and some norepinephrine) from the adrenals. Norepinephrine and epinephrine act on the cardiovascular system to constrict blood vessels, accelerate the heart, and increase the force of ventricular contraction. The net result is elevation of blood pressure and increased cardiac work. These effects underlie cardiovascular deaths.

Gastrointestinal Effects

Nicotine influences gastrointestinal (GI) function primarily by activating nicotinic receptors in *parasympathetic* ganglia, thereby increasing secretion of gastric acid and augmenting tone and motility of GI smooth muscle. In addition, nicotine can promote vomiting. Nicotine-induced vomiting results from a complex process that involves nicotinic receptors in the aortic arch, carotid sinus, and CNS.

Central Nervous System Effects

Nicotine is a CNS stimulant. The drug stimulates respiration and produces an arousal pattern on an electroencephalograph. Moderate doses can cause tremors, and high doses can cause convulsions.

Nicotine has multiple psychological effects. The drug increases alertness, facilitates memory, improves cognition, reduces aggression, and suppresses appetite. In addition, by promoting release of dopamine, nicotine activates the brain's "pleasure system" located in the mesolimbic area. The effects of nicotine on the pleasure system are identical to those of other highly addictive drugs, including cocaine, amphetamines, and opioids.

Effects During Pregnancy and Lactation

Nicotine exposure during gestation can harm the fetus, and nicotine in breast milk can harm the nursing infant. Nonetheless, because pharmaceutical nicotine is safer than tobacco smoke, it is reasonable to consider using nicotine therapy during pregnancy to help a patient quit smoking.

Tolerance and Dependence

Tolerance

Tolerance develops to some effects of nicotine but not to others. Tolerance does develop to nausea and dizziness, which are common in the novice smoker. In contrast, *very little tolerance develops to the cardiovascular effects:* long-term smokers continue to experience increased blood pressure and increased cardiac work whenever they smoke.

Dependence

Chronic cigarette smoking results in dependence. By definition, this means that individuals who discontinue smoking will experience an withdrawal syndrome. Prominent symptoms are craving, nervousness, restlessness, irritability, impatience, increased hostility, insomnia, impaired concentration, increased appetite, and weight gain. Symptoms begin approximately 24 hours after smoking has ceased and can last for weeks to months. Women report more discomfort than men. Experience has shown that abrupt discontinuation may be preferable to gradual reduction.

Acute Poisoning

Nicotine is highly toxic. Doses as low as 40 mg can be fatal. Toxicity is underscored by the use of nicotine as an insecticide. Common causes of nicotine poisoning include ingestion of tobacco by children and exposure to nicotine-containing insecticides.

Symptoms

The most prominent symptoms involve the cardiovascular, GI, and CNSs. Specific symptoms include nausea, salivation, vomiting, diarrhea, cold sweats, disturbed hearing and vision, confusion, and faintness; pulses may be rapid, weak, and irregular. Death results from respiratory paralysis, which is caused by direct effects of nicotine on the muscles of respiration, as well as by effects in the CNS.

Treatment

Management centers on reducing nicotine absorption and supporting respiration; there is no specific antidote to nicotine poisoning. Absorption of ingested nicotine can be reduced by giving activated charcoal. If respiration is depressed, ventilatory assistance is indicated. Because nicotine undergoes rapid metabolic inactivation, recovery from the acute phase of poisoning can occur within hours.

Chronic Toxicity From Smoking

Currently, it is clear that chronic smoking can injure nearly every organ of the body. Smoking causes cardiovascular disease including abdominal aortic aneurysm, chronic lung disease, and cancers of the larynx, cervix, kidney, pancreas, stomach, lung, esophagus, oral cavity, and bladder. Leukemia, cataracts, pneumonia, periodontal disease, and type 2 diabetes

are also related to smoking. Smoking during pregnancy increases the risk for low birth weight, preterm labor, stillbirth, miscarriage, spontaneous abortion, perinatal mortality, and sudden infant death. The leading causes of smoking-related death are lung cancer, ischemic heart disease, and chronic airway obstruction.

PROTOTYPE DRUGS

Drugs to Aid Smoking Cessation

Nicotine-Based Products
Nicotine patch (NicoDerm CQ)
Nicotine gum (Nicorette)
Nicotine lozenge (Nicorette lozenge)
Nicotine nasal spray (Nicotrol NS)
Nicotine inhaler (Nicotrol inhaler)

Nicotine-Free Products
Varenicline (Chantix)
Bupropion (Zyban)

PHARMACOLOGIC AIDS TO SMOKING CESSATION

Cigarettes are highly addictive, which makes giving them up very hard. Nonetheless, abstinence *can* be achieved. Every year, approximately 41% of Americans who smoke make one or more attempts to quit. Of those who try to quit without formal help, only 4% to 7% achieve long-term success. In contrast, when a combination of counseling and drugs is used, the 6-month abstinence rate approaches 25%. However, even with the aid of counseling and drugs, the first attempt usually fails. In fact, most people try quitting five to seven times before they ultimately succeed. As time without a cigarette increases, the chances of relapse get progressively smaller: Of those who quit for a year, only 15% smoke again; and of those who quit for 5 years, only 3% smoke again.

Long-term smokers should be assured that quitting offers important health benefits. Regardless of how long you have smoked, quitting can reduce the risk for developing a tobacco-related disease, slow the progression of an established tobacco-related disease, and increase life expectancy. These benefits apply not only to people who quit while they are young and healthy but also to people who quit after age 65 years and to those with established tobacco-related disease. Data from the Nurses' Health Study indicate that former smokers eventually achieve the same disease-risk status as never smokers, even with respect to lung cancer. The risk for chronic obstructive pulmonary disease or death from a heart attack declines to that of never smokers in 20 years, and the risk for lung cancer reaches that of never smokers in 30 years.

Seven drug products have been shown to aid smoking cessation (Table 34.1). Of these seven products, five contain nicotine and two do not. The nicotine-based products—nicotine gum, nicotine lozenge, nicotine patch, nicotine inhaler, and nicotine nasal spray—are used as nicotine replacement therapy (NRT). The nicotine-free products—sustained-release bupropion (bupropion SR; Zyban) and varenicline (Chantix, Champix ♣)—are taken to decrease nicotine craving and to suppress symptoms of withdrawal. The most effective drug therapies for smoking cessation are varenicline alone and the nicotine patch combined with a short-acting nicotine product (e.g., nasal spray or gum). At this time, we cannot predict who will respond best to a particular product. Accordingly, selection should be based on patient preference, success with a particular product in the past, and side effects.

TABLE 34.1 Pharmacologic Aids for Smoking Cessation

Product	Common Side Effects	Advantages	Disadvantages	Preparation	Usual Adult Use	Length of Use
Nicotine-Based Products						
Nicotine patch (NicoDerm CQ)	Transient itching, burning, and redness under the patch; insomnia	Nonprescription; provides a steady level of nicotine; easy to use; unobtrusive	User cannot adjust dose if craving occurs; nicotine released more slowly than in other products	See Table 34.3	See Table 34.3	See Table 34.3
Nicotine gum (Nicorette, others)	Mouth and throat irritation, aching jaw muscles, dyspepsia	Nonprescription; user controls dose	Unpleasant taste; requires proper chewing technique; cannot eat or drink while chewing the gum; can damage dental work and is difficult for denture wearers to use	2 mg/piece and 4 mg/piece	Low to moderate nicotine dependence: 2 mg >25 cigarettes daily: 4-mg piece 9–12 pieces a day is reasonable	Use beyond 6 months is not recommended
Nicotine lozenge (Nicorette Lozenge, Thrive ♣)	Hiccups, dyspepsia, mouth irritation, nausea	Nonprescription; user controls dose; easier to use than nicotine gum	Cannot eat or drink while the lozenge is in the mouth	2 mg/lozenge and 4 mg/lozenge	First cigarette 30 min or more after waking: 2 mg First cigarette within 30 min of waking: 4 mg No more than 5 lozenges every 6 h or 20 daily	Dosing should decrease over a period of 12 weeks Dosing should stop after 12 weeks
Nicotine nasal spray (Nicotrol NS)	During first week: mouth and throat irritation, rhinitis, sneezing, coughing, teary eyes	User controls dose; fastest nicotine delivery and highest nicotine levels of all nicotine-based products	Prescription required; most irritating nicotine-based product; device visible when used	10 mg within a sealed cartridge	Frequent puffs over 20 min 6–16 cartridges daily	After 3 months, taper use to complete cessation over additional 2–3 months
Nicotine inhaler (Nicotrol Inhaler, Nicorette Inhaler ♣)	Mouth and throat irritation, cough	User controls dose; mimics hand-to-mouth motion of smoking	Prescription required; slow onset and low nicotine levels; frequent puffing needed; device visible when used	0.5 mg per activation	One spray per nostril 1–2 times per hour No more than 40 doses per day	Decrease use after 4–6 weeks
Nicotine-Free Products						
Varenicline (Chantix, Champix ♣)	Nausea, sleep disturbances, headaches, abnormal dreams	Easy to use (pill); no nicotine; most effective pharmacologic aid to smoking cessation	Prescription required; may cause neuropsychiatric disturbances, including suicidal thoughts and actions	0.5 mg and 1 mg tablets	0.5 mg PO daily × 3 days, 0.5 mg PO twice daily × 3 days, then 1 mg PO twice daily × 12 weeks If abstinence is achieved, an additional 12 weeks of treatment is warranted Begin 8–35 days before smoking cessation	Decrease use after 12 weeks
Bupropion (Zyban, Buproban)	Insomnia, dry mouth, agitation	Easy to use (pill); no nicotine; promotes weight loss, which may limit cessation-related weight gain; first-choice drug for smokers with depression	Prescription required; carries a small risk for seizures	150 mg extended-release tablets	150 mg PO daily × 3 days, 150 mg PO twice daily × 7–12 weeks Begin 1–2 weeks before smoking cessation	Decrease use after 7–12 weeks

Interventions for smoking cessation can be found in *Treating Tobacco Use and Dependence: 2008 Update,* a clinical practice guideline issued by the U.S. Public Health Service. As stated in the guideline, tobacco dependence is a chronic condition that warrants repeated intervention until long-term abstinence is achieved. This is the same philosophy that guides treatment of dependence on other highly addictive substances, including cocaine and heroin. Tobacco dependence can be treated with two methods: drugs and counseling. Both methods are effective, but a combination of both is more effective than either one alone. Accordingly, the guidelines recommend that all patients who want to quit be offered (1) at least one smoking cessation drug (bupropion, varenicline, or a nicotine-based product) along with (2) counseling, be it one-on-one, in a group, or over the phone (dial 1-800-QUITNOW in the United States). The overall intervention strategy is summarized in the "5 A's" model for treating tobacco use and dependence:

Ask (screen all patients for tobacco use).

Advise tobacco users to quit.

Assess willingness to make a quit attempt.

Assist with quitting (offer medication and provide or refer to counseling).

Arrange follow-up contacts, beginning within the first week after the quit date.

For additional information on smoking cessation, visit the internet sites for Canada and the United States listed in Table 34.2.

Nicotine Replacement Therapy

NRT allows smokers to substitute a pharmaceutical source of nicotine for the nicotine in cigarettes—and then gradually withdraw the replacement nicotine. This is analogous to using methadone to wean addicts from heroin.

Five FDA-approved formulations are available: chewing gum, lozenges, transdermal patches, a nasal spray, and an inhaler (see Table 34.1). With the gum, lozenges, patches, and inhaler, blood levels of nicotine rise slowly and remain relatively steady. Because nicotine levels rise slowly, these delivery systems produce less pleasure than cigarettes but nonetheless do relieve symptoms of withdrawal. With the nasal spray, blood levels of nicotine rise rapidly, much as they do with smoking. Hence the nasal spray provides some of the subjective pleasure that smoking does.

Long-term quit rates are significantly greater with NRT than with placebo—although absolute success rates remain low. For example, the 1-year success with nicotine patches is approximately 25%, compared with 9% for placebo. Success rates are highest when replacement therapy is combined with counseling.

TABLE 34.2 Internet-Based Resources for Smoking Cessation

United States
- U.S. Department of Health and Human Services: http://www.surgeongeneral.gov/library/reports/50-years-of-progress/consumer-guide.pdf
- Centers for Disease Control and Prevention: http://www.cdc.gov/tobacco/quit_smoking/
- American Lung Association: http://www.lungusa.org/stop-smoking/

Canada
- Health Canada: http://www.hc-sc.gc.ca/hc-ps/tobac-tabac/index-eng.php
- The Lung Association: https://www.lung.ca/news/latest-news/latest-news/support-key-increase-your-chances-quitting-smoking-and-staying-smoke

Nicotine products should generally be avoided during pregnancy. However, because smoking is probably more harmful than NRT, use of NRT during pregnancy is worth consideration.

Nicotine Chewing Gum (Nicotine Polacrilex)

Nicotine chewing gum (Nicorette, others) is composed of a gum base plus nicotine polacrilex, an ion exchange resin to which nicotine is bound. The gum must be chewed to release the nicotine. After release, nicotine is absorbed across the oral mucosa into the systemic circulation. Like other forms of NRT, nicotine gum doubles the cessation success rate.

The most common adverse effects are mouth and throat soreness, jaw muscle ache, eructation (belching), and hiccups. Using optimal chewing technique minimizes these problems.

Patients should be advised to chew the gum slowly and intermittently for approximately 30 minutes. Rapid chewing can release too much nicotine at one time, resulting in effects similar to those of excessive smoking (e.g., nausea, throat irritation, hiccups). Because foods and beverages can reduce nicotine absorption, patients should not eat or drink while chewing or for 15 minutes before chewing (see Table 34.1).

After 3 months without cigarettes, patients should discontinue nicotine use. Withdrawal should be done gradually. Use of nicotine gum beyond 6 months is not recommended.

Nicotine Lozenges (Nicotine Polacrilex)

The pharmacology of nicotine lozenges (Nicorette Lozenge, Thrive ✦) is very similar to that of nicotine gum. Both products contain nicotine bound to polacrilex. Sucking on the lozenge releases nicotine, which is then absorbed across the oral mucosa into the systemic circulation. Like nicotine gum and other forms of NRT, nicotine lozenges double the cessation success rate.

The most common adverse effects are mouth irritation, dyspepsia, nausea, and hiccups—all of which can be made worse by taking two lozenges at once or by taking several lozenges in immediate succession.

Administration consists of placing the lozenge in the mouth and allowing it to dissolve, which takes 20 to 30 minutes. Users should not eat or drink for 15 minutes before dosing and while the lozenge is in the mouth. In addition, they should not chew or swallow the lozenge (see Table 34.1).

Nicotine Transdermal Systems (Patches)

Nicotine transdermal systems are nicotine-containing adhesive patches that, after application to the skin, slowly release their nicotine content. The nicotine is absorbed into the skin and then into the blood, producing steady blood levels. Use of the patch about doubles the cessation success rate.

NicoDerm CQ can be purchased without a prescription. As indicated in Table 34.3, the patches come in different sizes. The larger patches release more nicotine.

Nicotine patches are applied once a day to clean, dry, nonhairy skin of the upper body or upper arm. The site should be changed daily and not reused for at least 1 week. NicoDerm CQ patches are left in place for 24 hours and then immediately replaced with a fresh one. Most patients begin with a large patch and then use progressively smaller patches over several weeks. Starting patch size is typically determined based on the number of cigarettes smoked daily. Certain patients (those with cardiovascular disease, those who weigh less than 100 pounds, and those who smoke less than one-half pack of cigarettes a day) should begin with a smaller patch.

Adverse effects are generally mild. Short-lived erythema, itching, and burning occur under the patch in 35% to 50% of users. In 14% to 17% of users, persistent erythema occurs, lasting up to 24 hours after patch removal. Patients who experience severe, persistent local reactions (e.g., severe erythema, itching, edema) should discontinue the patch and contact a medical provider.

Nicotine Inhaler

The nicotine inhaler (Nicotrol inhaler, Nicorette inhaler ❧) differs from other NRT products in that it looks much like a cigarette. Puffing on it delivers the nicotine. Because of this delivery method, using the inhaler can substitute for the hand-to-mouth behavior of smoking. In addition to nicotine, the inhaler contains menthol, whose purpose is to create a sensation in the back of the throat reminiscent of that caused by smoke. Like other forms of NRT, the inhaler doubles cessation success rates.

The nicotine inhaler consists of a mouthpiece and a sealed, tubular cartridge. Inside the cartridge is a porous plug containing 10 mg of nicotine. Inserting the cartridge into the mouthpiece breaks the seal. Puffing on the mouthpiece draws air over the plug and thereby draws nicotine vapor into the mouth. Most of the nicotine is absorbed through the *oral mucosa*—not in the lungs. As a result, blood levels rise slowly and peak 10 to 15 minutes after puffing stops. Blood levels are less than half those achieved with cigarettes. Each cartridge can deliver 300 to 400 puffs (see Table 34.1).

Adverse effects are mild. The most frequent are dyspepsia, coughing, throat irritation, oral burning, and rhinitis. The inhaler should not be used by patients with asthma. Because the cartridges contain dangerous amounts of nicotine, they should be kept away from children and pets.

Nicotine Nasal Spray

Nicotine nasal spray (Nicotrol NS) differs from other NRT formulations in that blood levels of nicotine rise *rapidly* after each administration, thereby closely simulating smoking. Because nicotine levels rise rapidly, the spray provides some of the subjective pleasure associated with cigarettes. As with other forms of NRT, the spray doubles smoking cessation rates (see Table 34.1).

Quitting success with the spray has been good news and bad news. The good news, as reported in one study, is that 27% of users avoided smoking for 1 year—approximately twice the abstinence rate achieved with placebo. The bad news is that many patients continued to use the spray, being unwilling or unable to give it up. Nonetheless, because the spray delivers nicotine without the additional hazards in cigarettes, using the spray is clearly preferable to smoking but not ideal for long-term use.

Adverse effects are mild and temporary. At first, most users experience rhinitis, sneezing, coughing, watering eyes, and nasal and throat irritation. Fortunately, these effects abate in a few days. Nicotine nasal spray should be avoided by patients with sinus problems, allergies, or asthma.

Bupropion SR

Bupropion SR (Zyban), an atypical antidepressant, was the first non-nicotine drug approved as an aid to smoking cessation. The drug is structurally similar to amphetamine and, like amphetamine, causes CNS stimulation and suppresses appetite. In people trying to quit cigarettes, bupropion reduces the urge to smoke and reduces some symptoms of nicotine withdrawal (e.g., irritability, anxiety). The drug is effective in the presence and absence of depression. For use in depression, bupropion is sold under the trade name Wellbutrin. The basic pharmacology of bupropion is discussed in Chapter 27.

Like the NRT products, bupropion SR doubles the cessation success rate. In one trial, patients were given bupropion SR (100, 150, or 300 mg/day) or placebo. At 7 weeks, abstinence rates were 19% with placebo, and 29%, 39%, and 44% with increasing dosages of bupropion SR. At 12 weeks, abstinence rates were lower: 12% with placebo and 20%, 23%, and 23% with increasing dosages of bupropion SR. Combining a nicotine patch with bupropion SR is somewhat more effective than either treatment alone. Mechanism of action, pharmacokinetics, and adverse effects associated with bupropion are listed in Table 34.4.

TABLE 34.3 Nicotine Transdermal Systems (Patches)

Trade Name	Surface Area (cm²)	Hours/Day in Place	Dose Absorbed	Duration of Use Per Patch Size	Total
NicoDerm CQ Step 1	30	24	21 mg over 24 h	First 4–6 weeks	8–10 weeks
NicoDerm CQ Step 2	20	24	14 mg over 24 h	Next 2 weeks	
NicoDerm CQ Step 3	10	24	7 mg over 24 h	Next 2 weeks	
Nicorette Invisipatch Step 1 ❧	22.5	16	25 mg over 16 h	First 8 weeks	12 weeks
Nicorette Invisipatch Step 2 ❧	13.5	16	15 mg over 16 h	Next 2 weeks	
Nicorette Invisipatch Step 3 ❧	9	16	10 mg over 16 h	Next 2 weeks	

SUMMARY OF KEY PRESCRIBING CONSIDERATIONS

Bupropion SR

Therapeutic Goal: Continued tobacco cessation
Identifying High-Risk Patients: Use with caution in patients with history of seizure, anorexia nervosa, cocaine use, and alcohol withdrawal.
Minimizing Adverse Effects: Bupropion SR should not be given in conjunction with Wellbutrin (bupropion) or monoamine oxidase inhibitors.

TABLE 34.4 Nicotine-Free Products: Mechanism of Action, Pharmacokinetics, Adverse Effects, and Interactions

Drug	Mechanism of Action	Pharmacokinetics	Adverse Effects	Interactions
Bupropion SR (Zyban)	Potential blocks uptake of norepinephrine and dopamine.	Half-life: 8–24 h Metabolism: Hepatic Excretion: Urine	Dry mouth Insomnia Weight loss	MAOIs Wellbutrin
Varenicline (Chantix)	Partial agonist at the $\alpha_4\beta_2$ nicotinc receptors that promote release of dopamine.	Half-life: 17–24 h Metabolism: Minimal (8%) Excretion: Urine	Nausea Cardiovascular events Psychiatric events	None Significant

MAOI, Monoamine oxidase inhibitor.

Varenicline

Varenicline (Chantix, Champix), a partial agonist at nicotinic receptors, is our most effective aid to smoking cessation. In clinical trials, more patients achieved abstinence with varenicline than with bupropion SR or the nicotine patch. Estimated abstinence rates after 6 months were 33.2% with varenicline, 24.2% with bupropion SR, and 23.4% with a nicotine patch. The most common side effect is nausea. The most troubling side effects are psychological changes. Unlike bupropion SR and NRT, varenicline does *not* cause weight loss.

In 2011 the FDA warned that varenicline can increase the risk for cardiovascular events (e.g., angina pectoris, peripheral edema, hypertension, nonfatal myocardial infarction) in patients with stable cardiovascular disease. After that, a Canadian study revealed a similar risk in patients *without* cardiovascular disease. Fortunately, cardiovascular risk appears to be small—much smaller than the risk posed by smoking. Nonetheless, patients should be warned about cardiovascular risk and instructed to notify the prescriber if they experience new or worsening cardiovascular symptoms and should seek immediate medical attention if symptoms of myocardial infarction appear. Mechanism of action, pharmacokinetics, and other adverse effects associated with varenicline are listed in Table 34.4.

Owing to concerns about unpredictable physical and psychiatric adverse effects, U.S. authorities have banned use of varenicline by truck drivers, bus drivers, airplane pilots, and air traffic controllers.

Preparations, Dosage, and Administration

 BLACK BOX WARNING

Bupropion

Postmarketing reports indicate that bupropion can cause serious *neuropsychiatric effects,* including mood changes, erratic behavior, and suicidality. All patients should be advised to contact their prescriber if they experience a significant change in behavior or mental status. Bupropion should be used with caution in patients with a history of psychiatric disease.

SUMMARY OF KEY PRESCRIBING CONSIDERATIONS

Varenicline

Therapeutic Goal: Continued tobacco cessation

Identifying High-Risk Patients: Use of varenicline by truck drivers, bus drivers, airplane pilots, and air traffic controllers is banned. Monitor patients with known cardiovascular disease closely.

Minimizing Adverse Effects: Patients should be instructed to notify the prescriber if they experience new or worsening cardiovascular symptoms.

35

Substance Use Disorders IV: Major Drugs of Abuse Other Than Alcohol and Nicotine

In this chapter, we discuss all of the major drugs of abuse except alcohol (Chapter 32) and nicotine (Chapter 33). As indicated in Table 35.1, abused drugs fall into six major categories: (1) opioids, (2) psychostimulants, (3) depressants, (4) psychedelics, (5) anabolic steroids, and (6) miscellaneous drugs of abuse. The basic pharmacology of many of these drugs is presented in previous chapters, so their discussion here is brief. Agents that have not been addressed previously (e.g., marijuana, *d*-lysergic acid diethylamide [LSD]) are discussed in depth.

HEROIN, OXYCODONE, AND OTHER OPIOIDS

The opioids (e.g., heroin, oxycodone, meperidine) are major drugs of abuse. As a result, most opioids are classified as schedule II substances. The basic pharmacology of the opioids is discussed in Chapter 24.

Patterns of Use

For most people with opioid use disorder (OUD), initial exposure to opioids occurs either recreationally (i.e., illicitly) or in the context of pain management in a medical setting. The overwhelming majority of individuals who go on to abuse opioids begin their drug use illicitly. A small percentage of those exposed to opioids therapeutically develop a pattern of compulsive drug use.

Opioid abuse by health care providers deserves special consideration. It is well established that health care providers, nurses, and pharmacists, as a group, abuse opioids to a greater extent than all other groups with similar educational backgrounds. The vulnerability of health care professionals to opioid abuse is primarily due to drug access.

Subjective and Behavioral Effects

Moments after intravenous (IV) injection, heroin produces sensations of pleasure, relaxation, warmth, and thirst. This initial reaction, known as a "rush" or "kick," persists for approximately 45 seconds. After this, the user experiences a prolonged sense of euphoria. These extended effects, rather than the initial rush, are the primary reason for opioid abuse.

Interestingly, when individuals first use opioids, nausea and vomiting are prominent, and an overall sense of *dysphoria* may be felt. In many cases, were it not for peer pressure, individuals would not continue opioid use long enough to allow these unpleasant reactions to be replaced by a more agreeable experience.

Preferred Drugs and Routes of Administration

In the past, heroin was the most commonly abused opioid drug, but no longer, although its use is increasing. Prescription opioid analgesics were abused much more commonly than heroin, but with the opioid epidemic and increases in deaths from overdose, heroin is becoming more available and is cheaper than prescription opioids.

Heroin

Among street users, heroin is the traditional opioid of choice. Because of its high lipid solubility, heroin crosses the blood–brain barrier with ease, causing effects that are both immediate and intense. This combination of speed and intensity sets heroin apart from other opioids.

Heroin can be administered in several ways. The order of preference is IV injection, smoking, and nasal inhalation (known as sniffing or snorting). IV injection produces effects with the greatest intensity and fastest onset (7 to 8 seconds). When heroin is smoked or snorted, effects develop more slowly, peaking in 10 to 15 minutes. Among users who seek addiction treatment, injection is the predominant method of administration. However, because sniffing and smoking are safer and easier than injection, these routes have become increasingly popular.

It should be noted that, when heroin is administered orally or subcutaneously, as opposed to intravenously, its effects cannot be distinguished from those of morphine and other opioids. This observation is not surprising given that, once in the brain, heroin is rapidly converted into morphine, its active form.

Oxycodone

In some parts of the United States, people are abusing the *controlled-release* formulation of oxycodone (OxyContin), an opioid similar to morphine. The controlled-release tablets were designed to provide steady levels of oxycodone over an extended time and are safe and effective when swallowed intact. However, abusers do not ingest the tablets whole. Rather, they crush the tablets and then either snort the powder or dissolve it in water and then inject it intravenously. As a result, the entire dose is absorbed *immediately,* producing blood levels that are dangerously high. Hundreds of deaths have been reported. The risk for respiratory depression and death is greatest in people who have not developed tolerance to opioids.

In an effort to reduce OxyContin abuse, the controlled-release tablets were reformulated in 2010 (review Chapter 24 for more information).

Tolerance and Physical Dependence
Tolerance

With prolonged opioid use, tolerance develops to some pharmacologic effects but not others. Effects to which tolerance does develop include euphoria, respiratory depression, and nausea. In contrast, little or no tolerance develops to constipation and miosis. Because tolerance to respiratory depression develops in parallel with tolerance to euphoria, respiratory depression does not increase because higher doses are taken to produce desired subjective effects. Persons tolerant to one opioid are cross-tolerant to other opioids. However, there is no cross-tolerance between opioids and general central nervous system (CNS) depressants (e.g., barbiturates, benzodiazepines, alcohol).

TABLE 35.1 Pharmacologic Categorization of Abused Drugs

Category	Examples
Opioids	Heroin
	Hydromorphone
	Meperidine
	Morphine
	Oxycodone
Psychostimulants	Cocaine
	Dextroamphetamine
	Methamphetamine
	Methylphenidate
Depressants	
Barbiturates	Amobarbital
	Pentobarbital
	Phenobarbital
	Secobarbital
Benzodiazepines	Diazepam
	Flunitrazepam
	Lorazepam
Miscellaneous	Alcohol
	γ-Hydroxybutyrate
	Meprobamate
	Methaqualone
Psychedelics	Dimethyltryptamine
	LSD
	Mescaline
	Psilocybin
Anabolic steroids	Nandrolone
	Oxandrolone
	Testosterone
Miscellaneous	Dextromethorphan
	Marijuana
	Nicotine
	Nitrous oxide

LSD, Lysergic acid diethylamide.

Physical Dependence

Long-term use produces substantial physical dependence. The abstinence syndrome resulting from opioid withdrawal is described in Chapter 24. It is important to note that, although the opioid withdrawal syndrome can be extremely unpleasant, it is rarely dangerous.

After the acute abstinence syndrome, which fades in 10 days, opioid addicts may experience a milder but protracted phase of withdrawal. This second phase, which may persist for months, is characterized by insomnia, irritability, and fatigue. Gastrointestinal hyperactivity and premature ejaculation may also occur.

Treatment of Acute Toxicity

Overdose produces a classic triad of symptoms: *respiratory depression, coma,* and *pinpoint pupils. Naloxone* (Narcan), an opioid antagonist, is the treatment of choice. This agent rapidly reverses all signs of opioid poisoning. However, dosage must be titrated carefully because if too much is given, the patient will swing from a state of intoxication to one of withdrawal. Owing to its short half-life, naloxone must be readministered every few hours until opioid concentrations have dropped to nontoxic levels, which may take days. Failure to repeat naloxone dosing may result in the death of patients who had earlier been rendered symptom free.

In an effort to decrease the deaths from opioid overdose, the U.S. Food and Drug Administration (FDA) approved the first preparation of naloxone intended for outpatient use in 2014. Soon after in 2015, the FDA approved a nasal formulation. As of 2017, legislation has been passed in all 50 states in an attempt to increase public access to naloxone. These laws vary from state to state.

If the patient is in a setting outside the hospital, two options are currently available for caregivers: nasal spray or autoinjector. When using *Narcan Nasal Spray,* one spray is administered to one nostril, delivering 4 mg of naloxone. If there is no response, additional doses may be given every 2 to 3 minutes until emergency medical services arrive. The autoinjector *Evzio* is a cartridge containing one dose of naloxone that is delivered to the muscle or skin of the outer thigh. The cartridge uses and electronic voice instruction system and blinking lights to help guide the caregiver through proper administration. As with the nasal spray, additional doses may be administered every 2 to 3 minutes until additional medical support arrives.

Drugs for Long-Term Management of Opioid Use Disorder

Three kinds of drugs are used for long-term management: *opioid agonists, opioid agonist-antagonists,* and *opioid antagonists.* Opioid agonists (methadone) and agonist-antagonists (buprenorphine) substitute for the abused opioid and are given to patients who are not yet ready for detoxification. In contrast, opioid antagonists (naltrexone) are used to discourage renewed opioid use after detoxification has been accomplished. Drugs used for long-term management of OUD are shown in Table 35.2.

Methadone

In addition to its role in facilitating opioid withdrawal, methadone (Methadose, Diskets) can be used for *maintenance therapy* and *suppressive therapy.* These strategies are used to modify drug-using behavior in patients who are not ready to try withdrawal.

Methadone maintenance consists of transferring the addict from the abused opioid to oral methadone. By taking methadone, the addict avoids both withdrawal and the need to procure illegal drugs. Maintenance dosing is done once a day. Maintenance is most effective when done in conjunction with nondrug measures directed at altering patterns of drug use.

Suppressive therapy is done to prevent the reinforcing effects of opioid-induced euphoria. Suppression is achieved by giving the addict progressively larger doses of methadone until a very high dose (120 mg/day) is reached. Building up to this dose creates a high degree of tolerance, and hence no subjective effects are experienced from the methadone itself. Because cross-tolerance exists among opioids, after the patient is tolerant to methadone, taking street drugs, even in high doses, cannot produce significant desirable effects. As a result, individuals made tolerant with methadone will be less likely to seek out illicit opioids.

⏵⏵ BLACK BOX WARNING
Methadone

Methadone can cause life-threatening QT prolongation and severe respiratory depression. Because of the long half-life of methadone, it should be prescribed only by health care providers with special training in chronic pain management.

Use of methadone to treat opioid addicts is restricted to opioid treatment programs approved by the designated state authority and certified by the federal Substance Abuse and Mental Health Services Administration. These restrictions on the nonanalgesic use of methadone

TABLE 35.2 Drugs for Long-Term Management of Opioid Addiction

Drug	Trade Name	Formulation	Dosing Schedule	CSA Schedule	Comments
Opioid Agonist					
Methadone	Methadose, Diskets	Dispersible tablets used to make an oral suspension	Once a day	II	Methadone maintenance may be provided only by Opioid Treatment Programs certified by the federal Substance Abuse and Mental Health Services Administration and approved by the designated state authority.
	Methadose	Concentrated oral liquid	Once a day		
Opioid Agonist-Antagonist					
Buprenorphine	Generic	Sublingual tablet	Once a day	III	May be prescribed in a primary care setting by any health care provider or nurse practitioner who has received authorized training and has registered with the Substance Abuse and Mental Health Services Administration.
	Suboxone[a]	Sublingual tablet	Once a day		
	Suboxone[a]	Sublingual film	Once a day		
			Once a day		
	Sublocade	Solution for SubQ injection	Once a month		
	Bunavail[a]	Buccal film			
	Zubsolv[a]	Sublingual Tablet	Once a day		
	Probuphine	Subdermal Implant	Every 6 months		
Opioid Antagonist					
Naltrexone	Generic	Oral tablet	Once a day	NR	Naltrexone is not a controlled substance and hence prescribers do not require special training or certification. IM naltrexone (Vivitrol) is the only drug approved for opioid addiction that is given monthly, rather than daily. Before receiving naltrexone, patients must undergo opioid detoxification.
	Vivitrol	Extended-release suspension for IM injection	Once a month		

[a]In addition to buprenorphine, Suboxone, Zubsolv, and Bunavail contain naloxone, an opioid antagonist, to discourage intravenous dosing.
CSA, Controlled Substances Act; *SubQ*, subcutaneous; *IM*, intramuscular; *NR*, not regulated under the CSA.

are needed to control abuse of methadone, a schedule II drug with the same abuse liability as morphine and other strong opioids.

The basic pharmacology of methadone is presented in Chapter 24.

Buprenorphine

Buprenorphine (Suboxone, Bunavail) is an agonist-antagonist opioid. The drug is a partial agonist at μ-receptors and a full antagonist at κ-receptors. Buprenorphine can be used for maintenance therapy and to facilitate detoxification (see earlier). When used for maintenance, buprenorphine alleviates craving, reduces use of illicit opioids, and increases retention in therapeutic programs.

Unlike methadone, which is available only through certified opioid treatment programs, buprenorphine can be prescribed and dispensed in general medical settings, such as primary care offices. Prescribers must receive at least 8 hours of authorized training and must register with the Substance Abuse and Mental Health Services Administration.

Buprenorphine has several properties that make it attractive for treating OUD. Because it is a partial agonist at μ-receptors, it has a low potential for abuse—but can still suppress craving for opioids. If the dosage is sufficiently high, buprenorphine can completely block access of strong opioids to μ-receptors and can thereby prevent opioid-induced euphoria. With buprenorphine, there is a ceiling to respiratory depression, which makes it safer than methadone. Development of physical dependence is low, and hence withdrawal is relatively mild.

Buprenorphine is currently available in multiple formulations for treatment of OUD. Three formulations—sublingual tablets, solution for subcutaneous injection, and a subdermal implant—contain buprenorphine *alone*. The other three formulations—sublingual tablets, sublingual films, and buccal film, marketed as *Suboxone, Zubsolv* and *Bunavail*—contain buprenorphine *combined with naloxone*. The

newest film, *Bunavail*, is placed on the inside of each cheek and is used for long-term maintenance. The naloxone in Suboxone is there to discourage IV abuse. If taken intravenously, the naloxone in Suboxone will precipitate withdrawal. However, with sublingual administration, very little naloxone is absorbed, and hence when the drug is administered as intended, the risk for withdrawal is low. Nonetheless, because there *is* a small risk with sublingual Suboxone, treatment is initiated with buprenorphine alone. Thereafter Suboxone is taken for maintenance.

The basic pharmacology of buprenorphine is presented in Chapter 24.

Naltrexone

After a patient has undergone opioid detoxification, naltrexone (Vivitrol), a pure opioid antagonist, can be used to discourage renewed opioid abuse. Benefits derive from blocking euphoria and all other opioid-induced effects. By preventing pleasurable effects, naltrexone eliminates the reinforcing properties of opioid use. When the former addict learns that taking an opioid cannot produce the desired response, drug-using behavior will cease. Naltrexone is not a controlled substance, and hence prescribers require no special training or certification.

Naltrexone is available in oral and intramuscular (IM) formulations. The oral formulation is dosed once a day. The IM formulation, sold as Vivitrol, is dosed once a month.

The basic pharmacology of naltrexone is presented in Chapter 24.

KRATOM

Kratom (*Mitragyna speciose*) is a tree grown in Southeast Asia. Kratom is composed of two compounds, mitragynine and 7-hydroxymitragynine. The leaves of the tree interact with opioid receptors in the brain to produce euphoria, sedation, and decreased sensation of pain, especially when taken in large doses. In smaller doses, kratom has also been known to cause stimulation, increased energy, and alertness. Currently, kratom is not a scheduled drug and can be purchased easily over the internet or local shops in the form of capsules, liquids, and powders. Many users take kratom for relief of pain as a substitute for opioid therapy or in an attempt to ease withdrawal from opioid cessation. Anecdotal reports suggest that kratom may be a safer alternative to opioid use for pain and that kratom may be less addictive. The U.S. Drug Enforcement Administration (DEA) is investigating the use of kratom and considering categorizing it as a schedule I drug, stating kratom is an, "imminent hazard to public health." The DEA bases this statement citing more than 40 deaths related to the use of kratom. These deaths were often related to use of kratom in combination with other substances, including prescription medications and other illicit drugs. Because there are many proponents of the potential positive uses for kratom, the DEA is allowing a period for public commentary on the issue prior to releasing a final decision.

GENERAL CENTRAL NERVOUS SYSTEM DEPRESSANTS

The family of CNS depressants consists of barbiturates, benzodiazepines, alcohol, and other agents. With the exception of the benzodiazepines, all of these drugs are more alike than different. The benzodiazepines have properties that set them apart. The basic pharmacology of the benzodiazepines, barbiturates, and most other CNS depressants is presented in Chapter 29; the pharmacology of alcohol is presented in Chapter 33. Discussion here is limited to abuse of these drugs.

Barbiturates

The barbiturates embody all of the properties that typify general CNS depressants and hence can be considered prototypes of the group. Depressant effects are dose dependent and range from mild sedation to sleep to coma to death. With prolonged use, barbiturates produce tolerance and physical dependence.

The abuse liability of the barbiturates stems from their ability to produce subjective effects similar to those of alcohol. The barbiturates with the highest potential for abuse have a short to intermediate duration of action. These agents—amobarbital, pentobarbital, and secobarbital—are classified under schedule II of the Controlled Substances Act. Other barbiturates appear under schedules III and IV. Despite legal restrictions, barbiturates are available cheaply and in abundance.

Tolerance

Regular use of barbiturates produces tolerance to some effects but not to others. Tolerance to subjective effects is significant. As a result, progressively larger doses are needed to produce desired psychological responses. Unfortunately, very little tolerance develops to respiratory depression. Consequently, as barbiturate use continues, the dose needed to produce subjective effects moves closer and closer to the dose that can cause respiratory arrest. (Note that this differs from the pattern seen with opioids, in which tolerance to subjective effects and to respiratory depression develop in parallel.) Individuals tolerant to barbiturates show cross-tolerance with other CNS depressants (e.g., alcohol, benzodiazepines, general anesthetics). However, little or no cross-tolerance develops to opioids.

Physical Dependence and Withdrawal Techniques

Chronic barbiturate use can produce substantial physical dependence. Cross-dependence exists between barbiturates and other CNS depressants but not with opioids. When physical dependence is great, the associated abstinence syndrome can be severe—sometimes fatal. In contrast, the opioid abstinence syndrome, although unpleasant, is rarely life threatening.

One technique for easing barbiturate withdrawal uses phenobarbital, a barbiturate with a long half-life. Because of cross-dependence, substitution of phenobarbital for the abused barbiturate suppresses symptoms of abstinence. After the patient has been stabilized, the dosage of phenobarbital is gradually tapered off, thereby minimizing symptoms of abstinence.

Benzodiazepines

Benzodiazepines differ significantly from barbiturates. Benzodiazepines are much safer than the barbiturates, and overdose with *oral* benzodiazepines *alone* is rarely lethal. However, the risk for death is greatly increased when oral benzodiazepines are combined with other CNS depressants (e.g., alcohol, barbiturates) or when benzodiazepines are administered intravenously. If severe overdose occurs, signs and symptoms can be reversed with *flumazenil* (Romazicon, Anexate ✦), a benzodiazepine antagonist. As a rule, tolerance and physical dependence are only moderate when benzodiazepines are taken for legitimate indications but can be substantial when these drugs are abused. In patients who develop physical dependence, the abstinence syndrome can be minimized by withdrawing benzodiazepines very slowly—over a period of months. The abuse liability of the benzodiazepines is much lower than that of the barbiturates. As a result, all benzodiazepines are classified under schedule IV of the Controlled Substances Act. Benzodiazepines are discussed in Chapter 29.

PSYCHOSTIMULANTS

Discussion here focuses on two CNS stimulants that have a high potential for abuse: cocaine and methamphetamine. Because of their considerable abuse liability, these drugs are classified as schedule II agents.

Cocaine

Cocaine is a stimulant extracted from the leaves of the coca plant. The drug has CNS effects similar to those of the amphetamines. In addition, cocaine can produce local anesthesia, as well as vasoconstriction and cardiac stimulation. Among abusers, a form of cocaine known as "crack" is used widely. Crack is extremely addictive, and the risk for lethal overdose is high.

According to the National Survey on Drug Use and Health, cocaine use has declined. In 2015, 2.4 million Americans 18 years and older reported using cocaine in any form, compared with 5.5 million in 2005.

Forms

Cocaine is available in two forms: *cocaine hydrochloride* and *cocaine base* (alkaloidal cocaine, freebase cocaine, "crack"). Cocaine base is heat stable, whereas cocaine hydrochloride is not. Cocaine hydrochloride is available as a white powder that is frequently diluted ("cut") before sale. Cocaine base is sold in the form of crystals ("rocks") that consist of nearly pure cocaine. Cocaine base is widely known by the street name "crack," a term inspired by the sound the crystals make when heated.

Routes of Administration

Cocaine *hydrochloride* is usually administered *intranasally*. The drug is "snorted" and absorbed across the nasal mucosa into the bloodstream. A few users (approximately 5%) administer cocaine hydrochloride intravenously. Cocaine hydrochloride cannot be smoked because it is unstable at high temperature.

Cocaine *base* is administered by *smoking*, a process referred to as "freebasing." Smoking delivers large amounts of cocaine to the lungs, where absorption is very rapid. Subjective and physiologic effects are equivalent to those elicited by IV injection.

Subjective Effects and Cocaine Use Disorder

At usual doses, cocaine produces euphoria similar to that produced by amphetamines. In a laboratory setting, individuals familiar with the effects of cocaine are unable to distinguish between cocaine and amphetamine. Cocaine causes euphoria through inhibition of neuronal reuptake of dopamine and thereby increases activation of dopamine receptors in the brain's reward circuit.

As with many other psychoactive drugs, the intensity of subjective responses depends on the rate at which plasma drug levels rise. Because cocaine levels rise relatively slowly with intranasal administration and almost instantaneously with IV injection or smoking, responses produced by intranasal cocaine are much less intense than those produced by the other two routes.

When crack cocaine is smoked, desirable subjective effects begin to fade within minutes and are often replaced by dysphoria. In an attempt to avoid dysphoria and regain euphoria, the user may administer repeated doses at short intervals. This use pattern—termed *binging*—can rapidly lead to addiction.

Acute Toxicity: Symptoms and Treatment

Overdose is frequent, and deaths have occurred. Mild overdose produces agitation, dizziness, tremor, and blurred vision. Severe overdose can produce hyperpyrexia, convulsions, ventricular dysrhythmias, and hemorrhagic stroke. Angina pectoris and myocardial infarction may develop secondary to coronary artery spasm. Psychological manifestations of overdose include severe anxiety, paranoid ideation, and hallucinations (visual, auditory, and/or tactile). Because cocaine has a short half-life, symptoms subside in 1 to 2 hours.

Although there is no specific antidote to cocaine toxicity, most symptoms can be controlled with drugs. IV *diazepam* or *lorazepam* can reduce anxiety and suppress seizures. *Diazepam* may also alleviate hypertension and dysrhythmias because these result from increased central sympathetic activity. If hypertension is severe, it can be corrected with IV *nitroprusside*. Dysrhythmias associated with prolonging the QT interval may respond to *hypertonic sodium bicarbonate*. Although β-blockers can suppress dysrhythmias, they might further compromise coronary perfusion (by preventing β_2-mediated coronary vasodilation). Reduction of thrombus formation with aspirin can lower the risk for myocardial ischemia. Hyperthermia should be reduced with external cooling.

Chronic Toxicity

When administered intranasally on a long-term basis, cocaine can cause atrophy of the nasal mucosa and loss of sense of smell. In extreme cases, necrosis and perforation of the nasal septum occur. Nasal pathology results from local ischemia secondary to chronic vasoconstriction. Injury to the lungs can occur from smoking cocaine base.

Treatment of Cocaine Use Disorder

Although achieving complete abstinence from cocaine is extremely difficult, treatment *can* greatly reduce cocaine use. For the cocaine addict, psychosocial therapy is the cornerstone of treatment. This therapy is directed at motivating users to commit to a drug-free life and then helping them work toward that goal. A combination of individual therapy and group drug counseling is most effective, producing a 70% reduction in cocaine use at 12-month follow-up.

Can medication help with cocaine addiction? To date, no drug has been proven broadly effective in treating cocaine abuse. However, ongoing work with two agents is encouraging:

- *Anticocaine vaccine*—Subjects receiving the vaccine develop antibodies that bind with cocaine and thereby render the cocaine inactive. The higher the antibody titer, the greater the reduction in cocaine use. The vaccine has been tested in mice. Human testing may start in 2016.
- *Disulfiram* (Antabuse)—Subjects receiving a combination of disulfiram plus cognitive behavioral therapy reduced their cocaine use from two or three times daily to 0.5 times daily. Disulfiram is the same drug discussed in Chapter 33 for treating alcohol abuse.

Methamphetamine

The basic pharmacology of the amphetamine family is discussed in Chapter 31. Discussion here is limited to abuse of methamphetamine.

Description and Routes

Methamphetamine is a white, crystalline powder that readily dissolves in water or alcohol. The drug may be swallowed, "snorted," smoked, or injected intravenously. Owing to its potential for abuse, methamphetamine is classified as a schedule II drug.

Patterns of Use

Use of methamphetamine declined between the years of 2006 and 2012. Yet, we are currently seeing an increase in use. According to the 2016 National Survey on Drug Use and Health, use of methamphetamine within the past month by Americans age 12 years and older increased from 569,000 in 2014 to 667,000 in 2016.

Subjective and Behavioral Effects

As discussed in Chapter 31, amphetamines act primarily by increasing the release of norepinephrine and dopamine and partly by reducing the reuptake of both transmitters. By doing so, methamphetamine produces arousal and elevation of mood. Euphoria is likely, and talkativeness is prominent. A sense of increased physical strength and mental capacity occurs. Self-confidence rises. Users feel little or no need for food and sleep.

Adverse Psychological Effects

All amphetamines can produce a psychotic state characterized by delusions, paranoia, and auditory and visual hallucinations, making patients look like they have schizophrenia. Although psychosis can be triggered by a single dose, it occurs more commonly with long-term abuse. Methamphetamine-induced psychosis usually resolves spontaneously after drug withdrawal. If needed, an antipsychotic agent (e.g., haloperidol) can be given to suppress symptoms.

Adverse Cardiovascular Effects

Because of its sympathomimetic actions, methamphetamine can cause vasoconstriction and excessive stimulation of the heart, leading to hypertension, angina pectoris, and dysrhythmias. Vasoconstriction can be relieved with an α-adrenergic blocker (e.g., phentolamine). Cardiac stimulation can be reduced with a mixed α- and β-blocker (e.g., labetalol).

Other Adverse Effects

By suppressing appetite, methamphetamine can cause significant weight loss. Use during pregnancy increases the risk for preterm birth, hypertension, placental abruption, intrauterine growth restriction, and neonatal death. Heavy use can promote severe tooth decay, known informally as "meth mouth." Causes include reduced salivation, grinding and clenching of the teeth, increased consumption of sugary drinks, and neglect of oral hygiene. Lastly, methamphetamine can cause direct injury to dopaminergic nerve terminals in the brain, leading to prolonged deficits in cognition and memory.

Treatment

Amphetamine-type use disorder responds well to cognitive behavioral therapy. One such approach, known as the Matrix Model, combines group therapy, individual therapy, family education, drug testing, and encouragement to participate in non–drug-related activities. At this time, no medications are approved for treatment. However, encouraging results have been achieved with two drugs: *bupropion* (Wellbutrin, Zyban), currently approved for major depression and smoking cessation, and *modafinil* (Provigil, Alertec ♣), a nonamphetamine stimulant currently approved for narcolepsy, shift-work sleep disorder, and obstructive sleep apnea–hypopnea syndrome. An additional drug, ibudilast, is in clinical trials. Preliminary results indicate that ibudilast may dampen cravings for methamphetamine and improve cognitive functioning.

Synthetic Cathinones

Synthetic cathinones are drugs better known by their street name "bath salts." These drugs are closely related to the naturally occurring khat plant, found in East Africa and southern Arabia. Bath salts have appeared on the market within the past few years and are touted as substitutes to other psychostimulants, such as cocaine or methamphetamine.

Bath salts are consumed by injecting, swallowing, snorting, or smoking. Often, bath salts are sold in packets of white powder or tablets labeled "not for human consumption" or as plant food or cleaning substances. They are structurally related to amphetamines and are thought to increase dopamine, serotonin, and norepinephrine levels. This leads to feelings of euphoria and alertness. Onset of duration is fairly quick, with overall duration of 2 to 4 hours.

Multiple negative psychological effects have been noted with the use of bath salts, including paranoia, aggression, hallucinations, panic attacks, agitation, and delirium. Physical effects range from nose bleeds and sweating to renal failure and death. Bath salts were formerly available over the counter in gas stations and convenience stores, but due to their negative effects and many emergency room visits, bath salts are banned for sale in use in all 50 states.

MARIJUANA AND RELATED PREPARATIONS

Marijuana is the most commonly used federally deemed illicit drug in the United States. More than 128 million Americans have tried it at least once. In 2015 nearly 22 million Americans 12 years and older used marijuana. Among youth, rates of daily marijuana use are the highest since the 1970s. Results of the 2016 *Monitoring the Future* survey show that 5.4% of 8th graders and 14% of 10th graders reported using marijuana in the past month. Marijuana use among 12th graders has risen to 22.5%.

Cannabis Sativa, the Source of Marijuana

Marijuana is prepared from *C. sativa,* the Indian hemp plant—an unusual plant in that it has separate male and female forms. Psychoactive compounds are present in all parts of the male and female plants. However, the greatest concentration of psychoactive substances is found in the flowering tops of the female plants.

The two most common *Cannabis* derivatives are *marijuana* and *hashish.* Marijuana is a preparation consisting of leaves and flowers of male and female plants. Alternative names for marijuana include *grass, weed, pot,* and *dope.* The terms *joint* and *reefer* refer to marijuana cigarettes. Hashish is a dried preparation of the resinous exudate from female flowers. Hashish is considerably more potent than marijuana.

Psychoactive Component

The major psychoactive substance in *C. sativa* is delta-9-tetrahydro-cannabinol (THC), an oily chemical with high lipid solubility.

The THC content of *Cannabis* preparations is variable. The highest concentrations are found in the flowers of the female plant. The lowest concentrations are in the seeds. Depending on growing conditions and the strain of the plant, THC in marijuana preparations may range from 1% to 90%.

Mechanism of Action

Psychological effects of THC result from activating specific cannabinoid receptors in the brain. The endogenous ligand for these receptors appears to be *anandamide,* a derivative of arachidonic acid unique to the brain. The concentration of cannabinoid receptors is highest in brain regions associated with pleasure, memory, thinking, concentration, appetite, sensory perception, time perception, and coordination of movement.

There is evidence that marijuana may act in part through the same reward system as opioids and cocaine. Both heroin and cocaine produce pleasurable sensations by promoting release of dopamine in the brain's reward circuit. In rats, IV THC also causes dopamine release. Interestingly, release of dopamine by THC is blocked by naloxone, a drug that blocks the effects of opioids. This suggests that THC causes release of dopamine by first causing release of endogenous opioids.

Pharmacokinetics
Administration by Smoking

When marijuana or hashish is smoked, approximately 60% of the THC content is absorbed. Absorption from the lungs is rapid. Subjective effects begin in minutes and peak 10 to 20 minutes later. Effects from a single marijuana cigarette may persist for 2 to 3 hours. Termination results from metabolism of THC to inactive products.

Oral Administration

When marijuana or hashish is ingested, practically all of the THC undergoes absorption. However, most is inactivated on its first pass through the liver. Hence only 6% to 20% of absorbed drug actually reaches the systemic circulation. Because of this extensive first-pass metabolism, oral doses must be 3 to 10 times greater than smoked doses to produce equivalent effects. With oral dosing, effects are delayed and prolonged: responses begin in 30 to 50 minutes and persist up to 12 hours.

Behavioral and Subjective Effects

Marijuana produces three principal subjective effects: *euphoria, sedation,* and *hallucinations.* This set of responses is unique to marijuana; no other psychoactive drug causes all three. Because of this singular pattern of effects, marijuana is in a class by itself.

Effects of Low to Moderate Doses

Responses to low doses of THC are variable and depend on several factors, including dosage size and route, setting of drug use, and expectations and previous experience of the user. The following effects are common: euphoria and relaxation; gaiety and a heightened sense of the humorous; increased sensitivity to visual and auditory stimuli; enhanced sense of touch, taste, and smell; increased appetite and ability to appreciate the flavor of food; and distortion of time perception such that short spans seem much longer than they really are. In addition to these effects, which might be considered pleasurable (or at least innocuous), moderate doses can produce undesirable responses. Among these are impairment of short-term memory; decreased capacity to perform multistep tasks; slowed reaction time and impairment of motor coordination (which can make driving dangerous); altered judgment and decision making (which can lead to high-risk sexual behavior); temporal disintegration (inability to distinguish between past, present, and future); depersonalization (a sense of strangeness about the self); decreased ability to perceive the emotions of others; and reduced interpersonal interaction.

High-Dose Effects

In high doses, marijuana can have serious adverse psychological effects. The user may experience hallucinations, delusions, and paranoia. Euphoria may be displaced by intense anxiety, and a dissociative state may occur in which the user feels "outside of himself or herself." In extremely high doses, marijuana can produce a state resembling toxic psychosis, which may persist for weeks. Because of the widespread use of marijuana, psychiatric emergencies caused by the drug are relatively common.

Not all users are equally vulnerable to the adverse psychological effects of marijuana. Some individuals experience ill effects only at extremely high doses. In contrast, others routinely experience adverse effects at moderate doses.

Effects of Chronic Use

Amotivational syndrome. Chronic, excessive use of marijuana is associated with a behavioral phenomenon known as an *amotivational syndrome,* characterized by apathy, dullness, poor grooming, reduced interest in achievement, and disinterest in the pursuit of conventional goals. The precise relationship between marijuana and development of the syndrome is not known, nor is it certain what other factors may contribute. Available data do not suggest that the amotivational syndrome is due to organic brain damage.

Cannabinoid hyperemesis syndrome. Although this syndrome was first described in 2004, it was not commonly recognized until the increase in legalization of marijuana. Cannabinoid hyperemesis syndrome (CHS) is characterized by a pattern of cyclic nausea and vomiting often relieved by taking hot showers or baths and is diagnosed in chronic marijuana users. The mechanism behind CHS is unknown and thought to be quite paradoxical because many use marijuana for the relief of nausea and vomiting. The treatment for CHS is cessation of marijuana use.

Physiologic Effects
Cardiovascular Effects

Marijuana produces a dose-related increase in heart rate. Increases of 20 to 50 beats/min are typical. However, rates up to 140 beats/min are not uncommon. Pretreatment with propranolol prevents marijuana-induced tachycardia but does not block the drug's subjective effects. Marijuana causes orthostatic hypotension and pronounced reddening of the conjunctivae. These responses apparently result from vasodilation.

Respiratory Effects

When used *acutely,* marijuana produces *bronchodilation.* However, when smoked chronically, the drug causes airway constriction. In addition, chronic use is closely associated with development of bronchitis, sinusitis, and asthma. Lung cancer is another possible outcome. Animal studies have shown that tar from marijuana smoke is a more potent carcinogen than tar from cigarettes.

Effects on Reproduction

Research in animals has shown multiple effects on reproduction. In males, marijuana decreases spermatogenesis and testosterone levels. In females, the drug reduces levels of follicle-stimulating hormone, luteinizing hormone, and prolactin.

Multiple effects may be seen in babies and children who were exposed to marijuana in utero. Some babies present with trembling, altered responses to visual stimuli, and a high-pitched cry. Preschoolers may have a decreased ability to perform tasks that involve memory and sustained attention. Schoolchildren may exhibit deficits in memory, attentiveness, and problem solving.

Altered Brain Structure

Long-term marijuana use is associated with structural changes in the brain. Specifically, the volumes of the hippocampus and amygdala are reduced by an average of 12% and 7.1%, respectively. We do not know if volume reduction is due to reduced cell size, reduced synaptic density, or loss of glial cells or neurons. Interestingly, hippocampal volume loss occurs primarily in the left hemisphere.

Therapeutic use. In the United States there are no approved medical uses for marijuana. However, there *are* FDA-approved uses for three *purified* cannabinoids: THC, cannabidiol (CBD), and dronabinol, an analog of THC. An additional cannabinoid preparation—nabiximols—is approved in Canada.

Approved Uses for Cannabinoids

Suppression of emesis. Intense nausea and vomiting are common side effects of cancer chemotherapy. In certain patients, these responses can be suppressed more effectively with cannabinoids than with traditional antiemetics (e.g., prochlorperazine, metoclopramide). At this time, two cannabinoids—*dronabinol* (Marinol) and *nabilone* (Cesamet)—are available for antiemetic use. Dronabinol, a synthetic form of THC, is a schedule III drug. Nabilone, a THC derivative, is a schedule II drug. Dosage forms and dosages are presented in Chapter 66.

Appetite stimulation. Dronabinol is FDA approved for stimulating appetite in patients with acquired immunodeficiency disease (AIDS). By relieving anorexia, treatment may prevent or reverse loss of weight.

Treatment of seizure in lennox-gastaut and dravet syndromes. In 2018 the FDA approved the first CBD-based drug for the treatment of Lennox-Gastaut and Dravet syndrome, genetic conditions causing frequent seizures. Children with both Lennox-Gastaut and Dravet syndromes experience often difficult to control seizures that result in developmental delay and intellectual disability. Use of cannabidiol (Epidiolex) in children ages 2 years and older reduced the frequency of seizures. Epidiolex is an oral liquid dosed upon the weight of the child. It has been deemed a schedule V drug by the DEA.

Relief of neuropathic pain. Nabiximols (Sativex ♣), administered by oral spray, is approved in Canada for treating neuropathic pain caused by multiple sclerosis (MS). Nabiximols is a mixture of two cannabinoids: THC and cannabidiol. Because the cannabinoids in Sativex are absorbed through the oral mucosa, the product has a rapid onset (like smoked marijuana) while being devoid of the dangerous tars in marijuana smoke. In the United States nabiximols is under study for treating intractable cancer pain. However, the drug is not yet approved in the United States and cannot be legally imported, owing to its current classification as a schedule I substance.

Unapproved Uses for Cannabinoids

Glaucoma. In patients with glaucoma, smoking marijuana may reduce intraocular pressure. Unfortunately, marijuana may also reduce blood flow to the optic nerve. We do not know if the drug improves vision.

Multiple sclerosis. Whether smoked or ingested, marijuana appears to reduce spasticity and tremor of MS. Oral cannabinoids may also reduce urge incontinence. As discussed earlier, cannabinoids can reduce neuropathic pain of MS.

Pain. Certain strains of marijuana have been found useful in pain management. Specific types of pain include headache, joint pain, muscle

---

BOX 35.1   Current Marijuana Research

Effect of Cannabis and Endocannabinoids on HIV Neuropathic Pain NCT03099005
- Medical Marijuana and Its Effects on Motor Function in People With Multiple Sclerosis NCT02898974
- Effects of Vaporized Marijuana on Neuropathic Pain NCT01037088
- Vaporized Cannabis for Chronic Pain Associated With Sickle Cell Disease (Cannabis-SCD) NCT01771731
- Safety and Efficacy on Spasticity Symptoms of a Cannabis Sativa Extract in Motor Neuron Disease (CANALS) NCT01776970
- Investigation of Cannabis for Pain and Inflammation in Lung Cancer: NCT02675842
- Inhaled Cannabis Versus Fentanyl Buccal Tablets for Management of Breakthrough Pain in Cancer Patients: NCT03564548

HIV, Human immunodeficiency virus.

---

spasticity, and cancer-related pain. Limited research on the use of marijuana for pain is available but increasing (see next).

Medical Research on Marijuana

Proponents of making marijuana available by prescription argue that smoked marijuana can reduce chronic pain, suppress nausea caused by chemotherapy, improve appetite in patients with AIDS, lower intraocular pressure in patients with glaucoma, and suppress spasticity associated with MS and spinal cord injury. However, the evidence supporting most of these claims is weak—largely because federal regulations had effectively barred marijuana research.

In 2016 the DEA announced its intention to grant licenses to marijuana growers in the United States for use in research. Prior to that time, the University of Mississippi was the only contracted facility to grow marijuana for research. The FDA also released a statement that "Controlled clinical trials testing the safety and efficacy of a drug, along with careful review through the FDA's drug approval process, is the most appropriate way to bring marijuana-derived treatments to patients." Since that time, many studies have begun. Just a few of the many trials and research can be located at ClinicalTrials.gov and are listed in Box 35.1.

Legal Status of Marijuana

United States

Medical marijuana. Thirty-one states[a] and the District of Columbia have enacted laws that eliminate criminal penalties for medical use of marijuana, and more states are considering doing the same. Because of the new state laws, patients can currently possess and use small amounts of marijuana for medical purposes. In most of these states, qualified patients must have a debilitating medical condition plus documentation from their health care provider that medical use of marijuana "may be of benefit."

What about federal marijuana regulations? Because marijuana is classified by the DEA as a schedule I substance, health care providers still cannot *prescribe* the drug—all they can do is *suggest* it may be of benefit. Furthermore, in 2005, the U.S. Supreme Court ruled that DEA legislation trumps the new state laws, and hence people who use or provide medical marijuana can still be prosecuted under federal law, even in states where medical marijuana has been legalized. In a (delayed)

---

[a]Alaska, Arizona, Arkansas, California, Colorado, Connecticut, Delaware, Florida, Hawaii, Illinois, Louisiana, Maine, Maryland, Massachusetts, Michigan, Minnesota, Montana, Nevada, New Hampshire, New Jersey, New Mexico, New York, North Dakota, Ohio, Oklahoma, Oregon, Pennsylvania, Rhode Island, Vermont, Washington, and West Virginia.

TABLE 35.3   Potential[a] Drug Interactions With Marijuana

Drugs	Pathway	Potential Reaction
Warfarin	CYP450	Increased effects of warfarin
Chlorpromazine Theophylline	CYP1A2	Increased metabolism of chlorpromazine and theophylline
Ketoconazole Clarithromycin Erythromycin Cyclosporine Verapamil Itraconazole Voriconazole Boceprevir	CYP3A4	Increase peak concentrations of THC
Rifampin	CYP3A4	Reduce the serum levels of THC and CBD
Amiodarone, Cimetidine, Cotrimoxazole, Metronidazole, Fluoxetine, Fluvoxamine, Fluconazole Voriconazole	CYP2C9	Inhibit the elimination of THC

[a]Many of these are not research based.
CBD, Cannabidiol; *THC*, tetrahydrocannabinol.

---

response to this ruling, the Department of Justice, in 2009, instructed U.S. attorneys not to use federal resources to prosecute people whose actions comply with state laws that allow medical marijuana use. Hence although patients may be breaking federal law, the Department of Justice will not prosecute them.

Recreational marijuana. Nine[b] states and Washington, DC have passed legislation allowing the legal use of recreational marijuana. The first states to legalize the recreational use of marijuana were Colorado and Washington in 2012. Laws regarding growing, distribution, and use vary per individual state.

Canada. Medical use of marijuana has been legal in Canada since 2001, when the Marijuana Medical Access Regulations took effect. Patients with documentation from a health care provider can get their marijuana through Health Canada, or they can get a license to grow their own. According to the Government of Canada Department of Justice, recreational marijuana became legal for sale in Canada on October 17th, 2018.

Drug Interactions

Various drug interactions should be considered when prescribing medications to chronic marijuana users. THC is metabolized by the liver, specifically through the CYP2C9 and CYP3A4 pathways. CBD is processed through CYP3A4 and CYP2C19. In vitro studies demonstrate that both these substances can inhibit CYP450. Table 35.3 lists some of these potential interactions.

In addition, because of marijuana's ability to cause tachycardia, use with sympathomimetics or anticholinergics may increase this effect. Caution should also be used when combining marijuana with drugs that depress the CNS.

Synthetic Marijuana

Synthetic cannabis blends showed up on the market in the early 2000s. They became popular because of their availability and their lack of

---

[b]Alaska, California, Colorado, Maine, Massachusetts, Nevada, Oregon, Vermont, and Washington.

traces in drug tests. They were initially legal because they were thought to contain blends of natural herbs sprayed with chemicals that mimic the effects of THC. These chemicals come in two classes: THC analogs and other compounds.

Although synthetic marijuana was once thought harmless, the American Association of Poison Control Centers reported more than 7000 calls regarding synthetic marijuana in a 2-year period. In addition, several deaths and many episodes of florid psychosis and toxicity are possibly related to synthetic marijuana use. Side effects include hypertension, nausea, vomiting, anxiety, agitation, paranoid behavior, hallucinations, and catatonic state. By 2011 the FDA had placed many of these chemicals on the controlled substances list as schedule I drugs, making them illegal to possess. However, more than 500 compounds exist; therefore synthetic marijuana is still available. Many organizations, including the U.S. military, have banned all similar compounds.

PSYCHEDELICS

The psychedelics are a fascinating drug family for which LSD can be considered the prototype. Other family members include mescaline, dimethyltryptamine (DMT), psilocin, and salvia. The psychedelics are so named because of their ability to produce what has been termed a *psychedelic state*. Individuals in this state show an increased awareness of sensory stimuli and are likely to perceive the world around them as beautiful and harmonious; the normally insignificant may assume exceptional meaning, the "self" may seem split into an "observer" and a "doer," and boundaries between "self" and "nonself" may fade, producing a sense of unity with the cosmos.

Psychedelic drugs are often referred to as *hallucinogens* or *psychotomimetics*. These names reflect their ability to produce hallucinations and mental states that resemble psychoses.

Although psychedelics can cause hallucinations and psychotic-like states, these are not their most characteristic effects. The characteristic that truly distinguishes the psychedelics from other agents is their *ability to bring on the same types of alterations in thought, perception, and feeling that otherwise occur only in dreams*. In essence, the psychedelics seem able to activate mechanisms for dreaming without causing unconsciousness.

d-Lysergic Acid Diethylamide
History

The first person to experience LSD was a Swiss chemist named Albert Hofmann. In 1943, 5 years after LSD was first synthesized, Hofmann accidentally ingested a minute amount of the drug. The result was a dreamlike state accompanied by perceptual distortions and vivid hallucinations. The high potency and unusual actions of LSD led to speculation that it might provide a model for studying psychosis. Unfortunately, that speculation did not prove correct: extensive research has shown that the effects of LSD cannot be equated with idiopathic psychosis. With the realization that LSD did not produce a "model psychosis," medical interest in the drug declined. However, not everyone lost interest; during the 1960s, nonmedical experimentation flourished. This widespread use caused substantial societal concern, and, by 1970, LSD had been classified as a schedule I substance. Nonetheless, street use of LSD continues.

Mechanism of Action

LSD acts at multiple sites in the brain and spinal cord. However, effects are most prominent in the cerebral cortex and the locus coeruleus. Effects are thought to result from activation of serotonin-2 receptors. This concept has been reinforced by the observation that *ritanserin*, a selective blocker of serotonin-2 receptors, can prevent the effects of LSD in animals.

Time Course

LSD is usually administered orally but can also be injected or smoked. With oral dosing, initial effects can be felt in minutes. Over the next few hours, responses become progressively more intense and then subside 8 to 12 hours later.

Subjective and Behavioral Effects

Responses to LSD can be diverse, complex, and changeable. The drug can alter thinking, feeling, perception, sense of self, and sense of relationship with the environment and other people. LSD-induced experiences may be sublime or terrifying. Just what will be experienced during any particular "trip" cannot be predicted.

Perceptual alterations can be dramatic. Colors may appear iridescent or glowing, kaleidoscopic images may appear, and vivid hallucinations may occur. Sensory experiences may merge so that colors seem to be heard and sounds seem to be visible. Afterimages may occur, causing current perceptions to overlap with preceding perceptions. The LSD user may feel a sense of wonderment and awe at the beauty of commonplace things.

LSD can have a profound influence on affect. Emotions may range from elation, good humor, and euphoria to sadness, dysphoria, and fear. The intensity of emotion may be overwhelming.

Thoughts may turn inward. Attitudes may be reevaluated and old values assigned new priorities. A sense of new and important insight may be felt. However, despite the intensity of these experiences, enduring changes in beliefs, behavior, and personality are rare.

Physiologic Effects

LSD has few physiologic effects. Activation of the sympathetic nervous system can produce tachycardia, elevation of blood pressure, mydriasis, piloerection, and hyperthermia. Neuromuscular effects (tremor, incoordination, hyperreflexia, and muscular weakness) may also occur.

Tolerance and Dependence

Tolerance to LSD develops rapidly. Substantial tolerance can be seen after just three or four daily doses. Tolerance to subjective and behavioral effects develops to a greater extent than to cardiovascular effects. Cross-tolerance exists with mescaline and psilocybin but not with DMT. Because DMT is similar to LSD, the absence of cross-tolerance is surprising. There is no cross-tolerance with amphetamines or THC. On cessation of LSD use, tolerance rapidly fades. Abrupt withdrawal of LSD is not associated with an abstinence syndrome. Hence there is no evidence for physical dependence.

Toxicity

Toxic reactions are primarily psychological. LSD has never been a direct cause of death, although fatalities have occurred from accidents and suicides.

Acute panic reactions are relatively common and may be associated with a fear of disintegration of the self. Such "bad trips" can usually be managed by a process of "talking down" (providing emotional support and reassurance in a nonthreatening environment). Panic episodes can also be managed with an antianxiety agent, such as diazepam. Neuroleptics (e.g., haloperidol, chlorpromazine) may actually intensify the experience, and hence their use is questionable.

A small percentage of former LSD users experience episodic visual disturbances, referred to as *flashbacks* by users and *hallucinogen persisting perception disorder* (HPPD) by clinicians. These disturbances may manifest as geometric pseudohallucinations, flashes of color, or positive afterimages. Visual disturbances may be precipitated by several factors, including marijuana use, fatigue, stress, and anxiety. Phenothiazines exacerbate these experiences rather than providing relief. HPPD appears to be caused by permanent changes in the visual system.

In addition to panic reactions and visual disturbances, LSD can cause other adverse psychological effects. Depressive episodes, dissociative reactions, and distortions of body image may occur. When an LSD experience has been intensely terrifying, the user may be left with persistent residual fear. The drug may also cause prolonged psychotic reactions. In contrast to acute effects, which differ substantially from symptoms of schizophrenia, prolonged psychotic reactions mimic schizophrenia faithfully.

Salvia

Salvia divinorum is a hallucinogenic herb native to southern Mexico and to Central and South America. Its primary psychoactive component is *salvinorin A,* a potent activator of κ-opioid receptors. The genus *Salvia,* a part of the mint family, is commonly known as sage—hence the colorful street names for *S. divinorum:* magic mint, diviner's sage, and sage of the seers. Salvia is legal in some states, illegal in others, and not yet regulated under the Controlled Substances Act.

Salvia is used extensively in the United States, primarily by teens and young adults. In 2015, 1.8% of high school seniors reported using the drug in the past year. Approximately 15% of Americans older than 12 years report having used a hallucinogen such as salvia at least once in their lives.

How is salvia administered? Among Mexican Indians, the traditional method is to chew the leaves or drink a liquid extract. In contrast, recreational users usually smoke the dried leaves, either in a pipe or rolled in a joint. When the smoke is inhaled, salvinorin A undergoes rapid absorption from the lungs. As a result, psychological effects begin quickly (in less than 1 minute) and then quickly fade (typically in 5–10 minutes).

Like other psychedelic drugs, salvia induces a dreamlike state of unreality. Users may lose awareness of their own bodies and of the room they are in. They may feel they are floating, traveling through time and space, or merging with or transforming into objects. Some feel they are being twisted or pulled. There may be a sense of overlapping realities and of being in several places at once. Speech may become slurred, and sentences may lack fluent structure. Uncontrollable laughter may break out. Possible physical effects include chills, dizziness, nausea, incoordination, and bradycardia. Whether salvia poses long-term health risks has not been studied. However, we do know that Mexican Indians have used the drug for generations, with no apparent ill effects.

Mescaline, Psilocin, Psilocybin, and Dimethyltryptamine

In addition to LSD and salvia, the family of psychedelic drugs includes mescaline, psilocin, psilocybin, DMT, and several related compounds. Some psychedelics are synthetic, and some occur naturally. DMT and LSD represent the synthetic compounds. Mescaline, a constituent of the peyote cactus, and psilocin and psilocybin, constituents of "magic mushrooms," represent compounds found in nature.

The subjective and behavioral effects of the miscellaneous psychedelic drugs are similar to those of LSD. Like LSD, these drugs can elicit modes of thought, perception, and feeling that are normally restricted to dreams. In addition, they can cause hallucinations and induce mental states that resemble psychosis.

The miscellaneous psychedelics differ from LSD with respect to potency and time course. LSD is the most potent of the psychedelics, producing its full spectrum of effects at doses as low as 0.5 µg/kg. Psilocin and psilocybin are 100 times less potent than LSD, and mescaline is 4000 times less potent than LSD. Although the effects of LSD are prolonged (responses may last 12 or more hours), the effects of mescaline

and DMT are shorter: responses to mescaline usually fade within 8 to 12 hours, and responses to DMT fade within 1 to 2 hours.

Dissociative Drugs

The dissociative drugs phencyclidine (PCP) and ketamine were originally developed as surgical anesthetics. When taken recreationally, these drugs distort perception of sight and sound and produce feelings of dissociation (detachment) from the environment. High doses can produce sedation, immobility, analgesia, and amnesia.

Phencyclidine

PCP was originally developed as an anesthetic for animals. The drug was tried briefly as a general anesthetic for humans but was withdrawn, owing to severe emergence of delirium. Although rejected for therapeutic use, PCP has become widely used as a drug of abuse, largely because it can be synthesized easily by amateur chemists, making it cheap and abundant.

PCP produces a unique set of effects. Hallucinations are prominent. In addition, the drug can produce CNS depression, CNS excitation, and analgesia. At low doses, PCP produces effects like those of alcohol. Low-dose intoxication is characterized by euphoria, release of inhibitions, and emotional lability. As dosage increases, the clinical picture becomes more variable and complex. Symptoms include excitation, disorientation, and reduced perception of tactile and painful stimuli. High doses can cause severe adverse physiologic and psychological effects. Psychological effects include hallucinations, confusional states, combativeness, and psychosis.

DEXTROMETHORPHAN

Dextromethorphan (DXM) is a cough suppressant widely available in over-the-counter cough and cold remedies (see Chapter 63). At the low doses needed for cough suppression, DXM is devoid of psychological effects. However, at doses 5 to 10 times higher, DXM can cause euphoria, disorientation, paranoia, and altered sense of time, as well as visual, auditory, and tactile hallucinations. These effects are produced by dextrorphan, a metabolite of DXM that blocks receptors for *N*-methyl-D-aspartate. Note that this is the same mechanism used by PCP and ketamine. Many of the products that contain DXM also contain other drugs, including acetaminophen, antihistamines, phenylephrine, and pseudoephedrine. Therefore when excessive doses are taken, users are subject to toxicity from these compounds and from DXM itself. Many products contain DXM, including Coricidin HBP Cough & Cold, Robitussin DM, and Vicks NyQuil Cough Syrup.

3,4-METHYLENEDIOXYMETHAMPHETAMINE (MDMA, ECSTASY)

MDMA, also known as "ecstasy or Molly," is a complex drug with stimulant and psychedelic properties. The drug is structurally related to methamphetamine (a stimulant) and mescaline (a hallucinogen). Low doses produce mild LSD-like psychedelic effects; higher doses produce amphetamine-like stimulant effects. These effects result from (1) blocking reuptake of serotonin and (2) promoting the release of serotonin, dopamine, and norepinephrine. Although MDMA can produce effects that are clearly pleasurable, it can also be dangerous; the biggest concerns are neurotoxicity, seizures, excessive cardiovascular stimulation, and hyperthermia and its sequelae. MDMA is classified as a schedule I drug.

Time Course and Dosage

MDMA is usually dosed orally but may also be snorted, injected, or inserted as a rectal suppository. With oral administration, effects begin in 20 minutes, peak in 2 to 3 hours, and persist 4 to 5 hours. The usual dose is 100 mg or less.

Who Uses MDMA and Why?

MDMA is used primarily by adolescents and young adults. According to a survey conducted in 2015, the use of MDMA in school-age children has continued to steadily decline.

Why do people take MDMA? Because it makes them feel very good. The drug can elevate mood, increase sensory awareness, and heighten sensitivity to music. It can also facilitate interpersonal relationships: users report a sense of closeness with others, lowering of defenses, reduced anxiety, enhanced communication, and increased sociability.

Adverse Effects

MDMA is not free of risks. The drug can injure serotonergic neurons, stimulate the heart, and raise body temperature to a dangerous level. In addition, it can cause neurologic effects (e.g., seizures, spasmodic jerking, jaw clenching, teeth grinding) and a host of adverse psychological effects (e.g., confusion, anxiety, paranoia, panic attacks, visual hallucinations, and suicidal thoughts and behavior). Every year, MDMA is associated with several thousand admissions to emergency departments, mainly because of seizures.

MDMA can damage serotonergic neurons, perhaps irreversibly. When administered to rats and primates in doses only two to four times greater than those that produce hallucinations in humans, MDMA causes *irreversible destruction of serotonergic neurons,* resulting in passivity and insomnia. At least three lines of evidence suggest that MDMA is also neurotoxic in humans. First, MDMA causes dose-related impairment of memory, a brain function mediated in part by serotonin. Memory impairment persists long after MDMA was last taken. Second, the cerebrospinal fluid of long-term MDMA users contains abnormally low concentrations of serotonin metabolites, suggesting a loss of serotonergic neurons. And third, using positron emission tomography to study former MDMA users, researchers demonstrated decreased binding of a ligand selective for the serotonin transporter, indicating damage to serotonergic neurons. In this study, reductions in ligand binding correlated with the extent of MDMA use and not with the duration of abstinence.

MDMA can cause hyperthermia in association with dehydration, hyponatremia, and rhabdomyolysis. Treatment consists of rapid cooling, rehydration, and administering dantrolene (Dantrium), a drug that relaxes skeletal muscle, thereby reducing heat generation and the risk for rhabdomyolysis. The risk for hyperthermia and dehydration could be greatly reduced by providing ample fluids at dance parties known as "raves" and other events where MDMA is likely to be used.

Because of its amphetamine-like actions, MDMA can increase heart rate, blood pressure, and myocardial oxygen consumption. Remarkably, the increases in heart rate and blood pressure equal those produced by maximal doses of dobutamine, a powerful adrenergic agonist (see Chapter 15). Cardiovascular stimulation poses a special risk to users with heart disease.

INHALANTS

The inhalants are a diverse group of drugs that have one characteristic in common: administration by inhalation. These drugs can be divided into anesthetics and organic solvents.

Anesthetics

Provided that dosage is modest, anesthetics produce subjective effects similar to those of alcohol (euphoria, exhilaration, loss of inhibitions). The anesthetics that have been abused most are *nitrous oxide* ("laughing gas") and *ether.* One reason for the popularity of these drugs is ease of administration: both agents can be used without exotic equipment. For nitrous oxide, ready availability also promotes use: small cylinders of the drug, marketed for aerating whipping cream, can be purchased without restriction.

Organic Solvents

A wide assortment of solvents has been inhaled to induce intoxication. These compounds include *toluene, gasoline, lighter fluid, paint thinner, nail polish remover, benzene, acetone, chloroform,* and *model-airplane glue.* These agents are used primarily by children and the very poor—people who, because of age or insufficient funds, lack access to more conventional drugs of abuse. In recent years, use of inhalants by young children and teens has been rising.

Administration

Solvents are administered by three processes, referred to as "bagging," "huffing," and "sniffing." Bagging is performed by pouring solvent in a bag and inhaling the vapor. Huffing is performed by pouring the solvent on a rag and inhaling the vapor. Sniffing is performed by inhaling the solvent directly from its container.

Acute Pharmacologic Effects

The acute effects of organic solvents are somewhat like those of alcohol (euphoria, impaired judgment, slurred speech, flushing, CNS depression). In addition, these compounds can cause visual hallucinations and disorientation with respect to time and place. High doses can result in sudden death. Possible causes include anoxia, respiratory depression, vagal stimulation (which slows heart rate), and dysrhythmias.

Chronic Toxicity

Prolonged use is associated with multiple toxicities. For example, chloroform is toxic to the heart, liver, and kidneys, and toluene can cause severe brain damage and bone marrow depression. Many solvents can damage the heart; fatal dysrhythmias have occurred secondary to drug-induced heart block.

ANABOLIC STEROIDS

Many athletes take anabolic steroids (androgens) to enhance athletic performance. The principal benefit is increased muscle mass and strength. Because of the massive doses that are used, the risk for adverse effects is substantial. With long-term steroid use, an addiction syndrome develops. Because of their abuse potential, most androgens are now classified as schedule III drugs. The basic pharmacology of androgens and their abuse by athletes are discussed in Chapter 52.

Review of Hemodynamics

Hemodynamics is the study of the movement of blood throughout the circulatory system as well as the regulatory mechanisms and driving forces involved. Concepts introduced here reappear throughout the chapters on cardiovascular drugs, so we urge you to review these now. Because this is a pharmacology text and not a physiology text, discussion is limited to hemodynamic factors that have particular relevance to the actions of drugs.

OVERVIEW OF THE CIRCULATORY SYSTEM

The circulatory system has two primary functions: (1) delivery of oxygen, nutrients, hormones, electrolytes, and other essentials to cells; and (2) removal of carbon dioxide and metabolic wastes from cells. In addition, the system helps fight infection.

The circulatory system has two major divisions: the *pulmonary circulation* and the *systemic circulation*. The pulmonary circulation delivers blood to the lungs. The systemic circulation delivers blood to all other organs and tissues. The systemic circulation is also known as the *greater circulation* or *peripheral circulation.*

Components of the Circulatory System

The circulatory system is composed of the *heart* and *blood vessels.* The heart is the pump that moves blood through the arterial tree. The blood vessels have several functions:
- *Arteries* transport blood under high pressure to tissues.
- *Arterioles* are control vessels that regulate local blood flow.
- *Capillaries* are the sites for exchange of fluid, oxygen, carbon dioxide, nutrients, hormones, and wastes.
- *Venules* collect blood from the capillaries.
- *Veins* transport blood back to the heart. In addition, veins serve as a major reservoir for blood.

Arteries and veins differ with respect to distensibility (elasticity). Arteries are very muscular and hence do not readily stretch. As a result, large increases in arterial pressure (AP) cause only small increases in arterial diameter. Veins are much less muscular and hence are 6 to 10 times more distensible. As a result, small increases in venous pressure cause large increases in vessel diameter, which produce a large increase in venous volume.

Distribution of Blood

The adult circulatory system contains about 5 L of blood, which is distributed throughout the system. As indicated in Fig. 36.1, 9% is in the pulmonary circulation, 7% is in the heart, and 84% is in the systemic circulation. Within the systemic circulation, however, distribution is uneven: most (64%) of the blood is in veins, venules, and venous sinuses; the remaining 20% is in arteries (13%) and arterioles or capillaries (7%). The large volume of blood in the venous system serves as a reservoir.

What Makes Blood Flow?

Blood moves within vessels because the force that drives flow is greater than the resistance to flow. As shown in Fig. 36.2, the force that drives blood flow is the pressure gradient between two points in a vessel. Blood will flow from the point where pressure is higher toward the point where pressure is lower. Resistance to flow is determined by the diameter and length of the vessel and by blood viscosity. From a pharmacologic viewpoint, the most important determinant of resistance is vessel diameter: the larger the vessel, the smaller the resistance. Accordingly, when vessels dilate, resistance declines, causing blood flow to increase; and when vessels constrict, resistance rises, causing blood flow to decline. To maintain adequate flow when resistance rises, blood pressure must rise as well.

How Does Blood Get Back to the Heart?

As indicated in Fig. 36.3, pressure falls progressively as blood moves through the systemic circulation. Pressure is 120 mm Hg when blood enters the aorta, 30 mm Hg when blood enters capillaries, and only 18 mm Hg when blood leaves capillaries; it then drops to negative values (0 to 5 mm Hg) in the right atrium. (Negative atrial pressure is generated by expansion of the chest during inspiration.)

Given that pressure is only 18 mm Hg when blood leaves capillaries, we must ask, "How does blood get back to the heart?" In addition to the small pressure head in venules, three mechanisms help ensure venous return. First, negative pressure in the right atrium helps "suck" blood toward the heart. Second, constriction of smooth muscle in the venous wall increases venous pressure, which helps drive blood toward the heart. Third and most important, the combination of venous valves and skeletal muscle contraction constitutes an auxiliary "venous pump." As shown in Fig. 36.4A, the veins are equipped with a system of one-way valves. When skeletal muscles contract (see Fig. 36.4B), venous blood is squeezed toward the heart—the only direction the valves will permit.

REGULATION OF CARDIAC OUTPUT

In the average adult, cardiac output is about 5 L/min. Hence, every minute, the heart pumps the equivalent of all the blood in the body. In this section, we consider the major factors that determine how much blood the heart pumps.

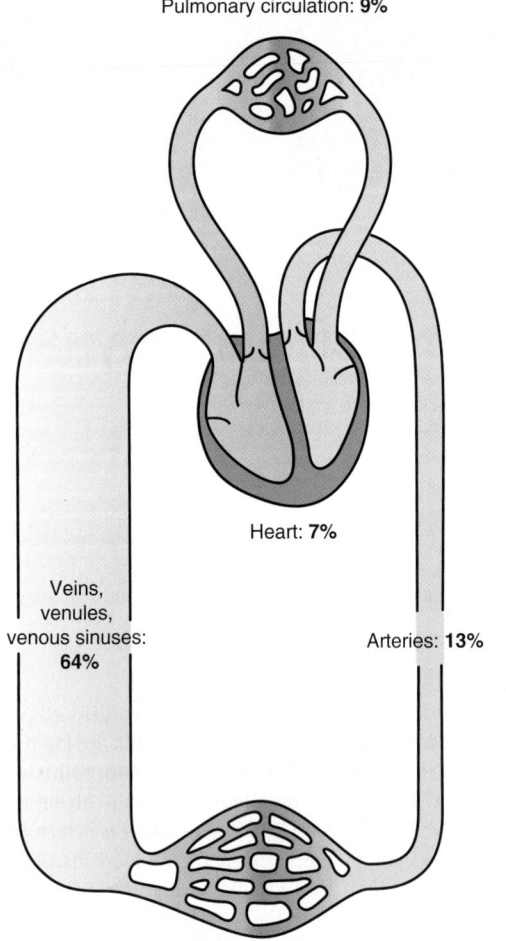

Fig. 36.1 Distribution of Blood in the Circulatory System. A large percentage of the blood resides in the venous system.

Fig. 36.2 Forces That Promote and Impede Flow of Blood. Blood flows from the point of higher pressure toward the point of lower pressure. Resistance to flow is determined by vessel diameter, vessel length, and blood viscosity.

Determinants of Cardiac Output

The basic equation for cardiac output is:

$$CO = HR \times SV$$

where CO is cardiac output, HR is heart rate, and SV is stroke volume. According to the equation, an increase in HR or SV will increase CO, whereas a decrease in HR or SV will decrease CO. For the average

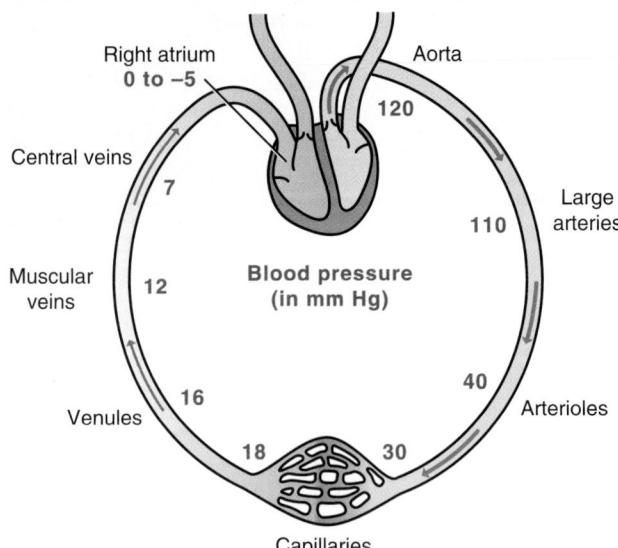

Fig. 36.3 Distribution of Pressure Within the Systemic Circulation. Pressure is highest when blood leaves the left ventricle, falls to only 18 mm Hg as blood exits capillaries, and reaches negative values within the right atrium.

person, heart rate is about 70 beats/min and stroke volume is about 70 mL. Multiplying these, we get 4.9 L/min—the average value for CO.

Heart Rate

Heart rate is controlled primarily by the autonomic nervous system (ANS). Rate is increased by the sympathetic branch acting through β_1-adrenergic receptors in the sinoatrial (SA) node. Rate is decreased by the parasympathetic branch acting through muscarinic receptors in the SA node. Parasympathetic impulses reach the heart through the vagus nerve.

Stroke Volume

Stroke volume is determined largely by three factors: (1) myocardial contractility, (2) cardiac afterload, and (3) cardiac preload. *Myocardial contractility* is defined as the force with which the ventricles contract. Contractility is determined primarily by the degree of cardiac dilation, which in turn is determined by the amount of venous return. The importance of venous return in regulating contractility and SV is discussed separately later. In addition to regulation by venous return, contractility can be increased by the sympathetic nervous system, acting through β_1-adrenergic receptors in the myocardium.

Preload

Preload is formally defined as the amount of tension (stretch) applied to a muscle before contraction. In the heart, stretch is determined by ventricular filling pressure—that is, the *force of venous return:* the greater filling pressure, the more the ventricles will stretch. Cardiac preload can be expressed as either *end-diastolic volume* or *end-diastolic pressure*. As discussed later, an increase in preload will increase SV, whereas a decrease in preload will reduce SV. Frequently the terms *preload* and *force of venous return* are used interchangeably—although they are not truly equivalent.

Afterload

Afterload is formally defined as the load against which a muscle exerts its force (i.e., the load a muscle must overcome in order to contract). For the heart, afterload is the *arterial pressure* that the left ventricle must overcome to eject blood. Common sense tells us that if afterload

Fig. 36.4 Venous Valves and the Auxiliary Venous "Pump." (A) Veins and their one-way valves in the leg. The configuration of these valves ensures that blood will move toward the heart. (B) Contraction of skeletal muscle pumps venous blood toward the heart.

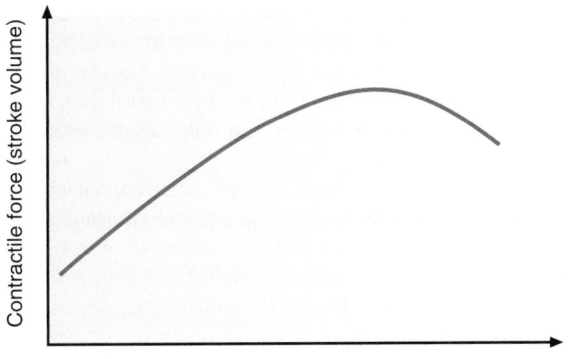

Fig. 36.5 The Starling Relationship Between Myocardial Fiber Length and Contractile Force. An increase in fiber length produces a corresponding increase in contractile force. Fiber length increases as the ventricles enlarge during filling. Increased contractile force is reflected by increased stroke volume.

increases, SV will decrease. Conversely, if afterload falls, SV will rise. Cardiac afterload is determined primarily by the degree of peripheral resistance, which in turn is determined by the constriction and dilation of arterioles. That is, when arterioles constrict, peripheral resistance rises, causing AP (afterload) to rise as well. Conversely, when arterioles dilate, peripheral resistance falls, causing AP to decline.

The Starling Law of the Heart

The *Starling law* states that the force of ventricular contraction is proportional to muscle fiber length (up to a point). Accordingly, as fiber length (ventricular diameter) increases, there is a corresponding increase in contractile force (Fig. 36.5). Because of this built-in mechanism, when more blood enters the heart, more is pumped out. As a result, the healthy heart is able to precisely match its output with the volume of blood delivered by veins. That is, when venous return increases, CO increases correspondingly. Conversely, when venous return declines, CO declines to precisely the same extent. Hence under normal, nonstressed conditions, SV is determined by factors that regulate venous return.

Why does contractile force change as a function of fiber length (ventricular diameter)? Recall that muscle contraction results from the interaction of two proteins: actin and myosin. As the heart stretches in response to increased ventricular filling, actin and myosin are brought into a more optimal alignment with each other, which allows them to interact with greater force.

Factors That Determine Venous Return

Having established that venous return is the primary determinant of SV (and hence CO), we need to understand the factors that determine venous return. With regard to pharmacology, the most important factor is *systemic filling pressure* (i.e., the force that returns blood to the heart). The normal value for filling pressure is 7 mm Hg. This value can be raised to 17 mm Hg by the constriction of veins. Filling pressure can also be raised by an increase in blood volume. Conversely, filling pressure, and hence venous return, can be lowered by venodilation or by reducing blood volume. Blood volume and venous tone can both be altered with drugs.

In addition to systemic filling pressure, three other factors influence venous return: (1) the auxiliary muscle pumps discussed previously, (2) resistance to flow between peripheral vessels and the right atrium, and (3) right atrial pressure, elevation of which will impede venous return. None of these factors can be directly influenced with drugs.

The Starling Law and Maintenance of Systemic-Pulmonary Balance

Because the myocardium operates in accord with the Starling law, the right and left ventricles always pump exactly the same amount of blood. When venous return increases, SV of the right ventricle increases, thereby increasing delivery of blood to the pulmonary circulation, which in turn delivers more blood to the left ventricle; this increases filling of the left ventricle, which causes *its* SV to increase. Because an increase in venous return causes the output of *both* ventricles to increase, blood flow through the systemic and pulmonary circulations is always in balance as long as the heart is healthy.

In the failing heart, the Starling law breaks down. That is, the force of contraction no longer increases in proportion to increased ventricular filling. As a result, blood backs up behind the failing ventricle (Fig. 36.6). In this example, output of the left ventricle is 1% less than the

Fig. 36.6 Systemic-Pulmonary Imbalance That Develops When the Output of the Left and Right Ventricles Is Not Identical. In this example, the output of the left ventricle *(LV)* is 1% less than the output of the right ventricle *(RV)*. Hence while the right ventricle pumps 5000 mL/min, the left pumps only 4950 mL/min—50 mL/min less than the right side. This causes blood to back up in the pulmonary circulation. After 20 minutes, 1000 mL of blood has shifted from the systemic circulation to the pulmonary circulation. Death would ensue in less than 40 minutes. Numbers in the pulmonary and systemic circulations indicate volume of blood in liters.

output of the right ventricle, which causes blood to back up in the pulmonary circulation. In only 20 minutes, this small imbalance between left and right ventricular output shifts a liter of blood from the systemic circulation to the pulmonary circulation. In less than 40 minutes, death from pulmonary congestion would ensue. This example underscores the importance of systemic-pulmonary balance and the critical role of the Starling mechanism in maintaining it.

REGULATION OF ARTERIAL PRESSURE

AP is the driving force that moves blood through the arterial side of the systemic circulation. The general formula for AP is:

$$AP = PR \times CO$$

where AP is arterial pressure, PR is peripheral resistance, and CO is cardiac output. Accordingly, an increase in PR or CO will increase AP, whereas a decrease in PR or CO will decrease AP. Peripheral resistance is regulated primarily through constriction and dilation of arterioles. Cardiac output is regulated by the mechanisms discussed previously. Regulation of AP through processes that alter PR and CO is discussed later.

Overview of Control Systems

Under normal circumstances, AP is regulated primarily by three systems: the ANS, the renin-angiotensin-aldosterone system (RAAS), and the kidneys. These systems differ greatly with regard to time frame of response. The ANS acts in two ways: (1) it responds rapidly (in seconds or minutes) to acute changes in blood pressure; and (2) it provides steady-state control. The RAAS responds more slowly, taking hours or days to influence AP. The kidneys are responsible for long-term control and hence may take days or weeks to adjust AP.

AP is also regulated by a fourth system: a family of natriuretic peptides. These peptides come into play primarily under conditions of volume overload.

Steady-State Control by the Autonomic Nervous System

The ANS regulates AP by adjusting CO and PR. Sympathetic tone to the heart increases HR and contractility, thereby increasing CO. In contrast, parasympathetic tone slows the heart and thereby reduces CO. As discussed in Chapter 13, constriction of blood vessels is regulated exclusively by the sympathetic branch of the ANS; blood vessels have no parasympathetic innervation. Steady-state sympathetic tone provides a moderate level of vasoconstriction. The resultant resistance to blood flow maintains AP. Complete elimination of sympathetic tone would cause AP to fall by 50%.

Rapid Control by the Autonomic Nervous System: The Baroreceptor Reflex

The baroreceptor reflex serves to maintain AP at a predetermined level. When AP changes, the reflex immediately attempts to restore AP to the preset value.

The reflex works as follows: Baroreceptors (pressure sensors) in the aortic arch and carotid sinus sense AP and relay this information to the vasoconstrictor center of the medulla. When AP changes, the vasoconstrictor center compensates by sending appropriate instructions to arterioles, veins, and heart. For example, when AP drops, the vasoconstrictor center causes (1) constriction of nearly all arterioles, thereby increasing PR; (2) constriction of veins, thereby increasing venous return; and (3) acceleration of HR (by increasing sympathetic impulses to the heart and decreasing parasympathetic impulses). The combined effect of these responses is to restore AP to the preset level. When AP rises too high, opposite responses occur: the reflex dilates arterioles and veins and slows the heart.

The baroreceptor reflex is poised for rapid action but not for sustained action. When AP falls or rises, the reflex acts within seconds to restore the preset pressure. However, when AP *remains* elevated or lowered, the system resets to the new pressure within 1 to 2 days. After this, the system perceives the new (elevated or reduced) pressure as "normal" and ceases to respond.

Drugs that lower AP will trigger the baroreceptor reflex. For example, if we administer a drug that dilates arterioles, the resultant drop in PR will reduce AP, causing the baroreceptor reflex to activate. The most noticeable response is *reflex tachycardia*. The baroreceptor reflex can temporarily negate efforts to lower AP with drugs.

The Renin-Angiotensin-Aldosterone System

The RAAS supports AP by causing (1) constriction of arterioles and veins and (2) retention of water by the kidneys. Vasoconstriction is mediated by a hormone named *angiotensin II*. Water retention is mediated in part by *aldosterone* through retention of sodium. Responses develop in hours (vasoconstriction) to days (water retention). The RAAS and its role in controlling blood pressure are discussed in Chapter 36.

Renal Retention of Water

When AP remains low for a long time, the kidneys respond by retaining water, which in turn causes AP to rise. Pressure rises because fluid retention increases blood volume, which increases venous pressure, which increases venous return, which increases CO, which increases AP. Water retention is a mechanism for maintaining AP over long periods (weeks, months, years).

Reduction in AP causes the kidneys to retain water, because low AP reduces renal blood flow (RBF), which in turn reduces glomerular filtration rate (GFR). Because less fluid is filtered, less urine is produced, and therefore more water is retained. Low AP activates the RAAS, causing levels of angiotensin II and aldosterone to rise. Angiotensin II causes constriction of renal blood vessels and thereby further decreases RBF and GFR. Aldosterone promotes renal retention of sodium, which causes water to be retained along with it.

Postural Hypotension

Postural hypotension, also known as *orthostatic hypotension,* is a reduction in AP that can occur when we move from a supine or seated position to an upright position. The cause of hypotension is pooling of blood in veins, which decreases venous return, which in turn decreases CO. Between 300 and 800 mL of blood can pool in veins when we stand, causing CO to drop by as much as 2 L/min. When we stand, gravity increases the pressure that blood exerts on veins. Because veins are not very muscular, they are unable to retain their shape when pressure increases; hence they stretch. The resultant increase in venous volume allows blood to pool.

Two mechanisms help overcome postural hypotension. One is the system of auxiliary venous pumps, which promote venous return. In fact, in healthy individuals, these auxiliary pumps usually prevent postural hypotension from occurring in the first place. When postural hypotension does occur, the baroreceptor reflex can restore AP by (1) constricting veins and arterioles and (2) increasing HR.

What would happen if we gave a drug that promoted dilation of veins (or prevented them from constricting)? In patients taking drugs that interfere with venoconstriction, postural hypotension is more intense and more prolonged. Hypotension is more intense because venous pooling is greater. Hypotension is more prolonged because there is no venoconstriction to help reverse venous pooling. As with drugs that reduce AP by dilating arterioles, drugs that reduce AP by relaxing veins can trigger the baroreceptor reflex and thereby cause reflex tachycardia.

Natriuretic Peptides

Natriuretic peptides serve to protect the cardiovascular system in the event of volume overload, a condition that increases preload and thereby increases CO and AP. Volume overload is caused by excessive retention of sodium and water. Natriuretic peptides work primarily by (1) reducing blood volume and (2) promoting dilation of arterioles and veins. Both actions lower AP.

The family of natriuretic peptides has three principal members: *atrial natriuretic peptide* (ANP), *B-* or *brain natriuretic peptide* (BNP), and *C-natriuretic peptide* (CNP). ANP is produced by myocytes of the atria; BNP is produced by myocytes of the ventricles (and to a lesser extent by cells in the brain, where BNP was discovered); and CNP is produced by cells of the vascular endothelium. When blood volume is excessive, all three peptides are released. (Release of ANP and BNP is triggered by stretching of the atria and ventricles, which occurs because of increased preload.)

ANP and BNP have similar actions. Both peptides reduce blood volume and increase venous capacitance and thereby reduce cardiac preload. Three processes are involved. First, ANP and BNP shift fluid from the vascular system to the extravascular compartment; the underlying mechanism is increased vascular permeability. Second, these peptides act on the kidney to cause diuresis (loss of water) and natriuresis (loss of sodium). Third, they promote dilation of arterioles and veins, in part by suppressing sympathetic outflow from the central nervous system. In addition to these actions, ANP and BNP help protect the heart during the early phase of heart failure by suppressing both the RAAS and sympathetic outflow and by inhibiting proliferation of myocytes. Although CNP shares some actions of ANP and BNP, its primary action is to promote vasodilation.

Diuretics

Diuretics have two major applications: in the treatment of hypertension and the mobilization of edematous fluid associated with heart failure, cirrhosis, or kidney disease. In addition, because of their ability to maintain urine flow, diuretics are used to prevent renal failure.

REVIEW OF RENAL ANATOMY AND PHYSIOLOGY

An understanding of the diuretic drugs requires a basic knowledge of the anatomy and physiology of the kidney. Therefore these topics are reviewed first before the diuretics themselves are discussed.

Anatomy

The basic functional unit of the kidney is the *nephron*. As indicated in Fig. 37.1, the nephron has four functionally distinct regions: (1) the *glomerulus*, (2) the *proximal convoluted tubule (PCT)*, (3) the *loop of Henle*, and (4a, 4b) the *distal convoluted tubule*. All nephrons are oriented within the kidney such that the upper portion of the loop of Henle is located in the renal cortex and the lower end of the loop descends toward the renal *medulla*. Without this orientation, the kidney could not produce concentrated urine.

In addition to the nephrons, the *collecting ducts* (the tubules into which the nephrons pour their contents) play a critical role in kidney function. The final segment of the distal convoluted tubule (4b) plus the collecting duct into which it empties (5) can be considered a single functional unit: the *distal nephron*.

Physiology
Overview of Kidney Functions
The kidney serves three basic functions: (1) cleansing of extracellular fluid (ECF) and maintenance of ECF volume and composition; (2) maintenance of acid–base balance; and (3) excretion of metabolic wastes and foreign substances (e.g., drugs, toxins). Of the three, maintenance of ECF volume and composition is the one that diuretics affect most.

The Three Basic Renal Processes
Effects of the kidney on ECF are the net result of three basic processes: (1) *filtration*, (2) *reabsorption*, and (3) *active secretion*. To cleanse the entire ECF, a huge volume of plasma must be filtered. Furthermore, to maintain homeostasis, practically everything that has been filtered must be reabsorbed, leaving behind only a small volume of urine for excretion.

Filtration. Filtration occurs at the *glomerulus* and is the first step in urine formation. Virtually all small molecules (electrolytes, amino acids, glucose, drugs, metabolic wastes) that are present in plasma undergo filtration. In contrast, cells and large molecules (lipids, proteins) remain behind in the blood. The most prevalent constituents of the filtrate are sodium ions and chloride ions. Bicarbonate ions and potassium ions are also present, but in smaller amounts.

The filtration capacity of the kidney is very large. Each minute, the kidney produces 125 mL of filtrate, which adds up to 180 L/day. Because the total volume of ECF is only 12.5 L, the kidneys can process the equivalent of all the ECF in the body every 100 minutes. Hence the ECF undergoes complete cleansing about 14 times each day.

Be aware that filtration is a *nonselective process* and therefore cannot regulate the composition of urine. Reabsorption and secretion—processes that display a significant degree of selectivity—are the primary determinants of what the urine ultimately contains. Of the two, reabsorption is by far the more important.

Reabsorption. More than 99% of the water, electrolytes, and nutrients filtered at the glomerulus undergo reabsorption. This conserves valuable constituents of the filtrate while allowing wastes to undergo excretion. Reabsorption of solutes (e.g., electrolytes, amino acids, glucose) takes place by way of *active transport*. Water then follows passively along the osmotic gradient created by solute reuptake. Specific sites along the nephron at which reabsorption takes place are discussed later. Diuretics work primarily by interfering with reabsorption.

Active tubular secretion. The kidney has two major kinds of "pumps" for active secretion. These pumps transport compounds from the plasma into the lumen of the nephron. One pump transports *organic acids* and the other transports *organic bases*. Together, these pumps can promote the excretion of a wide assortment of molecules, including metabolic wastes, drugs, and toxins. The pumps for active secretion are located in the *proximal convoluted tubule.*

Processes of Reabsorption That Occur at Specific Sites Along the Nephron
Because most diuretics act by disrupting solute reabsorption, to understand the diuretics, we must first understand the major processes by which nephrons reabsorb filtered solutes. Because sodium and chloride ions are the predominant solutes in the filtrate, reabsorption of these ions is of greatest interest. As we discuss reabsorption, numeric values are given for the percentage of solute reabsorbed at specific sites along the nephron. It is important to note that these values are only approximate. Fig. 37.2 depicts the sites of sodium and chloride reabsorption, indicating the amount of reabsorption that occurs at each site.

Proximal convoluted tubule. The PCT has a high reabsorptive capacity. *A large fraction (about 65%) of filtered sodium and chloride is reabsorbed at the PCT.* In addition, essentially all of the bicarbonate and potassium in the filtrate is reabsorbed here. As sodium, chloride, and other solutes are actively reabsorbed, water follows passively. Because solutes and water are reabsorbed to an equal extent, the tubular urine remains isotonic (300 mOsm/L). By the time the filtrate leaves the PCT, sodium and chloride are the only solutes that remain in significant amounts.

Loop of Henle. The *descending limb* of the loop of Henle is freely permeable to water. Hence, as tubular urine moves down the loop and

Fig. 37.1 Schematic Representation of a Nephron and Collecting Duct.

passes through the hypertonic environment of the renal medulla, water is drawn from the loop into the interstitial space. This process decreases the volume of the tubular urine and causes the urine to become concentrated (tonicity increases to about 1200 mOsm/L).

Within the thick segment of the *ascending limb* of the loop of Henle, about *20% of filtered sodium and chloride is reabsorbed* (see Fig. 37.2). Because, unlike the descending limb, the ascending limb is not permeable to water, water must remain in the loop as reabsorption of sodium and chloride takes place. This process causes the tonicity of the tubular urine to return to that of the original filtrate (300 mOsm/L).

Distal convoluted tubule (early segment). About 10% of filtered sodium and chloride is reabsorbed in the early segment of the distal convoluted tubule. Water follows passively.

Distal nephron: late distal convoluted tubule and collecting duct. The distal nephron is the site of two important processes. The first involves exchange of sodium for potassium and is under the influence of aldosterone. The second determines the final concentration of the urine and is regulated by antidiuretic hormone (ADH). Although sodium–potassium exchange is discussed in more detail, there will be no further discussion of ADH because it has little to do with the actions of diuretics.

Sodium–potassium exchange. Aldosterone, the principal mineralocorticoid of the adrenal cortex, stimulates reabsorption of sodium from the distal nephron. At the same time aldosterone causes potassium to be secreted. Although not directly coupled, these two processes—sodium retention and potassium excretion—can be viewed as an exchange

mechanism. This exchange is shown in Fig. 37.2. Aldosterone promotes sodium–potassium exchange by stimulating cells of the distal nephron to synthesize more of the pumps responsible for sodium and potassium transport.

INTRODUCTION TO DIURETICS

How Diuretics Work

Most diuretics share the same basic mechanism of action: blockade of sodium and chloride reabsorption. By blocking the reabsorption of these prominent solutes, diuretics create osmotic pressure within the nephron,

Fig. 37.2 Schematic Diagram of a Nephron Showing Sites of Sodium Absorption and Diuretic Action. The percentages indicate how much of the filtered sodium and chloride are reabsorbed at each site.

which prevents the passive reabsorption of water. Hence diuretics cause water and solutes to be retained within the nephron and thereby promote the excretion of both.

The increase in urine flow that a diuretic produces is directly related to the amount of sodium and chloride reabsorption that it blocks. Accordingly, drugs that block solute reabsorption to the greatest degree produce the most profound diuresis. Because the amount of solute in the nephron becomes progressively smaller as filtrate flows from the proximal tubule to the collecting duct, *drugs that act early in the nephron have the opportunity to block the greatest amount of solute reabsorption. As a result, these agents produce the greatest diuresis.* Conversely, because most of the filtered solute has already been reabsorbed by the time the filtrate reaches the distal parts of the nephron, diuretics that act at distal sites have very little reabsorption available to block. Consequently such agents produce relatively scant diuresis.

It is instructive to look at the quantitative relationship between blockade of solute reabsorption and production of diuresis. Recall that the kidneys produce 180 L of filtrate a day, practically all of which is normally reabsorbed. With filtrate production at this volume, a diuretic will increase daily urine output by 1.8 L for each 1% of solute reabsorption that is blocked. A 3% blockade of solute reabsorption will produce 5.4 L of urine a day—a rate of fluid loss that would reduce body weight by 12 pounds in 24 hours. Clearly, with only a small blockade

of reabsorption, diuretics can produce a profound effect on the fluid and electrolyte composition of the body.

Adverse Impact on Extracellular Fluid

To promote excretion of water, diuretics must interfere with the normal operation of the kidney. By doing so, diuretics can cause *hypovolemia* (from excessive fluid loss), *acid–base imbalance,* and *altered electrolyte levels.* These adverse effects can be minimized by using short-acting diuretics and by timing drug administration such that the kidney is allowed to operate in a drug-free manner between periods of diuresis. Both measures will give the kidney periodic opportunities to readjust the ECF to compensate for any undesired alterations produced under the influence of diuretics.

Classification of Diuretics

There are four major categories of diuretic drugs: (1) *loop diuretics* (e.g., furosemide); (2) *thiazide diuretics* (e.g., hydrochlorothiazide); (3) *osmotic diuretics* (e.g., mannitol); and (4) *potassium-sparing diuretics.* The last group, the potassium-sparing agents, can be subdivided into *aldosterone antagonists* (e.g., spironolactone) and *nonaldosterone antagonists* (e.g., triamterene).

In addition to the four major categories of diuretics, there is a fifth group: the *carbonic anhydrase inhibitors*. Although the carbonic anhydrase inhibitors are classified as diuretics, these drugs are employed primarily to lower intraocular pressure (IOP) and not to increase urine production. Therefore the carbonic anhydrase inhibitors are discussed in Chapter 87.

LOOP DIURETICS

The loop agents are the most effective diuretics available. These drugs produce more loss of fluid and electrolytes than any other diuretics. They are known as *loop diuretics* because their site of action is in the loop of Henle.

Furosemide

Furosemide (Lasix) is the most frequently prescribed loop diuretic and will serve as the prototype for the group.

Mechanism of Action

Furosemide acts in the thick segment of the ascending limb of the loop of Henle to block reabsorption of sodium and chloride (see Fig. 37.2). By blocking solute reabsorption, furosemide prevents passive reabsorption of water. Because a substantial amount (20%) of filtered NaCl is normally reabsorbed in the loop of Henle, interference with reabsorption here can produce profound diuresis.

Pharmacokinetics

With oral administration, diuresis begins in 60 minutes and persists for 8 hours. Oral therapy is used when rapid onset is not required. Furosemide undergoes hepatic metabolism followed by renal excretion.

Therapeutic Uses

Furosemide is a powerful drug that is generally reserved for situations that require rapid or massive mobilization of fluid. This drug should be avoided when less efficacious diuretics (thiazides) will suffice. Conditions that justify the use of furosemide include (1) pulmonary edema associated with congestive heart failure (CHF); (2) edema of hepatic, cardiac, or renal origin that has been unresponsive to less efficacious diuretics; and (3) hypertension that cannot be controlled with other diuretics. Furosemide is especially useful in patients with severe renal impairment because, unlike the thiazides (see later), the drug can promote diuresis even when renal blood flow and glomerular filtration rate (GFR) are low. If treatment with furosemide alone is insufficient, a thiazide diuretic may be added to the regimen. There is no benefit to combining furosemide with another loop diuretic.

Adverse Effects

Hyponatremia, hypochloremia, and dehydration. Furosemide can produce excessive loss of sodium, chloride, and water. Severe dehydration can result. Signs of evolving dehydration include dry mouth, unusual thirst, and oliguria. Impending dehydration can also be anticipated from excessive loss of weight. If dehydration occurs, furosemide should be withheld.

The risk for dehydration and its sequelae can be minimized by initiating therapy with low doses, adjusting the dosage carefully, and monitoring weight loss every day.

Hypotension. Furosemide can cause a substantial drop in blood pressure. At least two mechanisms are involved: (1) loss of volume and (2) relaxation of venous smooth muscle, which reduces venous return to the heart. Signs of hypotension include dizziness, lightheadedness, and fainting. If blood pressure falls precipitously, furosemide should be discontinued. Because of the risk for hypotension, blood pressure should be monitored routinely.

Hypotension

> Patients should be taught to monitor their blood pressure and instructed to notify the prescriber if it drops substantially. Also, patients should be informed about symptoms of postural hypotension (dizziness, lightheadedness) and advised to sit or lie down if these occur. Patients should be taught that postural hypotension can be minimized by rising slowly.

Hypokalemia. Potassium is lost through increased secretion in the distal nephron. If serum potassium falls below 3.5 mEq/L, fatal dysrhythmias may result. As discussed later, under "Drug Interactions," loss of potassium is of special concern for patients taking digoxin, a drug for heart failure. Hypokalemia can be minimized by consuming potassium-rich foods (e.g., dried fruits, nuts, spinach, potatoes, bananas), taking potassium supplements, or using a potassium-sparing diuretic.

Ototoxicity. Rarely, loop diuretics cause hearing impairment. With furosemide, deafness is transient. With ethacrynic acid (another loop diuretic), irreversible hearing loss may occur. The ability to impair hearing is unique to the loop diuretics. Diuretics in other classes are not ototoxic. Additional adverse effects of furosemide can be found in Table 37.2.

PATIENT-CENTERED CARE ACROSS THE LIFE SPAN

Diuretics

Life Stage	Patient Care Concerns
Infants	See later entry, "Breastfeeding women."
Children/adolescents	Diuretics can be used safely in children, just in smaller doses. Side-effect profiles are similar to those in adults.
Pregnant women	Animal studies have revealed that furosemide can cause maternal death, abortion, and fetal resorption. Risks and benefits must be considered for administration during pregnancy.
Breastfeeding women	Furosemide may decrease breast milk production through excessive diuresis. Data are lacking regarding transmission of drug from mother to infant through breast milk.
Older adults	Diuretics are the most common cause of adverse medication reactions and interactions in older adults. Patients must be monitored closely for dehydration and cardiac dysrhythmias.

Drug Interactions

Digoxin. In the presence of low potassium, the risk for serious digoxin-induced toxicity (ventricular dysrhythmias) is greatly increased. Because loop diuretics promote potassium loss, use of these drugs in combination with digoxin can increase the dysrhythmia risk. This interaction is unfortunate in that most patients who take digoxin for heart failure must also take a diuretic. To reduce the risk for toxicity, potassium levels should be monitored routinely and, when indicated, potassium supplements or a potassium-sparing diuretic should be given.

TABLE 37.1   Loop Diuretics: Routes, Time Course, and Dosage

Drug	Availability	Time Course Onset (min)	Duration (h)	Dosage (mg)	Doses/Day
Furosemide (Lasix)	20-, 40-, 80-mg tablets 40-mg/5-mL solution	Within 60	6–8	20–80	1–2
Ethacrynic acid (Edecrin)	25-mg tablets 1-mg/mL solution	Within 30	6–8	50–100	1–2
Bumetanide (Burinex ❧, generic only in the United States)	0.5-, 1-, 2-mg tablets 0.25-mg/mL solution	30–60	4–6	0.5–2	1
Torsemide (Demadex)	5-, 10-, 20-, 100-mg tablets	Within 60	6–8	5–20	1

❧ Available in Canada.

TABLE 37.2   Loop and Thiazide Diuretics: Adverse Effects and Drug Interactions

Adverse Effects	Drug Interactions
Hyponatremia, hypochloremia, and dehydration	Digoxin
Hypotension	Ototoxic drugs
Hypokalemia	Potassium-sparing diuretics
Ototoxicity (loop diuretics)	Lithium
Hyperglycemia	Antihypertensive agents
Hyperuricemia	NSAIDs
Reduction of HDL cholesterol	
Increase in LDL cholesterol and triglycerides	

HDL, High-density lipoprotein; *LDL*, low-density lipoprotein; *NSAIDs*, nonsteroidal antiinflammatory drugs.

   Ototoxic drugs. The risk for furosemide-induced hearing loss is increased by concurrent use of other ototoxic drugs, especially aminoglycoside antibiotics (e.g., gentamicin). Therefore combined use of these drugs should be avoided.
   Potassium-sparing diuretics. The potassium-sparing diuretics (e.g., spironolactone, triamterene) can help counterbalance the potassium-wasting effects of furosemide, thereby reducing the risk for hypokalemia. Additional drug interactions can be found in Table 37.2.

Other Loop Diuretics

In addition to furosemide, three other loop diuretics are available: ethacrynic acid (Edecrin), torsemide (Demadex), and bumetanide (Burinex, available in Canada; ❧, generic only in the United States). All three are much like furosemide. They all promote diuresis by inhibiting sodium and chloride reabsorption in the thick ascending limb of the loop of Henle. All are approved for edema caused by heart failure, chronic renal disease, and cirrhosis, but only torsemide, like furosemide, is also approved for hypertension. Routes, dosages, and time courses are shown in Table 37.1. Adverse effects and drug interactions are shown in Table 37.2.

BLACK BOX WARNING

Loop Diuretics

All loop diuretics can cause profound diuresis with water and electrolyte depletion.

SUMMARY OF KEY PRESCRIBING CONSIDERATIONS

Loop Diuretics

Therapeutic Goal: Loop diuretics are indicated for patients with (1) pulmonary edema associated with congestive heart failure; (2) edema of hepatic, cardiac, or renal origin that has been unresponsive to less effective diuretics; (3) hypertension that cannot be controlled with thiazide and potassium-sparing diuretics; and (4) low renal blood flow who need diuretic therapy.
Baseline Data: Weight, vital signs, electrolytes
Identifying High-Risk Patients: Use with caution in patients with cardiovascular disease, renal impairment, diabetes mellitus, or a history of gout and in patients who are pregnant or taking digoxin, lithium, ototoxic drugs, NSAIDs, or antihypertensive drugs.
Evaluating Therapeutic Effects: Monitor blood pressure and pulse rate; also, patients should weigh themselves daily and evaluate for decreased edema. Have patients monitor for signs or symptoms of hypokalemia.
Minimizing Adverse Effects: Initiate therapy with low doses, adjust doses carefully, monitor weight loss daily, and use an intermittent dosing schedule.

THIAZIDES AND RELATED DIURETICS

The thiazide diuretics have effects similar to those of the loop diuretics. Like the loop diuretics, thiazides increase renal excretion of sodium, chloride, potassium, and water. In addition, thiazides elevate plasma levels of uric acid and glucose. The principal difference between the thiazides and loop diuretics is that the maximal diuresis produced by the thiazides is considerably lower than the maximal diuresis produced by the loop diuretics. In addition, whereas loop diuretics can be effective even when urine flow is decreased, thiazides cannot.

Hydrochlorothiazide

Hydrochlorothiazide (Microzide) is the most widely used thiazide diuretic and will serve as the prototype for this group. Because of its use in hypertension, hydrochlorothiazide is one of the most widely used drugs.

Mechanism of Action

Hydrochlorothiazide promotes urine production by blocking the reabsorption of sodium and chloride in the *early segment of the distal convoluted tubule* (see Fig. 37.2). Retention of sodium and chloride in the nephron causes water to be retained as well, thereby producing an increased flow of urine. Because only 10% of filtered sodium and chloride is normally reabsorbed at the site where thiazides act, the maximal urine flow these drugs can produce is lower than that produced by the loop diuretics.

The ability of thiazides to promote diuresis is dependent on adequate kidney function. These drugs are ineffective when GFR is low (less than 15 to 20 mL/min). Hence, in contrast to the loop diuretics, thiazides cannot be used to promote fluid loss in patients with severe renal impairment.

Pharmacokinetics

Diuresis begins about 2 hours after oral administration. Effects peak within 4 to 6 hours and may persist up to 12 hours. Most of the drug is excreted unchanged in the urine (Table 37.3).

Therapeutic Uses

Essential hypertension. The primary indication for hydrochlorothiazide is hypertension, a condition for which thiazides are often drugs of first choice. For many hypertensive patients, blood pressure can be controlled with a thiazide alone, although many other patients require multiple-drug therapy. The role of thiazides in hypertension is discussed in Chapter 41.

Edema. Thiazides are preferred drugs for mobilizing edema associated with mild to moderate heart failure. They are also given to mobilize edema associated with hepatic or renal disease.

Adverse Effects and Drug Interactions

The adverse effects and drug interactions of thiazide diuretics are similar to those of the loop diuretics and are shown in Table 37.3. In fact, with the exception that thiazides are not ototoxic, the adverse effects of the thiazides and loop diuretics are nearly identical.

SUMMARY OF KEY PRESCRIBING CONSIDERATIONS

Thiazide Diuretics

Therapeutic Goal: Treatment of hypertension and edema
Baseline Data: Weight, vital signs, electrolytes
Identifying High-Risk Patients: Use with caution in patients with cardiovascular disease, renal impairment, diabetes mellitus, or a history of gout and in patients taking digoxin, lithium, or antihypertensive drugs.
Evaluating Therapeutic Effects: Monitor blood pressure and pulse rate; also, patients should weigh themselves daily and evaluate for decreased edema. Have patients monitor for signs or symptoms of hypokalemia.
Minimizing Adverse Effects: Initiate therapy with low doses, adjust doses carefully, monitor weight loss daily, and use an intermittent dosing schedule.

POTASSIUM-SPARING DIURETICS

The potassium-sparing diuretics can elicit two potentially useful responses. First, they produce a modest increase in urine production. Second, they produce a substantial *decrease in potassium excretion.* Because their diuretic effects are limited, the potassium-sparing drugs are rarely used alone to promote diuresis. However, because of their marked ability to decrease potassium excretion, these drugs are often used to counteract potassium loss caused by thiazide and loop diuretics.

There are two subcategories of potassium-sparing diuretics: *aldosterone antagonists* and *non–aldosterone antagonists.* In the United States, only one aldosterone antagonist—spironolactone—is used for diuresis. Two non–aldosterone antagonists—triamterene and amiloride—are currently employed.

Spironolactone
Mechanism of Action

Spironolactone (Aldactone) blocks the actions of aldosterone in the distal nephron. Because aldosterone acts to promote sodium uptake in exchange for potassium secretion (see Fig. 37.2), inhibition of aldosterone has the opposite effect: *retention of potassium and increased excretion of sodium.* The diuresis caused by spironolactone is scanty because most of the filtered sodium load has already been reabsorbed by the time the filtrate reaches the distal nephron.

The effects of spironolactone are delayed, taking up to 48 hours to develop (Table 37.4). Recall that aldosterone acts by stimulating cells of the distal nephron to synthesize the proteins required for sodium and potassium transport. By preventing aldosterone's action, spironolactone blocks the synthesis of *new* proteins but does not stop existing transport proteins from doing their job. Therefore effects are not visible until the existing proteins complete their normal life cycle—a process that takes 1 or 2 days.

▶▶ BLACK BOX WARNING
Spirolonactone

Spironolactone has been shown to be tumorigenic in rats. Avoid unnecessary use.

Therapeutic Uses

Hypertension and edema. Spironolactone is used primarily for hypertension and edema. Although it can be employed alone, the drug is used most commonly in combination with a thiazide or loop diuretic. The purpose of spironolactone in these combinations is to counteract

TABLE 37.3   Thiazides and Related Diuretics: Dosages and Time Course of Effects

Generic Name	Trade Name	Availability	Time Course Onset (h)	Time Course Duration (h)	Optimal Oral Adult Dosage (mg/day)
Thiazides					
Chlorothiazide	Diuril	250-, 500-mg tablets 250-mg/5 mL suspension	1–2	6–12	500–1000
Hydrochlorothiazide	Microzide	12.5-mg capsules 12.5-, 25-, 50-mg tablets	2	6–12	12.5–25
Methyclothiazide	Generic	5-mg tablets	2	24	2.5–5
Related Drugs					
Chlorthalidone	Generic	25-, 50-, 100-mg tablets	2	24–72	50–100
Indapamide	Lozide ♣, generic only in the United States	1.25-, 2.5-mg tablets	1–2	Up to 36	2.5–5
Metolazone	Zaroxolyn	2.5-, 5-, 10-mg tablets	1	12–24	2.5–20

♣ Available in Canada.

TABLE 37.4   Potassium-Sparing Diuretics: Names, Dosages, and Time Course of Effects

| Generic Name | Trade Name | Availability | Time Course | | Usual Adult Dosage (mg/day) |
			Onset (h)	Duration (h)	
Spironolactone	Aldactone	25-, 50-, 100-mg tablets	24–48	48–72	25–200
Triamterene	Dyrenium	50-, 100-mg capsules	2–4	12–16	50–300
Amiloride	Midamor	5-mg tablets	2	24	5–20

 Available in Canada.

the potassium-wasting effects of the more powerful diuretics. Spironolactone also makes a small contribution to diuresis.

Heart failure. In patients with severe heart failure, spironolactone reduces mortality and hospital admissions. Benefits derive from the protective effects of aldosterone blockade in the heart and blood vessels (see Chapter 42).

Adverse Effects

Hyperkalemia. The potassium-sparing effects of spironolactone can result in hyperkalemia, a condition that can produce fatal dysrhythmias. Although hyperkalemia is most likely when spironolactone is used alone, it can also develop when spironolactone is used in conjunction with potassium-wasting agents (thiazides and loop diuretics). If serum potassium rises above 5 mEq/L or if signs of hyperkalemia develop (e.g., abnormal heart rhythm), spironolactone should be discontinued and potassium intake restricted.

Endocrine effects. Spironolactone is a steroid derivative with a structure similar to that of steroid hormones (e.g., progesterone, estradiol, testosterone). As a result, spironolactone can cause a variety of endocrine effects, including *gynecomastia, menstrual irregularities, impotence, hirsutism,* and *deepening of the voice.*

Drug Interactions

Thiazide and loop diuretics. Spironolactone is frequently combined with thiazide and loop diuretics. The goal is to counteract the potassium-wasting effects of the more powerful diuretic.

Agents that raise potassium levels. Because of the risk for hyperkalemia, caution must be employed when spironolactone is combined with potassium supplements, salt substitutes (which contain potassium chloride), or another potassium-sparing diuretic. In addition, three groups of drugs—angiotensin-converting enzyme inhibitors (ACEIs), angiotensin receptor blockers (ARBs), and direct renin inhibitors—can elevate potassium levels (by suppressing aldosterone secretion) and hence should be combined with spironolactone only when clearly necessary.

Triamterene
Mechanism of Action

Like spironolactone, triamterene (Dyrenium) disrupts sodium–potassium exchange in the distal nephron. However, in contrast to spironolactone, which reduces ion transport *indirectly* through blockade of aldosterone, triamterene is a *direct inhibitor of the exchange mechanism itself.* The net effect of inhibition is a decrease in sodium reabsorption and a reduction in potassium secretion. Hence sodium excretion is increased, whereas potassium is conserved. Because it inhibits ion transport directly, triamterene acts much more quickly than spironolactone. Initial responses develop in hours, compared with days for spironolactone. As with spironolactone, diuresis with triamterene is minimal.

Therapeutic Uses

Triamterene can be used alone or in combination with other diuretics to treat *hypertension* and *edema.* When used alone, triamterene produces mild diuresis. When combined with other diuretics (e.g., furosemide, hydrochlorothiazide), triamterene augments diuresis and helps counteract

the potassium-wasting effects of the more powerful diuretic. It is the latter effect for which triamterene is principally employed.

Adverse Effects

Hyperkalemia. Excessive potassium accumulation is the most significant adverse effect. Hyperkalemia is most likely when triamterene is used alone but can also occur when the drug is combined with thiazides or loop diuretics. Caution should be employed when triamterene is used in conjunction with another potassium-sparing diuretic or with potassium supplements or salt substitutes. In addition, caution is needed if the drug is combined with an ACEI, ARB, or direct renin inhibitor.

⯈⯈ **BLACK BOX WARNING**
Triamterene and Amiloride

Triamterene and amiloride carry a risk for hyperkalemia, which is potentially fatal if uncorrected. Potassium levels should be monitored at treatment start, when the dosage is changed, and during illness affecting renal function.

Other adverse effects. Relatively common side effects include *nausea, vomiting, leg cramps,* and *dizziness.* Blood dyscrasias occur rarely.

Amiloride
Pharmacological Properties

Amiloride has actions similar to those of triamterene. Both drugs inhibit potassium loss by direct blockade of sodium–potassium exchange in the distal nephron. Also, both drugs produce only modest diuresis. Although it can be employed alone as a diuretic, amiloride is used primarily to counteract potassium loss caused by more powerful diuretics (thiazides, loop diuretics). The major adverse effect is hyperkalemia. Accordingly, concurrent use of other potassium-sparing diuretics or potassium supplements must be monitored closely. Caution is needed if the drug is combined with an ACEI, ARB, or direct renin inhibitor.

 SUMMARY OF KEY PRESCRIBING CONSIDERATIONS
Potassium-Sparing Diuretics

Therapeutic Goal: Counterbalance the potassium-losing effects of thiazide and loop diuretics.

Baseline Data: Weight, vital signs, electrolytes.

Identifying High-Risk Patients: Potassium-sparing diuretics are contraindicated in patients with hyperkalemia and should be used with caution in patients taking potassium supplements or another potassium-sparing diuretic. Use with caution in patients taking angiotensin-converting enzyme inhibitors, angiotensin receptor blockers, and direct renin inhibitors.

Evaluating Therapeutic Effects: Potassium levels should be monitored on a regular basis. The object is to maintain serum potassium levels between 3.5 and 5 mEq/L.

Minimizing Adverse Effects: Patients should be instructed to restrict their intake of potassium-rich foods.

Drugs Acting on the Renin-Angiotensin-Aldosterone System

In this chapter we consider four families of drugs: angiotensin-converting enzyme (ACE) inhibitors, angiotensin II receptor blockers (ARBs), direct renin inhibitors (DRIs), and aldosterone antagonists. With all four groups, effects result from interfering with the renin-angiotensin-aldosterone system (RAAS). The ACE inhibitors have established roles in the treatment of hypertension, heart failure, and diabetic nephropathy; in addition, these drugs are indicated for myocardial infarction (MI) and prevention of cardiovascular events in patients at risk. Indications for ARBs are limited to hypertension, heart failure, diabetic nephropathy, and prevention of cardiovascular events in patients at risk. The aldosterone antagonist eplerenone has only two indications: hypertension and heart failure; spironolactone is also used to prevent diuretic-induced hypokalemia and treat hyperaldosteronism. Current indications for DRIs are limited to hypertension. We begin by reviewing the physiology of the RAAS, and then we discuss the drugs that affect it.

PHYSIOLOGY OF THE RENIN-ANGIOTENSIN-ALDOSTERONE SYSTEM

The RAAS plays an important role in regulating blood pressure, blood volume, and fluid and electrolyte balance. In addition, the system appears to mediate certain pathophysiologic changes associated with hypertension, heart failure, and MI. The RAAS exerts its effects through angiotensin II and aldosterone.

Types of Angiotensin

Before considering the physiology of the RAAS, we need to introduce the angiotensin family, which consists of angiotensin I, angiotensin II, and angiotensin III. All three compounds are small polypeptides. Angiotensin I is the precursor of angiotensin II (Fig. 38.1) and has only weak biologic activity. In contrast, angiotensin II has strong biologic activity. Angiotensin III, which is formed by degradation of angiotensin II, has moderate biologic activity.

Actions of Angiotensin II

Angiotensin II participates in all processes regulated by the RAAS. The most prominent actions of angiotensin II are vasoconstriction and stimulation of aldosterone release. Both actions raise blood pressure. In addition, angiotensin II (as well as aldosterone) can act on the heart and blood vessels to cause pathologic changes in their structure and function.

Vasoconstriction

Angiotensin II is a powerful vasoconstrictor. The compound acts directly on vascular smooth muscle (VSM) to cause contraction. Vasoconstriction is prominent in arterioles and less so in veins. As a result of angiotensin-induced vasoconstriction, blood pressure rises. In addition to its direct action on blood vessels, angiotensin II can cause vasoconstriction indirectly by acting on (1) sympathetic neurons to promote norepinephrine release, (2) the adrenal medulla to promote epinephrine release, and (3) the central nervous system to increase sympathetic outflow to blood vessels.

Release of Aldosterone

Angiotensin II acts on the adrenal cortex to promote synthesis and secretion of aldosterone, whose actions are discussed later. The adrenal cortex is highly sensitive to angiotensin II, and hence angiotensin II can stimulate aldosterone release even when angiotensin II levels are too low to induce vasoconstriction. Aldosterone secretion is enhanced when sodium levels are low and when potassium levels are high.

Alteration of Cardiac and Vascular Structure

Angiotensin II may cause pathologic structural changes in the heart and blood vessels. In the heart, it may cause *hypertrophy* and *remodeling*. In hypertension, angiotensin II may be responsible for increasing the thickness of blood vessel walls. In atherosclerosis, it may be responsible for thickening the intimal surface of blood vessels, and in heart failure and MI, it may be responsible for causing cardiac hypertrophy and fibrosis. Known effects of angiotensin II that could underlie these pathologic changes include the following:
* Increased migration, proliferation, and hypertrophy of VSM cells
* Increased production of extracellular matrix by VSM cells
* Hypertrophy of cardiac myocytes
* Increased production of extracellular matrix by cardiac fibroblasts

Actions of Aldosterone
Regulation of Blood Volume and Blood Pressure

After being released from the adrenal cortex, aldosterone acts on distal tubules of the kidney to cause retention of sodium and excretion of potassium and hydrogen. Because retention of sodium causes water to be retained as well, aldosterone increases blood volume, which causes blood pressure to rise.

Pathologic Cardiovascular Effects

Like angiotensin II, aldosterone can promote cardiac remodeling and fibrosis. In addition, aldosterone can activate the sympathetic nervous system and suppress uptake of norepinephrine in the heart, thereby predisposing the heart to dysrhythmias. Furthermore, aldosterone can promote vascular fibrosis (which decreases arterial compliance), and it can disrupt the baroreceptor reflex. These adverse effects appear to be limited to states such as heart failure, in which levels of aldosterone can be extremely high.

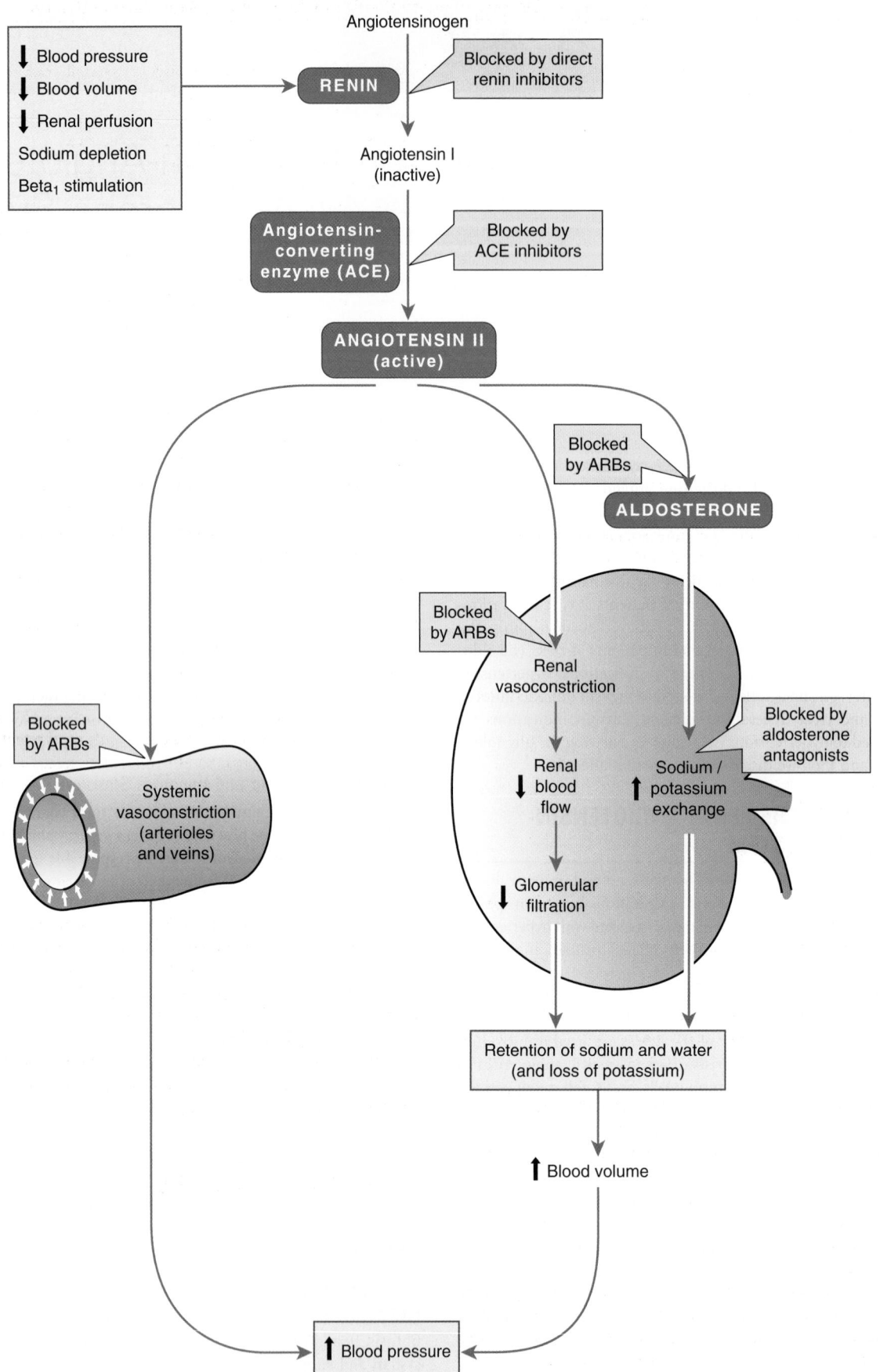

Fig. 38.1 Regulation of Blood Pressure by the Renin-Angiotensin-Aldosterone System. In addition to the mechanisms depicted, angiotensin II can raise blood pressure by (1) acting on the distal nephron to promote reabsorption of sodium and (2) increasing vasoconstriction by three mechanisms: promoting release of norepinephrine from sympathetic nerves; promoting release of epinephrine from the adrenal medulla; and acting in the central nervous system to increase sympathetic outflow to blood vessels. *ARBs*, Angiotensin receptor blockers.

PATIENT-CENTERED CARE ACROSS THE LIFE SPAN

RAAS Inhibitors

Life Stage	Patient Care Concerns
Infants	Captopril and enalapril have been used in infants safely for management of hypertension (HTN).
Children/ adolescents	Some ACE inhibitors and ARBs are approved for use in children older than 6 years for treatment of HTN.
Pregnant women	Animal studies revealed that drugs that block the RAAS should be avoided in pregnancy, especially in the second and third trimesters.
Breast-feeding women	Data are lacking regarding effects on the infant when breastfeeding. Caution is advised.
Older adults	The SCOPE and LIFE trials revealed a 25% decrease in stroke in patients 55 to 80 years old using losartan compared with atenolol. A 20% decreased risk for new-onset diabetes was seen with candesartan compared with placebo.

ACE, Angiotensin-converting enzyme; *ARBs*, angiotensin II receptor blockers; *DRIs*, direct renin inhibitors; *FDA*, U.S. Food and Drug Administration; *RAAS*, renin-angiotensin-aldosterone system.

Formation of Angiotensin II by Renin and Angiotensin-Converting Enzyme

Angiotensin II is formed through two sequential reactions. The first is catalyzed by renin, the second by ACE.

Renin

Renin catalyzes the formation of *angiotensin I* from *angiotensinogen*. This reaction is a rate-limiting step in angiotensin II formation. Renin is produced by juxtaglomerular cells of the kidney and undergoes controlled release into the bloodstream, where it cleaves angiotensinogen into angiotensin I.

Regulation of renin release. Because renin catalyzes the rate-limiting step in angiotensin II formation and because renin must be released into the blood to act, the factors that regulate renin release regulate the rate of angiotensin II formation.

Release of renin can be triggered by multiple factors (see Fig. 38.1). Release *increases* in response to a *decline* in blood pressure, blood volume, plasma sodium content, or renal perfusion pressure. Reduced renal perfusion pressure is an especially important stimulus for renin release and can occur in response to (1) stenosis of the renal arteries, (2) reduced systemic blood pressure, and (3) reduced plasma volume (brought on by dehydration, hemorrhage, or chronic sodium depletion). For the most part, these factors increase renin release through effects exerted locally in the kidney. However, some of these factors may also promote renin release through activation of the sympathetic nervous system. (Sympathetic nerves increase secretion of renin by causing stimulation of β_1-adrenergic receptors on juxtaglomerular cells.)

Release of renin is *suppressed* by factors opposite to those that cause release. That is, renin secretion is inhibited by elevation of blood pressure, blood volume, and plasma sodium content. Hence, as blood pressure, blood volume, and plasma sodium content increase in response to renin release, further release of renin is suppressed. In this regard, we can view release of renin as being regulated by a classical negative feedback loop.

Angiotensin-Converting Enzyme (Kinase II)

ACE catalyzes the conversion of angiotensin I (inactive) into angiotensin II (highly active). ACE is located on the luminal surface of all blood vessels. The vasculature of the lungs is especially rich in the enzyme. Because ACE is abundant, conversion of angiotensin I into angiotensin II occurs almost instantaneously after angiotensin I has been formed. ACE is a relatively nonspecific enzyme that can act on a variety of substrates in addition to angiotensin I.

Nomenclature regarding ACE can be confusing and requires comment. As just noted, ACE can act on several substrates. When the substrate is angiotensin I, we refer to the enzyme as ACE. However, when the enzyme is acting on other substrates, we refer to it by different names. Of importance to us, when the substrate is a hormone known as *bradykinin*, we refer to the enzyme as *kinase II*. So, please remember, whether we call it ACE or kinase II, we are talking about the same enzyme.

Regulation of Blood Pressure by the Renin-Angiotensin-Aldosterone System

The RAAS is poised to help regulate blood pressure. Factors that lower blood pressure turn the RAAS on; factors that raise blood pressure turn it off. However, although the RAAS does indeed contribute to blood pressure control, its role in *normovolemic, sodium-replete* individuals is only modest. In contrast, the system can be a major factor in maintaining blood pressure in the presence of *hemorrhage, dehydration,* or *sodium depletion*.

The RAAS, acting through angiotensin II, raises blood pressure through two basic processes: vasoconstriction and renal retention of water and sodium. Vasoconstriction raises blood pressure by increasing total peripheral resistance; retention of water and sodium raises blood pressure by increasing blood volume. Vasoconstriction occurs within minutes to hours of activating the system and hence can raise blood pressure quickly. In contrast, days, weeks, or even months are required for the kidney to raise blood pressure by increasing blood volume.

Angiotensin II acts in two ways to promote renal retention of water. First, by constricting renal blood vessels, angiotensin II reduces renal blood flow and thereby reduces glomerular filtration. Second, angiotensin II stimulates release of aldosterone from the adrenal cortex. Aldosterone then acts on renal tubules to promote retention of sodium and water and excretion of potassium.

Tissue (Local) Angiotensin II Production

In addition to the traditional RAAS that we have been discussing, in which angiotensin II is produced in the blood and then carried to target tissues, angiotensin II is produced in individual tissues. This permits discrete, local effects of angiotensin II independent of the main system. Interference with local production of angiotensin II may underlie some effects of the ACE inhibitors.

It should be noted that some angiotensin II is produced by pathways that *do not involve* ACE. As a result, drugs that inhibit ACE cannot completely block angiotensin II production.

PROTOTYPE DRUGS

Drugs Acting on the RAAS

Angiotensin-Converting Enzyme (ACE) Inhibitor
Lisinopril

Angiotensin II Receptor Blocker
Losartan

Direct Renin Inhibitor
Aliskiren

Aldosterone Antagonist
Eplerenone

RAAS, Renin angiotensin aldosterone system.

ANGIOTENSIN-CONVERTING ENZYME INHIBITORS

The ACE inhibitors are important drugs for *treating* hypertension, heart failure, diabetic nephropathy, and MI. In addition, they are used to *prevent* adverse cardiovascular events in patients at risk. Their most prominent adverse effects are cough, angioedema, first-dose hypotension, and hyperkalemia. For all of these agents, beneficial effects result largely from suppressing formation of angiotensin II. Because the similarities among ACE inhibitors are much more striking than their differences, we will discuss these drugs as a group, although lisinopril is listed above as our prototype.

Mechanism of Action and Overview of Pharmacologic Effects

As shown in Fig. 38.2, ACE inhibitors produce their beneficial effects and adverse effects by (1) reducing levels of angiotensin II (through inhibition of ACE) and (2) increasing levels of bradykinin (through inhibition of kinase II). By reducing levels of angiotensin II, ACE inhibitors can dilate blood vessels (primarily arterioles and to a lesser extent veins), reduce blood volume (through effects on the kidney), and, importantly, prevent or reverse pathologic changes in the heart and blood vessels mediated by angiotensin II and aldosterone. Inhibition of ACE can also cause hyperkalemia and fetal injury. Elevation of bradykinin causes vasodilation (secondary to increased production of prostaglandins and nitric oxide) and can also promote cough and angioedema.

Pharmacokinetics

Regarding pharmacokinetics, the following generalizations apply:
* Nearly all ACE inhibitors are administered *orally*. The only exception is enalaprilat (the active form of enalapril), which is given intravenously.

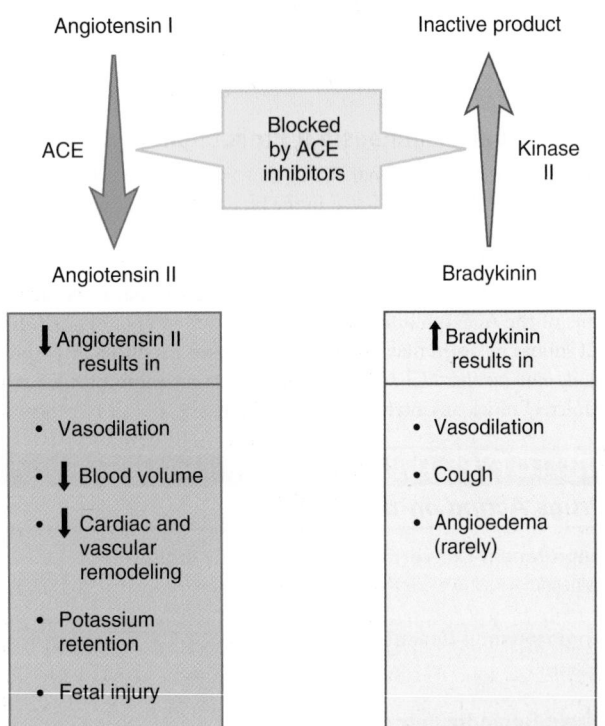

Fig. 38.2 Overview of Angiotensin-Converting Enzyme Inhibitor Actions and Pharmacologic Effects. *Angiotensin-converting enzyme (ACE)* and *kinase II* are two names for the same enzyme. When angiotensin II is the substrate, we call the enzyme ACE; when bradykinin is the substrate, we call it kinase II. Inhibition of this enzyme decreases *production* of angiotensin II (thereby *reducing* angiotensin II levels) and decreases *breakdown* of bradykinin (thereby *increasing* bradykinin levels).

* Except for captopril and moexipril, all oral ACE inhibitors can be administered with food.
* With the exception of captopril, all ACE inhibitors have prolonged half-lives and hence can be administered just once or twice a day. Captopril is administered two or three times a day.
* With the exception of lisinopril, all ACE inhibitors are *prodrugs* that must undergo conversion to their active form in the small intestine and liver. Lisinopril is active as given.
* All ACE inhibitors are *excreted by the kidneys*. As a result, nearly all can accumulate to dangerous levels in patients with kidney disease and hence *dosages must be reduced in these patients*. Only one agent—fosinopril—does not require a dosage reduction.

Therapeutic Uses

When the ACE inhibitors were introduced, their only indication was hypertension. Currently, they are also used for heart failure, acute MI, left ventricular (LV) dysfunction, and diabetic and nondiabetic nephropathy. In addition, they can help prevent MI, stroke, and death in patients at high risk for cardiovascular events. It should be noted that no single ACE inhibitor is approved for all of these conditions (Table 38.1). However, given that all ACE inhibitors are very similar, it seems likely that all may produce similar benefits.

Hypertension

All ACE inhibitors are approved for hypertension. They are useful against essential hypertension of mild to moderate intensity—although maximal benefits may take several weeks to develop.

In patients with essential hypertension, the mechanism underlying blood pressure reduction is not fully understood. *Initial* responses are proportional to circulating angiotensin II levels and are clearly related to reduced formation of that compound. (By lowering angiotensin II levels, ACE inhibitors dilate blood vessels and reduce blood volume; both actions help lower blood pressure.) However, with *prolonged* therapy, blood pressure often undergoes additional decline. During this phase, there is no relationship between reductions in blood pressure and reductions in *circulating* angiotensin II. It may be that the delayed response is due to reductions in *local* angiotensin II levels—reductions that would not be revealed by measuring angiotensin II in the blood.

ACE inhibitors offer several advantages over most other antihypertensive drugs. In contrast to the sympatholytic agents, ACE inhibitors do not interfere with cardiovascular reflexes. Hence exercise capacity is not impaired, and orthostatic hypotension is minimal after the initial dose. In addition, these drugs can be used safely in patients with bronchial asthma, a condition that precludes the use of β_2-adrenergic antagonists. ACE inhibitors do not promote hypokalemia, hyperuricemia, or hyperglycemia—side effects seen with thiazide diuretics. However, elevations in potassium levels are common and should be monitored. Furthermore, they rarely induce lethargy, weakness, or sexual dysfunction—responses that are common with other antihypertensive agents. Most important, *ACE inhibitors reduce the risk for cardiovascular mortality caused by hypertension*. The only other drugs proved to reduce hypertension-associated mortality are β-blockers and diuretics (see Chapter 41).

Heart Failure

ACE inhibitors produce multiple benefits in heart failure. By lowering arteriolar tone, these drugs improve regional blood flow, and by reducing cardiac afterload, they increase cardiac output. By causing venous dilation, they reduce pulmonary congestion and peripheral edema. By dilating blood vessels in the kidney, they increase renal blood flow and thereby promote excretion of sodium and water. This loss of fluid has two beneficial effects: (1) it helps reduce edema; and, (2) by lowering blood volume, it decreases venous return to the heart and thereby reduces

TABLE 38.1 **Angiotensin-Converting Enzyme Inhibitors: Approved Indications and Adult Dosages**

Generic Name	Trade Name	Approved Indications	Availability	Starting Dosage[a]	Usual Maintenance Dosage[a]
Benazepril	Lotensin	Hypertension	5-, 10-, 20-, 40-mg tablets	10 mg once/day	20–80 mg/day in 1 or 2 doses
Captopril	Generic only	Hypertension	12.5-, 25-, 50-, 100-mg tablets	25 mg 2 or 3 times/day	25–50 mg 2 or 3 times/day
		Heart failure		6.25–12.5 mg 3 times/day	50 mg 3 times/day
		LVD after MI		12.5 mg 3 times/day	50 mg 3 times/day
		Diabetic nephropathy		25 mg 3 times/day	25 mg 3 times/day
Enalapril	Vasotec	Hypertension	2.5-, 5-, 10-, 20-mg tablets	2.5–5 mg once/day	10–40 mg/day in 1 or 2 doses
		Heart failure		2.5 mg twice/day	10–20 mg twice/day
		Asymptomatic LVD		2.5 mg twice/day	10 mg twice/day
Fosinopril	Generil	Hypertension	10-, 20-, 40-mg tablets	10 mg once/day	20–40 mg/day in 1 or 2 doses
		Heart failure		5–10 mg once/day	20–40 mg once/day
Lisinopril	Prinivil, Zestril	Hypertension	2.5-, 5-, 10-, 20-, 30-, 40-mg tablets	10 mg once/day	10–40 mg once/d
		Heart failure		2.5–5 mg once/day	20–40 mg once/day
		Acute MI		5 mg once/day	10 mg once/day for at least 6 weeks
Moexipril	Generic only	Hypertension	7.5-, 15-mg tablets	7.5 mg once/day	7.5–30 mg/day in 1 or 2 doses
Perindopril	Aceon, Coversyl ♣	Hypertension	2-, 4-, 8-mg tablets	4 mg once/day	4–8 mg/day in 1 or 2 doses
		Stable CAD		4 mg once/day	8 mg once/day
Quinapril	Accupril	Hypertension	5-, 10-, 20-, 40-mg tablets	10–20 mg/day	20–80 mg/day in 1 or 2 doses
		Heart failure		5 mg twice/day	20–40 mg twice/day
Ramipril	Altace	Hypertension	1.25-, 2.5-, 5-, 10-mg capsules	2.5 mg once/day	2.5–20 mg/day in 1 or 2 doses
		Heart failure after MI		1.25–2.5 mg twice/day	5 mg twice/day
		Prevention of MI, stroke, and death in people at high risk for CVD		2.5 mg/day for 1 week	10 mg once/day
Trandolapril	Mavik	Hypertension	1-, 2-, 4-mg tablets	1 mg once/day in non-black patients and 2 mg once/day in black patients	2–4 mg once/day
		Heart failure after MI		1 mg once/day	4 mg once/day
		LVD after MI		1 mg once/day	4 mg once/day

[a]For all ACE inhibitors except fosinopril, dosage must be reduced in patients with significant renal impairment.
ACE, Angiotensin-converting enzyme; *CAD,* coronary artery disease; *CVD,* cardiovascular disease; *LVD,* left ventricular dysfunction; *MI,* myocardial infarction.

right-heart workload. Lastly, by suppressing aldosterone and reducing local production of angiotensin II in the heart, ACE inhibitors may prevent or reverse pathologic changes in cardiac structure. Although only seven ACE inhibitors are approved for heart failure (see Table 38.1), both the American Heart Association and the American College of Cardiology have concluded that the ability to improve symptoms and prolong survival is a class effect. The use of ACE inhibitors in heart failure is discussed further in Chapter 42.

Myocardial Infarction

ACE inhibitors can reduce mortality after acute MI (heart attack). In addition, they decrease the chance of developing overt heart failure. Treatment should begin as soon as possible after infarction and should continue for at least 6 weeks. In patients who develop overt heart failure, treatment should continue long term. As for patients who do not develop heart failure, there are no data to indicate whether continued treatment would be beneficial. At this time, only three ACE inhibitors—captopril, lisinopril, and trandolapril—are approved for patients with MI.

Diabetic and Nondiabetic Nephropathy

ACE inhibitors can benefit patients with diabetic nephropathy, the leading cause of end-stage renal disease in the United States.

In patients with overt nephropathy, as indicated by proteinuria of more than 500 mg/day, ACE inhibitors can slow progression of renal disease. In patients with less advanced nephropathy (30 to 300 mg proteinuria/day), ACE inhibitors can delay onset of overt nephropathy. These benefits were first demonstrated in patients with type 1 diabetes (insulin-dependent diabetes mellitus) and were later demonstrated in patients with type 2 diabetes (non–insulin-dependent diabetes mellitus). More recently, ACE inhibitors have been shown to provide similar benefits in patients with nephropathy unrelated to diabetes.

The principal protective mechanism appears to be reduction of glomerular filtration pressure. ACE inhibitors lower filtration pressure by reducing levels of angiotensin II, a compound that can raise filtration pressure by two mechanisms. First, angiotensin II raises systemic blood pressure, which raises pressure in the afferent arteriole of the glomerulus (Fig. 38.3). Second, it constricts the efferent arteriole, thereby generating back-pressure in the glomerulus. The resultant increase in filtration pressure promotes injury. By reducing levels of angiotensin II, ACE inhibitors lower glomerular filtration pressure and thereby slow development of renal injury.

At this time, the only ACE inhibitor approved for nephropathy is captopril. However, the American Diabetes Association considers benefits

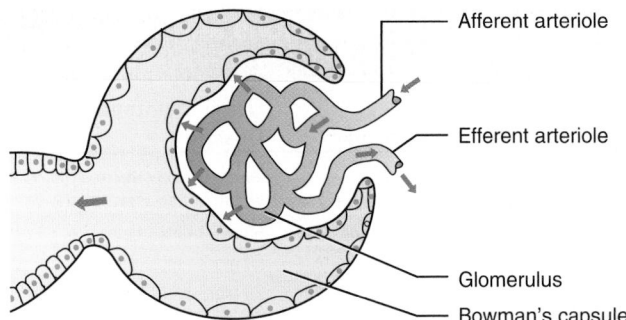

Fig. 38.3 Elevation of Glomerular Filtration Pressure by Angiotensin II. Angiotensin II increases filtration pressure by (1) increasing pressure in the afferent arteriole (secondary to increasing systemic arterial pressure) and (2) constricting the efferent arteriole, thereby generating back-pressure in the glomerulus.

in diabetic nephropathy to be a class effect and hence recommends choosing an ACE inhibitor based on its cost and likelihood of patient adherence.

Can ACE inhibitors be used for *primary prevention* of diabetic nephropathy? No. This conclusion is based on the *Renin-Angiotensin System Study* (RASS), which evaluated the effects of an ACE inhibitor—*enalapril* (Vasotec)—and an ARB—*losartan* (Cozaar)—in patients with type 1 diabetes who did not have hypertension or any signs of early kidney disease. Both drugs failed to protect the kidney: compared with patients receiving placebo, those receiving enalapril or losartan developed the same degree of microalbuminuria (an early sign of kidney damage), the same decline in kidney function, and the same changes in glomerular structure (as shown by microscopic analysis of kidney biopsy samples). Hence, although ACE inhibitors may slow progression of established nephropathy, they do not protect against early kidney damage.

Prevention of Myocardial Infarction, Stroke, and Death in Patients at High Cardiovascular Risk

One ACE inhibitor—*ramipril* (Altace)—is approved for reducing the risk for MI, stroke, and death (from cardiovascular causes) in patients at *high* risk for a major cardiovascular event—high risk being defined by (1) a history of stroke, coronary artery disease, peripheral vascular disease, or diabetes, combined with (2) at least one other risk factor, such as hypertension, high low-density lipoprotein cholesterol, low high-density lipoprotein cholesterol, or cigarette smoking. Ramipril was approved for this use based on results of the *Heart Outcomes Prevention Evaluation* (HOPE) trial, a large study in which patients at high cardiovascular risk took either ramipril (10 mg/day) or placebo. Follow-up time was 5 years. The combined end point of MI, stroke, or death from cardiovascular causes was significantly lower in the ramipril group (14% vs. 18%)—a 22% reduction in risk. Possible mechanisms underlying benefits include reduced vascular resistance and protection of the heart, blood vessels, and kidneys from the damage that angiotensin II and aldosterone can cause over time.

Like ramipril, *perindopril* (Aceon, Coversyl ♦) can reduce morbidity and mortality in patients at risk for major cardiovascular events. Benefits were demonstrated in the *EURopean trial On reduction of cardiac events with Perindopril in stable coronary Artery disease* (EUROPA). Patients in EUROPA were at lower risk than those in HOPE.

Can ACE inhibitors other than ramipril and perindopril also reduce cardiovascular risk? Possibly. However, at this time there is insufficient evidence to say for sure.

Diabetic Retinopathy

The RASS trial showed that at least one ACE inhibitor—*enalapril*—can reduce the risk for diabetic retinopathy in *some* patients. Specifically, in patients with *type 1 diabetes* who do not have hypertension, nephropathy, or established retinopathy, enalapril prevented or slowed development of retinal change. However, in patients with type 1 diabetes and *established* retinopathy, enalapril had no benefit. In patients with *type 2 diabetes*, enalapril had no benefit, regardless of retinopathy status.

Adverse Effects

ACE inhibitors are generally well tolerated. Some adverse effects (e.g., first-dose hypotension, hyperkalemia) are due to a reduction in angiotensin II, whereas others (cough, angioedema) are due to elevation of bradykinin.

First-Dose Hypotension

A precipitous drop in blood pressure may occur after the first dose of an ACE inhibitor. This reaction is caused by widespread vasodilation secondary to abrupt lowering of angiotensin II levels. First-dose hypotension is most likely in patients with severe hypertension, in patients taking diuretics, and in patients who are sodium depleted or volume depleted. To minimize the first-dose effect, initial doses should be low. Patients should be educated on the potential for light headedness associated with hypotension. If taking the first dose at home patients can use home blood pressure monitoring periodically after the first dose of an ACE inhibitor. If hypotension develops, the patient should assume a supine position and seek medical attention if symptoms do not resolve.

Cough

All ACE inhibitors can cause persistent, dry, irritating, nonproductive cough. Severity can range from a scratchy throat to severe hacking cough. The underlying cause is accumulation of bradykinin secondary to inhibition of kinase II (another name for ACE). Cough occurs in approximately 10% of patients and is the most common reason for discontinuing therapy. Factors that increase the risk for cough include advanced age, female sex, and Asian ancestry. Cough begins to subside 3 days after discontinuing an ACE inhibitor and is gone within 10 days.

Hyperkalemia

Inhibition of aldosterone release (secondary to inhibition of angiotensin II production) can cause potassium retention by the kidney. As a rule, significant potassium accumulation is limited to patients taking potassium supplements, salt substitutes (which contain potassium), or a potassium-sparing diuretic. For most other patients, hyperkalemia is rare. Patients should be instructed to avoid potassium supplements and potassium-containing salt substitutes unless they are prescribed.

Renal Failure

ACE inhibitors can cause severe renal insufficiency in patients with *bilateral renal artery stenosis or stenosis in the artery to a single remaining kidney*. In patients with renal artery stenosis, the kidneys release large amounts of renin. The resulting high levels of angiotensin II serve to maintain glomerular filtration by two mechanisms: elevation of blood pressure and constriction of efferent glomerular arterioles (see Fig. 38.3). When ACE is inhibited, causing angiotensin II levels to fall, the mechanisms that had been supporting glomerular filtration fail, causing urine production to drop precipitously. Not surprisingly, *ACE inhibitors are contraindicated for patients with bilateral renal artery stenosis (or stenosis in the artery to a single remaining kidney)*.

Are ACE inhibitors safe *early* in pregnancy? Possibly. Even though an article in the *New England Journal of Medicine* reported that among

▶▶ BLACK BOX WARNING

Fetal Injury

Use of angiotensin-converting enzyme (ACE) inhibitors during the *second* and *third* trimesters of pregnancy can injure the developing fetus. Specific effects include hypotension, hyperkalemia, skull hypoplasia, pulmonary hypoplasia, anuria, renal failure (reversible and irreversible), and death. Women who become pregnant while using ACE inhibitors should discontinue treatment as soon as possible. Infants who have been exposed to ACE inhibitors during the second or third trimester should be closely monitored for hypotension, oliguria, and hyperkalemia.

209 children exposed to ACE inhibitors during the first trimester, 18 (8.7%) had major congenital malformations, compared with 3.2% of controls, these data contrast with animal studies, which suggest that such malformations are not likely. Furthermore, no mechanism by which ACE inhibitors might disrupt early embryogenesis is known. It is currently thought that the malformations attributed to ACE inhibitors are more related to hypertension in pregnancy not the drug itself. However, because there is lack of complete data, the U.S. Food and Drug Administration still recommends avoiding their use in pregnancy.

Angioedema

Angioedema is a potentially fatal reaction that develops in up to 1% of patients. Symptoms, which result from increased capillary permeability, include giant wheals and edema of the tongue, glottis, lips, eyes, and pharynx. Severe reactions should be treated with subcutaneous epinephrine. If angioedema develops, ACE inhibitors should be discontinued and never used again. It is important to note that angioedema can occur at any point throughout use of the drug, not just at initiation of therapy. Angioedema is caused by accumulation of bradykinin secondary to inhibition of kinase II.

Neutropenia

Neutropenia, with its associated risk for infection, is a rare but serious complication. Neutropenia is most likely in patients with renal impairment and in those with collagen vascular diseases (e.g., systemic lupus erythematosus, scleroderma). These patients should be followed closely. Fortunately, neutropenia is reversible when detected early. If neutropenia develops, ACE inhibitors should be withdrawn immediately. Neutrophil counts should normalize in approximately 2 weeks. In the absence of early detection, neutropenia may progress to fatal agranulocytosis. Patients should be informed about early signs of infection (e.g., fever, sore throat) and instructed to report them immediately. Neutropenia is more common with captopril than with other ACE inhibitors.

Drug Interactions

Diuretics

Diuretics may intensify first-dose hypotension. To prevent this interaction, diuretics should be withdrawn 2 to 3 days before giving an ACE inhibitor. Diuretic therapy can be resumed later if needed.

Antihypertensive Agents

The hypotensive effects of ACE inhibitors are often additive with those of other antihypertensive drugs (e.g., diuretics, sympatholytics, vasodilators, calcium channel blockers). When an ACE inhibitor is added to an antihypertensive regimen, dosages of other drugs may require reduction.

Drugs That Raise Potassium Levels

ACE inhibitors increase the risk for hyperkalemia caused by *potassium supplements and potassium-sparing diuretics*. The risk for hyperkalemia is increased because, by suppressing aldosterone secretion, ACE inhibitors

TABLE 38.2 Angiotensin-Converting Enzyme Inhibitor Combination Drugs	
Generic Name	**Trade Name**
Benazepril/HCTZ	Lotensin HCT
Benazepril/amlodipine	Lotrel
Captopril/HCTZ	Generic only
Enalapril/HCTZ	Vaseretic
Fosinopril/HCTZ	Generic only
Lisinopril/HCTZ	Zestoretic
Moexipril/HCTZ	Generic only
Perindopril/indapamide	Coversyl Plus 🍁
Perindopril/amlodipine	Prestalia
Quinapril/HCTZ	Accuretic
Ramipril/HCTZ	Altace HCT 🍁
Trandolapril/verapamil	Tarka

HCT, Hydrochlorothiazide; *HCTZ,* hydrochlorothiazide.

can reduce excretion of potassium. To minimize the risk for hyperkalemia, potassium supplements and potassium-sparing diuretics should be used only when clearly indicated.

Lithium. ACE inhibitors can cause lithium to accumulate to toxic levels. Lithium levels should be monitored frequently.

Nonsteroidal antiinflammatory drugs. Aspirin, ibuprofen, and other nonsteroidal antiinflammatory drugs (NSAIDs) may reduce the antihypertensive effects of ACE inhibitors.

Preparations, Dosage, and Administration

Except for enalaprilat, all ACE inhibitors are administered orally. Of the oral products, all are available in single-drug formulations. Most are also available in fixed-dose combinations with hydrochlorothiazide, a thiazide diuretic, and one agent—perindopril—is available combined with indapamide (Table 38.2). Three ACE inhibitors—benazepril, perindopril, and trandolapril—are available combined with calcium channel blockers. Dosages for all ACE inhibitors (except fosinopril) should be reduced in patients with renal impairment. Dosages for specific indications are shown in Table 38.1.

SUMMARY OF KEY PRESCRIBING CONSIDERATIONS

Angiotensin-Converting Enzyme (ACE) Inhibitors

Therapeutic Goal: Reduce blood pressure in patients with hypertension, improve hemodynamics in patients with heart failure, slow progression of established diabetic nephropathy, reduce mortality, and treat heart failure after myocardial infarction.

Baseline Data: Determine blood pressure and renal function.

Monitoring: Consider checking creatinine 2–4 weeks after starting. Have patients track blood pressure values.

Identifying High-Risk Patients: Angiotensin-converting enzyme inhibitors are contraindicated during the second and third trimesters of pregnancy and in patients with bilateral renal artery stenosis.

Evaluating Therapeutic Effects: Monitor for reduced blood pressure. In patients with diabetic nephropathy, monitor proteinuria and glomerular filtration rate.

Minimizing Adverse Effects: Instruct patients to consult the prescriber if experiencing cough or facial swelling. Use caution in combinations with drugs that elevate potassium levels.

ANGIOTENSIN II RECEPTOR BLOCKERS

Initially, ARBs were approved only for hypertension. Currently, they also are approved for treating heart failure, diabetic nephropathy, and MI and for prevention of MI, stroke, and death in people at high risk for cardiovascular events.

Like the ACE inhibitors, ARBs decrease the influence of angiotensin II. However, the mechanisms involved differ: ACE inhibitors block *production* of angiotensin II, whereas ARBs block the *actions* of angiotensin II. Because both groups interfere with angiotensin II, they both have similar effects. They differ primarily in that ARBs pose a much lower risk for cough or hyperkalemia.

Even though ACE inhibitors and ARBs have very similar effects, these drugs are not clinically interchangeable. We have clear and extensive evidence that ACE inhibitors decrease cardiovascular morbidity and mortality. The evidence for ARBs is less convincing. Accordingly, until more is known, ACE inhibitors are preferred. For patients who cannot tolerate ACE inhibitors, ARBs are an appropriate second choice.

Eight ARBs are available. Although losartan is listed as our prototype, All eight are very similar—hence we will discuss them as a group, (Tables 38.3 and 38.4).

Mechanism of Action and Overview of Pharmacologic Effects

ARBs block access of angiotensin II to its receptors in blood vessels, the adrenals, and all other tissues. As a result, ARBs have effects much like those of the ACE inhibitors. By blocking angiotensin II receptors on blood vessels, ARBs cause dilation of arterioles and veins. By blocking angiotensin II receptors in the heart, ARBs can prevent angiotensin II from inducing pathologic changes in cardiac structure. By blocking angiotensin II receptors in the adrenals, ARBs decrease release of aldosterone and can thereby increase renal excretion of sodium and water. Sodium and water excretion is further increased through dilation of renal blood vessels.

In contrast to the ACE inhibitors, ARBs do *not* inhibit kinase II and hence do not increase levels of bradykinin in the lung. As a result, ARBs have a lower risk for cough, the most common reason for stopping ACE inhibitors.

Therapeutic Uses

Hypertension

All ARBs are approved for hypertension. Reductions in blood pressure equal those seen with ACE inhibitors. Evidence that ARBs share the ability of ACE inhibitors to reduce mortality is lacking.

Heart Failure

Currently, only two ARBs—*valsartan* (Diovan) and *candesartan* (Atacand)—are approved for heart failure. In clinical trials, these

---

TABLE 38.3 Angiotensin II Receptor Blocker Combination Drugs

Generic Name	Trade Name
Azilsartan/chlorthalidone	Edarbyclor
Candesartan/HCTZ	Atacand HCT
Eprosartan/HCTZ	Teveten HCT
Irbesartan/HCTZ	Avalide
Losartan/HCTZ	Hyzaar
Olmesartan/HCTZ	Benicar HCT
Olmesartan/amlodipine	Olmetec Plus ✤
Olmesartan/amlodipine/HCTZ	Azor
	Tribenzor
Telmisartan/HCTZ	Micardis HCT
Telmisartan/amlodipine	Twynsta
Valsartan/HCTZ	Diovan HCT
Valsartan/amlodipine	Exforge
Valsartan/amlodipine/HCTZ	Exforge HCT
Valsartan/nebivolol	Byvalson

HCT, Hydrochlorothiazide; *HCTZ*, hydrochlorothiazide.

TABLE 38.4 Angiotensin II Receptor Blockers: Approved Indications and Adult Dosages

Generic Name	Trade Name	Approved Indications	Availability	Initial Dosage	Maintenance Dosage
Azilsartan	Edarbi	Hypertension	40-, 80-mg tablets	40–80 mg once/day	80 mg once/day
Candesartan	Atacand	Hypertension	4-, 8-, 16-, 32-mg tablets	16 mg once/day	8–32 mg/day in 1 or 2 doses
		Heart failure		4 mg once/day	32 mg once/day
Eprosartan	Teveten	Hypertension	400-, 600-mg tablets	600 mg once/day	400–800 mg/day in 1 or 2 doses
Irbesartan	Avapro	Hypertension	75-, 150-, 300-mg tablets	150 mg once/day	150–300 mg once/day
		Diabetic nephropathy[a]		300 mg once/day	300 mg once/day
Losartan	Cozaar	Hypertension	25-, 50-, 100-mg tablets	25–50 mg once/day	25–100 mg/day in 1 or 2 doses
		Stroke prevention[b]		50 mg once/day	50–100 mg once/day
		Diabetic nephropathy[a]		50 mg once/day	100 mg once/day
Olmesartan	Benicar, Olmetec ✤	Hypertension	5-, 20-, 40-mg tablets	20 mg once/day	20–40 mg once/day
Telmisartan	Micardis	Hypertension	20-, 40-, 80-mg tablets	40 mg once/day	20–80 mg once/day
		Prevention of MI, stroke, and death in people at high risk for CVD but who cannot take an ACE inhibitor		80 mg once/day	80 mg once/day
Valsartan	Diovan	Hypertension	40-, 80-, 160-, 320-mg tablets	80–160 mg once/day	80–320 mg once/day
		Heart failure		40 mg twice/day	40–160 mg twice/day
		MI		20 mg twice/day	160 mg twice/day

[a]In patients with type 2 diabetes.
[b]In nonblack patients with hypertension and left ventricular hypertrophy.
ACE, Angiotensin-converting enzyme; *CVD*, cardiovascular disease; *MI*, myocardial infarction.

drugs reduced symptoms, decreased hospitalizations, improved functional capacity, and increased LV ejection fraction. More important, they prolonged survival. Because experience with these drugs is limited, they should be reserved for patients who cannot tolerate ACE inhibitors (because of cough). Although the other ARBs are not yet approved for heart failure, most authorities believe they are effective.

Diabetic Nephropathy

Two ARBs—*irbesartan* (Avapro) and *losartan* (Cozaar)—are approved for managing nephropathy in hypertensive patients with type 2 diabetes. In clinical trials, these drugs delayed development of overt nephropathy and slowed progression of established nephropathy. Benefits are due in part to reductions in blood pressure and in part to mechanisms that have not been determined. How do ARBs compare with ACE inhibitors? Although both groups of drugs can delay progression of nephropathy, only the ACE inhibitors have been shown to reduce mortality. As noted earlier, neither ARBs nor ACE inhibitors are effective for primary prevention of diabetic nephropathy.

Myocardial Infarction

One ARB—*valsartan* (Diovan)—is approved for reducing cardiovascular mortality in post-MI patients with heart failure or LV dysfunction. Approval was based on the results of a major trial—the *Valsartan in Acute Myocardial Infarction Trial* (VALIANT)—that showed that valsartan was as effective as captopril at reducing short-term and long-term mortality in these patients.

Stroke Prevention

One ARB—*losartan* (Cozaar)—is approved for reducing the risk for stroke in patients with hypertension and LV hypertrophy. In clinical studies, stroke prevention with losartan was better than with atenolol (a β-blocker), even though both drugs produced an equivalent decrease in blood pressure. This observation indicates that the benefits of losartan cannot be explained on the basis of reduced blood pressure alone.

Prevention of Myocardial Infarction, Stroke, and Death in Patients at High Cardiovascular Risk

One ARB—*telmisartan* (Micardis)—is approved for reducing the risk for MI, stroke, and death from cardiovascular causes in patients 55 years and older but only if they are intolerant of ACE inhibitors. (Recall that ramipril, an ACE inhibitor, is also approved for preventing MI, stroke, and death in high-risk patients.) Approval of telmisartan was based on the Ongoing Telmisartan Alone and in Combination with Ramipril Global Endpoint Trial (ONTARGET), which showed that telmisartan was similar to ramipril with regard to reducing cardiovascular morbidity and mortality. Of note, combining telmisartan with ramipril was no more effective than either agent alone but did increase the risk for adverse events. Can other ARBs reduce cardiovascular risk? Possibly, but proof is lacking.

Diabetic Retinopathy

In the RASS mentioned previously, benefits of the ARB *losartan* (Cozaar) were like those of enalapril: in patients with type 1 diabetes without established retinopathy, losartan slowed the development and progression of retinopathy—but had no benefit in patients with established retinopathy. In patients with type 2 diabetes, the drug offered no benefit at all, regardless of retinopathy status.

Adverse Effects

All of the ARBs are well tolerated. In contrast to ACE inhibitors, ARBs do not cause clinically significant hyperkalemia. Furthermore, because

ARBs do not promote accumulation of bradykinin in the lung, they have a lower incidence of cough.

Angioedema

Like the ACE inhibitors, ARBs can cause angioedema, although the incidence is much lower with ARBs. If angioedema occurs, ARBs should be withdrawn immediately and never used again. Severe reactions are treated with subcutaneous epinephrine.

ARBs cause angioedema possibly by increasing bradykinin availability. Unlike ACE inhibitors, ARBs do not inhibit bradykinin breakdown. However, through an indirect inhibition of ACE, ARBs may be able to increase local bradykinin synthesis.

Approximately 8% of patients who experience angioedema with an ACE inhibitor will also develop angioedema if given an ARB. Nonetheless, switching to an ARB may be worth the risk for specific patients, namely, those with a disorder for which ARBs are known to improve outcomes (i.e., heart failure, diabetes, and MI).

 BLACK BOX WARNING

Fetal Harm

Like the angiotensin-converting enzyme (ACE) inhibitors, angiotensin II receptor blockers (ARBs) can injure the developing fetus if taken during the second or third trimester of pregnancy and hence are contraindicated during this period. In addition, there is concern that ARBs and ACE inhibitors may harm the fetus earlier in pregnancy and hence should be discontinued as soon as pregnancy is discovered.

Renal Failure

Like the ACE inhibitors, ARBs can cause renal failure in patients with bilateral renal artery stenosis or stenosis in the artery to a single remaining kidney. Accordingly, ARBs must be used with extreme caution in patients with these conditions.

Drug Interactions

The hypotensive effects of ARBs are additive with those of other antihypertensive drugs. When an ARB is added to an antihypertensive regimen, dosages of the other drugs may require reduction.

SUMMARY OF KEY PRESCRIBING CONSIDERATIONS

Angiotensin II Receptor Blockers

Therapeutic Goal: Reduce blood pressure in patients with hypertension, improve hemodynamics in patients with heart failure, slow progression of established diabetic nephropathy, reduce mortality, and treat heart failure after myocardial infarction.

Baseline Data: Determine blood pressure and renal function.

Monitoring: Consider checking creatinine 2–4 weeks after starting. Have patients track blood pressure values.

Identifying High-Risk Patients: Angiotensin-converting enzyme inhibitors are contraindicated during the second and third trimesters of pregnancy and in patients with bilateral renal artery stenosis.

Evaluating Therapeutic Effects: Monitor for reduced blood pressure. In patients with diabetic nephropathy, monitor proteinuria and glomerular filtration rate.

Minimizing Adverse Effects: Instruct patients to consult the prescriber if experiencing cough or facial swelling. Use caution in combinations with drugs that elevate potassium levels.

ALISKIREN, A DIRECT RENIN INHIBITOR

DRIs are drugs that act on renin to inhibit the conversion of angiotensinogen into angiotensin I. By decreasing production of angiotensin I, DRIs can suppress the entire RAAS. Currently, only one DRI—*aliskiren* (Tekturna, Rasilez ✤)—is available.

Blood pressure reduction with aliskiren equals that seen with ACE inhibitors. Aliskiren causes less cough and angioedema than the ACE inhibitors but poses similar risks to the developing fetus.

Mechanism of Action

Aliskiren binds tightly with renin and thereby inhibits the cleavage of angiotensinogen into angiotensin I. Because this reaction is the first and rate-limiting step in the production of angiotensin II and aldosterone, aliskiren can reduce the influence of the entire RAAS. In clinical trials, the drug decreased plasma renin activity by 50% to 80%. Although aliskiren works at an earlier step than either the ACE inhibitors or ARBs, there is no proof that doing so results in superior clinical outcomes.

Therapeutic Use

Aliskiren is approved only for *hypertension*. It may be used alone or in combination with other antihypertensives. In clinical trials, aliskiren reduced blood pressure to the same extent as did ACE inhibitors, ARBs, or calcium channel blockers. Maximal effects developed within 2 weeks. Although aliskiren can reduce blood pressure in hypertensive patients, data are conflicting regarding reduction of negative outcomes (i.e., blindness, stroke, kidney disease, death). The Aliskiren in the Evaluation of Proteinuria in Diabetes (AVOID) study demonstrated a renoprotective effect in diabetic patients when combined with losartan. Yet in the Aliskiren Trial in type 2 Diabetes Using Cardiorenal Disease Endpoints (ALTITUDE), incidence of nonfatal stroke, renal dysfunction, and hypotension led to a premature closure of the study. Given these mixed results, more studies are currently underway. Until the long-term benefits and safety of aliskiren are known, older antihypertensives should be considered first.

Pharmacokinetics

Aliskiren is administered orally, and bioavailability is low (only 2.5%). Dosing with a *high-fat meal* makes availability much lower (approximately 0.8%). Aliskiren undergoes some metabolism by CYP3A4 (the 3A4 isozyme of cytochrome P450), but the extent of metabolism is not known. Approximately 25% of the drug is eliminated unchanged in the urine. The half-life is approximately 24 hours.

Adverse Effects

Aliskiren is generally well tolerated. At usual doses, the risk for angioedema, cough, or hyperkalemia is low. At high therapeutic doses, some patients experience diarrhea. Like other drugs that affect the RAAS, aliskiren should be avoided during pregnancy.

Angioedema and Cough

With ACE inhibitors, angioedema and cough result from inhibition of kinase II. Because aliskiren does not inhibit kinase II, the risk for these effects is low. In clinical trials, the incidence of cough was 1.1% with aliskiren, versus approximately 10% with an ACE inhibitor. Similarly, the incidence of angioedema was 0.06% with aliskiren, versus 1% with an ACE inhibitor. If angioedema does occur, aliskiren should be discontinued immediately.

Gastrointestinal Effects

Aliskiren causes dose-dependent diarrhea, seen in 2.3% of patients taking 300 mg/day. Women and older adults are most susceptible.

Excessive doses (600 mg/day) are associated with abdominal pain and dyspepsia.

Hyperkalemia

Like the ACE inhibitors, aliskiren rarely causes hyperkalemia when used alone. However, hyperkalemia might be expected if aliskiren were combined with an ACE inhibitor, a potassium-sparing diuretic, or potassium supplements.

 BLACK BOX WARNING
Fetal Injury and Death

> Although aliskiren has not been studied in pregnant women, the drug is likely to pose a risk for major congenital malformations and fetal death because the risk for these events is well established with other drugs that suppress the renin-angiotensin-aldosterone system. Therefore, like the angiotensin-converting enzyme inhibitors and angiotensin II receptor blockers, aliskiren is contraindicated during the second and third trimesters and should be discontinued as soon as possible when pregnancy occurs.

ALDOSTERONE ANTAGONISTS

Aldosterone antagonists are drugs that block receptors for aldosterone. Two such agents are available: eplerenone and spironolactone. Both drugs have similar structures and actions, and both are used for the same disorders: hypertension and heart failure. However, they differ in that spironolactone is less selective than eplerenone. As a result, spironolactone causes more side effects.

Eplerenone

Eplerenone (Inspra) is a first-in-class *selective aldosterone receptor blocker*. The drug is used for hypertension and heart failure and has one significant side effect: hyperkalemia.

Mechanism of Action

Eplerenone produces selective blockade of aldosterone receptors, having little or no effect on receptors for other steroid hormones (e.g., glucocorticoids, progesterone, androgens). In the kidney, activation of aldosterone receptors promotes excretion of potassium and retention of sodium and water. Receptor blockade has the opposite effect: retention of potassium and increased excretion of sodium and water. Loss of sodium and water reduces blood volume and hence blood pressure. Blockade of aldosterone receptors at nonrenal sites may prevent or reverse pathologic effects of aldosterone on cardiovascular structure and function.

Therapeutic Use

Hypertension. For treatment of hypertension, eplerenone may be used alone or in combination with other antihypertensive agents. Maximal reductions in blood pressure take approximately 4 weeks to develop. In clinical trials, reductions in blood pressure were equivalent to those produced by spironolactone and superior to those produced by losartan (an ARB). In patients already using an ACE inhibitor or an ARB, adding eplerenone produced a further reduction in blood pressure.

Although it is clear that eplerenone can lower blood pressure, we have no information on what really matters: the drug's ability to reduce morbidity and mortality in patients with isolated hypertension and lack of LV hypertrophy. Until more is known, eplerenone should be reserved for patients who have not responded to traditional antihypertensive drugs.

Heart failure. In patients with heart failure, eplerenone can improve symptoms, reduce hospitalizations, and prolong life. Benefits appear to derive from blocking the adverse effects of aldosterone on cardiovascular structure and function. Use of eplerenone in heart failure is discussed in Chapter 42.

Adverse Effects

Eplerenone is generally well tolerated. The incidence of adverse effects is nearly identical to that of placebo. A few adverse effects—diarrhea, abdominal pain, cough, fatigue, gynecomastia, flu-like syndrome—occur slightly (1% to 2%) more often with eplerenone than with placebo.

Hyperkalemia. The greatest concern is hyperkalemia, which can occur secondary to potassium retention. Because of this risk, combined use with potassium supplements, salt substitutes, or potassium-sparing diuretics (e.g., spironolactone, triamterene) is contraindicated. Combined use with ACE inhibitors or ARBs is permissible but should be done with caution. Eplerenone is contraindicated for patients with high serum potassium (>5.5 mEq/L) and for patients with impaired renal function or type 2 diabetes with microalbuminuria, both of which can promote hyperkalemia. Monitoring potassium levels is recommended for patients at risk (e.g., those taking ACE inhibitors or ARBs).

Drug Interactions

Inhibitors of CYP3A4 can increase levels of eplerenone, thereby posing a risk for toxicity. Weak inhibitors (e.g., erythromycin, saquinavir, verapamil, fluconazole) can double eplerenone levels. Strong inhibitors (e.g., ketoconazole, itraconazole) can increase levels fivefold. If eplerenone is combined with a weak inhibitor, eplerenone dosage should be reduced. Eplerenone should not be combined with a strong inhibitor.

Drugs that raise potassium levels can increase the risk for hyperkalemia. Eplerenone should not be combined with potassium supplements, salt substitutes, or potassium-sparing diuretics. Combining eplerenone with ACE inhibitors or ARBs should be done with caution.

Drugs similar to eplerenone (e.g., ACE inhibitors and diuretics) are known to increase levels of *lithium*. Although the combination of eplerenone and lithium has not been studied, caution is nonetheless advised. Lithium levels should be measured frequently.

Spironolactone

Spironolactone (Aldactone), a much older drug than eplerenone, blocks receptors for aldosterone but also binds with receptors for other steroid hormones (e.g., glucocorticoids, progesterone, androgens). Blockade of aldosterone receptors underlies beneficial effects in hypertension and heart failure, as well as the drug's major adverse effect: hyperkalemia. Binding with receptors for other steroid hormones underlies additional adverse effects: gynecomastia, menstrual irregularities, impotence, hirsutism, and deepening of the voice. The basic pharmacology of spironolactone and its use in heart failure are discussed in Chapters 41 and 42, respectively.

 BLACK BOX WARNING

Spironolactone

Use of spironolactone is tumorigenic in chronic toxicity studies in rats.

39

Calcium Channel Blockers

Calcium channel blockers (CCBs) are drugs that prevent calcium ions from entering cells. These agents have their greatest effects on the heart and blood vessels. CCBs are used widely to treat hypertension, angina pectoris, and cardiac dysrhythmias. Although they are helpful, there has been controversy about the safety of CCBs, especially in patients with hypertension and diabetes.

CALCIUM CHANNELS: PHYSIOLOGIC FUNCTIONS AND CONSEQUENCES OF BLOCKADE

Calcium channels are gated pores in the cytoplasmic membrane that regulate entry of calcium ions into cells. Calcium entry plays a critical role in the function of vascular smooth muscle (VSM) and the heart.

Vascular Smooth Muscle

In VSM, calcium channels regulate contraction. When an action potential travels down the surface of a smooth muscle cell, calcium channels open and calcium ions flow inward, thereby initiating the contractile process. If calcium channels are blocked, contraction will be prevented and vasodilation will result.

At therapeutic doses, CCBs act selectively on *peripheral arterioles* and *arteries and arterioles of the heart.* CCBs have no significant effect on veins.

Heart

In the heart, calcium channels help regulate the myocardium, the sinoatrial (SA) node, and the atrioventricular (AV) node. Calcium channels at all three sites are coupled to β_1-adrenergic receptors.

Myocardium

In cardiac muscle, calcium entry has a positive inotropic effect. That is, calcium increases force of contraction. If calcium channels in atrial and ventricular muscle are blocked, contractile force will diminish.

Sinoatrial Node

Pacemaker activity of the SA node is regulated by calcium influx. When calcium channels are open, spontaneous discharge of the SA node increases. Conversely, when calcium channels close, pacemaker activity declines. Hence the effect of calcium channel blockade is to reduce heart rate.

Atrioventricular Node

Impulses that originate in the SA node must pass through the AV node on their way to the ventricles. Because of this arrangement, regulation of AV conduction plays a critical role in coordinating contraction of the ventricles with contraction of the atria.

The excitability of AV nodal cells is regulated by calcium entry. When calcium channels are open, calcium entry increases and cells of the AV node discharge more readily. Conversely, when calcium channels are closed, discharge of AV nodal cells is suppressed. Hence the effect of calcium channel blockade is to decrease velocity of conduction through the AV node.

Coupling of Cardiac Calcium Channels to β_1-Adrenergic Receptors

In the heart, calcium channels are coupled to β_1-adrenergic receptors (Fig. 39.1). As a result, when cardiac β_1 receptors are activated, calcium influx is enhanced. Conversely, when β_1 receptors are blocked, calcium influx is suppressed. Because of this relationship, CCBs and β blockers have identical effects on the heart. That is, they both reduce force of contraction, slow heart rate, and suppress conduction through the AV node.

CALCIUM CHANNEL BLOCKERS: CLASSIFICATION AND SITES OF ACTION

Classification

The CCBs used in the United States belong to two families (Table 39.1). The largest family is the *dihydropyridines,* for which *nifedipine* is the prototype. The other family, the nondihydropyridines, includes the drugs: *verapamil* and *diltiazem.*

PROTOYTPE DRUGS

Calcium Channel Blockers

> **Nondihydropyridine: Agent That Affects the Heart and Blood Vessels**
> Verapamil
>
> **Dihydropyridine: Agent That Acts Mainly on Blood Vessels**
> Nifedipine

Sites of Action

At therapeutic doses, the dihydropyridines act primarily on arterioles; in contrast, verapamil and diltiazem act on arterioles *and* the heart (see Table 39.1). However, although dihydropyridines do not affect the heart at *therapeutic* doses, *toxic* doses can produce dangerous cardiac suppression (just as verapamil and diltiazem can). The differences in selectivity among CCBs are based on structural differences among the drugs themselves and structural differences among calcium channels.

NONDIHYDROPYRIDINES—VERAPAMIL AND DILTIAZEM: AGENTS THAT ACT ON VASCULAR SMOOTH MUSCLE AND THE HEART

Verapamil

Verapamil (Calan, Verelan, Covera-HS ✦) blocks calcium channels in blood vessels and in the heart. Major indications are angina pectoris,

Fig. 39.1 Coupling of Cardiac Calcium Channels With β1-Adrenergic Receptors. In the heart, β1 receptors are coupled to calcium channels. As a result, when cardiac β1 receptors are activated, calcium influx is enhanced. The process works as follows: binding of an agonist (e.g., norepinephrine) causes a conformational change in the β receptor, which in turn causes a change in G protein, converting it from an inactive state (in which guanosine diphosphate *[GDP]* is bound to the α subunit) to an active state (in which guanosine triphosphate *[GTP]* is bound to the α subunit). (G protein is so named because it binds guanine nucleotides: GDP and GTP.) After activation, the α subunit dissociates from the rest of G protein and activates adenylyl cyclase, an enzyme that converts adenosine triphosphate *(ATP)* to cyclic adenosine monophosphate *(cAMP)*. cAMP then activates protein kinase, an enzyme that phosphorylates proteins—in this case, the calcium channel. Phosphorylation changes the channel such that calcium entry is enhanced when the channel opens. (Opening of the channel is triggered by a change in membrane voltage [i.e., by passage of an action potential].) The effect of calcium entry on cardiac function is determined by the type of cell involved. If the cell is in the SA node, heart rate increases; if the cell is in the atrioventricular node, impulse conduction through the node accelerates; and if the cell is part of the myocardium, force of contraction is increased. Because binding of a single agonist molecule to a single β receptor stimulates the synthesis of many cAMP molecules—with the subsequent activation of many protein kinase molecules, causing the phosphorylation of many calcium channels—this system can greatly amplify the signal initiated by the agonist.

essential hypertension, and cardiac dysrhythmias. Verapamil was the first CCB available and will serve as our prototype for the group.

Hemodynamic Effects

The overall hemodynamic response to verapamil is the net result of (1) direct effects on the heart and blood vessels and (2) reflex responses.

Direct effects. By blocking calcium channels in the heart and blood vessels, verapamil has five direct effects:

- Blockade at peripheral arterioles causes dilation and thereby reduces arterial pressure.
- Blockade at arteries and arterioles of the heart increases coronary perfusion.
- Blockade at the SA node reduces heart rate.
- Blockade at the AV node decreases AV nodal conduction.
- Blockade in the myocardium decreases force of contraction.

Of the direct effects on the heart, reduced AV conduction is the most important.

Indirect (reflex) effects. Verapamil-induced lowering of blood pressure activates the baroreceptor reflex, causing increased firing of sympathetic nerves to the heart. Norepinephrine released from these nerves acts to increase heart rate, AV conduction, and force of contraction. However, because these same three parameters are suppressed by the direct actions of verapamil, the direct and indirect effects tend to neutralize each other.

Net effect. Because the direct effects of verapamil on the heart are counterbalanced by indirect effects, the drug has little or no net effect on cardiac performance: for most patients, heart rate, AV conduction, and contractility are not noticeably altered. Consequently the overall cardiovascular effect of verapamil is simply vasodilation accompanied by reduced arterial pressure and increased coronary perfusion.

Pharmacokinetics

Verapamil may be administered orally or intravenously. The drug is well absorbed after oral administration but undergoes extensive metabolism on its first pass through the liver. Consequently only about 20% of an oral dose reaches the systemic circulation. Effects begin 30 minutes after dosing and peak within 5 hours. Elimination is primarily by hepatic metabolism. Because the drug is eliminated by the liver, doses must be reduced substantially in patients with hepatic impairment.

TABLE 39.1   Calcium Channel Blockers: Classification, Sites of Action, and Indications

Classification	Sites of Action	Hypertension	Angina	Dysrhythmias	Migraine[a]	Others
Dihydropyridines						
Nifedipine (Adalat CC, Nifediac, Nifedical, Procardia)	Arterioles	✔	✔		✔	[b]
Amlodipine (Norvasc)	Arterioles	✔	✔			
Felodipine (Plendil, Renedil) 🍁	Arterioles	✔				
Isradipine (DynaCirc CR)	Arterioles	✔				
Nicardipine (Cardene SR)	Arterioles	✔	✔			
Nimodipine (Nymalize, Nimotop) 🍁	Arterioles				✔	[c]
Nisoldipine (Sular)	Arterioles	✔				
Nondihydropyridines						
Verapamil (Calan, Covera-HS 🍁, Verelan)	Arterioles/heart	✔	✔	✔	✔	
Diltiazem (Cardizem, Dilacor XR, Tiazac, others)	Arterioles/heart	✔	✔	✔	✔	

[a]Investigational use.
[b]Suppression of preterm labor (investigational use).
[c]Prophylaxis of neurologic injury after rupture of an intracranial aneurysm.

Therapeutic Uses

Angina pectoris. Verapamil is used widely to treat angina pectoris. The drug is approved for vasospastic angina and angina of effort. Benefits in both disorders derive from vasodilation. The role of verapamil in angina is discussed in Chapter 45.

Essential hypertension. Verapamil is a second-line agent for chronic hypertension, used after thiazide diuretics. The drug lowers blood pressure by dilating arterioles. The role of verapamil and other CCBs in hypertension is discussed in Chapter 41.

Cardiac dysrhythmias. Administered intravenously, verapamil is used to slow ventricular rate in patients with atrial flutter, atrial fibrillation, and paroxysmal supraventricular tachycardia. Benefits derive from suppressing impulse conduction through the AV node, thereby preventing the atria from driving the ventricles at an excessive rate. Antidysrhythmic applications are discussed in Chapter 43.

Adverse Effects

Common effects. Verapamil is generally well tolerated. *Constipation* occurs frequently and is the most common complaint. This problem, which can be especially severe in older adults, can be minimized by increasing dietary fluids and fiber. Constipation results from blockade of calcium channels in smooth muscle of the intestine. Other common effects—dizziness, facial flushing, headache, and edema of the ankles and feet—occur secondary to vasodilation.

Cardiac effects. Blockade of calcium channels in the heart can compromise cardiac function. In the SA node, calcium channel blockade can cause bradycardia; in the AV node, blockade can cause partial or complete AV block; and in the myocardium, blockade can decrease contractility. When the heart is healthy, these effects rarely have clinical significance. However, in patients with certain cardiac diseases, verapamil can seriously exacerbate dysfunction. Accordingly, the drug must be used with special caution in patients with cardiac failure and must not be used at all in patients with sick sinus syndrome or second-degree or third-degree AV block.

Drug and Food Interactions

Digoxin. Like verapamil, digoxin suppresses impulse conduction through the AV node. Accordingly, when these drugs are used

concurrently, the risk for AV block is increased. Patients receiving the combination should be monitored closely.

Verapamil increases plasma levels of digoxin by about 60%, thereby increasing the risk for digoxin toxicity. If signs of toxicity appear, digoxin dosage should be reduced.

β-adrenergic blocking agents. β blockers and verapamil have the same effects on the heart: they decrease heart rate, AV conduction, and contractility. Hence, when a β blocker and verapamil are used together, there is a risk for excessive cardiosuppression. To minimize risk, β blockers and intravenous verapamil should be administered several hours apart.

Grapefruit juice. Grapefruit juice can inhibit the intestinal and hepatic metabolism of many drugs and thus raise their levels. It was originally thought that grapefurit juice caused significant interactions with all calcium channel blockers. New evidence reveals that felodipine and nifedipine carry the highest risk. Although verapamil, amlodipine, and diltiazem may still interact with grapefruit juice, the interaction with these medications is less than originally thought.

Diltiazem
Actions and Uses

Similar to verapamil, diltiazem (Cardizem, Dilacor XR, Tiazac, others) blocks calcium channels in the heart and blood vessels. As a result, the actions and applications of verapamil and diltiazem are very similar. Diltiazem has the same effects on cardiovascular function as does verapamil. Both drugs lower blood pressure through arteriolar dilation and, because their direct suppressant actions are balanced by reflex cardiac stimulation, both have little net effect on the heart. Similar to verapamil, diltiazem is used for angina pectoris, essential hypertension, and cardiac dysrhythmias (atrial flutter, atrial fibrillation, and paroxysmal supraventricular tachycardia).

Pharmacokinetics

Oral diltiazem is well absorbed and then extensively metabolized on its first pass through the liver. As a result, bioavailability is only about 50%. Effects begin rapidly (within a few minutes) and peak within half an hour. The drug undergoes nearly complete metabolism before it is eliminated in the urine and feces.

Adverse Effects

The adverse effects of diltiazem are similar to those of verapamil except that diltiazem causes less constipation. The most common effects are dizziness, flushing, headache, and edema of the ankles and feet. Both drugs can exacerbate cardiac dysfunction in patients with bradycardia, sick sinus syndrome, heart failure, or second-degree or third-degree AV block. Similar to other CCBs, diltiazem may cause chronic eczematous rash in older adults.

PATIENT-CENTERED CARE ACROSS THE LIFE SPAN

Calcium Channel Blockers

Life Stage	Patient Care Concerns
Infants	Verapamil can be used in infants to convert certain heart dysrhythmias.
Children/ adolescents	Calcium channel blockers are used in children to treat hypertension, hypertensive emergencies, and hypertrophic cardiomyopathy.
Pregnant women	The risks and benefits of therapy must be discussed when considering use in pregnancy.
Breastfeeding women	Certain drugs, such as verapamil, may pose harm to the infant. For other drugs, such as nifedipine, data are lacking regarding transmission of drug from mother to infant via breast milk.
Older adults	In older patients, calcium channel blockers have been associated with chronic eczematous eruptions.

Drug and Food Interactions

Both verapamil and diltiazem can exacerbate digoxin-induced suppression of AV conduction and can intensify the cardiosuppressant effects of β blockers. Patients receiving diltiazem concurrently with digoxin or a β blocker should be monitored closely for cardiac status.

SUMMARY OF KEY PRESCRIBING CONSIDERATIONS

Verapamil and Diltiazem

Therapeutic Goal: Verapamil and diltiazem are indicated for hypertension, angina, and cardiac dysrhythmias.

Baseline Data: Determine blood pressure and pulse rate and obtain laboratory evaluations of liver and kidney function.

Monitoring: No routine blood monitoring required.

Identifying High-Risk Patients: These drugs are contraindicated in patients with hypotension, sick sinus syndrome, and second- or third-degree atrioventricular block.

Evaluating Therapeutic Effects: Monitor blood pressure periodically. For angina, the patient should keep ongoing records of time and intensity of anginal attacks.

Minimizing Adverse Effects: Initiate therapy with low doses, adjust doses carefully, monitor weight loss daily, and use an intermittent dosing schedule.

DIHYDROPYRIDINES: AGENTS THAT ACT MAINLY ON VASCULAR SMOOTH MUSCLE

All the drugs discussed in this section belong to the *dihydropyridine* family. At therapeutic doses, these drugs produce significant blockade of calcium channels in blood vessels and minimal blockade of calcium channels in the heart. The dihydropyridines are similar to verapamil in some respects but quite different in others.

Nifedipine

Nifedipine (Adalat CC, Nifedical XL, Procardia, Procardia XL) was the first dihydropyridine available and will serve as our prototype for the group. Similar to verapamil, nifedipine blocks calcium channels in VSM and thereby promotes vasodilation. However, in contrast to verapamil, nifedipine produces very little blockade of calcium channels in the heart. As a result, nifedipine cannot be used to treat dysrhythmias, does not cause cardiac suppression, and is less likely than verapamil to exacerbate preexisting cardiac disorders. Nifedipine also differs from verapamil in that nifedipine is more likely to cause reflex tachycardia. Contrasts between nifedipine and verapamil are shown in Table 39.2.

Hemodynamic Effects

Direct effects. The direct effects of nifedipine on the cardiovascular system are limited to blockade of calcium channels in VSM. Such blockade in peripheral arterioles causes vasodilation and thus lowers arterial

TABLE 39.2 Comparisons and Contrasts Between Nifedipine and Verapamil

Property	DRUG	
	Nifedipine	Verapamil
Direct Effects on the Heart and Arterioles		
Arteriolar dilation	Yes	Yes
Effects on the Heart		
Reduced automaticity	No	Yes
Reduced AV conduction	No	Yes
Reduced contractile force	No	Yes
Major Indications		
Hypertension	Yes	Yes
Angina pectoris (classical and variant)	Yes	Yes
Dysrhythmias	No	Yes
Adverse Effects		
Exacerbation of		
AV block	No	Yes
Sick sinus syndrome	No	Yes
Heart failure	No	Yes
Effects Secondary to Vasodilation		
Edema (ankles and feet)	Yes	Yes
Flushing	Yes	Yes
Headaches	Yes	Yes
Dizziness	Yes	Yes
Reflex tachycardia	Yes	No
Constipation	No	Yes
Drug Interactions		
Intensifies digoxin-induced AV block	No	Yes
Intensifies cardiosuppressant effects of β blockers	No	Yes
Often combined with a β blocker to suppress reflex tachycardia	Yes	No

AV, Atrioventricular

pressure; in arteries and arterioles of the heart, it increases coronary perfusion. Because nifedipine does not block cardiac calcium channels at usual therapeutic doses, the drug has no *direct* suppressant effects on automaticity, AV conduction, or contractile force.

Indirect (reflex) effects. By lowering blood pressure, nifedipine activates the baroreceptor reflex, thereby causing sympathetic stimulation of the heart. Because nifedipine lacks direct cardiosuppressant actions, cardiac stimulation is unopposed; hence heart rate and contractile force increase.

It is important to note that reflex effects occur primarily with the *immediate-release* (IR) formulation of nifedipine, not with the slow-release (SR) formulation. This is because the baroreceptor reflex is turned on only by a *rapid* fall in blood pressure; a gradual decline will not activate the reflex. With the IR formulation, blood levels of nifedipine rise quickly; hence blood pressure drops quickly and the reflex is turned on. Conversely, with the SR formulation, blood levels of nifedipine rise slowly, so blood pressure falls slowly and the reflex is blunted.

Net effect. The overall hemodynamic response to nifedipine is simply the sum of its direct effect (vasodilation) and indirect effect (reflex cardiac stimulation). Accordingly, nifedipine (1) lowers blood pressure, (2) increases heart rate, and (3) increases contractile force. Note, however, that the reflex increases in heart rate and contractile force are transient and occur primarily with the IR formulation.

Pharmacokinetics

Nifedipine is well absorbed after oral administration but undergoes extensive first-pass metabolism. As a result, only about 50% of an oral dose reaches the systemic circulation. With the IR formulation, effects begin rapidly and peak in 30 minutes; with the SR formulation, effects begin in 20 minutes and peak in 6 hours. Nifedipine is fully metabolized before excretion in the urine.

Therapeutic Uses

Angina pectoris. Nifedipine is indicated for vasospastic angina and angina of effort. The drug is usually combined with a β blocker to prevent reflex stimulation of the heart, which could intensify anginal pain. Long-term use reduces the rates of overt heart failure, coronary angiography, and coronary bypass surgery but not rates of stroke, myocardial infarction, or death. The role of nifedipine in angina is discussed in Chapter 45.

Hypertension. Nifedipine is used widely to treat *essential hypertension.* Only the SR formulation should be used. In the past, nifedipine was used for *hypertensive emergencies,* but it has largely been replaced by drugs that are safer. The use of CCBs in essential hypertension is discussed in Chapter 41.

Adverse Effects

Some adverse effects are similar to those of verapamil; others are quite different. Both verapamil and nifedipine can cause flushing, dizziness, headache, peripheral edema, and gingival hyperplasia and may pose a risk for chronic eczematous rash in older patients. In contrast to verapamil, nifedipine causes very little constipation. Also, because

nifedipine causes minimal blockade of calcium channels in the heart, the drug is not likely to exacerbate AV block, heart failure, bradycardia, or sick sinus syndrome. Accordingly nifedipine is preferred to verapamil for patients with these disorders.

A response that occurs with nifedipine that does not occur with verapamil is *reflex tachycardia.* This response is problematic in that it increases cardiac oxygen demand and can thereby increase pain in patients with angina. To prevent reflex tachycardia, nifedipine can be combined with a β blocker (e.g., metoprolol).

Immediate-Release Nifedipine

IR nifedipine has been associated with increased mortality in patients with myocardial infarction and unstable angina. Other IR CCBs have been associated with an increased risk for myocardial infarction in patients with hypertension. In both cases, however, a causal relationship has not been established. Nonetheless the National Heart, Lung, and Blood Institute has recommended that *IR* nifedipine, especially in higher doses, be used with great caution if at all. It is important to note that these adverse effects have not been associated with *SR* nifedipine or with any other long-acting CCB.

Drug Interactions

β-adrenergic blockers. β blockers are combined with nifedipine to prevent reflex tachycardia. It is important to note that whereas β blockers can *decrease* the adverse cardiac effects of *nifedipine,* they can *intensify* the adverse cardiac effects of *verapamil* and *diltiazem.*

Other Dihydropyridines

In addition to nifedipine, six other dihydropyridines are available (see Table 39.1). All are similar to nifedipine. Like nifedipine, these drugs produce greater blockade of calcium channels in VSM than in the heart.

 SUMMARY OF KEY PRESCRIBING CONSIDERATIONS

Dihydropyridines

Therapeutic Goal: Amlodipine, nifedipine, and nicardipine are approved for essential hypertension and angina. Isradipine, felodipine, and nisoldipine are approved for hypertension only.

Baseline Data: Determine blood pressure and pulse rate and obtain laboratory evaluations of liver and kidney function.

Monitoring: No routine blood monitoring required.

Identifying High-Risk Patients: Use with caution in patients with hypotension, sick sinus syndrome, heart failure, and second- or third-degree atrioventricular block.

Evaluating Therapeutic Effects: Monitor blood pressure periodically. Patients should keep an ongoing record of anginal attacks, including time and frequency.

Minimizing Adverse Effects: Reflex tachycardia can be suppressed with a β blocker. Peripheral edema can be reduced with a diuretic.

40

Vasodilators

Vasodilation can be produced by a variety of drugs. What sets vasodilators apart from other drugs that cause vasodilation is their mechanism of action: they act directly on the smooth muscles in arterioles and veins to produce vessel relaxation. Two agents—hydralazine and minoxidil—are introduced here. A third, sodium nitroprusside, is used in emergency situations in inpatient settings. This drug is discussed in Chapter 92 on drug therapy in acute care.

In approaching the vasodilators, concepts that apply to the vasodilators as a group are considered first, followed by a discussion of the pharmacology of individual agents.

BASIC CONCEPTS IN VASODILATOR PHARMACOLOGY

Selectivity of Vasodilatory Effects

Vasodilators differ from one another with respect to the types of blood vessels they affect. Both hydralazine and minoxidil produce selective dilation of arterioles. Nitroprusside dilates both arterioles *and* veins.

The selectivity of a vasodilator determines its hemodynamic effects. For example, drugs that dilate *resistance vessels* (arterioles) cause a decrease in cardiac *afterload* (the force the heart works against to pump blood). By decreasing afterload, arteriolar dilators reduce cardiac work while causing cardiac output and tissue perfusion to increase. In contrast, drugs that dilate *capacitance vessels* (veins) reduce the force with which blood is returned to the heart, which reduces ventricular filling. This reduction in filling decreases cardiac *preload* (the degree of stretch of the ventricular muscle before contraction), which in turn decreases the force of ventricular contraction. Hence, by decreasing preload, venous dilators cause a decrease in cardiac work along with a decrease in cardiac output and tissue perfusion.

Because hemodynamic responses to the dilation of arterioles and veins differ, the selectivity of a vasodilator is a major determinant of its effects, both therapeutic and undesired. Undesired effects related to selective dilation of arterioles and veins are discussed later. Therapeutic implications of selective dilation are discussed in Chapters 41, 42, and 45.

Overview of Therapeutic Uses

The vasodilators as a group have a broad spectrum of uses. Principal indications are *essential hypertension, hypertensive crisis, angina pectoris, heart failure,* and *myocardial infarction.* The specific applications of any particular agent are determined by its pharmacological profile. Important facets of that profile are route of administration, site of vasodilation (arterioles, veins, or both), and intensity and duration of effects.

Adverse Effects Related to Vasodilation
Postural Hypotension

The underlying cause of postural hypotension is relaxation of smooth muscle in *veins.* Because of venous relaxation, gravity causes blood to "pool" in veins, thereby decreasing venous return to the heart. Reduced venous return causes a decrease in cardiac output and a corresponding decrease in blood pressure. Hypotension from venous dilation is minimal in recumbent subjects because the effect of gravity on venous return is small when we are lying down.

PHARMACOLOGY OF INDIVIDUAL VASODILATORS

Hydralazine
Cardiovascular Effects

Hydralazine causes selective dilation of arterioles. The drug has little or no effect on veins. Arteriolar dilation results from a direct action on vascular smooth muscle (VSM). The exact mechanism is unknown. In response to arteriolar dilation, peripheral resistance and arterial blood pressure fall. In addition, heart rate and myocardial contractility increase, largely by reflex mechanisms. Because hydralazine acts selectively on arterioles, postural hypotension is minimal.

Pharmacokinetics

Absorption and time course of action. Hydralazine is readily absorbed after oral administration. Effects begin within 45 minutes and persist for 6 hours or longer. With parenteral administration, effects begin faster (within 10 minutes) and last 2 to 4 hours.

Metabolism. Hydralazine is inactivated by a metabolic process known as *acetylation.* The ability to acetylate drugs is genetically determined. Some people are rapid acetylators and others are slow acetylators. The distinction between rapid and slow acetylators can be clinically significant, because individuals who acetylate hydralazine slowly are likely to have higher blood levels of the drug, which can result in excessive vasodilation and other undesired effects. To avoid the accumulation of hydralazine, dosage should be reduced in slow acetylators.

Therapeutic Uses

Essential hypertension. Oral hydralazine can be used to lower blood pressure in patients with essential hypertension. The regimen almost always includes a β blocker (Table 40.1). Although commonly employed in the past, hydralazine has been largely replaced by newer antihypertensive agents (see Chapter 41).

Heart failure. As discussed in Chapter 42, hydralazine (usually in combination with isosorbide dinitrate) can be used short term to reduce afterload in patients with heart failure. With prolonged therapy, tolerance to hydralazine develops.

TABLE 40.1 Vasodilator Preparations, Dosage, and Administration

Drug	Forms	Usual Adult Doses
Hydralazine	Tablets 10, 25, 50, 100 mg	Low initially 10 mg PO four times daily. Gradually increase. Daily doses >200 mg are associated with increased adverse effects.
Hydralazine/isosorbide dinitrate [BiDil]	Tablet 20/37.5 mg	Start with 1 tablet PO three times daily. May increase to max of 6 tablets/day.
Minoxidil	Tablets 2.5 and 10 mg	Initial dose 5 mg PO daily. May increase to max of 100 mg/day.

PO, Oral administration.

Adverse Effects

Reflex tachycardia. By lowering arterial blood pressure, hydralazine can trigger reflex stimulation of the heart, thereby causing cardiac work and myocardial oxygen demand to increase. Because hydralazine-induced reflex tachycardia is frequently severe, the drug is usually combined with a β blocker.

Increased blood volume. Hydralazine-induced hypotension can cause sodium and water retention and a corresponding increase in blood volume. A diuretic can prevent volume expansion.

Systemic lupus erythematosus–like syndrome. Hydralazine can cause an acute rheumatoid syndrome that closely resembles systemic lupus erythematosus (SLE). Symptoms include muscle pain, joint pain, fever, nephritis, pericarditis, and the presence of antinuclear antibodies. The syndrome occurs most frequently in slow acetylators and is rare when dosage is kept below 200 mg/day. If an SLE-like reaction occurs, hydralazine should be discontinued. Symptoms are usually reversible but may take 6 or more months to resolve. In some cases, rheumatoid symptoms persist for years.

Drug Interactions

Hydralazine can be combined with a *β blocker* to protect against reflex tachycardia and with a *diuretic* to prevent sodium and water retention and expansion of blood volume. Drugs that lower blood pressure will intensify hypotensive responses to hydralazine. Accordingly, if hydralazine is used with other *antihypertensive agents*, care is needed to avoid excessive hypotension. In the treatment of heart failure, hydralazine is usually combined with *isosorbide dinitrate*, a drug that dilates veins.

Minoxidil

Minoxidil produces more intense vasodilation than hydralazine but also causes more severe adverse reactions. Because it is both very effective and very dangerous, minoxidil is reserved for patients with severe hypertension unresponsive to safer drugs.

Cardiovascular Effects

Like hydralazine, minoxidil produces selective dilation of *arterioles*. Little or no venous dilation occurs. Arteriolar dilation decreases peripheral resistance and arterial blood pressure. In response, reflex mechanisms increase heart rate and myocardial contractility. Both responses can increase cardiac oxygen demand and can thereby exacerbate angina pectoris.

Vasodilation results from a direct action on VSM. To relax VSM, minoxidil must first be metabolized to minoxidil sulfate. This metabolite then causes potassium channels in VSM to open. The resultant efflux of potassium hyperpolarizes VSM cells, thereby reducing their ability to contract.

Pharmacokinetics

Minoxidil is rapidly and completely absorbed after oral administration. Vasodilation is maximum within 2 to 3 hours and then gradually declines. Residual effects may persist for 2 days or more. Minoxidil is extensively metabolized. Metabolites and parent drug are eliminated in the urine. The drug's half-life is 4.2 hours.

Therapeutic Uses

The only cardiovascular indication for minoxidil is *severe hypertension*. Because of its significant adverse effects, minoxidil is reserved for patients who have not responded to safer drugs. To minimize adverse responses (reflex tachycardia, expansion of blood volume, pericardial effusion), minoxidil should be used with a β blocker plus intensive diuretic therapy.

Adverse Effects

Reflex tachycardia. Blood pressure reduction triggers reflex tachycardia, a serious effect that can be minimized by comcomitant treatment with a β blocker.

Sodium and water retention. Fluid retention is both common and serious. Volume expansion may be so severe as to cause cardiac decompensation. Management of fluid retention requires a loop diuretic (e.g., furosemide) used alone or in combination with a thiazide diuretic. If diuretics are inadequate, dialysis must be employed or minoxidil withdrawn.

Hypertrichosis. About 80% of patients taking minoxidil for 4 weeks or more develop hypertrichosis (excessive growth of hair). Hair growth begins on the face and later develops on the arms, legs, and back. Hypertrichosis appears to result from proliferation of epithelial cells at the base of the hair follicle; vasodilation may also be involved. Excessive hair growth is a cosmetic problem that can be controlled by shaving or using a depilatory. However, many patients find hypertrichosis both unmanageable and intolerable and refuse to continue treatment.

 BLACK BOX WARNING

Minoxidil

Minoxidil can cause pericardial effusion, occasionally progressing to tamponade, and may exacerbate angina pectoris.

SUMMARY OF KEY PRESCRIBING CONSIDERATIONS:

Vasodilators

Therapeutic Goal: Reduction of blood pressure in patients with hypertension. Reduce afterload for a short time in patients with heart failure.

Baseline Data: Weight, vital signs.

Monitoring: Blood pressure and heart rate should be recorded by the patient on a daily basis. Daily weight should be recorded in patients taking minoxidil.

Identifying High-Risk Patients: Avoid use in pregnant patients if possible.

Evaluating Therapeutic Effects: Monitor for reduced blood pressure. Monitor for a lessening of signs and symptoms of heart failure, including dyspnea.

Minimizing Adverse Effects: If being combined with other antihypertensives, low doses should be used to minimize hypotension. Patients should be cautioned to stand up slowly so as to avoid postural hypotension.

PATIENT-CENTERED CARE ACROSS THE LIFE SPAN

Vasodilators

Life Stage	Patient Care Concerns
Infants	Hydralazine is used in infants as young as 1 month of age for the management of chronic hypertension.
Children/adolescents	Hydralazine can be used safely in children, just in smaller doses. Side-effect profiles are similar to those of adults.
Pregnant women	When considering use of hydralazine and minoxidil in pregnancy, benefits should outweigh the risks.
Breastfeeding women	Data are lacking regarding transmission of drug from mother to infant via breast milk.
Older adults	Monitor for falls because there is increased risk with polypharmacy and associated orthostatic hypotension.

41

Drugs for Hypertension

Hypertension is a common, chronic disorder that affects about 2 million American children, 85 million American adults, and more than 1 billion people worldwide. According to the World Health Organization, hypertension is the leading global risk for mortality and has increased nearly 20% in the past 20 years. Left untreated, hypertension can lead to heart disease, kidney disease, and stroke. Conversely, a treatment program of lifestyle modifications and drug therapy can reduce blood pressure (BP) and the risk for long-term complications. However, although we can reduce symptoms and long-term consequences, we cannot cure hypertension. As a result, treatment must continue lifelong, making nonadherence a significant problem. Despite advances in management, hypertension remains undertreated: among Americans with the disease, only 74% undergo treatment, and only 48% take sufficient medicine to bring their BP under control.

In 2017, the American College of Cardiology, the American Heart Association, and the Task Force on Clinical Practice Guidelines issued a new guideline for hypertension entitled *2017 ACC/AHA/AAPA/ABC/ ACPM/AGS/AphA/ASH/ASPC/NMA/PCNA Guideline for the Prevention, Detection, Evaluation and Management of High Blood Pressure in Adults.* Throughout this chapter, clinical practice recommendations reflect those in the 2017 hypertension guidelines except where noted otherwise.[a]

BASIC CONSIDERATIONS IN HYPERTENSION

In this section, we consider three issues: (1) the classification of BP based on values for systolic and diastolic pressure, (2) the types of hypertension, and (3) the damaging effects of chronic hypertension.

Classification of Blood Pressure

Classifications of blood pressure have varied through the past decade. The latest categories of blood pressures in adults are shown in Table 41.1.

Types of Hypertension

There are two broad categories of hypertension: *primary hypertension* and *secondary hypertension.* Primary hypertension is by far the most common form of hypertensive disease. Less than 10% of people with hypertension have a secondary form.

Primary (Essential) Hypertension

Primary hypertension is defined as hypertension that has no identifiable cause. A diagnosis of primary hypertension is made by ruling out probable

---

[a]Although the 2017 hypertension guideline is the most influential guideline in the United States, it is not the only authoritative guideline available. Treatment guidelines have been released by several organizations, including the American Society of Hypertension, the Canadian Hypertension Education Program, the European Society of Hypertension in conjunction with the European Society of Cardiology, and the World Health Organization in conjunction with the International Society of Hypertension.

specific causes of BP elevation. Primary hypertension is a chronic, progressive disorder. In the absence of treatment, patients will experience a continuous, gradual rise in BP over the rest of their lives.

In the United States, primary hypertension affects about 30% of adults. However, not all groups are at equal risk: older people are at higher risk than younger people, African Americans are at higher risk than Caucasians, and postmenopausal women are at higher risk than premenopausal women.

Secondary Hypertension

Secondary hypertension is defined as an elevation of BP brought on by an identifiable primary cause. Because secondary hypertension results from an identifiable cause, it may be possible to treat that cause directly rather than relying on antihypertensive drugs for symptomatic relief. As a result, some individuals can actually be cured. For example, if hypertension occurs secondary to pheochromocytoma, surgical removal of the tumor may produce permanent cure. When cure is not possible, secondary hypertension can be managed with the same drugs used for primary hypertension.

MANAGEMENT OF CHRONIC HYPERTENSION

In this section we consider treatments for chronic hypertension. We begin by addressing patient evaluation and other basic issues, after which we discuss the two modes of management: lifestyle modifications and drug therapy.

Basic Considerations
Diagnosis

Diagnosis should be based on several BP readings, not just one. If an initial screen shows that BP is elevated (but does not represent an immediate danger), measurement should be repeated on two subsequent office visits. At each visit, two measurements should be made at least 5 minutes apart. The patient should be seated in a chair—not on an examination table—with his or her feet on the floor. High readings should be confirmed in the contralateral arm. If the mean of all readings shows that systolic BP (SBP) is indeed greater than 130 mm Hg or that diastolic BP (DBP) is greater than 80 mm Hg, a diagnosis of hypertension can be made.

Ideally diagnosis would be based on *ambulatory blood pressure monitoring* (ABPM) because office-based measurements are often abnormally high, causing individuals to be diagnosed with hypertension who may not truly have it have it. By contrast, when BP is measured with ABPM, false-positive diagnoses can be avoided. Accordingly some experts recommend that office-based measurements be used only for *screening* and that treatment be postponed until the diagnosis is confirmed using ABPM. In this way the risks and expense of unnecessary treatment will be avoided.

Patient Evaluation

Evaluation of patients with hypertension has two major objectives. Specifically, providers should assess for (1) identifiable causes of

TABLE 41.1   Categories of Blood Pressure in Adults

Classification	SBP	DBP
Normal	<120 mm Hg AND	<80 mm Hg
Elevated	120–129 mm Hg AND	<80 mm Hg
Hypertension		
Stage 1	130–139 mm Hg OR	80–89 mm Hg
Stage 2	≥140 mm Hg OR	≥ 90 mm Hg

American College of Cardiology, the American Heart Association. 2017 ACC/AHA/AAPA/ABC/ACPM/AGS/AphA/ASH/ASPC/NMA/PCNA Guideline for the Prevention, Detection, Evaluation and Management of High Blood Pressure in Adults.

hypertension and (2) factors that increase cardiovascular risk. To aid evaluation, diagnostic tests are required.

Hypertension with a treatable cause. As discussed previously, some forms of hypertension result from a treatable cause, such as Cushing syndrome, pheochromocytoma, and use of oral contraceptives. Patients should be evaluated for these causes and managed appropriately. In many cases, direct treatment of the underlying cause can control BP, eliminating the need for further antihypertensive therapy.

Factors that increase cardiovascular risk. Two types of factors—existing target-organ damage and major cardiovascular risk factors—increase the risk for cardiovascular events in people with hypertension. When these factors are present, aggressive therapy is indicated. Accordingly, to select appropriate interventions, we must identify patients with the following types of *target-organ damage:*

- Heart disease
- Left ventricular hypertrophy
- Angina pectoris
- Prior myocardial infarction (MI)
- Prior coronary revascularization
- Heart failure
- Stroke or transient ischemic attack
- Chronic kidney disease
- Peripheral arterial disease
- Retinopathy

We must also identify patients with the following *major cardiovascular risk factors* (other than hypertension):

- Cigarette smoking
- Physical inactivity
- Dyslipidemia
- Diabetes
- Microalbuminuria
- Advancing age (>55 years for men, >65 years for women)
- Family history of premature cardiovascular disease

Diagnostic tests. The following tests should be done in all patients: electrocardiogram; complete urinalysis; hemoglobin and hematocrit; and blood levels of sodium, potassium, calcium, creatinine, glucose, uric acid, triglycerides, and cholesterol (total, low-density lipoprotein, and high-density lipoprotein cholesterol).

Treatment Goals

The ultimate goal in treating hypertension is to reduce cardiovascular and renal morbidity and mortality. The hope is that this can be accomplished without decreasing quality of life with the drugs employed. For adult patients, the goal is to maintain SBP below 130 mm Hg and DBP below 80 mm Hg.

Therapeutic Interventions

We can reduce BP in two ways: by implementing healthy lifestyle changes and by treatment with antihypertensive drugs. For all patients, lifestyle changes are indicated. Lifestyle changes and drug therapy are discussed in detail next.

Lifestyle Modifications

Lifestyle changes offer multiple cardiovascular benefits with little cost and minimal risk. When implemented before hypertension develops, they may actually prevent hypertension. When implemented after hypertension has developed, they can lower BP, possibly decreasing or eliminating the need for drugs. Last, lifestyle modifications can decrease other cardiovascular risk factors. Therefore all patients should be strongly encouraged to adopt a healthy lifestyle. Key components include sodium restriction, inclusion of the Dietary Approaches to Stop Hypertension (DASH) eating plan, restricting alcohol consumption, participating in aerobic exercise, maintaining a healthy body weight, and smoking cessation for those patients that use tobacco.

Drug Therapy

Drug therapy together with lifestyle modifications can control BP in all patients with chronic hypertension. The decision to use drugs should be the result of collaboration between prescriber and patient. We have a wide assortment of antihypertensive drugs. For most patients, therefore, it should be possible to establish a program that is effective and yet devoid of objectionable side effects.

PROTOTYPE DRUGS
Drugs for Hypertension

Diuretics
Hydrochlorothiazide
Spironolactone

β-Adrenergic Blocker
Metoprolol

Inhibitors of the Renin-Angiotensin-Aldosterone System
Captopril (angiotensin-converting enzyme inhibitor)
Losartan (angiotensin II receptor blocker)
Aliskiren (direct renin inhibitor)
Eplerenone (aldosterone antagonist)

Calcium Channel Blockers
Verapamil
Nifedipine

Review of Blood Pressure Control

Before discussing the antihypertensive drugs, we must review the major mechanisms by which BP is controlled. This information will clarify the mechanisms by which drugs lower BP.

Principal determinants of blood pressure. The principal determinants of BP are shown in Fig. 41.1. As indicated, arterial pressure is the product of cardiac output and peripheral resistance. An increase in either will increase BP.

Cardiac output. Cardiac output is influenced by four factors: (1) heart rate, (2) myocardial contractility (force of contraction), (3) blood volume, and (4) venous return of blood to the heart. An increase in any of these will increase cardiac output, thereby causing BP to rise. Conversely, a decrease in these factors will make BP fall. Hence, to

Fig. 41.1 Primary Determinants of Arterial Blood Pressure.

reduce BP, we might give a β blocker to reduce cardiac output, or a diuretic to reduce blood volume, or a venodilator to reduce venous return.

Peripheral vascular resistance. Vascular resistance is increased by arteriolar constriction. Therefore we can reduce BP with drugs that promote arteriolar dilation.

Systems that help regulate blood pressure. Having established that BP is determined by heart rate, myocardial contractility, blood volume, venous return, and arteriolar constriction, we can now examine how these factors are regulated. Three regulatory systems are of particular significance: (1) the sympathetic nervous system, (2) the renin-angiotensin-aldosterone system (RAAS), and (3) the kidney.

Sympathetic baroreceptor reflex. The sympathetic nervous system employs a reflex circuit—the baroreceptor reflex—to keep BP at a preset level. This circuit operates as follows:

1. Baroreceptors in the aortic arch and carotid sinus sense BP and relay this information to the brain stem.
2. When BP is perceived as too low, the brain stem sends impulses along sympathetic nerves to stimulate the heart and blood vessels.
3. BP is then elevated by (a) activation of β_1 receptors in the heart, resulting in increased cardiac output; and (b) activation of vascular α_1 receptors, resulting in vasoconstriction.
4. When BP has been restored to an acceptable level, sympathetic stimulation of the heart and vascular smooth muscle subsides.

The baroreceptor reflex frequently opposes our attempts to reduce BP with drugs. Opposition occurs because the "set point" of the baroreceptors is high in people with hypertension. That is, the baroreceptors are set to perceive excessively high BP as "normal" (i.e., appropriate). As a result, the system operates to maintain BP at pathologic levels. Consequently, when we attempt to lower BP using drugs, the reduced (healthier) pressure is interpreted by the baroreceptors as below what it should be and, in response, signals are sent along sympathetic nerves to "correct" the reduction. These signals produce reflex tachycardia and vasoconstriction—responses that can counteract the hypotensive effects of drugs. Clearly, if treatment is to succeed, the regimen must compensate for the resistance offered by this reflex. Prescribing a *β blocker*, which will block reflex tachycardia, can be an effective method of compensation. Fortunately, when BP has been suppressed with drugs for an extended time, the baroreceptors become reset at a lower level. Consequently, as therapy proceeds, sympathetic reflexes offer progressively less resistance to the hypotensive effects of medication.

Renin-angiotensin-aldosterone system. The RAAS can elevate BP, negating the hypotensive effects of drugs. The RAAS is discussed in Chapter 38 and reviewed briefly here.

The RAAS elevates BP beginning with the release of renin from juxtaglomerular cells of the kidney. These cells release renin in response to reduced renal blood flow, reduced blood volume, reduced BP, and activation of β_1-adrenergic receptors on the cell surface. After its release, *renin* catalyzes the conversion of angiotensinogen into angiotensin I, a weak vasoconstrictor. After this, *angiotensin-converting enzyme*

(ACE) acts on angiotensin I to form *angiotensin II,* a compound that constricts systemic and renal blood vessels. Constriction of systemic blood vessels elevates BP by increasing peripheral resistance. Constriction of renal blood vessels elevates BP by reducing glomerular filtration, which causes retention of salt and water, which in turn increases blood volume and BP. In addition to causing vasoconstriction, angiotensin II causes release of *aldosterone* from the adrenal cortex. Aldosterone acts on the kidney to further increase the retention of sodium and water.

Because drug-induced reductions in BP can activate the RAAS, this system can counteract the effect we are trying to achieve. We have five ways to cope with this problem. First, we can suppress renin release with *β blockers.* Second, we can prevent conversion of angiotensinogen to angiotensin I with a *direct renin inhibitor* (DRI). Third, we can prevent the conversion of angiotensin I into angiotensin II with an *ACE inhibitor* (ACEI). Fourth, we can block receptors for angiotensin II with an *angiotensin II receptor blocker* (ARB). And fifth, we can block receptors for aldosterone with an *aldosterone antagonist.*

Renal regulation of blood pressure. As discussed in Chapter 36, the kidney plays a central role in the long-term regulation of BP. When BP falls, glomerular filtration rate (GFR) falls too, thereby promoting the retention of sodium, chloride, and water. The resultant increase in blood volume increases venous return to the heart, causing an increase in cardiac output, which in turn increases arterial pressure. We can neutralize renal effects on BP with *diuretics.*

Antihypertensive Mechanisms: Sites of Drug Action and Effects Produced

As discussed previously, drugs can lower BP by reducing heart rate, myocardial contractility, blood volume, venous return, and the tone of arteriolar smooth muscle. In this section we survey the principal mechanisms by which drugs produce these effects.

The major mechanisms for lowering BP are shown in Fig. 41.2 and Table 41.2. The figure depicts the principal sites at which antihypertensive drugs act. The table shows the effects elicited when drugs act at these sites. The numbering system used in the following text corresponds with the system used in Fig. 41.2 and Table 41.2.

1—Brain stem. Antihypertensive drugs acting in the brain stem suppress sympathetic outflow to the heart and blood vessels, resulting in decreased heart rate, decreased myocardial contractility, and vasodilation. Vasodilation contributes the most to reducing BP. Dilation of arterioles reduces BP by decreasing vascular resistance. Dilation of veins reduces BP by decreasing venous return to the heart.

2—Sympathetic ganglia. Ganglionic blockade reduces sympathetic stimulation of the heart and blood vessels. Antihypertensive effects result primarily from dilation of arterioles and veins. Ganglionic blocking agents produce such a profound reduction in BP that they are rarely used, and then only for hypertensive emergencies. Because their use is so limited, the last such agent available—mecamylamine—was voluntarily withdrawn from the US market in 2009.

3—Terminals of adrenergic nerves. Antihypertensive agents that act at adrenergic nerve terminals decrease the release of norepinephrine, resulting in decreased sympathetic stimulation of the heart and blood vessels. These drugs, known as *adrenergic neuron blocking agents,* are used only rarely.

4—β_1-Adrenergic receptors on the heart. Blockade of cardiac β_1 receptors prevents sympathetic stimulation of the heart. As a result, heart rate and myocardial contractility decline.

5—α_1-Adrenergic receptors on blood vessels. Blockade of vascular α_1 receptors promotes dilation of arterioles and veins. Arteriolar dilation reduces peripheral resistance. Venous dilation reduces venous return to the heart.

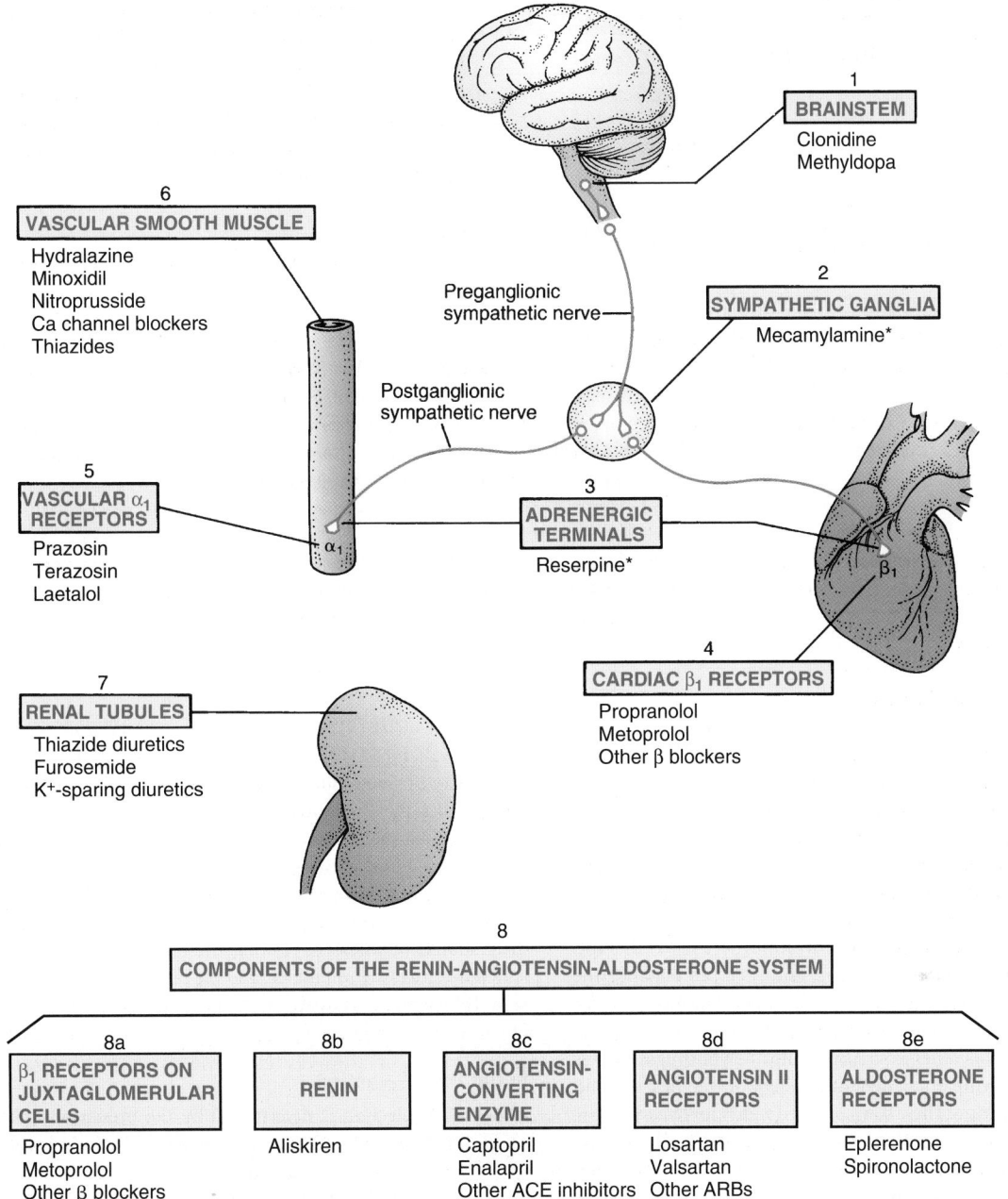

Fig. 41.2 Sites of Action of Antihypertensive Drugs. Note that some antihypertensive agents act at more than one site: β blockers act at sites 4 and 8a, and thiazides act at sites 6 and 7. The hemodynamic consequences of drug actions at the sites depicted are shown in Table 41.2. *ACE,* Angiotensin-converting enzyme; *ARB,* angiotensin II receptor blocker; *,* no longer available in the United States.

6—Vascular smooth muscle. Several antihypertensive drugs (see Fig. 41.2) act directly on vascular smooth muscle to cause relaxation. One of these agents—sodium nitroprusside—is used only for hypertensive emergencies. The rest are used for chronic hypertension.

7—Renal tubules. Diuretics act on renal tubules to promote salt and water excretion. As a result, blood volume declines, causing BP to fall.

Components of the renin-angiotensin-aldosterone system (8a–8e).

8a—β₁ Receptors on juxtaglomerular cells. Blockade of β₁ receptors on juxtaglomerular cells suppresses release of renin. The resultant decrease in angiotensin II levels has three effects: peripheral vasodilation, renal vasodilation, and suppression of aldosterone-mediated volume expansion.

8b—Renin. Inhibition of renin decreases the conversion of angiotensinogen into angiotensin I and thereby suppresses the entire RAAS. The result is peripheral vasodilation, renal vasodilation, and suppression of aldosterone-mediated volume expansion.

8c—Angiotensin-converting enzyme. Inhibitors of ACE suppress formation of angiotensin II. The result is peripheral vasodilation, renal vasodilation, and suppression of aldosterone-mediated volume expansion.

8d—Angiotensin II receptors. Blockade of angiotensin II receptors prevents the actions of angiotensin II. Hence blockade results in peripheral vasodilation, renal vasodilation, and suppression of aldosterone-mediated volume expansion.

TABLE 41.2   Antihypertensive Effects Elicited by Drug Actions at Specific Sites

Site of Drug Action[a]	Representative Drug	Drug Effects
Brain stem	Clonidine	Suppression of sympathetic outflow decreases sympathetic stimulation of the heart and blood vessels.
Sympathetic ganglia	Mecamylamine[b]	Ganglionic blockade reduces sympathetic stimulation of the heart and blood vessels.
Adrenergic nerve terminals	Reserpine[b]	Reduced norepinephrine release decreases sympathetic stimulation of the heart and blood vessels.
Cardiac β_1 receptors	Metoprolol	β_1 blockade decreases heart rate and myocardial contractility.
Vascular α_1 receptors	Prazosin	α_1 Blockade causes vasodilation.
Vascular smooth muscle	Hydralazine	Relaxation of vascular smooth muscle causes vasodilation.
Renal tubules	Hydrochlorothiazide	Promotion of diuresis decreases blood volume.
Components of the Renin-Angiotensin-Aldosterone System (8a–8e)		
8a. β_1 receptors on juxtaglomerular cells	Metoprolol	β_1 blockade suppresses renin release, resulting in) vasodilation secondary to reduced production of angiotensin II and prevention of aldosterone-mediated volume expansion.
8b. Renin	Aliskiren	Inhibition of renin suppresses formation of angiotensin I, which in turn decreases formation of angiotensin II and thereby reduces vasoconstriction and aldosterone-mediated volume expansion.
8c. Angiotensin-converting enzyme	Captopril	Inhibition of angiotensin-converting enzyme decreases formation of angiotensin II and thereby prevents vasoconstriction and aldosterone-mediated volume expansion.
8d. Angiotensin II receptors	Losartan	Blockade of angiotensin II receptors prevents angiotensin-mediated vasoconstriction and aldosterone-mediated volume expansion.
8e. Aldosterone receptors	Eplerenone	Blockade of aldosterone receptors in the kidney promotes excretion of sodium and water and thereby reduces blood volume.

[a]Site numbers in this table correspond with site numbers in Fig. 41.2.
[b]No longer available in the United States.

8e—Aldosterone receptors. Blockade of aldosterone receptors in the kidney promotes excretion of sodium and water and thereby reduces blood volume.

Classes of Antihypertensive Drugs

In this section we consider the principal drugs employed to treat chronic hypertension. Drugs for hypertensive emergencies and hypertensive disorders of pregnancy are considered separately.

Diuretics. Diuretics are a mainstay of antihypertensive therapy. These drugs reduce BP when used alone, and they can enhance the effects of other hypotensive drugs. The basic pharmacology of the diuretics is discussed in Chapter 37.

Sympatholytics (antiadrenergic drugs). Sympatholytic drugs suppress the influence of the sympathetic nervous system on the heart, blood vessels, and other structures. These drugs are used widely for hypertension.

There are four subcategories of sympatholytic drugs used regularly for hypertension: (1) β blockers (see Chapter 16), (2) α_1 blockers (Chapter 16), (3) α/β blockers (Chapter 16), and (4) centrally acting α_2 agonists (see Chapter 17).

Calcium channel blockers. The CCBs fall into two groups: dihydropyridines (e.g., nifedipine and amlodipine) and nondihydropyridines (verapamil and diltiazem). Drugs in both groups promote dilation of arterioles. In addition, verapamil and diltiazem have direct suppressant effects on the heart.

The basic pharmacology of the CCBs is discussed in Chapter 39.

Drugs that suppress the renin-angiotensin-aldosterone system. Because the RAAS plays an important role in controlling BP, drugs that suppress the system—especially the ACEIs—have a significant role in controlling hypertension. The basic pharmacology of these drugs is discussed in Chapter 38.

Fundamentals of Hypertension Drug Therapy
Treatment Algorithm

The basic approach to treating hypertension was published with the new 2017 guidelines in the *Journal of the American College of Cardiology* and can be found on online at http://www.onlinejacc.org/content/

early/2017/11/04/j.jacc.2017.11.006?_ga=2.176790566.2093167245.1516654950-136371117.1515608281. As shown in the algorithm at this link, lifestyle changes should be instituted first. If these fail to lower BP enough, drug therapy should be started—and the lifestyle changes should continue. Treatment often begins with a single drug. If needed, another drug may be *added* (if the initial drug was well tolerated but inadequate) or *substituted* (if the initial drug was poorly tolerated). However, before another drug is considered, possible reasons for failure of the initial drug should be assessed. Among these are insufficient dosage, poor adherence, excessive salt intake, and the presence of secondary hypertension. If treatment with two drugs is unsuccessful, a third and even a fourth may be added.

Initial Drug Selection

Initial drug selection is determined by the presence or absence of a *compelling indication,* defined as a comorbid condition for which a specific class of antihypertensive drugs has been shown to improve outcomes. Initial drugs for patients with and without compelling indications are discussed next.

Patients without compelling indications. For initial therapy in the absence of a compelling indication, a *thiazide diuretic* is currently recommended for most patients. This preference is based on long-term controlled trials showing conclusively that thiazides can reduce morbidity and mortality in hypertensive patients and are well tolerated and inexpensive. Other options for initial therapy—*ACEIs, ARBs,* and *CCBs*—equal diuretics in their ability to lower BP. However, they may not be as effective at reducing morbidity and mortality. Accordingly, these drugs should be reserved for special indications and for patients who have not responded to thiazides. Certain other alternatives—*centrally acting sympatholytics* and *direct-acting vasodilators*—are associated with a high incidence of adverse effects and hence are not well suited for initial monotherapy. One last alternative—α_1 *blockers*—is no longer recommended as first-line therapy. As noted, when the α blocker doxazosin was compared with the diuretic chlorthalidone, doxazosin was associated with a much higher incidence of adverse cardiovascular events.

Patients with compelling indications. For patients with hypertension plus certain comorbid conditions (e.g., heart failure, diabetes), there is strong evidence that specific antihypertensive drugs can reduce morbidity and mortality. Drugs shown to improve outcomes for six comorbid conditions are indicated in Table 41.3. Based on national guidelines, these drugs should be used for initial therapy. If needed, other antihypertensive agents can be added to the regimen. Management of hypertension in patients with diabetes and renal disease—two specific comorbid conditions—is discussed further under "Individualizing Therapy."

Adding Drugs to the Regimen

Rationale for drug selection. When two or more drugs are being used to treat hypertension, each drug should come from a different class. That is, each drug should have a different mechanism of action. In accord with this guideline, it would be appropriate to combine a β blocker, a diuretic, and a vasodilator because each lowers BP by a different mechanism. In contrast, it would be inappropriate to combine two thiazide diuretics or two β blockers or two vasodilators.

Benefits of multidrug therapy. Treatment with multiple drugs offers significant benefits. First, by employing drugs that have different mechanisms, we can increase the likelihood of attaining goal blood pressure: targeting BP control at several sites is likely to be more effective than targeting it at one site. Second, when drugs are used in combination, each can be administered in a lower dosage than would be possible if it were used alone. As a result, both the frequency and the intensity of side effects are reduced. Third, when proper combinations are selected, one agent can offset the adverse effects of another. For example, if a vasodilator is used alone, reflex tachycardia is likely to occur. However, if a vasodilator is combined with a β blocker, reflex tachycardia will be minimal.

Dosing. For each drug in the regimen, *dosage should be low initially and then gradually increased.* For most people with chronic hypertension, the disease poses no immediate threat. Hence there is no need to lower BP rapidly using high doses. Also, when BP is reduced slowly, baroreceptors gradually reset to the new lower pressure. As a result, sympathetic reflexes offer less resistance to the hypotensive effects of therapy. Finally, because there is no need to drop BP rapidly and higher doses carry a higher risk for adverse effects, use of high initial doses would needlessly increase the risk for adverse effects.

Step-Down Therapy

After BP has been controlled for at least 1 year, an attempt should be made to reduce dosages and the number of drugs in the regimen. Of course lifestyle modifications should continue. When reductions are made slowly and progressively, many patients are able to maintain BP control with less medication—and some can be maintained with no medication at all. If drugs are discontinued, regular follow-up is essential, because BP usually returns to hypertensive levels—although it may take years to do so.

Individualizing Therapy
Patients With Comorbid Conditions

Comorbid conditions complicate treatment. Two conditions that are especially problematic—renal disease and diabetes—are discussed here. Preferred drugs for patients with these and other comorbid conditions are shown in Table 41.3. Drugs to avoid in patients with specific comorbid conditions are summarized in Table 41.4.

Renal disease. Nephrosclerosis secondary to hypertension is among the most common causes of progressive renal disease. Pathophysiologic changes include degeneration of renal tubules and fibrotic thickening of the glomeruli, both of which contribute to renal insufficiency. Nephrosclerosis sets the stage for a downward spiral: renal insufficiency causes water retention, which in turn causes BP to rise higher, which in turn promotes even more renal injury, and so forth. Therefore early detection and treatment are essential. To slow the progression of renal damage, the most effective strategy is to lower BP. Although all classes of antihypertensive agents are effective in nephrosclerosis, ACEIs and ARBs work best. Hence, in the absence of contraindications, all patients should be prescribed one of these drugs. In most cases, a diuretic is also used. In patients with advanced renal insufficiency, thiazide diuretics are ineffective; hence a loop diuretic should be employed. Potassium-sparing diuretics should be avoided.

Diabetes. Preferred antihypertensive drugs in patients with diabetes are ACEIs, ARBs, CCBs, and diuretics (in low doses). In patients with diabetic nephropathy, ACEIs and ARBs can slow the progression of renal damage and reduce albuminuria. In diabetic patients as in nondiabetic patients, β blockers and diuretics can decrease morbidity and mortality. It is important to note, however, that β blockers can suppress glycogenolysis and mask early signs of hypoglycemia; therefore they must be used with caution. Thiazides and loop diuretics promote hyperglycemia and hence should also be used with care.

How do ACEIs compare with CCBs in patients with hypertension and diabetes? In one large study, patients taking nisoldipine (a CCB) had a higher incidence of MI than did patients taking enalapril (an ACEI). Because the study was not placebo-controlled, it was impossible to distinguish between two possible interpretations: (1) the CCB increased the risk for MI or (2) the ACEI protected against MI. Either way, it seems clear that ACEIs are better than CCBs for patients with hypertension and diabetes.

TABLE 41.3 Classes of Antihypertensive Drugs Recommended for Initial Therapy of Hypertension in Patients With Certain High-Risk Comorbid Conditions

High-Risk Comorbid Conditions that Constitute Compelling Indications for the Drugs Checked	Drug Classes Recommended for Initial Therapy of Hypertension					
	Diuretic	β Blocker	ACE Inhibitor	ARB	CCB	Aldosterone Antagonist
Heart failure	✔	✔	✔	✔		✔
Post–myocardial infarction		✔	✔			✔
High coronary disease risk	✔	✔	✔		✔	
Diabetes	✔	✔	✔	✔	✔	
Chronic kidney disease			✔	✔		
Prevention of recurrent stroke	✔		✔			

ACE, Angiotensin-converting enzyme; *ARB*, angiotensin II receptor blocker; *CCB*, calcium channel blocker.
Adapted from 2017 ACC/AHA/AAPA/ABC/ACPM/AGS/AphA/ASH/ASPC/NMA/PCNA Guideline for the Prevention, Detection, Evaluation and Management of High Blood Pressure in Adults.

TABLE 41.4   Comorbid Conditions That Require Cautious Use or Complete Avoidance of Certain Antihypertensive Drugs

Comorbid Condition	Drugs to Be Avoided or Used With Caution	Reason for Concern
Cardiovascular Disorders		
Heart failure	Verapamil Diltiazem	These drugs act on the heart to decrease myocardial contractility and can thereby further reduce cardiac output.
AV heart block	β Blockers Labetalol Verapamil Diltiazem	These drugs act on the heart to suppress AV conduction and can thereby intensify AV block.
Coronary artery disease	Hydralazine	Reflex tachycardia induced by hydralazine can precipitate an anginal attack.
Post–myocardial infarction	Hydralazine	Reflex tachycardia induced by hydralazine can increase cardiac work and oxygen demand.
Other Disorders		
Dyslipidemia	β Blockers Diuretics	These drugs may exacerbate dyslipidemia.
Renal insufficiency	K$^+$-sparing diuretics K$^+$ supplements	Use of these agents can lead to dangerous accumulations of potassium.
Asthma	β Blockers Labetalol	β$_2$ Blockade promotes bronchoconstriction.
Depression	Reserpine[a]	Reserpine can cause depression.
Diabetes mellitus	Thiazides Furosemide β Blockers	Thiazides and furosemide promote hyperglycemia, and β blockers suppress glycogenolysis and can mask signs of hypoglycemia.
Gout	Thiazides Furosemide	These diuretics promote hyperuricemia.
Hyperkalemia	K$^+$-sparing diuretics ACE inhibitors Direct renin inhibitors Aldosterone antagonists	These drugs cause potassium accumulation.
Hypokalemia	Thiazides Furosemide	These drugs cause potassium loss.
Collagen diseases	Hydralazine	Hydralazine can precipitate a lupus erythematosus–like syndrome.
Liver disease	Methyldopa	Methyldopa is hepatotoxic.
Preeclampsia	ACE inhibitors ARBs Direct renin inhibitors	These drugs can injure the fetus.

[a]No longer available in the United States.
ACE, Angiotensin-converting enzyme; *ARB*, angiotensin II receptor blocker; *AV*, atrioventricular.

Patients in Special Populations

African Americans. Hypertension is a major health problem for African American adults. Hypertension develops earlier, has a much higher incidence, and is likely to be more severe in this group. As a result, African Americans face a greater risk for heart disease, end-stage renal disease, and stroke. Compared with the general population, African Americans experience a 50% higher rate of death from heart disease, are twice as likely to die of stroke, and are six times more likely to experience hypertension-related end-stage renal disease.

With timely treatment, this disparity can be greatly reduced if not eliminated. We know that African Americans and Caucasians respond equally to treatment (although not always to the same drugs). The primary problem is that hypertension often goes untreated among African Americans until after significant organ damage has developed. If hypertension were diagnosed and treated earlier, the prognosis would be greatly improved. Accordingly it is important that African Americans undergo routine monitoring of BP. If hypertension is diagnosed,

treatment should begin at once. Because African Americans have a high incidence of salt sensitivity and cigarette use, lifestyle modifications are an important component of treatment.

African Americans respond better to some antihypertensive drugs than to others. Controlled trials have shown that *diuretics* can decrease morbidity and mortality in African Americans. Therefore diuretics are drugs of first choice. *CCBs* and *α/β blockers* are also effective. In contrast, monotherapy with β blockers or *ACEIs* is less effective in African Americans than in Caucasians. Nonetheless, β blockers and ACEIs should be used if they are strongly indicated for a comorbid condition. For example, ACEIs should be used in African American patients who have type 1 diabetes with proteinuria. Also, ACEIs should be used in patients with hypertensive nephrosclerosis, a condition for which ACEIs are superior to CCBs. When BP cannot be adequately controlled with a single drug, one of several two-drug combinations are recommended: an ACEI plus a thiazide diuretic, an ACEI plus a CCB, or a β blocker plus a thiazide.

Children and adolescents. The incidence of secondary hypertension in children is much higher than that in adults. Therefore efforts to diagnose and treat an underlying cause should be especially diligent. For children with primary hypertension, treatment is the same as for adults—although doses are lower and should be adjusted with care. Because ACEIs and ARBs can cause fetal harm, they should be avoided in young women who are sexually active or pregnant.

Older adults. By age 65 years, most Americans have hypertension. Furthermore, high BP in this group almost always presents as *isolated systolic hypertension;* DBP is usually normal or low. The good news, as shown in the Hypertension in the Very Elderly Trial (HYVET), is that treatment can reduce the incidence of heart failure, fatal stroke, and all-cause mortality among these individuals. Unfortunately, about 40% of older adults are not achieving blood pressure goals despite treatment.

PATIENT-CENTERED CARE ACROSS THE LIFE SPAN

Hypertension

Life Stage	Patient Care Concerns
Infants	See later entry, "Breastfeeding women."
Children/ adolescents	No data are available on the long-term effects of antihypertensive drugs on growth and development of children. Drugs recommended for treatment of hypertension in children 1–18 years old include ACEIs, diuretics, β blockers, and calcium channel blockers.
Pregnant women	Drugs of choice in treating pregnant women with mild preeclampsia include labetalol and methyldopa. Magnesium sulfate is used in the prevention of seizures in severe preeclampsia or for treatment of seizures in eclampsia.
Breastfeeding women	Effects of RAAS-blocking drugs have not been studied in breastfeeding; β blockers, such as metoprolol, appear safe for the breastfeeding infant. Diuretics appear safe but may suppress lactation.
Older adults	Treatment with ACEIs, diuretics, and/or β blockers is reasonable. Caution must be taken to avoid overdiuresis when using diuretics in the older-adult population. Central acting alpha agonists and peripheral alpha-1 antagonists should also be avoided.

ACEI, Angiotensin-converting enzyme inhibitor; *RAAS,* renin-angiotensin-aldosterone system: *SBP,* systolic blood pressure

Because cardiovascular reflexes are blunted in older adults, treatment carries a significant risk of orthostatic hypotension. Therefore initial doses should be low—about one-half those used for younger adults—and dosage escalation should be done slowly. Drugs that are especially likely to cause orthostatic hypotension (e.g., α_1 blockers, α/β blockers) should be used with caution.

Minimizing Adverse Effects

Antihypertensive drugs can produce many unwanted effects, including hypotension, sedation, and sexual dysfunction. Although not stressed previously, practically all antihypertensive drugs can interfere with sexual function.

The fundamental strategy for decreasing side effects is to tailor the regimen to the sensitivities of the patient. Simply put, if one drug causes effects that are objectionable, a more acceptable drug should be substituted. The best way to identify unacceptable responses is to encourage patients to report them.

Adverse effects caused by exacerbation of comorbid diseases are both predictable and avoidable. We know, for example, that β blockers can intensify AV block and hence should not be taken by people with these disorders. Other conditions that can be aggravated by antihypertensive drugs are listed in Table 41.4. To help avoid drug–disease mismatches, the medical history should identify all comorbid conditions. With this information, the prescriber can choose drugs that are least likely to make the comorbid condition worse.

High initial doses and rapid dosage escalation can increase the incidence and severity of adverse effects. Accordingly, doses should be low at first and then gradually increased. Remember, there is usually no need to reduce BP rapidly. Hence large initial doses that can cause a rapid fall in BP but also produce adverse effects should be avoided.

Promoting Adherence

The major cause of treatment failure in patients with chronic hypertension is lack of adherence to the prescribed regimen. In this section we consider the causes of nonadherence and discuss some solutions.

Why adherence is often hard to achieve. Much of the difficulty in promoting adherence stems from the nature of hypertension itself. Hypertension is a chronic, slowly progressing disease that, through much of its course, is devoid of overt symptoms. Because symptoms are absent, it can be difficult to convince patients that they are ill and need treatment. In addition, because there are no symptoms to relieve, drugs cannot produce an obvious therapeutic response. In the absence of such a response, it can be difficult for patients to believe that their medication is doing anything useful.

Because hypertension progresses very slowly, the disease tends to encourage procrastination. For most people, the adverse effects of hypertension will not become manifest for many years. Realizing this, patients may reason (incorrectly) that they can postpone therapy without significantly increasing risk.

The negative aspects of treatment also contribute to nonadherence. Antihypertensive regimens can be complex and expensive. In addition, treatment must continue lifelong. Last, antihypertensive drugs can cause a number of adverse effects, ranging from sedation to hypotension to impaired sexual function. It is difficult to convince people who are feeling good to take drugs that may make them feel worse. Some people may decide that exposing themselves to the negative effects of therapy today is paying too high a price to avoid the adverse consequences of hypertension at some indefinite time in the future.

Ways to promote adherence

Patient education. Adherence requires motivation, and patient education can help provide it. Patients should be taught about the consequences of hypertension and the benefits of treatment. Because hypertension does not cause discomfort, it may not be clear to patients that their condition is indeed serious. Patients must be helped to understand that, left untreated, hypertension can cause heart disease, kidney disease, and stroke. In addition, patients should appreciate that, with proper therapy, the risks for these long-term complications can be minimized, resulting in a longer and healthier life. Last, patients must understand that drugs do not cure hypertension—they only control symptoms. Hence, for treatment to be effective, medication must be taken lifelong.

PATIENT EDUCATION
Monitoring Blood Pressure

Patients should be taught the goal of treatment and to monitor and record their BP daily. This increases patient involvement and provides positive feedback that can help promote adherence.

Minimize side effects. If we expect patients to comply with long-term treatment, we must keep adverse effects to a minimum. As discussed earlier, adverse effects can be minimized by (1) encouraging patients to report side effects, (2) discontinuing objectionable drugs and substituting more acceptable ones, (3) avoiding drugs that can exacerbate comorbid conditions, and (4) using doses that are low initially and are then gradually increased.

Establish a collaborative relationship. The patient who feels like a collaborative partner in the treatment program is more likely to comply than is the one who feels that treatment is being imposed. Collaboration allows the patient to help set treatment goals, create the treatment program, and evaluate progress. In addition, a collaborative relationship facilitates communication about side effects.

Simplify the regimen. Antihypertensive regimens may consist of several drugs taken multiple times a day. Such complex regimens deter adherence. Therefore to promote adherence, the dosing schedule should be as simple as possible. After an effective regimen has been established, dosing just once or twice daily should be tried. If an appropriate combination product is available (e.g., a fixed-dose combination of a thiazide diuretic plus an ACEI), the combination product may be substituted for its components.

Other measures. Adherence can be promoted by giving positive reinforcement when therapeutic goals are achieved. Involvement of family members can be helpful. Also, adherence can be promoted by scheduling office visits at convenient times and by following up when appointments are missed. For many patients, antihypertensive therapy represents a significant economic burden; devising a regimen that is effective but inexpensive will help.

DRUGS FOR HYPERTENSIVE DISORDERS OF PREGNANCY

Hypertension is the most common complication of pregnancy, with an incidence of about 10%. When hypertension develops, it is essential to distinguish between chronic hypertension and preeclampsia. Chronic hypertension is relatively benign, whereas preeclampsia can lead to life-threatening complications for the patient and the fetus.

Chronic Hypertension

Chronic hypertension, seen in 5% of pregnancies, is defined as hypertension that was present before pregnancy or that developed before the 20th week of gestation. Persistent *severe* hypertension carries a risk to both the patient and the fetus. Potential adverse outcomes include placental abruption, maternal cardiac decompensation, premature birth, fetal growth delay, central nervous system hemorrhage, and renal failure. The goal of treatment is to minimize the risk for hypertension to the patient and fetus while avoiding drug-induced harm to the fetus. With the exception of ACEIs, ARBs, and DRIs, antihypertensive drugs that were being taken before pregnancy can be continued. *ACEIs, ARBs, and DRIs are contraindicated owing to their potential for harm* (fetal growth delay, congenital malformations, neonatal renal failure, neonatal death). When drug therapy is initiated *during* pregnancy, *methyldopa* and *labetalol* are the traditional agents of choice. These drugs have limited effects on uteroplacental and fetal hemodynamics and do not adversely affect the fetus or neonate. Regardless of the drug selected, treatment should

not be overly aggressive because an excessive drop in BP can compromise uteroplacental blood flow.

According to guidelines issued by the American College of Obstetricians and Gynecologists (ACOG), "severe" hypertension requires treatment, whereas "mild" hypertension generally does not. (The ACOG defines severe hypertension as SBP >160 mm Hg or DBP >110 mm Hg and mild hypertension as SBP 140 to 159 mm Hg or DBP 90 to 109 mm Hg.) There is good evidence that treating severe hypertension reduces risk. In contrast, there is little evidence that treating mild hypertension offers significant benefit.

Patients who have chronic hypertension during pregnancy are at increased risk for developing preeclampsia (see later). Unfortunately, reducing BP does *not* lower this risk.

Preeclampsia and Eclampsia

Preeclampsia is a multisystem disorder characterized by the combination of elevated BP (>140/90 mm Hg) and proteinuria (≥300 mg in 24 hours) that develops after the 20th week of gestation. The disorder occurs in about 5% of pregnancies. Rarely, women with preeclampsia develop seizures. If seizures do develop, the condition is then termed *eclampsia*. Risk factors for preeclampsia include black race, chronic hypertension, diabetes, collagen vascular disorders, and previous preeclampsia. The etiology of preeclampsia is complex and incompletely understood.

Preeclampsia poses serious risks for the fetus and mother. Risks for the fetus include intrauterine growth restriction, premature birth, and even death. The mother is at risk for seizures (eclampsia), renal failure, pulmonary edema, stroke, and death.

Management of preeclampsia is based on the severity of the disease, the status of mother and fetus, and the length of gestation. The objective is to preserve the health of the mother and deliver an infant who will not require intensive and prolonged neonatal care. Success requires close maternal and fetal monitoring. Although drugs can help reduce BP, delivery is the only cure.

Management of *mild* preeclampsia is controversial and depends on the duration of gestation. If preeclampsia develops near term and if fetal maturity is certain, induction of labor is advised. However, if mild preeclampsia develops earlier in gestation, experts disagree about appropriate intervention. Suggested measures include bed rest, prolonged hospitalization, treatment with antihypertensive drugs, and prophylaxis with an anticonvulsant. Studies to evaluate these strategies have generally failed to demonstrate benefits from any, including treatment with antihypertensive drugs.

The definitive intervention for *severe* preeclampsia is delivery. However, making the choice to induce labor presents a dilemma. Because preeclampsia can deteriorate rapidly, with grave consequences for the patient and fetus, immediate delivery is recommended. However, if the fetus is not sufficiently mature, immediate delivery can threaten its life. Do we deliver the fetus immediately, which would eliminate risk for the patient but present a serious risk for the fetus—or do we postpone delivery, which would reduce risk for the fetus but greatly increase risk for the patient? If the patient elects to postpone delivery, then BP can be lowered with drugs. Because severe preeclampsia can be life-threatening, treatment must be done in a tertiary care center to permit close monitoring. The major objective is to prevent maternal cerebral complications (e.g., hemorrhage, encephalopathy).

42

Drugs for Heart Failure

Heart failure (HF) is a disease with two major forms: (1) HF with left ventricular (LV) systolic dysfunction, now referred to as heart failure with reduced ejection fraction (HFrEF); and (2) diastolic HF, also known as heart failure with preserved LV ejection fraction (HFpEF). In this chapter discussion is limited to the first form. Accordingly, for the rest of this chapter, the term *heart failure* will be used to denote the first form only.

HF is a progressive, often fatal disorder characterized by ventricular dysfunction, reduced cardiac output, insufficient tissue perfusion, and signs of fluid retention (e.g., peripheral edema, shortness of breath). The disease affects nearly 6 million Americans and is responsible for 285,000 deaths every year. Of those who have HF, 20% are likely to die within 1 year and 50% within 5 years. HF is primarily a disease of older adults, affecting 4% to 8% of those at age 65 years and more than 9% to 12% of those older than 80 years. Direct and indirect health care costs of HF are estimated at more than $30 billion yearly. With improved evaluation and care, many hospitalizations could be prevented, quality of life could be improved, and life expectancy could be extended.

In the past, HF was commonly referred to as *congestive heart failure.* This term was used because HF frequently causes fluid accumulation (congestion) in the lungs and peripheral tissues. However, because many patients do not have signs of pulmonary or systemic congestion, the term *heart failure* is now preferred.

Drugs recommended for treatment include diuretics, inhibitors of the renin-angiotensin-aldosterone system (RAAS), β blockers, and digoxin. In this chapter, only digoxin is discussed at length. The other drugs are presented at length in previous chapters, so discussion here is limited to their use in HF.

To understand HF and its treatment, a basic understanding of hemodynamics is essential. In particular, you must understand the role of venous pressure, afterload, and the Starling mechanism in determining cardiac output. It is also important to understand the roles of the baroreceptor reflex, the RAAS, and the kidneys in regulating arterial pressure. These concepts can be reviewed by reading Chapter 36.

PATHOPHYSIOLOGY OF HEART FAILURE

HF is a syndrome in which the heart is unable to pump sufficient blood to meet the metabolic needs of tissues. The syndrome is characterized by signs of *inadequate tissue perfusion* (fatigue, shortness of breath, exercise intolerance) and/or signs of *volume overload* (venous distention, peripheral and pulmonary edema). The major underlying causes of HF are chronic hypertension and myocardial infarction. Other causes include valvular heart disease, coronary artery disease, congenital heart disease, dysrhythmias, and aging of the myocardium. In its earliest stage, HF is asymptomatic. As failure progresses, fatigue and shortness of breath develop. As cardiac performance declines further, blood backs up behind the failing ventricles, causing venous distention, peripheral edema, and pulmonary edema. HF is a chronic disorder that requires continuous treatment with drugs.

Cardiac Remodeling

In the initial phase of failure, the heart undergoes remodeling, a process in which the ventricles dilate, hypertrophy, and become more spherical. These alterations in cardiac geometry increase wall stress and reduce LV ejection fraction. Remodeling occurs in response to cardiac injury, brought on by infarction and other causes. The remodeling process is driven primarily by neurohormonal systems, including the sympathetic nervous system (SNS) and the RAAS. In addition to promoting remodeling, neurohormonal factors promote cardiac fibrosis and myocyte death. The net result of these pathologic changes—remodeling, fibrosis, and cell death—is a progressive decline in cardiac output. As a rule, cardiac remodeling precedes the development of symptoms and continues after they appear. As a result, cardiac performance continues to decline.

Physiologic Adaptations to Reduced Cardiac Output

In response to reductions in cardiac pumping ability, the body undergoes several adaptive changes. Some of these help improve tissue perfusion; others compound existing problems.

Cardiac Dilation

Dilation of the heart is characteristic of HF. Cardiac dilation results from a combination of increased venous pressure (see later) and reduced contractile force. Reduced contractility lowers the amount of blood ejected during systole, causing end-systolic volume to rise. The increase in venous pressure increases diastolic filling, which causes the heart to expand even further.

Because of the Starling mechanism, the increase in heart size that occurs in HF helps improve cardiac output. That is, as the heart fails and its volume expands, contractile force increases, causing a corresponding increase in stroke volume. However, note that the maximal contractile force that can be developed by the failing heart is considerably lower than the maximal force of the healthy heart. This limitation is reflected in the curve for the failing heart shown in Fig. 42.1.

If cardiac dilation is insufficient to maintain cardiac output, other factors come into play. As discussed later, these are not always beneficial.

Increased Sympathetic Tone

HF causes arterial pressure to fall. In response, the baroreceptor reflex increases sympathetic output to the heart, veins, and arterioles. At the same time, parasympathetic effects on the heart are reduced. The consequences of increased sympathetic tone are summarized here.
- *Increased heart rate.* Acceleration of heart rate increases cardiac output, thereby helping improve tissue perfusion. However, if the heart rate increases too much, there will be insufficient time for complete ventricular filling and cardiac output will fall.
- *Increased contractility.* Increased myocardial contractility has the obvious benefit of increasing cardiac output. The only detriment is an increase in cardiac oxygen demand.

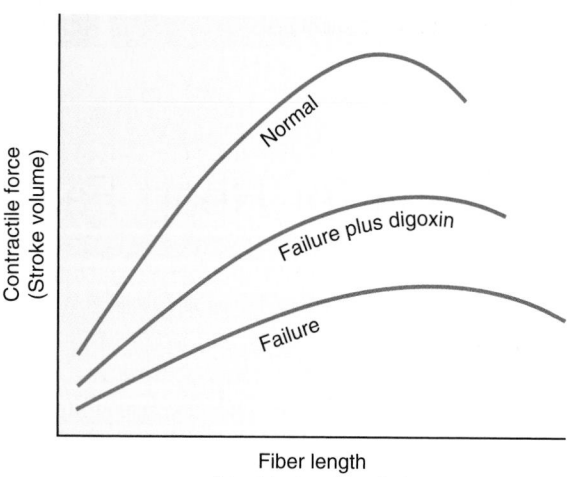

Fig. 42.1 Relationship of Ventricular Diameter to Contractile Force. In the normal heart and the failing heart, increased fiber length produces increased contractile force. However, for any given fiber length, contractile force in the failing heart is much less than in the healthy heart. By increasing cardiac contractility, digoxin shifts the relationship between fiber length and stroke volume in the failing heart toward that in the normal heart.

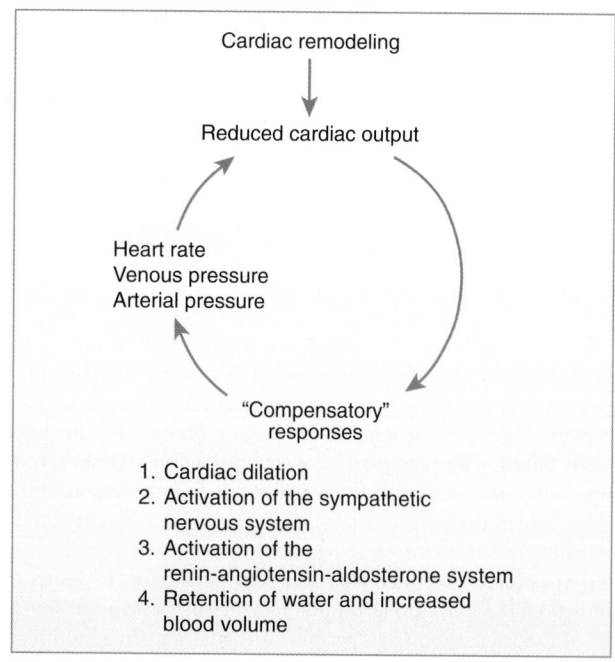

Fig. 42.2 The Vicious Cycle of Maladaptive Compensatory Responses to a Failing Heart.

- *Increased venous tone.* Elevation of venous tone increases venous pressure and thereby increases ventricular filling. Because of the Starling mechanism, increased filling increases stroke volume. Unfortunately, if venous pressure is excessive, blood will back up behind the failing ventricles, thereby aggravating pulmonary and peripheral edema. Furthermore, excessive filling pressure can dilate the heart so much that stroke volume will begin to decline.
- *Increased arteriolar tone.* Elevation of arteriolar tone increases arterial pressure, thereby increasing perfusion of vital organs. Unfortunately, increased arterial pressure also means that the heart must pump against greater resistance. Because cardiac reserve is minimal in HF, the heart may be unable to meet this challenge and output may fall.

Water Retention and Increased Blood Volume

Mechanisms. Water retention results from two mechanisms. First, reduced cardiac output causes a reduction in renal blood flow, which in turn decreases glomerular filtration rate (GFR). As a result, urine production is decreased and water is retained.

Second, HF activates the RAAS. Activation occurs in response to reduced blood pressure and reduced renal blood flow. When activated, the RAAS promotes water retention by increasing circulating levels of *aldosterone* and *angiotensin II*. Aldosterone acts directly on the kidneys to promote the retention of sodium and water. Angiotensin II causes constriction of renal blood vessels, which decreases renal blood flow and thereby further decreases urine production. In addition, angiotensin II causes constriction of systemic arterioles and veins and thereby increases venous and arterial pressure.

Consequences. As with other adaptive responses to HF, increased blood volume can be beneficial or harmful. Increased blood volume increases venous pressure and thereby increases venous return. As a result, ventricular filling and stroke volume are increased. The resultant increase in cardiac output can improve tissue perfusion. However, as noted, if venous pressure is too high, edema of the lungs and periphery may result. More important, *if the increase in cardiac output is insufficient to maintain adequate kidney function, renal retention of water will progress*

unabated. The resultant accumulation of fluid will cause severe cardiac, pulmonary, and peripheral edema—and ultimately death.

Natriuretic peptides. In response to stretching of the atria and dilation of the ventricles, the heart releases two natriuretic peptides: atrial natriuretic peptide (ANP) and brain natriuretic peptide (BNP). As discussed in Chapter 38, these hormones promote both dilation of arterioles and veins and loss of sodium and water through the kidneys. Hence they tend to counterbalance vasoconstriction caused by the SNS and angiotensin II as well as retention of sodium and water caused by the RAAS. However, as HF progresses, the effects of ANP and BNP eventually become overwhelmed by the effects of the SNS and RAAS.

The level of circulating BNP is an important index of cardiac status in HF patients and thus can be a predictor of long-term survival. High levels of BNP indicate poor cardiac health and can predict a lower chance of survival. Conversely, low levels of BNP indicate better cardiac health and can predict a higher chance of survival. This information can be helpful when a hospitalized patient is being assessed at discharge.

The Vicious Cycle of "Compensatory" Physiologic Responses

As discussed previously, reduced cardiac output leads to compensatory responses: (1) cardiac dilation, (2) activation of the SNS, (3) activation of the RAAS, and (4) retention of water and expansion of blood volume. Although these responses represent the body's attempt to compensate for reduced cardiac output, they can actually make matters worse: excessive heart rate can reduce ventricular filling, excessive arterial pressure can lower cardiac output, and excessive venous pressure can cause pulmonary and peripheral edema. Thus as depicted in Fig. 42.2, the "compensatory" responses can create a self-sustaining cycle of maladaptation that further impairs cardiac output and tissue perfusion. If cardiac output becomes too low to maintain a sufficient production of urine, the resultant accumulation of water will eventually be fatal. The actual cause of death is complete cardiac failure secondary to excessive cardiac dilation and cardiac edema.

ACC/AHA Stage   NYHA Functional Classification

A At high risk for HF but without structural heart disease or symptoms of HF	
B Structural heart disease but without symptoms of HF	I Asymptomatic
C Structural heart disease with prior or current symptoms of HF	II Symptomatic with moderate exertion
	III Symptomatic with minimal exertion
D Advanced structural heart disease with marked symptoms of HF at rest despite maximal medical therapy. Specialized interventions (e.g., heart transplant, mechanical assist device) required	IV Symptomatic at rest

Fig. 42.3 American College of Cardiology/American Heart Association (ACC/AHA) stages and New York Heart Association (NYHA) functional classification of heart failure. HF, Heart failure.

Signs and Symptoms of Heart Failure

The prominent signs and symptoms of HF are a direct consequence of the pathophysiology just described. Decreased tissue perfusion results in reduced exercise tolerance, fatigue, and shortness of breath; shortness of breath may also reflect pulmonary edema. Increased sympathetic tone produces tachycardia. Increased ventricular filling, reduced systolic ejection, and myocardial hypertrophy result in cardiomegaly (increased heart size). The combination of increased venous tone plus increased blood volume helps cause pulmonary edema, peripheral edema, hepatomegaly (increased liver size), and distention of the jugular veins. Weight gain results from fluid retention.

Classification of Heart Failure Severity

There are two major schemes for classifying HF severity. One scheme, established by the New York Heart Association (NYHA), classifies HF based on the functional limitations it causes. A newer scheme, proposed jointly by the American College of Cardiology (ACC) and the American Heart Association (AHA), is based on the observation that HF is a progressive disease that moves through stages of increasing severity.

The NYHA scheme, which has four classes, can be summarized as follows:
- Class I—no limitation of ordinary physical activity
- Class II—slight limitation of physical activity: normal activity produces fatigue, dyspnea, palpitations, or angina
- Class III—marked limitation of physical activity: even mild activity produces symptoms
- Class IV—symptoms occur at rest

The ACC/AHA scheme, which also has four stages, can be summarized as follows:
- Stage A—at high risk for HF but without structural heart disease or symptoms of HF
- Stage B—structural heart disease but without symptoms of HF
- Stage C—structural heart disease with prior or current symptoms of HF
- Stage D—refractory HF requiring specialized interventions

The ACC/AHA scheme was unveiled in treatment guidelines issued in 2001. The newest version of that document (2017 ACC/AHA/HFSA Focused Update of the 2013 ACCF/AHA Guideline for the Management

of Heart Failure—Executive Summary: A Report of the American College of Cardiology Foundation/American Heart Association Task Force on Practice Guidelines) is discussed later, under "Management of Heart Failure."

Note that the ACC/AHA scheme is intended to complement the NYHA scheme, not replace it. The relationship between the two is shown in Fig. 42.3.

OVERVIEW OF DRUGS USED TO TREAT HEART FAILURE

For routine therapy, HF is treated with three types of drugs: (1) diuretics, (2) agents that inhibit the RAAS, and (3) β blockers. Other agents (e.g., digoxin, dopamine, hydralazine) may be used as well.

Diuretics

Diuretics are first-line drugs for all patients with signs of volume overload or a history of volume overload. By reducing blood volume, these drugs can decrease venous pressure, arterial pressure (afterload), pulmonary edema, peripheral edema, and cardiac dilation. However, excessive diuresis must be avoided: if blood volume drops too low, cardiac output and blood pressure may fall precipitously, thereby further compromising tissue perfusion. For the most part, benefits of diuretics are limited to symptom reduction. As a rule, these drugs do not prolong survival. The basic pharmacology of the diuretics is discussed in Chapter 37.

Thiazide Diuretics

The thiazide diuretics (e.g., hydrochlorothiazide) produce moderate diuresis. These oral agents are used for long-term therapy of HF when edema is not too great. Because thiazides are ineffective when GFR is low (creatinine clearance <40 to 50 mL/min), these drugs cannot be used if cardiac output is greatly reduced. The principal adverse effect of the thiazides is *hypokalemia*, which increases the risk for *digoxin-induced dysrhythmias* (see later).

Loop Diuretics

The loop diuretics (e.g., furosemide) produce profound diuresis. In contrast to the thiazides, these drugs can promote fluid loss even when GFR is low. Therefore loop diuretics are preferred to thiazides when cardiac output is greatly reduced. Because they can mobilize large volumes of water and they work when GFR is low, loop diuretics are drugs of choice for patients with severe HF. Like the thiazides, these drugs can cause *hypokalemia*, thereby increasing the risk for *digoxin toxicity*. In addition, loop diuretics can cause severe *hypotension* secondary to excessive volume reduction.

Potassium-Sparing Diuretics

In contrast to the thiazides and loop diuretics, the potassium-sparing diuretics (e.g., spironolactone, triamterene) promote only scant diuresis. In patients with HF, these drugs are employed to counteract potassium loss caused by thiazide and loop diuretics, thereby lowering the risk for digoxin-induced dysrhythmias. Not surprisingly, the principal adverse effect of the potassium-sparing drugs is *hyperkalemia*. Because *angiotensin-converting enzyme inhibitors (ACEIs)* and *angiotensin II receptor blockers (ARBs)* also carry a risk for hyperkalemia, caution is needed if these drugs are combined with a potassium-sparing diuretic. Accordingly, when therapy with an ACEI or ARB is initiated, the potassium-sparing diuretic should be discontinued. It can be resumed later if needed.

One potassium-sparing diuretic—spironolactone—prolongs survival in patients with HF primarily by blocking receptors for aldosterone, not by causing diuresis. This drug and a related agent—eplerenone—are discussed later, under the section "Aldosterone Antagonists."

Drugs That Inhibit the Renin-Angiotensin-Aldosterone System

The RAAS plays an important role in both cardiac remodeling and the hemodynamic changes that occur in response to reduced cardiac output. Accordingly, agents that inhibit the RAAS can be highly beneficial. Four groups of drugs are available: ACEIs, ARBs, direct renin inhibitors (DRIs), and aldosterone antagonists. Of the four, the ACEIs have been studied most thoroughly in HF. The basic pharmacology of the RAAS inhibitors is presented in Chapter 38.

PROTOTYPE DRUGS

Drugs for Heart Failure

Inhibitors of the Renin-Angiotensin-Aldosterone System
Captopril (angiotensin-converting enzyme inhibitor)
Losartan (angiotensin II receptor blocker)
Eplerenone (aldosterone antagonist)

Diuretics
Hydrochlorothiazide
Furosemide

Inotropic Agent
Digoxin (a cardiac glycoside)

β Blocker
Metoprolol

Angiotensin-Converting Enzyme Inhibitors

ACEIs (e.g., captopril, enalapril) are the essential HF therapies; they can improve functional status and prolong life. In one trial, the 2-year mortality rate for patients taking enalapril was 47% lower than the rate for patients taking placebo. Other large controlled trials have shown similar benefits. Accordingly, in the absence of specific contraindications, all patients with HF should receive one of these drugs. Although ACEIs can be used alone, they are usually combined with a β blocker and a diuretic.

ACEIs block the production of angiotensin II, decrease the release of aldosterone, and suppress the degradation of kinins. As a result, they improve hemodynamics and favorably alter cardiac remodeling.

Hemodynamic benefits. By suppressing the production of angiotensin II, ACEIs cause dilation of arterioles and veins and decrease the release of aldosterone. Resulting benefits in HF are as follows:

- *Arteriolar dilation* improves regional blood flow in the kidneys and other tissues, and, by reducing afterload, it increases stroke volume and cardiac output. Increased renal blood flow promotes excretion of sodium and water.
- *Venous dilation* reduces venous pressure and thereby also pulmonary congestion, peripheral edema, preload, and cardiac dilation.
- *Suppression of aldosterone release* enhances the excretion of sodium and water while also causing the retention of potassium.

Interestingly, suppression of angiotensin II production diminishes over time, suggesting that long-term benefits are the result of some other action.

Influence on cardiac remodeling. With continued use, ACEIs have a favorable influence on cardiac remodeling. Elevation of kinins is largely responsible. This statement is based in part on the observation that, in experimental models, giving a kinin receptor blocker decreases beneficial effects on remodeling. Also, we know that suppression of angiotensin II production diminishes over time, so reduced angiotensin II cannot fully explain long-term benefits.

Adverse effects. The principal adverse effects of the ACEIs are *hypotension* (secondary to arteriolar dilation), *hyperkalemia* (secondary to decreased aldosterone release), *intractable cough*, and *angioedema*. In addition, these drugs can cause *renal failure in patients with bilateral renal artery stenosis*. Because of their ability to elevate potassium levels, ACEIs should be used with caution in patients taking potassium supplements or a potassium-sparing diuretic (e.g., spironolactone, triamterene).

▶▶ BLACK BOX WARNING

Risk With Angiotensin Converting Enzyme Inhibitors During Pregnancy

Use of angiotensin-converting enzyme inhibitors during pregnancy—especially during the second and third trimesters—can cause *fetal injury.* Accordingly, if pregnancy occurs, these drugs should be discontinued.

Dosage. Adequate dosage is still debated in the literature: higher dosages may be associated with increased survival, but conflicting evidence remains. Results of the Assessment of Treatment with Lisinopril and Survival (ATLAS) trial indicate that the doses needed to increase survival are higher than those needed to produce hemodynamic changes. In contrast to the ATLAS trial, the NETWORK trial and the High Dose Enalapril Study Group did not find a difference in mortality between patients on low-dose or high-dose ACEIs. Treatment with ACEIs should be initiated at low doses and slowly titrated upward if the patient tolerates treatment. Target dosages associated with disease modification are shown in Table 42.1. These dosages should be used unless side effects make them intolerable.

Angiotensin II Receptor Blockers

In patients with HF, the effects of ARBs are similar to those of ACEIs, but not identical. Hemodynamic effects of both groups are much the same. Clinical trials have shown that ARBs improve LV ejection fraction, reduce HF symptoms, increase exercise tolerance, decrease hospitalization, enhance quality of life, and—most important—reduce mortality. However, because ARBs do not increase levels of kinins, their effects on cardiac remodeling are less favorable than those of ACEIs. For this

TABLE 42.1 Inhibitors of the Renin-Angiotensin-Aldosterone System Used in Heart Failure

Drug	Initial Daily Dose	Maximum Daily Dose
Ace Inhibitors		
Captopril, generic only	6.25 mg 3 times	50 mg 3 times
Enalapril (Vasotec)	2.5 mg twice	10–20 mg twice
Fosinopril generic only	5–10 mg once	40 mg once
Lisinopril (Zestril)	2.5–5 mg once	20–40 mg once
Quinapril (Accupril)	5 mg twice	20 mg twice
Ramipril (Altace)	1.25–2.5 mg once	10 mg once
Trandolapril (Mavik)	1 mg once	4 mg once
Angiotensin II Receptor Blockers		
Candesartan (Atacand)	4–8 mg once	32 mg once
Losartan (Cozaar)	25–50 mg once	50–150 mg once
Valsartan (Diovan)	20–40 mg twice	160 mg twice
Sacubitril/Valsartan (Entresto)	24/26 mg twice	97/103 mg twice
Hyperpolarization-Activated Cyclic Nucleotide-Gated (Hcn) Channel Blocker		
Ivabradine (Corlanor)	5 mg twice	7.5 mg twice
Aldosterone Antagonists		
Eplerenone (Inspra)	25 mg once	50 mg once
Spironolactone (Aldactone)	12.5–25 mg once	25 mg once or twice

reason and because clinical experience with ACEIs is much greater than that with ARBs, ACEIs are generally preferred. For now, ARBs should be reserved for HF patients who cannot tolerate ACEIs, usually owing to intractable cough. (Because ARBs do not increase bradykinin levels, they do not cause cough.)

Angiotensin Receptor Neprilysin Inhibitor

Sacubitril/valsartan (Entresto). Sacubitril/valsartan (Entresto) is a newly approved drug that functions in two different manners. Sacubitril is a new class of drug, called an angiotensin receptor neprilysin inhibitor (ANRI). In simple terms, Entresto increases natriuretic peptides while suppressing the negative effects of the RAAS. As discussed earlier in the chapter, ANP and BNP are important indices of cardiac status in HF patients. Entresto is approved for patients with stages II to IV HF to be used in place of an ACEI or ARB.

In the PARADIGM-HF study, Entresto was superior to enalapril alone in terms of the overall end points of reduction in hospitalizations, risk for all-cause mortality, and risk for death from cardiovascular causes. In fact, the study was terminated early because of the overwhelmingly positive results.

Because Entresto contains an ARB, the contraindications and side effects are similar. Entresto can cause angioedema, hyperkalemia, and hypotension. Administration should be avoided in pregnancy, as such use can cause fetal harm.

Aldosterone Antagonists

In patients with HF, aldosterone antagonists—*spironolactone* (Aldactone) and *eplerenone* (Inspra)—can reduce symptoms, decrease hospitalizations, and prolong life. These benefits were first demonstrated with spironolactone in the Randomized Aldactone Evaluation Study (RALES). Similar results were later obtained with eplerenone. Current guidelines

recommend adding an aldosterone antagonist to standard HF therapy, but only in patients with persistent symptoms despite adequate treatment with an ACEI and a β blocker.

Aldosterone antagonists work primarily by blocking aldosterone receptors in the heart and blood vessels. To understand these effects, we need to review the role of aldosterone in HF. In the past, researchers believed that all aldosterone did was promote the renal retention of sodium (and water) in exchange for the excretion of potassium. However, we now know that aldosterone has additional—and more harmful—effects, including the following:

- Promotion of myocardial remodeling (which impairs pumping)
- Promotion of myocardial fibrosis (which increases the risk for dysrhythmias)
- Activation of the SNS and suppression of norepinephrine uptake in the heart (both of which can promote dysrhythmias and ischemia)
- Promotion of vascular fibrosis (which decreases arterial compliance)
- Promotion of baroreceptor dysfunction

During HF, activation of the RAAS causes levels of aldosterone to rise. In some patients, levels reach 20 times normal. As aldosterone levels grow higher, harmful effects increase and prognosis becomes progressively worse.

Drugs can reduce the effects of aldosterone by either decreasing aldosterone production or blocking aldosterone receptors. ACEIs, ARBs, and DRIs decrease aldosterone production; spironolactone and eplerenone block aldosterone receptors. Although ACEIs and ARBs can reduce aldosterone production, they do not block it entirely. Furthermore, production is suppressed only for a relatively short time. Hence when ACEIs or ARBs are used alone, the detrimental effects of aldosterone can persist. However, when an aldosterone antagonist is added to the regimen, any residual effects are eliminated. As a result, symptoms of HF are improved and life is prolonged.

Aldosterone antagonists have one major adverse effect: *hyperkalemia*. The underlying cause is renal retention of potassium. Risk is increased by renal impairment and by using an ACEI or ARB. To minimize risk, potassium levels and renal function should be measured at baseline and periodically thereafter. Potassium supplements should be discontinued.

Spironolactone—but not eplerenone—poses a significant risk for *gynecomastia* (breast enlargement) in men, a condition that can be both cosmetically troublesome and painful. In the RALES trial, 10% of males experienced painful breast enlargement.

▶▶ BLACK BOX WARNING

Spironolactone

Spironolactone is associated with tumorigenesis in studies completed on rats.

Direct Renin Inhibitors

As discussed in Chapter 38, DRIs can shut down the entire RAAS. In theory, their benefits in HF should equal those of the ACEIs and ARBs. At this time, only one DRI—*aliskiren* (Tekturna)—is available. In a recent trial, aliskiren did not improve outcomes in hospitalized patients with HF. Additional studies on aliskiren are being conducted currently. Because of these findings, aliskiren is approved for hypertension, but is not yet approved for HF.

β Blockers

The role of β blockers in HF continues to evolve. Until the mid-1990s, HF was considered an absolute contraindication to these drugs. After all, blockade of cardiac β_1-adrenergic receptors *reduces* contractility—an effect that is clearly detrimental, given that contractility is already compromised in the failing heart. However, it is now clear that, with careful control of dosage, β blockers can improve patient status. Controlled trials have shown that three β blockers—*carvedilol* (Coreg), *bisoprolol* (Zebeta), and *sustained-release metoprolol* (Toprol XL)—when added to conventional therapy, can improve LV ejection fraction, increase exercise tolerance, slow progression of HF, reduce the need for hospitalization and—most important—prolong survival. Accordingly, β blockers are now recommended as first-line therapy for most patients. These drugs can even be used in patients with severe disease (NYHA class IV) provided that the patient is euvolemic and hemodynamically stable. Although the mechanism underlying benefits is uncertain, likely possibilities include protecting the heart from both excessive sympathetic stimulation and dysrhythmias. Because excessive β blockade can reduce contractility, doses must be very low initially and then gradually increased. Full benefits may not be seen for 1 to 3 months. Among patients with HF, the principal adverse effects are (1) fluid retention and worsening of HF, (2) fatigue, (3) hypotension, and (4) bradycardia or heart block. The basic pharmacology of the β blockers is discussed in Chapter 16.

Ivabradine (Corlanor)

In 2015, the US Food and Drug Administration approved ivabradine (*Corlanor*) for use in patients with stable, symptomatic HF, LV ejection fraction less than 35% in sinus rhythm, and heart rate greater than 70 beats/min on maximally tolerated doses of β blockers, or who have a contraindication to β-blocker use. Because it is new and not included in the current treatment guidelines, we discuss ivabradine only briefly.

Ivabradine causes a dose-dependent reduction in heart rate by blocking channels responsible for cardiac pacemaker current. Although the drug slows heart rate, it does not possess negative inotropic effects or cause QTc prolongation. When used in recommended doses, heart rate reduction is approximately 10 beats/min.

The Systolic Heart failure treatment with the I^f inhibitor ivabradine Trial (SHIFT) was a randomized, double-blind study comparing ivabradine to placebo in 6558 adults. End results revealed that the use of ivabradine reduced risk of hospitalization for worsening HF or cardiovascular death. Given these findings, ivabradine may be a useful alternative to patients with HF who need additional β blockade above what is currently available.

Digoxin

Digoxin belongs to a class of drugs known as *cardiac glycosides,* agents best known for their *positive inotropic actions*—that is, their ability to increase myocardial contractile force. By increasing contractile force, digoxin can increase cardiac output. In addition, it can alter the electrical activity of the heart and can favorably affect neurohormonal systems. Unfortunately, although digoxin can reduce symptoms of HF, it does not prolong life. Used widely in the past, *digoxin is considered a second-line agent today.* The pharmacology of digoxin is discussed later.

Vasodilators Other Than Angiotensin-Converting Enzyme Inhibitors and Angiotensin II Receptor Blockers
Isosorbide Dinitrate Plus Hydralazine

For the treatment of HF, isosorbide dinitrate (ISDN) and hydralazine are usually combined. The combination represents an alternative to ACEIs or ARBs. However, ACEIs and ARBs are generally preferred.

BiDil, a fixed-dose combination of hydralazine and ISDN, is approved for treating HF—but only in blacks, making BiDil the first medication approved for a specific ethnic group. Can BiDil help people in other ethnic groups? Probably, but data are lacking: the manufacturer tested the product only in black patients. As discussed in Chapter 7, testing was limited primarily because of regulatory and market incentives, not because there were data suggesting that it would not work for others.

Of course now that BiDil is approved, clinicians may prescribe it for anyone they see fit.

DIGOXIN, A CARDIAC GLYCOSIDE

Digoxin (Lanoxin) belongs to a family of drugs known as *cardiac glycosides.* These drugs are prepared by extraction from *Digitalis purpurea* (purple foxglove) and *Digitalis lanata* (Grecian foxglove) and hence are also known as *digitalis glycosides.* In the United States digoxin is the only cardiac glycoside available.

Digoxin has profound effects on the mechanical and electrical properties of the heart. In addition, it has important neurohormonal effects. In patients with HF, benefits derive from increased myocardial contractility and from effects on neurohormonal systems.

Digitalis is a dangerous drug because it can cause severe dysrhythmias at doses close to therapeutic. Owing to its prodysrhythmic actions, digoxin must be used with respect, caution, and skill.

Digoxin is indicated for HF and for the control of dysrhythmias (see Chapter 43). When used for HF, digoxin can reduce symptoms, increase exercise tolerance, and decrease hospitalizations. However, the drug does *not* prolong life. Furthermore, when used by women, it may actually *shorten* life. Because benefits are limited to symptomatic relief and the risk for toxicity is substantial, *digoxin is now considered a second-line drug for treating HF.*

Mechanical Effects on the Heart

Digoxin exerts a *positive inotropic action* on the heart. That is, the drug *increases the force of ventricular contraction* and can thereby increase cardiac output (Fig. 42.4).

Mechanism of Inotropic Action

Digoxin increases myocardial contractility by inhibiting an enzyme known as *sodium-potassium adenosine triphosphatase* (Na^+,K^+-ATPase). By way of an indirect process described later, inhibition of Na^+,K^+-ATPase promotes calcium accumulation within myocytes. The calcium then augments contractile force by facilitating the interaction of actin and myosin, the myocardial contractile proteins.

Relationship of Potassium to Inotropic Action

Potassium ions compete with digoxin for binding to Na^+,K^+-ATPase. This competition is of great clinical significance. Because potassium competes with digoxin, when potassium levels are low, binding of digoxin to Na^+,K^+-ATPase increases. This increase can produce excessive inhibition of Na^+,K^+-ATPase, with resultant toxicity. Conversely, when levels of potassium are high, inhibition of Na^+,K^+-ATPase by digoxin is reduced, causing a reduction in the therapeutic response. Because an increase in potassium can impair therapeutic responses whereas a decrease in potassium can cause toxicity, it is imperative that potassium levels be kept within the normal physiologic range.

Hemodynamic Benefits in Heart Failure
Increased Cardiac Output

In patients with HF, increased myocardial contractility increases cardiac output. By increasing contractility, digoxin shifts the relationship of fiber length to stroke volume in the failing heart toward that in the healthy heart. Consequently, at any given heart size, the stroke volume of the failing heart increases, causing cardiac output to rise.

Consequences of Increased Cardiac Output

As a result of increased cardiac output, three major secondary responses occur: (1) sympathetic tone declines, (2) urine production increases, and (3) renin release declines. These responses can reverse virtually all

Fig. 42.4 Ion Fluxes Across the Cardiac Cell Membrane. During the action potential, Na^+ and Ca^{2+} enter the cardiac cell and K^+ exits. Following the action potential, Na^+, K^+-ATPase pumps Na^+ out of the cell and takes up K^+. Ca^{2+} leaves the cell in exchange for the uptake of Na^+. By inhibiting Na^+, K^+-ATPase, digoxin prevents the extrusion of Na^+, causing Na^+ to accumulate inside the cell. The resulting buildup of intracellular Na^+ suppresses the Na^+-Ca^{2+} exchange process, thereby causing intracellular levels of Ca^{2+} to rise.

signs and symptoms of HF. However, they do not correct the underlying problem of cardiac remodeling.

Decreased Sympathetic Tone

By increasing contractile force and cardiac output, digoxin increases arterial pressure. In response, sympathetic nerve traffic to the heart and blood vessels is reduced through the baroreceptor reflex. (Recall that a compensatory *increase* in sympathetic tone had taken place because of HF.)

The decrease in sympathetic tone has several beneficial effects. First, heart rate is reduced, thereby allowing more complete ventricular filling. Second, afterload is reduced (because of reduced arteriolar constriction), thereby allowing more complete ventricular emptying. Third, venous pressure is reduced (because of reduced venous constriction), thereby reducing cardiac distention, pulmonary congestion, and peripheral edema.

Increased Urine Production

The increase in cardiac output increases renal blood flow and thereby increases the production of urine. The resultant loss of water reduces blood volume, which in turn reduces cardiac distention, pulmonary congestion, and peripheral edema.

Decreased Renin Release

In response to increased arterial pressure, renin release declines, causing levels of aldosterone and angiotensin II to decline as well. The decrease in angiotensin II decreases vasoconstriction, thereby further reducing afterload and venous pressure. The decrease in aldosterone reduces the retention of sodium and water, which reduces blood volume, which in turn further reduces venous pressure.

Summary of Hemodynamic Effects

We can see that, through direct and indirect mechanisms, digoxin has the potential to reverse all of the overt manifestations of HF: cardiac output improves, heart rate decreases, heart size declines, constriction of arterioles and veins decreases, water retention reverses, blood volume declines, peripheral and pulmonary edema decrease, and water weight is lost. In addition, exercise tolerance improves and fatigue is reduced. There is, however, one important caveat: Although digoxin can produce substantial improvement in HF symptoms, it does not prolong life.

Neurohormonal Benefits in Heart Failure

At dosages below those needed for positive inotropic effects, digoxin can modulate the activity of neurohormonal systems. The underlying mechanism is inhibition of Na^+,K^+-ATPase.

In the kidney, digoxin can suppress renin release. By inhibiting Na^+,K^+-ATPase in renal tubules, digoxin decreases tubular absorption of sodium. As a result, less sodium is presented to the distal tubule, so renin release is suppressed.

Through effects on the vagus nerve, digoxin can decrease sympathetic outflow from the central nervous system (CNS). Specifically, by inhibiting Na^+,K^+-ATPase in vagal afferent fibers, digoxin increases the sensitivity of cardiac baroreceptors. As a result, these receptors discharge more readily, thereby signaling the CNS to reduce sympathetic traffic to the periphery.

How important are these effects on renin and sympathetic tone? No one knows for sure. However, they are probably just as important as inotropic effects and perhaps even more important.

Electrical Effects on the Heart

The effects of digoxin on the electrical activity of the heart are of therapeutic and toxicologic importance. It is because of its electrical effects that digoxin is useful for treating dysrhythmias (see Chapter 43). Ironically, these same electrical effects are responsible for *causing* dysrhythmias, the most serious adverse effect of digoxin.

The electrical effects of digoxin can be bewildering in their complexity. Through a combination of actions, digoxin can alter the electrical activity in noncontractile tissue (the sinoatrial [SA] node, atrioventricular [AV] node, and Purkinje fibers) as well as in ventricular muscle. In these various regions, digoxin can alter automaticity, refractoriness, and impulse conduction. Whether these parameters are increased or decreased depends on cardiac status, digoxin dosage, and the region involved.

Although the electrical effects of digoxin are many and varied, only a few are clinically significant. These are discussed next.

Adverse Effects I: Cardiac Dysrhythmias

Dysrhythmias are the most serious adverse effect of digoxin. They result from altering the electrical properties of the heart. Fortunately, when used in the dosages recommended today, dysrhythmias are uncommon.

Digoxin can mimic practically all types of dysrhythmias. AV block with escape beats is among the most common. Ventricular flutter and ventricular fibrillation are the most dangerous.

Because serious dysrhythmias are a potential consequence of therapy, all patients should be evaluated frequently for changes in heart rate and rhythm. If significant changes occur, digoxin should be withheld.

PATIENT EDUCATION
Monitoring Heart Rate

Patients should be taught to monitor their pulses and instructed to report any significant changes in rate or regularity. Many providers will instruct the patient to hold the medication if their heart rate is less than 50 just prior to taking the medication.

Predisposing Factors

Hypokalemia. The most common cause of dysrhythmias in patients receiving digoxin is hypokalemia secondary to the use of diuretics. Less common causes include vomiting and diarrhea. Hypokalemia promotes dysrhythmias by increasing digoxin-induced inhibition of Na^+,K^+-ATPase, which in turn leads to the increased automaticity of Purkinje fibers. Because low potassium can precipitate dysrhythmias, *it is imperative that serum potassium levels be kept within the normal range.* If diuretic therapy causes potassium levels to fall, a potassium-sparing diuretic (e.g., spironolactone) can be prescribed to correct the problem. Potassium supplements may also be used. Patients should be taught to recognize symptoms of hypokalemia (e.g., muscle weakness) and instructed to notify the prescriber if these develop.

Elevated digoxin levels. Digoxin has a narrow therapeutic range; *drug levels only slightly higher than therapeutic greatly increase the risk for toxicity.* Possible causes of excessive digoxin levels include (1) intentional or accidental overdose, (2) increased digoxin absorption, and (3) decreased digoxin elimination.

If digoxin levels are kept within the optimal therapeutic range—now considered to be 0.5 to 0.8 ng/mL—the chances of a dysrhythmia will be reduced. However, it is important to note that careful control of drug levels does not eliminate the risk. As discussed previously, there is only a loose relationship between digoxin levels and clinical effects. As a result, some patients may experience dysrhythmias even when drug levels are within what is normally considered a safe range.

Heart disease. The ability of digoxin to cause dysrhythmias is greatly increased by the presence of heart disease. Doses of digoxin that have no adverse effects on healthy volunteers can precipitate serious dysrhythmias in patients with HF. The probability and severity of a dysrhythmia are directly related to the severity of the underlying disease. Because heart disease is the reason for taking digoxin, it should be no surprise that people taking the drug are at risk for dysrhythmias.

Diagnosing digoxin-induced dysrhythmias. Diagnosis is not easy, largely because the failing heart is prone to spontaneous dysrhythmias. Hence when a dysrhythmia occurs, we cannot simply assume that digoxin is the cause: the possibility that the dysrhythmia is the direct result of heart disease must be considered. Compounding diagnostic difficulties is the poor correlation between plasma digoxin levels and dysrhythmia onset. Because of this loose association, the presence of an apparently excessive digoxin level does not necessarily indicate that digoxin is responsible for the problem. Laboratory data required for diagnosis include digoxin level, serum electrolytes, and an electrocardiogram (ECG). Ultimately, diagnosis is based on experience and clinical judgment. Resolution of the dysrhythmia after digoxin withdrawal confirms the diagnosis.

Managing digoxin-induced dysrhythmias. With proper treatment, digoxin-induced dysrhythmias can almost always be controlled. Basic management measures are as follows:

• *Withdraw digoxin and potassium-wasting diuretics.* For many patients, no additional treatment is needed. To help ensure that medication is stopped, a written order to withhold digoxin should be made.
• *Monitor serum potassium.* If the potassium level is low or nearly normal, potassium should be replaced. Potassium displaces digoxin from Na^+,K^+-ATPase and thereby helps reverse toxicity. However, if potassium levels are high or if AV block is present, no more potassium should be given. Under these conditions, more potassium may cause complete AV block.
• Some patients may require an antidysrhythmic drug. *Phenytoin* and *lidocaine* are most effective. Quinidine, another antidysrhythmic drug, can cause plasma levels of digoxin to rise and so should not be used.
• Patients who develop bradycardia or AV block can be treated with atropine. (Atropine blocks the vagal influences that underlie bradycardia and AV block.) Alternatively, electronic pacing may be employed.
• When overdose is especially severe, digoxin levels can be lowered using *Fab antibody fragments* (Digibind, Digifab). After intravenous (IV) administration, these fragments bind digoxin and thereby prevent it from acting. *Cholestyramine* and *activated charcoal*, agents that also bind digoxin, can be administered orally to suppress absorption of digoxin from the gastrointestinal (GI) tract.

Adverse Effects II: Noncardiac Adverse Effects

The principal noncardiac toxicities of digoxin concern the GI system and the CNS. Because adverse effects on these systems frequently precede the development of dysrhythmias, symptoms involving the GI tract and CNS can provide advance warning of more serious toxicity. Accordingly, patients should be taught to recognize these effects and instructed to notify the prescriber if they occur.

Anorexia, nausea, and *vomiting* are the most common GI side effects. These responses result primarily from stimulation of the chemoreceptor trigger zone of the medulla. Digoxin rarely causes diarrhea.

Fatigue is the most frequent CNS effect. *Visual disturbances* (e.g., blurred vision, yellow tinge to vision, appearance of halos around dark objects) are also relatively common.

Adverse Effects III: Measures to Reduce Adverse Effects

PATIENT EDUCATION
Digoxin Toxicity

Patients should be warned about digoxin-induced dysrhythmias and instructed to take their medication exactly as prescribed. In addition, they should be informed about symptoms of developing toxicity (altered heart rate or rhythm, visual or gastrointestinal disturbances) and instructed to notify the prescriber if these develop. If a potassium supplement or potassium-sparing diuretic is part of the regimen, it should be taken exactly as ordered.

Drug Interactions

Digoxin is subject to a large number of significant drug interactions. Some are pharmacodynamics, and some are pharmacokinetic. Several important interactions are discussed later. Interactions are shown in Table 42.2.

TABLE 42.2 Drug Interactions With Digoxin

Drug	Effect
Pharmacodynamic Interactions	
Thiazide diuretics	Promote potassium loss and thereby increase
Loop diuretics	the risk for digoxin-induced dysrhythmias
Succinylcholine	
β blockers	Decrease contractility and heart rate
Verapamil	
Diltiazem	
Sympathomimetics	Increase contractility and heart rate
Pharmacokinetic Interactions	
Cholestyramine	Decrease digoxin levels by decreasing digoxin
Kaolin-pectin	absorption or bioavailability
Metoclopramide	
Neomycin	
Sulfasalazine	
Aminoglycosides	Increase digoxin levels by increasing digoxin
Antacids	absorption or bioavailability
Azithromycin	
Clarithromycin	
Colestipol	
Erythromycin	
Omeprazole	
Tetracycline	
Alprazolam	Increase digoxin levels by decreasing
Amiodarone	excretion of digoxin, altering distribution of
Atorvastatin	digoxin, or both
Captopril	
Diltiazem	
Nifedipine	
Nitrendipine	
Propafenone	
Quinidine	
Verapamil	

Diuretics

Thiazide diuretics and *loop diuretics* promote loss of potassium and thereby increase the risk for digoxin-induced dysrhythmias. Accordingly, when digoxin and these diuretics are used concurrently, serum potassium levels must be monitored and maintained within the normal range. If hypokalemia develops, potassium levels can be restored with potassium supplements, a potassium-sparing diuretic, or both.

Angiotensin-Converting Enzyme Inhibitors and Angiotensin II Receptor Blockers

These drugs can increase potassium levels and can thereby decrease therapeutic responses to digoxin. Caution should be exercised if an ACEI or ARB is combined with potassium supplements or a potassium-sparing diuretic.

Sympathomimetics

Sympathomimetic drugs (e.g., dopamine, dobutamine) act on the heart to increase the rate and force of contraction. The increase in contractile force can add to the positive inotropic effects of digoxin. These complementary actions can be beneficial. In contrast, the ability of sympathomimetics to increase heart rate may be detrimental in that the risk for a tachydysrhythmia is increased.

Quinidine

Quinidine is an antidysrhythmic drug that can cause plasma levels of digoxin to rise. Quinidine increases digoxin levels by (1) displacing digoxin from tissue binding sites and (2) reducing renal excretion of digoxin. By elevating levels of free digoxin, quinidine can promote digoxin toxicity. Accordingly, concurrent use of quinidine and digoxin should be avoided.

Amiodarone

Amiodarone, a drug used to treat supraventricular dysrhythmias, may increase the serum concentration of digoxin. Consider reducing the digoxin dose by 30% to 50% when initiating therapy in conjunction with amiodarone.

Verapamil

Verapamil, a calcium channel blocker (CCB), can significantly increase plasma levels of digoxin. If the combination is employed, digoxin dosage must be reduced. In addition, verapamil can suppress myocardial contractility and thereby counteract the benefits of digoxin.

Pharmacokinetics

Absorption

Absorption with digoxin tablets is variable, ranging between 60% and 80%, and can be decreased by certain foods and drugs. Meals high in bran can decrease absorption significantly, as can cholestyramine, kaolin-pectin, and certain other drugs (see Table 42.2). Of note, taking digoxin with meals decreases the rate of absorption but not the extent.

In the past, there was considerable variability in the absorption of digoxin from tablets prepared by different manufacturers. This variability resulted from differences in the rate and extent of tablet dissolution. Because of this variable bioavailability, it had been recommended that patients not switch between different digoxin brands. Today, bioavailability of digoxin in tablets produced by different companies is fairly uniform, making brands of digoxin more interchangeable than in the past. However, given the narrow therapeutic range of digoxin, some authorities still recommend that patients not switch between brands of digoxin tablets—even when prescriptions are written generically—except with the approval and supervision of the prescriber.

Distribution

Digoxin is distributed widely and crosses the placenta. High levels are achieved in cardiac and skeletal muscle, owing largely to binding to Na^+,K^+-ATPase. About 23% of digoxin in plasma is bound to proteins, mainly albumin.

Elimination

Digoxin is eliminated primarily by *renal excretion*. Hepatic metabolism is minimal. Because digoxin is eliminated by the kidneys, renal impairment can lead to toxic accumulation. Accordingly, dosage must be reduced if kidney function declines. Because digoxin is not metabolized to a significant extent, changes in liver function do not affect digoxin levels.

Half-Life and Time to Plateau

The half-life of digoxin is about 1.5 days. Therefore, in the absence of a loading dose, about 6 days (four half-lives) are required to reach plateau. When use of the drug is discontinued, another 6 days are required for digoxin stores to be eliminated.

Single-Dose Time Course

Effects of a single oral dose begin 30 minutes to 2 hours after administration and peak within 4 to 6 hours.

A Note on Plasma Digoxin Levels

Levels above 1 ng/mL offer no additional benefits but do increase the risk for toxicity. Knowledge of plasma levels can be useful for the following:

- Establishing dosage
- Monitoring compliance
- Diagnosing toxicity
- Determining the cause of therapeutic failure

After a stable blood level has been achieved, routine measurement of digoxin levels can be replaced with an annual measurement. Additional measurements may be useful in the following circumstances:

- Digoxin dosage is changed
- Symptoms of HF intensify
- Kidney function deteriorates
- Signs of toxicity appear
- Drugs that can affect digoxin levels are added to or deleted from the regimen

Although knowledge of digoxin plasma levels can aid the clinician, it must be understood that the extent of this aid is limited. The correlation between plasma levels of digoxin and clinical effects—both therapeutic and adverse—is not very tight: drug levels that are safe and effective for patient A may be subtherapeutic for patient B and toxic for patient C. Because of interpatient variability, knowledge of digoxin levels does not permit precise predictions of therapeutic effects or toxicity. Hence information regarding drug levels must not be relied on too heavily. Rather, this information should be seen as but one factor among several to be considered when clinical responses are being evaluated.

 SUMMARY OF KEY PRESCRIBING CONSIDERATIONS

Digoxin

Therapeutic Goal: Digoxin is used to treat heart failure and dysrhythmias.

Baseline Data: Laboratory tests should include electrocardiogram, serum electrolytes, and evaluation of kidney function.

Monitoring: Measurement of plasma drug levels in patient with unchanged symptoms of heart failure after initiation or patient with symptoms of toxicity. Optimal rate for digoxin is 0.5–0.8 ng/mL.

Identifying High-Risk Patients: Digoxin is contraindicated in patients experiencing ventricular fibrillation or ventricular tachycardia. Caution must be exercised in patients with renal insufficiency or hypokalemia.

Evaluating Therapeutic Effects: Assess for reductions in orthopnea, dyspnea on exertion, jugular venous distention, edema, and crackles.

Minimizing Adverse Effects: Patients should be taught to report early signs of hypokalemia and to inform the provider regarding signs of toxicity, including visual disturbances or nausea and vomiting.

MANAGEMENT OF HEART FAILURE

Our discussion of HF management is based on recommendations in the 2017 ACC/AHA/HFSA Focused Update of the 2013 ACCF/AHA Guideline for the Management of Heart Failure: Executive Summary A Report of the American College of Cardiology Foundation/American Heart Association Task Force on Practice Guidelines. These guidelines can be viewed at https://www.ahajournals.org/doi/10.1161/CIR.0000000000000509. As noted earlier, these guidelines approach HF as a progressive disease that advances through four stages of increasing severity. Management of each stage is discussed next and in Fig. 42.5.

Stage A

By definition, patients in ACC/AHA stage A have no symptoms of HF and no structural or functional cardiac abnormalities, but they do have behaviors or conditions strongly associated with developing HF. Important among these are hypertension, coronary artery disease, diabetes, family history of cardiomyopathy, and a personal history of alcohol abuse, rheumatic fever, or treatment with a cardiotoxic drug (e.g., doxorubicin, trastuzumab).

Management is directed at reducing risk. Hypertension, hyperlipidemia, and diabetes should be controlled, as should ventricular rate in patients with supraventricular tachycardias. An ACEI or ARB can be useful for patients with diabetes, atherosclerosis, or hypertension. Patients should cease behaviors that increase HF risk, especially smoking and alcohol abuse. (Excessive, chronic consumption of alcohol is a leading cause of cardiomyopathy. In patients with HF, acute alcohol consumption can suppress contractility.) There is no evidence that getting regular exercise can prevent the development of HF, although exercise does have other health benefits. Routine use of dietary supplements to prevent structural heart disease is not recommended.

Stage B

Like patients in stage A, those in stage B have no signs or symptoms of HF, but they do have structural heart disease that is strongly associated with the development of HF. Among these structural changes are LV hypertrophy or fibrosis, LV dilation or hypocontractility, valvular heart disease, and previous myocardial infarction.

The goal of management is to prevent development of symptomatic HF. The approach is to implement measures that can prevent further cardiac injury, thus delaying the progression of remodeling and LV dysfunction. Specific measures include all those discussed earlier for stage A. In addition, treatment with an ACEI plus a β blocker is recommended for all patients with a reduced ejection fraction, history of myocardial infarction, or both. For patients who cannot tolerate ACEIs, an ARB may be used instead. As in stage A, there is no evidence that using dietary supplements or getting regular exercise can help prevent progression to symptomatic HF.

Stage C

Patients in stage C have symptoms of HF and also structural heart disease. As discussed earlier, symptoms include dyspnea, fatigue, peripheral edema, and distention of the jugular veins. Treatment has four major goals: (1) relief of pulmonary and peripheral congestive symptoms, (2) improvement of functional capacity and quality of life, (3) slowing of cardiac remodeling and progression of LV dysfunction, and (4) prolongation of life. Treatment measures include those recommended for stages A and B plus those discussed subsequently.

Drug Therapy

Drug therapy of HF has changed dramatically over the past 15 to 20 years. Formerly digoxin was a mainstay of treatment. Today its role is secondary. First-line therapy now consists of three drugs: a diuretic, an ACEI or ARB, and a β blocker. As a rule, digoxin is added only when symptoms cannot be managed with the preferred agents.

Diuretics. All patients with evidence of fluid retention should restrict salt intake and use a diuretic. Diuretics are the only reliable means of correcting fluid overload. Furthermore, these drugs produce symptomatic improvement faster than any other drugs. If renal function is good, a thiazide diuretic will work. However, if renal function is significantly impaired, as it is in most patients, a loop diuretic will be needed. Efficacy

At Risk for Heart Failure **Heart Failure**

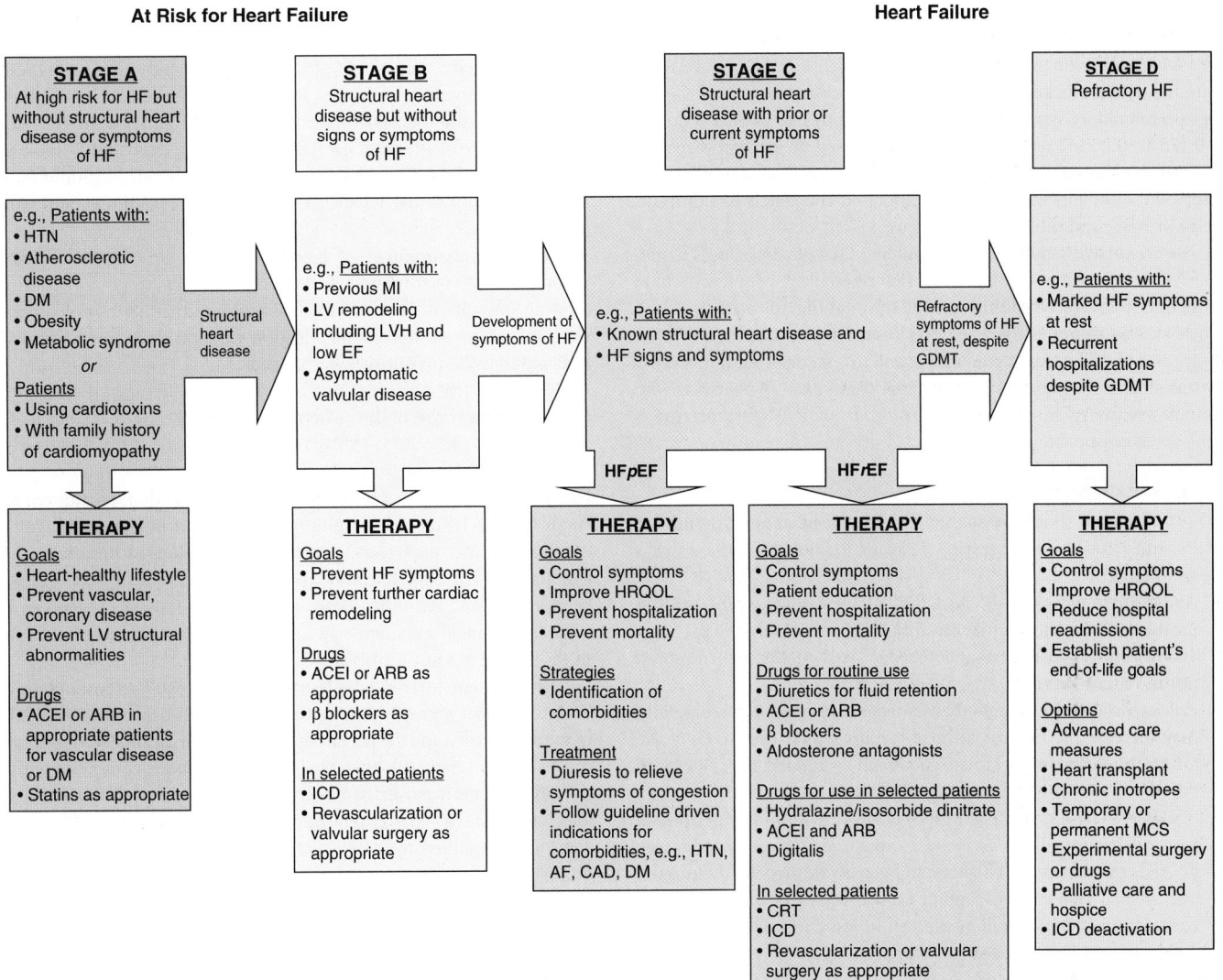

Fig. 42.5 Recommended Therapies for Varying Stages of Heart Failure. *ACEI,* Angiotensin-converting enzyme inhibitor; *AF,* atrial fibrillation; *ARB,* Angiotensin II receptor blocker; *CAD,* coronary artery disease; *CRT,* cardiac resynchronization therapy; *DM,* diabetes mellitus; *EF,* ejection fraction; *GDMT,* guideline directed medical therapy; *HF,* heart failure; *HFpEF,* heart failure with preserved ejection fraction; *HFrEF,* heart failure with reduced ejection fraction; *HTN,* hypertension; *HRQOL,* health-related quality of life; *ICD,* implantable cardioverter-defibrillator; *LV,* left ventricular; *LVH,* left ventricular hypertrophy; *MCS,* mechanical circulatory support; *MI,* myocardial infarction. (Adapted from Hunt SA, Abraham WT, Chin MH, et al. 2009 Focused update incorporated into the ACC/AHA 2005 guidelines for the diagnosis and management of heart failure in adults: a report of the American College of Cardiology Foundation/American Heart Association Task Force on Practice Guidelines. *J Am Coll Cardiol.* 2009;53:e1–e90.)

of diuresis is best assessed by daily measurement of body weight. After fluid overload has been corrected, diuretic therapy should continue to prevent recurrence. Diuretics should not be used alone. Rather, for most patients, they should be combined with an ACEI (or ARB) plus a β blocker. Because aspirin and other nonsteroidal antiinflammatory drugs (NSAIDs) can decrease the effects of diuretics and increase the incidence of acute kidney injury when used in combination with an ACEI and a diuretic, these agents should be avoided. As noted, although diuretics reduce symptoms, they do not prolong survival.

Angiotensin-converting enzyme inhibitors and angiotensin II receptor blockers. In the absence of specific contraindications (e.g., pregnancy), all patients with stage C HF should receive an ACEI. If fluid retention is evident, a diuretic should be used as well. Symptomatic improvement may take weeks or even months to develop. However, even in the absence

of symptomatic improvement, ACEIs may prolong life. Dosage should be sufficient to reduce mortality (see Table 42.1). For patients who cannot tolerate ACEIs (owing to intractable cough or angioedema), ARBs remain the recommended alternative.

β Blockers. In the absence of specific contraindications, all patients with stage C HF should receive an approved β blocker (e.g., carvedilol). As with ACEIs, symptomatic improvement may not be evident for months. Nonetheless, life may be prolonged even in the absence of clinical improvement.

Aldosterone antagonists. Adding an aldosterone antagonist (spironolactone or eplerenone) to standard therapy (i.e., diuretic, ACEI or ARB, and a β blocker) is reasonable in patients with moderately severe or severe symptoms of HF after a heart attack. However, aldosterone antagonists must not be used if kidney function is impaired or serum potassium is elevated. The monitoring of renal function and potassium levels is imperative.

Digoxin. Digoxin may be used in combination with ACEIs (or ARBs), diuretics, and β blockers to improve clinical status. However, although digoxin can reduce symptoms, it does not prolong life. The usual dosage is 0.125 to 0.25 mg/day. Adjustments are based on clinical response. Digoxin may be started early to help improve symptoms, or it may be reserved for patients who have not responded adequately to a diuretic, ACEI or ARB, and β blocker.

Isosorbide dinitrate/hydralazine. Adding ISDN/hydralazine is *recommended* to improve outcomes in self-described black people who have moderate to severe symptoms despite optimal therapy with ACEIs, β blockers, and diuretics. For all other patients who continue to have symptoms despite treatment with standard therapy, adding ISDN/hydralazine to the regimen is considered *reasonable*. For patients who cannot tolerate ACEIs or ARBs, *substitution* of ISDN/hydralazine is considered reasonable.

Drugs to Avoid

Patients in stage C should avoid three classes of drugs: antidysrhythmics, CCBs, and NSAIDs (e.g., aspirin). Reasons for not using these drugs are as follows:

- *Antidysrhythmic agents*—These drugs have cardiosuppressant and prodysrhythmic actions that can make HF worse. Only two agents—amiodarone (Cordarone) and dofetilide (Tikosyn)—have been proved not to reduce survival.
- *Calcium channel blockers*—These drugs can make HF worse and may increase the risk for adverse cardiovascular events. Only the long-acting dihydropyridine CCBs, such as amlodipine (Norvasc), have been shown not to reduce survival.
- *NSAIDs*—These drugs promote sodium retention and peripheral vasoconstriction. Both actions can make HF worse. In addition, NSAIDs can reduce the efficacy and intensify the toxicity of diuretics and ACEIs. Hence even though aspirin has beneficial effects on coagulation, it should still be avoided unless clinically indicated for conditions such as myocardial infarction.

Evaluating Treatment

Evaluation is based on symptoms and physical findings. Reductions in dyspnea on exertion, paroxysmal nocturnal dyspnea, and orthopnea indicate success. The physical examination should assess for reductions in jugular distention, edema, and crackles. Success is also indicated by increased capacity for physical activity. Accordingly, patients should be interviewed to determine improvements in the maximal activity they can perform without symptoms, the type of activity that regularly produces symptoms, and the maximal activity they can tolerate. Successful treatment should also improve health-related quality of life in general. Thus the interview should look for improvements in sleep, sexual function, outlook on life, cognitive function, and ability to participate in usual social, recreational, and work activities.

Routine measurement of ejection fraction or maximal exercise capacity is not recommended. Although the degree of reduction in ejection fraction measured at the beginning of therapy is predictive of outcome, improvement in the ejection fraction does not necessarily indicate that the prognosis has changed.

As noted earlier, a reduction in circulating BNP indicates improvement. The lower the BNP, the better the odds of long-term survival.

Stage D

Patients in stage D have advanced structural heart disease and marked symptoms of HF at rest despite treatment with maximal dosages of medications used in stage C. Repeated and prolonged hospitalization is common. For eligible candidates, the best long-term solution is a heart transplant. An implantable LV mechanical assist device can be used as a "bridge" in patients awaiting a transplant and to prolong life in those who are not transplant eligible.

Management focuses largely on control of fluid retention, which underlies most signs and symptoms. Intake and output should be monitored closely, and the patient should be weighed daily. Fluid retention can usually be treated with a loop diuretic, perhaps combined with a thiazide. If volume overload becomes severe, the patient should be hospitalized and given a diuretic intravenously. If needed, an IV inotropic agent can be added to increase renal blood flow, thereby enhancing diuresis. Patients should not be discharged until a stable and effective oral diuretic regimen has been established. These drugs are discussed further in Chapter 92.

β blockers and ACEIs may be tried, but doses should be low and responses monitored with care. In stage D, β blockers pose a significant risk for making HF worse, and ACEIs may induce profound hypotension or renal failure.

When severe symptoms persist despite application of all recommended therapies, options for end-of-life care should be discussed with the patient and family.

43

Antidysrhythmic Drugs

A *dysrhythmia* is defined as an abnormality in the rhythm of the heartbeat. In their mildest forms, dysrhythmias have only modest effects on cardiac output. However, in their most severe forms, dysrhythmias can disable the heart so that no blood is pumped at all. Because of their ability to compromise cardiac function, dysrhythmias are associated with a high degree of morbidity and mortality.

There are two basic types of dysrhythmias: *tachydysrhythmias* and *bradydysrhythmias*. Only the tachydysrhythmias are considered in this chapter. This is by far the largest group of dysrhythmias and the group that responds best to drugs. The bradydysrhythmias are not discussed because they are few in number and are commonly treated with electronic pacing. When drugs are indicated, atropine is usually the agent of choice.

It is important to appreciate that virtually all of the drugs used to treat dysrhythmias can also *cause* dysrhythmias. These drugs can create new dysrhythmias and worsen existing ones. Because of these prodysrhythmic actions, antidysrhythmic drugs should be employed only when the benefits of treatment clearly outweigh the risks.

For two reasons, use of antidysrhythmic drugs is declining. First, research has shown that some of these agents actually *increase* the risk for death. Second, nonpharmacologic therapies—especially implantable defibrillators and radiofrequency (RF) ablation—have begun to replace drugs as the preferred treatment for many types of dysrhythmia.

A note on terminology: dysrhythmias are also known as *arrhythmias*. Because the term *arrhythmia* denotes an *absence* of cardiac rhythm, whereas *dysrhythmia* denotes an *abnormal* rhythm, *dysrhythmia* is the more appropriate term.

INTRODUCTION TO CARDIAC ELECTROPHYSIOLOGY, DYSRHYTHMIAS, AND THE ANTIDYSRHYTHMIC DRUGS

This section discusses background information that will clarify the actions and uses of antidysrhythmic drugs. It begins by reviewing the electrical properties of the heart and the electrocardiogram (ECG). This is followed by a discussion of how dysrhythmias are generated. After that, the classification of the antidysrhythmic drugs as well as the ability of these drugs to *cause* dysrhythmias are considered. The chapter concludes by discussing the major dysrhythmias and the basic principles that guide antidysrhythmic therapy.

Electrical Properties of the Heart

Dysrhythmias result from alteration of the electrical impulses that regulate cardiac rhythm—and antidysrhythmic drugs control rhythm by correcting or compensating for these alterations. Accordingly, to understand both the generation and treatment of dysrhythmias, we must first understand the electrical properties of the heart. Therefore this section begins by

reviewing (1) pathways and timing of impulse conduction, (2) cardiac action potentials, and (3) basic elements of the ECG.

Impulse Conduction: Pathways and Timing

For the heart to pump effectively, contraction of the atria and ventricles must be coordinated. Coordination is achieved through precise timing and routing of impulse conduction. In the healthy heart, impulses originate in the sinoatrial (SA) node, spread rapidly through the atria, pass slowly through the atrioventricular (AV) node, and then spread rapidly through the ventricles by way of the His-Purkinje system (Fig. 43.1).

SA node. Under normal circumstances, the SA node serves as the pacemaker for the heart. Pacemaker activity results from spontaneous phase 4 depolarization (see later). Because cells of the sinus node usually discharge faster than other cells that display automaticity, the SA node normally dominates all other potential pacemakers.

After the SA node discharges, impulses spread rapidly through the atria along the *internodal pathways*. This rapid conduction allows the atria to contract in unison.

AV node. Impulses originating in the atria must travel through the AV node to reach the ventricles. In the healthy heart, impulses arriving at the AV node are delayed before going on to excite the ventricles. This delay provides time for blood to fill the ventricles before ventricular contraction.

His-Purkinje system. The fibers of the His-Purkinje system consist of specialized conducting tissue. The function of these fibers is to conduct electrical excitation very rapidly to all parts of the ventricles. Stimulation of the His-Purkinje system is caused by impulses leaving the AV node. These impulses are conducted rapidly down the bundle of His, enter the right and left bundle branches, and then distribute to the many fine branches of the Purkinje fibers (see Fig. 43.1). Because impulses travel quickly through this system, all regions of the ventricles are stimulated almost simultaneously, producing synchronized ventricular contraction with resultant forceful ejection of blood.

Cardiac Action Potentials

Cardiac cells can initiate and conduct action potentials, consisting of self-propagating waves of depolarization followed by repolarization. As in neurons, cardiac action potentials are generated by the movement of ions into and out of cells. These ion fluxes take place by way of specific channels in the cell membrane. In the resting cardiac cell, negatively charged ions cover the inner surface of the cell membrane, whereas positively charged ions cover the external surface. Because of this separation of charge, the cell membrane is said to be *polarized*. Under proper conditions, channels in the cell membrane open, allowing positively charged ions to rush in. This influx eliminates the charge difference across the cell membrane, and thus the cell is said to depolarize. After depolarization, positively charged ions are extruded from the cell, causing the cell to return to its original polarized state.

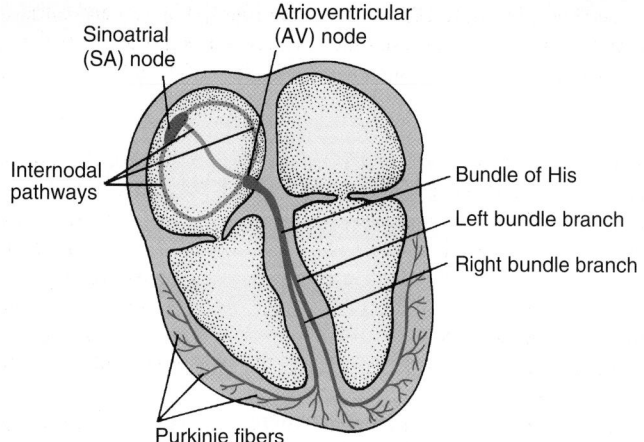

Sinoatrial (SA) node

Atrioventricular (AV) node

Internodal pathways

Bundle of His

Left bundle branch

Right bundle branch

Purkinje fibers

Fig. 43.1 Cardiac Conduction Pathways.

In the heart, two kinds of action potentials occur: *fast potentials* and *slow potentials*. These potentials differ with respect to the mechanisms by which they are generated, the kinds of cells in which they occur, and the drugs to which they respond.

Profiles of fast and slow potentials are depicted in Fig. 43.2. Note that action potentials in this figure represent the electrical activity of *single cardiac cells*. Such single-cell recordings, which are made using experimental preparations, should not be confused with the ECG, which is made using surface electrodes and thus reflects the electrical activity of the entire heart.

Fast potentials. Fast potentials occur in fibers of the *His-Purkinje system* and in *atrial and ventricular muscle*. These responses serve to conduct electrical impulses rapidly throughout the heart.

As shown in Fig. 43.2A, fast potentials have five distinct phases, labeled 0, 1, 2, 3, and 4. As each phase is discussed, the focus will be on its ionic basis and its relationship to the actions of antidysrhythmic drugs.

Phase 0. In phase 0, the cell undergoes *rapid depolarization* in response to *influx of sodium ions*. Phase 0 is important in that the speed of phase 0 depolarization determines the velocity of impulse conduction.

Myocardium and His-Purkinje system

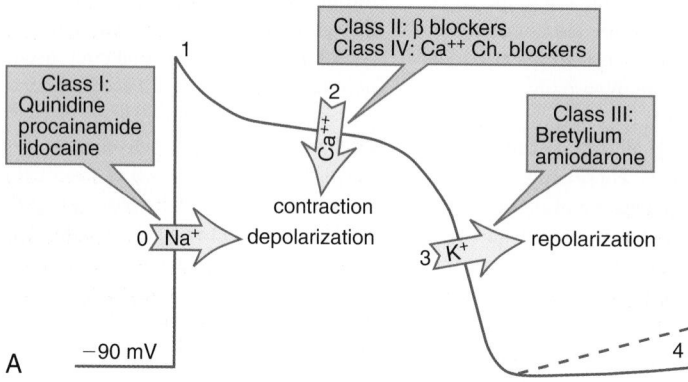

SA node and AV node

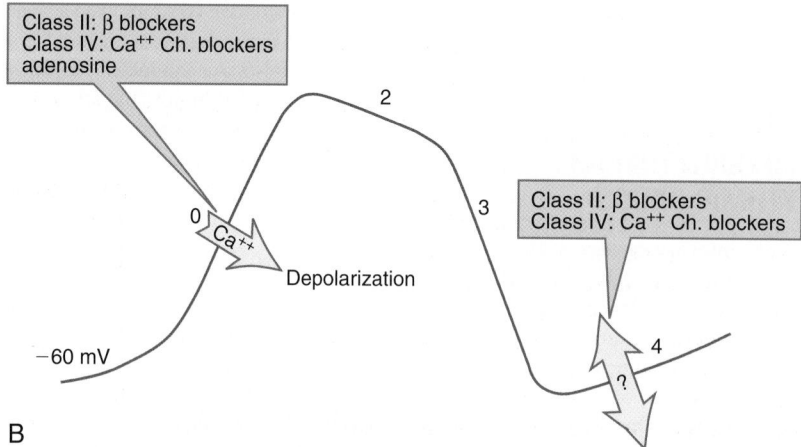

Fig. 43.2 Ion Fluxes During Cardiac Action Potentials and Effects of Antidysrhythmic Drugs. (A) Fast potential of the His-Purkinje system and atrial and ventricular myocardium. Blockade of sodium influx by class I drugs slows conduction in the His-Purkinje system. Blockade of calcium influx by β blockers and CCBs decreases contractility. Blockade of potassium efflux by class III drugs delays repolarization and thereby prolongs the effective refractory period. (B) Slow potential of the sinoatrial *(SA)* node and atrioventricular *(AV)* node. Blockade of calcium influx by β blockers, CCBs, and adenosine slows AV conduction. β blockers and CCBs decrease SA nodal automaticity (phase 4 depolarization); the ionic basis of this effect is not understood.

Drugs that decrease the rate of phase 0 depolarization (by blocking sodium channels) slow impulse conduction through the His-Purkinje system and myocardium.

Phase 1. During phase 1, rapid (but partial) repolarization takes place. Phase 1 has no relevance to antidysrhythmic drugs.

Phase 2. Phase 2 consists of a prolonged plateau in which the membrane potential remains relatively stable. During this phase, *calcium* enters the cell and promotes the contraction of atrial and ventricular muscle. Drugs that reduce calcium entry during phase 2 do *not* influence *cardiac rhythm.* However, because calcium influx is required for contraction, these drugs *can* reduce myocardial contractility.

Phase 3. In phase 3, rapid repolarization takes place. This repolarization is caused by *extrusion of potassium* from the cell. Phase 3 is relevant in that delay of repolarization prolongs the action potential duration and thereby prolongs the effective refractory period (ERP). (The ERP is the time during which a cell is unable to respond to excitation and initiate a new action potential. Therefore extending the ERP prolongs the minimal interval between two propagating responses.) Phase 3 repolarization can be delayed by drugs that block potassium channels.

Phase 4. During phase 4, two types of electrical activity are possible: (1) the membrane potential may remain *stable* (solid line in Fig. 43.2A) or (2) the membrane may undergo *spontaneous depolarization* (dashed line). In cells undergoing spontaneous depolarization, the membrane potential gradually rises until a threshold potential is reached. At this point, rapid phase 0 depolarization takes place, setting off a new action potential. Hence it is phase 4 depolarization that gives cardiac cells *automaticity* (i.e., the ability to initiate an action potential through self-excitation). The capacity for self-excitation makes potential pacemakers of all cells that have it.

Under normal conditions, His-Purkinje cells undergo very slow spontaneous depolarization and myocardial cells do not undergo any. However, under pathological conditions, significant phase 4 depolarization may occur in all of these cells and especially in Purkinje fibers. When this happens, a dysrhythmia can result.

Slow potentials. Slow potentials occur in cells of the *SA node* and *AV node.* The profile of a slow potential is depicted in Fig. 43.2B. Similar to fast potentials, slow potentials are generated by ion fluxes. However, the specific ions involved are not the same for every phase.

From a physiologic and pharmacologic perspective, slow potentials have three features of special significance: (1) phase 0 depolarization is slow and mediated by calcium influx, (2) these potentials conduct slowly, and (3) spontaneous phase 4 depolarization in the SA node normally determines heart rate.

Phase 0. Phase 0 (depolarization phase) of slow potentials differs significantly from phase 0 of fast potentials. As Fig. 43.2 shows, whereas phase 0 of fast potentials is caused by a *rapid influx of sodium,* phase 0 of slow potentials is caused by *slow influx of calcium.* Because calcium influx is slow, the rate of depolarization is slow; and because depolarization is slow, these potentials conduct slowly. This explains why impulse conduction through the AV node is delayed. Phase 0 of the slow potential is of therapeutic significance in that drugs that suppress calcium influx during phase 0 can slow (or stop) AV conduction.

Phases 2 and 3. Slow potentials lack a phase 1 (see Fig. 43.2B). Phases 2 and 3 of the slow potential are not significant with respect to the actions of antidysrhythmic drugs.

Phase 4. Cells of the SA node and AV node undergo spontaneous phase 4 depolarization. The ionic basis of this phenomenon is complex and incompletely understood.

Under normal conditions, the rate of phase 4 depolarization in cells of the SA node is faster than in all other cells of the heart. As a result, the SA node discharges first and determines heart rate. Hence the SA node is referred to as the cardiac *pacemaker.*

As shown in Fig. 43.2B, two classes of drugs (β blockers and calcium channel blockers [CCBs]) can suppress phase 4 depolarization. By doing so, these agents can decrease automaticity in the SA node.

The Electrocardiogram

The major components of an ECG are shown in Fig. 43.3. Here, three features are especially prominent: the P wave, the QRS complex, and the T wave. The P wave is caused by *depolarization in the atria.* Therefore the P wave corresponds to atrial contraction. The QRS complex is caused by *depolarization of the ventricles,* so the QRS complex corresponds to ventricular contraction. If conduction through the ventricles is slowed, the QRS complex will widen. The T wave is caused by *repolarization of the ventricles,* so this wave is not associated with overt physical activity of the heart.

In addition to the features just described, the ECG has three other components of interest: the PR interval, the QT interval, and the ST segment. The PR interval is defined as the time between the onset of the P wave and the onset of the QRS complex. Lengthening of this interval indicates a delay in conduction through the AV node. Several drugs increase the PR interval. The QT interval is defined as the time between the onset of the QRS complex and completion of the T wave. This interval is prolonged by drugs that delay ventricular repolarization. The ST segment is the portion of the ECG that lies between the end of the QRS complex and the beginning of the T wave. Digoxin depresses the ST segment.

Generation of Dysrhythmias

Dysrhythmias arise from two fundamental causes: *disturbances of impulse formation* (automaticity) and *disturbances of impulse conduction.* One or both of these disturbances underlie all dysrhythmias. Factors that may alter automaticity or conduction include hypoxia, electrolyte imbalance, cardiac surgery, reduced coronary blood flow, myocardial infarction, and antidysrhythmic drugs.

Disturbances of Automaticity

Disturbances of automaticity can occur in any part of the heart. Cells normally capable of automaticity (cells of the SA node, AV node, and His-Purkinje system) can produce dysrhythmias if their normal rate of discharge changes. In addition, dysrhythmias may be produced if tissues that do not normally express automaticity (atrial and ventricular muscle) develop spontaneous phase 4 depolarization.

Altered automaticity in the SA node can produce tachycardia or bradycardia. Excessive discharge of sympathetic neurons that innervate

Fig. 43.3 The Electrocardiogram.

the SA node can augment automaticity to such a degree that sinus tachycardia results. Excessive vagal (parasympathetic) discharge can suppress automaticity to such a degree that sinus bradycardia results.

Increased automaticity of Purkinje fibers is a common cause of dysrhythmias. The increase can be brought on by injury and by excessive stimulation of Purkinje fibers by the sympathetic nervous system. If Purkinje fibers begin to discharge faster than the SA node, they will escape control by the SA node; potentially serious dysrhythmias can result.

Under special conditions, automaticity may develop in cells of atrial and ventricular muscle. If these cells fire faster than the SA node, dysrhythmias will result.

PATIENT-CENTERED CARE ACROSS THE LIFE SPAN

Antidysrhythmic Drugs

Life Stage	Patient Care Concerns
Children/adolescents	Some antidysrhythmic drugs can be used safely in children, just in smaller doses. These include disopyramide, flecainide, and sotalol. Side-effect profiles are similar to those of adults.
Pregnant women	Many of the drugs discussed in this chapter are associated with adverse affects in both animal and human fetuses. Use of dronedarone is contraindicated in pregnant women.
Breastfeeding women	For most of the drugs discussed in this chapter, data are lacking regarding transmission of drug from mother to infant through breast milk. Breastfeeding is contraindicated in women taking dronederone. Amiodarone crosses the placental barrier and enters breast milk and can thereby harm the developing fetus and breastfeeding infant. Accordingly, pregnancy and breastfeeding should be avoided while the drug is being and for several months after stopping it.
Older adults	Aging alters the absorption, distribution, metabolism, and elimination of antidysrhythmic drugs. Liver and kidney function must be monitored, and antiarrhythmic dosing may need to be adjusted for age. Older-adult patients are also more susceptible to the side effects of many antidysrhythmics, including bradycardia, orthostatic hypotension, urinary retention, and falls.

Disturbances of Conduction

AV block. Impaired conduction through the AV node produces varying degrees of AV block. If impulse conduction is delayed (but not prevented entirely), the block is termed *first degree*. If some impulses pass through the node but others do not, the block is termed *second degree*. If all traffic through the AV node stops, the block is termed *third degree*.

Reentry (recirculating activation). Reentry, also referred to as recirculating activation, is a generalized mechanism by which dysrhythmias can be produced. Reentry causes dysrhythmias by establishing a localized, self-sustaining circuit capable of repetitive cardiac stimulation. Reentry results from a unique form of conduction disturbance. The mechanism of reentrant activation and the effects of drugs on this process are described next.

In normal impulse conduction, electrical impulses travel down both branches of the Purkinje fiber to cause excitation of the muscle at two locations (Fig. 43.4A). Impulses created within the muscle travel in both directions (to the right and to the left) away from their sites of origin. Those impulses that are moving toward each other meet midway

between the two branches of the Purkinje fiber. Because in the wake of both impulses the muscle is in a refractory state, neither impulse can proceed further, so both impulses stop.

In a reentrant circuit (see Fig. 43.4B), there is a region of one-way conduction block of one branch of the Purkinje fiber. This region prevents conduction of impulses downward (toward the muscle) but does not prevent impulses from traveling upward. (Impulses can travel back up the block because impulses in muscle are very strong and hence are able to pass the block, whereas impulses in the Purkinje fiber are weaker and so are unable to pass.) A region of one-way block is essential for reentrant activation.

How does one-way block lead to reentrant activation? As an impulse travels down the Purkinje fiber, it is blocked in one branch but continues unimpeded in the other. Upon reaching the tip of the second (unblocked) branch, the impulse stimulates the muscle. As described earlier, the impulse in the muscle travels to the right and to the left away from its site of origin. However, in this new situation, as the impulse travels toward the impaired branch of the Purkinje fiber, it meets no impulse coming from the other direction and continues on, resulting in stimulation of the terminal end of the first (blocked) branch. This stimulation causes an impulse to travel backward up the blocked branch of the Purkinje fiber. Because blockade of conduction in that branch is one-way (downward only), the impulse can pass upward through the region of block and then back down into the unblocked branch, causing reentrant activation of this branch. Under proper conditions, the impulse will continue to cycle indefinitely, resulting in repetitive ectopic beats.

There are two mechanisms by which drugs can abolish a reentrant dysrhythmia. First, drugs can improve conduction in the sick branch of the Purkinje fiber and can thereby eliminate the one-way block (see Fig. 43.4C). Alternatively, drugs can suppress conduction in the sick branch, thereby converting one-way block into two-way block (see Fig. 43.4D).

Classification of Antidysrhythmic Drugs

According to the Vaughan Williams classification scheme, the antidysrhythmic drugs fall into five groups (Table 43.1). There are four major classes of antidysrhythmic drugs (classes I, II, III, and IV) and a fifth group that includes adenosine and digoxin. Membership in classes I through IV is determined by effects on ion movements during slow and fast potentials (see Fig. 43.2).

Class I: Sodium Channel Blockers

Class I drugs block cardiac sodium channels (see Fig. 43.2A). By doing so, these drugs slow impulse conduction in the atria, ventricles, and His-Purkinje system. Class I constitutes the largest group of antidysrhythmic drugs.

Class II: β Blockers

Class II consists of β-adrenergic blocking agents. As suggested by Fig. 43.2, these drugs reduce calcium entry (during fast and slow potentials) and depress phase 4 depolarization (in slow potentials only). β blockers have three prominent effects on the heart:
- In the SA node, they reduce automaticity.
- In the AV node, they slow conduction velocity.
- In the atria and ventricles, they reduce contractility.

Cardiac effects of the β blockers are nearly identical to those of the CCBs.

Class III: Potassium Channel Blockers (Drugs That Delay Repolarization)

Class III drugs block potassium channels (see Fig. 43.2A) and thereby delay repolarization of fast potentials. By delaying repolarization, these drugs prolong both the action potential duration and the ERP.

Fig. 43.4 Reentrant Activation: Mechanism and Drug Effects. (A) In normal conduction, impulses from the branched Purkinje fiber stimulate the strip of ventricular muscle in two places. Within the muscle, waves of excitation spread from both points of excitation, meet between the Purkinje fibers, and cease further travel. (B) In the presence of one-way block, the strip of muscle is excited at only one location. Impulses spreading from this area meet no impulses coming from the left and therefore can travel far enough to stimulate branch 1 of the Purkinje fiber. This stimulation passes back up the fiber, past the region of one-way block, and then stimulates branch 2, causing reentrant activation. (C) Elimination of reentry by a drug that improves conduction in the sick branch of the Purkinje fiber. (D) Elimination of reentry by a drug that further suppresses conduction in the sick branch, thereby converting one-way block into two-way block.

Class IV: Calcium Channel Blockers

Only two CCBs—verapamil and diltiazem—are employed as antidysrhythmics. As indicated in Fig. 43.2, calcium channel blockade has the same effect on cardiac action potentials as does β blockade. Accordingly, verapamil, diltiazem, and β blockers have nearly identical effects on cardiac function—namely, reduction of automaticity in the SA node, delay of conduction through the AV node, and reduction of myocardial contractility. Antidysrhythmic benefits derive from suppressing AV nodal conduction.

Other Antidysrhythmic Drugs

Adenosine and digoxin do not fit into the four major classes of antidysrhythmic drugs. Both drugs suppress dysrhythmias by decreasing conduction through the AV node and reducing automaticity in the SA node.

Prodysrhythmic Effects of Antidysrhythmic Drugs

Virtually all of the drugs used to treat dysrhythmias have prodysrhythmic (proarrhythmic) effects. That is, *all of these drugs can worsen existing dysrhythmias and generate new ones.* This ability was documented dramatically in the Cardiac Arrhythmia Suppression Trial (CAST), in which use of class IC drugs (encainide and flecainide) to prevent dysrhythmias after myocardial infarction actually *doubled the rate of mortality.* Because of their prodysrhythmic actions, antidysrhythmic drugs should be used only when dysrhythmias are symptomatically significant and only when the potential benefits clearly outweigh the risks. Applying this guideline, it would be inappropriate to give antidysrhythmic drugs to a patient with nonsustained ventricular tachycardia (VT) because this dysrhythmia does not significantly reduce cardiac output. Conversely, when a patient is facing death from ventricular fibrillation, any therapy that might work must be tried. In this case the risk for prodysrhythmic effects is clearly outweighed by the potential benefits of stopping the fibrillation.

Overview of Common Dysrhythmias and Their Treatment

The common dysrhythmias can be divided into two major groups: *supraventricular dysrhythmias* and *ventricular dysrhythmias.* In general, ventricular dysrhythmias are more dangerous than supraventricular dysrhythmias. With either type, intervention is required only if the dysrhythmia interferes with effective ventricular pumping. Treatment often proceeds in two phases: (1) *termination* of the dysrhythmia (with

TABLE 43.1 Vaughan Williams Classification of Antidysrhythmic Drugs

Class I: Sodium Channel Blockers

Class IA
Quinidine
Procainamide (Procan ✦, generic in United States)
Disopyramide (Norpace, Rythmodan ✦)

Class IB
Phenytoin (Dilantin)
Mexiletine, generic only

Class IC
Flecainide, generic only
Propafenone (Rythmol, Rythmol SR)

Class II: β Blockers
Propranolol (Inderal LA)
Acebutolol (Sectral)

Class III: Potassium Channel Blockers (Drugs That Delay Repolarization)
Amiodarone (Cordarone, Pacerone)
Dronedarone (Multaq)
Sotalol (Betapace, Betapace AF)
Dofetilide (Tikosyn)

Class IV: Calcium Channel Blockers
Verapamil (Calan, Covera -HS ✦, Verelan)
Diltiazem (Cardizem, Dilacor-XR, Tiazac, others)

Other Antidysrhythmic Drugs
Digoxin (Lanoxin)

electrical countershock, drugs, or both), followed by (2) *long-term suppression* with drugs. Dysrhythmias can also be treated with an implantable cardioverter-defibrillator (ICD) or by destroying small areas of cardiac tissue using radiofrequency (RF) catheter ablation.

It is important to appreciate that drug therapy of dysrhythmias is highly empiric (i.e., based largely on the response of the patient and not on scientific principles). In practice, this means that even after a dysrhythmia has been identified, we cannot predict with certainty just which drugs will be effective. Frequently, trials with several drugs are required before control of rhythm is achieved. In the discussion that follows, only first-choice drugs are considered.

Supraventricular Dysrhythmias

Supraventricular dysrhythmias are dysrhythmias that arise in areas of the heart above the ventricles (atria, SA node, AV node). Supraventricular dysrhythmias per se are not especially harmful because dysrhythmic activity within the atria does not significantly reduce cardiac output except in patients with valvular disorders and heart failure (HF). Supraventricular tachydysrhythmias *can* be dangerous, however, in that atrial impulses are likely to traverse the AV node, resulting in excitation of the ventricles. If the atria drive the ventricles at an excessive rate, diastolic filling will be incomplete and cardiac output will decline. Hence, when supraventricular tachydysrhythmias are being treated, the objective is frequently slowing of ventricular rate (by blocking impulse conduction through the AV node) and not elimination of the dysrhythmia itself.

Of course, if treatment did abolish the dysrhythmia, this outcome would not be unwelcome. Acute treatment of supraventricular dysrhythmias is accomplished with vagotonic maneuvers, direct-current (DC) cardioversion, and certain drugs: class II agents, class IV agents, adenosine, and digoxin.

Atrial fibrillation. Atrial fibrillation is the most common sustained dysrhythmia, affecting about 4 million people in the United States. The disorder is caused by multiple atrial ectopic foci firing randomly; each focus stimulates a small area of atrial muscle. This chaotic excitation produces a highly irregular atrial rhythm. Depending on the extent of impulse transmission through the AV node, the ventricular rate may be very rapid or nearly normal.

In addition to compromising cardiac performance, atrial fibrillation carries a high risk for stroke because, in patients with atrial fibrillation, some blood can become trapped in the atria (rather than flowing straight through to the ventricles), thereby permitting formation of a clot. When normal sinus rhythm is restored, the clot may become dislodged and then may travel to the brain to cause stroke.

Treatment of atrial fibrillation has two goals: improvement of ventricular pumping and prevention of stroke. Pumping can be improved by either (1) restoring normal sinus rhythm or (2) slowing ventricular rate. The preferred method is to slow ventricular rate by *long-term* therapy with a β blocker (atenolol or metoprolol) or a cardioselective CCB (diltiazem or verapamil), both of which impede conduction through the AV node. For patients who elect to restore normal rhythm, options are DC cardioversion, short-term treatment with drugs (e.g., amiodarone, sotalol), or RF ablation of the dysrhythmia source.

To prevent stroke, patients are treated with warfarin or newer anticoagulants. For those undergoing treatment to restore normal sinus rhythm, warfarin should be taken for 3 weeks before the procedure and for 4 weeks after. For those taking an antidysrhythmic drug long term to control ventricular rate, warfarin or a direct oral anticoagulant must be taken long term too. Alternatives to warfarin include four direct oral anticoagulants—apixiban (Eliquis), dabigatran (Pradaxa), edoxaban (Savysa), and rivaroxaban (Xarelto)—and antiplatelet drugs (either aspirin alone or aspirin and clopidogrel).

Atrial flutter. Atrial flutter is caused by an ectopic atrial focus discharging at a rate of 250 to 350 times a minute. Ventricular rate is considerably slower, however, because the AV node is unable to transmit impulses at this high rate. Typically, one atrial impulse out of two reaches the ventricles. The treatment of choice is DC cardioversion, which almost always converts atrial flutter to normal sinus rhythm. Cardioversion may also be achieved with intravenous (IV) ibutilide. To prevent the dysrhythmia from recurring, patients may need long-term therapy with drugs—either a class IC agent (flecainide or propafenone) or a class III agent (amiodarone, dronedarone, sotalol, dofetilide).

There are two alternatives to cardioversion: (1) RF ablation of the dysrhythmic focus and (2) control of ventricular rate with drugs. As with atrial fibrillation, ventricular rate is controlled with drugs that suppress AV conduction: verapamil, diltiazem, or a β blocker.

Like atrial fibrillation, atrial flutter poses a risk for stroke, which can be reduced by treatment with anticoagulants.

Sustained supraventricular tachycardia (SVT). This is usually caused by an AV nodal reentrant circuit. Heart rate is increased to 150 to 250 beats per minute. SVT often responds to interventions that increase vagal tone, such as carotid sinus massage or the Valsalva maneuver. If these are ineffective, an intravenous β blocker or CCB can be tried. With these drugs, ventricular rate will be slowed even if the dysrhythmia persists. When the dysrhythmia has been controlled, β blockers and/or CCBs can be taken orally to prevent recurrence. As a last resort, amiodarone can be used for prevention.

Ventricular Dysrhythmias

In contrast to atrial dysrhythmias, which are generally benign, ventricular dysrhythmias can cause significant disruption of cardiac pumping. Accordingly, the usual objective is to abolish the dysrhythmia. Cardioversion is often the treatment of choice. When antidysrhythmic drugs are indicated, agents in class I or class III are usually employed.

Ventricular tachycardia. VT arises from a single, rapidly firing ventricular ectopic focus, typically located at the border of an old infarction. The focus drives the ventricles at a rate of 150 to 250 beats per minute. Because the ventricles cannot pump effectively at these rates, immediate intervention is required. Cardioversion is the treatment of choice. If cardioversion fails to normalize rhythm, intravenous amiodarone should be administered; lidocaine and procainamide are alternatives. For long-term management, drugs (e.g., sotalol, amiodarone) or an ICD may be employed.

Ventricular fibrillation. Ventricular fibrillation is a life-threatening emergency that requires immediate treatment. This dysrhythmia results from the asynchronous discharge of multiple ventricular ectopic foci. Because many different foci are firing, and each focus initiates contraction in its immediate vicinity, localized twitching takes place all over the ventricles, making coordinated ventricular contraction impossible. As a result, the pumping action of the heart stops. In the absence of blood flow, the patient becomes unconscious and cyanotic. If heartbeat is not restored rapidly, death soon follows. Electrical countershock (defibrillation) is applied to eliminate fibrillation and restore cardiac function. If necessary, intravenous lidocaine can be used to enhance the effects of defibrillation. Procainamide may also be helpful. Amiodarone can be used for long-term suppression. As an alternative, an ICD may be employed.

Premature ventricular complex (PVC). PVCs are beats that occur before they should in the cardiac cycle. These beats are caused by ectopic ventricular foci. PVCs may arise from a single ectopic focus or from several foci. In the absence of additional signs of heart disease, PVCs are benign and not usually treated. However, in the presence of acute myocardial infarction, PVCs may predispose the patient to ventricular fibrillation. In this case therapy is required. A β blocker is the agent of choice.

Digoxin-induced ventricular dysrhythmias. Digoxin toxicity can mimic practically all types of dysrhythmias. Varying degrees of AV block are among the most common. Ventricular flutter and ventricular fibrillation are the most dangerous. Digoxin causes dysrhythmias by increasing automaticity in the atria, ventricles, and His-Purkinje system and by decreasing conduction through the AV node.

With proper treatment, digoxin-induced dysrhythmias can almost always be controlled. Treatment is discussed in Chapter 42. If antidysrhythmic drugs are required, lidocaine and phenytoin are the agents of choice. In patients with digoxin toxicity, DC cardioversion may bring on ventricular fibrillation. Accordingly, this procedure should be used only when absolutely required.

Torsades de pointes. Torsades de pointes is an atypical, rapid, undulating ventricular tachydysrhythmia that can evolve into potentially fatal ventricular fibrillation. The main factor associated with the development of torsades de pointes is prolongation of the QT interval, which can be caused by a variety of drugs, including class IA and class III antidysrhythmic agents. Acute management consists of intravenous magnesium plus cardioversion for sustained VT.

Principles of Antidysrhythmic Drug Therapy
Balancing Risks and Benefits

Therapy with antidysrhythmic drugs is based on a simple but important concept: treat only if there is a clear benefit, and then only if the benefit outweighs the risks. As a rule, this means that intervention is needed only when the dysrhythmia interferes with ventricular pumping.

Treatment offers two potential benefits: reduction of symptoms and reduction of mortality. Symptoms that can be reduced include palpitations, angina, dyspnea, and faintness. For most antidysrhythmic drugs, there is little or no evidence of reduced mortality. In fact, mortality may actually increase.

Antidysrhythmic therapy carries considerable risk. Because of their *prodysrhythmic actions*, antidysrhythmic drugs can exacerbate existing dysrhythmias and generate new ones. Examples abound: toxic doses of digoxin can generate a wide variety of dysrhythmias; drugs that prolong the QT interval can cause torsades de pointes; many drugs can cause ventricular ectopic beats; several drugs (quinidine, flecainide, propafenone) can cause atrial flutter; and one drug—flecainide—can produce incessant VT. Because of their prodysrhythmic actions, antidysrhythmic drugs can *increase mortality*. Other adverse effects include HF and third-degree AV block (caused by CCBs and β blockers) as well as many noncardiac effects, including severe diarrhea (quinidine), a lupus-like syndrome (procainamide), and pulmonary toxicity (amiodarone).

Properties of the Dysrhythmia to Be Considered

Sustained versus nonsustained dysrhythmias. As a rule, nonsustained dysrhythmias require intervention only when they are symptomatic; in the absence of symptoms, treatment is usually unnecessary. In contrast, sustained dysrhythmias can be dangerous, so the benefits of treatment generally outweigh the risks.

Asymptomatic versus symptomatic dysrhythmias. No study has demonstrated a benefit to treating dysrhythmias that are asymptomatic or minimally symptomatic. In contrast, therapy may be beneficial for dysrhythmias that produce symptoms (palpitations, angina, dyspnea, faintness).

Supraventricular versus ventricular dysrhythmias. Supraventricular dysrhythmias are generally benign. The primary harm comes from driving the ventricles too rapidly to allow adequate filling. The goal of treatment is to either (1) terminate the dysrhythmia or (2) prevent excessive atrial beats from reaching the ventricles (using a β blocker, CCB, or digoxin). In contrast to supraventricular dysrhythmias, ventricular dysrhythmias frequently interfere with pumping. Accordingly, the goal of treatment is to terminate the dysrhythmia and prevent its recurrence.

Phases of Treatment

Treatment has two phases: acute and long term. The goal of acute treatment is to terminate the dysrhythmia. For many dysrhythmias, termination is accomplished with DC cardioversion (electrical countershock) or vagotonic maneuvers (e.g., carotid sinus massage) rather than drugs. The goal of long-term therapy is to prevent dysrhythmias from recurring. Quite often, the risks of using long-term prophylactic therapy outweigh the benefits.

Long-Term Treatment: Drug Selection and Evaluation

Selecting a drug for long-term therapy is largely empiric. There are many drugs that might be employed, and it is usually not possible to predict which one is going to work. Therefore finding an effective drug is done by trial and error.

Drug selection can be aided with electrophysiological testing. In these tests, a dysrhythmia is generated artificially by programmed electrical stimulation of the heart. If a candidate drug is able to suppress the electrophysiologically induced dysrhythmia, it may also work against the real thing.

Ambulatory ECG monitoring can be used to evaluate treatment. If monitoring indicates that dysrhythmias are still occurring with the present drug, a different drug should be tried.

Minimizing Risks

Several measures can help minimize risk, including the following:

- Starting with low doses and increasing them gradually.
- Using a Holter monitor during initial therapy to detect danger signs—especially QT prolongation, which can precede torsades de pointes.
- Monitoring plasma drug levels. Unfortunately, although drug levels can be good predictors of noncardiac toxicity (e.g., quinidine-induced nausea), they are less helpful for predicting adverse cardiac effects.

PHARMACOLOGY OF THE ANTIDYSRHYTHMIC DRUGS

As discussed earlier, the antidysrhythmic drugs fall into four main groups—classes I, II, III, and IV—plus a fifth group that includes adenosine and digoxin. The pharmacology of these drugs is presented next and in Table 43.2.

Class I: Sodium Channel Blockers

Class I antidysrhythmic drugs block cardiac sodium channels. By doing so, they decrease conduction velocity in the atria, ventricles, and His-Purkinje system.

There are three subgroups of class I agents. Drugs in all three groups block sodium channels. In addition, class IA agents delay repolarization, whereas class IB agents accelerate repolarization. Class IC agents have pronounced prodysrhythmic actions.

The class I drugs are similar in action and structure to the local anesthetics. In fact, one of these drugs—lidocaine—has both local anesthetic and antidysrhythmic applications. Because of their relationship to the local anesthetics, class I agents are sometimes referred to as *local anesthetic antidysrhythmic agents.*

Class IA Agents

Quinidine. Quinidine is the oldest, best-studied, and most widely used class IA drug. Accordingly, quinidine will serve as the prototype for the group. Similar to other antidysrhythmic agents, quinidine has prodysrhythmic actions.

PROTOTYPE DRUGS

Antidysrhythmic Drugs

Class I: Sodium Channel Blockers
Quinidine (class IA)
Lidocaine (class IB)

Class II: β Blocker
Propranolol

Class III: Drug That Delays Repolarization
Amiodarone

Class IV: Calcium Channel Blockers
Verapamil

Others
Digoxin

Chemistry and source. Quinidine is similar to quinine in structure and actions. The natural source of both drugs is the bark of the South American cinchona tree. Accordingly, these agents are referred to as cinchona alkaloids. Like quinine, quinidine has antimalarial and antipyretic properties.

Effects on the heart. By blocking sodium channels, quinidine *slows impulse conduction* in the atria, ventricles, and His-Purkinje system. In addition, the drug *delays repolarization* at these sites, apparently by blocking potassium channels. Both actions contribute to the suppression of dysrhythmias.

Quinidine is strongly *anticholinergic* (atropine-like) and blocks vagal input to the heart. The resultant *increase* in SA nodal automaticity and AV conduction can drive the ventricles at an excessive rate. To prevent excessive ventricular stimulation, patients are usually pretreated with digoxin, verapamil, or a β blocker, all of which suppress AV conduction.

Effects on the electrocardiogram. Quinidine has two pronounced effects on the ECG. The drug *widens the QRS complex* (by slowing depolarization of the ventricles) and *prolongs the QT interval* (by delaying ventricular repolarization).

Therapeutic uses. Quinidine is a broad-spectrum agent active against *supraventricular* and *ventricular dysrhythmias.* The drug's principal indication is long-term suppression of dysrhythmias, including SVT, atrial flutter, atrial fibrillation, and sustained VT. To prevent quinidine from increasing ventricular rate, patients are usually pretreated with an AV nodal blocking agent (digoxin, verapamil, β blocker).

▶▶ **BLACK BOX WARNING**

Quinidine

An analysis of older studies indicates that quinidine may actually *increase* mortality in patients with *atrial flutter* and *atrial fibrillation.*

Adverse effects

Cinchonism. Cinchonism is characterized by tinnitus (ringing in the ears), headache, nausea, vertigo, and disturbed vision. These can develop with just one dose.

Cardiotoxicity. At high concentrations, quinidine can cause severe cardiotoxicity (sinus arrest, AV block, ventricular tachydysrhythmias, asystole). These reactions occur secondary to increased automaticity of Purkinje fibers and reduced conduction throughout all regions of the heart.

As cardiotoxicity develops, the ECG changes. Important danger signals are *widening of the QRS complex* (by 50% or more) and *excessive prolongation of the QT interval.*

Drug interactions

Digoxin. Quinidine can double digoxin levels. The increase is caused by displacing digoxin from plasma albumin and by decreasing digoxin elimination. When these drugs are used concurrently, digoxin dosage must be reduced. Also, patients should be monitored closely for digoxin toxicity (dysrhythmias). Because of its interaction with digoxin, quinidine is a last-choice drug for treating digoxin-induced dysrhythmias.

Class IB Agents

As a group, class IB agents differ from quinidine and the other class IA agents in two respects: (1) whereas class IA agents *delay* repolarization, class IB agents *accelerate* repolarization; and (2) class IB agents have little or no effect on the ECG.

Mexiletine. Mexiletine is an oral analogue of lidocaine used for symptomatic ventricular dysrhythmias. Principal indications are PVCs and sustained VT. Like lidocaine, mexiletine does not alter the ECG. The drug is eliminated by hepatic metabolism, therefore effects may be prolonged in patients with liver disease or reduced hepatic blood flow. The most common adverse effects are GI (nausea, vomiting,

TABLE 43.2 Properties of Antidysrhythmic Drugs

Drug	Usual Route	Effects on the Heart	Effects on the ECG	Major Antidysrhythmic Applications	Adverse Effects
Class IA					
Quinidine	PO	Slows impulse conduction and delays repolarization in the atria, ventricles, and His-Purkinje system	Widens QRS, prolongs QT	Broad spectrum: used for long-term suppression of ventricular and supraventricular dysrhythmias	Diarrhea Cinconism Cardiotoxicity
Procainamide	PO		Widens QRS, prolongs QT	Broad spectrum: similar to quinidine, but toxicity makes it less desirable for long-term use	Systemic lupus erythematosus–like syndrome Cardiotoxicity
Disopyramide	PO		Widens QRS, prolongs QT	Ventricular dysrhythmias	Negative ionotropic effects— hypotension Anticholinergic symptoms
Class IB					
Phenytoin	PO	No significant change	No significant change	Digoxin-induced ventricular dysrhythmias	
Mexiletine	PO	Increases ration of refractory period to action potential duration	No significant change	Ventricular dysrhythmias	Blood dyscrasias Hepatotoxicity
Class IC					
Flecainide	PO	Decreases cardiac conduction and increases the effective refractory period	Widens QRS, prolongs PR	Maintenance therapy of supraventricular dysrhythmias	Decrease in myocardial contractility
Propafenone	PO	Decreases cardiac conduction in the atria, ventricles, and His-Purkinje system	Widens QRS, prolongs PR	Maintenance therapy of supraventricular dysrhythmias	Decreased myocardial contractility Nausea, vomiting, diarrhea
Class II					
Propranolol	PO	Decreased automaticity of the SA node Decreased velocity of conduction through the AV node	Prolongs PR, bradycardia	Dysrhythmias caused by excessive sympathetic activity; control of ventricular rate in patients with supraventricular tachydysrhythmias	Decreased myocardial contractility Potential to cause bronchospasm
Acebutolol	PO		Prolongs PR, bradycardia	Premature ventricular beats	
Class III					
Amiodarone	PO, IV	Delays repolarization Prolongs action potential duration	Prolongs QT and PR, widens QRS	Life-threatening ventricular dysrhythmias, atrial fibrillation[a]	Cardiotoxicity Thyrotoxicity Ophthalmic effects Dermatologic toxicity
Dronedarone	PO	Delays repolarization	Prolongs QT and PR, widens QRS	Atrial flutter, atrial fibrillation	Diarrhea, weakness, skin reactions Hepatotoxicity
Sotalol	PO, IV	Decreased AV nodal conduction Prolongation of atrial and ventricular action potentials	Prolongs QT and PR, bradycardia	Life-threatening ventricular dysrhythmias, atrial fibrillation/ flutter	Bradycardia, AV block, bronchospasm
Dofetilide	PO	Prolongs refractory period in His-Purkinje system and ventricles.	Prolongs QT	Highly symptomatic atrial dysrhythmias	Torsades de pointes
Class IV					
Verapamil	PO	Slows AV automaticity, Delays AV nodal conduction	Prolongs PR, bradycardia	Control of ventricular rate in patients with supraventricular tachydysrhythmias	Reduction of myocardial contractility Peripheral edema Bradycardia
Others					
Digoxin	PO, IV	Decreases conduction through the AV node Increases vagal impulses	Prolongs PR, depresses ST	Control of ventricular rate in patients with supraventricular tachydysrhythmias	Cardiotoxicity Nausea, vomiting Visual disturbances

[a]Amiodarone is widely used for atrial fibrillation but is not approved for this use.
AV, Atrioventricular; *ECG*, electrocardiogram; *IV*, intravenous; *PO*, per os (orally).

diarrhea, constipation) and neurologic (tremor, dizziness, sleep disturbances, psychosis, convulsions). About 40% of patients find these intolerable. Like other class I agents, mexiletine has prodysrhythmic properties. Mexiletine may also exacerbate heart failure.

 BLACK BOX WARNING

Mexiletine

> Mexiletine has been associated with increased risk for mortality when used to treat non–life-threatening arrhythmias.

Class IC Agents

Class IC antidysrhythmics block cardiac sodium channels and thereby reduce conduction velocity in the atria, ventricles, and His-Purkinje system. In addition, these drugs delay ventricular repolarization, causing a small increase in the ERP. All class IC agents can exacerbate existing dysrhythmias and create new ones. Currently, only two class IC agents are available: flecainide and propafenone (see Table 43.2).

Class II: β Blockers

Class II consists of β-adrenergic blocking agents. At this time only four β blockers—propranolol, acebutolol, esmolol, and sotalol—are approved for treating dysrhythmias. One of these drugs—sotalol—also blocks potassium channels and is discussed under class III. The basic pharmacology of the β blockers is presented in Chapter 16. Discussion here is limited to their antidysrhythmic use.

Propranolol

Propranolol (Inderal LA) is considered a nonselective β-adrenergic antagonist in that it blocks both β_1- and β_2-adrenergic receptors. β_1 blockade affects the heart and β_2 blockade affects the bronchi.

Effects on the heart and electrocardiogram. Blockade of cardiac β_1 receptors attenuates sympathetic stimulation of the heart. The result is (1) decreased automaticity of the SA node, (2) decreased velocity of conduction through the AV node, and (3) decreased myocardial contractility. The reduction in AV conduction velocity translates to a prolonged PR interval on the ECG.

It is worth noting that cardiac β_1 receptors are functionally coupled to calcium channels and that β_1 blockade causes these channels to close. Therefore the effects of β blockers on heart rate, AV conduction, and contractility all result from decreased calcium influx. Because β blockers and CCBs both decrease calcium entry, the cardiac effects of these drugs are very similar.

Therapeutic use. Propranolol is especially useful for treating dysrhythmias caused by excessive sympathetic stimulation of the heart. Among these are sinus tachycardia, severe recurrent VT, exercise-induced tachydysrhythmias, and paroxysmal atrial tachycardia evoked by emotion or exercise. In patients with supraventricular tachydysrhythmias, propranolol has two beneficial effects: (1) suppression of excessive discharge of the SA node and (2) slowing of ventricular rate by decreasing transmission of atrial impulses through the AV node.

Adverse effects. β blockers are generally well tolerated. Principal adverse effects concern the heart and bronchi. By blocking cardiac β_1 receptors, propranolol can cause *heart failure, AV block,* and *sinus arrest. Hypotension* can occur secondary to reduced cardiac output. In patients with asthma, blocking β_2 receptors in the lung can cause *bronchospasm.* Because of its cardiac and pulmonary effects, propranolol should be used cautiously in patients with asthma and is contraindicated in patients with sinus bradycardia, high-degree heart block, and HF.

Class III: Potassium Channel Blockers

Five class III antidysrhythmics are available: amiodarone, dronedarone, dofetilide, ibutilide, and sotalol (which is also a β blocker). All five delay repolarization of fast potentials. Hence all five prolong the action potential duration and ERP. By doing so, they prolong the QT interval. In addition, each drug can affect the heart in other ways; therefore they are not interchangeable. Four of the drugs are discussed further on. Ibutilide is available intravenously only and is therefore discussed in Chapter 92.

Amiodarone

Amiodarone (Cordarone, Pacerone) is a class III antidysrhythmic agent that has complex effects on the heart. The drug is highly effective against both atrial and ventricular dysrhythmias. Unfortunately, serious toxicities (e.g., lung damage, visual impairment) are common and may persist for months after treatment has stopped. Because of toxicity, amiodarone is *approved* only for life-threatening ventricular dysrhythmias that have been refractory to safer agents. Nonetheless, because of its efficacy, amiodarone is one of our most frequently prescribed antidysrhythmic drugs, used for atrial and ventricular dysrhythmias alike.

Amiodarone is available for oral and intravenous use. Indications, electrophysiologic effects, time course of action, and adverse effects differ for each route. Accordingly, oral and intravenous therapy are discussed separately.

Therapeutic Use

Although amiodarone is very effective, concerns about toxicity limit its indications. In the United States, oral amiodarone is *approved* only for long-term therapy of two life-threatening ventricular dysrhythmias: *recurrent ventricular fibrillation* and *recurrent hemodynamically unstable ventricular tachycardia.* Treatment should be reserved for patients who have not responded to safer drugs.

Amiodarone is our most effective drug for *atrial fibrillation* and is prescribed widely to treat this dysrhythmia—even though it is not approved for this use. The drug is given to convert atrial fibrillation to normal sinus rhythm and to maintain normal sinus rhythm after conversion.

Effects on the heart and electrocardiogram. Amiodarone has complex effects on the heart. Like all other drugs in this class, amiodarone delays repolarization and thereby prolongs the action potential duration and ERP. The underlying cause of these effects may be blockade of potassium channels. Additional cardiac effects include reduced automaticity in the SA node, reduced contractility, and reduced conduction velocity in the AV node, ventricles, and His-Purkinje system. These occur secondary to blockade of sodium channels, calcium channels, and β receptors. Prominent effects on the ECG are QRS widening and prolongation of the PR and QT intervals. Amiodarone also acts on coronary and peripheral blood vessels to promote dilation.

Pharmacokinetics. Amiodarone is highly lipid soluble and accumulates in many tissues, especially the liver and lungs. The drug is metabolized in the liver by CYP3A4 (the 3A4 isoenzyme of cytochrome P450) and then excreted in the bile. Amiodarone has an extremely long half-life, ranging from 25 to 110 days. Because of its slow elimination, amiodarone continues to act long after dosing has ceased.

Adverse effects. Amiodarone produces many serious adverse effects. Furthermore, because the drug's half-life is protracted, toxicity can continue for weeks or months after drug withdrawal. To reduce adverse events, the FDA requires that all patients using amiodarone be given a medication guide describing potential toxicities.

Amiodarone: Pulmonary Toxicity

Lung damage—hypersensitivity pneumonitis, interstitial/alveolar pneumonitis, pulmonary fibrosis—is the greatest concern. Symptoms (dyspnea, cough, chest pain) resemble those of heart failure and pneumonia. Pulmonary toxicity develops in 2% to 17% of patients and carries a 10% risk for mortality. Patients at highest risk are those receiving long-term, high-dose therapy. A baseline chest radiograph and pulmonary function test are recommended. Pulmonary function should be monitored throughout treatment. If lung injury develops, amiodarone should be withdrawn.

Thyroid toxicity. Amiodarone may cause hypothyroidism or hyperthyroidism. Accordingly, thyroid function should be assessed at baseline and periodically during treatment. Hypothyroidism can be treated with thyroid hormone supplements. Hyperthyroidism can be treated with an antithyroid drug (e.g., methimazole) or thyroidectomy. Discontinuation of amiodarone should be considered.

Amiodarone: Liver Toxicity

Amiodarone can injure the liver. Accordingly, tests of liver function should be obtained at baseline and periodically throughout treatment. If circulating liver enzymes exceed three times the normal level, amiodarone should be discontinued. Signs and symptoms of liver injury, which are seen only rarely, include anorexia, nausea, vomiting, malaise, fatigue, itching, jaundice, and dark urine.

Ophthalmic effects. Rarely, amiodarone has been associated with optic neuropathy and optic neuritis, sometimes progressing to blindness. However, a causal relationship has not been established. Patients who develop changes in visual acuity or peripheral vision should undergo ophthalmological evaluation. If optic neuropathy or neuritis is diagnosed, discontinuation of amiodarone should be considered.

Virtually all patients develop corneal microdeposits. Fortunately these deposits have little or no effect on vision and so rarely necessitate amiodarone cessation.

Dermatologic toxicity. Patients frequently experience *photosensitivity reactions* (skin reactions triggered by exposure to ultraviolet radiation). To reduce risk, patients should avoid sunlamps and should wear sunblock and protective clothing when outdoors. With frequent and prolonged sun exposure, exposed skin may turn *bluish gray*. Fortunately this discoloration resolves within months after amiodarone is discontinued.

Drug interactions. Amiodarone is subject to significant interactions with many drugs. The result can be toxicity or reduced therapeutic effects. Accordingly, combined use with these drugs should be avoided. When it cannot be, the patient should be monitored closely. Interactions of concern include the following:

- Amiodarone can *increase* levels of several drugs, including quinidine, procainamide, phenytoin, digoxin, diltiazem, warfarin, cyclosporine, and three statins: lovastatin, simvastatin, and atorvastatin. Dosages of these agents often require reduction.
- Amiodarone levels can be *increased* by grapefruit juice and by inhibitors of CYP3A4. Toxicity can result.
- Amiodarone levels can be *reduced* by cholestyramine (which decreases amiodarone absorption) and by agents that induce CYP3A4 (e.g., St. John's wort, rifampin).
- The risk for severe dysrhythmias is increased by diuretics (because they can reduce levels of potassium and magnesium) and by drugs that prolong the QT interval, of which there are many.

- Combining amiodarone with a β blocker, verapamil, or diltiazem can lead to excessive slowing of heart rate.

Class IV: Calcium Channel Blockers

Only two CCBs—*verapamil* (Calan, Covera-HS ♣,Verelan) and *diltiazem* (Cardizem, Dilacor-XR, Tiazac, others)—are able to block calcium channels in the heart. Accordingly, they are the only CCBs used to treat dysrhythmias. Their basic pharmacology is discussed in Chapter 39. Consideration here is limited to their use against dysrhythmias.

Effects on the Heart and the Electrocardiogram

Blockade of cardiac calcium channels has three effects:
- Slowing of SA nodal automaticity
- Delay of AV nodal conduction
- Reduction of myocardial contractility

Note that these are identical to the effects of β blockers, which makes sense in that β blockers promote calcium channel closure in the heart. The principal effect on the ECG is prolongation of the PR interval, reflecting delayed AV conduction.

Therapeutic Uses

Verapamil and diltiazem have two antidysrhythmic uses. First, they can slow ventricular rate in patients with atrial fibrillation or atrial flutter. Second, they can terminate SVT caused by an AV nodal reentrant circuit. In both cases, benefits derive from suppressing AV nodal conduction. With intravenous administration, effects can be seen in 2 to 3 minutes. Verapamil and diltiazem are not active against ventricular dysrhythmias.

Adverse Effects

Although generally safe, these drugs *can* cause undesired effects. Blockade of cardiac calcium channels can cause *bradycardia, AV block,* and *heart failure*. Blockade of calcium channels in vascular smooth muscle can cause vasodilation, resulting in *hypotension* and *peripheral edema*. Blockade of calcium channels in intestinal smooth muscle can produce *constipation*.

Drug Interactions

Both verapamil and diltiazem can elevate levels of *digoxin*, thereby increasing the risk for digoxin toxicity. Also, because digoxin shares with verapamil and diltiazem the ability to decrease AV conduction, combining digoxin with either drug increases the risk of AV block.

Because verapamil, diltiazem, and *β blockers* have nearly identical suppressant effects on the heart, combining verapamil or diltiazem with a β blocker increases the risk for bradycardia, AV block, and HF.

Other Antidysrhythmic Drugs
Digoxin

Although its primary indication is HF, digoxin (Lanoxin) is also used to treat supraventricular dysrhythmias. The basic pharmacology of digoxin is discussed in Chapter 42. Consideration here is limited to treatment of dysrhythmias.

Effects on the heart. Digoxin suppresses dysrhythmias by decreasing conduction through the AV node and automaticity in the SA node. The drug decreases AV conduction by (1) a direct depressant effect on the AV node and (2) acting in the CNS to increase vagal (parasympathetic) impulses to the AV node. Digoxin decreases automaticity of the SA node by increasing vagal traffic to the node and by decreasing sympathetic traffic. It should be noted that, although digoxin decreases automaticity in the SA node, it can increase automaticity in Purkinje fibers. The latter effect contributes to dysrhythmias caused by digoxin.

Effects on the electrocardiogram. By slowing AV conduction, digoxin prolongs the PR interval. The QT interval may be shortened, reflecting accelerated repolarization of the ventricles. Depression of the ST segment is common. The T wave may be depressed or even inverted. There is little or no change in the QRS complex.

Adverse effects and interactions. The major adverse effect is cardiotoxicity (dysrhythmias). Risk is increased by hypokalemia, which can result from concurrent therapy with diuretics (thiazides and loop diuretics). Accordingly, it is essential that potassium levels be kept within the normal range (3.5 to 5 mEq/L). The most common adverse effects are GI disturbances (anorexia, nausea, vomiting, abdominal discomfort). CNS responses (fatigue, visual disturbances) are also relatively common.

Antidysrhythmic uses. Digoxin is used only for supraventricular dysrhythmias. The drug is inactive against ventricular dysrhythmias.

44

Prophylaxis of Atherosclerotic Cardiovascular Disease: Drugs That Help Normalize Cholesterol and Triglyceride Levels

Our main topic for the chapter is drugs used to lower cholesterol. Drugs used to lower triglycerides (TGs) are considered as well. Cholesterol plays a role in atherosclerotic cardiovascular disease (ASCVD). ASCVD includes the vessels of the heart as well as the brain. Damage to these vessels can result in myocardial infarction (MI) or stroke. Moderate cardiac ASCVD usually manifests first as anginal pain. Severe cardiac ASCVD sets the stage for acute coronary syndrome (ACS) and MI. In the United States, cardiac ASCVD is the leading killer of men and women, causing 801,000 deaths in 2013. According to the American Heart Association (AHA), about 92 million Americans have a history of coronary events (angina, MI, or both). More than half of these people are women.

ASCVD begins as a fatty streak in the arterial wall. This is followed by deposition of fibrous plaque. As atherosclerotic plaque grows, it impedes coronary blood flow, causing anginal pain. Worse yet, atherosclerosis encourages formation of thrombi, which can block flow to the brain and heart entirely, thereby causing MI and stroke.

It is important to appreciate that atherosclerosis is not limited to arteries of the heart or brain: atherosclerotic plaque can develop in any artery and can thereby compromise circulation to any tissue. Furthermore, adverse effects can occur at sites distant from the original lesion: a ruptured lesion can produce a thrombus, which can travel downstream to block a new vessel.

The risk for developing ASCVD is directly related to increased levels of blood cholesterol, in the form of low-density lipoproteins (LDLs). By reducing levels of LDL cholesterol, we can slow progression of atherosclerosis, reduce the risk for serious ASCVD and its potential consequences, and prolong life. The preferred method for lowering LDL cholesterol is modification of diet combined with exercise. Drugs are employed only when diet modification and exercise are insufficient.

We approach our primary topic—cholesterol and its influence on ASCVD—in three stages. First, we discuss cholesterol itself, plasma lipoproteins (structures that transport cholesterol in blood), and the process of atherogenesis. Second, we discuss guidelines for cholesterol screening and management of high cholesterol. Third, we discuss the pharmacology of the cholesterol-lowering drugs, as well as drugs used to lower TGs.

CHOLESTEROL

Cholesterol has several physiologic roles. Of greatest importance, cholesterol is a component of all cell membranes and membranes of intracellular organelles. In addition, cholesterol is required for synthesis of certain hormones (e.g., estrogen, progesterone, testosterone) and for synthesis of bile salts, which are needed to absorb and digest dietary fats. Also, cholesterol is deposited in the stratum corneum of the skin, where it reduces evaporation of water and blocks transdermal absorption of water-soluble compounds.

Some of our cholesterol comes from dietary sources (exogenous cholesterol), and some is manufactured by cells (endogenous cholesterol), primarily in the liver. More cholesterol comes from endogenous production than from the diet. A critical step in hepatic cholesterol synthesis is catalyzed by an enzyme named *3-hydroxy-3-methylglutaryl coenzyme A reductase*, or simply *HMG-CoA reductase*. As discussed later, drugs that inhibit this enzyme—the statins—are our most effective and widely used cholesterol-lowering agents.

An increase in dietary cholesterol produces only a small increase in cholesterol in the blood, primarily because a rise in cholesterol intake inhibits endogenous cholesterol synthesis. Interestingly, an increase in dietary saturated fats produces a substantial (15% to 25%) increase in circulating cholesterol because the liver uses saturated fats to make cholesterol. Accordingly, when we want to reduce cholesterol levels, it is more important to reduce intake of saturated fats than to reduce intake of cholesterol itself, although cholesterol intake should definitely be lowered.

PLASMA LIPOPROTEINS

Structure and Function of Lipoproteins

Function

Lipoproteins serve as carriers for transporting lipids—cholesterol and TGs—in blood. Like all other nutrients and metabolites, lipids use the bloodstream to move throughout the body. However, being lipids, cholesterol and TGs are not water soluble and hence cannot dissolve directly in plasma. Lipoproteins provide a means of solubilizing these lipids, thereby permitting transport.

Basic Structure

The basic structure of lipoproteins is depicted in Fig. 44.1. As indicated, lipoproteins are tiny, spherical structures that consist of a *hydrophobic core*, composed of cholesterol and TGs, surrounded by a *hydrophilic shell*, composed primarily of phospholipids. Because the hydrophilic shell completely covers the lipid core, the entire structure is soluble in the aqueous environment of the plasma.

Apolipoproteins

All lipoproteins have one or more *apolipoprotein* molecules embedded in their shell (see Fig. 44.1). Apolipoproteins, which constitute the protein component of lipoproteins, have three functions:

- They serve as recognition sites for cell-surface receptors and thereby allow cells to bind with and ingest lipoproteins.
- They activate enzymes that metabolize lipoproteins.
- They increase the structural stability of lipoproteins.

Classes of Lipoproteins

There are six major classes of plasma lipoproteins. Distinctions among classes are based on size, density, apolipoprotein content, transport

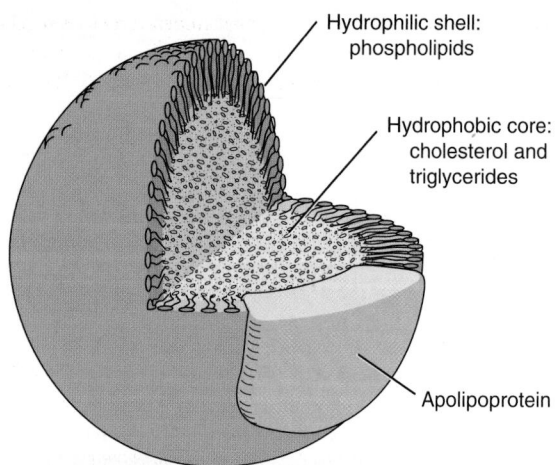

Hydrophilic shell:
phospholipids

Hydrophobic core:
cholesterol and
triglycerides

Apolipoprotein

Fig. 44.1 Basic Structure of Plasma Lipoproteins.

TABLE 44.1 **Properties of the Plasma Lipoproteins That Affect Atherosclerosis**			
Lipoprotein Class	**Major Core Lipids**	**Transport Function**	**Influence on Atherosclerosis**
VLDL	Triglycerides	Delivery of triglycerides to nonhepatic tissues	*Probably contribute* to atherosclerosis
LDL	Cholesterol	Delivery of cholesterol to nonhepatic tissues	*Definitely contribute* to atherosclerosis
HDL	Cholesterol	Transport of cholesterol from nonhepatic tissues back to the liver	*Protect* against atherosclerosis

Category	**Total Cholesterol (mg/dL)**	**LDL Cholesterol (mg/dL)**
Acceptable	<170	<110
Borderline	170–199	110–129
Elevated	≥200	≥130

HDL, High-density lipoprotein; *LDL,* low-density lipoprotein; *VLDL,* very-low-density lipoprotein.

function, and primary core lipids (cholesterol or TG). From a pharmacologic perspective, the features of greatest interest are *lipid content,* *apolipoprotein content,* and *transport function.*

Of the six major classes of lipoproteins, three are especially important in coronary atherosclerosis. These classes are named (1) very-low-density lipoproteins (VLDLs), (2) low-density lipoproteins (LDLs), and (3) high-density lipoproteins (HDLs). Properties of these classes are shown in Table 44.1.

Very-Low-Density Lipoproteins

VLDLs contain mainly *triglycerides* (and some cholesterol), and they account for nearly all of the TGs in blood. The main physiologic role of VLDLs is to *deliver triglycerides* from the liver to adipose tissue and muscle, which can use the TGs as fuel. Each VLDL particle contains one molecule of *apolipoprotein B-100,* which allows VLDLs to bind with cell-surface receptors and thereby transfer their lipid content to cells.

The role of VLDLs in atherosclerosis is unclear. Although several studies suggest a link between elevated levels of VLDLs and development

of atherosclerosis, this link has not been firmly established. However, we do know that elevation of TG levels (above 500 mg/dL) increases the risk for *pancreatitis.*

Low-Density Lipoproteins

LDLs contain *cholesterol* as their primary core lipid, and they account for the majority (60% to 70%) of all cholesterol in blood. The physiologic role of LDLs is *delivery of cholesterol to nonhepatic tissues.* LDLs can be viewed as byproducts of VLDL metabolism, in that the lipids and apolipoproteins that compose LDLs are remnants of VLDL degradation.

Cells that require cholesterol meet their needs through endocytosis (engulfment) of LDLs from the blood. The process begins with binding of LDL particles to LDL receptors on the cell surface. When cellular demand for cholesterol increases, cells synthesize more LDL receptors and thereby increase their capacity for LDL uptake. Accordingly, cells that are unable to make more LDL receptors cannot increase cholesterol absorption. Increasing the number of LDL receptors on cells is an important mechanism by which certain drugs increase LDL uptake and thereby reduce LDL levels in blood.

Of all lipoproteins, LDLs make the greatest contribution to coronary atherosclerosis. The probability of developing ASCVD is directly related to the level of LDLs in blood. Conversely, by reducing LDL levels, we decrease the risk for ASCVD. Accordingly, *when cholesterol-lowering drugs are used, the main goal is to reduce elevated LDL levels.* Multiple studies have shown that, by reducing LDL levels, we can arrest or perhaps even reverse atherosclerosis and can thereby reduce mortality from ASCVD. In fact, for each 1% reduction in the LDL level, there is about a 1% reduction in the risk for a major cardiovascular (CV) event.

High-Density Lipoproteins

Like LDLs, HDLs contain *cholesterol* as their primary core lipid, and they account for 20% to 30% of all cholesterol in the blood. In contrast to LDLs, whose function is delivery of cholesterol to peripheral tissues, HDLs carry cholesterol from peripheral tissues back to the liver. That is, *HDLs promote cholesterol removal.*

The influence of HDLs on ASCVD is dramatically different from that of LDLs. Whereas elevation of LDLs *increases* the risk for ASCVD, elevation of HDLs *reduces* the risk for ASCVD. That is, high HDL levels actively protect against ASCVD.

Low-Density Lipoprotein Versus High-Density Lipoprotein Cholesterol

The previous discussion shows that not all cholesterol in plasma has the same effect on ASCVD. As stated, a rise in cholesterol associated with LDLs increases the risk for ASCVD. In contrast, a rise in cholesterol associated with HDLs lowers the risk. Consequently, when speaking of plasma cholesterol levels, we need to distinguish between cholesterol that is associated with HDLs and cholesterol that is associated with LDLs. To make this distinction, we use the terms *HDL cholesterol* and *LDL cholesterol.* Because LDL cholesterol promotes atherosclerosis, it has been dubbed *bad cholesterol.* Conversely, because HDL seems to protect against atherosclerosis, it is often called *good cholesterol* or *healthy cholesterol.*

ROLE OF LOW-DENSITY LIPOPROTEIN CHOLESTEROL IN ATHEROSCLEROSIS

LDLs initiate and fuel development of atherosclerosis. The process begins with transport of LDLs from the arterial lumen into endothelial cells that line the lumens of blood vessels. From there, they move into the space that underlies the arterial epithelium. When in the subendothelial space, components of LDLs undergo *oxidation*. This step is critical in that oxidized LDLs do the following:

- Attract monocytes from the circulation into the subendothelial space, after which the monocytes are converted to macrophages (which are critical to atherogenesis)
- Inhibit macrophage mobility, thereby keeping macrophages at the site of atherogenesis
- Undergo uptake by macrophages (macrophages do not take up LDLs that have not been oxidized)
- Damage the vascular endothelium, as they are cytotoxic

As macrophages engulf more and more cholesterol, they become large and develop large vacuoles. When macrophages assume this form, they are referred to as *foam cells*. Foam cell accumulation beneath the arterial epithelium produces a *fatty streak*, which makes the surface of the arterial wall lumpy, causing blood flow to become turbulent. Continued accumulation of foam cells can eventually cause rupture of the endothelium, thereby exposing the underlying tissue to the blood. This results in platelet adhesion and formation of microthrombi. As the process continues, smooth muscle cells migrate to the site, synthesis of collagen increases, and there can be repeated rupturing and healing of the endothelium. The end result is a mature atherosclerotic lesion, characterized by a large lipid core and a tough *fibrous cap*. In less mature lesions, the fibrous cap is not strong, and hence the lesions are unstable and more likely to rupture. As a result, arterial pressure and shear forces (from turbulent blood flow) can cause the cap to rupture. Accumulation of platelets at the site of rupture can rapidly cause thrombosis and can thereby cause infarction. Infarction is less likely at sites of mature atherosclerotic lesions. The atherosclerotic process is depicted in Fig. 44.2.

It is important to appreciate that atherogenesis involves more than just deposition of lipids. In fact, atherogenesis is now considered primarily a chronic *inflammatory process*. When LDLs penetrate the arterial wall, they cause mild injury. The injury, in turn, triggers an inflammatory response that includes infiltration of macrophages, T lymphocytes, and other potentially noxious chemicals (e.g., C-reactive protein [CRP]). In the late stage of the disease process, inflammation can weaken atherosclerotic plaque, leading to plaque rupture and subsequent thrombosis.

2018 AMERICAN COLLEGE OF CARDIOLOGY/ AMERICAN HEART ASSOCIATION GUIDELINE ON THE MANAGEMENT OF BLOOD CHOLESTEROL

It is well established that high levels of cholesterol (primarily LDL cholesterol) cause substantial morbidity and mortality and that aggressive treatment can save lives. Accordingly, periodic cholesterol screening and risk assessment are recommended. If the assessment indicates ASCVD risk, lifestyle changes—especially diet and exercise—should be implemented. If ASCVD risk is high, LDL-lowering drugs should be added to the regimen.

In 1988, the National Cholesterol Education Program (NCEP) began issuing guidelines on cholesterol detection and management. The update of that original document was issued in 2001 and amended in 2004, and new guidelines were developed in 2013 in partnership with the American College of Cardiology (ACC) and the AHA. A summary of the most recent 2018 guidelines—*2018 AHA/ACC/ AACVPR/AAPA/ABC/ACPM/ADA/AGS/APhA/ASPC/NLA/PCNA Guideline on the Management of Blood Cholesterol*—was published in the *Journal of the American College of Cardiology* and is available at http://www.onlinejacc.org/content/73/24/3168.

Like earlier NCEP guidelines, the 2018 ACC/AHA cholesterol guideline focuses on the role of high cholesterol in ASCVD and stresses the

importance of treatment. However, the new guideline focuses specifically on identifying patients who are most likely to benefit from cholesterol-lowering therapy through calculation of ASCVD risk.

PATIENT-CENTERED CARE ACROSS THE LIFE SPAN

Treating Dyslipidemia

Life Stage	Patient Care Concerns
Children/adolescents	Lovastatin, simvastatin, pravastatin, and atorvastatin are approved for use in children. It is recommended to avoid statin use in children younger than 10 years.
Pregnant women	Statins are contraindicated in pregnancy. Ezetimibe and fibrates can be used in pregnancy, but benefit should outweigh risk.
Breastfeeding women	Effects of statins, ezetimibe, and fibrates have not been studied in breastfeeding. Given the possibility of harm, benefit should outweigh risk.
Older adults	In patients 65 years and older, statins, compared with placebo, significantly reduced the risk for myocardial infarction as well as the risk for stroke by 23.8%. However, the cost-benefit evaluation of treatment in older-adult people should be considered.

Atherosclerotic Cardiovascular Disease Risk Assessment

Under the 2018 ACC/AHA guidelines, ASCVD risk assessment is directed at determining the patient's *absolute risk for developing clinical coronary disease over the next 10 years*. The mode of intervention is then determined by the individual's degree of risk.

Factors in Risk Assessment

To assess the ASCVD risk for an individual, we need three kinds of information. Specifically, we need to (1) identify ASCVD risk factors, (2) calculate 10-year ASCVD risk, and (3) identify ASCVD risk equivalents.

Identifying atherosclerotic cardiovascular disease risk factors. Major risk factors that modify LDL treatment goals include positive risk factors (advancing age, black race, hypertension, cigarette smoking, and low HDL cholesterol) and one negative risk factor (high HDL cholesterol). (LDL itself is not listed because the reason for counting these risk factors is to modify treatment of high LDL.)

We know that diabetes is a very strong predictor of developing ASCVD. Accordingly, we no longer consider diabetes to be a risk *factor*. Instead, for the purpose of risk assessment, diabetes is now considered an ASCVD risk *equivalent*—that is, having diabetes is considered equivalent to having ASCVD as a predictor of a major coronary event.

Calculating 10-year atherosclerotic cardiovascular disease risk. The 2018 ACC/AHA cholesterol guideline defines high ASCVD risk as 20% or greater. Patients with existing clinical ASCVD are placed in a "very-high risk" category, despite their screening percentage. For all other people, 10-year risk must be calculated. The instrument employed most often is the Framingham Risk Prediction Score, which takes five factors into account: age, total cholesterol, HDL cholesterol, smoking status, and systolic blood pressure. These are similar to risk factors noted earlier.

**Damaged endothelium:
Chronic endothelial injury**

- Hypertension
- Smoking
- Hyperlipidemia
- Hyperhomocystinemia
- Hemodynamic factors
- Toxins
- Viruses
- Immune reactions

Endothelium
Tunica intima
Tunica media
Adventitia

A

Response to injury

Monocyte
Damaged endothelium
Platelets
Macrophage
Lipids

Fatty streak

B

Platelets attach to endothelium
Foamy macrophage ingesting lipids
Migration of smooth muscle into the intima
Lipid accumulation
Fibroblast

Fibrous plaque

C

Collagen cap (fibrous tissue)
Fibroblast
Fissure in plaque
Lipid pool

Complicated lesion

D

Thrombus
Thinning collagen cap
Lipid pool

Fig. 44.2 Progression of Atherosclerosis. (A) Damaged endothelium. (B) Diagram of fatty streak and lipid core formation. (C) Diagram of fibrous plaque. Raised plaques are visible: some are yellow and some are white. (D) Diagram of a complicated lesion, showing a thrombus (in red) and collagen (in blue). (From McCance KL, Huether SE. *Pathophysiology: The Biologic Basis for Disease in Adults and Children.* 7th ed. St. Louis: Elsevier; 2014.)

Framingham scores can be determined using either (1) the tables for men and women shown in Fig. 44.3 or (2) a web-based risk calculator, such as the one provided by the ACC/AHA at http://www.cvriskcalculator.com/.

Identifying an Individual's Atherosclerotic Cardiovascular Disease Risk Category

Under the 2018 ACC/AHA cholesterol guideline, there are four categories of patients who would benefit from statin treatment of cholesterol (Box 44.1). Category assignment is based on (1) the presence or absence of ASCVD (or an ASCVD risk equivalent, such as diabetes), (2) the number of risk factors the individual has (other than high LDL cholesterol), and (3) the individual's 10-year ASCVD score. An example of a risk calculator is found in Fig. 44.3.

Treatment of High Low-Density Lipoprotein Cholesterol

Treatment of high LDL cholesterol is based on the individual's ASCVD risk category or the presence of other comorbidities such as diabetes. Treatment may be started with a high-intensity statin or a moderate-intensity statin depending on the patient's risk factors (Table 44.2; see Fig. 44.4). To reduce LDL levels, the 2018 ACC/AHA guideline recommends two forms of intervention: (1) therapeutic lifestyle changes (TLCs) and (2) drug therapy. For some people, cholesterol can be reduced adequately with TLCs alone. Others require TLCs *plus* cholesterol-lowering drugs. Please note that drugs should be used only as an *adjunct* to TLCs—not as a *substitute*.

BOX 44.1 Statin Benefit Groups as Defined by the 2018 American College of Cardiology / American Heart Association Blood Cholesterol Guidelines

Individuals with clinical ASCVD

Individuals with primary elevations of LDL cholesterol ≥190 mg/dL

Individuals 40–75 years of age with diabetes and LDL cholesterol 70–189 mg/dL

Individuals without clinical ASCVD or diabetes who are 40–75 years of age with LDL cholesterol 70–189 mg/dL and an estimated 10-year ASCVD risk of 7.5% or higher

ASCVD, Atherosclerotic cardiovascular disease; *LDL,* low-density lipoprotein.
From the 2018 ACC/AHA Guideline on the Treatment of Blood Cholesterol available at http://www.onlinejacc.org/content/73/24/3168.

TABLE 44.2 High-, Moderate-, and Low-Intensity Statin Therapy

High-Intensity Therapy	Moderate-Intensity Therapy	Low-Intensity Therapy
Daily dose lowers LDL-C on average by ≥50%	Daily dose lowers LDL-C on average by ~30% to <50%	Daily dose lowers LDL-C on average by <30%
Atorvastatin: 40–80 mg	Atorvastatin: 10 mg	Simvastatin: 10 mg
Rosuvastatin: 20 mg	Rosuvastatin: 10 mg	Pravastatin: 10–20 mg
	Simvastatin: 20–40 mg	Lovastatin: 20 mg
	Pravastatin: 40 mg	
	Lovastatin: 40 mg	

LDL-C, Low-density lipoprotein cholesterol.
Adapted from 2018 ACC/AHA Guideline on the Treatment of Blood Cholesterol http://www.onlinejacc.org/content/73/24/3168.

Therapeutic Lifestyle Changes

Therapeutic lifestyle changes are nondrug measures used to lower LDL cholesterol. TLCs focus on four main issues: diet, exercise, weight control, and smoking cessation. These measures are first-line treatment for LDL reduction and should be implemented before drug therapy. However, TLCs can be a challenge because some people do not eat healthier diets or exercise. Physical conditions such as arthritis can limit attempts at exercise, and economic and time limitations can be a barrier to healthier eating.

Drug Therapy

Drugs are not the first-line therapy for lowering LDL cholesterol. Rather, drugs should be employed only if TLCs fail to reduce LDL cholesterol to an acceptable level—and then only if the combination of elevated LDL cholesterol and the patient's ASCVD risk category justify drug use. When drugs are used, it is essential that lifestyle modification continues because the beneficial effects of diet and drugs are additive; drugs alone may be unable to achieve the LDL goal. It is important to note that the principal benefit of drug therapy is *primary prevention:* Drugs are much better at preventing or slowing ASCVD than at promoting regression of established coronary atherosclerosis. Furthermore, because LDL cholesterol levels will return to pretreatment values if drugs are withdrawn, *treatment must continue lifelong.* Patients should be made aware of this requirement.

The most effective agents are the *HMG-CoA reductase inhibitors* (e.g., atorvastatin [Lipitor]), usually referred to simply as *statins.* A newer class of immunologics called *monoclonal antibodies* can also be used to treat high cholesterol. Lesser used alternatives are *bile acid sequestrants* (e.g., cholestyramine) and *niacin* (nicotinic acid). Treatment is initiated with a single drug, almost always a statin. If the statin is ineffective, a bile acid sequestrant can be added to the regimen.

In addition to lowering LDL cholesterol, drugs may be used to raise HDL cholesterol. The most effective agents are the fibrates. However, virtually all of the drugs that we use to lower LDL cholesterol have the added benefit of increasing HDL cholesterol, at least to some degree. This rise of HDL therefore can be considered a beneficial "side effect."

Secondary Treatment Targets
Metabolic Syndrome

The term *metabolic syndrome (also known as syndrome X)* refers to a group of metabolic abnormalities associated with an increased risk for ASCVD and type 2 diabetes. The metabolic abnormalities involved are high blood glucose, high TGs, high apolipoprotein B, low HDL, small LDL particles, a prothrombotic state, and a proinflammatory state. Hypertension is both common and important.

According to a joint scientific statement—issued by the International Diabetes Federation Task Force on Epidemiology and Prevention; the National Heart, Lung, and Blood Institute; the AHA; the World Heart Federation; the International Atherosclerosis Society; and the International Association for the Study of Obesity—the metabolic syndrome is diagnosed when three or more of the following are present:

- *High TG levels*—150 mg/dL or higher (or undergoing drug therapy for high TGs)
- *Low HDL cholesterol*—below 40 mg/dL for men or below 50 mg/dL for women (or undergoing drug therapy for reduced HDL)
- *Hyperglycemia*—fasting blood glucose 100 mg/dL or higher (or undergoing drug therapy for hyperglycemia/diabetes mellitus)
- *High blood pressure*—systolic 130 mm Hg or higher and/or diastolic 85 mm Hg or higher (or undergoing drug therapy for hypertension)
- *Waist circumference 40 inches or more for most men or 35 inches or more for most women.* (These limits can vary depending on ethnicity, country, or geographic region within a country.)

Estimate of 10-year risk for MEN

Age	Points
20–34	−9
35–39	−4
40–44	0
45–49	3
50–54	6
55–59	8
60–64	10
65–69	11
70–74	12
75–79	13

Total Cholesterol	Points Age 20–39	Age 40–49	Age 50–59	Age 60–69	Age 70–79
<160	0	0	0	0	0
160–199	4	3	2	1	0
200–239	7	5	3	1	0
240–279	9	6	4	2	1
≥280	11	8	5	3	1

	Points Age 20–39	Age 40–49	Age 50–59	Age 60–69	Age 70–79
Nonsmoker	0	0	0	0	0
Smoker	8	5	3	1	1

HDL (mg/dL)	Points
≥60	−1
50–59	0
40–49	1
<40	2

Systolic BP (mm Hg)	If Untreated	If Treated
<120	0	0
120–129	0	1
130–139	1	2
140–159	1	2
≥160	2	3

Point Total	10-Year Risk %
<0	<1
0	1
1	1
2	1
3	1
4	1
5	2
6	2
7	3
8	4
9	5
10	6
11	8
12	10
13	12
14	16
15	20
16	25
≥17	≥30

10-Year Risk _____%

Estimate of 10-year risk for WOMEN

Age	Points
20–34	−7
35–39	−3
40–44	0
45–49	3
50–54	6
55–59	8
60–64	10
65–69	12
70–74	14
75–79	16

Total Cholesterol	Points Age 20–39	Age 40–49	Age 50–59	Age 60–69	Age 70–79
<160	0	0	0	0	0
160–199	4	3	2	1	1
200–239	8	6	4	2	1
240–279	11	8	5	3	2
≥280	13	10	7	4	2

	Points Age 20–39	Age 40–49	Age 50–59	Age 60–69	Age 70–79
Nonsmoker	0	0	0	0	0
Smoker	9	7	4	2	1

HDL (mg/dL)	Points
≥60	−1
50–59	0
40–49	1
<40	2

Systolic BP (mm Hg)	If Untreated	If Treated
<120	0	0
120–129	1	3
130–139	2	4
140–159	3	5
≥160	4	6

Point Total	10-Year Risk %
<9	<1
9	1
10	1
11	1
12	1
13	2
14	2
15	3
16	4
17	5
18	6
19	8
20	11
21	14
22	17
23	22
24	27
≥25	≥30

10-Year Risk _____%

Fig. 44.3 Tables for Calculating Framingham Risk Prediction Scores. To determine an individual's 10-year risk for developing clinical coronary disease, simply circle the appropriate points for each of the five risk factors considered (age, total cholesterol, smoking status, high-density lipoproteins [HDL] cholesterol, and systolic blood pressure) and then add up the points. The point total indicates the 10-year risk. For example, a total of 13 points indicates a 10-year risk of 12% for men. *BP,* Blood pressure.

CENTRAL ILLUSTRATION: 2018 AHA/ACC/AACVPR/AAPA/ABC/ACPM/ADA/AGS/APhA/
ASPC/NLA/PCNA Guideline on the management of blood cholesterol

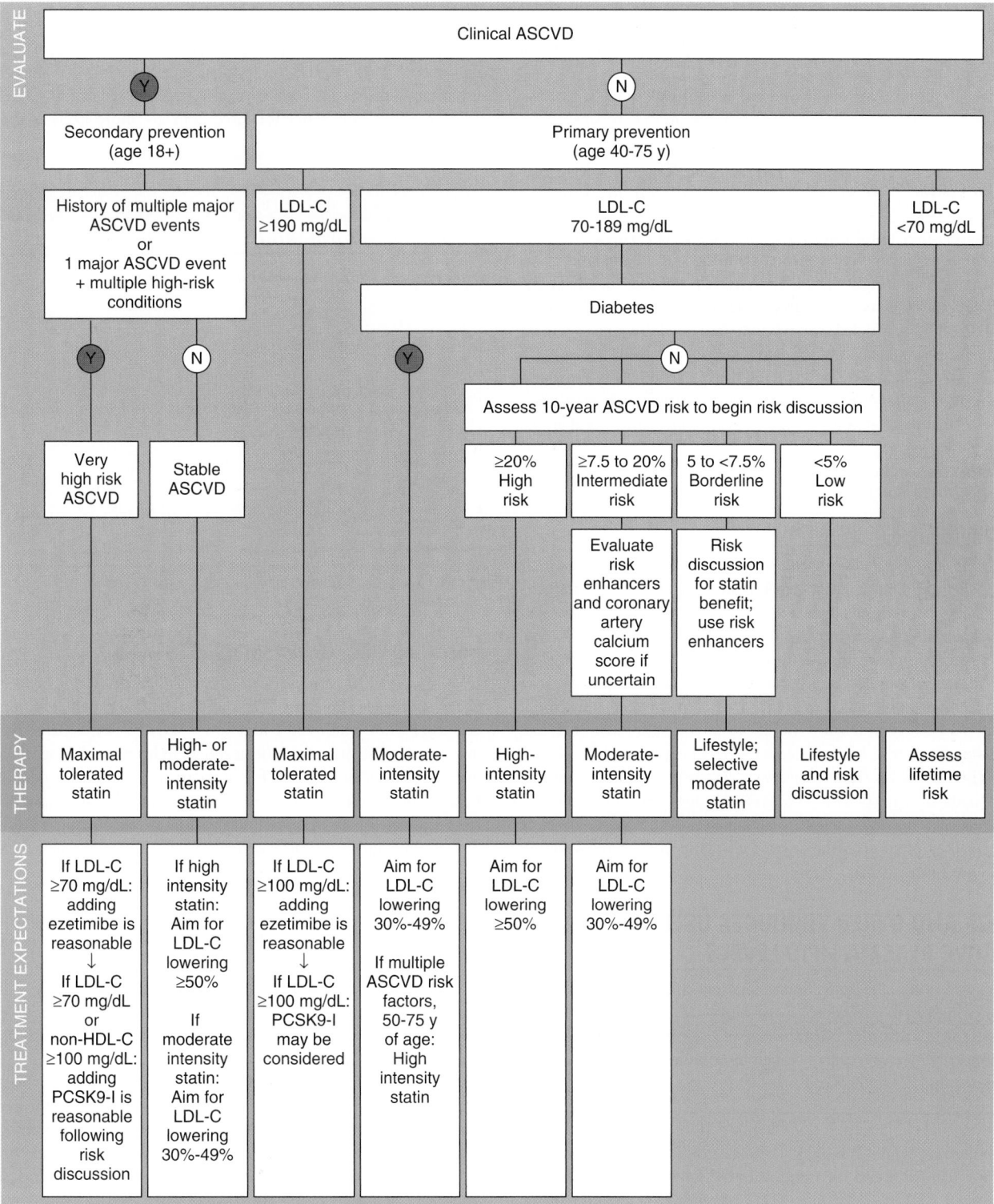

Grundy, S.M., et al. *J* Am Coll Cardiol. 10.1016/j.jacc.2018.11.003.

Fig. 44.4 Recommendations for statin therapy for atherosclerotic cardiovascular disease prevention. *ASCVD*, Atherosclerotic cardiovascular disease; *LDL-C*, low-density lipoprotein cholesterol. (From Gundy SM, et al. AHA/ACC/AACVPR/AAPA/ABC/ACPM/ADA/AGS/APhA/ASPC/NLA/PCNA guideline on the management of blood cholesterol. *J Am Coll Cardiol.* doi: 10.1016/j.jacc.2018.11.003.)

Treatment has two primary goals: reducing the risk for atherosclerotic disease and reducing the risk for type 2 diabetes. According to ATP III, basic therapy consists of weight control and increased physical activity, which, together, can reduce all symptoms of the metabolic syndrome. In addition, specific treatment should be directed at lowering blood pressure and TG levels. Patients should take low-dose aspirin to reduce the risk for thrombosis, unless they are at high risk for intracranial bleeds (hemorrhagic stroke).

Although the term *metabolic syndrome* is widely used, there is debate about its clinical relevance. In the CV community, most clinicians believe the term has great utility. By contrast, in the diabetes community, many clinicians feel the term is misleading, in that it implies the existence of a specific disease entity, even though it is defined only by a cluster of risk factors that may or may not have a common underlying cause. Furthermore, they point out that the risk associated with a diagnosis of metabolic syndrome is no greater than the sum of the risks of its components. Accordingly, until there is more proof that the metabolic syndrome actually exists, they believe the term serves no clinical purpose and hence should be avoided. This position was voiced in a joint statement from the American Diabetes Association and the European Association for the Study of Diabetes. The AHA and the National Heart, Lung, and Blood Institute countered with a joint statement of their own, reasserting their belief that the metabolic syndrome is an important clinical entity. Although the two camps disagree about whether the metabolic syndrome is an actual disease, both sides strongly agree that the risk factors that define the syndrome should be identified and treated.

High Triglycerides

High TG levels (above 200 mg/dL) may be an independent risk factor for ASCVD. In clinical practice, high TGs are seen most often in patients with metabolic syndrome. However, high levels may also be associated with inactive lifestyle, cigarette smoking, excessive alcohol intake, type 2 diabetes, certain genetic disorders, and high carbohydrate intake (when carbohydrates account for more than 60% of total caloric intake). In most patients with high TG levels, the first treatment goal is to achieve the original LDL goal. Dietary modification is always recommended. Statins being taken to lower cholesterol may help lower TGs as well, perhaps to a satisfactory level. However, if TG levels remain unacceptably high, medications specific to TGs—fibrates—may be needed. Unfortunately, when these drugs are combined with cholesterol-lowering drugs (as they often are), the adverse effects of cholesterol-lowering agents may be intensified.

DRUGS AND OTHER PRODUCTS USED TO IMPROVE PLASMA LIPID LEVELS

As discussed earlier, the lipid abnormality that contributes most to CV disease is high LDL cholesterol. Accordingly, we will focus primarily on drugs for this disorder. Nonetheless, we also need to consider other lipid abnormalities, especially (1) high total cholesterol,[a] (2) low HDL cholesterol, and (3) high TGs.

---

[a]Note that total cholesterol is slightly different from the simple sum of LDL cholesterol (LDL-C) plus HDL cholesterol (HDL-C); triglycerides (TGs) also contribute to the value, as in the following equation: total cholesterol = HDL-C + LDL-C + (TG/5) (provided TG levels are below 400 mg/dL). As we consider the drugs for lipid disorders, you should be aware of the following: although all of these drugs can improve lipid profiles, not all of them improve clinical outcomes (reduced morbidity and mortality). This leads us to question whether some of the lipid abnormalities are a true cause of pathophysiology and ultimate death, or whether they are simply "associated markers" of some other pathophysiology that we don't yet understand.

Some drugs for dyslipidemias are more selective than others. That is, whereas some drugs may improve just one dyslipidemia (e.g., high TGs), others may improve two or more dyslipidemias. The highly selective agents can be useful as add-ons, to "target" a particular lipid abnormality when other medications prove inadequate.

Drugs that lower *LDL cholesterol* levels include HMG-CoA reductase inhibitors (statins), bile acid sequestrants, monoclonal antibodies, and ezetimibe. All are effective to varying degrees. The HMG-CoA reductase inhibitors—the statins—are more effective than the others, cause fewer adverse effects, are better tolerated, and are more likely to improve clinical outcomes.

PROTOTYPE DRUGS

LDL Cholesterol- and Triglyceride-Lowering Drugs

HMG-CoA Reductase Inhibitor (Statin)
Lovastatin

Bile Acid Sequestrant
Colesevelam

Monoclonal Antibodies (Proprotein Convertase Subtilisin/ Kexin Type 9 [PCSK9] Inhibitors)
Alirocumab
Evolocumab

Others
Ezetimibe

PCSK9, Proprotein convertase subtilisin kexin type 9.

HMG-CoA Reductase Inhibitors (Statins)

HMG-CoA reductase inhibitors, commonly called *statins,* are the most effective drugs for lowering LDL and total cholesterol. In addition, they can raise HDL cholesterol and lower TGs in some patients. Most important, these drugs have been shown to improve clinical outcomes, including lowering the risk for heart failure, MI, and sudden death. Because of these benefits, and because so many people have ASCVD risks associated with dyslipidemias, statins are among our most widely prescribed drugs—and have earned 10s of billions for their makers.

Beneficial Actions

The statins have several actions that can benefit patients with (or at risk for) atherosclerosis. The most obvious and important are reductions of LDL cholesterol.

Reduction of low-density lipoproteins cholesterol. Statins have a profound effect on LDL cholesterol. Low doses decrease LDL cholesterol by about 25%, and larger doses decrease levels by as much as 63% (Table 44.3). Reductions are significant within 2 weeks and maximum within 4 to 6 weeks. Because cholesterol synthesis normally increases during the night, statins are most effective when given in the evening. If statin therapy is stopped, serum cholesterol will return to pretreatment levels within weeks to months. Therefore treatment should continue lifelong, unless serious adverse effects or specific contraindications (especially pregnancy or muscle damage) arise. The mechanism by which statins reduce cholesterol levels is discussed later.

Elevation of high-density lipoproteins cholesterol. Statins can increase levels of HDL cholesterol. Recall that low levels of HDL cholesterol (below 40 mg/dL) are an independent risk factor for ASCVD. Hence by raising HDL cholesterol, statins may help reduce the risk for CV events in yet another way. The objective is to raise levels to 50 mg/dL or more.

	% Change in Serum Lipids[a]			Effect of CYP3A4 Inhibitors on Statin Levels[b]	Effect of Renal or Hepatic Impairment on Statin Levels
Drug	**LDL-C**	**HDL-C**	**TGs**		
Atorvastatin (Lipitor)	↓ 25–60	↑ 5–15	↓ 15–50	Moderate ↑	No change with renal disease; significant ↑ with hepatic impairment
Fluvastatin (Lescol, Lescol XL)	↓ 20–40	↑ 2–11	↓ 10–25	None	No change with renal disease; possible ↑ with hepatic impairment
Lovastatin (Altoprev, Mevacor)	↓ 20–40	↑ 5–10	↓ 5–25	Significant ↑	↑ With significant renal impairment; no change with hepatic impairment
Pitavastatin (Livalo)	↓ 40–45	↑ 6–8	↓ 15–30	Little or none	↑ With significant renal impairment; little or no change with hepatic impairment
Pravastatin (Pravachol)	↓ 20–40	↑ 1–15	↓ 10–25	None	Potential ↑ with either renal or hepatic impairment
Rosuvastatin (Crestor)	↓ 30–60	↑ 3–20	↓ 10–40	None	↑ Levels with severe renal impairment or hepatic dysfunction
Simvastatin (Zocor)	↓ 25–50	↑ 7–15	↓ 8–40	Significant ↑	Potential ↑ with severe renal or hepatic impairment

TABLE 44.3 HMG-CoA Reductase Inhibitors: Selected Aspects of Clinical Pharmacology

[a]The values were obtained from a variety of studies, and do not reflect dose dependency of drug responses.
[b]Inhibitors of CYP3A4 (the 3A4 isoenzyme of P450) include itraconazole, ketoconazole, erythromycin, clarithromycin, HIV protease inhibitors, cyclosporine, nefazodone, and substances in grapefruit juice.
↑, Increase; ↓, decrease; *HDL-C*, high-density lipoprotein cholesterol; *LDL-C*, low-density lipoprotein cholesterol; *TGs*, triglycerides.

Reduction of triglyceride levels. Although statins mainly affect cholesterol synthesis and thereby lower LDL cholesterol levels, these drugs may also lower TGs. Just why these "anticholesterol" drugs lower TGs is unknown, but the response has been amply documented. Please note that, although statins may reduce TG levels, they are not actually prescribed for this action. Hence TG reduction is usually a beneficial side effect in patients taking statins to lower their LDL cholesterol. Of note, the ability to lower TGs seems to be short lived, and hence a drug designed to lower TGs eventually may need to be added.

Nonlipid beneficial cardiovascular actions. There is increasing evidence that statins do more than just alter lipid levels. Specifically, they can promote atherosclerotic plaque stability (by decreasing plaque cholesterol content), reduce inflammation at the plaque site, slow progression of coronary artery calcification, improve abnormal endothelial function, enhance the ability of blood vessels to dilate, reduce the risk for atrial fibrillation, and reduce the risk for thrombosis by (1) inhibiting platelet deposition and aggregation and (2) suppressing production of thrombin, a key factor in clot formation. All of these actions help reduce the risk for CV events.

Mechanism of Cholesterol Reduction

The mechanism by which statins decrease LDL cholesterol levels is complex and depends ultimately on *increasing the number of LDL receptors on hepatocytes*. The process begins with inhibition of hepatic HMG-CoA reductase, the rate-limiting enzyme in cholesterol biosynthesis. In response to decreased cholesterol production, hepatocytes synthesize more HMG-CoA reductase. As a result, cholesterol synthesis is largely restored to pretreatment levels. However—and for reasons that are not fully understood—inhibition of cholesterol synthesis causes hepatocytes to synthesize more LDL receptors. As a result, hepatocytes are better able to remove more LDLs from the blood. In patients who are genetically unable to synthesize LDL receptors, statins fail to reduce LDL levels, indicating that (1) inhibition of cholesterol synthesis, by itself, is not sufficient to explain cholesterol-lowering effects; and (2) for statins to be effective, synthesis of LDL receptors must increase.

In addition to inhibiting HMG-CoA reductase, statins decrease production of apolipoprotein B-100. As a result, hepatocytes decrease production of VLDLs. This lowers VLDL levels, and TG levels too,

because they're the main lipid in VLDLs. Also, statins raise HDL levels by 5% to 22%.

Clinical Trials

Statins slow progression of ASCVD and decrease the risk for stroke, hospitalization, cardiac events, peripheral vascular disease, and death. Benefits are seen in men and women, and in apparently healthy people as well as those with a history of CV events. Hence the statins are useful for both primary and secondary prevention. Furthermore, these drugs can even help people with *normal* LDL levels, in addition to those whose LDL level is high. Statins may also have some added protective effects in people with diabetes.

Therapeutic Uses

When the statins were introduced, they were approved only for hypercholesterolemia (elevated LDL cholesterol levels) in adults. As understanding of their benefits grew, so has the list of indications. Today the statins have nearly a dozen US Food and Drug Administration (FDA)–approved indications and can be prescribed for young patients as well as adults. Indications for individual statins are shown in Table 44.4. Major indications are discussed next.

Hypercholesterolemia. Statins are the most effective drugs we have for lowering LDL cholesterol. In sufficient dosage, statins can decrease LDL cholesterol by more than 60%. For many patients, the treatment goal is to drop LDL cholesterol to below 100 mg/dL. For patients at very high CV risk, a target of 70 mg/dL may be appropriate.

Primary and secondary prevention of cardiovascular events. As discussed, statins can reduce the risk for CV events (e.g., MI, angina, stroke) in patients who have never had one (primary prevention), and they can reduce the risk for a subsequent event after one has occurred (secondary prevention). Risk reduction is related to the reduction in LDL: the greater the LDL reduction, the greater the reduction in risk.

Primary prevention in people with normal low-density lipoproteins levels. One agent—*rosuvastatin* (Crestor)—is approved for reducing the risk for CV events in people with *normal* levels of LDL and no clinically evident ASCVD, but who do have an increased risk based on advancing age, high levels of *high-sensitivity C-reactive protein,* and at least one other risk factor for CV disease (e.g., hypertension, low HDL,

TABLE 44.4.   HMG-CoA Reductase Inhibitors: Food and Drug Administration-Approved Indications

Indication	Atorvastatin (Lipitor)	Fluvastatin (Lescol, Lescol XL)	Lovastatin (Altoprev, Mevacor)	Pitavastatin (Livalo)	Pravastatin (Pravachol)	Rosuvastatin (Crestor)	Simvastatin (Zocor)
Primary hypercholesterolemia	✔	✔	✔	✔	✔	✔	✔
Homozygous familial hyperlipidemia	✔					✔	✔
Heterozygous familial hypercholesterolemia in adolescents	✔		✔		✔	✔	✔
Mixed dyslipidemia	✔	✔	✔	✔	✔	✔	✔
Primary dysbetalipoproteinemia	✔				✔	✔	✔
Primary prevention of coronary events	✔		✔		✔	✔ᵃ	✔
Secondary prevention of CV events	✔	✔	✔		✔		✔
Increasing HDL cholesterol in primary hypercholesterolemia	✔		✔	✔		✔	✔
Prevention of MI and stroke in type 2 diabetes	✔		✔				
Slowing progression of coronary atherosclerosis		✔	✔		✔	✔	

ᵃRosuvastatin is approved for primary prevention in patients who have *normal* low-density lipoprotein cholesterol and no clinical evidence of atherosclerotic cardiovascular disease but who do have high levels of C-reactive protein combined with other risk factors for cardiovascular disease.
CV, Cardiovascular; *HDL*, high-density lipoproteins; *MI*, myocardial infarction.

smoking). Approval for this use was based in large part on results of the JUPITER trial.

Post-myocardial infarction therapy. Patients who have survived an MI, and who were not on statin therapy at the time of the event, are routinely started on a statin, the rationale being "better late than never." The current trend is to begin statins as soon as the patient is stabilized and able to take oral drugs. Other drugs for MI are discussed in Chapter 91.

Diabetes. CV disease is the primary cause of death in people with diabetes. Hence to reduce mortality, controlling CV risk factors—especially hypertension and high cholesterol—is as important as controlling high blood glucose. The American Diabetes Association recommends a statin for all patients older than 40 years whose LDL cholesterol is greater than 100 mg/dL. The American College of Physicians recommends a statin for (1) all patients with type 2 diabetes plus diagnosed ASCVD, *even if they don't have high cholesterol*; and (2) all adults with type 2 diabetes plus one additional risk factor (e.g., hypertension, smoking, age older than 55 years), *even if they don't have high cholesterol*. Taken together, these guidelines suggest that most patients with diabetes should receive a statin.

Pharmacokinetics

Statins are administered orally. The amount absorbed ranges between 30% and 90%, depending on the drug. Regardless of how much is absorbed, most of an absorbed dose is extracted from the blood on its first pass through the liver, the principal site at which statins act. Only a small fraction of each dose reaches the systemic circulation. Statins undergo rapid hepatic metabolism followed by excretion primarily in the bile. Only four agents—*lovastatin, pitavastatin, pravastatin,* and *simvastatin*—undergo clinically significant (10% to 20%) excretion in the urine.

Three statins—*atorvastatin, lovastatin,* and *simvastatin*—are metabolized by CYP3A4 (the 3A4 isoenzyme of cytochrome P450). As a result, levels of these drugs can be lowered by agents that induce CYP3A4 synthesis and speed up the metabolic inactivation of the statin. More important, statin levels can be increased—sometimes dramatically—by agents that inhibit CYP3A4 (see later).

One agent—*rosuvastatin*—reaches abnormally high levels in people of Asian heritage. At usual therapeutic doses, rosuvastatin levels in these people are about twice those in whites. Accordingly, if rosuvastatin is used by Asians, dosage should be reduced.

Adverse Effects

Statins are generally well tolerated. Side effects are uncommon. Some patients develop headache, rash, or gastrointestinal (GI) disturbances (dyspepsia, cramps, flatulence, constipation, abdominal pain). However, these effects are usually mild and transient. Serious adverse effects—hepatotoxicity and myopathy—are relatively rare. Some statins pose a greater risk than others, as noted subsequently.

Myopathy and rhabdomyolysis. Statins can injure muscle tissue. *Mild injury* occurs in 5% to 10% of patients. Characteristic symptoms are muscles aches, tenderness, or weakness that may be localized to certain muscle groups or diffuse. Rarely, mild injury progresses to *myositis,* defined as muscle inflammation associated with moderate elevation of creatine kinase (CK), an enzyme released from injured muscle. Release of potassium from muscle may cause blood potassium concentrations to rise. Rarely, myositis progresses to potentially fatal *rhabdomyolysis,* defined as muscle disintegration or dissolution. Release of muscle components leads to marked elevations of blood CK (greater than 10 times the upper limit of normal [ULN]) and elevations of free myoglobin. High levels of CK, in turn, may cause *renal impairment* because excess CK can plug up the glomeruli, thereby preventing normal filtration.

Fortunately, fatal rhabdomyolysis is extremely rare: the overall incidence is less than 0.15 case per 1 million prescriptions. Nonetheless, patients should be informed about the risk for myopathy and instructed to notify the prescriber if unexplained muscle pain or tenderness occurs. How statins cause myopathy is unknown.

Several factors increase the risk for myopathy. Among these are advanced age, small body frame, frailty, multisystem disease (e.g., chronic renal insufficiency, especially associated with diabetes), use of statins in high doses, low vitamin D and coenzyme Q levels, concurrent use of fibrates (which can cause myopathy too), and use of drugs that can raise statin levels (see later). In addition, hypothyroidism increases risk.

Accordingly, if muscle pain develops, thyroid function should be assessed. Measurement of CK levels can facilitate diagnosis. Levels should be determined at baseline and again if symptoms of myopathy appear. If the CK level is more than 10 times the ULN, the statin should be discontinued. If the level is less than 10 times the ULN, the statin can be continued, provided myopathy symptoms and the CK level are followed weekly. However, given that weekly blood tests are expensive and inconvenient, it may be best to stop the statin and reevaluate therapy, even when CK levels *are* less than 10 times the ULN. Routine monitoring of CK in asymptomatic patients is unnecessary.

Of the seven statins in current use, *rosuvastatin* (Crestor) poses the highest risk for rhabdomyolysis. But even with this drug, the absolute number of cases is extremely low. With the other statins, the risk is even lower. The risk for serious myopathy is extremely low, whereas the risk for untreated LDL cholesterol is very high. Accordingly, when statins are used to lower cholesterol, the benefits of therapy (reduction of CV events) far outweigh the small risk for myopathy. Additional strategies for management of myalgia include replacement of vitamin D and coenzyme Q and switching statins. Studies reveal that replacement of vitamin D and coenzyme Q can reduce myalgias in patients with low levels. Switching statins can be effective because patients may not have myalgias when taking a different drug, even if it is within the same class.

Hepatotoxicity. Liver injury, as evidenced by elevations in serum transaminase levels, develops in 0.5% to 2% of patients treated 1 year or longer. However, jaundice and other clinical signs are rare. Progression to outright liver failure occurs very rarely. Because of the risk for liver injury, product labeling recommends that liver function tests (LFTs) be done before treatment and then if clinically indicated after starting the drug. If serum transaminase levels rise to 3 times the ULN and remain there, statins should be discontinued. Transaminase levels decline to pretreatment levels after drug withdrawal.

In patients with viral or alcoholic hepatitis, statins should be avoided. However, in patients with the most common cause of hepatitis—nonalcoholic fatty liver disease—statins are acceptable therapy. In fact, in these patients, not only can statins reduce cholesterol levels; they may also decrease liver inflammation, improve LFTs, and reduce steatosis (fatty infiltration in the liver). LFTs should be monitored at baseline and as clinically indicated thereafter. If LFTs climb to three times the ULN, statin use should stop.

New-onset diabetes. The risk for developing new-onset diabetes while taking a statin is 1 in 500 patients prescribed a statin. Yet many of the patients in these studies had prediabetes before taking a statin. It is unclear whether taking a statin accelerates the advancement from prediabetes to diabetes. Despite the possibility, the CV benefits of taking a statin far outweigh the risk, and management should not change.

Drug Interactions

With other lipid-lowering drugs. Combining a statin with most other lipid-lowering drugs (except probably the bile acid sequestrants) can increase the incidence and severity of the most serious statin-related adverse events: muscle injury, liver injury, and kidney damage. Increased risk occurs primarily with fibrates (gemfibrozil, fenofibrate), which are commonly combined with statins. The bottom line: when statins are combined with other lipid-lowering agents, use extra caution and monitor for adverse effects more frequently.

With drugs that inhibit CYP3A4. Drugs that inhibit CYP3A4 can raise levels of *lovastatin* and *simvastatin* substantially and can raise levels of *atorvastatin* moderately, by slowing their inactivation. Important inhibitors of CYP3A4 include macrolide antibiotics (e.g., erythromycin), azole antifungal drugs (e.g., ketoconazole, itraconazole), HIV protease inhibitors (e.g., ritonavir), amiodarone (an antidysrhythmic drug), and cyclosporine (an immunosuppressant). If these drugs are combined

with a statin, increased caution is advised. Some authorities recommend an automatic reduction in statin dosage if these inhibitors are used.

As discussed in Chapter 5, chemicals in grapefruit and grapefruit juice can inhibit CYP3A4. Furthermore, the inhibition may persist for 3 days or more after eating the fruit or drinking its juice. Accordingly, statin users should avoid grapefruits and their juice.

Use in Pregnancy

Statins are contraindicated in pregnancy: the risks to the fetus outweigh any potential benefits of treatment. Some statins have caused fetal malformation in animal models—but only at doses far higher than those used in humans. To date, teratogenic effects in humans have not been reported. Nonetheless, because statins inhibit synthesis of cholesterol, and because cholesterol is required for synthesis of cell membranes as well as several fetal hormones, concern regarding human fetal injury remains. Moreover, there is no compelling reason to continue lipid-lowering drugs during pregnancy: stopping the statin for 9 months is not going to cause a sudden, dangerous rise in cholesterol levels or risk for ASCVD. Women of childbearing age should be informed about the potential for fetal harm and warned against becoming pregnant. If pregnancy occurs and the patient plans to continue the pregnancy, statins should be discontinued.

Drug Selection

Seven statins are available for use alone: atorvastatin, fluvastatin, lovastatin, pitavastatin, pravastatin, rosuvastatin, and simvastatin. Information on preparations, dosage, and administration is shown in Table 44.5.

Several factors bear on statin selection, including the LDL goal, drug interactions, kidney function, safety in Asian patients, and price.

Low-density lipoproteins goal. If a 30% to 40% reduction in LDL is deemed sufficient, any statin will do. However, if LDL must be lowered by more than 40%, then atorvastatin or simvastatin may be preferred. Furthermore, not only are these two drugs highly effective, but clinical experience with them is extensive.

Drug interactions. Drugs that inhibit CYP3A4 can raise levels of atorvastatin, lovastatin, and simvastatin, thereby increasing the risk for toxicity, especially myopathy and liver injury. Accordingly, in patients taking a CYP3A4 inhibitor, other statins may be preferred.

Kidney function. For patients with normal renal function, any statin is acceptable. However, for patients with significant renal impairment, atorvastatin and fluvastatin are preferred (because no dosage adjustment is needed).

Safety in asians. The same dose of *rosuvastatin*, when given to Asian and white subjects, may produce twofold higher blood levels in the Asians. Accordingly, when rosuvastatin is used in Asians, start with the lowest available dosage and monitor diligently.

A Word Regarding Niacin (Nicotinic Acid)

Niacin was once thought to be beneficial in the reduction of LDL and TG levels. However, despite these previously demonstrated favorable effects on lipid levels, niacin does little to improve outcomes and carries much potential harm. Therefore in 2016, a panel of experts recommended that niacin be removed from the guidelines for use in hypertriglyceridemia and in lowering LDL cholesterol.

Bile Acid Sequestrants

Bile acid sequestrants reduce LDL cholesterol levels. In the past, these drugs were a mainstay of lipid-lowering therapy. Today, they are used primarily as adjuncts to statins. Three agents are available: colesevelam, cholestyramine, and colestipol. Colesevelam is newer than the other two and is better tolerated.

TABLE 44.5   HMG-CoA Reductase Inhibitors: Preparations, Dosage, and Administration

Drug	Dosage	Administration With Regard to Meals	Dosage Changes in Special Populations	Preparations
Atorvastatin (Lipitor)	*Initial:* 10 mg at bedtime *Maximum:* 80 mg at bedtime	Take without regard to meals	No changes needed	*Lipitor (tablets):* 10, 20, 40, 80 mg
Atorvastatin/ Amlodipine (Caduet)	*Initial:* 10/5 at bedtime. *Maximum:* 80/10 mg at bedtime	Take without regard to meals	No changes needed	*Tablets:* 10/5, 20/5, 40/5, 80/5, 10/10, 20/10. 40/10, 80/10 mg
Fluvastatin (Lescol, Lescol XL)	*Initial:* 20–40 mg at bedtime *Maximum, Lescol:* 40 mg twice a day *Maximum, Lescol XL:* 80 mg at bedtime	Take without regard to meals	Reduce dosage for severe renal impairment	*Lescol (capsules):* 20, 40 mg *Lescol XL (extended-release tablets):* 80 mg
Lovastatin (Altoprev, Mevacor; generics)	*Initial:* 20 mg *Maximum:* 40 mg twice daily or 80 mg at bedtime	Take immediate-release tablets with evening meal to increase absorption. Take extended-release tablets at bedtime.	Reduce dosage for severe renal impairment	*Altoprev (extended-release tablets):* 20, 40, 60 mg *Mevacor and generics (tablets):* 10, 20, 40 mg
Pitavastatin (Livalo)	*Initial:* 2 mg once daily at any time of day *Maximum:* 4 mg once daily	Take without regard to meals	Reduce dosage for moderate to severe renal impairment	*Livalo (tablets):* 1, 2, 4 mg
Pravastatin (Pravachol; generics)	*Initial:* 40 mg at bedtime *Maximum:* 80 mg at bedtime	Take without regard to meals	Reduce dosage for moderate to severe renal impairment	*Pravachol and generics (tablets):* 10, 20, 40, 80 mg
Rosuvastatin (Crestor)	*Initial:* 5–20 mg at bedtime *Maximum:* 40 mg at bedtime	Take without regard to meals	Reduce dosage for severe renal impairment Reduce dosage in Asian patients	*Crestor (tablets):* 5, 10, 20, 40 mg
Simvastatin (Zocor; generics)	*Initial:* 20 mg at bedtime *Maximum:* 40 mg/d (Before 2011, the maximum recommended dosage was higher: 80 mg/d)	Take without regard to meals	Reduce dosage for severe renal impairment	*Zocor and generics (tablets):* 5, 10, 20, 40, 80 mg
Simvastatin/Ezetimibe (Vytorin)	*Initial:* 10/20 mg at bedtime *Maxiumum:* 10/80 mg	Take without regard to meals	Adjust dose for patients with renal impairment	*Tablets:* 10/10, 10/20, 10/40, 10/80-mg

 ## SUMMARY OF KEY PRESCRIBING CONSIDERATIONS

Statins

Therapeutic Goal: Primarily to lower levels of LDL cholesterol.

Baseline Data: Obtain laboratory values for total cholesterol, LDL, HDL, and TGs. Obtain baseline LFTs and a CK level.

Monitoring: Cholesterol levels should be monitored monthly early in treatment and at longer intervals thereafter.

Identifying High-Risk Patients: Statins are contraindicated in pregnant women and in patients with viral or alcoholic hepatitis. Exercise caution in patients with fatty liver disease and in those taking fibrates or ezetimibe.

Evaluating Therapeutic Effects: Improvement in serum cholesterol levels, including decrease in LDL and increase in HDL levels.

Minimizing Adverse Effects: Patients should report muscle pain or tenderness to the provider.

CK, Creatine kinase; *HDL,* high-density lipoproteins; *LDL,* low-density lipoproteins; *LFTS,* liver function tests; *TGs;* triglycerides.

Colesevelam

Colesevelam (Welchol) is the drug of choice when a bile acid sequestrant is indicated. Like the older sequestrants, colesevelam is a nonabsorbable resin that binds (sequesters) bile acids and other substances in the GI tract and thereby prevents their absorption and promotes their excretion. Colesevelam is preferred to the older sequestrants for three reasons: (1) The drug is better tolerated (less constipation, flatulence, bloating, and cramping); (2) it does not reduce absorption of fat-soluble vitamins (A, D, E, and K); and (3) it does not significantly reduce the absorption of statins, digoxin, warfarin, and most other drugs studied.

In addition to its beneficial effects on plasma lipids, colesevelam can help control hyperglycemia in patients with type 2 diabetes. The drug was approved for adjunctive therapy of diabetes in 2008. Diabetes and its management are the subject of Chapter 48.

Effect on plasma lipoproteins. The main response to bile acid sequestrants is a reduction in LDL cholesterol. LDL decline begins during the first week of therapy and becomes maximal (about a 20% drop) within about a month. When these drugs are discontinued, LDL cholesterol returns to pretreatment levels in 3 to 4 weeks.

Bile acid sequestrants may increase VLDL levels in some patients. In most cases, the elevation is transient and mild. However, if VLDL levels are elevated before treatment, the increase induced by the bile acid sequestrants may be sustained and substantial. Accordingly, bile acid sequestrants are not drugs of choice for lowering LDL cholesterol in patients with high VLDL levels.

Pharmacokinetics. Bile acid sequestrants are biologically inert. Also, they are insoluble in water, cannot be absorbed from the GI tract, and are not attacked by digestive enzymes. After oral administration, they simply pass through the intestine and are excreted in the feces.

Mechanism of action. The bile acid sequestrants lower LDL cholesterol through a mechanism that ultimately depends on increasing LDL receptors on hepatocytes. As background, you need to know that bile acids secreted into the intestine are normally reabsorbed and reused. Bile acid sequestrants prevent this reabsorption. After oral dosing, these drugs form an insoluble complex with bile acids in the intestine; this complex prevents the reabsorption of bile acids and thereby accelerates their excretion. Because bile acids are normally reabsorbed, the increase in excretion creates a demand for increased synthesis, which takes place in the liver. Because bile acids are made from cholesterol, liver cells require an increased cholesterol supply to increase bile acid production. The required cholesterol is provided by LDL. To avail themselves of more LDL cholesterol, liver cells increase their number of LDL receptors, thereby increasing their capacity for LDL uptake. The result is an increase in LDL uptake from plasma, which decreases circulating LDL levels. Individuals who are genetically incapable of increasing LDL receptor synthesis are unable to benefit from these drugs.

Therapeutic use. Colesevelam is indicated as adjunctive therapy to diet and exercise for reducing LDL cholesterol in patients with primary hypercholesterolemia. The drug may be used alone but usually is combined with a statin. On average, colesevelam alone can lower LDL cholesterol by about 20% (the typical range is between 15% and 30%). In contrast, combined therapy with a statin can reduce LDL cholesterol by up to 50%. Similar results can be obtained by combining a sequestrant with niacin.

Adverse effects. The bile acid sequestrants are not absorbed from the GI tract and hence are devoid of systemic effects. Accordingly, they are safer than all other lipid-lowering drugs.

Adverse effects are limited to the GI tract. *Constipation* is the main complaint. This can be minimized by increasing dietary fiber and fluids. If necessary, a mild laxative may be used. Other GI effects include *bloating*, *indigestion*, and *nausea*. The older agents—cholestyramine and colestipol—can decrease fat absorption and may thereby *decrease uptake of fat-soluble vitamins*. However, this does not seem to be a problem with colesevelam.

Drug interactions. The bile acid sequestrants can form insoluble complexes with other drugs. Medications that undergo binding cannot be absorbed and hence are not available for systemic effects. Drugs known to form complexes with the sequestrants include thiazide diuretics, digoxin, warfarin, and some antibiotics. To reduce formation of sequestrant-drug complexes, oral medications that are known to interact should be administered either 1 hour before the sequestrant or 4 hours after.

Ezetimibe

Ezetimibe (Zetia, Ezetrol) is a unique drug for reducing plasma cholesterol. Benefits derive from blocking cholesterol absorption.

Mechanism of Action and Effect on Plasma Lipoproteins

Ezetimibe acts on cells of the brush border of the small intestine to inhibit dietary cholesterol absorption. The drug also inhibits reabsorption of cholesterol secreted in the bile. Treatment reduces plasma levels of total cholesterol, LDL cholesterol, TGs, and apolipoprotein B. In addition, ezetimibe can produce a small *increase* in HDL cholesterol.

Therapeutic Use

Ezetimibe is indicated as an adjunct to diet modification for reducing total cholesterol, LDL cholesterol, and apolipoprotein B in patients with primary hypercholesteremia. The drug is approved for monotherapy and for combined use with a statin. In clinical trials, ezetimibe alone reduced LDL cholesterol by about 19%, increased HDL cholesterol by

---

HDL, High-density lipoproteins; *LDL*, low-density lipoproteins; *TG*, triglyceride.

1% to 4%, and decreased TGs by 5% to 10%. When ezetimibe was combined with a statin, the reduction in LDL cholesterol was about 25% greater than with the statin alone. Despite these desirable effects on blood lipids, there is no evidence that ezetimibe reduces atherosclerosis or improves clinical outcomes.

Pharmacokinetics

Ezetimibe is administered orally, and absorption is not affected by food. In the intestinal wall and liver, ezetimibe undergoes extensive conversion to ezetimibe glucuronide, an active metabolite. Both compounds—ezetimibe itself and its main metabolite—are eliminated primarily in the bile. The elimination half-life is about 22 hours.

Adverse Effects

Ezetimibe is generally well tolerated. During clinical trials, the incidence of significant side effects was nearly identical to that seen with placebo. However, during postmarketing surveillance, there have been reports of myopathy, rhabdomyolysis, hepatitis, pancreatitis, and thrombocytopenia. In contrast to the bile acid sequestrants, ezetimibe does not cause constipation and other adverse GI effects.

Drug Interactions

Statins. In patients taking a statin, adding ezetimibe slightly increases the risk for liver damage (as indicated by elevated transaminase levels). If the drugs are combined, transaminase levels should be monitored before starting therapy as well as whenever clinically indicated thereafter. Combining ezetimibe with a statin may also increase the risk for myopathy.

Fibrates. Both ezetimibe and fibrates (gemfibrozil and fenofibrate) can increase the cholesterol content of bile and can thereby increase the risk for gallstones. Both also increase the risk for myopathy. Accordingly, combined use is not recommended.

Bile acid sequestrants. Cholestyramine (and possibly colestipol) can significantly decrease the absorption of ezetimibe. To minimize effects on absorption, ezetimibe should be administered at least 2 hours before a sequestrant or more than 4 hours after.

Cyclosporine. Cyclosporine may greatly increase levels of ezetimibe. If the drugs are combined, careful monitoring is needed.

Caution

In patients with hepatic impairment, bioavailability of ezetimibe is significantly increased. At this time, we do not know whether increased availability is harmful. Until more is known, patients with moderate or severe hepatic insufficiency should not be given the drug.

Fibric Acid Derivatives (Fibrates)

The fibric acid derivatives, also known as *fibrates,* are the most effective drugs we have for lowering TG levels. In addition, these drugs can raise HDL cholesterol but have little or no effect on LDL cholesterol. Furthermore, there is no proof that fibrates reduce mortality from ASCVD. Fibrates can increase the risk for bleeding in patients taking warfarin (an anticoagulant) and the risk for rhabdomyolysis in patients taking statins. Because of these and other undesired effects, and because mortality is not reduced, fibrates are considered third-line drugs for managing lipid disorders. In the United States three preparations are available: gemfibrozil (Lopid), fenofibrate (Tricor, others), and fenofibric acid (TriLipix, Fibricor), a delayed-release preparation (Table 44.6).

Gemfibrozil

Gemfibrozil (Lopid) decreases TG (VLDL) levels and raises HDL cholesterol levels. The drug does not reduce LDL cholesterol to a significant degree. Its principal indication is hypertriglyceridemia.

Effect on plasma lipoproteins. Gemfibrozil decreases plasma TG content by lowering VLDL levels. Maximal reductions in VLDLs range from 40% to 55% and are achieved within 3 to 4 weeks of treatment. Gemfibrozil can raise HDL cholesterol by 6% to 10%. In patients with normal TG levels, the drug can produce a small reduction in LDL levels. However, if TG levels are high, gemfibrozil may actually increase LDL levels.

Therapeutic use. Gemfibrozil is used primarily to *reduce high levels of plasma triglycerides* (VLDLs). Treatment is limited to patients who have not responded adequately to weight control and diet modification. Gemfibrozil can also reduce LDL cholesterol slightly. However, other drugs (statins, cholestyramine, colestipol) are much more effective.

Gemfibrozil can be used to *raise HDL cholesterol,* although it is not approved for this application. When tested in patients with normal LDL cholesterol and low HDL cholesterol, gemfibrozil reduced the risk for major CV events—but did not reduce *mortality* from ASCVD. Because LDL cholesterol was normal, it appears that benefits were due primarily to elevation of HDL cholesterol, along with reduction of plasma TGs.

Adverse effects. Gemfibrozil is generally well tolerated. The most common reactions are rash and GI disturbances (nausea, abdominal pain, diarrhea).

Gallstones. Gemfibrozil increases biliary cholesterol saturation, thereby increasing the risk for gallstones. Patients should be informed about manifestations of gallbladder disease (e.g., upper abdominal discomfort, intolerance of fried foods, bloating) and instructed to notify the prescriber at once if these develop. Patients with preexisting gallbladder disease should not take the drug.

Myopathy. Like the statins, gemfibrozil and other fibrates can cause myopathy. Warn patients to report any signs of muscle injury, such as tenderness, weakness, or unusual muscle pain.

Liver injury. Gemfibrozil is hepatotoxic. The drug can disrupt liver function and may also pose a risk for liver cancer. Periodic tests of liver function are recommended.

Drug interactions. *Gemfibrozil displaces warfarin from plasma albumin,* thereby increasing anticoagulant effects. Prothrombin time (international normalized ratio) should be measured frequently to assess coagulation status. Warfarin dosage may need to be reduced.

As noted, gemfibrozil increases the risk for *statin-induced myopathy.* Accordingly, the combination of a statin with gemfibrozil should be used with great caution, if at all.

SUMMARY OF KEY PRESCRIBING CONSIDERATIONS

Fibrates

Therapeutic Goal: Reduction in elevated levels of TGs. May also be used to raise low levels of HDL cholesterol.

Baseline Data: Total cholesterol, LDL, HDL, and TG.

Monitoring: Obtain periodic tests of blood lipids

Identifying High-Risk Patients: These drugs are contraindicated in patients with liver disease and gallbladder disease.

Evaluating Therapeutic Effects: Decrease in LDL levels and/or increase in HDL cholesterol levels.

Minimizing Adverse Effects: Educate patients to report muscle tenderness or weakness. Have patients notify prescriber with symptoms of upper abdominal discomfort or intolerance of certain high-fat foods or fried foods.

HDL, High-density lipoproteins; *LDL,* low-density lipoproteins; *TG,* triglyceride.

MONOCLONAL ANTIBODIES (PROPROTEIN CONVERTASE SUBTILISIN/KEXIN TYPE 9 [PCSK9] INHIBITORS)

Alirocumab (Praluent) and Evolocumab (Repatha) compose a new type of drug class used for patients with high LDL levels, specifically in patients with heterozygous familial hypercholesterolemia or atherosclerotic heart problems who need additional lowering of LDL cholesterol. The PCSK9 inhibitors are indicated as an adjunct to diet modification and maximally tolerated statin therapy for reducing total LDL cholesterol.

TABLE 44.6   Fibrates

Drug	Actions and Uses	Pharmacokinetics	Adverse Effects	Usual Dosage
Gemfibrozil (Lopid)	Lowers TG by lowering VLDL levels. Indicated for hypertriglyceridemia and mixed dyslipidemia.	Hepatic metabolism Renal excretion	GI disturbances Gallstones Myopathy Liver injury	600 mg PO twice daily
Fenofibrate (Tricor)	Lowers TG by decreasing levels of VLDLs. Indicated for hypertriglyceridemia.	Hepatic metabolism Renal excretion	GI disturbances Gallstones Liver injury	40–160 mg PO daily
Fenofibric Acid (TriLipix)	Lowers TG by decreasing levels of VLDLs. Indicated for hypertriglyceridemia, mixed dyslipidemia, and hypercholesterolemia.	Hepatic metabolism Renal excretion	GI disturbances Myopathy	45–135 mg PO daily

GI, Gastrointestinal; *PO,* per os (orally); *TG;* triglyceride; *VLDL,* very-low-density lipoproteins.

Mechanism of Action and Effect on Plasma Lipoproteins

Proprotein convertase subtilisin kexin type 9 (PCSK9) is a protein that binds to low-density lipoprotein receptors (LDLRs) within the liver. LDLR is the primary receptor that clears circulating LDL. When PCSK9 binds to LDLRs, there is an increase in LDL cholesterol because LDLRs cannot clear LDL. By inhibiting PCSK9, we can free up LDLRs and decrease circulating levels of LDL in the blood.

Pharmacokinetics

PCSK9 inhibitors are administered subcutaneously. Because monoclonal antibodies are composed of protein, no specific metabolism studies were conducted. It is thought that the proteins degrade to small peptides and amino acids within the body. Both drugs have a long half-life of 11 to 20 days.

Adverse Effects

Hypersensitivity

Hypersensitivity reactions, including vasculitis, rash, and urticarial requiring hospitalization, have been noted with use of PCSK9 inhibitors.

Immunogenicity

Because this class of drug is composed of protein, there is risk for developing antibodies: 4.8% of patients treated with alirocumab and 0.1% treated with evolocumab developed antibodies to the drug after initiating treatment. These patients also had a higher incidence of injection site reactions compared with patients who did not develop antibodies.

Drug Interactions

Neither drug is noted to have any significant drug interactions.

45

Drugs for Angina Pectoris

Angina pectoris is defined as sudden pain beneath the sternum, often radiating to the left shoulder, left arm, and jaw. Anginal pain is precipitated when the oxygen supply to the heart is insufficient to meet oxygen demand. Most often, angina occurs secondary to atherosclerosis of the coronary arteries, so angina should be seen as a symptom of a disease and not as a disease in its own right. In the United States more than 10 million people have chronic stable angina; about 500,000 new cases develop annually.

Drug therapy of angina has two goals: (1) prevention of myocardial infarction (MI) and death and (2) prevention of myocardial ischemia and anginal pain. Two types of drugs are employed to decrease the risk for MI and death: cholesterol-lowering drugs and antiplatelet drugs. These agents are discussed in Chapters 44 and 46, respectively.

In this chapter, we focus on antianginal drugs (i.e., drugs that prevent myocardial ischemia and anginal pain). There are three main families of antianginal agents: *organic nitrates* (e.g., nitroglycerin), *β blockers* (e.g., metoprolol), and *calcium channel blockers* (CCBs; e.g., verapamil). In addition, a fourth agent—*ranolazine*—can be combined with these drugs to supplement their effects. Most of the chapter focuses on the organic nitrates. β blockers and CCBs are discussed at length in previous chapters, so consideration here is limited to their use in angina.

ANGINA PECTORIS: PATHOPHYSIOLOGY AND TREATMENT STRATEGY

Angina pectoris has three forms: (1) *chronic stable angina* (exertional angina), (2) *variant angina* (Prinzmetal or vasospastic angina), and (3) *unstable angina.* Our focus is on stable angina and variant angina. Consideration of unstable angina is discussed in the acute care chapter at the end of your text.

Chronic Stable Angina (Exertional Angina)
Pathophysiology
Stable angina is triggered most often by an increase in physical activity. Emotional excitement, large meals, and cold exposure may also precipitate an attack. Because stable angina usually occurs in response to strain, this condition is also known as *exertional angina* or *angina of effort.*

The underlying cause of exertional angina is coronary artery disease (CAD). If an artery is only partially blocked by plaque, blood flow will be reduced and angina pectoris will result. However, if complete vessel blockage occurs, blood flow will stop and MI will result.

The effect of CAD on the balance between myocardial oxygen demand and oxygen supply is shown in Fig. 45.1. In both the healthy heart and the heart with CAD, oxygen supply and oxygen demand are in balance during rest. In the presence of CAD, resting oxygen demand is met through dilation of arterioles distal to the partial occlusion. This dilation reduces resistance to blood flow, compensating for the increase in resistance created by plaque.

The picture is very different during exertion. In the healthy heart, as cardiac oxygen demand rises, coronary arterioles dilate, causing blood flow to increase. The increase keeps oxygen supply in balance with oxygen demand. By contrast, in people with CAD, arterioles in the affected region are already fully dilated during rest. Thus when exertion occurs, there is no way to increase blood flow to compensate for the increase in oxygen demand. The resultant imbalance between oxygen supply and oxygen demand causes anginal pain.

Treatment Strategy
The goal of antianginal therapy is to reduce the intensity and frequency of anginal attacks. Because anginal pain results from an imbalance between oxygen supply and oxygen demand, logic dictates two possible remedies: (1) increase cardiac oxygen supply or (2) decrease oxygen demand. Because the underlying cause of stable angina is occlusion of the coronary arteries, there is little we can do to increase cardiac oxygen supply. Therefore the first remedy is not a real option. Consequently, all we really can do is *decrease cardiac oxygen demand.* As discussed earlier, oxygen demand can be reduced with drugs that decrease heart rate, contractility, afterload, and preload.

Overview of Therapeutic Agents
Stable angina can be treated with three main types of drugs: *organic nitrates, β blockers,* and *calcium channel blockers.* As noted previously, *ranolazine* can be combined with these drugs for additional benefit. All four groups relieve the pain of stable angina primarily by decreasing cardiac oxygen demand (Table 45.1). Please note that drugs only provide symptomatic relief; they do not affect the underlying pathology. To reduce the risk for MI, all patients with known CAD should receive an antiplatelet drug (e.g., aspirin) unless it is contraindicated. Other measures to reduce the risk for infarction are discussed later in the section "Drugs Used to Prevent Myocardial Infarction and Death."

Nondrug Therapy
Patients should attempt to avoid factors that can precipitate angina. These include overexertion, heavy meals, emotional stress, and exposure to cold.

Risk factors for stable angina should be corrected. Important among these are smoking, hypertension, hyperlipidemia, and a sedentary lifestyle. Patients should be strongly encouraged to quit smoking. Patients with a sedentary lifestyle should be encouraged to establish a regular program of aerobic exercise. Hypertension and hyperlipidemia are major risk factors and should be treated. These disorders are discussed in Chapters 41 and 44, respectively.

Variant Angina (Prinzmetal Angina, Vasospastic Angina)
Pathophysiology
Variant angina is caused by *coronary artery spasm,* which restricts blood flow to the myocardium. Hence, as in stable angina, pain is secondary to insufficient oxygenation of the heart. In contrast to stable angina, whose symptoms occur primarily at times of exertion, variant angina

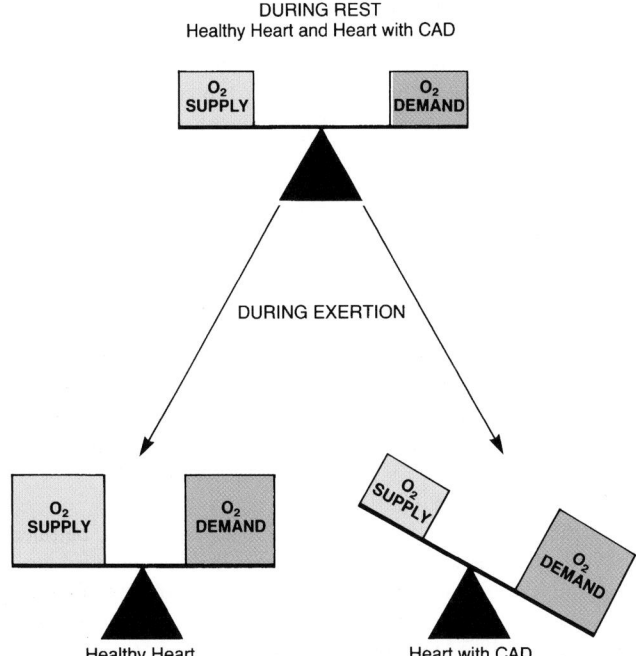

DURING REST
Healthy Heart and Heart with CAD

DURING EXERTION

Healthy Heart

Heart with CAD

Fig. 45.1 Effect of Exertion on the Balance Between Oxygen Supply and Oxygen Demand in the Healthy Heart and the Heart With Coronary Artery Disease *(CAD)*. In the healthy heart, O_2 supply and O_2 demand are always in balance; during exertion, coronary arteries dilate, producing an increase in blood flow to meet the increase in O_2 demand. In the heart with CAD, O_2 supply and O_2 demand are in balance only during rest. During exertion, dilation of coronary arteries cannot compensate for the increase in O_2 demand, and an imbalance results.

TABLE 45.1   Mechanisms of Antianginal Action

Drug Class	Mechanism of Pain Relief	
	Stable Angina	Variant Angina
Nitrates	*Decrease oxygen demand* by dilating veins, which decreases preload	*Increase oxygen supply* by relaxing coronary vasospasm
β blockers	*Decrease oxygen demand* by decreasing heart rate and contractility	Not used
Calcium channel blockers	*Decrease oxygen demand* by dilating arterioles, which decreases afterload (all calcium blockers), and by decreasing heart rate and contractility (verapamil and diltiazem)	*Increase oxygen supply* by relaxing coronary vasospasm
Ranolazine	*Appears to decrease oxygen demand,* possibly by helping the myocardium generate energy more efficiently	Not used

can produce pain at any time, even during rest and sleep. Frequently, variant angina occurs in conjunction with stable angina.

Treatment Strategy

The goal is to reduce the incidence and severity of attacks. In contrast to stable angina, which is treated primarily by reducing oxygen demand,

variant angina is treated by *increasing cardiac oxygen supply*. This makes sense in that the pain is caused by a reduction in oxygen supply, rather than by an increase in demand. Oxygen supply is increased with vasodilators, which prevent or relieve coronary artery spasm.

Overview of Therapeutic Agents

Vasospastic angina is treated with two groups of drugs: *calcium channel blockers* and *organic nitrates*. Both relax coronary artery spasm. β blockers and ranolazine, which are effective in stable angina, are not effective in variant angina. As with stable angina, therapy is symptomatic only; drugs do not alter the underlying pathology.

ORGANIC NITRATES

The organic nitrates are the oldest and most frequently used antianginal drugs. These agents relieve angina by causing vasodilation. Nitroglycerin, the most familiar organic nitrate, will serve as our prototype.

PROTOTYPE DRUGS

Drugs for Angina Pectoris

Organic Nitrate
Nitroglycerin

β Blockers
Propranolol
Metoprolol

Calcium Channel Blockers
Verapamil
Nifedipine

Drug That Increases Myocardial Efficiency
Ranolazine

Nitroglycerin

Nitroglycerin has been used to treat angina since 1879. The drug is effective, fast acting, and inexpensive. Despite availability of newer antianginal agents, nitroglycerin remains the drug of choice for relieving an acute anginal attack.

Vasodilator Actions

Nitroglycerin acts directly on vascular smooth muscle (VSM) to promote vasodilation. At usual therapeutic doses, the drug acts primarily on *veins*. Dilation of arterioles is only modest.

The biochemical events that lead to vasodilation begin with uptake of nitrate by VSM, followed by conversion of nitrate to its active form: *nitric oxide*. As indicated, conversion requires the presence of *sulfhydryl groups*. Nitric oxide then activates guanylyl cyclase, an enzyme that catalyzes the formation of cyclic guanosine monophosphate (cGMP). Through a series of reactions, elevation of cGMP leads to dephosphorylation of light-chain myosin in VSM. (Recall that, in all muscles, phosphorylated myosin interacts with actin to produce contraction.) As a result of dephosphorylation, myosin is unable to interact with actin, and thus VSM relaxes, causing vasodilation. For our purposes, the most important aspect of this sequence is the conversion of nitrate to its active form—nitric oxide—in the presence of a sulfhydryl source.

Mechanism of Antianginal Effects

Stable angina. Nitroglycerin decreases the pain of exertional angina primarily by *decreasing cardiac oxygen demand*. Oxygen demand is decreased as follows: by dilating veins, nitroglycerin decreases venous return to the heart and thereby decreases ventricular filling; the resultant decrease in wall tension (preload) decreases oxygen demand.

In patients with stable angina, nitroglycerin does not appear to increase blood flow to ischemic areas of the heart. This statement is based on two observations. First, nitroglycerin does not dilate atherosclerotic coronary arteries. Second, when nitroglycerin is injected directly into coronary arteries during an anginal attack, it does not relieve pain. Both observations suggest that pain relief results from effects of nitroglycerin on peripheral blood vessels—not from effects on coronary blood flow.

Variant angina. In patients with variant angina, nitroglycerin acts by relaxing or preventing spasm in coronary arteries. Hence the drug *increases oxygen supply.* It does not reduce oxygen demand.

Pharmacokinetics

Absorption. Nitroglycerin is *highly lipid soluble* and crosses membranes with ease. Because of this property, nitroglycerin can be administered by uncommon routes (sublingual, buccal, transdermal) as well as by more conventional routes (oral, intravenous).

Metabolism. Nitroglycerin undergoes *rapid inactivation* by hepatic enzymes (organic nitrate reductases). As a result, the drug has a plasma half-life of only 5 to 7 minutes. When nitroglycerin is administered orally, most of each dose is destroyed on its first pass through the liver.

Adverse Effects

Nitroglycerin is generally well tolerated. Principal adverse effects—headache, hypotension, and tachycardia—occur secondary to vasodilation.

Headache. Initial therapy can produce severe headache. This response diminishes over the first few weeks of treatment. In the meantime, headache can be reduced with aspirin, acetaminophen, or some other mild analgesic.

Orthostatic hypotension. Relaxation of VSM causes blood to pool in veins when the patient assumes an erect posture. Pooling decreases venous return to the heart, which reduces cardiac output, causing blood pressure to fall. Symptoms of orthostatic hypotension include light-headedness and dizziness. Patients should be instructed to sit or lie down if these occur. Lying with the feet elevated promotes venous return and can help restore blood pressure.

Reflex tachycardia. Nitroglycerin lowers blood pressure—primarily by decreasing venous return, and partly by dilating arterioles. By lowering blood pressure, the drug can activate the baroreceptor reflex, causing sympathetic stimulation of the heart. The resultant increase in both heart rate and contractile force increases cardiac oxygen demand, which negates the benefits of therapy. Pretreatment with a β blocker or verapamil (a CCB that directly suppresses the heart) can prevent sympathetic cardiac stimulation.

Drug Interactions

Hypotensive drugs. Nitroglycerin can intensify the effects of other hypotensive agents. Consequently, care should be exercised when nitroglycerin is used concurrently with β blockers, CCBs, diuretics, and all other drugs that can lower blood pressure, including inhibitors of phosphodiesterase type 5 (PDE-5). Also, patients should be advised to avoid alcohol.

β blockers, verapamil, and diltiazem. These drugs can suppress nitroglycerin-induced tachycardia. β blockers do so by preventing sympathetic activation of β_1-adrenergic receptors on the heart. Verapamil and diltiazem prevent tachycardia through direct suppression of pacemaker activity in the sinoatrial node.

Tolerance

Tolerance to nitroglycerin-induced vasodilation can develop rapidly (over the course of a single day). One possible mechanism is depletion of sulfhydryl groups in VSM: in the absence of sulfhydryl groups, nitroglycerin cannot be converted to nitric oxide, its active form. Another possible mechanism is reversible oxidative injury to mitochondrial aldehyde dehydrogenase, an enzyme needed to convert nitroglycerin into nitric oxide. Patients who develop tolerance to nitroglycerin display cross-tolerance to all other nitrates, and vice versa. Development of tolerance is most likely with high-dose therapy and uninterrupted therapy. To prevent tolerance, nitroglycerin and other nitrates should be used in the lowest effective dosages; long-acting formulations (e.g., patches, sustained-release preparations) should be used on an intermittent schedule that allows at least 8 drug-free hours every day, usually during the night (Tables 45.2 and 45.3). If pain occurs during the nitrate-free interval, it can be managed with sparing use of a short-acting nitrate (e.g., sublingual nitroglycerin) or by adding a β blocker or CCB to the regimen. Tolerance can be reversed by withholding nitrates for a short time.

Discontinuing Nitroglycerin

Long-acting preparations (transdermal patches, topical ointment, sustained-release oral tablets or capsules) should be discontinued slowly. If they are withdrawn abruptly, vasospasm may result.

Summary of Therapeutic Uses

Acute therapy of angina. For acute treatment of angina pectoris, nitroglycerin is administered in sublingual tablets and a translingual spray. Both formulations can be used to abort an ongoing anginal attack and to provide prophylaxis in anticipation of exertion.

Sustained therapy of angina. For sustained prophylaxis against angina, nitroglycerin is administered in the following formulations:

TABLE 45.2 Organic Nitrates: Time Course of Action		
Drug and Dosage Form	**Onset[a]**	**Duration[b]**
Nitroglycerin		
Sublingual tablets	Rapid (1–3 min)	Brief (30–60 min)
Translingual spray	Rapid (2–3 min)	Brief (30–60 min)
Oral capsules, SR	Slow (20–45 min)	Long (3–8 h)
Transdermal patches	Slow (30–60 min)	Long (24 h)[c]
Topical ointment	Slow (20–60 min)	Long (2–12 h)
Isosorbide Mononitrate		
Oral tablets, IR	Slow (30–60 min)	Long (6–10 h)
Oral tablets, SR	Slow (30–60 min)	Long (7–12 h)
Isosorbide Dinitrate		
Sublingual tablets	Rapid (2–5 min)	Long (1–3 h)
Oral tablets, IR	Slow (20–40 min)	Long (4–6 h)
Oral tablets, SR	Slow (30 min)	Long (6–8 h)
Oral capsules, SR	Slow (30 min)	Long (6–8 h)

[a]Nitrates with a *rapid* onset have two uses: (1) termination of an ongoing anginal attack and (2) short-term prophylaxis before anticipated exertion. Of the rapid-acting nitrates, nitroglycerin (sublingual tablet or translingual spray) is preferred to the others for terminating an ongoing attack.

[b]*Long-acting* nitrates are used for sustained prophylaxis (prevention) of anginal attacks. All cause tolerance if used without interruption.

[c]Although patches can release nitroglycerin for up to 24 hours, they should be removed after 12 to 14 hours to avoid tolerance.

IR, Immediate release; *SR,* sustained release.

TABLE 45.3   Organic Nitrates: Trade Names and Dosages

Drug and Formulation	Trade Name	Indication	Usual Dosage
Nitroglycerin			
Sublingual tablets	Nitrostat	Acute suppression of anginal attack	0.3–0.6 mg as needed every 5 min for maximum of three doses
Sublingual powder	GONITRO	Acute suppression of anginal attack	1–2 packets (400 mcg/packet, up to three packets in a 15-min period)
Translingual spray	Nitrolingual NitroMist	Acute suppression of anginal attack	1–2 sprays (up to 3 sprays in a 15-min period)
Oral capsules, SR	Nitro-Time	Long term anginal prophylaxis	2.5–6.5 mg 3 or 4 times daily; to avoid tolerance, administer only once or twice daily; do not crush or chew
Transdermal patches	Minitran, Nitro-Dur, Transderm Nitro , Trinipatch	Sustained anginal prophylaxis	1 patch a day; to avoid tolerance, remove after 12–14 h, allowing 10–12 patch-free hours each day. Patches come in sizes that release 0.1–0.8 mg/h.
Topical ointment	Nitro-Bid	Sustained protection against anginal attacks	1–2 inches (7.5–40 mg) every 4–6 h
Intravenous	Generic only	Acute suppression of anginal attack	5 mcg/min initially, then increased gradually as needed (max: 200 mcg/min); tolerance develops with prolonged continuous infusion
Isosorbide Mononitrate			
Oral tablets, IR	Generic only	Sustained protection against anginal attacks	20 mg twice daily; to avoid tolerance, take the first dose upon awakening and the second dose 7 h later
Oral tablets, SR	Imdur	Sustained protection against anginal attacks	60–240 mg once a day; do not crush or chew
Isosorbide Dinitrate			
Sublingual tablets	Generic only	Acute prophylaxis for anginal attacks	2.5–5 mg before activities that may cause angina. For acute angina, 2.5–5 mg every 5 min for maximum of three doses. Do not crush or chew
Oral tablets, IR	Isordil Oral Titradose	Sustained protection against anginal attacks	10–40 mg 2 or 3 times daily; to avoid tolerance, take the last dose no later than 7:00 PM
Oral tablets, SR	Generic only	Sustained protection against anginal attacks	40 mg every 6–12 h; to avoid tolerance, take only once or twice daily (at 8:00 AM and 2:00 PM)
Oral capsules, SR	Dilatrate-SR	Sustained protection against anginal attacks	40 mg every 6–12 h; to avoid tolerance, take only once or twice daily (at 8:00 AM and 2:00 PM)

IR, Immediate release; *SR*, sustained release.

transdermal patches, topical ointment, and sustained-release oral capsules.

Isosorbide Mononitrate and Isosorbide Dinitrate

Both of these drugs have pharmacologic actions identical to those of nitroglycerin. Both drugs are used for angina, both are taken orally, and both produce headache, hypotension, and reflex tachycardia. Differences between them relate only to route of administration and time course of action. Time course determines whether a particular drug or dosage form will be used for acute therapy, sustained prophylaxis, or both. As with nitroglycerin, tolerance can develop to long-acting preparations. To avoid tolerance, the dosing schedule for long-acting preparations should allow at least 12 drug-free hours a day. Time courses are shown in Table 45.2. Trade names and dosages are shown in Table 45.3. A fixed-dose combination of isosorbide dinitrate plus hydralazine is discussed in Chapter 42.

β BLOCKERS

β blockers (e.g., propranolol, metoprolol) are first-line drugs for *angina of effort*, but are *not* effective against vasospastic angina. When administered on a fixed schedule, β blockers can provide sustained protection against

SUMMARY OF KEY PRESCRIBING CONSIDERATIONS

Nitroglycerin

Therapeutic Goal: Reduction of the frequency and intensity of anginal attacks.

Baseline Data: Frequency and intensity of anginal attacks and the factors that precipitate anginal attacks. Blood pressure and heart rate should be noted.

Monitoring: No routine blood monitoring necessary.

Identifying High-Risk Patients: Use with caution in hypotensive patients and in patients taking drugs that can lower blood pressure.

Evaluating Therapeutic Effects: Instruct patients to keep a record of the frequency and intensity of anginal attacks and the factors that precipitate these attacks.

Minimizing Adverse Effects: Use with phosphodiesterase type 5 inhibitors (sildenafil) is contraindicated.

effort-induced anginal pain. Exercise tolerance is increased, and the frequency and intensity of anginal attacks are lowered. All of the β blockers appear equally effective. In addition to reducing anginal pain, β blockers decrease the risk for death, especially in patients with a prior MI.

β blockers reduce anginal pain primarily by *decreasing cardiac oxygen demand,* principally through blockade of β₁ receptors in the heart, which decreases heart rate and contractility. β blockers reduce oxygen demand further by causing a modest reduction in arterial pressure (afterload). In addition to decreasing oxygen demand, β blockers help increase oxygen supply. By slowing heart rate, they increase time in diastole and thereby increase the time during which blood flows through myocardial vessels. In patients taking vasodilators (e.g., nitroglycerin), β blockers provide the additional benefit of blunting reflex tachycardia.

For treatment of stable angina, dosage should be low initially and then gradually increased. The dosing goal is to reduce resting heart rate to 50 to 60 beats/min and limit exertional heart rate to about 100 beats/min. β blockers should not be withdrawn abruptly because doing so can increase the incidence and intensity of anginal attacks and may even precipitate MI.

β blockers can produce a variety of adverse effects. Blockade of cardiac β₁ receptors can produce *bradycardia, decreased atrioventricular (AV) conduction,* and *reduction of contractility.* Consequently, β blockers should not be used by patients with sick sinus syndrome, heart failure, or second-degree or third-degree AV block. Blockade of β₂ receptors in the lung can promote bronchoconstriction. Accordingly, β blockers should be used with caution by patients with asthma. If an asthmatic individual absolutely must use a β blocker, a β₁-selective agent (e.g., metoprolol) should be chosen. β blockers can mask signs of hypoglycemia and therefore must be used with caution in patients with diabetes.

The basic pharmacology of the β blockers is discussed in Chapter 16.

CALCIUM CHANNEL BLOCKERS

The CCBs used most frequently are *verapamil, diltiazem,* and *nifedipine* (a dihydropyridine-type calcium channel blocker). Accordingly, our discussion focuses on these three drugs. *All three* can block calcium channels in VSM, primarily in arterioles. The result is arteriolar dilation and reduction of peripheral resistance (afterload). In addition, all three can relax coronary vasospasm. *Verapamil* and *diltiazem* also block calcium channels in the heart and can thereby decrease heart rate, AV conduction, and contractility.

CCBs are used to treat both stable and variant angina. In *variant angina,* these drugs promote relaxation of coronary artery spasm, *increasing cardiac oxygen supply.* In *stable angina,* they promote relaxation of peripheral arterioles; the resultant decrease in afterload *reduces cardiac oxygen demand.* Verapamil and diltiazem can produce modest additional reductions in oxygen demand by suppressing heart rate and contractility.

The major adverse effects of the CCBs are cardiovascular. Dilation of peripheral arterioles lowers blood pressure and can thereby induce *reflex tachycardia.* This reaction is greatest with nifedipine and minimal with verapamil and diltiazem. Because of their suppressant effects on the heart, verapamil and diltiazem must be used cautiously in patients taking β blockers and in patients with bradycardia, heart failure, or AV block. These precautions do not apply to nifedipine or other dihydropyridines.

The basic pharmacology of the CCBs is discussed in Chapter 39.

RANOLAZINE

Actions and Therapeutic Use

Ranolazine (Ranexa) represents the first new class of antianginal agents to be approved in more than 25 years. In clinical trials, the drug reduced the number of angina episodes per week and increased exercise tolerance. However, these benefits were modest and were smaller in women than in men. Unlike most other antianginal drugs, ranolazine does not reduce heart rate, blood pressure, or vascular resistance. However, it *can* prolong the QT interval and is subject to multiple drug interactions. Ranolazine works by reducing accumulation of sodium and calcium in myocardial cells, which might help the myocardium use energy more efficiently. However, the exact mechanism of action is unknown. Despite limited efficacy, many drug interactions, and a risk for dysrhythmias (see later), ranolazine is now approved as a first-line drug for angina. It may be combined with nitrates, β blockers, amlodipine (a CCB), and other drugs used for angina treatment.

Pharmacokinetics

Absorption from the GI tract is highly variable but not affected by food. Plasma levels peak 2 to 5 hours after dosing. In the liver, ranolazine undergoes rapid and extensive metabolism, mainly by CYP3A4 (the 3A4 isoenzyme of cytochrome P450). The drug has a plasma half-life of 7 hours and is excreted in the urine (75%) and feces (25%), almost entirely as metabolites.

Adverse Effects
QT Prolongation
Ranolazine can cause a dose-related increase in the QT interval and may thereby increase the risk for torsades de pointes, a serious ventricular dysrhythmia. Accordingly, the drug is contraindicated for patients with preexisting QT prolongation and for those taking other drugs that can increase the QT interval. In addition, ranolazine is contraindicated for patients at risk for developing high levels of the drug—namely, patients with hepatic impairment or those taking drugs that inhibit CYP3A4. The issue of drug-induced QT prolongation is discussed in Chapter 5.

Elevation of Blood Pressure
In patients with severe renal impairment, ranolazine can raise blood pressure by about 15 mm Hg. Accordingly, blood pressure should be monitored often in these people.

Drug Interactions
CYP3A4 Inhibitors
Agents that inhibit CYP3A4 can increase levels of ranolazine and can thereby increase the risk for torsades de pointes. Accordingly, moderate or strong CYP3A4 inhibitors should be avoided. Among these agents are grapefruit juice, HIV protease inhibitors (e.g., ritonavir), macrolide antibiotics (e.g., erythromycin), azole antifungal drugs (e.g., itraconazole), and some CCBs.

QT Drugs
Drugs that prolong the QT interval (e.g., quinidine, sotalol) can increase the risk for torsades de pointes in patients taking ranolazine and hence should be avoided. Chapter 5 presents a comprehensive list of QT drugs.

Calcium Channel Blockers
Most CCBs—but not amlodipine—can inhibit CYP3A4 and thus increase levels of ranolazine. Accordingly, when use of ranolazine plus a CCB is indicated, amlodipine is the only CCB that should be used.

Preparations, Dosage, and Administration
Ranolazine (Ranexa) is formulated in extended-release tablets (500 and 1000 mg) that should be swallowed intact, with or without food. Dosing begins at 500 mg twice daily and may be increased to a maximum of 1000 mg twice daily. Ranolazine may be used in combination with a nitrate, β blocker, or amlodipine (a CCB), and other drugs for angina.

TREATMENT MEASURES

Guidelines for Management of Chronic Stable Angina

In 1999, three organizations—the American Heart Association (AHA), the American College of Cardiology (ACC), and the American College of Physicians–American Society of Internal Medicine—joined forces to produce the first national guidelines on the management of chronic stable angina. The 1999 guidelines were updated in 2002 and again in 2007. In addition, the guideline, *2012 ACCF/AHA/ACP/AATS/PCNA/SCAI/STS Guideline for the Diagnosis and Management of Patients With Stable Ischemic Heart Disease*, echoed many of the same recommendations made previously for this population. Guidelines including a 2014 focused update of the 2012 original, are available free online at www.circ.ahajournals.org. The following discussion reflects recommendations in these guidelines.

Treatment of stable angina has two objectives: (1) prevention of MI and death, and (2) reduction of cardiac ischemia and associated anginal pain. Although both goals are desirable, prevention of MI and death is clearly more important. If two treatments are equally effective at decreasing anginal pain, but one also decreases the risk for death, then the latter is preferred.

Drugs Used to Prevent Myocardial Infarction and Death

We now have medical treatments that can decrease the risk for MI and death in patients with chronic stable angina. Therapy directed at preventing MI and death is a new paradigm in the management of stable angina, and all practitioners should become familiar with it.

Antiplatelet drugs. These agents decrease platelet aggregation and thereby decrease the risk for thrombus formation in coronary arteries. The most effective agents are *aspirin* and *clopidogrel*. In patients with stable angina, low-dose aspirin produces a 33% decrease in the risk for adverse cardiovascular events. Benefits of clopidogrel seem equal to those of aspirin, although they are not as well documented. The guidelines recommend that all patients with stable angina take 75 to 162 mg of aspirin daily, unless there is a specific reason not to. Aspirin, clopidogrel, and other antiplatelet drugs are discussed in Chapter 46.

Cholesterol-lowering drugs. Elevated cholesterol is a major risk factor for coronary atherosclerosis. Drugs that lower cholesterol can slow the progression of CAD, stabilize atherosclerotic plaques, and even cause plaque regression. Therapies that reduce cholesterol are associated with decreased mortality from coronary heart disease. For example, in patients with established CAD, taking simvastatin can decrease the risk for mortality by 35%. Because of the well-established benefits of cholesterol-lowering therapy, the guidelines recommend that all patients with stable angina receive a cholesterol-lowering drug. The pharmacology of the cholesterol-lowering drugs is discussed in Chapter 44.

Angiotensin-converting enzyme inhibitors. There is strong evidence that, in patients with CAD, ACE inhibitors greatly reduce the incidence of adverse outcomes. In the Heart Outcomes Prevention Evaluation (HOPE) trial, for example, ramipril reduced the incidence of stroke, MI, and cardiovascular death. Among one subset of patients—those with diabetes—benefits were particularly striking. Ramipril decreased the risk for stroke by 33%, MI by 22%, and cardiovascular death by 37%. In addition, ramipril reduced the risk for nephropathy, retinopathy, and other microvascular complications of diabetes. Because of these well-documented benefits, the guidelines recommend angiotensin-converting enzyme (ACE) inhibitors for most patients with established CAD, and especially for those with diabetes. The pharmacology of the ACE inhibitors is discussed in Chapter 38.

Antianginal Agents: Drugs Used to Reduce Anginal Pain

The goal of antianginal therapy is to achieve complete (or nearly complete) elimination of anginal pain, along with a return to normal activities. This should be accomplished with a minimum of adverse drug effects.

The basic strategy of antianginal therapy is to provide baseline protection using one or more long-acting drugs (β blocker, CCB, long-acting nitrate) supplemented with sublingual nitroglycerin when breakthrough pain occurs. A flow plan for drug selection is shown in Fig. 45.2. As indicated, treatment is approached sequentially. Progression from one step to the next is based on patient response. Some patients can be treated with a single long-acting drug, some require two or three, and some require revascularization.

Initial treatment consists of sublingual nitroglycerin plus a long-acting antianginal drug. β blockers are the preferred agents for baseline therapy because they can decrease mortality, especially in patients with a prior MI. In addition to providing prophylaxis, β blockers suppress nitrate-induced reflex tachycardia.

Fig. 45.2 Flow Plan for Antianginal Drug Selection in Patients With Chronic Stable Angina. *(1)* Avoid short-acting dihydropyridines. *(2)* At any point in this process, based on coronary anatomy, severity of angina symptoms, and patient preference, it is reasonable to consider evaluation for coronary revascularization with either percutaneous coronary intervention *(PCI)* or coronary artery bypass graft *(CABG)*. Unless a patient is documented to have left main, three-vessel, or two-vessel coronary artery disease with significant stenosis of the proximal left anterior descending coronary artery, there is no demonstrated survival advantage associated with CABG or PCI in low-risk patients with chronic stable angina. Accordingly, medical therapy should be attempted in most patients before considering PCI or CABG. (Adapted from Fihn SD, Gardin J, Abrams J, et al. 2012 ACCF/AHA/ACP/AATS/PCNA/SCAI/STS Guideline for the Diagnosis and Management of Patients with Stable Ischemic Heart Disease. 2012. Available online at www.circ.ahajournals.org.)

If a β blocker is inadequate, or if there are contraindications to β blockade, a long-acting CCB should be added or substituted. Dihydropyridine-type CCBs (e.g., nifedipine) lack cardiosuppressant actions and thus are safer than β blockers for patients with bradycardia, AV block, or heart failure. When a CCB is to be *combined* with a β blocker, a dihydropyridine is preferred to verapamil or diltiazem because verapamil and diltiazem will intensify the cardiosuppressant actions of the β blocker, whereas a dihydropyridine CCB will not.

If a CCB is inadequate, or if there are contraindications to calcium channel blockade, a long-acting nitrate (e.g., transdermal nitroglycerin) should be added or substituted. However, because tolerance can develop quickly, these nitrate preparations are less well suited than β blockers or CCBs for continuous protection.

Note that, as we proceed along the drug selection flow plan, drugs are *added* to the regimen, resulting in treatment with two or more agents. Combination therapy increases our chances of success because

oxygen demand is decreased by multiple mechanisms: β blockers reduce heart rate and contractility, CCBs reduce afterload (by dilating arterioles) and nitrates reduce preload (by dilating veins).

If combined treatment with a β blocker, CCB, and long-acting nitrate fails to provide relief, coronary artery bypass graft (CABG) surgery or percutaneous coronary intervention (PCI) may be indicated. Note that these invasive procedures should be considered only after more conservative treatment has been tried.

How should we treat angina in patients who have a coexisting condition? The antianginal drugs employed—nitrates, β blockers, and CCBs—are the same ones used in patients who have angina alone. However, when selecting among these drugs, we must consider the coexisting disorder as well as the angina. For example, as noted previously, in patients with asthma, CCBs are preferred to β blockers (because β blockers promote bronchoconstriction, whereas CCBs do not). Table 45.4 shows more than 20 coexisting conditions and indicates which antianginal agents to use as well as which ones to avoid.

TABLE 45.4   Choosing Between β Blockers and Calcium Channel Blockers for Treating Angina in Patients Who Have a Coexisting Condition

Coexisting Condition	Recommended Treatment (Alternative Treatment)	Drugs to Avoid
Medical Conditions		
Systemic hypertension	β blockers (long-acting, slow-release CCBs)	
Migraine or vascular headache	β blockers (verapamil or diltiazem)	
Asthma or COPD with bronchospasm	Verapamil or diltiazem	β blockers
Hyperthyroidism	β blockers	
Raynaud disease	Long-acting, slow-release CCBs	β blockers
Type 1 diabetes	β blockers, particularly if prior MI, or long-acting, slow-release CCBs	
Type 2 diabetes	β blockers or long-acting, slow-release CCBs	
Depression	Long-acting, slow-release CCBs	β blockers
Mild peripheral vascular disease	β blockers or long-acting, slow-release CCBs	
Severe peripheral vascular disease with ischemia at rest	Long-acting, slow-release CCBs	β blockers
Cardiac Dysrhythmias and Conduction Abnormalities		
Sinus bradycardia	Long-acting, slow-release CCBs that do not decrease heart rate	β blockers, diltiazem, verapamil
Sinus tachycardia (not due to heart failure)	β blockers	
Supraventricular tachycardia	Verapamil, diltiazem, or β blockers	
AV block	Long-acting, slow-release CCBs that do not slow AV conduction	β blockers, diltiazem, verapamil
Rapid atrial fibrillation (with digoxin)	Verapamil, diltiazem, or β blockers	
Ventricular dysrhythmias	β blockers	
Left Ventricular Dysfunction		
Congestive heart failure		
Mild (LVEF ≥40%)	β blockers	
Moderate to severe (LVEF <40%)	Amlodipine or felodipine (nitrates)	Diltiazem, verapamil
Left-sided valvular heart disease		
Mild aortic stenosis	β blockers	
Aortic insufficiency	Long-acting, slow-release dihydropyridine CCBs	
Mitral regurgitation	Long-acting, slow-release dihydropyridine CCBs	
Mitral stenosis	β blockers	
Hypertrophic cardiomyopathy	β blockers, verapamil, diltiazem	Dihydropyridine CCBs, nitrates

AV, Atrioventricular; *CCB,* calcium channel blocker; *COPD,* chronic obstructive pulmonary disease; *LVEF,* left ventricular ejection fraction; *MI,* myocardial infarction.
Adapted from Fihn SD, Gardin J, Abrams J, et al. 2012 ACCF/AHA/ACP/AATS/PCNA/SCAI/STS Guideline for the Diagnosis and Management of Patients with Stable Ischemic Heart Disease. 2012. Available online at www.circ.ahajournals.org/.

Reduction of Risk Factors

The treatment program should reduce anginal risk factors: smokers should quit; sedentary patients should get aerobic exercise; and patients with diabetes, hypertension, or high cholesterol should receive appropriate therapy.

Smoking. Smoking increases the risk for cardiovascular mortality by 50%. Fortunately, smoking cessation greatly decreases cardiovascular risk. Accordingly, all patients who smoke should be strongly encouraged to quit. Smoking cessation is discussed in Chapter 34.

High cholesterol. As noted, high cholesterol levels increase the risk of adverse cardiovascular events, and therapies that reduce cholesterol reduce that risk. Accordingly, most patients with high cholesterol levels should receive cholesterol-lowering therapy.

Hypertension. High blood pressure increases the risk for cardiovascular mortality, and lowering blood pressure reduces the risk. Accordingly, all patients with hypertension should receive treatment. Blood pressure should be reduced to 130/80 mm Hg or less. Management of hypertension is discussed in Chapter 41.

Diabetes. Both type 1 (insulin-dependent) and type 2 (non-insulin-dependent) diabetes increase the risk for cardiovascular mortality. Type 1 increases the risk 3- to 10-fold; type 2 increases the risk 2- to 4-fold.

Although there is good evidence that tight glycemic control decreases the risk for microvascular complications of diabetes, there is little evidence to show that tight glycemic control decreases the risk for cardiovascular complications and in fact, may be harmful. Nonetheless, it is prudent to strive for optimal glycemic control which may vary slightly with each individual.

Physical inactivity. Increased physical activity has multiple benefits. In patients with chronic stable angina, exercise increases exercise tolerance and the sense of well-being and decreases anginal symptoms, cholesterol levels, and objective measures of ischemia. Accordingly, the guidelines recommend that patients perform 30 to 60 minutes of a moderate-intensity activity 3 to 4 times a week. Such activities include walking, jogging, cycling, and other aerobic exercises. Exercise by moderate- to high-risk patients should be medically supervised.

Management of Variant Angina

Treatment of vasospastic angina can proceed in three steps. For initial therapy, either a calcium channel blocker or a long-acting nitrate is selected. If either drug alone is inadequate, then combined therapy with a CCB *plus* a nitrate should be tried. If the combination fails to control symptoms, CABG surgery may be indicated. β blockers are not effective in vasospastic angina.

46

Anticoagulant and Antiplatelet Drugs

The drugs discussed here are used to prevent the formation of thrombi and dissolve thrombi that have already formed. These drugs act in several ways: some suppress coagulation, some inhibit platelet aggregation, and some promote clot degradation. They all interfere with normal hemostasis. As a result, they all carry a significant risk for bleeding.

COAGULATION: PHYSIOLOGY AND PATHOPHYSIOLOGY

Hemostasis

Hemostasis is the physiologic process by which bleeding is stopped. Hemostasis occurs in two stages: (1) formation of a platelet plug, followed by (2) reinforcement of the platelet plug with fibrin. Both processes are set in motion by blood vessel injury.

Stage One: Formation of a Platelet Plug

Platelet aggregation is initiated when platelets come in contact with collagen on the exposed surface of a damaged blood vessel. In response to contact with collagen, platelets adhere to the site of vessel injury. Adhesion initiates platelet *activation,* which in turn leads to massive platelet *aggregation.*

Platelet aggregation is a complex process that ends with formation of *fibrinogen bridges* between *glycoprotein IIb/IIIa (GP IIb/IIIa) receptors* on adjacent platelets (Fig. 46.1). For these bridges to form, GP IIb/IIIa receptors must first undergo activation—that is, they must undergo a configurational change that allows them to bind with fibrinogen. As indicated in Fig. 46.1A, activation of GP IIb/IIIa can be stimulated by multiple factors, including thromboxane A_2 (TXA_2), thrombin, collagen, platelet-activating factor (PAF), and adenosine diphosphate (ADP). Under the influence of these factors, GP IIb/IIIa changes its shape, binds with fibrinogen, and thereby causes aggregation (see Fig. 46.1B). The aggregated platelets constitute a plug that stops bleeding. This plug is unstable, however, and must be reinforced with *fibrin* if protection is to last.

Stage Two: Coagulation

Coagulation is defined as the production of *fibrin,* a thread-like protein that reinforces the platelet plug. Fibrin is produced by two convergent pathways (Fig. 46.2), referred to as the *contact activation pathway* (also known as the *intrinsic pathway*) and the *tissue factor pathway* (also known as the *extrinsic pathway*). These two pathways converge at factor Xa, after which they employ the same final series of reactions. In both pathways, each reaction in the sequence amplifies the reaction that follows. Hence, after this sequence is initiated, it becomes self-sustaining and self-reinforcing.

The *tissue factor pathway* is turned on by trauma to the vascular wall, which triggers release of tissue factor,[a] also known as *tissue*

[a]The term *tissue factor* refers not to a single compound but rather to a complex of several compounds, including a proteolytic enzyme and phospholipids released from tissue membranes.

thromboplastin. Tissue factor then combines with and thereby activates factor VII, which in turn activates factor X, which then catalyzes the conversion of *prothrombin* (factor II) into *thrombin* (factor IIa). Thrombin then does three things. First, it catalyzes the conversion of fibrinogen into fibrin. Second, it catalyzes the conversion of factor V into *its* active form (Va), a compound that greatly increases the activity of factor Xa, even though it has no direct catalytic activity of its own. Third, thrombin catalyzes the conversion of factor VIII into *its* active form (VIIIa), a compound that greatly increases the activity of factor IXa in the contact activation pathway.

The *contact activation pathway* is turned on when blood makes contact with collagen that has been exposed as a result of trauma to a blood vessel wall. Collagen contact stimulates conversion of factor XII into its active form, XIIa (see Fig. 46.2). Factor XIIa then activates factor XI, which activates factor IX, which activates factor X. After this, the contact activation pathway is the same as the tissue factor pathway. As noted, factor VIIIa, which is produced under the influence of thrombin, greatly increases the activity of factor IXa, even though it has no direct catalytic activity of its own. Important to our understanding of anticoagulant drugs is the fact that *four coagulation factors—factors VII, IX, X, and II (prothrombin)—require vitamin K for their synthesis.* These factors appear in green boxes in Fig. 46.2. The significance of the vitamin K–dependent factors will become apparent when warfarin, an oral anticoagulant, is discussed.

Keeping Hemostasis Under Control

To protect against widespread coagulation, the body must inactivate any clotting factors that stray from the site of vessel injury. Inactivation

Fig. 46.1 Mechanism of Platelet Aggregation and Actions of Antiplatelet Drugs. (A) Multiple factors—thromboxane A$_2$ *(TXA$_2$)*, thrombin, collagen, platelet-activating factor *(PAF)*, and adenosine diphosphate *(ADP)*—promote activation of the glycoprotein *(GP)* IIb/IIIa receptor. Each platelet has 50,000 to 80,000 GP IIb/IIIa receptors, although only one is shown. (B) Activation of the GP IIb/IIIa receptor permits binding of fibrinogen, which causes aggregation by forming cross-links between platelets. After aggregation occurs, the platelet plug is reinforced with fibrin (not shown). *AA*, Arachidonic acid; *P2Y$_{12}$*, P2Y$_{12}$ ADP receptor.

is accomplished with *antithrombin,* a protein that forms a complex with clotting factors and thereby inhibits their activity. The clotting factors that can be neutralized by antithrombin appear in yellow in Fig. 46.2. As to be discussed, antithrombin is intimately involved in the action of *heparin,* an injectable anticoagulant drug.

Physiological Removal of Clots

As healing of an injured vessel proceeds, removal of the clot is eventually necessary. The body accomplishes this with *plasmin,* an enzyme that degrades the fibrin meshwork of the clot. Plasmin is produced through the activation of its precursor, *plasminogen.* The *fibrinolytic*

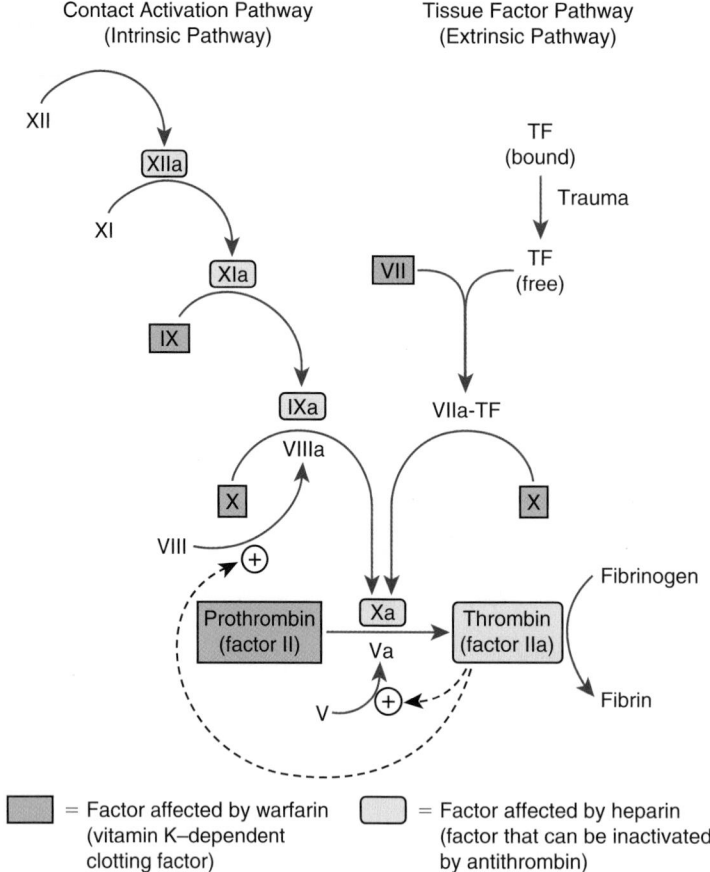

Contact Activation Pathway
(Intrinsic Pathway)

Tissue Factor Pathway
(Extrinsic Pathway)

▢ = Factor affected by warfarin
(vitamin K–dependent
clotting factor)

▢ = Factor affected by heparin
(factor that can be inactivated
by antithrombin)

Fig. 46.2 Outline of Coagulation Pathways Showing Factors Affected by Warfarin and Heparin. *TF,* Tissue factor. Common names for factors are shown in roman numerals: V, proaccelerin; VII, proconvertin; VIII, antihemophilic factor; IX, Christmas factor; X, Stuart factor; XI, plasma thromboplastin antecedent; and XII, Hageman factor. The letter "a" after a factor's name (e.g., factor VIIIa) indicates the active form of the factor.

drugs (e.g., alteplase) act by promoting the conversion of plasminogen to plasmin.

Thrombosis

A thrombus is a blood clot formed in a blood vessel or the heart. Thrombosis (thrombus formation) reflects pathological functioning of hemostatic mechanisms.

Arterial Thrombosis

Formation of an arterial thrombus begins with the adhesion of platelets to the arterial wall. (Adhesion is stimulated by damage to the wall or rupture of an atherosclerotic plaque.) After adhesion, platelets release adenosine diphosphate (ADP) and TXA₂, thereby attracting additional platelets to the evolving thrombus. With continued platelet aggregation, occlusion of the artery takes place. As blood flow comes to a stop, the coagulation cascade is initiated, causing the original plug to undergo reinforcement with fibrin. The consequence of an arterial thrombus is localized tissue injury owing to lack of perfusion.

Venous Thrombosis

Venous thrombi develop at sites where blood flow is slow. Stagnation of blood initiates the coagulation cascade, resulting in the production of fibrin, which enmeshes red blood cells and platelets to form the thrombus. The typical venous thrombus has a long tail that can break

off to produce an *embolus.* Such emboli travel within the vascular system and become lodged at faraway sites, frequently the pulmonary arteries. Hence, unlike an arterial thrombus, whose harmful effects are localized, injury from a venous thrombus occurs secondary to embolization at a site distant from the original thrombus.

OVERVIEW OF DRUGS FOR THROMBOEMBOLIC DISORDERS

The drugs considered fall into three major groups: (1) anticoagulants, (2) antiplatelet drugs, and (3) thrombolytic drugs, also known as fibrinolytic drugs. *Anticoagulants* (e.g., heparin, warfarin, dabigatran) disrupt the coagulation cascade and thereby suppress the production of fibrin. *Antiplatelet drugs* (e.g., aspirin, clopidogrel) inhibit platelet aggregation. *Thrombolytic drugs* (e.g., alteplase) promote the lysis of fibrin, causing the dissolution of thrombi. Because these drugs are used only in a hospital setting, discussion of thrombolytics occurs in Chapter 92. Drugs that belong to these groups are shown in Table 46.1.

Although the anticoagulants and antiplatelet drugs both suppress thrombosis, they do so by different mechanisms. As a result, they differ in their effects and applications. The *antiplatelet drugs* are most effective at preventing *arterial* thrombosis, whereas *anticoagulants* are most effective against *venous* thrombosis.

TABLE 46.1   Overview of Drugs for Thromboembolic Disorders

Generic Name	Trade Name	Route	Action	Therapeutic Use
Anticoagulants *Vitamin K Antagonist*			Anticoagulants decrease formation of fibrin	Used primarily to prevent thrombosis in *veins* and the *atria of the heart*
Warfarin	Coumadin	PO		
Heparin and Its Derivatives: Drugs That Activate Antithrombin				
Heparin (unfractionated)		SC, IV		
LMW heparins				
Dalteparin	Fragmin	SC		
Enoxaparin	Lovenox	SC		
Fondaparinux	Arixtra	SC		
Direct Oral Anticoagulants (DOACs) *Direct Thrombin Inhibitors*				
Dabigatran	Pradaxa, Pradax 🍁	PO		
Direct Factor Xa Inhibitors				
Rivaroxaban	Xarelto	PO		
Apixaban	Eliquis	PO		
Betrixaban	Bevyxxa	PO		
Edoxaban	Savaysa	PO		
Antiplatelet Drugs *Cyclooxygenase Inhibitor*			Antiplatelet drugs suppress platelet aggregation	Used primarily to prevent thrombosis in *arteries*
Aspirin		PO		
P2Y$_{12}$ Adenosine Diphosphate Receptor Antagonists				
Clopidogrel	Plavix	PO		
Prasugrel	Effient	PO		
Ticagrelor	Brilinta	PO		
Protease-Activated Receptor-1 (PAR-1) Antagonists				
Vorapaxar	Zontivity	PO		
Other Antiplatelet Drugs				
Dipyridamole	Persantine	PO		
Cilostazol	Pletal	PO		

DOACs, Direct oral anticoagulants; *LMW*, low molecular weight.

ANTICOAGULANTS

By definition, anticoagulants are drugs that *reduce the formation of fibrin*. Two basic mechanisms are involved. One anticoagulant—warfarin—inhibits the *synthesis* of clotting factors, including factor X and thrombin. All other anticoagulants inhibit the *activity* of clotting factors: factor Xa, thrombin, or both.

Anticoagulants are in three pharmacologic classes—vitamin K antagonists, direct factor Xa inhibitors, and direct thrombin inhibitors (see Table 46.1).

Heparin and Its Derivatives: Drugs That Activate Antithrombin

All drugs in this group share the same mechanism of action. Specifically, they greatly enhance the activity of *antithrombin*, a protein that inactivates two major clotting factors: *thrombin* and *factor Xa*. In the absence of thrombin and factor Xa, production of fibrin is reduced; hence clotting is suppressed.

This discussion focuses on three preparations: *unfractionated heparin,* the *low-molecular-weight (LMW) heparins,* and *fondaparinux.* Although all three activate antithrombin, they do not have equal effects on thrombin and factor Xa. Specifically, heparin reduces the activity of thrombin and factor Xa more or less equally; the LMW heparins reduce the activity of factor Xa more than they reduce the activity of thrombin; fondaparinux causes selective inhibition of factor Xa, having no effect on thrombin. Properties of the three preparations are shown in Table 46.2.

Heparin (Unfractionated)

Heparin is a rapid-acting anticoagulant administered only by injection. Heparin differs from warfarin (an oral anticoagulant) in several respects, including mechanism, time course, indications, and management of overdose.

Chemistry level. Heparin is not a single molecule but rather a mixture of long polysaccharide chains with molecular weights that range from 3000 to 30,000. The active region is a unique pentasaccharide (five-sugar) sequence found randomly along the chain. An important feature of

TABLE 46.2	Comparison of Drugs That Activate Antithrombin		
Property	Unfractionated Heparin	Low-Molecular-Weight Heparins	Fondaparinux
Molecular weight range	3000–30,000	1000–9000	1728
Mean molecular weight	12,000–15,000	4000–5000	1728
Mechanism of action	Activation of antithrombin, resulting in the inactivation of factor Xa and thrombin	Activation of antithrombin, resulting in preferential inactivation of factor Xa, plus some inactivation of thrombin	Activation of antithrombin, resulting in selective inactivation of factor Xa
Routes	IV, SC	SC only	SC only
Nonspecific binding	Widespread	Minimal	Minimal
Laboratory monitoring	aPTT monitoring is essential	No aPTT monitoring required	No aPTT monitoring required
Dosage	Dosage must be adjusted on the basis of aPTT	Dosage is fixed	Dosage is fixed
Setting for use	Hospital	Hospital or home	Hospital or home
Cost	$3/day for heparin itself, but hospitalization and aPTT monitoring greatly increase the real cost	$35/day for LMW heparin (enoxaparin [Lovenox]), but home use and absence of aPTT monitoring greatly reduce the real cost	$59/day for fondaparinux, but home use and absence of aPTT monitoring greatly reduce the real cost

aPTT, Activated partial thromboplastin time; *LMW,* low molecular weight.

heparin's structure is the presence of many negatively charged groups. Because of these negative charges, heparin is highly polar and hence cannot readily cross membranes.

Mechanism of anticoagulant action. Heparin suppresses coagulation by helping antithrombin inactivate clotting factors, primarily thrombin and factor Xa. As shown in Fig. 46.3, binding of heparin to antithrombin produces a conformational change in antithrombin that greatly enhances its ability to inactivate both thrombin and factor Xa. However, the process of inactivating these two clotting factors is distinct. To inactivate thrombin, heparin must simultaneously bind with both thrombin and antithrombin, thereby forming a ternary complex. In contrast, to inactivate factor Xa, heparin binds only with antithrombin; heparin itself does not bind with factor Xa.

By activating antithrombin and thereby promoting the inactivation of thrombin and factor Xa, heparin ultimately suppresses the formation of fibrin. Because fibrin forms the framework of thrombi in *veins,* heparin is especially useful for prophylaxis of *venous thrombosis.* Because thrombin and factor Xa are inhibited as soon as they bind with the heparin-antithrombin complex, the anticoagulant effects of heparin develop *quickly* (within minutes of intravenous administration). This contrasts with warfarin, whose full effects are not seen for *days.*

Therapeutic uses. Heparin is a preferred anticoagulant for use during *pregnancy* (because it does not cross the placenta) and in situations that require rapid onset of anticoagulant effects, including *pulmonary embolism* (PE) and *massive deep vein thrombosis* (DVT). In addition, heparin is used for patients undergoing *open heart surgery* and *renal dialysis;* during these procedures, heparin serves to prevent coagulation in devices of extracorporeal circulation (heart-lung machines, dialyzers). Low-dose therapy is used to *prevent postoperative venous thrombosis.* Heparin may also be useful for treating *disseminated intravascular coagulation,* a complex disorder in which fibrin clots form throughout the vascular system and in which bleeding tendencies may be present; bleeding can occur because massive fibrin production consumes available supplies of clotting factors. Heparin is also used as an adjunct to thrombolytic therapy of *acute myocardial infarction* (MI).

Adverse effects

Hemorrhage. All the drugs in this chapter increase the risk for bleeding. Bleeding develops in about 10% of patients and is the principal complication of treatment. Hemorrhage can occur at any site and may be fatal. Patients should be monitored closely for signs of blood loss. These include reduced blood pressure, increased heart rate, bruises,

petechiae, hematomas, red or black stools, cloudy or discolored urine, pelvic pain (suggesting ovarian hemorrhage), headache or faintness (suggesting cerebral hemorrhage), and lumbar pain (suggesting adrenal hemorrhage). If bleeding develops, heparin should be withdrawn.

The risk for hemorrhage can be decreased in several ways. First, dosage should be carefully controlled so that the activated partial thromboplastin time (see later) does not exceed twice the control value. In addition, candidates for heparin therapy should be screened for risk factors (see Warnings and Contraindications, further on). Finally, antiplatelet drugs (e.g., aspirin, clopidogrel) should be avoided.

⏩ **BLACK BOX WARNING**

Spinal or Epidural Hematoma

Heparin and all other anticoagulants pose a risk for spinal or epidural hematoma in patients undergoing spinal puncture or spinal or epidural anesthesia. Pressure on the spinal cord caused by the bleed can result in prolonged or permanent paralysis.

Risk for hematoma is increased by the following:
- Use of an indwelling epidural catheter
- Use of other anticoagulants (e.g., warfarin, dabigatran)
- Use of antiplatelet drugs (e.g., aspirin, clopidogrel)
- History of traumatic or repeated epidural or spinal puncture
- History of spinal deformity, spinal injury, or spinal surgery

Patients should be monitored for signs and symptoms of neurologic impairment. If impairment develops, immediate intervention is needed.

Heparin-induced thrombocytopenia. This is a potentially fatal immune-mediated disorder characterized by reduced platelet counts (thrombocytopenia) and a seemingly paradoxical *increase* in thrombotic events. The underlying cause is the development of antibodies against heparin–platelet protein complexes. These antibodies activate platelets and damage the vascular endothelium, thereby promoting both thrombosis and a rapid loss of circulating platelets. Thrombus formation poses a risk for DVT, PE, cerebral thrombosis, and MI. Ischemic injury secondary to thrombosis in the limbs may require amputation of an arm or leg. Coronary thrombosis can be fatal. The primary treatment for heparin-induced thrombocytopenia (HIT) is discontinuation of heparin and, if anticoagulation is still needed, substitution of a non-heparin anticoagulant (e.g., argatroban). The incidence of HIT is

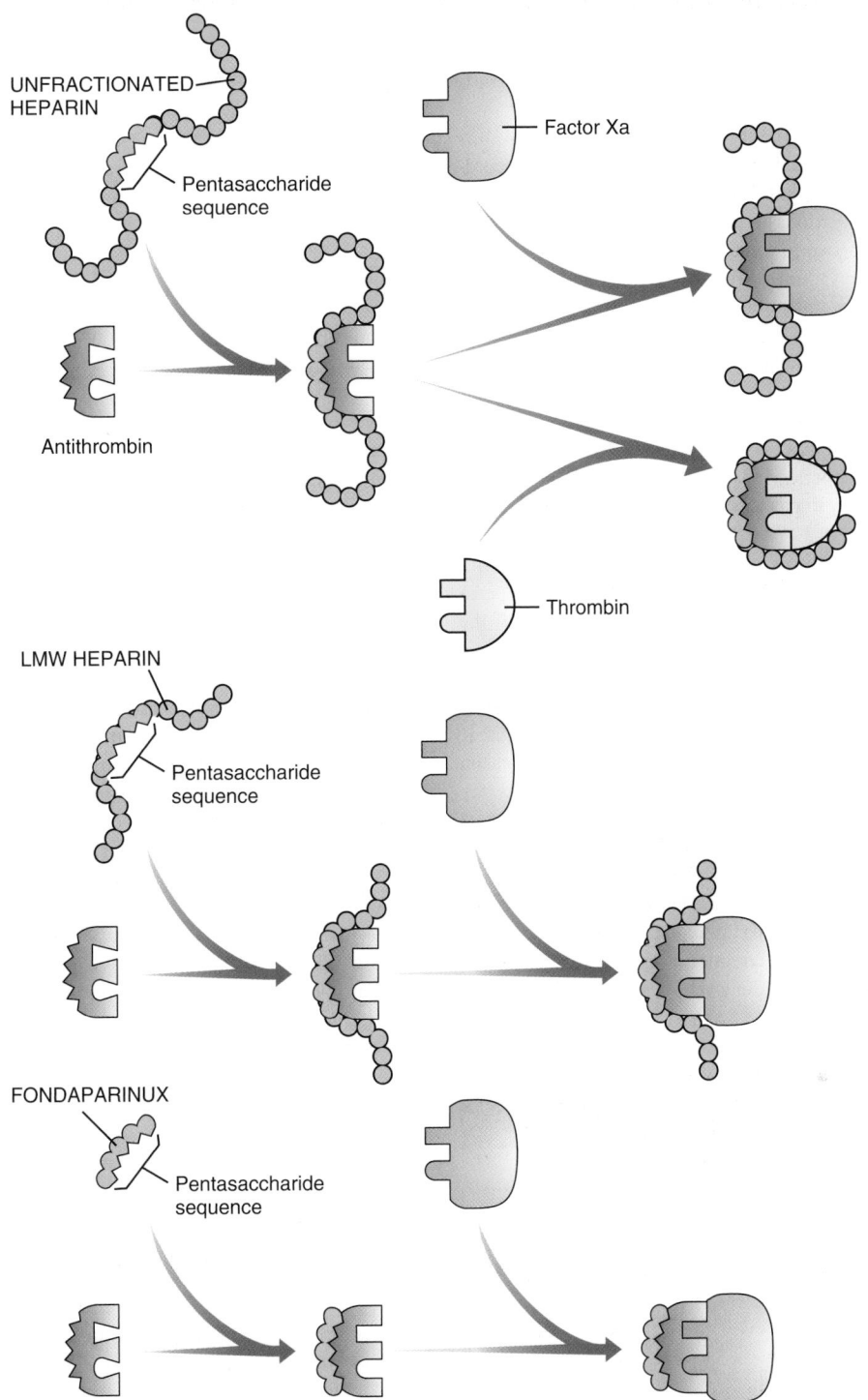

Fig. 46.3 Mechanism of Action of Heparin, Low-Molecular-Weight *(LMW)* Heparins, and Fondaparinux. All three drugs share a pentasaccharide sequence that allows them to bind with—and activate—antithrombin, a protein that inactivates two major clotting factors: thrombin and factor Xa. All three drugs enable antithrombin to inactivate factor Xa, but only heparin also facilitates inactivation of thrombin. *Upper panel:* Unfractionated heparin binds with antithrombin, causing a conformational change in antithrombin that greatly increases its ability to interact with factor Xa and thrombin. When the heparin-antithrombin complex binds with thrombin, heparin changes its conformation so that both heparin and antithrombin come in contact with thrombin. Formation of this ternary complex is necessary for thrombin inactivation. Inactivation of factor Xa is different: it only requires contact between activated antithrombin and factor Xa; contact between heparin and factor Xa is unnecessary. *Middle panel:* LMW heparins have the same pentasaccharide sequence as unfractionated heparin and can bind with and activate antithrombin. However, in contrast to unfractionated heparin, most molecules of LMW heparin can inactivate only factor Xa. They are unable to inactivate thrombin because most molecules of LMW heparin are too small to form a ternary complex with thrombin and antithrombin. *Lower panel:* Fondaparinux is a synthetic pentasaccharide identical in structure to the antithrombin binding sequence found in unfractionated heparin and LMW heparins. Being even smaller than LMW heparins, fondaparinux is too small to form a ternary complex with thrombin and can only inactivate factor Xa. *LMW,* Low molecular weight.

between 0.2% and 5% among patients who receive heparin for more than 4 days.

HIT should be suspected whenever platelet counts fall significantly or when thrombosis develops despite adequate anticoagulation. Accordingly, to reduce the risk for HIT, patients should be monitored for signs of thrombosis and for reductions in platelets. Platelet counts should be determined frequently (two to three times a week) during the first 3 weeks of heparin use and monthly thereafter. If severe thrombocytopenia develops (platelet count below 100,000/mm³), heparin should be discontinued.

Warnings and contraindications

Warnings. Heparin must be used with extreme caution in all patients who have a high likelihood of bleeding. Among these are individuals with hemophilia, increased capillary permeability, dissecting aneurysm, peptic ulcer disease, severe hypertension, or threatened abortion. Heparin must also be used cautiously in patients with severe disease of the liver or kidneys.

Contraindications. Heparin is contraindicated for patients with thrombocytopenia and uncontrollable bleeding. In addition, heparin should be avoided both during and immediately after surgery of the eye, brain, or spinal cord. Lumbar puncture and regional anesthesia are additional contraindications.

Drug interactions. In heparin-treated patients, platelet aggregation is the major remaining defense against hemorrhage. Aspirin and other drugs that depress platelet function or affect coagulation will weaken this defense and hence must be employed with caution.

Laboratory monitoring. The objective of anticoagulant therapy is to reduce blood coagulability to a level that is low enough to prevent thrombosis but not so low as to promote spontaneous bleeding. Because heparin levels can be highly variable, achieving this goal is difficult and requires careful control of dosage based on frequent tests of coagulation. The laboratory tests employed most commonly are the *activated partial thromboplastin time* (aPTT) or anti-Xa level.

PATIENT-CENTERED CARE ACROSS THE LIFE SPAN

Anticoagulants

Life Stage	Patient Care Concerns
Infants	Heparin is commonly used in infants needing anticoagulation. Argatroban has been used successfully in infants with HIT. Warfarin is also administered to infants.
Children/adolescents	Many anticoagulants can be used safely in children, just in smaller doses. Side-effect profiles are similar to those of adults.
Pregnant women	Warfarin is contraindicated in pregnancy. LMW heparins and unfractionated heparin are commonly used in pregnancy. In pregnant women with HIT, argatroban is a safe alternative.
Breastfeeding women	Data are lacking regarding safety of these medications in breastfeeding. Warfarin and heparin are both safe to use.
Older adults	In older adults, embolic stroke from atrial fibrillation is more common. Usually anticoagulation is recommended to reduce the risk, however therapy should be individualized based on bleeding risk.

FDA, US Food and Drug Administration; *HIT*, heparin-induced thrombocytopenia; *LMW*, low-molecular-weight

Low-Molecular-Weight Heparins

Group properties. LMW heparins are simply heparin preparations composed of molecules that are shorter than those found in unfractionated heparin. LMW heparins are as effective as unfractionated heparin and are easier to use because they can be given using a fixed dosage and do not require aPTT monitoring. As a result, LMW heparins can be used at home, whereas unfractionated heparin must be given in a hospital when it is administered intravenously. Because of these advantages, LMW heparins are now considered first-line therapy for the prevention and treatment of DVT. In the United States, two LMW heparins are available: enoxaparin (Lovenox) and dalteparin (Fragmin). Differences between LMW heparins and unfractionated heparin are shown in Table 46.3.

Mechanism of action. The anticoagulant activity of LMW heparin is mediated by the same active pentasaccharide sequence that mediates the anticoagulant action of unfractionated heparin. However, because LMW heparin molecules are short, they do not have quite the same effect as unfractionated heparin. Specifically, whereas unfractionated heparin is equally good at inactivating factor Xa *and* thrombin, *LMW heparins preferentially inactivate factor Xa,* being much less able to inactivate thrombin. Why the difference? To inactivate thrombin, a heparin chain must not only contain the pentasaccharide sequence that activates antithrombin but also be long enough to provide a binding site for thrombin. This binding site is necessary because inactivation of thrombin requires simultaneous binding of thrombin with heparin and antithrombin (see Fig. 46.3). In contrast to unfractionated heparin chains, most (but not all) LMW heparin chains are too short to allow thrombin binding; hence LMW heparins are less able to inactivate thrombin.

Therapeutic use. LMW heparins are *approved* for (1) the prevention of DVT after abdominal surgery, hip replacement surgery, or knee replacement surgery; (2) the treatment of established DVT, with or without PE; and (3) the prevention of ischemic complications in patients with unstable angina, non–Q-wave MI, and ST-elevation MI (STEMI). In addition, these drugs have been used extensively *off label* to prevent DVT after general surgery and in patients with multiple trauma and acute spinal injury. When used for prophylaxis or treatment of DVT, LMW heparins are at least as effective as unfractionated heparin and possibly more effective.

Administration, dosing, and monitoring. All LMW heparins are administered by subcutaneous (SC) injection. Dosage is sometimes based on body weight, depending on indication. Because plasma levels of LMW heparins are predictable for any given dose, these drugs can be employed using a fixed dosage without laboratory monitoring. This contrasts with unfractionated heparin, which requires dosage adjustments on the basis of aPTT or anti-Xa measurements. Adjustments should also be made for patients with a creatinine clearance less than 30 mL/min. Because LMW heparins have an extended half-life, dosing can be done once or twice daily. For prophylaxis of DVT, dosing is begun in the perioperative period and continued 5 to 10 days.

Adverse effects and interactions. *Bleeding* is the major adverse effect. However, the incidence of bleeding complications is less than with unfractionated heparin. Despite the potential for bleeding, LMW heparins are considered safe for outpatient use. Like unfractionated heparin, LMW heparins can cause immune-mediated *thrombocytopenia.* As with unfractionated heparin, overdose with LMW heparins can be treated with protamine sulfate.

Like unfractionated heparin, LMW heparins can cause *severe neurologic injury,* including permanent paralysis, when given to patients undergoing *spinal puncture* or *spinal or epidural anesthesia.* The risk for serious harm is increased by concurrent use of antiplatelet drugs (e.g., aspirin, clopidogrel) or anticoagulants (e.g., warfarin, dabigatran). Patients should be monitored closely for signs of neurologic impairment.

TABLE 46.3   Unfractionated Heparin, Low-Molecular-Weight Heparin, and Fondaparinux Pharmacokinetics, Doses, Indications

Drug	Class	Metabolism	Excretion	Time Course	Availability	Usual Dosing for Specified Indications
Heparin	Unfractionated heparin (UFH)	Hepatic	Renal	Immediate effects Lasts hours and varies with dosage	IV SC	VTE Ppx: 5000 units q 8–12 h VTE treatment: Varies per hospital protocol NSTEMI and STEMI: Start at 12 units/kg per hour with initial bolus
Dalteparin (Fragmin)	Low-molecular-weight heparin (LMWH)	Hepatic	Renal	Half-Life 3–5 h	SC prefilled syringes 2500 U/0.2 mL, 5000 U/0.2 mL, 7500 U/0.3 mL, 10,000 U/1 mL, 12,500 U/0.5 mL, 15,000 U/0.6 mL, 18,000 U/0.72 mL	DVT Ppx surgery and restricted mobility: 5000 units qd VTE in cancer patients: 200 units/kg per day for first month, then 150 units/kg per day Unstable angina, NSTEMI: 120 units/kg q 12 h
Enoxaparin (Lovenox)	Low-molecular-weight heparin (LMWH)	Hepatic	Renal	Half-life 4.5–7 h	SC prefilled syringes 30 mg/0.3 mL, 40 mg/04 mL, 60 mg/0.6 mL, 80 mg/0.8 mL, 100 mg/1 mL, 120 mg/0.8 mL, 150 mg/1 mL	DVT Ppx—hip or knee replacement: 30–40 mg qh (depending on patient weight) DVT Ppx—abdominal surgery and limited mobility: 40 mg qd to q 12 h depending on patient weight VTE Tx: 1 mg/kg q 12 h Unstable angina, NSTEMI: 1 mg/kg q 12 h STEMI as PCI adjunct: 1 mg/kg q 12 h with initial 30-mg bolus
Fondaparinux (Arixtra)	Selective Xa inhibitor	Hepatic	Renal	Half-life 17–21 h	SC prefilled syringes 2.5 mg/0.5 mL, 5 mg/0.4 mL, 7.5 mg/0.6 mL, 10 mg/0.8 mL	DVT Ppx orthopedic or abdominal surgery: 2.5 mg qd VTE Tx: 5–10 mg qd depending on patient weight

NSTEMI, Non–Q wave myocardial infarction; *PCI,* percutaneous coronary intervention; *Ppx,* prophylaxis; *STEMI,* ST-elevation myocardial infarction; *Tx,* treatment; *VTE,* venous thromboembolism.

Individual preparations. In the United States, two LMW heparins are available: enoxaparin and dalteparin (see Table 46.3). Additional LMW heparins are available in other countries. Each preparation is unique, so clinical experience with one may not apply fully to the other.

 SUMMARY OF KEY PRESCRIBING CONSIDERATIONS

Heparins

Therapeutic Goal: Prevention of thrombosis

Baseline Data: partial thromboplastin time (PTT), platelets, complete blood count (CBC)

Monitoring: Use of unfractionated heparin for treatment of venous thromboembolism (VTE) requires frequent monitoring of PTT or anti-Xa levels

Identifying High-Risk Patients: Heparin is contraindicated in patients with severe thrombocytopenia or uncontrollable bleeding. Use with caution in patients at high risk for bleeding.

Evaluating Therapeutic Effects: PTT or anti-Xa levels should be within therapeutic range, according to facility policy.

Minimizing Adverse Effects: Limit use with other anticoagulants or medications that can increase the risk of bleeding.

Fondaparinux

Actions. Fondaparinux (Arixtra) is a synthetic, SC anticoagulant that enhances the activity of antithrombin to cause selective inhibition of factor Xa. The result is reduced production of thrombin and hence reduced coagulation. Note that fondaparinux differs from the heparin preparations, which cause inactivation of thrombin as well as factor Xa.

Fondaparinux is closely related in structure and function to heparin and the LMW heparins. Structurally, fondaparinux is a pentasaccharide identical to the antithrombin-binding region of the heparins. Hence, like the heparins, fondaparinux is able to induce a conformational change in antithrombin, thereby increasing antithrombin's activity—but only against factor Xa, not against thrombin. Why is fondaparinux selective for factor Xa? Because the drug is quite small—even smaller than the LMW heparins. As a result, it is too small to form a complex with both antithrombin and thrombin and hence cannot reduce thrombin activity (see Fig. 46.3).

Therapeutic use. Fondaparinux is approved for (1) preventing DVT after hip fracture surgery, hip replacement surgery, knee replacement surgery, or abdominal surgery; (2) treating acute PE (in conjunction with warfarin); and (3) treating acute DVT (in conjunction with warfarin). The drug is somewhat more effective than enoxaparin (an LMW heparin) at preventing DVT but may cause slightly more bleeding.

Anticoagulation may persist for 2 to 4 days after the last dose. Fondaparinux is administered using a fixed dosage and does not require routine laboratory monitoring.

Adverse effects. As with other anticoagulants, bleeding is the biggest concern. The risk is increased by advancing age and renal impairment. Fondaparinux should be used with caution in patients with moderate renal impairment, defined as creatinine clearance (CrCl) of 30 to 50 mL/min, and avoided in patients with severe renal impairment, defined as CrCl below 30 mL/min. The drug should also be avoided for prophylactic use in patients weighing less than 50 kg because low body weight increases bleeding risk. After surgery, at least 6 hours should elapse before starting fondaparinux. Aspirin and other drugs that interfere with hemostasis should be used with caution. In contrast to overdose with heparin or LMW heparins, overdose with fondaparinux cannot be treated with protamine sulfate.

Fondaparinux does not promote immune-mediated HIT, although it can still lower platelet counts. During clinical trials, thrombocytopenia developed in 3% of patients. Platelet counts should be monitored; if they fall below 100,000/mm³, fondaparinux should be discontinued.

In patients undergoing anesthesia using an epidural or spinal catheter, fondaparinux (as well as other anticoagulants) can cause a spinal or epidural hematoma, which can result in permanent paralysis. However, in clinical trials, when fondaparinux was administered no sooner than 2 hours after catheter removal, no hematomas were reported.

Warfarin, a Vitamin K Antagonist

Warfarin (Coumadin, Jantoven), a vitamin K antagonist, is our oldest *oral* anticoagulant. The drug is similar to heparin in some respects and quite different in others. Like heparin, warfarin is used to prevent thrombosis. In contrast to heparin, warfarin has a delayed onset, which makes it inappropriate for emergencies. However, because it does not require injection, warfarin is well suited for long-term prophylaxis. As in the case of heparin, warfarin carries a significant risk for hemorrhage, which is amplified by the many drug interactions to which warfarin is subject.

History

The history of warfarin underscores its potential for harm. Warfarin was discovered after a farmer noticed that his cattle bled after eating spoiled clover silage. The causative agent was identified as bishydroxycoumarin (dicumarol). Research into derivatives of dicumarol led to the synthesis of warfarin. When warfarin was first developed, clinical use was ruled out owing to concerns about hemorrhage. So, instead of becoming a medicine, warfarin was used to kill rats. The drug proved especially effective in this application and remains one of our most widely used rodenticides. Clinical interest in warfarin was renewed after the report of a failed suicide attempt using huge doses of a warfarin-based rat poison. The clinical trials triggered by that event soon demonstrated that warfarin could be employed safely to treat humans.

Mechanism of Action

Warfarin suppresses coagulation by decreasing production of four clotting factors—factors VII, IX, X, and prothrombin. These factors are known as *vitamin K–dependent clotting factors* because an active form of vitamin K is needed to make them. Warfarin works by inhibiting *vitamin K epoxide reductase complex 1* (VKORC1), the enzyme needed to convert vitamin K to the required active form. Because of its mechanism, warfarin is referred to as a *vitamin K antagonist*, a term that is somewhat misleading because it implies antagonism of vitamin K *actions*, not antagonism of vitamin K *activation*. In therapeutic doses, warfarin reduces the production of vitamin K–dependent clotting factors by 30% to 50%. The pharmacokinetics of warfarin is shown in Table 46.4.

Therapeutic Uses

Overview of uses. Warfarin is employed most frequently for the long-term prophylaxis of thrombosis. Specific indications are (1) the prevention of venous thrombosis and associated PE, (2) the prevention of thromboembolism in patients with prosthetic heart valves, and (3) the prevention of thrombosis in patients with atrial fibrillation. The drug has also been used to reduce the risk for recurrent transient ischemic attacks (TIAs) and recurrent MI. Because onset of effects is delayed, warfarin is not useful in emergencies. When rapid action is needed, anticoagulant therapy can be initiated with heparin.

Atrial fibrillation. As discussed in Chapter 43, atrial fibrillation carries a high risk for stroke secondary to clot formation in the atrium. When people have atrial fibrillation, anticoagulant therapy is given long term to prevent clot formation. Until recently, warfarin was the only oral anticoagulant available and hence has been the reference standard for stroke prevention. However, five direct oral anticoagulants (DOACs)— dabigatran (Pradaxa, Pradax ✦), apixaban (Eliquis), betrixaban (Bevyxxa), edoxaban (Savaysa), and rivaroxaban (Xarelto)—which are much easier to use than warfarin, are likely to replace warfarin as the treatment of choice for many patients.

Monitoring Treatment

The objective of treatment is to raise the international normalized ration (INR) to an appropriate value. Recommended INR ranges are shown in Table 46.5. As indicated, an INR of 2 to 3 is appropriate for most patients—although for some patients, the target INR is 2.5 to 3.5. Unfortunately, because warfarin has a delayed onset and prolonged duration of action, the INR cannot be altered quickly: after the dosage has been changed, it may take a week or more to reach the desired INR.

INR must be determined frequently during warfarin therapy. Prothrombin time (PT) should be measured daily during the first 5 days of treatment, twice a week for the next 1 to 2 weeks, once a week for the next 1 to 2 months, and every 2 to 4 weeks thereafter. In addition, PT should be determined whenever a drug that interacts with warfarin is added to or deleted from the regimen.

Adverse Effects

Hemorrhage. Bleeding is the major complication of warfarin therapy. Hemorrhage can occur at any site. Patients should be monitored closely for signs of bleeding. If bleeding develops, warfarin should be discontinued. Severe overdose can be treated with *vitamin K* (see later). Patients should be encouraged to carry identification (e.g., a Medic

TABLE 46.4	**Warfarin Pharmacokinetics**		
Absorption	**Distribution**	**Elimination**	**Time Course**
Readily absorbed after oral dosing	Bound to albumin, 99% Unbound molecules readily cross membranes, including placenta and milk-producing glands	Renal and gastrointestinal (feces)	Half-life 6 h–2.5 days; Peak effects take several days to develop

TABLE 46.5 Monitoring Warfarin Therapy: Recommended Ranges of Prothrombin Time–Derived Values

Condition Being Treated	RECOMMENDED RANGES	
	Observed PT Ratio[a]	INR[b]
Atrial fibrillation[c]	1.3–1.5	2–3
Valvular heart disease[c]	1.3–1.5	2–3
Pulmonary embolism	1.3–1.5	2–3
Venous thrombosis[d]	1.3–1.5	2–3
Tissue heart valves[c]	1.3–1.5	2–3
Mechanical heart valves	1.5–2	3–4.5
Systemic embolism		
Prevention	1.3–1.5	2–3
Recurrent	1.5–2	2–3

[a]Observed prothrombin time (PT) ratio = ratio of patient's PT to a control PT value. In this table, the reagent used to determine the control PT value is one of the preparations of rabbit brain thromboplastin employed in the United States. Had a different preparation of thromboplastin been used, the observed PT ratio could be very different.
[b]International normalized ratio (INR) is calculated from the observed PT ratio. The INR is equivalent to the PT ratio that would have been obtained if the patient's PT has been compared with a PT value obtained using the international reference preparation, a standardized human brain thromboplastin prepared by the World Health Organization. In contrast to PT ratios, INR values are comparable from one laboratory to the next throughout the United States and the rest of the world.
[c]For prevention of ischemic stroke and systemic embolism.
[d]Prophylaxis in high-risk surgery; treatment.

Alert bracelet) to inform emergency personnel of warfarin use. Of note, compared with warfarin, the direct oral anticoagulants—apixaban, rivaroxaban, betrixaban, edoxaban, and dabigatran—pose a significantly lower risk for serious bleeds.

Several measures can reduce the risk for bleeding. Candidates for treatment must be carefully screened for risk factors (see Warnings and Contraindications further on). INR must be measured frequently. A variety of drugs can potentiate warfarin's effects (see later) and hence must be used with care.

PATIENT EDUCATION

Risk for Bleeding With Warfarin

Patients should be given detailed verbal and written instructions regarding signs of bleeding, dosage size and timing, and scheduling of INR tests. When a patient is incapable of accurate self-medication, a responsible individual must supervise treatment. Patients should be advised to make a record of each dose rather than relying on memory. A soft toothbrush can reduce gingival bleeding. An electric razor can reduce cuts from shaving.

Warfarin intensifies bleeding during surgery. Accordingly, surgeons must be informed of warfarin use. Patients anticipating elective procedures should discontinue warfarin at least 5 days before the appointment. If an emergency procedure must be performed, injection of vitamin K can help suppress bleeding.

Fetal hemorrhage and teratogenesis from use during pregnancy. Warfarin can cross the placenta and affect the developing fetus. Fetal hemorrhage and death have occurred. In addition, warfarin can cause gross malformations, central nervous system defects, and optic atrophy. Accordingly, use of warfarin during pregnancy is contraindicated. Women of childbearing age should be informed about the potential for teratogenesis and advised to postpone pregnancy. If pregnancy occurs, the possibility of termination should be discussed. If an anticoagulant is needed during pregnancy, heparin or LMW heparin, which do not cross the placenta, should be employed.

Use during lactation. Warfarin enters breast milk. Women should be advised against breastfeeding.

Drug Interactions

General considerations. Warfarin is subject to a large number of clinically significant adverse interactions—perhaps more than from any other drug. As a result of interactions, anticoagulant effects may be reduced to the point of permitting thrombosis, or they may be increased to the point of causing hemorrhage. Patients must be informed about the potential for hazardous interactions and instructed to avoid *all* drugs not specifically approved by the prescriber. This prohibition includes prescription drugs and over-the-counter products.

Interactions between warfarin and other drugs are shown in Table 46.6. As indicated, the interactants fall into three major categories: (1) *drugs that increase anticoagulant effects,* (2) *drugs that promote bleeding,* and (3) *drugs that decrease anticoagulant effects.* The major mechanisms by which anticoagulant effects can be *increased* are (1) displacement of warfarin from plasma albumin, (2) inhibition of the hepatic enzymes that degrade warfarin, and (3) decreased synthesis of clotting factors. The major mechanisms for *decreasing* anticoagulant effects are (1) acceleration of warfarin degradation through the induction of hepatic drug-metabolizing enzymes, (2) increased synthesis of clotting factors, and (3) inhibition of warfarin absorption. Mechanisms by which drugs can *promote bleeding,* and thereby complicate anticoagulant therapy, include (1) inhibition of platelet aggregation, (2) inhibition of clotting factors, and (3) generation of gastrointestinal (GI) ulcers.

The existence of an interaction between warfarin and another drug does not absolutely preclude using the combination. The interaction does mean, however, that the combination must be used with due caution. The potential for harm is greatest when an interacting drug is being added to or withdrawn from the regimen. At these times, PT must be monitored and the dosage of warfarin adjusted to compensate for the effect of removing or adding an interacting drug.

Warnings and Contraindications

Like heparin, warfarin is contraindicated for patients with severe thrombocytopenia or uncontrollable bleeding and for those undergoing lumbar puncture, regional anesthesia, or surgery of the eye, brain, or spinal cord. Also like heparin, warfarin must be used with extreme caution in patients at high risk for bleeding, including those with hemophilia, increased capillary permeability, dissecting aneurysm, GI ulcers, and severe hypertension and in women anticipating abortion. In addition, warfarin is contraindicated in the presence of vitamin K deficiency, liver disease, and alcoholism—conditions that can disrupt the hepatic synthesis of clotting factors. Warfarin is also contraindicated during pregnancy and lactation.

Vitamin K_1 for warfarin overdose. The effects of warfarin overdose can be overcome with vitamin K_1 (phytonadione). Vitamin K_1 antagonizes warfarin's actions and can thereby reverse the warfarin-induced inhibition of clotting factor synthesis. (Vitamin K_3—menadione—has no effect on warfarin action.)

TABLE 46.6   Interactions Between Warfarin and Other Drugs

Drug Category	Mechanism of Interaction	Representative Interacting Drugs
Drugs that *increase* the effects of warfarin	Displacement of warfarin from albumin	Aspirin and other salicylates
		Sulfonamides
	Inhibition of warfarin degradation	Acetaminophen
		Amiodarone
		Azole antifungal agents
		Cimetidine
		Disulfiram
		Leflunomide
		Trimethoprim-sulfamethoxazole
	Decreased synthesis of clotting factors	Certain parenteral cephalosporins, including cefoperazone and cefamandole
Drugs that *promote bleeding*	Inhibition of platelet aggregation	Abciximab
		Aspirin and other salicylates
		Cilostazol
		Clopidogrel
		Dipyridamole
		Eptifibatide
		Prasugrel
		Ticagrelor
		Ticlopidine
		Tirofiban
	Inhibition of clotting factors and/or thrombin	Antimetabolites
		Apixaban
		Argatroban
		Bivalirudin
		Dabigatran
		Desirudin
		Fondaparinux
		Heparins
		Rivaroxaban
	Promotion of ulcer formation	Aspirin
		Glucocorticoids
		Indomethacin
		Phenylbutazone
Drugs that *decrease* the effects of warfarin	Induction of drug-metabolizing enzymes	Carbamazepine
		Phenobarbital
		Phenytoin
		Rifampin
	Promotion of clotting factor synthesis	Oral contraceptives
		Vitamin K_1
	Reduction of warfarin absorption	Cholestyramine
		Colestipol

As a rule, small doses—2.5 mg by oral administration (PO)—are preferred. Large doses (e.g., 10 mg PO) can cause prolonged resistance to warfarin, thereby hampering restoration of anticoagulation after bleeding is under control.

If vitamin K fails to control bleeding or if life or organ threatening bleeding occurs, levels of clotting factors can be raised quickly by infusing fresh whole blood, fresh-frozen plasma, or plasma concentrates of vitamin K–dependent clotting factors.

What about dietary vitamin K? Like medicinal vitamin K, dietary vitamin K can reduce the anticoagulant effects of warfarin. Dietary sources include mayonnaise, canola oil, soybean oil, and green leafy vegetables. Patients need not avoid these foods, but instead should keep their intake of vitamin K constant. If vitamin K intake does increase,

warfarin dosage should be increased as well. Conversely, if vitamin K intake decreases, the warfarin dosage should also decrease.

Contrasts between warfarin and heparin. Although heparin and warfarin are both anticoagulants, they differ in important ways (Table 46.7). Whereas warfarin is given orally, heparin is given by injection. Although both drugs decrease fibrin formation, they do so by different mechanisms: heparin inactivates thrombin and factor Xa, whereas warfarin inhibits the synthesis of clotting factors. Heparin and warfarin differ with respect to time course of action: effects of heparin begin and fade rapidly, whereas effects of warfarin begin slowly but persist for several days. Different tests are used to monitor therapy: changes in aPTT are used to monitor heparin treatment; changes in PT are used to monitor warfarin. Finally, these drugs differ with respect to

TABLE 46.7 Contrasts Between Heparin and Warfarin

	Heparin	Warfarin
Mechanism of action	Activates antithrombin, which then inactivates thrombin and factor Xa	Inhibits synthesis of vitamin K–dependent clotting factors, including prothrombin and factor X
Route	IV or SC	PO
Onset	Rapid (minutes)	Slow (hours)
Duration	Brief (hours)	Prolonged (days)
Monitoring	aPTT	PT (INR)[a]
Antidote for overdose	Protamine	Vitamin K$_1$

[a]Test results are reported as an INRinternational normalized ratio.
aPTT, Activated partial thromboplastin time; *INR*, international normalized ratio; *IV*, intravenous; *PO*, by mouth; *PT*, prothrombin time; *SC*, subcutaneous.

management of overdose: protamine is given to counteract heparin; vitamin K$_1$ is given to counteract warfarin.

SUMMARY OF KEY PRESCRIBING CONSIDERATIONS

Warfarin

Therapeutic Goal: Prevention of thrombosis.
Baseline Data: PT, CBC. Genetic testing for variants of CYP2C9 and VKORC1 may be done to identify patients who may require a reduction in warfarin dosage.
Monitoring: PT/INR should be monitored frequently at the onset of therapy (daily to every few days). Once the INR goal has been obtained and is stable on a weekly basis, monthly monitoring is reasonable.
Identifying High-Risk Patients: Warfarin is contraindicated in pregnancy and in patients with uncontrollable bleeding. Use with caution in patients with vitamin K deficiency or liver disease and in those with a high risk of bleeding.
Evaluating Therapeutic Effects: PT/INR should be within target range for the specified patient goal.
Minimizing Adverse Effects: Counsel patients on diet and medication interactions.

DIRECT ORAL ANTICOAGULANTS

Direct Thrombin Inhibitors

The anticoagulants discussed in this section work by the direct inhibition of thrombin. Hence they differ from the heparin-like anticoagulants, which inhibit thrombin indirectly (by enhancing the activity of antithrombin). The pharmacokinetics of these drugs are located in Table 46.9. One of the direct thrombin inhibitors—dabigatran—is administered orally; and two others—bivalirudin and argatroban—are administered by continuous intravenous infusion. Only the PO drugs are suitable for outpatient use.

Dabigatran Etexilate

Dabigatran etexilate (Pradaxa, Pradax) is an *oral* prodrug that undergoes rapid conversion to *dabigatran,* a reversible direct thrombin inhibitor. Compared with warfarin—our oldest oral anticoagulant—dabigatran has

five major advantages: rapid onset; no need to monitor anticoagulation; few drug–food interactions; lower risk for major bleeding; and, because responses are predictable, the same dose can be used for all patients regardless of age or weight. Contrasts between dabigatran and warfarin are shown in Table 46.8.

Mechanism of action. Dabigatran is a direct, reversible inhibitor of thrombin. The drug binds with and inhibits thrombin that is free in the blood as well as thrombin that is bound to clots. In contrast, heparin inhibits only free thrombin. By inhibiting thrombin, dabigatran (1) prevents the conversion of fibrinogen into fibrin and (2) prevents the activation of factor XIII, thereby also preventing the conversion of soluble fibrin into insoluble fibrin.

Therapeutic use

Atrial fibrillation. In the United States, dabigatran was first approved for the prevention of stroke and systemic embolism in patients with nonvalvular atrial fibrillation. Approval was based on the Randomized Evaluation of Long-Term Anticoagulation Therapy (RE-LY) trial, in which more than 18,000 patients were randomized to receive either dabigatran (110 or 150 mg twice daily) or warfarin (dosage adjusted to produce an INR of 2 to 3). At the lower dabigatran dose (110 mg twice daily), the incidence of bleeding with dabigatran was less than that with warfarin, but protection against stroke was also less. By contrast, at the higher dose (150 mg twice daily), the incidence of bleeding with dabigatran equaled that with warfarin, but the incidence of stroke or embolism was significantly lower. On the basis of these results, the US Food and Drug Administration (FDA) concluded that, for patients with atrial fibrillation, the benefit/risk profile of dabigatran was better at 150 mg twice daily than at 110 mg twice daily; hence the FDA approved the higher dose for these patients.

Knee or hip replacement. Dabigatran is approved for the prevention of VTE after knee or hip replacement surgery. The dosage is 220 mg qd after an initial dose of 110 mg.

Treatment of deep venous thrombosis and pulmonary embolism. In 2014, the FDA approved dabigatran for the treatment of DVT and PE in patients who have been treated with a parenteral anticoagulant for 5 to 10 days and to reduce the risk for recurrent DVT and PE in patients who have been previously treated. The dose for treatment is 150 mg twice daily.

Adverse effects

Bleeding. Like all other anticoagulants, dabigatran can cause bleeding. In the RE-LY trial, about 17% of patients taking 150 mg of dabigatran twice daily experienced bleeding of any intensity, and 3% experienced major bleeding. Patients who develop pathologic bleeding should stop taking the drug. Compared with warfarin, dabigatran is safer, posing a much lower risk for hemorrhagic stroke and other major bleeds.

Because dabigatran is not highly protein-bound, dialysis can remove much of the drug (about 60% over 2 to 3 hours). Because dabigatran is eliminated primarily in the urine, maintaining adequate diuresis is important.

Owing to bleeding risk, dabigatran should be stopped before elective surgery. For patients with normal renal function (CrCl 50 mL/min or higher), dosing should stop 1 or 2 days before surgery. For patients with renal impairment (CrCl below 50 mL/min), dosing should stop 3 to 5 days before surgery.

Gastrointestinal disturbances. About 35% of patients experience *dyspepsia* (abdominal pain, bloating, nausea, vomiting) and/or *gastritis-like symptoms* (esophagitis, gastroesophageal reflux disease, gastric hemorrhage, erosive gastritis, hemorrhagic gastritis, GI ulcer). Symptoms of *dyspepsia* can be reduced by taking dabigatran with food and by using an acid-suppressing drug (proton pump inhibitor or histamine-2 receptor blocker). If these measures do not help, patients may try a switch to warfarin, which carries a much lower risk for adverse GI effects.

TABLE 46.8   Properties of Oral Anticoagulants

	Warfarin (Coumadin)	Rivaroxaban (Xarelto)	Apixaban (Eliquis)	Betrixaban (Bevyxxa)	Edoxaban (Savaysa)	Dabigatran Etexilate (Pradaxa, Pradax ✦)
Mechanism	Decreased synthesis of vitamin K–dependent clotting factors	Inhibition of factor Xa	Inhibition of factor Xa	Inhibition of factor Xa	Inhibition of factor Xa	Direct inhibition of thrombin
Indications and Usual Dosing						
Atrial fibrillation	Yes Varies per INR	Yes 20 mg qd	Yes 5 mg bid	No	Yes 60 mg qd	Yes 150 mg bid
Heart valve replacement	Yes Varies per INR	No	No	No	No	No
Knee or hip replacement	Yes Varies per INR	Yes 10 mg qd	Yes 2.5 mg bid	No	No	Yes 220 mg qd
Onset	Delayed (days)	Rapid (hours)	Rapid (hours)	Rapid (hours)	Rapid (hours)	Rapid (hours)
Duration	Prolonged	Short	Short	Short	Short	Short
Antidote available	Yes (oral/parenteral vitamin K)	Yes (Andexanet alfa)	Yes (Andexanet alfa)	No	No	Yes (Idaricuzumab)
Drug-food interactions	Many	Few	Few	Few	Few	Few
INR testing needed	Yes	No	No	No	No	No
Dosage	Adjusted based on INR	Fixed	Fixed	Fixed	Fixed	Fixed
Doses/day	One	One	Two	One	One	Two
Clinical experience	Extensive	Limited	Limited	Limited	Limited	Limited
Advantages, summary	• Decades of clinical experience • Precise dosage timing not critical, owing to long duration • Antidote available for overdose	• Rapid onset • Fixed dosage • No blood tests needed • Less bleeding and hemorrhagic stroke • Few drug–food interactions • Antidote available for overdose	Same as rivaroxaban	Same as rivaroxaban but no antidote	Same as rivaroxaban but no antidote	Same as rivaroxaban
Disadvantages, summary	• Delayed onset • Blood tests required • No fixed dosage • Many drug–food interactions	• Dosing on time is important, owing to short duration	Same as rivaroxaban	Approved only for VTE prophylaxis in patients with moderate to severe restricted mobility	Same as rivaroxaban but no antidote to overdose	Same as rivaroxaban *plus* gastrointestinal disturbances are common

TABLE 46.9   Pharmacokinetics of the Direct Oral Anticoagulants

Drug	Absorption	Distribution	Metabolism	Elimination
Rivaroxaban (Xarelto)	Readily absorbed with high bioavailability (80%–100%).	92%–95% Protein bound.	Hepatic	Renal and GI (feces)
Apixaban (Eliquis)	Moderate (50%) bioavailability	87% protein bound	Hepatic	Renal and GI (feces)
Betrixaban (Bevyxxa)	Low to moderate (35%) bioavailability	60% protein bound	Hepatic	GI (feces) and renal
Edoxaban (Savaysa)	Moderate (62%) bioavailability	55% protein bound	Minimal	Renal
Dabigatran (Pradaxa)	Well absorbed from GI tract	35% protein bound	Minimal	Renal

Drug interactions. Dabigatran is not metabolized by hepatic P450 enzymes, nor is it an inhibitor or inducer of these enzymes. Accordingly, dabigatran does not have metabolic interactions with other drugs.

Dabigatran etexilate is a substrate for intestinal *P-glycoprotein,* the transporter protein that can pump dabigatran and other drugs back into the intestine. Drugs that inhibit P-glycoprotein can increase dabigatran absorption and blood levels, and drugs that induce P-glycoprotein can decrease dabigatran absorption and blood levels. Combined use with a P-glycoprotein *inhibitor* (e.g., ketoconazole, amiodarone, verapamil, quinidine) can cause bleeding from excessive dabigatran levels; hence patients taking these combinations should be monitored closely. Combined use with a P-glycoprotein *inducer* appears to be safe, even though it might reduce the beneficial effects somewhat.

Bleeding risk is increased by other drugs that impair hemostasis.

Direct Factor Xa Inhibitors
Rivaroxaban

Actions and uses. Rivaroxaban (Xarelto) is an *oral* anticoagulant that causes selective inhibition of factor Xa (activated factor X). Unlike fondaparinux, which acts indirectly (see earlier), rivaroxaban binds directly with the active center of factor Xa and thereby inhibits the production of thrombin. Compared with warfarin, our oldest oral anticoagulant, rivaroxaban and the other direct oral anticoagulants have several advantages: rapid onset, fixed dosage, lower bleeding risk, few drug interactions, and no need for INR monitoring. Rivaroxaban has four approved uses: (1) prevention of DVT and PE after total hip or knee replacement surgery, (2) prevention of stroke in patients with atrial fibrillation, (3) prevention of recurrent DVT and PE, and (4) treatment of DVT and PE unrelated to orthopedic surgery. Contrasts with warfarin are shown in Table 46.8.

Adverse effects

Bleeding. Bleeding is the most common adverse effect and can occur at any site. Patients have experienced epidural hematomas as well as major intracranial, retinal, adrenal, and GI bleeds. Some people have died. Bleeding risk is increased by other drugs that impede hemostasis. How does rivaroxaban compare with warfarin? The risk for hemorrhagic stroke and other major bleeds is significantly lower with rivaroxaban. Drug reversal is discussed later.

Spinal or epidural hematoma. Like all other anticoagulants, rivaroxaban poses a risk for spinal or epidural hematoma in patients undergoing spinal puncture or epidural anesthesia. Prolonged or permanent paralysis can result. Rivaroxaban should be discontinued at least 18 hours before removing an epidural catheter; after the catheter is out, another 6 hours should elapse before rivaroxaban is restarted. If a traumatic puncture occurs, rivaroxaban should be delayed for at least 24 hours. Anticoagulant-related spinal or epidural hematoma was discussed further earlier (see Adverse Effects, under Heparin).

Drug interactions. Levels of rivaroxaban can be altered by drugs that inhibit or induce CYP3A4 and P-glycoprotein. Specifically, in patients with *normal renal function,* drugs that inhibit CYP3A4 strongly *and also* inhibit P-glycoprotein (e.g., ketoconazole, itraconazole, ritonavir) can raise rivaroxaban levels enough to increase the risk for bleeding. Similarly, in patients with *renal impairment,* drugs that inhibit CYP3A4 moderately *and also* inhibit P-glycoprotein (e.g., amiodarone, dronedarone, quinidine, diltiazem, verapamil, ranolazine, macrolide antibiotics) can raise rivaroxaban levels enough to increase the risk for bleeding. Conversely, drugs that induce CYP3A4 strongly *and also* induce P-glycoprotein (e.g., carbamazepine, phenytoin, rifampin, St. John's wort) may reduce rivaroxaban levels enough to increase the risk for thrombotic events. Of note, rivaroxaban itself does not inhibit or induce cytochrome P450 enzymes or P-glycoprotein and hence is unlikely to alter the effects of other drugs.

Owing to the risk for bleeding, rivaroxaban should not be combined with other anticoagulants. Concurrent use with antiplatelet drugs and fibrinolytics should be done with caution.

Precautions

Renal impairment. Renal impairment can delay the excretion of rivaroxaban and can thereby increase the risk for bleeding. Accordingly, rivaroxaban should be avoided in patients with *severe* renal impairment, indicated by a CrCl below 30 mL/min. In patients with moderate renal impairment (CrCl 30 to 50 mL/min), rivaroxaban should be used with caution. If renal failure develops during treatment, rivaroxaban should be discontinued.

Hepatic impairment. In clinical trials, rivaroxaban levels and anticoagulation were excessive in patients with moderate hepatic impairment. Accordingly, in patients with moderate or severe hepatic impairment, rivaroxaban should not be used.

Pregnancy. Rivaroxaban appears to be unsafe in pregnancy. The drug increases the risk for pregnancy-related hemorrhage and may have detrimental effects on the fetus. When pregnant rabbits were given high doses (10 mg/kg or more) during organogenesis, rivaroxaban increased fetal resorption, decreased fetal weight, and decreased the number of live fetuses. However, dosing of rats and rabbits early in pregnancy was not associated with gross fetal malformations. Rivaroxaban should be used only if the benefits are deemed to outweigh the risks to the mother and fetus.

Reversal of the Direct Oral Anticoagulants

Although the risk of bleeding is less than with warfarin, the main concern with use of the DOACs remains bleeding. When these drugs first emerged, there were no known specific antidotes. Lack of an antidote led to an uneasiness regarding care of the patient with bleeding, overdose or of patients requiring emergent surgical procedures. As the use of DOACs increased, two antidotes have been approved; idarucizumab and andexanet alfa. These and other options for reversal are shown in Tables 46.10 and 46.11. To assist in decision making, the American College of Cardiology published a decision pathway in 2017 titled, *2017 ACC Expert Consensus Decision Pathway on Management of Bleeding in Patients on Oral Anticoagulants.*

ANTIPLATELET DRUGS

Antiplatelet drugs suppress platelet aggregation. Because a platelet core constitutes the bulk of an *arterial thrombus,* the principal indication

---

TABLE 46.10 Approved Direct Oral Anticoagulant Reversal Agents

Drug	Reversal Agent	Mechanism of Reversal Agent	Suggested Dosing	Approved Indication
Apixaban (Eliquis) Rivaroxaban (Xarelto)	Andexanet alfa (Andexxa)	Binds and sequesters the Xa inhibitors. Also binds and inhibits the activity of tissue factor pathway inhibitor.	400–800 mg IV bolus followed by 4–8 mg/min infusion depending on last DOAC dose	For life-threatening or uncontrolled bleeding
Dabigatran (Pradaxa)	Idarucizumab (Praxbind)	Monoclonal antibody fragment that binds to dabigatran	5 g IV once, may repeat dose ×1	Emergency surgery or urgent procedures Life-threatening or uncontrolled bleeding

DOAC, Direct oral anticoagulant; *IV,* intravenous.

SUMMARY OF KEY PRESCRIBING CONSIDERATIONS

DOACs

> **Therapeutic Goal:** Prevention and treatment of thrombosis.
> **Baseline Data:** PTT, CBC, renal function.
> **Monitoring:** No routine monitoring is required with these drugs.
> **Identifying High-Risk Patients:** Use is contraindicated in patients with uncontrolled bleeding. Use with caution in patients with high risk for bleeding or renal dysfunction.
> **Evaluating Therapeutic Effects:** Patients should remain free of stroke symptoms or worsening signs of VTE.
> **Minimizing Adverse Effects:** Educate patients on the increased risk of bleeding and tell them to inform health care providers of the use of such an agent prior to any procedures or surgery.

for the antiplatelet drugs is the prevention of thrombosis in *arteries*. In contrast, the principal indication for anticoagulants (e.g., heparin, warfarin) is the prevention of thrombosis in veins.

There are four major groups of antiplatelet drugs: aspirin (a "group" with only one member), P2Y$_{12}$ ADP receptor antagonists,

PAR-1 antagonists, and GP IIb/IIIa receptor antagonists. As indicated in Fig. 46.1, aspirin and the P2Y$_{12}$ ADP receptor antagonists affect only one pathway in platelet activation; hence their antiplatelet effects are limited. In contrast, the GP IIb/IIIa antagonists block the final common step in platelet activation; hence they have powerful antiplatelet effects. Properties of the major classes of antiplatelet drugs are shown in Table 46.12. Because GP IIb/IIIa antagonists are given only in the hospital setting, they are discussed further in Chapter 92.

Aspirin

The basic pharmacology of aspirin is discussed in Chapter 57. Consideration here is limited to aspirin's role in preventing arterial thrombosis.

Mechanism of Antiplatelet Action

Aspirin suppresses platelet aggregation by causing *irreversible inhibition of cyclooxygenase*, an enzyme required by platelets to synthesize TXA$_2$. As noted, TXA$_2$ is one of the factors that can promote platelet activation. In addition to activating platelets, TXA$_2$ acts on vascular smooth muscle to promote vasoconstriction. Both actions promote hemostasis. By inhibiting cyclooxygenase, aspirin suppresses both TXA$_2$-mediated vasoconstriction and platelet aggregation, thereby reducing the risk for arterial thrombosis. Because inhibition of cyclooxygenase by aspirin is irreversible and platelets lack the machinery to synthesize new cyclooxygenase, the effects of a single dose of aspirin persist for the life of the platelet (7 to 10 days).

In addition to inhibiting the synthesis of TXA$_2$, aspirin can inhibit synthesis of *prostacyclin* by the blood vessel wall. Because prostacyclin has effects that are exactly opposite to those of TXA$_2$—namely, suppression of platelet aggregation and promotion of vasodilation—suppression of prostacyclin synthesis can partially offset the beneficial effects of aspirin therapy. Fortunately, aspirin is able to inhibit synthesis of TXA$_2$ at doses that are lower than those needed to inhibit synthesis of prostacyclin. Accordingly, if we keep the dosage of aspirin *low* (325 mg/day or less), we can minimize inhibition of prostacyclin production while maintaining inhibition of TXA$_2$ production.

TABLE 46.11   Factor Products for the Reversal of Direct Oral Anticoagulants

Factor Product	Factors
Recombinant factor VII (NovoSeven)	FVII
Three-factor PCC (Bebulin, Profilnine)	FII, FIX, FX, heparin
Four-factor PCC (KCentra)	FII, FVII, FIX, FX, proteins C and S, heparin
Activated PCC (FEIBA)	FII, activated FVII, FIX, FX, protein C

PCC, Prothrombin complex concentrate.
Adapted from Jariwala A, Hamman K. Stop bleeding! Oral anticoagulation and options for reversal. *JNP.* 2018;14(1):54–55.

TABLE 46.12   Properties of the Major Classes of Antiplatelet Drugs and Usual Dosing

	Aspirin, a Cyclooxygenase Inhibitor	P2Y$_{12}$ ADP Receptor Blockers	PAR-1 Antagonists
Representative drug	Aspirin	Clopidogrel (Plavix) Prasugrel (Effient) Ticagrelor (Brilinta)	Vorapaxar (Zontivity)
Mechanism of antiplatelet action	Irreversibly inhibits cyclooxygenase and thereby blocks synthesis of thromboxane A$_2$	Irreversibly blocks receptors for ADP[a]	Reversibly blocks the PAR-1 expressed on platelets
Route	PO	PO	PO
Duration of effects	Effects persist 7–10 days after the last dose	Effects persist 7–10 days after the last dose[a]	Effects persist 7–10 days after the last dose
Usual dosing	Primary prevention of cardiovascular disease or colorectal cancer: 81 mg daily Acute coronary syndrome 162–325 mg	Clopidogrel: Prevention of thrombosis: 75 mg/day Acute coronary syndrome: 300 mg once followed by 75 mg/day Prasugrel: Acute coronary syndrome: 60 mg once followed by 10 mg/day Ticagrelor: Prevention of thrombosis: 60 mg bid Acute coronary syndrome: 180 mg once followed by 90 mg qd	Prevention of thrombosis: 2.08 mg/day
Cost	$3/month	$87/month	$320/month

[a]ADP receptor blocker—ticagrelor (Brilinta)—causes reversible ADP receptor blockade, so effects wear off faster than with clopidogrel.
ADP, Adenosine diphosphate; *PAR-1,* protease-activated receptor-1.

Indications for Antiplatelet Therapy

Antiplatelet therapy with aspirin has multiple indications of proven efficacy:

- *Ischemic stroke* (to reduce the risk for death and nonfatal stroke)
- *Transient ischemic attacks* (*TIAs*) (to reduce the risk for death and nonfatal stroke)
- *Chronic stable angina* (to reduce the risk for MI and sudden death)
- *Unstable angina* (to reduce the combined risk for death and nonfatal MI)
- *Coronary stenting* (to prevent reocclusion)
- *Acute MI* (to reduce the risk for vascular mortality)
- *Previous MI* (to reduce the combined risk for death and nonfatal MI)
- *Primary prevention of MI* (to prevent a first MI in men and in women aged 65 and older)

In all of these situations, prophylactic therapy with aspirin can reduce morbidity and possibly mortality. Primary prevention of MI is discussed further next.

Primary prevention of myocardial infarction. Currently, the US Preventive Services Task Force (USPSTF) recommends the use of low-dose aspirin for prevention of cardiovascular disease and colorectal cancer in adults aged 50 to 59 years who have a 10% or greater 10-year cardiovascular disease (CVD) risk, are not at increased risk for bleeding, have a life expectancy of at least 10 years, and are willing to take low-dose aspirin daily for at least 10 years. In patients younger than 50 years or older than 70 years, the evidence regarding risk versus benefit is inconclusive. In patients between the ages of 60 and 69 years, the assessment of benefit should outweigh the risk of bleeding. A recent study in the *New England Journal of Medicine* showed an increased mortality with use of aspirin in healthy older adults and no reduction in disability, cardiovascular disease, or dementia. There was also an increase in GI bleeding. Ultimately each patient should be treated individually after completion of a CVD risk assessment and discussion.

Cardiovascular risk is based on five factors—age, gender, cholesterol levels, blood pressure, and smoking status—and can be calculated using an online risk assessment tool, such as those at www.med-decisions.com. Although the optimal aspirin dosage for primary prevention is unknown, low doses (e.g., 81 mg/day) appear to be as effective as higher ones.

Adverse Effects

Even in low doses, aspirin increases the risk for GI bleeding and hemorrhagic stroke. Among middle-aged people taking aspirin for 5 years, the estimated rate of major GI bleeding episodes is 2 to 4 per 1000 patients, and the rate of hemorrhagic stroke is 0 to 2 episodes per 1000 patients. Use of enteric-coated or buffered aspirin may *not* reduce the risk for GI bleeding. Benefits of treatment must be weighed against bleeding risks. If GI bleeding occurs, adding a proton pump inhibitor (e.g., omeprazole [Prilosec]) to reduce gastric acidity can help.

P2Y₁₂ Adenosine Diphosphate Receptor Antagonists

Drugs in this class block $P2Y_{12}$ ADP receptors on the platelet surface, preventing ADP-stimulated aggregation (see Fig. 46.1). Three $P2Y_{12}$ ADP receptor antagonists are available. Two of them—clopidogrel and prasugrel—cause *irreversible* receptor blockade, and the third—ticagrelor—causes *reversible* receptor blockade. Clopidogrel, prasugrel, and ticagrelor are used for secondary prevention of atherothrombotic events in patients with acute coronary syndrome (ACS), defined as unstable angina or MI. All three drugs are taken orally and can cause serious bleeding.

Clopidogrel

Clopidogrel (Plavix) is an oral antiplatelet drug with effects much like those of aspirin. The drug is taken to prevent stenosis of coronary stents and for secondary prevention of MI, ischemic stroke, and other vascular events.

Antiplatelet actions. Clopidogrel blocks $P2Y_{12}$ ADP receptors on platelets and thereby prevents ADP-stimulated platelet aggregation. As with aspirin, antiplatelet effects are irreversible and hence persist for the life of the platelet. Effects begin 2 hours after the first dose and plateau after 3 to 7 days of treatment. At the recommended dosage, platelet aggregation is inhibited by 40% to 60%. Platelet function and bleeding time return to baseline 7 to 10 days after the last dose.

Pharmacokinetics. Clopidogrel is rapidly absorbed from the GI tract, both in the presence and absence of food. Bioavailability is about 50%. Clopidogrel is a *prodrug* that undergoes metabolism to its active form, primarily by hepatic CYP2C19 (the 2C19 isoenzyme of cytochrome P450). People with variant forms of the CYP2C19 gene are *poor metabolizers* of clopidogrel and hence may not benefit adequately from the drug.

Therapeutic use. Clopidogrel is used widely to prevent blockage of coronary artery stents and to reduce thrombotic events—MI, ischemic stroke, and vascular death—in patients with ACS and in those with atherosclerosis documented by recent MI, recent stroke, or established peripheral arterial disease. In patients with ACS, clopidogrel should always be combined with aspirin (75 to 325 mg once daily).

▶▶ BLACK BOX WARNING

Clopidogrel

Clopidogrel should not be used in poor metabolizers. Patients with variant forms of the *CYP2C19* gene cannot reliably convert clopidogrel to its active form. When treated with standard dosages of clopidogrel, these poor metabolizers exhibit a higher rate of cardiovascular events compared with normal metabolizers.

Poor metabolizers can be identified by testing a blood or saliva sample for CYP2C19 variants or by simply measuring the platelet response to treatment. Unfortunately, even with this information, the course of action is not clear. Yes, poor metabolizers could be given higher doses, but doses that might be safe and effective have not been established. As an alternative, poor metabolizers could be treated with either prasugrel (Effient) or ticagrelor (Brilinta), two other $P2Y_{12}$ ADP receptor antagonists, which are discussed later.

Adverse effects. Clopidogrel is generally well tolerated. Adverse effects are about the same as with aspirin. The most common complaints are abdominal pain, dyspepsia, diarrhea, and rash.

Bleeding. Like all other antiplatelet drugs, clopidogrel poses a risk for serious bleeding. However, compared with aspirin, clopidogrel causes less GI bleeding (2% vs. 2.7%) and less intracranial hemorrhage (ICH) (0.4% vs. 0.5%). Owing to bleeding risk, clopidogrel should be discontinued 5 days before elective surgery. If possible, major bleeding should be managed without discontinuing clopidogrel because discontinuation would increase the risk of a thrombotic event.

Patients should be told about the risk for bleeding and warned that they may bruise or bleed more easily and that bleeding will take longer than usual to stop. Also, patients should be informed about signs of bleeding (e.g., blood in the urine, black tarry stools, vomitus that looks like coffee grounds) and instructed to contact the prescriber if these develop. Finally, patients who develop these symptoms should be warned not to stop clopidogrel until the prescriber says they should.

Thrombotic thrombocytopenic purpura. Rarely, patients develop thrombotic thrombocytopenic purpura (TTP), a potentially fatal condition characterized by thrombocytopenia, hemolytic anemia, neurological symptoms, renal dysfunction, and fever. Most cases occur during the first 2 weeks of treatment. TTP is a serious disorder that requires urgent treatment, including plasmapheresis.

Drug interactions

Drugs that promote bleeding. Clopidogrel should be used with caution in patients taking other drugs that promote bleeding (e.g., heparin, warfarin, aspirin, and nonsteroidal antiinflammatory drugs [NSAIDs]).

Proton pump inhibitors. Omeprazole (Prilosec, Losec✚) and other proton pump inhibitors (PPIs) suppress the secretion of gastric acid (see Chapter 64) and hence are often combined with clopidogrel to protect against GI bleeding. Unfortunately, PPIs may also reduce the antiplatelet effects of clopidogrel. PPIs inhibit CYP2C19, the enzyme that converts clopidogrel to its active form. Hence the dilemma: if clopidogrel is used alone, there is a significant risk for GI bleeding; however, if clopidogrel is combined with a PPI to reduce the risk for GI bleeding, antiplatelet effects may be reduced as well. After considering the available evidence, three organizations—the American College of Cardiology, the American Heart Association, and the American College of Gastroenterology—issued a consensus document on the problem. This document concludes that although PPIs may reduce the antiplatelet effects of clopidogrel somewhat, there is no evidence that the reduction is large enough to be clinically relevant. Accordingly, for patients who have risk factors for GI bleeding (e.g., advanced age, use of NSAIDs or anticoagulants), the benefits of combining a PPI with clopidogrel probably outweigh any risk from reduced antiplatelet effects; hence combining a PPI with clopidogrel is probably acceptable for these people. Conversely, for patients who lack risk factors for GI bleeding, combined use of clopidogrel with a PPI may reduce the benefits of clopidogrel without offering any meaningful GI protection; hence combining a PPI with clopidogrel in these patients should probably be avoided. When a PPI *is* used with clopidogrel, pantoprazole (Protonix) would be a good choice because, compared with other PPIs, pantoprazole causes less inhibition of CYP2C19.

CYP2C19 inhibitors other than proton pump inhibitors. As in the case of the PPIs, several other drugs can inhibit CYP2C19. Among these are cimetidine, fluoxetine, fluvoxamine, fluconazole, ketoconazole, voriconazole, etravirine, felbamate, and ticlopidine. Because these drugs may reduce the antiplatelet effects of clopidogrel (by reducing its activation), use of alternative drugs is preferred.

Protease-Activated Receptor-1 Antagonists
Vorapaxar

Uses. Vorapaxar (Zontivity) is approved for use in conjunction with aspirin and/or clopidogrel in the reduction of thrombotic CV events in patients with a history of MI or peripheral arterial disease (PAD). When used with other antiplatelet agents, vorapaxar reduces the rate of CV death, MI, stroke, and urgent coronary revascularization.

Mechanism of action. PAR-1 mediates the effects of thrombin, and these receptors are located on the surface of platelets. By reversibly antagonizing these receptors, vorapaxar inhibits thrombin-induced and thrombin receptor agonist peptide (TRAP)-induced platelet aggregation. Vorapaxar does not work on ADP receptors.

Pharmacokinetics. Vorapaxar is well absorbed after oral administration. Antiplatelet effects begin within 1 hour. The drug undergoes extensive hepatic metabolism followed by excretion in the feces. Vorapaxar has a long half-life (8 days). Effects persist for 7 to 10 days after drug withdrawal (i.e., until new platelets have been synthesized).

Adverse effects

Bleeding. Like all other antiplatelet drugs, vorapaxar poses a risk for serious bleeding. In the Global Utilization of Streptokinase and Tissue Plasminogen Activator for Occluded Coronary Arteries (GUSTO) study, serious non–coronary artery bypass graft (CABG) bleeding developed in 3% of patients taking vorapaxar. This is similar to the rates seen with ticagrelor in the study of Platelet Inhibition and Patient Outcomes (PLATO) trial.

📄 SUMMARY OF KEY PRESCRIBING CONSIDERATIONS

Antiplatelet Medications

Therapeutic Goal: Prevent blockage of coronary artery stents and reduce thrombotic events.

Baseline Data: CBC, consider testing for variants of the CYP2C19 gene when initiating clopidogrel.

Monitoring: No routine monitoring required.

Identifying High-Risk Patients: Antiplatelet therapy is contraindicated in patients with active pathological bleeding. Should be used with caution in patients taking other drugs that promote bleeding.

Evaluating Therapeutic Effects: Important to monitor for signs of thrombotic events, including TIAs, CVAs, or MI.

Minimizing Adverse Effects: When aspirin is being used, important to weigh the risks and benefits of treatment as well as to use the lowest effective dose. Educate patients to inform providers if starting an over-the-counter PPI.

Other Antiplatelet Drugs
Dipyridamole

Dipyridamole [Persantine] suppresses platelet aggregation, perhaps by increasing plasma levels of adenosine. The drug is approved only for prevention of thromboembolism after heart valve replacement. For this application, dipyridamole is always combined with warfarin. The recommended dosage is 75 to 100 mg qid. A fixed-dose combination of dipyridamole and aspirin is indicated for recurrent stroke (see next).

Dipyridamole plus aspirin

Actions and use. Dipyridamole combined with aspirin is available in a fixed-dose formulation sold as Aggrenox. The product is used to prevent recurrent ischemic stroke in patients who have had a previous stroke or TIA. Both drugs—aspirin and dipyridamole—suppress platelet aggregation. However, because they do so by different mechanisms, the combination is more effective than either drug alone.

Cilostazol

Actions and therapeutic use. Cilostazol (Pletal), a platelet inhibitor and vasodilator, is indicated for intermittent claudication. (Intermittent claudication is a syndrome characterized by pain, cramping, and weakness of the calf muscles brought on by walking and relieved by resting for a few minutes. The underlying cause is atherosclerosis in the legs.) Cilostazol suppresses platelet aggregation by inhibiting phosphodiesterase type 3 (PDE-3) in platelets, and promotes vasodilation by inhibiting PDE-3 in blood vessels (primarily in the legs). Inhibition of platelet aggregation is greater than with aspirin, ticlopidine, or dipyridamole. Full effects take up to 12 weeks to develop but reverse quickly (within 48 h) after drug withdrawal.

47

Drugs for Deficiency Anemias

Most deficiency anemias result from deficiency of iron, vitamin B$_{12}$, or folic acid. Accordingly, this chapter focuses on anemias caused by these deficiencies. To facilitate discussion, the development of red blood cells (RBCs) is reviewed first.

RED BLOOD CELL DEVELOPMENT

RBCs begin developing in the bone marrow and then mature in the blood. As developing RBCs grow and divide, they evolve through four stages (Fig. 47.1). In their earliest stage, RBCs lack hemoglobin and are known as *proerythroblasts.* In the next stage, they gain hemoglobin and are called *erythroblasts.* Both the erythroblasts and the proerythroblasts reside in bone marrow. After the erythroblast stage, RBCs evolve into *reticulocytes* (immature erythrocytes) and enter the systemic circulation. After the reticulocyte stage, circulating RBCs reach full maturity and are referred to as *erythrocytes.*

The development of RBCs requires the cooperative interaction of several factors: bone marrow must be healthy; erythropoietin (a stimulant of RBC maturation) must be present; iron must be available for hemoglobin synthesis; and other factors, including vitamin B$_{12}$ and folic acid, must be available to support the synthesis of DNA. If any of these is absent or amiss, anemia will result.

IRON DEFICIENCY

Iron deficiency is the most common nutritional deficiency and the most common cause of nutrition-related anemia. Worldwide, people with iron deficiency number in the hundreds of millions. In the United States, about 5% of the population is iron deficient.

Biochemistry and the Physiology of Iron

To understand the consequences of iron deficiency as well as the rationale behind iron therapy, we must first understand the biochemistry and physiology of iron. This information is reviewed next.

Metabolic Functions

Iron is essential to the function of hemoglobin, myoglobin (the oxygen-storing molecule of muscle), and a variety of iron-containing enzymes. Most (70% to 80%) of the body's iron is present in hemoglobin. A much smaller amount (10%) is present in myoglobin and iron-containing enzymes.

Fate in the Body

The major pathways for iron movement and utilization are shown in Fig. 47.2. In the discussion that follows, the numbers in parentheses refer to the circled numbers in the figure.

Uptake and distribution. The life cycle of iron begins with (1) uptake of iron into mucosal cells of the small intestine. These cells absorb 5% to 20% of dietary iron. Their maximal absorptive capacity is 3 to 4 mg/day. Iron in the ferrous form (Fe^{2+}) is absorbed more readily than iron

in the ferric form (Fe^{3+}). Vitamin C enhances absorption and food reduces absorption.

After uptake, iron can either (2a) undergo storage within mucosal cells in the form of *ferritin* (a complex consisting of iron plus a protein used to store iron) or (2b) undergo binding to *transferrin* (the iron transport protein) for distribution throughout the body.

Utilization and storage. Iron that is bound to transferrin can undergo one of four fates. Most transferrin-bound iron (3a) is taken up by cells of the bone marrow for incorporation into hemoglobin. Small amounts (3b) are taken up by the liver and other tissues for storage as ferritin. Last (3c), some of the iron in plasma is taken up by muscle (for production of myoglobin) and some is taken up by all other tissues (for production of iron-containing enzymes).

Recycling. As Fig. 47.2 depicts, iron associated with hemoglobin undergoes continuous recycling. After hemoglobin is made in bone marrow, iron reenters the circulation (4) as a component of hemoglobin in erythrocytes. (The iron in circulating erythrocytes accounts for about 70% of total body iron.) After 120 days of useful life, RBCs are catabolized (5). Iron released by this process reenters the plasma bound to transferrin (6), and then the cycle begins anew.

Elimination. Excretion of iron is minimal. Under normal circumstances, only 1 mg of iron is excreted each day. At this rate, if none of the lost iron were replaced, body stores would decline by only 10% a year.

Iron leaves the body by several routes. Most excretion occurs through the bowel. Iron in ferritin is lost as mucosal cells slough off, and iron also enters the bowel in bile. Small amounts are excreted in urine and sweat.

Note that, although very little iron leaves the body as a result of excretion (i.e., normal physiological loss), substantial amounts can leave because of blood loss. Hence menorrhagia, hemorrhage, and blood donations can all cause iron deficiency.

Regulation of body iron content. The amount of iron in the body is regulated through control of intestinal absorption. As noted, most of the iron that enters the body stays in the body. If all dietary iron were readily absorbed, body iron content would rapidly accumulate to a toxic level. However, *excessive buildup is prevented through control of iron uptake: as body stores rise, uptake of iron declines; conversely, as body stores become depleted, uptake increases.* For example, when body stores of iron are high, only 2% to 3% of dietary iron is absorbed. In contrast, when body stores are depleted, as much as 20% may be absorbed.

Daily Requirements

Requirements for iron are determined largely by the rate of erythrocyte production. When RBC production is low, iron needs are low too. Conversely, when RBC production is high, iron needs rise. Accordingly, among infants and children—individuals whose rapid growth rate requires massive RBC synthesis—iron requirements are high (relative to body weight). In contrast, the daily iron needs of adults are relatively low. Adult men need only 8 mg of dietary iron each day. Adult women need considerably more (15 to 18 mg/day) to replace iron lost through menstruation.

During pregnancy, requirements for iron increase dramatically, owing to (1) expansion of maternal blood volume and (2) production of RBCs by the fetus. In most cases, the iron needs of pregnant women are too great to be met by diet alone. Consequently iron supplements (about 27 mg/day) are recommended during pregnancy and for 2 to 3 months after delivery.

Table 47.1 shows the recommended dietary allowances (RDAs) of iron as a function of age. The RDA values in the table are about 10 times greater than actual physiologic need because, on average, only 10% of dietary iron is absorbed. Therefore if physiologic requirements are to be met, the diet must contain 10 times more iron than is needed.

Iron Deficiency: Causes, Consequences, and Diagnosis
Causes
Iron deficiency results when there is an imbalance between iron uptake and iron demand. As a rule, the imbalance results from increased demand, not from reduced uptake. The most common causes of increased iron demand are (1) blood volume expansion during pregnancy coupled with RBC synthesis by the growing fetus; (2) blood volume expansion during infancy and early childhood; and (3) chronic blood loss, usually of gastrointestinal (GI) or uterine origin. Rarely, iron deficiency results from reduced iron uptake; potential causes include gastrectomy and sprue.

Consequences
Iron deficiency has multiple effects, the most conspicuous being *iron deficiency anemia.* In the absence of iron for hemoglobin synthesis, red blood cells become *microcytic* and *hypochromic.* The reduced oxygen-carrying capacity of blood results in listlessness, fatigue, and pallor of the skin and mucous membranes. If tissue oxygenation is severely compromised, tachycardia, dyspnea, and angina may result. In addition to causing anemia, iron deficiency impairs myoglobin production and the synthesis of iron-containing enzymes. In young children, iron deficiency can cause developmental problems; in school-aged children, iron deficiency may impair cognition.

Diagnosis
The hallmarks of iron deficiency anemia are (1) the presence of microcytic, hypochromic erythrocytes and (2) the absence of hemosiderin (aggregated ferritin) in bone marrow (Table 47.2). Additional laboratory

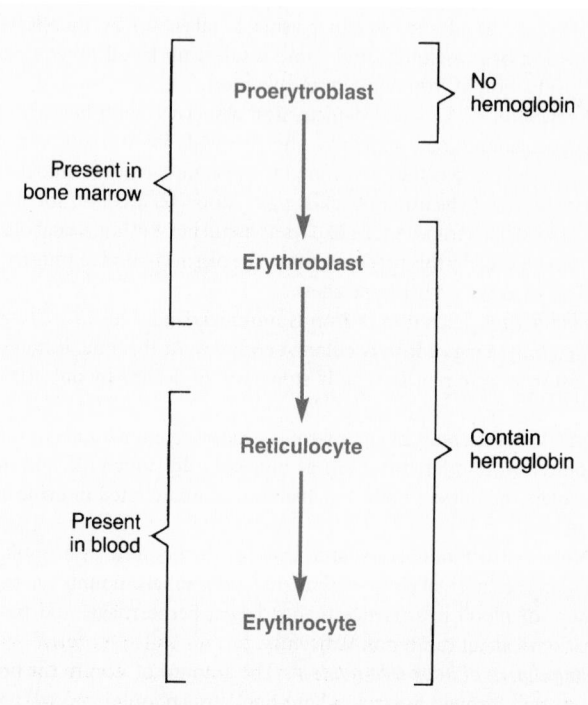

Fig. 47.1 Stages of Red Blood Cell Development.

TABLE 47.1 Recommended Dietary Allowances for Iron

Life Stage	Age	RDA for Iron (mg/day)
Infants	7–12 months	11
Children	1–3 years	7
	4–8 years	10
Males	9–13 years	8
	14–18 years	11
	≥19 years	8
Females: nonpregnant, nonlactating	9–13 years	8
	14–18 years	15
	19–50 years	18
	≥51 years	8
Females: pregnant	14–50 years	27[a]
Females: lactating	14–18 years	10
	19–50 years	9

[a]Iron requirements during pregnancy cannot be met through dietary sources alone, so supplements are recommended.
RDA, Recommended dietary allowances.

TABLE 47.2 Diagnosing Anemia

	Red Cell Size	Classification	Laboratory Values	Common Causes
Microcytic anemia	Microcytic <80 fL	Iron deficiency anemia	Serum iron <60 µg/dL Iron-binding capacity <300 µg/dL Ferritin (male) <50 µg/mL Ferritin (female) <12 µg/mL	Poor diet Chronic blood loss • Menorrhagia • Colon polyp • Hemorrhoids
Megaloblastic Anemia	Macrocytic >100 fL	Vitamin B₁₂ deficiency	Vitamin B₁₂ <200 pg/mL	Celiac disease Lack of intrinsic factor Enteritis
		Folate deficiency	Folate <2 ng/mL	Low dietary intake

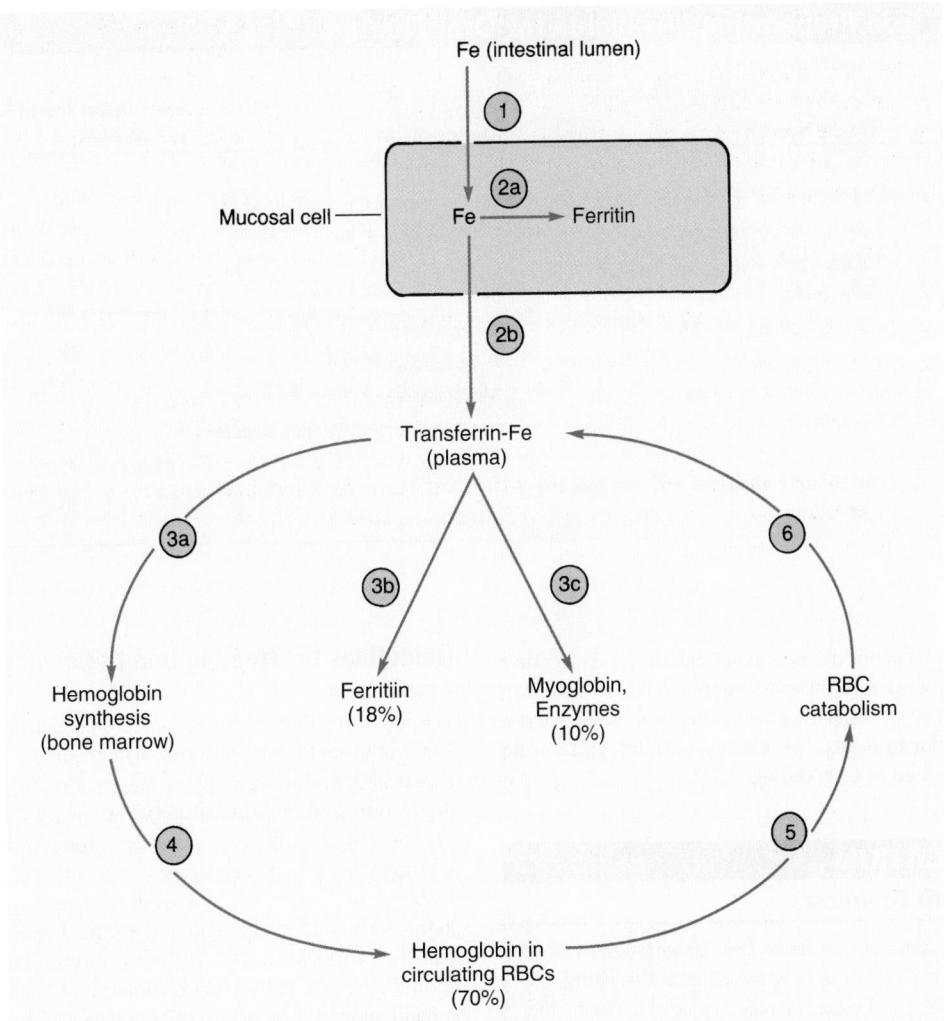

Fe (intestinal lumen)

①

Mucosal cell — Fe ②ᵃ→ Ferritin

②ᵇ

Transferrin-Fe
(plasma)

③ᵃ   ③ᵇ   ③ᶜ   ⑥

Hemoglobin   Ferritiin   Myoglobin,   RBC
synthesis   (18%)   Enzymes   catabolism
(bone marrow)   (10%)

④   ⑤

Hemoglobin in
circulating RBCs
(70%)

Fig. 47.2 Fate of Iron in the Body. Pathways labeled with circled numbers are explained in the text. Values in parentheses indicate percentage of total body stores. Elimination of iron is not shown because most iron is rigidly conserved. *Fe,* Iron; *RBC,* red blood cell.

data that can help confirm a diagnosis include reduced RBC count, reduced reticulocyte hemoglobin content, reduced hemoglobin and hematocrit values, reduced serum iron content, and increased serum iron-binding capacity (IBC).[a]

When a diagnosis of iron deficiency anemia is made, it is imperative that the underlying cause be determined. This is especially true when the suspected cause is GI-related blood loss, because GI blood loss may be indicative of peptic ulcer disease or GI cancer, conditions that demand immediate treatment.

Oral Iron Preparations

As shown in Table 47.3, iron for oral therapy is available in multiple forms. Of these, the ferrous salts (especially ferrous sulfate) and carbonyl iron are used most often. Accordingly, the following discussion is limited to these iron preparations.

---

[a]Serum IBC measures iron binding by transferrin. An *increase* in IBC indicates an increase in the amount of transferrin that is *not* carrying any iron and signals reduced iron availability.

Ferrous Iron Salts

We have two basic types of iron salts: ferrous salts and ferric salts. Discussion here is limited to the ferrous iron salts because they are absorbed three times more readily than the ferric salts and thus are more widely used. Four ferrous iron salts are available: ferrous sulfate, ferrous gluconate, ferrous fumarate, and ferrous aspartate. All four are equally effective and with all four, GI disturbances are the major adverse effect.

Ferrous sulfate

Indications. Ferrous sulfate is the treatment of choice for iron deficiency anemia. It is also the preferred drug for *preventing* deficiency when iron needs cannot be met by diet alone (e.g., during pregnancy or chronic blood loss). Ferrous sulfate costs less than ferrous gluconate or ferrous fumarate but has equal efficacy and tolerability.

Adverse effects

Gastrointestinal disturbances. The most significant adverse effects involve the GI tract. These effects, which are dose-dependent, include nausea, heartburn, bloating, constipation, and diarrhea. Gastrointestinal reactions are most intense during initial therapy and become less disturbing with continued drug use. Because of their GI effects, oral iron

TABLE 47.3   Iron Preparations Available for Oral Therapy

Iron Preparation	Trade Names	Description	Elemental Iron (% by Weight)	Dose Providing 100 mg Elemental Iron
Ferrous Iron Salts				
Ferrous sulfate	Feosol, FeroSul, Ferodan 🍁, Slow FE, others	All four compounds are salts of the ferrous form of iron.	20	500 mg
Ferrous gluconate	Fergon, Floradix, others		11.6	860 mg
Ferrous fumarate	Ferro-Sequels, Hemocyte, Palafer 🍁, others		33	300 mg
Ferrous aspartate	FE Aspartate		16	625 mg
Ferrous bisglycinate	Ferrochel, others	An iron–amino acid chelate.		
Ferric ammonium citrate	Iron Citrate	A ferric iron salt.		
Carbonyl iron	Feosol, Ircon, Icar, others	Microparticles of elemental iron.	100	100 mg
Heme iron polypeptide	Proferrin	Hemoglobin extracted from porcine RBCs.		
Polysaccharide iron complex	Niferex-150 Forte, Ferrex 150, Triferexx 150 🍁, others	Ferric iron complexed to hydrolyzed starch.		

preparations can aggravate peptic ulcers, regional enteritis, and ulcerative colitis. Accordingly, patients with these disorders should not take iron by mouth. In addition to its other GI effects, oral iron may impart a dark green or black color to stools. This effect is harmless and should not be interpreted as a sign of GI bleeding.

PATIENT EDUCATION

Preventing Tooth Staining

Liquid iron preparations can stain the teeth. This can be prevented by (1) diluting liquid preparations with juice or water, (2) administering the iron through a straw or with a dropper, and (3) rinsing the mouth after administration.

Toxicity. Iron in large amounts is toxic. Poisoning is almost always the result of accidental or intentional overdose, not from therapeutic doses. Death from iron ingestion is rare in adults. By contrast, *in young children, iron-containing products remain among the leading causes of poisoning fatalities.* For children, the lethal dose of elemental iron is 2 to 10 g. To reduce the risk for pediatric poisoning, iron should be stored in childproof containers and kept out of a child's reach.

Drug interactions. Interaction of iron with other drugs can alter the absorption of iron, the other drug, or both. *Antacids* reduce the absorption of iron. Coadministration of iron with tetracyclines decreases the absorption of both. *Ascorbic acid* (vitamin C) promotes iron absorption but also increases its adverse effects. Accordingly, attempts to enhance iron uptake by combining iron with ascorbic acid offer no advantage over a simple increase in iron dosage.

Carbonyl Iron

Carbonyl iron is pure elemental iron in the form of microparticles, which confer good bioavailability. Therapeutic efficacy equals that of the ferrous salts. Because of the microparticles, iron is absorbed slowly, so the risk for toxicity is reduced. Compared with ferrous sulfate, carbonyl iron requires a much higher dosage to cause serious harm. Because of this increased margin of safety, carbonyl iron should pose a reduced risk to children in the event of accidental ingestion.

Guidelines for Treating Iron Deficiency
Assessment

Before starting therapy, the cause of iron deficiency must be determined. Without this information, appropriate treatment is impossible. Potential causes of deficiency include pregnancy, bleeding, inadequate diet, and, rarely, impaired intestinal absorption.

The objective is to increase the production of hemoglobin and erythrocytes. When therapy is successful, reticulocytes will increase within 4 to 7 days; within 1 week, increases in hemoglobin and the hematocrit will be apparent; and within 1 month, hemoglobin levels will rise by at least 2 g/dL. If these responses fail to occur, the patient should be evaluated for (1) compliance, (2) continued bleeding, (3) inflammatory disease (which can interfere with hemoglobin production), and (4) malabsorption of oral iron.

Routes of Administration

Oral iron is preferred because it is safer than parenteral iron and just as effective. Parenteral iron should be used only when oral iron is ineffective or intolerable. Of the two parenteral routes, the intravenous route is safer and preferred. These medications are discussed in Chapter 92.

Duration of Therapy

Therapy with oral iron should be continued until hemoglobin levels become normal (about 15 g/dL). This phase of treatment may require 1 to 2 months. After this, continued treatment can help replenish stores of ferritin. However, for most patients, dietary iron alone is sufficient.

Therapeutic Combinations

As a rule, combinations of antianemic agents should be avoided. Combining oral iron with parenteral iron can lead to iron toxicity. Accordingly, the use of oral iron should cease before iron injections are given. Combinations of iron with vitamin B_{12} or folic acid should be avoided; as discussed in the following sections, use of these combinations can confuse the interpretation of hematologic responses.

VITAMIN B_{12} DEFICIENCY

The term *vitamin B_{12}* refers to a group of compounds with similar structures. These compounds are large molecules that contain an atom

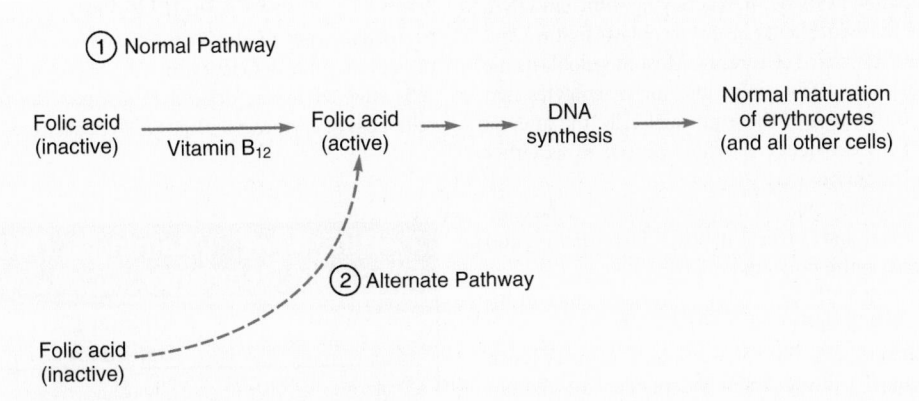

Fig. 47.3 Relationship of Folic Acid and Vitamin B₁₂ to DNA Synthesis and Cell Maturation. Folic acid requires activation to be of use. Normally, activation occurs through a vitamin B₁₂-dependent pathway. However, when folic acid is present in large amounts, activation can occur via an alternate pathway, bypassing the need for B₁₂.

of cobalt. Because of the cobalt atom, members of the vitamin B_{12} family are known as *cobalamins*.

The most prominent consequences of vitamin B_{12} deficiency are *anemia* and *injury to the nervous system*. Anemia reverses rapidly after vitamin B_{12} administration. Neurologic damage takes longer to repair and in some cases may never fully resolve. Additional effects of B_{12} deficiency include GI disturbances and impaired production of white blood cells and platelets.

Biochemistry and Physiology of Vitamin B_{12}

To understand the consequences of vitamin B_{12} deficiency and the rationale behind therapy, the normal biochemistry and physiology of B_{12} must first be understood. This information is reviewed next.

Metabolic Function

Vitamin B_{12} is essential for the synthesis of DNA and hence is required for the growth and division of virtually all cells. The mechanism by which the vitamin influences DNA synthesis is depicted in Fig. 47.3. As indicated, vitamin B_{12} helps catalyze the conversion of folic acid to its active form. Active folic acid then participates in several reactions that are essential for DNA synthesis. Hence *it is by permitting the utilization of folic acid that vitamin B_{12} influences cell growth and division,* and it is the absence of usable folic acid that underlies the blood cell abnormalities seen during B_{12} deficiency.

Fate in the Body
Absorption

Efficient absorption of B_{12} requires *intrinsic factor,* a compound secreted by parietal cells of the stomach. After ingestion, vitamin B_{12} forms a complex with intrinsic factor. Upon reaching the ileum, the B_{12}–intrinsic factor complex interacts with specific receptors on the intestinal wall, causing the complex to be absorbed. In the absence of intrinsic factor, absorption of vitamin B_{12} is greatly reduced. However, about 1% of the amount present can still be absorbed by passive diffusion; no intrinsic factor is needed.

Distribution and Storage

After absorption, the vitamin B_{12}–intrinsic factor complex dissociates. Free B_{12} then binds to *transcobalamin II* for transport to tissues. Most vitamin B_{12} goes to the liver and is stored. Total body stores of B_{12} are tiny, ranging from 2 to 3 mg by most estimates.

Elimination

Excretion of vitamin B_{12} takes place very slowly: each day, about 0.1% of the total body store is lost. Because B_{12} is excreted so slowly, years are required for B_{12} deficiency to develop, even when none of the lost B_{12} is replaced.

Vitamin B_{12} Deficiency: Causes, Consequences, and Diagnosis
Causes

In most cases, vitamin B_{12} deficiency is the result of *impaired absorption.* Only rarely is insufficient B_{12} in the diet the cause. Potential causes of poor absorption include (1) regional enteritis, (2) celiac disease (a malabsorption syndrome involving abnormalities in the intestinal villi), (3) development of antibodies directed against the vitamin B_{12}–intrinsic factor complex, and (4) bariatric surgery. In addition, because stomach acid is required to release vitamin B_{12} from foods, the vitamin cannot be absorbed if acid secretion is significantly reduced, as often happens in older adults and in those taking acid-suppressing drugs.

Most frequently, impaired absorption of vitamin B_{12} occurs secondary to a lack of intrinsic factor. The usual causes are atrophy of gastric parietal cells and surgery of the stomach (total gastric resection).

When vitamin B_{12} deficiency is caused by an absence of intrinsic factor, the resulting syndrome is called *pernicious anemia*—a term suggesting a highly destructive or fatal condition. Pernicious anemia is an old term that refers back to the days when, for most patients, vitamin B_{12} deficiency had no effective therapy and the condition was uniformly fatal. Today, vitamin B_{12} deficiency secondary to lack of intrinsic factor can be managed successfully, so the label *pernicious* no longer has its original ominous connotation.

Consequences

Many of the consequences of B_{12} deficiency result from the disruption of DNA synthesis. The tissues affected most are those with a high proportion of cells undergoing growth and division. Accordingly, B_{12} deficiency has profound effects on the bone marrow (the site where blood cells are produced) and the epithelial cells lining the mouth and GI tract.

Megaloblastic anemia. The most conspicuous consequence of B_{12} deficiency is an anemia in which large numbers of *megaloblasts* (oversized erythroblasts) appear in the bone marrow and in which *macrocytes* (oversized erythrocytes) appear in the blood. These strange cells are produced because of impaired DNA synthesis. Lacking sufficient DNA, growing cells are unable to divide; hence, as erythroblasts mature and their division is prevented, oversized cells result. Most megaloblasts die within the bone marrow; only a few evolve into the macrocytes that can be seen in the blood. Because of these unusual cells, the anemia associated with vitamin B_{12} deficiency is often referred to as either *megaloblastic* or *macrocytic* anemia.

Severe anemia is the principal cause of mortality from B_{12} deficiency. Anemia produces peripheral and cerebral hypoxia. Heart failure and dysrhythmias are the usual cause of death.

It is important to note that the hematologic effects of vitamin B_{12} deficiency can be reversed with large doses of *folic acid*. As indicated in Fig. 47.3, when folic acid is present in large amounts, some of it can be activated by an alternate pathway that is independent of vitamin B_{12}. This pathway bypasses the metabolic block caused by B_{12} deficiency, permitting DNA synthesis to proceed.

Neurological damage. Deficiency of vitamin B_{12} causes demyelination of neurons, primarily in the spinal cord and brain. A variety of signs and symptoms can result. Early manifestations include paresthesias of the hands and feet and a reduction in deep tendon reflexes. Late-developing responses include loss of memory, mood changes, hallucinations, and psychosis. If vitamin B_{12} deficiency is prolonged, neurologic damage can become permanent.

The precise mechanism by which B_{12} deficiency results in neuronal damage is unknown. We do know, however, that *neuronal damage is not related to effects on folic acid or DNA*. That is, the mechanism that underlies neuronal damage is different from the mechanism that underlies disruption of hematopoiesis. Consequently, although administering large doses of folic acid can correct the hematologic consequences of B_{12} deficiency, folic acid will not improve the neurologic picture.

Other effects. As noted, vitamin B_{12} deficiency can adversely affect virtually all tissues in which a high proportion of cells are undergoing growth and division. Therefore in addition to disrupting the production of erythrocytes, lack of B_{12} also prevents the bone marrow from making leukocytes (white blood cells) and thrombocytes (platelets). Loss of these blood elements can lead to infection and spontaneous bleeding. Disruption of DNA synthesis can also suppress division of the cells that form the epithelial lining of the mouth, stomach, and intestine, causing oral ulceration and a variety of GI disturbances.

Diagnosis

When megaloblastic anemia occurs, it may be due to vitamin B_{12} deficiency or other causes, especially a lack of folic acid. Hence if therapy is to be appropriate, a definitive diagnosis must be made. The combination of megaloblastic anemia plus low plasma vitamin B_{12} plus evidence of B_{12} malabsorption leads to a clear diagnosis of vitamin B_{12} deficiency (Table 47.4).

Guidelines for Treating Vitamin B_{12} Deficiency
Route of B_{12} Administration

As discussed previously, oral therapy can be used for most patients, including those with conditions that impair B_{12} absorption (Table 47.5). The major exception is patients with severe neurologic deficits caused by B_{12} deficiency. For these people, parenteral cyanocobalamin is indicated.

Treatment of Moderate B_{12} Deficiency

The primary manifestations of moderate B_{12} deficiency are megaloblasts in the bone marrow and macrocytes in peripheral blood. Moderate deficiency does not cause leukopenia, thrombocytopenia, or neurologic complications. Moderate deficiency can be managed with vitamin B_{12} alone; no other measures are required.

Treatment of Severe B_{12} Deficiency

Severe deficiency produces multiple effects, all of which must be attended to. Unlike mild deficiency, in which erythrocytes are the only blood cells affected, severe deficiency disrupts the production of all blood cells. Loss of erythrocytes leads to hypoxia, cerebrovascular insufficiency,

TABLE 47.4 Vitamin B_{12} Deficiency Versus Folic Acid Deficiency

	Vitamin B_{12} Deficiency	Folic Acid Deficiency
Usual cause	Vitamin B_{12} malabsorption from lack of intrinsic factor	Low dietary folic acid
Primary hematological effect	Megaloblastic anemia	Megaloblastic anemia
Neurological effect	Damage to brain and spinal cord	None[a]
Diagnosis	Low plasma vitamin B_{12}; low B_{12} absorption (Schilling test)	Low plasma folic acid
Treatment (usual route)	Cyanocobalamin (PO or IM)	Folic acid (PO)
Usual duration of therapy	Lifelong	Short term

[a]Folic acid deficiency early in pregnancy can cause neural tube defects in the fetus.
IM, Intramuscular; *PO*, by mouth

TABLE 47.5 Vitamin B_{12} Preparations and Dosage

Preparation	Usual Daily Dosage for Deficiency[a]
Capsules: 1000 mcg, 3000 mcg, 5000 mcg	Initial treatment: 1000-2000 mcg daily for 1-2 weeks
Tablets: 50 mcg, 100 mcg, 250 mcg, 500 mcg, 1000 mcg, 2000 mcg, 2500 mcg	Maintenance treatment: 1000 mcg daily
ER Tablets: 1000 mcg, 1500 mcg, 5000 mcg	
Oral Disintegrating Tablet: 1500 mcg	
Sublingual Tablet: 500 mcg, 1000 mcg, 2500 mcg, 3000 mcg, 5000 mcg, 6000 mcg	
Chewable Tablets: 250 mcg, 500 mcg, 750 mcg	
Sublingual Solution: 5000 mcg/mL	
Solution for Injection: 1000 mcg/mL	Initial treatment: 1000 mcg IM/SC daily for one week. Then weekly for one month. Maintenance: 1000 mcg IM/SC monthly.
Intranasal [Nascobal]: 500 mcg per actuation	1 spray in one nostril weekly

[a]Supplementation doses are usually lower.
ER, Extended release, *IM*, intramuscular, *SC*, subcutaneous.

and heart failure. Loss of leukocytes encourages infection, and loss of thrombocytes promotes bleeding. In addition to causing serious hematologic deficits, severe B_{12} deficiency has adverse effects on the nervous system and GI tract.

Treatment of severe deficiency involves the following: (1) IM injection of vitamin B_{12} and folic acid (the folic acid accelerates recovery of hematologic deficits); (2) administration of two to three units of packed RBCs (to correct anemia quickly); (3) transfusion of platelets; and (4) therapy with antibiotics if infection has developed.

After treatment with vitamin B_{12} plus folic acid, recovery from anemia occurs quickly. Within 1 to 2 days, megaloblasts disappear from the bone marrow; within 3 to 5 days, reticulocyte counts become elevated; by day 10, the hematocrit begins to rise; and within 14 to 21 days, the hematocrit becomes normal.

Recovery from neurologic damage is slow and depends on how long the damage had been present. When deficits have been present for only 2 to 3 months, recovery is relatively fast. When deficits have been present for many months or for years, recovery is slow; months may pass before any improvement is apparent and complete recovery may never occur.

Long-Term Treatment

For patients who lack intrinsic factor or who suffer from some other permanent cause of vitamin B_{12} malabsorption, lifelong treatment is required. Traditional therapy consists of monthly IM or SC injections of cyanocobalamin. However, *large daily oral doses can be just as effective, as can weekly intranasal doses.* During prolonged therapy, treatment should be assessed periodically: plasma levels of vitamin B_{12} should be measured every 3 to 6 months, blood samples should be examined for the return of macrocytes, and blood counts should be performed.

Potential Hazard of Folic Acid

Treatment with folic acid can exacerbate the neurologic consequences of B_{12} deficiency. Recall that folic acid by itself can reverse the *hematologic* effects of B_{12} deficiency but will not alleviate *neurologic* deficits. So, by correcting the most obvious manifestation of B_{12} deficiency (anemia), folic acid can mask the fact that deficiency of B_{12} still exists. As a result, *use of folic acid can lead to undertreatment with B_{12} itself* and thereby permit neurologic damage to progress. Clearly, folic acid is not a substitute for vitamin B_{12}, and vitamin B_{12} deficiency should never be treated with folic acid alone. Whenever folic acid is employed during treatment of vitamin B_{12} deficiency, extra care must be taken to ensure that periodically B_{12} dosage is adequate.

FOLIC ACID DEFICIENCY

In one respect, folic acid deficiency is identical to vitamin B_{12} deficiency: in both states, *megaloblastic anemia* is the most conspicuous pathology. However, in other important ways, folic acid deficiency and vitamin B_{12} deficiency are dissimilar (see Table 47.4). Consequently, when a patient presents with megaloblastic anemia, it is essential to determine whether the cause is deficiency of folic acid, vitamin B_{12}, or both.

Physiology and Biochemistry of Folic Acid
Metabolic Function

As noted in the discussion of vitamin B_{12}, folic acid (also known as *folate* in its natural form) is an essential factor for DNA synthesis. Without folic acid, DNA replication and cell division cannot proceed.

To be usable, dietary folic acid must first be converted to an active form. Under normal conditions, activation occurs through a pathway that employs vitamin B_{12} (see Fig. 47.3). However, when large amounts of folate are ingested, some can be activated through an alternate pathway—one that does not employ vitamin B_{12}. Hence even in the absence of vitamin B_{12}, if sufficient amounts of folic acid are consumed, active folate will be available for DNA synthesis.

Fate in the Body

Folic acid is absorbed in the early segment of the small intestine and then transported to the liver and other tissues, where it is either used or stored.

Folic acid in the liver undergoes extensive enterohepatic recirculation. That is, folate from the liver is excreted into the intestine, after which it is reabsorbed and then returned to the liver through the hepatic-portal circulation. This enterohepatic recirculation helps salvage up to 200 µg of folate per day. Accordingly, the process is an important way to maintain folate stores.

In contrast to vitamin B_{12}, folic acid is not conserved rigidly: every day, significant amounts are excreted. As a result, if intake of folic acid were to cease, signs of deficiency would develop rapidly (within weeks if body stores were already low).

Folic Acid Deficiency: Causes, Consequences, and Diagnosis
Causes

Folic acid deficiency has two principal causes: (1) poor diet (especially in patients who abuse alcohol) and (2) malabsorption secondary to intestinal disease. An increase in folic acid requirements may also cause deficiency. This may be seen in pregnancy and lactation, patients undergoing hemodialysis, and those with chronic hemolytic anemias. Rarely, certain drugs may cause folate deficiency.

Alcohol use disorder. Alcohol use disorder may be the most common cause of folate deficiency. Deficiency results for two reasons: (1) insufficient folic acid in the diet and (2) derangement of enterohepatic recirculation secondary to alcohol-induced injury to the liver. Fortunately, with improved diet and reduced alcohol consumption, alcohol-related folate deficiency will often reverse.

Sprue. Sprue is an intestinal malabsorption syndrome that decreases folic acid uptake. Because sprue does not block folate absorption entirely, deficiency can be corrected by giving large doses of folic acid orally.

Consequences

With the important exception that folic acid deficiency does not injure the nervous system, the effects of folate deficiency are identical to those of vitamin B_{12} deficiency. As with B_{12} deficiency, the most prominent consequence of folate deficiency is *megaloblastic anemia.* In addition, similar to B_{12} deficiency, lack of folic acid may result in leukopenia, thrombocytopenia, and injury to the oral and GI mucosa. Because it has already been noted that many of the consequences of vitamin B_{12} deficiency result from depriving cells of active folic acid, the similarities between folate deficiency and vitamin B_{12} deficiency should be no surprise.

The developing fetus. Folic acid deficiency *very early* in pregnancy can cause neural tube defects (e.g., spina bifida, anencephaly). Accordingly, it is imperative that all women of reproductive age ensure adequate folate levels *before* pregnancy occurs. To accomplish this, the US Preventive Services Task Force now recommends that *all women who may become pregnant consume 400 to 800 µg of supplemental folic acid each day—in addition to the folate they get from food.*

Other consequences. As discussed in Chapter 67, folic acid deficiency may increase the risk for colorectal cancer and atherosclerosis.

Guidelines for Treating Folic Acid Deficiency
Choice of Treatment Modality

The modality for treating folic acid deficiency should be matched with the cause. If the deficiency is due to poor diet, it should be corrected by dietary measures—not with supplements except for women who

TABLE 47.6   Folic Acid Preparations and Dosage

Preparations	Usual Adult Dosage for Deficiency[a]
Tablets: 0.4, 0.8, 1 mg	Initial treatment: 1-5 mg daily Maintenance: 400 mcg daily
Solution for Injection: 5 mg/mL	Initial treatment: 1-5 mg daily Maintenance: 400 mcg daily

[a]Supplementation doses are usually lower.

may become pregnant. Ingestion of one serving of a fresh vegetable or one glass of fruit juice a day will often suffice. In contrast, when folate deficiency is the result of malabsorption, diet alone cannot correct the deficiency, so supplemental folate will be needed.

Route of Administration

Oral administration is preferred for most patients (Table 47.6). Unlike vitamin B_{12}, folic acid is rarely administered by injection. Even in the presence of intestinal disease, oral folic acid can be effective provided that the dosage is high enough.

Prophylactic Use of Folic Acid

Folic acid should be taken prophylactically only when clearly appropriate. The principal candidates for prophylactic folate are women who might become pregnant and those who are pregnant or lactating. Because folic acid may mask vitamin B_{12} deficiency, indiscriminate use of folate should be avoided.

Treatment of Severe Deficiency

Folic acid deficiency can produce severe megaloblastic anemia. To ensure a rapid response, therapy should be initiated with an IM injection of folic acid and vitamin B_{12}. (Because of the metabolic interrelationship between folic acid and vitamin B_{12}, the combination of these agents accelerates recovery.) After the initial injection, treatment should be continued with folic acid alone. Folic acid should be given orally in a dosage of 1000 to 2000 µg/day for 1 to 2 weeks. After this, maintenance doses of 400 µg/day may be required.

Therapy is evaluated by monitoring the hematologic picture. When treatment has been effective, megaloblasts will disappear from the bone marrow within 48 hours; the reticulocyte count will increase measurably within 2 to 3 days; and the hematocrit will begin to rise in the second week.

48

Drugs for Diabetes Mellitus

DIABETES MELLITUS: BASIC CONSIDERATIONS

The term *diabetes mellitus* is derived from the Greek word for *fountain* and the Latin word for *honey*. The term describes one of the prominent symptoms of untreated diabetes: production of large volumes of glucose-rich urine. Indeed, long ago, the disease we currently call diabetes was "diagnosed" by the sweet smell of urine—and, yes, by its sweet taste, too. In this chapter we use the terms *diabetes mellitus* and *diabetes* interchangeably.

Diabetes is primarily a disorder of carbohydrate metabolism. Symptoms mainly result from a deficiency of insulin or from cellular resistance to insulin's actions. The principal sign of diabetes is *sustained hyperglycemia*, which results from impaired glucose uptake by cells and from increased glucose production. When hyperglycemia develops, it can quickly lead to polyuria, polydipsia, ketonuria, and weight loss. Over time, hyperglycemia can lead to heart disease, renal failure, blindness, neuropathy, amputations, impotence, and stroke. There is an often-overlooked point about diabetes: in addition to affecting carbohydrate metabolism, insulin deficiency disrupts metabolism of proteins and lipids. We refer to regulation of blood glucose levels as *glycemic control*.

In the United States, diabetes is the most common endocrine disorder and the seventh leading cause of death by disease. According to the 2017 National Diabetes Fact Sheet, compiled by the Centers for Disease Control and Prevention, approximately 30 million Americans have diabetes, and nearly one-fourth of them have not been diagnosed. Another 84 million or so Americans are estimated to have prediabetes and are at increased risk for developing diabetes in the future.

We need to do a better job of diagnosing diabetes and treating it—and we need to do what we can to reduce the risk for developing the disease in the first place. Unfortunately, the risk for developing diabetes is largely genetic, a factor that cannot be modified. Nonetheless, we can still reduce risk significantly by adopting a healthy lifestyle, centered on engaging in physical activity and establishing a healthy diet.

Types of Diabetes Mellitus

There are two main forms of diabetes mellitus: type 1 diabetes mellitus (often abbreviated as T1DM) and type 2 diabetes mellitus (often abbreviated as T2DM). Both forms have similar signs and symptoms. Major differences concern etiology, prevalence, treatments, and outcomes (illness severity and deaths). The distinguishing characteristics of type 1 and type 2 diabetes are shown in Table 48.1 and discussed later. Another important form—gestational diabetes—is discussed later under "Diabetes and Pregnancy." Although there are additional forms of diabetes, they are relatively rare and will not be discussed specifically here.

Type 1 Diabetes

Type 1 diabetes accounts for approximately 5% of all diabetes cases. In the past, type 1 diabetes was called *juvenile-onset diabetes mellitus* or *insulin-dependent diabetes mellitus (IDDM)*. However, these terms have fallen out of favor because type 2 diabetes is becoming more common in children, and many people with type 2 diabetes use insulin to manage their diabetes. In general, type 1 diabetes develops during childhood or adolescence, and symptom onset is relatively abrupt. That being said, type 1 diabetes can develop during adulthood.

The primary defect in type 1 diabetes is destruction of pancreatic β cells—the cells responsible for insulin synthesis and release into the bloodstream. Insulin levels are reduced early in the disease and usually fall to zero later. β cell destruction is the result of an autoimmune process (i.e., the patient's immune system inappropriately wages war against its own β cells). The trigger for this immune response is not entirely known, but genetic, environmental, and infectious factors likely play a role.

Type 2 Diabetes

Type 2 diabetes is the most prevalent form of diabetes, accounting for 90% to 95% of all diagnosed cases. In the past, type 2 diabetes was called *non–insulin-dependent diabetes mellitus (NIDDM)* or *adult-onset diabetes mellitus*. As discussed previously for type 1 diabetes, these terms are no longer clinically useful because insulin is commonly used by people with type 2 diabetes and type 2 diabetes can occur in all age groups. The disease most commonly begins in middle age and progresses gradually. In contrast to type 1 diabetes, type 2 diabetes carries little risk for ketoacidosis. However, type 2 diabetes does carry the same long-term risks as type 1 diabetes (see later).

Symptoms of type 2 diabetes usually result from a combination of *insulin resistance* and *impaired insulin secretion*. In contrast to patients with type 1 diabetes, those with type 2 diabetes are capable of insulin synthesis. In fact, early in the disease, insulin levels tend to be normal or slightly elevated, a state known as *hyperinsulinemia*. However, although insulin is still produced, its secretion is no longer tightly coupled to plasma glucose level: release of insulin is delayed, and peak output is subnormal. More important, the target tissues of insulin (liver, muscle, adipose tissue) exhibit insulin resistance: for a given blood insulin level, cells in these tissues are less able to take up and metabolize the glucose available to them. Insulin resistance appears to result from three causes: reduced binding of insulin to its receptors, reduced receptor numbers, and reduced receptor responsiveness. Over time, hyperglycemia leads to diminished pancreatic β cell function, and hence insulin production and secretion eventually decline as the β cells work harder to overcome insulin resistance within the tissues.

TABLE 48.1   Characteristics of Type 1 and Type 2 Diabetes Mellitus

| Characteristics | TYPE OF DIABETES MELLITUS | |
	Type 1	Type 2
Age of onset	Usually childhood or adolescence	Usually older than 40 years
Speed of onset	Abrupt	Gradual
Family history	Frequently negative	Frequently positive
Prevalence	Approximately 5% of people with diabetes have type 1 diabetes	90%–95% of people with diabetes have type 2 diabetes
Etiology	Autoimmune process	Unknown—but there is a strong familial association, suggesting that heredity is a risk factor
Primary defect	Loss of pancreatic β cells	Insulin resistance and inappropriate insulin secretion
Insulin levels	Reduced early in the disease and completely absent later	Levels may be low (indicating deficiency), normal, or high (indicating resistance)
Treatment	Insulin replacement is mandatory, along with strict dietary control	Treat with an oral antidiabetic or noninsulin injectable agent and/or insulin, but always in combination with a reduced-calorie diet and appropriate exercise
Blood glucose	Levels fluctuate widely in response to infection, exercise, and changes in caloric intake and insulin dose	Levels are generally more stable than in type 1 diabetes
Symptoms	Polyuria, polydipsia, polyphagia, weight loss	May be asymptomatic initially
Body composition	Usually thin and undernourished at diagnosis	Frequently obese
Ketosis	Common, especially if insulin dosage is insufficient	Uncommon

TABLE 48.2   Criteria for the Diagnosis of Diabetes Mellitus

Fasting plasma glucose ≥126 mg/dL[a]
Or
Random plasma glucose ≥ 200 mg/dL *plus* symptoms of diabetes[b]
Or
Oral glucose tolerance test (OGTT): 2-h plasma glucose ≥200 mg/dL[c]
or
Hemoglobin A$_{1c}$ 6.5% or higher

[a]*Fasting* is defined as no caloric intake for at least 8 hours.
[b]*Random* is defined as any time of day without regard to meals. Classical symptoms of diabetes include polyuria, polydipsia, and unexplained weight loss.
[c]In this OGTT, plasma glucose content is measured 2 hours after ingesting the equivalent of 75 g of anhydrous glucose dissolved in water. The OGTT is not recommended or needed for routine clinical use.
Data from Position Statement Standards of Medical Care in Diabetes—2019. Abridged for Primary Care Providers. American Diabetes Association Clinical Diabetes 2019 Jan; 37(1):11-34. https://clinical.diabetesjournals.org/content/37/1/11.

Although the underlying causes of type 2 diabetes are not entirely known, there is a strong familial association, suggesting that genetics play a role. This possibility was reinforced by a study that implicated the gene for *insulin receptor substrate-2* (IRS-2), a compound that helps mediate intracellular responses to insulin.

Diabetes and Pregnancy

Although insulin therapy has greatly improved outcomes, successful management of the diabetic pregnancy remains a challenge. Three factors contribute to the problem. First, the placenta produces hormones that antagonize insulin's actions. Second, production of cortisol, a hormone that promotes hyperglycemia, increases threefold during pregnancy. Both factors increase the body's need for insulin. And third, because glucose can pass freely from the maternal circulation to the fetal circulation, hyperglycemia in the mother will stimulate excessive secretion of insulin in the fetus. The resultant hyperinsulinism can have multiple adverse effects on the fetus.

Successful management of diabetes during pregnancy demands that proper glucose levels be maintained in both the mother and fetus; failure to do so may be teratogenic or may otherwise harm the fetus. Achieving glucose control requires diligence on the part of the mother and her prescriber. Some experts on diabetes in pregnancy advise that blood glucose levels must be monitored six to seven times a day. Insulin dosage and food intake must be adjusted accordingly.

Gestational diabetes is defined as diabetes that appears in the pregnant patient during pregnancy and then subsides rapidly after delivery. Gestational diabetes is managed in much the same manner as any other diabetic pregnancy: blood glucose should be monitored and then controlled with diet and insulin. In most cases the diabetic state disappears almost immediately after delivery, permitting discontinuation of insulin. However, if the diabetic state persists beyond parturition, it is no longer considered gestational and should be rediagnosed and treated accordingly.

In women taking an oral drug for type 2 diabetes, current practice is to discontinue the oral drug and switch to insulin. The only exception is the oral agent metformin, which is often satisfactory for managing type 2 diabetes in pregnancy. Women who discontinue oral medications can resume oral therapy after delivery.

Diagnosis

Diagnosis of diabetes was once made solely by measuring blood levels of glucose. However, hemoglobin A$_{1c}$—a test that provides an estimate of glycemic control over the previous 2 to 3 months is now considered a standard test as well. For all of these tests, diagnostic values of diabetes are shown in Table 48.2.

Tests Based on Blood Levels of Glucose

Excessive plasma glucose is diagnostic of diabetes. Several tests may be used: a fasting plasma glucose (FPG) test, a casual plasma glucose test, and an oral glucose tolerance test (OGTT). To make a definitive diagnosis, the patient must be tested on two separate days, and both tests must be positive. Any combination of two tests (e.g., two FPG tests; one FPG test and one OGTT) may be used.

Fasting plasma glucose test. To determine FPG levels, blood is drawn at least 8 hours after the last meal. In normoglycemic individuals, FPG levels are less than 100 mg/dL. If FPG glucose levels are 126 mg/dL or higher, diabetes is present.

Random plasma glucose test. For this test, blood can be drawn at any time, without regard to meals. Fasting is not required. Of note, the test can be performed in the office, using a finger-stick blood sample and the same type of test device used by patients at home. A plasma glucose level that is 200 mg/dL or greater suggests diabetes. However, to make a definitive diagnosis, the patient must also display classic signs of diabetes: polyuria, polydipsia, and rapid weight loss. Ketonuria may also be present, but only if blood glucose is extremely high.

Oral glucose tolerance test. This test is often used when diabetes is suspected but could not be definitively diagnosed by measuring fasting or casual plasma glucose levels. The OGTT is performed by giving an oral glucose load (equivalent to 75 g of anhydrous glucose) and measuring plasma glucose levels 2 hours later. In individuals who do not have diabetes, 2-hour glucose levels will be less than 140 mg/dL. Diabetes is suggested if 2-hour plasma glucose levels are 200 mg/dL or greater. The OGTT test is more expensive and time consuming than the alternatives and is not used routinely.

Hemoglobin A$_{1c}$

As described later under "Monitoring Treatment," levels of hemoglobin A$_{1c}$, or simply A$_{1c}$, reflect average blood glucose levels over the previous 2 to 3 months. Accordingly, if a patient's A$_{1c}$ is high, we know that the patient's glucose levels have been high for a relatively long time. In other words, we know that the patient has diabetes. An A$_{1c}$ value of 6.5% or higher is considered diagnostic.

It is important to note that the A$_{1c}$ test is not necessarily accurate in all patients because some people have conditions that can affect hemoglobin levels, thus skewing the results of this test. Among these are pregnancy, chronic kidney or liver disease, recent severe bleeding or blood transfusion, and certain blood disorders, including thalassemia, iron deficiency anemia, and anemia related to vitamin B$_{12}$ deficiency.

Increased Risk for Diabetes (Prediabetes)

Increased risk for diabetes (sometimes referred to as prediabetes) is a state defined by *impaired FPG* (between 100 and 125 mg/dL) or *impaired glucose tolerance* (2-hour OGTT result of 140 to 199 mg/dL). These values are below those that define diabetes but are too high to be considered normal. People with "prediabetes" are at increased risk for developing type 2 diabetes and cardiovascular disease (CVD)—but not the microvascular complications associated with diabetes (i.e., retinopathy, nephropathy, neuropathy). The risk for CVD can be reduced by dietary modifications, increased physical activity, and, if indicated, use of appropriate drugs to control blood lipids and blood pressure. The risk for progression to diabetes may be reduced by diet and exercise and possibly by certain oral antidiabetic drugs (such as metformin).

It is important to note that many people who meet the criteria for prediabetes never go on to develop diabetes—even if they *do not* modify their lifestyle, and even if they *do not* take antidiabetic drugs. Hence, although prediabetes indicates an increased *risk* for diabetes, it by no means guarantees that diabetes will occur.

Overview of Treatment

The primary goal of treating type 1 or type 2 diabetes is prevention of long-term complications. To minimize complications, treatment must keep glucose levels as close to "normal" as safely possible. In addition, treatment must keep blood pressure and blood lipids within an acceptable range. In both type 1 and type 2 diabetes, proper diet and adequate physical activity are central components of management.

Type 1 Diabetes

Preventing complications of diabetes requires a comprehensive plan directed at glycemic control and reduction of cardiovascular risk factors. Glycemic control is accomplished with an integrated program of diet, self-monitoring of blood glucose (SMBG), physical activity, and insulin replacement. Of importance, glycemic control must be achieved *safely,* that is, adequately controlling glycemia while minimizing the risk for hypoglycemia.

Insulin replacement. Among patients with type 1 diabetes, survival requires daily dosing with insulin. Before insulin replacement became available, people with type 1 diabetes invariably died within a few years after disease onset. The cause of death was usually ketoacidosis. It is essential to coordinate insulin dosage with carbohydrate intake. If carbohydrate intake is too great or too small with respect to insulin dosage, hyperglycemia or hypoglycemia will result.

Although insulin is the cornerstone to the management of type 1 diabetes, the use of other medications as add-on therapy to insulin is currently under study.

Managing hypertension and dyslipidemia. An angiotensin-converting enzyme (ACE) inhibitor (e.g., lisinopril) or an angiotensin II receptor blocker (ARB; e.g., losartan) can reduce the risk for diabetic nephropathy, a long-term consequence of poor glycemic control. These same drugs are preferred agents for managing diabetic hypertension. The current goal, as set by the American Diabetes Association (ADA), is to keep blood pressure at or less than 140/90 mm Hg, with lower systolic blood pressure targets (<140 mm Hg) appropriate for some individuals (see Chapter 38).

To reduce high levels of low-density lipoprotein (LDL) cholesterol, statins (e.g., atorvastatin) are preferred drugs. Not only do statins reduce cardiovascular events in patients with high cholesterol, they reduce cardiovascular events in patients with normal or low cholesterol. See Chapter 44 for a discussion of lipid-lowering therapies.

Type 2 Diabetes

As with type 1 diabetes, preventing long-term complications requires a comprehensive treatment plan. Lifestyle measures (diet and physical activity) and drug therapy are the foundation of glycemic control. Physical activity provides the additional benefit of promoting glucose uptake by muscle, even when insulin levels are low. In addition to glycemic control, the plan should address other factors that can increase morbidity and mortality. Accordingly, all patients should be screened and treated for hypertension, nephropathy, retinopathy, and neuropathy. In addition, dyslipidemias (high LDL cholesterol, low high-density lipoprotein [HDL] cholesterol, and high triglycerides) should be corrected.

Recommendations for glycemic control have changed. Until recently, treatment was started with lifestyle measures *alone;* drugs were added only if these measures failed. Currently, treatment is started with lifestyle measures *plus* drug therapy. As a result, glycemic control is established sooner, and the risk for long-term complications is lowered.

Type 2 diabetes can be treated with a variety of oral and injectable drugs. Among the oral drugs, metformin is used most widely. Among the injectable drugs, insulin is used most widely. As type 2 diabetes progresses, less and less insulin is produced. As a result, it is common for people with type 2 diabetes to eventually require insulin therapy.

Given the many drugs available for type 2 diabetes, how does one decide which drugs to use for a given patient? As recommended in the 2019 ADA Standards of Medical Care in Diabetes, there are a number of patient-specific considerations that come into play when deciding

TABLE 48.3 General Glycemic Treatment Targets for Nonpregnant Adults With Diabetes

A_{1c}	<7.0%[a]
Premeal plasma glucose	70–130 mg/dL[a]
Peak postmeal plasma glucose	<180 mg/dL[a]

[a]Goals should be individualized based on
- Duration of diabetes
- Age/life expectancy
- Comorbid conditions
- Known cardiovascular disease or advanced microvascular complications
- Hypoglycemia unawareness
- Other individualized considerations

Data from the American Diabetes Association.

TABLE 48.4 Hemoglobin A_{1c} Levels and Their Corresponding eAG Levels

A_{1c} Level (% of Total Hb)	CORRESPONDING eAG LEVEL	
	mg/dL	mmol/L
6	126	7.0
7	154	8.6
8	183	10.2
9	212	11.8
10	240	13.4
11	269	14.9
12	298	16.5

The formula to convert from A_{1c} (%) to average glucose concentration equivalents (expressed in mg/dL) is: eAG = (A_{1c} × 28.7) − 46.7.

eAG, Estimated average glucose in blood; *Hb*, hemoglobin.
Data from the American Diabetes Association.

on a course of treatment. To treat type 2 diabetes, the position statement recommends a four-step approach:

Step 1. At diagnosis, initiate lifestyle changes *plus* metformin.

Step 2. Continue lifestyle changes plus metformin, and *add* a second drug, either a thiazolidinedione, a dipeptidyl peptidase-4 (DPP-4) inhibitor, a sodium-glucose cotransporter 2 (SGLT-2) inhibitor, a glucagon-like peptide-1 (GLP-1) receptor agonist. A sulfonylurea or basal insulin should be considered if the patient does not achieve goal with these drugs. The choice of agent is made in light of relative efficacy, hypoglycemia risk, tolerability, weight-related considerations, and cost.

Step 3. Progress from step 2 to a three-drug combination (inclusive of metformin). Again, the choice of regimen used is determined based on drug- and patient-specific considerations.

Step 4. If three-drug combination therapy that includes basal insulin fails to achieve treatment goals after 3 to 6 months, it is recommended to proceed to a combination injectable regimen inclusive of insulin and possibly a GLP-1 receptor agonist.

Treatment should start at step 1 and then progress to steps 2, 3, and 4 if needed. The exception to this stepwise approach is in patients who have an A_{1c} of 9% or greater at the time of diagnosis, in which case it is recommended to consider dual therapy (i.e., start at step 2). In addition, patients who have an A_{1c} of 10% or greater, have a fasting blood glucose of 300 or more, or are markedly symptomatic may be started on combination injectable therapy immediately.

Determining Appropriate Glycemic Goals

In both type 1 and type 2 diabetes, it is important to determine appropriate glycemic goals for the individual based on his or her lifestyle and other patient-specific considerations. The process of maintaining glucose levels within a normal range, around the clock, is often referred to as "tight glycemic control." Maintaining tight glycemic control is difficult but can be worth the trouble, especially for young patients with type 1 diabetes. However, for many patients with type 2 diabetes, the risks of tight control may be greater than the benefits. Table 48.3 shows current recommendations regarding glycemic goals.

Monitoring Treatment

We need monitoring (1) to determine whether glucose levels are being maintained in a safe range, both short term and long term; and (2) to guide changes in treatment when the range is not satisfactory or safe. SMBG levels are the standard method for day-to-day monitoring. As mentioned previously, A_{1c} is measured to assess long-term glycemic control.

Self-Monitoring of Blood Glucose

SMBG is recommended for all patients who use insulin. That is, SMBG is recommended for all patients with type 1 diabetes and for all patients with type 2 diabetes receiving insulin. It is additionally used by most patients with type 2 diabetes using other therapies as well. Information on blood glucose concentration provides a guide for "fine-tuning" dosages of insulin and other antidiabetic drugs. The frequency of SMBG for any given patient can vary widely based on the therapies the patient uses and how active he or she is. A patient on metformin monotherapy may need to check his or her blood sugar only once per week, whereas a patient with type 1 diabetes on an intensive insulin regimen may check eight times per day or more. Frequently used target values for blood glucose are 70 to 130 mg/dL before meals and 100 to 140 mg/dL at bedtime.

Monitoring of Hemoglobin A_{1c}

As mentioned previously, Measurement of hemoglobin A_{1c}—also called *glycosylated hemoglobin* or *glycated hemoglobin*—provides an index of *average glucose levels* over the prior 2 to 3 months. Glucose interacts spontaneously with hemoglobin in red blood cells to form glycosylated derivatives, the most prevalent being A_{1c}. With prolonged hyperglycemia, levels of A_{1c} gradually increase. Because red blood cells have a long life span (120 days), levels of A_{1c} reflect average glucose levels over an extended time. Hence, by measuring A_{1c} every 3 to 6 months, we can get a picture of long-term glycemic control. However, please note that measuring A_{1c} tells us nothing about acute, hour-to-hour swings in blood glucose. Accordingly, although measuring A_{1c} is an important part of diabetes management, it is clearly no substitute for SMBG.

Results are usually reported as a *percentage of total hemoglobin in blood* (e.g., 7%). In addition, they may be reported as a value for *estimated average glucose* (eAG), expressed as mg of glucose/dL of blood (i.e., the same units patients see every day when doing SMBG). Selected A_{1c} values and their eAG equivalents are shown in Table 48.4.

The general goal is to keep the A_{1c} less than 7%. Although an A_{1c} goal of less than 7% is good for most patients, a less stringent goal (e.g., less than 8%) may be appropriate for some patients, such as those with a history of severe hypoglycemia, limited life expectancy, or advanced microvascular or macrovascular complications. According to a 2014 statement issued jointly by the ADA and the European Association for the Study of Diabetes, A_{1c} should be measured every 3 months until the value drops to 7% and at least every 6 months thereafter. As noted previously, a value of 6.5% or greater is considered diagnostic of diabetes.

PROTOTYPE DRUGS

Drugs for Diabetes Mellitus

Insulin Preparations
Insulin lispro (short duration, rapid acting)
Regular insulin (short duration, short acting)
Neutral protamine Hagedorn insulin (intermediate duration)
Insulin glargine (long duration)
Insulin degludec (ultralong duration)

Biguanides
Metformin

Sulfonylureas
Glyburide

Meglitinides (Glinides)
Repaglinide

Thiazolidinediones (Glitazones)
Pioglitazone

α-Glucosidase Inhibitors
Acarbose

Gliptins (Dipeptidyl Peptidase-4 Inhibitors)
Sitagliptin

Sodium-Glucose Cotransporter 2 Inhibitors
Canagliflozin

Glucagon-like Peptide-1 Receptor Antagonists
Exenatide

INSULIN

Insulin is used to treat all patients with type 1 diabetes and many patients with type 2 diabetes. Our discussion of insulin is divided into three sections: physiology, preparations and administration, and therapeutic use.

Physiology

Structure

The structure of insulin is shown in Fig. 48.1. As indicated, insulin consists of two amino acid chains: the "A" (acidic) chain and the "B" (basic) chain. The A and B chains are linked to each other by two disulfide bridges.

Biosynthesis

Insulin is synthesized in the pancreas by β cells within the islets of Langerhans. The immediate precursor of insulin is called proinsulin.

Proinsulin consists of insulin itself plus a peptide loop that runs from the A chain to the B chain. This loop is named *connecting peptide* or *C-peptide*. In the final step of insulin synthesis, C-peptide is enzymatically clipped from the proinsulin molecule.

Measurement of plasma C-peptide levels offers a way to assess residual capacity for insulin synthesis. Because commercial insulin preparations lack C-peptide and because endogenous C-peptide is present only as a by-product of insulin biosynthesis, the presence of C-peptide in the blood indicates the pancreas is still producing some insulin of its own.

Secretion

The principal stimulus for insulin release is a rise in blood glucose, and the most common cause of glucose elevation is eating a meal, especially one rich in carbohydrates. Under normal conditions, there is tight coupling between rising levels of blood glucose and increased secretion

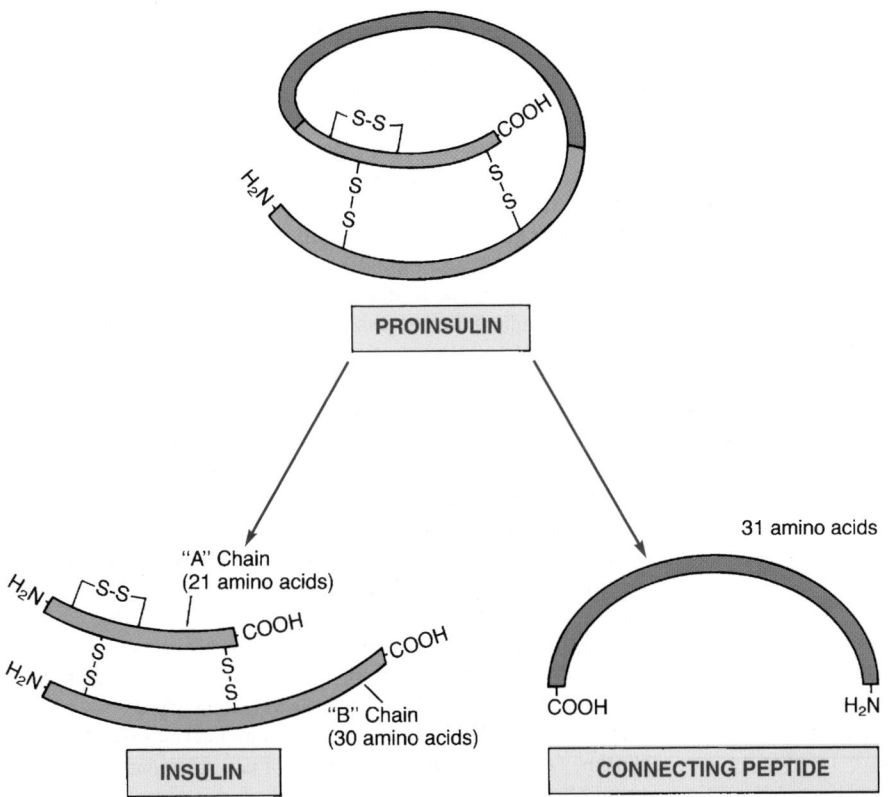

Fig. 48.1 Conversion of Proinsulin to Insulin. Proinsulin is the immediate precursor of the insulin secreted by human pancreas. Enzymes clip off connecting peptide *(C-peptide)* to release active insulin, composed of two peptide chains (A and B) connected by two disulfide *(S–S)* bonds. Because C-peptide arises only from endogenous insulin, its presence in blood indicates that at least some pancreatic insulin is being made.

of insulin. Insulin release may also be triggered by amino acids, fatty acids, ketone bodies, and gut hormones such as GLP-1 (more on this later).

The sympathetic nervous system provides additional control of release. Activation of β_2-adrenergic receptors in the pancreas *promotes* secretion of insulin. Conversely, activation of α-adrenergic receptors in the pancreas *inhibits* insulin release. Of the two modes of regulation, activation of β receptors is more important.

Metabolic Actions

The metabolic actions of insulin are primarily *anabolic* (i.e., conservative, constructive). Insulin promotes conservation of energy and buildup of energy stores, such as glycogen. The hormone also promotes cell growth and division.

Insulin acts in two ways to promote anabolic effects. First, it stimulates cellular transport (uptake) of glucose, amino acids, nucleotides, and potassium. Second, insulin promotes synthesis of complex organic molecules. Under the influence of insulin and other factors, glucose is converted into glycogen, amino acids are assembled into proteins, and fatty acids are incorporated into triglycerides. The principal metabolic actions of insulin are shown in Table 48.5.

Metabolic Consequences of Insulin Deficiency

Insulin deficiency puts the body into a *catabolic* mode. Hence, in the absence of insulin, glycogen is converted into glucose, proteins are degraded into amino acids, and fats are converted to glycerol (glycerin) and free fatty acids. These catabolic effects contribute to the signs and symptoms of diabetes. Note that the catabolic effects resulting from insulin deficiency are opposite to the anabolic effects when insulin levels are normal.

Insulin deficiency promotes *hyperglycemia* by three mechanisms: (1) increased glycogenolysis, (2) increased gluconeogenesis, and (3) reduced glucose utilization. *Glycogenolysis,* by definition, generates free glucose by breaking down glycogen. The raw materials that allow increased *gluconeogenesis* are the amino acids and fatty acids produced by metabolic breakdown of proteins and fats. *Reduced glucose utilization* occurs because insulin deficiency decreases cellular uptake of glucose and decreases conversion of glucose to glycogen.

TABLE 48.5	Metabolic Actions of Insulin	
Substance Affected	**Insulin Action**	**Site of Action**
Carbohydrates	↑ Glucose uptake	Muscle, adipose tissue
	↑ Glucose oxidation	Muscle
	↑ Glucose storage	Muscle, liver
	↑ Glycogen synthesis	
	↓ Glycogenolysis	
	Gluconeogenesis[a]	Liver
Amino acids and proteins	↑ Amino acid uptake	Muscle
	↓ Amino acid release	Muscle
	↑ Protein synthesis	Muscle
Lipids	↑ Triglyceride synthesis	Adipose tissue
	↓ Release of FFA and glycerol	Adipose tissue
	↓ Oxidation of FFA to ketoacids[b]	Liver

[a]Because of decreased delivery of substrate (fatty acids and amino acids) to the liver.
[b]Because of decreased delivery of FFAs to the liver.
FFAs, Free fatty acids.

Preparations and Administration

There are many insulin preparations or formulations. Major differences concern time course, appearance, concentration, and route of administration. Because of these differences, insulin preparations cannot be used interchangeably. In fact, if a patient is given the wrong preparation, the consequences can be dire. Unfortunately, medication errors with insulins remain all too common, which explains why insulin appears on all lists of "high-alert" agents.

Sources of Insulin

All forms of insulin currently manufactured in the United States are produced using recombinant DNA technology. Some products, referred to as *human insulin,* are identical to insulin produced by the human pancreas. Other products, referred to as *human insulin analogs,* are modified forms of human insulin. The analogs have the same pharmacologic actions as human insulin but have different time courses.

Types of Insulin

There are multiple types of insulin: "natural" insulin (also known as regular insulin or native insulin) and six modified insulins. Three of the modified insulins—insulin lispro, insulin aspart, and insulin glulisine—act more rapidly than regular insulin but have a shorter duration of action. The exception to this is a formulation of regular insulin that is administered via inhalation, which also acts more rapidly than injectable regular insulin. The other modified insulins act more slowly than regular insulin but have a longer duration of action. Two processes are used to prolong insulin effects: (1) complexing natural insulin with a protein and (2) altering the insulin molecule itself. When the insulin molecule has been altered, we refer to the product as a *human insulin analog.*

When classified according to time course, insulin preparations fall into four major groups: short duration, intermediate duration, long duration, and ultralong duration (Table 48.6). The short-duration insulins can be subdivided into two groups: rapid acting (insulin lispro, insulin aspart, and insulin glulisine, and inhaled human insulin) and short acting (regular or "natural" insulin). Time courses for different insulin types are shown in Fig. 48.2. Selected properties of insulin types are shown in Table 48.7.

Short duration: rapid acting. Short-duration insulins are administered in association with meals to control the postprandial rise in blood glucose. To provide glycemic control between meals and at night, short-acting insulins must be used in conjunction with an intermediate- or long-acting agent in people with type 1 diabetes.

Insulin lispro. Insulin lispro (Humalog) is a rapid-acting analog of regular insulin. Effects begin within 15 to 30 minutes of subcutaneous (subQ) injection and persist for 3 to 6 hours. Insulin lispro acts faster than regular insulin but has a shorter duration of action. Because of its rapid onset, insulin lispro can be administered immediately before eating or even after eating. In contrast, regular insulin is generally administered 30 to 60 minutes before meals.

The structure of insulin lispro is nearly identical to that of natural insulin. The only difference is that the positions of two amino acids have been switched. Because of this switch, molecules of insulin lispro aggregate less than do molecules of regular insulin, which explains why insulin lispro acts more rapidly.

Insulin aspart. Insulin aspart (NovoLog) is an analog of human insulin with a rapid onset (10 to 20 minutes) and short duration (3 to 5 hours). Insulin aspart is very similar to insulin lispro.

Insulin glulisine. Like insulin lispro and insulin aspart, insulin glulisine (Apidra) is a synthetic analog of natural human insulin with a rapid onset (10 to 15 minutes) and short duration (3 to 5 hours).

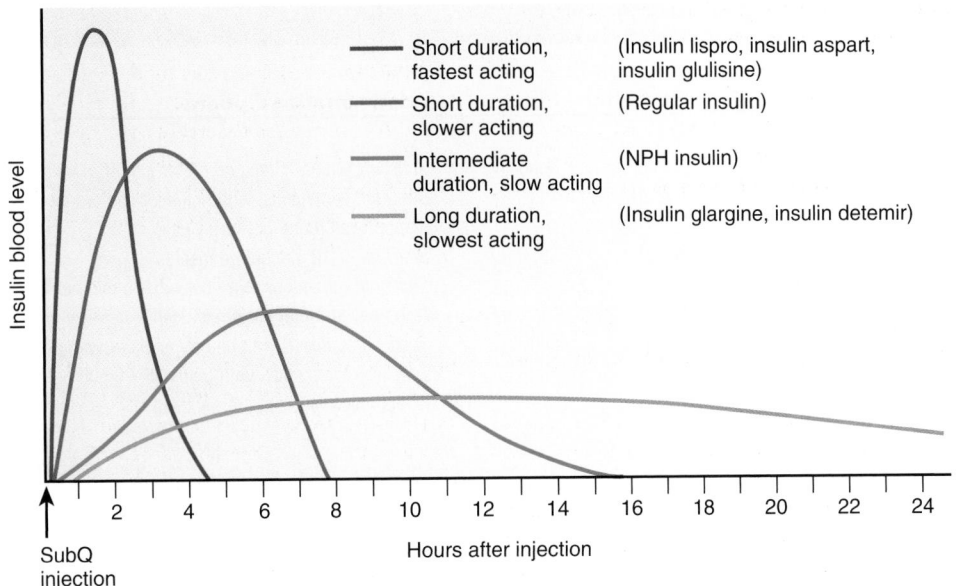

Fig. 48.2 Time-effect Relationship for Different Types of Insulin After Subcutaneous Injection. *NPH,* Neutral protamine Hagedorn.

TABLE 48.6 Types of Insulin: Time Course of Action After Subcutaneous Injection

Generic Name	Trade Name	TIME COURSE		
		Onset (min)	Peak (h)	Duration (h)
Short Duration: Rapid Acting				
Insulin lispro	Humalog	15–30	0.5–2.5	3–6
Insulin aspart	NovoLog	10–20	1–3	3–5
Insulin glulisine	Apidra	10–15	1–1.5	3–5
Short Duration: Short Acting				
Regular insulin	Humulin R, Novolin R	30–60	1–5	6–10
Intermediate Duration				
Neutral protamine Hagedorn insulin	Humulin N, Novolin N	60–120	6–14	16–24
Long Duration				
Insulin glargine (U-100)	Lantus	70	None[a]	18–24
Insulin detemir	Levemir	60–120	12–24	Varies[b]
Ultralong Duration				
Insulin glargine (U-300)	Toujeo	360	None[a]	>24
Insulin degludec	Tresiba	30–90	None[a]	>24

[a]Levels are steady with no discernible peak.
[b]Duration is dose dependent: at 0.2 units/kg, duration is 12 hours; at 0.4 units/kg, duration is 20 to 24 hours.

Owing to its rapid onset, the drug should be administered close to the time of eating.

Inhaled human insulin. As mentioned briefly before, when regular human insulin is inhaled, the time action profile is altered such that the regular insulin works more quickly and has a shorter duration when compared with regular insulin when injected subQ. Inhaled human insulin (Afrezza) is a mealtime insulin product that can be used in people with type 1 and type 2 diabetes. The insulin product is available commercially in cartridges that contain 4, 8, or 12 units each.

Short duration: short acting

Regular insulin injection. Regular insulin (Humulin R, Novolin R) is unmodified human insulin. The product has four approved routes: subQ injection, subQ infusion, and intramuscular (IM) injection (used rarely).

For routine treatment of diabetes, regular insulin can be (1) injected before meals to control postprandial hyperglycemia and (2) infused subcutaneously via insulin pump to provide basal glycemic control. After *subQ injection,* molecules of regular insulin form small aggregates at the injection site. As a result, absorption is slightly delayed. Effects begin in 30 to 60 minutes, peak in 1 to 5 hours, and last up to 10 hours. Onset is slower than with the rapid-acting insulins and faster than with the longer acting insulins. Because of this delay, most people using insulin pumps use a rapid-acting insulin analog instead of regular insulin.

Intermediate duration

Neutral protamine Hagedorn insulin suspension. Neutral protamine Hagedorn (NPH) insulin (Humulin N, Novolin N), also known as *isophane insulin,* is prepared by conjugating regular insulin with protamine (a large protein). The presence of protamine decreases the solubility of NPH insulin and thus delays absorption. As a result, onset of action is delayed and duration of action is extended. Because onset is delayed, NPH insulin cannot be administered at mealtime to control postprandial hyperglycemia. Rather, the drug is injected twice or three times daily to provide glycemic control between meals and during the night. Of the longer-acting insulins in current use, NPH insulin is the only one suitable for mixing with short-acting insulins. Because protamine is a foreign protein, allergic reactions are possible.

Long duration

Insulin glargine (U-100). U-100 insulin glargine (Lantus, Basaglar) is a modified human insulin with a prolonged duration of action (up to 24 hours). The drug is indicated for once-daily subQ dosing to treat adults and children with type 1 diabetes and adults with type 2 diabetes. That being said, some patients require twice-daily administration to achieve the full 24 hours of basal coverage. Dosing may be done any time of day (morning, afternoon, or evening) but should be done at the same time every day, if possible.

TABLE 48.7 Properties of Insulin Types

Generic Name (Trade Name)	Class	Rx or OTC	Strength	Route	Administration Options
Short Duration: Rapid Acting					
Insulin lispro (Humalog)	HA	Rx	U-100, U-200	SubQ, IV	*SubQ inj:* within 15 min before or just after meals *SubQ inf:* continuous, with bolus just before meals *IV:* approved route, but rarely used
Insulin aspart (NovoLog)	HA	Rx	U-100	SubQ, IV	*SubQ inj:* 5–10 min before meals *SubQ inf:* continuous, with bolus 5–10 min before meals *IV:* approved route, but rarely used
Insulin glulisine (Apidra)	HA	Rx	U-100	SubQ, IV	*SubQ inj:* within 15 min before meals or within 20 min after *SubQ inf:* continuous, with bolus 15–20 min before meals *IV:* approved route, but rarely used
Short Duration: Short Acting					
Regular insulin (Humulin R, Novolin R)	H	OTC[a]	U-100, U-500	SubQ, IV, IM	*SubQ inj:* 30 min before meals *SubQ inf:* continuous, with bolus 20–30 min before meals *IV:* for emergencies and glycemic management in the inpatient setting (never use U-500 IV) *IM:* approved route but rarely used
Intermediate Duration					
NPH insulin (Humulin N, Novolin N)	H	OTC	U-100	SubQ	*SubQ inj:* twice daily at the same times each day; gently agitate before use
Long Duration					
U-100 Insulin glargine (Lantus)	HA	Rx	U-100	SubQ	*SubQ inj:* once or twice daily at the same time each day
Insulin detemir (Levemir)	HA	Rx	U-100	SubQ	*SubQ inj:* once or twice daily at the same time each day
Ultralong Duration					
U-300 Insulin glargine (Toujeo)	HA	Rx	U-300	SubQ	*SubQ inj:* once daily at the same time each day
Insulin degludec (Tresiba)	HA	Rx	U-100, U-200	SubQ	*SubQ inj:* once daily at the same time each day

[a]U-100 formulations are OTC, the U-500 formulation is Rx.

H, Human insulin; *HA*, human insulin analog; *inj*, injection; *inf*, infusion; *Rx*, prescription needed; *NPH*, neutral protamine Hagedorn; *OTC*, over the counter (no prescription needed); *U-100*, 100 units/mL; *U-200*, 200 units/mL; *U-300*, 300 units/mL; *U-500*, 500 units/mL.

U-100 insulin glargine differs from natural human insulin by four amino acids. Hence, when injected subcutaneously, it forms microprecipitates that slowly dissolve and thereby release insulin glargine in small amounts over an extended time. In contrast to other long-acting insulins (e.g., insulin detemir), which cause blood levels to rise to a peak and then fall to a trough, insulin glargine achieves blood levels that are relatively steady.

Insulin detemir. Insulin detemir (Levemir) is a human insulin analog with a slow onset and dose-dependent duration of action. At low doses (0.2 units/kg), effects persist about 12 hours. At higher doses (0.4 units/kg), effects persist for up to 20 to 24 hours. Because of its slow onset and prolonged duration, insulin detemir is used to provide basal glycemic control. It is not given before meals to control postprandial hyperglycemia. Compared with NPH insulin, insulin detemir has a slower onset and longer duration.

Ultralong duration

Insulin glargine (U-300). U-300 insulin glargine (Toujeo) is similar to U-100 insulin glargine except that it is three times concentrated, which prolongs its duration of action to be in excess of 24 hours. The drug is indicated for once-daily subQ dosing to treat both type 1 and type 2 diabetes. Because U-300 insulin glargine has a longer duration of action than U-100 insulin glargine, use of this product is an option for those individuals who do not realize a full 24 hours of effect with the U-100 product.

Insulin degludec. Insulin degludec (Tresiba) is the only human insulin analog with effects that persist for up to 42 hours. Because of its prolonged duration, insulin degludec is used to provide basal glycemic control. Similarly to insulin glargine, insulin degludec does not have a peak.

PATIENT EDUCATION

Mixing Insulins

Mixing should be done only with insulins of proven compatibility. Of the three longer-acting insulins in current use, *only NPH insulin is appropriate for mixing with short-acting insulins* (i.e., regular, lispro, aspart, and glulisine insulins). When a mixture is prepared, the short-acting insulin should be drawn into the syringe first to avoid contaminating the stock vial of the short-acting insulin with NPH insulin.

Commercially available premixed combinations are described in Table 48.8.

TABLE 48.8   Premixed Insulin Combinations

Description	Trade Name	TIME COURSE		
		Onset (min)	Peak (h)	Duration (h)
70% NPH insulin/30% regular insulin	Humulin 70/30	30–60	1.5–16	10–16
	Novolin 70/30	30–60	2–12	10–16
50% NPH insulin/50% regular insulin	Humulin 50/50	30–60	2–12	10–16
70% insulin aspart protamine/30% insulin aspart	NovoLog Mix 70/30	10–20	1–4	15–18
75% insulin lispro protamine/25% insulin lispro	Humalog Mix 75/25	15–30	1–6.5	10–16
50% insulin lispro protamine/50% insulin lispro	Humalog Mix 50/50	15–30	0.8–4.8	10–16

Use only after the dosages and ratios of the components have been established as correct for the patient.
NPH, Neutral protamine Hagedorn.

B = Breakfast, L = Lunch, S = Supper, HS = Bedtime

Fig. 48.3 Examples of Insulin Dosing Schedules. (A) Twice daily premixed regimen. (B) Continuous subcutaneous insulin infusion.

Therapeutic Use

Indications

The principal indication for insulin is *diabetes mellitus.* Insulin is required by all patients with type 1 diabetes and by many patients with type 2 diabetes. In fact, most of the insulin sold is used by people with type 2 diabetes—largely because type 2 diabetes accounts for 90% to 95% of all cases of diabetes.

Insulin Therapy of Diabetes

Insulin is given to all patients who have type 1 diabetes and to many who have type 2 diabetes. In addition, insulin is the preferred drug to manage gestational diabetes. In treating these disorders, the objective is to prevent complications by keeping blood glucose within an acceptable range. When therapy is successful, both hyperglycemia and hypoglycemia are minimized and the long-term complications of diabetes are avoided.

Dosage. To achieve optimal glucose control, insulin dosage must be closely matched with insulin needs. If carbohydrate intake is increased, insulin dosage must be increased, too. When a meal is missed or is low in carbohydrates, or when physical activity levels increase, the dosage of insulin must be decreased. Dosing requires additional adjustments to meet specialized needs. For example, insulin needs are *increased* by infection, stress, obesity, the adolescent growth spurt, and pregnancy after the first trimester. Conversely, insulin needs are *decreased* by exercise and during the first trimester of pregnancy. To ensure that insulin dosage is coordinated with insulin requirements, the patient and the health care team must work together to establish an integrated program of nutrition, exercise, insulin replacement therapy, and appropriate blood glucose monitoring.

Total daily dosages may range from 0.1 unit/kg body weight to more than 2.5 units/kg. For patients with type 1 diabetes, initial dosages typically range from 0.5 to 0.6 units/kg/day. For patients with type 2 diabetes, initial dosages typically range from 0.2 to 0.6 units/kg/day.

Dosing schedules. The schedule of insulin administration helps determine the extent to which glucose control can be achieved. Two dosing schedules are compared here. These example regimens include use of a twice-daily premixed insulin regimen and an intensive basal/bolus strategy. Although three example regimens are discussed, it should be

noted that practitioners can use available insulin products in a number of ways and combinations to meet patient-specific needs and treatment goals.

Twice-daily premixed regimen. There are several premixed insulin products on the market. As shown in Fig. 48.3A, a twice-daily regimen of such a premixed insulin product can be used to provide both basal and prandial insulin coverage. The advantage of this strategy is that patients have to give only two injections per day. However, a disadvantage is that if given with breakfast and dinner, there is no mealtime coverage at lunch. In addition, using a fixed combination does not allow for adjustments of the long-acting or short-acting insulin individually; if the dose is changed, both components are altered.

Intensive basal/bolus strategy. For patients with type 1 diabetes, an intensive basal/bolus strategy is often used. As shown in Fig. 48.3B, this strategy involves the use of a long-acting insulin (such as insulin glargine [Lantus]) in addition to a short-acting insulin (such as regular insulin, insulin aspart, insulin lispro, or insulin glulisine). This insulin dosing strategy allows for very good basal coverage and the ability to dose a short-acting insulin with each meal and as needed to cover snacks or elevated blood glucose levels.

Achieving optimal glucose control. As we have seen, the primary requirement for achieving tight glucose control is a method of insulin delivery that permits dosage adjustments that accommodate ongoing variations in insulin needs. Intensive basal/bolus therapy and continuous subcutaneous insulin infusion (CSII) meet this criterion. In addition to an adaptable method of insulin delivery, achieving tight glucose control requires the following:

- Careful attention to all elements of the treatment program (diet, exercise, insulin replacement therapy)
- Defined glycemic targets
- Self-monitoring of blood glucose in concordance with the patient's individualized management plan
- A high degree of patient motivation
- Extensive patient education

Tight glucose control cannot be achieved without the informed participation of the patient. Accordingly, patients must receive thorough instruction on the following:

- The nature of diabetes
- The importance of optimal glucose control

- The major components of the treatment routine (insulin replacement, SMBG, diet, exercise)
- Procedures for purchasing insulin, syringes, and needles
- The importance of avoiding arbitrary changes between insulins from different manufacturers
- Methods of insulin storage
- Procedures for mixing insulins (if applicable)
- Calculation of dosage adjustments
- Techniques of insulin administration
- Methods for monitoring blood glucose

In the final analysis, responsibility for managing diabetes rests with the patient. The health care team can design a treatment program and provide education and guidance. However, optimal glucose control can be achieved only if the patient is actively involved in his or her own therapy.

Complications of Insulin Treatment

Hypoglycemia. Hypoglycemia (blood glucose less than 70 mg/dL) occurs when insulin levels exceed insulin needs. A major cause of insulin excess is overdose. Imbalance between insulin levels and insulin needs can also result from reduced intake of food, vomiting and diarrhea (which reduce absorption of nutrients), excessive consumption of alcohol (which promotes hypoglycemia), unusually intense exercise (which promotes cellular glucose uptake and metabolism), and childbirth (which reduces insulin requirements).

PATIENT EDUCATION

Hypoglycemia

Patients with diabetes and their families should be familiar with the signs and symptoms of hypoglycemia. Establishing whether patients are experiencing hypoglycemia and whether they recognize hypoglycemic symptoms is recommended as a critical component of an encounter with a patient with diabetes. Some symptoms result from activation of the sympathetic nervous system; others arise from a lack of glucose within the central nervous system (CNS). When glucose levels fall *rapidly*, activation of the sympathetic nervous system occurs, resulting in tachycardia, palpitations, sweating, and nervousness. However, if glucose declines *gradually*, symptoms may be limited to those of CNS origin. Mild CNS symptoms include headache, confusion, drowsiness, and fatigue. If hypoglycemia is severe, convulsions, coma, and death may follow.

Rapid treatment of hypoglycemia is mandatory: if hypoglycemia is allowed to persist, irreversible brain damage or even death may result. In conscious patients, glucose levels can be restored with a fast-acting oral sugar (e.g., glucose tablets, orange juice, sugar cubes, honey, corn syrup, nondiet soda). However, if the swallowing reflex or the gag reflex is suppressed, nothing should be administered by mouth. In cases of severe hypoglycemia, intravenous (IV) glucose is the preferred treatment. Parenteral *glucagon* is an alternative treatment. (The pharmacology of glucagon is discussed at the end of the chapter.)

In anticipation of hypoglycemic episodes, people with diabetes should always have an oral carbohydrate available (e.g., sugared candy, sugar cubes, glucose tablets). Some prescribers recommend that patients keep glucagon on hand too—particularly people on insulin therapy. Patients should carry some sort of identification (e.g., a medical alert bracelet) to inform emergency personnel of their condition.

In some patients, hypoglycemia occurs without producing the symptoms noted previously. This is known as *hypoglycemia unawareness*.

As a result, the patient remains unaware of hypoglycemia until blood sugar has become dangerously low. Hypoglycemia unawareness is a particular problem among patients practicing tight glucose control. This is because as patients experience more frequent hypoglycemia, they start to have diminished symptoms over time. The risk for dangerous hypoglycemia can be minimized by frequently monitoring blood glucose. In addition, current recommendations state that treatment goals should be temporarily loosened (such as for several weeks) for people experiencing hypoglycemia unawareness so that they can regain hypoglycemia awareness.

Hypoglycemia can result in coma. The most definitive diagnosis is made by measuring plasma glucose levels: in hypoglycemic coma, glucose levels are very low.

Drug Interactions

Hypoglycemic agents. Drugs that lower blood glucose levels can intensify hypoglycemia induced by insulin. Among these drugs are *sulfonylureas, glinides*, and *alcohol* (used acutely or long term in excessive doses). When these drugs are combined with insulin, special care must be taken to ensure as best as possible that blood glucose does not fall too low.

Hyperglycemic agents. Drugs that raise blood glucose (e.g., *thiazide diuretics, glucocorticoids, sympathomimetics*) can counteract the desired effects of insulin. When these agents are combined with insulin, insulin dosage may need to be increased.

β-Adrenergic blocking agents. β-Blockers can delay awareness of and response to hypoglycemia by masking signs that are associated with stimulation of the sympathetic nervous system (e.g., tachycardia, palpitations) that hypoglycemia normally causes. Furthermore, because β-blockade impairs glycogenolysis and because glycogenolysis is one means by which the body can respond to and counteract a fall in blood glucose, β-blockers can make insulin-induced hypoglycemia even worse by preventing the body's natural counterregulatory response.

SUMMARY OF KEY PRESCRIBING CONSIDERATIONS

Insulin

Therapeutic Goal: Maintain plasma levels of glucose and A$_{1c}$ within an acceptable range

Baseline Data: Random plasma glucose, fasting plasma glucose, A$_{1c}$, serum electrolytes, urinary glucose and ketones

Monitoring: Patients should monitor glucose levels multiple times daily. A$_{1c}$ can be measured two to four times yearly.

Identifying High-Risk Patients: Patients taking additional medications that may raise (sympathomimetics, glucocorticoids) or lower (sulfonylureas) blood glucose should be monitored more extensively.

Evaluating Therapeutic Effects: Improvement in symptoms, including decrease in urination, fatigue, and decrease in plasma glucose levels and A$_{1c}$.

Minimizing Adverse Effects: Educate patients and families on the signs and symptoms of hypoglycemia as well as extreme hyperglycemia.

NONINSULIN MEDICATIONS FOR THE TREATMENT OF DIABETES

The noninsulin medications for the treatment of diabetes fall into two major groups: oral drugs and injectable drugs. Their actions and major adverse effects are shown in Table 48.9.

TABLE 48.9 Drugs for Type 2 Diabetes

Class and Specific Agents	Actions	Major Adverse Effects
Oral Drugs		
Biguanide		
Metformin (Fortamet, Glucophage, Glumetza, Riomet)	Decreases glucose production by the liver, increases tissue response to insulin	Gastrointestinal (GI) symptoms: decreased appetite, nausea, diarrhea Lactic acidosis (rarely)
Second-Generation Sulfonylureas		
Glimepiride (Amaryl) Glipizide (Glucotrol) Glyburide[a] (DiaBeta, Glynase PresTab)	Promote insulin secretion by the pancreas; may also increase tissue response to insulin	Hypoglycemia Weight gain
Meglitinides (Glinides)		
Nateglinide (Starlix) Repaglinide (Prandin, GlucoNorm ♦)	Promote insulin secretion by the pancreas	Hypoglycemia Weight gain
Thiazolidinediones (Glitazones)		
Pioglitazone (Actos) Rosiglitazone (Avandia)	Decrease insulin resistance and thereby increase glucose uptake by muscle and adipose tissue and decrease glucose production by the liver	Hypoglycemia but only in the presence of excessive insulin Heart failure Bladder cancer Fractures (in women) Ovulation and thus possible unintended pregnancy
α-Glucosidase Inhibitors		
Acarbose (Precose, Glucobay ♦) Miglitol (Glyset)	Delay carbohydrate digestion and absorption, thereby decreasing the postprandial rise in blood glucose	GI symptoms: flatulence, cramps, abdominal distention, borborygmus
Dipeptidyl Peptidase-4 (DPP-4) Inhibitors (Gliptins)		
Alogliptin (Nesina) Linagliptin (Tradjenta) Saxagliptin (Onglyza) Sitagliptin (Januvia)	Enhance the activity of incretins (by inhibiting their breakdown by DPP-4) and thereby increase insulin release, reduce glucagon release, and decrease hepatic glucose production	Pancreatitis Hypersensitivity reactions
Sodium-Glucose Cotransporter 2 (SGLT-2) Inhibitors		
Canagliflozin (Invokana) Dapagliflozin (Farxiga)	Increase glucose excretion via the urine by inhibiting SGLT-2 in the kidney tubules, decreasing glucose levels and inducing weight loss by caloric loss through the urine	Genital mycotic infections Orthostasis
Dopamine Agonist		
Bromocriptine (Cycloset)	Activates dopamine receptors in the central nervous system; how it improves glycemic control is unknown	Orthostatic hypotension Exacerbation of psychosis
Noninsulin Injectable Drugs		
Glucagon-like Peptide-1 (GLP-1) Receptor Agonists (Incretin Mimetics)		
Exenatide (Byetta) Exenatide extended release (Bydureon) Liraglutide (Victoza) Dulaglutide (Trulicity) Lixisenatide (Adlyxin)	Lower blood glucose by slowing gastric emptying, stimulating glucose-dependent insulin release, suppressing postprandial glucagon release, and reducing appetite	Hypoglycemia GI symptoms: nausea, vomiting, diarrhea Pancreatitis Renal insufficiency Thyroid cancer? (liraglutide, exenatide extended-release)
Amylin Mimetics		
Pramlintide (Symlin)	Delays gastric emptying and suppresses glucagon secretion, decreasing the postprandial rise in glucose	Hypoglycemia Nausea Injection-site reactions

[a]Commonly known as *glibenclamide* outside the United States.

Oral Drugs

There are seven main families of oral antidiabetic drugs: biguanides, sulfonylureas, meglitinides (glinides), thiazolidinediones (glitazones), α-glucosidase inhibitors, DPP-4 inhibitors (gliptins), and SGLT-2 inhibitors. These agents are approved for use in type 2 diabetes, but agents such as the SGLT-2 inhibitors are used off-label in combination with insulin for the treatment of type 1 diabetes—with clinical studies in progress. In the past, the oral agents were used only after a program of diet modification and exercise had failed to yield sufficient glycemic control. Currently, one oral agent—metformin—is usually started immediately after type 2 diabetes has been diagnosed.

The oral agents work in a variety of ways. Some of them—notably the sulfonylureas, and glinides (collectively referred to as "insulin secretagogues")—actively drive blood glucose down by increasing insulin release from β cells of the pancreas. Others—notably metformin (a biguanide), the α-glucosidase inhibitors, and SGLT-2 inhibitors—do not drive blood glucose down; rather, they simply modulate the rise in glucose that happens after a meal. This distinction is not just academic: if taken when blood glucose is normal or low, agents that drive glucose down can cause *hypoglycemia*. Hypoglycemia is not a large risk with the drugs that simply impair the postprandial rise in blood glucose.

Biguanides: Metformin

Metformin (Glucophage, Glucophage XR, Fortamet, Glumetza, Riomet), classified chemically as a biguanide, is the drug of choice for initial therapy in most patients with type 2 diabetes (Table 48.10). Typically, metformin is started immediately after the diagnosis of type 2 diabetes. The most common side effects are gastrointestinal (GI) disturbances. Lactic acidosis, a potentially fatal complication, is rare.

Mechanism of action. Metformin lowers blood glucose and improves glucose tolerance in three ways. First, it inhibits glucose production in the liver. Second, it reduces (slightly) glucose absorption in the gut. And third, it sensitizes insulin receptors in target tissues (fat and skeletal muscle) and thereby increases glucose uptake in response to whatever insulin may be available. In contrast to the sulfonylureas (see later), metformin does not stimulate insulin release from the pancreas. As a result, metformin does not actively drive blood glucose levels down and hence poses little if any added risk for hypoglycemia when used alone.

Pharmacokinetics. After oral dosing, metformin is slowly absorbed from the small intestine. Of particular interest, metformin is not metabolized. Rather, it is excreted unchanged by the kidneys. Hence, in the event of renal impairment, metformin can accumulate to toxic levels.

Therapeutic uses

Glycemic control. Metformin is used to lower blood sugar in patients with type 2 diabetes. In the past, treatment was reserved for patients who had not responded adequately to a program of diet modification and exercise. Currently, however, treatment is usually begun as soon as type 2 diabetes is diagnosed.

Metformin may be used alone or in combination with other agents. When used alone, metformin lowers fasting and postprandial blood glucose levels. When metformin is used as a component of combination therapy, the combination lowers blood sugar more effectively than either drug alone—which is to be expected because other available agents act through different mechanisms.

Metformin is well suited for patients who tend to skip meals. When meals are skipped, blood sugar can drop below a level that is healthy. Because metformin does not lower blood glucose any further, it will not make the situation any worse. In contrast, drugs that actively lower blood glucose, such as the sulfonylureas, can drop a normal or slightly low blood glucose into clinically significant hypoglycemia.

Prevention of type 2 diabetes. Data from the Diabetes Prevention Program (DPP), a large study sponsored by the National Institutes of Health, indicate that metformin can delay development of type 2 diabetes in high-risk individuals. The DPP enrolled 3234 people aged 25 to 85 years. All participants had impaired glucose tolerance (as determined by an OGTT), and all were severely overweight. Participants were randomly assigned to one of three protocols: (1) intensive lifestyle changes with the aim of reducing body weight by 7% through moderate exercise (e.g., vigorous walking 30 minutes a day, 5 days a week) combined with a low-fat diet, (2) treatment with metformin (850 mg twice daily), or (3) treatment with placebo. The results? Metformin reduced the risk for developing type 2 diabetes by 31%. However, benefits were limited primarily to younger patients and to those who were most overweight; the drug was relatively ineffective in older patients and those less overweight. However, it must be stressed that metformin is not a substitute for diet and exercise. In fact, the DPP showed that lifestyle changes are even more effective than metformin: the combination of moderate exercise plus weight loss (5% to 7% of initial weight) reduced the average risk for type 2 diabetes by 58%. Benefits were greatest (71%) for people older than 60 years.

Gestational diabetes. For decades, insulin was considered the preferred, if not the only, antidiabetic drug for managing diabetes during pregnancy, whether the mother had type 1 or type 2 diabetes. Recent clinical studies have compared metformin with insulin in pregnant women with type 2 diabetes. Multiple outcomes were assessed, including glycemic control in the mother, and blood glucose and Apgar scores in the neonate. The result? Outcomes with metformin were essentially the same as those with insulin, the traditional agent for managing gestational diabetes—suggesting that metformin may become an acceptable alternative for many women. (*Note:* The data obtained with metformin do *not* apply to other classes of oral agents, such as the sulfonylureas and glitazones.)

Polycystic ovary syndrome. Polycystic ovary syndrome (PCOS) is a combined endocrine-metabolic disorder characterized by androgen excess and insulin resistance. It affects approximately 5% to 10% of women of reproductive age. Symptoms include irregular periods, anovulation, infertility, acne, and hirsutism. Although not approved for PCOS, metformin can be very helpful. Metformin treatment increases insulin sensitivity and decreases insulin levels, which, through an indirect mechanism, lowers androgen levels. The net result is improved glucose tolerance, improved ovulation, and increased pregnancy rates.

Side effects. The most common side effects are decreased appetite, nausea, and diarrhea. These generally subside over time. However, in 3% to 5% of patients, *GI side effects* lead to discontinuation of treatment.

TABLE 48.10	Metformin Availability and Usual Dosing	
Name	**Formulations**	**Usual Initial Adult Dosing**
Generic	IR Tablets: 500, 850, 100 mg	IR- 850–1000 mg daily
	ER tablets: 500, 750, 1000 mg	ER- 500 mg nightly
Fortamet	ER tablets: 500, 1000 mg	500 mg nightly
Glucophage	IR Tablets: 500, 850, 1000 mg	850 mg daily or 500 mg twice daily
Glucophage XR	ER tablets: 500, 750 mg	500 mg nightly
Glumetza	ER tablets: 500, 1000 mg	1000 mg nightly
Riomet	Solution: 500 mg/mL	850 mg daily or 500 mg twice daily

ER, Extended release; *IR,* immediate release.

Therefore the dose of metformin must be titrated up to the target dose to minimize the severity of GI side effects.

Metformin decreases absorption of vitamin B_{12} and folic acid and can thereby cause deficiencies of both. Deficiency of B_{12}, in turn, can contribute to peripheral neuropathy, a common long-term consequence of diabetes. However, there is no proof (yet) that metformin actually makes diabetic neuropathy worse. Likewise, there is no current recommendation about prescribing vitamin B_{12} for patients who are taking the drug. As discussed in Chapter 67, deficiency of folic acid during pregnancy can impair development of the CNS, resulting in neural tube defects, which manifest as anencephaly or spina bifida. Nonetheless, metformin appears to be a safe drug for use during pregnancy.

In contrast to sulfonylureas (see later), metformin does not cause weight gain. In fact, patients maintain or possibly *lose* weight with metformin therapy. As a result, metformin is considered a "weight-neutral" antidiabetic drug, in contrast to several other antidiabetic drugs that tend to increase weight ("weight-positive" drugs). Appetite suppression and weight loss in response to metformin can occur both in the presence and absence of nausea, indicating that reduced food intake because of metformin-induced nausea is not the only reason for weight loss in those patients who lose weight.

BLACK BOX WARNING

Metformin

> Severe metabolic acidosis can occur with accumulation of metformin. Highest risk occurs in diabetic patients with significant renal impairment.

Metformin and other biguanides inhibit mitochondrial oxidation of lactic acid and can thereby cause lactic acidosis. This condition is a medical emergency and has a mortality rate of approximately 50%. Fortunately, lactic acidosis is rare (approximately 3 cases/100,000 patient-years) when metformin is used at recommended doses in patients with good renal function. However, in patients with renal insufficiency, metformin can rapidly accumulate to toxic levels. Accordingly, the drug must never be used by these people. In addition, metformin must be avoided in patients who are prone to increased lactic acid production. Among these are patients with liver disease, severe infection, or a history of lactic acidosis; patients who consume alcohol to excess; and patients with shock and other conditions that can result in hypoxemia.

All patients taking metformin should be informed about early signs of lactic acidosis—hyperventilation, myalgia, malaise, and unusual somnolence—and instructed to report these to the prescriber. Metformin should be withdrawn until lactic acidosis has been ruled out. If lactic acidosis is diagnosed, hemodialysis can correct the condition and remove accumulated metformin.

Because heart failure (HF) can predispose to lactic acidosis, metformin is contraindicated for people with failing hearts. However, in one study, patients with HF who took the drug were *less* likely to die than those who took a sulfonylurea. These data suggest that use of metformin in HF is much safer than previously believed.

Sulfonylureas

The sulfonylureas, introduced in the 1950s, were the first oral antidiabetic drugs available. They work by promoting insulin release and hence are to be used only in type 2 diabetes. The sulfonylureas were a major advance in diabetes therapy: for the first time, some patients could be treated with an oral medication, rather than with daily injections of insulin. The major side effects with these drugs are hypoglycemia and weight gain.

The sulfonylureas fall into two groups: *first-generation agents* and *second-generation agents*. Both generations reduce glucose levels to the same extent. How do the generations differ? The second-generation

agents are *much more potent* than the first-generation agents, and hence dosages are much lower (as much as 1000 times lower in some cases). More important, with the second-generation agents, *significant drug–drug interactions are less common*, and the outcomes tend to be milder. Because of these differences, the second-generation agents have nearly completely replaced the first-generation agents in clinical practice. Accordingly, our discussion in this chapter is limited to the second-generation agents.

Three second-generation sulfonylureas are currently available (Table 48.11). All have similar actions and side effects, and they all share the same application: treatment of type 2 diabetes.

Mechanism of action. Sulfonylureas act primarily by stimulating the release of insulin from pancreatic islets. If the pancreas is incapable of insulin synthesis, sulfonylureas will be ineffective—which is why they do not work in patients with type 1 diabetes. With prolonged use, sulfonylureas may increase target cell sensitivity to insulin.

Sulfonylureas promote insulin release by binding with and thereby blocking adenosine triphosphate (ATP)-sensitive potassium channels in the cell membrane. As a result, the membrane depolarizes, thereby permitting influx of calcium, which in turn causes insulin release. The extent of release is glucose dependent and diminishes when plasma glucose declines.

Therapeutic use. Sulfonylureas are indicated only for type 2 diabetes. These drugs are of no help to patients with type 1 diabetes. Like all other drugs for type 2 diabetes, the sulfonylureas should be used in conjunction with a lifestyle program inclusive of dietary and physical activity interventions. The sulfonylureas may be used alone or together with other antidiabetic drugs.

Adverse effects

Hypoglycemia. Sulfonylureas cause a dose-dependent reduction in blood glucose and can thereby cause *hypoglycemia*. Importantly, regardless of what the glucose level is—high, normal, or low—sulfonylureas will make it go lower. If the level is high, reducing it will be therapeutic. However, if the level is normal, reducing it will cause mild hypoglycemia. And if the level is already low, reducing it can cause severe hypoglycemia.

Although sulfonylurea-induced hypoglycemia is usually mild, severe and even fatal cases have occurred. Hypoglycemia is sometimes persistent, requiring infusion of dextrose for several days. Hypoglycemic reactions are more likely in patients with kidney or liver dysfunction because sulfonylureas are eliminated by hepatic metabolism and renal excretion and hence may accumulate to dangerous levels when liver or kidney function is impaired. If signs of hypoglycemia develop (fatigue, excessive hunger, profuse sweating, palpitations), the patient should treat the hypoglycemia and notify the prescriber.

SUMMARY OF KEY PRESCRIBING CONSIDERATIONS

Sulfonylureas

> **Therapeutic Goal:** Maintain glycemic control in patients with type 2 diabetes in conjunction with diet and exercise.
> **Baseline Data:** Random plasma glucose, fasting plasma glucose, A_{1c}, serum electrolytes, urinary glucose and ketones
> **Monitoring:** Patients should monitor blood glucose at home regularly.
> **Identifying High-Risk Patients:** Sulfonylureas are contraindicated during pregnancy and breast-feeding. Use these drugs with caution in patients with renal or hepatic dysfunction.
> **Evaluating Therapeutic Effects:** Improvement in symptoms, including decrease in urination, fatigue, and decrease in plasma glucose levels and A_{1c}.
> **Minimizing Adverse Effects:** Educate patients about signs and symptoms of hypoglycemia.

TABLE 48.11 Sulfonylureas: Time Course and Dosage

Generic Name (Trade Name)	Duration (h)	Dosage[a]	Approximate Equivalent Dose (mg/24 h)[b]
First-Generation Agents[c]			
Tolbutamide (generic only)	6–12	*Initial:* 1–2 g/day in 1–2 doses *Maximum:* 2–3 g/day in 1–2 doses	1000–1500
Tolazamide (generic only)	12–24	*Initial:* 100–250 mg/day with breakfast *Maximum:* 0.75–1 g/day in 2 doses	250–375
Chlorpropamide (generic only)	24–60	*Initial:* 125 mg/day with breakfast *Maximum:* 750 mg once a day	250–375
Second-Generation Agents **Glipizide**			
Immediate release (Glucotrol)	10–24	*Initial:* 5 mg/day with breakfast *Maximum:* 40 mg/day in 2 doses	10
Sustained release (Glucotrol XL)	24	*Initial:* 5 mg/day with breakfast *Maximum:* 20 mg/day with breakfast	10
Glyburide			
Nonmicronized (DiaBeta)	16–24	*Initial:* 2.5–5 mg day with breakfast *Maximum:* 20 mg/day in 1 or 2 doses	5
Micronized (Glynase PresTab)	12–24	*Initial:* 1.5–3 mg/day with breakfast *Maximum:* 12 mg/day in 1 or 2 doses	3
Glimepiride (Amaryl)	24	*Initial:* 1–2 mg/day with breakfast *Maximum:* 8 mg/day with breakfast	2

[a]Older adults should use a smaller dose than those noted here.
[b]These values reflect differences in potency and can be used to estimate what dose to use when switching from one sulfonylurea to another.
[c]The first-generation agents are used only rarely.

TABLE 48.12 Metlitinides (Glinides)

Drug	Mechanism of Action	Metabolism and Excretion	Peak and Half-Life in Hours	Preparations	Usual Initial Adult Dosage
Repaglinide (Prandin)	Facilitates calcium influx in pancreatic β cells, which leads to increased insulin release	Metabolism: Hepatic Excretion: Gastrointestinal (bile)	Peak: 1 Half-life 1	Tablets 0.5, 1, 2 mg	0.5 mg 15–30 min before each meal
Nateglinide (Starlix)	Facilitates calcium influx in pancreatic β cells, which leads to increased insulin release	Metabolism: Hepatic Excretion: Urine	Peak: 0.5–1 Half-life 1.5	Tablets 60, 120 mg	120 mg 1–30 min prior to meals.

Meglitinides (Glinides)

Meglitinides—also known as *glinides*—are antidiabetic agents that have the same mechanism as the sulfonylureas: stimulation of pancreatic insulin release. The main difference between the glinides and the sulfonylureas is their pharmacokinetic profile—the glinides are shorter acting and are taken with each meal. Only two glinides are available: repaglinide and nateglinide.

Repaglinide

Actions and uses. Like the sulfonylureas, repaglinide (Prandin, GlucoNorm ✦) blocks ATP-sensitive potassium channels on pancreatic β cells and thereby facilitates calcium influx, which leads to increased insulin release. In clinical trials, repaglinide was about as effective as glyburide and glipizide (second-generation sulfonylureas). The drug is approved for type 2 diabetes only. Because repaglinide has the same mechanism as the sulfonylureas, patients who do not respond to sulfonylureas will not respond to this agent either. Repaglinide is approved for monotherapy or combined therapy with metformin or a glitazone (Table 48.12).

Adverse effects. Repaglinide is generally well tolerated. The main significant adverse effect is *hypoglycemia*. In patients with liver dysfunction, metabolism of repaglinide may be slowed, and hence the risk for hypoglycemia may be increased. Because of possible hypoglycemia, it is imperative that patients eat no later than 30 minutes after taking the drug.

Thiazolidinediones (Glitazones). The thiazolidinediones, also known as *glitazones* or simply *TZDs*, reduce glucose levels primarily by decreasing insulin resistance. These drugs are not related chemically or functionally to sulfonylureas or biguanides. Their only indication is type 2 diabetes, mainly as an add-on to metformin (Table 48.13).

Pioglitazone

Actions and use. Pioglitazone (Actos) reduces insulin resistance and may also decrease glucose production. The underlying mechanism is activation of a specific receptor type in the cell nucleus, known as the *peroxisome proliferator–activated receptor* γ (PPAR γ). By activating PPAR γ, pioglitazone turns on insulin-responsive genes that help regulate carbohydrate and lipid metabolism. As a result, cellular responses to insulin are increased, thereby promoting (mainly) increased glucose

TABLE 48.13   Thiazolidinediones (Glitazones)

Drug	Mechanism of Action	Metabolism and Excretion	Peak and Half-Life	Preparations	Usual Initial Adult Dosage
Pioglitazone (Actos)	Turn on insulin-responsive genes that help regulate carbohydrate and lipid metabolism.	Metabolism: Hepatic Excretion: Gastrointestinal (bile)	Peak: 2 Half-life: 3–7 Metabolites: 16–24	Tablets: 15, 30, 45 mg	15–30 mg daily
Rosiglitazone (Avandia)	Increases insulin sensitivity by turning on insulin-responsive genes that help regulate carbohydrate and lipid metabolism.	Metabolism: Hepatic Excretion: Renal	Peak: 1 Half-Life: 3–4	Tablets 2, 4 mg	4 mg daily or 2 mg twice daily

SUMMARY OF KEY PRESCRIBING CONSIDERATIONS

Meglitinides (Glinides)

Therapeutic Goal: Maintain glycemic control in patients with type 2 diabetes in combination with diet and exercise.

Baseline Data: Random plasma glucose, fasting plasma glucose, A_{1c}, serum electrolytes, urinary glucose and ketones

Monitoring: Patients should monitor blood glucose regularly

Identifying High-Risk Patients: Use with caution in patients with liver impairment and those taking gemfibrozil.

Evaluating Therapeutic Effects: Improvement in symptoms, including decrease in urination, fatigue, and decrease in plasma glucose levels and A_{1c}.

Minimizing Adverse Effects: Educate patients about signs and symptoms of hypoglycemia.

uptake by skeletal muscle and adipose cells and (partly) decreased glucose production by the liver. Because pioglitazone enhances responses to insulin, insulin must be present for the drug to work.

Pioglitazone is approved as an adjunct to diet and exercise to improve glycemic control in adults with type 2 diabetes. The drug can be used as monotherapy but is usually combined with metformin, a sulfonylurea, and/or supplemental insulin. Because insulin is required for pioglitazone to work, the drug is not effective in patients with type 1 diabetes.

Adverse effects. Pioglitazone is generally well tolerated. The most common reactions are upper respiratory tract infection, headache, sinusitis, and myalgia.

BLACK BOX WARNING

Pioglitazone

Pioglitazone is associated with *heart failure* (HF) secondary to renal *retention of fluid*. If HF is diagnosed, pioglitazone should be discontinued or used in reduced dosage.

Although HF can precipitate, for most patients, fluid retention is not clinically significant. However, for patients with HF, especially severe or uncompensated HF, increased fluid retention can make HF worse. In these individuals, fluid retention is exacerbated when pioglitazone is used in combination with insulin therapy. Accordingly, pioglitazone should be used with caution in patients with *mild* HF and should be avoided by those with *severe* failure. Patients should be informed about signs of HF (dyspnea, edema, fatigue, rapid weight gain) and instructed to consult the prescriber immediately if these develop. Unlike rosiglitazone, pioglitazone has not been associated with myocardial infarction.

Although TZDs have a low risk for *hypoglycemia* when used as monotherapy, the risk is increased when pioglitazone is combined with insulin or with drugs that inhibit pioglitazone metabolism. Use these combinations with caution.

Pioglitazone can cause *ovulation* in anovulatory premenopausal women, thereby posing a risk for unintended pregnancy. This effect has not been studied in clinical trials, and hence the incidence is unknown. Women should be informed about the potential for ovulation and educated about contraceptive options.

Postmarketing data indicate an increased risk for *bladder cancer*, associated mainly with long-term, high-dose pioglitazone therapy. Package labeling warns against using pioglitazone in patients with active bladder cancer or with a history of bladder cancer. Patients should be informed about signs of bladder cancer (e.g., blood in the urine, worsening urinary urgency, painful urination) and instructed to contact their prescriber if these develop.

Pioglitazone appears to increase the risk for *fractures* in women but not in men. Most fractures have occurred in the foot, hand, or upper arm, not the spine. Risk appears greater with long-term, high-dose therapy. Fracture risk can be reduced through measures to maintain bone health. Among these are exercise, assuring adequate intake of calcium and vitamin D, and, if indicated, use of drugs for osteoporosis (see Chapter 61).

Although pioglitazone has been associated with rare cases of hepatic failure, a causal relationship has not been established. Nonetheless, serum alanine aminotransferase (ALT), a marker of liver function, should be measured at baseline and periodically thereafter (e.g., every 3 to 6 months). If ALT levels increase to more than three times the upper limit of normal or if jaundice develops, pioglitazone should be withdrawn. Patients should be informed about symptoms of liver injury (nausea, vomiting, abdominal pain, fatigue, anorexia, dark urine, jaundice) and instructed to notify the prescriber if these develop.

Pioglitazone has mixed effects on *plasma lipids*. One effect—elevation of LDL cholesterol—increases cardiovascular risk. Two other effects—elevation of HDL cholesterol and reduction of triglycerides—reduce cardiovascular risk. The net effect appears to be either (1) a reduction in cardiovascular risk or, at worst, (2) no increase in cardiovascular risk. However, the HF risk mentioned previously must not be overlooked.

α-Glucosidase Inhibitors

The α-glucosidase inhibitors—acarbose and miglitol—act in the intestine to delay absorption of carbohydrates. These drugs are indicated for type 2 diabetes (Table 48.14).

Acarbose

Mechanism of action. Acarbose (Precose, Glucobay ✦) delays absorption of dietary carbohydrates and thereby reduces the rise in blood glucose after a meal. To be absorbed, oligosaccharides and complex

TABLE 48.14 α-Glucosidase Inhibitors

Drug	Mechanism of Action	Metabolism and Excretion	Peak and Half-Life	Preparations	Usual Initial Adult Dosage
Acarbose (Precose)	Delays absorption of dietary carbohydrates	Metabolism: Minimal–Completed by bacteria in the gastrointestinal (GI) tract Excretion: GI (feces) and renal	Peak: 1 Half-life 2	Tablets 25, 50, 100 mg	25 mg three times daily
Miglitol (Glyset)	Delays absorption of dietary carbohydrates	Metabolism: None Excretion: Urine	Peak: 1 Half-life 2	Tablets 25, 50, 100 mg	25 mg three times daily

TABLE 48.15 Dipeptidyl Peptidase-4 Inhibitors

Drug	Mechanism of Action	Metabolism and Excretion	Peak and Half-Life	Preparations	Usual Initial Adult Dosage
Sitagliptin (Januvia)	Enhances actions of incretin hormones to stimulate glucose dependent insulin and suppresses glucagon release	Metabolism: Minimal Excretion: Renal	Peak 1–4 Half-Life: 12	Tablets 25, 50, 100 mg	100 mg daily
Saxagliptin (Onglyza)		Metabolism: Hepatic Excretion: Renal	Peak 2 Half-Life: 2.5	Tablets 2.5, 5 mg	2.5–5 mg daily
Linagliptin (Tradjenta)		Metabolism: Minimal Excretion: Gastrointestinal (feces)	Peak 1.5 Half-Life: 12	Tablets 5 mg	5 mg daily
Alogliptin (Nesina)		Metabolism: Minimal Excretion: Renal	Peak 2–3 Half-Life: 21	Tablets 6.25, 12.5, 25 mg	25 mg daily

 ## SUMMARY OF KEY PRESCRIBING CONSIDERATIONS

Thiazolidinediones

Therapeutic Goal: Maintain glycemic control in patients with type 2 diabetes in conjunction with diet and exercise.

Baseline Data: Random plasma glucose, fasting plasma glucose, A$_{1c}$, serum electrolytes, urinary glucose and ketones

Monitoring: Patients should monitor blood glucose regularly.

Identifying High-Risk Patients: Thiazolidinediones are contraindicated in patients with severe heart failure and should be used with caution in patients with mild heart failure or symptoms of heart failure. These drugs are also contraindicated in patients with bladder cancer or history of bladder cancer.

Evaluating Therapeutic Effects: Improvement in symptoms, including decrease in urination, fatigue, and decrease in plasma glucose levels and A$_{1c}$.

Minimizing Adverse Effects: Educate patients on signs and symptoms of heart failure as well as hypoglycemia.

carbohydrates must be broken down to monosaccharides by α-glucosidase, an enzyme located on the brush border of cells that line the intestine. Acarbose inhibits this enzyme and thereby slows digestion of carbohydrates, which reduces the postprandial rise in blood glucose.

Therapeutic use. Acarbose is indicated for patients with type 2 diabetes in conjunction with a program of diet modification and exercise. The drug may be used alone or in combination with insulin, metformin, or a sulfonylurea. In clinical trials, 24 weeks of therapy with acarbose alone reduced mean peak postprandial glucose levels by 57 mg/dL, compared with 71 mg/dL for tolbutamide (a sulfonylurea) alone and 85 mg/dL for acarbose plus tolbutamide. In addition to lowering glucose levels after meals, acarbose lowers A$_{1c}$ levels, indicating an overall improvement in glycemic control.

Adverse effects and interactions. Acarbose frequently causes *flatulence, cramps, abdominal distention, borborygmus* (rumbling bowel sounds), and *diarrhea*. These responses result from bacterial fermentation of unabsorbed carbohydrates in the colon. Because of the common occurrence of these GI-related side effects, this class of medication is not often used in the United States. In addition to its GI effects, acarbose can decrease absorption of iron, thereby posing a risk for *anemia*.

Hypoglycemia does not occur with acarbose alone but may develop when acarbose is combined with *insulin* or a *sulfonylurea*. When hypoglycemia develops, sucrose cannot be used for oral therapy because acarbose will impede its hydrolysis and thereby delay absorption. Accordingly, in patients taking acarbose, oral therapy of hypoglycemia must be accomplished with glucose itself.

Long-term, high-dose therapy may cause *liver dysfunction.* Asymptomatic elevation of plasma transaminases (which come from damaged liver cells) occurs in approximately 15% of patients. However, overt jaundice is rare. Liver function tests should be monitored every 3 months for the first year, and periodically thereafter. Liver dysfunction reverses when acarbose is discontinued.

Dipeptidyl Peptidase-4 Inhibitors (Gliptins)

DPP-4 inhibitors promote glycemic control by enhancing the actions of incretin hormones. Reduction in A$_{1c}$ are modest. Hypoglycemia is uncommon when these drugs are used alone. Pancreatitis and severe hypersensitivity reactions occur rarely.

The ADA considers the DPP-4 inhibitors to be an optional second-line therapy as an add-on to metformin in the treatment of type 2 diabetes (Table 48.15). When added to the regimen, the resulting decrease in A$_{1c}$ is about 0.5%. However, for some patients, even this small improvement can be clinically significant.

Sitagliptin

Mechanism of action. Sitagliptin (Januvia) enhances the actions of *incretin hormones*, endogenous compounds that (1) stimulate glucose-dependent release of insulin and (2) suppress postprandial release of glucagon (a hormone that increases glucose production in the liver). Both actions help keep blood glucose from climbing too high. How does sitagliptin boost incretin actions? It inhibits DPP-4, an enzyme that inactivates the incretin hormones. As discussed later, another class of drugs—GLP-1 receptor agonists—also boost incretin actions, but by a different mechanism: rather than preventing incretin breakdown, they mimic incretin actions.

Therapeutic use. Sitagliptin is indicated for type 2 diabetes, either as monotherapy or combined with another antidiabetic drug (e.g., metformin, sulfonylurea, or a glitazone). Like all the other agents for managing diabetes, sitagliptin should be used as an adjunct to diet and exercise.

Adverse effects and interactions. Sitagliptin is generally well tolerated. In clinical trials, the most common side effects were upper respiratory tract infection, headache, and inflammation of the nasal passages and throat—at rates similar to those seen with placebo. The incidence of hypoglycemia was approximately 1.2%, compared with 0.9% with placebo—again a nonsignificant difference.

Rarely, patients have developed *pancreatitis*, including fatal hemorrhagic or necrotizing pancreatitis according to postmarketing reports. Patients should be informed about signs and symptoms of pancreatitis (e.g., severe and persistent abdominal pain, with or without vomiting) and instructed to stop sitagliptin immediately. If pancreatitis is confirmed, sitagliptin should not be resumed. We do not know if patients with a history of pancreatitis are at increased risk, although the U.S. Food and Drug Administration recommends cautious use of these agents in such patients.

There have been postmarketing reports of serious *hypersensitivity reactions*, including anaphylaxis, angioedema, and Stevens-Johnson syndrome. However, a causal relationship has not been established. Nonetheless, if a hypersensitivity reaction is suspected, sitagliptin should be discontinued.

Sitagliptin has no known clinically relevant drug interactions and no contraindications, including pregnancy.

SUMMARY OF KEY PRESCRIBING CONSIDERATIONS

Dipeptidyl Peptidase-4 Inhibitors (Gliptins)

Therapeutic Goal: Management of glucose control as an adjuvant treatment for type 2 diabetes.

Baseline Data: Random plasma glucose, fasting plasma glucose, A$_{1c}$, serum electrolytes, urinary glucose and ketones

Monitoring: Patients should monitor blood glucose regularly.

Identifying High-Risk Patients: Use with caution in patients that have a history of pancreatitis.

Evaluating Therapeutic Effects: Improvement in symptoms, including decrease in urination, fatigue, and decrease in plasma glucose levels and A$_{1c}$.

Minimizing Adverse Effects: Educate patients on signs and symptoms of hypoglycemia.

Sodium-Glucose Cotransporter 2 Inhibitors

The kidney plays a major role in glucose homeostasis owing to its role in the filtration and reabsorption of glucose in the renal tubules. The transport of glucose from the tubule into the tubular epithelial cells is accomplished by SGLTs. SGLT-2 is a high-capacity, low-affinity transporter expressed chiefly in the kidney that accounts for approximately 90% of glucose reabsorption in the kidney. SGLT-2 inhibitors have been shown to block the reabsorption of filtered glucose, leading to glucosuria. This mechanism of action has proved clinically useful in patients with type 2 diabetes in terms of improving glycemic control. In addition, the glucosuria associated with SGLT-2 inhibition is associated with caloric loss, thus providing a potential benefit of weight loss. Although currently approved agents hold an indication for the management of type 2 diabetes only, these agents are being studied and used off-label in people with type 1 diabetes (Table 48.16).

Canagliflozin

Actions and therapeutic use. Canagliflozin (Invokana) was the first SGLT-2 inhibitor approved in the United States. By inhibiting SGLT-2 in the kidney, canagliflozin reduces the reabsorption of glucose, thereby increasing urinary glucose excretion. Clinical studies of canagliflozin have shown benefits in terms of improved glycemic control and weight loss.

Adverse effects. The most common side effects noted with canagliflozin in clinical trials were female genital fungal infections, urinary tract infections, and increased urination. Because SGLT-2 inhibitors increase the amount of sugar present in the urine, the increased risk for such infections is not much of a surprise. In addition, particularly in older adults, use of canagliflozin can lead to postural hypotension and dizziness, particularly if used in combination with diuretics.

Drug interactions. Coadministration of canagliflozin with Uridine 5'-diphospho-glucuronosyltransferase inducers—such as rifampin, phenytoin, or phenobarbital—can decrease canagliflozin efficacy. Accordingly, if used with such an agent, the 300-mg canagliflozin dose should be considered. Because canagliflozin causes a diuretic effect, the risk for dehydration and hypotension may be increased when used in combination with thiazide and loop diuretics.

SUMMARY OF KEY PRESCRIBING CONSIDERATIONS

Sodium-Glucose Cotransporter 2 Inhibitors

Therapeutic Goal: Management of blood glucose in patients with type 2 diabetes.

Baseline Data: Random plasma glucose, Fasting plasma glucose, A$_{1c}$, serum electrolytes, urinary glucose and ketones

Monitoring: Patients should monitor blood glucose regularly.

Identifying High-Risk Patients: Use with caution in patients prone to vulvovaginal and urinary tract infections.

Evaluating Therapeutic Effects: Improvement in symptoms, including decrease in fatigue, plasma glucose levels, and A$_{1c}$.

Minimizing Adverse Effects: Educate patients on signs and symptoms of hypoglycemia. These drugs also cause a diuretic effect; therefore patients should stay hydrated and monitor for signs and symptoms of urinary tract or vulvovaginal infections.

TABLE 48.16	Sodium-Glucose Cotransporter 2 Inhibitors				
Drug	**Mechanism of Action**	**Metabolism and Excretion**	**Peak and Half-Life**	**Preparations**	**Usual Initial Adult Dosage**
Canagliflozin (Invokana)	Reduces the reabsorption of glucose, increasing urinary excretion of glucose	Metabolism: Minimal hepatic Excretion: Gastrointestinal (GI) (feces), renal	Peak 1–2 Half-Life: 12	Tablets 100, 300 mg	100 mg daily
Dapagliflozin (Farxiga)		Metabolism: Minimal hepatic Excretion: Renal	Peak 2 Half-Life: 12	Tablets 5, 10 mg	5 mg daily
Empagliflozin (Jardiance)		Metabolism: Hepatic Excretion: Renal, GI (feces)	Peak 1.5 Half-Life: 12	Tablets 10, 25 mg	10 mg daily

Oral Combination Products

As noted previously, many patients with type 2 diabetes must take several medications with complementary mechanisms of action to meet glycemic goals. Accordingly, to help minimize the number of pills that patients must take on a daily basis, several oral combination products are commercially available. Because metformin is the recommended first-line agent in combination with lifestyle interventions, most combination products contain metformin with a second antidiabetic agent. Table 48.17 shows combination products available in the United States. Keep in mind, however, that combination products have drawbacks. First, they are often more expensive than taking the components separately. And second, they limit dosing flexibility.

Noninsulin Injectable Agents

In addition to insulin, we currently have two additional classes of injectable agents available for the treatment of diabetes. In the amylin mimetic class, pramlintide—the only amylin mimetic currently on the market—is indicated for type 1 *and* type 2 diabetes. The other class of drugs—GLP-1 receptor agonists (or incretin mimetics)—is indicated for type 2 diabetes only, yet these drugs are increasingly being used off-label for people with type 1 diabetes. Because all of these agents are injectable, they are often mistaken for insulin products, but they work very differently than insulin. See Table 48.18 for injectable combination drug therapies.

Glucagon-like Peptide-1 Receptor Agonists

GLP-1 receptor agonists, often referred to as *incretin mimetics*, work by augmenting the effects of the incretin hormone GLP-1. Under physiologic conditions, GLP-1 and other incretins are released from cells of the GI tract after a meal. Incretin mimetics activate receptors for GLP-1 and thereby cause the same effects as endogenous incretins. That is, they slow gastric emptying, stimulate glucose-dependent release of insulin, inhibit postprandial release of glucagon, and suppress appetite. Owing to augmentation of these effects, incretin mimetics are effective in improving glucose control and can induce weight loss. You will recall that DPP-4 inhibitors "boost" the effects of incretin hormones by slowing their degradation by the enzyme DPP-4. In contrast, GLP-1 receptor agonists are structurally related to the native GLP-1 hormone but are resistant to metabolism by DPP-4. There are currently six GLP-1 receptor agonist products approved in the United States (Table 48.19).

Exenatide. Exenatide (Byetta) was the first *incretin mimetic*. The drug is used to improve glucose control in patients with type 2 diabetes. A longer-acting formulation of exenatide known as Exenatide Once Weekly (Bydureon) is also currently available and is dosed once weekly (compared with twice daily with Byetta). Nausea is common, and hypoglycemia can occur, particularly if used in combination with a sulfonylurea.

Description and actions. Exenatide is a synthetic analog of GLP-1, a peptide hormone in the *incretin* family. Exenatide activates receptors for GLP-1 and thereby causes the same effects as endogenous incretins. That is, it slows gastric emptying, stimulates glucose-dependent release of insulin, inhibits postprandial release of glucagon, and suppresses appetite.

Therapeutic use. Exenatide is indicated as adjunctive therapy to improve glycemic control in patients with type 2 diabetes. In clinical trials, subQ injection of exenatide (Byetta) 5 or 10 μg twice daily before

TABLE 48.17 Combination Oral Agents for the Treatment of Type 2 Diabetes

Trade Name	Generic Name
Metaglip	Glipizide-metformin
Glucovance	Glyburide-metformin
Jentadueto	Linagliptin-metformin
Kombiglyze XR	Saxagliptin-metformin
Janumet, Janumet XR	Sitagliptin-metformin
Kazano	Alogliptin-metformin
Oseni	Alogliptin-pioglitazone
Duetact	Pioglitazone-glimepiride
ActoPlus Met, ActoPlus Met XR	Pioglitazone-metformin
PrandiMet	Repaglinide-metformin
Synjardy, Synjardy XR	Empagliflozin-metformin
Glyxambi	Empagliflozin-linagliptin
Invokamet, Invokamet XR	Canagliflozin-metformin
Xigduo XR	Dapagliflozin-metformin
Qtern	Dapagliflozin-saxagliptin

TABLE 48.18 Injectable Combination Drug Therapies

Drug Combination	Availability
Liraglutide/degludec (Xultophy 100/3.6)	Injection 100/3.6 mg/mL
Insulin glargine/lixisenatide (Soliqua 100/33)	Injection 100/33 μg/mL

TABLE 48.19 Glucagon-like Peptide-1 Receptor Agonists

Drug	Mechanism of Action	Metabolism and Excretion	Peak and Half-Life	Preparations	Usual Initial Adult Dosage
Exenatide (Byetta, Bydureon)	Activates receptors for GLP-1- slowing gastric emptying, inhibits glucagon, suppresses appetite, and stimulates glucose-dependent release of insulin	Metabolism: Minimal Excretion: Renal	Peak 2[a] Half-Life: 2.5[a]	Prefilled syringe for injection 5, 10 mcg per injection ER suspension for injection 2 mg per injection	5 mcg subQ twice daily 2 mg subQ weekly
Liraglutide (Victoza)		Metabolism: Minimal Excretion: Renal, GI (feces)	Peak 8–12 Half-Life: 13	Solution for injection 6 mg/mL	0.6 mg subQ daily
Dulaglutide (Trulicity)		Metabolism: Minimal Excretion: Unknown	Peak 48 Half-Life: 120	ER Suspension for injection 0.75, 1.5 mg per injection	0.75 subQ weekly

[a]Does not include extended release suspensions.

ER, Extended release; *GI*, gastrointestinal; *subQ*, subcutaneous.

the two largest meals of the day produced a modest decrease in fasting blood glucose and a large decrease in postprandial blood glucose. Patients did not gain any weight, and many lost weight. In contrast, exenatide ER for injectable suspension (Bydureon) 2 mg given by subQ injection once weekly has a greater effect on fasting glucose as opposed to postprandial blood glucose. These differences are related to the varying pharmacokinetic profiles of these two products.

Adverse effects. Dose-related *hypoglycemia* is common when exenatide is combined with a sulfonylurea (but not when combined with metformin). To minimize hypoglycemia, sulfonylurea dosage may need a reduction. *GI effects*—nausea, vomiting, and diarrhea—are common with exenatide (Byetta). Exenatide ER suspension (Bydureon) is better tolerated in terms of nausea and vomiting but can result in injection-site irritation and pruritus. In some patients, *antiexenatide antibodies* develop. These antibodies do not cause adverse effects, but they can reduce exenatide's effects.

Exenatide poses a risk for *pancreatitis*. Severe cases have led to pancreatic necrosis, pancreatic hemorrhage, and even death. Patients should be informed about signs and symptoms of pancreatitis—typically severe and persistent abdominal pain, with or without vomiting—and instructed to stop exenatide immediately. If pancreatitis is confirmed, exenatide should not be resumed. Patients with a history of pancreatitis should probably not use this drug.

Exenatide can cause *renal impairment,* sometimes requiring hemodialysis or a kidney transplant. Fortunately, the incidence is low—approximately 1 case for every 13,000 patients. Risk for renal impairment may be increased by nausea, vomiting, diarrhea, or any other event that can cause dehydration. Exenatide should be avoided in patients with severe renal impairment and should be used with caution in kidney transplant recipients.

In pregnant animals, doses of exenatide only three times the human dose caused *fetal harm,* manifesting as reduced growth and skeletal abnormalities. At this time, the drug should be used only if the benefits are believed to outweigh the fetal risk. Furthermore, given the established safety and efficacy of insulin in pregnancy, there seems to be little reason to even try exenatide.

There have been postmarketing reports of serious *hypersensitivity reactions,* including anaphylaxis and angioedema. If severe reaction occurs, patients should stop taking exenatide and seek immediate medical attention.

SUMMARY OF KEY PRESCRIBING CONSIDERATIONS

Glucagon-like Peptide-1 (GLP-1) Receptor Agonists

Therapeutic Goal: Improvement of glucose control in patients with type 2 diabetes.

Baseline Data: Random plasma glucose, fasting plasma glucose, A_{1c}, serum electrolytes, urinary glucose and ketones

Monitoring: Patients should monitor blood glucose regularly.

Identifying High-Risk Patients: GLP-1 Agonists should be used with caution in pregnancy; benefits should clearly outweigh risks. Avoid use in patients with renal dysfunction or patients that have undergone renal transplant. Use with caution in patients with a history of pancreatitis.

Evaluating Therapeutic Effects: Improvement in symptoms, including decrease in urination, fatigue, weight loss, and decrease in plasma glucose levels and A_{1c}.

Minimizing Adverse Effects: Educate patients on the signs and symptoms of hypoglycemia. These drugs also delay gastric emptying, so may delay the absorption of other drugs if taken simultaneously.

Amylin Mimetic: Pramlintide

Pramlintide (Symlin) is an amylin mimetic. The drug is used to complement the effects of insulin in patients with type 1 or type 2 diabetes. Severe hypoglycemia is a concern, and nausea is common.

Description and actions. Pramlintide is a synthetic analog of amylin, a peptide hormone made in the pancreas and coreleased with insulin. Both amylin and pramlintide, which mimics the effects of amylin, reduce postprandial levels of glucose, mainly by delaying gastric emptying and suppressing glucagon secretion. In addition, both agents act in the brain to increase the sense of satiety, helping lower caloric intake.

Therapeutic use. Pramlintide is indicated as a supplement to mealtime insulin in patients with type 1 or type 2 diabetes who have failed to achieve glucose control despite optimal insulin therapy. Patients with type 2 diabetes may combine insulin and pramlintide with metformin and/or a sulfonylurea. In clinical trials, adding subQ pramlintide to mealtime insulin decreased postprandial glucose levels, smoothed out glucose fluctuations, and reduced the needed mealtime dose of insulin. Mean reductions in A_{1c} were approximately 0.39% for those with type 1 diabetes and 0.55% for those with type 2 diabetes.

Pharmacokinetics. Blood levels peak approximately 20 minutes after subQ injection and decline with a half-life of 49 minutes. Unlike most drugs, pramlintide is metabolized in the kidneys rather than the liver. One active metabolite has been identified.

Adverse effects. Hypoglycemia is the biggest concern. Pramlintide does not cause hypoglycemia when used alone but poses a risk for severe hypoglycemia when combined with insulin, especially in patients with type 1 diabetes. As a rule, hypoglycemia develops within 3 hours of dosing. To reduce risk, insulin dosage must be decreased, at least initially. In addition, pramlintide should not be given to patients who have hypoglycemia unawareness, a history of poor adherence to their insulin regimen, poor adherence to SMBG, or recurrent hypoglycemia needing assistance.

▶▶ BLACK BOX WARNING

Pramlintide

Pramlintide poses a risk for severe hypoglycemia when combined with insulin, especially in patients with type 1 diabetes.

Nausea occurs early in therapy and is more common in patients with type 1 diabetes (37%–48%) than type 2 diabetes (28%–30%). The incidence and severity of nausea can be reduced by gradual titration of dosage.

Injection-site reactions—redness, swelling, or itching—may occur but generally resolve within a few days to weeks.

49

Drugs for Thyroid Disorders

Thyroid hormones have profound effects on metabolism, cardiac function, growth, and development. These hormones stimulate the metabolic rate of most cells and increase the force and rate of cardiac contraction. During infancy and childhood, thyroid hormones promote maturation; severe deficiency can produce extreme short stature and permanent mental impairment. Fortunately, most abnormalities of thyroid function can be effectively treated.

We begin our study of thyroid drugs by reviewing thyroid physiology. Next we review the pathophysiology of hypothyroid and hyperthyroid states. Finally, we discuss the agents used for thyroid disorders.

THYROID PHYSIOLOGY

Chemistry and Nomenclature

The thyroid gland produces two active hormones: triiodothyronine (T_3) and thyroxine (T_4, tetraiodothyronine). These hormones have nearly identical structures. The only difference is that T_4 contains four atoms of iodine, whereas T_3 contains three. The biologic effects of T_3 and T_4 are qualitatively similar. However, when compared on a molar basis, T_3 is much more potent.

Preparations of T_3 and T_4 used clinically, although synthetic, are identical in structure to the naturally occurring hormones. The generic name of synthetic T_3 is *liothyronine,* and the generic name of synthetic T_4 is *levothyroxine.* A fixed-ratio mixture of T_3 plus T_4, known as *liotrix,* is also available.

Synthesis and Fate of Thyroid Hormones
Synthesis
Synthesis of thyroid hormones takes place in four steps (Fig. 49.1). The circled numbers in the figure correspond with these steps:
- *Step 1.* Formation of thyroid hormone begins with the active transport of *iodide* into the thyroid. Under normal conditions, this process produces concentrations of iodide within the thyroid that are 20 to 50 times greater than the concentration of iodide in plasma. When plasma iodide levels are extremely low, intrathyroid iodide content may reach levels that are more than 100 times greater than those in plasma.
- *Step 2.* After uptake, iodide undergoes oxidation to *iodine,* the active form of iodide. Iodide oxidation is catalyzed by an enzyme called *peroxidase.*
- *Step 3.* In this step, activated iodine becomes incorporated into tyrosine residues that are bound to *thyroglobulin,* a large glycoprotein. One tyrosine molecule may receive either one or two iodine atoms, resulting in the production of monoiodotyrosine (MIT) or diiodotyrosine (DIT), respectively.
- *Step 4.* In this final step, iodinated tyrosine molecules are coupled. Coupling of one DIT with one MIT forms T_3 (step 4A); coupling of one DIT with another DIT forms T_4 (step 4B).

Fate
Thyroid hormones are released from the thyroid gland by a proteolytic process. The amount of T_4 released is substantially greater than the amount of T_3 released. However, much of the T_4 that is released undergoes conversion to T_3 by enzymes in peripheral tissues. In fact, conversion of T_4 to T_3 accounts for the majority (approximately 80%) of the T_3 found in plasma.

More than 99.5% of the T_3 and T_4 in plasma is bound to plasma proteins. Consequently, only a tiny fraction of circulating thyroid hormone is free to produce biologic effects.

Thyroid hormones are eliminated primarily by hepatic metabolism. Because T_3 and T_4 are extensively bound to plasma proteins, metabolism is slow. As a result, the half-lives of these hormones are prolonged—approximately 1 day for T_3 and 7 days for T_4.

Thyroid Hormone Actions

Thyroid hormones have three principal actions: (1) stimulation of energy use, (2) stimulation of the heart, and (3) promotion of growth and development. Stimulation of energy use elevates the basal metabolic rate, resulting in increased oxygen consumption and increased heat production. Stimulation of the heart increases both the rate and force of contraction, resulting in increased cardiac output and increased oxygen demand. Thyroid effects on growth and development are profound: thyroid hormones are essential for normal development of the brain and other components of the nervous system, and they have a significant effect on maturation of skeletal muscle.

Thyroid hormones produce their effects by modulating the activity of specific genes. Furthermore, it appears that most, if not all, of the effects of thyroid hormones are mediated by T_3, not by T_4. There is good evidence that T_3 penetrates to the cell nucleus and binds with high affinity to nuclear receptors, which in turn bind to specific DNA sequences. The result is modulation of gene transcription, causing production of proteins that mediate thyroid hormone effects. Although T_4 also binds with nuclear receptors, its affinity is low, and gene transcription is not altered. Hence it would seem that T_4 serves only as a source of T_3, having little or no physiologic effects of its own.

Regulation of Thyroid Function by the Hypothalamus and Anterior Pituitary

The functional relationship between the hypothalamus, anterior pituitary, and thyroid is shown in Fig. 49.2. As indicated, thyrotropin-releasing hormone (TRH), secreted by the hypothalamus, acts on the pituitary to cause secretion of thyrotropin (thyroid-stimulating hormone [TSH]). TSH then acts on the thyroid to stimulate all aspects of thyroid function: thyroid size is enlarged, iodine uptake is augmented, and synthesis and release of thyroid hormones are increased. In response to rising plasma levels of T_3 and T_4, further release of TSH is suppressed. The stimulatory effect of TSH on the thyroid, followed by the inhibitory effect of thyroid hormones on the pituitary, constitutes a negative feedback loop.

Effect of Iodine Deficiency on Thyroid Function

When iodine availability is diminished, production of thyroid hormones decreases. The ensuing drop in thyroid hormone levels promotes release of TSH, which acts on the thyroid to increase its size (causing goiter)

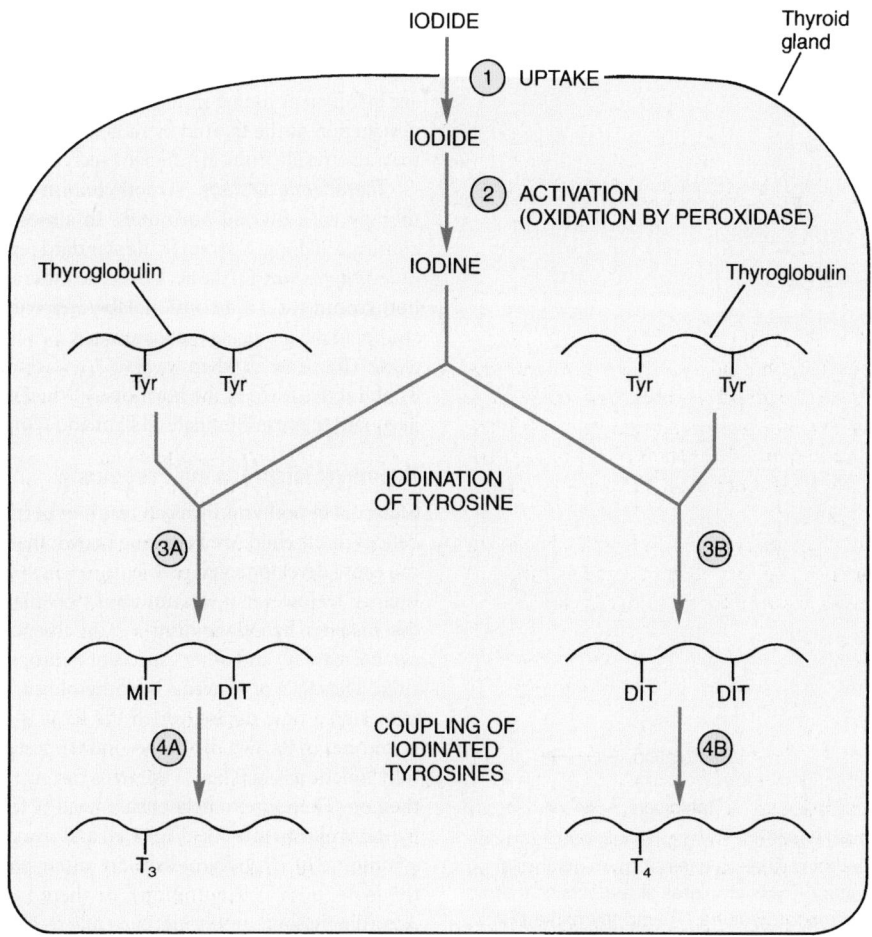

Fig. 49.1 Steps in Thyroid Hormone Synthesis. The reactions at each step *(circled numbers)* are explained in the text. *DIT,* Diiodotyrosine; *MIT,* monoiodotyrosine; T_3, triiodothyronine; T_4, thyroxine; *Tyr,* tyrosine.

and ability to concentrate iodine. If iodine deficiency is not too severe, the increased capacity for iodine uptake will restore normal production of T_3 and T_4.

THYROID FUNCTION TESTS

Several laboratory tests can be used to evaluate thyroid function. Three are described here. Values indicating euthyroid (normal), hypothyroid, and hyperthyroid states are shown in Table 49.1.

Serum Thyroid-Stimulating Hormone Test

Serum TSH determinations are used primarily for screening and diagnosis of hypothyroidism and for monitoring replacement therapy in hypothyroid patients.

Measurement of serum TSH is the most sensitive method for diagnosing hypothyroidism because the anterior pituitary is exquisitely sensitive to changes in thyroid hormone levels. As a result, very small reductions in serum T_3 and T_4 can cause a dramatic rise in serum TSH. Therefore even when the degree of hypothyroidism is minimal, it will be reflected by an abnormally high level of TSH. When replacement therapy is instituted, the TSH level should return to normal.

Serum TSH determinations can also be used to distinguish primary hypothyroidism from secondary hypothyroidism. In primary (thyroidal) hypothyroidism, TSH levels are *high*. However, in secondary hypothyroidism (hypothyroidism resulting from anterior pituitary dysfunction),

TABLE 49.1 **Serum Values for Thyroid Function Tests**			
	SERUM VALUES		
Thyroid Test	**Normal**	**Hypothyroid**	**Hyperthyroid**
Total T_4 (μg/dL)	4.5–12.5	Under 4.5	Over 12.5
Free T_4 (ng/dL)	0.9–2	Under 0.9	Over 2
Total T_3 (ng/dL)	80–220	Under 80	Over 220
Free T_3 (pg/dL)	230–620	Under 230	Over 620
TSH (milli-international units/L)	0.3–6	Over 6	Under 0.3

Laboratory studies have different reference ranges. These are relative ranges and are not absolute.
T_3, Triiodothyronine; T_4, thyroxine; *TSH,* thyroid-stimulating hormone.

TSH levels are low, normal, or even slightly elevated—despite the presence of low levels of T_3 and T_4.

Serum Thyroxine Test

Testing can measure either *total T_4* (bound plus free) or *free T_4*. Measurement of free T_4 is preferred. The T_4 test can be used to monitor thyroid hormone replacement therapy and to screen for thyroid dysfunction. However, in both cases, measurement of TSH is preferred.

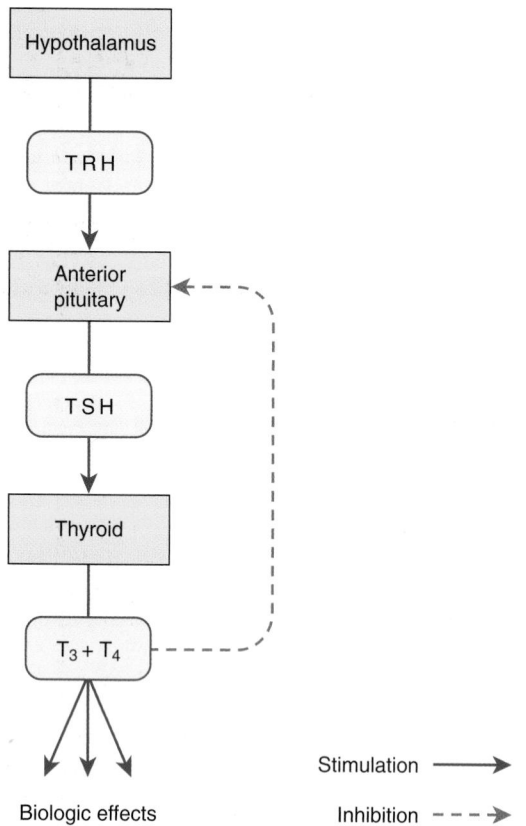

Fig. 49.2 Regulation of Thyroid Function. Thyrotropin-releasing hormone *(TRH)* from the hypothalamus stimulates release of thyroid-stimulating hormone *(TSH)* from the pituitary. TSH stimulates all aspects of thyroid function, including release of triiodothyronine *(T₃)* and thyroxine *(T₄)*. T₃ and T₄ act on the pituitary to suppress further TSH release.

Serum Triiodothyronine Test

As with T_4, we can measure either total or free T_3. Measurement of free T_3 is preferred. This test is useful for diagnosing hyperthyroidism. In this disorder, levels of T_3 often rise sooner and to a greater extent than do levels of T_4. T_3 determinations can also be used to monitor thyroid hormone replacement therapy (all thyroid preparations should increase levels of T_3).

THYROID PATHOPHYSIOLOGY

Hypothyroidism

Hypothyroidism can occur at any age. In adults, mild deficiency of thyroid hormone is referred to simply as *hypothyroidism*. Severe deficiency is called *myxedema*. When hypothyroidism occurs in infants, the resulting condition is called *congenital hypothyroidism*.

Hypothyroidism in Adults

Clinical presentation. Signs and symptoms of hypothyroidism depend on disease severity. With mild hypothyroidism, symptoms are subtle and may go unrecognized for what they are. In contrast, with moderate to severe disease, characteristic signs and symptoms emerge. The face is pale, puffy, and expressionless. The skin is cold and dry. The hair is brittle, and hair loss occurs. Heart rate and temperature are lowered. The patient may complain of lethargy, fatigue, and intolerance to cold. Mentation may be impaired. Thyroid enlargement may occur if reduced levels of T_3 and T_4 promote excessive release of TSH.

Causes. Hypothyroidism in the adult is usually due to malfunction of the thyroid itself. In iodine-sufficient countries, the principal cause is *chronic autoimmune thyroiditis* (Hashimoto thyroiditis). Other causes are insufficient iodine in the diet, surgical removal of the thyroid, and destruction of the thyroid by radioactive iodine. Adult hypothyroidism may also result from insufficient secretion of TSH and TRH.

Therapeutic strategy. Hypothyroidism in adults requires replacement therapy with thyroid hormones. In almost all cases, treatment must continue lifelong. Currently, the standard replacement regimen consists of *levothyroxine* (T_4) alone. Combined therapy with levothyroxine plus liothyronine (T_3) is an option. However, with only three exceptions, all studies to date indicate that combined T_3/T_4 offers no advantage over T_4 alone. (Remember, when we give T_4, much of it is rapidly converted to T_3, the active form of the hormone.) When replacement doses of T_4 are adequate, they can eliminate all signs and symptoms of thyroid deficiency.

Hypothyroidism During Pregnancy

Maternal hypothyroidism can result in permanent neuropsychological deficits in the child. We have long known that *congenital* hypothyroidism can cause developmental problems (see next section "Hypothyroidism in Infants"). However, it was not until 1999 that researchers demonstrated that *maternal* hypothyroidism—in the absence of fetal hypothyroidism—can decrease IQ and other aspects of neuropsychological function in the child. The effect of maternal hypothyroidism is limited largely to the first trimester, a time during which the fetus is unable to produce thyroid hormones of its own. By the second trimester, the fetal thyroid gland is fully functional, and hence the fetus can supply its own hormones from then on. Therefore to help ensure healthy fetal development, maternal hypothyroidism must be diagnosed and treated very early. Unfortunately, symptoms of hypothyroidism are often nonspecific (e.g., irritability, tiredness, poor concentration), or there may be no symptoms at all. Accordingly, some authorities currently recommend routine screening for hypothyroidism as soon as pregnancy is confirmed. If hypothyroidism is diagnosed, replacement therapy should begin immediately.

When women taking thyroid supplements become pregnant, dosage requirements usually increase—often by as much as 50%. The need for increased dosage begins between weeks 4 and 8 of gestation, levels off at approximately week 16, and then remains steady until parturition. To ensure adequate hormone levels, some authorities increase T_4 dosage by 30% as soon as pregnancy is confirmed. Further adjustments are based on serum TSH levels, which should be monitored closely.

Hypothyroidism in Infants

Clinical presentation. Hypothyroidism in newborns may be permanent or transient. In either case, congenital hypothyroidism can cause delay in mental development and derangement of growth. In the absence of thyroid hormones, the child develops a large and protruding tongue, potbelly, and dwarfish stature. Development of the nervous system, bones, teeth, and muscles is impaired.

Causes. Congenital hypothyroidism usually results from a failure in thyroid development. Other causes include autoimmune disease, severe iodine deficiency, TSH deficiency, and exposure to radioactive iodine in utero.

Therapeutic strategy. Hypothyroidism in newborns requires replacement therapy with thyroid hormones. If treatment is initiated within a few days of birth, physical and mental development will be normal. However, if therapy is delayed beyond 3 to 4 weeks, some permanent disability will be evident, although the physical effects of thyroid deficiency will reverse.

In all children, replacement therapy should continue for 3 years, after which it should be stopped for 4 weeks. The objective is to determine whether thyroid deficiency is permanent or transient. If TSH rises, indicating thyroid hormone production is low, we know the deficiency is permanent, so replacement therapy should resume. If TSH and T_4 normalize, we know the deficiency was transient, and hence further replacement therapy is unnecessary.

Hyperthyroidism

There are two major forms of hyperthyroidism: *Graves disease* and *toxic nodular goiter* (also known as *Plummer disease*). Of the two disorders, Graves disease is more common. Signs and symptoms of both disorders are similar. The principal difference is that Graves disease may cause exophthalmos, whereas toxic nodular goiter does not.

Graves Disease

Graves disease is the most common cause of excessive thyroid hormone secretion. This disorder occurs most frequently in women aged 20 to 40 years. The incidence in females is 6 times greater than in males.

Clinical presentation. Most clinical manifestations result from elevated levels of thyroid hormone. Heartbeat is rapid and strong, and dysrhythmias and angina may develop. The central nervous system is stimulated, resulting in nervousness, insomnia, rapid thought flow, and rapid speech. Skeletal muscles may weaken and atrophy. Metabolic rate is raised, resulting in increased heat production, increased body temperature, intolerance to heat, and skin that is warm and moist. Appetite is increased. However, despite increased food consumption, weight loss occurs if caloric intake fails to match the increase in metabolic rate. Collectively, the previous signs and symptoms are referred to as *thyrotoxicosis*.

In addition to thyrotoxicosis, patients with Graves disease often present with *exophthalmos*. The underlying cause is an immune-mediated infiltration of the extraocular muscles and orbital fat by lymphocytes, macrophages, plasma cells, mast cells, and mucopolysaccharides.

Cause. Thyroid stimulation in Graves disease is caused by thyroid-stimulating immunoglobulins (TSIs), which are antibodies produced by an autoimmune process. TSIs increase thyroid activity by stimulating receptors for TSH on the thyroid gland. That is, TSIs mimic the effects of TSH on thyroid function. TSIs are not responsible for exophthalmos.

Treatment. Treatment for Graves disease is directed at decreasing the production of thyroid hormones. Three modalities are used: (1) surgical removal of thyroid tissue, (2) destruction of thyroid tissue with radioactive iodine, and (3) suppression of thyroid hormone synthesis with an antithyroid drug (methimazole or propylthiouracil). Radiation is the preferred treatment for adults, whereas antithyroid drugs are preferred for younger patients.

β-Blockers and nonradioactive iodine may be used as adjunctive therapy. β-Blockers suppress tachycardia by blocking β-receptors on the heart. Nonradioactive iodine inhibits synthesis and release of thyroid hormones.

Because exophthalmos is not the result of hyperthyroidism per se, this condition is not improved by lowering thyroid hormone production. If exophthalmos is severe, it can be treated with surgery or with high doses of oral glucocorticoids.

Toxic Nodular Goiter (Plummer Disease)

Toxic nodular goiter is the result of a thyroid adenoma. Clinical manifestations are much like those of Graves disease, except exophthalmos is absent. Toxic nodular goiter is a persistent condition that rarely undergoes spontaneous remission. Treatment modalities are the same as for Graves disease. However, if an antithyroid drug is used, symptoms return rapidly when the drug is withdrawn. Accordingly, surgery and radiation, which provide long-term control, are often preferred.

Thyrotoxic Crisis (Thyroid Storm)

Thyrotoxic crisis can occur in patients with severe thyrotoxicosis when they undergo major surgery or develop a severe intercurrent illness (e.g., infection, sepsis). The syndrome is characterized by profound hyperthermia (105°F or even higher), severe tachycardia, restlessness, agitation, and tremor. Unconsciousness, coma, hypotension, and heart failure may ensue. These symptoms are produced by excessive levels of thyroid hormones.

Thyrotoxic crisis can be life threatening and requires immediate treatment. High doses of potassium iodide or strong iodine solution are given to suppress thyroid hormone release. Methimazole is given to suppress thyroid hormone synthesis. A β-blocker is given to reduce heart rate. Additional measures include sedation, cooling, and giving glucocorticoids and intravenous (IV) fluids.

THYROID HORMONE PREPARATIONS FOR HYPOTHYROIDISM

Thyroid hormones are available as pure, synthetic compounds and as extracts of animal thyroid glands. All preparations have qualitatively similar effects. The synthetic preparations are more stable and better standardized than the animal gland extracts. As a result, the synthetics are preferred to the natural products. Properties of thyroid hormone preparations are shown in Table 49.2.

Levothyroxine (T_4)

Levothyroxine (Synthroid) is a synthetic preparation of thyroxine, a naturally occurring thyroid hormone. The structure of levothyroxine is identical to that of the natural hormone. Levothyroxine is the drug of choice for most patients who require thyroid hormone replacement. Consequently, levothyroxine will serve as our prototype for the thyroid hormone preparations.

TABLE 49.2 Thyroid Hormone Preparations

Generic Name	Trade Names	Dosage Forms	Approximate Equivalent Dosage[a]	Description
Levothyroxine	Levoxyl, Synthroid	Tablets, injection	50–60 µg	Synthetic preparation of T_4 identical to the naturally occurring hormone
Liothyronine	Cytomel, Triostat	Tablets, injection	15–37 µg	Synthetic preparation of T_3 identical to the naturally occurring hormone
Liotrix	Thyrolar	Tablets	60 µg	Synthetic T_4 plus synthetic T_3 in a 4:1 fixed ratio
Thyroid	Armour Thyroid, Nature-Throid, Thyroid USP, Westhroid	Tablets, capsules	60 mg	Desiccated animal thyroid glands (currently rarely used)

[a]Approximate dosage needed to produce equivalent effects.
T_3, Triiodothyronine; T_4, thyroxine; *USB*, United States Pharmacopeia.

PROTOTYPE DRUGS
Drugs for Thyroid Disorders

Drugs for Hypothyroidism
Levothyroxine (T_4)

Drugs for Hyperthyroidism
Methimazole (a thionamide)

Pharmacokinetics

Absorption. Absorption of oral levothyroxine is reduced by food. Accordingly, to minimize variability in blood levels, levothyroxine should be taken on an empty stomach in the morning, at least 30 to 60 minutes before breakfast.

Conversion to triiodothyronine (T_3). Much of an administered dose of levothyroxine is converted to T_3 in the body. As a result, levothyroxine can produce nearly normal levels of both T_3 and T_4. Hence for most patients, there is no need to give T_3 along with levothyroxine.

Half-life and plasma levels. Because levothyroxine is highly protein bound (approximately 99.97%), the hormone has a prolonged half-life (approximately 7 days). From a clinical perspective, this long half-life is good news and bad news. The good news is that hormone levels remain fairly steady, even with once-a-day dosing, which makes levothyroxine well suited for lifelong therapy. The bad news is that it takes approximately 1 month (four half-lives) for plasma levels of levothyroxine to reach plateau (steady state). As a result, onset of full effects is delayed.

Therapeutic Uses

Levothyroxine is indicated for all forms of hypothyroidism, regardless of cause. The drug is used for congenital hypothyroidism, myxedema coma, simple goiter, and primary hypothyroidism in adults and children. Levothyroxine is also used to treat hypothyroidism resulting from insufficient TSH (secondary to pituitary malfunction) and from insufficient TRH (secondary to hypothalamic malfunction). In addition, levothyroxine is used to maintain proper levels of thyroid hormones after thyroid surgery, irradiation, and treatment with antithyroid drugs.

Adverse Effects

When administered in appropriate dosage, levothyroxine rarely causes adverse effects. With an acute overdose, *thyrotoxicosis* may result. Signs and symptoms include tachycardia, angina, tremor, nervousness, insomnia, hyperthermia, heat intolerance, and sweating. The patient should be informed about these signs and instructed to notify the prescriber if they develop. Chronic overdosage is associated with accelerated bone loss and increased risk for atrial fibrillation, especially in older adults. Loss of bone increases the risk for fractures.

Drug Interactions

Drugs that reduce levothyroxine absorption. Absorption of levothyroxine can be reduced by the following drugs:
- Histamine 2 (H_2) receptor blockers (e.g., cimetidine [Tagamet])
- Proton pump inhibitors (e.g., lansoprazole [Prevacid])
- Sucralfate (Carafate)
- Cholestyramine (Questran)
- Colestipol (Colestid)
- Aluminum-containing antacids (e.g., Maalox, Mylanta)
- Calcium supplements (e.g., Tums, Os-Cal)
- Iron supplements (e.g., ferrous sulfate)
- Magnesium salts
- Orlistat (Xenical)

To ensure adequate absorption of levothyroxine, patients should separate administration of levothyroxine and these drugs by 4 hours. As noted earlier, food also reduces absorption.

Drugs that accelerate levothyroxine metabolism. Several drugs can accelerate the metabolism of levothyroxine. Among these are phenytoin (Dilantin), carbamazepine (Tegretol, Carbatrol), rifampin (Rifadin), sertraline (Zoloft), and phenobarbital. Accordingly, to maintain adequate levothyroxine levels, patients taking these drugs may need to increase their levothyroxine dosage.

Warfarin. Levothyroxine accelerates the degradation of vitamin K–dependent clotting factors. As a result, effects of warfarin are enhanced. If thyroid hormone replacement therapy is started in a patient taking warfarin, the dosage of warfarin may need to be reduced.

Catecholamines. Thyroid hormones increase cardiac responsiveness to catecholamines, thereby increasing the risk for catecholamine-induced dysrhythmias. Caution must be exercised when administering catecholamines to patients receiving levothyroxine and other thyroid preparations.

Other interactions. Levothyroxine can increase requirements for insulin and digoxin. When converting patients from a hypothyroid to a euthyroid state, dosages of insulin and digoxin may need to be increased.

Are Levothyroxine Preparations Interchangeable?

Levothyroxine is available in several brand-name and generic formulations. Whether any of these are interchangeable is in dispute.

Levothyroxine has a narrow therapeutic range, so tight control of plasma drug levels is important. Otherwise, symptoms of hypothyroidism or toxicity will develop. To maintain good control, all pills a patient takes must produce the same levothyroxine levels. Accordingly, if a patient switches from one product to another, the new product must be bioequivalent to the old one.

Whether or not any levothyroxine products—brand name or generic—are truly equivalent is a point of contention. According to the U.S. Food and Drug Administration (FDA), certain formulations of levothyroxine are therapeutically equivalent to others. For example, the FDA maintains that generic levothyroxine made by Mylan is equivalent to two brand-name products: Levoxyl and Synthroid. However, three medical organizations—the American Association of Clinical Endocrinologists (AACE), The Endocrine Society (TES), and the American Thyroid Association (ATA)—*strongly* disagree, as expressed in a position statement. They believe the FDA's testing procedure was seriously flawed. First, the FDA measured only blood levels of levothyroxine; they did not measure serum TSH, the favored clinical test for assessing thyroid status. Second, and more important, testing was done in *normal* (euthyroid) volunteers. Hence when blood levels of levothyroxine were measured, the values reflected the sum of endogenous thyroxine plus levothyroxine contributed by the drug—making it impossible to state with precision how much of the total was truly due to the drug. As a result, conclusions regarding the equivalence of levothyroxine products are questionable. Nonetheless, pharmacists may switch patients from one product to another, often without the knowledge of the patient or prescriber—a practice with the potential for causing toxicity or therapeutic failure.

Given the debate about whether certain levothyroxine products are clinically interchangeable, what should the clinician do? In their position statement, the AACE, TES, and ATA recommend the following:
- Maintain patients on the same brand-name levothyroxine product.
- If a switch *is* made (from one branded product to another, from a branded product to a generic product, or from one generic product to another), retest serum TSH in 6 weeks and adjust the levothyroxine dosage as indicated.

- Advise patients to check with their prescriber before allowing a pharmacist to switch to a different levothyroxine product.

Dosage and Administration I: General Considerations

Routes of administration. Levothyroxine is almost always administered by mouth. Oral doses should be taken once daily on an empty stomach (to enhance absorption). *Dosing is usually done in the morning, at least 30 to 60 minutes before eating.*

IV administration is used for myxedema coma and for patients who cannot take levothyroxine orally for an extended period of time. IV doses are approximately 50% of the size of oral doses.

Evaluation. The goal of replacement therapy is to provide a dosage that compensates precisely for the existing thyroid deficit. This dosage is determined using a combination of clinical judgment and laboratory tests. When therapy is successful in adults, clinical evaluation should reveal a reversal of the signs and symptoms of thyroid deficiency—and an absence of signs of thyroid excess. Successful therapy of infants is reflected in normalization of intellectual function and normalization of growth and development. Monthly determinations of height provide a good index of success.

Measurement of serum TSH is an important means of evaluation. Successful replacement therapy causes elevated TSH levels to fall. However, TSH will not normalize quickly and often lags behind normalization of serum T_3 and T_4. Hence evaluation should not be done until 6 to 8 weeks after starting treatment. A TSH target of 0.5 to 2 milli-international units/L is appropriate for most patients. When an adequate replacement dosage is established, TSH levels will remain suppressed for the duration of treatment.

In some cases, serum T_4 must be used to evaluate therapy because TSH secretion remains high in some patients even though levels of thyroid hormones have been restored to normal. When this happens, success is indicated by levels of T_4 in the normal to high-normal range—whether or not TSH values are normal.

Duration and administration of therapy. For most hypothyroid patients, replacement therapy must be continued for life. Treatment provides symptomatic relief but does not produce cure. Patients must be made fully aware of the chronic nature of their condition. In addition, they should be forewarned that, although therapy will cause symptoms to improve, these improvements do not constitute a reason to interrupt or discontinue drug use. Additional information on doses and administration of levothyroxine are located in Table 49.3

DRUGS FOR HYPERTHYROIDISM

Antithyroid Drugs: Thionamides

The thionamide drugs—methimazole and propylthiouracil (PTU)—suppress synthesis of thyroid hormones. These agents can be used long

term to treat hyperthyroidism or short term as preparation for subtotal thyroidectomy or therapy with radioactive iodine. Methimazole and PTU are similar in most respects. Primary differences concern pharmacokinetics (Tables 49.4 and 49.5), dosing, and adverse effects.

Methimazole

Methimazole (Tapazole) is a first-line drug for hyperthyroidism. Benefits derive from inhibiting thyroid hormone synthesis. Methimazole is safer and more convenient than PTU and hence is preferred for most patients—except women who are pregnant or breastfeeding, and perhaps patients who are in thyrotoxic crisis.

Mechanism of action. Therapeutic effects result from blocking synthesis of thyroid hormones. Two mechanisms are involved. First, methimazole prevents the oxidation of iodide, thereby inhibiting incorporation of iodine into tyrosine. Second, methimazole prevents iodinated tyrosines from coupling. Both effects result from inhibiting peroxidase, the enzyme that catalyzes both reactions.

Please note that, although methimazole prevents thyroid hormone synthesis, it does not destroy existing stores of thyroid hormone. Hence after therapy has begun, it may take 3 to 12 weeks to produce a euthyroid state.

Pharmacokinetics. Methimazole is well absorbed after oral dosing. Binding to plasma proteins is minimal. The drug readily crosses membranes, including those of the placenta. Levels in breast milk are

SUMMARY OF KEY PRESCRIBING CONSIDERATIONS

Levothyroxine

Therapeutic Goal: Resolution of signs and symptoms of hypothyroidism and restoration of normal laboratory values for serum thyroid-stimulating hormone (TSH) and free thyroxine (T_4).

Baseline Data: Obtain serum levels of TSH and free T_4.

Monitoring: Check TSH 6-8 weeks after initiating therapy and after any dosage change. Check TSH at least once a year after serum TSH is stabilized.

Identifying High-Risk Patients: Use with caution in those patients with cardiovascular disease, and start with lower doses in older adult patients.

Evaluating Therapeutic Effects: Clinical evaluation should reveal reversal of signs of thyroid deficiency and an absence of signs of thyroid excess. In children, normalization of intellectual function, growth, and development should occur. Monthly measurements of height provide a good index of thyroid sufficiency. Laboratory tests should indicate normal plasma levels of TSH and T_4. Measure TSH levels at least once a year.

Minimizing Adverse Effects: Overdose may cause thyrotoxicosis. Symptoms include tachycardia, angina, tremor, nervousness, insomnia, sweating, and heat intolerance.

TABLE 49.3 Dosage and Administration of Levothyroxine: Specific Applications			
Condition	**Average Daily Dose**	**Dosage Forms**	**Additional Considerations for Administration**
Hypothyroidism in adults	100–125 µg for 70 kg adult	Oral	Older adults have lower starting doses of 25–50 µg daily
Myxedema coma	200–500 µg once	Injection	Additional dose of 100–300 µg can be given a day later
Congenital hypothyroidism	Age: <3 months: 10–15 mg/kg 3–5 months: 8–10 mg/kg 6–11 months: 6–8 mg/kg 1–5 years: 5–6 mg/kg 6–12 years: 4–5 mg/kg	Oral	Dose decreases with age. Doses adjusted to normalize TSH and free T_4.
Simple goiter	100–200 µg	Oral	—

TSH, Thyroid stimulating hormone; *T4,* thyroxine.

sufficient to affect the nursing infant. The plasma half-life is 6 to 13 hours—long enough to permit once-a-day dosing.

Therapeutic uses. Methimazole has four applications in hyperthyroidism:

- It can be used as the sole form of therapy for Graves disease.
- It can be used as an adjunct to radiation therapy until the effects of radiation become manifest.
- It can be given to suppress thyroid hormone synthesis in preparation for thyroid gland surgery (subtotal thyroidectomy).
- It can be given to patients experiencing thyrotoxic crisis.

Adverse effects. Methimazole is generally well tolerated but should be avoided by women who are pregnant or breastfeeding. Agranulocytosis is the most dangerous toxicity. The reaction is rare (approximately 3 cases per 10,000 patients) and usually develops during the first 2 months of therapy. Sore throat and fever may be the earliest indications, and patients should be instructed to report these immediately. Because agranulocytosis often develops rapidly, periodic blood counts cannot guarantee early detection. If agranulocytosis occurs, methimazole should be discontinued. Agranulocytosis will then reverse. Treatment with granulocyte colony-stimulating factor (filgrastim [Neupogen]) may accelerate recovery.

Hypothyroidism. When given in high doses, methimazole can convert the patient from a hyperthyroid state to a hypothyroid state. If this occurs, dosage should be reduced. Temporary treatment with thyroid hormone may be required.

Effects in pregnancy. Methimazole can cause neonatal hypothyroidism, goiter, and even congenital hypothyroidism. Accordingly, the drug should be avoided during the first trimester. Use in the second and third trimesters is considered safe. Compared with methimazole, PTU crosses the placenta poorly, and hence risk to the fetus is low. Accordingly, if a thionamide is needed during the first trimester of pregnancy, PTU is the preferred drug.

TABLE 49.4 Pharmacokinetics of Methimazole and Propylthiouracil

	Methimazole	Propylthiouracil
Bioavailability	80%–95%	80%–95%
Plasma protein binding	0	75%–80%
Levels in breast milk	Low	Low
Transplacental passage	Higher	Low
Half-life	6–13 h	1–2 h
Dosing frequency		
Initial therapy	1–3 times a day	3 or 4 times a day
Maintenance therapy	Once a day	2 or 3 times a day

Effects in lactation. Methimazole therapy does not affect thyroid function or intellectual development in breastfed infants with doses up to 20 mg daily.

Radioactive Iodine
Physical Properties

Iodine-131 (^{131}I) is a radioactive isotope of stable iodine that emits a combination of β particles and γ rays. Radioactive decay of ^{131}I takes place rapidly, with a half-life of 8 days. Hence after 56 days (seven half-lives), less than 1% of the radioactivity in a dose of ^{131}I remains.

Use in Graves Disease

^{131}I can be used to destroy thyroid tissue in patients with hyperthyroidism. The objective is to produce clinical remission without causing complete destruction of the gland. Unfortunately, delayed hypothyroidism, due to excessive thyroid damage, is a frequent complication.

Effect on the thyroid. Like stable iodine, ^{131}I is concentrated in the thyroid gland. Destruction of thyroid tissue is produced primarily by emission of beta particles. (The gamma rays from ^{131}I are relatively harmless.) Because β particles have a very limited ability to penetrate any type of physical barrier, they do not travel outside the thyroid. Hence damage to surrounding tissue is minimal.

Reduction of thyroid function is gradual. Initial effects become apparent in days or weeks. Full effects develop in 2 to 3 months.

Not all patients respond satisfactorily to a single treatment. Approximately 66% of patients with Graves disease are cured with a single exposure to ^{131}I. Others require two or more treatments.

Advantages and disadvantages of ^{131}I therapy. The advantages of ^{131}I treatment are considerable: (1) it has a relatively low cost; (2) patients are spared the risks, discomfort, and expense of thyroid surgery; (3) death from ^{131}I treatment is extremely rare; and (4) no tissue other than the thyroid is injured (patients should be reassured of this).

Treatment with ^{131}I is not without drawbacks. First, the effect of treatment is delayed, taking several months to become maximal. Second, and more important, treatment is associated with a significant incidence of delayed hypothyroidism. Hypothyroidism results from excessive dosage and occurs in up to 90% of patients within the first year after ^{131}I exposure.

Who should be treated and who should not. ^{131}I is indicated for adults with hyperthyroidism, as well as patients who have not responded adequately to antithyroid drugs or to subtotal thyroidectomy.

As a rule, very young children are considered inappropriate candidates. The likelihood of delayed hypothyroidism is higher than in adults. In addition, there is concern that administration of ^{131}I to young patients may carry a slight risk for cancer. However, it should be noted that there is no evidence that the use of ^{131}I in Graves disease has ever caused

TABLE 49.5 Antithyroid Drug Preparations

Generic Name	Trade Names	Dosage Forms	Daily Dosage	Therapeutic Uses	Additional Considerations for Administration
Methimazole	Tapazole	Tablets	Initial: 30–40 mg Maintenance: 5–15 mg	Graves disease Adjunct to radiation therapy Suppression of thyroid hormone prior to thyroid surgery Thyrotoxic crisis	Treatment continues for 1–2 years
Propylthiouracil (PTU)	Generic	Tablets	Initial: 300–900 mg Maintenance: 150 mg	Pregnant women in the first trimester Thyroid storm Intolerance to methimazole	Treatment continues for 1–2 years PTU has caused rare cases of liver injury. Onset is sudden and progression is rapid.

SUMMARY OF KEY PRESCRIBING CONSIDERATIONS
Methimazole

Therapeutic Goal: Methimazole has four indications: (1) reduction of thyroid hormone production in Graves' disease, (2) control of hyperthyroidism until the effects of radiation on the thyroid become manifest, (3) suppression of thyroid hormone production before subtotal thyroidectomy, and (4) treatment of thyrotoxic crisis.

Baseline Data: Obtain serum levels of thyroid-stimulating hormone (TSH), free triiodothyronine (T_3), and free thyroxine (T_4). Check baseline CBC and LFTs prior to initiation.

Monitoring: Check CBC with differential if signs or symptoms of infection. Check LFTs if signs or symptoms of liver dysfunction.

Identifying High-Risk Patients: Methimazole should be avoided in the first trimester of pregnancy.

Evaluating Therapeutic Effects: Monitor for weight gain, decreased heart rate, and other indications that levels of thyroid hormone have declined. Laboratory tests should indicate a decrease in serum free T_3 and free T_4.

Minimizing Adverse Effects

Agranulocytosis: Inform patients about early signs of agranulocytosis, including fever or sore throat. If follow-up blood tests reveal leukopenia, methimazole should be stopped.

Hypothyroidism: Methimazole may cause excessive reductions in thyroid hormone synthesis. If signs of hypothyroidism develop or if plasma levels of T_3 and T_4 become subnormal, dosage should be reduced.

PATIENT-CENTERED CARE ACROSS THE LIFE SPAN
Thyroid Drugs

Life Stage	Patient Care Concerns
Infants	Thyroid hormone preparation is used to treat hypothyroidism in infants. Treatment should continue for 3 years.
Children/ adolescents	Thyroid hormone preparations are used in children and adolescents. Doses are based on clinical response. Antithyroid drugs (methimazole and propylthiouracil [PTU]) are also safe in children. Iodine-131 is not generally used in children.
Pregnant women	Iodine-131 is contraindicated in pregnancy. Methimazole should be avoided in the first trimester of pregnancy.
Breastfeeding women	Thyroid hormone preparations and antithyroid medications are generally safe in breastfeeding women.
Older adults	Thyroid gland dysfunction is common in the older adult. This is associated with increased morbidity if not treated. Thyroid hormone preparations and antithyroid medications can be used successfully to treat thyroid dysfunction in the older adult.

cancer of the thyroid or any other tissue. Although ^{131}I is generally avoided in young children, is it commonly used in postpubertal adolescents and young adults.

^{131}I is *contraindicated in pregnancy and lactation.* Exposure of the fetus to ^{131}I after the first trimester may damage the immature thyroid, and exposure to radiation at any point in fetal life carries a risk for generalized developmental harm. Accordingly, a negative pregnancy test is required before giving ^{131}I. Because ^{131}I enters breast milk, women receiving this agent should not breastfeed.

Dosage. Dosage of ^{131}I is determined by thyroid size and by the rate of thyroidal iodine uptake. For Graves disease, the dosage usually ranges between 4 and 10 millicuries (mCi).

Nonradioactive Iodine: Lugol Solution
Description
Lugol solution, also known as strong iodine solution, is a mixture containing 5% elemental iodine and 10% potassium iodide. The iodine undergoes reduction to iodide within the gastrointestinal (GI) tract before absorption.

Mechanism of Action
When present in high concentrations, iodide has a paradoxical suppressant effect on the thyroid. Three mechanisms are involved. First, high concentrations of iodide decrease iodine uptake by the thyroid. Second, high concentrations of iodide inhibit thyroid hormone synthesis by suppressing both the iodination of tyrosine and the coupling of iodinated tyrosine residues. Third, high concentrations of iodine inhibit release of thyroid hormone into the blood. All three actions combine to decrease circulating levels of T_3 and T_4.

Unfortunately, the effects of iodide on thyroid function cannot be sustained indefinitely. With long-term iodide administration, suppressant effects become weaker. Accordingly, iodide is rarely used alone for thyroid suppression.

Therapeutic Use
Strong iodine solution can be given to hyperthyroid individuals to suppress thyroid function in preparation for thyroidectomy. Initial effects develop within 24 hours. Peak effects develop in 10 to 15 days. In most cases, plasma levels of thyroid hormone are reduced with methimazole before initiating strong iodine solution. Then strong iodine solution (along with more PTU) is administered for the last 10 days before surgery. In addition to its use before thyroidectomy, strong iodine solution is used in thyrotoxic crisis.

Dosage and Administration
When used to prepare hyperthyroid patients for thyroidectomy, strong iodine solution is administered in a dosage of 5 to 7 drops 3 times daily for 10 days immediately preceding surgery. Iodine solution should be mixed with juice or some other beverage to mask its unpleasant taste. The dosage for thyrotoxic crisis is 10 drops every 8 hours.

SUMMARY OF KEY PRESCRIBING CONSIDERATIONS
Radioactive Iodine

Therapeutic Goal: Suppression of thyroid hormone production in preparation for subtotal thyroidectomy. Also used to suppress thyroid hormone release in patients experiencing thyroid storm.

Baseline Data: Obtain serum levels of thyroid-stimulating hormone (TSH), free triiodothyronine (T_3), and free thyroxine (T_4).

Minimizing Adverse Effects: Inform patients about symptoms of iodism, including brassy taste, burning sensations in the mouth, and soreness of gums and teeth. Iodine can also cause corrosive injury to the GI tract. Instruct patients to notify the prescriber if severe abdominal distress develops.

50

Estrogens and Progestins: Basic Pharmacology and Noncontraceptive Applications

To understand pharmacologic properties of manufactured estrogens and progestins, it is important to first understand properties and actions of the endogenous hormones. We begin this chapter with a discussion of how estrogens and progestins regulate physiologic processes.

Estrogens and progestins (also known as *progestogens*) are hormones with multiple actions. They promote female maturation and help regulate the ongoing activity of female reproductive organs. In addition, they affect bone mineralization and lipid metabolism. The principal endogenous estrogen is estradiol. The principal endogenous progestational hormone (i.e., progestin) is progesterone. Both hormones are produced by the ovaries. During pregnancy, large amounts are produced by the placenta. In addition, small amounts of estrogens and progestins are produced in peripheral tissues.

THE MENSTRUAL CYCLE

Because much of the clinical pharmacology of the estrogens and progestins is related to their actions during the menstrual cycle, understanding the menstrual cycle is central to understanding these hormones. Accordingly, we begin by reviewing the menstrual cycle. The anatomic and hormonal changes that take place during the cycle are shown in Fig. 50.1. As indicated, the first half of the cycle (days 1 through 14) is called the *follicular phase,* and the second half is called the *luteal phase.* One full cycle typically takes approximately 28 days.

Ovarian and Uterine Events

The menstrual cycle consists of a coordinated series of ovarian and uterine events. In the ovary, the following sequence occurs: (1) several ovarian follicles ripen; (2) one of the ripe follicles ruptures, causing ovulation; (3) the ruptured follicle evolves into a corpus luteum; and (4) if fertilization does not occur, the corpus luteum atrophies. As these ovarian events are taking place, parallel events take place in the uterus: (1) while ovarian follicles ripen, the endometrium prepares for nidation (implantation of a fertilized ovum) by increasing in thickness and vascularity; (2) after ovulation, the uterus continues its preparation by increasing secretory activity; and (3) if implantation fails to occur, the thickened endometrium breaks down, causing menstruation, and the cycle begins anew.

Roles of Estrogens and Progesterone

The uterine changes that occur during the cycle are brought about under the influence of estrogens and progesterone produced by the ovaries. During the first half of the cycle, estrogens are secreted by the maturing ovarian follicles. As suggested by Fig. 50.1, these estrogens act on the uterus to cause proliferation of the endometrium. At midcycle, one of the ovarian follicles ruptures and then evolves into a corpus luteum. For most of the second half of the cycle, estrogens and progesterone are produced by the newly formed corpus luteum. These hormones maintain the endometrium in its hypertrophied state. At the end of the cycle, the corpus luteum atrophies, causing production of estrogens and progesterone to decline. In response to the diminished supply of ovarian hormones, the endometrium breaks down.

Role of Pituitary Hormones

Two anterior pituitary hormones—follicle-stimulating hormone (FSH) and luteinizing hormone (LH)—play central roles in regulating the menstrual cycle. Precisely timed alterations in the secretion of these hormones are responsible for coordinating the structural and secretory changes that occur throughout the menstrual cycle. During the first half of the cycle, FSH acts on the developing ovarian follicles, causing them to mature and secrete estrogens. The resultant rise in estrogen levels exerts a negative feedback influence on the pituitary, thereby suppressing further FSH release. At midcycle, LH levels rise abruptly (see Fig. 50.1). This LH surge causes the dominant follicle to swell rapidly, burst, and release its ovum. After ovulation, the ruptured follicle becomes a corpus luteum and, under the influence of LH, begins to secrete progesterone.

ESTROGENS

Biosynthesis and Elimination

Females

In premenopausal women, the ovary is the principal source of estrogen. During the follicular phase of the menstrual cycle, estrogens are synthesized by ovarian follicles; during the luteal phase, estrogens are synthesized by the corpus luteum. The major estrogen produced by the ovaries is *estradiol.* In the periphery, some of the estradiol secreted by the ovaries is converted into *estrone* and *estriol,* hormones that are less potent than estradiol. Estrogens are eliminated by a combination of hepatic metabolism and urinary excretion.

During pregnancy, large quantities of estrogens are produced by the placenta. Excretion of these hormones results in high levels of estrogens in the urine.

Males

Estrogen production is not limited to females. In the human male, small amounts of testosterone are converted into estradiol and estrone

Fig. 50.1 The Menstrual Cycle: Anatomic and Hormonal Changes. *FSH,* Follicle-stimulating hormone; *LH,* luteinizing hormone.

by the testes. Enzymatic conversion of testosterone in peripheral tissues (e.g., liver, fat, skeletal muscle) results in additional estrogen production.

Mechanism of Action

Like other steroidal hormones (e.g., testosterone, cortisol), estrogen acts primarily through receptors in the cell nucleus, not on the cell surface. Hence to produce its effects, estrogen must diffuse into cells, migrate to the nucleus, and then bind with an estrogen receptor (ER). The estrogen-ER complex then binds with an estrogen response element on a target gene, altering the rate of gene transcription. It is important to note that not all ERs are found in the nucleus: some ERs are found on cell membranes. Activating these surface receptors produces a rapid response—more rapid than can be produced by activating nuclear receptors.

There are two forms of ERs, termed ER α and ER β. ER α is highly expressed in the vagina, uterus, ovaries, mammary glands, vascular epithelium, and hypothalamus. ER β is expressed in the ovary and prostate and to less extent in the lungs, brain, bones, and blood vessels. Some cells have both types of ER receptor.

Physiologic and Pharmacologic Effects
Effects on Primary and Secondary Sex Characteristics of Females

Estrogens support the development and maintenance of the female reproductive tract and secondary sex characteristics. These hormones are required for the growth and maturation of the uterus, vagina, fallopian tubes, and breasts. In addition, estrogens direct pigmentation of the nipples and genitalia.

Estrogens have a profound influence on physiologic processes related to reproduction. During the follicular phase of the menstrual cycle, estrogens promote (1) ductal growth in the breast, (2) thickening and cornification of the vaginal epithelium, (3) proliferation of the uterine epithelium, and (4) copious secretion of thickened mucus from endocervical glands. In addition, estrogens increase vaginal acidity (by promoting local deposition of glycogen, which is then acted on by lactobacilli and corynebacteria to produce lactic acid). At the end of the menstrual cycle, a decline in estrogen levels can bring on menstruation. However, it is the fall in progesterone levels at the end of the cycle that normally causes breakdown of the endometrium and resultant menstrual bleeding. After menstruation, estrogens promote endometrial restoration.

During pregnancy, the placenta produces estrogen in large amounts. This estrogen stimulates uterine blood flow and growth of uterine muscle. In addition, it acts on the breast to continue ductal proliferation. However, final transformation of the breast for milk production requires the combined influence of estrogen, progesterone, and human placental lactogen.

Metabolic Actions

Endogenous estrogens affect various nonreproductive tissues. Important among these are bone, cardiovascular, blood, and neural tissue. Estrogens also have an important roles glucose homeostasis.

Bone. Estrogens have a positive effect on bone mass. Under normal conditions, bone undergoes continuous remodeling, a process in which bone mineral is resorbed and deposited in equal amounts. The principal effect of estrogens on the process is to block bone resorption, although estrogens may also promote mineral deposition.

During puberty, the long bones grow rapidly under the combined influence of growth hormone, adrenal androgens, and *low* levels of ovarian estrogens. When estrogen levels grow high enough, they promote epiphyseal closure and thereby bring linear growth to a stop.

Cardiovascular effects. Cardiovascular disease is much less common in premenopausal women compared with postmenopausal women. Estrogens have several roles in lowering this risk. For example, ERs in the vascular smooth muscle respond to activation by decreasing vasoconstriction. Activation of ERs in vessel endothelium results in the production of nitric oxide, which results in vasodilation and increased perfusion. Estrogens also decrease atherosclerosis through favorable effects on cholesterol levels: levels of low-density lipoprotein (LDL) cholesterol are reduced, whereas levels of high-density lipoprotein (HDL) cholesterol are elevated.

Blood coagulation. Estrogens both promote and suppress blood coagulation. Estrogens promote coagulation by (1) increasing levels of coagulation factors (e.g., factors II, VII, IX, X, and XII) and (2) decreasing levels of factors that suppress coagulation (e.g., antithrombin). Estrogens suppress coagulation by increasing the activity of factors that promote breakdown of fibrin, a protein that reinforces blood clots. The net effect—increased or decreased coagulation—may be determined by a hereditary defect in one of these targets.

Central nervous system effects. In the central nervous system (CNS), estrogens have a neuroprotective effect by defending neurons from the effects of oxidative stress and injury. They also have a role in neuronal growth and repair through stimulation of nerve growth factors. Estrogen-induced synaptic changes, coupled with estrogen-promoted increases in synaptic serotonin, dopamine, and norepinephrine, are thought to preserve cognitive function, enhance short-term memory, and regulate mood. Cerebral perfusion is also enhanced by the release of nitric acid and the resulting vasodilation.

Glucose homeostasis. Estrogens play an active role in maintaining glucose levels. In conditions that lead to insulin resistance due to impaired transport, estrogen has been shown to increase insulin sensitivity to promote glucose uptake. Estrogens also have a role in insulin secretion and are believed to protect pancreatic islet beta cells from certain types of injury.

Physiologic Alterations Accompanying Menopause

Menopause and the associated loss of estrogen typically begin at approximately age 51 to 52 years, with 95% of women entering menopause between the ages of 45 and 55 years. During the initial phase, the menstrual cycle becomes irregular, anovulatory cycles may occur,

and periods of amenorrhea may alternate with menses. Eventually, ovulation and menstruation cease entirely. Production of ovarian estrogens decreases gradually, coming to a complete stop several years after menstruation has ceased.

Loss of estrogen has multiple effects. Prominent symptoms experienced by the patient include vasomotor symptoms, sleep disturbances, and urogenital atrophy. Additional physiologic changes include bone loss and altered lipid metabolism. Alterations in cognition and sexual response are manifestations of physiologic changes.

Vasomotor Symptoms

Vasomotor symptoms (hot flashes and night sweats) develop in approximately 70% of postmenopausal women. Episodes are characterized by sudden skin flushing, sweating, and a sensation of uncomfortable warmth. These episodes can occur at night, resulting in drenching sweats. Severe episodes can cause sleep disturbances, fatigue, and irritability. In most women, hot flashes abate within several months to a few years; in others, they may persist for a decade or more.

Genitourinary Syndrome of Menopause

Of all structures in the body, the urethra and vagina have the highest concentrations of ERs. Activation of these receptors maintains the functional integrity of the urethra and vaginal epithelium. Hence when estrogen levels decline during menopause, these structures undergo degenerative change.

Genitourinary syndrome of menopause encompasses a constellation of symptoms due to atrophic changes that accompany loss of estrogen. Atrophy of the urethra causes urge incontinence and urinary frequency. Urethritis and urinary tract infections can also occur. Atrophy of the vaginal epithelium can lead to dryness and dyspareunia (pain with intercourse). In addition, alterations in vaginal secretions result in decreased acidity, which can allow the growth of pathogenic bacteria, resulting in and increased risk for vaginal infections.

Female Sexual Interest-Arousal Disorder

Female sexual interest-arousal disorder (FSIAD) is not unique to women in menopause; however, its occurrence is more common during this stage of life. FSIAD presents as a decrease in libido or decreased arousal during sexual activity. Although dyspareunia can be a contributing factor, these changes often occur in the absence of dyspareunia. Some women do not perceive these alterations as a disorder at all, but for others, it can cause considerable personal distress. (discussed later).

Mental Changes

Many women report cognitive changes such as difficulty in problem solving and short-term memory loss around the time when menopause begins. Others experience depression or an increase in anxiety. These changes tend to occur during the time of transition and often compounded sleep disturbances.

Bone Loss

In the absence of estrogen, bone resorption accelerates, leading to a 12% loss of bone density shortly after menopause. Osteoporosis is characterized by bone demineralization, altered bone architecture, and reduced bone strength. Compression fractures of the vertebrae are common and can decrease height and produce a hump. In osteoporotic women, fractures of the hip and wrist can result from minimal trauma.

Altered Lipid Metabolism

Studies have demonstrated slight, but significant, increases in LDL cholesterol with concomitant decreases in HDL cholesterol. These are thought to have a role in the increase in cardiovascular disease that increases after menopause.

Clinical Pharmacology

Now that we have reviewed the effects of endogenous estrogens and their loss, let's examine how estrogen preparations are used clinically. We will begin with a discussion of therapeutic uses.

Therapeutic Uses

Estrogens have contraceptive and noncontraceptive applications. In this chapter, discussion is limited to the noncontraceptive applications. Use of estrogens for contraception is discussed in Chapter 51.

Menopausal hormone therapy. Hormone therapy (HT) in post-menopausal women is the most common noncontraceptive use of estrogens. When estrogen is used for this purpose, it is usually accompanied by the use of progestins. For this reason, we will cover HT after the discussion of progestins.

Female hypogonadism. In the absence of ovarian estrogens, pubertal transformation will not take place. Causes of estrogen deficiency include primary ovarian failure, hypopituitarism, bilateral oophorectomy (removal of both ovaries), and Turner syndrome (a genetic disorder that impairs gonadal function). In girls with estrogen insufficiency, puberty can be induced by giving exogenous estrogens. This treatment promotes breast development, maturation of the reproductive organs, and development of pubic and axillary hair. To simulate normal patterns of estrogen secretion, the regimen should consist of continuous low-dose therapy (for approximately a year) followed by cyclic administration of estrogen in higher doses. Estrogen therapy for these conditions is typically managed by specialists.

Acne. Estrogens, in the form of oral contraceptives, can help control acne. Treatment is limited to patients at least 14 or 15 years old who want contraception. Use of estrogen for acne is discussed in Chapter 88.

Cancer palliation. Estrogens are sometimes used for palliative therapy in management of advanced prostate cancer in men and in a select type of metastatic breast cancer in both men and women. This use is directed by an oncologist or other specialist in this field.

Gender-affirmation therapy for transgender women. Although not approved by the U.S. Food and Drug Administration (FDA) for this purpose, estrogens are prescribed off-label as part of gender-affirmation drug therapy. (discussed later).

Adverse Effects

The principal concerns with estrogen therapy are the potential for endometrial hyperplasia, endometrial cancer, breast cancer, and cardiovascular thromboembolic events. Of these, the potential for endometrial hyperplasia and endometrial cancer can be resolved by prescribing a progestin, if indicated.

Estrogens have been associated with gallbladder disease, jaundice, and headache. Use during menopause may produce or uncover gallbladder disease. Jaundice may develop in women with preexisting liver dysfunction, especially those who experienced cholestatic jaundice of pregnancy.

Nausea is the most frequent undesired response to the estrogens. Fortunately, nausea diminishes with continued use and is rarely so severe as to necessitate treatment cessation.

Estrogens can increase the risk for headache, especially migraine headache. Fluid retention with edema commonly occurs. Chloasma, a patchy brown facial discoloration, though not dangerous, may cause significant distress for some women.

Contraindications

Estrogens should not be taken by patients with a history of deep vein thrombosis (DVT), pulmonary embolus, or conditions such as stroke or myocardial infarction (MI) that occurred secondary to a thromboembolic event. They should not be prescribed to women who are pregnant or who have vaginal bleeding without a known cause. Patients with a history of liver disease, estrogen-dependent tumors, or breast cancer (except when indicated for management) also should not take estrogens.

Interactions

Estrogens are major substrates of CYP1A2 and CYP3A4. Inducers of these isoenzymes may lower estrogen levels, whereas drugs that are inhibitors may raise estrogen levels. In addition, they may decrease the effectiveness of some antidiabetic drugs and thyroid preparations. Estrogens can also interact with anticoagulants and other drugs that affect clotting.

Preparations

Estrogen is available in conjugated and esterified forms. Esterified estrogens are plant based; conjugated estrogens are natural preparations derived from the urine of pregnant horses. Until mid-2016, synthetic conjugated estrogens A (Cenestin) and B (Enjuvia) were available; however, the manufacturer has withdrawn them from the market. At the time of this writing, there is no generic substitution for these synthetic conjugated estrogens.

Routes of Administration

Oral. Owing to convenience, the oral route is used more than any other. The most active estrogenic compound—estradiol—is available alone and in combination with progestins.

Transdermal. Transdermal estradiol is available in four formulations:
- Emulsion (Estrasorb)
- Spray (Evamist)
- Gels (EstroGel, Elestrin, Divigel)
- Patches (Alora, Climara, Estraderm, Menostar, Vivelle-Dot, Oesclim ♣)

Application is specific to certain body regions. The emulsion is applied once daily to the top of both thighs and the back of both calves. The spray is applied once daily to the forearm. The gel is applied once daily to one arm, from the shoulder to the wrist or to the thigh (Divigel). The patches are applied to the skin of the trunk (but not the breasts). Rates of estrogen absorption with transdermal formulations range from 14 to 60 μg/24 hours, depending on the product used.

Compared with oral formulations, the transdermal formulations have four advantages:
- The total dose of estrogen is greatly reduced (because the liver is bypassed).
- There is less nausea and vomiting.
- Blood levels of estrogen fluctuate less.
- There is a lower risk for DVT, pulmonary embolism, and stroke.

Intravaginal. Estrogens for intravaginal administration are available as inserts, creams, and vaginal rings. The intravaginal inserts (Imvexxy, Vagifem, Yuvafem), creams (Estrace Vaginal, Premarin Vaginal), and one of the two available vaginal rings (Estring) are used only for local effects, primarily treatment of vulval and vaginal atrophy associated with menopause. The other vaginal ring (Femring) is used for systemic effects (e.g., control of hot flashes and night sweats) as well as local effects (e.g., treatment of vulval and vaginal atrophy).

Parenteral. Although estrogens are formulated for intravenous (IV) and intramuscular (IM) administration, use of these routes is rare. IV administration is generally limited to acute, emergency control of heavy uterine bleeding.

PATIENT EDUCATION
Estrogen Administration

Transdermal Patch

Give the patient the following instructions for using estradiol transdermal patches:

- Apply to an area of clean, dry, intact skin on the abdomen or some other region of the trunk (but not the breasts or waistline) by pressing the patch firmly in place for 10 s.
- If the patch falls off, reapply the same patch or, if necessary, apply a new patch.
- Remove the old patch and apply a new patch once or twice weekly according to the product specifications.
- Rotate the application site such that the same site is not used more than once each week.

Transdermal Emulsion

Instruct the patient to apply the emulsion each morning to the top of both thighs and the back of both calves.

Transdermal Gel

Instruct the patient to apply the gel once daily after showering to one arm, from the shoulder to the wrist.

Transdermal Spray

Instruct the patient to apply 1, 2, or 3 sprays once daily to the inner forearm, and then let it dry at least 2 min before dressing and at least 30 min before washing.

Intravaginal Cream

Instruct the patient to apply estrogen cream high into the vagina, usually at bedtime, using the applicator provided.

Intravaginal Ring

Instruct the patient to insert the ring as deeply as possible, and to leave it in place for 3 months, after which it should be removed, and then replaced with a new ring if indicated.

Intravaginal Insert

Inform patients that dosing consists of 1 insert daily for 2 weeks, followed by 1 insert twice a week thereafter. Instruct patients to place each insert as deep as comfortably possible using the applicator supplied.

PHYTOESTROGENS

Phytoestrogens are plant-based compounds that have weak estrogenic activity. There are three types: isoflavones, lignins, and coumestans. The most commonly used and studied phytoestrogens are the isoflavones which are derived from plants such as soy beans and red clover.

Phytoestrogens are commonly used by women as a "natural" way to manage symptoms associated with menopause. There is strong anecdotal support for phytoestrogen therapy; however, findings from randomized controlled trials are inconsistent. Because there is inadequate supporting evidence, their use is not recommended. That being said, their use also is not necessarily discouraged, either.

Phytoestrogens are not as potent as estradiol, but they carry some of the same risks. Women should not use phytoestrogens if they have a history of thromboembolic events or a personal or family history of breast, uterine, or ovarian cancer.

The American Association of Clinical Endocrinologists suggest that women preferring to use phytoestrogens should be encouraged

SUMMARY OF KEY PRESCRIBING CONSIDERATIONS
Estrogens

Therapeutic Goal: Management of symptoms and structural changes associated with decreased endogenous estrogen. (Other uses include palliation of metastatic breast cancer in selected cases.)

Baseline Data: Heart rate, blood pressure, weight. Pregnancy test, thyroid-stimulating hormone (TSH), serum triglyceride (or full lipid panel, if indicated). Screening for breast cancer and cardiovascular disease. Gynecologic exam, if indicated.

Monitoring: Blood pressure, weight. Serum triglycerides, TSH if thyroid replacement required, Regular breast and pelvic exams as recommended for age. Schedule endometrial biopsy for unscheduled bleeding that continues for 6 months.

Identifying High-Risk Patients: Estrogen therapy should not be prescribed for patients with:

- Abnormal vaginal bleeding of unknown cause
- Estrogen-dependent cancer or breast cancer (except when used as treatment for certain metastatic cancers)
- History of deep vein thrombosis or pulmonary embolism
- Stroke, myocardial infarction, or other arterial thromboembolism occurring within the past year
- Abnormal liver function or disease
- Pregnancy

Evaluating Therapeutic Effects: Therapeutic effects depend on the reason prescribed. For menopausal HT, patients report relief of symptoms and the vagina is pink and moist on gynecologic exam.

Minimizing Adverse Effects:

- Nausea is common early in treatment. Advise patients that this adverse effect diminishes with time. In the meantime, avoidance of cooking odors and warm, stuffy environments may help. Dry foods and raw fruits and vegetables are less likely to provoke nausea. Guided imagery with muscle relaxation, yoga, and music therapy may be helpful.
- Menopausal HT with estrogen alone increases the risk for endometrial carcinoma. Adding a progestin lowers this risk to the pretreatment level.
- Adverse effects similar to those caused by oral contraceptives (e.g., abnormal vaginal bleeding, hypertension, benign hepatic adenoma, reduced glucose tolerance) are summarized in Chapter 51.

to obtain these ingredients from whole food sources to avoid overdosage. One gram of soy yields approximately 1.5 mg of isoflavones. (For reference purposes, 1 g = 0.035 ounce and 1 ounce = 28.35 g.) If they will be using supplements, a daily dose of 40 to 80 mg is the typical dose used in research. It may take several weeks before effects are noticed.

SELECTIVE ESTROGEN RECEPTOR MODULATORS

Selective estrogen receptor modulators (SERMs) are drugs that activate ERs in some tissues and block them in others. These drugs were developed in an effort to provide the benefits of estrogen (e.g., protection against osteoporosis, maintenance of the urogenital tract, reduction of LDL cholesterol) while avoiding its drawbacks (e.g., promotion of breast cancer, uterine cancer, and thromboembolism). Four SERMs are available in the United States: tamoxifen (Nolvadex-D), toremifene (Fareston), raloxifene (Evista), and bazedoxifene (Duavee). None of these offers all of the benefits of estrogen, and none avoids all of the drawbacks.

Tamoxifen was the first SERM to be widely used. By blocking ERs, tamoxifen (and its active metabolite, endoxifen) can inhibit cell growth in the breast. As a result, the drug is used extensively to prevent and treat breast cancer. Unfortunately, blockade of ERs also produces hot flashes. By activating ERs, tamoxifen protects against osteoporosis and has a favorable effect on serum lipids. However, receptor activation also increases the risk for endometrial cancer and thromboembolism. The pharmacology of tamoxifen and toremifene (a close relative of tamoxifen) is discussed in Chapter 85.

Raloxifene is very similar to tamoxifen. The principal difference is that raloxifene does not activate ERs in the endometrium and hence does not pose a risk for uterine cancer. Like tamoxifen, raloxifene protects against breast cancer and osteoporosis, increases the risk for thromboembolism, and induces hot flashes. Raloxifene is approved only for prevention and treatment of osteoporosis and for prevention of breast cancer in high-risk women. Raloxifene is discussed at length in Chapter 61.

In 2013 the FDA approved *Duavee* (conjugated estrogens/bazedoxifene) for prevention of vasomotor symptoms and osteoporosis in postmenopausal women with a uterus. Duavee is the first drug to combine estrogen with an estrogen agonist/antagonist (bazedoxifene). The bazedoxifene component of Duavee reduces the risk for excessive growth of the lining of the uterus that can occur with the estrogen component. Contraindications to taking Duavee are the same as for other estrogen-containing products.

PROGESTINS

Estrogens and progestins are often prescribed together. Before we discuss these uses, it will be helpful to discuss progesterone. As previously mentioned, progesterone is the principal endogenous progestational hormone. As its name implies, progesterone acts before gestation to prepare the uterus for implantation of a fertilized ovum. In addition, progesterone helps maintain the uterus throughout pregnancy.

Biosynthesis

Progesterone is produced by the ovaries *and* the placenta. Ovarian production occurs during the second half of the menstrual cycle. During this period, progesterone is synthesized by the corpus luteum, in response to LH released from the anterior pituitary. If implantation of a fertilized ovum does not occur, progesterone production by the corpus luteum ceases and menstrual flow begins. However, if implantation *does* take place, the developing trophoblast will produce its own luteotropic hormone—human chorionic gonadotropin (hCG)—that will stimulate the corpus luteum to continue making progesterone. For the first 7 weeks of gestation, the placenta depends entirely on progesterone from the corpus luteum. However, between weeks 7 and 10, production of progesterone is shared between the corpus luteum and placenta. After 10 weeks of gestation, progesterone made by the placenta is sufficient to support pregnancy, and hence ovarian progesterone production declines. Placental synthesis of progesterone and estrogen continues throughout the pregnancy.

Mechanism of Action

As with estrogen, receptors for progesterone are found in the cell nucleus. Hence to produce an effect, progesterone must diffuse across the cell membrane, migrate to the nucleus, and then bind with a progesterone receptor (PR). The progesterone-PR complex then binds with a progesterone regulatory element on a target gene, thereby rapidly increasing gene transcription. As with estrogen, there are two types of receptors for progesterone, designated PR-A and PR-B. In general, the stimulatory actions of progesterone are mediated by PR-B, whereas inhibitory actions are mediated by PR-A.

Physiologic Effects
Effects During the Menstrual Cycle

Progesterone is secreted during the second half of the menstrual cycle from a proliferative state into a secretory state. If implantation does not occur, progesterone production by the corpus luteum declines. The resultant fall in progesterone levels is the principal stimulus for the onset of menstruation.

In addition to affecting the endometrium, progesterone affects the endocervical glands, breasts, body temperature, respiration, and mood. Under the influence of progesterone, secretions from endocervical glands become scant and viscous. (In contrast, estrogen makes these secretions profuse and watery.) In addition, progesterone causes the epithelium of the breast to divide and grow. Actions in the CNS may cause depression and sleepiness. By increasing the sensitivity of the respiratory center to CO_2, progesterone causes the partial pressure of carbon dioxide (P_{CO_2}) in blood to fall. At midcycle, when ovulation occurs, progesterone raises body temperature by 0.6°C (1°F).

Effects During Pregnancy

As noted, progesterone levels increase during pregnancy. These high levels suppress contraction of *uterine smooth muscle* and thereby help sustain pregnancy. Unfortunately, progesterone also suppresses contraction of *gastrointestinal smooth muscle,* which leads to prolonged transit time and constipation. In the *breast,* progesterone promotes growth and proliferation of alveolar tubules (acini), the structures that produce milk. Metabolic effects include suppression of arterial P_{CO_2}, altered serum bicarbonate content, and elevation of serum pH. Finally, progesterone may help suppress the maternal immune system, thereby preventing immune attack on the fetus.

Clinical Pharmacology

Now that we have reviewed the effects of endogenous progesterone, let's examine how progestins are used clinically. We will begin with a discussion of therapeutic uses.

Therapeutic Uses

Discussion in this chapter is limited to the noncontraceptive uses of progestins. Use for contraception is considered in Chapter 51.

Menopausal hormone therapy. The primary noncontraceptive use of progestins is to counteract the adverse effects of estrogen on the endometrium in women undergoing menopausal HT. This application is discussed later in this chapter.

Dysfunctional uterine bleeding. This condition, characterized by heavy irregular bleeding, occurs when progesterone levels are insufficient to balance the stimulatory influence of estrogen on the endometrium. In the absence of sufficient progesterone, estrogen puts the endometrium in a state of continuous proliferation. Because progesterone is unavailable to induce monthly endometrial breakdown, the excessively proliferative endometrium undergoes spontaneous sloughing at irregular intervals. The result is periodic episodes of severe bleeding.

Treatment has two objectives: the initial goal is cessation of hemorrhage, and the long-term goal is to establish a regular monthly cycle. Excessive bleeding can be stopped by administering a progestin for 10 to 14 days. When dosing is stopped, withdrawal bleeding takes place. Bleeding is likely to be profuse and associated with cramping. Giving an oral contraceptive twice daily for 5 to 7 days can help stabilize the endometrium and thereby reduce bleeding duration.

Cyclic therapy is used to establish a regular monthly cycle. In one regimen, oral dosing is started 10 to 14 days after the onset of each menstrual period and continued for the next 10 days. Alternatively, a progestin can be given for the first 10 days of each month. Both approaches can promote regular endometrial breakdown and menstruation.

Amenorrhea. Progestins can induce menstrual flow in selected women who are experiencing amenorrhea. If endogenous estrogen levels are adequate, treatment with a progestin for 5 to 10 days will be followed by withdrawal bleeding when the progestin is stopped. If estrogen levels are low, it may be necessary to induce endometrial proliferation with an estrogen before giving the progestin.

Endometrial hyperplasia and carcinoma. Progestins can provide palliation in women with metastatic endometrial carcinoma, but these drugs do not prolong life. Several months of treatment may be required for a response. Management is by specialists.

Endometrial hyperplasia, a potentially precancerous condition, can be suppressed with progestins. Benefits derive from counteracting the proliferative effects of estrogen. Treatment options include oral therapy with megestrol acetate (Megace) or medroxyprogesterone acetate (Provera) and local delivery of a levonorgestrel using the Mirena intrauterine device (IUD).

Other uses. Progestins are used to support an early pregnancy in women with corpus luteum deficiency syndrome and in women undergoing in vitro fertilization (IVF). One progestin—hydroxyprogesterone acetate (Makena)—is approved for preventing preterm birth in women with a singleton pregnancy and a history of preterm delivery.

Adverse Effects

Up to 20% of patients may experience breast tenderness, headache, abdominal discomfort, arthralgias, and depression. When used continuously for birth control, progestins greatly decrease production of cervical mucus and cause involution of the endometrial layer. Effects on the endometrium lead to spotting, breakthrough bleeding, and irregular menses. Progestins, in combination with estrogen, increase the risk for breast cancer in postmenopausal women.

Preparations and Routes of Administration

Progestins are available in oral, IM, subcutaneous (subQ), intravaginal, intrauterine, and transdermal formulations. Older oral progestins include medroxyprogesterone acetate (Provera), norethindrone (Micronor, Nor-QD, others), norethindrone acetate (Aygestin), megestrol acetate (Megace), levonorgestrel (Plan B One-Step, Next Choice), and a micronized formulation of progesterone (Prometrium). Newer oral progestins— norgestimate and drospirenone—are available in fixed-dose combinations with estradiol sold as Prefest and Angeliq, respectively. IM progestins are medroxyprogesterone acetate (Depo-Provera) and progesterone (in oil). Medroxyprogesterone acetate is also available in a formulation for subQ injection (Depo-SubQ Provera 104). Micronized progesterone for intravaginal use is available as progesterone gel (Crinone) and a vaginal insert (Endometrin). Transdermal products are limited to norethindrone (formulated with estradiol under the name CombiPatch) and levonorgestrel (formulated with estradiol under the name Climara Pro). A second-generation progestin—etonogestrel—used for contraception is available by itself as a subQ implant (Nexplanon) and combined with estradiol in a vaginal ring (NuvaRing). (See Chapter 51.)

MENOPAUSAL HORMONE THERAPY

Menopausal HT, formerly known as *hormone replacement therapy* (HRT), consists of low doses of estrogen (with or without a progestin) taken to compensate for the loss of estrogen that occurs during menopause. There are two basic regimens for HT: estrogen alone (ET) and estrogen plus a progestin (estrogen/progestin therapy [EPT]). The purpose of estrogen in both regimens is to control menopausal symptoms by replacing estrogen that was lost owing to menopause. The progestin is present for one reason only: to counterbalance estrogen-mediated stimulation of the endometrium, which can lead to endometrial

SUMMARY OF KEY PRESCRIBING CONSIDERATIONS

Progestins

Therapeutic Goal: Goals for noncontraceptive uses are to counteract endometrial hyperplasia caused by unopposed estrogen during hormone therapy; management of dysfunctional uterine bleeding, amenorrhea, and endometriosis; and support of pregnancy in women with corpus luteum deficiency. Progestins are also used in in vitro fertilization cycles and to prevent prematurity in women at high risk for preterm birth.

Baseline Data: Heart rate, blood pressure, and weight. Pregnancy test. Screening for breast and cardiovascular disease. Pelvic exam as indicated for age.

Monitoring: Blood pressure. Assessment for fluid retention, including weight. Consider referral for transvaginal ultrasound or hysteroscopy for occurrence of undiagnosed bleeding that continues for 6 months.

Identifying High-Risk Patients: Progestins are *contraindicated* in the presence of undiagnosed abnormal vaginal bleeding. *Relative contraindications* include active thrombophlebitis or a history of thromboembolic disorders, active liver disease, and carcinoma of the breast.

Minimizing Adverse Effects: Progestins can cause breakthrough bleeding, spotting, and amenorrhea. Warn patients that this may occur, and instruct them to report any abnormal or prolonged vaginal bleeding.

hyperplasia and cancer. (Progestins should not be prescribed for women who have undergone hysterectomy.)

It is typically the vasomotor symptoms that compel most women to seek HT. Hot flashes and the drenching sweats that accompany them can interfere with daily life and cause sleepless nights. Not only are they uncomfortable, but they also may create embarrassing situations, especially for women working with the public when appearances can be important. When vasomotor symptoms are severe, HT can be truly life changing.

Women who take HT often report an improved quality of life as well. In addition to controlling vasomotor symptoms, they report improved sleep, restoration of libido, improved cognition, and enhanced mood. Although there have been insufficient studies to quantify quality-of-life issues, the anecdotal evidence supports this as an added benefit.

From the medical perspective, HT confers three primary benefits: suppression of vasomotor symptoms, prevention of urogenital atrophy, and prevention of osteoporosis and related fractures. For all three, treatment is highly effective. (Unfortunately, the benefits of urogenital atrophy and osteoporosis prevention are not sustained and will decline after HT is withdrawn.)

Given the positive physiologic effects of estrogen and the detrimental physiologic changes that occur with estrogen loss, it might seem logical to prescribe HT for all women experiencing menopause. Indeed, this was once common practice with therapy that began during perimenopause and continued into later years of life. Then, in the early 2000s, data from two landmark studies, the Women's Health Initiative (WHI) and the Heart and Estrogen/progestin Replacement Study and its follow-up (HERS and HERS II), demonstrated that, contrary to popular assumptions, use of HT could increase, rather than prevent, cardiovascular events. Women taking HT in the study also had an increase in thromboembolic events such as DVT and stroke. For women receiving EPT (but not ET), there was a significant increase in the incidence of breast cancer. The reaction in the medical community was strong and swift as many providers stopped prescribing HT altogether and use of HT declined by 80%.

More recently, increased scrutiny of these early studies yielded concerns that have resulted in a reexamination of these risks. Subjects in those studies tended to be older. For example, only 3.5% of women in the WHI study were in the 50- to 54-year age range, which is the age at which most women currently begin HT. Furthermore, the therapy in those studies was at a higher dose, and use was prolonged beyond that of recommended current practice. When WHI data for women aged 50 to 59 years taking HT for less than 10 years were examined, it was discovered that the increase in venous thromboembolic episodes was only between 1.1 to 5 out of 1000 women taking ET and 5.1 to 10 out of 1000 women taking EPT. For women taking ET, there was no increase in coronary heart disease (CHD), and for women taking EPT, CHD increase was 1.1 to 5 out of 1000 women and venothrombotic episode increase was 5.1 to 10 out of 1000 women. Moreover, when benefits were examined, *for both ET and EPT, 5.1 to 10 out of 1000 women experienced a reduction in overall mortality compared with women not taking HT.*

Subsequent and ongoing research has provided more insight into the relationships of HT to dosage, time of initiation, length of use, and patient age, which were not adequately accounted for in the original reports from these studies. The more informed view of HT has evolved to a more reasoned approach to HT.

Benefits and Risks of Hormone Therapy

As with any drug, prescribing decisions require weighing the benefits and risks. It is important to keep in mind that our understanding of the benefits and risks of HT continues to evolve as current research focuses on the new demographic of younger woman taking HT at lower doses over fewer years.

PROTOTYPE DRUGS

Estrogens and Progestins

Estrogens
Conjugated estrogens (Premarin)
Estradiol

Progestins
Medroxyprogesterone acetate
Norethindrone

Recognizing that findings based on women older than 60 years taking high-dose, long-term HT for more than a decade could not be generalized to younger women taking low-dose HT for shorter time intervals, the Endocrine Society undertook an extensive review of published research to determine the benefits and risk of HT in women recently menopausal (i.e., less than 10 years postmenopausal) and aged 50 to 59. Significant findings are summarized in Table 50.1. Not included in the table are results of benefits related to the vasomotor and urogenital symptoms because the benefit (90% reduction in symptoms) is firmly established. Also not included are many of the previously assumed risks that were not supported in the data.

Based on these findings, especially considering the benefits of overall mortality, it certainly seems unreasonable to refuse HT for younger women desiring it once individual risks are assessed. Unfortunately, this does not address concerns of older women who have indications for therapy. More studies are needed; however, in the meantime, it is important to recognize that risk for complications increases with age. Furthermore, research findings suggest that use of HT in women older than 65 years may increase the risk for dementia.

Recommendations on Hormone Therapy Use

When making decisions regarding whether or not to prescribe HT, risk factors for the individual must be inventoried, and the hoped-for benefits

TABLE 50.1 Benefits and Risks of Menopausal Hormone Therapy

Benefits Over 5 Years	NUMBER OF FEWER CASES PER 1000 WOMEN AGED 50–59 YEARS	
	Estrogen + Progestin (EPT)	Estrogen Only (ET)
Coronary heart disease	0.9	3.8
Osteoporotic fractures	4.9	5.9
Breast cancer	—	1.5
Colorectal cancer	1.2	—
Type 2 diabetes mellitus	11	11
Mortality for all causes	5.3 fewer deaths	5 fewer deaths

Risk Over 5 Years	NUMBER OF INCREASED CASES PER 1000 WOMEN AGED 50–59 YEARS	
	Estrogen + Progestin (EPT)	Estrogen Only (ET)
Thromboembolism	5	2
Stroke	1.0	1.2
Breast cancer	6.8	—
Cholecystitis[a]	9.6	14.2

[a]Data specific for cholecystitis are based on a larger demographic because data specific to ages 50 to 59 years were not available.

should be clearly defined. For women with significant baseline risks (e.g., personal or family history of breast cancer, cardiovascular disease), the risk for harm from HT goes up.

Recently, several expert sources have issued revised recommendations on HT. The recommendations that follow represent a composite of those offered by four groups: the North American Menopause Society, The Endocrine Society, the FDA, and the U.S. Preventive Services Task Force (USPSTF). Fig. 50.2 provides additional guidance.

General Recommendations

To balance benefits and risks, an individual risk profile should be compiled for every woman considering HT. All candidates for HT should be informed of known risks. Women with multiple risk factors should consider alternative therapies. For most women, the benefits of *long-term* HT for disease prevention do not outweigh the risks and hence long-term HT should generally be avoided. Conversely, the benefits of short-term therapy (<5 years) to treat menopausal symptoms often *do* justify the risks. To keep risk as low as possible, HT should be used in the lowest dosage and for the shortest time needed to accomplish treatment goals.

Use for approved indications. HT has only three approved indications:
- Treatment of moderate to severe vasomotor symptoms associated with menopause
- Treatment of genitourinary syndrome of menopause
- Prevention of postmenopausal osteoporosis

With the first two indications, duration of treatment is relatively short (typically 3 to 4 years), and hence the risk for harm is relatively low—except for women with established heart disease. In contrast, prevention of osteoporosis requires lifelong HT, and hence the risk for harm is higher.

The only approved indication for long-term *progestin* therapy is protection against endometrial cancer, which could be caused by unopposed estrogen. Accordingly, use of EPT should be limited to women

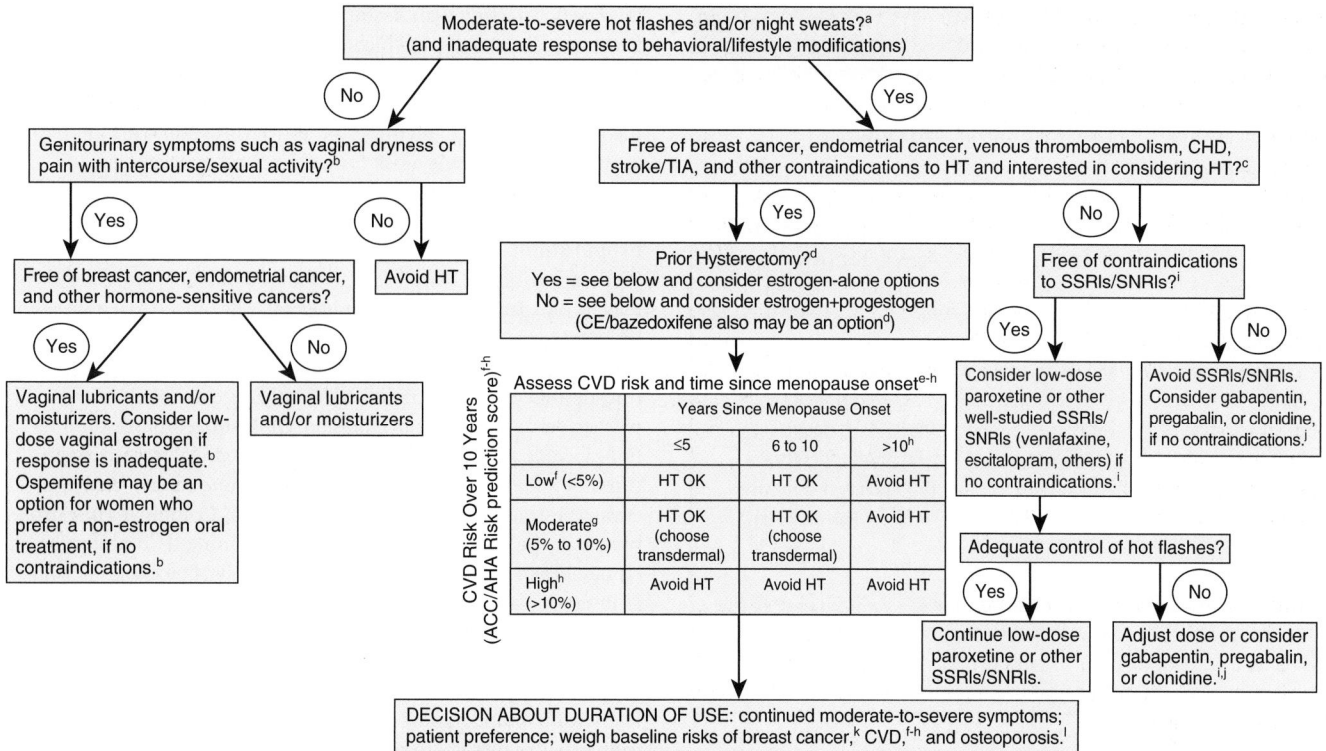

Fig. 50.2 Algorithm for Menopausal Symptom Management. *ACC/AHA,* American College of Cardiology/American Heart Association; *ASCVD,* atherosclerotic cardiovascular disease; *CE,* conjugated estrogens; *CHD,* coronary heart disease; *CVD,* cardiovascular disease; *EPT,* estrogen plus progestogen therapy; *ET,* estrogen therapy; *FDA,* U.S. Food and Drug Administration; *FSH,* follicle-stimulating hormone; *hCG,* human chorionic gonadotropin; *HT,* hormone therapy; *NAMS,* North American Menopause Society; *PRL,* prolactin; *SNRI,* serotonin-norepinephrine reuptake inhibitor; *SSRI,* selective serotonin reuptake inhibitors; *TIA,* transient ischemic attack; *TSH,* thyroid-stimulating hormone. (From the North American Menopause Society, http://www.menopause.org/docs/default-source/2014/menopro-app-algorithm-2014.pdf.)

with an intact uterus. For women who have had a hysterectomy, ET should be used.

Treatment of vasomotor symptoms. HT is the most effective treatment for vasomotor symptoms. To increase safety, the lowest effective dosage should be used. Furthermore, because vasomotor symptoms subside over time, the need for continued HT should be reassessed at regular intervals.

For women determined to be at too high risk for HT, other options are available, but they are less effective than estrogen. Trials have shown that two antidepressants—*escitalopram* (Lexapro) and *desvenlafaxine* (Pristiq)—can produce a modest but meaningful reduction in both the frequency and severity of hot flashes. Escitalopram is a selective serotonin reuptake inhibitor (SSRI); desvenlafaxine is a serotonin-norepinephrine reuptake inhibitor (SNRI). Other SSRIs and SNRIs are likely to be effective as well. *Paroxetine* (Brisdelle), an SSRI, was approved in 2013 for the treatment of vasomotor symptoms in menopause. SSRIs and SNRIs are discussed further in Chapter 27. Other drugs that have demonstrated some success are clonidine, a centrally-acting alpha2 agonist (see Chapter 17), and pregabalin. a gamma-aminobutyric acid [GABA] analog (see Chapter 21).

By contrast, controlled trials have shown that soy isoflavones do *not* reduce hot flashes. In fact, these preparations may make symptoms worse. Similarly, black cohosh, once commonly recommended for vasomotor symptoms, has fallen out of favor and presents a risk for harm without substantial benefit (see Chapter 69).

Treatment of genitourinary syndrome of menopause. Estrogen is the most effective treatment for genitourinary syndrome of menopause,

characterized by dryness, irritation, and uncomfortable intercourse. Because systemic estrogen carries significant risks, the FDA recommends that, if HT is being used solely to manage vulvar and vaginal symptoms, a topical estrogen formulation should be considered. Options include vaginal creams, vaginal inserts, and vaginal rings (Table 50.2). Although long-term data are lacking, it seems likely that topical estrogen is safer than oral estrogen because, with nearly all topical formulations, blood levels of estrogen remain low. The notable exception is the Femring, which releases enough estrogen to cause significant systemic effects.

Prevention of osteoporosis. HT reduces postmenopausal bone loss and thereby decreases the risk for osteoporosis and related fractures. Unfortunately, when HT is stopped, bone mass rapidly decreases by approximately 12%. Hence to maintain bone health, HT must continue lifelong. As a result, the risk for harm is increased. Accordingly, alternative treatments are preferred. In fact, labeling of HT products currently must carry the following advice: *When this product is prescribed solely to prevent postmenopausal osteoporosis, approved nonestrogen treatments should be carefully considered. Furthermore, HT should be considered only for women with significant risk for osteoporosis, and only when that risk outweighs the risks of HT.* As discussed in Chapter 61, effective alternatives to HT include raloxifene (Evista), bisphosphonates (e.g., alendronate [Fosamax]), calcitonin (Miacalcin), and teriparatide (Forteo). Of course, all women (not to mention men) should practice primary prevention of bone loss by ensuring adequate intake of calcium and vitamin D, performing regular weight-bearing exercise, and avoiding smoking and excessive alcohol use.

TABLE 50.2 Intravaginal Estrogens for Menopausal Hormone Therapy

Generic Name	Trade Name	Usual Maintenance Dosage
Vaginal Creams		
Conjugated estrogens	Premarin	Apply 0.5–2 g/day (625 µg conjugated estrogens/g).[a]
Estradiol	Estrace	Apply 1–2 g 1–3 times/week (100 µg estradiol/g)
Vaginal Rings		
Estradiol	Estring	This 2-mg ring releases 7.5 µg/day for 90 days.
Estradiol acetate	Femring	The 12.4-mg ring releases 50 µg/day for 90 days.[a]
		The 24.8-mg ring releases 100 µg/day for 90 days.[a]
Vaginal Inserts		
Estradiol hemihydrate	Imvexxy, Vagifem, Yuvafem	Place 1 insert (4 µg–10 µg) intravaginally every day for 2 weeks, then 1 insert twice a week thereafter.

[a]Administer cyclically (3 weeks on and 1 week off). For short-term use only.

All intravaginal estrogens are used to treat urogenital atrophy. Imvexxy has a specific indication for dyspareunia. With one product—Femring—estradiol is absorbed in amounts sufficient to cause systemic effects, both beneficial (e.g., suppression of vasomotor symptoms) and adverse (e.g., increased risk for thrombosis).

Inappropriate uses

Heart disease. HT should *not* be prescribed for the express purpose of preventing CHD. For most women, HT confers no protection and may increase the risk for CHD and MI in some women.

To reduce risk for cardiovascular events, postmenopausal women should be counseled about alternative ways to promote cardiovascular health. Among these are avoiding smoking, performing regular aerobic exercise, decreasing intake of saturated fats, and taking prescribed drugs to treat hypertension, diabetes, and high cholesterol.

Dementia. HT should not be used to prevent dementia, including Alzheimer disease. There is no evidence that either EPT or ET can protect against dementia, whereas there *is* evidence that EPT may *cause* dementia and that ET can increase the combined risk for dementia and mild cognitive impairment.

Discontinuing Hormone Therapy

Unfortunately, discontinuation may cause vasomotor symptoms to return; typically, this occurs within 4 days of the last HT dose. Women who had severe symptoms before initiating HT are at highest risk for developing intolerable symptoms when they stop.

No firm guidelines exist for stopping HT. There are two basic methods: immediate cessation and tapering slowly. However, there are no controlled studies to indicate which option might result in fewer symptoms. For women who choose to taper slowly, again there are two basic options, referred to as "dose tapering" and "day tapering." With dose tapering, dosing is done every day, but the size of the daily dose is gradually reduced. If intense symptoms return after a dosage reduction, further reductions should be delayed until symptoms improve. With day tapering, the daily dose remains unchanged, but the number of days between doses is gradually

increased—starting with dosing every other day, then every third day, and so on. Regardless of which method is used—dose tapering or day tapering—only the dosage of *estrogen* should be lowered. For women on EPT, the *progestin dosage should remain unchanged* because lowering the progestin dosage might permit estrogen to stimulate endometrial growth, thereby posing a risk for endometrial hyperplasia.

Drug Products for Hormone Therapy
Preparations

Preparations for HT are listed in Tables 50.2, 50.3, and 50.4. Dosing may be oral, transdermal, or intravaginal. The oral estrogens used most often are conjugated equine estrogens (Premarin) (prepared by extraction from pregnant mares' urine), estradiol (Estrace), and estropipate. For transdermal therapy, estradiol is the only estrogen used, formulated in patches, gels, a spray, and an emulsion. Oral estrogen/progestin combinations include conjugated equine estrogens/medroxyprogesterone acetate (Prempro, Premphase), estradiol/norethindrone acetate (Activella), and ethinyl estradiol/norethindrone (Femhrt). Combination estrogen/progestin patches are estradiol/norethindrone (CombiPatch) and estradiol/levonorgestrel (Climara Pro). Intravaginal products—formulated as inserts, creams, and rings—are used primarily to manage symptoms of urogenital atrophy.

Dosing Schedules

Every woman undergoing systemic HT receives an estrogen, and every woman with a uterus also receives a progestin to counteract the stimulant effects of estrogen on the endometrium. Several dosing schedules may be used. Estrogen and progestin are commonly administered *continuously*. An alternative is to give estrogen continuously but give the progestin cyclically (e.g., on calendar days 15 through 28). However, cyclic progestin has the disadvantage of promoting monthly bleeding, which may explain why most women prefer continuous dosing.

Vaginal estrogens can be given continuously for 1 to 2 weeks, followed by dosing 1 to 3 times per week, titrating the dosing schedule based on symptoms. Estring remains in the vagina for 3 months, after which it is removed and replaced with a new ring.

▶ BLACK BOX WARNING
Estrogen Therapy

Endometrial cancer risk is increased in women with a uterus who take unopposed estrogen.
Estrogen may increase the risk for deep vein thrombosis and stroke.
Estrogen is not indicated for cardiovascular disease or dementia and may increase the risk for dementia in women aged 65 years and older.

PATIENT EDUCATION
Estrogens

Inform the patient that nausea can be reduced by taking estrogens with food and by dosing at night. Explain that nausea diminishes over time.

Remind patients that estrogens present a small risk of breast cancer and endometrial cancer. To minimize risk of undetected breast cancer, remind patients of the need to receive periodic mammograms. Instruct the patient to report any persistent or recurrent vaginal bleeding, so that the possibility of endometrial carcinoma can be evaluated.

To reduce cardiovascular risk, advise women to avoid smoking, perform regular exercise, decrease intake of saturated fats, and take appropriate drugs to treat hypertension, diabetes, and high cholesterol.

TABLE 50.3   Oral Drugs for Menopausal Hormone Therapy

Generic Name	Trade Name	Usual Dosage
Estrogens		
Conjugated estrogens, equine	Premarin	0.3–1.25 mg/day
Esterified estrogens	Menest, Estragen ♦	0.3–2.5 mg/day
Estradiol, micronized	Estrace	0.5–2 mg/day
Estropipate	Generic only	0.75–6 mg/day
Progestins[a]		
Medroxyprogesterone acetate	Provera	2.5–10 mg
Progesterone (micronized)	Prometrium	200 mg
Estrogen/Progestin Combinations[a]		
Conjugated estrogens/ medroxyprogesterone acetate	Prempro	0.3/1.5, 0.45/1.5, 0.625/2.5, or 0.625/5 mg daily
Conjugated estrogens/ medroxyprogesterone acetate	Premphase	Days 1–14: 0.625 mg estrogen (alone) daily Days 15–28: 0.625/5 mg estrogen/progesterone daily
Estradiol/drospirenone	Angeliq	0.5/0.25 or 1/0.5 mg daily
Estradiol/norethindrone acetate	Activella	0.5/0.1 or 1/0.5 mg daily
Estradiol/norgestimate	Prefest	1 mg estradiol every day; 0.09 mg norgestimate in a repeating cycle of 3 days on and 3 days off
Ethinyl estradiol/ norethindrone	Femhrt	2.5 μg/0.5 mg or 5 μg/1 mg daily
Other Estrogen Combinations		
Esterified estrogens/ methyltestosterone	Covaryx	1.25 mg/2.5 mg daily
Esterified estrogens/ methyltestosterone	Covaryx HS	0.625/1.25 mg daily
Conjugated estrogens/ bazedoxifene[b]	Duavee	0.45 mg/20 mg twice daily

[a]Progestins are used to counteract the effects of estrogen on the uterus. The progestins listed can be used when the regimen calls for taking estrogen and progestin separately, rather than using a combination product. In estrogen/progestin regimens, the estrogen is taken daily, and the progestin is taken daily or intermittently (e.g., 14 days on, 14 days off).
[b]Bazedoxifene is an estrogen antagonist/selective estrogen receptor modulator that acts to reduce excessive growth of the uterine lining that can occur with the estrogen component.

DRUG THERAPY FOR TRANSGENDER WOMEN

Transgender people have a gender identity that is different from their gender assignment (i.e., the gender they were assigned at birth). Therefore a transgender woman is a woman who is phenotypically male (i.e., born with male sex organs) but her internal experience is that of a woman.

TABLE 50.4   Transdermal Drugs for Menopausal Hormone Therapy

Generic Name	Trade Name	Strength (μg absorbed/day)	Application
Estrogens			
Transdermal Patches			
Estradiol	Menostar	14	Once weekly
	Climara	25, 37.5, 50, 60, 75, 100	Once weekly
	Alora	25, 50, 75, 100	Twice weekly
	Oesclim ♦	25, 37.5, 50, 75, 100	Twice weekly
	Vivelle-Dot	25, 37.5, 50, 75, 100	Twice weekly
	Estraderm	50, 100	Twice weekly
Topical Emulsion			
Estradiol hemihydrate	Estrasorb	50	Once daily
Transdermal Spray			
Estradiol	Evamist	1.53–4.6 mg is applied[a]	Once daily
Topical Gel			
Estradiol	EstroGel	0.75 mg is applied[a]	Once daily
	Elestrin	0.52 or 1.04 mg is applied[a]	Once daily
	Divigel	0.25, 0.5, or 1 mg is applied[a]	Once daily
Estrogen/Progestin Combinations			
Transdermal Patches			
Estradiol/ norethindrone	CombiPatch	50/140, 50/250	Twice weekly
Estradiol/ levonorgestrel	Climara Pro	45/15	Once weekly

[a]Application of this dose produces blood levels of estrogen and estrone similar to those seen in the follicular phase of the ovulatory cycle.

🕐 PATIENT-CENTERED CARE ACROSS THE LIFE SPAN

Estrogens

Life Stage	Considerations or Concerns
Children	Estrogens are not indicated for prepubertal children.
Pregnant women	Estrogens are contraindicated during pregnancy.
Breastfeeding women	Estrogens may affect infant development and may decrease both the quantity and quality of milk produced.
Older adults	Beers Criteria include estrogens among those identified as potentially inappropriate for use in geriatric patients.

To promote development of sexual characteristics that match her gender identity, the transgender woman needs hormonal therapy (HT).

Treatment for transgender women requires medication to decrease testosterone levels (if testes are present) coupled with estrogen to promote female characteristics. Management is highly individualized. Many patients want to maintain fertility, for example, so their therapy must be different from that of the patient for whom this is not a concern. Furthermore, people who self-identify as nonbinary (i.e., those who

BLACK BOX WARNING
Estrogen and Progestin Therapy

Estrogen plus progestin may increase the risk for thromboembolic events such as deep vein thrombosis, stroke, myocardial infarction, and pulmonary embolism.

Estrogen plus progestin is not indicated for cardiovascular disease or dementia and may increase the risk for dementia in women aged 65 years and older.

Estrogen plus progestin may increase breast cancer risk.

PATIENT-CENTERED CARE ACROSS THE LIFE SPAN
Progestins

Life Stage	Considerations or Concerns
Children	Progestins are not indicated for prepubertal children.
Pregnant women	High-dose therapy during the first 4 months of pregnancy has been associated with an increased incidence of birth defects (limb reductions, heart defects, masculinization of the female fetus).
Breastfeeding women	Progestins may contribute to neonatal jaundice.
Older adults	Progestins are only indicated if the patient is taking estrogen and has a uterus.

do not subscribe to a single gender of male or female) may want therapy that either maintains or downplays features of both genders.

Monitoring of therapy must include not only the effects of estrogen on developing female sex characteristics but also the effectiveness of medications (antiandrogens, gonadotropin-releasing hormone (GnRH) agonists, or others) in decreasing male sex characteristics. Laboratory monitoring includes serum estrogen (estradiol) and testosterone levels, as well as prolactin and triglycerides. Potassium levels should be included if spironolactone is prescribed as the antiandrogen of choice. HT risks are the same as for nontransgender patients. For estrogen, thrombo-embolic events remain the greatest risk factor. However, this is uncommon unless the patient has other risk factors such as smoking.

Finally, it is important to continue to assess for risk factors associated with both male and female genders. For example, transgender women will continue to be at risk for prostate cancer regardless of whether she has undergone gender confirming surgery. She will also need to be screened for breast cancer following the same guidelines as all women.

Pharmacologic therapy should be initiated and managed by endo-crinologists or other specialists in transgender health. Because you are likely to have transgender women as patients for general care of common illnesses and preventive medicine, it is important to have a familiarity with their therapy. Authoritative guidelines have been developed by the following organizations.

The following clinical guidelines provide additional information.

- The World Professional Association for Transgender Health's *Standards of Care for the Health of Transsexual, Transgender, and Gender Nonconforming People* available at https://www.wpath.org/publications/soc
- Center of Excellence for Transgender Health's *Guidelines for the Primary and Gender-Affirming Care of Transgender and Gender Nonbinary Peoples* available at http://transhealth.ucsf.edu/pdf/Transgender-PGACG-6-17-16.pdf
- The Endocrine Society's *Endocrine Treatment of Gender-Dysphoric/Gender-Incongruent Persons: An Endocrine Society Clinical Practice Guideline* available at https://academic.oup.com/jcem/article/102/11/3869/4157558

MANAGEMENT OF FEMALE SEXUAL INTEREST-AROUSAL DISORDER

Research indicates that approximately 10%–40% of women experience female sexual interest-arousal disorder (FSIAD), (formerly hypoactive sexual desire disorder). The incidence is greatly increased following hormonal changes associated with menopause. Although this is not a always treated with HT, this appears to be an appropriate chapter to discuss new treatments.

In centuries past, treatments to increase a woman's interest in sex have ranged from dangerous (e.g., cantharidin, or Spanish fly, the toxic chemical from a beetle that causes irritation and blistering of the mucosa) to ridiculous (e.g., filling the vagina with various horrid substances). More recent management has focused on addressing psychological issues and on off-label use of drugs such as sildenafil and testosterone (both with varying degrees of success). Some women report that "self-medicating" with recreational drugs such as cocaine and methylphenidate (Ritalin) increase libido, although we would never recommend these drugs for that purpose.

Flibanserin

In 2015 the US Food and Drug Administration approved the first drug to manage FSIAD. The drug, flibanserin (Addyi) is available by prescription for women with low libido not associated with medical or mental health problems, relationship problems, or medication side effects. Unfortunately, it is not indicated for treatment of women who are postmenopausal.

Unlike drugs for males with sexual dysfunction, which are predictably rapid following administration of a single dose, flibanserin requires daily doses for several weeks before benefits are seen. (Prescribing information recommends discontinuing the drug if improvement is not seen after 8 weeks.)

Flibanserin has several serious risks. CNS depression and hypotension, with or without syncope, are the most common adverse effects. Flibanserin is a substrate of multiple isoenzymes, most notably CYP3A4, so drug interactions are common. It is also expensive: a month's supply is approximately $960.

There are a couple of restrictions on prescribers and pharmacies as well. Flibanserin is available only through a Risk Evaluation and Mitigation Strategy (REMS). The Addyi REMS program requires enrollment and training for any providers wanting to prescribe the drug. In addition, only pharmacies certified with the Addyi REMS program may dispense flibanserin.

Additional information on flibanserin is available at http://www.addyi.com/hcp. Information on the Addyi REMS program is available at https://addyirems.com/AddyiUI/rems/home.action.

Bremelanotide

In 2019, bremelanotide (Vyleesi) became the most recent drug approved for this condition. Bremelanotide activates melanocortin receptors; however, the mechanism of action for improving sexual desire is unknown.

Bremelanotide is administered by subcutaneous injection at least 45 minutes before sexual activity occurs. Dosing is limited to one dose in 24 hours and no more than eight doses a month.

In clinical trials, 25% of subjects experienced improved sexual desire compared to 17% of those receiving a placebo. The most common side effects were nausea (40%), vomiting, flushing, headache, and injection site reactions. A transient rise in blood pressure can occur lasting up to 12 hours after taking bremelanotide. An uncommon (1%) reaction was a permanent darkening of gums and portions of skin. As with all newly-approved drugs, we will probably learn more following postmarketing trials and reports.

Birth control can be accomplished by interfering with the reproductive process at any step from gametogenesis to nidation (implantation of a fertilized ovum). Pharmacologic methods of contraception include oral contraceptives, etonogestrel implants, injectable medroxyprogesterone acetate, intrauterine devices, vaginal rings, and transdermal patches.

Most of this chapter focuses on combination oral contraceptive pills—the most widely used *reversible* form of contraception. Sterilization is used more often but is not reversible. In preparing to study these agents and other forms of contraception, a review of Chapter 50 is recommended, with special attention to information on the menstrual cycle and the physiologic and pharmacologic effects of estrogens and progestins.

EFFECTIVENESS OF BIRTH CONTROL METHODS

The effectiveness of a birth control method can be expressed as the percentage of unplanned pregnancies that occur while the method is being used. Employing this criterion, Table 51.1 compares the effectiveness of the major birth control methods. As it shows, the most effective methods are an etonogestrel implant (Nexplanon), an intrauterine device (IUD), and sterilization. Oral contraceptives (OCs), medroxyprogesterone (Depo-Provera), the contraceptive ring, and the contraceptive patch are close behind. The least reliable methods include barrier methods, periodic abstinence, spermicides, and withdrawal.

Table 51.1 contains two columns of figures, one labeled *theoretical use* and the other *actual use*. The *perfect use* figures represent pregnancy rates when a method of birth control is employed exactly as it should be (i.e., consistently and with proper technique). The *typical use* figures represent pregnancy rates observed in actual practice. The higher pregnancy rates reported in the *typical use* column are largely an indication that methods of birth control are not always used when and as they should be.

SELECTING A BIRTH CONTROL METHOD

The method of contraception chosen most frequently is sterilization: female sterilization (tubal ligation) plus male sterilization (vasectomy) are selected by 19% of birth control users. OCs or male condoms are chosen by most of the remaining birth control users. Diaphragms, periodic abstinence, IUDs, and other techniques account for a small fraction of birth control use.

Several factors should be considered when a method of birth control is being chosen. Chief among these are *effectiveness, safety,* and *personal preference*. As shown in Table 51.1, the most effective methods are etonogestrel subdermal implants (Nexplanon), intramuscular medroxyprogesterone acetate (Depo-Provera), sterilization, and IUDs. Three other methods—OCs, the contraceptive ring (NuvaRing), and the contraceptive patch (Ortho Evra)—are close behind. The remaining methods—condoms, the sponge, diaphragm, cervical cap, spermicides,

and periodic abstinence—must be used in a near-perfect fashion to afford any reasonable level of protection.

When safety is factored into the selection equation, several guidelines apply. Combination OCs should be avoided by women with certain cardiovascular disorders (see later) as well as by women older than 35 years who smoke. For women in these categories, an alternative method (e.g., diaphragm, progestin-only pill, or IUD) is preferable. Although OCs are effective and relatively convenient, they can also cause significant side effects. Accordingly, women who consider the benefit/risk ratio unfavorable should be advised about alternative contraceptive techniques.

Personal preference is a major factor in providing the motivation needed for consistent implementation of a birth control method. Because even the best form of contraception will be less effective if improperly practiced, the importance of personal preference cannot be overemphasized. Practitioners should take pains to educate patients about the contraceptive methods available so that selection and use can be based on understanding.

Additional factors that bear on selecting a birth control method include family planning goals, age, frequency of sexual intercourse, and the individual's capacity for adherence. If family planning goals have already been met, sterilization of either the male or female partner may be desirable. For women who engage in coitus frequently, OCs or a long-term method (e.g., Nexplanon, Depo-Provera, IUD) are reasonable choices. Conversely, when sexual activity is limited, use of a spermicide, condom, or diaphragm may be more appropriate. Because barrier methods combined with spermicides can offer some protection against STDs (as well as providing contraception), these combinations may be of special benefit to individuals who have multiple partners. If adherence is a problem (as it can be with OCs, condoms, and diaphragms), use of a long-term method (e.g., vaginal contraceptive ring, IUD, Nexplanon, Depo-Provera) can confer more reliable protection.

To help women select the birth control method that suits them best, Planned Parenthood has created a step-by-step computerized selection tool that is accessible online at https://tools.plannedparenthood.org/bc/birth_control_quiz. This tool accounts for all of the factors noted previously.

ORAL CONTRACEPTIVES

There are two main categories of OCs: (1) those that contain an estrogen *plus* a progestin, known as *combination OCs,* and (2) those that contain just a progestin, known as "minipills" or *progestin-only OCs*. Of the two groups, combination OCs are by far the more widely used.

Combination Oral Contraceptives

Since their introduction in the late 1950s, combination OCs have become one of the most widely prescribed families of drugs. These drugs are both safe and effective, although minor side effects are common.

TABLE 51.1 Effectiveness of Birth Control Methods

Birth Control Method	FAILURE RATE[a] (%)	
	Actual Use[b]	Theoretical Use[c]
No method	85	85
Extremely Effective		
Etonogestrel subdermal implant (Nexplanon)	0.05	0.05
Surgical sterilization		
Female: tubal ligation	0.5	0.5
Male: vasectomy	0.15	0.1
Intrauterine devices		
Copper T 380A (ParaGard)	0.8	0.6
Levonorgestrel T (Mirena)	0.2	0.2
Very Effective		
Oral contraceptives		
Combination pills	8	0.3
Progestin-only pills	8	0.3
Intramuscular medroxyprogesterone acetate (Depo-Provera)	3	0.3
Vaginal contraceptive ring (NuvaRing)	8	0.3
Contraceptive patch (Ortho Evra)	8	0.3
Effective		
Condoms		
Male	15	2
Female (FC2 Female Condom)	21	5
Diaphragm with spermicide	16	6
Least Effective		
Contraceptive sponge (Today Sponge)		
Parous	32	20
Nulliparous	16	9
Spermicide alone	29	18
Periodic abstinence	25	3–5
Withdrawal	27	4

[a]Failure rate: percentage of women who have an unplanned pregnancy during the first year of use.
[b]Actual use: failure rate usually observed in actual practice.
[c]Theoretical use: failure rate that would be expected if the birth control method were practiced exactly as it should be.

PROTOTYPE DRUGS

Drugs for Birth Control

Combination Oral Contraceptive
Ethinyl estradiol/norethindrone

Progestin-Only Oral Contraceptive
Norethindrone

Long-Acting Contraceptives
Subdermal etonogestrel implant (Nexplanon)
Depot medroxyprogesterone acetate (Depo-Provera)

Drugs for Emergency Contraception
Levonorgestrel alone (Plan B One-Step)
Ulipristal acetate (ella)

TABLE 51.2 Progestins Used in Combination Oral Contraceptives

Progestins	Comments
First Generation Ethynodiol diacetate Norethindrone	• Lower risk for thrombosis than with other progestins • Mildly androgenic
Second Generation Levonorgestrel Norgestrel	• Greater risk for thrombosis than with FGPs • More androgenic than FGPs • Prolonged half-life
Third Generation Desogestrel Norgestimate	• Greater risk for thrombosis than with FGPs (especially desogestrel) • Less androgenic than FGPs
Fourth Generation Dienogest Drospirenone	For drospirenone *and* dienogest: • Greater risk for thrombosis than with other progestins (especially drospirenone) • Less androgenic than FGPs • Low risk for acne and hirsutism For drospirenone only: • Risk for hyperkalemia

FGPs, First-generation progestins.

Mechanism of Action

Combination OCs reduce fertility primarily by *inhibiting ovulation*. The estrogen in combination OCs suppresses release of follicle-stimulating hormone from the pituitary (and thereby inhibits follicular maturation), and progestin in combination OCs acts in the hypothalamus and pituitary to suppress the midcycle luteinizing hormone surge, which normally triggers ovulation. Secondary mechanisms include thickening of the cervical mucus (creating a barrier to the penetration of sperm) and alteration of the endometrium, making it less hospitable for implantation.

Components

Estrogens. Only three estrogens are employed: *ethinyl estradiol, mestranol,* and *estradiol valerate.* Most combination OCs use ethinyl estradiol. A few older products use mestranol, which undergoes conversion to ethinyl estradiol in the body. One new product—*Natazia*—uses estradiol valerate, which undergoes conversion to estradiol in the body.

Progestins. Combination OCs employ eight different progestins that can be grouped into four generations (Table 51.2). Progestins in all four generations are equally effective. Differences relate to side effects, especially thrombotic events, androgenic effects (acne, hirsutism, dyslipidemia), and hyperkalemia.

Effectiveness

As shown in Table 51.1, OCs can be very effective. With perfect use, the failure rate is only 0.3%. However, with typical use, the failure rate is significantly higher: about 8%. Among women of higher weight, efficacy is somewhat reduced. Possible reasons include decreased blood levels of the hormones, sequestration in adipose tissue, and altered metabolism. However, even though the efficacy of OCs is slightly reduced in higher-weight women, these drugs are still more reliable than most of the alternatives.

Overall Safety

Determining the relative safety of combination OCs is complex. Part of the difficulty lies with the fact that much of our information on the adverse effects of OCs was gathered when these agents were employed in higher doses than are used today. Newer data show that today's OCs as currently prescribed are considerably safer than indicated by older studies. An additional complication stems from the fact that the risk for mortality associated with OCs is much smaller than the risk associated with pregnancy and delivery. Keeping the previous provisos in mind, we can make the following observations on OC safety: Of the contraceptive methods available, OCs produce the broadest spectrum of adverse effects, ranging from nausea to menstrual irregularity to rare thromboembolic disorders. However, despite their wide variety of undesired actions, OCs when used by healthy women produce no greater mortality than any other form of birth control.

Adverse Effects

Combination OCs can cause a variety of adverse effects. However, although many types of effects may occur, severe effects are rare. Hence, compared with the serious risks associated with pregnancy and childbirth, the risks of OCs are low. Nonetheless, because OCs are usually taken by women who are healthy and OCs represent a potential health hazard (albeit small), we must take steps to minimize risk. To this end a full medical history should be obtained. If the history reveals an *absolute* contraindication to OC use (Table 51.3), OCs should not be prescribed. In women with *relative* contraindications, OCs should be used with caution. Current consensus by the World Health Organization and the American College of Obstetrics and Gynecology suggest that birth control can be safely prescribed after a thorough medical history and blood pressure is taken. A full examination with pelvic exam is not needed to prescribe OCs. Some states in the United States are allowing pharmacists to prescribe OCs, thus eliminating the need for a healthcare visit.

Thromboembolic disorders. Combination OCs have been associated with an increased risk for venous thromboembolism (VTE), arterial thromboembolism, pulmonary embolism, myocardial infarction (MI), and thrombotic stroke. Among OC users, the *relative* risk for a thrombotic event is two to three times the risk in nonusers. However, the *absolute*

risk is still very small: about 8 to 10 events per 10,000 woman-years of OC use. Furthermore, the risk for thrombosis associated with OCs is considerably lower than the risk associated with pregnancy and delivery. OCs promote thrombosis in part by raising levels of clotting factors. Thrombosis is not due to atherosclerosis.

Until the mid-1990s, it was believed that thrombotic events were caused solely by the estrogen in combination OCs. However, it is now clear that the progestin can contribute too. Two progestins—*drospirenone* and *desogestrel*—appear to carry the greatest risk.

Fortunately the risk for thrombotic events with OCs used today is much lower than that with the OCs used in the past because the amount of estrogen in OCs has been reduced. When combination OCs first became available, they contained high doses of estrogens (e.g., 100 µg of ethinyl estradiol). Today's OCs contain no more than 50 µg of ethinyl estradiol (and usually less), so the risk for thromboembolism is quite low.

Major factors that increase the risk for thromboembolism are *heavy smoking, a history of thromboembolism,* and *thrombophilias*. Additional risk factors include diabetes, hypertension, cerebrovascular disease, coronary artery disease, and surgery, where immobilization increases the risk for postoperative thrombosis.

In the past OCs were not recommended for women above 35 years of age because earlier studies indicated an increase in the risk for MI for this group. However, reanalysis has shown that the risk was limited to older women who smoked. With today's low-estrogen OCs, nonsmokers may continue use OCs until menopause with no greater risk for MI than among younger women.

Several measures can help minimize thromboembolic phenomena:
- The estrogen dose in OCs should be no greater than required for contraceptive efficacy.
- OCs containing drospirenone or desogestrel should generally be avoided because they may pose a higher risk for developing VTE.
- OCs should not be prescribed for heavy smokers, women with a history of thromboembolism, or those with other risk factors for thrombosis.
- OCs should be discontinued at least 4 weeks before surgery in which postoperative thrombosis might be expected.

PATIENT EDUCATION
Thrombosis and Thromboembolism

Women should be informed about the symptoms of thrombosis and thromboembolism (e.g., leg tenderness or pain, sudden chest pain, shortness of breath, severe headache, sudden visual disturbance) and instructed to consult the prescriber if these occur.

What about the cardiovascular risk for *former* OC users? Data from the Women's Health Initiative suggest that use of OCs in the past may *protect* against cardiovascular disease. Among women with a history of OC use, there was an 8% decrease in the overall incidence of cardiovascular disease, including a reduced risk for angina, MI, peripheral vascular disease, transient ischemic attacks, and elevation of cholesterol.

Women with a history of thrombosis should avoid estrogen/progestin products but can still use a progestin-only method. Options include the levonorgestrel intrauterine system (Mirena), medroxyprogesterone acetate injection (Depo-Provera), the etonogestrel subdermal implant (Nexplanon), and the "minipill"—all of which are discussed later.

► BLACK BOX WARNING
Oral Contraceptive Pills

Cigarette smoking increases the risk of serious cardiovascular side effects from combination oral contraceptive pills.

TABLE 51.3 Absolute and Relative Contraindications to the Use of Combination Oral Contraceptives

Absolute contraindications	Thrombophlebitis, thromboembolic disorders, cerebral vascular disease, coronary occlusion, *or* a past history of these conditions, *or* a condition that predisposes to these disorders
	Abnormal liver function
	Known or suspected breast cancer
	Undiagnosed abnormal vaginal bleeding
	Known or suspected pregnancy
	Smokers older than 35 years
Relative contraindications	Hypertension
	Cardiac disease
	Diabetes
	History of cholestatic jaundice of pregnancy
	Gallbladder disease
	Uterine leiomyoma
	Epilepsy
	Migraine

Cancer. OCs present no known risk for cancer—with the important exception of promoting (not causing) breast cancer growth. The effects of OCs on cancers of the ovaries, endometrium, cervix, and breast have been studied extensively. Effects on three of these cancers are clear: OCs *protect* against ovarian and endometrial cancer and have *no effect* (positive or negative) on cervical cancer, which is caused by human papillomaviruses.

What about breast cancer? Until a decade ago the question was unresolved—some studies found a link between OC use and breast cancer, others did not. A recent study of 1.8 million women in Denmark, published in the *New England Journal of Medicine* in 2017, concluded that women who used hormonal contraceptives did have an increased risk over those who never used hormonal therapy, but the overall increase in risk was small. It was also noted that the longer the duration of use, the higher the risk. Although in this study the use of hormonal contraception increased the risk for breast cancer slightly, the individual patient must always be taken into account. Risk is also affected by the patient's age, personal risk of cancer, and overall health.

Another large study showed that OCs *do* increase risk for *some* women, specifically women who have the *BRCA1* gene mutation. Even without taking OCs, these women have a very high—50% to 80%—lifetime risk for breast cancer. OCs increase this risk by one-third. The same study found that OCs do *not* increase risk in women with the *BRCA2* mutation.

It is important to note that, although OCs do not *cause* breast cancer, estrogens can promote the growth of *existing* breast carcinoma. Accordingly, women with this disease should not take OCs.

Hypertension. Combination OCs can cause hypertension, but the risk with today's low-estrogen preparations is very low. OCs raise blood pressure by increasing blood levels of two compounds: angiotensin and aldosterone. If hypertension develops and OCs are determined to be the cause, two options are open: (1) discontinue the OC or (2) continue the OC and manage the hypertension with drugs.

Abnormal uterine bleeding. By altering the endometrium, OCs may decrease or eliminate menstrual flow. In addition, breakthrough bleeding and spotting may occur, especially with the use of extended-cycle OCs (e.g., Seasonique, Seasonale). Spotting and bleeding can also occur with monthly cycle OCs, most often during the first 3 months when low-estrogen OCs are used. If a woman misses her period while taking monthly cycle OCs, the possibility of pregnancy should be assessed. After discontinuation of OCs, normal menstruation usually resumes, although the first period may be delayed. Women with a pretreatment history of irregular menses will return to their previous pattern when OCs are discontinued.

Use in pregnancy and lactation. OCs have no therapeutic role during pregnancy and hence are *contraindicated for use by pregnant women.* Pregnancy should be ruled out before starting OC use; if pregnancy should occur despite OC use, use should stop immediately. Woman should be assured, however, that inadvertent use of OCs during early pregnancy poses no risk for fetal harm.

Combination OCs enter breast milk and reduce milk production, especially in the early stages of lactation. In contrast, progestin-only OCs have little or no effect on milk production and hence are preferred for contraception during lactation, at least early on. (Later, when the milk supply is well established and especially with the addition of solids to the infant's diet, use of combination OCs may resume.)

Stroke in women with migraine. When used by women who experience migraine headaches, OCs may increase the risk for thrombotic stroke. However, the absolute increase is low: only 8 cases per 100,000 women at age 20 years, rising to 80 cases per 100,000 women at age 40 years. Because the risk is low, OCs are generally considered safe for women with migraine provided that they are younger than 35 years, do not smoke, and are healthy, and provided their headaches are not preceded by a visual change known as an aura (migraine with aura has a greater risk for stroke than migraine without aura). Migraine and its management are discussed in Chapter 25.

Effects related to estrogen or progestin imbalance. Many of the mild side effects of combination OCs result from an excess or deficiency of estrogen or progestin. Effects that can result from an excess of estrogen include nausea, breast tenderness, and edema. Progestin excess can increase appetite and cause fatigue and depression. A deficiency in either hormone can cause menstrual irregularities. Side effects related to hormonal imbalance are shown in Table 51.4.

Quite often these effects can be reduced by adjusting the estrogen/progestin balance of an OC regimen. With most women, therapy is initiated with an OC containing 30 to 35 µg of ethinyl estradiol. If significant nausea occurs, it can be managed by dosing at bedtime or, if needed, switching to an OC with less estrogen. Using less estrogen can also reduce breast discomfort. During the first 3 months of use, spotting and breakthrough bleeding are common and usually resolve on their own. If they do not, they can be managed by increasing the estrogen dosage or using a product that contains a different progestin.

TABLE 51.4 **Side Effects Caused by an Excess of or Deficiency in the Estrogen or Progestin Content of an Oral Contraceptive Regimen**

ESTROGEN		PROGESTIN	
Excess	**Deficiency**	**Excess**	**Deficiency**
Nausea	Early or midcycle breakthrough bleeding	Increased appetite	Late breakthrough bleeding
Breast tenderness		Weight gain	Amenorrhea
Edema	Increased spotting	Depression	Hypermenorrhea
Bloating	Hypomenorrhea	Tiredness	
Hypertension		Fatigue	
Migraine		Hypomenorrhea	
Cervical mucorrhea		Breast regression	
Polyposis		Monilial vaginitis	
		Acne, oily scalp[a]	
		Hair loss[a]	
		Hirsutism[a]	

[a]Caused by progestins that have strong androgenic activity.

For women who experience androgenic effects (e.g., acne, hirsutism), switching to an OC that has drospirenone or dienogest can help. Other side effects can be reduced by making similar adjustments. When one combination OC is being substituted for another, the change is best made at the beginning of a new cycle.

Glucose intolerance. OCs can elevate blood glucose levels. This diabetogenic effect is caused by the progestin in OCs. Glucose intolerance is most likely in patients who are already diabetic or have experienced gestational diabetes. Because hypoglycemic agents (e.g., insulin) can control glucose elevations induced by OCs, the presence of diabetes does not preclude OC use. Prediabetic women should be monitored for the development of hyperglycemia. Glucose intolerance may be less likely to occur with OCs that contain desogestrel or norgestimate.

Noncontraceptive Benefits of Oral Contraceptives

OCs decrease the risk for several disorders, including ovarian cancer, endometrial cancer, ovarian cysts, pelvic inflammatory disease (PID), benign breast disease, iron deficiency anemia, and acne. In addition, OCs favorably affect menstrual symptoms: cramps are reduced, menstrual flow is reduced in volume and duration, and menses are more predictable. In women with premenstrual disorder or premenstrual dysphoric disorder, OCs can reduce symptom intensity. In some women with menstrual-associated migraine, OCs can reduce migraine frequency. Surprisingly, OCs may even benefit women with rheumatoid arthritis.

Drug Interactions

Drugs and herbs that reduce the effects of oral contraceptives. Products that induce hepatic cytochrome P3A4 can accelerate OC metabolism and thereby reduce OC effects. See Chapter 4 for a list of common drugs that induce CYP450 enzyme families. Women taking OCs in combination with any of these agents should be alert for indications of reduced OC blood levels, such as breakthrough bleeding or spotting. If these signs appear, it may be necessary to either (1) increase the estrogen dosage of the OC, (2) combine the OC with a second form of birth control (e.g., condom), or (3) switch to an alternative form of birth control.

Drugs whose effects are reduced by oral contraceptives. OCs can decrease the benefits of warfarin and hypoglycemic agents. By increasing levels of clotting factors, OCs can decrease the effectiveness of *warfarin*, an anticoagulant. By increasing levels of glucose, OCs can counteract the benefits of insulin and other hypoglycemic agents used in diabetes. Accordingly, when combined with OCs, warfarin and hypoglycemic agents may require increased dosage.

Drugs whose effects are increased by oral contraceptives. OCs can impair the hepatic metabolism of several agents, including *theophylline, tricyclic antidepressants, diazepam,* and *chlordiazepoxide.* Because of reduced clearance, these drugs may accumulate to toxic levels. If signs of toxicity appear, the dosages of these drugs should be reduced.

Preparations

Nearly all the combination OCs in current use contain the same estrogen: ethinyl estradiol. In contrast, eight different progestins are employed. The OCs with low estrogen are safer. As a rule, high-estrogen OCs are reserved for women taking drugs that induce P450. Usual dosing combinations are provided in Table 51.5. Products with unique properties are discussed next.

Levomefolate. In addition to an estrogen and a progestin, Beyaz, Safyral, Tydemy, and YAZ Plus (maple leaf after YAZ Plus) all contain levomefolate, a metabolite of folic acid. The purpose is to reduce the risk for fetal neural tube defects—anencephaly and spina bifida—if

TABLE 51.5 Common Combinations of Oral Contraceptives[a]

Regimen	Estrogen	μg	Progestin	mg
28-Day Cycle				
Monophasic				
	Ethinyl estradiol	20	Norethindrone	1
			Levonorgestrel	0.8
			Drospirenone	3
	Ethinyl estradiol	30	Levonorgestrel	0.15
			Norethindrone	1.5
			Desogestrel	0.15
			Drospirenone	3
	Ethinyl estradiol	35	Norethindrone	0.4
				0.5
				1
			Norgestimate	0.25
Biphasic	Ethinyl estradiol	20 (Phase 1)	Desogestrel	0.15 (Phase 1)
		10 (Phase 2)		0 (Phase 2)
Triphasic	Ethinyl estradiol	35	Norgestimate	0.18 (Phase 1)
				0.215 (Phase 2)
				0.25 (Phase 3)
Extended Cycle	Ethinyl estradiol	30	Levonorgestrel	0.15

[a]This list contains the most common combinations; thus it is not all-inclusive.

pregnancy should occur despite contraceptive use. As discussed in Chapter 67, neural tube defects can result if folic acid is low early in pregnancy.

Natazia. Natazia has two unique components: estradiol valerate and dienogest, a fourth-generation progestin. Estradiol valerate is a prodrug that undergoes rapid conversion to estradiol, the predominant endogenous estrogen. Dienogest, which is much like drospirenone (see previous discussion under "Components"), has strong progestational activity and antiandrogenic activity. However, in contrast to drospirenone, dienogest does not cause potassium retention; hence there is no need to monitor potassium levels. Unlike all other combination OCs, Natazia employs a four-phase dosing schedule in which the amount of estradiol decreases over the monthly cycle and the amount of progestin (dienogest) increases. Because of this schedule, the duration of withdrawal bleeding is shorter than that with other combination OCs and the intensity of bleeding is lighter. In women who normally experience heavy or prolonged menstrual bleeding, Natazia can reduce blood loss.

Dosing Schedules

With only one exception, combination OCs are dosed in a *cyclic pattern.* For most products, each cycle is *28 days long.* However, with a few newer products, the cycle is either *extended* (to 91 days) or *continuous* (Amethyst).

28-day-cycle schedules. The 28-day regimens are subdivided into four groups: *monophasic, biphasic, triphasic,* and *quadriphasic (four-phasic)* (see Table 51.5). In a monophasic regimen, the daily doses of estrogen and progestin remain constant throughout the cycle of use. In the other regimens, the estrogen, progestin, or both change as the cycle progresses. The biphasic, triphasic, and quadriphasic schedules reflect efforts to more closely simulate ovarian production of estrogens and progestins. However, these preparations appear to offer little or no advantage over monophasic OCs.

Most 28-day cycle products are taken in a repeating sequence consisting of 21 days of an active pill followed by 7 days on which either (1) no pill is taken, (2) an inert pill is taken, or (3) an iron-containing pill is taken. The sequence is begun on either the first day of the menstrual cycle or the first Sunday after the onset of menses. With the first option, protection is conferred immediately; hence no backup contraception is needed. With a Sunday start, which is done to have menses occur on weekdays rather than the weekend, protection may not be immediate; hence an alternate form of birth control should be used during the first 7 days of the pill pack. With both options, each dose should be taken at the same time every day (e.g., with a meal or at bedtime). Successive dosing cycles should commence every 28 days even if there is breakthrough bleeding or spotting.

Extended-cycle and continuous schedules. Many health care providers recommend taking combination OCs for an extended time rather than following the traditional 28-day cycle because doing so decreases episodes of withdrawal bleeding, with the associated menstrual pain, premenstrual symptoms, headaches, and other problems. Prolonged use of OCs is possible because these drugs suppress endometrial thickening, hence monthly bleeding is not required to slough off hypertrophied tissue. At this time, 14 products are packaged and marketed for prolonged use.

It is important to note that there is nothing special about the estrogen/progestin combinations used in these extended-cycle products. In other words, we could get the same results with other combination OCs provided that they are *monophasic*. To achieve an extended schedule, the user would simply purchase four packets of a 28-day product (each of which contains 21 active pills) and then take the active pills for 84 days straight.

What to Do If Doses Are Missed

The chances of ovulation (and hence pregnancy) from missing one OC dose are small. However, the risk for pregnancy becomes progressively greater with each successive omission.

For products that use a *28-day cycle*, the following recommendations from the Centers for Disease Control apply:

- If *one or more pills* are missed in the *first week*, take one pill as soon as possible and then continue with the pack. Use an additional form of contraception for 7 days.
- If *one or two pills* are missed during the *second or third week*, take one pill as soon as possible and then continue with the *active* pills in the pack but skip the placebo pills and go straight to a new pack once all the active pills have been taken.
- If *three or more pills* are missed during the *second or third week*, follow the same instructions given for missing one or two pills but use an additional form of contraception for 7 days.

Important note: the response to a missed dose of Natazia, as described in the package insert, is more complex than that with other combination OCs.

For combination OCs that use an *extended or continuous cycle*, up to 7 days can be missed with little or no increased risk for pregnancy provided that the pills had been taken *continuously for the prior 3 weeks*.

It should be noted that although these are general guidelines for missed doses, suggestions for individual drugs may differ. Providers can refer to package inserts if there is concern for variation in information. For additional information, visit https://www.cdc.gov/reproductivehealth/contraception/mmwr/spr/combined.html#Fig2

Progestin-Only Oral Contraceptives

Progestin-only OCs, also known as "minipills," contain a progestin but no estrogen. Because they lack estrogen, minipills do not cause thromboembolic disorders, headaches, nausea, or most of the other adverse effects associated with combination OCs. Unfortunately, although slightly safer than combination OCs, the progestin-only preparations are less effective and are more likely to cause irregular bleeding (breakthrough bleeding, spotting, amenorrhea, inconsistent cycle length, variations in the volume and duration of monthly flow). Irregular bleeding is the major drawback of these products and the principal reason that women discontinue them.

Contraceptive effects of the minipill result largely from altering cervical secretions. Under the influence of progestins, cervical glands produce a thick, sticky mucus that acts as a barrier to penetration by sperm. Progestins also modify the endometrium, making it less favorable for implantation. Compared with combination OCs, minipills are weak inhibitors of ovulation; hence this mechanism contributes little to their effects. For these reasons, taking the pill at the same time every day is important to their effectiveness. Taking a pill even 3 hours late can reduce their efficacy and use of back up protection or emergency contraception is recommended if unprotected sexual intercourse occurred. Unlike combination OCs, whose administration is cyclic, progestin-only OCs are taken continuously. Use is initiated on day 1 of the menstrual cycle, and one pill is taken daily thereafter. A backup contraceptive method should be used for the first 7 days.

If one or more doses is missed or taken greater than 3 hours after the scheduled dose, the following guidelines apply: If one pill is missed, it should be taken as soon as remembered and backup contraception should be used for at least 2 days. The pills should be resumed as scheduled on the next day. If two pills are missed, the regimen should be restarted and backup contraception should be used for at least 2 days. In addition, if two or more pills are missed and no menstrual bleeding occurs, a pregnancy test should be done.

COMBINATION CONTRACEPTIVES WITH NOVEL DELIVERY SYSTEMS

Two combination contraceptives—*a transdermal patch* and a *vaginal ring*—have the same mechanism as combination OCs but they deliver hormones in novel ways. Like combination OCs, both of these contraceptives contain two hormones—an estrogen and a progestin—that undergo absorption into the systemic circulation and then prevent pregnancy primarily by suppressing ovulation. What is different is how the hormones are delivered: with the patch, the hormones are absorbed through the skin, and with the vaginal ring, the hormones are absorbed through the vaginal mucosa. Otherwise the pharmacology of these contraceptives is essentially identical to that of combination OCs.

Transdermal Contraceptive Patch

The Xulane transdermal contraceptive patch has the same mechanism as combination OCs. Furthermore, the patch has the same contraceptive efficacy and the same incidence of breakthrough bleeding and spotting. The principal difference between them lies with their dosing schedules: whereas combination OCs must be taken every day, the patch is applied just once a week. As a result, the patch is more convenient than OCs and adherence is better.

The Xulane patch contains 0.53 mg of µg of ethinyl estradiol (the estrogen found in most combination OCs) and 4.86 mg of norelgestromin (the active metabolite of norgestimate, a progestin found in some OCs). Each day the patch releases 35 µg of ethinyl estradiol and 150 µg of norelgestromin. After release, these hormones penetrate the skin, enter capillaries, and undergo distribution throughout the body. Plasma levels plateau 2 days after the first patch is applied.

For women not currently using OCs, the first patch should be applied during the first 24 hours of the menstrual period. For women switching from OCs, the first patch should be applied on the first day of withdrawal bleeding.

In clinical trials, 4.6% of patches became partially or completely detached. When this occurs, the patch should be reattached or replaced. If the patch has been off less than 24 hours, backup contraception is unnecessary. However, if the patch has been off more than 24 hours, a new cycle should be started, accompanied by backup contraception during the first 7 days.

The most common adverse effects are breast discomfort, headache, local irritation, nausea, and menstrual cramps. Compared with Triphasil (a combination OC), the patch produces a higher incidence of breast discomfort and dysmenorrhea. Contraindications and drug interactions are the same as for combination OCs.

Does the patch cause more VTE than OCs do? Possibly. Three epidemiologic studies have examined the question. In two of the studies, the risk for VTE in women using the patch was double the risk in women using combination OCs. However, there was no difference in risk in the third study. Of note, women who use the patch are exposed to 60% more estrogen than those who use an OC containing 35 µg of estrogen. The higher estrogen exposure may increase the risk for VTE.

Vaginal Contraceptive Ring

NuvaRing is a hormonal contraceptive device designed for vaginal insertion. Like combination OCs, the ring contains an estrogen/progestin combination that prevents pregnancy largely by suppressing ovulation. Adverse effects, drug interactions, warnings, and contraindications for the ring are the same as for combination OCs. The ring is made of transparent, flexible material and looks like a very skinny doughnut, with an overall diameter of 2.1 in and a cross-sectional diameter of 1/8 in. Insertion is done by the user.

The NuvaRing contains 2.7 mg of ethinyl estradiol and 11.7 mg of etonogestrel (the active metabolite of desogestrel, a progestin found in some OCs). Each day, the ring releases 15 µg of ethinyl estradiol and 120 µg of etonogestrel. After release, the hormones penetrate the vaginal mucosa, undergo absorption into the blood, and then distribute throughout the body. Contraception results from systemic effects, not from local effects in the vagina.

One ring is inserted once each month, left in place for 3 weeks, and then removed; a new ring is inserted 1 week later. During the ring-free week, withdrawal bleeding occurs. The new ring should be inserted on schedule even if bleeding is still ongoing. If a ring is expelled before 3 weeks have passed, it can be washed off in warm water (not hot water) and reinserted. If the expelled ring cannot be reused, a new one should be inserted. If more than 3 hours elapse between ring expulsion and reinsertion, contraceptive effects may be diminished; hence backup contraception should be used for 7 days.

The most common adverse effects are vaginitis, headaches, upper respiratory infection, leukorrhea, sinusitis, weight gain, and nausea. Common reasons for discontinuing the ring include a foreign body sensations, coital problems, ring expulsion, vaginal symptoms, headache, and emotional lability. The risk for serious adverse effects—thrombosis, embolism, and hypertension—is the same as that with combination OCs.

LONG-ACTING CONTRACEPTIVES

Subdermal Etonogestrel Implants

A subdermal system (Nexplanon) for delivery of etonogestrel is available for long-term reversible contraception. As shown in Table 51.1, Nexplanon is among the most effective contraceptives available.

Description

Nexplanon consists of a single 4-cm rod that contains 68 mg of etonogestrel, a synthetic progestin. The rod is implanted subdermally in the groove between the biceps and triceps in the nondominant arm.

Etonogestrel then diffuses slowly and continuously, providing blood levels sufficient for contraception for 3 years, after which the rod is removed. If continued contraception is desired, a new rod is implanted. While currently FDA approved for 3 years, recent studies have shown that Nexplanon continues to be effective for up to 5 years post insertion.

Mechanism of Action

Etonogestrel suppresses ovulation and thickens cervical mucus. In addition, it causes the endometrium to become involuted and hence hostile to implantation.

Pharmacokinetics

Daily release of etonogestrel is 60 to 70 µg initially; it then gradually declines to 25 to 30 µg over 3 years. Absorbed drug is slowly metabolized by the liver. When the rod is removed, etonogestrel becomes undetectable within 5 to 7 days.

Drug Interactions

Agents that induce hepatic enzymes—such as barbiturates, phenytoin, rifampin, carbamazepine, topiramate, HIV protease inhibitors, and St. John's wort—may reduce the efficacy of Nexplanon. Accordingly, Nexplanon should not be used by women taking these drugs.

Adverse Effect: Irregular Bleeding

In women using Nexplanon, bleeding episodes are irregular and unpredictable. In clinical trials, amenorrhea occurred in 22% of women; infrequent bleeding (less than three bleeding or spotting episodes in 90 days) occurred in 34% of women; frequent bleeding (more than five bleeding or spotting episodes in 90 days) occurred in 7% of women, and prolonged bleeding (more than 14 days of bleeding in 90 days) occurred in 18% of women. Despite effects on bleeding, levels of hemoglobin were unaffected over 3 years. The general pattern of irregular and unpredictable bleeding does not change while Nexplanon is being used. Bleeding irregularities are the leading reason for discontinuing the device.

Use During Breastfeeding

Nexplanon is safe to use during breastfeeding after the 21st postpartum day. Very little etonogestrel is excreted in breast milk. In a controlled clinical trial, there were no significant effects on the physical or psychomotor development of infants. Nexplanon also had no effect on the production or quality of milk, even when the rod was implanted just a few days postpartum.

Depot Medroxyprogesterone Acetate

Depot medroxyprogesterone acetate (DMPA) is given by injection intramuscularly or subcutaneously. It protects against pregnancy for 3 months or longer by inhibiting the secretion of gonadotropins. The drug thereby (1) inhibits follicular maturation and ovulation, (2) thickens the cervical mucus, and (3) causes thinning of the endometrium, making implantation unlikely. When injections are discontinued, return of fertility is delayed by an average of 9 months.

Most adverse effects are like those seen with other progestin-only contraceptives. Menstrual disturbances are common; menstruation may be irregular at first and then, after 6 to 12 months, may cease entirely. Mild weight gain (about 3.5 lb) is likely during the first year. Women may also experience abdominal bloating, headache, depression, and decreased libido. However, it is unclear that DMPA is the cause. Although DMPA has produced uterine and mammary cancers in animals, a large-scale study has shown no increase in the risk for cervical, ovarian, or breast cancer in women, and the risk for endometrial cancer is actually reduced.

DMPA poses a risk for reversible bone loss, but this risk does not outweigh the benefits of treatment. During the first 1 to 2 years of DMPA use, bone mineral density (BMD) declines rapidly, at a rate of 1% to 2% per year. After this time, however, the rate of bone loss slows. Importantly, when DMPA is discontinued, BMD returns to pretreatment levels, typically within 30 months. Whether DMPA-induced bone loss increases the risk for fractures is unclear. While this story was still evolving, the US Food and Drug Administration (FDA) revised the label for DMPA to include a black box warning that recommends against using the drug for more than 2 years. However, in the light of the data gathered, this warning appears unwarranted. Accordingly, in 2008, an American College of Obstetricians and Gynecologists committee counseled that practitioners should not let concerns about bone loss deter them from prescribing DMPA or cause them to limit prescriptions to 2 years. In addition, the committee recommended against routine testing of BMD in women on DMPA. When patients are being counseled about this issue, practitioners should point out that any risk for fracture with DMPA is theoretical, whereas the risks associated with pregnancy are very real.

Intrauterine Devices

IUDs are among the most reliable forms of reversible birth control (see Table 51.1). In addition, the IUDs available today are very safe when used by appropriate patients. Worldwide, more than 85 million women use these devices.

With proper counseling and patient selection, IUDs are very safe. Historically, due to the wicking ability of the old IUD strings, the increased risk of pelvic inflammatory disease related to IUD use was a concern. However, recent studies, clinical trials, and systematic reviews of the IUDs currently in use do not support this concern. Gonorrhea and chlamydia infection are associated with the risk of pelvic inflammatory disease, therefore, screening should be done prior to or at the point of insertion. Rates of pelvic inflammatory diseases are similar among women with and without an IUD. The risk for PID is highest during the first 20 days after insertion, with a rate of 9.7 cases per 1000 woman-years of use. One month after insertion, the risk declines to only 1.4 cases per 1000 woman-years of use.

IUDs can cause cramping and alteration of menses. Cramping is most intense upon IUD insertion and can be minimized by applying a topical anesthetic (2% lidocaine intracervical gel) or by premedicating with ibuprofen.

Two main classes of intrauterine devices are currently in use: a hormone-free copper IUD (TCu380A or Paragard) and a levonorgestrel containing IUD (various dosages exist). The TCu380A IUD causes a foreign body reaction and chemical changes which are toxic to sperm, thereby interfering with fertilization. The TCu380A is a great option for women who desire a highly effective form of birth control but are sensitive to hormones. Main side effects of the TCu380A include heavier menstrual bleeding and cramping. The TCu380A can be used for up to 10 years and likely longer.

The levonorgestrel containing IUDs work to prevent pregnancy by thickening cervical mucus, inhibition of ovulation, and alterations to the endometrium which prevents implantation. Main side effects include bleeding irregularities including spotting, irregular menstrual cycles, and oligomenorrhea/amenorrhea. The levonorgestrel containing IUDs can be used for 3 to 7 years depending on the dose form.

SPERMICIDES

Spermicides are chemical surfactants that kill sperm by destroying their cell membranes. These drugs are available in the form of a foam, gel, jelly, suppository, vaginal film, and contraceptive sponge. All formulations can be purchased without a prescription. When used alone, spermicides are only moderately effective (see Table 51.1). Combined use with a diaphragm or condom increases efficacy. As shown in Table 51.6, spermicidal preparations contain either nonoxynol 9 or octoxynol 9.

Spermicides are generally devoid of serious side effects. Studies show no relationship between spermicides and birth defects. However, there is some evidence that nonoxynol 9 may increase the risk for HIV transmission. The apparent mechanism is the promotion of vaginal, cervical, anal, and rectal lesions that facilitate HIV penetration to cells. Allergic reactions (to the drug or vehicle) occur in some women.

Correct use is required for contraceptive efficacy. The spermicide must be applied before intercourse but no more than 1 hour in advance (when used alone). Containers for foam preparations must be shaken thoroughly before each use to ensure dispersal of the spermicide. Suppositories should be inserted at least 10 to 15 minutes before intercourse to allow time for dissolution. Spermicides should be reapplied each time intercourse is anticipated. Douching should be postponed for at least 6 hours after coitus.

The contraceptive sponge (Today Sponge) is a soft, porous, polyurethane disk impregnated with 1000 mg of nonoxynol 9. When inserted to cover the cervix, it protects against conception by (1) releasing spermicide, (2) absorbing seminal fluid, and (3) blocking penetration of sperm. Unlike other spermicide products, which must be reapplied before each act of intercourse, a single sponge is effective for 24 hours regardless of how often coitus takes place. After 24 hours, the sponge should be removed. The rates of unintended pregnancy with the sponge are high: 16% among typical nulliparous users and 32% among parous users. The most common adverse effects are vaginal irritation and dryness.

EMERGENCY CONTRACEPTION

Emergency contraception (EC) is defined as contraception that is implemented *after* intercourse. Women can use EC to prevent pregnancy after unprotected intercourse, which can result from sexual assault, contraceptive failure (e.g., broken condom), or other reasons. Safe and effective methods of EC have been available for decades. However, products marketed specifically for EC are relatively new.

EC can be accomplished in two basic ways: taking an *emergency contraceptive pill* (ECP), also known as a *morning-after pill;* or inserting a copper-T IUD. Taking an ECP is most common. Furthermore, of the three basic types of ECPs—progestin-only pills, ulipristal-containing pills, and estrogen/progestin pills—the progestin-only pills are used most widely.

TABLE 51.6	Spermicides	
Formulation	**Active Ingredient**	**Trade Name**
Foam	Nonoxynol 9 (12.5%)	Delfen Contraceptive
Jelly	Nonoxynol 9 (3%)	Gynol II Extra Strength Contraceptive[a]
Gel	Nonoxynol 9 (4%)	Conceptrol Disposable Contraceptive
	Nonoxynol 9 (3.5%)	Advantage 24[a]
	Nonoxynol 9 (2.2%)	K-Y Plus[a]
	Nonoxynol 9 (2%)	Shur Seal[a]
Suppository	Nonoxynol 9 (2.27%)	Encare
	Nonoxynol 9 (100 mg)	Semicid
Sponge	Nonoxynol 9 (1000 mg)	Today Sponge
Vaginal film	Nonoxynol 9 (28%)	VCF

[a]Intended for use only in combination with a vaginal diaphragm.

Progestin-Only Emergency Contraception Pills

Three progestin-only products are available: Plan B One-Step, Next Choice One Dose, and Next Choice. All three contain *levonorgestrel*. These products are packaged and marketed specifically for EC. This contrasts with the estrogen/progestin products, which are marketed as OCs but can be used off-label for EC.

Plan B One-Step and Next Choice One Dose

Plan B One-Step and Next Choice One Dose consist of a single high-dose (1.5-mg) tablet of levonorgestrel, a progestin found in many combination OCs. The package insert calls for taking the tablet within 72 hours of unprotected intercourse. However, although early implementation is best, Plan B One-Step, Next Choice One Dose, and other ECPs can still be effective when started up to 5 days after intercourse. Success is indicated by the onset of menstrual bleeding in about 21 days.

Plan B One-Step reduces the odds of pregnancy by 89% and Next Choice One Dose prevented 84% of expected pregnancies, which is better than it may seem. In the absence of these two medications, the pregnancy rate from a single act of unprotected intercourse is about 8% (i.e., 8 women in 100 would become pregnant). However, among women using Plan B One-Step or Next Choice One Dose, only 1 and 1.3 in 100 are likely to become pregnant—a reduction of 89% and 84%, respectively.

Plan B One-Step and Next Choice One Dose work primarily by delaying or stopping ovulation. Inhibition of fertilization may also contribute. Of note, levonorgestrel is *not* effective after fertilization has occurred.

The major side effects of Plan B One-Step are heavier menstrual bleeding, nausea, abdominal pain, headache, and dizziness. Nausea can be reduced by taking an antiemetic (e.g., prochlorperazine) 1 hour before dosing. Importantly, if pregnancy does occur, having used levonorgestrel will not increase the risk for major congenital malformations, pregnancy complications, or any other adverse pregnancy outcomes.

These drugs will not terminate an existing pregnancy and will not harm a fetus if present. Recall that pregnancy is defined as implantation of a fertilized egg. Because Plan B One-Step and Next Choice One Dose act before fertilization and implantation, they cannot be considered abortifacients.

Plan B One-Step and Next Choice One Dose are now available over the counter. No prescription is required.

Next Choice

Next Choice consists of two 0.75-mg tablets of levonorgestrel (one half the amount in a single Plan B One-Step or Next Choice One Dose tablet). According to the package insert, women should take 1 tablet within 72 hours of intercourse and a second tablet 12 hours later. However, taking both tablets at the same time is just as effective. (This is equivalent to taking one tablet of Plan B One-Step or Next Choice One Step.) As with Plan B One-Step and Next Choice One Dose, these ECPs can still be effective when started up to 5 days after intercourse but are most effective when taken earlier. Adverse effects are similar to those of Plan B One-Step and Next Choice One Dose. If vomiting occurs within 2 hours of dosing, a repeat dose may be required. Like Plan B One-Step, Next Choice can be obtained without a prescription.

Ulipristal Acetate Emergency Contraception Pill

Ulipristal acetate (ella) acts as an agonist-antagonist at receptors for progestin. Like levonorgestrel, ulipristal acetate prevents conception primarily by suppressing ovulation. Despite this similarity, ulipristal acetate and levonorgestrel differ in two important ways. First, ulipristal acetate remains highly effective when taken up to 5 days (120 hours) after intercourse, whereas levonorgestrel is most effective when taken within 3 days (72 hours) of intercourse. Second, whereas levonorgestrel (Plan B One-Step, Next Choice, Next Choice One Dose) is available without a prescription for women 15 years of age and older, ulipristal acetate (ella) requires a prescription for all women regardless of age. The dosage for ulipristal acetate is 1 tablet (30 mg) taken up to 5 days after unprotected intercourse. Principal adverse effects are headache, nausea, dysmenorrhea, and abdominal pain. If vomiting occurs within 3 hours of dosing, an additional dose may be required.

Estrogen/Progestin Emergency Contraception Pills (Yuzpe Regimen)

The *Yuzpe regimen*, first described in 1974 by Professor A. Alfred Yuzpe, consists of two doses of an OC that contains an estrogen (ethinyl estradiol) plus a progestin (levonorgestrel or norgestrel). The first dose should be taken within 72 hours of unprotected intercourse and the second dose 12 hours later. Pregnancy is prevented by interfering with ovulation, fertilization, and implantation. Similar to other ECPs, this regimen will not cause abortion. Compared with Plan B One-Step, this regimen is less effective (75% vs 89%) and causes more nausea (50% vs 13.3%) and vomiting (19% vs 6%). However, because other ECPs are more effective, better tolerated, and readily available, the Yuzpe regimen is used infrequently.

Mifepristone as an Emergency Contraception Pill

One drug—mifepristone (RU 486)—can prevent pregnancy *or* cause abortion, depending on when it is taken. If mifepristone is taken within 5 days of unprotected intercourse, it will prevent pregnancy from occurring and thus can be considered an ECP. However, if mifepristone is taken after this time, it may terminate a pregnancy that has already begun and thus can be considered an abortifacient. When used as an ECP, mifepristone is 100% effective. The drug is available in the United States but is not approved for use as an EC.

The Copper Intrauterine Device

Insertion of a *copper IUD* within 5 days of unprotected intercourse can prevent pregnancy in most women. The method is more than 99.9% effective, allowing less than 1 pregnancy for every 1000 IUD recipients. IUD insertion has the additional benefit of providing ongoing contraception for up to 10 years. Although using an IUD for EC is highly effective, the technique does have drawbacks: the IUD is expensive, not all women are candidates, and obtaining one quickly may be difficult.

DRUGS FOR MEDICAL ABORTION

Mifepristone (RU 486) With Misoprostol

Mifepristone (RU 486) (Mifeprex) is a synthetic steroid that blocks receptors for progesterone and glucocorticoids. In the United States the drug has one approved indication: termination of early intrauterine pregnancy; cotreatment with misoprostol is usually required. Investigational uses include breast cancer, ovarian cancer, meningiomas, Cushing syndrome, uterine fibroids, and endometriosis. In addition, mifepristone is the most effective drug known for EC, although it is not used routinely for this purpose.

Mifepristone, followed by misoprostol, is a safe and effective alternative to surgery for termination of early pregnancy. Together, these drugs terminate pregnancy in about 95% of women. Principal adverse effects are abdominal pain and vaginal bleeding, which are unavoidable aspects of abortion. There is also a small risk for infection. In contrast to surgical abortion, which is generally unavailable before 8 weeks of gestation, abortion with mifepristone is performed early—within 7 weeks of conception.

Mechanism of Action

Mifepristone acts through blockade of progesterone receptors. Although it also blocks receptors for glucocorticoids, this action does not contribute to abortion. In the pregnant uterus, the drug has three effects. First, blockade of progesterone receptors leads to decidual breakdown and detachment of the conceptus. Second, mifepristone promotes cervical softening and dilation. Third, mifepristone increases uterine production of prostaglandins and renders the myometrium more responsive to the contractile effects of these prostaglandins. All three effects lead to expulsion of the conceptus. If mifepristone alone fails to induce abortion, the patient is given 400 μg of oral misoprostol, a synthetic prostaglandin that reinforces the uterine contractions induced by mifepristone. The pharmacology of misoprostol is discussed separately later.

Adverse Effects

The most common side effects are bleeding, cramping, nausea, vomiting, diarrhea, and headache. The most serious adverse effects are severe bleeding and sepsis.

Successful abortion necessarily causes abdominal pain (cramping) and bleeding. Nearly all women experience these events. About 80% of patients experience transient cramping beginning 1 hour after taking misoprostol; most women require an opioid analgesic for relief. Bleeding and spotting typically last 9 to 16 days. However, in some women bleeding persists for 30 days or more. About 1% of women experience severe bleeding; treatment measures include curettage, uterotonic drugs (e.g., methylergonovine, ergonovine), and infusion of fluids, blood, or both.

Mifepristone/misoprostol has been associated with a few cases of serious bacterial infection, including very rare cases of fatal septic shock. Accordingly, patients and providers should be alert for typical signs of sepsis (sustained fever of 100.4°F or higher, severe abdominal pain, pelvic tenderness). However, in two confirmed cases of sepsis caused by *Clostridium sordellii*, these signs were absent. Instead, the patients presented with nausea, vomiting, and diarrhea but without fever or abdominal pain. In patients with typical or atypical presentation, the possibility of infection should be evaluated immediately.

The bleeding caused by mifepristone/misoprostol could mask bleeding due to a ruptured ectopic pregnancy. Accordingly, before mifepristone/ misoprostol is used, ectopic pregnancy must be ruled out. This is best done by a routine ultrasound examination.

Misoprostol (but not mifepristone), a proven teratogen, can cause Möbius syndrome, a rare fetal anomaly. Hence if the mifepristone/ misoprostol fails to induce abortion, performing surgical abortion should be considered.

Contraindications

Major contraindications to mifepristone/misoprostol are ectopic pregnancy, hemorrhagic disorders, or use of anticoagulant drugs. Because mifepristone blocks receptors for glucocorticoids, it should not be used in women with adrenal insufficiency and those on long-term glucocorticoid therapy.

SUMMARY OF KEY PRESCRIBING CONSIDERATIONS

Combination Oral Contraceptives

Therapeutic Goal: Prevention of unwanted pregnancy.

Baseline Data: Assess for history of hypertension, diabetes, thromboembolism, cerebrovascular or cardiovascular disease, breast cancer. Urine pregnancy test.

Monitoring: No routine monitoring required.

Identifying High-Risk Patients: Contraindications to use include current pregnancy, history of thromboembolus, breast cancer, and women over 35 years of age who continue to smoke tobacco. Use with caution in women with diabetes, hypertension, and cardiac disease.

Evaluating Therapeutic Effects: If combination oral contraceptives are being used for menstrual symptoms, it is important to evaluate for decrease in cramping, menstrual flow, or duration of menses.

Minimizing Adverse Effects: Educate patients on proper protocol for missed doses (depending on medication type and cycle). Effectiveness of oral contraceptives can be reduced with some medications, including certain common antibiotics.

52

Androgens

Androgen hormones are produced by the testes, ovaries, and adrenal cortex. The major endogenous androgen is testosterone. Androgens are noted most for their ability to promote expression of male sex characteristics. However, androgens also influence sexuality in females. In addition, androgens have significant physiologic and pharmacologic effects unrelated to sexual expression or function. The primary clinical application of the androgens is management of androgen deficiency in males. Principal adverse effects are virilization (development of male secondary sex characteristics) and hepatotoxicity.

TESTOSTERONE

Testosterone is the prototype of the androgen hormones. This compound is the principal endogenous androgen in both males and females. In addition to its physiologic role, testosterone is representative of the androgens employed clinically.

Biosynthesis and Secretion
Males

Testosterone is made by Leydig cells of the testes. Daily production in men ranges from 2.5 to 10 mg. Synthesis is promoted by two hormones of the anterior pituitary: follicle-stimulating hormone (FSH) and luteinizing hormone (LH), also known as interstitial cell–stimulating hormone. Production of testosterone is regulated by negative feedback control: rising plasma levels of testosterone act on the pituitary to suppress further release of FSH and LH, thereby decreasing the stimulus for further testosterone formation.

Some of the testosterone present in plasma is produced by the adrenal glands. However, androgenic activity of adrenal origin is much less than that of testicular origin. Hence, in males, adrenal androgens have minimal functional significance.

Testosterone production changes over time. Peak production occurs around age 17 years. Production then remains steady until age 30 or 40 years, after which it slowly declines. By the time a man reaches 80 years, testosterone production is only half what it was in his youth.

Females

In women, preandrogens (precursors of testosterone) are secreted by the adrenal cortex and ovaries. Conversion into testosterone takes place in peripheral tissues. Synthesis of preandrogens by the adrenal glands is regulated by adrenocorticotropic hormone, whereas synthesis of preandrogens by the ovaries is regulated by LH. Daily testosterone production is about 300 µg (150 µg from the ovaries and 150 µg from the adrenal glands). The total is 10 to 40 times less than the amount produced in men. In the event of ovarian or adrenocortical pathology (e.g., adenoma, carcinoma, hyperplasia), secretion of androgens can increase greatly and may be sufficient to produce virilization. At menopause, testosterone production decreases.

Mechanism of Action

Effects of testosterone on its target tissues are mediated by specific receptors located in the cell cytoplasm. After binding of testosterone to its receptor, the hormone-receptor complex migrates to the cell nucleus and then acts on DNA to promote synthesis of specific messenger RNA molecules. These, in turn, serve as templates for production of specific proteins, which then mediate testosterone effects. It should be noted that in some tissues—prostate, seminal vesicles, and hair follicles—androgen receptors do not interact with testosterone itself. Rather, they interact with dihydrotestosterone, a testosterone metabolite.

Physiologic and Pharmacologic Effects
Effects on Sex Characteristics in Males

Pubertal transformation. Increased production of testosterone promotes the transformations that signal puberty in males. Under the influence of testosterone, the testes enlarge, after which the penis and scrotum enlarge. Pubic and axillary hair appears, and hair on the trunk, arms, and legs assumes adult male patterns. Testosterone stimulates growth of bone and skeletal muscle, causing height and weight to increase rapidly. Testosterone also accelerates epiphyseal closure, causing bone growth to cease within a few years. The larynx enlarges, thereby deepening the voice. Sebaceous glands increase in number, causing the skin to become oily; acne results if the glands become clogged and infected. The final pubertal change is beard development. Several years are required for all of these changes to occur.

Spermatogenesis. Androgens are necessary for production of sperm by the seminiferous tubules and for maturation of sperm as they pass through the epididymis and vas deferens. Androgen deficiency causes sterility.

Effects on Sex Characteristics in Females

Under physiologic conditions, endogenous androgens have only moderate effects in females. Principal among these are promotion of clitoral growth and, perhaps, maintenance of normal libido. However, when production of androgens becomes excessive (e.g., in girls with congenital adrenal hyperplasia), virilization can take place. Virilization can also occur in response to therapeutic use of androgens or to androgen abuse.

Anabolic Effects

Testosterone promotes growth of skeletal muscle. This anabolic effect results from binding of androgens to the same type of receptor that mediates androgen actions in other tissues. Effects in young males and in females of any age can be dramatic. In contrast, effects in healthy adult males are modest. The testes of adult males already produce enough testosterone to cause near-maximal stimulation of the musculature; therefore the increment in muscle mass that can be achieved with exogenous androgens in adult males is relatively small.

Erythropoietic Effects

Testosterone promotes synthesis of erythropoietin, a hormone that acts on bone marrow to increase production of erythrocytes. This action of testosterone, together with the high levels of testosterone present in males, explains why men have a higher hematocrit than women. When women are given testosterone, the hematocrit rises and hemoglobin levels increase by an average of 4.3 g/dL. In contrast, because men have high testosterone levels to begin with, the increase in plasma hemoglobin that can be elicited with exogenous androgens is smaller—only 1 g/dL.

CLINICAL PHARMACOLOGY OF THE ANDROGENS

In addition to testosterone, a few other androgens are employed clinically. All of these agents can bind to androgen receptors, and therefore all can elicit similar responses. Major differences among individual androgens pertain to route of administration, pharmacokinetics, adverse effects, and specific applications.

Classification

The androgens used clinically fall into two basic groups: (1) testosterone and testosterone esters and (2) 17-α-alkylated compounds (noted for their hepatotoxicity). Androgens belonging to each group are shown in Table 52.1.

When one is speaking of testosterone-like compounds, it is traditional to distinguish between "androgens" and "anabolic steroids." However, we will not make this distinction because it is now clear that the receptor type that mediates the androgenic actions of the androgens is the same receptor type that mediates the anabolic actions of these hormones. Consequently it has not been possible to separate anabolic activity from androgenic activity: virtually all anabolic hormones are also androgenic. Accordingly, rather than creating two categories—androgens versus anabolic steroids—and assigning some agents to one category and some to the other, we will refer to all testosterone-like drugs as androgens.

Therapeutic Uses

In 2018, the US Food and Drug Administration (FDA) published a required label change for testosterone (see https://www.fda.gov/drugs/drugsafety/ucm436259.htm). The new labeling approves testosterone use only for those patients with confirmed testosterone deficiency due to hypogonadism. The FDA further emphasized that lowered testosterone due to aging did not meet the criteria for hypogonadism.

Also in 2018, the Endocrine Society published updated clinical guidelines for managing testosterone therapy. These are available at https://academic.oup.com/jcem/article/103/5/1715/4939465. Their algorithm to guide diagnosis of low testosterone due to hypogonadism is included in this article.

Individual androgens differ in their applications. No single androgen is employed for all uses discussed here. Specific applications of individual androgens are shown in Table 52.1.

Male Hypogonadism

Hypogonadism is a condition in which the testes fail to produce adequate amounts of testosterone. Male hypogonadism may be hereditary, or it may result from other causes, including pituitary failure, hypothalamic failure, and primary dysfunction of the testes.

Replacement Therapy

Androgen replacement therapy is beneficial when testicular failure occurs in adult males. Some studies demonstrate that treatment restores libido, increases ejaculate volume, and supports expression of secondary sex characteristics. However, treatment will not restore fertility. The principal drugs employed for testosterone replacement are testosterone itself and two testosterone esters: testosterone enanthate and testosterone cypionate. Preparations and dosages for replacement therapy are shown in Table 52.2.

Delayed Puberty

In some boys, puberty fails to occur at the usual age (i.e., before age 15 years). Most often, this failure reflects a familial pattern of delayed puberty and does not indicate pathology. Puberty can be expected to occur spontaneously but later than usual. Hence treatment is not an absolute necessity. However, some providers will prescribe a limited course of androgen therapy off label if the psychologic pressures of delayed sexual maturation are causing a boy significant distress. In these cases, a limited course of androgen therapy is indicated. Both fluoxymesterone (Androxy, Halotestin) and methyltestosterone (Methitest) are approved for this purpose.

If delayed puberty is the result of true hypogonadism, long-term replacement therapy is indicated (see later section titled Androgen Preparations for Male Hypogonadism).

Testosterone Therapy in Menopausal Women

Testosterone therapy can alleviate some menopausal symptoms, especially fatigue, reduced libido, and reduced genital sensitivity. The North American Menopause Society notes that testosterone can have a positive effect on sexual function and that women with no other identifiable

TABLE 52.1　Approved Uses of Individual Androgens

Androgen	Hypogonadism (Male)	Replacement Therapy (Male)	Delayed Puberty (Male)	Catabolic States
Testosterone and Testosterone Esters				
Testosterone	✓	✓		
Testosterone cypionate	✓	✓		
Testosterone enanthate	✓	✓		
17-α-Alkylated Androgens				
Fluoxymesterone	✓	✓	✓	
Methyltestosterone	✓	✓	✓	
Oxandrolone				✓

TABLE 52.2 Preparations and Dosages for Androgen Replacement Therapy in Hypogonadism

Drug	Preparation	Dosage	Considerations
Fluoxymesterone (Androxy, Halotestin)	Oral tablet: 2, 5, and 10 mg	5–20 mg once daily	These 17-α-alkylated androgens are hepatotoxic and androgenic effects are erratic.
Methyltestosterone (Methitest)	Oral tablet: 10 mg	10–50 mg/day	
Testosterone cypionate (Depo-Testosterone)	Solution for IM injection: 100 and 200 mg/mL	50–400 mg every 2–4 weeks	Requires an office visit every 2–4 weeks. Blood levels fluctuate widely (high after dosing and low before the next dose) and thereby can cause variations in libido, energy, and mood.
Testosterone enanthate (Delatestryl)	Solution for IM injection: 200 mg/mL	50–400 mg every 2–4 weeks	
Testosterone transdermal (Androderm)	Transdermal patch: 2 mg/24 h, 4 mg/h	2–6 mg/day	Rash at patch site is common.
Testosterone gel (AndroGel, Testim, Vogelxo)	AndroGel 1% gel: 15 mg/2.5 g Testim 1% gel: 50 mg/5 mL Vogelxo 1% 50 mg/5 g AndroGel 1.62% gel	5–10 g of 1% gel once daily (delivers 50–100 mg/day) 20.25–81 mg/day	It may be difficult to attain adequate levels. Easier to use and better tolerated than testosterone patches. Can transfer to others via intimate contact.
Testosterone metered dose pump (Androgel Pump, Axiron, Fortesta, Vogelxo Pump)	Androgel 1.62% gel: 20.25 mg/actuation Axiron 2% solution: 30 mg/actuation Fortesta 2% gel: 10 mg/actuation Vogelxo Pump 1%: 12.5 mg/actuation	20.25–81 mg/day 30–120 mg/day 10–70 mg/day	
Testosterone buccal (Striant)	Buccal tablet: 30 mg	30 mg q 12 h	Provides fairly steady testosterone levels but may cause mouth or gum irritation.
Testosterone nasal (Natesto)	Nasal pump: 5.5 mg/actuation	11 mg per nostril 3 times daily	May cause local adverse effects (e.g., epistaxis, scabbing, nasopharyngitis, rhinorrhea).
Testosterone implants (Testopel)	Pellets: 75 mg	150–450 mg (2–6 pellets) subQ every 3–6 months	Provides steady levels but requires invasive procedure.

IM, Intramuscular; *subQ,* subcutaneous.

cause of decreased desire may be candidates for testosterone therapy provided that estrogen is taken as well. Regardless, testosterone is not approved for replacement in women in the United States, although it is approved in the United Kingdom. When prescribed off label, it must be prescribed at doses lower than those used for men. The goal is to mimic premenopausal testosterone production—about 300 µg/day.

Cachexia

Cachexia is a wasting of the body associated with severe illnesses such as AIDS, severe trauma, and chronic systemic infections. Testosterone levels often decline in these patients, putting them at risk for wasting and loss of muscle mass. Testosterone therapy decreases this risk. Oxandrolone (Oxandrin) is FDA-approved for this purpose. Oxandrolone is an anabolic steroid that is a synthetic derivative of testosterone.

BLACK BOX WARNING

Oxandrolone (Oxandrin)

Oxandrolone can cause peliosis hepatitis, a condition in which blood-filled cysts form in the liver, leading to liver failure or intra-abdominal hemorrhage. It can also contribute to the development of highly vascular liver tumors.

An increased risk for atherosclerosis can occur secondary to marked elevations in low-density lipoprotein (LDL) and decreases in high-density lipoprotein (HDL).

Anemias

Androgens are sometimes used in men and women to treat anemias that have been refractory to other therapy. Anemias most likely to respond include aplastic anemia, anemia associated with renal failure, Fanconi anemia, and anemia caused by cancer chemotherapy. Androgens help relieve anemia by promoting synthesis of erythropoietin, the renal hormone that stimulates production of red blood cells, and possibly white blood cells and platelets. With the emergence of other therapies

such as erythropoietin-stimulating agents, however, androgens have fallen out of favor for off-label treatment of anemia.

Drug Therapy for Transgender Men

Although not approved by the FDA for this purpose, testosterone is prescribed off label as part of gender-affirmation drug therapy. This use is discussed further in *Drug Therapy for Transgender Men* at the end of this chapter.

PATIENT-CENTERED CARE ACROSS THE LIFE SPAN

Androgens

Life Stage	Considerations or Concerns
Children	Androgens can cause virilization in children. They can also accelerate epiphyseal closure, thereby decreasing adult height.
Pregnant women	The ability of androgens to cause fetal harm outweighs any possible therapeutic benefit. Potential fetal changes include vaginal malformation, clitoral enlargement, and formation of a structure resembling the male scrotum. Virilization is most likely when androgens are taken during the first trimester. Women who become pregnant while using androgens should be informed about the possible effect on the fetus.
Breastfeeding women	Testosterone is excreted in breast milk. Breastfeeding is contraindicated.
Older adults	Older patients are at an increased risk for thromboembolic conditions such as myocardial infarction or stroke. The Beers criteria identify testosterone and methyltestosterone as potentially inappropriate for patients 65 years and older.

Adverse Effects

Virilization in Women, Girls, and Boys

Virilization is the most common complication of androgen therapy. When taken in high doses by women, androgens can cause acne, deepening of the voice, proliferation of facial and body hair, male-pattern baldness, increased libido, clitoral enlargement, and menstrual irregularities. Clitoral growth, hair loss, and lowering of the voice may be irreversible. Masculinization can also occur if taken by children (e.g., for sports performance enhancement). Boys may experience growth of pubic hair, penile enlargement, increased frequency of erections, and even priapism (persistent erection). In girls, growth of pubic hair and clitoral enlargement may occur. To prevent irreversible masculinization, androgens must be discontinued when virilizing effects first appear.

Premature Epiphyseal Closure

When given to children, androgens can accelerate epiphyseal closure, thereby decreasing adult height. To evaluate androgen effects on the epiphyses, radiographic examination of the hand and wrist should be performed every 6 months.

Hepatotoxicity

Androgens can cause *cholestatic hepatitis* and other disorders of the liver. Clinical *jaundice* may occur but is rare. Patients receiving androgens should undergo periodic tests of liver function. If jaundice develops, it will reverse after discontinuation of androgen use. Androgens may also be carcinogenic: *hepatocellular carcinoma* has developed in some patients after prolonged use of these drugs.

It must be emphasized that not all androgens are hepatotoxic: liver damage is associated primarily with the *17-α-alkylated androgens*. These androgens all share a structural feature in common: an alkyl group substituted on carbon 17 of the steroid nucleus. Because of their capacity to cause liver damage, *the 17-α-alkylated compounds should not be used long term*. In contrast to the 17-α-alkylated androgens, testosterone and the testosterone esters (testosterone cypionate, testosterone enanthate) are not associated with liver disease.

Effects on Cholesterol Levels

Androgens can lower plasma levels of HDL cholesterol and elevate plasma levels of LDL cholesterol. These actions may increase the risk for atherosclerosis and related cardiovascular events.

Prostate Cancer

Androgens do not cause prostate cancer, but they can promote the growth of this cancer after it occurs. Accordingly, androgens are contraindicated for men with diagnosed prostate cancer. Men without diagnosed prostate cancer should be monitored for the emergence of covert cancer.

Edema

Edema can result from androgen-induced retention of salt and water. This complication is a concern for patients with heart failure and those with a predisposition to developing edema from other causes. Treatment consists of discontinuing the androgen and giving a diuretic if needed.

Abuse Potential

As discussed later, androgens are frequently misused (abused) to enhance athletic performance. Because of their abuse potential, nearly all androgens are regulated as schedule III controlled substances.

Risk for Thromboembolic Events

There have been postmarketing reports of thromboembolic events including stroke, myocardial infarction, deep venous thrombosis, and pulmonary embolism. These events are believed to have been the result of testosterone's erythropoietic effects. To address this potentially life-threatening concern, the FDA has issued a Testosterone Product Safety Alert requiring labeling changes in 2018. (See https://www.fda.gov/drugs/drugsafety/ucm436259.htm.)

Androgen Preparations for Male Hypogonadism

Treatment options for androgen replacement therapy have expanded in recent years. In the past, intramuscular (IM) therapy with a long-acting testosterone ester was the major treatment mode. Today, there are six attractive alternatives: a nasal gel, transdermal patch, transdermal gel, topical solution, buccal tablet, and implantable subcutaneous pellets. All formulations are regulated as schedule III controlled substances.

Oral Androgens

Only two androgens are approved for oral therapy of male hypogonadism. Despite the advantages of cost and ease of administration, these are not first-line agents. The androgenic effects of oral androgens are erratic. Furthermore, both fluoxymesterone and methyltestosterone are 17-α-alkylated androgens and therefore pose a risk for hepatotoxicity. Accordingly they should not be used long term.

Transdermal Testosterone

Testosterone is available in three transdermal formulations: patch, gel, and liquid. With all three formulations, testosterone is absorbed through the skin and then slowly absorbed into the blood.

Patches. Testosterone patches (Androderm) are indicated for male hypogonadism. Two strengths are available, delivering 2 or 4 mg of testosterone in 24 hours. Patches are applied once daily to the upper arm, thigh, back, or abdomen. The principal adverse effect is rash at the site of application.

Gels. Testosterone is available in four gel formulations sold as AndroGel, Testim, Fortesta, and Vogelxo. AndroGel contains 1% or 1.62% of testosterone; Testim contains 1% of testosterone and Fortesta 2% of testosterone. Compared with transdermal patches, the gels have three advantages: they (1) cause less local irritation, (2) cannot fall off, and (3) produce more consistent testosterone levels.

The principal disadvantage of the gels is that testosterone can be transferred to others by skin-to-skin contact. This is possible because only 10% of an applied dose is absorbed; the other 90% remains on the skin after the gel dries. In one study, blood levels of testosterone were doubled in female partners of gel users after 15 minutes of intimate contact that occurred within 2 to 12 hours after the gel had been applied. Testosterone transfer is a concern because the drug can cause virilization of female partners and can also cause fetal harm. In children, contact transfer can cause genital enlargement, premature development of pubic hair, advanced bone age, increased libido, and aggressive behavior. In most cases these effects regress after testosterone exposure stops. To reduce the risk for unintended gel transfer, the following guidelines should be observed:

- Gel users should wash their hands with soap and warm water after every application.
- Gel users should cover the application site with clothing once the gel has dried.

▶▶ BLACK BOX WARNING
Testosterone Gel and Topical Solution

Secondary exposure to testosterone gel on uncovered skin and to testosterone gel on unwashed clothing has resulted in virilization in children.

- Gel users should wash the application site before skin-to-skin contact with another person.
- Women and children should avoid skin-to-skin contact with application sites on gel users.
- Women and children who make accidental contact with a gel application site should wash contaminated skin immediately.

AndroGel is supplied in a metered-dose pump that delivers 12.25 mg per actuation (1%) or 20.25 mg per actuation (1.62%) and in unit-dose foil packets containing 20.25 mg of testosterone (of which 2.5 mg becomes absorbed) and 40.5 mg of testosterone (of which 5 mg becomes absorbed). The gel is applied once daily (preferably in the morning) to clean, dry skin of the shoulders, upper arms, or abdomen but not the genitalia. Patients should be instructed to squeeze the entire contents of the packet into the palms and then immediately apply the gel to the skin and rub it in. To prevent the transfer of testosterone to others, patients should wash their hands and, after the gel has dried, keep the treated area covered with clothing. Because testosterone can be washed off, patients should wait 5 to 6 hours before showering or swimming. To ensure safe and effective dosing, blood levels of testosterone should be measured 14 days after the initiation of therapy and periodically thereafter.

Testim is available in 5-g tubes that contain 50 mg of testosterone, of which 10% (5 mg) is absorbed. It is applied once daily to skin of the shoulders or upper arms but not to the abdomen or scrotum. As with AndroGel, patients should wash their hands immediately after application and keep the treated area covered. They should also avoid showering for at least 2 hours. Testosterone levels should be checked after 14 days and periodically thereafter.

Fortesta is supplied in a metered-dose pump that delivers 10 mg of testosterone per actuation. All doses are applied to the front or inner thigh. As with AndroGel, patients should wash their hands immediately and keep the treated area covered. Also, they should avoid swimming or showering for at least 2 hours. Fortesta is a flammable, alcohol-based formulation; hence patients should avoid flames or smoking until the gel has dried. Testosterone levels should be checked after days 14 and 35 and periodically thereafter.

Vogelxo in the tube formulation is applied in the same manner as Testim. Vogelxo in the metered-dose pump is applied in the same way as Fortesta. For both, the same advice and precautions apply.

Topical solution. Testosterone topical solution for underarm application (Axiron) is much like the testosterone gels. The principal difference is the application site: Axiron liquid is formulated specifically for application to the axilla, whereas Testim is applied to the shoulder or upper arm, and AndroGel is applied to the shoulder, upper arm, or abdomen. After application, testosterone is absorbed rapidly into the skin and then slowly into the blood. Steady-state levels are reached in 14 days. After application stops, blood levels take 7 to 10 days to decline to baseline.

Axiron is supplied as an alcohol-based solution in a metered-dose pump that delivers 30 mg of testosterone per actuation. Dosing is done by pumping the liquid onto an applicator (supplied with the pump) and then applying the liquid to clean, dry, intact skin of the underarm—and not anywhere else. Patients should not swim or bathe for 2 hours after application. If an underarm deodorant or antiperspirant is used, it should be applied before applying the testosterone (to avoid contaminating the deodorant or antiperspirant dispenser). Because of its alcohol content, Axiron liquid is flammable. Accordingly, users should stay away from flames until the solution has dried.

Axiron is applied to each axilla at the same time every morning. After 14 days or longer, blood levels of testosterone are measured and dosage is adjusted up or down as indicated.

Like the testosterone gels, testosterone topical solution can be transferred to others through skin-to-skin contact, posing a risk to women and children. Accordingly, the same guidelines noted previously to prevent drug transfer should be followed.

Nasal gel. Testosterone nasal gel (Natesto) is the newest formulation approved for testosterone administration. It comes in a metered-dose pump that sprays 5.5 mg of testosterone each time the pump is actuated.

Because the drug is administered nasally, patients with nasal disorders or abnormalities (e.g., chronic sinusitis, a severely deviated nasal septum) should not take this drug. There has not been adequate testing for interactions with other nasally administered drugs. Currently, only adrenergic agonists (e.g., oxymetazoline nasal spray) are approved for administration with Natesto.

The nasal route of administration can cause localized reactions. These include rhinorrhea, epistaxis, and nasopharyngitis; however, these tend to be modest effects.

Administration instructions are supplied with the drug; however, it is important that the provider be aware of these in order to answer patient questions.

1. The pump should be primed before use and excess gel should be removed.
2. The patient should blow his nose before administration.
3. The pump is inserted into the nostril with the tip aimed toward the lateral nostril wall.
4. The pump should be depressed slowly until it stops.
5. As the tip is withdrawn, it should be wiped against the lateral nostril wall to ensure that any remaining gel is distributed to the nostril.
6. After administration in both nostrils, the nose should be lightly massaged below the nasal bridge.
7. The patient should avoid blowing or sniffing for at least 1 hour after administration.

Implantable testosterone pellets. Testosterone pellets (Testopel) are long-acting formulations indicated for male hypogonadism and delayed puberty. The pellets are implanted subdermally in the hip area or abdominal wall lateral to the umbilicus. Each pellet contains 75 mg of testosterone. The usual dosage is 150 to 450 mg (two to six pellets) every 3 to 6 months. About one-third of the dose is absorbed the first month, one-fourth the second month, and one-sixth the third month. For patients switching from IM testosterone propionate or IM testosterone enanthate, the recommended dosage is two pellets for each 25 mg of IM testosterone used weekly. For example, a patient receiving 75 mg of IM testosterone enanthate each week would switch to six pellets every 3 to 4 months.

Testosterone buccal tablets. Testosterone buccal tablets (Striant), approved for male hypogonadism, produce steady blood levels of testosterone. Tablets are applied to the gum area just above the incisor tooth and are designed to stay in place until removed. To ensure good adhesion, tablets should be held in place (with a finger over the lip) for 30 seconds. The recommended dosage is 1 tablet every 12 hours, alternating sides of the mouth with each dose. If a tablet falls out before 8 hours, it should be replaced with a new one for the remainder of the dosing interval. If a tablet falls out after 8 hours, it should be replaced with a new one, and the next scheduled dose should be skipped (i.e., the replacement tablet should remain in place for 16 hours or so). The tablets are not affected by eating, drinking, chewing gum, or brushing teeth. Adverse effects, which are usually transient, include local irritation, bitter taste, and taste distortion. Treatment for up to 1 year has not caused serious gum changes. It has been hypothesized that transfer of testosterone from buccal routes may occur through saliva transfer during kissing.

Intramuscular testosterone esters. Two IM testosterone esters are available: testosterone cypionate (Depo-Testosterone) and testosterone enanthate (Delatestryl). Both drugs are formulated in oil and both are long-acting. After IM injection, these drugs are slowly absorbed and then hydrolyzed to release free testosterone. Unfortunately these preparations produce testosterone blood levels that vary widely: testosterone levels are higher than normal immediately after dosing and decline to lower than normal before the next dose. As a result, patients may experience significant variations in libido, energy, and mood.

ANDROGEN (ANABOLIC STEROID) ABUSE

Many athletes take androgens (anabolic steroids) and androgen precursors to enhance athletic performance. The potential benefits of this practice, although substantial, are accompanied by significant risks. Drugs commonly used by athletes include nandrolone, stanozolol, and methenolone. All of these drugs are regulated as controlled substances, making their use without a prescription illegal.

What can anabolic steroids do for the athlete? Exogenous androgens can significantly increase muscle mass and strength in males and females of all ages when given in sufficiently large doses. One study showed that after 10 weeks, testosterone treatment produced a 7-lb increase in muscle mass in subjects who did not exercise and a 13-lb increase in subjects who exercised and took the drug. In contrast, exercise in the absence of exogenous testosterone produced only a 4-lb increase in muscle mass. Similar increases were shown in the subjects' ability to bench-press weights.

The potential for adverse effects of androgens is substantial. Salt and water retention can lead to hypertension. When administered in the high doses used by athletes, androgens suppress the release of LH and FSH, resulting in testicular shrinkage, sterility, and gynecomastia. Acne is common. Reduction of HDL cholesterol and elevation of LDL cholesterol may theoretically accelerate the development of atherosclerosis. Because most of the androgens that athletes take are 17-α-alkylated compounds, hepatotoxicity (cholestatic hepatitis, jaundice, hepatocellular carcinoma) is an ever-present risk. Most recently, androgens have been linked with kidney damage. In females, androgens can cause menstrual irregularities and virilization. In boys and girls, androgens may reduce attainable adult height.

What about psychologic effects? Androgens are reputed to cause depression, manic episodes, and aggressiveness. There have been very few controlled studies to measure psychologic effects of androgens; however, in the controlled studies undertaken, dosages of androgens were often less than those typically taken by athletes. Surveys of athletes who engage in anabolic steroid use indicate an association with risky behavior and aggression; however, it is possible that these were inherent traits of the surveyed athletes regardless of steroid use.

Long-term androgen use can lead to an abuse syndrome. Characteristics include preoccupation with androgen use and difficulty in stopping it. When androgens are finally are discontinued, an abstinence syndrome can develop similar to that produced by the withdrawal of alcohol, opioids, and cocaine.

Because of their abuse potential, anabolic steroids are classified as schedule III substances under an amendment to the Controlled Substances Act. (Schedule III drugs are defined as those with a low to moderate potential for dependence.) For more information on drug abuse in sports, a good place to start is www.wada-ama.org, the website of the World Anti-Doping Agency. This organization is dedicated to promoting, coordinating, and monitoring the fight against the use of anabolic steroids and other banned substances in sports. Other good resources include the US Anti-Doping Agency (http://www.usada.org) and the National Center for Drug-Free Sport (http://www.drugfreesport.com/index.asp).

Drug Therapy for Transgender Men

The term *transgender* is used to denote a person who self-identifies as having a gender that is different from the gender assigned at birth. Transgender men therefore are men who were identified as female at birth based on external sexual anatomy but who self-identify as male.

In order for transgender men to more fully experience their lives as men, they may choose to undergo hormone therapy so that their gender expression (i.e., how their gender is presented to others) matches their gender identity. This gender identity–affirming care is initiated and managed by endocrinologists or other specialists in transgender health, but because any physician may have transgender men as patients for general care of common illnesses and preventive medicine, it is important to have a familiarity with their therapy.

The goal of hormone therapy is twofold: (1) to stop menstruation and (2) to stimulate the development of male secondary sex characteristics. Testosterone therapy accomplishes both goals. Treatment is similar as that used to treat hypogonadism. To assure appropriate dosage, serum testosterone levels are assessed periodically (e.g., every 3 months as dosage is optimized and then once or twice yearly). It is also important to monitor hematocrit, hemoglobin, and serum cholesterol.

Successful therapy achieves the following outcomes:
- The voice deepens
- Male-pattern hair growth and distribution occurs
- There is a decrease in glandular breast tissue (the degree of decrease, if it occurs, varies)
- The clitoris enlarges
- The patient experiences an improved quality of life (of note, mental health issues and psychologic symptoms typically improve following gender affirmation therapy)

 SUMMARY OF KEY PRESCRIBING CONSIDERATIONS

Androgens

Therapeutic Goal: To manage hypogonadism and subsequent testosterone deficiency through testosterone supplementation.

Baseline Data: Serum testosterone concentration, complete blood count (CBC), lipid panel, liver function, prostate specific antigen (PSA).

Monitoring: Serum testosterone concentration, lipids, liver function, and PSA after 1 year (refer to urologist for evaluation if PSA is greater than 4.0 ng/mL or greater than 1.4 ng/mL above baseline)

Identifying High-Risk Patients: Androgens are contraindicated for pregnant women, for men who have prostate cancer or breast cancer, and for enhancing athletic performance.

Evaluating Therapeutic Effects: Development of secondary sex characteristics and restoration of energy, libido, and other symptoms of testosterone deficiency.

Minimizing Adverse Effects:
- Virilization may occur in women who want to avoid this affect. Assess for deepening voice, chest and facial hair, acne, and menstrual irregularities at each clinical encounter. Irreversible changes may be avoided if androgens are withdrawn early.
- Accelerated bone maturation in children can decrease attainable adult height. Monitor effects on epiphyses with radiographs of the hand and wrist twice yearly.
- The 17-α-alkylated androgens can cause cholestatic hepatitis, jaundice, and other liver disorders. Rarely, liver cancer develops. Monitor for signs and symptoms of liver dysfunction such as jaundice, fatigue, and malaise. Obtain periodic tests of liver function. Liver function normalizes after the cessation of drug use. Avoid long-term use of 17-α-alkylated preparations.
- Salt and water retention may result in edema. Assess for edema and weight gain at each clinical encounter. Treatment consists of androgen withdrawal if indicated or use of a diuretic.
- Androgens can cause masculinization of the female fetus. Rule out pregnancy before androgen use. Ensure that female patients of child-bearing age are using adequate contraception and engaging in consistent use.

PATIENT EDUCATION

Topical Testosterone

To minimize the risk for accidental skin-to-skin transfer, advise users of testosterone gel or testosterone topical solution to (1) wash their hands after every application, (2) cover the application site with clothing after the gel has dried, and (3) wash the application site before anticipated contact with another person. Also, warn women and children to avoid contact with the user's skin where testosterone was applied and advise them to wash contaminated skin if accidental contact with an application site should occur.

PATIENT EDUCATION

Androgens

Tell female patients about signs of virilization (deepening of the voice, acne, changes in body and facial hair, menstrual irregularities). Instruct them to report these if they occur.

Apprise patients of the signs of liver dysfunction (yellow tint to skin and eyes, fatigue, loss of appetite, nausea, dark-colored urine, light-colored stools). Advise them to report the occurrence of these changes.

Inform patients that swelling of the extremities or unusual weight gain may be evidence of salt and water retention. Counsel them to report these events.

Remind patients of child-bearing age that this drug can cause fetal malformations. If the patient is capable of becoming pregnant, emphasize the need for consistent use of reliable contraception.

Adverse effects of testosterone therapy are the same as those accompanying testosterone therapy for other reasons. These include

- Acne
- Possible male-pattern hair loss
- Polycythemia
- Hypercholesterolemia
- Liver impairment
- Thromboembolic disorders with increased risk of myocardial infarction and stroke

There is also a theoretical increase in risk for endometrial cancer in patients who have not had a hysterectomy. This complication has not been demonstrated in practice, however.

Despite hormone therapy, transgender men who have not had gender-affirming (formerly sexual reassignment) surgery remain at risk for conditions affecting women. It will therefore be important to continue screening for breast, cervical, and uterine cancer.

The following websites offer additional information on this topic, including clinical guidelines:

- The World Professional Association for Transgender Health, https://www.wpath.org/publications/soc
- Center of Excellence for Transgender Health, http://transhealth.ucsf.edu/pdf/Transgender-PGACG-6-17-16.pdf
- The Endocrine Society—Transgender Health, https://www.endocrine.org/guidelines-and-clinical-practice/clinical-practice-guidelines/gender-dysphoria-gender-incongruence

53

Male Sexual Dysfunction and Benign Prostatic Hyperplasia

MALE SEXUAL DYSFUNCTION

There are several types of male sexual dysfunction. This chapter focuses on the two most common types treated by advanced practice providers: erectile dysfunction (ED) and premature ejaculation.

ERECTILE DYSFUNCTION

ED is defined as a persistent inability to achieve or sustain an erection suitable for satisfactory sexual performance. In the United States, ED affects up to 30 million men. ED is commonly associated with chronic illness, especially diabetes, hypertension, and depression. Among men with diabetes, the incidence of ED is between 35% and 75%. In approximately one-fourth of ED cases, the identified cause is medications. Commonly used drugs that can cause ED are shown in Table 53.1.

The risk for ED increases with advancing age. According to the National Institutes of Health, ED affects approximately 4% of men in their 50s. Just a decade later, 17% of men in their 60s are unable to achieve any erection at all. This total inability to achieve erection affects 47% of men older than 75 years. Fortunately new advances in medicine can rectify this problem for most patients.

First-line treatments for ED are lifestyle measures (increased exercise, smoking cessation), changing drug regimens to remove the drugs that may cause ED, and drug therapy with sildenafil (Viagra) or another drug in its class. Other interventions include psychotherapy and surgical implantation of a penile prosthesis.

Physiology of Erection

Before discussing drugs for ED, it is important to review the physiology of erection. As shown in Fig. 53.1, the process begins with sexual arousal; it increases parasympathetic nerve traffic to the penis, causing local release of nitric oxide. Nitric oxide then activates guanylyl cyclase, an enzyme that makes cyclic guanosine monophosphate (cGMP). Through a series of steps, cGMP promotes relaxation of arterial and trabecular smooth muscle. The resultant arterial dilation increases local blood flow and blood pressure, which, in combination with relaxation of trabecular smooth muscle, causes expansion and engorgement of sinusoidal spaces in the corpus cavernosum. This, in turn, causes venous occlusion and thereby reduces venous outflow. The combination of increased arterial pressure and arterial inflow plus reduced venous outflow causes sufficient engorgement to produce erection. Erection subsides when cGMP is removed by phosphodiesterase type 5 (PDE-5), an enzyme that converts cGMP into guanosine monophosphate.

Oral Drugs for Erectile Dysfunction: Phosphodiesterase-5 Inhibitors

Drugs for ED fall into two major groups: oral and nonoral. The oral agents—PDE-5 inhibitors—are by far the most common treatments for ED. These constitute our primary focus. The nonoral agents—papaverine plus phentolamine, alprostadil—are considered briefly. These drugs are summarized in Table 53.2.

Four PDE-5 inhibitors are available: sildenafil, tadalafil, vardenafil, and avanafil. All are considered first-line therapy for ED. Current guidelines recommend that, in the absence of a specific contraindication, all men with ED be offered one of these drugs. Which drug is preferred? Only a few trials have compared them head to head, so there is insufficient evidence to recommend one over the others. Accordingly, selection among them should be based on patient preference and prescriber judgment.

Sildenafil

Sildenafil was introduced in 1998 as the first oral treatment for ED. The drug is reliable and easy to use. Benefits derive from enhancing the natural response to sexual stimuli; sildenafil does not cause erection directly. Although sildenafil is generally well tolerated, it can be dangerous for men taking certain vasodilators, specifically α-adrenergic blockers, nitroglycerin, and other nitrates used for angina pectoris.

PATIENT EDUCATION
Phosphodiesterase-5 Inhibitors

Inform patients that dosing may be done with or without food, although a high-fat meal will delay absorption of avanafil, sildenafil, or vardenafil (but not tadalafil). Be sure to warn them that grapefruit juice should be avoided because this can raise PDE-5 inhibitor levels.

Advise patients to take avanafil approximately 15–30 min before sexual activity. All other PDE-5 inhibitors should be taken about 1 h before sexual activity.

Counsel men with preexisting cardiovascular disease regarding the cardiac risk for sexual activity (irrespective of a PDE-5 inhibitor). Advise men who experience symptoms (e.g., anginal pain, lightheadedness) during sex to refrain from further sexual activity and discuss the event with their prescriber.

Warn patients to seek immediate medical attention if an erection lasts more than 4 h. Prolonged priapism can cause permanent damage.

Advise patients to stop their PDE-5 inhibitor and seek immediate medical attention if they experience sudden loss of vision in one or both eyes or if hearing loss develops.

Instruct patients to avoid nitrates for at least 12 h after taking avanafil, for at least 24 h after taking sildenafil or vardenafil, and for at least 48 h after taking tadalafil.

The erection-enhancing effects of sildenafil were discovered by accident. The drug was developed as a cardiac medicine, but benefits were minimal. However, in the course of testing, some men noticed a surprising side effect: their ED had been cured! The rest, as they say, is history. Sildenafil has been wildly popular. First-year sales were the hottest in pharmaceutical history. By now, tens of millions of men in more than 100 countries have used the drug. In addition to ED, sildenafil is approved for pulmonary arterial hypertension (PAH). When used for this purpose, sildenafil is sold as *Revatio*.

TABLE 53.1   Commonly Used Drugs That Can Cause Sexual/Erectile Dysfunction

Drug Class	Representative Drug	Incidence of SD/ED[a]
Renal/Cardiovascular Drugs		
Cardiac glycosides	Digoxin (Lanoxin)	36%
Central α_2-adrenergic agonists	Clonidine (Catapres)	1%–10%
β Blockers	Propranolol (Inderal)	10%–15%
Thiazide diuretics	Hydrochlorothiazide	10%–20%
Aldosterone antagonists	Spironolactone (Aldactone)	4%–30%
CNS Drugs		
Selective serotonin reuptake inhibitors	Fluoxetine (Prozac)	Up to 70%
Monoamine oxidase inhibitors	Isocarboxazid (Marplan)	16%–31%
Tricyclic antidepressants	Amitriptyline (Elavil)	7%–30%
Antipsychotics	Chlorpromazine (Thorazine)	30%–60%
Mood stabilizers	Lithium (Lithobid)	5%–50%
Social lubricant/intoxicant	Alcohol	50%–75%
Urogenital Drugs		
5-α-Reductase inhibitors	Finasteride (Proscar)	33%

[a]Values for sexual dysfunction/erectile dysfunction (SD/ED) incidence are estimates based on patient reports, not on carefully controlled trials.
CNS, Central nervous system.

Mechanism of action. Sildenafil causes selective inhibition of PDE-5. By doing so, it increases and preserves cGMP levels in the penis, thereby making the erection harder and longer lasting. Note that the drug only enhances the normal erectile response to sexual stimuli (e.g., erotic imagery, fantasies, physical contact). In the absence of sexual stimuli, nothing happens.

Preparations, dosing, and pharmacokinetics. Preparations and dosing for sildenafil and other PDE-5 inhibitors are provided in Table 53.2. Pharmacokinetics is provided in Table 53.3.

Sexual benefits

In men with erectile dysfunction. Sildenafil has been evaluated in several thousand men (aged 19 to 87 years) with ED of organic, psychogenic, or mixed-cause origin. At least some improvement in erection hardness and duration was seen in 70% of men taking the drug compared with 20% taking placebo. Benefits were dose-related and lasted up to 4 hours, although they began to fade after 2 hours. Sildenafil was able to help a wide range of patients, including those with ED resulting from diabetes, spinal cord injury, and transurethral prostate resection as well as ED of no known physical cause.

In men without erectile dysfunction. Despite anecdotal reports to the contrary, sildenafil has little or no effect on erection quality or duration in men who do not have ED. Any apparent benefits in healthy men are likely the result of a placebo response.

In women. Sildenafil is not approved for use in women and probably will not be. Although several large-scale studies showed the drug to be safe in women, they failed to show much enhancement of sexual arousal. Thus the manufacturer decided not to seek US Food and Drug Administration (FDA) approval for treating female sexual interest-arousal disorder (formerly hypoactive sexual desire disorder) or any other condition in women.

Adverse effects

Hypotension. At recommended doses, sildenafil produces a small (8.4/5.5 mm Hg) reduction in blood pressure. However, in men taking nitrates or α blockers, severe hypotension can develop.

PATIENT-CENTERED CARE ACROSS THE LIFE SPAN

Drugs for Erectile Dysfunction

Life Stage	Considerations or Concerns
Children	Safety for PDE-5 inhibitors has not been established. PDE-5 inhibitors are not indicated for children. Alprostadil is indicated for the treatment of patent ductus arteriosus in neonates and sildenafil is indicated for the treatment of pulmonary hypertension; however, the formulations for ED would not apply.
Pregnant women	PDE-5 inhibitors are considered safe in pregnant women; however, they are not indicated for use in women and therefore should not be taken by pregnant women. Alprostadil urethral pellets and injectable alprostadil or papaverine with phentolamine would not be used by people without a penis. It is recommended that men taking these drugs use a condom if their partner is a pregnant woman.
Breastfeeding women	Excretion in breast milk is unknown; however, drugs for erectile dysfunction are not indicated for use in women.
Older adults	Consider lower dosing when prescribing for adults age 65 and older.

Priapism. A few cases of priapism (painful erection lasting more than 6 hours) have been reported. If an erection persists more than 4 hours, immediate medical intervention is required. Left untreated, priapism can cause permanent damage of penile tissue. If priapism persists longer than 24 hours, chances are very high that the patient will never be able to have sexual intercourse again. Persistent erection can be relieved by aspirating blood from the corpus cavernosum, followed by irrigation with a solution containing a vasoconstrictor (e.g., epinephrine, phenylephrine, metaraminol). If this is unsuccessful, surgery is required.

Nonarteritic ischemic optic neuropathy. Very rarely, men taking sildenafil have developed NAION, resulting in irreversible blurring or loss of vision. The cause is blockage of blood flow to the optic nerve. In most cases there were underlying anatomic or vascular risk factors for NAION. Furthermore, although NAION developed during sildenafil use, a direct causal relationship has not been established. Nonetheless, patients with NAION in one eye should not use sildenafil owing to a potential risk for developing NAION in the other eye.

Sudden hearing loss. Very rarely, men taking sildenafil have experienced sudden hearing loss, usually in one ear, sometimes in association with dizziness, vertigo, and tinnitus. Such loss may be partial or complete. In one-third of cases, hearing had returned by the time the loss was reported, but it had not returned in the remaining two-thirds. To date a direct causal relationship between sildenafil and hearing loss has not been established. Nonetheless the drug is suspected because (1) sudden hearing loss is unusual and (2) it developed when sildenafil was being taken. Men who experience sudden hearing loss should discontinue the drug, but only if they are taking it for ED; men taking the drug for PAH should continue treatment.

Other adverse effects. The most common adverse effects are headache, flushing, and dyspepsia. Sildenafil may also cause nasal congestion, diarrhea, rash, and dizziness. About 3% of patients experience mild transient visual disturbances (a blue tinge to vision, increased sensitivity to light, blurring). In addition, sildenafil may intensify symptoms of obstructive sleep apnea (perhaps by relaxing pharyngeal muscles or dilating pulmonary blood vessels).

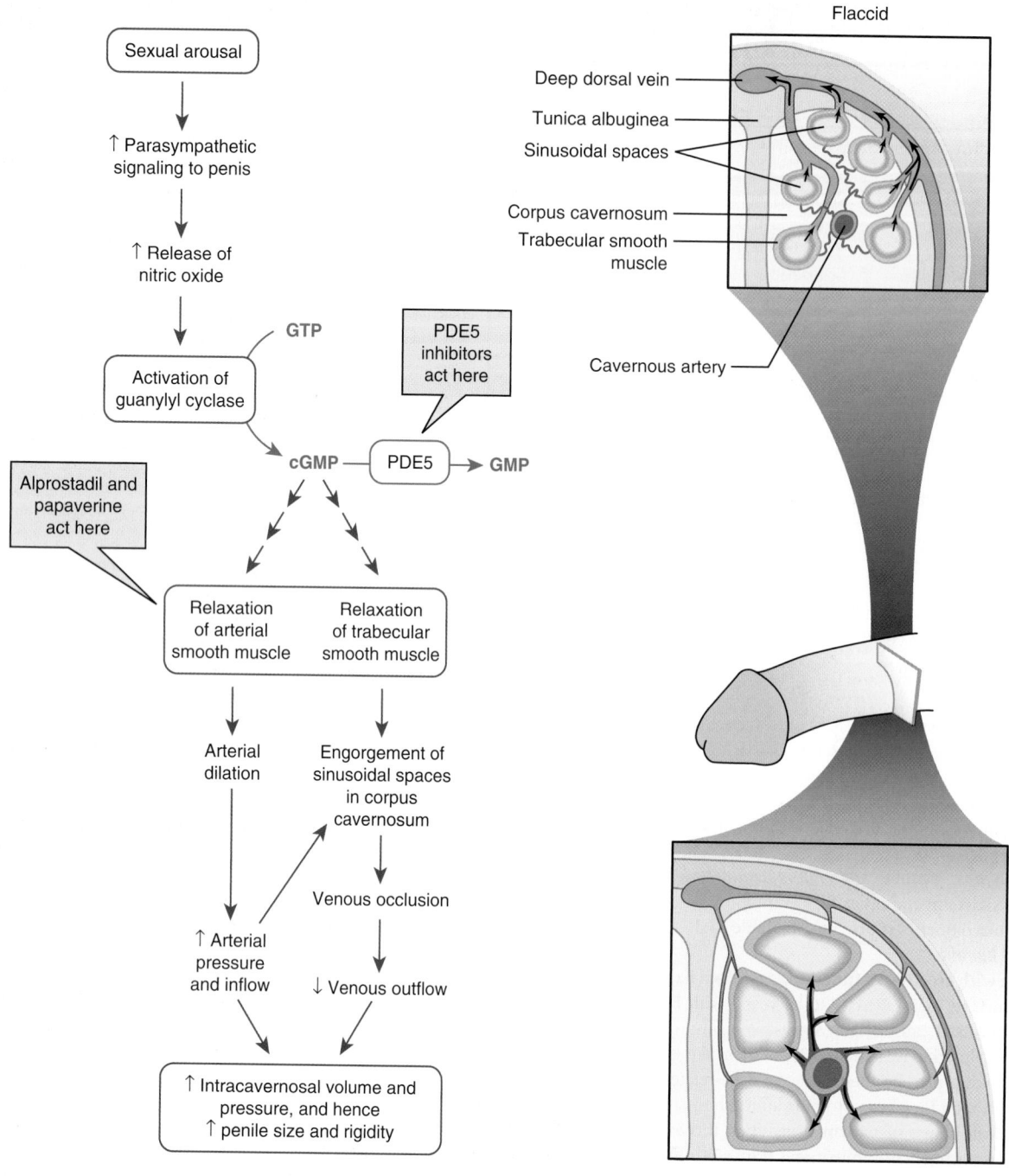

Fig. 53.1 Physiology of Penile Erection. In the flaccid state, there is free outflow of venous blood and restricted inflow of arterial blood. During sexual arousal, cyclic guanosine monophosphate *(cGMP)* relaxes arterial and trabecular smooth muscle, permitting free inflow of arterial blood and subsequent engorgement of sinusoidal spaces, whose expansion compresses penile veins and thus restricts blood outflow. The resultant accumulation of blood at elevated pressure increases penile size and rigidity. Removal of cGMP by PDE-5 restores penile smooth muscle to the nonaroused state and detumescence ensues. *GTP,* Guanosine triphosphate; *PDE-5,* phosphodiesterase type 5.

TABLE 53.2 Drugs for Erectile Dysfunction: Preparation, Dosage, and Considerations

Drug Class and Drug	Preparation	Dosage for ED	Considerations
PDE-5 Inhibitors			
Avanafil (Stendra)	Tablets: 50, 100, 200 mg	100 mg taken approximately 15 min before sexual activity. May be increased to 200 mg if needed. Decrease to lowest effective dose.	Reduce dosage if patient is taking CYP3A4 inhibitors (e.g., ketoconazole, ritonavir). Grapefruit juice can elevate drug levels. Use caution when combining with an α blocker; may cause serious drop in BP. Concurrent use of nitrates is contraindicated. High-fat foods delay absorption and can double the time to onset. Limit to once a day.
Sildenafil (Viagra)	Tablets: 25, 50, 100 mg	50 mg once daily approximately 60 min before sexual activity. May be increased to 100 mg if needed. Decrease to lowest effective dose.	Reduce dosage if patient is taking CYP3A4 inhibitors (e.g., ketoconazole, ritonavir). Grapefruit juice can elevate drug levels. Use caution when combining with an α blocker—may cause serious drop in BP. Concurrent use of nitrates is contraindicated. High-fat foods may delay onset by as much as 60 min. Limit to once a day.
Tadalafil (Cialis)	Tablets: 2.5, 5, 10, 20 mg	PRN use: 10 mg before sexual activity. May be increased to 20 mg if needed. Decrease to lowest effective dose. Daily use: 2.5 mg orally once daily; timing unrelated to sexual activity. May increase to 5 mg if needed.	Reduce dosage if patient is taking CYP3A4 inhibitors (e.g., ketoconazole, ritonavir). Grapefruit juice can elevate drug levels. Concurrent use of nitrates is contraindicated. If taken daily, should be taken at the same time each day. To prevent dangerous drop in blood pressure, do not combine with α blockers except tamsulosin.
Vardenafil (Levitra, Staxyn)	Tablets (Levitra): 2.5, 5, 10, 20 mg Orally disintegrating tablets (Staxyn): 10 mg	Levitra: 10 mg taken approximately 60 min before sexual activity. May be increased to 20 mg if needed. Decrease to lowest effective dose. Decrease starting dose to 5 mg for patients age 65 and older. Staxyn: 10 mg taken approximately 60 min before sexual activity. Do not increase dosage.	Fatty drugs can delay onset of action. Do not combine with α blockers; doing so can cause serious decrease in blood pressure. Reduce dosage if patient is taking CYP3A4 inhibitors (e.g., ketoconazole, ritonavir). Grapefruit juice can elevate drug levels. Concurrent use of nitrates is contraindicated. Vardenafil prolongs the QT interval. Do not prescribe for men taking class I or III antidysrhythmic drugs.
Prostaglandin E₁			
Alprostadil intracavernosal injection (Caverject, Caverject Impulse, Edex)	Intracavernosal kit (Caverject Impulse): 10 and 20 μg Intracavernosal Kit (Edex): 10, 20, 40 μg Solution for intracavernosal injection (Caverject): 20 and 40 μg	Typical dosages range from 5–40 μg. Dosing is individualized; determination is made in the health care setting. Maximum dosing is 60 μg for Caverject and 40 μg for Edex.	Patients self-administer injection into the penis. Limit total dosing to three times a week, not to exceed once in 24 h.
Alprostadil intraurethral insertion (Muse)	Urethral pellets (Muse): 125, 250, 500, 1000 μg	Intraurethral insertion: Initial dosing is 125–250 μg 5–10 min before sexual activity. (Effect lasts 30–60 min.) Increase if needed to lowest effective dose.	Patients self-insert the pellet into the urethra. Limit use to twice daily.
Vasodilator Plus α-Adrenergic Antagonist			
Papaverine with phentolamine	Papaverine 30 mg/mL with phentolamine 1 mg/mL	Dosing is individualized; determination is made in the health care setting. As little as 0.1 mL may be sufficient.	Patients self-administer injection into the penis.

TABLE 53.3   Comparison of Phosphodiesterase-5 Inhibitors

Parameter	DRUG			
	Sildenafil (Viagra)	Tadalafil (Cialis)	Vardenafil (Levitra, Staxyn)	Avanafil (Stendra)
Dosing schedule	PRN only	PRN *or* once daily	PRN only	PRN
Median time to peak level	1 h	2 h	1 h	30–45 min
Half-life	4 h	17.5 h	4–5 h	5 h
Duration of action	4 h	36 h	4 h	4 h
Major mode of metabolism	CYP3A4	CYP3A4	CYP3A4	CYP3A4
Drug Interactions				
Nitrates	Contraindicated: Wait 24 h before giving a nitrate	Contraindicated: Wait 48 h before giving a nitrate	Contraindicated: Wait 24 h before giving a nitrate	Contraindicated: Wait 12 h before giving a nitrate
α blockers	Use with caution	Contraindicated (except for tamsulosin, 0.4 mg once daily)	Contraindicated	Use with caution
CYP3A4 inhibitors	Reduce sildenafil dosage	Reduce tadalafil dosage to no more than 10 mg every 72 h	Reduce vardenafil dosage	Do not take with strong CYP3A4 inhibitors; reduce dosage with moderate inhibitors
Class I and III antidysrhythmic drugs	No interaction	No interaction	Vardenafil prolongs the QT interval—avoid class I and III antidysrhythmics	No interaction

Drug interactions

Nitrates. Both sildenafil and nitrates (e.g., nitroglycerin, isosorbide dinitrate) promote hypotension, and they both do so by increasing cGMP (nitrates increase cGMP formation, and sildenafil slows cGMP breakdown). If these drugs are combined, life-threatening hypotension can result. Therefore *sildenafil is absolutely contraindicated for men taking nitrates.* At least 24 hours should elapse between the last dose of sildenafil and administration of a nitrate. If elimination of sildenafil is slowed (owing to a CYP3A4 inhibitor or hepatic or renal impairment), an even longer time should elapse before nitrate use.

PROTOTYPE DRUGS

Drugs for Erectile Dysfunction and Benign Prostatic Hyperplasia

Drugs for Erectile Dysfunction
Phosphodiesterase-5 Inhibitor
Sildenafil

Nonoral Drugs
Papaverine/phentolamine
Alprostadil

Drugs for Benign Prostatic Hyperplasia
5-α-Reductase Inhibitor
Finasteride

α-Adrenergic Antagonist
Tamsulosin

αBlockers. α-Adrenergic antagonists—including doxazosin (Cardura) and other α blockers used for prostatic hyperplasia (see later)—dilate arterioles and can thereby lower blood pressure. Combined use with sildenafil has caused symptomatic postural hypotension. Accordingly these combinations should be used with caution.

Inhibitors of CYP3A4. Inhibitors of CYP3A4 (e.g., ketoconazole, itraconazole, erythromycin, cimetidine, saquinavir, ritonavir, grapefruit juice) can suppress the metabolism of sildenafil, thereby increasing its level. These combinations should be used with caution.

Safety concerns for men with coronary heart disease. Reports of adverse cardiovascular events, including at least 130 cardiac deaths, raised concern about the safety of sildenafil in men with coronary heart disease (CHD). However, there was a question as to what caused the adverse events: sildenafil or the sexual activity that sildenafil permitted. As they attempted to answer this question, researchers made two important observations: First, giving sildenafil to resting men with severe CHD produced no harmful effects on coronary blood flow or any other hemodynamic parameter. Second, in men with stable CHD who were performing exercise, sildenafil had no effect on CHD symptoms, exercise tolerance, or exercise-induced ischemia. Taken together, these results suggest that in men with CHD, sexual activity—and not sildenafil—is the likely cause of ischemic events. However, even though sildenafil itself appears to be safe for men with CHD, sexual activity may not be. Accordingly the drug should be used with caution by men with the following conditions:

- Myocardial infarction, stroke, or life-threatening dysrhythmia within the last 6 months
- Resting hypotension (blood pressure below 90/50 mm Hg)
- Resting hypertension (blood pressure above 170/110 mm Hg)
- Heart failure
- Unstable angina

In addition, sildenafil should not be used at all by men taking nitroglycerin or any other drug in the nitrate family.

To reduce the risk for adverse events, candidates for sildenafil therapy should undergo a careful evaluation of cardiovascular function. Those with impaired function should be counseled about the risks posed by sexual activity and all other moderate to intense physical activity.

Vardenafil, Tadalafil, and Avanafil

Vardenafil, tadalafil, and avanafil are very similar to sildenafil. All three drugs inhibit PDE-5 and all three are approved for oral therapy of ED. Vardenafil is unique in that it prolongs the QT interval, and tadalafil is unique in that its effects last for 36 hours. Avanafil is unique in that it has the fastest onset of action. Otherwise the clinical effects of all four PDE-5 inhibitors appear to be about equal, although some patients may respond better to one than to the others. Properties of all four are shown in Table 53.3.

Vardenafil

Actions and use. Vardenafil (Levitra, Staxyn) was the second selective PDE-5 inhibitor approved for ED. As with sildenafil, benefits derive from relaxing arterial and trabecular smooth muscle in the penis. Effects begin about 60 minutes after dosing and persist about 4 hours. There is no evidence that vardenafil works faster, longer, or better than sildenafil.

Adverse effects. The most common adverse effects are headache, flushing, and rhinitis. Like other PDE-5 inhibitors, vardenafil can lower blood pressure. Like sildenafil, vardenafil can cause visual changes and has been associated with sudden hearing loss and vision loss from NAION.

Vardenafil can prolong the cardiac QT interval and might thereby pose a risk for serious dysrhythmias. However, dysrhythmias have not been reported. Nonetheless, to reduce risk, vardenafil should be used with caution in patients taking other drugs that cause QT prolongation.

Drug interactions. Vardenafil is contraindicated for use with α-adrenergic blockers and with nitroglycerin and other nitrates. Plasma levels can be increased by inhibitors of CYP3A4 (e.g., ketoconazole, ritonavir), hence such combinations must be used with caution. As noted, caution is needed in patients taking drugs that prolong the QT interval.

Tadalafil

Actions and use. Tadalafil (Cialis) was approved mere months after vardenafil. Like sildenafil and vardenafil, the drug is indicated for oral therapy of ED. As with other PDE-5 inhibitors, benefits derive from relaxation of penile arterial and trabecular smooth muscle brought on by accumulation of cGMP. On average, therapeutic levels of the drug are reached by 2 hours after dosing and persist for about 36 hours—much longer than with sildenafil or vardenafil. As a result, timing of dosing and sexual activity need not be tightly coupled. Furthermore, in addition to being approved for dosing as needed (similar to sildenafil and vardenafil), tadalafil is also approved for daily dosing (but only for men who anticipate sexual activity at least twice a week).

As discussed later in this chapter, tadalafil is also used for the treatment of benign prostatic hyperplasia (BPH). In addition, similar to sildenafil, tadalafil (sold as Adcirca) is used for the treatment of PAH.

Adverse effects. The most common adverse effects are headache, dyspepsia, back pain, myalgia, limb pain, flushing, and nasal congestion. As in the case of other PDE-5 inhibitors, tadalafil can lower blood pressure. Very rarely, the drug alters color vision. A few cases of NAION and sudden hearing loss have been reported, but a causal relationship has not been established. Because tadalafil has a long duration of action, adverse effects may persist for many hours.

Drug interactions. Tadalafil is contraindicated for use with nitrates or α blockers (except tamsulosin [Flomax]). As with sildenafil and vardenafil, CYP3A4 inhibitors can cause levels of tadalafil to rise. To avoid toxicity, men taking CYP3A4 inhibitors should limit tadalafil dosage to 10 mg every 72 hours.

"As needed" dosing. The manufacturer does not identify a minimum time between dosing and sexual activity. However, because blood levels peak more slowly than with sildenafil or vardenafil, allowing at least 1 hour for absorption would seem reasonable. Dosage should be reduced in men with moderate renal or hepatic insufficiency. Men with severe hepatic insufficiency should not use the drug. For men taking CYP3A4 inhibitors, the maximal dosage is 10 mg every 72 hours.

Daily dosing. Daily dosing is recommended only for men who anticipate sexual activity at least twice a week. The medication should be taken at the same time each day.

Avanafil

Actions and use. Avanafil (Stendra), approved in 2012, is the latest selective PDE-5 inhibitor approved for ED. Actions are the same as for the other PDE-5 inhibitors; however, effects begin about 15 minutes after dosing and last about 2 hours.

Adverse effects. Headache is the only adverse effect, occurring in at least 10% of patients. A few patients will experience flushing, nasal congestion, and nasopharyngitis. Similar to other PDE-5 inhibitors, avanafil can lower blood pressure.

Drug interactions. Avanafil is contraindicated for use with nitroglycerin and other nitrates. It can increase the hypotensive effects of alcohol and antihypertensive drugs, especially α-adrenergic antagonists. A starting dose of 50 mg (the lowest strength available) is recommended if the drug is prescribed for patients taking antihypertensive drugs. Plasma levels can be increased when the drug is taken with CYP3A4 inhibitors (e.g., ketoconazole, ritonavir, and erythromycin). For this reason dosing should not exceed 50 mg in 24 hours for patients taking CYP3A4 inhibitors.

Nonoral Drugs for Erectile Dysfunction

Unlike the PDE-5 inhibitors, which are administered orally, the drugs discussed in this section—alprostadil and papaverine/phentolamine—are administered by nonoral routes. Specifically they are administered either by injection into the penis or by insertion into the urethra. Because of this inconvenient method of dosing, these drugs are second-line agents for ED.

Alprostadil (Prostaglandin E₁)

Mechanism of action. Alprostadil's active ingredient has the same chemical structure as prostaglandin E_1 (PGE_1), which has vasodilating properties. Relaxation of smooth muscle (arterial, venous, and trabecular), causes a rapid inflow of arterial blood. As explained regarding the physiology of erection, the blood fills the vascular sinusoidal spaces of the corpus cavernosum, resulting in an erection. Pressure from the engorged penis helps block venous outflow to promote maintenance of the erect state.

Adverse effects. The most common adverse effect, a dull ache in the penis, occurs in 32% of users. Another 12% report urethral burning. Minor bleeding or spotting and testicular pain occur in about 5% of patients. Systemic symptoms are rare when the drug is taken as directed and approximate those of placebo use.

Transurethral. Alprostadil pellets (Muse), the only ED drug that is approved for twice-daily use, is inserted into the urethra. Administration is accomplished by loading a pellet into a small plastic applicator, which is then inserted 1½ inches into the urethra. Detailed instructions for insertion are available in the package insert. Both the package insert and a training video are available online at http://www.muserx.com/how-to-use-muse.

Erection develops 5 to 10 minutes after drug insertion and lasts 30 to 60 minutes. Dosage is determined in the provider's office; the objective is to employ the smallest dose required to produce an erection sufficient for intercourse.

Intracavernous. Alprostadil (Caverject, Caverject Impulse, Edex) is also available in a form for direct injection into the corpus cavernosum. A training video demonstrating how to inject the medication plus a link to access written instructions is available online at http://www.caverject.com/how-inject-caverject-impulse.

The response is rapid, and the injections are relatively painless. Optimal dosage is determined in the prescriber's office. The dosing end point is an erection that is sufficient for intercourse but that does not last for more than 1 hour. Injectable alprostadil should be used no more than three times a week and not more than once in 24 hours. Acute adverse effects are burning sensations, prolonged erection, and priapism. Penile fibrosis may develop with the continued use of injections; this complication has not been reported with the pellets.

Papaverine Plus Phentolamine

The combination of papaverine (a vasodilator) plus phentolamine (an α-adrenergic blocking agent) can provide tumescence (engorgement due to vascular congestion) when injected directly into the corpus cavernosum. Erection develops within 10 minutes and lasts 2 to 4 hours. In clinical trials, an erection suitable for intercourse was produced in 65% to 100% of males with ED of neurological or vascular origin.

Mechanism of action. As with the other drugs for ED, papaverine and phentolamine produce erection by increasing arterial inflow to the penis and decreasing venous outflow. Arterial inflow is augmented by α-adrenergic blockade (causing arterial dilation) and by the direct relaxant action of papaverine on arterial smooth muscle.

Adverse effects. Priapism occurs in about 10% of patients. Development of painless fibrotic nodules in the corpus cavernosum is common. Other adverse effects include orthostatic hypotension with dizziness, transient paresthesias, ecchymosis (extravasation of blood into subcutaneous tissue), and difficulty in achieving orgasm or ejaculation.

Papaverine and phentolamine are not approved by the FDA for treatment of erectile dysfunction, and many experts in the field do not recommend their use. As mentioned, there are some significant adverse effects. Also, these drugs come from compounding pharmacies. In light of numerous FDA recalls from compounding pharmacies in recent years, some providers have concerns about safety and quality issues as well.

Nonpharmacological Interventions for Erectile Dysfunction

Drug therapy does not benefit all patients. For these individuals, other options include vacuum-assisted devices, penile prostheses, revascularization surgery, and psychotherapy.

Vacuum-assisted devices promote erections by increasing arterial blood flow to the penis. Erections are maintained by applying a constrictive ring at the base of the penis to sustain engorgement. Penile prostheses come in two basic types: inserted rods, which result in a permanent erection; and inflatable prostheses that are inflated by use of a pump placed within the scrotum. Penile revascularization is less frequently used because good outcomes are low compared with other options. For those with erectile dysfunction related to psychological concerns (e.g., past sexual trauma, performance anxiety, relationship issues, depression), psychotherapy is an appropriate intervention.

Clinical Guidelines for the Management of Erectile Dysfunction

In 2018, the American Urological Association updated their clinical guidelines for male sexual dysfunction and erectile dysfunction. They are unique in that they do not begin with a trial of pharmacological interventions but rather offer all options, including surgery, as a first option (Fig. 53.2), guideline statements. These are available at http://www.auanet.org/guidelines/male-sexual-dysfunction-erectile-dysfunction-(2018).

The Canadian Urologic Association also developed and published updated clinical guidelines for treatment of erectile dysfunction. These guidelines offer a step-by-step process to guide management and adjustment of therapy and are available at http://www.ncbi.nlm.nih.gov/pmc/articles/PMC4336024/pdf/cuaj-1-2-23.pdf. Both guidelines are evidence-based.

SUMMARY OF KEY PRESCRIBING CONSIDERATIONS

Phosphodiesterase-5 Inhibitors

This summary pertains only to the use of PDE-5 inhibitors for ED, not for their use in PAH.

Therapeutic Goal: PDE-5 inhibitors are used to enhance both the hardness and duration of erection in men with ED.

Baseline Data: Heart rate, blood pressure. Thorough eye examination. Assess hearing. Evaluate patients for cardiovascular disorders, including stroke, hypotension, hypertension, heart failure, unstable angina, myocardial infarction, and recent history of a severe dysrhythmia.

Monitoring: Heart rate, blood pressure. Eye examination to include visual acuity, assessment of color vision, pupillary response, and fundoscopic exam. Assess for tinnitus, vertigo, and hearing loss. Assess for signs or symptoms of pulmonary edema.

Identifying High-Risk Patients: PDE-5 inhibitors are contraindicated for men taking nitrates (e.g., nitroglycerin) and should generally be avoided by men taking α blockers. Avoid vardenafil—but not sildenafil or tadalafil—in men taking class I or class III antidysrhythmic drugs.

For men with preexisting cardiovascular disease, consider carefully the cardiac risk associated with sexual activity before prescribing a PDE-5 inhibitor or any drug for ED. Use PDE-5 inhibitors with caution in men taking CYP3A4 inhibitors and in those with NAION, coronary heart disease, and other cardiovascular disorders.

Evaluating Therapeutic Effects: Evaluate patient satisfaction with therapy.

Minimizing Adverse Effects: Variability in response can be a problem if diet and timing are not considered. High-fat meals will delay absorption of avanafil, sildenafil, or vardenafil (but not tadalafil), thus delaying onset of action. Timing is important: Avanafil should be taken approximately 15–30 min before sexual activity. All other PDE-5 inhibitors should be taken about 1 h before sexual activity. Only tadalafil is approved for daily dosing.

Stress the importance of having an examination for development of vision or hearing changes. Explain that prolonged priapism lasting longer than 4 h is a surgical emergency; present to the local emergency department if this occurs.

PREMATURE EJACULATION

Defining Premature Ejaculation

Premature ejaculation is considered by many to be the most common type of male sexual dysfunction; however, this depends on how one defines PE. There are several definitions. The definition used by most lay people is simply ejaculation that occurs earlier than a man or his partner want it to occur. Using this definition, PE affects approximately 30% of the male population.

This definition was not sufficiently restrictive for research purposes; consequently, the International Society of Sexual Medicine (ISSM) proposed an operationalized definition that has become generally accepted. This definition includes three criteria for PE:

- Ejaculation that occurs before or within 1 minute of vaginal penetration[1] from the first sexual experience (lifelong PE) or within 2 to 3 minutes (acquired PE)
- An inability to delay ejaculation in all (or almost all) vaginal penetrations
- Psychological distress due to inability to delay ejaculation

Using these more restrictive criteria, approximately 4% of the male population has PE.

[1]The ISSM expert panel agreed that PE can occur in situations other than vaginal intercourse; however, the definition has not been changed

ERECTILE DYSFUNCTION ALGORITHM

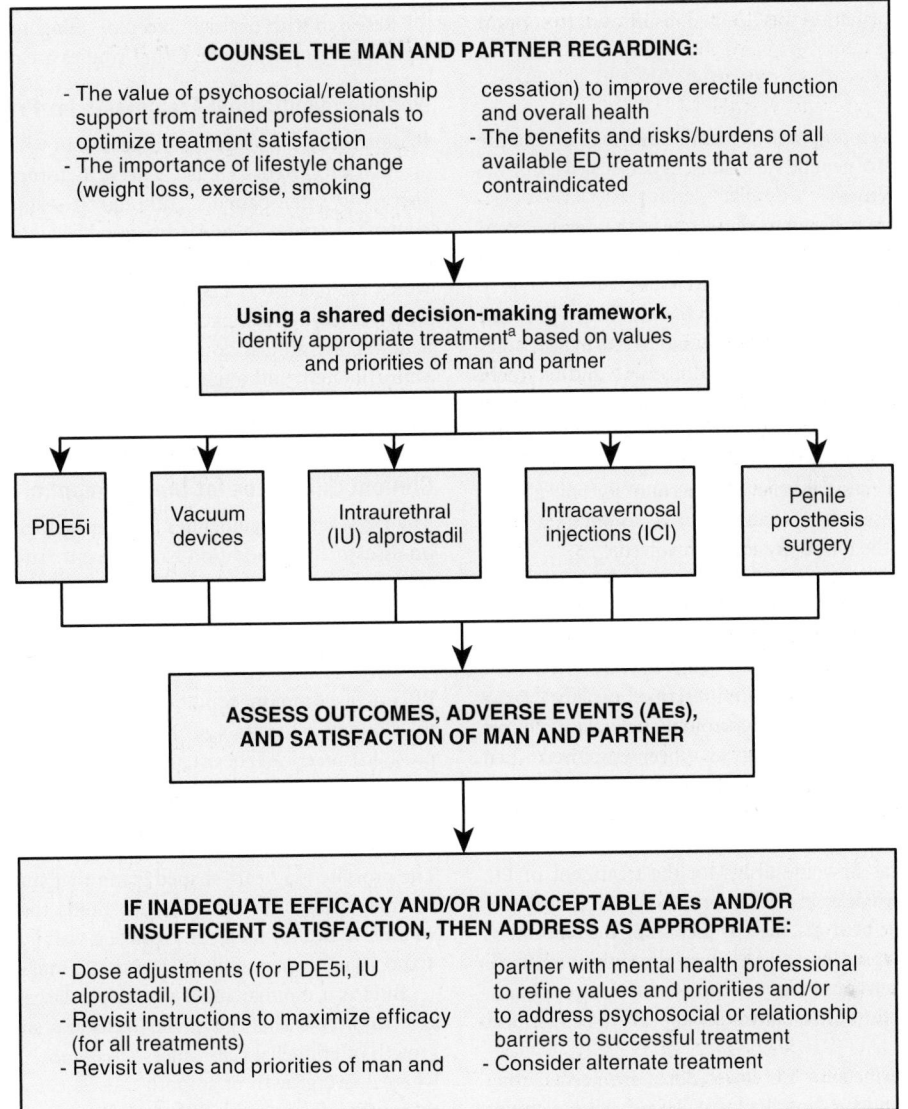

COUNSEL THE MAN AND PARTNER REGARDING:

- The value of psychosocial/relationship support from trained professionals to optimize treatment satisfaction
- The importance of lifestyle change (weight loss, exercise, smoking cessation) to improve erectile function and overall health
- The benefits and risks/burdens of all available ED treatments that are not contraindicated

Using a shared decision-making framework, identify appropriate treatment[a] based on values and priorities of man and partner

PDE5i

Vacuum devices

Intraurethral (IU) alprostadil

Intracavernosal injections (ICI)

Penile prosthesis surgery

ASSESS OUTCOMES, ADVERSE EVENTS (AEs), AND SATISFACTION OF MAN AND PARTNER

IF INADEQUATE EFFICACY AND/OR UNACCEPTABLE AEs AND/OR INSUFFICIENT SATISFACTION, THEN ADDRESS AS APPROPRIATE:

- Dose adjustments (for PDE5i, IU alprostadil, ICI)
- Revisit instructions to maximize efficacy (for all treatments)
- Revisit values and priorities of man and partner with mental health professional to refine values and priorities and/or to address psychosocial or relationship barriers to successful treatment
- Consider alternate treatment

[a]For men with testosterone deficiency, defined as the presence of symptoms and signs and a total testosterone <300 ng/dl, counseling should emphasize that restoration of testosterone levels to theraputic levels is likely to increase efficacy of ED treatments other than prosthesis surgery.

Fig. 53.2 American Urological Association: Management of Erectile Dysfunction. *ED*, Erectile dysfunction; *PDE-5*, phosphodiesterase type 5; (From Burnett AL, Nehra A, Breau RH, et al. *2018 Erectile Dysfunction: AUA Guideline (2018)*. American Urological Association; http://www.auanet.org/Documents/Guidelines/PDF/ED%20Algorithm.pdf; Clinical guidelines at http://www.auanet.org/guidelines/male-sexual-dysfunction-erectile-dysfunction-(2018).)

due to inconsistent correlations between vaginal intercourse, oral sex, and masturbation. They did not include penetration occurring between men because available information was deemed insufficient to support its inclusion.

Pathophysiology

Several suggestions have been proposed as possible causes of premature ejaculation. Among these are genetic variations, hypersensitivity of the glans penis, and overexcitement.

Psychological factors are believed to play a role in the development and persistence of PE. These factors include performance anxiety, body image concerns, and interpersonal relationship issues.

The role of neurotransmitter dysregulation has also been proposed as a possible cause of PE. Serotonin, dopamine, and oxytoxin have roles in ejaculation. Serotonin delays ejaculation; dopamine and oxytocin are believed to stimulate ejaculation. Consequently alterations in neurotransmitter synthesis and release or alterations in neurotransmitter receptor sensitivity may play a role in PE.

Each of these proposed causes is believed to account for only a small percentage of PE. More research is needed in order to obtain a more precise understanding of the pathophysiology involved.

Drug Therapy for Premature Ejaculation

PE is managed with psychotherapy, behavioral therapy, medications, or a combination of these modalities. No drugs have received FDA approval for treatment of PE, so drugs are prescribed off label. Drug therapy typically includes the use of selective serotonin reuptake inhibitors (SSRIs) or topical anesthetics. Other drugs have been employed when these are ineffective.

Selective Serotonin Reuptake Inhibitors

SSRIs are recommended as first-line drugs for the treatment of PE. Recall that serotonin causes a delay in ejaculation. SSRIs prevent reuptake of serotonin by presynaptic neurons, thereby increasing the amount of serotonin in neuronal synapses. As a result, more serotonin is available to stimulate postsynaptic serotonin receptors, thus enhancing serotonin neurotransmission. Of all the SSRIs, paroxetine appears to be the most effective.

When SSRIs are prescribed for PE, lower doses are needed than when they are prescribed for depression. Typical daily dosing is citalopram (Celexa) 20 to 40 mg, fluoxetine (Prozac, Sarafem) 20 to 40 mg, paroxetine (Brisdelle, Paxil, Paxil CR, Pexeva) 10 to 40 mg, and sertraline (Zoloft) 50 to 200 mg. With daily dosing, it takes about 2 to 3 weeks before most patients achieve maximal response. SSRIs are discussed in depth in Chapter 27.

Topical Anesthetics

Topical anesthetics such as lidocaine (Maxilene) and prilocaine (Citanext Plain Dental, an anesthetic commonly used in dental procedures) decrease sensitivity of the glans penis. Although this is effective in some cases, it presents a problem in that it may be transferred to the partner. In women, this transfer results in vaginal numbness and, not surprisingly, delay in orgasm. For this reason, desensitizing agents should be used with a condom.

Other Drugs

Clomipramine (Anafranil), a tricyclic antidepressant that affects serotonin uptake, has demonstrated success and is considered a second-line drug when SSRIs cannot be taken. When used, dosage is 12.5 to 50 mg daily.

Tramadol, an opioid analgesic, has demonstrated positive results in several studies. Unfortunately the risk of addiction and harmful adverse effects make it less attractive. Opioids are discussed in Chapter 24.

Sometimes PE accompanies ED. PDE-5 inhibitors have shown success in these instances.

Research with oxytocin receptor antagonists has not demonstrated significant improvement. Other studies are ongoing.

Nonpharmacological Treatments for Premature Ejaculation

Radiofrequency ablation, a procedure in which a radio wave produces an electrical current to "burn" a nerve to disrupt signals, has demonstrated success in some patients. Although it seems promising, randomized controlled trials are needed to establish utility. Needless to say, it is challenging to recruit subjects into a randomized controlled trial in which the placebo is a sham ablation procedure.

In a study comparing acupuncture with sham acupuncture, acupuncture almost doubled the amount of time before ejaculation. Unfortunately, although the increase was significant, the amount of time to ejaculation was only 65.7 seconds compared to with 33.1 seconds.

Clinical Guidelines for Management of Premature Ejaculation

The ISSM clinical guidelines for management of PE include guidance on assessment in addition to treatment. These are available at http://www.issm.info/images/uploads/PE_Guidelines_v12_-_FEB_2014.pdf/

BENIGN PROSTATIC HYPERPLASIA

BPH is a common condition that develops in more than 50% of men by age 60 years and 90% by age 85 years. Although BPH and prostate cancer can coexist, there is no evidence that one predisposes to the other.

Pathophysiology

The prostate is a heart-shaped gland that surrounds the male urethra. Its major function is to produce fluids that contribute to ejaculate volume. In healthy men, the prostate is walnut-sized and weighs between 4 and 20 g. In men with BPH, prostate mass may reach 50 to 80 g.

BPH is a nonmalignant prostate enlargement caused by excessive growth of epithelial (glandular) cells and smooth muscle cells. Overgrowth of epithelial cells causes *mechanical obstruction* of the urethra, whereas overgrowth of smooth muscle causes *dynamic obstruction* of the urethra. In men with BPH, the ratio of epithelium to smooth muscle varies from 1:3 to 4:1; in general, the larger the prostate, the higher the percentage of epithelium.

Signs and symptoms of BPH include urinary hesitancy, urinary urgency, increased frequency of urination, dysuria, nocturia, straining to void, postvoid dribbling, decreased force and caliber of the urinary stream, and a sensation of incomplete bladder emptying. There is no direct correlation between symptoms and prostate size. Therefore some men with only moderate enlargement may be highly symptomatic, whereas others with substantial enlargement may have no symptoms. Long-term complications of BPH include obstructive nephropathy, bladder stones, and recurrent urinary tract infections.

Treatment Modalities

BPH can be managed in three ways: invasive treatments, drug therapy, and "watchful waiting." Invasive options include transurethral resection of the prostate, laser prostatectomy, transurethral electrovaporization of the prostate, and transurethral microwave therapy. These procedures are most appropriate for men with severe symptoms or complications. Drugs are indicated for men with moderate symptoms. Watchful waiting, which consists of annual reevaluation with reconsideration of management based on results, is appropriate for men with minimal symptoms.

Drug Therapy for Benign Prostatic Hyperplasia

BPH can be treated with two major classes of drugs: *5-α-reductase inhibitors* and *α₁-adrenergic antagonists*. With both the goal is to relieve bothersome urinary symptoms and delay disease progression. The 5-α-reductase inhibitors are most appropriate for men with very large prostates (mechanical obstruction), whereas α blockers are preferred for men with relatively small prostates (dynamic obstruction). Major drugs for BPH are shown in Tables 53.4 and 53.5. Preparation and dosing of drugs for BPH is provided in Table 53.5.

5-α-Reductase Inhibitors

Two 5-α-reductase inhibitors are available: finasteride and dutasteride. Both drugs can reduce prostate size, although several months are required for a noticeable effect. There is no proof that one drug works better than the other.

Finasteride

Mechanism of action. Finasteride (Proscar) acts in reproductive tissue to inhibit 5-α-reductase, an enzyme that converts testosterone to dihydrotestosterone (DHT), the active form of testosterone in the prostate. Treatment reduces levels of DHT in blood by 70% (but does not decrease testosterone levels). By decreasing DHT availability, finasteride promotes regression of prostate epithelial tissue and thereby decreases *mechanical obstruction* of the urethra. Because the percentage of epithelial tissue is highest in very large prostates, finasteride is most effective in men whose prostates are highly enlarged. Conversely, the drug confers less benefit if the degree of enlargement is small. One should be aware that prostate shrinkage occurs slowly—over a period of 6 to 12 months.

Adverse reactions. By reducing levels of DHT, finasteride can protect against prostate cancer—but only cancers classified as low grade. Finasteride does not protect against high-grade prostate cancer. In fact, when given to healthy men to prevent prostate cancer, finasteride actually *increased* the likelihood of a high-grade tumor. Accordingly, the Oncologic Drugs Advisory Committee of the FDA recommends against allowing the manufacturer to label finasteride as a drug for prostate cancer prevention.

Finasteride is generally well tolerated. However, in 5% to 10% of patients, it decreases ejaculate volume and libido. In addition, gynecomastia develops in some men.

Finasteride is teratogenic to the male fetus; therefore it is contraindicated for women who are pregnant or may become pregnant. In addition, because finasteride can be absorbed through the skin, pregnant women should not handle tablets that have been broken or crushed. Men are also advised not to donate blood if taking finasteride or until at least 1 month after stopping the drug to avoid the risk of having a pregnant woman as the blood recipient.

Finasteride decreases serum levels of prostate-specific antigen (PSA), a marker for prostate cancer. The expected decline is 30% to 50%. PSA levels should be determined before treatment and 6 months later. If PSA levels do not fall as expected, the patient should be evaluated for cancer of the prostate.

Preparation and dosage of 5-α-reductase inhibitors are provided in Table 53.5. For treatment of BPH, therapy continues for life. As discussed in Chapter 88, the drug is also available in 1-mg tablets, sold as *Propecia*, for treatment of male-pattern baldness.

Dutasteride. Dutasteride (Avodart) is similar to finasteride in most respects. However, there are two important differences. First, with dutasteride, the reduction in circulating DHT is more complete.

TABLE 53.4 Drugs for Benign Prostatic Hyperplasia

Generic Name	Trade Name	Actions in BPH	Adverse Effects
5-α-Reductase Inhibitors			
Dutasteride	Avodart	Reduce dihydrotestosterone production, which causes the prostate to shrink, which reduces mechanical obstruction of the urethra. May also delay BPH progression. Benefits take months to develop.	Decreased ejaculate volume and libido. Teratogenic to the male fetus.
Finasteride	Proscar		
α₁ Blockers			
Selective α₁ₐ Blockers			
Silodosin	Rapaflo	Blockade of α₁ₐ receptors relaxes smooth muscle in the bladder neck, prostate capsule, and prostatic urethra, and thereby decreases dynamic obstruction of the urethra. Benefits develop rapidly.	Abnormal ejaculation (ejaculation failure, reduced ejaculate volume, retrograde ejaculation). Risk of floppy-iris syndrome during cataract surgery.
Tamsulosin	Flomax		
Nonselective α₁ Blockers			
Alfuzosin	Uroxatral, Xatral ♦	Same as the selective α₁ₐ blockers.	Hypotension, fainting, dizziness, somnolence, and nasal congestion (from blocking α₁ receptors on blood vessels)
Doxazosin	Cardura, Cardura XL		
Terazosin	Hytrin		
Phosphodiesterase-5 Inhibitor			
Tadalafil	Cialis	Smooth muscle relaxation in the bladder, prostate, and urethra.	Hypotension, priapism
α₁ₐ Blocker/5-α-Reductase Inhibitor			
Tamsulosin/ dutasteride	Jalyn	Combination of the effects of 5-α-reductase inhibitors and selective α₁ₐ blockers	Decreased libido and abnormal ejaculation (ejaculation failure, reduced ejaculate volume, retrograde ejaculation)

BPH, Benign prostatic hyperplasia.

TABLE 53.5 Drugs for Benign Prostatic Hyperplasia: Preparations and Dosage

Drug Class and Drug	Preparation	Dosage for BPH	Considerations
α₁-Adrenergic Antagonists			
Alfuzosin (Uroxatral, Xatral)	ER Tablet: 10 mg	10 mg once daily.	
Doxazosin (Cardura, Cardura XL)	IR Tablet: 1, 2, 4, 8 mg (scored) ER Tablet: 4 and 8 mg	IR Tablet: 1 mg once daily. May increase gradually to a maximum of 8 mg once daily. ER Tablet: 4 mg once daily. May increase to 8 mg once daily.	
Silodosin (Rapaflo)	Capsule: 4 and 8 mg	8 mg once daily. Reduce to 4 mg once daily with moderate renal impairment. Contraindicated in severe renal or hepatic impairment.	
Terazosin (Hytrin)	Capsule: 1, 2, 5, 10 mg Tablet: 1, 2, 5, 10 mg	Initial: 1 mg once daily Typical: 10 mg once daily. Maximum: 20 mg once daily.	
Tamsulosin (Flomax)	Capsule: 0.4 mg	0.4 mg once daily May increase to 0.8 mg daily.	
5-α-Reductase Inhibitors			
Dutasteride (Avodart)	Capsule: 0.5 mg	0.5 mg once a day	
Finasteride (Proscar)	Tablets: 5 mg	5 mg once a day	
Phosphodiesterase-5 Inhibitor			
Tadalafil (Cialis)	Tablets: 2.5, 5, 10, 20 mg	5 mg once a day If taking an α blocker, dosing should start at 2.5 mg once a day, and then increase to 5 mg once a day as needed and tolerated.	
Combination Products: α₁-Adrenergic Antagonist plus 5-α-Reductase Inhibitor			
Tamsulosin plus dutasteride (Jalyn)	Capsule: Tamsulosin 0.4 mg plus dutasteride 0.5 mg	1 capsule daily	

BPH, Benign prostatic hyperplasia; *ER,* extended release; *IR,* immediate release.

Second, dutasteride has an extremely long half-life (about 5 weeks); therefore it takes months to clear the drug after dosing has stopped.

Mechanism of action. Similar to finasteride, dutasteride inhibits 5-α-reductase and thereby suppresses production of DHT. However, whereas finasteride inhibits only the form of 5-α-reductase found in reproductive tissues, dutasteride also inhibits the form found in the skin and liver. As a result, dutasteride produces a greater reduction in circulating DHT (93% vs. 70%). Whether this translates to a greater clinical response has not been established because dutasteride and finasteride have not been directly compared. However, an examination of data from separate (non-comparative) clinical trials found both drugs produced a significant reduction in the size of the prostate gland, coupled with decreased symptoms and improved long-term outcomes.

Adverse effects. Dutasteride is generally well tolerated. However, similar to finasteride, dutasteride reduces ejaculate volume and libido in some men and causes a decline in PSA in all men.

Dutasteride is teratogenic. It can be absorbed through the skin, so pregnant women should not handle the drug. Men should not donate blood while using dutasteride or for at least 6 months after stopping it to avoid transmission to women through administration of blood products.

Like finasteride, dutasteride can reduce the likelihood of a low-grade prostate tumor, but it increases the likelihood of a high-grade prostate tumor. Accordingly, the drug should not be used for prostate cancer prevention.

Although many capsules can be opened and sprinkled on food, this is not the case with dutasteride. The capsule contents can be irritating to the oropharyngeal mucosa; therefore the capsule must be swallowed whole with a full glass of water.

📄 SUMMARY OF KEY PRESCRIBING CONSIDERATIONS

5-α Reductase-Inhibitors

Therapeutic Goal: Reduction in prostate size relieves symptoms of bladder outlet obstruction

Baseline Data: PSA

Monitoring: Repeat PSA at 6 months; if there is no decrease, evaluate for prostate cancer. Repeat PSA periodically.

Identifying High-Risk Patients: Do not prescribe for patients suspected to have prostate cancer

Evaluating Therapeutic Effects: Anticipate symptom improvement after 6–12 months.

Minimizing Adverse Effects: The most common adverse effect is sexual dysfunction. Because these changes can be permanent, the patient should return for possible dosage adjustment or change in medications if this concerns the patient.

α₁-Adrenergic Antagonists

Five α₁ blockers are approved for BPH: alfuzosin (Uroxatral, Xatral), terazosin (Hytrin), doxazosin (Cardura), silodosin (Rapaflo), and tamsulosin (Flomax). These drugs have not been directly compared in clinical trials, so we cannot say whether one is more effective than the others. However, two newer ones—silodosin and tamsulosin—may be better tolerated. The pharmacology of these drugs is discussed in Chapter 16. Discussion here is limited to their use in BPH.

Mechanism of action. Blockade of α₁ receptors relaxes smooth muscle in the bladder neck (trigone and sphincter), prostate capsule, and prostatic urethra, thereby decreasing *dynamic obstruction* of the urethra. Symptomatic improvement and increased urinary flow develop *rapidly*. Because dynamic obstruction is the major contributor to symptoms in patients with relatively mild prostatic enlargement, α blockers are preferred to 5-α-reductase inhibitors for these men. To maintain benefits, α blockers must be taken lifelong. Unlike the 5-α-reductase inhibitors, the α_1 blockers do not reduce prostate size.

Receptor specificity and impact on blood pressure. The α blockers differ regarding specificity of receptor blockade and resultant effect on blood pressure. Specifically, whereas silodosin and tamsulosin are *selective for α_{1a} receptors* (the type of α_1 receptors found in the prostate), alfuzosin, terazosin, and doxazosin are *nonselective α_1 blockers* and hence block α_1 receptors in blood vessels as well as α_{1a} receptors in the prostate. By blocking α_1 receptors in blood vessels, the three nonselective agents promote vasodilation and can thereby lower blood pressure. In fact, two of these drugs—doxazosin and terazosin—were developed as antihypertensive agents; their use in BPH came later. Because of their effect on blood pressure, the nonselective α_1 blockers are especially useful for patients who have hypertension in addition to BPH but may be dangerous for men with reduced blood pressure. Conversely, because silodosin and tamsulosin have little or no effect on blood pressure, they are of no benefit to men with hypertension but are preferred if reducing blood pressure would be a problem.

PATIENT-CENTERED CARE ACROSS THE LIFE SPAN

Drugs for Benign Prostatic Hyperplasia

Life Stage	Considerations or Concerns
Children	These drugs are not approved for children.
Pregnant women	The α1-adrenergic antagonists are considered relatively safe during pregnancy with the exception of doxazosin and terazosin. Animal reproduction studies have identified adverse effects with doxazosin and, at high doses, with terazosin. Finasteride and dutasteride are teratogens; they cause feminization of the male fetus. Because these drugs can be absorbed through the skin, pregnant women should not handle finasteride or dutasteride tablets that have been broken or crushed. Men taking finasteride or dutasteride should not donate blood to avoid the risk of exposing a pregnant recipient. To donate blood after stopping the drug, a wait of at least 1 month is required after stopping finasteride and at least 6 months after stopping dutasteride.
Breast-feeding women	It is not known if 5-α-reductase inhibitors are excreted in breast milk. Women taking these drugs for off-label uses (e.g., hirsutism) should not breastfeed.
Older adults	Beers Criteria includes the peripheral α-1 blockers doxazosin and terazosin among its listing of potentially inappropriate medications for patients age 65 and older.

Adverse effects. The α_1 blockers are generally well tolerated. For the nonselective agents (alfuzosin, doxazosin, and terazosin), principal adverse effects are hypotension, fainting, dizziness, somnolence, and nasal congestion. Because *silodosin* and *tamsulosin* have minimal effects on vascular smooth muscle, these drugs are less likely to cause hypotension, fainting, dizziness, or nasal congestion. However, silodosin and tamsulosin *can* cause abnormal ejaculation (ejaculation failure, reduced volume, retrograde ejaculation), whereas the nonselective agents do

not. In contrast to dutasteride and finasteride, the α blockers do not reduce levels of PSA.

For men undergoing cataract surgery, α blockade increases the risk for intraoperative *floppy-iris syndrome,* a complication that can increase postoperative pain, delay recovery, and reduce the hoped-for improvement in vision acuity. In severe cases, the syndrome can cause defects to the iris that may lead to blindness. Men anticipating cataract surgery should postpone α blocker therapy until after the procedure. Men already taking an α blocker should be sure to tell their ophthalmologist.

Drug interactions. Exercise caution when nonselective α blockers are being combined with other drugs that lower blood pressure; excessive hypotension could result. Drugs of concern include organic nitrates (e.g., nitroglycerin), antihypertensive drugs, and PDE-5 inhibitors used for ED (e.g., sildenafil [Viagra]).

Strong inhibitors of CYP3A4—such as erythromycin, itraconazole, nefazodone, and HIV protease inhibitors (e.g., ritonavir)—can dramatically increase levels of alfuzosin and silodosin. Accordingly alfuzosin and silodosin must not be combined with these drugs.

Use in women. Tamsulosin and other α blockers are being used off label to treat women with urinary hesitancy or urinary retention associated with bladder outlet obstruction or insufficient contraction of the bladder detrusor muscle. Benefits derive from relaxing smooth muscle in the bladder neck and urethra. Maximal improvement may take several weeks to develop.

α_1 Blocker/5-α-Reductase Inhibitor Combination

In clinical trials, combining an α blocker with a 5-α-reductase inhibitor has been superior to treatment with either agent alone. Because α blockers and 5-α-reductase inhibitors work by different mechanisms, it is not surprising that combining them can be helpful: the α blocker can provide rapid symptomatic relief (by relaxing prostate-related smooth muscle) while, over time, the 5-α-reductase inhibitor can provide additional symptomatic relief (by shrinking the prostate) and may also delay disease progression.

Research has demonstrated effectiveness with tamsulosin plus dutasteride and doxazosin plus finasteride. Presumably, other combinations of an α blocker with a 5-α-reductase inhibitor would also be effective. If a single dose is preferred, tamsulosin plus dutasteride (Jalyn) is available.

Tadalafil, a PDE-5 Inhibitor

Tadalafil (Cialis) is approved for men who have BPH by itself or BPH combined with ED. In men with BPH, tadalafil produces a modest decrease in symptoms (urinary frequency, urinary urgency, straining) but does not improve urinary flow rate. Furthermore, only 1 in 6 men benefit. Initial improvement is seen in 2 weeks. How does tadalafil help? Possibly by relaxing smooth muscle in the prostate, bladder, and urethra. Although tadalafil is the only PDE-5 inhibitor approved for ED, other PDE-5 inhibitors can reduce symptoms too. Owing to the risk for hypotension, tadalafil should be used with caution in men taking an α blocker and should be avoided in men taking nitrates.

Other Drugs for Benign Prostatic Hyperplasia

Anticholinergics. Symptoms of overactive bladder (OAB), such as urgency and frequency, are often experienced by men with BPH. Anticholinergic drugs (specifically antimuscarinics) are helpful when this occurs. Those approved for OAB include darifenacin, fesoterodine, oxybutynin, solifenacin, tolterodine, and trospium. These may be used alone or in combination with an α blocker such as tamsulosin to improve urinary symptoms (see Chapter 14).

Botulinum toxin. Botulinum toxin (Botox, others), a well-known remedy for facial wrinkles, can also help men with BPH. A single injection into the prostate can relieve urinary symptoms for up to 1 year. Benefits derive in part from blocking the release of acetylcholine from neurons that innervate urinary tract smooth muscle. However, because the drug also reduces both prostate size and blood levels of PSA, other mechanisms must also be involved.

Complementary and Alternative Medication for Benign Prostatic Hyperplasia

Saw palmetto is an herbal preparation used widely to treat BPH despite numerous randomized control trials (RCTs) refuting the findings of earlier less rigorous studies. In 2012 a Cochrane review of 32 RCTs involving 5666 men found no significant difference between saw palmetto and a placebo even at doses two and three times the usual dose.

What about other CAMs? In their latest clinical guidelines, the American Urological Association declined to recommend any dietary supplement or herbal treatment, including saw palmetto, until there is a sufficient body of evidence from rigorous clinical trials to support their use.

Review of the Immune System

The immune system protects us from invading organisms (viruses, bacteria, fungi, and parasites) and can destroy cancer cells before they destroy us. Unfortunately, the immune system does not always act in our best interest: it can attack transplanted organs and tissues and can turn on the cells it normally protects.

To study the immune system, we begin with an overview. After that, we discuss the two major types of specific immune responses: antibody-mediated immunity (humoral immunity) and cell-mediated immunity.

INTRODUCTION TO THE IMMUNE SYSTEM

Our objective in this section is to establish an overview of immune system components and how they function. Much of the information introduced here is amplified later.

Natural Immunity Versus Specific Acquired Immunity

Our bodies can mount two types of immune responses, referred to as *natural immunity* (innate or native immunity) and *specific acquired immunity*. Factors that confer natural immunity include physical barriers (e.g., skin), phagocytic cells, and natural killer cells. All of these factors are present before exposure to a particular infectious agent, and all respond nonspecifically. In contrast, specific acquired immune responses occur only after exposure to a foreign substance. The foreign substances that induce specific responses are called *antigens,* and the objective of the immune response is to destroy them. With each succeeding reexposure to a particular antigen, the specific immune response to that antigen becomes more rapid and more intense. Specific immune responses are possible because certain cells of the immune system (T lymphocytes and B lymphocytes) possess receptors that can recognize individual antigens. Our focus here is on specific acquired immunity, not on natural immunity.

Cell-Mediated Immunity Versus Antibody-Mediated (Humoral) Immunity

Specific acquired immune responses can be classified as either cell mediated or humoral. *Cell-mediated immunity* refers to immune responses in which targets are attacked directly by immune system cells—specifically, cytolytic T cells and macrophages. *Humoral immunity* refers to immune responses that are mediated by *antibodies.* (The term *humoral*—defined as "pertaining to elements dissolved in blood or body fluids"—connotes that antibodies dissolved in the blood.)

Introduction to Cells of the Immune System

Immune responses are mediated by several types of cells, some of which play a bigger role than others. The major actors are the *lymphocytes* (B cells, cytolytic T cells, helper T cells), *macrophages,* and *dendritic cells.* Accessory cells include neutrophils and basophils. With the exception of some dendritic cells, all of the cells involved in the immune response arise from pluripotent stem cells in the bone marrow (Fig. 54.1) and, for at least part of their life cycle, circulate in the blood. Defining characteristics of individual immune system cells are shown in Table 54.1.

B Lymphocytes (B Cells)

B lymphocytes have the job of making *antibodies.* Hence B cells mediate humoral immunity. As discussed later, antibody specificity is determined by the structure of highly specific receptors found on the surface of B cells. Like all other lymphocytes, B cells circulate in the blood and lymph. B cells are so named because in chickens, where B cells were discovered, these cells are produced in the *bursa of Fabricius,* a structure not found in mammals. In humans and other mammals, B cells are produced in the bone marrow.

Cytolytic T Lymphocytes (Cytolytic T Cells, CD8 Cells)

Cytolytic T cells are key players in cellular immunity. These cells do not produce antibodies. Rather, they attack and kill target cells directly. Specificity of attack is determined by the presence of antigen molecules on the surface of the target cell and specific receptors for that antigen on the surface of the T cell. Cytolytic T cells are also known as *CD8 cells* and *cytotoxic T cells.* The designation "CD8" refers to the presence of cell-surface marker molecules known as *cell differentiation complex 8.* The "T" in T cell stands for thymus, the organ in which cytolytic T cells and helper T cells mature. Like B cells, cytolytic T cells circulate in the blood and lymph.

Helper T Lymphocytes (Helper T Cells, CD4 Cells)

Helper T cells contribute to the immune response in three ways: (1) they have an essential role in antibody production by B cells; (2) they release factors that promote type IV sensitivity reactions, also known as delayed-type hypersensitivity (DTH); and (3) they participate in the activation of cytolytic T cells. Specificity of helper T cells is achieved through highly specific cell-surface receptors that recognize individual antigens. Like other lymphocytes, helper T cells circulate in the blood and lymph. Helper T cells carry CD4 (cell differentiation complex 4) marker molecules on their surface and hence are referred to as *CD4 cells.*

467

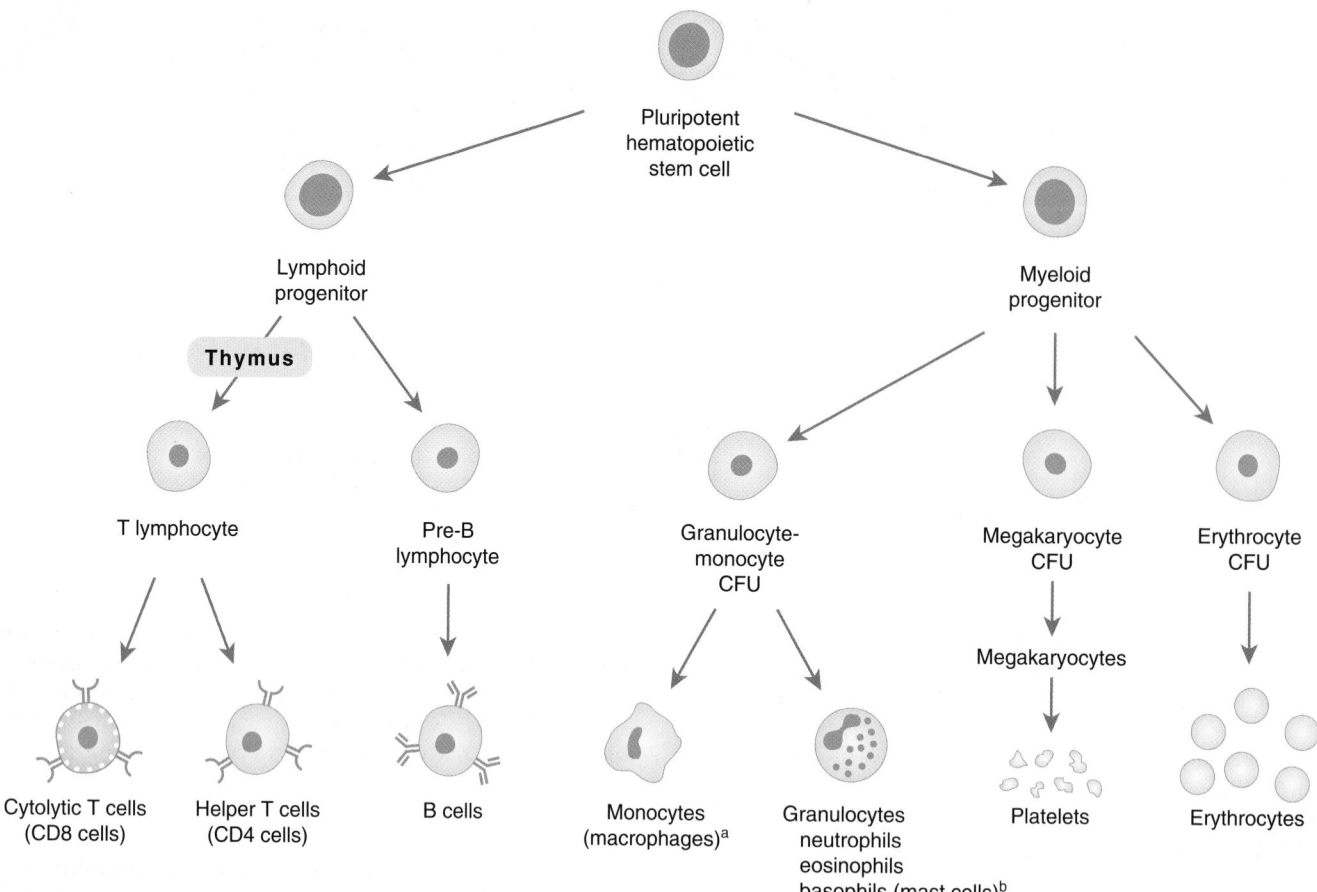

Fig. 54.1 Maturation of Blood Cells. With the exception of platelets and erythrocytes, all of the mature blood cells shown participate in immune responses. However, only cells of lymphoid origin (cytolytic T cells, helper T cells, B cells) possess receptors that can recognize specific antigens. Monocytes that have moved into tissues are called macrophages. [a]Basophils that have moved into tissues are called mast cells. [b]*CFU*, Colony-forming unit.

TABLE 54.1	Cells of the Immune System	
Cell Type	**Synonyms**	**Primary Immune-Related Actions**
Major Cell Types		
B lymphocytes	B cells	• Produce antibodies
CTLs	Cytolytic T cells, cytotoxic T cells, CD8 cells	• Lyse target cells
Helper T lymphocytes	Helper T cells, CD4 cells	• Promote proliferation and differentiation of B cells and CTLs
		• Initiate delayed-type hypersensitivity
Macrophages		• Promote proliferation and differentiation of helper T cells and CTLs by serving as APCs
		• Participate in delayed-type hypersensitivity
		• Phagocytize cells tagged with antibodies
		• Phagocytize cells in the effector stage of delayed-type hypersensitivity
Dendritic cells		• Promote proliferation of CTLs and helper T cells by serving as APCs
Accessory Cells		
Mast cells		• Mediate immediate hypersensitivity reactions
Basophils		• Mediate immediate hypersensitivity reactions
Neutrophils	Polymorphonuclear leukocytes	• Phagocytize foreign particles (e.g., bacteria), especially those tagged with IgG
		• Mediate inflammation
Eosinophils		• Attack helminths and foreign particles that have been coated with IgE
		• Contribute to immediate hypersensitivity reactions

APC, Antigen-presenting cell; *CTL,* cytolytic T lymphocyte; *Ig,* immunoglobulin.

Fig. 54.2 Antibody Structure. The basic antibody structure depicting heavy and light chains is shown on the left. Variable regions of the heavy and light chains, which form the antigen-binding site, appear in green. As shown on the right, papain digestion of antibodies produces two types of fragments: Fab fragments, which retain the ability to bind antigen; and Fc fragments, which do not bind antigen and tend to crystallize in the test tube.

The term *helper* is somewhat misleading in that it connotes a useful but dispensable role. Nothing could be further from reality. Helper T cells are not simply nice to have around; they are absolutely required for an effective immune response. The critical nature of their contribution—and the grim consequences of their absence—are manifested in people with human immunodeficiency virus (HIV)/acquired immunodeficiency syndrome (AIDS): helper T cells are the immune cells that HIV attacks. Because of helper T cell loss, AIDS patients are at high risk for death from opportunistic infection.

Macrophages

Macrophages begin their existence in the bone marrow, enter the blood as monocytes, and then infiltrate tissues, where they evolve into macrophages. Macrophages are present in all organs and tissues.

The primary function of macrophages is *phagocytosis* (i.e., ingestion of microbes, other foreign material, and cellular debris). In their role as phagocytes, macrophages are the principal scavengers of the body. Although their major job is phagocytosis, macrophages also have an important role in specific acquired immunity, natural immunity, and inflammation.

In specific acquired immunity, macrophages have three functions: (1) they are required for activation of T cells (both helper T cells and cytolytic T cells), (2) they are the final mediators of DTH, and (3) they phagocytize cells that have been tagged with antibodies. Of these three immune-related roles, activation of T cells is arguably the most critical. When performing this function, macrophages are referred to as *antigen-presenting cells* (APCs). Because antigen presentation is an absolute requirement for specific immune responses (see later), you can appreciate how important macrophages are.

Dendritic Cells

Dendritic cells perform the same antigen-presenting task as do macrophages. However, unlike macrophages, dendritic cells do not also serve as scavengers. Dendritic cells are found in lymph nodes and other lymphoid tissues.

Mast Cells and Basophils

These cells mediate immediate hypersensitivity reactions. Mast cells, which are derived from basophils, are concentrated in the skin and other soft tissues. Basophils circulate in the blood. Both cell types release histamine, heparin, and other compounds that cause the symptoms of immediate hypersensitivity. Release of these mediators is triggered when an antigen binds to antibodies on the cell surface. The role of mast cells and basophils in allergic reactions is discussed in Chapter 63.

Neutrophils

Neutrophils, also known as polymorphonuclear leukocytes, phagocytize bacteria and other foreign particles. As discussed later, neutrophils avidly devour cells that have tagged with antibodies of the immunoglobulin G (IgG) class. Accordingly, neutrophils can be viewed as important effectors in humoral immunity. Neutrophils are also major contributors to inflammation.

Eosinophils

Eosinophils attack and destroy foreign particles that have been coated with antibodies of the IgE class. Their usual target is helminths (parasitic worms). Eosinophils also contribute to tissue injury and inflammation associated with immediate hypersensitivity reactions.

Antibodies

Antibodies are a family of structurally related glycoproteins that mediate humoral immunity. The most characteristic feature of antibodies is their ability to recognize and bind with specific antigens. Alternative names for antibodies are *immunoglobulins* and *globulins*.

All antibodies are produced by B lymphocytes. Some of the antibodies that B cells produce are retained on the surface of the B cell, where they serve as the receptors whereby B cells recognize specific antigens. However, most of the antibodies that B cells produce are secreted from the cell, after which they bind to their specific antigen, thereby initiating the effector phase of humoral immunity. The process of antibody production is discussed in detail later.

All antibodies are composed of units that have the same basic structure. As shown in Fig. 54.2, antibodies have four chains: two heavy chains and two light chains. Disulfide bridges connect the four chains to form a unit. Each heavy chain and each light chain has two regions, one in which the sequence of amino acids is *constant* and one in which the sequence is highly *variable*. The variable regions form the antigen-binding site.

There are five classes of antibodies (immunoglobulins), known as IgA, IgD, IgE, IgG, and IgM. All are constructed from the same basic parts just described. However, the heavy chains differ for each class. Primary functions of the five classes are shown in Table 54.2.

When antibodies are subjected to digestion by papain in the laboratory, they break down into three pieces (see Fig. 54.2). Two of the pieces retain the ability to bind antigen and hence are called *Fab fragments* (fragment, antigen binding). The third piece does not bind antigen and tends to form crystals in the test tube and hence is called the *Fc fragment* (fragment, crystalline).

Antigens

Antigens are molecules that induce specific immune responses and, as a result, become the targets of those responses. By way of analogy, an antigen is like the child who pokes a stick in a hornet's nest, at once triggering a response and becoming its target. An antigen may trigger production of antibodies, cytotoxic T cells, or both—all of which can then attack the antigen.

Most antigens are large molecules. Because antigens are big, the antigen-binding region of the resultant antibodies cannot recognize and bind the entire antigen molecule. Rather, the antibodies recognize and bind selected small portions of the antigen, referred to as *epitopes* or *antigenic determinants*. All antigens have multiple epitopes. As a result, more than one antibody can bind the antigen.

In research and in clinical practice, we may want to generate antibodies to molecules that are too small to induce an immune response. To overcome this obstacle, we can link the small molecule to a larger molecule, usually a protein. When this is done, the small molecule is referred to as a *hapten*, and the large molecule is referred to as a *carrier*. At least some of the resultant antibodies will be selective for the hapten.

Characteristic Features of Immune Responses

Cell-mediated immunity and humoral immunity share five characteristic features: specificity, diversity, memory, time limitation, and selectivity for antigens of nonself origin (i.e., the ability to discriminate between self and nonself).

Specificity

Cell-mediated and humoral immune responses are triggered by specific antigens, and their purpose is to destroy the antigen that triggered the response. The ability to respond to a specific antigen (i.e., the ability to make subtle distinctions among related molecules) is conferred by highly specific receptors on B cells and T cells.

Diversity

Our immune systems can respond to millions of different antigenic determinants. This is possible because our immune systems have millions of clones of B and T lymphocytes—each of which is preprogrammed to recognize a different antigenic determinant. As noted, this ability to discriminate between antigens is the result of having unique cell-surface receptors.

Memory

Exposure to an antigen affects the immune system such that reexposure produces a faster, larger, and more prolonged response compared with the initial exposure (Fig. 54.3). During the initial response, B and T lymphocytes that recognize the antigen undergo proliferation. Most of the new cells participate in the attack against the antigen. However, some of the new cells become *memory cells*, thereby increasing the pool of antigen-specific cells available to respond in the future. Hence, when the antigen is encountered again, the memory cells mobilize and thereby accelerate and intensify the response.

Time Limitation

Immune responses do not last indefinitely. They are time limited. The reasons are twofold. First, as the immune response proceeds, it greatly decreases the level of antigen that initiated the response, thereby attenuating the stimulus for continuing. Second, activated B cells and T cells function only for a short time, after which they become quiescent

TABLE 54.2	Functions of Antibody Classes
Class	**Function**
IgA	• Located in mucous membranes of the GI tract and lungs and in many secretions, where it serves as the first line of defense against microbes entering the body via these routes • Transferred to infants via breast milk; is not absorbed from the GI tract but does protect the infant against microbes *in the GI tract*
IgD	• Found only on the surface of mature B cells, where it serves as a receptor for antigen recognition (along with IgM)
IgE	• Binds to the surface of mast cells; subsequent binding of antigen to IgE stimulates release of histamine, heparin, and other mediators from the mast cells, thereby causing symptoms of allergy (e.g., hives, hay fever) • Binds to parasitic worms, after which eosinophils bind to IgE and release compounds that lyse the worms
IgG	• Produced in copious amounts in response to antigenic stimulation and hence is the major antibody in blood • Fixes complement and thereby promotes target-cell lysis • Binds target cells and thereby enhances phagocytosis • Transferred across the placenta to the fetal circulation, thereby providing neonatal immunity
IgM	• First class of antibody produced in response to an antigen • Fixes complement and thereby promotes target-cell lysis • Present on the surface of mature B cells, where it serves as a receptor for antigen recognition (along with IgD)

GI, Gastrointestinal tract; *Ig,* immunoglobulin.

Fig. 54.3 Memory and Time Limitation of Immune Responses. After the initial exposure to antigen X, antibody levels rise slowly, peak at a low level, and then decline rapidly. After the second exposure to antigen X, antibody levels rise more rapidly, reach a higher peak, persist longer, and then slowly decline.

or die. Hence, in the absence of a continuing stimulus to generate more active B cells and T cells, the immune response fades.

Selectivity for Antigens of Nonself Origin

Under normal conditions, our immune systems target only foreign antigens, leaving potentially antigenic molecules on our own cells untouched. Sparing of self is possible because, as T cells develop in the thymus, cells that are able to react with antigens of self origin are eliminated. As discussed later, this discrimination between self and nonself is made possible by *major histocompatibility complex* (MHC) molecules.

When the ability to discriminate between self and nonself fails, our immune systems can attack our own cells. The result is an *autoimmune disease*. There are many diseases of autoimmune origin, including psoriasis, multiple sclerosis, rheumatoid arthritis, myasthenia gravis, type 1 diabetes, systemic lupus erythematosus, two inflammatory bowel diseases (ulcerative colitis and Crohn disease), and two thyroid diseases (Graves disease and Hashimoto thyroiditis).

Phases of the Immune Response

Specific immune responses can be viewed as having three main phases: recognition, activation, and effector.

Recognition Phase

The recognition phase occurs when a mature lymphocyte encounters its matching antigen. All specific immune responses begin with antigen recognition by B cells and T cells. Antigen recognition is possible because of antigen-specific receptors on the lymphocyte surface.

Activation Phase

Antigen recognition activates the lymphocyte, which then undergoes proliferation and differentiation. Some of the daughter cells differentiate into cells that actively participate in the immune response, attacking the source of the antigen. Other daughter cells differentiate into memory cells, thereby preparing the host for a more intense, rapid, and prolonged response in the event of antigen reexposure.

Effector Phase

In this stage, the immune system attempts to eliminate the specific antigen that initiated the response. With cell-mediated or antibody-mediated immunity, several effector mechanisms can be involved. In cell-mediated immunity, antigen-bearing target cells can be lysed by cytolytic T cells, or they can be ingested by macrophages. In antibody-mediated immunity, target cells may be primed for attack by phagocytes or by the complement system.

Major Histocompatibility Complex Molecules

The *MHC* is a group of *genes* that codes for *MHC molecules*, which become expressed on the surface of all cells. MHC molecules are critical to immune system function. They play a key role in the activation of helper and cytotoxic T lymphocytes, they guide cytotoxic T lymphocytes toward target cells, and they provide the basis for distinguishing between self and nonself.

There are two classes of MHC gene products, referred to as *class I MHC molecules* and *class II MHC molecules*. Class I MHC molecules are found on virtually all cells except erythrocytes; class II MHC molecules are found primarily on B cells and APCs (macrophages and dendritic cells). As discussed later, *class I MHC molecules* on the surface of APCs help to initiate immune responses by "presenting" antigen to *cytotoxic T cells*. In contrast, *class II MHC molecules* on the surface of APCs help initiate immune responses by presenting antigen to *helper T cells*.

As a rule, the sequence of amino acids in MHC molecules produced by one individual differs from the sequence of amino acids in MHC molecules produced by everyone else. That is, it is rare for two individuals to have MHC molecules that are identical. As a result, MHC molecules from one individual are recognized as foreign (nonself) by the immune systems of nearly everyone else. Hence, when we attempt to transplant organs between individuals who are not identical twins, immune rejection of the transplant is likely. To reduce the risk for rejection, we can treat patients with immunosuppressant drugs.

Cytokines, Lymphokines, and Monokines

The terms *cytokine*, *lymphokine*, and *monokine* are encountered frequently when discussing the immune system and can be a source of confusion. The term *cytokine* refers to any mediator molecule (other than an antibody) released by *any* immune system cell. A *lymphokine* is simply a cytokine released by a *lymphocyte*, and a *monokine* is simply a cytokine released by a *mononuclear phagocyte* (monocyte or macrophage). Put another way, *cytokine* is a generic term for the whole class of nonantibody mediators released by immune cells, whereas the terms *lymphokine* and *monokine* are more restrictive, referring only to nonantibody mediators released by lymphocytes and mononuclear phagocytes, respectively. Examples of cytokines and their functions are listed in Table 54.3.

ANTIBODY-MEDIATED (HUMORAL) IMMUNITY

As noted, there are two types of immune responses: humoral immunity and cell-mediated immunity. In this section, we review humoral immunity, focusing on (1) how antibodies are produced and (2) the mechanisms by which antibodies protect us. Cell-mediated immunity is discussed in the section that follows.

TABLE 54.3   Functions of Selected Cytokines

Cytokine	Function
IL-1	Stimulates lymphocyte progenitor cells
IL-2	Stimulates proliferation and differentiation of helper T cells and cytolytic T cells
IL-3	Stimulates proliferation of bone marrow lineage cells, B cells, and T cells
IL-4	Activates B cells, T cells, and macrophages
IL-5	Stimulates generation of eosinophils
IL-6	Stimulates proliferation of bone marrow cells and plasma cells
IL-7	Stimulates B cells and T cells
IL-8	Attracts neutrophils, B cells, and T cells
IL-9	Stimulates proliferation of mast cells
IL-10	Inhibits some T cells
IL-11	Enhances actions of IL-3
IL-12	Enhances actions of IL-2
Interferon α	Activates macrophages, cytolytic T cells, and natural killer cells
Interferon γ	Activates macrophages and T cells and enhances expression of MHC molecules
Tumor necrosis factor	Kills tumor cells; promotes inflammation
Granulocyte-macrophage colony-stimulating factor	Stimulates proliferation of monocytes, macrophages, and granulocytes (neutrophils, eosinophils, basophils)

IL, Interleukin; *MHC*, major histocompatibility complex.

Production of Antibodies

Antibody production requires the cooperative interaction of three types of cells: *B cells,* which actually make the antibodies; *helper T cells* (CD4 cells), which stimulate the B cells; and an *APC* (either a macrophage or a dendritic cell), which activates the CD4 cells so that they can then help the B cells. The major steps in the process are depicted in Fig. 54.4.

Overview of Antibody Production

Production of antibodies begins with binding of a specific antigen to two types of cells: a virgin B cell and an APC. The APC may be either a macrophage or a dendritic cell. After processing the antigen, the APC is able to bind with a specific CD4 cell, thereby causing the CD4 cell to proliferate and differentiate into active CD4 cells and memory CD4 cells. The active CD4 cells then bind with processed antigen on B cells, thereby causing the B cells to proliferate and differentiate into (1) plasma cells, which manufacture the antibodies and (2) memory B cells, which await the next antigen exposure.

Specific Cellular Events in Antibody Production

B cells. Participation of B cells in the immune response begins with recognition and binding of a *specific antigen.* The receptor that B cells use for antigen recognition is actually an antibody (IgD or IgM). For any given B cell, this antibody (receptor) is highly specific for just one antigenic determinant. After the antigen binds the B cell receptor, the receptor-antigen complex is internalized and the antigen is broken down into small peptide fragments. Each fragment is then complexed with a *class II MHC molecule,* after which the *antigen–MHC II complexes* are transported to the cell surface. (In Fig. 54.4, only one such complex is shown. However, in a real cell, many such complexes, each with a different piece of the antigen, would appear on the cell surface.) The final step of B cell activation occurs when a CD4 helper T cell recognizes and binds with an antigen–MHC II complex on the B cell. This binding

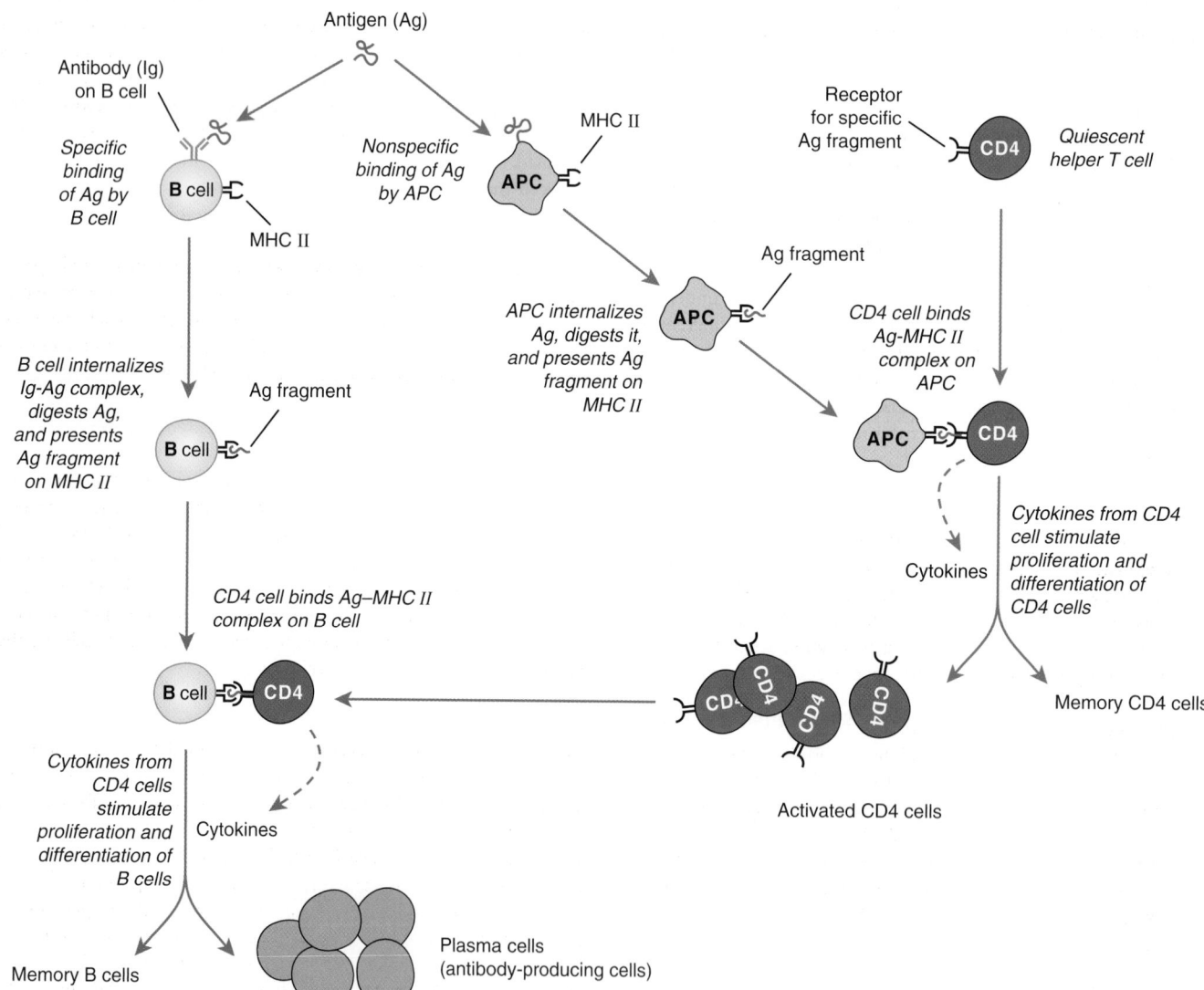

Fig. 54.4 Major Events in Antibody-Mediated (Humoral) Immunity. Humoral immunity requires three types of cells: B cells, antigen-presenting cells *(APCs),* and helper T cells (CD4 cells). Binding of a CD4 cell with an APC activates the CD4 cell, which then binds with a B cell and releases cytokines, which then stimulate the B cell. *Ig,* Immunoglobulin (antibody); *MHC II,* class II MHC molecule.

causes the CD4 cell to secrete cytokines, which then stimulate the B cell to proliferate and differentiate into two types of cells: plasma cells and memory B cells. The plasma cells are the cells that make antibodies. The memory cells serve to hasten, intensify, and prolong the immune response if antigen exposure should recur.

Antigen-presenting cells. APCs are essential for activation of CD4 helper T cells because CD4 cells cannot recognize antigen that is free in solution. Rather, they can recognize only antigen that has been complexed with an MHC II molecule.

Participation of APCs in the immune response begins with nonspecific binding of antigen to the APC (see Fig. 54.4). Next, as in B cells, the antigen is internalized and broken into fragments, which are then complexed with MHC II molecules and transported to the cell surface, where they are available for interaction with CD4 cells.

Helper T cells (CD4 cells). The job of CD4 cells in humoral immunity is to activate B cells. In the absence of activation by CD4 cells, B cells are unable to proliferate and produce antibodies.

Participation of CD4 cells in the immune response begins when these cells bind with an antigen–MHC II complex on the surface of an APC. Binding is mediated by a receptor on the CD4 cell that is specific for the particular antigen in the antigen–MHC II complex. (As noted, for the CD4 cell to recognize the antigen, the antigen must be complexed with an MHC II molecule, which is why the APC is essential for CD4 cell activation.) Upon binding with the antigen–MHC II complex, the CD4 cell releases cytokines, which then cause the CD4 cell itself to proliferate and differentiate into memory CD4 cells and activated CD4 cells. The activated CD4 cells then bind with their corresponding antigen–MHC II complexes on B cells, release cytokines, and thereby cause proliferation and differentiation of the B cells.

Antibody Effector Mechanisms

Antibodies are simply molecules with the ability to bind to other molecules. Antibodies have no special destructive powers. To rid the body of antigens, which is what antibodies are for, antibodies usually work in conjunction with other factors, namely *phagocytic cells* and the *complement system*. The only antigens that antibodies can neutralize without help are bacterial toxins and viruses.

Opsonization of Bacteria

One mechanism for ridding the body of pathogenic bacteria is phagocytosis by macrophages and neutrophils. However, because of their structures, some bacteria are difficult for phagocytes to grab hold of, and hence these bacteria are resistant to ingestion. Antibodies help promote phagocytosis of these bacteria by acting as *opsonins*. (An opsonin is a molecule that binds to a bacterium or other target particle and thereby promotes phagocytosis by providing a handle for phagocytes to grab.)

Bacterial opsonization by antibodies occurs in two steps. First, the antigen-binding region of the antibody binds with antigen on the bacterial surface, which leaves the Fc portion of the antibody projecting away from the bacterial surface. Second, phagocytes link up with the Fc portion of the antibody, which brings them in close contact with the bacterium, and hence enables them to commence phagocytosis. Phagocytes are able to bind the Fc fragment because they have high-affinity receptors for Fc on their surface. Most of the antibodies that act as opsonins belong to the IgG class.

Activation of the Complement System

The complement cascade is a complex system consisting of at least 20 serum proteins that, when activated, can cause multiple effects, including cell lysis, opsonization, degranulation of mast cells, and infiltration of phagocytes. The system can be activated in two ways, known as the *classical pathway* and the *alternative pathway*. The classical pathway is activated by *antibodies;* the alternative pathway is not. However, with both pathways, the end results are essentially the same. Consideration here is limited to the classical pathway.

The classical pathway is turned on when C1 (the first component of the complement system) encounters an antigen-antibody complex and then binds with the Fc region of the antibody. C1 will not bind with antibody that is free in solution, and hence free antibodies cannot activate the system. Activation of the complement system triggers a cascade of reactions that amplify the response at each stage. The result is production of compounds that can injure target cells.

Lysis of target cells that have been tagged with antibodies is the most dramatic effect of the complement system. Lysis is caused by cylindrical *membrane attack complexes,* which are formed by the complement cascade. After their insertion into the target-cell membrane, the attack complexes act as pores through which fluid can enter the cell. Fluid influx causes the target cell to swell and then burst.

Neutralization of Viruses and Bacterial Toxins

Neutralization of toxins and viruses is the only protective action that antibodies can perform unassisted. To hurt us, bacterial toxins must first bind with receptors on our cells. Likewise, to infect us, viruses must first bind with cell-surface receptors. By binding with antigenic determinants on toxins and viruses, antibodies make it impossible for toxins and viruses to bind with cellular receptors. As a result, these agents can no longer hurt us.

CELL-MEDIATED IMMUNITY

Cell-mediated immunity has two branches, one mediated by *helper T lymphocytes* (CD4 cells) plus *macrophages,* and one mediated primarily by *cytolytic T lymphocytes* (CTLs, CD8 cells). In the branch mediated by CD4 cells and macrophages, the result is called *DTH.* In the branch mediated by CD8 cells, the result is *target-cell lysis.*

Delayed-Type Hypersensitivity (Type IV Hypersensitivity)

The object of DTH is to rid the body of bacteria that replicate primarily within macrophages (e.g., *Listeria monocytogenes, Mycobacterium tuberculosis*). For DTH to occur, two cells are needed: an *infected macrophage* and a *CD4 helper T cell.* The macrophage serves to activate the CD4 cell, which in turn activates the macrophage, thereby enabling the macrophage to kill the bacteria residing within. Hence the same cell (i.e., the macrophage) is both the activator of the CD4 cell and the recipient of the activated CD4 cell's help.

Activation of Helper T Cells

Activation of CD4 cells in DTH is essentially identical to the activation of CD4 cells in humoral immunity. As shown in Fig. 54.5, the process begins when a macrophage becomes infected with intracellular bacteria. As in humoral immunity, the macrophage breaks down the antigen to small peptides, combines each peptide with a class II MHC molecule, and then presents the antigen–MHC II complexes on its surface. In the next step, a CD4 cell binds with an antigen–MHC II complex on the macrophage. As discussed earlier, selectivity of binding is determined by receptors on the CD4 cell that recognize a specific antigen fragment— but only when the fragment is bound to a class II MHC molecule. Binding of the CD4 cell with the APC causes the CD4 cell to release (1) cytokines that cause the CD4 cell itself to proliferate and differentiate into memory cells and (2) mediators of DTH, including interferon γ and tumor necrosis factor.

Fig. 54.5 Cell-Mediated Immunity: Delayed-Type Hypersensitivity. Delayed-type hypersensitivity requires two cells: an infected macrophage and a CD4 cell. Binding of the CD4 cell to the macrophage activates the CD4 cell, which then releases interferon γ and several cytokines. Interferon γ activates the macrophage. The cytokines cause the CD4 cell to proliferate and differentiate into memory cells. *Ag,* Antigen; *MHC II,* class II MHC molecule.

Activation of Macrophages

Interferon γ, released from the activated CD4 cell, is the major stimulus for macrophage activation. In response to interferon γ, macrophages increase production of lysosomes and reactive oxygen. The reactive oxygen is ultimately responsible for killing bacteria inside the macrophage. In addition to ridding macrophages of bacteria, DTH produces local inflammation.

Cytolytic T Lymphocytes

CTLs (CD8 cells) kill other cells. Their principal job is to kill self cells that are infected with viruses, thereby halting viral replication. In addition, CTLs participate in rejection of transplants. Here our discussion is limited to killing virally infected cells.

The process by which CTLs kill other cells has two stages: activation of CTLs, followed by recognition and killing of the target cell. The process is depicted in Fig. 54.6.

Activation of Cytolytic T Cells

Activation of CTLs requires the participation of an *APC* and a *helper T cell* (CD4 cell). The process is very similar to the activation of CD4 cells discussed earlier. However, there is one important difference: CD4 cells specifically recognize antigen that is bound to a *class II* MHC molecule on an APC, whereas CTLs specifically recognize antigen that is bound to a *class I* MHC molecule on an APC.

In viral infections, activation of CTLs begins with processing of viral antigens by an APC. As shown in Fig. 54.6, the APC combines the antigen with a class I MHC molecule and then presents the antigen–MHC I complex on its surface. Next, a pre-CTL binds to the

antigen–MHC I complex. (Like CD4 cells, each pre-CTL has receptors that are specific for a particular antigen–MHC I complex.) Linking of the pre-CTL with the APC primes the pre-CTL for the next stage of activation: stimulation by cytokines (interleukin-2, interferon γ, and probably others) provided by an activated CD4 cell. (Activation of the CD4 cell, which is not shown in Fig. 54.6, occurs when the CD4 cell encounters an APC that has a viral antigen–MHC II complex.) In response to the cytokines released by the CD4 cell, the pre-CTL undergoes proliferation and differentiation into memory CTLs and activated CTLs.

Recognition of Virally Infected Target Cells

CTLs recognize their targets by the presence of an antigen–MHC I complex. This is the same process by which CTLs recognize APCs. As noted earlier, virtually all cells in the body carry class I MHC molecules. (Class II molecules are limited to APCs and B cells.) Hence when a cell is infected with a virus, viral antigens form intracellular complexes with MHC I molecules, after which the antigen–MHC I complexes are presented on the cell surface. As shown in Fig. 54.6, activated CTLs recognize the antigen–MHC I complex and hence bind with the target cell. Because only cells that are infected with the virus will bear viral antigens on their class I MHC molecules, attack by CTLs is limited to infected cells; all others are spared.

Mechanisms of Cell Kill

Binding of a CTL to its target cell causes the CTL to release mediators that kill the target. Two mechanisms of cell kill are involved: *lysis* and *apoptosis* (programmed cell death). The mediator of lysis is called *perforin,*

Fig. 54.6 Cell-Mediated Immunity: Cytolytic T Cells. This branch of cell-mediated immunity requires three types of cells: cytolytic T lymphocytes *(CTLs)*, antigen-presenting cells *(APCs)*, and CD4 cells. Binding of the pre-CTL with the APC begins the activation of the CTL. Stimulation of the CTL by cytokines from the CD4 cell completes the activation of the CTL, which then binds with and kills its target. Activation of the CD4 cells, which is not shown, takes place as depicted in Figs. 54.4 and 54.5. *Ag,* Antigen; *MHC I,* class I MHC molecule.

a molecule that forms pores in the target-cell membrane; the resultant influx of fluid causes the cell to swell and then burst. (This mechanism is very similar to one by which the complement system causes cell lysis.) The mediators of apoptosis have not been identified with certainty. However, their effects are very clear. The initial effect is activation of intracellular enzymes that digest the cell's own DNA. This is followed by fragmentation of the nucleus and cell death. Only the target cell is harmed; bystander cells and the CTL itself are not touched. In fact, after releasing its mediators, the CTL disconnects from the doomed target and goes on to seek another target cell.

55

Childhood Immunization

Thanks to widespread immunization, the incidence of several infectious diseases has been dramatically reduced, and one disease—smallpox—has been eliminated from the planet. Of all the advances in medicine, none has reduced sickness and death more than immunization.

Experience has shown that the most effective way to reduce vaccine-preventable diseases (VPDs) is to create a highly immune population. Accordingly, universal vaccination is a national goal. Although immunization carries some risk, the risks from failing to vaccinate are much greater. Discussion in this chapter is limited to childhood immunization.

GENERAL CONSIDERATIONS

Definitions

To discuss immunization, we must use special terminology. Accordingly, we begin by defining some terms.

Vaccine

A vaccine is a preparation containing whole or fractionated microorganisms. Administration causes the recipient's immune system to manufacture antibodies directed against the microbe from which the vaccine was made. Most of the preparations discussed in this chapter are vaccines.

Killed Vaccines Versus Live Vaccines

There are two major classes of vaccines: killed and live (albeit attenuated). Killed vaccines are composed of whole, killed microbes or isolated microbial components (e.g., the polysaccharide of *Haemophilus influenzae* type b or the surface antigen of hepatitis B). In contrast, live, attenuated vaccines are composed of live microbes that have been weakened or rendered completely avirulent. Live vaccines can be dangerous in recipients who are immunocompromised because these people are unable to mount an effective immune response, even against an avirulent organism.

Toxoid

A toxoid is a bacterial toxin that has been changed to a nontoxic form. Administration causes the recipient's immune system to manufacture antitoxins (i.e., antibodies directed against the natural bacterial toxin). Antitoxins protect against injury from toxins but do not kill the bacteria that produce them. In this chapter, only two toxoids are considered: tetanus toxoid and diphtheria toxoid.

Vaccination

The terms *vaccination* and *vaccine* derive from *vaccinia,* a virus whose name in turn derives from *vacca* (Latin for cow). At one time, vaccinia virus was used as a vaccine against smallpox. (Vaccinia itself causes cowpox—a mild sickness—and in the process induces synthesis of smallpox antibodies.) Hence, when the term *vaccination* was originally coined, it had the limited meaning of giving vaccinia to generate immunity against smallpox. Currently, vaccination refers broadly to giving any vaccine or toxoid.

Specific Immune Globulins

These preparations contain a high concentration of antibodies directed against a specific antigen (e.g., hepatitis B virus). Administration provides immediate passive immunity. These preparations are made from donated blood.

Reporting Vaccine-Preventable Diseases

Public health officials rely on health care providers to report cases of VPDs. Nearly all VPDs that occur in the United States are notifiable. Health care providers should report individual cases to their local or state health department. Each week, the state health departments make a report to the Centers for Disease Control and Prevention (CDC). The information is used to (1) determine whether an outbreak is occurring, (2) evaluate prevention and control strategies, and (3) evaluate the effect of national immunization policies and practices.

Immunization Records

The *National Childhood Vaccine Act* requires a permanent record of each mandated vaccination a child receives. The information should be recorded in either (1) the permanent medical record of the recipient or (2) a permanent office log or file. The following data are required:
- Date of vaccination
- Route and site of vaccination
- Vaccine type, manufacturer, lot number, and expiration date
- Name, address, and title of the person administering the vaccine

The purpose of these records is twofold. First, they help ensure that children receive appropriate vaccinations. Second, they help avoid overvaccination and thereby reduce the risk for possible hypersensitivity reactions. To promote uniformity in record keeping, an official immunization card has been adopted by every state and the District of Columbia.

Adverse Effects of Immunization

Vaccines are generally very safe. Although mild reactions are common, serious events are rare. Many children experience local reactions (discomfort, swelling, and erythema at the injection site). Fever is also common. Very rare but severe effects include *anaphylaxis* (e.g., in response to measles, mumps, and rubella virus vaccine); acute *encephalopathy* (caused by diphtheria and tetanus toxoids and pertussis vaccine); and vaccine-associated *paralytic poliomyelitis* (caused by oral poliovirus vaccine). In 2011 the safety of vaccines was reaffirmed in a lengthy report—*Adverse Effects of Vaccines: Evidence and Causality*—issued by the Institute of Medicine of the National Academies.

Vaccinations can hurt. This pain, in turn, can lead to needle fears, procedural anxiety, and avoiding additional immunizations. Accordingly, minimizing pain is a primary goal. Strategies to reduce pain and anxiety include holding the child upright during the vaccination, applying a topical anesthetic, providing tactile stimulation, performing intramuscular injections rapidly without prior aspiration, and injecting the most painful vaccine last. Pain can be further reduced by use of microneedles, needle-free devices, and intranasal vaccines. What about giving analgesic-antipyretics, such as acetaminophen and ibuprofen? Evidence from a study in Russia indicates that giving these drugs before or shortly after vaccination can reduce the immune response. In addition, studies show that prophylactic administration of antipyretics does not significantly reduce the incidence of fever or pain. Accordingly, routine prophylactic use of these drugs to prevent pain or fever should be discouraged. The American Academy of Pediatrics (AAP) still condones their use for children who experience fever after the immunization is given.

Immunocompromised children are at special risk from live vaccines. The reason is that, in the absence of an adequate immune response, the viruses or bacteria in these normally safe vaccines are able to multiply in profusion, thereby causing serious infection. Accordingly, live vaccines should generally be avoided in children who are severely immunosuppressed. Causes of immunosuppression include congenital immunodeficiency, human immunodeficiency virus (HIV) infection, leukemia, lymphoma, generalized malignancy, and therapy with radiation, cytotoxic anticancer drugs, and high-dose glucocorticoids.

Some parents are concerned that *thimerosal,* a mercury-based preservative found in some vaccines, might cause *autism.* For two reasons, this concern is unfounded. First, several large, high-quality studies conducted in Denmark, Britain, and the United States have failed to show a causal link between childhood immunization using thimerosal-containing vaccines and development of autism. Second, thimerosal is being phased out of vaccines made in the United States (owing to concerns about mercury exposure, not concerns about autism). At this time, the amount of thimerosal in most routinely used childhood vaccines is either zero or extremely low (less than 0.5 µg per 0.5-mL dose). The only exceptions are certain flu vaccines, which still contain thimerosal as a preservative. However, even if these flu vaccines are used, total mercury exposure from childhood vaccination will still be well below the limit considered safe by the U.S. Food and Drug Administration (FDA) and the Environmental Protection Agency.

The risk for serious adverse reactions can be minimized by observing appropriate *precautions* and *contraindications.* Table 55.1 lists contraindications that apply to all vaccines. Precautions and contraindications that apply to specific vaccines are discussed in the context of those preparations. Certain conditions, such as diarrhea and mild illness, may be inappropriately regarded as contraindications by some practitioners. As a result, vaccination may be needlessly postponed. Conditions that are often considered contraindications, although they are not, are also listed in Table 55.1.

Practitioners are required to report certain adverse events to the *Vaccine Adverse Event Reporting System* (VAERS). The information is used to help determine whether (1) a particular event that occurs after vaccination is actually caused by the vaccine and (2) what the risk factors might be. In addition to reporting events that they are required to report, practitioners should report all other serious or unusual adverse events, regardless of whether they believe the event was caused by the vaccine. Forms for reporting adverse events can be obtained from the VAERS website (www.vaers.hhs.gov) or by calling 1-800-822-7967.

The *National Vaccine Injury Compensation Program* (NVICP), established by the *National Childhood Vaccine Injury Act,* was created to provide compensation for injury or death resulting from vaccination. The program is intended as an alternative to civil litigation in that negligence need not be proved. As a provision of the law, a table was created listing the vaccines covered by the program and the injuries, disabilities, illness, and conditions—including death—for which compensation may be paid. Compensation may also be paid for injuries not listed in the table, provided that (1) a listed vaccine is involved and (2) causality can be demonstrated. Injuries related to vaccines not listed

TABLE 55.1 Contraindications That Apply to All Vaccines and Conditions Often Incorrectly Regarded as Contraindications

True Contraindications (Vaccine Should Not Be Administered)	Not Contraindications (Vaccine May Be Administered)
Anaphylactic reaction to a specific vaccine: contraindicates further doses of that vaccine Anaphylactic reaction to a vaccine component: contraindicates use of all vaccines that contain that substance Moderate or severe illnesses with or without a fever	Mild to moderate local reaction (soreness, erythema, swelling) after a dose of an injectable vaccine Mild acute illness with or without low-grade fever Diarrhea Current antimicrobial therapy Convalescent phase of illnesses Prematurity (same dosage and indications as for normal, full-term infants) Recent exposure to an infectious disease Personal or family history of either penicillin allergy or nonspecific allergies

in the table are not covered under the program. Additional information can be obtained by calling 1-800-338-2382.

Vaccine Information Statements

The National Childhood Vaccine Injury Act requires that Vaccine Information Statements (VISs) be given to all vaccinated patients (or their parents or legal representatives) before certain vaccines are administered. The VISs, produced by the CDC, are one-page, two-sided documents that describe the benefits and risks of specific vaccines. For vaccines that require a series of shots, a VIS must be given *before each dose,* not just the first dose. The VISs are available in more than 30 languages and can be obtained online at https://www.cdc.gov/vaccines/hcp/vis/index.html.

Childhood Immunization Schedule

Each year, the CDC Advisory Committee on Immunization Practices (ACIP), in cooperation with the American Academy of Family Physicians (AAFP) and the AAP, issues revised recommendations for childhood immunization in the United States. You can find the yearly schedule recommendations and catch-up immunization schedule for persons aged 4 months through 18 years, as well as the most recent updates, online at www.cdc.gov/vaccines/. Please note that adult immunization schedules can also be found there.

TARGET DISEASES

Routine childhood vaccination is currently recommended for protection against 16 infectious diseases: diphtheria, tetanus, pertussis, measles, mumps, rubella, invasive *H. influenzae* type b, (Hib), hepatitis A, hepatitis B, polio, varicella (chickenpox), influenza, invasive pneumococcal disease, meningococcal disease, rotavirus gastroenteritis, and genital human papillomavirus (HPV) infection. In the following discussion, certain VPDs are considered in a group (e.g., measles, mumps, rubella) because vaccination against these VPDs is traditionally done simultaneously using a combination vaccine.

Measles, Mumps, and Rubella

Measles

Measles is a highly contagious viral disease characterized by rash and high fever (103°F to 105°F). Infection is spread by inhalation of aerosolized sputum or by direct contact with nasal or throat secretions. Initial symptoms include fever, cough, headache, sore throat, and conjunctivitis. Three days later, rash develops. Rash begins at the hairline, spreads to the rest of the body in 36 hours, and then fades in a few days. Secondary infections can result in pneumonia and otitis media (inner-ear infection). However, of the potential complications of measles, encephalitis is by far the most serious. Sequelae of encephalitis include blindness, deafness, and convulsions. Although encephalitis is rare (0.1% incidence), it carries a 10% risk for death.

Mumps

Mumps is a viral disease that primarily affects the parotid glands (the largest of the three pairs of salivary glands). Although mumps can occur in adults, it usually occurs in children aged 5 to 15 years. As a rule, the first symptom is swelling in one of the parotid glands, often accompanied by local pain and tenderness. The patient may also experience fever (100°F to 104°F). Swelling increases for 2 to 3 days and then fades entirely by day 6 or 7. Swelling in the second parotid gland often develops after swelling in the first but may also occur simultaneously or not at all. Painful *orchitis* (inflammation of the testes) develops in approximately one-third of adult and adolescent males. Acute *aseptic meningitis* develops in approximately 10% of all patients; symptoms, which resolve completely, include dizziness, headache, and vomiting.

Rubella

Rubella, also known as German measles, is a generally mild viral infection. However, if it occurs during pregnancy, the consequences can be severe. Initial symptoms include sore throat, mild fever, and swelling in lymph nodes located behind the ears and in the back of the neck. Shortly after, a rash develops on the face and scalp, spreads rapidly to the torso and arms, and then fades in 2 or 3 days. Arthritis may also develop, mainly in women. In pregnant women, rubella can cause miscarriage, stillbirth, and congenital defects, especially if the disease occurs during the first trimester. Possible birth defects include cataracts, heart disease, developmental delay, and hearing loss. In the United States rubella has been eliminated: since 2002, all cases reported here have been traceable to foreigners who brought the disease from abroad.

Diphtheria, Tetanus, and Pertussis

Diphtheria

Diphtheria is a potentially fatal infection caused by *Corynebacterium diphtheriae*, a gram-positive bacillus. The bacterium colonizes the throat and nasal passages and produces a toxin that spreads throughout the body. Initial symptoms include sore throat, fever, headache, and nausea. Colonization of the airway begins as patches of gray or dirty-yellow membrane that eventually grow together, forming a thick coating. This coating, combined with swelling, can impede swallowing and breathing; in severe cases a tracheostomy is needed. The toxin produced by *C. diphtheriae* can damage the heart and nerves, resulting in heart failure and paralysis. Diphtheria treatment includes giving diphtheria antitoxin and antibiotics (e.g., erythromycin, penicillin G).

Tetanus

Tetanus is a frequently fatal disease characterized by painful spasm of all skeletal muscles. The cause is a potent endotoxin elaborated by *Clostridium tetani*, a gram-positive bacillus. Infection with *C. tetani* typically results from puncturing the skin with a nail, splinter, or other object that is contaminated with soil, street dust, or animal or human feces. The first symptom is often stiffness of the jaw. As infection progresses, the patient may experience stiff neck, difficulty swallowing, restlessness, irritability, headache, chills, fever, and convulsions. Eventually, spasm develops in muscles of the abdomen, back, neck, and face. Treatment options include tetanus antitoxin, a booster dose of tetanus toxoid, and antibiotics (e.g., metronidazole, penicillin G, doxycycline).

Pertussis

Pertussis occurs primarily in infants and young children. The cause is *Bordetella pertussis*, a gram-negative bacillus. Initial symptoms include rhinorrhea, mild fever, and persistent cough. As infection worsens, coughing becomes more intense. The acute phase of the disease can last 4 to 6 weeks. During this time, infants experience difficulty eating, drinking, and breathing. Deaths have occurred. Complications of pertussis include pneumonia, seizures, ear infections, and, rarely, permanent neurologic injury. Azithromycin is the treatment of choice.

Poliomyelitis

Poliomyelitis, also known as polio, is a serious disease in which the poliovirus attacks neurons of the central nervous system that control muscle movement. The result is skeletal muscle paralysis, usually in the legs. However, muscles of respiration and muscles of the arms may be affected, too. In approximately 10% of cases, polio is fatal. The disease is caused by three different polioviruses. Paralytic polio is usually caused by type 1 poliovirus. Polio has no cure. However, proper symptomatic treatment can improve comfort and reduce or prevent some crippling effects. Vaccination against polio has eliminated the disease from the Western hemisphere, except for eight to nine cases annually caused by the vaccine itself. To prevent vaccine-induced polio, use of the live virus vaccine (oral polio vaccine) was discontinued in the United States.

Haemophilus influenzae Type b

H. influenzae type b is a gram-negative bacterium that can cause meningitis, pneumonia, and serious throat and ear infections. The bacterium is the leading cause of serious illness in children under the age of 5 years, and the most common cause of bacterial meningitis, which has a mortality rate of 5%. Among children who survive meningitis, between 25% and 35% suffer lasting neurologic deficits. As a result of childhood vaccination, the annual incidence of infection has dropped significantly. Of the cases that occurred, almost all were in unvaccinated children. Infection with *H. influenzae* can be treated successfully with antibiotics.

Varicella

Varicella is a common, highly contagious, and potentially serious disease of childhood. The causative organism is varicella-zoster virus, a member of the herpesvirus group. Patients typically develop 250 to 500 maculopapular or vesicular lesions, usually on the face, scalp, or trunk. Other symptoms include fever, malaise, and loss of appetite. Among children, the most common complications are bacterial suprainfection and acute cerebellar ataxia. Reye syndrome and encephalitis develop rarely. Among adults, the most serious common complication is varicella pneumonia. As a rule, symptoms in adults are more severe than in children: hospitalization is 10 times more likely in adults, and death is 20 times more likely. Although adults account for only 2% of varicella cases, they account for 50% of varicella-related deaths.

Herpes zoster, also known as *shingles* or simply *zoster,* develops in 15% of patients years after childhood chickenpox has resolved. The cause is reactivation of varicella-zoster viruses that had been dormant within sensory nerve roots. Episodes of zoster begin with neurologic pain in the area of skin supplied by the affected nerve roots. Blister-like lesions develop within 3 to 4 days and usually disappear 2 to 3 weeks later. However, in approximately 14% of patients, neurologic pain persists for a month or more—and in a few cases, pain lasts for years.

Hepatitis B

Hepatitis B is a serious liver infection caused by the hepatitis B virus. Acute infection can cause anorexia, malaise, diarrhea, vomiting, jaundice, pain (in muscles, joints, and stomach), and death. Chronic infection can result in cirrhosis, liver cancer, and death.

Although hepatitis B is found in virtually all body fluids, only blood, serum-derived fluids, saliva, semen, and vaginal fluids are infectious. The most common modes of transmission are needle-stick accidents, sexual contact with an infected partner, maternal-child transmission during birth, and use of contaminated intravenous equipment or solutions.

Hepatitis B is discussed further in Chapter 80.

Hepatitis A

Hepatitis A is a serious liver infection caused by the hepatitis A virus. Symptoms of hepatitis A include fever, malaise, nausea, jaundice, anorexia, diarrhea, and stomach pain. However, not all infected persons become symptomatic. Among children younger than 6 years, only 30% develop symptoms. In contrast, symptoms are present in most older infected children and adults. When symptoms do occur, they develop rapidly and then usually fade in less than 2 months. However, between 10% and 15% of patients experience prolonged or relapsing disease that persists up to 6 months. During the course of the infection, the virus undergoes replication in the liver, passage into the bile, and then excretion in the feces. As a result, the usual mode of transmission is fecal-oral in the context of close personal contact with an infected person. In addition, hepatitis A can be contracted by ingesting contaminated food or water. Blood-borne transmission is rare. Individuals at risk include household and sexual contacts of infected individuals, international travelers, and people living in areas where hepatitis A is endemic (e.g., American Indian reservations, Alaskan Native villages).

Pneumococcal Infection

In the United States, *Streptococcus pneumoniae* (pneumococcus) is the leading bacterial cause of childhood meningitis, sepsis, pneumonia, and otitis media. Among children with pneumococcal meningitis, up to 50% suffer permanent brain damage or hearing loss and approximately 10% die. The risk for acquiring pneumococcal infection is highest for children younger than 2 years. Factors that increase infection risk include sickle cell disease, immunodeficiency, asplenia, chronic diseases, attending a group child care center, and being a Native American, African American, or Alaskan Native or a socially disadvantaged person. Worldwide, pneumococcal infection ranks among the leading causes of death from infectious disease.

Meningococcal Infection

Meningococcal infection is a serious disease caused by *Neisseria meningitidis*, also known as meningococcus. Invasive meningococcal disease is a leading cause of meningitis in American children. Worldwide, most infections are caused by five *N. meningitidis* serogroups—designated A, B, C, Y, and W-135—identified on the basis of antigenic differences in surface polysaccharides. In the United States, only three serogroups—B, C, and Y—cause most cases. Meningococcal infection is readily transmitted through direct contact with respiratory secretions from patients and from asymptomatic carriers. Injury results from a meningococcal endotoxin, which is produced so quickly that death can result within hours of infection onset. Although only a few hundred cases occur here each year, the disease is clearly of great concern, with a fatality rate of 10% to 14% despite antibiotic therapy. Furthermore, of those who

survive, 11% to 19% suffer severe and permanent sequelae, including neurologic disability, deafness, developmental delay, and limb amputations. Infection rate is highest during infancy, with a second peak during adolescence and early adulthood. Outbreaks can occur in child care centers, schools, and colleges. Risk factors for acquiring the disease include immunodeficiency, antecedent viral infection, household crowding, chronic underlying disease, active and passive smoking, and anatomic and functional asplenia.

Influenza

Influenza is a serious infection of the respiratory tract and a major cause of morbidity and mortality worldwide. Characteristics of the influenza virus and of influenza itself (mode of transmission, symptoms, time course, methods of prevention and treatment) are discussed in Chapter 80.

Rotavirus Gastroenteritis

Rotavirus, which infects the intestinal mucosa, is the most common diarrheal pathogen worldwide. Infection presents initially as upset stomach and vomiting, usually with fever, and then progresses to several days of diarrhea, which can be mild to severe. The combination of vomiting and severe diarrhea can result in life-threatening dehydration. Virtually all children become infected repeatedly within the first 5 years of life. However, the first episode is generally the worst. As a result, severe diarrhea and dehydration are most likely in the very young—children 3 to 35 months old. Infected children shed large amounts of rotavirus in their stool, and hence transmission is usually fecal-oral, resulting from touching the stool or a contaminated object.

Genital Human Papillomavirus Infection

HPV infection is the cause of virtually all anogenital warts and cervical cancers. Transmission occurs most often by direct genital contact during vaginal or anal intercourse. The types of HPV that infect the anogenital region can also cause cancers of the vulva, vagina, urethra, tongue, tonsils, penis, and anus. Cancer of the anus in men and women who have anal intercourse is currently as common as cervical cancer was before the Papanicolaou (Pap) test was introduced. The discussion that follows focuses on the role of HPV in cervical cancer and genital warts. Treatment of genital warts is discussed in Chapter 88.

Genital HPV is the most common sexually transmitted infection. Among sexually active males and females, approximately 50% will be infected at some time during their life. Fortunately, although HPV infections are common, most are benign and clear spontaneously, usually within a few months to a year. As a result, most men and women never get genital warts and most women never get precancerous cervical lesions or cervical cancer.

Approximately 100 types of HPV are known to exist, approximately 40 of which infect the anogenital region. The types of HPV associated with malignancy are referred to as *oncogenic* or *high risk,* whereas the types associated with genital warts are called *low risk.* Approximately 95% of genital warts are caused by just two HPV types, known as HPV-6 and HPV-11. Approximately 70% of cervical cancers are caused by two other types, known as HPV-16 and HPV-18. Fortunately, only 2.2% of women carry high-risk strains.

Respiratory Syncytial Virus

Respiratory syncytial virus (RSV), an enveloped virus of the Paramyxoviridae family, was first identified in 1956. In the United States, RSV infection is the most common cause of bronchiolitis (inflammation of small airways in the lungs) and pneumonia in children younger than 1 year and remains among the most common causes for hospitalization in children younger than 5 years.

All children are at risk for RSV, but the incidence of severe disease is highest in children born prematurely and in those with cardiopulmonary disease. Children at high risk account for nearly half of RSV-related hospital admissions in the United States. An additional at-risk population is older adults, who often suffer from flulike symptoms caused by RSV.

SPECIFIC VACCINES AND TOXOIDS

The following discussion is limited to the vaccines and toxoids used for routine childhood immunization. The major preparations employed are listed in Table 55.2. Their adverse effects are shown in Table 55.3.

Childhood immunization schedules, catch-up schedules, and recent changes—as recommended by the ACIP, the AAP, and the AAFP—are available online at www.cdc.gov/vaccines/.

Measles, Mumps, and Rubella Virus Vaccine
Description

Measles, mumps, and rubella vaccine (MMR), marketed under the trade name *M-M-R II*, is a combination product composed of three live virus vaccines. Administration induces synthesis of antibodies directed against measles, mumps, and rubella viruses. Immunization with MMR is preferred to immunization with the three vaccines separately.

TABLE 55.2	Vaccines and Toxoids Available in the United States				
Preparation Name (Synonym)	**Trade Name**	**Type of Preparation**	**Route and Site**	**Number and Timing**	
Measles, mumps, and rubella virus vaccine (MMR)	M-M-R II	Live virus	SubQ, in outer aspect of upper arm	Two doses: #1: between 12 and 16 months #2: between 4 and 6 years	
Measles, mumps, and rubella, and varicella virus vaccine (MMRV)	ProQuad[a]	Live virus	SubQ, in anterolateral thigh or outer aspect of upper arm		
Diphtheria and tetanus toxoids and acellular pertussis vaccine (DTaP)	Tripedia, DAPTACEL, Infanrix, Boostrix,[b] Adacel[b]	Toxoids (diphtheria and tetanus) plus inactivated bacteria components (pertussis)	IM, in deltoid or mediolateral thigh	Five doses: #1: 2 months #2: 4 months #3: 6 months #4: between 15 and 18 months #5: between 4 and 6 years Booster every 10 years thereafter starting at age 11 years	
Diphtheria and tetanus toxoids and acellular pertussis adsorbed, hepatitis B (recombinant), and inactivated poliovirus vaccine	PEDIARIX	Toxoids (diphtheria and tetanus) plus inactivated bacteria components (pertussis) plus inactive viral antigen (hepatitis B) plus inactivated viruses (poliovirus)	IM, in deltoid or anterolateral thigh		
Tetanus and diphtheria toxoids	Tenivac Decavac	Toxoids	IM, in deltoid or mediolateral thigh		
Haemophilus influenzae type b (Hib) conjugate vaccine	ActHIB, PedvaxHIB, Hiberix, Comvax[c]	Bacterial polysaccharide conjugated to protein	IM, in midthigh or outer aspect of upper arm	Four doses: #1: 2 months #2: 4 months #3: 6 months #4: between 12 and 15 months	
Poliovirus vaccine, inactivated (IPV, Salk vaccine)	IPOL	Inactivated viruses of all three polio serotypes	SubQ, in anterolateral thigh	Four doses: #1: 2 months #2: 4 months #3: between 6 and 18 months #4: between 4 and 6 years	
Varicella virus vaccine	Varivax	Live virus	SubQ, in deltoid or anterolateral thigh	Two doses: #1: between 12 and 15 months #2: between 4 and 6 years	
Hepatitis A vaccine (HepA)	Havrix, VAQTA	Inactive viral antigen	IM, in deltoid	Two doses: #1: 12 months #2: 6–12 months after	
Hepatitis B vaccine (HepB)	Recombivax HB, Engerix-B, Comvax[c]	Inactive viral antigen	IM, in deltoid or anterolateral thigh	Three doses: #1: within 12 hours of birth #2: between 1 and 2 months #3: after an additional 6 months	

TABLE 55.2   Vaccines and Toxoids Available in the United States—cont'd

Preparation Name (Synonym)	Trade Name	Type of Preparation	Route and Site	Number and Timing
Pneumococcal conjugate vaccine (PCV13)	Prevnar 13	Bacterial polysaccharide conjugated to protein	IM, in deltoid or anterolateral thigh	Four doses: #1: 2 months #2: 4 months #3: 6 months #4: between 12 and 15 months
Pneumococcal polysaccharide vaccine (PPSV)	Pneumovax 23	Bacterial polysaccharide (unconjugated)	IM, in deltoid or anterolateral thigh	
Influenza vaccine (inactivated)	Fluzone, Fluvirin, others	Inactive viral antigen	IM, in deltoid or anterolateral thigh	Yearly after age 6 months
Influenza vaccine (live)	FluMist	Live virus	Intranasal	Approved after age 2 years
Meningococcal conjugate vaccine (MCV4)	Menactra, Menveo	Bacterial polysaccharide conjugated to protein	IM, in deltoid	Two doses: #1: between 11 and 12 years #2: age 16 years
Meningococcal subgroup B recombinant vaccine	Bexsero, Trumenba.	Recombinant protein solution	IM, in deltoid	Two doses: #1: between 11 and 12 years #2: at least 1 month after
Rotavirus vaccine	Rotarix, RotaTeq	Live virus	Oral	RotaTeq Three Doses: #1: 6–12 weeks #2: 4–10 weeks after #3: 4–10 weeks after second dose Rotarix Two doses: #1: 6–12 weeks #2: 4 weeks later
Human papillomavirus vaccine	Gardasil 9	DNA-free virus-like particles	IM, in deltoid or anterolateral thigh	Prior to age 15: Two doses: #1 as early as age 9. #2 between 6-12 months after first dose. After age 15: Three doses: #1: as early as age 15 years #2: 1-2 months after #3: 6 months after the first dose

[a]ProQuad combines two older vaccines: M-M-R II and Varivax.
[b]Boostrix and Adacel are indicated for *booster* immunization, *not* for the *initial* immunization series. Boostrix is for patients 11 to 18 years old. Adacel is for patients 11 to 64 years old.
[c]Comvax is a combination vaccine for immunization against *H. influenzae* type b and hepatitis B.
IM, Intramuscular; *SubQ,* subcutaneous.

TABLE 55.3   Adverse Effects of Some Vaccines and Toxoids

Preparation	Mild Effects	Serious Effects
Measles, mumps, and rubella virus vaccine	Local reactions; rash; fever; swollen glands in cheeks and neck and under the jaw; pain, stiffness, and swelling in joints	Anaphylaxis, thrombocytopenia[a]
Diphtheria and tetanus toxoids and acellular pertussis vaccine	Local reactions, fever, fretfulness, drowsiness, anorexia, persistent crying	Acute encephalopathy, convulsions, shock-like state
Haemophilus influenzae type b conjugate vaccine	Local reactions, fever, crying, diarrhea, vomiting	None
Varicella virus vaccine	Local reactions, fever, mild varicella-like rash (local or generalized)	None
Hepatitis A vaccine	Local soreness, headache, anorexia, fatigue	Anaphylaxis
Hepatitis B vaccine	Local discomfort, fever	Anaphylaxis
Pneumococcal conjugate vaccine	Local reactions, fever, irritability	None
Influenza vaccine (inactivated)	Local reactions, fever	None
Influenza vaccine (live attenuated)	Runny nose, headache, cough, fever	None
Meningococcal conjugate vaccine	Local reactions, headache, fatigue	None
Rotavirus vaccine	Diarrhea, vomiting, ear infection, runny nose, sore throat	Intussusception (rare)
Human papillomavirus vaccine	Local reactions, fainting	None

[a]A study showing a connection with autism was disproved.

Efficacy

After a single dose of MMR, an effective response develops in 97% of vaccinated patients within 2 to 6 weeks. A second dose increases protection.

Adverse Effects

Mild. Local soreness, erythema, and swelling may develop soon after vaccination. Within 1 to 2 weeks, some children experience glandular swelling in the cheeks and neck and under the jaw. Transient rash develops in 5% to 15% of vaccinated patients. Fever (103°F or higher) that persists for several days occurs in 5% to 15% of vaccinated patients 5 to 12 days after vaccination. MMR-induced fever poses a small risk for febrile seizures, but these seizures do *not* increase the risk for developing epilepsy. Within 1 to 3 weeks of the first dose, approximately 1% of vaccinated patients experience pain, stiffness, and swelling in one or more joints; these symptoms usually subside in a few days but occasionally persist for a month or more. Fever can be reduced with acetaminophen or a nonaspirin, nonsteroidal antiinflammatory drug, such as ibuprofen. However, as noted earlier, these drugs should not be given before vaccination to *prevent* discomfort. Rather, they should be reserved for managing discomfort after it develops.

Severe. Transient thrombocytopenia occurs very rarely (0.0025% incidence). MMR-induced thrombocytopenia is generally benign, but hemorrhage has developed in a few vaccinated patients.

MMR can induce anaphylactic reactions. However, the incidence is extremely low: only a handful of cases have occurred in more than 70 million vaccinations. In the past, MMR-induced anaphylaxis was thought to result from allergy to eggs (the measles component of the vaccine is produced in chick embryo fibroblasts). However, it now appears that egg allergy is not involved. Rather, the leading suspect is a hydrolysis product of gelatin. Until more is known, authorities recommend that MMR be used with extreme caution in children with a known allergy to gelatin. The AAP states that most children with a history of anaphylactic reactions to eggs have no adverse reactions to the MMR. If children have egg allergies other than anaphylaxis, they should be vaccinated in the usual manner.

The Institute of Medicine and the AAP have organized several panels of independent scientists that have determined that there is no causal link between MMR and development of autism, Crohn disease, or any other serious long-term illness.

Precautions and Contraindications

MMR is *contraindicated* during pregnancy and should be used with *caution* in children with a history of (1) thrombocytopenia or thrombocytopenic purpura or (2) anaphylactic-like reactions to gelatin, eggs, or neomycin (MMR contains a small amount of this antibiotic).

MMR can be administered to children with *mild febrile illness* (e.g., upper respiratory infection with or without low-grade fever). However, for children with *moderate or severe febrile illness,* vaccination should be postponed until the illness has resolved.

Products that contain *immune globulins* (e.g., whole blood, serum, specific immune globulins) contain antibodies against the viruses in MMR and therefore can inhibit the immune response to the vaccine. Accordingly, in children who have received immune globulins, vaccination with MMR should be postponed for at least 3 months.

In vaccinated patients who are *immunocompromised,* replication of the viruses in MMR may be much greater than normal. If the immunodeficiency is severe, death may occur. However, of the more than 200 million people who have received MMR in the United States, only five such deaths have been reported. Nonetheless, ***children with severe immunodeficiency should NOT be given MMR.*** Severe immunodeficiency may result from immunosuppressive drugs

(e.g., glucocorticoids, cytotoxic anticancer drugs), certain cancers (e.g., leukemia, lymphoma, generalized malignancy), and advanced HIV infection. However, it is important to note that if HIV infection is *asymptomatic,* MMR should be given. In this situation, there is no risk for serious adverse events from MMR, whereas there *is* a risk for severe complications from measles should the disease develop. Vaccination with MMR early in the course of HIV infection is preferred because the immune response to vaccination diminishes as HIV infection progresses.

Diphtheria and Tetanus Toxoids and Acellular Pertussis Vaccine

Preparations

Primary vaccination against diphtheria, tetanus, and pertussis is usually done simultaneously using a combination product composed of diphtheria toxoid, tetanus toxoid, and *acellular* pertussis vaccine (DTaP). Vaccination with DTaP produces antibodies against diphtheria toxin, tetanus toxin, and *B. pertussis.* DTaP is available under several trade names, including *DAPTACEL* and *Infanrix.*

After children have received a full series of DTaP shots, they will need subsequent booster shots. Two booster products are available: *Tdap* and *Td.* Tdap—sold as *Boostrix* and *Adacel*—is composed of tetanus toxoid, reduced diphtheria toxoid, and acellular pertussis vaccine—and hence boosts protection against all three diseases. By contrast, Td boosts protection against only two diseases: tetanus and diphtheria. A booster shot with Tdap is currently recommended for all children 11 to 18 years old. Boosters with Td are given every 10 years thereafter.

Products used for immunization against diphtheria, tetanus, and pertussis are shown in Table 55.4.

TABLE 55.4 Products for Immunization Against Diphtheria, Tetanus, and Pertussis

Symbol	Description	Trade Names	Comments
Vaccines for Children Younger Than 10 Years			
DTaP	Diphtheria toxoid, tetanus toxoid, and acellular pertussis vaccine	DAPTACEL, Infanrix	Used for routine vaccination against diphtheria, tetanus, and pertussis
DT	Diphtheria toxoid and tetanus toxoid	Generic only	Used for children younger than 7 years who should not get pertussis vaccine
Vaccines for Adolescents and Adults			
Tdap	Tetanus toxoid, reduced diphtheria toxoid, and acellular pertussis vaccine, adolescent preparation	Boostrix, Adacel	Used as a *booster* in adolescents and adults to protect against all three diseases
Td	Tetanus toxoid and diphtheria toxoid	Tenivac Decavac	Used as a *booster* for adolescents and adults to protect against tetanus and diphtheria, but not pertussis

Efficacy

Immunization with DTaP reduces the risk for disease by 80% to 90%. Protection begins after the third dose and persists 4 to 6 years (against pertussis) and 10 years (against diphtheria and tetanus).

Adverse Effects

Mild. Mild reactions are common. The reactions seen most often are low fever, fretfulness, drowsiness, anorexia, and local reactions: pain, swelling, and redness. Mild reactions usually develop a few hours to 48 hours after vaccination and then resolve in 1 to 2 days. Ibuprofen can decrease fever and pain. However, as noted earlier, ibuprofen should not be given before vaccination to *prevent* discomfort. It should be reserved for managing discomfort after it develops.

Moderate. Moderate reactions occur less often than mild reactions. Persistent, inconsolable crying lasting 3 hours or longer occurs in 1% of vaccinated patients. Crying is most likely with the first dose of DTaP and is not associated with long-term sequelae. Fever (105°F or higher) occurs in 0.3% of vaccinated patients; the pertussis component appears responsible. Approximately 0.06% of vaccinated patients develop convulsions (with or without fever). These seizures have no permanent sequelae and do not increase the risk for subsequent febrile or afebrile seizures. A shocklike state develops in 0.06% of vaccinated patients and has no lasting sequelae.

Severe: encephalopathy. Very rarely, DTaP causes acute encephalopathy. The incidence is between 0 and 10.5 episodes per million doses. Most cases occur within 3 days of vaccination. Some of the children who experience acute encephalopathy develop chronic neurologic dysfunction later in life. However, the contribution of acute encephalopathy to long-term neurologic deficits is unclear.

Precautions and Contraindications

DTaP can be administered to children with *mild febrile illness* (e.g., upper respiratory infection with or without low-grade fever). However, for children with *moderate or severe febrile illness*, administration should be postponed until the illness has resolved.

DTaP is *contraindicated* if a prior vaccination with DTaP produced (1) an immediate anaphylactic reaction or (2) encephalopathy within 7 days of vaccination.

DTaP should be administered with *caution* (if at all) if a prior vaccination with DTaP produced any of the following:

- A shocklike state
- Fever (105°F or higher) occurring within 48 hours of vaccination and not attributable to another identifiable cause
- Persistent, inconsolable crying lasting 3 or more hours and occurring within 48 hours of vaccination
- Seizures (with or without fever) occurring within 3 days of vaccination

Poliovirus Vaccine
Preparations

Poliovirus is composed of inactivated polioviruses, hence the name *inactivated poliovirus vaccine* (IPV, Salk vaccine). The trade name for IPV is *IPOL*.

Efficacy

Between 97.5% and 100% of children receiving IPV develop antibodies to poliovirus types 1, 2, and 3. Antibodies develop after two or more doses and persist for many years.

Adverse Effects of Inactivated Poliovirus Vaccine

IPV is devoid of serious adverse effects. As with other injected drugs, local soreness may occur. IPV contains trace amounts of streptomycin, neomycin, and bacitracin. Children with an allergy to these drugs should be monitored.

Haemophilus influenzae Type b Conjugate Vaccine
Preparations

Vaccines directed against Hib are prepared by conjugating (covalently binding) a Polyribosylribitol Phosphate (PRP) from *H. influenzae* to either (1) tetanus toxoid or (2) an outer membrane protein (OMP) isolated from *N. meningitidis*. The reason for conjugating PRP to these other compounds is to enhance antigenicity. The vaccines made with OMP—marketed as *PedvaxHIB* and *Comvax*[a] and abbreviated PRP-OMP—elicit a stronger immune response than the vaccines made with tetanus toxoid, marketed as *ActHIB* and *Hiberix*.

Efficacy

Immunization with Hib vaccine decreases the risk for disease by 88% to 98%. When PedvaxHIB is used, protection begins 1 week after the first dose. However, when ActHIB is used, protection is delayed, beginning 1 to 2 weeks after the fourth dose. With both vaccines, protection persists for several years.

Adverse Effects

Hib vaccine is among the safest of all vaccines. Serious adverse effects have not been reported. The few adverse effects that do occur are generally transient and mild. Between 2% and 5% of vaccinated patients develop local reactions (swelling, erythema, warmth, and tenderness). Approximately 1% experience fever (temperature above 101°F), crying, diarrhea, or vomiting.

Varicella Virus Vaccine
Description

Varicella virus vaccine is composed of live, attenuated varicella viruses. Two subcutaneously delivered products are available: varicella vaccine by itself, sold as *Varivax*, and varicella vaccine combined with MMR (MMRV), sold as *ProQuad*.

Efficacy

Varicella vaccine, given as a two-dose series, confers full protection in approximately 99% of vaccinated patients. Furthermore, among those who get varicella despite vaccination, symptoms are always mild: these children develop fewer lesions (less than 50, compared with 250 to 500 for unvaccinated children), experience less fever, and recover more quickly. In Japan, herpes zoster (shingles) has not been observed in any adult who received varicella vaccine as a child, even if breakthrough varicella had occurred.

Adverse Effects

Varicella vaccine is very safe; no serious adverse events have been reported. Approximately 25% of vaccinated patients experience erythema, soreness, and swelling at the injection site; 15% develop fever (temperature greater than 102°F); and 3% develop a mild, local varicella-like rash, consisting of just a few lesions. Approximately 5% of healthy children develop a sparse, generalized varicella-like rash within a month of the injection. In children with leukemia, the incidence of generalized rash is much higher—approximately 50%. For all vaccinated patients, rates of fever and rash are higher when MMRV is used than when MMR and varicella vaccine are given separately.

In theory, children receiving the vaccine can transmit vaccine viruses to others. However, among otherwise healthy vaccinated patients, such transmission has not been reported. In contrast, among leukemic children who developed a rash after vaccination, a few cases of viral transmission have occurred. To reduce the risk for transmission, vaccinated patients

[a]Comvax is a combination vaccine for immunization against *H. influenzae* type b and hepatitis B.

should temporarily avoid close contact with susceptible, high-risk individuals (e.g., neonates, pregnant women, immunocompromised people).

Precautions and Contraindications

Varicella vaccine is *contraindicated* for pregnant patients, individuals with certain cancers (e.g., leukemia, lymphomas), and individuals with hypersensitivity to neomycin or gelatin, both of which are in the vaccine. In addition, the vaccine should generally be avoided by individuals who are immunocompromised, including those with HIV infection or congenital immunodeficiency and those taking immunosuppressive drugs.

Children receiving the vaccine should avoid aspirin and other salicylates for 6 weeks. This precaution is based on the theoretical risk for developing Reye syndrome: if the child develops varicella (albeit a mild case) in response to the vaccine, the very small risk for developing Reye syndrome is somewhat increased by concurrent use of salicylates.

Hepatitis B Vaccine
Preparations

Hepatitis B vaccine (HepB) contains *hepatitis B surface antigen* (HBsAg), the primary antigenic protein in the viral envelope. Administration of HepB promotes synthesis of specific antibodies directed against hepatitis B virus. Because HepB is made from a viral component, rather than from a live virus, it cannot cause disease.

HepB is available in pediatric and adult formulations. The pediatric formulation, marketed as *Recombivax HB*, contains 10 μg of HBsAg/mL. The adult formulation, marketed as *Engerix-B*, contains 20 μg of HBsAg/mL. A combination vaccine for adults, marketed as *Twinrix*, protects against hepatitis A *and* hepatitis B. In all three products, the HBsAg is produced in yeast using recombinant DNA technology.

Efficacy

Greater than 85% of vaccinated patients are protected after the second dose of HepB, and more than 90% are protected after the third dose. Although the duration of protection has not been determined with precision, it appears to be at least 5 to 7 years.

Adverse Effects and Contraindications

HepB is one of our safest vaccines. The most common reactions are soreness at the injection site and mild to moderate fever. Acetaminophen or ibuprofen may be used to relieve discomfort, but aspirin should be avoided. The only contraindication to HepB is a prior anaphylactic reaction either to HepB itself or to baker's yeast.

Hepatitis A Vaccine
Preparations

Hepatitis A vaccine (HepA) is prepared from inactivated hepatitis A virus. In the United States, two products are available: *Havrix* and *VAQTA*.

Efficacy

Immunization with HepA decreases the risk for clinical disease by 94% to 100%. Protective levels of antibodies are seen in 94% to 100% of adults and children 1 month after the first dose and in 100% of vaccinated patients 1 month after the second dose. Protection appears to be long lasting: among vaccinated children who were followed for 7 years, no cases of hepatitis A were detected.

Who Should Be Vaccinated?

Hepatitis A vaccination is recommended for *all* children 12 through 23 months old and for children older than 23 months who live in areas where vaccination programs target older children (owing to increased risk for infection). In addition, HepA is recommended for the following:

- People at least 1 year old traveling to places with high rates of hepatitis A, including Central or South America, Mexico, the Caribbean islands, Africa, Asia (except Japan), and southern or eastern Europe
- People in communities that have frequent outbreaks of hepatitis A
- Men who have sex with men
- People who use illegal drugs
- People with chronic liver disease
- People who receive clotting factor concentrates
- People who work with nonhuman primates or who work with hepatitis A in research laboratories
- People who expect to have close personal contact with an international adoptee from a country where hepatitis A is common

Adverse Effects

Mild reactions are common. Soreness at the injection site occurs in approximately 54% of adults and 18% of children. Headache occurs in 14% of adults and 9% of children. Other mild reactions include loss of appetite and malaise. When mild reactions occur, they usually begin 3 to 5 days after vaccination and last only 1 to 2 days.

Pneumococcal Conjugate Vaccine

There are two vaccines for use in prevention of pneumococcal disease; a *13-valent pneumococcal conjugate vaccine* (PCV13), sold as *Prevnar 13*, for prevention of invasive pneumococcal disease in infants and children, and an unconjugated vaccine—*pneumococcal polysaccharide vaccine* (PPSV), sold as *Pneumovax 23*—for adults and high-risk children older than 2 years. PPSV does not work in children younger than 2 years.

Description

PCV13 consists of 13 pneumococcal capsular polysaccharide antigens that have been conjugated to a protein carrier—specifically, CRM197, a nontoxic variant of diphtheria toxin. The protein carrier increases antigenicity, especially in infants. The 13 antigens in the vaccine are from the 13 serotypes of *S. pneumoniae* that cause the majority of invasive pneumococcal infections in American children younger than 6 years. PPSV23, like PCV13, contains polysaccharides, but it covers 23 serotypes of pneumococcal disease.

Efficacy

PCV13 and PPSV23 are highly effective. PCV13 vaccination was 100% effective in preventing invasive disease caused by the *S. pneumoniae* serotypes that the vaccine was designed to protect against. Vaccination was also 89% effective at preventing invasive disease caused by *all* serotypes of *S. pneumoniae*. In addition to preventing invasive pneumococcal disease, vaccination with PCV13 caused a modest reduction in cases of otitis media (see Chapter 89). PPSV23 is most effective in the adult population.

Adverse Effects

Both PCV13 and PPSV23 appear very safe. No serious adverse effects have been reported. Approximately 50% to 70% of vaccinated patients get drowsy after the shot, lose their appetite, or develop erythema or tenderness at the injection site. Mild fever develops in 33%, and a higher fever (temperature above 102.2°F) develops in 5%. Approximately 80% become irritable or fussy.

Who Should Be Vaccinated?

The ACIP recommends vaccinating children in the following groups:

- All children younger than 2 years
- All healthy children between their second and fifth birthdays who have not completed the PCV series

- All children between their second and fifth birthdays who have conditions that put them at high risk for serious pneumococcal disease. In this group are children with sickle cell anemia, injury to the spleen, cochlear implants, chronic heart or lung disease, or immunosuppression of any cause (e.g., diabetes, cancer, liver disease, HIV infection, use of immunosuppressive drugs)

Meningococcal Conjugate Vaccine

In the United States, we have two *meningococcal conjugate polysaccharide vaccines* (MCVs): *Menactra* and *Menveo*. Both vaccines protect against the same four meningococcal serotypes—hence their abbreviation *MCV4*. Menactra is indicated for people 9 months to 55 years old, and Menveo is indicated for people 2 to 55 years old.

An unconjugated vaccine—*meningococcal polysaccharide vaccine* (MPSV4) (Menomune)—has been available since the 1970s but is not very effective in children. Accordingly, MCV4 is currently preferred. MPSV4 is active against the same meningococcal serotypes as MCV4.

There are also two recombinant vaccines directed at serotype B meningococci: *Bexsero* and *Trumenba*. Both are approved for use in patients 10 to 25 years of age.

Description

Menactra is a tetravalent conjugate vaccine directed against four meningococcal serogroups: A, C, Y, and W-135. Each dose consists of 4 µg of capsular polysaccharide from each of the four serogroups conjugated with 48 µg of a protein carrier, specifically, diphtheria toxoid. The carrier protein increases immunogenicity.

Menveo is nearly identical to Menactra. However, there are two differences. First, the amount of capsular polysaccharide in each dose of Menveo is greater (10 µg of polysaccharide from serogroup A, and 5 µg of polysaccharide from serogroups C, Y, and W-135). Second, in Menveo, the polysaccharides are conjugated to a different diphtheria protein.

Bexsero and *Trumenba* are newer vaccines directed specifically at B subgroups of meningococcal disease. *Bexsero* contains 50 µg of each NHBA, NadA, fHbp, and PorA proteins found on the surface of meningococci. *Trumenba* is composed of 60 µg of each fHBP protein subtypes A and B.

Efficacy

The efficacy of MCV4 at preventing meningococcal disease has not been evaluated in clinical trials. However, we do know the vaccine is highly immunogenic. For example, when 423 adolescents were vaccinated, rates of seroconversion for serogroups A, C, Y, and W-135 were 100%, 99%, 98%, and 99%, respectively, as measured by bactericidal antibody assay. FDA approval of MCV4 was based on its documented immunogenicity and the documented ability of other vaccines to prevent meningococcal infection.

Bexsero was studied in adolescents within Canada, Australia, and the United Kingdom. Composite antibody response rates (fHbo, NadA, PorA) rose from a baseline of 24% to 66% at 11 months after the second dose in the United Kingdom and from 0% to 63% in the Canadian and Australian populations. In a controlled trial completed in the United States with children between the ages of 11 and 18 years, *Trumenba* increased rates of serum antibody titer in adolescents from 0.7% to 83% after the third dose.

Adverse Effects

The most common reactions are local pain, headache, and fatigue. Local redness, swelling, and induration are also common.

Concerns that MCV4 might cause *Guillain-Barré syndrome* (GBS) appear to be unfounded, as shown by two large studies. In one study, there were 99 confirmed cases of GBS among 12,589,910 vaccinated patients. In the other study, there were 5 cases among 889,684 vaccinated patients. In both studies the incidence of GBS was no higher than would be expected in the absence of vaccination. In light of this information, the CDC and ACIP have removed precautionary language regarding a risk for GBS after meningococcal vaccination.

Who Should Be Vaccinated?

The ACIP recommends routine meningococcal vaccination for all children and adolescents aged 11 to 12 years with a booster dose at age 16 years. Children who were not vaccinated at this time should be vaccinated as soon as possible. Vaccination is also recommended for people at increased risk for meningococcal disease, including the following:

- College freshmen living in dormitories
- U.S. military recruits
- Microbiologists who are routinely exposed to meningococcal bacteria
- Anyone traveling to (or living in) a part of the world where meningococcal disease is common
- Anyone who has an injured spleen or whose spleen has been removed
- Anyone who has an immune disorder known as terminal complement component deficiency
- Anyone who might have been exposed to meningitis during an outbreak
- Persons with persistent complement component deficiency, anatomic or functional asplenia, and certain other risk factors

MCV4 is the preferred vaccine for people 2 to 55 years old in these risk groups, but MPSV4 can be used if MCV4 is not available. Only MPSV4 should be used for adults older than 55 years (not because MPSV4 is more effective but because it is approved for use in this age group, whereas MCV4 is not). The newer subgroup B vaccines may be used in addition to the MCV4 vaccinations, preferably between the ages of 16 and 18 years. These are only recommended for use in children older than 10 years if they are high risk (functional asplenia, complement deficiency).

For more details on dosing, refer to the Meningococcal VIS and the Adult Immunization Schedule, available online at www.cdc.gov/vaccines, and to Healthcare Personnel Vaccination Recommendations, available online at www.immunize.org/catg.d/p2017.pdf.

Influenza Vaccine

Annual vaccination against influenza is currently recommended for all children between ages 6 months and 18 years (as well as all adults). Properties of intramuscular, intradermal, and intranasal influenza vaccines (composition, efficacy, adverse effects, contraindications, preparations, dosage, route), along with information on adult vaccination, are presented in Chapter 80.

Rotavirus Vaccine
Preparations and Efficacy

In the United States two rotavirus vaccines are available: *RotaTeq* and *Rotarix*. Both contain live, attenuated viruses. To induce a strong immune response, these viruses must replicate within the infant's gut. Accordingly, the vaccine is administered orally. RotaTeq and Rotarix differ in composition and dosing schedule.

RotaTeq is a *pentavalent* vaccine directed against the five most common serotypes of human rotavirus, termed G1, G2, G3, G4, and P1A. In trials in the United States and Finland, RotaTeq prevented 74% of *all* rotavirus gastroenteritis cases and 98% of *severe* cases. Vaccination also reduced the need for diarrhea-related hospitalization by 96%.

Rotarix is a *monovalent* vaccine developed from a rotavirus with the most common serotype found in humans. However, although Rotarix is monovalent, it confers protection against four rotavirus serotypes: G1, G3, G4, and G9. In clinical trials, Rotarix prevented 79% of *all* rotavirus gastroenteritis cases, 90% of *severe* cases, and 96% of diarrhea-related hospitalizations.

Safety

Although generally very safe, both RotaTeq and Rotarix may carry a small risk for *intussusception,* a rare, life-threatening form of bowel obstruction that occurs when the bowel folds in on itself, like a collapsing telescope. Of note, during prelicensure testing in more than 130,000 infants, no cases of intussusception were seen. However, with both vaccines, several cases were reported during postmarketing surveillance. Fortunately, the estimated risk is very low: approximately 1 case for each 50,000 to 70,000 vaccinated patients.

Who Should Be Vaccinated?

The ACIP recommends that all infants receive rotavirus vaccine, beginning at approximately age 8 weeks.

Who Should Not Be Vaccinated?

Rotarix, but not RotaTeq, is contraindicated for infants with any uncorrected congenital malformation of the gastrointestinal tract that could predispose to intussusception. Both vaccines are contraindicated for children with a history of intussusception.

Some vaccinated patients with *severe combined immunodeficiency (SCID),* a rare inherited disorder, have developed vaccine-acquired rotavirus infection. Accordingly, these vaccines are contraindicated for infants with SCID. Rotavirus vaccines have not been evaluated in children who are immunocompromised for other reasons. Nonetheless, because these vaccines contain live viruses, it would seem prudent to use them with caution in all immunocompromised infants, regardless of the cause.

Infants with moderate to severe diarrhea or vomiting should probably not be vaccinated until they recover.

Human Papillomavirus Vaccine

Two HPV vaccines are available: Gardasil ♣ and Gardasil 9. In the United States, the Gardasil 9 is the only HPV vaccine currently in use. These vaccines differ in composition, indications, and immunogenicity. Gardasil ♣ is a quadrivalent vaccine, and Gardasil 9 is a 9-valent vaccine. Gardasil protects against cervical, vulvar, and vaginal cancer in females, as well as anal cancer and genital warts in females and males. Gardasil was the first vaccine licensed in the United States for the specific purpose of protecting against cancer of any type.

Quadrivalent and 9-Valent HPV Vaccines: Gardasil ♣ and Gardasil 9

Composition. Gardasil ♣ is a quadrivalent vaccine designed to stimulate production of neutralizing antibodies directed at four types of HPV—specifically, types 16 and 18 (which cause 70% of cervical cancers) and types 6 and 11 (which cause 95% of genital warts). Gardasil 9 protects against HPV types 6, 11, 16, 18, 31, 33, 45, 52, and 58. The vaccines consist of *virus-like particles* (VLPs), which are virus-sized, empty spheres composed of viral capsid proteins. To the immune system, VLPs look like the actual virus, and hence VLPs can evoke an immune response. Because VLPs are empty (and hence do not contain viral DNA), VLPs cannot cause infection.

Indications. Gardasil ♣ and Gardasil 9 are used to prevent cancers, precancerous lesions, and genital warts in females and males.

Cancers and precancerous lesions in female patients. Gardasil ♣ and Gardasil 9 are indicated for girls and women 9 to 45 years old to prevent the following cancers caused by HPV types 16, 18, 31, 33, 45, 52, and 58:

- Cervical cancer
- Vulvar cancer
- Vaginal cancer

In addition, Gardasil ♣ and Gardasil 9 are indicated for prevention of the following precancerous and dysplastic lesions caused by HPV types 6, 11, 16, 18, 31, 33, 45, 52, and 58:

- Cervical adenocarcinoma in situ
- Cervical intraepithelial neoplasia grades 1, 2, and 3
- Vulvar intraepithelial neoplasia grades 2 and 3
- Vaginal intraepithelial neoplasia grades 2 and 3
- Anal intraepithelial neoplasia grades 1, 2, and 3

Genital warts in females and males. Gardasil is indicated for females and males 9 to 45 years old to prevent genital warts caused by HPV types 6 and 11.

Anal cancer in females and males. Gardasil is indicated for females and males 9 to 26 years old to prevent anal cancer and precancerous lesions caused by HPV types 6, 11, 16, 18, 31, 33, 45, 52, and 58.

Efficacy. Gardasil is highly effective, as demonstrated in Females United to Unilaterally Reduce Endo/Ectocervical Disease II (FUTURE II), a phase 3, randomized, double-blind, placebo-controlled trial. Researchers enrolled 12,167 healthy women, aged 16 to 23 years, and gave them three intramuscular injections of Gardasil or placebo over a 6-month interval. During 2 years of follow-up, Gardasil was nearly 100% effective at preventing precancerous cervical lesions, precancerous vaginal and vulvar lesions, and genital warts caused by HPV types 6, 11, 16, and 18. However, although Gardasil protected against new HPV infection, it did not eliminate infection that was already present. Furthermore, although Gardasil prevented precancerous cervical lesions, the study period was too short to tell whether vaccination prevents cervical cancer. Nonetheless, given that HPV infection causes more than 99% of cervical cancers, it seems highly likely that protection against this cancer will be conferred. At this time, the estimated duration of protection against HPV is 5 to 10 years. Studies are underway to determine whether and when booster vaccination may be needed.

Safety. Gardasil appears to be very safe. Injection-site reactions—pain, erythema, swelling, and itching—although common, are mild and short lived. Fainting has occurred in teenage girls, sometimes resulting in hospitalization. However, the incidence of fainting is no greater than with other vaccines. Vaccinated patients who feel faint should sit or lie down to prevent falling.

Who should be vaccinated? Given that HPV infection is sexually transmitted and that HPV infects males and females, universal vaccination would be required to achieve maximal protection in the community. Accordingly, ACIP now recommends *routine* vaccination for males *and* females with HPV vaccine.

Females: routine vaccination. The ACIP recommends routine vaccination for all girls 11 to 12 years old. Why girls this young? Because the vaccine protects only against *acquiring* HPV infection. It cannot clear infection that already exists. Therefore vaccination is most beneficial when done before vaccinated patients become sexually active, which is the case for most girls in this age group.

Vaccination with the HPV vaccine remains voluntary, not compulsory, throughout most of the United States. Reasons for objection to vaccination include expense (approximately $390 for the three-dose series), concerns about safety, and concerns that conferring protection against a sexually transmitted infection might encourage promiscuity (a concern that has no basis in fact). Parents who are considering withholding vaccination would do well to ask this question: does protecting my daughter against developing cervical cancer later in life outweigh my concerns about vaccination? If the answer is yes, then vaccination should not be withheld.

Males: routine vaccination. ACIP recommends the HPV vaccine for all males 11 to 12 years old. Vaccination of males can help to protect them from genital warts and HPV-related cancers and may help to prevent spread of HPV to females.

Females and males: catch-up vaccination. ACIP recommends the HPV vaccine for females and males 13 to 21 years old who did not receive the vaccine when they were younger.

Who should not be vaccinated? HPV vaccine is not recommended for patients who are pregnant. Those who are breastfeeding may receive the vaccine.

Respiratory Syncytial Virus Vaccine (Experimental)

Scientists are currently testing experimental vaccines to prevent RSV. In animal tests, an RSV vaccine elicited high levels of RSV-specific antibodies.

56

Antihistamines

Histamine is a small molecule produced in specialized cells throughout the body. The compound plays an important role in allergic reactions and regulation of gastric acid secretion. The antihistamines, a widely used family of drugs, block histamine actions.

To understand the antihistamines, we must first understand histamine itself. Accordingly, the chapter begins with a discussion of histamine, emphasizing its contribution to allergic responses.

HISTAMINE

Histamine is a locally acting compound with prominent and varied effects. In the vascular system, histamine dilates small blood vessels and increases capillary permeability. In the bronchi, histamine produces constriction of smooth muscle. In the stomach, histamine stimulates secretion of acid. In the central nervous system (CNS), histamine acts as a neurotransmitter. Despite this impressive spectrum of actions, clinical use of histamine is limited to diagnostic procedures. However, although its clinical utility is minimal, histamine is still of great interest owing to its involvement in two common pathologic states: allergic disorders and peptic ulcer disease.

Distribution, Synthesis, Storage, and Release
Distribution
Histamine is present in practically all tissues. Levels are especially high in the skin, lungs, and the gastrointestinal (GI) tract. The histamine content of plasma is low.

Synthesis and Storage
In the periphery, histamine is synthesized and stored in two types of cells: *mast cells* and *basophils.* Mast cells are present in the skin and other soft tissues. Basophils are present in blood. In both mast cells and basophils, histamine is stored in secretory granules.

In the CNS, histamine is produced by neurons with cell bodies in the posterior hypothalamus and with axonal projections to the frontal and temporal cortices and other brain regions.

Release
Release of histamine from mast cells and basophils is produced by allergic and nonallergic mechanisms.

Allergic Release
The initial requirement for allergic release is production of antibodies of the immunoglobulin E class. These antibodies are generated after exposure to specific allergens (e.g., pollens, insect venoms, certain drugs). Once made, the antibodies become attached to the outer surface of mast cells and basophils (Fig. 56.1). When the individual is reexposed to the allergen, the allergen becomes bound by the antibodies. Binding of allergen to adjacent antibodies creates a bridge between those antibodies. By a mechanism that is not fully understood, this bridging process mobilizes intracellular calcium. The calcium, in

turn, causes the histamine-containing storage granules to fuse with the cell membrane and disgorge their contents into the extracellular space. Note that allergic release of histamine requires *prior exposure* to the allergen; an allergic reaction cannot occur during initial allergen exposure.

Nonallergic Release
Several agents (certain drugs, radiocontrast media, plasma expanders) can act directly on mast cells to trigger histamine release. With these agents, no prior sensitization is needed. Cell injury can also cause direct release.

Physiologic and Pharmacologic Effects
Histamine acts primarily through two types of receptors, named histamine-1 (H_1) and histamine-2 (H_2). The response produced depends on which of these receptors is involved.

Effects of Histamine-1 Stimulation
Vasodilation. Activation of H_1 receptors causes dilation of small blood vessels (arterioles and venules). Vasodilation is prominent in the skin of the face and upper body, causing the area to become warm and flushed. If extensive vasodilation occurs, total peripheral resistance declines and blood pressure falls.

Increased capillary permeability. Activation of H_1 receptors increases capillary permeability. Receptor activation causes capillary endothelial cells to contract, creating openings between these cells through which fluid, protein, and platelets can escape. Escape of fluid and protein into the interstitial space produces edema. If loss of intravascular fluid is substantial, blood pressure may fall.

Bronchoconstriction. H_1 activation causes constriction of the bronchi. If histamine is administered to an individual with asthma, severe bronchoconstriction will follow. However, although *exogenous* histamine can induce bronchial constriction, histamine is not the cause of bronchoconstriction that occurs during a spontaneous asthma attack. Consequently, antihistamines are of no use for treating asthma.

Central nervous system effects. In the CNS, H_1 receptors have a role in cognition, memory, and the cycle of sleeping and waking. In addition, H_1 receptors appear to have a role in seizure suppression, modulation of neurotransmitter release, and regulation of energy and endocrine homeostasis.

Other effects. Activation of H_1 receptors on sensory nerves produces *itching* and *pain.* H_1 activation also promotes *secretion of mucus.*

Effects of Histamine-2 Stimulation
The major response to activation of H_2 receptors is *secretion of gastric acid.* Histamine acts directly on parietal cells of the stomach to promote acid release. Although acetylcholine and gastrin also help regulate acid release, histamine has a dominant role. We know this because, in the presence of H_2 blockade, acetylcholine and gastrin are unable to elicit acid secretion.

Fig. 56.1 Release of Histamine by Allergen-Antibody Interaction. *IgE,* Immunoglobulin E.

Role of Histamine in Allergic Responses

Allergic reactions are mediated by histamine and other compounds (e.g., prostaglandins, leukotrienes, tryptase). The intensity of an allergic reaction is determined by which mediator is involved. The symptoms of mild allergy (e.g., rhinitis, itching, localized edema) are caused largely by histamine acting at H_1 receptors. As a result, mild allergic conditions (e.g., hay fever, acute urticaria, mild transfusion reactions) are generally responsive to antihistamine therapy.

THE TWO TYPES OF ANTIHISTAMINES: HISTAMINE-1 ANTAGONISTS AND HISTAMINE-2 ANTAGONISTS

Antihistamines fall into two basic categories: H_1 receptor antagonists and H_2 receptor antagonists. The principal use of H_1 blockers is treatment of mild allergic disorders. The principal use of H_2 blockers is treatment of gastric and duodenal ulcers. Because H_2 antagonists do not block H_1 receptors, these drugs are of no use for treating allergies. In this chapter, we focus on H_1 antagonists. The H_2 blockers, which are widely used, are discussed in Chapter 64.

Histamine-1 Antagonists
Basic Pharmacology

The H_1 antagonists are the classic antihistamines. Because of its historical use, the term *antihistamines* is still used as a synonym for the subgroup of histamine antagonists that produce selective H_1 blockade. Here we continue to use the term *antihistamine* interchangeably with H_1 blocker and H_1 antagonist.

Although all H_1 antagonists available have similar antihistaminic actions, these drugs differ significantly in side effects. Because of these differences, selection of a prototype to represent the group is not feasible. Thus rather than structuring discussion around one prototypic drug, we discuss the H_1 antagonists collectively. Differences among individual antihistamines are addressed as appropriate.

Classification

The H_1 antagonists fall into two major groups: *first-generation H_1 antagonists* and *second-generation H_1 antagonists*. The principal difference between the groups is that first-generation antihistamines are highly sedating, whereas second-generation antihistamines do not tend to do so.

Mechanism of Action

H_1 blockers bind selectively to H_1-histaminic receptors, thereby blocking the actions of histamine at these sites. H_1 antagonists do not block H_2 receptors. In addition, they do not block release of histamine from mast cells or basophils.

It should be noted that, although interaction of the classic antihistamines with *histaminic* receptors is limited to the H_1 receptor subtype, these drugs can also bind to *nonhistaminic* receptors. Most notably, certain antihistamines can bind to and block *muscarinic* receptors. This action underlies several important side effects.

Pharmacologic Effects

Peripheral effects. The major therapeutic effects of the H_1 antagonists can be attributed to preventing the actions of histamine at H_1 receptors. In arterioles and venules of the skin, H_1 blockers inhibit the dilator actions of histamine and thereby reduce localized flushing. In capillary beds, the antihistamines prevent histamine-induced increases in permeability and thereby reduce edema. By blocking histamine at sensory nerves, H_1 antagonists reduce itching and pain. Blockade of H_1 receptors in mucous membranes suppresses secretion of mucus.

Effects on the central nervous system. Antihistamines can cause both excitation and depression of the CNS. At therapeutic doses, antihistamines produce CNS depression: reaction time is slowed, alertness is diminished, and drowsiness is likely. These effects are more pronounced with some antihistamines than with others. With most second-generation antihistamines (e.g., fexofenadine), CNS depression is negligible.

Overdose with antihistamines can produce *CNS stimulation.* Seizures frequently result. Very young children are especially sensitive to CNS stimulation by these drugs.

Other pharmacologic effects. Blockade of muscarinic cholinergic receptors by antihistamines can produce typical *anticholinergic* responses. These are discussed later under "Adverse Effects." Several antihistamines can suppress nausea and vomiting, as discussed later under "Motion Sickness."

Therapeutic Uses

All of the H_1 antagonists are useful in treating allergic disorders. Some are also indicated for other conditions (e.g., motion sickness, insomnia).

Mild allergy. Antihistamines can reduce symptoms of mild allergies. In people with *seasonal allergic rhinitis,* H_1 blockers can reduce sneezing, rhinorrhea, and itching of the eyes, nose, and throat. In patients with

🔹 PATIENT-CENTERED CARE ACROSS THE LIFE SPAN

Antihistamines

Life Stage	Patient Care Concerns
Infants	Antihistamines can cause sedation in infants. Although they can be used in small doses in children older than 6 months, caution should be used.
Children/ adolescents	Antihistamines can be used safely in children, just in smaller doses. Side effect profiles are similar to those of adults. Promethazine is contraindicated in children younger than 2 years because deaths have occurred in this population.
Pregnant women	There has been debate regarding whether antihistamines cause fetal harm when used in pregnancy. Many of these drugs are classified in U.S. Food and Drug Administration Pregnancy Risk Category C and should be avoided unless absolutely necessary.
Breastfeeding women	Occasional, small doses of antihistamines do not appear to cause sedation in infants. Caution should be used.
Older adults	Many of the antihistamines are listed within the Beers Criteria and should be avoided in older adults. Because antihistamines can cause sedation, smaller doses should be used initially and titrated up if needed. In addition, these medications can make glaucoma or benign prostatic hyperplasia worse.

TABLE 56.1 Pharmacologic Effects of Histamine-1 Antagonists Used for Systemic Therapy

Drug	H_1-Blocking Activity	Sedative Effects	Anticholinergic Effects
First-Generation Agents			
Alkylamines			
Brompheniramine	+++	+	++
Chlorpheniramine	++	+	++
Dexchlorpheniramine	+++	+	++
Ethanolamines			
Clemastine	+ to ++	++	+++
Diphenhydramine	+ to ++	+++	+++
Phenothiazine			
Promethazine[a]	+++	+++	+++
Piperazine			
Hydroxyzine	++ to +++	+++	++
Second-Generation (Nonsedating) Agents			
Cetirizine[b]	+++	+	±
Levocetirizine[b]	+++	+	±
Fexofenadine	+++	±	±
Loratadine	++ to +++	±	±
Desloratadine	++ to +++	±	±

[a]Promethazine is contraindicated in children younger than 2 years owing to a risk for fatal respiratory depression. *Parenteral* promethazine can cause severe local tissue injury.
[b]Cetirizine and levocetirizine have mild sedative effects.
H_1, Histamine-1; ±, low to none; +, low; ++, moderate; +++, high.

acute urticaria, these drugs can reduce redness, itching, and edema. The antihistamines can also reduce symptoms of *allergic conjunctivitis* and urticaria associated with *mild transfusion reactions*. In all these conditions, benefits result from H_1 receptor blockade—not from preventing allergen-induced release of histamine from mast cells and basophils. Because mild allergic reactions may be mediated by substances in addition to histamine, antihistamines often fail to produce complete relief.

Motion sickness. Some antihistamines, such as promethazine (Phenergan) and dimenhydrinate (Dramamine), are labeled for use in motion sickness. Benefits derive from blocking H_1 receptors and muscarinic receptors in the neuronal pathway leading from the vestibular apparatus of the inner ear to the vomiting center of the medulla. Motion sickness and its treatment are discussed in Chapter 66.

Insomnia. The ability of antihistamines to cause drowsiness has been exploited in the treatment of insomnia. Practically every over-the-counter (OTC) sleep aid contains an H_1 antagonist—diphenhydramine or pyrilamine—as its active ingredient. However, although antihistamines can induce sleep when used in sufficient dosage, the doses recommended for OTC preparations are usually too low to be effective.

Adverse Effects

All of the H_1 blockers can produce undesired effects. As a rule, these responses are more of a nuisance than a source of serious discomfort or danger. Frequently, side effects subside with continued drug use. Because individual antihistamines differ in their abilities to produce particular side effects (Table 56.1), adverse responses can be minimized by judicious drug selection.

Sedation. Sedation is the most common side effect of the antihistamines and can lead to serious consequences. In fact, the degree of impairment seen with antihistamines equals that seen when blood levels of alcohol exceed the legal limit. Worse yet, impairment can occur without feeling tired. Accordingly, patients should exercise extreme caution when driving or performing other hazardous activities. They should also avoid alcohol and other CNS depressants, which will intensify the depressant effects of the H_1 antagonist. Fortunately, tolerance to sedation often develops within a few days or weeks. If a preparation with a long half-life is being used, daytime sedation can be minimized by administering the entire daily dose at night.

The second-generation antihistamines exert little or no sedative effect. First, these drugs are relatively large molecules with low lipid solubility, so they cannot cross the blood–brain barrier. Second, these drugs have low affinity to the type of H_1 receptor found in the brain. In contrast, the first-generation antihistamines are relatively small molecules with high lipid solubility and hence can readily cross the blood–brain barrier. In addition, these drugs have a high affinity for H_1 receptors of the CNS.

For patients who experience disabling sedation with a first-generation H_1 antagonist, therapy with a second-generation (nonsedating) antihistamine is likely to help.

Nonsedative central nervous system effects. In addition to sedation, antihistamines can cause dizziness, incoordination, confusional states, and fatigue. Older patients are especially sensitive to these actions. In some patients, paradoxical excitation occurs, resulting in insomnia, nervousness, tremors, and even seizures. CNS stimulation is most common in children and after an overdose.

Gastrointestinal effects. GI disturbances are common. Responses include nausea, vomiting, loss of appetite, and diarrhea or constipation. These reactions can be minimized by administering antihistamines with food.

Anticholinergic effects. The H_1 antagonists possess weak atropine-like properties. These antimuscarinic actions can produce drying of mucous membranes in the mouth, nasal passages, and throat. Cholinergic blockade may also result in urinary hesitancy, constipation, and palpitations. If dry mouth becomes distressing, discomfort can be minimized by using hard sugarless candy and by taking frequent sips of liquid. Antihistamines should be used with caution in patients with asthma because thickening of bronchial secretions may impair breathing. Care is also needed in patients with other conditions that can be made worse by muscarinic blockade (e.g., urinary retention, benign prostatic hyperplasia, hypertension). The second-generation antihistamines are the least anticholinergic.

⟫ BLACK BOX WARNING

Promethazine

Promethazine (Phenergan) can cause severe respiratory depression, especially in very young patients. Deaths have occurred. Accordingly, the drug is now contraindicated for use in children younger than 2 years and should be used with caution in children older than 2 years.

Drug Interactions: Central Nervous System Depressants

Alcohol and other CNS depressants (e.g., barbiturates, benzodiazepines, opioids) can intensify the depressant effects of H_1 antagonists. Patients should be advised against drinking alcoholic beverages. If medications with CNS-depressant properties are combined with H_1 blockers, dosage of the depressant may need to be lowered.

Use in Pregnancy and Lactation

Pregnancy. The margin of safety of antihistamines in pregnancy is unknown. There have been reports of fetal malformation, but direct involvement of H_1 antagonists has not been proved. Given the uncertainty over the safety of these drugs, it is recommended that antihistamines be used only when clearly necessary and only when the benefits of treatment outweigh the potential risks to the fetus. Antihistamines should be avoided late in the third trimester because newborns are particularly sensitive to the adverse actions of these drugs.

Lactation. The H_1 antagonists can be excreted in breast milk, thereby posing a risk to the nursing infant. Because infants, and especially

TABLE 56.2 H_1 Antagonists Used for Systemic Therapy: Trade Names, Routes, and Dosage

Generic Name	Trade Names	Routes	Usual Adult Oral Dosage
First-Generation Agents			
Alkylamines			
Brompheniramine	Bromfed DM, others	PO	10 mg every 4–6 h
Chlorpheniramine	Chlor-Trimeton, others	PO	4 mg every 4–6 h
Dexchlorpheniramine	Generic only	PO	2 mg every 4–6 h
Ethanolamines			
Clemastine	Tavist Allergy	PO	1.34 mg every 12 h
Diphenhydramine	Benadryl	PO, IV, IM	25–50 mg every 6–8 h
Phenothiazine			
Promethazine[a]	Phenergan, others	PO, IV, IM, rectal suppository	12.5–25 mg every 6 h
Piperazine			
Hydroxyzine	Vistaril	PO	25–100 mg every 4–8 h
Piperidine			
Cyproheptadine	Generic only	PO	4 mg every 6–8 h
Second-Generation (Nonsedating) Agents			
Cetirizine[b]	Zyrtec, Reactine 🍁	PO	5–10 mg every 24 h Children 2–5 years: 2.5 mg every 24 h
Levocetirizine[b]	Xyzal	PO	5 mg every 24 h Children 6–11 years: 2.5 mg every 24 h Children 6 months–5 years: 1.25 mg every 24 h
Fexofenadine	Allegra, Allegra ODT	PO	180 mg every 24 h Children 6–11 years: 30 mg every 12 h Children 6 months–2 years: 15 mg every 12 h
Loratadine	Alavert, Claritin	PO	10 mg every 24 h Children 2–5 years: 5 mg every 24 h
Desloratadine	Clarinex, Clarinex RediTabs, Aerius 🍁	PO	5 mg every 24 h Children 6–11 years: 2.5 mg every 24 h Children 1–5 years: 1.25 mg every 24 h Children 2–11 months: 1 mg every 24 h

[a]Promethazine is contraindicated in children younger than 2 years owing to a risk for fatal respiratory depression.
[b]Cetirizine and levocetirizine have mild sedative effects.
PO, Per os; *IV,* intravenously; *IM,* intramuscularly.

newborns, are unusually sensitive to antihistamines, these drugs should be avoided by women who are breastfeeding. If necessary, small, occasional doses will likely not cause harm.

Preparations

As noted previously, the H_1 antagonists can be divided into two major groups: first-generation H_1 antagonists and second-generation H_1 antagonists. The first-generation agents can cause significant sedation. In contrast, the second-generation agents cause little or no sedation. All of the H_1 blockers can be administered by mouth. In addition, some can be given parenterally, by nasal spray, or by rectal suppository. Routes and dosages for individual H_1 antagonists are shown in Table 56.2.

First-generation histamine-1 antagonists. The first-generation antihistamines can be grouped into five major categories (see Table 56.1). These groups differ in antihistaminic efficacy and the ability to cause sedation and muscarinic blockade. Given these differences, it may be possible, through judicious drug selection, to produce effective H_1 blockade while minimizing undesired effects.

Sedation can be a significant problem. Among the first-generation agents, CNS depression is most prominent with the ethanolamines (e.g., diphenhydramine) and phenothiazines (e.g., promethazine) and least prominent with the alkylamines (e.g., chlorpheniramine). For many patients, the alkylamines can provide effective H_1 blockade while causing only a modest reduction in alertness. If sedation remains excessive with an alkylamine, a second-generation agent should be tried.

Most first-generation agents have significant anticholinergic properties. As a result, they can cause dry mouth, urinary hesitancy, and other typical anticholinergic side effects.

Second-generation (nonsedating) histamine-1 antagonists. Second-generation antihistamines produce much less sedation than first-generation agents because (1) the second-generation agents cross the blood–brain barrier poorly and (2) they have a low affinity for H_1 receptors of the CNS. Synergism with alcohol and other CNS depressants is low. Nonetheless, combined use of CNS depressants and the second-generation agents should be avoided. In addition to lacking sedative effects, the second-generation agents are largely devoid of anticholinergic actions. Because all of these drugs are very similar, initial selection can usually be based on price. If a cheaper agent proves ineffective, a more expensive agent can be tried.

Although there are five second-generation agents that are used for oral therapy, we will discuss only the prototype, fexofenadine. The remainder can be found in Table 56.2. Two other second-generation agents, azelastine (Astepro) and olopatadine (Patanase), both used for local effects in the nose, are discussed in Chapter 63.

Fexofenadine. Fexofenadine (Allegra, Allegra Allergy) is approved for oral therapy of seasonal allergic rhinitis and for chronic idiopathic urticaria. Of the second-generation antihistamines currently available, fexofenadine appears to offer the best combination of efficacy and safety. In clinical trials, the incidence of drowsiness and other side effects was nearly the same as with placebo. Fexofenadine has a half-life of 14.4 hours and is excreted unchanged in the urine. The drug is available in standard tablets (30, 60, and 180 mg) and a suspension (6 mg/mL), marketed as Allegra Children's Liquid, and in orally disintegrating tablets (30 mg), marketed as Allegra Children's Meltable Tablets. For all formulations, dosage should be reduced in patients with renal impairment.

Certain fruit juices (e.g., apple juice, orange juice, grapefruit juice) can reduce fexofenadine absorption, possibly reducing therapeutic effects. The mechanism is inhibition of organic anion transporting polypeptides, which contribute to absorption of fexofenadine from the GI tract. To ensure fexofenadine absorption, patients should not drink fruit juices within 4 hours before dosing or 1 to 2 hours after dosing.

 SUMMARY OF KEY PRESCRIBING CONSIDERATIONS

Antihistamines

Therapeutic Goal: Relief of symptoms of mild to moderate allergic disorders

Baseline Data: Description of current symptoms

Monitoring: No laboratory monitoring is required with use of these medications.

Identifying High-Risk Patients: Exercise caution when treating young children, older adults, and patients with conditions that may be aggravated by muscarinic blockade, including asthma, urinary retention, open-angle glaucoma, and prostatic hypertrophy.

Minimizing Adverse Effects: If sedation is an issue, have patient take the medication at night prior to sleep. Gastrointestinal upset can be minimized by taking with meals. Frequent sips of liquid can help reduce dry mouth.

57

Cyclooxygenase Inhibitors: Nonsteroidal Antiinflammatory Drugs and Acetaminophen

The family of cyclooxygenase inhibitors consists of aspirin and related drugs. Most of these agents have three useful effects: they can suppress inflammation, relieve pain, and reduce fever. In addition, aspirin—and only aspirin—can protect against myocardial infarction (MI) and stroke. All of these effects are produced through one central mechanism: inhibition of cyclooxygenase, the enzyme responsible for the synthesis of prostanoids (prostaglandins and related compounds). This same mechanism underlies their principal adverse effects: gastric ulceration, bleeding, and renal impairment. Cyclooxygenase inhibition also underlies MI and stroke, which can occur with most of these drugs but *not* with aspirin.

MECHANISM OF ACTION

All of the drugs discussed here work by inhibiting *cyclooxygenase* (COX), the enzyme that converts arachidonic acid into *prostanoids: prostaglandins* and related compounds (prostacyclin, thromboxane A_2 [TXA_2]). To understand the drugs that inhibit COX, we must first understand COX itself.

Cyclooxygenase is found in all tissues and helps regulate multiple processes. At sites of tissue injury, COX catalyzes the synthesis of prostaglandin E_2 (PGE_2) and prostaglandin I_2 (PGI_2, also called prostacyclin), which promote inflammation and sensitize receptors to painful stimuli. In the stomach, COX promotes synthesis of PGE_2 and PGI_2, which help protect the gastric mucosa. Three mechanisms are involved: reduced secretion of gastric acid, increased secretion of bicarbonate and cytoprotective mucus, and maintenance of submucosal blood flow. In platelets, COX promotes synthesis of TXA_2, which stimulates platelet aggregation. In blood vessels, COX promotes synthesis of prostacyclin, which causes vasodilation. In the kidney, COX catalyzes synthesis of PGE_2 and PGI_2, which promote vasodilation and thereby maintain renal blood flow. In the brain, COX-derived prostaglandins mediate fever and contribute to perception of pain. In the uterus, COX-derived prostaglandins help promote contractions at term. It is important to appreciate that prostaglandins, prostacyclin, and TXA_2 act *locally;* these compounds do not affect sites distant from where they were made.

Cyclooxygenase has two forms, named cyclooxygenase-1 (COX-1) and cyclooxygenase-2 (COX-2). COX-1 is found in practically all tissues, where it mediates "housekeeping" chores. Important among these are protecting the gastric mucosa, supporting renal function, and promoting platelet aggregation. In contrast, COX-2 is produced mainly at sites of *tissue injury,* where it mediates inflammation and sensitizes receptors to painful stimuli. COX-2 is also present in the *brain* (where it mediates fever and contributes to perception of pain), the *kidneys* (where it supports renal function), *blood vessels* (where it promotes vasodilation), and the *colon* (where it can contribute to colon cancer). Because COX-1 primarily mediates beneficial processes whereas COX-2 primarily mediates harmful processes, COX-1 has been dubbed the "good COX" and COX-2 the "bad COX." Some important functions of COX-1 and COX-2 are shown in Table 57.1.

Having established the roles of COX-1 and COX-2, we can now predict the effects of drugs that inhibit these enzymes. Inhibition of COX-1 (good COX) results largely in harmful effects:
- Gastric erosion and ulceration
- Bleeding tendencies
- Renal impairment
  Inhibition of COX-1 also has one very beneficial effect:
- Protection against MI and stroke (secondary to reduced platelet aggregation)
  Inhibition of COX-2 (bad COX) results largely in beneficial effects:
- Suppression of inflammation
- Alleviation of pain
- Reduction of fever
- Protection against colorectal cancer
  Inhibition of COX-2 also has two adverse effects:
- Renal impairment
- Promotion of MI and stroke (secondary to suppressing vasodilation)

CLASSIFICATION OF CYCLOOXYGENASE INHIBITORS

The cyclooxygenase inhibitors fall into two major categories: (1) drugs that have antiinflammatory properties and (2) drugs that lack antiinflammatory properties. Agents in the first group are referred to as *nonsteroidal antiinflammatory drugs* (NSAIDs). Representative members include aspirin, ibuprofen (Advil, Motrin, others), naproxen (Aleve, others), and celecoxib (Celebrex). The second class consists of just one drug: *acetaminophen* (Tylenol, others). Acetaminophen can reduce pain and fever but cannot suppress inflammation.

The NSAIDs can be subdivided into two groups: (1) *first-generation NSAIDs* (conventional NSAIDs, traditional NSAIDs) and (2) *second-generation NSAIDs* (selective COX-2 inhibitors, coxibs). The first-generation agents inhibit COX-1 *and* COX-2. The second-generation agents inhibit COX-2 only. Because the first-generation agents inhibit both COX isoforms, they are unable to suppress pain and inflammation without posing a risk for serious side effects (gastric ulceration, bleeding, renal impairment). In contrast, because of their selectivity for COX-2, the second-generation NSAIDs, *in theory,* can suppress pain and inflammation while (possibly) causing fewer adverse effects than the first-generation NSAIDs. However, *in reality,* COX-2 inhibitors appear even less safe than the first-generation agents, owing to an increased risk for MI and stroke.

Table 57.2 shows the principal indications and adverse effects of the first-generation NSAIDs, second-generation NSAIDs, and acetaminophen.

FIRST-GENERATION NONSTEROIDAL ANTIINFLAMMATORY DRUGS

The first-generation NSAIDs—a large and widely used group of drugs—inhibit COX-1 and COX-2. The traditional NSAIDs are used

TABLE 57.1   Cyclooxygenase-1 and -2: Functions and Effect of Inhibition

Location	COX Isoform	COX Reaction Product	Response to COX Reaction Product	Effect of COX Inhibition
Stomach	COX-1	PGE_2, PGI_2	Gastric protection: Increased bicarbonate secretion Increased mucus production Decreased acid secretion Maintenance of submucosal blood flow	Gastric ulceration
Platelets	COX-1	TXA_2	Platelet aggregation	Bleeding tendencies Protection against MI
Blood vessels	COX-2	Prostacyclin	Vasodilation	Vasoconstriction (which can promote MI)
Kidney	COX-1, COX-2	PGE_2, PGI_2	Maintenance of renal function: Renal vasodilation Maintenance of renal perfusion	Renal impairment
Injured tissue	COX-2	PGE_2	Inflammation Pain	Reduced inflammation Analgesia
Brain	COX-2	Unknown	Fever Pain	Reduced fever Analgesia
Colon/rectum	COX-2	Unknown	Colorectal cancer promotion	Colorectal cancer protection

COX-1, Cyclooxygenase-1; *COX-2*, cyclooxygenase-2; *MI*, myocardial infarction; *PGE$_2$*, prostaglandin E$_2$; *PGI$_2$*, prostaglandin I$_2$, (prostacyclin); *TXA$_2$*, thromboxane A$_2$.

TABLE 57.2   Principal Indications and Adverse Effects of the Four Major Types of Cyclooxygenase Inhibitors

	First-Generation NSAIDs: Aspirin	First-Generation NSAIDs: All Others	Second-Generation NSAIDs (Coxibs)	Acetaminophen
Indications				
Inflammation	Yes	Yes	Yes	No
Pain	Yes	Yes	Yes	Yes
Fever	Yes	Yes	No	Yes
Prevention of MI and stroke	Yes	No	No	No
Adverse Effects				
Gastric ulceration	Yes	Yes	Yes[a]	No
Renal impairment	Yes	Yes	Yes	No
Bleeding	Yes	Yes	No	No
MI and stroke	No	Yes	Yes	No
Liver damage with overdose	No	No	No	Yes

[a]Despite their selectivity for cyclooxygenase-2, coxibs can still cause gastric ulceration, although it may be less than with other nonsteroidal antiinflammatory drugs (NSAIDs).

to treat inflammatory disorders (e.g., rheumatoid arthritis, osteoarthritis, bursitis), alleviate mild to moderate pain, suppress fever, and relieve dysmenorrhea. Because they cannot inhibit COX-2 without inhibiting COX-1, first-generation NSAIDs cannot suppress inflammation without posing a risk for serious harm: NSAID-induced ulcers are responsible for more than 100,000 hospitalizations and 7000 to 10,000 deaths each year. Aspirin is the oldest member of the family and prototype for the group.

Aspirin

Aspirin is a highly valuable and effective medication. It provides excellent relief of mild to moderate pain, reduces fever, protects against thrombotic disorders, and remains a drug of choice for rheumatoid arthritis and other inflammatory conditions. Despite the introduction of many new NSAIDs, aspirin remains one of the most widely used members of the group and is the standard against which the others must be compared.

PROTOTYPE DRUGS

Cyclooxygenase Inhibitors (Aspirin-Like Drugs)

First-Generation Nonsteroidal Antiinflammatory Drugs (NSAIDs)
Aspirin
Ibuprofen

Second-Generation NSAID (Selective Cyclooxygenase-2 Inhibitor)
Celecoxib

Drug That Lacks Antiinflammatory Actions
Acetaminophen

Chemistry

Aspirin belongs to a chemical family known as *salicylates.* All members of this group are derivatives of salicylic acid. Aspirin is produced by substituting an acetyl group onto salicylic acid. Because of this acetyl group, aspirin is commonly known as *acetylsalicylic acid,* or simply ASA.

Mechanism of Action

Aspirin is a nonselective inhibitor of cyclooxygenase. Most beneficial effects—reductions of inflammation, pain, and fever—result from inhibiting COX-2. One beneficial effect—protection against MI and ischemic stroke—results from inhibiting COX-1. Major adverse effects—gastric ulceration, bleeding, and renal impairment—result from inhibiting COX-1.

It is important to note that aspirin is an *irreversible* inhibitor of cyclooxygenase. In contrast, all other NSAIDs are *reversible* (competitive) inhibitors. Because inhibition of cyclooxygenase by aspirin is irreversible, duration of action depends on how quickly specific tissues can synthesize new molecules of COX-1 and COX-2. With other NSAIDs, effects decline as soon as drug levels fall.

Pharmacokinetics

Absorption. Aspirin is absorbed rapidly and completely after oral dosing. The principal site of absorption is the small intestine. When administered by rectal suppository, aspirin is absorbed slowly, and blood levels are lower than with oral dosing.

Metabolism. Aspirin has a very short half-life (15 to 20 minutes) owing to rapid conversion to *salicylic acid,* an *active* metabolite. The rate of inactivation of salicylic acid depends on the amount present: at low therapeutic levels, salicylic acid has a half-life of approximately 2 hours, but at high therapeutic levels, the half-life may exceed 20 hours.

Distribution. Salicylic acid is extensively bound to plasma albumin. At therapeutic levels, binding is between 80% and 90%. Aspirin undergoes distribution to all body tissues and fluids, including breast milk, fetal tissues, and the central nervous system (CNS).

Excretion. Salicylic acid and its metabolites are excreted by the kidneys. Excretion of salicylic acid is highly dependent on urinary pH. Accordingly, by raising the pH of urine from 6 to 8, we can increase the rate of excretion fourfold.

Plasma drug levels. Low therapeutic doses of aspirin produce plasma salicylate levels less than 100 μg/mL. Antiinflammatory doses produce salicylate levels of about 150 to 300 μg/mL. Signs of salicylism (toxicity) begin when plasma salicylate levels exceed 200 μg/mL. Severe toxicity occurs at levels above 400 μg/mL.

Therapeutic Uses

Suppression of inflammation. Aspirin is an initial drug of choice for rheumatoid arthritis, osteoarthritis, and juvenile arthritis. It is also indicated for other inflammatory disorders, including rheumatic fever, tendinitis, and bursitis. The dosages employed to suppress inflammation are considerably larger than dosages used for analgesia or reduction of fever. The use of aspirin and other NSAIDs to treat arthritis is discussed further in Chapter 59.

The precise mechanisms by which aspirin decreases inflammation have not been established. We do know that prostanoids contribute to several components of the inflammatory process; hence inhibition of COX-2 provides a partial explanation of aspirin's antiinflammatory effects. Other possible mechanisms include modulation of T-cell function, suppression of inflammatory cell infiltration, and stabilization of lysosomes.

Analgesia. Aspirin is used widely to relieve mild to moderate pain. The degree of analgesia produced depends on the type of pain. Aspirin

is most active against joint pain, muscle pain, and headache. Aspirin can be more effective than opioids for some forms of postoperative pain. However, aspirin is relatively ineffective against severe pain of visceral origin. In contrast to opioid analgesics, aspirin produces neither tolerance nor physical dependence.

Aspirin relieves pain primarily through actions in the periphery. At sites of injury, prostanoids sensitize pain receptors to mechanical and chemical stimulation. Aspirin reduces pain by inhibiting COX-2, thereby suppressing prostanoid production. In addition to this peripheral mechanism, aspirin works in the CNS to help relieve pain.

Reduction of fever. Aspirin is a drug of choice for reducing temperature in febrile *adults.* However, because of the risk for Reye syndrome (see later), *aspirin should not be used to treat fever in children.* Although aspirin readily reduces fever, it will not lower normal body temperature, nor will it lower temperature that has become elevated in response to physical activity or to a rise in environmental temperature.

Body temperature is regulated by the hypothalamus, which maintains a balance between heat production and heat loss. Fever occurs when the set point of the hypothalamus becomes elevated, causing the hypothalamus to increase heat production and decrease heat loss. Set-point elevation is triggered by local synthesis of prostaglandins in response to endogenous pyrogens (fever-promoting substances). Aspirin lowers the set point by inhibiting COX-2 and thereby inhibits pyrogen-induced synthesis of prostaglandins.

Suppression of platelet aggregation. Synthesis of TXA_2 in platelets promotes aggregation. Aspirin suppresses platelet aggregation by causing *irreversible* inhibition of COX-1, the enzyme that makes TXA_2. Because platelets lack the machinery to synthesize new COX-1, the effects of a single dose persist for the life of the platelet (about 8 days).

There is a large body of evidence demonstrating that aspirin, through its antiplatelet actions, can benefit a variety of patients. Accordingly, the US Food and Drug Administration (FDA) recommended wider use of aspirin for antiplatelet effects. Professional labeling now recommends daily aspirin for men and women with the following:

- *Ischemic stroke* (to reduce the risk for death and nonfatal stroke)
- *Transient ischemic attacks* (to reduce the risk for death and nonfatal stroke)
- *Acute MI* (to reduce the risk for vascular mortality)
- *Previous MI* (to reduce the combined risk for death and nonfatal MI)
- *Chronic stable angina* (to reduce the risk of MI and sudden death)
- *Unstable angina* (to reduce the combined risk for death and nonfatal MI)
- *Angioplasty and other revascularization procedures* (in patients who have a preexisting condition for which aspirin is already indicated)

According to a review published in the *Journal of the American Medical Association*—"Aspirin Dose for the Prevention of Cardiovascular Disease"—a dose of 75 to 81 mg/d for these indications is adequate. Higher doses, which are commonly prescribed in these circumstances, offer no greater protection but will increase the risk for gastrointestinal (GI) bleeding.

In addition to these applications, aspirin can be taken by healthy people for *primary prevention* of MI and stroke. However, more recent studies show that aspirin provides less protection against cardiovascular disease than once thought. The potential small benefit must be weighed against the major risk of aspirin use, namely GI hemorrhage. Hence to determine the *net* benefit of primary prevention for any man or woman, we must determine his or her individual risk for a GI bleed and compare that risk with his or her individual risk for a cardiovascular event (i.e., the risk for MI in men or the risk for ischemic stroke in women).[a] Many organizations—including the American Heart Association (AHA), the American Thoracic Society, and the European Society of Cardiology—recommend against the use of aspirin for primary prevention of cardiovascular disease unless the patient has a 10-year risk greater than 10%.

How do we calculate 10-year risk for a cardiovascular event? Risk for an MI or stroke can be assessed using the calculator at http://www.cvriskcalculator.com/.

Cancer prevention

Colorectal cancer. There is good evidence that regular use of aspirin decreases the risk for colorectal cancer, even when the dosage is low. For example, results of a study reported in *The Lancet* in 2010 indicate that taking low-dose aspirin (75 to 300 mg/d) for more than 5 years reduces the incidence of colorectal cancer (by 24%) as well as mortality from colon cancer (by 35%). It appears that prevention occurs as effectively in patients taking 81 mg as in patients taking larger doses. At these low doses, the benefits of cancer protection may well outweigh the risk for possible bleeding and other adverse events.

Aspirin protects against colorectal cancer probably by inhibiting COX-2. In animal models, COX-2 promotes tumor growth and metastases, and inhibition of COX-2 slows tumor growth. In humans, most colorectal cancers express COX-2. Furthermore, protection by aspirin is limited to colon cancers that have high COX-2 levels. Aspirin does not protect against colon cancers with little or no COX-2.

Other cancers. Available data suggest that protection may not be limited to colorectal cancer. Results of a meta-analysis reported in *The Lancet*, "Effect of daily aspirin on long-term risk of death due to cancer: analysis of individual patient data from randomised trials," show that daily low-dose aspirin reduces the risk for death from *all* solid tumors (by 34%) but does not reduce the risk for death from hematologic cancers. In addition, *The Lancet* published an additional article in 2012 that analyzed five randomized controlled trials. This analysis determined that use of aspirin may also prevent distant metastasis of tumors that already exist. Earlier studies have shown protection against specific cancers. In a study involving men older than 60 years, daily use of aspirin and other NSAIDs was associated with a 50% decrease in the incidence of prostate cancer. In a study involving 2884 women, aspirin appeared to reduce the risk for breast cancer, especially among women with hormone receptor–positive tumors and among those who took seven or more aspirin tablets a week. In another study, taking aspirin at least three times a week for at least 6 months was associated with a 40% reduction in the incidence of ovarian cancer. In contrast to these positive results, results from the Women's Health Study found no protection with low-dose aspirin against cancer of the breast, colon, or any other tissue. The reasons for this discrepancy are not clear. Four additional studies are currently under way to examine various effects of aspirin on cancer prevention.

Adverse Effects

When administered short term in analgesic or antipyretic (fever-reducing) doses, aspirin rarely causes serious adverse effects. However, toxicity is common in the case of inflammatory disorders, which require long-term high-dose treatment.

Gastrointestinal effects. The most common side effects are *gastric distress, heartburn,* and *nausea.* These can be reduced by taking aspirin with food or a full glass of water.

Occult GI bleeding occurs often. In most cases the amount of blood lost each day is insignificant. However, with chronic aspirin use, cumulative blood loss can produce anemia.

Long-term aspirin—*even in low doses*—can cause life-threatening *gastric ulceration, perforation,* and *bleeding.* Ulcers result from four causes:

- Increased secretion of acid and pepsin
- Decreased production of cytoprotective mucus and bicarbonate
- Decreased submucosal blood flow
- The direct irritant action of aspirin on the gastric mucosa

The first three occur secondary to inhibition of COX-1. Direct injury to the stomach is most likely with aspirin preparations that dissolve slowly: owing to slow dissolution, particulate aspirin becomes entrapped in folds of the stomach wall, causing prolonged exposure to high concentrations of the drug. Because aspirin-induced ulcers are often asymptomatic, perforation and upper GI hemorrhage can occur without premonitory signs. (Hemorrhage is due in part to erosion of the stomach wall and in part to suppression of platelet aggregation.) Factors that increase the risk for ulceration include the following:

- Advanced age
- A history of peptic ulcer disease
- Previous intolerance to aspirin or other NSAIDs
- Cigarette smoking
- History of alcohol abuse (Alcohol intensifies the irritant effects of aspirin and should not be consumed.)

What can we do to *prevent* ulcers? According to an expert panel—convened by the American College of Gastroenterology, the AHA, and the American College of Cardiology—prophylaxis with a *proton pump inhibitor* (PPI) is recommended for patients at risk, including those with a history of peptic ulcers, those taking glucocorticoids, and older adults. PPIs (e.g., omeprazole, lansoprazole) reduce ulcer generation by suppressing production of gastric acid. In addition to PPIs, other drugs that may be considered include histamine-2 receptor antagonists (H$_2$RAs) and misoprostol. COX-2 inhibitors may also be tried instead of traditional NSAIDs because they are thought to produce fewer GI side effects. Because many ulcers are caused by infection with *Helicobacter pylori* (see Chapter 64), the panel recommends that patients with ulcer histories undergo testing and treatment for *H. pylori* before starting long-term aspirin use. *Treatment* of NSAID-induced ulcers is discussed in Chapter 64.

Bleeding. Aspirin promotes bleeding by inhibiting platelet aggregation. Taking just two 325-mg aspirin tablets can double bleeding time for about 1 week. (Recall that platelets are unable to replace aspirin-inactivated cyclooxygenase; hence bleeding time is prolonged for the life of the platelet.) Because of its effects on platelets, *aspirin is contraindicated for patients with bleeding disorders* (e.g., hemophilia, vitamin K deficiency, hypoprothrombinemia). To minimize blood loss during childbirth and elective surgery, *high-dose* aspirin should be discontinued at least 1 week before these procedures. There is no need to stop aspirin before procedures with a low risk for bleeding (e.g., dental, dermatologic, or cataract surgery). In most cases use of *low-dose* aspirin to protect against thrombosis should *not* be interrupted for elective surgery and dental procedures. Caution is needed when aspirin is used in conjunction with anticoagulants.

In patients taking daily aspirin, high blood pressure increases the risk for hemorrhagic stroke, even though aspirin protects against ischemic stroke. To reduce risk for hemorrhagic stroke, blood pressure should be 150/90 mm Hg (and preferably lower) before starting daily aspirin.

---

[a]Major factors that increase the risk for a GI bleed are use of NSAIDs and a history of ulcers. Major risk factors for an MI are advancing age, diabetes, high total cholesterol, low HDL cholesterol, and smoking. Major risk factors for an ischemic stroke are advancing age, hypertension, diabetes, smoking, atrial fibrillation, left ventricular hypertrophy, and a history of cardiovascular disease.

Renal impairment. Aspirin can cause acute, reversible impairment of renal function, resulting in salt and water retention and edema. Clinically significant effects are most likely in patients with additional risk factors: advanced age, existing renal impairment, hypovolemia, hepatic cirrhosis, or heart failure. Aspirin impairs renal function by inhibiting COX-1, thereby depriving the kidney of prostaglandins needed for normal function.

Development of renal impairment is signaled by reduced urine output, weight gain despite use of diuretics, and a rapid rise in serum creatinine and blood urea nitrogen. If any of these occurs, aspirin should be withdrawn immediately. In most cases kidney function then returns to baseline.

The risk for acute renal impairment can be reduced by identifying high-risk patients and treating them with the smallest dosages possible.

In addition to its acute effects on renal function, aspirin may pose a risk for renal papillary necrosis and other types of renal injury when used long term.

Salicylism. Salicylism is a syndrome that begins to develop when aspirin levels climb just slightly above therapeutic. Overt signs include *tinnitus, sweating, headache,* and *dizziness.* Acid–base disturbance may also occur (see later). If salicylism develops, aspirin should be withheld until symptoms subside. Aspirin should then resume, but with a small reduction in dosage. In some cases, development of tinnitus can be used to adjust aspirin dosage: when tinnitus occurs, the maximal acceptable dose has been achieved. However, this guideline may be inappropriate for older patients because they may fail to develop tinnitus even when aspirin levels become toxic.

Acid–base disturbance results from the effects of aspirin on respiration. When it is administered in high therapeutic doses, aspirin acts on the CNS to stimulate breathing. The resultant increase in CO_2 loss produces *respiratory alkalosis.* In response, the kidneys excrete more bicarbonate. There is also a subsequent buildup of acids, producing a resultant metabolic acidosis. Thus many patients who present with salicylate toxicity will have a mixed acid–base imbalance.

Reye syndrome. Use of aspirin in children younger than 18 years is associated with Reye syndrome.

This syndrome is a rare but serious illness of childhood that has a mortality rate of 20% to 30%. Characteristic symptoms are encephalopathy and fatty liver degeneration. Epidemiologic data have suggested a relationship between Reye syndrome and use of aspirin by children who have influenza or chickenpox. Although a direct causal link between aspirin and Reye syndrome was never established, the Centers for Disease Control and Prevention recommended that aspirin (and other NSAIDs) be avoided by children and teenagers suspected of having influenza or chickenpox. In response to this recommendation, aspirin was removed from most products intended for children, and aspirin use by children declined sharply. As a result, Reye syndrome essentially vanished. If a child with chickenpox or influenza needs an analgesic-antipyretic, acetaminophen can be used safely.

Adverse effects associated with use during pregnancy. Aspirin poses risks to the pregnant patient and her fetus. The principal risks to pregnant women are (1) anemia (from GI blood loss) and (2) postpartum hemorrhage. In addition, by inhibiting prostaglandin synthesis, aspirin may suppress spontaneous uterine contractions and thereby prolong labor.

Aspirin crosses the placenta and may adversely affect the fetus. Because prostaglandins help keep the ductus arteriosus patent, inhibition of prostaglandin synthesis by aspirin may induce premature closure of the ductus arteriosus. Aspirin use has also been associated with low birth weight, stillbirth, renal toxicity, intracranial hemorrhage in preterm infants, and neonatal death.

Summary of Precautions and Contraindications

Aspirin is contraindicated in patients with *peptic ulcer disease, bleeding disorders* (e.g., hemophilia, vitamin K deficiency, hypoprothrombinemia), and *hypersensitivity to aspirin itself or other NSAIDs.* In addition, the drug should be used with extreme caution by *pregnant women and by children who have chickenpox or influenza.* Caution should also be exercised when treating *older adult patients, patients who smoke cigarettes,* and *patients with H. pylori infection, heart failure, hepatic cirrhosis, hypovolemia, renal dysfunction, asthma, hay fever, chronic urticaria, nasal polyps,* or *a history of alcoholism.* Aspirin should be withdrawn 1 week before elective surgery or the anticipated date of childbirth.

PATIENT-CENTERED CARE ACROSS THE LIFE SPAN

Nonsteroidal Antiinflammatory Drugs

Life Stage	Patient Care Concerns
Infants	Because of the risk for Reye syndrome, aspirin should be avoided in infants. Acetaminophen and ibuprofen can be used safely in small doses for fever.
Children/ adolescents	Because of the risk for Reye syndrome, aspirin should be avoided in children and adolescents. Acetaminophen and ibuprofen can be used safely in small doses for fever.
Pregnant women	NSAIDs may result in premature closure of the ductus arteriosus. Therefore their use is contraindicated in the third trimester of pregnancy.
Breastfeeding women	NSAIDs and acetaminophen appear safe for use in breastfeeding mothers.
Older adults	NSAIDs are the most common drugs used to treat chronic pain in older adults. These drugs have been shown to increase hospital admissions in this population. NSAIDS also contribute to elevated BP, precipitate CHF decompensation and can provoke renal failure. Caution should be used with NSAIDs in older adults.

Drug Interactions

Because of its widespread use, aspirin has been reported to interact with many other medications. However, most of these interactions have little clinical significance. Significant interactions are discussed next.

Anticoagulants: warfarin, heparin, and others. Aspirin's most important interactions are with anticoagulants. Because aspirin suppresses platelet function and can decrease prothrombin production, it can intensify the effects of warfarin, heparin, and other anticoagulants. Furthermore, because aspirin can initiate gastric bleeding, augmenting anticoagulant effects can increase the risk for gastric hemorrhage. Accordingly, the combination of aspirin with anticoagulants must be used with care, even when aspirin is taken in low doses, to reduce the risk for thrombotic events.

Glucocorticoids. Like aspirin, glucocorticoids promote gastric ulceration. As a result, the risk for ulcers is greatly increased when these drugs are combined—as may happen when treating arthritis. To reduce the risk for gastric ulceration, patients can be given a PPI or H_2RA for prophylaxis.

Alcohol. Combining alcohol with aspirin and other NSAIDs increases the risk for gastric bleeding. To alert the public to this risk, the FDA now requires that labels for aspirin include the following statement: *Stomach Bleeding Warning: This product contains an NSAID, which may cause severe stomach bleeding. The chance is higher if you have 3 or more alcoholic drinks every day while using this product.* A similar label is required for all other NSAIDs and acetaminophen.

Nonaspirin nonsteroidal antiinflammatory drugs. Ibuprofen, naproxen, and other nonaspirin NSAIDs can reduce the antiplatelet effects of aspirin by blocking access of aspirin to COX-1 in platelets. This interaction is important because, in patients taking low-dose aspirin to prevent MI or ischemic stroke, other NSAIDs could negate aspirin's benefits. Since immediate-release aspirin produces complete platelet inhibition about 1 hour after dosing, we can prevent interference by giving aspirin about 2 hours before giving other NSAIDs. Of course we could eliminate interference entirely by using high-dose aspirin rather than another NSAID when conditions call for NSAID therapy.

Angiotensin-converting enzyme inhibitors and angiotensin receptor blockers. Like aspirin, angiotensin-converting enzyme inhibitors (ACEIs) and angiotensin receptor blockers (ARBs) can impair renal function. In susceptible patients, combining aspirin with drugs in either class can increase the risk for acute renal failure. High-dose aspirin should be avoided in patients taking these drugs. However, low-dose aspirin taken for antiplatelet effects should be continued.

Vaccines. Aspirin and other NSAIDs may blunt the immune response to vaccines. Accordingly, these drugs should not be used routinely to prevent vaccination-associated fever and pain.

Dosage and Administration

Aspirin is almost always administered by mouth. Gastric irritation can be minimized by dosing with water or food. Dosage depends on the age of the patient and the condition being treated. Adult and pediatric dosages for major indications are shown in Table 57.3.

Nonaspirin First-Generation Nonsteroidal Antiinflammatory Drugs

In attempts to produce an aspirin-like drug with fewer GI, renal, and hemorrhagic effects than aspirin, the pharmaceutical industry has produced a large number of drugs with actions much like those of aspirin. In the United States more than 20 nonaspirin NSAIDs are available (Table 57.4). Like aspirin, all other first-generation NSAIDs inhibit both COX-1 and COX-2. However, in contrast to aspirin, which causes *irreversible* inhibition of cyclooxygenase, the other traditional NSAIDs cause *reversible* inhibition. All of these drugs have antiinflammatory, analgesic, and antipyretic properties. In addition, they all can cause gastric ulceration, bleeding, and renal impairment—although the intensity of these effects may be less with some agents. Patients who

are hypersensitive to aspirin are likely to experience cross-hypersensitivity with other NSAIDs. For most NSAIDs, safety during pregnancy has not been established; hence use by pregnant women is discouraged.

The principal indications for the nonaspirin NSAIDs are rheumatoid arthritis and osteoarthritis. In addition, certain NSAIDs are used to treat fever, bursitis, tendinitis, mild to moderate pain, and dysmenorrhea (see Table 57.4).

In contrast to aspirin, the nonaspirin NSAIDs *do not* protect against MI and stroke. In fact, they *increase* the risk for thrombotic events. For the NSAIDs as a group, the increase in cardiovascular risk is relatively low—about 12%. Risk is highest with indomethacin (71%), sulindac (41%), and meloxicam (37%). However, although the increase in risk with these drugs appears high, it pales in comparison with smoking, which increases cardiovascular risk by 200% to 300%. To minimize cardiovascular risk, nonaspirin NSAIDs should be used in the lowest effective dosage for the shortest time needed. Also, these drugs should not be used before coronary artery bypass graft (CABG) surgery or for 14 days after. Other measures to reduce risk are discussed later, under "American Heart Association Statement on Cyclooxygenase Inhibitors in Chronic Pain."

Although individual NSAIDs differ chemically, pharmacokinetically, and to some extent pharmacodynamically, all are similar clinically: they all produce essentially equivalent antiinflammatory effects, and they all present a similar risk for serious adverse effects (gastric ulceration, bleeding, renal impairment, MI, and stroke). However, for reasons that are not understood, individual patients may respond better to one agent than another. Furthermore, individual patients may tolerate one NSAID better than another. Therefore, to optimize therapy for each patient, trials with more than one NSAID may be needed.

Ibuprofen

Basic pharmacology. Ibuprofen (Advil, Motrin, Caldolor, others) is the prototype of the propionic acid derivatives. Other members of the family are shown in Table 57.4 and discussed individually in the following paragraphs. Like aspirin, ibuprofen inhibits cyclooxygenase and has antiinflammatory, analgesic, and antipyretic actions. The drug is used to treat fever, mild to moderate pain, and arthritis. In addition, ibuprofen appears superior to most other NSAIDs for relief of primary dysmenorrhea, presumably because it produces good inhibition of cyclooxygenase in uterine smooth muscle. In clinical trials, ibuprofen was highly effective at promoting closure of the ductus arteriosus in preterm infants, a condition for which indomethacin is the current treatment of choice.

Ibuprofen is generally well tolerated, and the incidence of adverse effects is low. The drug produces less gastric bleeding than aspirin and less inhibition of platelet aggregation as well. Consequently ibuprofen is among the safer NSAIDs for use with anticoagulants. Very rarely, ibuprofen has been associated with Stevens-Johnson syndrome (SJS), a severe hypersensitivity reaction that causes blistering of the skin and mucous membranes and can result in scarring, blindness, and even death. Like other nonaspirin NSAIDs, ibuprofen may pose a risk for MI and stroke.

Nonacetylated Salicylates: Magnesium Salicylate, Sodium Salicylate, and Salsalate

Similarities to aspirin. The nonacetylated salicylates are similar to aspirin (an acetylated salicylate) in most respects. Like aspirin, these drugs inhibit COX-1 and COX-2 and are employed to treat arthritis, moderate pain, and fever. The most common adverse effects are GI disturbances. As with aspirin, these drugs should not be given to children with chickenpox or influenza owing to the possibility of precipitating Reye syndrome.

Contrasts with aspirin. In contrast to aspirin, the nonacetylated salicylates cause little or no suppression of platelet aggregation. As a

TABLE 57.3 Aspirin Dosage

Indication	Adult Dosage	Pediatric Dosage[a]
Aches and pains, fever	325–650 mg q 4 h as needed	Children <50 kg: 10-15 mg/kg/dose every 4-6 hours as needed Children 12 years and older and weighing >50 kg: 325-650 mg every 4-6 hours
Acute rheumatic fever	5–8 g/d in divided doses	100 mg/kg per day (initially), then 75 mg/kg qd for 4–6 weeks
Rheumatoid arthritis	3.6–5.4 g/d in divided doses	90–130 mg/kg per day in divided doses q 4–6 h
Suppression of Platelet Aggregation		
Initial therapy	325 mg once a day	
Chronic therapy	80 mg once a day	

[a]Owing to the risk for Reye syndrome, aspirin is usually avoided in patients younger than 18 years.

TABLE 57.4 Clinical Pharmacology of the Oral Nonsteroidal Antiinflammatory Drugs

Drug	Maximal Daily Dosage (mg)	Plasma Half-Life (h)	MAJOR INDICATIONS[a]				
			Arthritis	Moderate Pain	Fever	Dysmenorrhea	Bursitis/ Tendinitis
First-Generation NSAIDs							
Salicylates							
Aspirin (many trade names)	8000	0.2–0.3	A	A	A		
Magnesium salicylate (Doan's Tablets, others)	4640	2–30[b]	A	A	A		
Sodium salicylate[c] (generic)	3900	2–30[b]	A	A	A		
Salsalate	3000	2–30[b]	A	A	A		
Propionic Acid Derivatives							
Fenoprofen (Nalfon)	3200	3	A	A			
Flurbiprofen (generic)	300	5.7	A	I	I	I	I
Ibuprofen (Advil, Motrin, others)[d]	3200	1.8–2	A	A	A	A	
Ketoprofen (generic)	300	2	A	A		A	
Naproxen (Aleve, others)[e]	1375	12–17	A	A	A	A	A
Oxaprozin (Daypro)	1800	42–50	A				
Others							
Diclofenac (Cambia, Cataflam, Voltaren XR, Zipsor, Zorvolex)[f]	200	2	A	A		A	
Diflunisal (generic)	1500	11–15	A	A			
Etodolac (generic)	1200	7.3	A	A			I
Indomethacin (Indocin)	200	4.5	A				A
Ketorolac (generic)[g]	40 PO 120 IV	5–6	A[h]				
Meclofenamate (generic)	400	1.3	A	A		A	
Mefenamic acid (Ponstel, Ponstan ♦)	1000	2		A		A	
Meloxicam (Mobic, Mobicox ♦)	15	15–20	A				
Nabumetone (generic)	2000	22	A				
Piroxicam (Feldene)	20	50	A				
Sulindac (generic)	400	7.8	A				A
Tolmetin (generic)	1800	2–7	A				
Second-Generation NSAIDs (COX-2 Inhibitors)							
Celecoxib (Celebrex)	800	11	A	A		A	

[a]A, US Food and Drug Administration–approved indication; I, investigational use.
[b]Half-life increases with increasing dosage.
[c]Available as a combination pill with methenamine, sold as Cystex.
[d]Ibuprofen is also available in two *intravenous* formulations, sold as Caldolor and NeoProfen.
[e]Naproxen is also available in a fixed-dose combination with esomeprazole, sold as Vimovo.
[f]Diclofenac is also available in three *topical* formulations—sold as Flector Patch, Pennsaid, and Voltaren Gel—and in a fixed-dose combination with misoprostol, sold as Arthrotec.
[g]Ketorolac is also available in an *intravenous* formulation, sold generically, and in an *intranasal* formulation, sold as Sprix.
[h]Ketorolac is approved only for *acute* pain; use should not exceed 5 days.
COX-2, Cyclooxygenase-2; *IV,* intravenous; *NSAID,* nonsteroidal antiinflammatory drug; *PO,* oral.

result, these drugs cannot protect against MI and stroke and may actually increase risk.

Because of its sodium content, sodium salicylate should be avoided in patients on a sodium-restricted diet (e.g., patients with hypertension or heart failure).

Magnesium salicylate may accumulate to toxic levels in patients with chronic renal insufficiency and hence should not be used by these people.

Salsalate is a prodrug that breaks down to release two molecules of salicylate in the alkaline environment of the small intestine. Because the stomach is not exposed to salicylate, salsalate produces less gastric irritation than aspirin.

▶ BLACK BOX WARNING

First-Generation Nonsteroidal Antiinflammatory Drugs

All first-generation NSAIDs are associated with increased risk for gastrointestinal bleeding and cardiovascular events that can lead to hospitalization or death.

SECOND-GENERATION NONSTEROIDAL ANTIINFLAMMATORY DRUGS (CYCLOOXYGENASE-2 INHIBITORS, COXIBS)

The COX-2 inhibitors, also known as coxibs, were developed on the theory that selective inhibition of COX-2 should be able to suppress pain and inflammation while posing little or no risk for gastric ulceration. To some degree, theory and reality agree: coxibs are just as effective as traditional NSAIDs at suppressing inflammation and pain, and they pose a somewhat lower risk for GI side effects. However, even with coxibs, patients can develop clinically significant gastroduodenal ulceration and bleeding. Furthermore, like traditional NSAIDs, coxibs can impair renal function and thereby cause hypertension and edema. Coxibs also increase the risk for MI and stroke.

Celecoxib
Therapeutic Use

Celecoxib (Celebrex) was the first selective COX-2 inhibitor to reach the market. The drug is indicated for osteoarthritis, rheumatoid arthritis, ankylosing spondylitis, juvenile idiopathic arthritis, acute pain, and dysmenorrhea. In addition, celecoxib is used off label for a rare genetic disorder known as familial adenomatous polyposis, which predisposes to development of colorectal cancer. For patients with arthritis, celecoxib is equal to naproxen (an NSAID) at relieving joint pain, stiffness, and swelling. Owing to concerns about cardiovascular safety, celecoxib is considered a last-choice drug for long-term management of pain (see later under "American Heart Association Statement on Cyclooxygenase Inhibitors in Chronic Pain").

It is important to note that celecoxib does *not* provide the cardiovascular benefits of aspirin because celecoxib does not inhibit COX-1 in platelets and hence does not suppress platelet aggregation.

Mechanism of Action

Celecoxib causes selective inhibition of COX-2, the COX isoform whose products mediate inflammation and pain. At therapeutic doses, celecoxib does not inhibit COX-1, the COX isoform whose products protect the stomach, help maintain renal function, and promote platelet aggregation.

Pharmacokinetics

Celecoxib is well absorbed after oral administration. Plasma levels peak in 3 hours. Binding to plasma proteins is extensive (97%). The drug undergoes hepatic metabolism followed by renal excretion. The half-life is 11 hours.

Adverse Effects

In premarketing trials, celecoxib was well tolerated. The discontinuation rate owing to adverse effects was 7.1% for celecoxib versus 6.1% for placebo. The most common complaints were *dyspepsia* and *abdominal pain*. Celecoxib does not decrease platelet aggregation and hence does not promote bleeding. Possible cardiovascular events are the biggest concern.

Gastroduodenal ulceration. Because celecoxib does not inhibit COX-1, the isoform of COX that protects the stomach, a low incidence of gastroduodenal ulceration would be expected. Some data support this expectation; others do not. When celecoxib was first approved, conclusions about its safety were based on 6-month data from the Celecoxib Arthritis Safety Study (CLASS), which indicated that celecoxib caused less GI toxicity than conventional NSAIDs (diclofenac, naproxen, ibuprofen). However, longer-term (12-month) data from the same study showed *no difference* in GI toxicity between celecoxib and conventional NSAIDs. Other studies have shown that, compared with patients taking conventional NSAIDs, those taking celecoxib

had a lower incidence of endoscopically detectable ulcers and of hospitalization for GI bleeding. What's the bottom line? Celecoxib *may* be safer than conventional NSAIDs, especially when used short term. However, convincing data of superior safety are lacking. Like traditional NSAIDs, celecoxib can be combined with a PPI to reduce GI complications.

Cardiovascular events. There is strong evidence that coxibs, like other nonaspirin NSAIDs, increase the risk for MI, stroke, and other serious cardiovascular events. In the Adenoma Prevention with Celecoxib (APC) trial, patients who took 400 or 800 mg of celecoxib a day experienced more major fatal or nonfatal cardiovascular events than did patients who took placebo. To minimize risk, celecoxib should be used in the lowest effective dosage for the shortest time needed. Also, the drug should be avoided in patients with existing heart disease and those who have just undergone CABG surgery, and it should be used with caution in patients with cardiovascular risk factors such as hypertension, diabetes, and dyslipidemia. Other measures to reduce risk are discussed later under "American Heart Association Statement on Cyclooxygenase Inhibitors in Chronic Pain."

Why is the risk for MI and stroke increased? First, because celecoxib does not inhibit COX-1, platelet aggregation is not suppressed. Second, because celecoxib inhibits COX-2 in blood vessels, vasoconstriction is increased. These two factors—unimpeded platelet aggregation and increased vasoconstriction—increase the likelihood of vessel blockage after the process of thrombosis has begun.

Renal impairment. Like conventional NSAIDs, celecoxib can impair renal function, thereby posing a risk to patients with hypertension, edema, heart failure, or kidney disease. Renal impairment apparently results from inhibiting COX-2.

Sulfonamide allergy. Celecoxib contains a sulfur molecule and hence can precipitate an allergic reaction in patients allergic to sulfonamides. Accordingly, the drug should be avoided by patients with sulfa allergy.

Use in pregnancy. Celecoxib and other NSAIDs can cause premature closure of the ductus arteriosus. Accordingly, these drugs are contraindicated during the third trimester of pregnancy.

Drug Interactions

Warfarin. Celecoxib may increase the anticoagulant effects of warfarin and may thereby increase the risk for bleeding. Celecoxib itself does not inhibit platelet aggregation and does not promote bleeding. However, the drug may enhance the anticoagulant effects of warfarin (perhaps by increasing warfarin levels). Celecoxib may be combined with warfarin, but effects of warfarin should be monitored closely, especially during the first few days of treatment.

Other interactions. Information on the interactions of celecoxib with other drugs is limited. Celecoxib may decrease the diuretic effects of furosemide as well as the antihypertensive effects of ACEIs. Conversely, celecoxib may increase levels of lithium (a drug for bipolar disorder). Levels of celecoxib may be increased by fluconazole (an antifungal drug).

ACETAMINOPHEN

Acetaminophen (Tylenol, Ofirmev, many others) is like aspirin in some respects but different in others. Acetaminophen has *analgesic* and *antipyretic* properties equivalent to those of aspirin. However, in contrast to aspirin and the other NSAIDs, *acetaminophen is devoid of clinically useful antiinflammatory and antirheumatic actions*. In addition, acetaminophen does not suppress platelet aggregation, does not cause gastric ulceration, and does not decrease renal blood flow or cause renal impairment. However, acetaminophen overdose can cause severe liver injury. In the United States acetaminophen is used more than any other analgesic.

SUMMARY OF KEY PRESCRIBING CONSIDERATIONS

NSAIDs

Therapeutic Goal: Major indications for the NSAIDs are inflammatory disorders, mild to moderate pain, fever, and primary dysmenorrhea. In addition, aspirin is used to prevent MI and stroke.

Baseline Data: Consider checking renal function prior to starting scheduled or long-term NSAID therapy.

Monitoring: No suggested routine laboratory monitoring

Identifying High-Risk Patients: Use with extreme caution in patients with peptic ulcer disease, bleeding disorders, and those taking anticoagulants. Caution is also needed when treating older adult patients with heart failure, renal dysfunction, or angina pectoris.

Evaluating Therapeutic Effects: Monitor pain levels and functional ability.

Minimizing Adverse Effects: If initiating long-term therapy, start NSAIDs with a proton pump inhibitor to decrease risk of GI bleeding.

Mechanism of Action

Differences between the effects of acetaminophen and aspirin are thought to result from selective inhibition of cyclooxygenase, the enzyme needed to make prostaglandins and related compounds. Whereas aspirin can inhibit cyclooxygenase in both the CNS and the periphery, inhibition by acetaminophen is limited to the CNS; acetaminophen has only minimal effects on cyclooxygenase at peripheral sites. By decreasing prostaglandin synthesis in the CNS, acetaminophen is able to reduce fever and pain. The inability to inhibit prostaglandin synthesis outside the CNS may explain the absence of antiinflammatory effects, gastric ulceration, and adverse effects on the kidneys and platelets.

Pharmacokinetics

Acetaminophen is readily absorbed after oral dosing and undergoes wide distribution. Most of each dose is metabolized by the liver, and the metabolites are excreted in the urine. The plasma half-life is approximately 2 hours.

Acetaminophen can be metabolized by two pathways; one is major and the other minor (Fig. 57.1). In the major pathway, acetaminophen undergoes conjugation with glucuronic acid and other compounds to form nontoxic metabolites. In the minor pathway, acetaminophen is oxidized by a cytochrome P450–containing enzyme into a highly reactive toxic metabolite: N-acetyl-p-benzoquinone imine. At therapeutic doses, practically all of the drug is converted to nontoxic metabolites through the major pathway. Only a small fraction is converted into the toxic metabolite through the minor pathway. Furthermore, under normal conditions, the toxic metabolite undergoes rapid conversion to a nontoxic form; glutathione is required for the conversion. In the

event of acetaminophen overdose, a larger than normal amount is processed through the minor pathway; hence a large quantity of the toxic metabolite is produced. As the liver attempts to clear the metabolite, glutathione is rapidly depleted and further detoxification stops. As a result, the toxic metabolite accumulates, causing damage to the liver (see later).

Adverse Effects

Adverse effects are extremely rare at therapeutic doses. Acetaminophen does not cause gastric ulceration or renal impairment and does not inhibit platelet aggregation. In addition, there is no evidence linking acetaminophen with Reye syndrome. Individuals who are hypersensitive to aspirin only rarely experience cross-hypersensitivity with acetaminophen. Overdose can cause severe *liver injury* (see later).

Data from the Nurses' Health Study show an association between daily use of *acetaminophen* (500 mg/d or more) and development of *hypertension*. Additional studies that examined a possible relationship between acetaminophen and hypertension in both men and women found conflicting results. Until more data become available, it would be prudent to monitor blood pressure in patients who take acetaminophen daily. The mechanism by which acetaminophen might raise blood pressure is unknown.

Acetaminophen use has also been associated with SJS, acute generalized exanthematous pustulosis (AGEP), and toxic epidermal necrolysis (TEN). SJS and TEN are characterized by painful rash, blistering of the skin and mucous membranes, and detachment of the epidermis. These are considered medical emergencies because they can result in death. Recovery can take weeks to months. AGEP is characterized by pustular lesions that predominately affect the upper trunk and body folds. It usually resolves within 2 weeks of onset. These reactions can occur at any time, even if the patient has taken acetaminophen previously. If rash appears while a patient is taking acetaminophen, the drug should be stopped and medical attention sought.

Drug and Vaccine Interactions

Alcohol

Regular alcohol consumption increases the risk for liver injury from acetaminophen—but only if acetaminophen dosage is excessive. Three mechanisms are involved. First, alcohol induces synthesis of the P450-containing enzyme in the minor metabolic pathway, thereby increasing production of acetaminophen's toxic metabolite (see Fig. 57.1). Second, stores of glutathione are depleted in chronic alcoholics. As a result, the liver is unable to convert the toxic metabolite to a nontoxic form. Third, chronic alcohol abusers often have preexisting liver damage, which renders them less able to tolerate injury from acetaminophen.

Alcohol in combination with acetaminophen can increase the risk for liver and kidney damage. Although information regarding liver

Fig. 57.1 Metabolism of Acetaminophen.

disease and acetaminophen has existed for some time, newer data reveal that even low-dose combinations of alcohol and acetaminophen can lead to renal dysfunction. Authorities recommend that if you drink alcohol on a regular basis, you should consume no more than 3000 mg of acetaminophen a day.

Although therapeutic doses of acetaminophen may be safe for alcohol drinkers, *high* doses certainly are not. Accordingly, to alert the public to the potential risk of combining alcohol with acetaminophen, the FDA requires that acetaminophen labels bear the following statement: *Liver Warning: This product contains acetaminophen. Severe liver damage may occur if you take 3 or more alcoholic drinks every day while using this product.*

Warfarin

There is evidence that acetaminophen may increase the risk for bleeding in patients taking warfarin. This is surprising because, unlike NSAIDs, acetaminophen does not suppress platelet aggregation and so should not promote bleeding. Yes, acetaminophen may inhibit warfarin metabolism, which would cause warfarin levels to rise. Accordingly, for patients taking more than 1 g of acetaminophen daily for several days, responses to warfarin should be monitored closely.

Vaccines

Acetaminophen and other analgesics-antipyretics can blunt the immune response to childhood vaccines. Accordingly, routine use of these drugs to prevent vaccination-associated pain or fever should be discouraged.

Therapeutic Uses

Acetaminophen is indicated for relief of pain and fever. Because acetaminophen is not associated with Reye syndrome, the drug is preferred to NSAIDs for use by children suspected of having chickenpox or influenza. Because it does not cause GI injury, acetaminophen is preferred to NSAIDs for patients with peptic ulcer disease. In addition, acetaminophen may be a safe alternative to aspirin for patients who have experienced aspirin hypersensitivity reactions. Because of its weak antiinflammatory actions, acetaminophen is *not* useful for treating arthritis or rheumatic fever.

Acute Toxicity: Liver Damage

Overdose with acetaminophen can cause severe liver injury and death. The cause is accumulation of the toxic metabolite discussed earlier. In the United States acetaminophen overdose—intentional or unintentional—is the leading cause of acute liver failure, accounting for about 50% of all cases. Risk for liver injury is increased by fasting, chronic alcohol use, and taking more than 4000 mg of acetaminophen per day.

Signs and Symptoms

The principal feature of acetaminophen overdose is *hepatic necrosis*. Severe poisoning can progress to hepatic failure, coma, and death. Early symptoms of poisoning (nausea, vomiting, diarrhea, sweating, abdominal discomfort) belie the severity of intoxication. It is not until 48 to 72 hours after drug ingestion that overt indications of hepatic injury appear.

Treatment

Liver damage can be minimized by giving *acetylcysteine* (Mucomyst , Acetadote), a specific antidote to acetaminophen. Acetylcysteine reduces injury by substituting for depleted glutathione in the reaction that converts the toxic metabolite of acetaminophen to its nontoxic form. When given within 8 to 10 hours of acetaminophen overdose, acetylcysteine is 100%

effective at preventing severe liver injury. Even when administered as much as 24 hours after poisoning, it can still provide significant protection. Acetylcysteine may be administered orally or intravenously.

Minimizing Risk

Risk for liver failure is very low with normal therapeutic doses (up to 4000 mg/d) except in people who drink alcohol, are undernourished, or have liver disease. Patient education can help reduce injury. Accordingly, you should do the following:

- Inform patients about the risk for liver toxicity.
- Advise patients to consume no more than 4000 mg of acetaminophen a day, including the amount in combination prescription products (e.g., Vicodin, Percocet) as well as over-the-counter products.
- Advise patients who are undernourished (e.g., owing to fasting or illness) to consume no more than 3000 mg of acetaminophen a day. Undernourished people are at risk because they have low stores of glutathione, the cofactor needed to convert the toxic metabolite of acetaminophen to a nontoxic form.
- Advise patients not to drink alcohol while taking acetaminophen.
- Advise patients who won't stop drinking alcohol (more than 3 drinks a day) to take no more than 3000 mg of acetaminophen a day.
- Advise patients with liver disease to ask their prescriber if acetaminophen is safe.

📄 SUMMARY OF KEY PRESCRIBING CONSIDERATIONS

Acetaminophen

Therapeutic Goal: To relieve pain and to reduce fever.

Baseline Data: Consider checking hepatic function prior to starting scheduled or long-term therapy.

Monitoring: No suggested routine laboratory monitoring.

Identifying High-Risk Patients: Use with caution in patients with alcohol use disorder, patients who consume moderate amounts of alcohol daily, or in patients taking warfarin.

Evaluating Therapeutic Effects: Monitor pain levels and functional ability.

Minimizing Adverse Effects: Acetaminophen is largely devoid of significant adverse effects at usual therapeutic doses except possibly in patients who routinely consume alcohol. Providers should educate patients to read medication labels carefully, as many over the counter medications may contain acetaminophen and should not be used in combination.

AMERICAN HEART ASSOCIATION STATEMENT ON CYCLOOXYGENASE INHIBITORS IN CHRONIC PAIN

Because most COX inhibitors—and especially COX-2 inhibitors—increase the risk for MI and stroke, the AHA recommends a stepped-care approach to their use, as discussed in an article titled, "Use of Nonsteroidal Antiinflammatory Drugs: An Update for Clinicians: A Scientific Statement from the American Heart Association." Recommendations in the article apply specifically to managing musculoskeletal pain in patients with or at high risk for cardiovascular disease. However, the recommendations may also apply to patients who lack documented cardiovascular risk. The approach has four basic steps:

Step 1. Begin with nondrug measures. Options include physical therapy, exercise, weight loss, orthotics, and application of heat or cold.

Step 2. If nondrug measures don't work, initiate drug therapy using *acetaminophen* or *aspirin,* which do not increase cardiovascular risk. If these drugs can't control pain, an opioid or tramadol can be tried, but only in the short term.

Step 3. If step 2 drugs are ineffective or intolerable, try other nonselective NSAIDs, such as naproxen, ibuprofen, or a nonacetylated salicylate (e.g., magnesium salicylate).

Step 4. As a *last resort,* try the selective COX-2 inhibitor celecoxib. Of all the NSAIDs, COX-2 inhibitors pose the greatest risk for cardiovascular harm; hence celecoxib is a last-choice drug for chronic pain.

Whenever these drugs are employed, patients should use the lowest effective dosage for the shortest possible time. During steps 2, 3, and 4, if the patient is considered at high risk for a thrombotic event, low-dose aspirin (81 mg/d) plus a PPI or H$_2$RA should be *added* to the regimen (except, of course, if high-dose aspirin is already in use).

58

Glucocorticoids in Nonendocrine Disorders

In the body, the adrenal cortex produces corticosteroids. These include mineralocorticoids, which modulate salt and water balance; and glucocorticoids, which influence carbohydrate metabolism and other processes discussed in this chapter.

The glucocorticoid drugs are nearly identical to the glucose-regulating steroids produced by the adrenal cortex. We can look on the glucocorticoid drugs as having two kinds of effects: physiologic and pharmacologic. *Physiologic* effects (i.e., those used to maintain normal physiologic function) are elicited by *low* doses of glucocorticoids. In contrast, *pharmacologic* effects require *high* doses. In high doses, glucocorticoids are used to treat inflammatory disorders (e.g., asthma, rheumatoid arthritis) and certain cancers. High doses are also used to suppress immune responses in organ transplant recipients.

Glucocorticoids are devoid of toxicity when used in physiologic doses. However, when taken in pharmacologic doses, especially for extended periods, glucocorticoids can cause an array of serious adverse effects.

All of the glucocorticoid drugs can produce the same spectrum of therapeutic effects. Because the similarities among these drugs are much more striking than the differences, we do not focus on a prototypical agent but rather discuss the glucocorticoids as a group.

REVIEW OF GLUCOCORTICOID PHYSIOLOGY

In order to understand glucocorticoid drugs, it is important to understand glucocorticoid physiology. The discussion that follows focuses on physiologic effects. This forms the foundation for understand pharmacologic effects of glucocorticoids.

Physiologic Effects

Endogenous glucocorticoids have an essential role in many physiologic processes. As we discuss these, keep in mind that these physiologic responses are elicited by low amounts of glucocorticoids.

Metabolism

Glucocorticoids influence the metabolism of carbohydrates, proteins, and fats. The principal effect on carbohydrate metabolism is elevation of blood glucose. Glucocorticoids do this by promoting synthesis of glucose from amino acids and lipids, reducing peripheral glucose utilization, and reducing glucose uptake by muscle and adipose tissue. Glucocorticoids also promote storage of glucose in the form of glycogen.

Glucocorticoids have a negative effect on protein metabolism. Specifically, these drugs suppress synthesis of proteins from amino acids and divert amino acids for production of glucose.

The most consistent effect of glucocorticoids on fat metabolism is stimulation of lipolysis (fat breakdown).

Cardiovascular and Hematologic Systems

Glucocorticoids are required to maintain the functional integrity of the vascular system. When levels of endogenous glucocorticoids are low, capillaries become more permeable, vasoconstriction is suppressed, and blood pressure falls.

Glucocorticoids have interesting effects on blood cells. They *increase* the number of circulating red blood cells and neutrophils. In contrast, they *decrease* counts of lymphocytes, eosinophils, basophils, and monocytes.

Central Nervous System

Glucocorticoids have essential roles in central nervous system (CNS) function, including a role in neural excitability. When homeostatic mechanisms are disrupted, lower glucocorticoid levels can cause depression and higher levels can cause excitation and even mania.

Stress Response

At times of physiologic stress (e.g., surgery, infection, trauma), the adrenal glands secrete larger quantities of glucocorticoids and epinephrine. Working together, these hormones help maintain blood pressure and blood glucose levels. If glucocorticoid release is insufficient, hypotension and hypoglycemia will occur. If the stress is especially severe, glucocorticoid insufficiency can result in circulatory failure and death.

Fluids and Electrolytes

To varying degrees, individual glucocorticoids can exert actions similar to aldosterone, the major mineralocorticoid released by the adrenal glands. Accordingly, glucocorticoids can act on the kidney to promote retention of sodium and water while increasing urinary excretion of potassium.

Neonatal Respiratory System

During labor and delivery, the adrenal glands of the full-term infant release a burst of glucocorticoids, which act to hasten maturation of the lungs. In the preterm infant, production of glucocorticoids is low, resulting in a high incidence of respiratory distress syndrome.

Control of Glucocorticoid Synthesis and Secretion

Synthesis and release of glucocorticoids are regulated by a negative feedback loop. The principal components of the loop are the hypothalamus, anterior pituitary, and adrenal cortex (Fig. 58.1). The loop is turned on when stress or some other stimulus from the CNS acts on the hypothalamus to cause release of corticotropin-releasing hormone (CRH). CRH then stimulates the pituitary to release adrenocorticotropic hormone (ACTH), which in turn acts on the adrenal cortex to promote synthesis and release of cortisol (the principal endogenous glucocorticoid). Cortisol has two basic effects: first, it stimulates physiologic responses; second, it acts on the hypothalamus and pituitary to suppress further release of CRH and ACTH. By inhibiting release of CRH and ACTH, cortisol suppresses its own production. As a result, this negative feedback loop keeps glucocorticoid levels within an appropriate range. When glucocorticoids are administered chronically in large doses, the feedback loop remains continuously suppressed. As discussed later, persistent suppression can be dangerous.

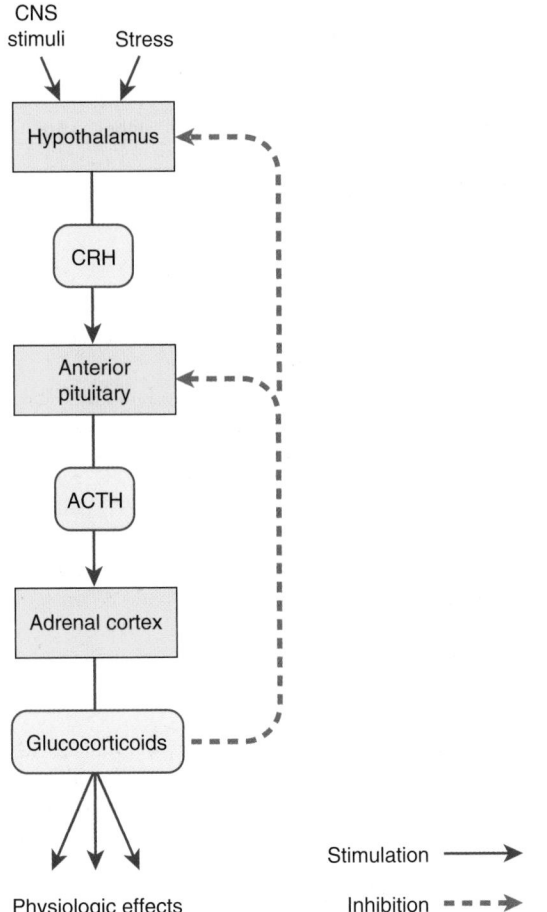

Fig. 58.1 Feedback Regulation of Glucocorticoid Synthesis and Secretion. *ACTH,* Adrenocorticotropic Hormone; *CNS,* Central Nervous System; *CRH,* Corticotropin-Releasing Hormone.

PHARMACOLOGY OF GLUCOCORTICOIDS

Molecular Mechanism of Action

Mechanistically, glucocorticoids differ from most drugs in two ways: (1) glucocorticoid receptors are located *inside* the cell rather than on the cell surface, and (2) glucocorticoids modulate the production of regulatory proteins rather than the activity of signaling pathways.

Here is how they do it: First, glucocorticoids penetrate the cell membrane and then bind with receptors in the cytoplasm, thereby converting the receptor from an inactive form to an active form. Next, the receptor–steroid complex migrates to the cell nucleus, where it binds to chromatin in DNA, thereby altering the activity of target genes. In most cases, activity of the target gene is increased, causing increased transcription of messenger RNA molecules that code for specific regulatory proteins. However, in some cases, activity of the target gene is suppressed; hence synthesis of certain regulatory proteins declines.

Pharmacologic Effects

When administered in the high doses employed to treat nonendocrine disorders, glucocorticoids produce antiinflammatory and immunosuppressive effects—effects not seen at physiologic doses. Of course these high doses also produce the physiologic effects seen at low doses.

Effects on Metabolism and Electrolytes

The effects of high-dose therapy on metabolism and electrolytes are like those seen with physiologic doses, but they are more intense. With high doses, glucose levels rise, protein synthesis is suppressed, and fat deposits are mobilized. As noted, most glucocorticoids have very little mineralocorticoid activity. Accordingly, these drugs do not usually induce significant sodium retention or potassium loss. However, these effects do occur in some patients and can be hazardous. In all patients, high-dose therapy can inhibit the intestinal absorption of calcium, an effect not seen at physiologic doses.

Antiinflammatory and Immunosuppressant Effects

The major clinical applications of the glucocorticoids stem from their ability to suppress immune responses and inflammation. Effects on the immune system and inflammation are interrelated; therefore they are considered together.

Before discussing the actions of glucocorticoids, we must review the process of inflammation. Characteristic symptoms of inflammation are pain, swelling, redness, and warmth. These are initiated by chemical mediators (prostaglandins, histamine, leukotrienes) and are amplified by the actions of lymphocytes and phagocytic cells (neutrophils and macrophages). Prostaglandins and histamine promote several symptoms of inflammation—swelling, redness, and warmth—by causing vasodilation and increasing capillary permeability. Prostaglandins and histamine contribute to pain, histamine stimulates pain receptors directly, and prostaglandins sensitize pain receptors to stimulation by histamine and other mediators. Neutrophils and macrophages heighten inflammation by releasing lysosomal enzymes, which cause tissue injury. Lymphocytes, which are important elements of the immune system, intensify inflammation by (1) causing direct cell injury and (2) promoting the formation of antibodies that help perpetuate the inflammatory response.

Glucocorticoids act through several mechanisms to interrupt the inflammatory processes. These drugs can inhibit synthesis of chemical mediators, thus reducing swelling, warmth, redness, and pain. In addition, they suppress infiltration of phagocytes, so damage from lysosomal enzymes is averted. Lastly, glucocorticoids suppress the proliferation of lymphocytes and thereby reduce the immune component of inflammation.

It is important to appreciate that the mechanisms by which glucocorticoids suppress inflammation are more diverse than the mechanisms by which nonsteroidal antiinflammatory drugs (NSAIDs) act. As discussed in Chapter 57, NSAIDs suppress inflammation primarily by inhibiting prostaglandin production. The glucocorticoids share this mechanism and act in other ways too. Because they act by multiple mechanisms, glucocorticoids have much greater antiinflammatory effects than do NSAIDs.

Pharmacokinetics

Glucocorticoids share similar pharmacokinetic properties. These properties are summarized next.

Absorption. The rate of glucocorticoid absorption depends on the route of administration and the specific glucocorticoid. With oral administration, absorption of all glucocorticoids is rapid and nearly complete. After intramuscular (IM) injection, absorption is rapid with two types of glucocorticoid esters (sodium phosphates and sodium succinates) and relatively slow with other derivatives (e.g., acetates, acetonides). Absorption from local sites of injection (e.g., intraarticular, intralesional) is slower than from IM sites.

Duration of action. Duration depends on dosage, route, and drug solubility. For glucocorticoids administered orally or intravenously, duration is determined largely by biologic half-life (Table 58.1). With IM administration, duration is a function of water solubility: highly soluble preparations have a shorter duration than do less soluble

TABLE 58.1 Systemic Glucocorticoids: Half-Lives, Relative Potencies, and Equivalent Doses

Drug	Biologic Half-Life (h)	Relative Mineralocorticoid Potency[a]	Relative Glucocorticoid (Antiinflammatory) Potency[b]	Equivalent Antiinflammatory Dose (mg)[c]
Short Acting				
Cortisone	8–12	2	0.8	25
Hydrocortisone	8–12	2	1	20
Intermediate Acting				
Prednisolone	18–36	1	4	5
Prednisone	18–36	1	4	5
Methylprednisolone	18–36	0	5	4
Triamcinolone	18–36	0	5	4
Long Acting				
Betamethasone	36–54	0	20–30	0.75
Dexamethasone	36–54	0	20–30	0.75

[a]Relative mineralocorticoid activity (sodium and water retention; potassium depletion): 0, very low; 1, moderate; 2, high.
[b]Glucocorticoid potency values are relative to the potency of hydrocortisone.
[c]Approximate *oral* or *intravenous* dose needed to produce equivalent antiinflammatory effects.

preparations. For locally administered glucocorticoids, duration is determined by solubility and the specific site of administration.

Metabolism and excretion. Glucocorticoids are metabolized primarily by the liver. As a rule, the resulting metabolites are inactive. Excretion of metabolites is renal.

Therapeutic Uses in Nonendocrine Disorders

As has been mentioned, high-dose therapy is required for the management of nonendocrine conditions. For some conditions, long-term therapy is required as well. Because prolonged high-dose therapy can produce serious adverse effects, the potential benefits of treatment must be weighed carefully against the very real risks.

Rheumatoid Arthritis

Glucocorticoids are indicated for adjunctive treatment of acute exacerbations of rheumatoid arthritis. These drugs can reduce inflammation and pain but do not alter the course of the disease. Because of the risk for serious complications, prolonged systemic use should be avoided when possible.

When arthritis is limited to just a few joints, intra-articular injections may be advantageous. Local injections can be highly effective and cause less toxicity than systemic therapy does. Frequently reductions in pain and inflammation can be so dramatic as to prompt vigorous use of joints that were previously immobile. Because excessive use of diseased joints can cause injury, patients should be warned against overactivity even though symptoms have eased.

The use of glucocorticoids in rheumatoid arthritis is discussed further in Chapter 59.

Systemic Lupus Erythematosus

Systemic lupus erythematosus (SLE) is a chronic disease similar in many ways to rheumatoid arthritis. However, in SLE, inflammation is not limited to joints. Rather, it occurs throughout the body. Symptoms frequently include pleuritis, pericarditis, and nephritis. A severe episode can be fatal. Fortunately, manifestations of SLE can usually be controlled with prompt and aggressive glucocorticoid therapy.

Inflammatory Bowel Disease

Glucocorticoids are used to treat severe cases of ulcerative colitis and Crohn disease, the two most common forms of inflammatory bowel disease. Administration may be oral or intravenous. Glucocorticoid therapy of these disorders is considered further in Chapter 66.

Miscellaneous Inflammatory Disorders

Glucocorticoids are useful in a variety of inflammatory disorders in addition to those discussed previously. Conditions that respond include bursitis, tendinitis, synovitis, osteoarthritis, gouty arthritis, and inflammatory disorders of the eye.

Allergic Conditions

Glucocorticoids can control symptoms of allergic reactions. Responsive conditions include allergic rhinitis (see Chapter 63), bee stings, and drug-induced allergies. Because glucocorticoid responses are delayed, these drugs have little value as *sole* therapy for severe allergic reactions (e.g., anaphylaxis). For life-threatening allergic reactions, epinephrine is the treatment of choice.

Asthma

Glucocorticoids are the most effective antiasthma agents available. For treatment of asthma, they may be administered orally or by inhalation. Adverse effects are minimal with inhaled glucocorticoids. In contrast, oral therapy can cause serious toxicity and hence should be reserved for patients who have failed to respond to safer treatments (e.g., inhaled glucocorticoids, inhaled cromolyn sodium). The use of glucocorticoids in asthma is discussed at length in Chapter 62.

Dermatologic Disorders

Glucocorticoids are beneficial in a wide variety of skin diseases, including pemphigus, psoriasis, mycosis fungoides, seborrheic dermatitis, contact dermatitis, and exfoliative dermatitis. For mild disease, topical administration is usually adequate. For severe disorders, systemic therapy may be needed. It should be noted that topical glucocorticoids can be absorbed in amounts sufficient to produce systemic toxicity. Topical therapy is discussed further in Chapter 88.

Prevention of Respiratory Distress Syndrome

A single course of glucocorticoid therapy may be administered to women who are a risk of preterm labor and delivery in order to reduce the risk of respiratory distress syndrome in the neonate. Use in this way can accelerate lung development which improves lung mechanics, gas exchange, and surfactant production.

PATIENT-CENTERED CARE ACROSS THE LIFE SPAN

Glucocorticoids

Life Stage	Patient Care Concerns
Children	Long-term use of steroid medications can cause inhibition of bone growth, which can result in decreased stature. Use during this period of increased bone growth increases the risk for lifetime osteoporosis.
Pregnant women	Inadequate studies of pharmacologic doses of glucocorticoids have been conducted in pregnant women; however, studies in animals have demonstrated both teratogenic and physiologic effects. Observational studies in humans suggest that use during the first trimester may contribute to cleft palate. Administration later in pregnancy places the neonate at risk for hypoadrenalism. For some conditions (e.g., severe persistent asthma), the risk of not using corticosteroids may cause more harm than using them. It is essential to weigh risk versus benefits, use the smallest dose for the shortest period of time to control symptoms, and use inhaled or other nonsystemic formulations when possible. When systemic use is needed, hydrocortisone is preferred over other glucocorticoids.
Breastfeeding women	When physiologic doses or low pharmacologic doses are used, the concentration achieved in milk is probably too low to affect the nursing infant. However, when large pharmacologic doses are employed, the amount ingested by the infant may be sufficient to cause growth delay and other adverse effects. Breastfeeding is not recommended for women taking large doses of glucocorticoids.
Older adults	Long-term use of glucocorticoids can cause osteoporosis, adrenal insufficiency, and gastrointestinal (GI) ulceration. These conditions may affect older adults disproportionately.

Adverse Effects

The adverse effects discussed next occur in response to *pharmacologic* (as opposed to *physiologic*) doses of glucocorticoids. The intensity of these effects increases with dosage size and treatment duration. These effects are not seen when dosage is physiologic. Furthermore, most are not seen when treatment is brief (a few days or less), even when doses are high.

Osteoporosis

Osteoporosis with resultant fractures is a frequent and serious complication of prolonged *systemic* glucocorticoid therapy. (It is uncommon when glucocorticoids are inhaled or administered topically, even when used for prolonged therapy.) The ribs and vertebrae are affected most. In some patients on high-dose glucocorticoids, vertebral compression fractures occur within weeks of beginning glucocorticoid use. Patients should be observed for signs of compression fractures (back and neck pain) and for indications of fractures in other bones.

There are three primary causes of osteoporosis: (1) The most important mechanism is suppression of bone formation by osteoblasts. (2) In addition, glucocorticoids accelerate bone resorption by osteoclasts. (3) Glucocorticoids also reduce intestinal absorption of calcium, causing hypocalcemia. In response to hypocalcemia, release of parathyroid hormone increases, which increases mobilization of calcium from bone.

Infection

By suppressing host defenses, glucocorticoids can increase susceptibility to infection. The risk for acquiring a new infection is increased, as is the risk for reactivating a latent infection (e.g., tuberculosis). In addition, because suppression of both the immune system and neutrophils reduces inflammation and other manifestations of infection, a fulminant infection may develop without detection. Hence glucocorticoids not only increase susceptibility to infection but can also mask the presence of an infection as it progresses.

Impaired Wound Healing

The inflammatory response to injury has a prominent role in wound healing. Because glucocorticoid therapy interferes with normal inflammatory responses, these agents can impair and delay wound healing.

Hyperglycemia

Because of their effects on glucose production, glucocorticoids can increase plasma glucose levels, thereby causing hyperglycemia and glycosuria. This presents a challenge for managing diabetes.

Myopathy

High-dose glucocorticoid therapy can cause myopathy, manifesting as weakness. The proximal muscles of the arms and legs are affected most. Damage to muscle may be sufficient to inhibit ambulation.

Fluid and Electrolyte Disturbance

Because of their mineralocorticoid activity, glucocorticoids can cause sodium and water retention and potassium loss. Retention of water and sodium can cause hypertension and edema. Hypokalemia can predispose to dysrhythmias and toxicity from digitalis. Fortunately most of the glucocorticoids in current use have minimal mineralocorticoid activity; therefore serious fluid and electrolyte disturbance is rare.

Growth Delay

Glucocorticoids can suppress growth in children. Growth delay is probably the result of reduced DNA synthesis and decreased cell division.

Psychologic Disturbances

Systemic glucocorticoids can cause psychologic disturbances. About 60% of patients experience a mild reaction: insomnia, anxiety, agitation, or irritability. Another 6% experience a severe reaction: delirium, hallucinations, depression, euphoria, or mania. Of these, up to one-third may become suicidal. Of note, previous psychiatric illness does not seem to predispose patients to psychologic reactions and a history of good mental health does not confer protection.

Cataracts and Glaucoma

Cataracts are a common complication of long-term glucocorticoid therapy. Risk factors are in dispute; cataract development may be related to age, dosage, or individual susceptibility.

Systemic glucocorticoids can cause open-angle glaucoma. Onset of ocular hypertension develops rapidly and reverses within 2 weeks of glucocorticoid cessation.

Peptic Ulcer Disease

Glucocorticoids have actions that can lead to peptic ulcer disease. By inhibiting prostaglandin synthesis, glucocorticoids can augment secretion of gastric acid and pepsin, inhibit production of cytoprotective mucus, and reduce gastric mucosal blood flow. These actions predispose to GI ulceration. Making matters worse, glucocorticoids can decrease gastric pain, thereby masking ulcer development. As a result, perforation and hemorrhage can occur without warning. The risk for ulceration is increased by concurrent use of other ulcerogenic drugs, such as aspirin and other NSAIDs.

Iatrogenic Cushing Syndrome

Long-term glucocorticoid therapy can induce a cushingoid syndrome with symptoms identical to those of naturally occurring Cushing syndrome. Prominent symptoms are hyperglycemia, glycosuria, fluid and electrolyte disturbances, osteoporosis, muscle weakness, cutaneous striations, and lowered resistance to infection. Redistribution of fat to the abdomen, face, and posterior neck produces the central obesity, rounded face, and fat pad at the cervical spine that are characteristic of Cushing syndrome and Cushing disease.

Adrenal Suppression

Development of adrenal suppression. Adrenal suppression is perhaps the most dangerous adverse effect of long-term glucocorticoid therapy if not managed properly. Like cortisol and other endogenous glucocorticoids, the glucocorticoids administered as drugs suppress release of CRH from the hypothalamus and ACTH from the anterior pituitary. By doing so, exogenous glucocorticoids inhibit the synthesis and release of endogenous glucocorticoids by the adrenal glands. During long-term therapy, the pituitary loses much of its ability to manufacture ACTH and, in response to the prolonged absence of ACTH, the adrenal glands atrophy and lose their ability to synthesize cortisol and other glucocorticoids. As a result, when prolonged glucocorticoid therapy is discontinued, there is a period during which the adrenal glands are unable to produce glucocorticoids. The subsequent adrenal insufficiency can be life-threatening. Patient responses are highly individualized; however, we should consider any patient who has received pharmacologic doses of glucocorticoids for over 3 weeks to be at risk for adrenal suppression.

The time needed for adrenal recovery is highly variable: it may be as short as 5 days or as long as a year. The extent of adrenal suppression and the time required for recovery are determined primarily by the duration of glucocorticoid use; dosage size is less important.

Adrenal suppression and physiologic stress. Adrenal suppression can be dangerous at times of physiologic stress even though glucocorticoid therapy is ongoing. Recall that when stress occurs, the adrenal glands normally secrete larger amounts of glucocorticoids than usual. If the stress is sufficiently severe (e.g., trauma, surgery), these glucocorticoids are essential for supporting life. Accordingly, because of adrenal suppression, *it is imperative that patients receiving long-term glucocorticoid therapy be given increased doses at times of stress* (unless the dosage is already very high). Furthermore, *after glucocorticoid use has ceased, supplemental doses are required whenever stress occurs until recovery of adrenal function is complete.*

Drug Interactions

Interactions Related to Potassium Loss

As noted, glucocorticoids can increase urinary loss of potassium and can thereby induce hypokalemia. Consequently, glucocorticoids must be used with caution when combined with *digoxin* (because hypokalemia increases the risk for digoxin-induced dysrhythmias) and when combined with *thiazide* or *loop diuretics* (because these potassium-depleting diuretics

will increase the risk for hypokalemia). When glucocorticoids are given together with any of the previously mentioned drugs, it is advisable to monitor plasma potassium levels and be alert for signs and symptoms of digoxin toxicity and fluid and electrolyte imbalance.

Nonsteroidal Antiinflammatory Drugs

NSAIDs have the same effects on the GI tract as do glucocorticoids. Accordingly, concurrent use of these agents increases the risk for ulceration and GI bleeding.

Insulin and Oral Hypoglycemics

As noted, glucocorticoids promote hyperglycemia. To maintain glycemic control, patients with diabetes may require increased doses of a glucose-lowering drug (insulin or another hypoglycemic agent).

Vaccines

Because of their immunosuppressant actions, glucocorticoids can decrease antibody responses to vaccines. Furthermore, if a live virus vaccine is employed, the immunosuppressant action of glucocorticoids increases the risk for developing (and spreading) viral disease.

Precautions and Contraindications

Contraindications

Glucocorticoids are contraindicated for patients with *systemic fungal infections* and those receiving *live virus vaccines.*

Precautions

Glucocorticoids must be used with caution in *pediatric patients* and in *women who are pregnant or breastfeeding.* Caution is also required in patients with *hypertension, heart failure, renal impairment, esophagitis, gastritis, peptic ulcer disease, diabetes mellitus, osteoporosis, open-angle glaucoma,* and *infections that are resistant to treatment.* In addition, caution is required during concurrent therapy with *potassium-depleting diuretics, digoxin, insulin, oral hypoglycemics,* and *NSAIDs.*

Preparations and Routes of Administration

Preparations

The glucocorticoids employed clinically include hydrocortisone (cortisol) and synthetic derivatives of hydrocortisone. Individual glucocorticoids differ with respect to (1) biologic half-life, (2) mineralocorticoid potency, and (3) glucocorticoid (antiinflammatory) potency (see Table 58.1).

The term *biologic half-life* refers to the time required for glucocorticoids to leave body tissues. In most cases, these drugs are cleared from tissues more slowly than from the blood. Hence the biologic half-life is usually longer than the plasma half-life. When glucocorticoids are administered by mouth or intravenous injection, it is the biologic half-life and not the plasma half-life that determines duration of action. Because of differences in their biologic half-lives, individual glucocorticoids can be classified as short acting, intermediate acting, or long acting.

Glucocorticoids with high *mineralocorticoid potency* (cortisone, hydrocortisone) can cause significant retention of sodium and water coupled with depletion of potassium. These effects can be especially hazardous for patients with hypertension or heart failure and for those taking digoxin. Because of the potential dangers of sodium retention and potassium loss, glucocorticoids with high mineralocorticoid activity should not be administered systemically for long periods.

The differences in *glucocorticoid potency* are reflected in the doses required to produce antiinflammatory effects—not mineralocorticoid effects. As with other drugs, potency is relatively unimportant. However, it is important to appreciate that, in order to produce equivalent therapeutic effects, dosages for some glucocorticoids must be much larger than for others.

TABLE 58.2   Glucocorticoid Routes of Administration

Drug	Systemic			Local				
	PO	IM	IV	IA	IB	IL	IS	ST
Betamethasone	✓							
Betamethasone sodium phosphate		✓	✓	✓		✓		✓
Betamethasone acetate/sodium phosphate		✓		✓		✓	✓	✓
Cortisone acetate	✓	✓						
Dexamethasone	✓							
Dexamethasone sodium phosphate		✓	✓	✓		✓	✓	✓
Hydrocortisone	✓							
Hydrocortisone acetate				✓	✓	✓	✓	✓
Hydrocortisone sodium succinate		✓	✓					
Methylprednisolone	✓							
Methylprednisolone acetate		✓		✓		✓		✓
Methylprednisolone sodium succinate		✓	✓					
Prednisolone	✓							
Prednisolone acetate	✓							
Prednisolone acetate/sodium phosphate		✓		✓	✓		✓	✓
Prednisolone sodium phosphate	✓							
Prednisone	✓							
Triamcinolone acetonide		✓		✓	✓	✓		
Triamcinolone hexacetonide				✓		✓		

IA, Intra-articular; *IB*, intrabursal; *IL*, intralesional; *IM*, intramuscular; *IS*, intrasynovial; *IV*, intravenous; *PO*, oral; *ST*, soft tissue

Routes of Administration

Glucocorticoids can be administered *orally, parenterally* (IV, IM, subQ), *topically,* and *intranasally* and by *local injection* (e.g., intra-articular, intralesional) or *inhalation.* Topical application is used for dermatologic disorders (see Chapter 88), inhalation therapy is used for asthma (see Chapter 62), and intranasal therapy is used for allergic rhinitis (see Chapter 63). Because local therapy (topical, intranasal, inhalation, local injection) minimizes systemic toxicity, this form of treatment is preferred to systemic therapy (oral, parenteral). When systemic effects are needed, oral administration is preferred to parenteral. It is important to note that even when glucocorticoids are administered for local effects, absorption can be sufficient to produce systemic effects. That is, local administration does not eliminate toxicity risk.

Individual glucocorticoids are available as various esters (e.g., prednisolone *acetate,* prednisolone *sodium phosphate*). When glucocorticoids are administered by routes other than oral or intravenous, the particular ester employed is a major determinant of duration of action. As indicated in Table 58.2, not all esters can be administered by all routes. Therefore, before giving a glucocorticoid, you should verify that the ester ordered is appropriate for the intended route.

Initiating and Withdrawing Therapy
General Guidelines for Dosing

For most patients, the therapeutic objective is to reduce symptoms to an acceptable level. Complete relief is not usually an appropriate goal.

Dosages are highly individualized and, for any patient with any disorder, dosage must be determined by trial and error. For patients whose disorder is not an immediate threat to life, the dosage should be low initially and then increased gradually until symptoms are under control. In the event of a life-threatening disorder, a large initial dose should be used; if a response does not occur rapidly, the dose should be doubled or even tripled. When glucocorticoids are used for a long time, the dosage should be reduced until the smallest effective amount has been established. Prolonged treatment with high doses should be done only if the disorder (1) is life-threatening or (2) has the potential to cause permanent disability. During long-term treatment, an increase in dosage will be needed at times of stress unless the dosage is very high to begin with. If disease status changes, appropriate adjustment of dosage must be made.

As noted, abrupt termination of long-term therapy may unmask adrenal insufficiency. To minimize the effects of adrenal insufficiency, glucocorticoid withdrawal should be gradual. Patients must be warned against abrupt discontinuation.

Alternate-Day Therapy

In alternate-day therapy, a large dose (of an intermediate-acting glucocorticoid) is given every other morning. This dosing schedule contrasts with traditional therapy, in which multiple smaller doses are administered daily. Benefits of alternate-day therapy are (1) reduced adrenal suppression, (2) reduced risk for growth delay, and (3) reduced toxicity overall. Adrenal insufficiency is decreased because, over the extended interval between doses, plasma glucocorticoids decline to a level that is low enough to permit some production of ACTH, thereby promoting some synthesis of cortisol by the adrenal glands. To allow maximal recovery of endocrine function, doses should be administered before 9:00 AM, and long-acting agents should be avoided. Early-morning administration is also helpful in that it mimics the burst of glucocorticoids normally released by the adrenal glands at dawn.

Unfortunately, alternate-day therapy does have one drawback: in the long interval between doses, drug levels may fall to a subtherapeutic value, thus permitting the flaring up of symptoms. Symptoms are likely to be most intense late on the second day after a dose is given. If symptoms become intolerable, switching to a single daily dose may be sufficient to provide control. As with alternate-day treatment, patients taking single daily doses should administer their medicine before 9:00 AM.

Glucocorticoid Withdrawal

To allow time for recovery of adrenal function, withdrawal of glucocorticoids should be done slowly. The withdrawal schedule is determined by the degree of adrenal suppression. A representative schedule is as follows: (1) taper the dosage to a physiologic range over 7 days; (2) switch from multiple daily doses to single doses administered each morning; (3) taper the dosage to 50% of physiologic values over the next month; and (4) monitor for production of endogenous cortisol and, when basal levels have returned to normal, cease routine glucocorticoid dosing (but be prepared to give supplemental doses at times of stress). As a rule, tapering is unnecessary when oral glucocorticoids have been used for less than 2 to 3 weeks.

In addition to unmasking adrenal insufficiency, stopping glucocorticoids may produce a withdrawal syndrome. Symptoms include hypotension, hypoglycemia, myalgia, arthralgia, and fatigue. In patients being treated for arthritis and certain other disorders, these symptoms may be confused with return of the underlying disease. Discomfort of withdrawal can be minimized by gradual dosage reduction.

PATIENT EDUCATION
Glucocorticoids

Instruct patients to take their medicine in the morning to mimic natural physiologic timing of hormone release. Administration with milk or a snack may decrease GI distress.

Warn patients against abrupt discontinuation of treatment when therapy is with high or prolonged dosing. Adrenal suppression may be life-threatening. Withdrawal symptoms may also occur.

Advise the patient to carry identification (e.g., Medic Alert bracelet) to ensure proper dosing in emergencies. Trauma and other emergencies will require higher doses of glucocorticoids to mimic the normal stress response.

Explain that glucocorticoids can increase the risk for infection. Inform patients about early signs of infection (e.g., fever, malaise), and instruct them to call the clinic if these occur.

Educate patients about signs and symptoms of fluid retention (e.g., weight gain, swelling of the lower extremities) and hypokalemia (e.g., muscle weakness, irregular pulses, cramping), and instruct them to notify the prescriber if these develop.

To decrease the risk of cataracts and glaucoma, reinforce the need for eye examinations during therapy. Instruct patients to call the clinic if vision becomes cloudy or blurred.

Explain that these drugs can cause GI bleeding. It is important to avoid over-the-counter drugs without first checking with the provider. Instruct patients to call the clinic if stools become black and tarry.

Inform patients about possible psychologic reactions and instruct them to report disturbing symptoms. Explain that dosage adjustments or other medications may be needed to manage these symptoms.

SUMMARY OF KEY PRESCRIBING CONSIDERATIONS
Glucocorticoids for Nonendocrine Disorders

Therapeutic Goal: The goal depends on the purpose of treatment. These drugs are prescribed primarily to reduce and control harmful inflammatory and allergic responses and to modulate immune responses in patients with autoimmune diseases and organ transplants. They also have a role in adjunctive therapy for blood cancers characterized by elevated lymphocytes and for management of certain types of cancer pain, especially neuropathic pain and pain due to expanding pressure within areas with limited capability for expansion (e.g., bowel obstruction, intracranial pressure).

Baseline Data: Obtain a history and physical exam with particular attention to neuromuscular examination and ophthalmologic examination. Assess for signs and symptoms of infection. Check blood pressure (BP) and body mass index (BMI). Assess height for pediatric patients. For conditions where use is anticipated beyond a few weeks, check complete blood count (CBC) with white blood cell (WBC) cell differential, serum glucose, electrolytes, lipid panel, and bone mineral density (BMD). Consider testing for latent tuberculosis (TB), especially if a patient is at risk.

Monitoring: Assess CBC, glucose, electrolytes, and lipids in 1 month then every 6 to 12 months if condition is stable; assess sooner for signs or symptoms of complications (e.g., hyperglycemia). An eye exam should be done every 6 months. Ask about muscle weakness at each visit and assess proximal muscle strength of extremities if weakness is present. Stools tested periodically (with Hemoccult) and as needed if GI ulceration is suspected or for any report of GI discomfort or black or red stools. Check BMD in 1 year and, if stable compared with baseline, every 2 to 3 years thereafter. If BMD decreased from baseline, assess annually. Periodically assess serum glucose and metabolic panel as guided by patient presentation. Assess BP and BMI at every visit. Check pediatric height every 6 months.

Identifying High-Risk Patients: Patients at risk for an increase in adverse effects when on long-term or high-dose glucocorticoid therapy include those with immune disorders, diabetes mellitus, cardiovascular disease, impaired renal function, osteoporosis, open-angle glaucoma, and GI disorders. Those who have recently received live virus vaccines are also at risk. Patients with infections should first be placed on antimicrobial therapy if feasible. Medication adjustments may be needed for patients taking potassium-depleting diuretics, digoxin, NSAIDs, or hypoglycemic drugs (including insulin).

Evaluating Therapeutic Effects: Depending on the purpose of therapy, evaluate the ability of glucocorticoids to control the problems for which they are prescribed.

Minimizing Adverse Effects:
Osteoporosis:
- Although osteoporosis is likely with prolonged systemic glucocorticoid therapy, it is uncommon when glucocorticoids are inhaled or administered topically; therefore nonsystemic glucocorticoid formulations should be administered when possible (e.g., inhalers for asthma; topical formulations for skin conditions). BMD should be monitored and dosage adjusted for evidence of bone loss.
- Before glucocorticoid treatment, BMD of the lumbar spine should be measured. This will identify patients at highest risk and provide a baseline for evaluating bone loss during treatment. If subsequent BMD evaluations show bone loss, the risks and benefits of decreasing glucocorticoid therapy should be considered.
- All patients should receive calcium and vitamin D supplements. Sodium restriction combined with a thiazide diuretic can enhance intestinal absorption of calcium and decrease the urinary excretion of calcium. There is solid evidence that a bisphosphonate can prevent glucocorticoid-induced bone loss by inhibiting

SUMMARY OF KEY PRESCRIBING CONSIDERATIONS—cont'd

bone resorption by osteoclasts. Calcitonin (Miacalcin), which also inhibits osteoclasts, is another option. For patients with significant bone loss, teriparatide (Forteo) may be preferred because, unlike bisphosphonates and calcitonin, which only prevent bone resorption, teriparatide actively promotes new bone formation. In postmenopausal women, estrogen therapy is an effective way to reduce bone loss. However, as discussed in Chapter 50, the risks of estrogen therapy generally outweigh the benefits. The roles of calcium, vitamin D, bisphosphonates, calcitonin, teriparatide, and estrogen in the prophylaxis and treatment of osteoporosis are discussed fully in Chapter 61.

Infection:
- Patients should avoid close contact with people who have a communicable disease and avoid crowds during times when communicable diseases (e.g., influenza) are high.
- If a significant infection occurs, glucocorticoids should be continued only if absolutely necessary and then only in combination with appropriate antimicrobial or antifungal therapy.
- *Pneumocystis jirovecii* pneumonia, commonly known as an opportunistic infection in people with AIDS, occurs with alarming frequency in people receiving high doses of glucocorticoids. Accordingly, it has been suggested that prophylaxis be considered for all people taking glucocorticoids long term in high doses.

Glucose Intolerance:
- Patients with diabetes may need an increased dosage of hypoglycemic medication. (For patients with normal pancreatic function, a significant elevation of blood glucose is unlikely.)
- Because glucocorticoids can unmask latent diabetes, even patients without a diagnosis of diabetes should undergo periodic evaluation of blood glucose levels.

Myopathy:
- Muscle weakness should be monitored closely to identify changes early.
- If myopathy develops, the glucocorticoid dosage should be reduced. Myopathy gradually resolves over several months.

Fluid and Electrolyte Disturbance:
- Select glucocorticoids that have low mineralocorticoid activity (see Table 58.1)
- Limit sodium intake.
- Promote consumption of potassium-rich foods (e.g., potatoes, sweet potatoes, white beans, bananas).
- Prescribe potassium supplements if hyperkalemia develops despite dietary changes.

Growth Delay:
- Plot growth trends to identify delays early.
- Growth suppression can be minimized with alternate-day therapy.

Psychologic Disturbances:
- Psychologic reactions are dependent on the dosage and duration of treatment. Long-term low-dose therapy is more likely to cause depression. In contrast, short-term high-dose therapy is more likely to cause mania and other psychoses. Cognitive impairment (e.g., distractibility, memory loss) can occur with either dosing pattern.
- Psychologic effects reverse when glucocorticoids are withdrawn. Delirium and hallucinations usually resolve quickly—within a few days to a week. Mood disturbances (depression, mania) resolve more slowly—over 6 weeks or longer.
- Drugs typically used to manage mood disorders and psychosis have demonstrated success in managing the psychologic adverse effects in many patients. Occasionally, though, psychologic effects are unresponsive to the usual drugs used to manage these conditions.

Cataracts and Glaucoma:
- Refer to ophthalmologist for abnormal ophthalmologic examination.
- Assess benefits versus risks and be prepared to wean off glucocorticoids if indicated.

Peptic Ulcer Disease:
- Avoid treatment with other drugs that promote GI bleeding or ulceration (e.g., NSAIDs).
- If GI ulceration occurs, glucocorticoids should slowly be withdrawn (unless their continued use is considered essential to support life).
- Prescribe antiulcer medication (see Chapter 64).

Cushing Syndrome:
- Carefully weigh benefits versus risks of continuing current glucocorticoid dosage.
- Consult with endocrinologist regarding optimal management.

Adrenal Suppression:
- If therapy will be prolonged, consider that alternate-day dosing can minimize the development of adrenal suppression.
- Do not suddenly stop treatment; wean carefully while monitoring response. Consultation with an endocrinologist is advisable.
- See section on glucocorticoid withdrawal.

59

Drug Therapy of Rheumatoid Arthritis

Rheumatoid arthritis (RA) is an autoimmune inflammatory disorder that affects more than 1.3 million Americans. Although RA can develop at any age, initial symptoms usually appear during the third and fourth decades of life. Among younger patients, the incidence of RA among females is three times greater than that among males. However, among patients older than 60 years, the incidence in men and women is equal. RA follows a progressive course and can eventually cause joint deformities and functional limitations. In many cases, drug therapy can delay disease progression. In others, benefits are limited to symptomatic relief. Some of the drugs used for RA were introduced in preceding chapters. Additional drugs are introduced here.

PATHOPHYSIOLOGY OF RHEUMATOID ARTHRITIS

The onset of RA is heralded by symmetric joint stiffness and pain. Symptoms are most intense in the morning and abate as the day advances. Joints become swollen, tender, and warm. For some patients, periods of spontaneous remission occur. For others, injury progresses steadily. In addition to joint injury, RA has systemic manifestations, including fever, weakness, fatigue, weight loss, thinning of the skin, scleritis (inflammation of the sclera), corneal ulcers, vasculitis (which can be severe), and nodules under the skin and periosteum (connective tissue that surrounds all bones).

The progression of joint deterioration is shown in Fig. 59.1. Inflammation begins in the synovium—the membrane that encloses the joint cavity. As inflammation intensifies, the synovial membrane thickens and begins to envelop the articular cartilage. This overgrowth is referred to as *pannus*. Damage to the cartilage is caused by enzymes released from the pannus and by chemicals and enzymes produced by the inflammatory process raging within the synovial space. Ultimately, the articular cartilage undergoes total destruction, resulting in direct contact between bones of the joint, followed by eventual bone fusion. After this, inflammation subsides.

Joint destruction is caused by an autoimmune process in which the immune system mounts an attack against synovial tissue. During the attack, mast cells, macrophages, and T lymphocytes produce cytokines and cytotoxins—compounds that promote inflammation and joint destruction. The cytokines of greatest importance are tumor necrosis factor (TNF), interleukin-1 (IL-1), IL-6, interferon γ, platelet-derived growth factor, and granulocyte-macrophage colony-stimulating factor. Why the immune system attacks joints is unclear.

OVERVIEW OF THERAPY

Treatment is directed at (1) relieving symptoms (pain, inflammation, and stiffness), (2) maintaining joint function and range of motion, (3) minimizing systemic involvement, and (4) delaying disease progression. To achieve these goals, a combination of pharmacologic and nonpharmacologic measures is used.

Nondrug Measures

Nondrug measures for managing RA include physical therapy, exercise, and surgery. Physical therapy may consist of massage, warm baths, and applying heat to the affected regions. These procedures can enhance mobility and reduce inflammation. A balanced program of rest and exercise can decrease joint stiffness and improve function. However, excessive rest and excessive exercise should be avoided: too much rest will foster stiffness, and too much activity can intensify inflammation.

Orthopedic surgery has made marked advances. For patients with severe disease of the hip or knee, total joint replacement can be performed. When joints of the hands or wrists have been damaged severely, function can be improved through removal of the diseased synovium and repair of ruptured tendons. Plastic implants can help correct deformities.

A complete program of treatment should include patient education and counseling. The patient should be informed about the nature of RA, the possible consequences of joint degeneration, management measures, and the benefits and limitations of drug therapy. If loss of mobility limits function at home, on the job, or in school, consultation with a social worker, occupational therapist, or specialist in vocational rehabilitation may be appropriate.

Drug Therapy

Antiarthritic drugs can produce symptomatic relief, and some drugs, if started very early in the disease process, can induce protracted remission. However, remission is rarely complete, and the disease typically advances steadily. As a result, drug therapy must be lifelong.

Classes of Antiarthritic Drugs

The antirheumatic drugs fall into three major groups:
- Nonsteroidal antiinflammatory drugs (NSAIDs)
- Glucocorticoids
- Disease-modifying antirheumatic drugs (DMARDs)

These major groups differ with respect to time course of effects, toxicity, and ability to slow RA progression.

The NSAIDs provide rapid relief of symptoms but do not prevent joint damage and do not slow disease progression. The NSAIDs are safer than DMARDs and glucocorticoids; thus treatment with NSAIDs requires less vigorous monitoring.

Like the NSAIDs, glucocorticoids provide rapid relief of symptoms. In addition, they can slow disease progression. Unfortunately, although glucocorticoids are effective, with long-term use they can cause serious toxicity. As a result, treatment is usually limited to short courses.

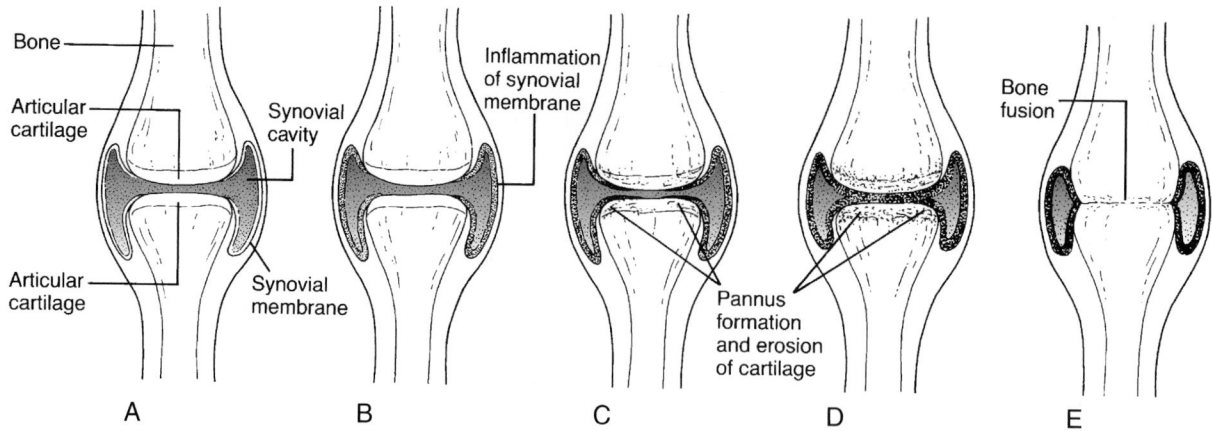

Fig. 59.1 Progressive Joint Degeneration in Rheumatoid Arthritis. (A) Healthy joint. (B) Inflammation of synovial membrane. (C) Onset of pannus formation and cartilage erosion. (D) Pannus formation progresses and cartilage deteriorates further. (E) Complete destruction of joint cavity together with fusion of articulating bones.

DMARDs are drugs that reduce joint destruction and slow disease progression. They accomplish this by interfering in immune and inflammatory responses. (See Chapter 84.) DMARDs are subdivided into three basic categories—*conventional (traditional) DMARDs, biologic DMARDs,* and *targeted DMARDs.* The conventional DMARDs are small molecules that are synthesized using conventional chemical techniques. These drugs have extensive effects on the immune system. The biologic DMARDs are large molecules produced through recombinant DNA technology. These drugs work on cytokines. The targeted DMARDs, the latest of the three categories, are synthetically developed small molecules that block specific pathways inside cells of the immune system. DMARDs from each of the three categories are provided in Table 59.2. All DMARDs have significant adverse effects; therefore close monitoring is required.

Drug Selection

Management of RA is usually overseen by a rheumatologist or other specialist.

Life Stage	Considerations or Concerns
Children	*Biologic DMARDs:* Children and adolescents taking TNF antagonists have developed lymphoma and other malignancies.
Pregnant women	*Biologic DMARDs:* TNF antagonists are US Food and Drug Administration (FDA) Pregnancy Risk Category B. Rituximab and abatacept are Pregnancy Risk Category C. *Nonbiologic DMARDs:* Azathioprine is teratogenic. Both leflunomide and methotrexate can cause fetal death and congenital abnormalities. Hydroxychloroquine may cause fetal ocular toxicity; however, in some conditions, such as maternal lupus or malaria, the drug decreases fetal risk associated with the conditions it treats. Sulfasalazine is Pregnancy Risk Category B.
Breastfeeding women	Breastfeeding is not recommended for mothers taking DMARDs.
Older adults	Elderly patients may be at a greater risk for infection secondary to the immunosuppressive effects of DMARDs.

The management of RA is aggressive. Current guidelines recommend starting a DMARD *early*—within 3 months of RA diagnosis for most patients (Fig. 59.2). When DMARD therapy is instituted early, it can be possible to delay or even prevent serious joint injury.

Because the effects of DMARDs take weeks or months to develop, whereas the effects of NSAIDs are immediate, an NSAID is given until the DMARD has had time to act, after which the NSAID can be withdrawn. Glucocorticoids are generally reserved for short-course management of symptom flareups and to control symptoms until the DMARD takes effect. If joint injury progresses despite treatment with an initial DMARD (typically methotrexate), another DMARD can be added or substituted.

Detailed information on pharmacologic management of RA can be found in clinical guidelines developed by the American College of Rheumatology (ACR). The document, *2015 American College of Rheumatology Guideline for the Treatment of Rheumatoid Arthritis,* is available at http://www.rheumatology.org/Portals/0/Files/ACR%20 2015%20RA%20Guideline.pdf. The discussion that follows is centered on these guidelines.

NONSTEROIDAL ANTIINFLAMMATORY DRUGS

The basic pharmacology of the NSAIDs is discussed in Chapter 57. Consideration here is limited to their role in RA.

Therapeutic Role

NSAIDs are prescribed for their antiinflammatory and analgesic actions. Both actions result from inhibiting cyclooxygenase (COX). NSAIDs provide only symptomatic relief; they do not slow disease progression. Accordingly, they are usually combined with a DMARD.

Nonsteroidal Antiinflammatory Drug Classification

There are two main classes of NSAIDs: (1) *first-generation NSAIDs,* which inhibit COX-1 *and* COX-2; and (2) *second-generation NSAIDs* (coxibs), which selectively inhibit COX-2. Anti inflammatory and analgesic effects result from inhibiting COX-2, whereas major adverse effects—especially gastroduodenal ulceration—result from inhibiting COX-1. Therefore the selectivity of this drug class results in less gastrointestinal (GI) ulceration than the first-generation NSAIDs while producing equal therapeutic effects.

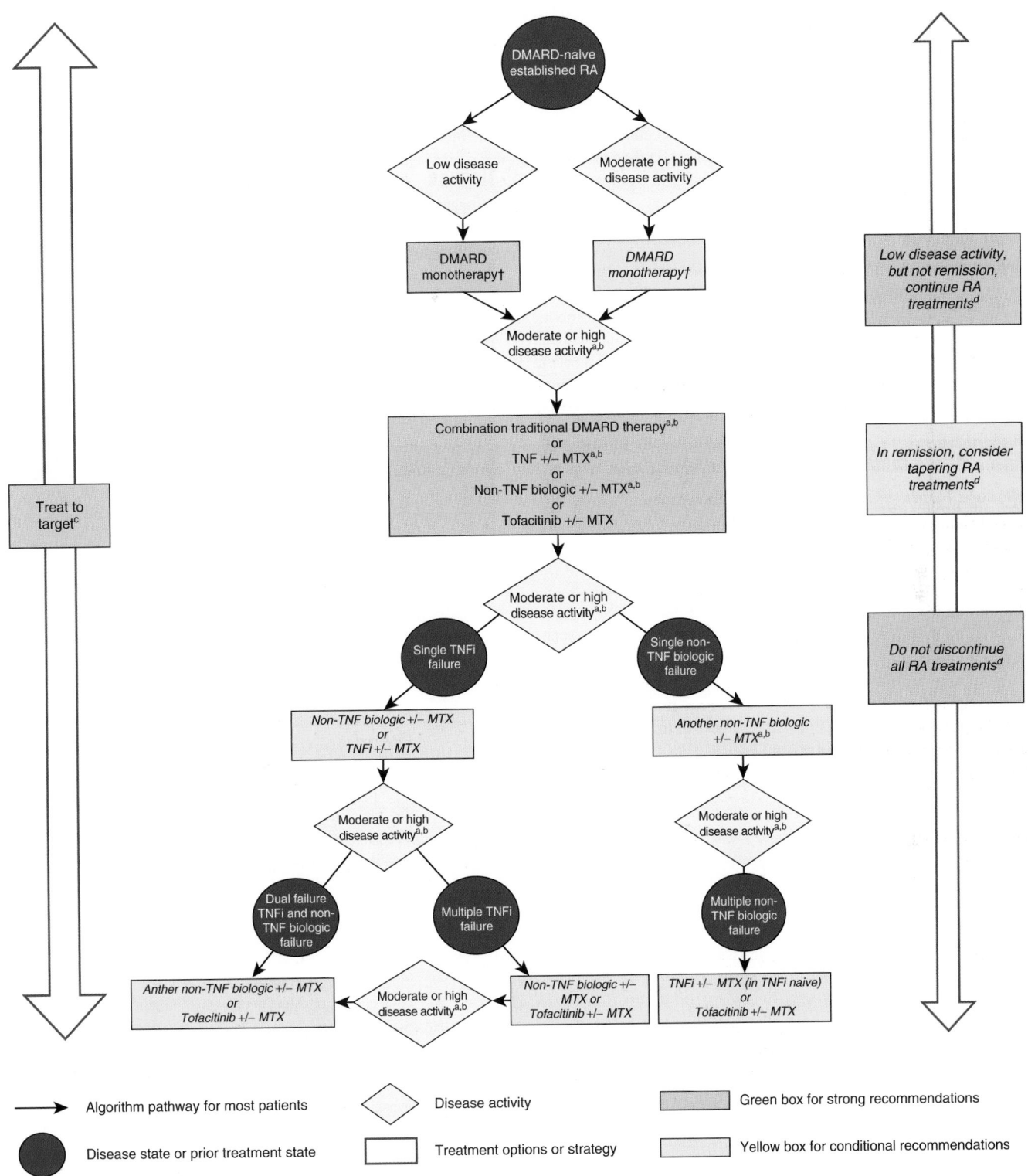

Fig. 59.2 Algorithm for Rheumatoid Arthritis Management. *DMARDs,* disease-modifying antirheumatic drugs; *RA,* rheumatoid arthritis; *TNF,* tumor necrosis factor. (From 2015 American College of Rheumatology Guidelines for the Treatment of Rheumatoid Arthritis. http://www.rheumatology.org/Portals/0/Files/ACR%20 2015%20RA%20Guideline.pdf.)

aconsider adding low-dose glucocorticoids (<10 mg/day of prednisone or equivalent) in patients with moderate or high RA disease activity when starting disease-modifying antirheumatic drugs (DMARDs) and in patients with DMARD failure or biologic failure.
bconsider using short-term glucocorticoids (defined as < 3 months treatment) for RA disease flares. Glucocorticoids should be used at the lowest possible dose and for the shortest possible duration to provide the best benefit-risk ratio for the patient.
ctreatment target should ideally be low disease activity or remission.
dtapering denotes scaling back therapy (reducing dose or dosing frequency), not discontinuing it and if done, must be conducted slowly and carefully.

Drug Selection

Selection of an NSAID is based largely on efficacy, safety, and cost.

Efficacy

All NSAIDs have essentially equal antirheumatic effects; however, individual patients may respond better to one NSAID than to another. Accordingly, it may be necessary to try more than one agent to achieve an optimal response.

Safety and Cost

All prescription-strength NSAIDs carry a boxed warning regarding risk for thrombotic events, GI ulceration, and bleeding. Although the risk for GI problems is lessened with COX-2 inhibitors, the risk for thrombotic events may be increased because coxibs inhibit COX-1 to a far lesser degree than first-generation NSAIDs. (Recall that COX-1 has a role in the production of thromboxane A_2, which participates in blood clotting.) Selection must balance these factors. Coxibs are more expensive than first-generation NSAIDs. If symptoms are controlled with a first-generation NSAID and the drug is well tolerated, cost considerations will dictate using that drug. However, if a first-generation NSAID produces serious gastric ulceration and the patient is at low risk for thrombosis, then switching to celecoxib might be appropriate—despite the increased cost.

Dosage

Dosages employed for antiinflammatory effects are considerably higher than those required for analgesia or fever reduction. For example, the treatment of RA may require 5.2 g (16 standard tablets) of aspirin a day compared with only 2.6 g for aches, pain, and fever. Typical dosages for RA are shown in Table 59.1.

GLUCOCORTICOIDS

The glucocorticoids are powerful antiinflammatory drugs that can relieve symptoms of severe RA and may also delay disease progression. For

---

TABLE 59.1   Nonsteroidal Antiinflammatory Drugs: Oral Dosage for Rheumatoid Arthritis

Generic Name	Trade Name	Daily Dosage
First-Generation NSAIDs		
Salicylates		
Aspirin	Multiple trade names	3.6–5.4 g/d in divided doses
Magnesium salicylate	Doan's Extra Strength	650–1160 mg q 6 h as needed
Salsalate	Generic only	3 g/d (in 2 or 3 doses)
Nonsalicylates		
Diclofenac (salt)	Cambia, Cataflam, Voltaren, Zipsor	Immediate release: 150–200 mg/d (in 3 or 4 doses)
		Delayed release: 150–200 mg.d (in 2–4 divided doses)
		Extended release: 100 or 200 mg/d (in 2 divided doses)
Diclofenac (free acid)	Zorvolex	18–35 mg tid
Diclofenac/misoprostol	Arthrotec	50 mg diclofenac/200 μg misoprostol 3 or 4 times daily
Diflunisal	Generic only	250–500 mg bid
Etodolac	Generic only	Immediate release: 400 mg bid *or* 300 mg bid/tid *or* 500 mg bid
		Extended release: 400–1000 mg once daily
Fenoprofen	Nalfon	300–600 mg tid/qid
Flurbiprofen	Generic only	200–300 mg/d (in 2–4 doses)
Ibuprofen	Motrin, Advil, others	400–800 mg tid/qid
Indomethacin	Indocin	25–50 mg tid
Ketoprofen	Generic only	Immediate release: 150–300 mg/d (in 3 or 4 doses)
		Extended release: 100–200 mg once a day
Meclofenamate	Generic only	200–400 mg/d (in 3 or 4 doses)
Meloxicam	Mobic, Mobicox ♦	7.5 mg once a day
Nabumetone	Generic only	1–2 g/d (in 1 or 2 doses)
Naproxen	Naprosyn	Immediate release: 250–500 mg bid
	Naprelan	Extended release: 750–1500 mg/d
	EC-Naprosyn	Delayed release: 375–500 mg bid
Naproxen sodium	Aleve, others	250–500 mg bid
Naproxen/esomeprazole	Vimovo	375–500 mg (naproxen) bid
Oxaprozin	Daypro	1.2 g once a day
Piroxicam	Feldene	10 mg twice daily *or* 20 mg once a day
Sulindac	Clinoril	150–200 mg bid
Tolmetin	Generic only	200–600 mg tid
Second-Generation NSAIDs (COX-2 Inhibitors)		
Celecoxib	Celebrex	100–200 mg bid

COX, Cyclooxygenase; *NSAID*, nonsteroidal anti-inflammatory drug

TABLE 59.2 Disease-Modifying Antirheumatic Drugs

Conventional DMARDs

Major drugs	Methotrexate (Trexall, Otrexup, Rasuvo, Xatmep)
	Sulfasalazine (Azulfidine)
	Leflunomide (Arava)
	Hydroxychloroquine (Plaquenil)
Minor drugs	Azathioprine (Imuran)
	Cyclosporine (Neoral, Sandimmune)
	Minocycline (Minocin)
	Penicillamine (Cuprimine, Depen)
	Protein A (Prosorba)
	Gold salts:
	Gold sodium thiomalate (Aurolate, Myochrysine)
	Auranofin (Ridaura)

Biologic DMARDs

Tumor necrosis factor inhibitors	Adalimumab (Humira)
	Certolizumab pegol (Cimzia)
	Etanercept (Enbrel)
	Golimumab (Simponi, Simponi Aria)
	Infliximab (Remicade)
B-lymphocyte–depleting agent	Rituximab (Rituxan)
T-cell activation inhibitor	Abatacept (Orencia)
Interleukin-6 receptor antagonist	Sarilumab (Kevzara)
	Tocilizumab (Actemra)
Interleukin-1 receptor antagonist	Anakinra (Kineret)

Targeted DMARDs

Janus kinase inhibitor	Baricitinib (Olumiant)
	Tofacitinib (Xeljanz, Xeljanz XR)

DMARDs, disease-modifying antirheumatic drugs

patients with generalized symptoms, *oral* glucocorticoids are indicated. However, if only one or two joints are affected, *intra-articular injections* may be employed. Because long-term oral therapy can cause serious toxicity (e.g., osteoporosis, gastric ulceration, adrenal suppression), short-term therapy should be used whenever possible. Most often glucocorticoids are used for temporary relief until drugs with more slowly developing effects (methotrexate and other DMARDs) can provide control. They may also be employed for flares, which are disease exacerbations that occur in patients whose condition was previously controlled. Long-term therapy should be limited to patients who have failed to respond adequately to all other options. Both NSAIDs and glucocorticoids place a patient at risk for GI ulceration and GI bleeding. When prescribed together, the risk for adverse GI effects may be increased fourfold; therefore NSAID therapy is usually discontinued whenever the patient is taking glucocorticoids. The pharmacology of the glucocorticoids is discussed in Chapter 58.

CONVENTIONAL DISEASE-MODIFYING ANTIRHEUMATIC DRUGS

The conventional DMARDs were the first to be developed for the management of RA.

Benefits of conventional DMARDs result from immunosuppression. Because RA is an autoimmune disease, suppression of the immune response (and the associated inflammation) can slow disease progression.

Clinical responses develop slowly, however. The conventional DMARDs cost much less than the biologic and targeted DMARDS, largely because the conventional agents are easier to make.

Commonly Used Disease-Modifying Antirheumatic Drugs

Methotrexate

Actions and uses. Many rheumatologists consider methotrexate (Trexall, Otrexup, Rasuvo) the DMARD of first choice owing to its efficacy, relative safety, low cost, and extensive use in RA. At least 80% of patients improve with this drug. Methotrexate acts faster than all other DMARDs. Therapeutic effects may develop in 3 to 6 weeks.

Methotrexate is a folate antagonist. Because folate is necessary for DNA synthesis and cellular replication, it inhibits these processes. Although this explains its mechanism of action for treatment of cancer, for RA, the exact mechanism of action is elusive. Benefits appear to be the result of immunosuppression secondary to reducing the activity of B and T lymphocytes.

Methotrexate is also approved for management of severe psoriasis after other treatments have been tried and found to be ineffective. Methotrexate, under the brand name Xatmep, is approved for the treatment of some cases of acute lymphoblastic leukemia and the management of polyarticular juvenile idiopathic arthritis in pediatric patients who do not respond adequately to other therapy.

Adverse effects. Major toxicities of methotrexate are hepatic fibrosis, bone marrow suppression, GI ulceration, and pneumonitis. To reduce GI and hepatic toxicity, supplementing dosing with folic acid (at least 5 mg/wk) is recommended. Supplemental folic acid enters the cell passively and does not compete with methotrexate. Periodic tests of liver and kidney function are mandatory, as are complete blood cell and platelet counts.

Methotrexate can cause fetal death and congenital abnormalities and therefore is contraindicated during pregnancy. (See Patient Centered Care Across the Life Span.) Recent data suggest that patients using methotrexate for RA may have a reduced life expectancy owing to increased deaths from cardiovascular disease, infection, and certain cancers (melanoma, lung cancer, and non-Hodgkin lymphoma).

Methotrexate is contraindicated for women who are pregnant or nursing. It is also contraindicated for patients with blood dyscrasias, immunodeficiency, and liver disease.

Preparations, dosage, and pharmacokinetics. Dosages for methotrexate and other DMARDs are provided in Table 59.3. Pharmacokinetic properties are provided in Table 59.4.

▶▶ BLACK BOX WARNING
Methotrexate (Trexall, Otrexup, Rasuvo, Xatmep)

Methotrexate can cause numerous and potentially fatal toxicities of the bone marrow, liver, lungs, and kidneys. Other fatalities have occurred associated with skin reactions and due to hemorrhagic enteritis and gastrointestinal perforation.

Drug interactions. Methotrexate increases the risk for hepatotoxicity when other drugs that contribute to liver injury (including alcohol) are taken. Similarly, methotrexate greatly increases the risk for serious myelosuppression when it is prescribed for patients taking other drugs that can decrease bone marrow function.

As would be expected with an immunosuppressant, methotrexate reduces the response to vaccines, thus decreasing their efficacy. Live vaccines are contraindicated for patients taking methotrexate. If it is necessary to give inactivated (killed) vaccines to patients receiving

PATIENT-CENTERED CARE ACROSS THE LIFE SPAN

Disease-Modifying Antirheumatic Drugs

Life Stage	Considerations or Concerns
Children	*Biologic DMARDs:* Children and adolescents taking TNF inhibitors have developed lymphoma and other malignancies.
Pregnant women[a]	*Conventional DMARDs:* Azathioprine is teratogenic. Both leflunomide and methotrexate can cause fetal death and congenital abnormalities. Hydroxychloroquine does not appear to cause fetal ocular toxicity, as once suspected; research is ongoing. In some conditions, such as maternal lupus or malaria, hydroxychloroquine decreases fetal risk associated with the conditions it treats. Sulfasalazine inhibits the absorption and metabolism of folic acid, thus increasing the risk for neural tube defects.
	Biologic DMARDs: Research is limited for all biologic DMARDs. Thus far we know that use of rituximab may result in B-cell lymphocytopenia lasting up to 6 months. Agranulocytosis has occured in neonates born to women taking infliximab. Animal reproduction studies have produced abnormalities for tocilizumab but *not* for etanercept or golimumab. Pregnancy registry data for adalimumab have not identified adverse outcomes; however, the number of subjects has been small (74 patients with RA taking adalimumab and 80 patients with RA not taking adalimumab).
	Targeted DMARDs: Fetal death and congenital abnormalities have occurred in animal studies. Until more is known, targeted DMARDs are not recommended for pregnant women.
Breastfeeding women	Breastfeeding is not recommended for mothers taking DMARDs.
Older adults	Elderly patients may be at a greater risk for infection secondary to the immunosuppressive effects of DMARDs.

[a]Research data related to human pregnancy outcomes for patients on DMARDs is limited. The Organization of Teratology Information Specialists (OTIS) is conducting the OTIS Vaccines and Medications in Pregnancy Surveillance Study as part of the Rheumatoid Arthritis and Pregnancy Study. Providers should encourage pregnant women with RA taking DMARDs (or other drugs) to join this study. Information is available at https://mothertobaby.org/ongoing-study/rheumatoid-arthritis or by calling 1-877-311-8972.

methotrexate, patients should be revaccinated within 3 months after therapy is discontinued. Ideally, needed vaccines should be administered prior to starting methotrexate. The ACR recommends that patients receive vaccines for the following communicable diseases prior to beginning therapy with a DMARD: pneumonia, influenza, hepatitis B, HPV, and herpes zoster.

Leflunomide

Actions and uses. Leflunomide (Arava) is a powerful immunosuppressant indicated for adults with active RA. In clinical trials, the drug decreased signs and symptoms and slowed disease progression. Compared with methotrexate, leflunomide is about equally effective but is potentially more hazardous and more expensive. Accordingly, the drug is often reserved for second-line use.

Leflunomide is a prodrug that undergoes conversion to its active form—metabolite 1 (M1)—in the body. M1 inhibits dihydro-orotate dehydrogenase, a mitochondrial enzyme needed for de novo synthesis of pyrimidines, which in turn are needed for T-cell proliferation and antibody production. In vitro, leflunomide inhibits T-cell proliferation. In animals, it suppresses inflammation.

Adverse effects. The most common adverse effects occur in at least 10% of patients: diarrhea, respiratory infection, reversible alopecia, and rash. The drug has also been associated with much more serious reactions: pancytopenia, Stevens-Johnson syndrome (SJS), peripheral neuropathy, interstitial lung disease, and severe hypertension.

Leflunomide is hepatotoxic. Elevation of liver enzymes occurs in about 10% of patients. In postmarketing reports, the drug has been associated with instances of severe liver injury, including some that were fatal. Leflunomide should be avoided in patients with liver impairment, hepatitis B, or hepatitis C. Patients should be informed about signs and symptoms of liver injury—abdominal pain, fatigue, dark urine, and jaundice—and advised to report them immediately.

Leflunomide may increase the risk for serious infection. The drug is immunosuppressive and can suppress the bone marrow. Rarely, patients experience sepsis and other severe infections, including tuberculosis (TB). Deaths have occurred. If an infection develops, it may be necessary to interrupt leflunomide use. If evidence of bone marrow suppression is detected, leflunomide should be discontinued. Patients should be screened for TB before starting this drug.

Leflunomide is carcinogenic in animals but has not been associated with cancer in humans.

Because it is a teratogen, leflunomide is contraindicated during pregnancy. Patients who wish to become pregnant must first clear leflunomide from the body. A three-step protocol is followed:

Step 1: Discontinue leflunomide.

Step 2: Take cholestyramine (8 g tid) for 11 days. (Cholestyramine binds leflunomide and its metabolites in the intestine, accelerating their excretion. Without cholestyramine, safe levels might not be achieved for 2 years.)

Step 3: Verify that plasma drug levels are below 20 μg/L.

To minimize any risk for fetal injury, men using leflunomide who wish to father a child should undergo the same clearance procedure.

Drug interactions. Leflunomide can inhibit the metabolism of certain NSAIDs (e.g., ibuprofen, diclofenac), causing their levels to rise. In addition, leflunomide can intensify liver damage from other hepatotoxic drugs (e.g., methotrexate) and hence should not be combined with such agents. Rifampin (a drug for TB) can raise leflunomide levels by 40%. Conversely, two other agents—cholestyramine and activated charcoal—can rapidly lower leflunomide levels.

Sulfasalazine

Sulfasalazine (Azulfidine, Azulfidine EN-tabs) has been used for decades to treat inflammatory bowel disease. Benefits for RA may result from antiinflammatory and immunomodulatory actions. In patients with RA, sulfasalazine can slow the progression of joint deterioration, sometimes with just 1 month of treatment. GI reactions (nausea, vomiting, diarrhea, anorexia, abdominal pain) are the most common reasons for stopping treatment. These reactions can be minimized by using an enteric-coated formulation and dividing the daily dosage. Dermatologic reactions (pruritus, rash, urticaria) are also common; rarely, fatal dermatologic conditions (e.g., SJS, toxic epidermal necrolysis [TEN]) have occurred. Fortunately, serious adverse effects—hepatitis

TABLE 59.3 Disease-Modifying Antirheumatic Drugs: Common Dosages for Rheumatoid Arthritis

Drug Name	Preparation	Dosage
Conventional (Traditional) DMARDS		
Methotrexate (Trexall, Otrexup, Rasuvo, Xatmep)	Tablet: 2.5 mg, 5 mg, 7.5 mg, 10 mg, 15 mg Solution: 25 mg/mL Autoinjector: 15 different dosages ranging from 7.5 mg/0.15 mL to 30 mg/0.6 mL	Oral, subQ, and IM: 7.5 mg/wk initially then adjusted upward until optimal response is achieved or a maximal dose of 20–30 mg/wk is reached. Optional oral dosing: 10–15 mg/wk initially, then increased by 5 mg/wk every 2–4 wk up to a maintenance level of 20–30 mg/wk.
Sulfasalazine (Azulfidine, Azulfidine EN-tabs)	IR tablet: 500 mg (scored) ER tablet: 500 mg	Initial: 0.5–1 g/d Maintenance: 1 g given 2 or 3 times a day.
Leflunomide (Arava)	Tablets: 10 mg, 20 mg	Initial: loading doses of 100 mg once a day for 3 days. Maintenance: 10–20 mg/d.
Hydroxychloroquine (Plaquenil)	Tablet: 200 mg	Initially: 400–600 mg/d increased slowly to achieve optimal response over 1–3 months. Maintenance: 200–400 mg/d.
Biologic DMARDS		
Adalimumab (Humira)	Prefilled syringe: 20 mg/0.4 mL, 40 mg/0.8 mL Autoinjector: 40 mg/0.8 mL	40 mg every 2 weeks. If used without methotrexate: 40 mg once a week.
Certolizumab pegol (Cimzia)	Prefilled syringe: 200 mg/mL	Initial: 400 mg repeated at 2 and 4 weeks. Maintenance: 200 mg every 2 weeks or 400 mg every month.
Etanercept (Enbrel)	Prefilled syringe: 25 mg/0.5 mL, 50 mg/mL Autoinjector: 50 mg/mL Powder: 25-mg for reconstitution in 1 mL of sterile bacteriostatic water	Adult: 50 mg subQ once a week. Children ages 4–17 years: 0.8 mg/kg (up to a maximum of 50 mg) once a week.
Golimumab (Simponi, Simponi Aria)	Prefilled syringe: 50 mg/0.5 mL, 100 mg/mL Autoinjector: 50 mg/0.5 mL, 100 mg/mL Solution for IV administration: 50 mg/4 mL	SubQ (Simponi): 50 mg once a month IV. (Simponi Aria): 2 mg/kg repeated at 4 weeks and then every 8 weeks for maintenance.
Infliximab (Remicade)	Powder: 100 mg in single-use vials to be dissolved in 10 mL of sterile water, followed by dilution in 0.9% sodium chloride to a final volume of 250 mL.	Initial: 3 mg/kg repeated at 2 weeks and 6 weeks. Maintenance: 3 mg/kg every 8 weeks.
Rituximab (Rituxan)	Solution: 10 mg/mL in 10-mL and 50-mL vials	Initial: 1000 mg IV infusion repeated in 2 weeks. Subsequent treatment: 1000 mg every 24 weeks if needed.
Abatacept (Orencia)	Prefilled syringe: 125 mg/mL IV: 250-mg powder for reconstitution in sterile water	SubQ: 125 mg/wk, preferably after a single IV loading dose of 10 mg/kg. IV for adults <60 kg, give 500 mg; 60–100 kg, give 750 mg; >100 kg, give 1000 mg. Repeat at 2 weeks and 4 weeks after first infusion and then repeat every 4 weeks. IV for polyarticular juvenile idiopathic arthritis: <75 kg, give 10 mg/kg; 75–100 kg, give 750 mg; >100 kg, give 1000 mg. As in adults, dosing is done on days 0, 14, and 28, and every 4 weeks thereafter.
Tocilizumab (Actemra)	Prefilled syringe: 162 mg/0.9 mL IV: 80 mg, 300 mg, and 400 mg as a concentrated solution (20 mg/mL) for dilution in 0.9% sodium chloride to a final volume of 100 mL	SubQ: <100 kg, give 162 mg every 2 weeks; may increase if response suboptimal >100 kg, give 162 mg weekly. IV: 4 mg/kg every 4 weeks, given as a single 60-min IV drip infusion. The dosage can be increased to 8 mg/kg every 4 weeks based on the clinical response. The maximal single dose is 800 mg.
Sarilumab (Kevzara)	Auto-injector: 150 mg/1.14 mL, 200 mg/1.14 mL Prefilled syringe: 150 mg/1.14 mL, 200 mg/1.14 mL	SubQ: 200 mg every 2 weeks
Anakinra (Kineret)	Prefilled syringe: 100 mg/0.67 mL	SubQ: 100 mg once daily.
Targeted DMARDS		
Tofacitinib	IR tablet: 5 mg ER tablet: 11 mg	IR: 5 mg twice daily. ER: 11 mg once daily.
Baricitinib	Tablet: 2 mg	2 mg once daily.

ER, Extended release; *GI*, gastrointestinal; *IM*, intramuscular; *IR*, immediate release; *IV*, intravenous; *subQ*, subcutaneous

TABLE 59.4 Pharmacokinetics: Disease-Modifying Antirheumatic Drugs

Conventional DMARDS	Peak	Protein Binding	Metabolism	Half-Life	Elimination
Methotrexate (Trexall, Otrexup, Rasuvo, Xatmep)					
Sulfasalazine (Azulfidine, Salazopyrin)	6 h (range 3–12 h)	>99%	Intestinal flora to sulfapyridine (and 5-aminosalicylic acid); acetylation postabsorption	7.6 h (range 4.2–11 h)	Urine
Leflunomide (Arava)	6–12 h	>99%	Primarily hepatic	2 weeks	Urine Feces
Hydroxychloroquine (Plaquenil)	UK	40%	Primarily hepatic	40 days	Urine
Biologic DMARDS					
Etanercept (Enbrel, Brenzys, Erelzi)	69 h (range 35–103 h)	UK	UK	102 h (range 72–132 h)	UK
Infliximab (Remicade)	UK	UK	UK	7.7–9.5 days	Presumed metabolized to peptides and amino acids that can be re-used for protein synthesis or renally excreted
Adalimumab (Humira)	131 h (range 75–187 h)	UK	Presumed opsonization via the reticuloendothelial system	2 weeks (range 10–20 days)	UK
Golimumab (Simponi, Simponi Aria)	2–6 days	UK	UK	2 weeks	UK
Certolizumab Pegol (Cimzia)	54–171 h	UK	UK	14 days	UK
Rituximab (Rituxan)	UK	UK	Presumed opsonization of bound drug via the reticuloendothelial system	18 days (range 5–78 days)	UK
Abatacept (Orencia)	UK	UK	UK	13 days (range 8–25 days)	Renal and hepatic
Tocilizumab (Actemra)	3–4.5 days (dose dependent)	UK	UK	10–18 days (dose dependent)	Biphasic elimination from circulation
Sarilumab (Kevzara)	2–4 days	UK	UK	8–10 days (dose dependent)	Lower doses: Nonlinear target-mediated pathways Higher doses: Linear proteolytic pathways
Anakinra (Kineret)	3–7 h	UK	UK	4–6 h	NA
Targeted DMARDS					
Tofacitinib (Xeljanz, Xeljanz XR)	IR: 0.5–1 h ER: 4 h	40%	Hepatic via CYP3A4 and CYP2C19	IR: 3 h ER: 6 h	Urine
Baricitinib (Olumiant)	1 h	50%	Hepatic via CYP3A4	12 h	Urine (75%) Feces

IR, Immediate release; *ER*, extended release; *UK*, unknown

and bone marrow suppression—are rare. To ensure early detection, periodic monitoring for hepatitis and bone marrow function (complete blood counts, platelet counts) should be performed. Because of its structure, sulfasalazine should not be prescribed for patients with sulfa allergy. Sulfasalazine is discussed in Chapter 66.

Hydroxychloroquine

Hydroxychloroquine (Plaquenil), a drug with antimalarial actions, is considered a preferred DMARD in the 2015 ACR treatment guidelines. How hydroxychloroquine works in RA is unknown. As a rule, the drug is usually combined with methotrexate. By itself, hydroxychloroquine does not slow disease progression, but early use can improve long-term outcomes.

Like other DMARDs, hydroxychloroquine has a delayed onset; full therapeutic effects take 3 to 6 months to develop. Concurrent therapy

with antiinflammatory agents (NSAIDs or glucocorticoids) is indicated during the latency period.

Retinal damage, which is rare, is the most serious toxicity. Retinopathy may be irreversible and can produce blindness. Visual loss is directly related to dosage. Low doses may be used in long-term treatment with little risk. When dosage has been excessive, retinal damage may appear after treatment has ceased and may progress in the absence of continued drug use. Patients should undergo a thorough ophthalmologic examination before treatment. Product labeling recommends annual evaluations for those with risk factors; however, annual exams can be deferred until after 5 years of therapy in patients without risk factors. Hydroxychloroquine should be discontinued at the first sign of retinal injury.

Cardiac problems, some fatal, have occurred when higher dosing is used. These include cardiomyopathy and varying degrees of atrioventricular heart block and bundle branch block. Because hydroxychloroquine can prolong the QT interval, the risk for ventricular dysrhythmias is also increased.

Other concerning adverse effects include hypoglycemia, proximal myopathy and neuropathy, and worsening of psoriasis. Hydroxychloroquine can also cause GI distress; however, this can be relieved by taking the drug with food or milk.

Other Conventional Disease-Modifying Antirheumatic Drugs

Several drugs that are FDA-approved for RA are used infrequently, largely because of adverse effects. Some (azathioprine, cyclosporine, minocycline, and gold) are no longer recommended; however, they may still be used as a last resort when other drugs fail to meet therapeutic objectives. These drugs are discussed briefly next.

Penicillamine

Penicillamine (Cuprimine, Depen) can relieve symptoms of RA and can delay disease progression. Unfortunately, treatment may be associated with serious toxicity, especially bone marrow suppression and autoimmune disorders. Because it is associated with fatalities, the use of penicillamine should be restricted to cases where RA is severe and unresponsive to other treatment. Therapeutic effects take 3 to 6 months to develop.

Gold Salts

Gold salts—auranofin (Ridaura)—have been used in RA for decades. Treatment can relieve pain and stiffness and may also delay disease progression. The mechanism underlying these benefits is unknown. Unfortunately, adverse effects are common. Potential reactions include intense pruritus, rashes, stomatitis, kidney damage, severe blood dyscrasias, encephalitis, hepatitis, peripheral neuritis, pulmonary infiltrates, and profound hypotension.

 BLACK BOX WARNING

Auranofin (Ridaura)

Gold compounds can cause gold toxicity manifested by serious blood dyscrasias, stomatitis, profuse diarrhea, proteinuria, hematuria, and rash.

Azathioprine

Azathioprine (Imuran) is an older DMARD with immunosuppressive and antiinflammatory actions. Serious toxicities include hepatitis and blood dyscrasias (leukopenia, thrombocytopenia, anemia). The drug may also pose a small risk for malignancy.

Cyclosporine

Cyclosporine (Neoral, Sandimmune), an immunosuppressive drug used to prevent rejection of transplanted organs, can reduce symptoms of RA. Because it can cause kidney damage and other serious adverse effects, cyclosporine should be reserved for severe, progressive RA that has not responded to safer DMARDs. In patients with an inadequate response to methotrexate, adding cyclosporine may produce significant improvement.

Minocycline

Minocycline (Minocin), an antibiotic in the tetracycline family, has been used experimentally in RA management. It can improve morning stiffness, joint pain and tenderness, and activities of daily living. In addition, it may delay disease progression in some patients. The precise mechanism by which it accomplishes this is unknown. The ACR did not include minocycline in the 2015 guidelines because of its infrequent use and the lack of new data since 2012.

Protein A Column (Prosorba)

The Prosorba column, used in combination with plasmapheresis, decreases the titer of circulating immune complexes that promote symptoms of RA. The column contains an adsorbent compound—protein A—that binds to antibodies of the immunoglobulin G (IgG) class and to IgG-antigen complexes. When the patient's plasma is passed through the column, these antibodies and immune complexes are removed. Treatment should be reserved for patients with moderate to severe RA who have been refractory to or intolerant of methotrexate and other DMARDs. The most common adverse effects are transient increases in joint swelling, joint pain, and fatigue.

BIOLOGIC DISEASE-MODIFYING ANTIRHEUMATIC DRUGS

The biologic DMARDs are immunosuppressive drugs that target specific components of the inflammatory process. These drugs are usually combined with methotrexate. Because they suppress immune function, all biologic DMARDs pose a risk for serious infections and perhaps cancer.

Compared with the small-molecule DMARDs, the large-molecule biologic DMARDs have unique physical and chemical properties. As a result, biologic DMARDs are processed in alternative ways that result in distinctive pharmacokinetic properties. For many, precise pharmacokinetics are still unknown. (Biologics are discussed further in Chapter 86.)

As noted earlier, the biologic DMARDs are so named because they are manufactured using recombinant DNA technology. This is an expensive process that is reflected in the cost of these drugs, which can range from $14,000 to more than $65,000 a year.

Tumor Necrosis Factor Inhibitors

The drugs in this group work by inhibiting the actions of TNF, an important immune mediator of joint injury in RA. Five TNF inhibitors (TNF antagonists) are available. In patients with RA, all five are highly and equally effective. Unfortunately, all five pose a risk for serious infections, including bacterial sepsis, invasive fungal infections, hepatitis B infection, and TB. Rarely, patients experience severe allergic reactions, heart failure, liver failure, hematologic disorders, neurologic disorders, or cancer. The principal differences among these drugs concern dosing schedule and route of administration.

In addition to their use in RA, these drugs are approved for other inflammatory disorders, including psoriatic arthritis, ankylosing spondylitis, and Crohn disease (Table 59.5).

Etanercept

Etanercept (Enbrel) was the first TNF antagonist available and will serve as our prototype for the group. Like all other TNF inhibitors, etanercept is highly effective at reducing RA symptoms and disease progression but may also promote serious infections and other adverse effects.

Actions and uses. Etanercept suppresses inflammation by inhibiting TNF. As noted earlier, TNF is an important contributor to the pathophysiology of RA. In patients with RA, TNF binds with receptors on cells in the synovium and thereby stimulates production of chemotactic factors and endothelial adhesion molecules, which in turn promote infiltration of neutrophils and macrophages. The result is inflammation and joint destruction.

How does etanercept neutralize TNF? Etanercept is a large molecule composed of two receptors for TNF that are linked to the Fc component

TABLE 59.5 Approved Indications for Tumor Necrosis Factor Inhibitors

Approved Indications	Etanercept (Enbrel)	Infliximab (Remicade)	Adalimumab (Humira)	Golimumab (Simponi)	Certolizumab (Cimzia)
Rheumatoid arthritis	✓	✓	✓	✓	✓
Ankylosing spondylitis	✓	✓	✓	✓	✓
Juvenile idiopathic arthritis	✓		✓	✓	✓
Psoriatic arthritis	✓	✓	✓	✓	
Plaque psoriasis	✓	✓	✓	✓	✓
Crohn disease		✓	✓		✓
Ulcerative colitis		✓	✓	✓	

PROTOTYPE DRUGS

Drugs for Rheumatoid Arthritis

Nonsteroidal Antiinflammatory Drugs
Aspirin (a first-generation NSAID)
Celecoxib (a COX-2 inhibitor)

Glucocorticoids
Prednisone

Disease-Modifying Antirheumatic Drugs
Methotrexate (conventional DMARD)
Etanercept (biologic DMARD)
Tofacitinib (targeted DMARD)

of IgG. The TNF receptors, which are produced through recombinant DNA technology, are identical to the TNF receptors found on human cells. Like the TNF receptors on our cells, etanercept binds tightly with TNF and thereby prevents TNF from interacting with its natural receptors on cells.

Etanercept is indicated for patients with moderately to severely active RA. In clinical trials, the drug was slightly superior to methotrexate at delaying the progression of joint damage, and it suppressed signs and symptoms of RA more rapidly. Among patients who had failed to respond to methotrexate, the addition of etanercept for 6 months reduced symptoms in 61%, compared with 27% who continued taking methotrexate alone.

In addition to RA, etanercept is approved for ankylosing spondylitis, plaque psoriasis, psoriatic arthritis, and juvenile idiopathic arthritis.

 BLACK BOX WARNING

Tumor Necrosis Factor Inhibitors

Patients taking tumor necrosis factor inhibitors (adalimumab, certolizumab pegol, etanercept, golimumab, and infliximab) are at an increased risk for developing serious systemic infections and sepsis.

Adverse effects. Children and adolescents taking TNF inhibitors have developed lymphoma and other malignancies.

Injection-site reactions—itching, erythema, swelling, pain—occur in 37% of patients but usually subside in a few days. Other mild but less common reactions include headache, rhinitis, dizziness, cough, and abdominal pain.

Etanercept increases the risk for several serious adverse effects. These include serious infections, severe allergic reactions, heart failure, cancer, hematologic disorders, liver injury, and central nervous system (CNS) demyelinating disorders.

Serious infections. Under normal conditions, TNF plays a crucial role in our immune response to infections, especially those caused by *Mycobacterium tuberculosis* and other intracellular pathogens. Accordingly, when we inhibit TNF with etanercept, the risk for infections goes up. Infection risk is further increased by diabetes, HIV infection, and concurrent use of immunosuppressant drugs, including glucocorticoids and methotrexate.

TB is a special concern. When TB develops in patients taking etanercept, the disease is often extrapulmonary and disseminated. To reduce risk, potential users should be tested for latent TB and, if the test is positive, should undergo TB treatment before etanercept is used. During etanercept treatment, patients should be monitored closely for TB development.

Etanercept may promote reactivation of latent infection with hepatitis B virus (HBV). Fatalities have occurred. Candidates for etanercept therapy should be tested for latent HBV, and those who test positive should be monitored closely. If reactivation of HBV infection occurs, etanercept should be stopped and the patient given antiviral drugs.

To reduce infection risk, etanercept should not be given to patients with active infection, including infections that are chronic or localized. Patients who develop a new infection should be monitored closely. Etanercept should be used with caution in patients with a history of recurrent infection or any condition that predisposes them to acquiring infection (e.g., advanced or poorly controlled diabetes). If a severe infection develops, etanercept should be discontinued.

Severe allergic reactions. Rarely, etanercept has been associated with severe allergic reactions, including SJS, erythema multiforme, and TEN. The median onset of symptoms in known cases was 28 days after starting etanercept. Patients and providers should be alert for these reactions.

Heart failure. Etanercept may pose a risk for heart failure. In patients using the drug, existing cases of heart failure have gotten worse, and new cases have developed. Exercise caution in patients with existing heart failure and monitor them closely for disease progression.

Cancer. Etanercept and other TNF inhibitors may increase the risk for lymphoma and other malignancies primarily in children, adolescents, and young adults.

Hematologic disorders. Etanercept may pose a small risk for hematologic disorders, including neutropenia, thrombocytopenia, and aplastic anemia, which can be fatal. Advise patients who develop signs or symptoms of a blood disorder (persistent fever, bruising, bleeding, pallor) to seek immediate medical attention. If a significant hematologic abnormality is diagnosed, discontinuation of etanercept should be considered.

Liver injury. Rarely, etanercept has been associated with severe liver injury, including acute liver failure. Some patients have required a liver transplant and some have died. Patients should be informed about symptoms of liver injury—fatigue, yellow skin, yellow eyes, anorexia, right-sided abdominal pain, dark brown urine—and advised to seek medical attention if these develop. If severe liver injury is diagnosed, discontinuation of etanercept should be considered. Etanercept should be used with caution in patients with preexisting liver dysfunction.

Central nervous system demyelinating disorders. Etanercept has been associated with rare cases of CNS demyelinating disorders, including multiple sclerosis, myelitis, and optic neuritis. However, a causal relationship has not been established. Nonetheless, caution is advised, especially in patients with a preexisting or recent-onset demyelinating disorder.

Drug interactions. In addition to decreasing the efficacy of vaccines, etanercept, by inhibiting TNF, may increase the risk for acquiring or transmitting infection after immunization with a *live virus vaccine.* Accordingly, live virus vaccines should be avoided. Vaccinations should be updated before starting the drug.

Immunosuppressant drugs—including glucocorticoids, methotrexate, tocilizumab, anakinra, and abatacept—increase the risk for serious infection. Use these combinations with caution.

Infliximab

Infliximab (Remicade), formulated for intravenous use, was the second TNF antagonist approved for RA. Like etanercept, infliximab binds to and thereby inhibits TNF. However, the two drugs are structurally different: whereas etanercept is composed of two TNF receptors, infliximab is a TNF antibody.

In patients with RA, infliximab is approved for combined use with methotrexate to reduce symptoms and delay disease progression. Infliximab is also approved for psoriasis (see Chapter 88), psoriatic arthritis, ankylosing spondylitis, and two intestinal disorders: Crohn disease and ulcerative colitis (see Chapter 66).

Like etanercept, infliximab has immunosuppressant actions that can increase the risk for serious infection, including bacterial sepsis, invasive fungal infections, HBV infection, and TB. Accordingly, the drug should not be given to patients with chronic infections and should be temporarily withdrawn if an acute infection develops. Patients should receive a TB test and HBV test to rule out latent infection before treatment.

Like other TNF inhibitors, infliximab has been associated with rare cases of heart failure, liver failure, hematologic disorders, neurologic disorders, severe allergic reactions, and cancer.

Infliximab is administered by slow intravenous infusion. Infusion reactions are common, manifesting with flu-like symptoms, headache, fever, chills, dyspnea, hypotension, skin reactions, and GI disturbance. Rarely, patients experience anaphylaxis. Symptoms can be reduced by pretreatment with an antihistamine, acetaminophen, or a glucocorticoid.

 BLACK BOX WARNING

Infliximab (Inflectra. Remicade, Renflexis, Remsima)

Infliximab may cause an increased risk for developing serious and potentially fatal infections.

Adalimumab

Like infliximab, adalimumab (Humira) is a monoclonal antibody that binds to and thereby neutralizes TNF. The drug is indicated for adults with moderate to severe RA who have not responded adequately to one or more DMARDs. In these patients, adalimumab can reduce symptoms and slow the progression of joint damage. The drug may be used alone or in combination with methotrexate or other DMARDs. In addition to RA, adalimumab is approved for ankylosing spondylitis, juvenile idiopathic arthritis, plaque psoriasis, psoriatic arthritis, ulcerative colitis, and Crohn disease.

Adalimumab is generally well tolerated. The most common side effects are injection-site reactions (rash, erythema, itching, pain, swelling), which develop in about 20% of patients. Like other TNF inhibitors, adalimumab can promote serious infections (e.g., bacterial sepsis, invasive fungal infections, HBV infection, TB) and has been associated with rare cases of heart failure, liver failure, hematologic disorders, neurologic disorders, severe allergic reactions, and cancer.

Golimumab

Golimumab (Simponi, Simponi Aria) is approved for RA, but only in combination with methotrexate. Like infliximab, golimumab is a monoclonal antibody that binds with and thereby neutralizes TNF. In addition to RA, golimumab is approved for the treatment of ulcerative colitis, ankylosing spondylitis, and psoriatic arthritis.

In clinical trials, the most common adverse effects were injection-site reactions, upper respiratory tract infections, and nasopharyngitis. However, except for injection-site reactions, the incidence of these adverse effects was only slightly higher than in patients receiving placebo. Like other TNF inhibitors, golimumab can promote serious infections (e.g., bacterial sepsis, invasive fungal infections, HBV infection, TB) and has been associated with rare cases of heart failure, liver failure, hematologic disorders, neurologic disorders, severe allergic reactions, and cancer.

Certolizumab Pegol

Certolizumab pegol (Cimzia) is a monoclonal antibody derivative designed to neutralize TNF. The drug consists of a recombinant humanized Fab antibody fragment that has been covalently bound to polyethylene glycol (PEG). Because of this "pegylation," the drug is eliminated slowly. Certolizumab is approved for treatment of adults with moderate to severe RA, Crohn disease, ankylosing spondylitis, and psoriatic arthritis. In patients with RA, the combination of certolizumab plus methotrexate is more effective than certolizumab alone.

Certolizumab can cause serious adverse effects. In clinical trials, the most common events were upper respiratory tract infections, urinary tract infections, and arthralgia. Like other TNF inhibitors, certolizumab can promote serious infections (e.g., bacterial sepsis, invasive fungal infections, HBV infection, TB) and has been associated with rare cases of heart failure, liver failure, hematologic disorders, neurologic disorders, severe allergic reactions, and cancer.

B-Lymphocyte–Depleting Agents

These agents reduce the number of B lymphocytes—cells that play an important role in the autoimmune attack on joints. As a result, they can reduce symptoms of RA and slow disease progression. Currently there is only one drug in this category: rituximab (Rituxan).

Rituximab

Actions and uses. Rituximab (Rituxan) is a monoclonal antibody directed against CD20, an antigen found exclusively on the surface of B lymphocytes. When rituximab binds with CD20, the immune system attacks the rituximab–B-cell complex, causing B-cell lysis and death.

Rituximab, in combination with methotrexate, is indicated for intravenous therapy of adults with moderate to severe RA who have not responded to one or more TNF inhibitors. In addition, rituximab is indicated for two inflammatory disorders of blood vessels—Wegener granulomatosis and microscopic polyangiitis—and for two types of cancer: B-cell non-Hodgkin lymphoma and B-cell chronic lymphocytic leukemia.

Adverse effects

Infusion reactions. Rituximab can cause severe infusion-related hypersensitivity reactions beginning within 30 to 120 minutes. The immediate reaction and its sequelae include hypotension, bronchospasm, angioedema, hypoxia, pulmonary infiltrates, myocardial infarction, and cardiogenic shock. Postinfusion renal toxicity may lead to renal failure. Deaths have occurred within 24 hours. To reduce the risk for these events, patients should be premedicated with an antihistamine and acetaminophen. Additionally, premedication with an intravenous glucocorticoid such as methylprednisolone is also recommended by some experts. If a severe reaction occurs, management includes giving glucocorticoids, epinephrine, bronchodilators, and oxygen.

▶▶ **BLACK BOX WARNING**
Rituximab (Rituxan)

Rituximab administration has resulted in severe and sometimes fatal reactions; approximately 80% occur during the first infusion.

Rituximab may cause severe mucocutaneous reactions, which may be fatal. It may also cause HBV reactivation and progressive multifocal leukoencepthalopathy (PML); both may be fatal.

Mucocutaneous reactions. Rituximab has been associated with severe mucocutaneous reactions, including SJS, lichenoid dermatitis, vesiculobullous dermatitis, and TEN. Deaths have occurred. Reaction onset is typically 1 to 3 weeks after rituximab exposure. Patients who experience these reactions should seek immediate medical attention and should not receive rituximab again.

Hepatitis B reactivation. There have been reports of HBV reactivation, which can lead to fulminant hepatitis, hepatic failure, and death. Patients at high risk for HBV should be screened before getting rituximab. Asymptomatic carriers should be closely monitored for clinical and laboratory signs of active HBV infection while taking rituximab and for several months after stopping.

Progressive multifocal leukoencephalopathy. Rituximab has been associated with rare cases of PML, a severe infection of the CNS caused by reactivation of the JC virus, an opportunistic pathogen resistant to all available drugs. Most cases have occurred in patients being treated for non-Hodgkin lymphoma. Patients and prescribers should be alert for any new neurologic signs and symptoms. If PML is diagnosed, rituximab should be discontinued immediately.

Other adverse effects. Like other monoclonal antibodies, rituximab can cause a flu-like syndrome, especially during the initial infusion. Symptoms include fever, chills, nausea, vomiting, and myalgia. Rituximab causes transient neutropenia.

Drug interactions. Rituximab should not be prescribed for patients taking T-cell activation inhibitors or targeted DMARDs. If rituximab is prescribed for patients taking leflunomide, it will be important to closely monitor for bone marrow suppression. Rituximab can enhance the immunosuppressant activity of other drugs, and it can decrease the efficacy of inactivated vaccines. Live vaccines should be avoided in patients taking rituximab.

T-Cell Activation Inhibitors

Activated T cells (T lymphocytes) inhabit the synovium of patients with RA. These activated T cells play a key role in the autoimmune attack on joints. T-cell activation inhibitors prevent T-cell activation. Currently there is only one drug in this class: abatacept (Orencia).

Atabacept

Action and uses. For T cells to achieve full activity, they must be stimulated by antigen-presenting cells (APCs). Abatacept—a complex molecule composed of a ligand (cytotoxic T-lymphocyte–associated

antigen 4) linked to IgG1 (an isotype of IgG)—binds with receptors on APCs and thereby prevents the APCs from activating T cells. The results are reduced T-cell proliferation and reduced production of interferon γ, interleukins, and TNF.

Abatacept has two approved indications: to reduce symptoms and delay disease progression in adults with moderately to severely active RA, and to decrease symptoms of moderately to severely active polyarticular juvenile idiopathic arthritis in children 6 years of age and older. Patients with RA who have not responded adequately to methotrexate or TNF inhibitors may experience significant improvement with abatacept.

Adverse effects. Abatacept is generally well tolerated. The most common adverse effects are headache, upper respiratory infection, nasopharyngitis, and nausea.

Because abatacept suppresses immune function, the drug can increase the risk for serious infections. Infections seen most often are pneumonia, cellulitis, bronchitis, diverticulitis, pyelonephritis, and urinary tract infections. Patients should be told about infection risk and advised to report suspected infection immediately. If a serious infection develops, abatacept should be discontinued.

Abatacept may blunt the effect of all vaccines and may increase the risk for infection from live virus vaccines. Before abatacept is given to children, all vaccinations should be up to date. Live virus vaccines should not be used in children or adults during abatacept use and for 3 months after stopping.

Drug interactions. Abatacept may be used in combination with other DMARDs but not with TNF inhibitors, targeted DMARDs, or IL-1 receptor antagonists. These combinations increase the risk for serious infection and offer no clinically significant benefit over abatacept alone.

Interleukin-6 Receptor Antagonists

In patients with RA, IL-6 helps amplify the autoimmune attack on joints. Accordingly, drugs that block the actions of IL-6 can reduce RA symptoms and disease progression. At this time, there are two IL-6 receptor antagonists: tocilizumab (Actemra) and sarilumab (Kevzara).

Tocilizumab

Actions and uses. Tocilizumab (Actemra) is a first-in-class IL-6 receptor antagonist. Although it received FDA approval for treatment of moderately to severely active RA, owing to the risk for infection and other serious adverse effects, tocilizumab is typically used only for those patients with RA who have not responded adequately to other DMARDs. Tocilizumab may be combined with methotrexate but not with TNF inhibitors or other DMARDs that increase the risk for infection. In addition to the treatment of RA, tocilizumab has also received FDA approval for the management of polyarticular juvenile idiopathic arthritis and systemic juvenile idiopathic arthritis.

How does tocilizumab work? The drug is a monoclonal antibody that blocks receptors for IL-6, a proinflammatory cytokine that helps mediate the autoimmune attack against the joints of patients with RA. By blocking IL-6 receptors, tocilizumab prevents IL-6 from promoting injury. Tocilizumab is the first drug to work by this mechanism.

Adverse effects. The most serious adverse effects are infections, GI perforation, liver injury, and hematologic effects: neutropenia and thrombocytopenia. Other adverse effects include headache, nasopharyngitis, hypertension, and increased cholesterol levels.

Serious infections. Owing to its immunosuppressant actions, tocilizumab increases the risk for life-threatening infections. Before starting tocilizumab, patients should be tested for latent TB and treated as indicated. During tocilizumab therapy, patients should be closely monitored for signs and symptoms of infection. For milder infections, tocilizumab should be given in reduced dosage or discontinued, depending on the magnitude of the change. Treatment should be interrupted if the patient develops a serious infection.

►► BLACK BOX WARNING
Tocilizumab (Actemra)

> Tocilizumab may cause an increased risk for developing serious and potentially fatal infections.

Gastrointestinal perforation. In clinical trials, perforation of the colon occurred rarely. Most cases were complications of preexisting diverticulitis. Patients at high risk for perforation—especially those with diverticulitis—should be closely monitored. Patients should be instructed to seek medical assistance in the event of severe, persistent abdominal pain.

Liver injury. Tocilizumab can cause elevation of circulating liver transaminases (aspartate aminotransferase and alanine aminotransferase). In clinical trials, this was not associated with apparent liver injury; however, in postmarketing studies, acute liver injury has occurred. Tocilizumab should not be initiated if transaminase levels are more than twice the upper limit of normal (ULN). Transaminase levels should be monitored every 4 to 8 weeks during treatment; if the levels exceed 5 times the ULN, tocilizumab should be discontinued.

Neutropenia and thrombocytopenia. Tocilizumab can reduce counts of neutrophils and platelets. Neutrophil reduction increases the risk for infection. In clinical trials, reduction of platelets was not associated with increased bleeding. Neutrophil and platelet counts should be determined at baseline and every 4 to 8 weeks during treatment. Tocilizumab should not be initiated if the absolute neutrophil count (ANC) is below 2000/mm^3 or if the platelet count is below 100,000/mm^3. Patients taking tocilizumab should discontinue the drug if the ANC falls below 500/mm^3 or if the platelet count falls below 50,000/mm^3.

Drug interactions. In general, tocilizumab should not be combined with other strong immunosuppressants owing to an increased risk for serious infections. Antirheumatic drugs to avoid include the TNF inhibitors (e.g., etanercept), T-cell inhibitors (e.g., abatacept), IL-1 antagonists (e.g., anakinra), and drugs that block the CD20 antigen (e.g., rituximab).

Tocilizumab can reduce blood levels of some drugs. Under normal circumstances, IL-6 suppresses the activity of several cytochrome P450 drug-metabolizing isoenzymes. By blocking receptors for IL-6, tocilizumab can negate that suppression. As a CYP3A4 inducer, tocilizumab increases the rate of metabolism and can thereby decrease serum drug levels of CYP3A4 substrates such as oral contraceptives and HMG-CoA reductase inhibitors. Dosages for all of these agents may have to be increased.

Tocilizumab should not be prescribed for patients taking biologic or targeted DMARDs. Administration with leflunomide is not contraindicated; however, myelosuppressant activity should be monitored closely. Care should be taken with administering with other drugs that have immunosuppressant and myelosuppressant activity.

Patients taking tocilizumab should not receive live vaccines. If inactivated vaccines are given, their efficacy may be decreased because of tocilizumab's immunosuppressant effect. For this reason, those vaccinated while taking tocilizumab should be revaccinated if tocilizumab is discontinued. Ideally, if vaccines are indicated (e.g., annual influenza vaccine), they should be administered at least 2 weeks before beginning therapy with tocilizumab.

Sarilumab

In 2017, sarilumab (Kevzara) received FDA approval for treatment of patients with moderately to severely active RA who do not have adequate response to or cannot take other DMARDs. It inhibits IL-6 mediated signaling by binding to IL-6 receptors.

Adverse effects of sarilumab mirror those of tocilizumab. In clinical studies, the most serious adverse reactions were immunosuppression, infections, GI perforation, and hypersensitivity reactions. Laboratory alterations included neutropenia, thrombocytopenia, and hyperlipidemia. Liver enzyme elevations were common, but no clinically apparent liver injury was detected. Because similar findings occurred with tocilizumab yet liver injury occurred following licensure and marketing, it is prudent to assume that this may also occur with sarilumab.

►► BLACK BOX WARNING
Sarilumab (Kevzara)

> Sarilumab may cause an increased risk for developing serious and potentially fatal infections.

Drug interactions with sarilumab mirror those of tocilizumab. It is particularly important to take care when drugs needed have the potential to enhance the immunosuppressive and hematologic effects of sarilumab.

Interleukin-1 Receptor Antagonists
Anakinra

Anakinra (Kineret) is currently the only DMARD in this category. It reduces symptoms of RA by blocking receptors for IL-1, a proinflammatory cytokine that plays a central role in synovial inflammation and joint destruction. The drug is indicated for patients with moderate to severe RA that have not responded to one or more conventional DMARDs (e.g., methotrexate). It is also approved for treatment of neonatal-onset multisystem inflammatory disease.

Like the TNF antagonists, anakinra poses a risk for serious infections. Accordingly, the drug should not be given to patients with active infection and should be stopped if a serious infection develops. Because both anakinra and the TNF antagonists increase infection risk, these drugs should not be combined.

TARGETED DISEASE-MODIFYING ANTIRHEUMATIC DRUG: JANUS KINASE INHIBITORS

Targeted DMARDs do not fit in either the conventional or biologic DMARD categories. However, like other DMARDs, they act on the immune system and pose a risk for serious and sometimes life-threatening infections.

Janus Kinase Inhibitors

The newest drugs developed to modulate the destructive effects of RA are the janus kinase (JAK) inhibitors. JAKs are intracellular enzymes that have a role in initiating cytokine signaling as part of the signal transducer and activation of transcription (STAT) pathway. This pathway is involved in inflammatory and immune responses; therefore, by inhibiting JAKs, these DMARDs reduce immune and inflammatory responses that underlie the pathology of RA.

Two JAK inhibitors are currently available: baricitinib (Olumiant) and tofacitinib (Xeljanz, Xeljanz XR).

Tofacitinib

Tofacitinib (Xeljanz, Xeljanz XR) is a synthetic JAK inhibitor. It was the first JAK inhibitor approved for treatment of RA.

Actions and uses. Tofacitinib prevents activation of the STAT pathway by preventing JAK enzyme signaling.

Tofacitinib is indicated for treatment of moderately to severely active RA in patients who cannot take methotrexate and for patients who have not experienced an adequate response to methotrexate. It is usually selected after trials of other DMARDs because, as a relatively newer drug, its long-term safety has not been established. In addition to its role in management of RA, it is also approved for treatment of psoriatic arthritis and ulcerative colitis.

Adverse effects. Approximately 20% of people taking tofacitinib develop infection. The most common infection in clinical trials was nasopharyngitis (up to 14% in one study), but other infections such as herpes zoster (5%) and gastroenteritis (4%) were documented. Other common adverse effects include headache, increased serum cholesterol, increased creatine phosphokinase, and skin rashes.

Less common but serious adverse effects have occurred. One of the most concerning is bone marrow suppression. Decreases in lymphocytes, neutrophils, and erythrocytes occur most often, but significant decreases in platelets were also observed.

Multiple systems may be affected. These have included bradycardia with prolonged PR intervals, interstitial lung disease, GI perforations, drug-induced liver injury, hyperlipidemia, and increased occurrence of malignancies.

 BLACK BOX WARNING

Tofacitinib (Xeljanz, Xeljanz XR)

> Tofacitinib increases the risk for developing serious and potentially fatal infections, including tuberculosis.

Patients taking tofacitinib have developed lymphoma and other malignancies.

Drug interactions. Tofacitinib is metabolized by CYP3A4 and CYP2C19 isoenzymes; therefore drugs that act as CYP3A4 or CYP2C19 inhibitors can increase tofacitinib levels, whereas drugs that are CYP3A4 or CYP2C19 inducers can lower tofacitinib levels.

Biologic DMARDS have an additive toxic effect when combined with tofacitinib; therefore patients taking these drugs should not have tofacitinib added to the therapeutic regimen.

Tofacitinib can increase immunosuppression when combined with other drugs having immunosuppressant effects.

Tofacitinib can decrease the efficacy of inactivated (killed) vaccines. If vaccinations are needed, they should be given 2 weeks before starting tofacitinib. Herpes zoster vaccinations are recommended for older patients. Live (attenuated) vaccines can cause serious complications and adverse reactions when administered to patients taking tofacitinib.

Baricitinib

Baricitinib (Olumiant) was approved in 2018 to treat moderately and severely active RA when adequate control was not achieved with TNF antagonists. It has no other indications at this time.

Like tofacitinib, baricitinib increases the risk for infections. In clinical trials, 16% of participants developed upper respiratory infections. Also, as in the case of tofacitinib, patients taking baricitinib developed GI perforations, lymphopenia, neutropenia, anemia, and drug-induced liver injury. Additionally, baricitinib was associated with thrombosis and lipid abnormalities.

BLACK BOX WARNING

Baricitinib (Olumiant)

> Baricitinib increases the risk for developing serious and potentially fatal infections.

Patients taking baricitinib have developed lymphoma and other malignancies.

Venous and arterial thrombosis has occurred in patients taking baricitinib; fatalities have occurred.

PATIENT EDUCATION

Disease-Modifying Antirheumatic Drugs

> Inform patients about the risk for infection and myelosuppression. Advise them to avoid close contact with people having a communicable disease. Instruct them to seek medical attention for signs or symptoms of infection or evidence of myelosuppression (bruising, bleeding, pallor, fatigue, fever). Advise patients to report signs of heart failure, such as shortness of breath and orthopnea, fatigue, and edema.
>
> For DMARDs that can cause liver injury, instruct patients to report fatigue, jaundice, anorexia, right-sided abdominal pain, and dark brown urine. Patients should also know about the increased risk of cancer and other drug-specific adverse effects.
>
> Inform patients that vaccinations should be current before therapy with a DMARD is begun. Once therapy begins, live virus vaccines must be avoided.

📄 SUMMARY OF KEY PRESCRIBING CONSIDERATIONS

Disease-Modifying Antirheumatic Drugs (DMARDs)

Therapeutic Goal: (1) Relieve RA symptoms (pain, inflammation, and stiffness), (2) maintain joint function and range of motion, (3) minimize systemic involvement, and (4) delay disease progression.

Baseline Data:

All DMARDs: CBC with WBC differential; assess for signs and symptoms of infection (especially TB and hepatitis) and malignancies (including skin examination). Rule out pregnancy for women of childbearing age. Screen for TB. A complete history and physical exam are also needed to establish pretherapy status. Emphasis should be placed on risks to immunocompetence and on liver and renal status.

Additional baseline data and areas of emphasis by specific drugs or classification:

All conventional DMARDs[a]: See All DMARDs under Baseline Data. Also, liver transaminases (alanine aminotransferase [ALT], aspartate aminotransferase [AST]) and serum creatinine. Baseline data for specific drugs follow.

- Methotrexate: Consider chest x-ray (CXR). Emphasis on pulmonary and GI status.
- Hydroxychloroquine: Ophthalmologic exam; cardiac exam with electrocardiography (ECG) if indicated.
- Leflunomide: Consider CXR. Emphasis on BP and pulmonary status.
- Sulfasalazine: Consider CXR. Emphasis on pulmonary and neurologic status.

All Biologic DMARDs: See All DMARDs under Baseline Data. Also, HBV screen, TB screen.

- TNF inhibitors (etanercept, infliximab, adalimumab, golimumab, certolizumab pegol): See All Biologic DMARDs. Also, emphasis on baseline cardiac status; obtain cardiology consult as indicated by assessment findings. Screen for complicating factors: demyelinating disorders, severe heart failure, and active infections.
- B-lymphocyte–depleting agents (rituximab): See All Biologic DMARDs. Also, ECG, BMP. Emphasis on baseline cardiac, renal, and neurologic status.
- IL-1 receptor antagonists (anakinra): See All Biologic DMARDs. Also, serum creatinine to screen renal function (renal dysfunction alters dosing).
- IL-6 receptor antagonists (tocilizumab, sarilumab): See All Biologic DMARDs. Also, liver function tests (LFTs), lipid panel. Neutrophil and platelet counts every 4 to 8 weeks.
- T-cell activation inhibitors (atabacept): See All Biologic DMARDs.

All Targeted DMARDs (tofacitinib, baricitinib): See All DMARDs listed under Baseline Data. Also, heart rate (HR) and blood pressure (BP); lipid panel, ALT and AST. Emphasis on baseline cardiac, pulmonary, and GI status.

Monitoring:

All DMARDs: CBC with WBC differential, assess for signs and symptoms of infection (especially TB) and development of new problems or worsening of previous problems.

Additional monitoring by specific drugs or classification:

All conventional DMARDs: See All DMARDS under Monitoring. Also, for all except hydroxychloroquine, the ACR recommends CBC with WBC differential, liver transaminases, and serum creatinine every 2 to 4 weeks for the first 3 months, every 8 to 12 weeks for months 3 to 6, and every 12 weeks for the duration of therapy. No follow-up on these laboratory studies is recommended for hydroxychloroquine; however, it would be prudent to do this if there were any baseline abnormalities. One should always ask about development of new symptoms. Additional monitoring for specific conventional DMARDs is as follows:

- Methotrexate: Evaluate pulmonary and GI status at each clinic visit.
- Hydroxychloroquine: Ophthalmologic exam (annually if at risk; annually after 5 years if not at risk), cardiac status with ECG if indicated, proximal muscle strength and deep tendon reflexes.
- Leflunomide: Evaluate BP and pulmonary status at every visit. Ask about signs and symptoms of peripheral neuropathy.
- Sulfasalazine: Evaluate skin condition and pulmonary and neurologic status at each clinic visit

Biologic DMARDs: See All DMARDS under Monitoring. Also, pulmonary and GI assessment.

- TNF inhibitors (etanercept, infliximab, adalimumab, golimumab, certolizumab pegol): Biologic DMARDs. Also, TB testing, AST, ALT, HBV testing for HBV carriers; Assess for signs and symptoms of heart failure, hypersensitivity.
- B-lymphocyte–depleting agents (rituximab): See Biologic DMARDs. Also, HBV testing, AST, ALT. Assess cardiac, renal, skin and mucous membranes, and neurological status at each visit. For HbsAg–negative or anti-HBc–positive patients, monitor for HBV reactivation with HBV DNA and ALT testing every 3 months during treatment. HR, BP, and cardiac monitoring during intravenous administration. Postinfusion, assess cardiac, pulmonary, and renal status. BMP if renal status questionable or if evidence of F&E imbalance.
- IL-1 receptor antagonists (anakinra): See Biologic DMARDs. Also, CBC with WBC differential monthly for 3 months and then every 3 months for 1 year.
- IL-6 receptor antagonists (tocilizumab, sarilumab): See Biologic DMARDs. TB screening, AST, ALT, lipid panel. Assessment emphasis on GI status.
- T-cell activation inhibitors (atabacept): See Biologic DMARDs.

Targeted DMARDs: See All DMARDs under Monitoring. Also, HR (for bradycardia) and BP, ECG if indicated (for prolonged PR interval); lipid panel, AST, ALT at 4 to 8 weeks and then every 3 months. Evaluate cardiac, pulmonary, and GI status at each clinic visit.

Identifying High-Risk Patients: High-risk patients are those who are immunosuppressed (e.g., owing to HIV infection or immunosuppressant drugs) and who have diabetes, heart failure, liver dysfunction, latent TB, latent HBV infection, renal failure, a history of recurrent infection, and any condition that predisposes to acquiring an infection.

Evaluating Therapeutic Effects: Evaluate control of RA symptoms and joint function and range of motion. Assess for systemic involvement and evidence of disease control or progression.

Minimizing Adverse Effects: Infections make up the most common adverse effects. The ACR recommends that patients receive vaccines for the following communicable diseases prior to beginning therapy with a DMARD: pneumonia, influenza, hepatitis B, HPV, and herpes zoster.

Patient education and close monitoring is essential to identify adverse effects in early stages, when they can be easily managed.

ACR, American College of Rheumatology; *ALT*, alanine aminotransferase; *AST*, aspartate aminotransferase; *BMP*, basic metabolic panel; *BUN*, blood urea nitrogen; *CXR*, chest x-ray; *DMARD*, disease-modifying antirheumatic drug; *DTRs*, deep tendon reflexes; *ECG*, electrocardiogram; *F&E*, fluids and electrolytes; *HBV*, hepatitis B virus; *HPV*, human papilloma virus; *HR*, heart rate; *LFTs*, liver function tests; *RA*, rheumatoid arthritis; *s/s*, signs and symptoms; *TB*, tuberculosis

[a]Laboratory monitoring protocols for conventional DMARDs are those of the American College of Rheumatology, 2015. They elected not to address monitoring for other DMARDs at the time of publication.

60

Drug Therapy for Gout

Gout is a painful inflammatory disorder seen mainly in men. Symptoms result from the deposition of uric acid crystals in joints. First, the pathophysiology of gout is discussed, followed by the drugs used for treatment.

PATHOPHYSIOLOGY OF GOUT

Gout is a recurrent inflammatory disorder characterized by *hyperuricemia* (high blood levels of uric acid) and episodes of *severe joint pain*, typically in the large toe. Hyperuricemia—defined as a blood uric acid above 7 mg/dL in men or 6 mg/dL in women—can occur through two mechanisms: (1) excessive production of uric acid and (2) impaired renal excretion of uric acid. Acute attacks are precipitated by crystallization of sodium urate (the sodium salt of uric acid) in the synovial space. Deposition of urate crystals promotes inflammation by triggering a complex series of events. A key feature of the inflammatory process is the infiltration of leukocytes, which, when inside the synovial cavity, phagocytize urate crystals and then break down, causing the release of destructive lysosomal enzymes. When hyperuricemia is chronic, large and gritty deposits, known as *tophi*, may form in the affected joint. Also, deposition of urate crystals in the kidney may cause renal damage. Fortunately, when gout is detected and treated early, the disease can be arrested, and these chronic sequelae avoided.

OVERVIEW OF DRUG THERAPY

Drugs are used in two ways in patients with gout. First, they are given short term to relieve symptoms of an acute gouty attack. Second, they are given long term to lower blood levels of uric acid.

In patients with infrequent flareups (less than three per year), treatment of symptoms may be all that is needed. Nonsteroidal antiinflammatory drugs (NSAIDs) are considered first-line agents for relieving the pain of an acute gouty attack. Glucocorticoids are an acceptable option. In the past, colchicine was considered a drug of choice for acute gout—even though it has a poor risk/benefit ratio. Today, colchicine is generally reserved for patients who are unresponsive to or intolerant of safer agents.

In patients with chronic gout, tophaceous gout, or frequent gouty attacks (three or more per year), drugs for hyperuricemia are indicated. Three types of drugs may be employed: agents that decrease uric acid production, agents that increase uric acid excretion (*uricosuric* drugs), and agents that convert uric acid to allantoin. A discussion of drugs used to treat gout follows. Drug preparations, dosage, and administration are presented in Table 60.1. Life span considerations are provided in the following table.

DRUGS FOR ACUTE GOUTY ARTHRITIS

Nonsteroidal Antiinflammatory Drugs

For acute gouty arthritis, NSAIDs are considered agents of first choice. Compared with colchicine, NSAIDs are better tolerated and their effects

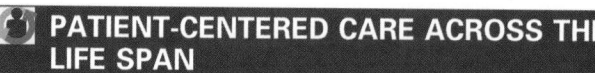

PATIENT-CENTERED CARE ACROSS THE LIFE SPAN

Drugs for Gout

Life Stage	Considerations or Concerns
Children	US labeling for indomethacin recommends using the lowest dose that is effective at the shortest possible duration. Canadian labeling contraindicates its use for patients younger than 14 years.
	When given for gout prophylaxis (as opposed to familiar Mediterranean fever), colchicine is not recommended for patients younger than 16 years.
	Febuxostat is not recommended for children. Allopurinol may be given to children younger than 6 years for the purpose of treating hyperuricemia associated with cancer therapy.
	Probenecid has been given to children as young as 2 years for purposes unrelated to gout. Safety of lesinurad has not been established for children and is only recommended for patients older than 18 years.
Pregnant women	NSAIDs should be avoided in the third trimester. Some studies have demonstrated fetal cardiovascular abnormalities and cleft palate after NSAID exposure. Exposure to indomethacin after 30 weeks of gestation has resulted in a number of abnormalities.
	Colchicine is associated with abnormal outcomes in animal reproduction studies; however, this has not been demonstrated in humans.
	Xanthine oxidase inhibitors and recombinant uric acid oxidases are associated with abnormal outcomes in animal studies.
	Probenecid has not been associated with increased fetal risk. Animal reproduction studies using lesinurad did not result in adverse developmental effects; the effects on fetal development in humans is unknown.
Breastfeeding women	US labeling recommends against breastfeeding by mothers taking indomethacin and naproxen. Canadian labeling contraindicates breastfeeding by mothers taking these drugs.
	Breastfeeding is not recommended for other drugs taken for gout.
	For patients taking xanthine oxidase inhibitors, Canadian labeling contraindicates breastfeeding.
Older adults	The Beers criteria list both indomethacin and naproxen among those drugs considered potentially inappropriate for patients 56 years and older, and note that indomethacin carries the greatest risk of all NSAIDs.
	Colchicine can be dangerous if the older patient has renal impairment.

FDA, US Food and Drug Administration; *NSAID*, nonsteroidal antiinflammatory drug.

TABLE 60.1 Preparations and Dosages of Antigout Drugs

Name	Preparation	Dosage
Nonsteroidal Antiinflammatory Drugs		
Indomethacin (Indocin and Tivorbex)	Indocin: 50-mg rectal suppository, 25 mg/5 mL oral suspension Tivorbex: 20-mg, 40-mg capsule Generic: 25-mg, 50-mg capsule Generic ER: 75-mg capsule	50 mg tid initially until pain is tolerable, then reduce dosage and continue dosing for 3–5 days.
Naproxen (Anaprox🍁, Naprosyn, Naprelan, and many others)	Anaprox: 275 mg 🍁 Anaprox DS: 550 mg Naprosyn: 500-mg scored tablets EC-Naprosyn: 375-mg, 500-mg enteric-coated tablets Generic: 250-, 375-, 500-mg tablets Naprelan (ER): 375-, 500-, 750-mg controlled-release tablets	Naprosyn: 750 mg initially, then 250 mg q 8 h until attack subsides. Naprosyn ER: one tablet initially, then one tablet daily until attack subsides. Anaprox: 825 mg initially, then 275 mg q 8 h until attack subsides.
Antigout Antiinflammatory Drug		
Colchicine (Colcrys and Mitigare)	Colcrys: 0.6-mg scored tablet Mitigare: 0.6-mg capsule	Acute attack (Colcrys only): 1.2 mg at first sign of the flare, followed by 0.6 mg 1 h later (maximum, 1.8 mg/24 h). Prophylaxis (Colcrys, Mitigare): 0.6 mg once or twice daily (maximum, 1.2 mg/24 h).
Glucocorticoids		
Prednisone (oral) (Deltasone)	Deltasone: 20-mg (scored) tablets	30–50 mg once daily or in two divided doses until pain is tolerable; then gradually tapered over 7–10 days.
Triamcinolone acetate (IM) (Aristospan and Kenalog)	Aristospan: 20 mg/mL in 1-mL and 5-mL vials Kenalog: 10 mg/mL in 5-mL vial; 40 mg/mL in 1-mL, 5-mL, and 10-mL vials	40–60 mg; may repeat after 1–4 days if flare continues.
Xanthine Oxidase Inhibitors		
Allopurinol (Zyloprim)	100- and 300-mg tablets	Dosages should be individualized to decrease plasma urate to 6 mg/dL.[a] Chronic tophaceous gout: 100 mg once a day, then increase by 50- to 100-mg increments every few weeks until urate target level is reached. Standard maintenance dose: 300 mg/day up to a maximum of 800 mg/day. Secondary hyperuricemia in adults: 100–800 mg/day.
Febuxostat (Uloric)	40- and 80-mg tablets	40 mg/day initially, increase to 80 mg/day if needed.
Uricosuric Agents		
Probenecid (generic only)	500-mg tablets	250 mg bid for 1 week. The maintenance dosage is 500 mg bid.
Lesinurad (Zurampic)	200 mg tablets	200 mg once daily in combination with a xanthine oxidase inhibitor
Recombinant Uric Acid Oxidase		
Pegloticase (Krystexxa)	8 mg/mL	8 mg IV every 2 weeks.
Combination Drugs		
Colchicine and probenecid (generic)	Colchicine 0.5 mg + probenecid 500 mg	One tablet daily for 1 week, then 1 tablet twice daily.

[a]Dosage should be reduced in patients with renal disease.
EC, Enteric coated; *ER*, extended release; *GI*, gastrointestinal; *IV*, intravenous; *NS*, normal saline.

are more predictable. Benefits derive from suppressing inflammation. Treatment should start as soon as possible after symptom onset. Most patients experience marked relief within 24 hours; swelling subsides over the next few days. Adverse effects of NSAIDs include gastrointestinal (GI) ulceration, impaired renal function, fluid retention, and increased risk for cardiovascular events. However, because the duration of treatment is brief, the risk for these complications is low. Which NSAID should be used? There is no good evidence that any NSAID is superior to the others for treatment of gout. Commonly used NSAIDs include

⟫ BLACK BOX WARNING
Nonsteroidal Antiinflammatory Drugs

NSAIDs may increase the risk for myocardial infarction, stroke, and other thromboembolic events.
NSAIDs increase the risk for dangerous gastrointestinal adverse effects such as bleeding, ulceration, and perforation.

NSAIDs, Nonsteroidal antiinflammatory drugs.

indomethacin (Indocin) and naproxen (Naprosyn, Anaprox ✦, and others) and diclofenac sodium (Voltaren). NSAIDs are discussed in Chapter 57.

Glucocorticoids

Glucocorticoids (e.g., prednisone), given orally or intramuscularly, are highly effective for relieving an acute gouty attack—although NSAIDs are generally preferred. Candidates for glucocorticoid therapy include patients who are hypersensitive to NSAIDs, patients who have medical conditions that contraindicate the use of NSAIDs, and patients with severe gout that is unresponsive to NSAIDs. Because of their effects on carbohydrate metabolism, glucocorticoids should be avoided, when possible, in patients prone to hyperglycemia. For oral therapy, prednisone can be used. For intramuscular (IM) therapy, triamcinolone acetonide can be used. Glucocorticoids are discussed in Chapter 58.

Colchicine

Colchicine (Colcrys, Mitigare) is an antiinflammatory agent with effects specific for gout. In the past, colchicine was considered a first-line drug for gout. However, owing to the common occurrence of GI toxicity and the availability of safe and effective alternatives, its use has been declined.

Therapeutic Use

Colchicine has two applications in gout. First, it can be used short term to treat an acute gouty attack. Second, it can be used long term to prevent attacks from recurring. Colcrys is approved for both uses. Mitigare is approved only for prophylaxis. (On a side note, conclusions of a 2015 Cochrane review of 39 trials with 4992 participants were that colchicine may also decrease the risk for myocardial infarction [MI] and improve outcomes post-MI.)

Acute gouty arthritis. High-dose colchicine can produce dramatic relief of an acute gouty attack. Within hours, patients whose pain had made movement impossible are able to walk. Inflammation disappears completely within 2 to 3 days.

Prophylaxis of gouty attacks. When taken during asymptomatic periods, low-dose colchicine can decrease the frequency and intensity of acute flareups. Colchicine may also be given for prophylaxis when urate-lowering therapy is initiated because there is a tendency for gouty episodes to increase at this time.

Mechanism of Action

How colchicine relieves or prevents episodes of gout is not fully understood. It *is* known that colchicine does not decrease urate production or removal. It may work, at least in part, by inhibiting leukocyte infiltration. It accomplishes this by disrupting microtubules, the structures required for cellular motility.

Pharmacokinetics

The pharmacokinetics of colchicine and urate-lowering drugs is provided in Table 60.2.

Adverse Effects

Colchicine has a narrow therapeutic index. As mentioned earlier, it disrupts cellular microtubules. Because microtubules are also required for cell division, colchicine is toxic to any tissue that has a large percentage of proliferating cells. Disruption of cell division in the GI tract and bone marrow underlies the drug's major toxicities.

Gastrointestinal effects. The most characteristic side effects are nausea, vomiting, diarrhea, and abdominal pain. These responses, which occur during the treatment of acute gouty attacks, result from injury to the rapidly proliferating cells of the GI epithelium. With the high doses used in the past, these GI effects were developed in nearly all patients. However, with the lower doses used today, GI toxicity is less common but still develops in 25% of patients. If GI symptoms occur, colchicine should be discontinued immediately regardless of the status of joint pain.

Myelosuppression. Injury to rapidly proliferating cells can suppress bone marrow function and thereby cause leukopenia, granulocytopenia, thrombocytopenia, and pancytopenia. Accordingly, colchicine should be used with caution in patients with hematologic disorders.

Myopathy. Colchicine can cause rhabdomyolysis (muscle breakdown) during long-term low-dose therapy. Risk is increased in patients with renal and hepatic impairment and in those taking statin drugs (e.g., atorvastatin and simvastatin), which can cause rhabdomyolysis on their own. Patients should be monitored for signs of muscle injury (tenderness, pain, and weakness).

Drug Interactions

Statins. As noted, atorvastatin, simvastatin, and other statins can increase the risk for colchicine-induced muscle injury. If possible, combined use of statins and colchicine should be avoided.

Drugs that can increase colchicine levels. Life-threatening reactions have occurred when colchicine was combined with two classes of drugs: P-glycoprotein (PGP) inhibitors and inhibitors of CYP3A4. Recall from Chapter 4 that PGP is a transporter protein that can reduce plasma drug levels through effects in the liver, kidney, and intestine. Hence, by inhibiting PGP, drugs such as cyclosporine and ranolazine can cause colchicine to accumulate to toxic levels. Similarly, by inhibiting CYP3A4, drugs such as ketoconazole, clarithromycin, and the HIV protease inhibitors (e.g., nelfinavir and ritonavir) can cause colchicine levels to

TABLE 60.2 Pharmacokinetics of Antigout Drugs

Drug Class and Drugs	Peak	Protein Binding	Metabolism	Half-Life	Elimination
Xanthine Oxidase Inhibitors					
Allopurinol (Aloprim and Zyloprim)	1.5 h	0%	Oxidation	1–2 h	Urine (76%) Feces
Febuxostat (Uloric)	1–1.5 h	99%	Hepatic	5–8 h	Urine (49%) Feces (46%)
Uricosuric Agents					
Probenecid (generic only in the United States, Benuryl)	2–4 h	85%–95%	Hepatic	6–12 h	Urine
Recombinant Uric Acid Oxidase					
Pegloticase (Krystexxa)	UK	UK	UK	14 days	Urine

UK, Unknown.

Fig. 60.1 Drugs That Lower Plasma Levels of Uric Acid. These drugs lower plasma urate by three mechanisms: allopurinol and febuxostat reduce uric acid formation, pegloticase catalyzes conversion of uric acid to allantoin, and probenecid facilitates uric acid excretion by the kidney.

rise. Accordingly, combined use of colchicine with strong inhibitors of either PGP or CYP3A4 should generally be avoided and is contraindicated in patients with hepatic or renal impairment.

Precautions and Contraindications

Colchicine should be used with care in older adults and debilitated patients and in patients with cardiac, renal, hepatic, and GI disease.

As noted, combined use of colchicine with strong inhibitors of PGP or CYP3A4 should generally be avoided. For both acute therapy and long-term prophylaxis, dosage should be adjusted on the basis of liver function, kidney function, and use of interacting drugs. Prescribing information for Mitigare but not Colcrys includes contraindications for hepatic or renal impairment.

Colchicine should be avoided during pregnancy unless the perceived benefits outweigh the potential risks.

DRUGS FOR HYPERURICEMIA (URATE-LOWERING THERAPY)

Urate-lowering therapy (ULT) is indicated for patients who experience relatively frequent acute gouty attacks. The purpose of therapy is to promote dissolution of urate crystals, prevent new crystal formation, prevent disease progression, reduce the frequency of acute attacks, and improve quality of life. The goal is to maintain a serum uric acid level lower than 6 mg/dL. For most patients, ULT must continue lifelong.

Six drugs—*allopurinol, febuxostat, lesinurad, probenecid, pegloticase,* and *rasburicase*[a]—are used to reduce uric acid levels. Three mechanisms are involved. Allopurinol and febuxostat inhibit uric acid formation. Probenecid and lesinurad accelerate uric acid excretion. Pegloticase and rasburicase convert uric acid to allantoin, a compound that is readily excreted by the kidney. These drugs lack antiinflammatory and analgesic

actions, so they are not useful against an acute gouty attack. The effects of all six drugs on uric acid are shown in Fig. 60.1.

Xanthine Oxidase Inhibitors

Two xanthine oxidase inhibitors are now available: allopurinol and febuxostat. Both seem equally effective. Allopurinol has been in use for decades, whereas febuxostat is relatively new. Because experience with allopurinol is more extensive, and febuxostat is much more expensive, allopurinol is often preferred.

Allopurinol

Therapeutic uses. Allopurinol (Zyloprim) is the current drug of choice for *chronic tophaceous gout.* By reducing blood uric acid levels, allopurinol prevents the formation of new tophi and causes regression of tophi that have already formed, thereby allowing joint function to improve. Reversal of hyperuricemia also decreases the risk for nephropathy from the deposition of urate crystals in the kidney.

Allopurinol can be used to treat hyperuricemia that develops secondary to cancer chemotherapy and to certain blood dyscrasias, such as polycythemia vera, myeloid metaplasia, and leukemia. Hyperuricemia develops during chemotherapy because when cells die, the breakdown of DNA releases uric acid. To minimize hyperuricemia, allopurinol should be administered before chemotherapy is begun.

Mechanism of action. Allopurinol and its major metabolite (alloxanthine) inhibit *xanthine oxidase* (XO), an enzyme required for uric acid formation. XO catalyzes the final two reactions that lead to the formation of uric acid from breakdown products of DNA.

Adverse effects. Allopurinol is generally well tolerated. Mild side effects include GI reactions (nausea, vomiting, diarrhea, and abdominal discomfort) and neurologic effects (drowsiness, headache, and metallic taste). Prolonged use (more than 3 years) may lead to the formation of cataracts.

Serious but less common adverse effects include bone marrow suppression, hepatotoxicity, and hypersensitivity. The most serious toxicity is a rare but potentially fatal hypersensitivity syndrome

---

[a]Rasburicase is approved to decrease uric acid levels associated with chemotherapy-related hyperuricemia. and not for management of gout.

characterized by rash, fever, eosinophilia, and dysfunction of the liver and kidneys. Severe cutaneous adverse reaction (SCAR) syndrome is more likely to occur in people of Korean, Chinese, and Thai ancestry. For patients at risk for SCAR, HLA-B*5801 testing is recommended. If rash or fever develops, allopurinol should be discontinued immediately. Many patients recover spontaneously, whereas others may require hemodialysis or glucocorticoid therapy.

Initial therapy may elicit an acute gouty attack. This can be prevented by giving colchicine or a low-dose NSAID.

The risk for drug accumulation can be a problem if allopurinol is administered to patients with renal impairment. This can be minimized by decreasing the dosage.

Drug interactions. Allopurinol can inhibit hepatic drug-metabolizing enzymes, thereby delaying the inactivation of other drugs. This interaction is of particular concern for patients taking warfarin, whose dosage should be reduced. If possible, combined use with mercaptopurine or azathioprine should be avoided because both of these anticancer drugs are substrates for XO and hence could accumulate to toxic levels in the presence of allopurinol. If combined use cannot be avoided, dosages of mercaptopurine and azathioprine should be greatly reduced (by as much as 75%). Theophylline, a drug for asthma, is also a substrate for XO and hence should not be combined with allopurinol. The combination of allopurinol plus ampicillin is associated with a high incidence of rash; if rash develops, allopurinol should be discontinued immediately.

PROTOTYPE DRUGS

Drugs for Gout

Xanthine Oxidase Inhibitor
Allopurinol

Uricosuric Agent
Probenecid

Recombinant Uric Acid Oxidase
Pegloticase

Febuxostat

Febuxostat (Uloric) is an alternative to allopurinol. Like allopurinol, febuxostat lowers urate levels by inhibiting XO. As with allopurinol, symptoms of gout may flare during initial therapy. Accordingly, patients should receive prophylactic NSAIDs or colchicine for up to 6 months after starting treatment. Adverse effects of febuxostat, which are uncommon, include liver function abnormalities, nausea, arthralgia, and rash. High doses (80 mg/day) are associated with a small increase in cardiovascular events. Similar to allopurinol, febuxostat should not be combined with drugs that are substrates for XO, especially theophylline, mercaptopurine, and azathioprine.

Uricosuric Agents
Probenecid

Therapeutic uses. Probenecid (Benuryl) treats gout by increasing the excretion of uric acid. By lowering plasma urate levels, probenecid also prevents formation of new tophi and facilitates regression of existing tophi. In addition to its use in gout, probenecid may be employed to prolong the effects of penicillin and cephalosporin by delaying their excretion by the kidneys.

Mechanism of action. Probenecid (generic only in the United States) acts on renal tubules to inhibit the reabsorption of uric acid. As a result, excretion of uric acid is increased and hyperuricemia is reduced.

PATIENT EDUCATION
Urate-Lowering Drugs

It may take weeks or even months to lower serum uric acid to the desired level.

Uric acid can crystallize in urine, which can cause kidney injury and kidney stones. It will be important to drink a lot of fluids—as much as 2.5 to 3 L each day—while uric acid levels are being lowered.

Report development of an acute gouty attack but do not stop taking your medicines. Temporary adjustments may be made in the dosage.

Report any new problems that develop. These may include decrease in the number of blood cells (pallor, fatigue, infections, bruising, and easy bleeding), liver problems (yellow skin and eyes, clay-colored stools, and dark urine), and kidney problems (fatigue, nausea, decreased urination, swelling in your feet and ankles, trouble sleeping flat in the bed, and flank pain).

Adverse effects. Probenecid is well tolerated by most patients. Mild GI effects (nausea, vomiting, and anorexia) occur occasionally. These can be reduced by taking the drug with food. *Hypersensitivity reactions,* usually manifesting as rash, develop in about 4% of patients. *Renal injury* may occur from the deposition of uric acid crystals in the kidney. The risk for kidney damage can be minimized by alkalinizing the urine and consuming 2.5 to 3 L of fluid daily until a serum uric acid level less than 6 mg/dL is achieved. Rarely, *liver injury* has been reported.

Product labeling for probenecid cautions that blood disorders (e.g., hemolytic anemia, pancytopenia) may be attributable to *glucose-6-phosphate dehydrogenase* (G6PD) *deficiency,* an inherited disorder. Patients at higher risk (e.g., those of African or Mediterranean ancestry) should be screened for G6PD deficiency before receiving the drug.

Probenecid should not be initiated at the beginning of an acute gout attack. The drug may exacerbate acute episodes of gout; hence treatment should be delayed until the acute attack has been controlled. Probenecid may induce acute attacks of gout during the initial months of therapy after gout appears to be controlled. If an attack occurs, colchicine or indomethacin can be added for relief.

Drug interactions. Aspirin and other *salicylates* interfere with the uricosuric action of probenecid. Accordingly, probenecid should not be used concurrently with these drugs. Probenecid inhibits the renal excretion of several drugs, including *indomethacin* and *sulfonamides;* dosages of these agents may require reduction.

Lesinurad

Lesinurad (Zurampic) is the latest drug approved for the treatment of gout. It increases excretion of uric acid by inhibiting the function of two transporter proteins that are responsible for reabsorption of uric acid that has been filtered from the renal tubules.

The most serious adverse effect is renal failure. The risk is increased with monotherapy; therefore, lesinurad should always be given in combination with a xanthine oxidase inhibitor such as allopurinol or febuxostat. Other than renal failure, few adverse effects were identified in clinical trials; approximately 5% developed headache and 3% developed gastroesophageal reflux disease. Cardiovascular events occurred in some patients during drug trials, but no relationship was identified between the drug and the event. Still, it is wise to err on the side of caution and consider this a possibility until more is known from postmarketing surveillance. As with other drugs that lower uric acid levels, gout flares may occur as urate is mobilized from tissue deposits. Prophylactic therapy to prevent these flares is recommended.

Lesinurad is a substrate of CYP2C9 isoenzymes. Therefore lesinurad levels may increase when given with CYP2C9 inhibitors and decrease when given with CYP2C9 inducers.

BLACK BOX WARNING

Lesinurad (Zurampic)

Lesinurad can cause acute renal failure when prescribed as monotherapy. It should be used with a xanthine oxidase inhibitor to decrease this complication

Recombinant Uric Acid Oxidase
Pegloticase

Therapeutic use. Pegloticase (Krystexxa) is indicated for intravenous therapy of chronic gout in patients who have not responded to oral ULT (e.g., allopurinol and probenecid). Although pegloticase is quite effective, the drug costs $22,299 for a single 8-mg (1 mL) dose and carries a significant risk for severe adverse effects. Accordingly, pegloticase is considered a treatment of last resort. (Rasburicase, another recombinant form of uric acid oxidase, is approved only for hyperuricemia associated with chemotherapy used to treat malignancy.)

Mechanism of action. How does pegloticase reduce urate levels? The drug is a recombinant form of *uricase* (urate oxidase), an enzyme that catalyzes the conversion of uric acid to allantoin, an inert, water-soluble compound that is readily excreted by the kidney. Uricase is present in nearly all mammals but not in humans and higher primates.

Adverse effects. As with other drugs for ULT, patients are likely to experience *gout flares* during the first few months of treatment. To reduce the intensity of such events, patients should take colchicine or an NSAID during treatment with pegloticase.

During premarketing trials, pegloticase triggered *anaphylaxis* in 6.5% of patients. Symptoms included wheezing, perioral or lingual edema, hemodynamic instability, and rash. To reduce risk, patients should be pretreated with an antihistamine and a glucocorticoid. Administration should be done in a setting equipped to manage a severe reaction.

During premarketing trials, *infusion reactions* were seen in 26% to 41% of patients. Symptoms include urticaria, dyspnea, chest discomfort, erythema, and pruritus. These reactions were seen despite pretreatment with an antihistamine, acetaminophen, and an intravenous glucocorticoid. If a reaction develops, slowing the infusion rate may reduce symptom intensity.

Pegloticase is *contraindicated* for patients with inherited G6PD deficiency owing to a risk for hemolysis and methemoglobinemia. Patients at higher risk should be screened for G6PD deficiency before receiving the drug.

BLACK BOX WARNING

Pegloticase (Krystexxa)

Anaphylaxis and infusion reactions may occur. These typically occur within 2 h after infusion but may be delayed. Administration should take place in health care facilities prepared for the management of life-threatening reactions.

Patients should be premedicated with an antihistamine and a glucocorticoid and monitored closely during the infusion.

PHARMACOLOGIC MANAGEMENT OF GOUT

As already mentioned, treatment of an acute gout attack or flare varies from prophylactic management to prevent joint and tissue damage as

SUMMARY OF KEY PRESCRIBING CONSIDERATIONS

Urate-Lowering Drugs

Therapeutic Goal: To control pain associated with acute gouty attacks and prevent future attacks. To alleviate signs and symptoms of gout, including tophi and other visible evidence.

Baseline Data: Serum uric acid and pain assessment on all patients

Additional baseline data for allopurinol: CBC, liver, and renal function. Consider HLA-B*5801 for patients with Korean, Chinese, or Thai ancestry.

Additional baseline data for febuxostat: LFTs. Assess cardiovascular risk factors.

Additional baseline data for probenecid: CBC, LFTs, renal function, G6PD screening for at-risk patients, and assure absence of current gouty attack.

Additional baseline data for lesinurad: Renal function.

Additional baseline data for pegloticase: G6PD screening for at-risk patients.

Monitoring: The ACR recommends monitoring serum uric acid every 2 to 5 weeks during drug titration until a uric acid level less than 6 mg/dL is achieved, then monitor every 6 months.

For all antigout drugs: Evaluate for improvement in signs and symptoms of gout.

Additional monitoring for allopurinol: Check CBC every 2 to 5 weeks until the desired uric acid level is attained, then monitor every 6 months and as needed for signs and symptoms of anemia, leukopenia, or thrombocytopenia. Check LFTs as needed for signs and symptoms of liver injury and periodically if patient has a history of liver disease. Check serum creatinine and BUN if there is a concern for decreased renal function. Monitor for signs and symptoms of hepatotoxicity and hypersensitivity reactions.

Additional monitoring for febuxostat: Check LFTs periodically. Monitor for signs and symptoms of hepatotoxicity, cardiovascular events (angina, MI, and stroke) and hypersensitivity reactions.

Additional monitoring for probenecid: Check CBC, serum creatinine, and BUN periodically. Check LFTs for signs and symptoms of liver injury. Monitor urine pH. Inquire about fluid intake and frequency of gout exacerbations.

Additional monitoring for lesinurad: Check renal function every 2-3 weeks initially then every 6 months.

Additional monitoring for pegloticase: Assess for hypersensitivity and infusion reactions during and following administration.

Identifying High-Risk Patients: Look for a history of abnormal blood, liver, or renal function. Additionally, for allopurinol, check HLA-B*5801-positive patients; for probenecid and pegloticase, look for G6PD deficiency.

Evaluating Therapeutic Effects: Serum uric acid less than 6 mg/dL, decreased frequency of acute gouty attacks.

Minimizing Adverse Effects: Close monitoring and appropriate screening will detect many problems in early stages when they are more manageable. For probenecid, alkalinizing urine (e.g., with potassium citrate or sodium bicarbonate) and promoting hydration until serum uric acid is decreased will help prevent uric acid from crystallizing out of acidic urine. For pegloticase, premedication with an antihistamine and a glucocorticoid can decrease the risk for infusion reactions. For lesinurad, administer with a xanthine oxidase inhibitor

ACR, American College of Rheumatology; *BUN,* blood urea nitrogen; *CBC,* complete blood count; *G6PD,* glucose-6-phosphate dehydrogenase; *LFTs,* liver function tests; *MI,* myocardial infarction.

Recommended Therapy for Patients With Gout

```
┌─────────────────────────────┐
│  Establish diagnosis of gout │
└─────────────────────────────┘
              │
              ▼
```

Baseline recommendations for patients with diagnosis of gout
- Patient education, with initiation of diet, lifestyle recommendations
- Consider secondary causes of hyperuricemia
- Consider elimination of <u>nonessential</u> prescription medications that induce hyperuricemia*
- Clinically evaluate gout disease burden (palpable tophi, frequency and severity of acute and chronic symptoms and signs)

Indications for pharmacologic ULT
Any patient with established diagnosis of gouty arthritis and
- Tophus or tophi by clinical exam or imaging study
- Frequent attacks of acute gouty arthritis (≥2 attacks/year)
- CKD stage 2 or worse
- Past urolithiasis

If pharmacologic ULT is indicated

Treat to serum urate target defined for individual patient
- The <u>minimum</u> serum urate target is <6 mg/dL
- Serum urate lowering below 5 mg/dL may be needed to improve gout signs and symptoms

Select first line ULT agent

Xanthine oxidase inhibitor (XOI):

| Allopurinol | OR | Febuxostat |

If at least one XOI is contra-indicated or not tolerated

Alternative first line ULT:

| Probenecid[a] |

Acute gout prophylaxis

Initiate concomitant pharmacologic antiinflammatory gout attack prophylaxis (See Fig. 59.4)

Treat to target serum urate target achieved? — No → **Increase intensity of ULT Reevaluate serum urate**

Yes

Long-term management of gout:
- Continuing gout attack prophylaxis if there are ongoing gout symptoms and/or signs (≥1 tophus on physical exam)
- Continue to regularly monitor serum urate <u>and</u> monitor for ULT side effects
- After palpable tophi and all acute and chronic gouty arthritis gout symptoms have resolved, continue all measures (including pharmacologic ULT) needed to maintain serum urate <6 mg/dL indefinitely
- Gout case scenarios, where referral to a specialist is considered, include: (i) Unclear etiology of hyperuricemia; (ii) Refractory signs or symptoms of gout; (iii) Difficulty in reaching target serum urate, particularly with renal impairment and a trial of XOI treatment; (iv) Multiple and/or serious adverse events from pharmacologic ULT

Examples of serum urate-elevating drugs that might be non-essential in a given patient, and potentially replaced by alternative agents that do not elevate serum urate:
- Niacin for management of hyperlipidemia
- Thiazide and loop diuretics for hypertension. However, in discussion, and without a specific vote, the TFP recognized the value of thiazide treatment in many patients with hypertension, and cautioned against imprudent cessation of thiazide treatment to lessen hyperuricemia at the cost of worsened control of blood pressure in difficult to control hypertension.
- Calcineurin inhibition with cyclosporine or tacrolimus, if it is not essential for immune suppression.
[a] Probenecid is not recommended as a first line or alternative first line ULT agent if the CrCl is <50.
CKD, Chronic kidney disease; *CrCl*, creatinine clearance; *ULT*, urate-lowering therapy.

Fig. 60.2 Baseline Recommendations for Patients With Gout. *TPF,* Task force panel; *ULT,* urate-lowering therapy. (Adapted from https://www.rheumatology.org/Portals/0/Files/ACR%20Guidelines%20for%20 Management%20of%20Gout_Part%201.pdf.)

Management of an Acute Gout Attack

General principles:
- Acute gouty arthritis attacks should be treated with pharmacologic therapy
- To provide optimal care, pharmacologic treatment should be initiated within 24 h of acute gout attack onset
- Ongoing pharmacologic ULT should not be interrupted during an acute gout

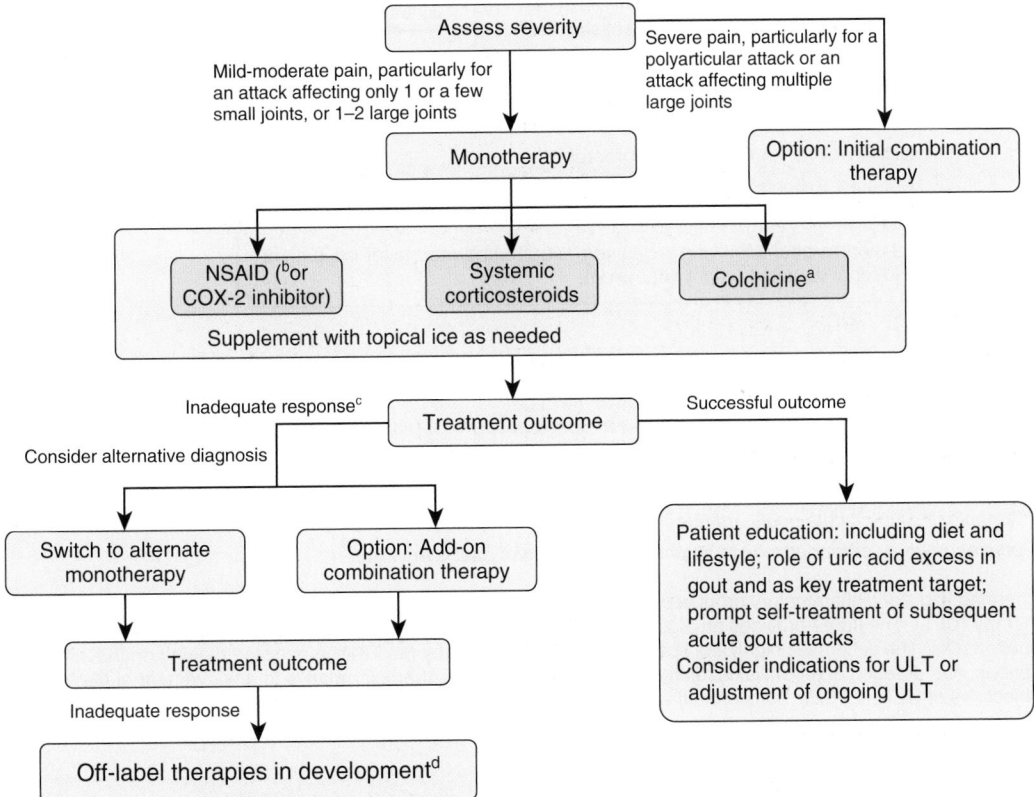

[a] Colchicine was recommended as an appropriate option for acute gout if started within 36 h of symptom onset.
[b] Selective COX-2 inhibition with agents available outside the United States such as etoricoxib was recommended as an option in patients with GI contra-indications or intolerance to NSAIDs, but selective COX-2 inhibition shares many adverse events with NSAID therapy. COX-2 inhibition therapy with celecoxib requires high doses and has unclear risk-benefit ratio at this time.
[c] Inadequate response is defined as
   <20% improvement in pain score within 24 h or
   <50% at ≥ 24 h
[d] Off-label use of biologic interleukin-1 inhibitor treatment has been investigated for acute gout when nonbiologic therapeutic categories are ineffective or contraindicated, but this approach is not approved for gout by medical regulatory agencies at the time this is written.

Fig. 60.3 Management of an Acute Gout Attack. *COX,* Cyclooxygenase; *NSAID,* nonsteroidal antiinflammatory drugs; *ULT,* urate-lowering therapy. (Adapted from http://www.rheumatology.org/Portals/0/Files/Gout_Part_2_ACR-12.pdf.)

Antiinflammatory Prophylaxis of Gout

Initiate Prophylaxis:
- With, or just prior to initiating ULT
- Medication choices

            Low dose colchicine[a]: Low dose colchicine, 0.6 mg once or twice daily
First line: OR   (Outside United States, 0.5 mg once or twice a day)
            Low dose NSAIDs: With proton pump inhibitor (where indicated)
                e.g., naproxen 250 mg twice daily

[b]Second line: Low dose prednisone or prednisolone[c] (≤10 mg/day)
      (if colchicine and NSAIDs <u>both</u> are not tolerated, contra-indicated, or ineffective)

Evaluate gout symptoms while on ULT

Activity of gout signs/symptoms[d] → **Continue pharmacologic anti-inflammatory prophylaxis**

No signs/symptoms

DURATION: Treatment for the greater of:
- At least 6 months

      OR

- 3 months after achieving target serum urate appropriate for the patient (No tophi detected on physical exam)

[a] *The TFP did not specifically address case scenarios involving renal impairment adjusted colchicine dosing for gout attack prophylaxis.*

[b] *Lack of consensus: Prednisone/prednisolone at doses above 10 mg/day.*

[c] *Without specific task force panel (TFP) vote, the TFP advised that this measure requires particular, continued attention to risk-benefit ratio.*

[d] *Examples include: acute gouty arthritis in the past 3 months, presence of palpable tophus or tophi, chronic tophaceous gouty arthropathy (with chronic synovitis) in the past 3 months.*

Pharmacologic antiinflammatory prophylaxis of gout attacks and its relationship to pharmacologic urate-lowering therapy (ULT). The figure provides an algorithm for use of antiinflammatory prophylaxis agents to prevent acute gout attacks. The schematic highlights specific recommendations by the TFP on decision making on the initiation, options, and duration of prophylaxis relative to pharmacologic ULT therapy, relative to achievement of the treatment objectives of ULT. *NSAIDs,* nonsteroidal antiinflammatory drugs.

Fig. 60.4 Antiinflammatory Prophylaxis of Gout. (From http://www.rheumatology.org/Portals/0/Files/Gout_Part_2_ACR-12.pdf.)

well as recurrent gout attacks. In 2012, the American College of Rheumatology (ACR) released guidelines for both situations.[a] These are summarized in the ACR algorithms. (Fig. 60.2 provides guidance for baseline management of gout and Fig. 60.3 details recommendations for an acute gout attack. A third algorithm, Fig. 60.4, illustrates antiinflammatory prophylaxis.) The full articles are available online at http://www.rheumatology.org/Practice-Quality/Clinical-Support/Clinical-Practice-Guidelines/Gout.

---

[a]The ACR is currently updating their guidelines for management of gout. The anticipated release date is 2020. Once released, these will be available on the ACR website at http://www.rheumatology.org.

61

Drugs Affecting Calcium Levels and Bone Mineralization

It is difficult to exaggerate the biologic importance of calcium, an element critical to blood coagulation and to the functional integrity of bone, nerve, muscle, and the heart. Because these calcium-dependent processes can be seriously disrupted by alterations in calcium availability, calcium levels must stay within narrow limits. To regulate calcium, the body employs three factors: parathyroid hormone (PTH), vitamin D, and calcitonin. Failure in these regulatory mechanisms results in hypercalcemia or hypocalcemia.

Our discussion of calcium and related drugs has four parts. First, we review calcium physiology. Second, we discuss the syndromes produced by disruption of calcium metabolism. Third, we discuss the pharmacologic agents used to treat calcium-related disorders. And fourth, we consider osteoporosis, the most common calcium-related disorder.

CALCIUM PHYSIOLOGY

Functions, Sources, and Daily Requirements

Functions

Calcium is critical to the function of the skeletal system, nervous system, muscular system, and cardiovascular system. In the skeletal system, calcium is required for the structural integrity of bone. In the nervous system, calcium helps regulate axonal excitability and transmitter release. In the muscular system, calcium participates in excitation-contraction coupling and contraction. In the cardiovascular system, calcium plays a role in myocardial contraction, vascular contraction, and blood coagulation.

Dietary Sources

Dairy products are good sources of calcium. For example, we can get about 300 mg from 1 cup of milk, 6 ounces of yogurt, or 1.5 ounces of cheese. Good nondairy sources include tofu (240 mg/0.5 cup), broccoli (180 mg/cup), and cooked spinach (240 mg/cup). Additionally, many processed foods are calcium fortified. Examples include fortified orange juice (300 mg/8 oz) and fortified cereals (250 to 1000 mg/serving). Information on the calcium content of other foods is available at www.ucsfhealth.org/education/calcium_content_of_selected_foods/index.html.

Daily Requirements

In 2010, the Institute of Medicine (IOM), later renamed the National Academy of Medicine, issued updated recommendations in a report titled *Dietary Reference Intakes for Calcium and Vitamin D* (Table 61.1). These remain the current standard.

Are North Americans getting enough calcium? According to the IOM report, some of us get adequate calcium from our diets. However, there is a concern that two groups—adolescent girls and postmenopausal women—may not get enough calcium from diet alone and may need calcium supplements. How much supplemental calcium should be taken? Only enough to make up the difference between what the diet provides (about 600 to 900 mg/day) and the recommended dietary allowance (RDA). Taking too much supplemental calcium increases the risk for vascular calcification, myocardial infarction, stroke, and kidney stones.

Body Stores
Calcium in Bone

Most calcium in the body (more than 98%) is present in bone. It is important to appreciate that bone—and the calcium it contains—is not static. Rather, bone undergoes continuous remodeling, a process in which old bone is resorbed, after which new bone is laid down (Fig. 61.1). The cells that resorb (break down) old bone are called *osteoclasts*, and the cells that deposit new bone and increase bone mass are called *osteoblasts*. Both cell types originate in the bone marrow. In adults, about 25% of trabecular bone (the honeycomb-like material in the center of bones) is replaced each year. In contrast, only 3% of cortical bone (the dense material that surrounds trabecular bone) is replaced each year.

Calcium in Blood

The normal value for total serum calcium is 10 mg/dL (2.5 mmol/L and 5 mEq/L). Of this total, about 50% is bound to proteins and other substances and hence is unavailable for use. The remaining 50% is present as free, ionized calcium—the form that participates in physiologic processes.

Absorption and Excretion
Absorption

Absorption of calcium takes place in the small intestine. Under normal conditions, about one-third of the ingested calcium is absorbed. Absorption is increased by parathyroid hormone (PTH) and vitamin D. In contrast, glucocorticoids decrease calcium absorption. Also, foods with insoluble fiber and phytic acid, such as whole-grain cereals and wheat bran, and foods containing oxalates, such as spinach, can interfere with calcium absorption.

Excretion

Calcium excretion is primarily renal. The amount lost is determined by glomerular filtration and the degree of tubular reabsorption. Excretion can be reduced by PTH, vitamin D, and thiazide diuretics (e.g., hydrochlorothiazide). Conversely, excretion can be increased by loop diuretics (e.g., furosemide), calcitonin, and loading with sodium. In addition to calcium lost in urine, substantial amounts can be lost in breast milk.

Physiologic Regulation of Calcium Levels

Blood levels of calcium are tightly controlled. Three processes are involved:

- Absorption of calcium from the intestine
- Excretion of calcium by the kidney
- Resorption or deposition of calcium in bone

Regulation of these processes is under the control of three factors: *PTH, vitamin D,* and *calcitonin,* as shown in Table 61.2. Note that preservation of calcium levels in blood takes priority over preservation of calcium in bone. Therefore if serum calcium is low, calcium will be

Fig. 61.1 Bone Remodeling Cycle. (A) Quiescent bone with lining cells covering the surface. (B) Resorption of old bone by multinucleated osteoclasts. (C) Osteoblasts migrate to the absorption site. (D) Osteoblasts deposit osteoid, a matrix of collagen and other proteins. (E) Osteoid undergoes calcification.

TABLE 61.1   Daily Calcium Intake by Life-Stage Group

Life-Stage Group[a]	Calcium Intake (mg/day)		
	AI[b]	RDA	UL[c]
0–6 months	200	—	1000
6–12 months	260	—	1500
1–3 years	—	700	2500
4–8 years	—	1000	2500
9–18 years	—	1300	3000
19–50 years	—	1000	2500
51–70 years			
Males	—	1000	2000
Females	—	1200	2500
Older than 70 years	—	1200	2000

[a]All values apply to males and females, except in the 51- to 70-year-old group. Calcium requirements do not change during pregnancy or lactation.
[b]Values for adequate intake (AI) are derived through experimental or observational data that show a mean calcium intake that appears to sustain a desired indicator of health, such as calcium retention in bone, for most members of the population group. AI values are employed for young children because there are insufficient data to derive a recommended dietary allowance (RDA).
[c]The tolerable upper intake level (UL) is defined as the maximal intake that is not likely to pose a risk for adverse health effects in almost all healthy individuals in a specified group. The UL is not intended to be a recommended level of intake. There is no established benefit to consuming calcium above the RDA.
Data from the Institute of Medicine of the National Academies.
Dietary reference intakes for calcium and vitamin D. Washington, DC: The National Academies Press; 2010.

TABLE 61.2   Effects of Parathyroid Hormone, Vitamin D, and Calcitonin on Calcium and Phosphate

	PTH	Vitamin D	Calcitonin
Calcium			
Plasma calcium level	Increase	Increase	Decrease
Intestinal calcium absorption	Increase	Increase	No effect
Renal calcium excretion	Decrease	Decrease	Increase
Calcium resorption from bone	Increase	Increase	Decrease
Phosphate			
Plasma phosphate level	Decrease	Increase	

PTH, Parathyroid hormone.

resorbed from bone and transferred to the blood—even if resorption compromises the structural integrity of bone.

Parathyroid Hormone

Release of PTH is regulated primarily by calcium, acting through calcium-sensing receptors on cells of the parathyroid gland. When calcium levels are *high*, activation of the calcium-sensing receptors is *increased*, causing secretion of PTH to be *suppressed*. Conversely, when calcium levels are low, receptor activation is reduced, causing PTH release to rise. PTH then restores calcium to normal levels by three mechanisms:
• PTH promotes calcium resorption from bone.
• PTH promotes tubular reabsorption of calcium that had been filtered by the kidney glomerulus.

- PTH promotes activation of vitamin D, thereby promoting increased absorption of calcium from the intestine.

  In addition to its effects on calcium, PTH reduces plasma levels of phosphate.

Vitamin D

The effect of Vitamin D is similar to that of PTH, in that both agents increase plasma calcium levels, and they do so by the same mechanisms: (1) increasing calcium resorption from bone, (2) decreasing calcium excretion by the kidney, and (3) increasing calcium absorption from the intestine. Vitamin D differs from PTH in that vitamin D elevates plasma levels of phosphate, whereas PTH reduces levels of phosphate.

Calcitonin

Calcitonin, a hormone produced by the thyroid gland, decreases plasma levels of calcium. Hence calcitonin acts in opposition to PTH and vitamin D. Calcitonin is released from the thyroid gland when calcium levels in blood rise too high. Calcitonin lowers calcium levels by inhibiting the resorption of calcium from bone and increasing calcium excretion by the kidney. Unlike PTH and vitamin D, calcitonin does not influence calcium absorption.

CALCIUM-RELATED PATHOPHYSIOLOGY

Hypercalcemia
Clinical Presentation

Mild hyperglycemia is usually asymptomatic. Early symptoms include weakness, fatigue, nausea, vomiting, anorexia, abdominal cramping, and constipation. With persistent and more severe hypercalcemia, kidney function is affected, resulting in polyuria, nocturia, and proteinuria, in addition to neurologic symptoms such as seizures, confusion, and ataxia. Cardiac dysrhythmia and coma may occur. Calcium deposition in soft tissues can damage the heart, blood vessels, and lungs; calcium deposition in the kidneys can cause nephrolithiasis.

Causes

Hypercalcemia may arise from a variety of causes. Life-threatening elevations in calcium are most often the result of cancer. Hyperparathyroidism is another common cause of severe hypercalcemia. Additional causes include vitamin D intoxication, sarcoidosis, and use of thiazide diuretics.

Treatment

Calcium levels can be lowered with drugs that (1) promote urinary excretion of calcium, (2) decrease mobilization of calcium from bone, (3) decrease intestinal absorption of calcium, and (4) form complexes with free calcium in blood. For severe hypercalcemia, initial therapy consists of replacing lost fluid with intravenous (IV) saline, followed by diuresis using IV saline and a loop diuretic (e.g., furosemide). Other agents for lowering calcium include inorganic phosphates (which promote calcium deposition in bone and reduce calcium absorption); edetate disodium (which binds calcium and promotes its excretion); glucocorticoids (which reduce intestinal absorption of calcium); and a group of drugs—calcitonin, bisphosphonates (e.g., zoledronic acid and pamidronate), denosumab (Prolia, Xgeva), and gallium nitrate—that inhibit resorption of calcium from bone. Cinacalcet (Sensipar), an oral calcimimetic drug that suppresses PTH secretion, can be used for hypercalcemia associated with hyperparathyroidism. In 2017, the FDA approved a second calcimimetic, etelcalcetide (Parsabiv) with this drug currently approved only for use in patients with chronic kidney disease on chronic hemodialysis.

Hypocalcemia
Clinical Presentation

Hypocalcemia increases neuromuscular excitability. As a result, tetany, convulsions, and spasm of the pharynx and other muscles may occur.

Cause

Hypocalcemia is caused most often by a deficiency of either PTH, vitamin D, or dietary calcium. Other causes include chronic renal failure and long-term use of certain medications, such as magnesium-based laxatives and drugs, used to manage osteoporosis (e.g., bisphosphonates and denosumab).

Treatment

Severe hypocalcemia is corrected by infusing an IV calcium preparation, usually calcium gluconate (see Chapter 92). After calcium levels have been restored, an oral calcium salt (e.g., calcium citrate) can be given for maintenance. Vitamin D should be included in the regimen if there is a coexisting deficiency.

Osteomalacia

Osteomalacia results from insufficient vitamin D. In the absence of vitamin D, mineralization of bone is impaired, resulting in bowing of the legs, fractures of the long bones, and kyphosis. In addition, patients may experience diffuse, dull, and aching bone pain. Treatment consists of vitamin D replacement therapy.

Osteoporosis

Osteoporosis, the most common disorder of calcium metabolism, is characterized by low bone mass and increased bone fragility. Osteoporosis is discussed at length later in this chapter.

Paget Disease of Bone
Clinical Presentation

Paget disease of bone is a chronic condition seen most frequently in adults older than 40 years. After osteoporosis, Paget disease is the most common disorder of bone in the United States. The disease is characterized by increased bone resorption and replacement of the resorbed bone with abnormal bone. Increased bone turnover causes elevation in serum alkaline phosphatase (reflecting increased bone deposition) and increased urinary hydroxyproline (reflecting increased bone resorption). It is important to note that alterations in bone homeostasis do not occur evenly throughout the skeleton. Rather, alterations occur locally, most often in the pelvis, femur, spine, skull, and tibia. Although most people with Paget disease are asymptomatic, about 10% experience bone pain and osteoarthritis. Skeletal deformity may also occur. Bone weakness may lead to fractures. Neurologic complications may occur secondary to compression of the spinal cord, spinal nerves, and cranial nerves. If bone associated with hearing is affected, deafness may result.

Treatment

Asymptomatic patients are usually not treated. Mild pain can be managed with analgesics and antiinflammatory agents. When the disease is more severe, a bisphosphonate is the treatment of choice. Benefits derive from suppressing bone resorption.

Hypoparathyroidism

Reductions in PTH usually result from inadvertent removal of the parathyroid glands during surgery on the thyroid gland. Lack of PTH causes hypocalcemia, which, in turn, may produce paresthesias, tetany, skeletal muscle spasm, laryngospasm, and convulsions. Symptoms can be relieved with calcium supplements and vitamin D.

Hyperparathyroidism
Primary Hyperparathyroidism

Primary hyperparathyroidism usually results from a benign parathyroid adenoma. The resulting increase in PTH secretion causes hypercalcemia and lowers serum phosphate. Hypercalcemia can cause skeletal muscle weakness, constipation (from decreased smooth muscle tone), and CNS symptoms (lethargy and depression). Hypercalciuria and hyperphosphaturia are also present and may cause renal calculi. Mobilization of calcium and phosphate from bone may produce bone abnormalities. Management of hyperparathyroidism is typically overseen by an endocrinologist. The only definitive treatment for primary hyperparathyroidism is surgical resection of the parathyroid glands. Hypercalcemia can be managed with calcium-lowering drugs, including cinacalcet (Sensipar), a drug that suppresses PTH secretion.

Secondary Hyperparathyroidism

Secondary hyperparathyroidism is a common complication of chronic kidney disease that occurs in nearly all patients with end-stage renal disease on dialysis. The disorder is characterized by high levels of PTH and disturbances of calcium and phosphorus homeostasis. Traditionally, the disorder has been managed with a vitamin D analog (e.g., calcitriol, paricalcitol, doxercalciferol) and phosphate-binding agents. However, these treatments frequently make mineral homeostasis worse. Cinacalcet (Sensipar) has been advocated by some experts because of its ability to reduce PTH levels while having a positive effect on calcium and phosphorus; however, others (e.g., the Kidney Disease: Improving Global Outcomes [KDIGO] working group) recommend against its use in the early or predialysis stages of kidney disease.

DRUGS FOR DISORDERS INVOLVING CALCIUM AND BONE MINERALIZATION

Calcium Salts

Calcium salts are available in oral and parenteral formulations for treating hypocalcemic states. These salts differ in their percentages of elemental calcium, which must be accounted for when determining dosage.

Oral formulations are presented here. Information on parenteral calcium preparations are available in Chapter 92.

Therapeutic Uses

Oral calcium preparations are used to treat *mild hypocalcemia*. In addition, calcium salts are taken as *dietary supplements*. Calcium supplements may have the added benefit of reducing symptoms of *premenstrual syndrome*. Also, data indicate that calcium supplements can produce a significant, albeit modest, reduction in recurrence of *colorectal adenomas*.

Adverse Effects

When calcium is taken chronically in high doses (3 to 4 g/day), *hypercalcemia* can result. Hypercalcemia is most likely in patients who are also receiving large doses of vitamin D. Signs and symptoms include GI disturbances (nausea, vomiting, and constipation), renal dysfunction (polyuria and nephrolithiasis), and CNS effects (lethargy and depression). In addition, hypercalcemia may cause cardiac dysrhythmias and deposition of calcium in soft tissue. Hypercalcemia can be minimized with frequent monitoring of plasma calcium content.

Drug Interactions

Glucocorticoids (e.g., prednisone) reduce absorption of oral calcium, leading to osteoporosis with long-term use. Calcium reduces absorption of several drugs when administered together. These drugs include tetracycline and quinolone antibiotics, thyroid hormone, the anticonvulsant phenytoin, and bisphosphonates. Thiazide diuretics decrease renal calcium

excretion and thus may cause hypercalcemia; however, loop diuretics increase calcium excretion and may cause hypocalcemia.

Food Interactions

Certain foods contain substances that can suppress calcium absorption. One such substance—oxalic acid—is found in spinach, rhubarb, Swiss chard, and beets. Phytic acid, another depressant of calcium absorption, and insoluble fiber, which also hampers absorption, are present in bran and whole-grain cereals. Oral calcium supplements should not be administered with these foods.

Preparations and Dosage

The calcium salts available for oral administration are shown in Table 61.3. Note that the dosage required to provide a specific amount of elemental calcium differs among preparations. Calcium carbonate, for example, has the highest percentage of calcium. Chewable tablets are preferred to standard tablets because of more consistent bioavailability. Bioavailability of calcium citrate appears especially good, owing to high solubility, and appears to be better absorbed in patients taking proton pump inhibitors. When calcium supplements are taken, total daily calcium intake (dietary plus supplemental) should equal the values in Table 61.1. To help ensure adequate absorption, no more than 600 mg should be consumed at one time.

PATIENT EDUCATION
Calcium Salts

Individual calcium salts differ with respect to percentage of elemental calcium. As a result, the dose required to provide a specific amount of calcium differs among the salts. Advise patients against switching to a different preparation.

Advise patients to take oral calcium salts with a large glass of water. Dosing with or shortly after meals promotes absorption. Advise patients to avoid taking calcium with foods that can suppress calcium absorption (e.g., spinach, Swiss chard, beets, bran, and whole-grain cereals).

Inform patients about signs of hypercalcemia (nausea, vomiting, constipation, frequent urination, lethargy, and depression) and instruct them to notify the prescriber if these occur.

Calcium binds to tetracyclines, thereby reducing tetracycline absorption. Instruct patients to separate administration of these agents by at least 1 h.

Calcium interferes with absorption of thyroid hormone. Instruct patients to separate administration of these agents by several hours.

TABLE 61.3 Oral Calcium Salts

Generic Name	Trade Name	Calcium Content (%)	Dose Providing 1000 mg of Calcium
Calcium acetate	PhosLo, Calphron, and Eliphos	25	4 g
Calcium carbonate	Tums, Rolaids, and others	40	2.6 g
Calcium citrate	Citracal and Cal-Cee	21	4.8 g
Calcium glubionate	Calcionate	6.6	15.2 g
Calcium gluconate[a]	Cal-G	9	11 g
Calcium lactate	Cal-Lac	13	7.6 g
Tricalcium phosphate	Posture	39	2.6 g

[a]Also available in parenteral form.

SUMMARY OF KEY PRESCRIBING CONSIDERATIONS

Oral Calcium Salts

Therapeutic Goal: Maintain serum calcium levels within normal reference range (typically 8.4–10.2 mg/dL but this may vary according to laboratory).

Baseline Data: Serum calcium (or serum ionized calcium for hypoalbuminemia or acid–base imbalance). Depending on patient status and severity, also check ECG, albumin, phosphate, and magnesium. (Often not needed for oral calcium preparations, which are indicated for mild hypocalcemia.)

Monitoring: Check serum calcium periodically. Other laboratory tests may be needed according to patient status.

Identifying High-Risk Patients: Calcium salts are *contraindicated* for patients with hypercalcemia, renal calculi, and hypophosphatemia.

Evaluating Therapeutic Effects: Symptoms of hypocalcemia abate and calcium levels return to within the normal range.

Minimizing Adverse Effects: Prolonged therapy can cause hypercalcemia. Hypercalcemia can be minimized with frequent monitoring of serum calcium.

Vitamin D

The term *vitamin D* refers to two compounds: *ergocalciferol* (vitamin D_2) and *cholecalciferol* (vitamin D_3). Vitamin D_3 is the form of vitamin D produced naturally in humans when our skin is exposed to sunlight. Vitamin D_2 is a form of vitamin D that occurs in plants. Vitamin D_2 is used as a prescription drug and to fortify foods. Both forms are used in over-the-counter supplements. It is important to note that both forms of vitamin D produce nearly identical biologic effects. Therefore, rather than distinguishing between them, we will use the term *vitamin D* to refer to vitamins D_2 and D_3 collectively.

Therapeutic Uses

Vitamin D is essential for bone health, owing to its effects on calcium utilization. The primary indications for vitamin D are vitamin D deficiency and associated conditions such as rickets, osteomalacia, and hypoparathyroidism.

Some studies suggest that vitamin D may also protect against diabetes, arthritis, cardiovascular disease, autoimmune disorders, and cancers of the breast, colon, prostate, and ovary. However, according to the IOM report on calcium and vitamin D, the available data are insufficient to support health claims beyond bone health. Until more definitive data are available, the possibility of additional benefits remains open but not proved.

Physiologic Actions

Vitamin D is an important regulator of calcium and phosphorus homeostasis. Vitamin D increases blood levels of both elements, primarily by increasing their absorption from the intestine and promoting their resorption from bone. In addition, vitamin D reduces renal excretion of calcium and phosphate (although the quantitative significance of this effect is not clear). With usual doses of vitamin D, there is no net loss of calcium from bone. However, vitamin D *can* promote bone decalcification if serum calcium concentrations cannot be maintained by increasing intestinal calcium absorption.

Sources and Daily Requirements

Sources. Vitamin D is obtained through the diet, supplements, and exposure to sunlight. Except for shiitake mushrooms and oily fish (e.g., salmon, tuna), natural foods have very little vitamin D. Accordingly, dietary vitamin D is obtained mainly through vitamin D-fortified foods, especially cereals, milk, yogurt, margarine, cheese, and orange juice.

Requirements. In 2010, the IOM issued revised guidelines for vitamin D intake. They now recommend the following:
- For children younger than 1 year, 400 international units (IU)/day
- For all people aged 1 through 70 years, 600 IU/day
- For adults aged 71 years and older, 800 IU/day

These recommendations are based on the assumption that people get very little of their vitamin D from exposure to sunlight.

According to the IOM report, most people in North America have blood levels of vitamin D in the range needed to support good bone health and, hence, do not need vitamin D supplements. Whether taking supplements would confer other benefits is yet to be proved.

Vitamin D Deficiency

Vitamin D is best measured by the serum concentration of 25-hydroxyvitamin D (25-[OH]D). Vitamin D is converted to 25(OH)D (also known as calcidol) by the liver; therefore the serum level of 25(OH)D provides a good representation of deficiency. Vitamin D deficiency is defined by a 25(OH)D concentration below 20 ng/mL. (Levels above 20 ng/mL are sufficient to maintain bone health.) In actual practice, the target level of 25-(OH)D is usually 30 to 60 ng/mL.

How much vitamin D is needed to *treat deficiency*? In 2011, The Endocrine Society made the following recommendations:
- For children less than 1 year, 2000 IU/day
- For children aged 1 to 18 years, 4000 IU/day
- For adults 19 years and older, up to 10,000 IU/day

Much higher doses are needed for patients who are obese and for those taking glucocorticoids and other drugs that suppress calcium absorption or that increase calcium excretion.

Screening for vitamin D deficiency is recommended for patients at risk, including those who are pregnant, obese, or have dark skin (because, compared with light-skinned people, they make less vitamin D in response to sunlight). For others, the US Preventive Services Task Force (USPSTF), in its 2014 update, declined to recommend for or against vitamin D deficiency screening for nonpregnant adults of 18 years and older.

Activation of Vitamin D

To affect calcium and phosphate metabolism, vitamin D must first undergo activation. The extent of activation is carefully regulated and is determined by calcium availability; when plasma calcium falls, activation of vitamin D is increased. The pathways for activating vitamins D_2 and D_3 are shown in Fig. 61.2.

Let's begin by focusing on vitamin D_3, the natural human vitamin. Vitamin D_3 (cholecalciferol) is produced in the skin through the action of sunlight on provitamin D_3 (7-dehydrocholesterol). Neither provitamin D_3 nor vitamin D_3 possesses significant biologic activity. In the next reaction, enzymes in the liver convert cholecalciferol into calcifediol, which serves as a transport form of vitamin D_3 and possesses only slight biologic activity. In the final step, calcifediol is converted into the highly active calcitriol. This reaction occurs in the kidney and can be stimulated by (1) PTH, (2) a drop in dietary vitamin D, and (3) a fall in plasma levels of calcium.

Vitamin D_2 is activated by the same enzymes that activate vitamin D_3. As we saw with vitamin D_3, only the last compound in the series (in this case 1,25-dihydroxyergocalciferol) has significant biologic activity.

Pharmacokinetics

As a rule, vitamin D is administered orally and then absorbed from the small intestine. Bile is essential for absorption. In the absence of adequate bile, intramuscular (IM) dosing may be required. In the blood, vitamin D is transported complexed with vitamin D-binding protein. Storage of vitamin D occurs primarily in the liver. As discussed, vitamin D undergoes metabolic activation. Reactions that occur in the liver produce the major transport form of vitamin D. A later reaction (in the kidney)

VITAMIN D₂	VITAMIN D₃	ACTIVITY

Fig. 61.2 Vitamin D Activation. Ergosterol is found in yeasts and fungi. 7-Dehydrocholesterol is present in the skin. Green boxes indicate forms of vitamin D used therapeutically.

produces the fully active form. Excretion of vitamin D is through the bile. Urinary excretion is minimal.

Viewing Vitamin D as a Hormone

Although referred to as a vitamin, vitamin D has all the characteristics of a hormone. With sufficient exposure to sunlight, the body can manufacture all the vitamin D it needs. Hence, under ideal conditions, external sources of vitamin D appear unnecessary. After its production in the skin, vitamin D travels to other locations (liver and kidney) for activation. Like other hormones, activated vitamin D then travels to various sites in the body (bone, intestine, and kidney) to exert regulatory actions. Also, like other hormones, vitamin D undergoes feedback regulation: as plasma levels of calcium fall, activation of vitamin D increases; when plasma levels of calcium return to normal, activation of vitamin D declines.

Toxicity (Hypervitaminosis D)

Serious vitamin D toxicity (hypervitaminosis D) can be produced by vitamin D doses that exceed 1000 IU/day (in infants) and 50,000 IU/day (in adults). Poisoning occurs most commonly in children; causes include accidental ingestion by the child and excessive dosing with vitamin D by parents. Doses of potentially toxic magnitude are also encountered clinically. When huge therapeutic doses are used, the margin of safety is small, and patients should be monitored closely for signs of poisoning.

Clinical presentation. Most signs and symptoms of vitamin D toxicity occur secondary to hypercalcemia. (See earlier discussion of hypercalcemia.) Very large doses of vitamin D can cause decalcification of bone, resulting in osteoporosis; mobilization of bone calcium can occur despite the presence of high calcium concentrations in blood. In children, vitamin D poisoning can suppress growth for 6 months or longer.

Treatment. Treatment consists of stopping vitamin D intake, reducing calcium intake, and increasing fluid intake. Glucocorticoids may be given to suppress calcium absorption. If hypercalcemia is severe, renal excretion of calcium can be accelerated using a combination of IV saline and furosemide.

Preparations, Dosage, and Administration

There are five preparations of vitamin D. Three of these—ergocalciferol, cholecalciferol, and calcitriol—are identical to forms of vitamin D that occur naturally. The other two—paricalcitol and doxercalciferol—are synthetic derivatives of natural vitamin D. (The naturally occurring preparations are highlighted in green boxes in Fig. 61.2.) Individual vitamin D preparations differ in their clinical applications.

Two forms of vitamin D—vitamin D₃ (cholecalciferol) and vitamin D₂ (ergocalciferol)—are used routinely as dietary supplements. Of the two, vitamin D₃ is preferred because it is more effective than vitamin D₂ at raising blood levels of 25-(OH)D, the active form of vitamin D in the body.

Vitamin D is almost always administered by mouth. Dosage is usually prescribed in international units (IU). (One IU is equivalent to the biologic activity in 0.025 mcg of vitamin D₃.) Daily dosages

PATIENT EDUCATION

Vitamin D

Instruct the patient to swallow oral preparations intact, without crushing or chewing.

Therapeutic responses to vitamin D require adequate calcium intake. Encourage intake of foods that are high in calcium.

of vitamin D range from 400 IU (for dietary supplementation) to as high as 500,000 IU (for vitamin D-resistant rickets). Additional information on preparation, dosage, and administration is available in Table 61.4.

Cinacalcet

Actions and Therapeutic Use

Cinacalcet (Sensipar) is a calcimimetic drug approved for primary hyperparathyroidism for those unable to undergo a parathyroidectomy and for those with hypercalcemia caused by parathyroid carcinoma. It is also approved to treat secondary hyperparathyroidism caused by chronic kidney disease [CKD]. This drug is typically prescribed by specialists (e.g., endocrinologists and nephrologists), so our discussion here will be brief.

Benefits of cinacalcet derive from decreasing secretion of PTH. How is secretion suppressed? Recall that extracellular calcium regulates PTH secretion by binding with calcium-sensing receptors on cells of the parathyroid gland, thereby signaling those cells to reduce PTH secretion.

SUMMARY OF KEY PRESCRIBING CONSIDERATIONS

Vitamin D

Therapeutic Goal: Purpose is to promote adequate levels of vitamin D in patients with rickets, osteomalacia, and hypoparathyroidism.

Baseline Data: Obtain serum 25(OH)D, calcium, phosphorus, and alkaline phosphatase as well as a 24-h urinary calcium determination.

Monitoring: Monitor serum 25(OH)D, calcium, serum phosphorus, and urinary calcium.

Identifying High-Risk Patients: Vitamin D is contraindicated in patients with hypercalcemia, hypervitaminosis D, and malabsorption syndrome. Exercise caution in patients taking digoxin.

Evaluating Therapeutic Effects: Improvement of osteomalacia and rickets.

Minimizing Adverse Effects: Vitamin D-induced hypercalcemia can cause dysrhythmias in patients taking digoxin. Monitor serum calcium and ensure it remains within normal range.

Large therapeutic doses may cause hypervitaminosis D, a syndrome characterized by hypercalcemia, hypercalciuria, decalcification of bone, and deposition of calcium in soft tissues. Monitor serum calcium content (levels should stay below 10 mg/dL) along with serum phosphorus and urinary calcium. If vitamin D toxicity develops, instruct the patient to discontinue vitamin D immediately, increase fluid intake, and institute a low-calcium diet. In severe cases, calcium excretion can be accelerated with IV saline plus furosemide.

TABLE 61.4   Indications, Preparation, and Dosage of Vitamin D Preparations[a]

Drug Name	Indications	Preparation	Dosage
Ergocalciferol (vitamin D$_2$ [Calciferol Drops, Drisdol])	Hypoparathyroidism, vitamin D-resistant rickets, familial hypophosphatemia	Capsules: 50,000 IU Oral solution: 8000 IU/mL	Vitamin D-resistant rickets: 12,000–500,000 IU daily Hypoparathyroidism: 25,000–200,000 IU daily (together with 4 g of calcium lactate 6 times/day)
Cholecalciferol (vitamin D$_3$ [Delta-D])	Prophylaxis and treatment of vitamin D deficiency	Capsules: 1000, 2000, 5000, 10,000, 25,000, and 50,000 IU Liquid: 400 and 5000 units/mL Tablets: 2000, 3000, 5000, and 50,000 IU	Prophylaxis: varies depending on risk Deficiency: • <1 year old, 2000 IU/day • 1–18 years old, 4000 IU/day • Age 19 years and older, up to 10,000 IU/day
Calcitriol (1,25-Dihydroxy-D$_3$ [Rocaltrol, Vectical, Calcijex ♦, and Silkis ♦])	Hypoparathyroidism and management of hypocalcemia in patients undergoing chronic renal dialysis	Capsules: 0.25 and 0.5 mcg Oral solution: 1 mcg/mL Solution for injection: 1 mcg/mL	Dialysis: daily oral doses of 0.5–1 mcg usually adequate Hypoparathyroidism: Initial dosage 0.25 mcg/day administered orally
Doxercalciferol (Hectorol)	Prevention and treatment of secondary hyperparathyroidism in patients undergoing chronic renal dialysis	Capsules: 0.5, 1, and 2.5 mcg[b]	Dosage carefully tailored to the patient Initial dosing: 10 mcg 3 times weekly administered at dialysis Adjusting dosage: gradually increase to a maximum of 20 mcg 3 times a week
Paricalcitol (Zemplar)	Prevention and treatment of secondary hyperparathyroidism in patients undergoing chronic renal dialysis	Capsules: 1, 2, and 4 mcg[a]	Initial dosing: 1–2 mcg/dose (with the once-daily schedule) or 2–4 mcg/dose (with the 3-times-weekly schedule) Adjusting dosage: gradually increase every 2–4 weeks based on the PTH level

[a]Typical dosing is provided. In practice, adjustments must be individualized to accommodate for patient status (e.g., chronic kidney disease).
[b]Also available for IV administration.
IU, International unit; *PTH*, parathyroid hormone.

Cinacalcet increases the sensitivity of the calcium-sensing receptors to activation by extracellular calcium. As a result, the ability of calcium to suppress PTH release is amplified.

Clinical trials have shown that, in patients with hyperparathyroidism secondary to CKD, cinacalcet decreases serum PTH by 23% to 46% and improves calcium and phosphorus homeostasis. Similarly, in patients with primary hyperparathyroidism, the drug decreases serum PTH and normalizes serum calcium.

Adverse Effects

The most common adverse effects are nausea, vomiting, and diarrhea. Because cinacalcet lowers calcium levels, hypocalcemia is an obvious concern. Accordingly, calcium levels should be monitored, and patients should be informed about possible manifestations of hypocalcemia (e.g., cramping, convulsions, myalgias, paresthesias, and tetany) and instructed to report them.

Drug Interactions

Cinacalcet is metabolized in part by cytochrome P450 isoenzyme 3A4, so inhibitors of this enzyme (e.g., ketoconazole, itraconazole, and erythromycin) can raise cinacalcet levels. If cinacalcet is used with one of these drugs, cinacalcet dosage may need an adjustment.

Monitoring

In patients with hyperparathyroidism from parathyroid carcinoma, measure serum calcium within 1 week of the first dose and each dosage change. After a maintenance dosage has been established, measure serum calcium every 2 months.

In patients with secondary hyperparathyroidism, measure serum calcium and phosphorus within 1 week of the first dose and each dosage change, and measure PTH within 4 weeks of the first dose and each dosage change. After a maintenance dosage has been established, measure calcium and phosphorus monthly and PTH every 1 to 3 months.

Calcitonin

Calcitonin-salmon (Miacalcin), more commonly called simply calcitonin, a form of calcitonin derived from salmon, is similar in structure to calcitonin synthesized by the human thyroid. Salmon calcitonin produces the same metabolic effects as human calcitonin but has a longer half-life and greater milligram potency. The drug is usually given by nasal spray but can also be given by injection. Intranasal calcitonin was removed from the Canadian market in 2013 because of an increased risk for malignancy associated with this formulation. Calcitonin remains available in the United States after the FDA failed to identify a causal relationship between calcitonin and elevated cancer risk; however, the FDA still recommends weighing the benefits and risk of calcitonin before prescribing it. In their clinical guidelines, the AACE and ACE note that there are more effective drugs on the market; therefore, calcitonin is not a drug of choice.

Actions

Calcitonin has two principal actions: (1) it inhibits the activity of osteoclasts and thus decreases bone resorption, and (2) it inhibits tubular resorption of calcium, thereby increasing calcium excretion. As a result of decreasing bone turnover, calcitonin decreases alkaline phosphatase in blood and increases hydroxyproline in urine. Preparations and dosages for the different indications are presented in Table 61.5.

Therapeutic Uses

Calcitonin has three indications. It is used to treat (1) postmenopausal osteoporosis, (2) Paget disease, and (3) hypercalcemia.

TABLE 61.5 Indications, Preparations, and Dosages of Nonbisphosphonate Drugs for Osteoporosis

Drug Name	Indications	Preparation	Dosage
Calcitonin, intranasal (Miacalcin)	Management of postmenopausal osteoporosis	Intranasal metered dose spray device delivers 200 IU per activation	200 IU (1 spray) each day, alternating nares daily
Calcitonin, injection (Miacalcin)	Postmenopausal osteoporosis, Paget disease of bone, and hypercalcemia	2-mL vials containing 200 IU/mL Administration is IM or subQ. Dosages are the same for both routes.	Postmenopausal osteoporosis: 100 IU every other day Paget disease of bone: 100 IU/day initially, followed by 50 IU (daily or 3 times a week) Hypercalcemia: initial dosage is 4 IU/kg every 12 h; maximal dosage is 8 IU/kg every 6 h
Denosumab (Prolia and Xgeva)	Prolia: Osteoporosis in women and men Xgeva: Hypercalcemia of malignancy, multiple myeloma, giant cell tumor of bone, and cancer metastasis to bone	Solution: Prolia—60 mg/mL Xgeva—120 mg/1.7 mL	Prolia: 60 mg subQ once every 6 months Xgeva: For all indications, 120 mg subQ every 4 weeks
Raloxifene (Evista)	Postmenopausal osteoporosis and risk reduction for estrogen-positive breast cancer	Tablet: 60 mg	For both indications, 60 mg daily
Teriparatide (Forteo)	Postmenopausal osteoporosis, osteoporosis in men, and GIOP	US: 2.4 mL multi-use injector containing 600 mcg—delivers 20 mcg on activation Canada: 3 mL multi-use injector containing 250 mcg/mL—delivers 20 mcg on activation	For all indications: 20 mcg subQ daily administered in abdomen or thigh
Abaloparatide [Tymlos]	Postmenopausal osteoporosis	1.56 mL injector containing 3120 mcg—delivers 80 mcg on activation	80 mcg subQ daily administered in periumbilical area

GIOP, Glucocorticoid-induced osteoporosis; *IM*, intramuscular; *IU*, international unit; *subQ*, subcutaneous.

Calcitonin, given by nasal spray or injection, is indicated for *treatment* of established postmenopausal osteoporosis—but not for prevention. Benefits derive from suppressing bone resorption. Unfortunately, these benefits subside within 1 or 2 years after the drug is discontinued. The treatment program should include supplemental calcium and adequate intake of vitamin D.

Calcitonin is helpful in moderate to severe Paget disease and is the drug of choice for rapid relief of pain associated with the disorder. Benefits occur secondary to inhibition of osteoclasts. Neurologic symptoms caused by spinal cord compression may be reduced.

Calcitonin can lower plasma calcium levels in patients with hypercalcemia secondary to hyperparathyroidism, vitamin D toxicity, and cancer. Levels of calcium (and phosphorus) are reduced owing to inhibition of bone resorption and increased renal excretion of calcium. Although calcitonin is effective against hypercalcemia, it is not a preferred treatment.

Adverse Effects

With intranasal dosing, nasal dryness and irritation are the most common complaints. As previously mentioned, studies demonstrating an increase in malignancies associated with nasal administration prompted withdrawal of this drug in Canada. After parenteral (IM, subcutaneous [subQ]) administration, about 10% of patients experience nausea, which diminishes with time. An additional 10% have inflammatory reactions at the injection site. Flushing of the face and hands may also occur. When calcitonin is taken for a year or longer, neutralizing antibodies often develop. In some patients, these antibodies bind enough calcitonin to prevent therapeutic effects.

PATIENT EDUCATION
Calcitonin

Instruct patients using Miacalcin to prime the metered-dose pump by holding the bottle upright and depressing the two white sidearms toward the bottle 6 times, which should produce a faint initial spray. The drug is then administered by placing the nozzle in the nostril and depressing the pump handle.

Teach patients how to inject calcitonin subcutaneously. Instruct them to rotate sites of injection.

SUMMARY OF KEY PRESCRIBING CONSIDERATIONS
Calcitonin

Therapeutic Goal: To maintain or improve bone mineral density (BMD) in patients with postmenopausal osteoporosis and Paget disease of bone.

Baseline Data: Check axial (spine and hip) dual-energy X-ray absorptiometry (DXA). Obtain serum levels of calcium, alkaline phosphatase, and 25(OH)D.

Monitoring: Check DXA every 1 to 2 years until stable, then every 2 years (or less, depending on patient status). Check height annually. Monitor for increased back pain and, if present, consider spinal radiographs to determine vertebral fractures. Monitor serum calcium and phosphorous.

Identifying High-Risk Patients: Salmon calcitonin is *contraindicated* for patients allergic to fish. Hypocalcemia must be corrected prior to initiating therapy.

Evaluating Therapeutic Effects: For osteoporosis, BMD increases, or at least remains constant, and fractures are prevented. For Paget disease of bone, bone pain is also decreased.

Minimizing Adverse Effects: For intranasal spray, discontinue the drug if nasal ulcerations occur, especially if accompanied by heavy bleeding. For minor ulceration, withdrawal may be temporary.

Bisphosphonates

Bisphosphonates are structural analogs of pyrophosphate, a normal constituent of bone. These drugs undergo incorporation into bone, and then inhibit bone resorption by decreasing the activity of osteoclasts. Principal indications are postmenopausal osteoporosis, osteoporosis in men, glucocorticoid-induced osteoporosis (GIOP), Paget disease of bone, and hypercalcemia of malignancy. Bisphosphonates may also help prevent and treat bone metastases in patients with cancer (see Chapter 85).

Bisphosphonates differ with respect to indications, routes, and dosing schedules. Some bisphosphonates are given by oral (PO) route, some by IV route, and some by both routes. Dosing schedules vary from as often as once a day (with oral agents) to as seldom as once every 2 years (with IV zoledronic acid). As with many drugs for osteoporosis and similar bone disorders, calcium and vitamin D supplements are recommended if there is inadequate dietary intake.

Four bisphosphonates approved for management of osteoporosis and GIOP are currently available in the United States. These are alendronate (Fosamax, Fosamax Plus D, and Binosto), ibandronate (Boniva), risedronate (Actonel and Atelvia), and zoledronic acid (Reclast, Zometa, and generic only). Additional bisphosphonates have been approved for the treatment of Paget disease (e.g., tiludronate [Skelid] and etidronate [generic only]) or complications of malignancy (e.g., pamidronate [generic only]); however, because these conditions are typically managed by endocrinologists, rheumatologists, and oncologists, they are not addressed in this chapter.

Alendronate is the most widely used oral bisphosphonate. It will serve as our prototype for the family.

PROTOTYPE DRUGS
Drugs Affecting Calcium Levels and Bone Mineralization

Antiresorptive Agents
Conjugated equine estrogens (Premarin)
Raloxifene (selective estrogen receptor modulator)
Alendronate (bisphosphonate)
Calcitonin nasal spray
Denosumab (RANKL inhibitor)

Bone-Forming Agent
Teriparatide (parathyroid hormone)

Alendronate

Therapeutic use. The primary purpose of alendronate is the prevention and treatment of osteoporosis in postmenopausal women, in whom benefits derive from decreasing bone resorption by osteoclasts. It is also approved for treating osteoporosis in men. In this group, the drug increases BMD, reduces vertebral fractures, and decreases loss of height.

Alendronate is considered a first-choice drug for the prevention and treatment of GIOP, a common complication of glucocorticoid therapy. Studies indicate that alendronate helps restore lost bone and may reduce the risk for fractures in this instance.

It is also a first-line treatment for Paget disease. Continuous daily therapy for 3 months produces a 50% decrease in serum alkaline phosphatase, indicating a substantial reduction in bone turnover. As in osteoporosis, benefits derive from inhibiting bone resorption by osteoclasts.

Mechanism of action. Approximately 50% of alendronate is taken up rapidly by bone. After alendronate has become incorporated into bone, it remains there for years and sometimes decades.

Alendronate suppresses resorption of bone by decreasing both the number and activity of osteoclasts. Several mechanisms are involved. As osteoclasts begin to resorb alendronate-containing bone, they ingest some of the drug, which then acts on the osteoclasts to inhibit their activity. In addition, alendronate reduces the *number* of osteoclasts by (1) acting directly to decrease their recruitment and (2) acting on osteoblasts, which then produce an inhibitor of osteoclast formation.

Adverse effects. Alendronate is generally well tolerated. Esophagitis is the principal concern. Rarely, the drug causes musculoskeletal pain, ocular inflammation, atypical femur fractures, and osteonecrosis of the jaw (ONJ). The risk for these adverse effects increases with long-term use. Fortunately, because bisphosphonates remain in bone for extensive periods of time, they continue to prevent fractures for years, and possibly for decades, after being discontinued.

Esophagitis. Esophagitis, sometimes resulting in ulceration, is the most serious adverse effect. Fortunately, esophagitis is rare, occurring in only 1 of every 10,000 patients. The cause of injury is prolonged contact with the esophageal mucosa, which can occur if alendronate fails to pass completely through the esophagus. Reasons for incomplete passage include taking the drug with insufficient water, taking the drug in a supine position, lying down after taking the drug, and having a preexisting esophageal disorder that impedes drug passage. Because of the risk for esophagitis, alendronate is contraindicated for patients with esophageal disorders that could prevent successful swallowing and for patients who are unable to sit or stand for at least 30 minutes. If symptoms of esophageal injury occur during treatment (e.g., difficulty swallowing, pain on swallowing, or new or worsening heartburn), patients should be instructed to discontinue alendronate and contact the prescriber.

Atypical femoral fractures. Alendronate and other bisphosphonates have been associated with atypical fractures of the femur, which occur with little or no trauma. Why do these fractures occur? One explanation is that excessive suppression of bone turnover reduces bone remodeling, and, as a result, repair of microcracks is suppressed and bone strength is reduced. Fortunately, the absolute risk for atypical fractures is low—about five additional cases for every 10,000 patient-years of bisphosphonate use. Risk increases with duration of treatment.

Do the benefits of preventing typical fractures (which are common) outweigh the risk of causing atypical fractures (which are rare)? The answer is clearly "Yes"—but only for women with osteoporosis who are deemed at high risk for a typical fracture. For women without osteoporosis who are at low risk for a typical fracture, the benefits of bisphosphonates may not justify the risks.

What can be done to reduce the risk for an atypical fracture? In 2010, a task force assembled by the American Society for Bone and Mineral Research recommended the following:

- Do not prescribe bisphosphonates for patients considered at low risk for osteoporosis-related fractures.
- Consider alternative treatments, such as raloxifene or teriparatide, for patients with osteoporosis of the spine and normal (or only moderately reduced) BMD of the femoral neck or hip.
- After 5 years of bisphosphonate use, evaluate annually the need for continued treatment.

Esophageal cancer. Alendronate and other oral bisphosphonates may—or may not—increase the risk for esophageal cancer. Studies have reached conflicting conclusions. If the risk is real, it is small (about 1 additional case for every 1000 patients older than 60 years treated for 5 years) and probably due to esophageal injury caused during oral dosing. Measures that might reduce risk include reducing the dosing frequency (i.e., dosing weekly rather than daily), taking the drug with a full glass of water, and staying upright for 30 to 60 minutes after dosing.

Musculoskeletal pain. Musculoskeletal pain, sometimes severe, has been reported during postmarketing surveillance. So far, a causal link with alendronate has not been established. Onset may occur shortly after the first dose or months later. Pain can be managed with analgesics, including short-term opioids and ketorolac when pain is severe. In most cases, discomfort gradually resolves after stopping alendronate. Interestingly, among patients who resume alendronate use, only 11% experience a return of pain. If pain does return, patients taking the drug for osteoporosis can switch to a different nonbisphosphonate agent.

Ocular problems. Ocular problems are rare but can be serious. Possible effects include conjunctivitis, scleritis, blurred vision, and eye pain. Drug-induced release of inflammatory cytokines may be the cause. Advise patients to report any vision changes or eye pain.

Osteonecrosis of the jaw. Very rarely, patients have developed ONJ, a potentially severe complication. This is seen mostly with IV bisphosphonates.

Hyperparathyroidism. In patients with Paget disease, alendronate can induce hyperparathyroidism. By inhibiting accelerated bone resorption, alendronate causes blood levels of calcium to fall; in response, secretion of PTH is increased. To prevent hyperparathyroidism, patients should receive calcium supplements.

Atrial fibrillation. Because an intravenous bisphosphonate (zoledronic acid) has been associated with rare cases of atrial fibrillation (AF), there has been an ongoing concern that oral alendronate may also cause the disorder. In 2008, the US Food and Drug Administration (FDA), based on data from clinical trials, determined there was no significant AF risk with oral formulations of bisphosphonates. Data from more recent research, however, have raised the issue once again. In 2014, the American Journal of Cardiology published a report of findings from a meta-analysis of randomized controlled trials and observational studies that contradicts earlier findings. Those authors assert that there is increased, although low, risk for new-onset AF with both oral and IV bisphosphonates.

Administration. Proper administration is necessary to maximize bioavailability and minimize the risk for esophageal injury. Alendronate absorption is dramatically diminished when taken with food; practically none is absorbed in this instance. Even taking the drug with a fluid such as coffee or orange juice can decrease absorption by 60%. To maximize bioavailability, alendronate should be taken in the morning before breakfast (i.e., on an empty stomach). No food or drink, other than water, should be consumed for at least 30 minutes after administration. Because minerals such as calcium, magnesium, and iron bind with alendronate and all other bisphosphonates, many experts advise waiting at least 2 hours after administration before taking calcium products, mineral supplements, or antacids.

Additional information on preparation and dosage of alendronate and other bisphosphonates is available in Table 61.6. Pharmacokinetics for alendronate and other drugs for osteoporosis are addressed in Table 61.7.

Risedronate

Actions and uses. Risedronate (Actonel, Atelvia, and Actonel DR) is an oral bisphosphonate approved for postmenopausal osteoporosis, male osteoporosis, GIOP, and Paget disease of bone. After absorption, most of the drug becomes incorporated into bone where it persists for years. As with other bisphosphonates, benefits derive from inhibiting osteoclast-mediated resorption of bone. In postmenopausal women with osteoporosis, risedronate increases BMD and reduces the risk for vertebral and nonvertebral fractures.

Adverse effects. The most common adverse effects are arthralgia, diarrhea, headache, rash, nausea, and a flu-like syndrome. Like alendronate, risedronate poses a significant risk for esophagitis and a very small risk for atypical femoral fractures. Ocular problems and musculoskeletal pain are rare. If risedronate poses a risk for esophageal cancer, ONJ, or AF, the risk is very small.

Administration. Like other oral bisphosphonates, risedronate is poorly absorbed from the GI tract. Absorption is only 1% under fasting conditions. The effect of food depends on the formulation used. With Actonel (an immediate-release [IR] formulation), food greatly reduces absorption. By contrast, with Atelvia (an enteric-coated, delayed-release [DR] formulation), food does not reduce absorption. In fact, Atelvia should be taken with food to reduce stomach pain.

With the IR tablets, each dose should be taken in the morning before ingesting the first food or fluids of the day (except for water). With the DR tablets, each dose should be taken in the morning after breakfast. (Atelvia, the enteric-coated DR tablet, is currently the only oral bisphosphonate that can be taken after eating, rather than before.) With both formulations, dosing should be done with a full glass of water. Also, the patient should be upright when swallowing and should not lie down for at least 30 minutes. Like alendronate, risedronate binds to divalent cations such as calcium, iron, and magnesium; therefore calcium products, mineral supplements, and antacids should not be administered within 2 hours of administering either of the risedronate formulation.

Ibandronate

Actions and uses. Ibandronate (Boniva) is approved for prevention and treatment of postmenopausal osteoporosis. Dosing may be done once a month (PO) or once every 3 months (IV). As with other bisphosphonates, it is incorporated into bone where it remains for years. Benefits derive from inhibiting osteoclast-mediated resorption of bone. In clinical trials, ibandronate increased BMD in the lumbar spine and other sites and reduced the risk for vertebral fractures. Although comparative studies have not been done, the drug is probably as effective as alendronate and risedronate, the only other bisphosphonates approved for oral therapy of osteoporosis.

Adverse effects. With oral administration, ibandronate is generally well tolerated. Like other oral bisphosphonates, it can cause adverse GI effects, including esophagitis, dyspepsia, and abdominal pain. Ocular inflammation, atypical fractures, and ONJ are rare. Musculoskeletal

---

TABLE 61.6 Indications, Preparations, and Dosages of Bisphosphonates

Drug Name	Indications	Preparation	Dosage
Alendronate (Fosamax and Binosto) Alendronate + vitamin D (Fosamax Plus D)	Prevention and treatment of osteoporosis in postmenopausal women, osteoporosis in men, Paget disease, and GIOP	Tablets (Fosamax): 70 mg Tablets (generic): 5, 10, 35, 40, and 70 mg Effervescent tablet (Binosto): 70 mg Oral solution (generic): 70 mg/75 mL Tablets (Fosamax D): 70 mg alendronate: 2800 IU vitamin D_3, 70 mg alendronate: 5600 IU vitamin D_3	Osteoporosis in postmenopausal women, prevention: 5-mg tablet daily or 35 mg once weekly Osteoporosis in postmenopausal women, treatment: 10-mg tablet daily or 70 mg once weekly Osteoporosis in men: 10-mg tablet once daily or 70 mg once weekly Paget disease: 40 mg once daily for 6 months for men or women GIOP for men, premenopausal women, and postmenopausal women taking estrogen: 5 mg once daily GIOP for postmenopausal women not taking estrogen: 10 mg once daily
Risedronate [Actonel, Atelvia]	IR: Prevention and treatment of osteoporosis in postmenopausal women, osteoporosis in men, prevention or treatment of GIOP, and Paget disease of bone DR: postmenopausal osteoporosis	IR (Actonel): 5-, 30-, 35-, and 100-mg tablets DR: (Atelvia): 35-mg enteric-coated tablets	Postmenopausal osteoporosis, Actonel: 5 mg once daily, 35 mg once weekly, or 150 mg once a month Postmenopausal osteoporosis, Atelvia: 35 mg once weekly Osteoporosis in men, Actonel: 35 mg once a week GIOP, Actonel: 5 mg once daily Paget disease of bone: 30 mg once daily
Ibandronate (Boniva)	Prevention and treatment of postmenopausal osteoporosis	Tablets: 150 mg IV: 3 mg/3 mL prefilled syringes	Prevention and treatment of osteoporosis, tablets: 150 mg once a month on the same day each month Treatment of osteoporosis, IV: 3 mg every 3 months
Zoledronic acid (Aclasta ♣, Reclast, and Zometa)	Aclasta ♣: Treatment of osteoporosis in postmenopausal women, patients >50 years with history of low trauma hip fracture, osteoporosis in men, prevention and treatment of GIOP, and Paget disease of bone Reclast: Prevention and treatment of osteoporosis in postmenopausal women, osteoporosis in men, GIOP, and Paget disease Zometa: hypercalcemia of malignancy	Aclasta ♣: 5 mg/100 mL Reclast: 5 mg/100 mL	Aclasta ♣: For all indications *except Paget disease:* 5 mg IV once a year Paget disease: one 5 mg dose Treatment of postmenopausal osteoporosis: 5 mg once a year Prevention of postmenopausal osteoporosis: 5 mg once every 2 years Osteoporosis in men: 5 mg once a year GIOP: 5 mg once a year, infused over 15 min or longer Paget disease: 5 mg (one dose produces extended remission; specific retreatment data not available)

DR, Delayed release; *GIOP*, glucocorticoid-induced osteoporosis; *IR*, immediate release.

TABLE 61.7   Pharmacokinetics: Drugs for Osteoporosis

Drug Class and Drugs	Peak	Protein Binding	Metabolism	Half-Life[a]	Elimination
Bisphosphonates					
Alendronate (Binosto and Fosamax)	NK	78%	Not metabolized	>10 years	Urine and feces
Risendronate (Actonel, Actonel DR, and Atelvia)	1–3 h	24%	Not metabolized	480–461 h	Urine (85%) Feces
Ibandronate (Boniva)	0.5–2 h	85.7%–99.5%	Not metabolized	Oral: 37–157 h IV: 5–25 h	Urine (50%–60%) Feces
Zoledronic acid (Reclast, Zometa, and Aclasta)	NK	23%–53%	Not metabolized	146 h	Urine (23%–55%) Feces
Recombinant Parathyroid Hormone and Parathyroid Hormone Analog					
Teriparatide (Forteo)	30 min	NK	Hepatic via proteolysis	1 h	Urine
Abaloparatide (Tymlos)	15–30 min	70%	Hepatic via proteolysis	1.7 h	Urine
Miscellaneous					
Calcitonin (Miacalcin)	23 min	NK	Renal, blood, and tissues	1 h	
Denosumab	3–21 days (average 10 days)	NK	NK	25–28 days	NK
Raloxifene	NK	95%	Hepatic	27–28 h	Feces

[a]Terminal half-life provided when available
h, Hour(s); *min*, minutes; *NK*, not known.

pain has not been reported. Whether ibandronate increases the risk for esophageal cancer is unknown. As with other bisphosphonates, divalent cations (e.g., calcium, magnesium, iron) can greatly decrease absorption.

With IV administration, ibandronate and other bisphosphonates can cause renal damage. Intravenous ibandronate should not be used by patients taking other nephrotoxic drugs or by those with severe renal impairment, defined as serum creatinine above 2.3 mg/dL or creatinine clearance less than 30 mL/min. Kidney function should be determined before each dose, and, if severe renal impairment is detected, the dose should be withheld. In addition to causing renal damage, IV ibandronate may cause an acute reaction characterized by fever, joint pain, and myalgia, primarily with the first dose.

Administration. With oral dosing, bioavailability is extremely low—only 0.6%. Food decreases this availability by another 90%! Oral dosing must be done on an empty stomach in the morning. Patients should swallow tablets whole with a full glass of water, while standing or sitting upright. For 60 minutes after dosing, patients must remain upright and must not eat or drink anything, including medications and dietary supplements.

IV administration carries a risk for renal damage if ibandronate is administered rapidly. Accordingly, ibandronate should be administered by slow IV push over an interval of 15 to 30 seconds.

Zoledronic Acid

Actions and uses. Zoledronic acid (Reclast, Zometa, and Aclasta ✤), also called zoledronate, is an IV bisphosphonate with approved indications for postmenopausal osteoporosis, osteoporosis in men, Paget disease of bone, GIOP, multiple myeloma or metastatic bone lesions from solid tumors, and hypercalcemia of malignancy (HCM). In addition, the drug is used off-label to prevent bone loss, fractures, and other skeletal-related events (SREs) in patients receiving any of a variety of therapies that create a risk for bone loss. Like other bisphosphonates, zoledronic acid undergoes incorporation into bone, where it remains for years. When osteoclasts ingest the drug, it inhibits their activity, preventing bone resorption.

For management of postmenopausal osteoporosis, zoledronic acid differs from all other bisphosphonates, in that dosing is done just once a year or once every 2 years. Compared with placebo treatment, once-yearly zoledronic acid decreases the incidence of vertebral fractures by 70%, hip fractures by 41%, and nonvertebral fractures by 25%. In addition, zoledronic acid improves BMD and markers of bone metabolism.

Adverse effects. The most common reaction is transient fever with flu-like symptoms, followed by nausea, constipation, dyspnea, abdominal pain, and bone and joint pain. In addition, zoledronic acid can cause clinically significant reductions in serum levels of calcium, phosphorus, and magnesium. Accordingly, levels of these elements should be followed and corrected when indicated.

Zoledronic acid has been associated with bone injury, most often *ONJ*, a condition characterized by local bone death and decreased bone strength. The underlying cause is impaired blood perfusion. (Bisphosphonates impair perfusion by inhibiting growth of blood vessels.) Among patients using zoledronic acid most cases of ONJ developed after tooth extractions and other dental procedures, which can increase risk by promoting infection. Other risk factors include cancer, cancer chemotherapy, use of systemic glucocorticoids, and poor oral hygiene. To reduce ONJ risk, a dental examination with appropriate preventive dentistry should be conducted before giving zoledronic acid, especially in patients with ONJ risk factors.

Zoledronic acid can cause dose-dependent *kidney damage*, which can progress to acute renal failure and, rarely, to death. Risk is increased by the following:
- Chronic renal impairment
- Advanced age
- Dehydration (e.g., secondary to fever, sepsis, diarrhea)
- Use of diuretics (which can cause dehydration)
- Use of nephrotoxic drugs (e.g., cyclosporine, amphotericin B, and aminoglycoside antibiotics)
- Use of nonsteroidal antiinflammatory drugs (NSAIDs)
- Rapid infusion of zoledronic acid

Owing to the risk for renal failure, zoledronic acid may be contraindicated in patients with significant renal impairment. When not contraindicated, dosage varies depending on the underlying condition and creatinine clearance.

Rarely, zoledronic acid has been associated with serious *AF*, resulting in hospitalization. In one trial, the incidence was 1.3% compared with 0.5% in patients taking placebo. Most cases developed more than 30 days after zoledronic acid infusion.

Administration. To minimize the risk for renal failure, zoledronic acid dosage should be kept low (5 mg or less per infusion), and the infusion should be slow (30 minutes or longer). In addition, the patient should be adequately hydrated before each infusion. To monitor for renal damage, creatinine clearance should be determined at baseline, before each dose, and periodically after each infusion. If renal impairment develops, Zoledronic acid dosage should be reduced or discontinued.

Estrogen

The basic pharmacology of estrogen, as well as postmenopausal estrogen therapy, is discussed in Chapter 50. Discussion here focuses on the role of estrogen in osteoporosis.

When estrogen levels decline, either because of natural menopause or surgical removal of the ovaries, osteoclasts increase in number, causing bone resorption to increase dramatically. Estrogen replacement can restore the brake on osteoclast proliferation and can therefore suppress resorption.

Low-dose estrogen (e.g., 0.3 mg/day) is recommended for the purpose of osteoporosis prevention. Women with an intact uterus should also receive a progestin (e.g., medroxyprogesterone) to minimize the risk for estrogen-induced endometrial cancer. For women without a uterus, the progestin is unnecessary.

For years, hormone therapy (HT)—estrogen with or without a progestin— had been considered the treatment of choice for preventing postmenopausal bone loss. Today, however, the benefits do not always outweigh the risks. Yes, HT does reduce bone loss and the risk for osteoporotic fractures; however, HT increases the risk for breast cancer, cholecystitis, and thromboembolic events such as myocardial infarction and stroke.

PATIENT EDUCATION

Bisphosphonates

> To minimize the risk for esophagitis, instruct patients to swallow the tablet whole with a full glass of water while sitting or standing upright. Explain that it is important to remain upright for at least 30 min (60 min with ibandronate).
>
> Intake of food, even in small amounts, prevents absorption of bisphosphonates. Instruct patients to take these drugs in the morning before eating or drinking anything other than water. (This applies to all oral bisphosphonates except Atelvia, a delayed-release brand of risedronate, which can and should be administered after eating.) After dosing, postpone ingesting anything—including orange juice, coffee, antacids, and calcium, iron, or magnesium supplements—for at least 30 min (60 min with ibandronate).

📄 SUMMARY OF KEY PRESCRIBING CONSIDERATIONS

Bisphosphonates

Therapeutic Goal: The goal is to prevent and treat osteoporosis by improving bone density and preventing bone loss.

Baseline Data: Obtain baseline axial DXA and height. Check serum calcium and 25(OH)D. Check creatinine level to assess for renal function. Conduct a pregnancy test, if indicated.

Monitoring: Check DXA every 1 to 2 years until stable, then every 2 years (or less, depending on patient status). Periodic monitoring of calcium, 25(OH)D, and creatinine is needed to assess ongoing status.

Identifying High-Risk Patients: *Oral* bisphosphonates are *contraindicated* for patients with esophageal disorders that can impede swallowing and for patients who cannot sit or stand for at least 30 min (60 min with ibandronate). They should also not be prescribed for patients with active upper GI problems. Bisphosphonates are not recommended for patients with creatinine levels below 30–35 mL/min. Low serum calcium and vitamin D should be corrected before instituting therapy and adequate levels should be maintained during therapy.

Zoledronic acid an IV bisphosphonate, is *contraindicated* for patients with acute renal failure or creatinine clearance below 35 mL/min and should be used with *caution* in patients who are older or dehydrated and in those with chronic renal impairment and those taking other nephrotoxic drugs.

Evaluating Therapeutic Effects: BMD increases, or at least remains constant, and fractures are prevented.

Minimizing Adverse Effects: Oral bisphosphonates can cause severe esophagitis, sometimes resulting in ulceration. Avoid these drugs in patients with esophageal disorders that could impede swallowing and in patients who are unable to sit or stand for 30 min (60 min with ibandronate).

Rarely, long-term bisphosphonate therapy has been associated with atypical fractures of the femur. To reduce risk, prescribers should do the following:

• Use these drugs only when needed (i.e., avoid bisphosphonates in patients considered at low risk for osteoporosis-related fractures).

• Consider alternative treatments, such as raloxifene or teriparatide, for patients with osteoporosis of the spine and normal (or only moderately reduced) BMD of the femoral neck or hip.

• Perform an annual reevaluation of the need for continued therapy in patients who have taken bisphosphonates for 5 years.

Oral bisphosphonates may (or may not) increase the risk for *esophageal cancer*. Reducing the dosing frequency (e.g., dosing monthly or weekly rather than daily) may reduce risk. It is also important to use precautions instituted to prevent esophagitis (i.e., taking the drug with a full glass of water and staying upright for 30–60 min after dosing.)

Rarely, bisphosphonates cause muscle, bone, and joint pain. NSAIDs will help with join discomfort as well as the flu-like symptoms that occur with some bisphosphonates. If pain is severe, opioids may be needed for short-term (a couple of days) relief. As a rule, pain gradually diminishes when bisphosphonates are withdrawn. In most cases, pain does not return when bisphosphonates are resumed. If it does resume, osteoporosis should be managed with a different drug (e.g., calcitonin, teriparatide, and raloxifene).

ONJ occurs primarily with IV bisphosphonates. To reduce ONJ risk, a dental examination with appropriate preventive dentistry should be conducted before giving bisphosphonates.

Intravenous *zoledronic acid* can damage the kidney, leading to acute renal failure. Carefully weigh benefits versus risks before prescribing to patients at increased risk (advanced age, chronic renal impairment, dehydration, or use of diuretics or nephrotoxic drugs). Before dosing, ensure the patient has adequate hydration and a creatinine clearance above 35 mL/min. To reduce risk, infuse zoledronic acid slowly (over 30 min or more). Monitor renal function by determining creatinine clearance at baseline, before each dose, and periodically after each infusion. If renal impairment develops, zoledronic acid dosage should be reduced or discontinued.

Despite the risks, estrogen is still approved for preventing and treating bone loss after menopause or surgical removal of the ovaries, because treatment reduces the overall risk for fractures by 24%. Estrogen is most effective when initiated immediately after menopause; however, treatment begun later in life can still offer significant protection. If estrogen is discontinued, a period of accelerated bone loss will ensue.

 BLACK BOX WARNING

Estrogen

Estrogen therapy is associated with an increased risk for endometrial cancer in women with a uterus who take unopposed estrogen as well as an increased risk for venous thromboembolic events (e.g., deep vein thrombosis and pulmonary embolism [PE]). It also may increase the risk for dementia in women 65 years and older.

Raloxifene

Raloxifene (Evista) belongs to a class of agents known as *selective estrogen receptor modulators* (SERMs). These are drugs that exert estrogenic effects in some tissues and antiestrogenic effects in others.

Like estrogen, raloxifene preserves BMD and reduces plasma levels of cholesterol. However, in contrast to estrogen, which promotes cancer of the breast and endometrium, raloxifene protects against these cancers. Because of its effects on bone, raloxifene is used to prevent and treat postmenopausal osteoporosis. Because of its effects on breast tissue, the drug is used to reduce the risk for breast cancer. Another SERM—tamoxifen—is used to *treat* breast cancer as well as prevent it (see Chapter 85).

Therapeutic Uses

Raloxifene has two indications: (1) prevention and treatment of osteoporosis in postmenopausal women and (2) protection against estrogen receptor-positive breast cancer.

Raloxifene can preserve or increase BMD, although not as effectively as estrogen. Raloxifene reduces the risk for *spinal* fractures by 55% but does not reduce the risk for fractures at other sites.

Raloxifene protects against estrogen receptor-positive breast cancer. It is approved for reducing the risk for invasive breast cancer in postmenopausal women who either (1) have osteoporosis or (2) are at high risk for breast cancer, even if they don't have osteoporosis.

Mechanism of Action

Raloxifene and other SERMs are structurally similar to estrogen, so they can bind to estrogen receptors. However, unlike estrogen, which functions as an agonist in all tissues, SERMs function as agonists in some tissues and antagonists in others. Hence SERMs can either mimic or block the actions of estrogen, depending on the SERM and the tissue involved. Raloxifene mimics the effects of estrogen on bone, lipid metabolism, and blood clotting and blocks estrogen effects in the breast and endometrium.

Adverse Effects and Interactions

Thromboembolic events. Like estrogen, raloxifene increases the risk for thromboembolic events such as deep vein thrombosis (DVT), pulmonary embolus (PE), and stroke. Because inactivity promotes DVT, patients should discontinue raloxifene at least 72 hours before prolonged immobilization (e.g., postsurgical recovery and extended bed rest) and should not resume the drug until full mobility has been restored. Also, patients should minimize periods of restricted activity, as can happen when traveling for long distances. Raloxifene is contraindicated for patients with a history of venous thrombotic events.

 BLACK BOX WARNING

Raloxifene

Raloxifene is associated with an increased risk for venous thromboembolic events (e.g., deep vein thrombosis and PE) and an increased risk for death from stroke when given to postmenopausal women who have a history or risk for coronary heart disease.

Fetal harm. Raloxifene should not be prescribed for pregnant women. In animal studies, doses below those used in humans have resulted in abortion, delayed fetal development, decreased neonatal survival, and anatomic abnormalities, including hydrocephaly and uterine hypoplasia. Although its use during pregnancy is obviously no concern for postmenopausal patients, it can be a concern for younger women taking the drug to prevent breast cancer.

Other adverse effects. Almost 10% of women taking raloxifene gain weight. Up to a third of patients experience hot flashes similar to those in women with menopause.

Comparison With Estrogen

The SERMs were developed in hope of creating a drug with all the benefits of estrogen and none of its drawbacks. Raloxifene partly fulfills this hope. Table 61.8 shows the ways in which estrogen and raloxifene are alike and different.

TABLE 61.8 Comparison of Estrogen and Raloxifene

Drug Target	Estrogen	Raloxifene
Bone	Increases BMD and reduces fracture risk	Increases BMD (but not as much as estrogen) and reduces fracture risk
Breast	Increases risk for breast cancer; causes breast enlargement and pain	Protects against breast cancer; does *not* cause breast enlargement or pain
Endometrium	Increases risk for endometrial cancer	Does *not* promote endometrial cancer and *may* offer protection
Plasma lipids	Lowers LDL cholesterol and raises HDL cholesterol	Lowers LDL cholesterol, but does not raise HDL cholesterol
Menopausal symptoms	Alleviates menopausal symptoms (e.g., hot flashes, vaginal dryness, and itching)	Does *not* alleviate menopausal symptoms and may actually increase hot flashes
Menstruation	Causes bleeding in 45% of postmenopausal women	Causes bleeding in 3%–5% of postmenopausal women
Blood clotting	Increases risk for DVT and pulmonary embolism	Increases risk for DVT and pulmonary embolism
Coronary heart disease	Black box warning related to cardiovascular disease	Black box warning related to cardiovascular disease
Developing fetus	Contraindicated during pregnancy because of possible fetal harm	Contraindicated during pregnancy because of possible fetal harm

BMD, Bone mineral density; *DVT,* deep vein thrombosis; *HDL,* high-density lipoprotein; *LDL,* low-density lipoprotein.

Preparations, Dosage, and Administration

Information on preparations, dosage, and administration for raloxifene and other non-bisphosphonates for osteoporosis are provided in Table 61.5.

PATIENT EDUCATION

Raloxifene

Advise women taking raloxifene for osteoporosis to ensure adequate intake of calcium and vitamin D.

Because raloxifene increases the risk for DVT, PE, and thrombotic stroke, advise patients to discontinue raloxifene at least 72 hours before prolonged immobilization (e.g., postsurgical recovery and extended bed rest) and to resume treatment only after full mobility has been restored. Instruct patients to avoid extended periods of restricted activity, as can happen when traveling.

Patients need to know that raloxifene can cause weight gain in some patients. Planning for reasonable intake and activity can prevent this adverse effect.

SUMMARY OF KEY PRESCRIBING CONSIDERATIONS

Raloxifene

Therapeutic Goal: Goals include prevention and treatment of postmenopausal osteoporosis and reduction of risk for invasive breast cancer in postmenopausal women who have osteoporosis or a high risk for breast cancer.

Baseline Data: Check axial DXA and height. Check serum calcium and 25(OH) D. Obtain a mammogram. Conduct a pregnancy test, if indicated.

Monitoring: Check DXA every 1 to 2 years until stable, then every 2 years (or less, depending on patient status). Check height annually. Monitor for increased back pain and, if present, consider spinal radiographs to determine vertebral fractures. Check weight periodically. Obtain yearly mammograms for patients taking raloxifene.

Identifying High-Risk Patients: Raloxifene is *contraindicated* for use by patients who are pregnant or have a history of venous thrombotic events.

Evaluating Therapeutic Effects: BMD increases, or at least remains constant, and fractures are prevented.

Minimizing Adverse Effects: Raloxifene increases the risk for DVT, PE, and thrombotic stroke. Do not give raloxifene to patients with a history of venous thrombotic events. Do not prescribe this drug for patients who require prolonged inactivity such as bed rest.

Small studies have determined that relaxation therapy can be effective in relieving hot flashes. Other interventions for hot flashes include maintaining a cool environment, avoidance of hot spicy foods, and losing weight, if needed.

Advise patients of the risk for weight gain. Instituting an exercise program and reasonable diet can help the patient be proactive in preventing this complication.

Bazedoxifene and Estrogen

Bazedoxifene, a SERM, and estrogen are available in a combination tablet (Duavee). It is available as 20 mg bazedoxifene and 0.45 mg conjugated estrogens to be taken once a day for postmenopausal osteoporosis. Additional information regarding this drug is available in Chapter 50.

Recombinant Parathyroid Hormone and Parathyroid Analog

Earlier we discussed the role of PTH in maintaining the serum calcium level within a narrow range. Two drugs take advantage of these actions to improve bone density: teriparatide, a form of PTH, and abaloparatide, a parathyroid analog. For both drugs, a lifetime limit of 2 years is recommended because the occurrence of osteosarcoma is dose-dependent in animal testing. (See Black Box Warning.)

BLACK BOX WARNING

Teriparatide and Abaloparatide

Teriparatide causes osteosarcoma in animal testing. This may indicate a potential increased risk for osteosarcoma in humans.

Teriparatide

Therapeutic uses. Teriparatide (Forteo) is a form of PTH produced by recombinant DNA technology. The drug has three indications: (1) treatment of osteoporosis in postmenopausal women, (2) treatment of osteoporosis in men, and (3) treatment of GIOP.

In postmenopausal women with documented osteoporosis, daily subQ injections of teriparatide for 18 months increased BMD of the lumbar spine and femoral neck and reduced the risk for vertebral fractures by 65%. Similar responses are seen in men. Teriparatide-induced increases in BMD are twice those seen with alendronate.

Mechanism of action. How does teriparatide parathyroid hormone (PTH) affect bone? The drug has two actions: it (1) increases bone resorption by osteoclasts and (2) increases bone deposition by osteoblasts. The net effect—resorption or deposition—depends on how the drug is administered. When given by continuous IV infusion, which produces a *steady* elevation of serum PTH, teriparatide *decreases* BMD, primarily by accelerating calcium resorption by osteoclasts. In contrast, when given by daily subQ injections, which produce *transient* elevations in serum PTH, the drug *increases* BMD, primarily by increasing bone deposition by osteoblasts.

Adverse effects. Adverse effects of teriparatide include nausea, headache, arthralgias, back pain, and leg cramps and injection site discomfort. Orthostatic hypotension and associated dizziness may occur within 4 hours of injection, so the patient should be in a location where it is possible to lie down, if needed. This adverse effect decreases after the first few doses. Temporary increases in serum levels of calcium and uric acid may occur.

Administration and storage. Teriparatide (Forteo) is supplied in special prefilled pen injectors that are designed to deliver a predetermined amount of drug with each activation. Each pen can be used up to 28 days after the first injection, after which it should be discarded, even if some drug remains. Patients should store the pens in a cold environment—2°C to 8°C (36°F to 46°F)—but not frozen, and should take them out of the cold only to make an injection. The cost for each injector (a 28-day supply) in the United States is greater than $3500, so treatment can be very expensive.

PATIENT EDUCATION

Teriparatide and Abaloparatide

Advise patients taking teriparatide and abaloparatide for osteoporosis to ensure adequate intake of calcium and vitamin D.

Instruct the patient to report a development of weakness, excessive tiredness, confusion, or bone pain because these can indicate a significant rise in calcium levels.

Explain that feeling dizzy or faint is common the first few hours after taking the first few doses. Instruct the patient to sit or lie down if this occurs.

Be certain that the patient understands that there is a potential risk for osteosarcoma with prolonged use; therefore there is a lifetime limit of 2 years for taking these drugs. If the patient changes providers in the future, it is important to inform new providers of a history of taking teriparatide or abaloparatide and the length of time it was taken.

Abaloparatide

Therapeutic uses. Abaloparatide (Tymlos) was approved in 2017 for the treatment of postmenopausal osteoporosis. This is currently its only indication, but additional indications are anticipated in the future.

Mechanism of action. Abaloparatide is an analog of PTH that acts as a PTH agonist at PTH1 receptors. This activation stimulates osteoblast activity. Osteoblasts build bone; therefore bone mass is increased.

Adverse effects. Adverse effects resemble those of teriparatide. The most common adverse effects of abaloparatide are increased uric acid levels, hypercalcemia, and erythema at the injection site. Antibody development increases by almost 50% (compared to 3% for patients taking teriparatide); however, no clinical significance has been identified.

Unlike teriparatide, special storage is not required. However, like teriparatide, this drug is expensive. Cost is greater than $2000 for a single month's supply.

 SUMMARY OF KEY PRESCRIBING CONSIDERATIONS

Recombinant Parathyroid Hormone and Parathyroid Analog (Teriparatide and Abaloparatide)

Therapeutic Goal: The goal is to prevent fracture and improve bone density in patients with osteoporosis.

Baseline Data: Check axial DXA and height. Obtain calcium and 25(OH)D levels. Consider uric acid level. Check pregnancy test, if indicated.

Monitoring: Check DXA every 1 to 2 years until stable, then every 2 years (or less, depending on patient status). Check height annually. Monitor for increased back pain and, if present, consider spinal radiographs to determine vertebral fractures. Monitor for signs and symptoms of kidney stones, which may increase due to elevated calcium levels.

Identifying High-Risk Patients: Patients with a history of urinary calculi may be at increased risk for recurrence. Patients taking drugs that decrease blood pressure may be at increased risk for orthostatic hypotension.

Evaluating Therapeutic Effects: BMD increases, or at least remains constant, and fractures are prevented.

Minimizing Adverse Effects: For approximately 4 h after injection, ensure the ability to lie down if orthostatic hypotension occurs. This side effect usually ends after several doses.

NSAIDs can help alleviate arthralgias and discomfort. Consider ketorolac over other NSAIDs if pain is severe.

Denosumab
Therapeutic Uses

Denosumab (Prolia and Xgeva) is a first-in-class receptor activator of nuclear factor kappa-B ligand (RANKL) inhibitor with four indications: (1) treatment of osteoporosis in men and postmenopausal women at high risk for fractures; (2) treatment of bone loss in men and women receiving certain anticancer therapy (e.g., androgen deprivation therapy for prostate cancer and aromatase inhibitor therapy for breast cancer); (3) GIOP; and (4) prevention of SREs in patients with bone metastases from solid tumors. Dosage is much higher in patients with bone metastases than in patients with osteoporosis; thus side effects are more severe in patients with bone metastases.

Denosumab is marketed under two trade names: Prolia and Xgeva. *Prolia* is used for men and women with a high risk for fractures or who have bone loss due to glucocorticoid anticancer therapy. *Xgeva* is used for bone metastases.

Denosumab was tested in a 3-year study that enrolled 7868 postmenopausal women with osteoporosis. Half the women received denosumab (60 mg injected subQ every 6 months), and the other half received placebo injections. All subjects also received at least 1000 mg of calcium daily and at least 400 IU of vitamin D daily. Compared with the women who got placebo injections, those who got denosumab had 68% fewer vertebral fractures, 40% fewer hip fractures, and 20% fewer fractures at other sites (wrist, leg, or shoulder). In a separate 12-month study, denosumab (60 mg subQ every 6 months) increased BMD at multiple sites (lumbar spine, femoral neck, trochanter, and radius) more effectively than oral alendronate (70 mg once a week). Taken together, these data suggest that denosumab is equal to bisphosphonates for treating postmenopausal osteoporosis.

Mechanism of Action

Denosumab is a monoclonal antibody (see Chapter 84) that decreases the formation and function of osteoclasts, thereby decreasing bone resorption and increasing BMD and bone strength. What's the underlying mechanism? Denosumab prevents the activation of a receptor known as receptor activator of nuclear factor kappa (RANK), found on the surface of osteoclasts and their precursor cells. Under normal conditions, RANK is activated by binding with an endogenous compound known as the *RANK ligand,* or simply RANKL. When activated by RANKL, RANK stimulates the formation and activity of osteoclasts. Denosumab binds with RANKL and prevents RANKL from activating RANK.

Adverse Effects

In postmenopausal women with osteoporosis, the most common adverse effects are back pain, pain in the extremities, musculoskeletal pain, hypercholesterolemia, and urinary bladder infection. In cancer patients with bone metastases, the most common adverse effects are fatigue, hypophosphatemia, and nausea. In all patients, suppression of bone turnover may delay fracture healing and increase the risk for new fractures and ONJ. The most serious adverse effects—hypocalcemia, infections, skin reactions, and ONJ—are discussed next.

Hypocalcemia. Denosumab can exacerbate preexisting hypocalcemia, presumably by reducing osteoclast activity. If hypocalcemia is present, it must be corrected before starting denosumab. The risk for hypocalcemia is elevated in patients with impaired renal function (including those on dialysis) and patients with other risk factors (e.g., a history of hypoparathyroidism, thyroid surgery, malabsorption syndromes, or excision of the small intestine). The manufacturer recommends monitoring levels of calcium, magnesium, and phosphorus in this at-risk group. To help prevent hypocalcemia when taking denosumab, all patients should take 1000 mg of calcium every day and at least 400 IU of vitamin D every day.

Serious infections. Denosumab increases the risk for serious infections, although the absolute risk is low. In clinical trials, some patients developed endocarditis, serious skin infections, and infections of the abdomen, urinary tract, and ear. Patients who develop signs of severe infection should seek immediate medical attention. Infection risk is increased in patients who are immunocompromised (e.g., owing to HIV infection or treatment with immunosuppressant drugs).

Dermatologic reactions. Denosumab increases the risk for dermatitis, eczema, rashes, and other skin reactions. Of note, these are not limited to the injection site. If a severe reaction occurs, discontinuation of denosumab should be considered.

Osteonecrosis of the jaw. Like the bisphosphonates, denosumab increases the risk for ONJ. Risk is further increased by invasive dental procedures (e.g., tooth extractions, dental implants, and oral surgery), and hence these should be conducted before starting denosumab. Patients who develop ONJ should be under the care of a dentist or oral surgeon. Maintaining good oral hygiene reduces ONJ risk.

Storage

Solutions should be stored under refrigeration and then warmed before use (by standing at room temperature for 15–30 minutes). All preparations should be clear and colorless (or pale yellow). Preparations that have particles or are cloudy or discolored should not be used.

PATIENT EDUCATION

Denosumab

Advise patients to ensure adequate intake of calcium and vitamin D. A dosage of 1000 mg of calcium with at least 400 IU of vitamin D daily is commonly recommended.

Instruct patients that denosumab may decrease their ability to fight infections. They should avoid contact with people who have a contagious disease and should practice good handwashing, especially when using public facilities.

Explain the need to report plans to have dental surgery. Maintain a routine plan for excellent dental hygiene. Report symptoms such as jaw pain and signs or symptoms of infection.

Emphasize the need to avoid stopping denosumab without first discussing this with the provider. The risk for bone fracture is increased after denosumab is discontinued.

SUMMARY OF KEY PRESCRIBING CONSIDERATIONS

Denosumab

Therapeutic Goal: The goal is to prevent fracture and improve bone density in patients with osteoporosis and to prevent bone injury in patients with metastatic bone lesions. In patients with hypercalcemia of malignancy, the goal is to maintain calcium serum levels within normal limits.

Baseline Data: Obtain axial DXA and height. Conduct a thorough oral exam. Obtain baseline calcium and 25(OH)D levels. Check a pregnancy test.

Monitoring: Check DXA every 1 to 2 years until stable, then every 2 years (or less, depending on patient status). Check height annually. Monitor for increased back pain and, if present, consider spinal radiographs to determine vertebral fractures. Check serum calcium, serum creatinine, and serum magnesium within the first 2 weeks of therapy and periodically thereafter.

Identifying High-Risk Patients: Patients with immunodeficiencies are at an increased risk for infection if taking denosumab. Patients with serious infections, even those with immunocompetence, should not take denosumab until the infection has resolved. Patients with hypocalcemia must have calcium levels corrected before receiving denosumab. Those with an increased risk for hypocalcemia have impaired renal function, a history of hypoparathyroidism or thyroid surgery, and malabsorption syndromes.

Evaluating Therapeutic Effects: BMD increases, or at least remains constant, and fractures are prevented.

Minimizing Adverse Effects: Supplemental calcium is important to prevent hypocalcemia.

NSAIDs, especially ketorolac, may help alleviate bone pain. Other pharmacologic and nonpharmacologic interventions for pain may be necessary. Excellent dental hygiene may have a role in reducing ONJ risk.

Drugs for Hypercalcemia

Furosemide

Furosemide, a loop diuretic, promotes renal excretion of calcium. This action is useful for treating hypercalcemic emergencies. In managing such emergencies, isotonic saline (IV) must be given before furosemide. The dosage of furosemide for adults is 80 to 100 mg every 1 to 2 hours as needed, infused no faster than 4 mg/min. To avoid fluid and electrolyte imbalance, urinary losses must be measured and replaced. The basic pharmacology of furosemide is discussed in Chapter 37.

Glucocorticoids

Glucocorticoids reduce intestinal absorption of calcium and can thereby reduce hypercalcemia. For severe hypercalcemia, parenteral glucocorticoid therapy is indicated (e.g., 100 to 500 mg hydrocortisone sodium succinate IV daily). Because glucocorticoids can produce serious adverse effects when taken chronically, the risks for long-term treatment must be carefully weighed against the benefits. The basic pharmacology of the glucocorticoids is discussed in Chapter 58.

Bisphosphonates

Pamidronate, etidronate, and zoledronic acid are approved for HCM. The mechanism is suppression of bone resorption by osteoclasts. The pharmacology of these agents is discussed previously.

Inorganic Phosphates

Phosphates reduce plasma levels of calcium and thus can be used to treat hypercalcemia. Suggested mechanisms for reducing plasma calcium include (1) decreased bone resorption, (2) increased bone formation, and (3) decreased intestinal absorption of calcium (secondary to decreased renal activation of vitamin D). Intravenous use of phosphates is hazardous and limited to patients with life-threatening hypercalcemia. Oral administration is considerably safer.

Oral phosphates are used for mild to moderate hypercalcemia. These agents should not be given to patients with renal impairment or elevated serum phosphate. Oral phosphates should not be combined with antacids that contain aluminum, magnesium, or calcium—agents that bind phosphate and prevent its absorption. Initial treatment should provide 1 to 2 g of phosphorus/day. Doses are reduced when serum calcium levels normalize.

Edetate Disodium

Edetate disodium (Endrate) is a chelating agent that binds calcium in the blood. As a result, it can rapidly reduce plasma levels of free calcium. The edetate disodium-calcium complex is filtered by the glomerulus but not reabsorbed by kidney tubules; hence renal excretion of calcium is increased. Although edetate disodium is highly effective at reducing hypercalcemia, it can be dangerous: It can cause profound hypocalcemia, resulting in tetany, convulsions, dysrhythmias, and possibly death. Severe nephrotoxicity can also occur. Because of its toxicity, edetate disodium is reserved only for life-threatening hypercalcemic crisis.

OSTEOPOROSIS

General Considerations

Osteoporosis is a serious medical problem characterized by low bone mass, altered bone architecture, and increased bone fragility. Because of bone fragility, patients are susceptible to fractures from minor traumatic events, such as coughing, rolling over in bed, or falling from a standing position.

Osteoporosis is the most common bone disease in humans. More than 10 million Americans have osteoporosis—80% of them older women—and another 34 million have reduced bone mass, a risk factor for osteoporosis. Every year, osteoporosis leads to 1.5 million fractures. The most common fracture sites are the vertebrae (spine), distal forearm (wrist), and femoral neck (hip). Vertebral fractures can result in loss of height, spinal deformity, chronic back pain, and impaired breathing. Complications from hip fractures are a significant cause of mortality: of the 300,000 Americans who get hip fractures each year, about 50,000 die of complications.

The economic burden of osteoporosis is high. Each year in the United States, osteoporosis-related fractures lead to more than 432,000 hospital admissions, nearly 2.5 million medical office visits, and about 180,000 admissions to nursing homes—at an estimated cost of $17 billion or $47 million a day.

Bone Mass

In men and women, bone mass changes across the life span. Bone mass peaks in the third decade, remains stable to age 50 years, and then slowly declines—at a rate that is usually less than 1% a year. In addition to this slow, aging-related decline, women go through a phase of *accelerated* bone loss (2%–3% a year) that begins after menopause and continues for several years. In both the slow and accelerated phases of decline, bone is lost because resorption of old bone outpaces deposition of new bone.

PATIENT-CENTERED CARE ACROSS THE LIFE SPAN

Drugs Affecting Bone Mineralization

Life Stage	Patient Care Concerns
Infants, children, and adolescents	With the exception of calcium and vitamin D, these drugs are not recommended for children, except denosumab when taken for bone cancer. In this instance, it is advised only for "skeletally mature" adolescents who are 13-17 years old.
Pregnant women	The drugs denosumab, estrogen, and raloxifene should not be prescribed for pregnant women. There is a theoretical concern that bisphosphonates could cause harm that has not yet been verified owing to inadequate long-term studies. Teriparatide and abaloparatide have not been sufficiently tested and should not be prescribed to pregnant women. Nasal spray formulations of calcitonin are not recommended during pregnancy. Vitamin D and calcium supplements are generally considered to be a concern only if the intake exceeds recommendations.
Breastfeeding women	Estrogen decreases both the quality and quantity of milk and may affect infant growth and development. For the remaining drugs, with the exception of calcium and vitamin D, breastfeeding is not recommended because of inadequate studies.
Older adults	Estrogen meets Beers Criteria (strength of recommendation: strong) for potentially inappropriate use in older patients. Because frail older adults commonly have difficulty swallowing, those who take bisphosphonates may be at an increased risk for esophagitis. Owing to occurrences of low-impact atypical femur fractures in older women who have had long-term bisphosphonate therapy, some orthopedists recommend against continuing bisphosphonate therapy beyond 5 years.

Primary Prevention: Calcium, Vitamin D, and Lifestyle

The risk for osteoporosis can be reduced by lifelong implementation of measures that can help maximize bone strength. Specifically, we need to ensure adequate intake of calcium and vitamin D, and we need to adopt a lifestyle that promotes bone health. Calcium is needed to maximize bone growth early in life and to maintain bone integrity later in life. Vitamin D is needed to ensure calcium absorption. The amount of calcium needed for optimal bone health is indicated in Table 61.1. Note that calcium requirements are greatest for adolescents and teens (1300 mg/day), then drop for younger adults (1000 mg/day), and then rise for older adults (1200 mg/day). If diet alone cannot meet calcium needs, supplements should be employed. Lifestyle measures that promote bone health include the following:

* Performing regular weight-bearing exercise (walking, yoga, dancing, racquet sports, weight lifting, and stair climbing)
* Avoiding excessive alcohol
* Avoiding smoking

Diagnosing Osteoporosis and Assessing Fracture Risk

Osteoporosis is diagnosed by measuring BMD, an important predictor of fracture risk. Both the National Osteoporosis Foundation (NOF) and the USPSTF recommend routine BMD testing for *all women* aged 65 years and above and for *younger postmenopausal women* deemed at increased risk for osteoporotic fractures. In addition, the NOF recommends testing of *all men* aged 70 years and older. (The USPSTF makes no recommendation regarding men.) BMD testing is not recommended for children or adolescents nor is routine testing indicated for premenopausal women or healthy young men.

The standard technique for measuring BMD is *dual-energy x-ray absorptiometry* (DEXA). DEXA scans only take a few minutes, and exposure to radiation is minimal—about $\frac{1}{10}$ that of a standard chest radiograph. Results of DEXA scans are reported in terms of *standard deviations* (SD) below mean BMD values in young adults. A BMD value that is 1 SD below the mean indicates 10% bone loss, a value that is 2 SD below the mean indicates 20% bone loss, and so forth. Using this system, the World Health Organization (WHO) has defined *normal* BMD for women as being no more than 1 SD below the mean for young adults. BMD values between 1 SD below the mean and 2.5 SD below the mean define *low bone mass* (also known as *osteopenia*). BMD values 2.5 SD or greater below the mean define *osteoporosis*. To simplify communication, we can talk about DEXA results in terms of a *T-score*, rather than using the phrase *SD above (or below) the mean*. For example, instead of saying that a BMD reading was 2.5 SD below the mean, we can simply say the T-score was −2.5.

Although loss of bone at one site (e.g., wrist) can predict the risk for fractures at other sites (e.g., hip and spine), it is preferable to measure BMD at specific sites to predict the risk for those sites. Accordingly, a thorough evaluation would include BMD measurements in the wrist, spine, and hip—the sites at which osteoporotic fractures occur most often.

Although we use BMD values to diagnose osteoporosis, it is important to understand that low BMD is not the only predictor of fractures. Other important predictors include a family history of hip fractures, a personal history of fractures, low body mass index, and use of oral glucocorticoids. To account for these risk factors, the WHO developed an important tool, called FRAX, which can assess an *individual*'s 10-year risk for experiencing a fracture. This web-based, interactive program is available online at www.shef.ac.uk/FRAX/. Individual risk is calculated after entering the following data:

* Age
* Gender
* Weight
* Height
* Previous fracture
* Hip fracture in a parent
* Secondary osteoporosis (i.e., malnutrition, hyperthyroidism, diabetes, and other disorders associated with osteoporosis)
* Rheumatoid arthritis
* Glucocorticoid use
* Current smoking

- Alcohol consumption
- Hip BMD

Of note, FRAX is tailored to specific countries and, for the United States, to four specific subgroups: African-Americans, Hispanics, Caucasians, and Asians.

Who Should Be Treated?

In 2016, the American Association of Clinical Endocrinologists (AACE) and the American College of Endocrinology (ACE) released joint clinical practice guidelines for diagnosis and treatment of postmenopausal osteoporosis. (See https://www.aace.com/files/postmenopausalguidelines.pdf.) According to this document, postmenopausal women and men 50 years and older should be considered for treatment if they present with any of the following:

- A hip fracture or vertebral fracture.
- Osteoporosis (T-score of −2.5 or less at the femoral neck or spine).
- Low bone mass (T-score between −1 and −2.5 at the femoral neck or spine) *plus either* a 10-year probability of a hip fracture of 3% or more *or* a 10-year probability of another major osteoporosis-related fracture of 20% or more, based on a US-adapted FRAX calculation.

Treating Osteoporosis in Women

The objective of osteoporosis treatment is to reduce the occurrence of fractures by maintaining or increasing bone strength.

Two types of drugs can be used: (1) agents that decrease bone resorption and (2) agents that promote bone formation. Antiresorptive drugs—estrogen, raloxifene, bisphosphonates, calcitonin, and denosumab—are used most often. These agents effectively prevent bone loss by reducing osteoclast activity but are largely unable to reverse bone loss that has already occurred. Accordingly, antiresorptive drugs are most beneficial when used early—before substantial loss has occurred. With all antiresorptive drugs, success requires a sufficiency of calcium and vitamin D. Currently, teriparatide (Forteo) is the only drug that effectively promotes bone formation. Of the drugs employed for osteoporosis, three agents—teriparatide, denosumab, and zoledronic acid (a bisphosphonate)—are most likely to reduce fractures.

Treating Osteoporosis in Men

In the United States, about 2 million men have aging-related osteoporosis and another 3 million are at risk. Hip fractures occur in 80,000 American men annually, compared with 269,000 American women. Of the men who get a hip fracture, 36% die within a year. Although rates of osteoporosis and fractures in men are significant, they are still much lower than in women. As discussed, bone mass in men peaks in the third decade and progressively declines at the age of 50 years. The rate of decline in men is about equal to that in women—except that in men, there is no counterpart to the accelerated phase of bone loss that occurs after menopause. If men and women lose bone mass at similar rates, why do men experience less osteoporosis? The main reason is that bones in men, at their peak, are larger and stronger than bones in women. Hence, after decline begins, male bones can tolerate more loss before fractures are likely. Factors that contribute to the risk for osteoporosis in men include low testosterone, prolonged use of glucocorticoids, white race, calcium deficiency, vitamin D deficiency, smoking, excessive alcohol consumption, and insufficient exercise. As in women, 10-year fracture risk can be assessed using the FRAX calculator developed by the WHO.

Treatment of male osteoporosis is confounded by a paucity of research. (Osteoporosis is one of the few areas of therapeutics in which research in women has greatly exceeded research in men.) At this time, only five drugs—*alendronate* (Fosamax), *risedronate* (Actonel),[a] *zoledronic acid* (Reclast), *teriparatide* (Forteo), and *denosumab* (Prolia)—are approved for osteoporosis in men. In one study, 2 years of alendronate increased BMD of the lumbar spine and hip and significantly decreased the incidence of vertebral fractures. Benefits with risedronate, zoledronic acid and teriparatide are similar. For alendronate, zoledronic acid and teriparatide, dosages are the same as those used in women. For risedronate, the only approved dosage is 35 mg once a week. Calcitonin has been tried in men, but proof of efficacy is lacking. If testosterone deficiency underlies osteoporosis, testosterone replacement therapy is indicated, unless the patient has testicular cancer or some other disorder that contraindicates testosterone use. All men should ensure adequate intake of calcium and vitamin D.

---

[a]The delayed-release formulation of risedronate, sold as *Atelvia,* is not approved for osteoporosis in men, although it *is* approved for osteoporosis in women.

62

Drugs for Asthma and Chronic Obstructive Pulmonary Disease

BASIC CONSIDERATIONS

Asthma is a common, chronic disorder that occurs in 1 in 11 children and 1 in 12 adults in the United States. Characteristic signs and symptoms are a sense of breathlessness and tightness in the chest, together with wheezing, dyspnea, and cough. The underlying cause is immune-mediated airway inflammation. According to the Centers for Disease Control and Prevention (CDC), more than 26.5 million people in the United States have the disease, representing an increase of 15% since the early 2000s. However, despite these increasing numbers, asthma management appears to be improving. This is reflected in the fact that, although the number of people with an asthma diagnosis has been increasing, the number of acute asthma episodes they experience is declining. With proper treatment, most patients can lead full lives with no limitations.

Chronic obstructive pulmonary disease (COPD) is a chronic, progressive, largely irreversible disorder characterized by airflow restrictions and inflammation. In most cases, COPD is preventable; the most common cause is smoking cigarettes. Symptoms include chronic cough, excessive sputum production, wheezing, dyspnea, and poor exercise tolerance. In the United States, COPD affects approximately 12 million, but an additional 12 million are estimated to be undiagnosed. In the most recent report by the CDC, chronic lower respiratory diseases were listed as the third leading cause of death in the United States. Unfortunately, although drug therapy is highly effective in asthma, benefits in COPD are minimal and limited to a small improvement in symptoms. Drug therapy does not slow disease progression, reduce hospitalizations, or prolong life.

Pathophysiology of Asthma

Asthma is a *chronic inflammatory* disorder of the airways. In approximately 50% of children with asthma and in some adults, airway inflammation results from an immune response to known allergens. In the remaining children and in most adults, the cause of airway inflammation is unknown—although as-yet unidentified allergens are suspected.

Fig. 62.1 depicts the events that lead to inflammation and bronchoconstriction in patients whose asthma is caused by specific allergens. Although this model may not apply completely to all asthma patients, it provides a basis for understanding the drugs used for treatment. The inflammatory process begins with binding of allergen molecules (e.g., house dust mite feces) to immunoglobulin E (IgE) antibodies on mast cells. This causes mast cells to release an assortment of mediators, including histamine, leukotrienes, prostaglandins, and interleukins.

These mediators have two effects. They act immediately to cause *bronchoconstriction*. In addition, they promote infiltration and activation of inflammatory cells (eosinophils, leukocytes, macrophages). These inflammatory cells then release mediators of their own. The end result is *airway inflammation,* characterized by edema, mucus plugging, and smooth muscle hypertrophy, all of which obstruct airflow. In addition, inflammation produces a state of *bronchial hyperreactivity.* Because of this state, mild trigger factors (e.g., cold air, exercise, tobacco smoke) are able to cause intense bronchoconstriction.

Pathophysiology of Chronic Obstructive Pulmonary Disease

Symptoms of COPD result largely from a combination of two pathologic processes: *chronic bronchitis* and *emphysema.* In most cases, both processes are caused by an exaggerated inflammatory reaction to cigarette smoke. Chronic bronchitis—defined by chronic cough and excessive sputum production—results from hypertrophy of mucus-secreting glands in the epithelium of the larger airways. Emphysema is defined as enlargement of the air space within the bronchioles and alveoli brought on by deterioration of the walls of these air spaces. Among individuals with COPD, the relative contribution of these two processes can vary. That is, some patients may suffer primarily from chronic bronchitis and some primarily from emphysema.

In addition to considerations of history and signs and symptoms of COPD, diagnosis of COPD requires spirometry testing. Patients who have signs and symptoms of COPD should be tested to measure the degree of airway obstruction. A postbronchodilator forced expiratory volume in 1 second (FEV_1)/forced vital capacity (FVC) of less than 0.7 is needed to confirm the COPD diagnosis.

Fig. 62.2 depicts the events that lead to inflammation, airway obstruction, and air trapping in patients with COPD. Irritants such as tobacco smoke initiate an inflammatory response in the airways. As a result of the frequent and recurrent irritation and the subsequent response by various leukocytes and inflammatory mediators, pathologic changes result in the bronchial edema and increase in mucus secretion that characterize chronic bronchitis. In addition, the continuous inflammation inhibits the production of protease inhibitors, which have a protective role in maintaining alveolar integrity. As a result of the inhibition, the protease enzymes break down elastin, resulting in the destruction of alveolar walls and the decrease in elastic recoil that characterize emphysema. In a small percentage of the population, emphysema results from a genetic alteration that results in α-1 antitrypsin deficiency. (α-1 Antitrypsin is a protease inhibitor that protects the lungs from enzymatic destruction by proteases.)

Fig. 62.1 Allergen-Induced Inflammation and Bronchospasm in Asthma.

Overview of Drugs for Asthma and Chronic Obstructive Pulmonary Disease

The major drugs for asthma and COPD are shown in Table 62.1. They fall into two main pharmacologic classes: *antiinflammatory agents* and *bronchodilators*. The principal antiinflammatory drugs are the *glucocorticoids*. The principal bronchodilators are the *β₂ agonists*. For chronic asthma and stable COPD, glucocorticoids are administered on a fixed schedule, almost always by inhalation. β₂ Agonists may be administered on a fixed schedule for long-term control or as needed (PRN) to manage an acute attack. Like the glucocorticoids, β₂ agonists are usually inhaled.

Administering Drugs by Inhalation

Most antiasthma drugs can be administered by inhalation. This route has three advantages: (1) therapeutic effects are enhanced by delivering drugs directly to their site of action, (2) systemic effects are minimized, and (3) relief of acute attacks is rapid. Three types of inhalation devices are usually used: metered-dose inhalers (MDIs), dry-powder inhalers (DPIs), and nebulizers. Some pharmaceutical companies also have developed specialized inhaler devices for their products.

Metered-Dose Inhalers

MDIs are small, hand-held, pressurized devices that deliver a measured dose of drug with each actuation. Dosing is usually accomplished with one or two inhalations. When two inhalations are needed, an interval of at least 1 minute should separate the first inhalation from the second.

PROTOTYPE DRUGS

Drugs for Asthma and Chronic Obstructive Pulmonary Disease

Antiinflammatory Drugs: Glucocorticoids
Beclomethasone (inhaled)
Prednisone (oral)

Antiinflammatory Drugs: Others
Cromolyn (mast cell stabilizer, inhaled)
Zafirlukast (leukotriene modifier, oral)

Antiinflammatory Drugs: Monoclonal Antibodies
Omalizumab (anti-IgE antibody)

Antiinflammatory Drugs: Phosphodiesterase-4 Inhibitors
Roflumilast (oral)

Bronchodilators: Anticholinergic Drugs
Ipratropium (inhaled, short acting)
Tiotropium (inhaled, long acting)

Bronchodilators: β₂-Adrenergic Agonists
Albuterol (inhaled, short acting)
Salmeterol (inhaled, long acting)

Bronchodilators: Methylxanthine
Theophylline (oral)

Fig. 62.2 Pathogenesis of Chronic Bronchitis and Emphysema.

When using most MDIs, the patient must begin to inhale before activating the device. This requires hand-breath coordination, making MDIs difficult to use correctly. Accordingly, patients will need a demonstration as well as written and verbal instruction. Even with optimal use, only approximately 10% of the dose reaches the lungs. Approximately 80% affects the oropharynx and is swallowed, and the remaining 10% is left in the device or exhaled.

Spacers are devices that attach directly to the MDI to increase delivery of drug to the lungs and decrease deposition of drug on the oropharyngeal mucosa (Fig. 62.3). Several kinds of spacers are available for use with MDIs. Some spacers contain a one-way valve that activates on inhalation, obviating the need for good hand-breath coordination. Some spacers also contain an alarm whistle that sounds off when inhalation is too rapid, thus maximizing effective drug administration. They can also prevent bronchospasm that may occur with sudden intake of an inhaled drug.

Dry-Powder Inhalers

DPIs are used to deliver drugs in the form of a dry, micronized powder directly to the lungs. Unlike MDIs, DPIs are breath activated. As a result, DPIs do not require the hand-breath coordination needed with MDIs, and so DPIs are much easier to use. Compared with MDIs, DPIs deliver more drug to the lungs (20% of the total released vs. 10%) and less to the oropharynx. In addition, spacers are not used with DPIs.

Nebulizers

A nebulizer is a small machine used to convert a drug solution into a mist. The droplets in the mist are much finer than those produced by inhalers, resulting in less drug deposit on the oropharynx and increased delivery to the lung. Inhalation of the nebulized mist can be done through a face mask or through a mouthpiece held between the teeth. Because the mist produced by a nebulizer is inhaled with each breath, hand-breath coordination is not a concern. Nebulizers take several

TABLE 62.1   Overview of Major Drugs for Asthma and Chronic Obstructive Pulmonary Disease

Antiinflammatory Drugs

Glucocorticoids

Inhaled

Beclomethasone dipropionate (QVAR)

Budesonide (Pulmicort Flexhaler, Pulmicort Respules, Pulmicort Turbuhaler 🍁)

Ciclesonide (Alvesco)

Flunisolide (Aerospan)

Fluticasone propionate (Flovent HFA, Flovent Diskus)

Mometasone furoate (Asmanex Twisthaler)

Oral

Methylprednisolone (A-Methapred, Depo-Medrol, Medrol, Medrol Dose-Pak)

Prednisolone (Flo-Pred, Orapred ODT, Millipred, Pediapred, Prelone, 🍁)

Prednisone (Deltasone, Winpred 🍁)

Leukotriene Receptor Antagonists

Montelukast, oral (Singulair)[a]

Zafirlukast, oral (Accolate)[a]

Zileuton, oral (Zyflo, Zyflo CR)[a]

Cromolyn

Cromolyn, inhaled (Nasalcrom)[a]

Immunoglobulin E Antagonist

Omalizumab, subcutaneous (Xolair)[a]

Phosphodiesterase-4 Inhibitors

Roflumilast, oral (Daliresp, Daxas 🍁)

Bronchodilators

β₂-Adrenergic Agonists

Inhaled: Short Acting

Albuterol (ProAir HFA, ProAir RespiClick, Proventil HFA, Ventolin HFA, Airomir 🍁, Apo-Salvent MDI 🍁)

Levalbuterol (Xopenex, Xopenex HFA)

Inhaled: Long Acting[b]

Arformoterol (Brovana)[c]

Formoterol (Foradil Aerolizer, Perforomist, Oxeze Turbuhaler 🍁)[b]

Indacaterol (Arcapta Neohaler, Onbrez Breezhaler 🍁)[c]

Olodaterol (Striverdi Respimat) [c]

Salmeterol (Serevent Diskus)[b]

Oral

Albuterol (VoSpire ER)

Terbutaline (generic only)

Methylxanthines

Aminophylline, oral (generic)

Theophylline, oral (Theo-24, Elixophyllin, Theolair 🍁, Theolair-SR, Pulmophylline, Theo ER 🍁)

Anticholinergics

Aclidinium bromide, inhaled (Tudorza Pressair) [c]

Glycopyrronium bromide, inhaled (Seebri Neohaler, Seebri Breezhaler 🍁)[c]

Ipratropium, inhaled (Atrovent HFA)

Tiotropium, inhaled (Spiriva, Spiriva HandiHaler, Spiriva Respimat)

Umeclidinium, inhaled (Incruse Ellipta)[c]

Antiinflammatory/Bronchodilator Combinations

Budesonide/formoterol, inhaled (Symbicort)

Fluticasone/salmeterol, inhaled (Advair Diskus, Advair HFA)

Fluticasone/vilanterol, inhaled (Breo Ellipta)

Mometasone/formoterol, inhaled (Dulera, Zenhale 🍁)

β Agonist/Cholinergic Antagonist Combinations

Albuterol/ipratropium, inhaled (Combivent Respimat, Combivent UDV 🍁)[c]

Indacaterol/glycopyrronium, inhaled (Utibron Neohaler, Ultibro Breezhaler 🍁)[c]

Olodaterol/tiotropium, inhaled (Stiolto Respimat)[c]

Vilanterol/umeclidinium, inhaled (Anoro Ellipta)[c]

[a]Approved only for asthma, not for chronic obstructive pulmonary disease.
[b]For treatment of asthma, must always be combined with an inhaled glucocorticoid.
[c]Approved only for chronic obstructive pulmonary disease, not for asthma.

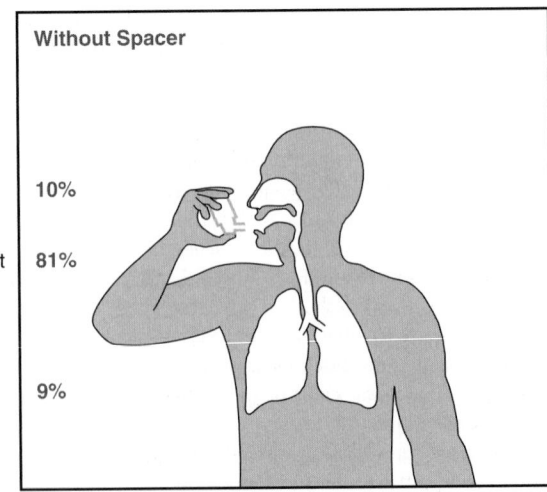

	With Spacer		Without Spacer
Inhaler device	57%		10%
Mouth and throat	22%		81%
Lungs	21%		9%

Fig. 62.3 Effect of a Spacer Device on the Distribution of Inhaled Medication. Note that, when a spacer is used, more medication reaches its site of action in the lungs and less is deposited in the mouth and throat.

minutes to deliver the same amount of drug contained in 1 inhalation from an inhaler, but for some patients, a nebulizer may be more effective than an inhaler. Although nebulizers are usually used at home or in a clinic or hospital, these devices, which weigh less than 10 pounds, are sufficiently portable for use in other locations.

ANTIINFLAMMATORY DRUGS

Antiinflammatory drugs—especially inhaled glucocorticoids—are the foundation of asthma and COPD therapy. These drugs are taken daily for long-term control. Most people with asthma require these drugs for management at some point.

PATIENT-CENTERED CARE ACROSS THE LIFE SPAN

Antiinflammatory Agents

Life Stage	Patient Care Concerns
Children	Inhaled glucocorticoids are the preferred long-term treatment for children of all ages, including infants. Face masks are recommended for administration of inhaled glucocorticoids to children younger than 4 years. Alternative treatments include cromolyn and leukotriene receptor antagonists (e.g., montelukast), but evidence supporting these drugs for asthma management is lower than that supporting inhaled glucocorticoids. Montelukast is the only leukotriene modifier approved for children aged 1–5 years.
Pregnant women	Inhaled glucocorticoids are preferred for uncontrolled asthma in pregnant women because uncontrolled asthma is associated with greater fetal risks. Of the leukotriene receptor antagonists, montelukast and zafirlukast are have a better safety profile than zileuton.
Breastfeeding women	Inhaled glucocorticoids are not a contraindication to breastfeeding. Women taking systemic glucocorticoids should not breastfeed.
Older adults	Benefits exceed risk. Inhaled glucocorticoids are much safer than systemic formulations.

Glucocorticoids

Glucocorticoids (e.g., budesonide, fluticasone) are the most effective drugs available for long-term control of airway inflammation. Administration is usually by inhalation but may also be intravenous (IV) or oral. Adverse reactions to inhaled glucocorticoids are generally minor, as are reactions to systemic glucocorticoids taken *acutely*. However, when *systemic* glucocorticoids are used *long term*, severe adverse effects are likely. The basic pharmacology of the glucocorticoids is presented in Chapter 58. Discussion here is limited to their use in asthma and COPD.

Mechanism of Action

Glucocorticoids reduce respiratory symptoms by *suppressing inflammation*. Specific antiinflammatory effects include the following:
- Decreased synthesis and release of inflammatory mediators (e.g., leukotrienes, histamine, prostaglandins)
- Decreased infiltration and activity of inflammatory cells (e.g., eosinophils, leukocytes)
- Decreased edema of the airway mucosa (secondary to a decrease in vascular permeability)

By suppressing inflammation, glucocorticoids reduce bronchial hyperreactivity and decrease airway mucus production. There is also some evidence that glucocorticoids may increase the number of bronchial β_2 receptors as well as their responsiveness to β_2 agonists.

Therapeutic Use

Glucocorticoids are used to control inflammation in both asthma and COPD. Although they are especially effective for asthma prophylaxis and for management of COPD exacerbations, glucocorticoids do not alter the natural course of these conditions, even when used in young children with asthma. However, they provide significant long-term control and management of symptoms, so the role they play is an important one.

Inhalation use. Inhaled glucocorticoids are very effective and are much safer than systemic glucocorticoids. Inhaled glucocorticoids are first-line therapy for management of the inflammatory component of asthma. Most patients with persistent asthma should use these drugs daily. There is conflicting evidence to support routine glucocorticoid use in COPD. Their primary use in COPD is in management of exacerbations.

Oral use. Oral glucocorticoids may be required for patients with moderate to severe persistent asthma or for management of acute exacerbations of asthma or COPD. Because of their potential for toxicity, these drugs are prescribed only when symptoms cannot be controlled with safer medications (inhaled glucocorticoids, inhaled β_2 agonists). Because the risk for toxicity increases with duration of use, treatment should be as brief as possible.

Adverse Effects

Inhaled glucocorticoids. Inhaled glucocorticoid preparations are largely devoid of serious toxicity, even when used in high doses.

The most common adverse effects are *oropharyngeal candidiasis* and *dysphonia* (hoarseness, speaking difficulty). Both effects result from local deposition of inhaled glucocorticoids. To minimize these effects, patients should rinse the mouth with water and gargle after each administration. Using a spacer device can help too. If candidiasis develops, it can be treated with an antifungal drug.

With long-term, high-dose therapy, some *adrenal suppression* may develop, although the degree of suppression is generally low for most patients. Children, especially those with a low body mass index (BMI) are at increased risk. For young children who have used inhaled glucocorticoids for longer than 6 months, the Pediatric Endocrine Society Drugs and Therapeutics Committee recommends monitoring for signs of adrenal insufficiency (hypoglycemia, hypotension, mental status alterations) and testing for adrenal insufficiency.

Glucocorticoids can *slow* growth in children and adolescents—but these drugs do *not* decrease final adult height. *Short-term* studies have shown that inhaled glucocorticoids slow growth; however, *long-term* studies indicate that adult height, although delayed, is not reduced. Less is known regarding whether glucocorticoids suppress growth and development of the brain, lungs, and other organs, in part because having asthma alone can affect organ growth. Because the benefits of inhaled glucocorticoids tend to be much greater than the risks, current guidelines for asthma management recommend these drugs for children while monitoring for evidence of complications.

Long-term use of inhaled glucocorticoids may promote *bone loss*. Fortunately, the amount of loss is much lower than the amount caused by oral glucocorticoids. To minimize bone loss, patients should (1) use the lowest dose that controls symptoms, (2) ensure adequate intake of calcium and vitamin D, and (3) participate in weight-bearing exercise.

There has been concern that prolonged therapy might increase the risk for *cataracts* and *glaucoma*. Although this may be an issue of concern with continuous use of high-dose inhaled glucocorticoids, this problem is not associated with long-term use of low to medium doses of inhaled glucocorticoids.

PATIENT EDUCATION

Glucocorticoids

Inform patients that glucocorticoids are intended for preventive therapy—not for aborting an ongoing attack. Instruct patients to administer glucocorticoids on a regular schedule—not as needed.

Instruct patients on the proper use of inhalers. Have patients demonstrate proper technique. If patients are prescribed both a short-acting β₂ agonist (SABA) and a glucocorticoid, explain that delivery of glucocorticoids to the airways can be enhanced by inhaling a SABA 5 minutes before inhaling the glucocorticoid.

Teach patients with chronic asthma to monitor and record peak expiratory flow (PEF), symptom frequency and symptom intensity, nighttime awakenings, effect on normal activity, and SABA use.

Advise patients to rinse their mouth and gargle after dosing to minimize dysphonia and oropharyngeal candidiasis.

Counsel patients to contact the clinic if they develop complications following a change from oral to inhaled glucocorticoids. Wearing a medical alert bracelet is advisable for patients who are at risk of adrenal insufficiency associated with long-term systemic use.

Advise patients to ensure adequate intake of calcium and vitamin D to decrease risk of bone loss. Performing weight-bearing exercise provides additional protection.

Oral glucocorticoids. When used acutely (less than 10 days), even in very high doses, oral glucocorticoids do not cause significant adverse effects. However, prolonged therapy, even in moderate doses, can be hazardous. Potential adverse effects include *adrenal suppression, osteoporosis, hyperglycemia, peptic ulcer disease,* and, in young patients, *growth suppression.*

Adrenal suppression is of particular concern. As discussed in Chapter 58, prolonged glucocorticoid use can decrease the ability of the adrenal cortex to produce glucocorticoids of its own. This can be life-threatening at times of severe physiologic stress (e.g., surgery, trauma, or systemic infection). Because high levels of glucocorticoids are required to survive severe stress and because adrenal suppression prevents production of endogenous glucocorticoids, *patients must be given increased doses of oral or IV glucocorticoids at times of stress. Failure to do so can prove fatal.*

Compensating for adrenal insufficiency. When patients have been on prolonged systemic glucocorticoid therapy, the adrenal glands decrease their endogenous production of glucocorticoids. If systemic therapy is stopped suddenly, as when switching from oral therapy to inhalation therapy, the patient can die. Similarly, during times of severe physical stress when the body would normally produce high levels of glucocorticoids, if the dose of systemic glucocorticoids is not increased to compensate, the patient can die. What important lesson can you take from this? When discontinuing a systemic glucocorticoid, you must be sure it is done gradually to allow the body to resume producing the endogenous hormone. On the other hand, if a patient taking systemic glucocorticoids experiences severe physical stress, such as a motor vehicle crash, or is scheduled for a stressful procedure, such as surgery, you must prescribe additional glucocorticoids to supplement for the endogenous hormone that the patient cannot produce.

Adrenal suppression is also a concern when discontinuing prolonged use of oral glucocorticoids or when transferring from an oral route to an inhaled route. Several months are required for recovery of adrenocortical function, so it is important to decrease the dosage gradually. Throughout this time, all patients—including those switched to inhaled glucocorticoids—must be given supplemental oral or IV glucocorticoids at times of severe stress.

Preparations, Dosage, and Administration

Inhaled glucocorticoids. Six glucocorticoids are available for inhalation (Table 62.2). Four are available in MDIs, three are available in DPIs, and one is available in suspension for nebulization. Inhaled glucocorticoids are administered on a regular schedule—not PRN. Pediatric and adult dosages are shown in Table 62.2. The dosage should be kept as low as possible to minimize adrenal suppression, possible bone loss, and other adverse effects.

Nebulized budesonide. Budesonide suspension (Pulmicort Respules) is the first inhaled glucocorticoid formulated for nebulized dosing. The product is approved for maintenance therapy of persistent asthma in children 1 to 8 years old. Improvement should begin in 2 to 8 days; maximal benefits may take 4 to 6 weeks to develop. Budesonide suspension is available in 2-mL ampules containing 250 or 500 μg of the drug. Administration is done with a jet nebulizer equipped with a mouthpiece or face mask; ultrasonic nebulizers should not be used. Administration

TABLE 62.2 Inhaled Glucocorticoids: Formulations and Dosages

Drug	Formulation	DOSAGE Adults	Children
Beclomethasone dipropionate (QVAR)	MDI: 40 or 80 μg/inhalation	40–320 μg twice daily	40–80 μg twice daily (5–11 years)
Budesonide			
(Pulmicort Flexhaler)	DPI: 90 or 180 μg/inhalation	360–720 μg twice daily	180–360 μg twice daily (6–17 years)
(Pulmicort Respules)	Suspension for nebulization	250–500 μg once or twice daily *or* 1000 μg once daily	500–1000 μg/day (1–8 years)
Ciclesonide (Alvesco)	MDI: 80 or 160 μg/inhalation	80–320 μg twice daily	80–320 μg twice daily (12 years and up)
Flunisolide (Aerospan)	MDI: 80 μg/inhalation	160–320 μg twice daily	80–320 μg twice daily (6–11 years)
Fluticasone propionate			
(Flovent HFA)	MDI: 44, 110, or 220 μg/inhalation	88–440 μg twice daily	88 μg twice daily (4–11 years)
(Flovent Diskus)	DPI: 50, 100, or 250 μg/inhalation	100–1000 μg twice daily	50–100 μg twice daily (4–11 years)
Mometasone furoate (Asmanex Twisthaler)	DPI: 110 or 220 μg/inhalation	220–440 μg once or twice daily	110 μg once daily (4–11 years)

DPI, Dry-powder inhaler; *MDI,* metered-dose inhaler.

takes 5 to 10 minutes. For children who are not taking an oral gluco-corticoid, the initial dosage is 500 μg/d in one or two doses. For children who are taking an oral glucocorticoid, the initial dosage is 1000 μg/d in one or two doses. After 1 week, dosage of the oral glucocorticoid should be tapered off.

Oral glucocorticoids. Methylprednisolone, prednisone, and prednisolone are preferred glucocorticoids for oral therapy of asthma. The dosage is the same regardless of the drug.

When beginning therapy with oral glucocorticoids, dosing initially focuses on bringing symptoms under control. For this reason, a higher dose is given initially followed by a gradually decreasing dosage. The goal is to use the lowest dosage that can keep the patient free of symptoms. For long-term treatment, alternate-day dosing is often used to minimize adrenal suppression.

 ## SUMMARY OF KEY PRESCRIBING CONSIDERATIONS

Inhaled Glucocorticoids

Therapeutic Goal: To achieve symptom control through suppression of airway inflammation

Baseline Data: History and physical with emphasis on respiratory system. Pulmonary function studies. Baseline height for children. Consider bone mineral density for older patients or others at risk.

Monitoring: Forced expiratory volume in 1 second (FEV$_1$), peak flow. Assess for oral candidiasis and glaucoma. Monitor for evidence of adrenal insufficiency (hypoglycemia, hypotension, mental status changes), especially in times of stress. For children: trend growth patterns; check for adrenal suppression if taking inhaled glucocorticoids for greater than 6 months.

Identifying High-Risk Patients: Inhaled glucocorticoids are contraindicated for patients with persistently positive sputum cultures for *Candida albicans.* (They are not contraindicated for oral candidiasis; however, they create an environment that supports growth of *C. albicans.*)

Evaluating Therapeutic Effects: Monitor peak expiratory flow, symptom frequency and symptom intensity, nighttime awakenings, effect on normal activity, and short-acting β$_2$ agonist use.

Minimizing Adverse Effects: If candidiasis develops, it can be treated with antifungal medication. In addition, using a spacer will decrease deposits onto the oropharynx, thereby decreasing the risk of developing this condition.

Adrenal suppression is a potentially life-threatening adverse effect of long-term glucocorticoid use. Although this is primarily a concern with systemic glucocorticoids, it can occur with long-term high-dose inhaled corticoids, especially at extremes of the life span. If it is discontinued or if the patient goes through a period of physical stress, observe for signs and symptoms of adrenal suppression. During times of severe physical stress when the body would normally produce high levels of glucocorticoids, systemic glucocorticoids should be given if adrenal suppression is suspected.

Leukotriene Receptor Antagonists

Leukotriene receptor antagonists (LTRAs) suppress the effects of leukotrienes, which are compounds that promote smooth muscle constriction, blood vessel permeability, and inflammatory responses through direct action as well as through recruitment of eosinophils and other inflammatory cells. In patients with asthma, these drugs can decrease bronchoconstriction and inflammatory responses such as edema and mucus secretion.

Three LTRAs are currently available: zileuton, zafirlukast, and montelukast. Zileuton blocks leukotriene synthesis; zafirlukast and montelukast block leukotriene receptors. All three drugs are dosed orally. (See Table 62.3 for preparations and dosages.) Current guidelines recommend using these agents as second-line therapy when an inhaled glucocorticoid cannot be used and as add-on therapy when an inhaled glucocorticoid alone is inadequate. Although generally well tolerated, all of the LTRAs can cause adverse neuropsychiatric effects, including depression, suicidal thinking, and suicidal behavior.

Zileuton

Zileuton (Zyflo, Zyflo CR), an inhibitor of leukotriene synthesis, is approved for asthma prophylaxis and maintenance therapy in adults and children 12 years and older. Symptomatic improvement can be seen within 1 to 2 hours of dosing. Because effects are not immediate, zileuton cannot be used to abort an ongoing attack. Zileuton is less effective than an inhaled glucocorticoid alone and appears to be less effective than a long-acting inhaled β$_2$ agonist as adjunctive therapy in patients not adequately controlled with an inhaled glucocorticoid.

Mechanism of action. Benefits derive from inhibiting 5-lipoxygenase, the enzyme that converts arachidonic acid into leukotrienes. This decreases the amount of leukotrienes available to induce inflammation.

Pharmacokinetics. Zileuton is given orally and undergoes rapid absorption, in both the presence and absence of food. Plasma levels peak 2 to 3 hours after dosing. Zileuton is rapidly metabolized by the liver, and the metabolites are excreted in the urine. Its plasma half-life is 2.5 hours.

Adverse effects. Zileuton can injure the liver, as evidenced by increased plasma levels of alanine aminotransferase (ALT) activity. A few patients have developed symptomatic hepatitis, which reversed after drug withdrawal. To reduce the risk for serious liver injury, ALT activity should be monitored. The recommended schedule is once a month for 3 months, then every 2 to 3 months for the remainder of the first year, and periodically thereafter.

Postmarketing reports indicate that zileuton and the other LTRAs can cause adverse neuropsychiatric effects, including depression, anxiety, agitation, abnormal dreams, hallucinations, insomnia, irritability, restlessness, and suicidal thinking and behavior. If these develop, switching to a different medication should be considered.

Zileuton is metabolized by cytochrome P450, where it acts as an inhibitor of CYP1A2 isoenzymes and can slow metabolism of drug substrates metabolized by this pathway, increasing their levels. Combined use with theophylline can markedly increase theophylline levels, so dosage of theophylline should be reduced. Zileuton can also increase levels of warfarin and propranolol.

Zafirlukast

Zafirlukast (Accolate) was the first representative of a unique group of antiinflammatory agents, the LTRAs. The drug is approved for maintenance therapy of chronic asthma in adults and children 5 years and older.

Mechanism of action. Benefits derive in part from reduced infiltration of inflammatory cells, resulting in decreased bronchoconstriction.

Pharmacokinetics. Zafirlukast is administered orally, and absorption is rapid. Food reduces absorption by 40%; therefore the drug should be administered at least 1 hour before meals or 2 hours after. Zafirlukast undergoes hepatic metabolism followed by fecal excretion. The half-life is approximately 10 hours but may be as long as 20 hours in older adults.

Adverse effects. The most common side effects of zafirlukast are headache and gastrointestinal (GI) disturbances, both of which are infrequent. Arthralgia and myalgia may also occur. Like zileuton, zafirlukast can cause depression, suicidal thinking, hallucinations, and other neuropsychiatric effects. A few patients have developed Churg-Strauss syndrome, a potentially fatal disorder characterized by weight

TABLE 62.3 Leukotriene Receptor Antagonists: Preparations and Dosages

Drug (Trade Name)	Preparation	Dosage
Montelukast (Singulair)	Granules: 4 mg/pkt Chewable tablets: 4 mg, 5 mg Tablets: 10 mg	12–23 months: one pkt of 4 mg granules daily 2–5 years: one pkt of 4 mg granules or one 4 mg tablet every evening 6–14 years: one 5 mg chewable tablet every evening 15 years and older: one 10 mg tablet every evening EIB prophylaxis: one 10-mg tablet at least 2 hours before exercising[a]
Zafirlukast (Accolate)	Tablets 10 mg, 20 mg	5–11 years: 10 mg tablet twice daily 12 years and older: 20 mg twice daily
Zileuton (Zyflo, Zyflo CR)	IR tablet: 600 mg ER tablet: 600 mg	12 years and older: • IR tablet: one 600 mg tablet 4 times daily • ER tablet: two 600 mg tablets twice daily

[a]No additional dose should be taken for at least 24 hours. Patients already taking montelukast daily should not take any more to prevent EIB.
EIB, Exercise-induced bronchospasm; *ER*, extended release; *IR*, immediate release; *Pkt*, Packet.

loss, flulike symptoms, and pulmonary vasculitis (blood vessel inflammation). However, in most cases, symptoms developed when glucocorticoids were being withdrawn, suggesting that glucocorticoid withdrawal may be a contributing factor.

Rarely, patients develop clinical signs of liver injury (e.g., abdominal pain, jaundice, fatigue). If these occur, zafirlukast should be discontinued, and liver function tests (especially serum ALT) should be performed immediately. If test results are consistent with liver injury, zafirlukast should not be resumed. Curiously, signs of liver injury have developed mainly in females.

Zafirlukast inhibits several isoenzymes of cytochrome P450 and can suppress metabolism of other drugs, causing their levels to rise. Concurrent use can raise serum theophylline to toxic levels. Theophylline levels should be closely monitored, especially when zafirlukast is started or stopped. Zafirlukast can also raise levels of warfarin and thus may cause bleeding.

Montelukast

Montelukast (Singulair), a leukotriene receptor blocker, is the most commonly used leukotriene modulator. The drug has three approved indications: (1) prophylaxis and maintenance therapy of asthma in patients at least 1 year old; (2) prevention of exercise-induced bronchospasm (EIB) in patients at least 15 years old; and (3) relief of allergic rhinitis (see Chapter 63). Montelukast cannot be used for quick relief of an asthma attack because effects develop too slowly. For prophylaxis and maintenance therapy of asthma, maximal effects develop within 24 hours of the first dose and are maintained with once-daily dosing in the evening. In clinical trials, montelukast decreased asthma-related nocturnal awakening, improved morning lung function, and decreased the need for a short-acting inhaled β_2 agonist throughout the day. Although montelukast is approved for preventing EIB, a SABA is preferred.

Mechanism of action. Montelukast has a high affinity for leukotriene receptors in the airway and on proinflammatory cells such as eosinophils. By occupying these receptors, the drug blocks receptor activation by the body's leukotrienes.

Pharmacokinetics. Montelukast is rapidly absorbed after oral administration. Bioavailability is approximately 64%. Blood levels peak 3 to 4 hours after ingestion. The drug is highly bound (more than 99%) to plasma proteins. Montelukast undergoes extensive metabolism by hepatic cytochrome P450 enzymes followed by excretion in the bile. The plasma half-life ranges from 2.7 to 5.5 hours.

Adverse effects. Montelukast is generally well tolerated. In clinical trials, adverse effects were equivalent to those of placebo. In contrast

to zileuton and zafirlukast, montelukast does not seem to cause liver injury. As with zafirlukast, Churg-Strauss syndrome has occurred when glucocorticoid dosage was reduced. Postmarketing reports suggest a link between montelukast and neuropsychiatric effects, especially mood changes and suicidality. Fortunately, these effects are rare.

Montelukast appears devoid of serious drug interactions. Unlike zileuton and zafirlukast, it does not increase levels of theophylline or warfarin. Concurrent use of phenytoin (an anticonvulsant that induces P450 isoenzymes) can decrease levels of montelukast.

Cromolyn

Cromolyn is an inhalational agent that suppresses bronchial inflammation. The drug is used for prophylaxis—not quick relief—in patients with mild to moderate asthma. Antiinflammatory effects are less than with glucocorticoids; therefore cromolyn is not a preferred drug for asthma therapy. However, when glucocorticoids create problems, cromolyn may be prescribed as alternative therapy.

Mechanism of Action

Cromolyn suppresses inflammation; it does not cause bronchodilation. The drug acts in part by stabilizing the cytoplasmic membrane of mast cells, preventing release of histamine and other mediators. In addition, cromolyn inhibits eosinophils, macrophages, and other inflammatory cells.

Pharmacokinetics

Cromolyn is administered by nebulizer. The fraction absorbed from the lungs is small and rarely produces significant systemic effects. Absorbed cromolyn is excreted unchanged in the urine.

Therapeutic Uses

Chronic asthma. Cromolyn is an alternative to inhaled glucocorticoids for prophylactic therapy of asthma. When administered on a fixed schedule, cromolyn reduces both the frequency and intensity of asthma attacks. Maximal effects may take several weeks to develop. No tolerance to effects is seen with long-term use. Cromolyn is especially effective for prophylaxis of seasonal allergic attacks and for acute allergy prophylaxis immediately before allergen exposure (e.g., before mowing the lawn).

Exercise-induced bronchospasm. Cromolyn can prevent bronchospasm in patients at risk for EIB. For best results, cromolyn should be administered 10 to 15 minutes before anticipated exertion but no longer than 1 hour before exercise.

Allergic rhinitis. Intranasal cromolyn (NasalCrom) can relieve symptoms of allergic rhinitis (see Chapter 63).

PATIENT EDUCATION
Cromolyn

Instruct patients on the proper use and care of nebulizers.

For acute prophylaxis, instruct patients to administer cromolyn 15 minutes before exercise and exposure to other precipitating factors (e.g., cold, environmental agents).

For long-term use, instruct patients to administer cromolyn on a regular schedule. Be sure to inform them that full therapeutic effects may take several weeks to develop.

Teach patients with chronic asthma to monitor and record peak expiratory flow, symptom frequency and symptom intensity, nighttime awakenings, effect on normal activity, and short-acting β_2 agonist use.

Adverse Effects

Cromolyn is the safest of all antiasthma medications. Significant adverse effects occur in fewer than 1 of every 10,000 patients. Occasionally, cough or bronchospasm occurs in response to cromolyn inhalation.

Preparations, Dosage, and Administration

Cromolyn is administered using a power-driven nebulizer. The initial dosage for adults and children is 20 mg 4 times a day. For maintenance therapy, the lowest effective dosage should be established.

Monoclonal Antibodies

Monoclonal antibodies form the newest drug category for management of airway inflammation. There are currently five drugs available in the United States: benralizumab, dupilumab, omalizumab, and mepolizumab, and reslizumab. None of these are approved as first-line agents, and none are approved for management of acute asthmatic episodes. (For additional information on monoclonal antibodies and other immunomodulators, see Chapter 84.)

Anti-IgE Antibody

Omalizumab. Omalizumab (Xolair) was the first monoclonal antibody to receive U.S. Food and Drug Administration (FDA) approval. Omalizumab is a monoclonal antibody with a unique mechanism of action: antagonism of the antibody IgE. The drug is a second-line agent indicated only for allergy-related asthma and only when preferred options have failed. Omalizumab offers modest benefits and has significant drawbacks: the drug poses a risk for anaphylaxis and cancer, must be given subcutaneously at a health care facility (due to a risk for serious reactions), and costs more than $10,000 a year. Furthermore, its long-term safety is unknown.

Mechanism of action. Omalizumab forms complexes with free IgE in the blood and thereby reduces the amount of IgE available to bind with its receptors on mast cells. This greatly reduces the number of IgE molecules on the mast cell surface and thus limits the ability of allergens to trigger release of histamine, leukotrienes, and other mediators that promote bronchospasm and airway inflammation. At recommended doses, omalizumab decreases free IgE in serum by 96%. When treatment stops, approximately 1 year is required for free IgE to return to its pretreatment level.

Therapeutic use. Omalizumab is approved for patients age 6 years and older with moderate to severe asthma that (1) is allergy related and that (2) cannot be controlled with an inhaled glucocorticoid. In clinical trials, the drug produced a modest decrease in the number of exacerbations and often permitted a reduction in glucocorticoid use. Because of its mechanism of action, omalizumab can help only patients whose asthma is caused by a specific allergen (e.g., pet dander, dust mite feces). Accordingly, a skin test or blood test proving allergen

reactivity is required. Unless instructed otherwise, patients should continue all asthma medications they were using before starting omalizumab.

Pharmacokinetics. Omalizumab is administered by subcutaneous (subQ) injection, and absorption is slow, producing peak plasma levels in 7 to 8 days. Degradation occurs in the liver. The drug's half-life is prolonged, approximately 26 days.

▶ BLACK BOX WARNING
Omalizumab (Xolair)

Omalizumab carries a risk for anaphylaxis that may occur at any time during the course of treatment. Patients should be notified of signs or symptoms that necessitate seeking medical care. Patients should be routinely monitored after administration in health care settings.

Adverse effects. Omalizumab can cause a variety of adverse effects. The most common are injection-site reactions, viral infection, upper respiratory infection, sinusitis, headache, and pharyngitis. Early clinical trials suggested a very small risk for cardiovascular problems and malignancy. A meta-analysis of postmarketing studies revealed no significant increase in cardiovascular events between subjects taking omalizumab and a placebo. There was a small increase in rare malignancy occurrence in subjects taking omalizumab; however, a clear relationship to the drug has not been established. Possible adverse consequences of long-term IgE suppression are unknown.

Life-threatening anaphylaxis—characterized by urticaria and edema of the throat and/or tongue—has occurred rarely (in less than 0.1% of patients). Anaphylaxis is most likely with the first dose but can also occur after receiving repeated doses with no apparent sensitivity. To minimize injury from anaphylaxis, patients should be observed for 2 hours after the first three doses and for 30 minutes after all subsequent doses. Facilities for managing anaphylaxis should be immediately available. Patients who experience a severe reaction should not be given omalizumab again.

Preparations, dosage, and administration. Omalizumab (Xolair) is available as a powder (202.5 mg) in single-use vials for reconstitution with 1.4 mL of sterile water. Dissolving the powder, which can take 20 minutes or longer, yields a final solution of 150 mg/1.2 mL. Administration is by subQ injection, which may take 5 to 10 seconds because the solution is somewhat viscous. The reconstituted solution should be used within 4 hours (if stored at room temperature) or within 8 hours (if stored cold). Omalizumab powder should be kept refrigerated.

The size of each dose and the dosing interval are determined by body weight and total serum IgE, measured at baseline. Dosages range from 150 to 300 mg every 4 weeks, to 225 to 375 mg every 2 weeks. No more than 150 mg should be injected at any site. If a dose exceeds 150 mg, it should be divided among two or more sites. Additional information on preparations and dosage of omalizumab and the other monoclonal antibodies for asthma is provided in Table 62.4.

Interleukin-5 Receptor Antagonists
Benralizumab, mepolizumab, and reslizumab

Actions and uses. Interleukin-5 (IL-5) is a selective cytokine that is responsible for the differentiation and maturation of eosinophils in the bone marrow. By inhibiting IL-5, IL-5 receptor antagonists decrease the production of eosinophils. Because these drugs are targeted specifically toward eosinophils, their approved use is restricted for the treatment of severe eosinophilic asthma. They are not indicated for first-line asthma

TABLE 62.4   Preparations and Dosages of Monoclonal Antibodies for Asthma

Drug Class and Drug	Preparation	Dosage	Cost
Interleukin-4 Receptor Antagonist			
Dupilumab (Dupixent)	Prefilled syringe: 200 mg/1.14 mL, 300 mg/2 mL	Two 200 mg doses subQ initially, then 200 mg every other week Or Two 300 mg doses subQ initially, then 300 mg every other week.	$1,542.92 per 200 mg dose $1,758.92 per 300 mg dose
Interleukin-5 Receptor Antagonist			
Benralizumab (Fasenra)	Prefilled syringe: 30 mg/mL	30 mg subQ every 4 weeks for 3 doses, then once every 8 weeks	$5,702.53 per dose
Mepolizumab (Nucala)	Solution (reconstituted): 100 mg	100 mg subQ once every 4 weeks	$3,442.40 per dose
Reslizumab (Cinqair)	Solution (IV): 100 mg/10 mL	3 mg/kg IV every 4 weeks	$1935.36 per dose for patient weighing 132 lb (60 kg)
Anti-IgE Antibody			
Omalizumab (Xolair)	Prefilled syringe: 75 mg/0.5 mL, 150 mg/mL Solution (reconstituted): 100 mg	150–375 mg subQ every 2 or 4 weeks[a]	$1,301.59–$3,253.98 per dose

[a]Dosage is based on pretreatment IgE and patient weight.

IgE, Immunoglobulin E; *IV*, intravenous; *SubQ*, subcutaneous.

PATIENT-CENTERED CARE ACROSS THE LIFE SPAN

Monoclonal Antibodies for Asthma

Life Stage	Considerations or Concerns
Children	Omalizumab was recently approved for children as young as 6 years. Benralizumab, dupilumab, and mepolizumab are approved for children age 12 years and older. Reslizumab is not approved for children.
Pregnant women	No adverse events have been reported in animal reproduction studies, but little is known about their effects in humans. For omalizumab, pregnancy registry data did not demonstrate an increase in fetal anomalies or poor pregnancy outcomes.
Breastfeeding women	The amount of these drugs that is excreted into breast milk is unknown. Manufacturers of these drugs urge consideration of risks to infant versus benefits of drug therapy for mother.
Older adults	No additional complications have been reported for older adults. No dosage adjustments are required for renal or hepatic impairment.

management but are indicated for add-on management when traditional therapy is inadequate.

There are currently three approved IL-5 receptor antagonists: benralizumab (Fasenra), mepolizumab (Nucala), and reslizumab (Cinqair). Benralizumab and mepolizumab are administered subcutaneously; reslizumab is administered intravenously.

Adverse effects. In clinical trials, there were few adverse effects noted. For benralizumab and mepolizumab, headache was the most common adverse effect (8% and 20%, respectively). This was followed by

pharyngitis (5%) for benralizumab and injection site reaction (8%), back pain (5%), and fatigue (5%) for mepolizumab. Other adverse effects occurred at less than 1%. For reslizumab, 3% developed sore throat. Transient increases in creatinine phosphokinase (CPK) occurred in 14% of those taking reslizumab, but the significance in this increase is unknown. (Interestingly, CPK elevations occurred in 9% of those receiving the placebo.)

Reslizumab carries a black box warning related to the anaphylaxis events that occurred among 0.3% of subjects in clinical trials. A variety of malignancies occurred among 0.6% of subjects who participated in clinical trials (compared with 0.3% taking a placebo); however, there is no common type. Whether this occurrence was related to reslizumab is not proven.

BLACK BOX WARNING

Reslizumab (Cinqair)

Anaphylaxis occurred during clinical trials. These episodes occurred as early as the second dose and either during administration or within 20 minutes of completion. Patients should be routinely monitored after administration in health care settings.

A potential for immunogenicity was noted during clinical trials. Among subjects receiving benralizumab, 13% developed antibenralizumab antibodies. In trials with mepolizumab, 6% developed antimepolizumab antibodies. Antireslizumab antibodies developed in 5% of subjects treated in clinical studies.

Hypersensitivity is currently the only contraindication for IL-5 receptor antagonists. It is not known whether these drugs have a significant effect in helminth infections because this was among the exclusion criteria for clinical trials. However, because eosinophils play a vital role in the immune response to helminth (worm) infections, it is recommended that patients be treated for any known helminth infections prior to beginning these drugs.

Interleukin-4 Receptor Alpha Antagonists

Dupilumab. Dupilumab (Dupixent) received FDA approval for management of moderate-to-severe asthma in late 2018. It is currently the only approved IL-4 α-antagonist for management of asthma.

Actions and uses. IL-4 is an inflammatory cytokine. Many types of cells express IL-4 receptor α (IL-4Rα) subunits. These include eosinophils, mast cells, macrophages, and other cells involved in the inflammatory process.

Dupilumab is a monoclonal IgG4 antibody that binds to the IL-4Rα subunit. Blocking IL-4Rα signaling inhibits IL-4 cytokine-induced inflammatory responses. In addition, because IL-13 receptor complexes are also on the IL-4Rα subunit, IL-13 inflammatory responses are also decreased.

Dupilumab is not a first-line drug. Its use is restricted to patients with either eosinophilic asthma or with dependence on oral glucocorticoids. Dupilumab is also approved for management of moderate to severe atopic dermatitis.

Adverse effects. In clinical trials, 14% to 18% of patients using dupilumab developed a local injection site reaction. adverse effects included conjunctivitis (9% to 10%) and oral herpes (3% to 4%). Eosinophilia occurred in 2% of subjects. Development of antidupilumab antibodies occurred in approximately 9% of subjects.

There are no contraindications for dupilumab other than hypersensitivity. For patients with helminth infestation, treatment of the infection is warranted prior to starting therapy with dupilumab.

Phosphodiesterase-4 Inhibitors

Roflumilast

One phosphodiesterase 4 (PDE4) inhibitor, Roflumilast (Daliresp. Daxas) is approved for management of COPD. In patients with severe, chronic COPD with a primary chronic bronchitis component, the risk for exacerbations may be reduced with this drug.

Mechanism of action. Roflumilast is a selective inhibitor of PDE, an enzyme that inactivates cyclic adenosine monophosphate (cAMP). By raising levels of cAMP in lung cells, the drug reduces inflammation by suppressing cytokine release and by decreasing pulmonary infiltration by neutrophils and other white blood cells. As a result, cough and excessive mucus production are reduced and mucociliary clearance is improved.

Therapeutic use. Romflumilast is approved only for management of COPD. It is not a first-line drug; rather, it is used for exacerbation prophylaxis in patients with severe COPD with a primary chronic bronchitis component and a history of frequent exacerbations.

Pharmacokinetics. Romflumilast has a bioavailability approximating 80%. It peaks in approximately 1 hour, although this is delayed if taken with food. It is 99% protein bound with a half-life of 17 hours. Metabolism to its active metabolite is via CYP3A4 and CYP1A2 isoenzymes. Excretions is primarily through urine.

Adverse effects. Adverse effects include diarrhea, reduced appetite, weight loss, nausea, headache, back pain, and insomnia. It should be prescribed with caution for patients with depression. Safety in pregnancy has not been established; however, adverse events occurred in animal reproduction studies. Breastfeeding is not recommended when taking this drug. That being said, because COPD is uncommonly among women of child-bearing age, this is not typically a concern.

Preparations, dosage, and administration. Romflumilast is available in oral tablets containing 250 and 500 µg. Recommended dosing is 250 µg daily for 4 weeks and then 500 µg daily. It may be administered with or without food. Administering with food will delay the time of absorption but not the extent.

BRONCHODILATORS

Bronchodilators provide symptomatic relief in patients with asthma and COPD but do not alter the underlying inflammation that is part of the disease process. This is why most patients who require a bronchodilator also use an inhaled glucocorticoid for long-term suppression of inflammation. Monotherapy with a bronchodilator is appropriate only when asthma is very mild and attacks are infrequent.

β₂-Adrenergic Agonists

Inhaled β₂ agonists are the most effective drugs available for relieving acute bronchospasm and preventing EIB. Virtually all patients with asthma use these first-line drugs as a component of an asthma management regimen. The basic pharmacology of the β₂ agonists is presented in Chapter 15. Discussion here is limited to their use in asthma.

PATIENT-CENTERED CARE ACROSS THE LIFE SPAN

Bronchodilators

Life Stage	Patient Care Concerns
Children	Although they may be used for younger children, short-acting β₂ agonists are approved for children 2 years and older. Special delivery devices such as nebulizers may be used for very young children. Safety and efficacy of anticholinergics has not been established for children younger than 11 years. Methylxanthines are approved for children of all ages, including neonates. It is important to consider variable drug clearance across age ranges when dosing.
Pregnant women	β₂ Agonists may cause uterine relaxation; however, expert guidelines note that benefits are greater than risks. Pregnant women must have adequate respiratory exchange to ensure adequate oxygenation of the developing fetus. Inhaled anticholinergics are among the safer drugs for pregnant women. Methylxanthines have been associated with adverse effects in some animal reproduction studies.
Breastfeeding women	Breastfeeding is not contraindicated with β₂ agonists or anticholinergics; however, manufacturers of both drugs recommend caution. Labeling for methylxanthines warns against breastfeeding only if the mother may have toxic levels.
Older adults	Benefits exceed risks for β-agonists and anticholinergics. Systemic anticholinergics are included in Beers Criteria for Potentially Inappropriate Use in Older Adults; they should not be substituted for inhaled anticholinergics. Older patients are at much higher risk for toxicity when taking methylxanthines.

Mechanism of Action

The β₂ agonists are sympathomimetic drugs that activate β₂-adrenergic receptors. By activating β₂ receptors in smooth muscle of the lung, these drugs promote *bronchodilation* and thus relieve bronchospasm. In addition, β₂ agonists have a limited role in suppressing histamine release in the lung and increasing ciliary motility.

Classification by Route and Time Course

β₂ Agonists may be administered orally or by inhalation, and their effects may be brief or prolonged. All of the oral agents are long acting.

Among the inhaled agents, some are short acting and some are long acting. With the short-acting inhaled preparations, effects begin almost immediately, peak in 30 to 60 minutes, and persist for 3 to 5 hours. Because of this time course, the SABAs can be used to abort an ongoing attack but cannot be used for prolonged prophylaxis. With the inhaled long-acting β₂ agonists (LABAs), onset depends on the drug: with formoterol and arformoterol, onset is relatively rapid, whereas with salmeterol, onset is delayed. However, because these drugs are used on a fixed schedule for long-term control, the difference in onset is not very important.

Inhaled short-acting β₂ agonists. SABAs are taken PRN to abort an ongoing attack. In patients with EIB, they are taken before exercise to prevent an attack from occurring. For hospitalized patients undergoing a severe acute attack, a nebulized SABA is the traditional treatment of choice. However, delivery with an MDI in the outpatient setting may be equally effective.

Long-acting inhaled β₂ agonists. Patients who experience frequent attacks may be prescribed a LABA for long-term control. Dosing is done on a fixed schedule, not PRN. LABAs are preferred over SABAs for patients with stable COPD. However, in patients with asthma, LABAs are not first-line therapy, and they must always be *combined with a glucocorticoid.* In fact, their use *alone* in asthma is *contraindicated* because LABA monotherapy has been associated with increased incidence of asthma-associated death.[a] For combined LABA-glucocorticoid therapy, the FDA recommends using a product that contains both drugs in the same inhaler.

 BLACK BOX WARNING

Long-Acting β₂-Adrenergic Agonists

All long-acting β₂ agonists (LABAs) carry a risk for asthma-related deaths. To attenuate this risk, the use of LABAs as monotherapy is contraindicated. LABAs should only be prescribed as a component of long-term therapy with medications such as inhaled glucocorticoids.

Oral β₂ agonists. These drugs are used only for long-term control. Onset is too slow to abort an ongoing attack. Like the long-acting inhaled β₂ agonists, the oral agents are not first-line therapy.

Adverse Effects

Inhaled preparations: short acting. Inhaled SABAs are well tolerated. Systemic effects—tachycardia, angina, and tremor—can occur but are usually minimal.

Inhaled preparations: long acting. Inhaled LABAs may increase the risk for severe asthma and asthma-related death when used as monotherapy for long-term control. To minimize risk, LABAs should be used only in patients taking a recommended medication for long-term control and only if that medication has been inadequate by itself. LABAs should never be used as first-line therapy for prolonged control and should never be used alone.

Oral preparations. The selectivity of the β₂-adrenergic agonists is only relative, not absolute. Accordingly, when these drugs are administered orally, they are likely to produce some activation of β₁ receptors in the heart. If dosage is excessive, stimulation of cardiac β₁ receptors can cause *angina pectoris* and *tachydysrhythmias.* Patients should be instructed to report chest pain or changes in heart rate or rhythm.

---

[a]Although using a LABA alone is contraindicated for patients with asthma, LABAs can still be used alone in patients with COPD.

PATIENT EDUCATION
β₂-Adrenergic Agonists

Instruct patients on the proper use of this inhalers. Have patients demonstrate proper technique.

For patients who have difficulty with hand-breath coordination, using a spacer with a one-way valve may improve results.

Advise patients with asthma to assess peak expiratory flow daily and compare with personal best. Counsel patients to keep a record of these assessments along with symptom frequency and symptom intensity, nighttime awakenings, effect on normal activity, and short-acting β₂ agonist (SABA) use.

Inform patients who are using metered-dose inhalers or dry-powder inhalers that, when two inhalations are needed, an interval of at least 1 minute should elapse between inhalations.

Instruct patients to report chest pain associated with changes in heart rate or rhythm. This could indicate cardiac stress secondary to adrenergic effects.

Warn patients against exceeding recommended dosages. If worsening symptoms require more frequent use of a SABA, the provider should be notified.

Inform patients that inhaled LABAs (formoterol, arformoterol, and salmeterol) should be taken on a fixed schedule—not as needed (PRN)—and always in combination with an inhaled glucocorticoid.

Instruct patients to take oral β₂ agonists on a fixed schedule—not PRN. Sustained-release preparations should be swallowed intact, without crushing or chewing.

Oral β₂ agonists often cause *tremor* by activating β₂ receptors in skeletal muscle. Tremor can be reduced by lowering the dosage. With continued drug use, tremor declines spontaneously.

Preparations, Dosage, and Administration

Nine selective β₂ agonists are available (Table 62.5). Some are used for quick relief and some for long-term control.

Inhaled preparations for quick relief. To provide quick relief, β₂ agonists must be administered by inhalation. Three types of devices may be used: MDIs, DPIs, and nebulizers.

For drugs administered with an MDI or DPI, the initial dosing schedule is one or two inhalations 3 or 4 times a day.

When two inhalations are needed, an interval of 1 minute or longer should separate them. During this interval, some bronchodilation develops, facilitating penetration of the second inhalation.

For certain patients, nebulizers may be superior to inhalers. Some patients who have become unresponsive to a β₂ agonist delivered with an inhaler may respond to the same drug when it is given with a nebulizer. The nebulizer delivers the dose slowly (over several minutes); as the bronchi gradually dilate, the drug gains deeper and deeper access to the lungs.

Inhaled preparations for long-term control. Three single-agent inhaled LABAs are approved for treatment of asthma: salmeterol (Serevent Diskus), formoterol (Foradil Aerolizer), and arformoterol (Brovana), the *(R,R)*-enantiomer of formoterol. Vilanterol, another LABA, is available only in combination with a glucocorticoid (fluticasone/vilanterol [Breo Ellipta] and umeclidinium/vilanterol [Anoro Ellipta]). LABAs have a long duration of action and thus are suited for long-term control. Dosing is every 12 hours. If supplemental bronchodilation is needed between doses, a SABA should be used. As discussed previously, LABAs are not first-choice agents for long-term control, and they should not be used alone. Rather, they should always be combined with an inhaled glucocorticoid, preferably in the same inhaler device.

TABLE 62.5   β₂-Adrenergic Agonists

Drug (Trade Name)	Formulation	INITIAL DOSAGE	
		Adults	Children
Inhaled Agents: Short Acting			
Albuterol			
(ProAir HFA, ProAir RespiClick, Proventil HFA, Ventolin HFA)	MDI (90 µg/inhalation)	2 inhalations every 4–6 h PRN	2 inhalations every 4–6 h PRN
(Proventil)	Solution for nebulization	1.25–5 mg every 4–8 h PRN	0.63–2.5 mg/kg every 4–6 h PRN
Levalbuterol			
(Xopenex HFA)	MDI (45 µg/inhalation)	2 inhalations every 4–6 h PRN	2 inhalations every 4–6 h PRN
(Xopenex)	Solution for nebulization	0.63 mg every 6–8 h PRN	0.31–1.25 mg every 4–6 h PRN
Inhaled Agents: Long Acting[a]			
Aclidinium bromide[b] (Tudorza Pressair)	DPI (400 µg/inhalation)	1 inhalation every 12 h	Safety and efficacy not established
Arformoterol[b] (Brovana)	Solution for nebulization	15 µg every 12 h	Safety and efficacy not established
Formoterol			
(Foradil Aerolizer)[a]	DPI (12 µg/inhalation)	1 inhalation every 12 h	1 inhalation every 12 h
(Perforomist)[b]	Solution for nebulization	20 µg every 12 h	Safety and efficacy not established
Indacaterol[b] (Arcapta Neohaler)	DPI (75 µg/inhalation)	1 inhalation every 24 h	N/A
Olodaterol (Striverdi Respimat)[b]	Respimat: 2.5 µg/inhalation	2 inhalations once daily	Safety and efficacy not established
Salmeterol[a] (Serevent Diskus)	DPI (50 µg/inhalation)	1 inhalation every 12 h	1 inhalation every 12 h
Oral Agents			
Albuterol			
Generic	Tablets, syrup	2 or 4 mg 3–4 times/d	2 mg 3–4 times/d
(VoSpire ER)	Tablets (extended release)	8 mg every 12 h	4 mg every 12 h
Terbutaline (generic only)	Tablets	5 mg 3 times/d	2.5 mg 3 times/d

[a]When used to treat asthma, must always be combined with an inhaled glucocorticoid.
[b]Approved only for chronic obstructive pulmonary disease, not asthma.
DPI, Dry-powder inhaler; *ER*, extended release; *HFA*, hydrofluoroalkane propellant; *MDI*, metered-dose inhaler; *PRN*, as needed.

📄 SUMMARY OF KEY PRESCRIBING CONSIDERATIONS

β Agonists

Therapeutic Goal: Short-acting inhaled β₂ agonists are used as needed (PRN) for prophylaxis of exercise-induced bronchospasm and to relieve ongoing asthma attacks and chronic obstructive pulmonary disease exacerbations. Oral and inhaled long-acting β₂ agonists are used for maintenance therapy.

Baseline Data: Forced expiratory volume in 1 second (FEV₁), frequency and severity of attacks. Attempt to identify trigger factors.

Monitoring: FEV₁, peak flow. Monitor home assessments of peak expiratory flow (PEF) at each clinic encounter.

Identifying High-Risk Patients: Systemic (oral, parenteral) β₂ agonists are *contraindicated* for patients with tachydysrhythmias or tachycardia associated with digitalis toxicity.

Use systemic β₂ agonists with *caution* in patients with diabetes, hyperthyroidism, organic heart disease, hypertension, or angina pectoris.

Evaluating Therapeutic Effects: Asthma control should be assessed at each clinic encounter. Monitor PEF, symptom frequency and symptom intensity, nighttime awakenings, effect on normal activity, and short-acting β₂ agonist use. It is also important to discuss medication adherence or deviation from the management plan. Because patients may forget some of the finer points of inhaled medication administration, this is a good time to have the patient demonstrate their technique for using inhalers.

Minimizing Adverse Effects

Inhaled short-acting β₂ agonists: When used at recommended doses, SABAs are generally devoid of significant adverse effects.

Inhaled long-acting β₂ agonists: When used correctly, LABAs are safe; however, when used *alone* for prophylaxis, they may increase the risk for severe asthma attacks and asthma-related death. (This is not a concern for COPD.) To minimize risk, these drugs should always be combined with an inhaled glucocorticoid, preferably in the same inhalation device.

Oral β₂ agonists: Excessive dosing can activate β₁ receptors on the heart, resulting in anginal pain and tachydysrhythmias. For this reason, selective β₂-adrenergic agonists should be prescribed (see Table 62.5) rather than nonselective β-adrenergic drugs (e.g., isoproterenol).

Although salmeterol is usually inhaled twice daily (every 12 hours), with continuous use, more frequent dosing may be needed because benefits seem to persist for a shorter time as the duration of treatment increases.

Oral preparations for long-term control. Two oral β₂ agonists—albuterol and terbutaline—are approved for long-term control of asthma. Dosing is 3 or 4 times a day. (In Canada, terbutaline is also available in an inhaled form as Bricanyl Turbuhaler offering 500 µg/actuation for PRN dosing.)

Tremor is common with systemic β₂ agonists and usually subsides with continued drug use. If necessary, tremor can be reduced by lowering the dosage.

Methylxanthines

We first encountered the methylxanthines (theophylline, caffeine, others) in Chapter 31. As discussed there, the most prominent actions of these drugs are (1) central nervous system (CNS) excitation and (2) bronchodilation. Other actions include cardiac stimulation, vasodilation, and diuresis.

Theophylline

Theophylline (Theo-24, Theochron, Elixophyllin, Theolair ♣, Uniphyl ♣) is the principal methylxanthine employed in asthma. Benefits derive primarily from bronchodilation. Theophylline has a narrow therapeutic range, so dosage must be carefully controlled. The drug is usually administered by mouth but may also be administered intravenously.

Mechanism of action. Theophylline produces bronchodilation by relaxing smooth muscle of the bronchi. Although the mechanism of bronchodilation has not been firmly established, the most probable is blockade of receptors for adenosine.

Therapeutic use. Oral theophylline is used for maintenance therapy of chronic stable asthma. Although less effective than β_2 agonists, theophylline has a longer duration of action (when administered in a sustained-release formulation). With regular use, theophylline can decrease the frequency and severity of asthma attacks. Because its effects are prolonged, theophylline may be most appropriate for patients who experience nocturnal attacks.

Once standard therapy in management of COPD, theophylline is no longer routinely recommended. Evidence-based guidelines recommend its use only if β_2 agonists and anticholinergics are not available or if the patient cannot afford long-term therapy with other drugs.

IV theophylline has been used in emergencies. However, the drug is no more effective than β_2 agonists and glucocorticoids and is clearly more dangerous.

Pharmacokinetics. Oral theophylline is available in sustained-release formulations and as an elixir. Absorption from sustained-release preparations is slow, but the resulting plasma levels are stable, being free of the wide fluctuations associated with the immediate-release products. Absorption from some sustained-release preparations can be affected by food.

Theophylline is metabolized in the liver. Rates of metabolism are affected by multiple factors—age, disease, drugs—and show wide individual variation. As a result, the plasma half-life of theophylline varies considerably among patients. For example, although the average half-life in nonsmoking adults is approximately 8 hours, the half-life can be as short as 2 hours in some adults and as long as 15 hours in others. Smoking either tobacco or marijuana accelerates metabolism and decreases the half-life. The average half-life in children is 4 hours. Metabolism is slowed in patients with certain pathologies (e.g., heart disease, liver disease, prolonged fever). Some drugs (e.g., cimetidine, fluoroquinolone antibiotics) decrease theophylline metabolism. Other drugs (e.g., phenobarbital) accelerate metabolism. Because of these variations in metabolism, dosage must be individualized.

Toxicity

Drug levels. Safe and effective therapy requires periodic measurement of theophylline blood levels. Traditionally, dosage has been adjusted to produce theophylline levels between 10 and 20 µg/mL. However, many patients respond well at 5 µg/mL, and, as a rule, there is little benefit to increasing levels to greater than 15 µg/mL. Therefore levels between 5 and 15 µg/mL are appropriate for most patients. At levels greater than 20 µg/mL, the risk for adverse effects is high.

Symptoms. Symptoms of toxicity are related to theophylline levels. At 20 to 25 µg/mL, relatively mild reactions occur (e.g., nausea, vomiting, diarrhea, insomnia, restlessness). Serious adverse effects are most likely at levels greater than 30 µg/mL. These reactions include severe dysrhythmias (e.g., ventricular fibrillation) and convulsions that can be highly resistant to treatment. Death may result from cardiorespiratory collapse.

PATIENT EDUCATION
Theophylline

Warn patients that, if a dose is missed, the following dose should not be doubled.

Instruct patients to swallow enteric-coated and sustained-release formulations intact, without crushing or chewing.

Warn patients against consuming caffeine-containing beverages (e.g., coffee, many soft drinks) and other sources of caffeine. Explain that caffeine can intensify adverse effects while decreasing theophylline breakdown.

Instruct patients to call the clinic if they start to develop symptoms of nausea, vomiting, abdominal discomfort, diarrhea, insomnia, restlessness, or palpitations, because these may signify theophylline toxicity.

Warn patients that smoking tobacco or marijuana can increase theophylline clearance, resulting in ineffective dosing.

Treatment. At the first indication of toxicity, dosing with theophylline should stop, and a theophylline level should be obtained. Absorption can be decreased by administering activated charcoal together with a cathartic in the event of an acute overdose. Ventricular dysrhythmias respond to lidocaine (most often recommended for methylxanthines) or amiodarone. IV benzodiazepines such as diazepam may help control seizures.

Drug interactions

Caffeine. Caffeine is a methylxanthine with pharmacologic properties like those of theophylline (see Chapter 31). Accordingly, caffeine can intensify the adverse effects of theophylline on the CNS and heart. In addition, caffeine can compete with theophylline for drug-metabolizing enzymes, causing theophylline levels to rise. Because of these interactions, individuals taking theophylline should avoid caffeine-containing beverages (e.g., coffee, many soft drinks) and other sources of caffeine.

Tobacco and marijuana smoke. Smoking tobacco or marijuana can induce theophylline metabolism, resulting in increased drug clearance of up to 50% in adults and 80% in older adults. (Secondhand smoke can result in similarly decreased drug levels.) Consequently, if a smoking patient stops smoking but the dose of theophylline is not decreased, the patient is at risk for developing theophylline toxicity over time.

Drugs that reduce theophylline levels. Several agents—including phenobarbital, phenytoin, and rifampin—can lower theophylline levels by inducing hepatic drug-metabolizing enzymes. Concurrent use of these agents may necessitate an increase in theophylline dosage.

Drugs that increase theophylline levels. Several drugs—including cimetidine and the fluoroquinolone antibiotics (e.g., ciprofloxacin)—can elevate plasma levels of theophylline, primarily by inhibiting hepatic metabolism. To avoid theophylline toxicity, the dosage of theophylline should be reduced when the drug is combined with these agents.

Formulations. Theophylline is available for IV and oral use. For IV use, generic solutions are available in concentrations of 400 mg/250 mL, 400 mg/500 mL, or 800 mg/500 mL of solution.

For oral use, the following concentrations are available:
- Elixophyllin oral elixir: 80 mg/15 mL
- Generic oral solution: 80 mg/15 mL
- Theochron 12-hour extended-release tablets: 100, 200, and 300 mg
- Generic 12-hour extended-release tablets: 100, 200, 300, and 450 mg
- Theo-24 24-hour extended-release capsule: 100, 200, 300, and 400 mg
- Generic 24-hour extended release tablets: 400 and 600 mg

Unlike the elixir and oral solution, the sustained-release tablets and capsules produce drug levels that are relatively stable. Accordingly, the sustained-release formulations are preferred for routine therapy.

Dosage and administration

Oral. Dosage must be individualized. To minimize chances of toxicity, doses should be low initially and then gradually increased. If a dose is missed, the following dose should not be doubled because doing so could produce toxicity. Smokers require higher than average doses. Conversely, patients with heart disease, liver dysfunction, or prolonged fever are likely to require lower doses. Patients should be instructed not to chew the sustained-release tablets or capsules. Product information should be consulted for compatibility with food.

The initial dosage is based on the age and weight of the patient and on the presence or absence of factors that can impair theophylline elimination. Specific initial dosages are described in the prescribing information in the package insert. As noted previously, maintenance doses should be adjusted to produce drug levels in the therapeutic range—typically 5 to 15 μg/mL.

Intravenous. IV theophylline is reserved for emergencies. Administration must be done slowly because rapid injection can cause fatal cardiovascular reactions. IV theophylline is incompatible with many other drugs. Accordingly, compatibility should be verified before mixing theophylline with other IV agents. For specific IV dosages, refer to the discussion of aminophylline next.

Other Methylxanthines

Aminophylline. Aminophylline is a theophylline salt that is considerably more soluble than theophylline itself. In solution, each molecule of aminophylline dissociates to yield two molecules of theophylline. Hence the pharmacologic properties of aminophylline and theophylline are identical. Aminophylline is available in formulations for oral and IV dosing. IV administration is employed most often.

Administration and dosage. Because of its relatively high solubility, aminophylline is the preferred form of theophylline for IV use. Infusions should be done slowly (no faster than 25 mg/min) because rapid injection can produce severe hypotension and death. The usual loading dose is 5.7 mg/kg. The maintenance infusion rate should be adjusted to provide plasma levels of theophylline that are within the therapeutic range (10 to 20 μg/mL). Aminophylline solutions are incompatible with a number of other drugs. Therefore compatibility must be verified before mixing aminophylline with other IV agents.

Aminophylline is available in 100- and 200-mg tablets for oral administration. Dosing guidelines are the same as for theophylline.

Anticholinergic Drugs

Anticholinergic drugs improve lung function by blocking muscarinic receptors in the bronchi, reducing bronchoconstriction. These drugs have FDA approval only for COPD but are recommended by expert panels for alternative management of asthma. They are administered by inhalation; therefore systemic effects are minimal. The basic pharmacology of the anticholinergic drugs is presented in Chapter 14.

Ipratropium was the first inhaled anticholinergic. In addition to ipratropium, we have three long-acting inhaled anticholinergic drugs. The long-acting formulations, more commonly referred to as long-acting muscarinic antagonists (LAMAs) are aclidinium, tiotropium, and umeclidinium.

Ipratropium

Therapeutic use. Ipratropium (Atrovent HFA) is an atropine derivative administered by inhalation to relieve bronchospasm. The drug has FDA approval only for bronchospasm associated with COPD but is often used off-label for asthma and is included in current evidence-based guidelines for asthma management.

Mechanism of action. Like atropine, ipratropium is a muscarinic antagonist. By blocking muscarinic cholinergic receptors in the bronchi,

SUMMARY OF KEY PRESCRIBING CONSIDERATIONS

Methylxanthines

Therapeutic Goal: Bronchodilation to decrease the intensity and frequency of moderate to severe asthma attacks and to control chronic obstructive pulmonary disease exacerbations

Baseline Data: Forced expiratory volume in 1 second (FEV₁)

Monitoring: FEV_1 and the frequency and severity of attacks. Close check of heart rate and rhythm, ECG if needed. Monitor levels to ensure that they are in the therapeutic range (for theophylline: 5 to 15 μg/mL for most patients). Check drug levels before making any dosage changes, for signs or symptoms of toxicity, and after adding or discontinuing drugs that affect methylxanthine levels.

Identifying High-Risk Patients: These drugs are *contraindicated* for patients with untreated seizure disorders or peptic ulcer disease.

Use with *caution* in patients with heart disease (can exacerbate dysrhythmias), liver dysfunction (increased risk for toxicity), peptic ulcer disease (can exacerbate condition), or seizure disorders (can exacerbate seizures).

Evaluating Therapeutic Effects: Control is improved, and toxicity does not develop

Minimizing Adverse Effects: Check a drug level if the patient develops signs or symptoms of toxicity. This should be done even if another cause is suspected. Prevent complications due to toxicity by routinely checking drug levels and adjusting dosage as needed to maintain levels within a therapeutic range.

Minimizing Adverse Interactions

Caffeine: Caffeine can intensify the adverse effects of theophylline on the heart and CNS and can decrease theophylline metabolism.

Smoking Tobacco or Marijuana: Tobacco and marijuana smoking can increase clearance to 50% in adults and 80% in older adults. Secondhand smoke also increases theophylline clearance. Accordingly, it is important to inquire regarding smoking habits to optimize dosing. If smoking is discontinued during therapy, it will be important to decrease the dosage of methylxanthines to avoid toxicity.

Drugs that Reduce Theophylline Levels: Phenobarbital, phenytoin, rifampin, and other drugs can lower theophylline levels. In the presence of these drugs, the dosage of theophylline may need to be increased.

Drugs that Increase Theophylline Levels: Cimetidine, fluoroquinolone antibiotics, and other drugs can elevate theophylline levels. When combined with these drugs, theophylline should be used in reduced dosage.

Management of Toxicity: Theophylline overdose can cause severe dysrhythmias and convulsions. Death from cardiorespiratory collapse may occur. Management of toxicity is discussed earlier in the chapter. Manage toxicity by (1) discontinuing theophylline and (2) administering activated charcoal (to decrease theophylline absorption) plus a cathartic (to accelerate fecal excretion). Preferred drugs to control ventricular dysrhythmias (most common dysrhythmia to occur) and seizures are IV lidocaine (amiodarone is an alternative) and IV benzodiazepines (e.g., diazepam).

ipratropium prevents bronchoconstriction. Therapeutic effects begin within 30 seconds, reach 50% of their maximum in 3 minutes, and persist approximately 6 hours. Ipratropium is effective against allergen-induced asthma and EIB but is less effective than the β₂ agonists. However, because ipratropium and the β₂-adrenergic agonists promote bronchodilation by different mechanisms, their beneficial effects are additive.

Adverse effects. Systemic effects are minimal because ipratropium is a quaternary ammonium compound and therefore always carries a positive charge. As a result, the drug is not readily absorbed from the lungs or from the digestive tract. The most common adverse reactions are dry mouth and irritation of the pharynx. If systemic absorption is sufficient, the drug may raise intraocular pressure in patients with glaucoma. Adverse cardiovascular events (heart attack, stroke, death) have occurred in people taking ipratropium; however, because absorption is minimal, it seems unlikely that ipratropium is the cause.

Preparations, dosage, and administration. Preparations, dosage, and administration information for ipratropium and other anticholinergics is provided in Table 62.6.

Tiotropium

Actions and use. Tiotropium (Spiriva, Spiriva Respimat) is a LAMA approved for maintenance therapy of bronchospasm associated with COPD. The drug is not approved for asthma but has been used off-label for patients who have not responded to other medications. Like ipratropium, tiotropium relieves bronchospasm by blocking muscarinic receptors in the lungs. Therapeutic effects begin approximately 30 minutes after inhalation, peak in 3 hours, and persist about 24 hours. With subsequent doses, bronchodilation gets better and better, reaching a plateau after eight consecutive doses (8 days). Compared with ipratropium, tiotropium is more effective, and its dosing schedule is more convenient (once daily vs. 4 times daily). Tiotropium is indicated only for long-term maintenance. For rapid relief of ongoing bronchospasm, patients should inhale a SABA.

Adverse effects. The most common adverse effect is dry mouth, which develops in 16% of patients. Fortunately, this response is generally mild and diminishes over time. Patients can suck on sugarless hard candy for relief, but should we warned that high intake of candy containing sorbitol and xylitol can cause diarrhea. Saliva substitutes (Aquoral, Biotene, others) are available over the counter.

Systemic anticholinergic effects (e.g., constipation, urinary retention, tachycardia, blurred vision) are minimal. Like ipratropium, tiotropium is a quaternary ammonium compound, and thus absorption into the systemic circulation is very limited. Like ipratropium, tiotropium has been associated with adverse cardiovascular events; however, because absorption is low, tiotropium is unlikely to be the cause.

TABLE 62.6 Anticholinergics: Preparations and Dosages

Drug (Trade Name)	Preparation	Formulation	Dosage
Short-Acting Anticholinergic			
Ipratropium (Atrovent HFA)	Solution	500 µg/vial	500 µg 3–4 times daily by nebulizer
	MDI	17 µg per actuation	2 inhalations 4 times daily (maximum dosage 12 inhalations/ 24 h)
Long-Acting Muscarinic Antagonist			
Aclidinium (Tudorza Pressair)	DPI	400 µg per actuation	400 µg twice daily
Tiotropium (Spiriva)	Handihaler DPI	18 µg capsules[a]	18 µg once daily
Umeclidinium (Incruse Ellipta)	DPI	62.5 µg per actuation	62.5 µg once daily

[a]Capsules are for insertion into DPI device and must not be swallowed.
DPI, Dry-powder inhaler; *HFA*, hydrofluoroalkane propellant; *MDI*, metered-dose inhaler.

Aclidinium

Actions and use. Aclidinium (Tudorza Pressair) is another LAMA indicated for management of bronchospasm associated with COPD. It relieves bronchospasm by blocking muscarinic receptors in the lung. Peak levels have occurred within 10 minutes of drug delivery; however, it is intended only for maintenance therapy and not for acute symptom relief.

Adverse effects. The most common adverse reactions reported in clinical trials were headache, nasopharyngitis, and cough. As with any anticholinergic, there is a theoretical risk for worsening narrow-angle glaucoma, urinary retention, and other systemic anticholinergic effects; however, these have not been reported.

Umeclidinium

Actions and use. Umeclidinium (Incruse Ellipta) is the newest LAMA indicated for management of bronchospasm associated with COPD. In addition to its availability as a single agent, it is also available in combination with the LABA vilanterol as the Anoro Ellipta. Both the single and combination drugs are indicated for COPD maintenance therapy only; they are not approved for asthma treatment.

Adverse effects. Umeclidinium contains lactose as a component of the powder mix. Theoretically, it may cause severe hypersensitivity reactions when taken by people who have milk protein allergies. In clinical trials, adverse effects were negligible: nasopharyngitis was reported by 8% of subjects; however, this was reported by 7% of those taking a placebo. Similarly, 5% reported upper respiratory tract infections; yet this was reported by 4% of those taking a placebo. Although it is possible for this anticholinergic drug to cause typical anticholinergic adverse effects because it is inhaled, the likelihood of this occurrence is markedly decreased.

COMBINATION DRUGS

Glucocorticoid/Long-Acting β₂ Agonist Combinations

Fluticasone/salmeterol (Advair Diskus, Advair HFA), fluticasone/vilanterol (Breo Ellipta), *budesonide/formoterol* (Symbicort), and *mometasone/formoterol* (Dulera) are available in fixed-dose combinations for inhalational therapy of asthma and COPD. The glucocorticoids (fluticasone, budesonide, and mometasone) provide antiinflammatory benefits, and the LABAs (salmeterol and formoterol) provide bronchodilation. All four products are indicated for long-term maintenance in adults and children. These combinations are more convenient than taking a glucocorticoid and LABA separately but have the disadvantage of restricting dosage flexibility. These products carry a black box warning about possible increased risk for asthma severity or asthma-related death (from the LABA in the combination). However, because the LABA is combined with a glucocorticoid, risk should be minimal. The four combination products have not been directly compared. Nonetheless, when used in equivalent dosages, they are likely to be equally effective. Formulations and dosages are presented in Table 62.7.

β₂-Adrenergic Agonist/Anticholinergic Combinations

The combination of a β₂ agonist with a cholinergic antagonist optimizes bronchodilation by capitalizing on the unique action of the individual agents. As mentioned previously, β₂ agonists promote bronchodilation by stimulating adrenergic receptors. In the lung, this relaxes smooth muscle in the airways. Cholinergic antagonists (anticholinergics) promote bronchodilation by blocking cholinergic receptors. This relaxes smooth muscle tone by preventing stimulation of cholinergic receptors. In addition, β₂ agonists primarily affect the bronchioles, whereas anticholinergics primarily affect the bronchi. This action on different areas of the airways further enhances bronchodilation.

All β agonist/anticholinergic combinations are inhaled. Four combinations are available: Albuterol/ipratropium (Combivent Respimat, Combivent UDV), indacaterol/glycopyrronium (Utibron Neohaler, Ultibro Breezhaler ♣), olodaterol/tiotropium (Stiolto Respimat), and vilanterol/umeclidinium, inhaled (Anoro Ellipta). These are only approved for management of COPD; however, Combivent (the only combination with a SABA) has been used off-label for management of asthma. See Table 62.8 for a listing of these combinations and recommended dosages.

Management of Asthma and Chronic Obstructive Pulmonary Disease

Before beginning a discussion of asthma and COPD therapy, we need to address a few tests of lung function. These are used in diagnosing pulmonary conditions and monitoring therapy outcomes.

FEV_1 is the single most useful test of lung function. To determine FEV_1, the patient inhales completely and then exhales as completely and forcefully as possible into the spirometer. The spirometer measures how much air was expelled during the first second of exhalation. Results are then compared with a "predicted normal value" for a healthy person of similar age, sex, height, and weight. Patients with obstructive pulmonary disease will have a decreased FEV_1 because there is obstruction to airflow on exhalation.

FVC, also measured with a spirometer, is defined as the total volume of air the patient can exhale after a full inhalation.

FEV_1/FVC (i.e., FEV_1 divided by FVC) is the fraction (percentage) of vital capacity exhaled during the first second of forced expiration. For patients with pulmonary problems, the FEV_1/FVC is used to distinguish obstructive from restrictive causes. Obstructive pulmonary conditions are those that prevent adequate exhalation. Recall that the FEV_1 measures forced exhalation. If there is obstruction to exhalation, the FEV_1 will be decreased; therefore the FEV_1/FVC will be decreased. Restrictive pulmonary conditions are those that prevent adequate inhalation. This can occur due to a variety of conditions: lung diseases such as pulmonary fibrosis, conditions of decreased intercostal or diaphragmatic strength such as myasthenia gravis, skeletal muscle deformities such as pectus excavatum, and conditions such as obesity or trauma to the thoracic area. For restrictive pulmonary conditions, the FVC is usually decreased, as well, so the FEV_1/FVC is normal or even increased.

PEF is defined as the maximal rate of airflow during expiration. This measurement is used to monitor, but not diagnose, asthma. To determine PEF, the patient exhales as forcefully as possible into a *peak flowmeter*, a relatively inexpensive, hand-held device. Results are approximately equal to the FEV_1. Although the FEV_1 is more accurate than the PEF (it measures airflow in large and small airways, whereas the PEF measures airflow in the large airways only), the measures correlate well and so the PEF is an excellent way to monitor therapy. Patients should measure their peak flow every morning. Often these readings can identify when patients are developing complications before symptoms develop.

MANAGEMENT OF ASTHMA

In 2007 the National Asthma Education and Prevention Program (NAEPP) of the National Heart, Lung, and Blood Institute issued *Expert Panel Report 3 (EPR-3): Guidelines for the Diagnosis and Management of Asthma*. These remain the most current U.S. recommendations for asthma management and are widely used to guide practice decisions. These are available online at https://www.nhlbi.nih.gov/health-topics/guidelines-for-diagnosis-management-of-asthma.

For several years, the NAEPP have been posting plans to update their guidelines, but the projected dates for these revisions keep getting

TABLE 62.7 Glucocorticoids and Long-Acting β₂ Agonists: Formulations and Dosages

Drug (Trade Name)	Inhaler	Formulation	Dosage[a]
Budesonide/formoterol (Symbicort)	HFA	80 µg/4.5 µg 160 µg/4.5 µg	2 inhalations twice daily 2 inhalations twice daily
Fluticasone/vilanterol (Breo Ellipta)	DPI	100 µg/25 µg 200 µg/25 µg	1 inhalation once daily 1 inhalation once daily
Fluticasone/salmeterol (Advair Diskus)	DPI	100 µg/50 µg 250 µg/50 µg 500 µg/50 µg	1 inhalation twice daily 1 inhalation twice daily 1 inhalation twice daily
Fluticasone/salmeterol (Advair HFA)	HFA	45 µg/21 µg 115 µg/21 µg 230 µg/21 µg	2 inhalations twice daily 2 inhalations twice daily 2 inhalations twice daily
Mometasone/formoterol (Dulera)	HFA	100 µg/5 µg 200 µg/5 µg	2 inhalations twice daily 2 inhalations twice daily

[a]Dosing is the same for children and adults when prescribed as recommended for age. These drugs are not approved for children younger than 12 years. Fluticason/vilanterol is not approved for children younger than 18 years.
DPI, Dry-powder inhaler; *HFA*, hydrofluoroalkane propellant.

TABLE 62.8 β₂ Agonist and Anticholinergic Combinations: Formulations and Dosages

Drug (Classification)	Trade Name	Preparation	Formulation Per Inhalation	Dosage
Ipratropium/albuterol (anticholinergic + SABA)	Duoneb	Solution	500 µg ipratropium/2,500 µg of albuterol	3 mL 4 times daily using a nebulizer
	Combivent Respimat	Inhaler	20 µg ipratropium/100 µg albuterol	1 inhalation 4 times daily (maximum 6 inhalations in 24 h)
Indacaterol/glycopyrronium (LABA + anticholinergic)	Utibron Neohaler	Inhaler	27.5 µg indacaterol/15 µg glycopyrronium (glycopyrrolate)	1 inhalation twice daily
Olodaterol/tiotropium (LABA + anticholingeric)	Stiolto Respimat	Inhaler	2.5 µg of olodaterol/2.5 µg tiotropium	2 inhalations once daily
Umeclidinium/vilanterol (Anticholingergic + LABA)	Anora Elipta	Inhaler	62.5 µg umeclidinium/25 µg vilanterol	1 inhalation once daily

LABA, Long-acting β₂ agonists; *SABA*, short-acting β₂ agonist pushed forward. Because over a decade has passed without an update, we recognize that a supplemental resource is necessary. For this purpose, we have chosen a comprehensive report by the Global Initiative for Asthma (GINA). This report, *Global Strategy for Asthma Management and Prevention* (GINA Report), is available at https://ginasthma.org/2018-gina -report-global-strategy-for-asthma-management-and-prevention. The GINA Report is updated yearly; the most current reports are posted to https://ginasthma.org.

The following discussion reflects EPR-3 recommendations. Where recommendations differ significantly from the GINA Report, we include GINA's additional recommendations.

Classification of Asthma Severity

Chronic asthma has four classes of increasing severity: (1) intermittent, (2) mild persistent, (3) moderate persistent, and (4) severe persistent. Diagnostic criteria for these classes are shown in Table 62.9. Note that severity classification is based on two separate domains: *impairment* and *risk*. Impairment refers to the effect of asthma on quality of life and functional capacity *in the present.* Risk refers to possible adverse events *in the future,* such as exacerbations and progressive loss of lung function. As we progress from intermittent asthma to severe persistent asthma, both impairment and risk increase: asthma symptoms occur more often and last longer, use of SABAs for symptomatic control increases, limitations on physical activity become more substantial, FEV_1 decreases, FEV_1/FVC drops, and the number of exacerbations that require oral glucocorticoids gets larger. It is important to note that the two domains of asthma—impairment and risk—may respond differently to drugs. Furthermore, patients can be at high risk for future events, even if their current level of impairment is low.

Treatment Goals

Treatment of chronic asthma is directed at two basic goals: reducing impairment and reducing risk. Components of each goal are listed here.

Reducing Impairment

- Preventing chronic and troublesome symptoms (e.g., coughing or breathlessness after exertion and at all other times)
- Reducing use of SABAs for symptom relief to 2 days a week or less
- Maintaining normal (or near-normal) pulmonary function
- Maintaining normal activity levels, including exercise and attendance at school or work
- Meeting patient and family expectations regarding asthma care

Reducing Risk

- Preventing recurrent exacerbations
- Minimizing the need for emergency department visits or hospitalizations
- Preventing progressive loss of lung function (for children, preventing reduced lung growth)
- Providing maximal benefits with minimal adverse effects

Chronic Drug Therapy

In patients with chronic asthma, drugs are used in two ways: some agents are taken to establish *long-term control,* and some are taken for *quick relief* of an ongoing attack (Table 62.10). Long-term control drugs are taken every day, whereas the quick-relief drugs are taken PRN. Of the long-term control agents in current use, inhaled glucocorticoids are by far the most important. With regular dosing, these drugs reduce the frequency and severity of attacks, as well as the need for quick-relief medications. Of the quick-relief drugs in current use, inhaled SABAs are the most important. These drugs act promptly to reverse

bronchoconstriction and provide rapid relief from cough, chest tightness, and wheezing.

For chronic drug therapy, both the EPR-3 and the GINA Report recommend a *stepwise* approach, in which drug dosages and drug classes are stepped up as needed and stepped down when possible. Six steps are described (Table 62.11). The basic concept is simple. First, all patients, starting with step 1, should use an inhaled SABA as needed for quick relief. Second, all patients—except those on step 1—should use a long-term control medication (preferably an inhaled glucocorticoid) to provide baseline control. Third, when patients move up a step, owing to increased impairment and risk, dosage of the control medication is increased, or another control medication is added, or both. And fourth, after a period of sustained control, moving down a step should be tried.

For patients just beginning drug therapy, the step they start on is determined by the pretreatment classification of asthma severity (Table 62.12). For example, a patient diagnosed with intermittent asthma would begin at step 1 (PRN use of an inhaled SABA), whereas a patient diagnosed with moderate persistent asthma would begin at step 3 (daily inhalation of a low-dose glucocorticoid plus daily inhalation of a LABA, supplemented with an inhaled SABA as needed).

After treatment has been ongoing, stepping up or down is based on *assessment of asthma control.* Like the diagnosis of pretreatment severity, assessment of control is based on two domains. Three categories of control are defined: well controlled, not well controlled, and very poorly controlled. Determinants for control, along with recommended actions for each category, are shown in Table 62.12 along with recommended actions for treatment.

Drugs for Acute Severe Exacerbations

Acute severe exacerbations of asthma require immediate attention. The goals are to relieve airway obstruction and hypoxemia and normalize lung function as quickly as possible. Initial therapy consists of the following:

- Giving oxygen to relieve hypoxemia
- Giving a systemic glucocorticoid to reduce airway inflammation
- Giving a nebulized high-dose SABA to relieve airflow obstruction
- Giving nebulized ipratropium to further reduce airflow obstruction

After resolution of the crisis and hospital discharge, an oral gluco-corticoid is taken for 5 to 10 days. All patients should also take a medium-dose inhaled glucocorticoid. Full recovery of lung function may take weeks.

Drugs for Exercise-Induced Bronchospasm

Exercise increases airway obstruction in practically all people with chronic asthma. The cause is bronchospasm secondary to loss of heat or water from the lung. EIB usually starts either during or immediately after exercise, peaks in 5 to 10 minutes, and resolves 20 to 30 minutes later.

With proper medication, most people with asthma can be as active as they wish. To prevent EIB, patients can inhale a SABA or cromolyn prophylactically. Inhaled SABAs, which prevent EIB in more than 80% of patients, are generally preferred over cromolyn, which is less effective. β_2 agonists should be inhaled immediately before exercise; cromolyn should be inhaled 15 minutes before exercise.

Reducing Exposure to Allergens and Triggers

For patients with chronic asthma, the treatment plan should include measures to control allergens and other factors that can cause airway inflammation and exacerbate symptoms. Important sources of asthma-associated allergens include the house dust mite, warm-blooded pets, cockroaches, and molds. Factors that can exacerbate asthma include tobacco smoke, wood smoke, and household sprays. To the extent possible, exposure to these factors should be reduced or eliminated.

TABLE 62.9 Classification of Asthma Severity and Recommendation for Initial Treatment

	Intermittent	Mild Persistent	Moderate Persistent	Severe Persistent
0–4 Years				
Symptoms	2 d/wk or less	More than 2 d/wk but less than daily	Daily	Several times daily
Nighttime awakenings	0	1–2 times/month	3–4 times/month	More than once/week
SABA use[a]	2 d/wk or less	More than 2 d/wk but less than daily	Daily	Several times a day
Effect on activity	None	Minimal activity limitation	Some activity limitation	Severe activity limitation
FEV₁ percent of predicted	N/A	N/A	N/A	N/A
FEV₁/FVC	N/A	N/A	N/A	N/A
Risk for exacerbations requiring systemic glucocorticoids	0–1 time/year	2 or more exacerbations in 6 months or wheezing lasting more than 1 day 4 or more times/year	Increased frequency and intensity of exacerbations or wheezing	Even greater increased frequency and intensity of exacerbations or wheezing
Recommended step for initial treatment[b]	Step 1	Step 2	Step 3	Step 3
5–11 Years				
Symptoms	2 d/wk or less	More than 2 d/wk but less than daily	Daily	Several times daily
Nighttime awakenings	2 times/month or less	3–4 times/month	More than once/week but less than nightly	Often nightly
SABA use[a]	2 d/wk or less	More than 2 d/wk but less than daily and no more than 1 time on any day	Daily	Several times a day
Effect on activity	None	Minimal activity limitation	Some activity limitation	Severe activity limitation
FEV₁ predicted	>80%	>80%	60%–80%	<60%
FEV₁/FVC	>85%	>80%	75%–80%	<75%
Risk for exacerbations requiring systemic glucocorticoids	0–1 time/year	2 or more times/year	Increased frequency and intensity of exacerbations	Even greater increased frequency and intensity of exacerbations
Recommended step for initial treatment[b]	Step 1	Step 2	Step 3	Step 3 or 4
12 Years and Older				
Symptoms	2 d/wk or less	More than 2 d/wk but less than daily	Daily	Several times daily
Nighttime awakenings	2 times/month or less	3–4 times/month	More than once/week but less than nightly	Often nightly
SABA use[a]	2 d/wk or less	More than 2 d/wk but less than daily and no more than 1 time on any day	Daily	Several times a day
Effect on activity	None	Minimal activity limitation	Some activity limitation	Severe activity limitation
FEV₁ predicted	>80%	>80%	60%–80%	<60%
FEV₁/FVC	Within normal limits for age[c]	Within normal limits for age[c]	Normal limits for age reduced by 5%[c]	Normal limits for age reduced by 5%[c]
Risk for exacerbations requiring systemic glucocorticoids	0–1 time/year	2 or more times/year	Increased frequency and intensity of exacerbations	Even greater increased frequency and intensity of exacerbations
Recommended step for initial treatment[b]	Step 1	Step 2	Step 3	Step 4 or 5

[a]Use for control of symptoms, not prophylaxis for exercise-induced bronchospasm.
[b]Steps of asthma management are detailed in Table 62.12.
[c]Normal FEV₁/FVC by age: 5% for age 8–19 years; 80% for 20–39 years; 75% for 40–59 years; 70% for 60–80 years.
FEV₁, Forced expiratory volume in 1 second; *FVC,* forced vital capacity; *N/A,* Not applicable; *SABA,* short-acting β₂ agonist.
From National Heart, Lung, and Blood Institute. (2012). Asthma Care Quick Reference: Diagnosing and managing asthma. Available at https://www.nhlbi.nih.gov/files/docs/guidelines/asthma_qrg.pdf

TABLE 62.10 Drugs for Asthma: Agents for Long-Term Control Versus Quick Relief

Long-Term Control Medications (Controllers)

Antiinflammatory drugs	Glucocorticoids (inhaled or oral)
	Leukotriene receptor antagonists
	Cromolyn
	Monoclonal Antibodies
Bronchodilators	Long-acting inhaled β₂ agonists[a]
	Long-acting oral β₂ agonists
	Theophylline

Quick-Relief Medications (Relievers)

Bronchodilators	Short-acting inhaled β₂ agonists
	Anticholinergics
Antiinflammatory drugs	Glucocorticoids, systemic[b]

[a]For treatment of asthma, should always be combined with an inhaled glucocorticoid.
[b]Considered quick-relief drugs when used in a short burst (3–10 days) at the start of therapy or during a period of gradual deterioration. Glucocorticoids are not used for immediate relief of an ongoing attack.

MANAGEMENT OF CHRONIC OBSTRUCTIVE PULMONARY DISEASE

Each year the Global Initiative for Chronic Obstructive Lung Disease (GOLD) updates and publishes the *Global Strategy for the Diagnosis, Management, and Prevention of Chronic Obstructive Pulmonary Disease* (GOLD Report). The current document, available at https://goldcopd.org/gold-reports, informs our discussion on COPD.

Classification of Airflow Limitation Severity

Severity of airflow limitation is based on FEV_1 spirometry following use of a bronchodilator. The four classes of increasing severity are (1) mild, (2) moderate, (3) severe, and (4) very severe. *Remember that, for all patients, a diagnosis of COPD requires an FEV_1/FVC less than 0.70; therefore this criterion must be met before the criteria for classification can be applied* (Table 62.13).

Treatment Goals

There are two primary goals of COPD management. The first is to reduce symptoms, improve the patient's health status, and increase exercise tolerance. The second goal is to reduce risks and mortality. The

TABLE 62.11 Stepwise Approach to Managing Asthma

	Quick Relief[a]	Preferred Long-Term Control	Alternate Long-Term Control
0–4 Years			
STEP 1	SABA prn	–	–
STEP 2	SABA prn	Low-dose IGC	Cromolyn *or* montelukast
STEP 3	SABA prn	Medium-dose IGC	–
STEP 4	SABA prn	Medium-dose IGC *plus* LABA *or* montelukast	–
STEP 5	SABA prn	High-dose IGC *plus* LABA *or* montelukast	–
STEP 6	SABA prn	High-dose IGC *plus* LABA *or* montelukast *plus* Oral glucocorticoids	–
5–11 Years			
STEP 1	SABA prn	–	–
STEP 2	SABA prn	Low-dose IGC	Cromolyn *or* LTRA *or* theophylline *AND* Consider allergen immunotherapy ("allergy shots") for patients with allergic asthma
STEP 3	SABA prn	Low-dose IGC *plus* LABA *or* LTRA *or* theophylline *OR* Medium-dose IGC	Consider allergen immunotherapy for patients with allergic asthma
STEP 4	SABA prn	Medium-dose IGC *plus* LABA *or* montelukast	Medium-dose IGC *plus* LTRA *or* theophylline *AND* Consider allergen immunotherapy ("allergy shots") for patients with allergic asthma
STEP 5	SABA prn	High-dose IGC *plus* LABA	High-dose IGC *plus* LTRA *or* theophylline
STEP 6	SABA prn	High-dose IGC *plus* LABA *plus* Oral glucocorticoids	High-dose IGC *plus* LTRA *or* theophylline *plus* Oral glucocorticoids

TABLE 62.11 Stepwise Approach to Managing Asthma—cont'd

	Quick Relief[a]	Preferred Long-Term Control	Alternate Long-Term Control
12 Years and Older			
STEP 1	SABA prn	–	–
STEP 2	SABA prn	Low-dose IGC	Cromolyn *or* LTRA *or* theophylline *and* Consider allergen immunotherapy ("allergy shots") for patients with allergic asthma
STEP 3	SABA prn	Low-dose IGC *plus* LABA *OR* Medium-dose IGC	Consider allergen immunotherapy for patients with allergic asthma
STEP 4	SABA prn	Medium-dose IGC *plus* LABA	Medium-dose IGC *plus* LTRA *or* theophylline *AND* Consider allergen immunotherapy ("allergy shots") for patients with allergic asthma
STEP 5	SABA prn	High-dose IGC *plus* LABA *AND* Consider omalizumab for patients with allergies	Consider add-on therapy (e.g., tiotropium, monoclonal antibody)
STEP 6	SABA prn	High-dose IGC *plus* LABA *plus* Oral glucocorticoids *AND* Consider omalizumab for patients with allergies	Consider add-on therapy (e.g., tiotropium, monoclonal antibody)

[a]Use of SABA more than 2 d/wk for symptom relief indicates inadequate control and the need for step-up therapy.

IGC, Inhaled glucocorticoid; *LABA*, long-acting β_2 agonist; *LTRA*, leukotriene receptor antagonist; *prn*, as needed; *SABA*, short-acting β_2 agonist. From National Heart, Lung, and Blood Institute. (2012). Asthma care quick reference: Diagnosing and managing asthma. Available at https://www.nhlbi.nih.gov/files/docs/guidelines/asthma_qrg.pdf; and Global Initiative for Asthma. (2018). Global strategy for asthma management and prevention. Available at https://ginasthma.org/gina-reports

TABLE 62.12 Assessment of Asthma Control and Recommended Action for Treatment

	Well Controlled	Not Well Controlled	Very Poorly Controlled
0–4 Years			
Symptoms	2 d/wk or less	More than 2 d/wk	Several times daily
Nighttime awakenings	Once/month or less	More than once/month	More than once/week
SABA use[a]	2 d/wk or less	More than 2 d/wk	Several times/day
Effect on activity	None	Some activity limitation	Severe activity limitation
FEV$_1$ percent of predicted	N/A	N/A	N/A
FEV$_1$/FVC	N/A	N/A	N/A
Questionnaires	N/A	N/A	N/A
• ATAQ[b]			
• ACQ[c]			
• ACT[d]			
Risk for exacerbations requiring systemic glucocorticoids[e]	0–1 time/year	2–3 times/year	More than 3 times/year
Risk for reduction in lung growth or progressive loss of lung function	N/A	N/A	N/A
Risk for adverse effects of treatment[f]	Variable[f]	Variable[f]	Variable[f]
Recommendation[g]	Continue current therapy. Reevaluate in 1–6 months. May step down after control well maintained for 3 months.	Step up therapy by 1 step. Reevaluate in 2–6 weeks. If no improvement in 4–6 weeks, consider adjusting therapy or consider alternative diagnoses.	Step up therapy by 1–2 steps. Consider short course of oral systemic glucocorticoids. Reevaluate in 2 weeks.

Continued

TABLE 62.12   Assessment of Asthma Control and Recommended Action for Treatment—cont'd

	Well Controlled	Not Well Controlled	Very Poorly Controlled
5–11 Years			
Symptoms	2 d/wk or less and no more than once a day	More than 2 d/wk or occurs several times/day on 1–2 d/wk	Several times/day
Nighttime awakenings	Once/month or less	2 times/month or more	2 times/week or more
SABA use[a]	2 d/wk or less	More than 2 d/wk	Several times/day
Effect on activity	None	Some activity limitation	Severe activity limitation
FEV$_1$ percent of predicted	>80%	60%–80%	<60%
FEV$_1$/FVC	>80%	75–80%	<75%
Questionnaires	N/A	N/A	N/A
• ATAQ[b]			
• ACQ[c]			
• ACT[d]			
Risk for exacerbations requiring systemic glucocorticoids[e]	0–1 time/year	2 or more times/year	2 or more times/year
Risk for reduction in lung growth or progressive loss of lung function	Long-term follow-up care required for evaluation	Long-term follow-up care required for evaluation	Long-term follow-up care required for evaluation
Risk for adverse effects of treatment[f]	Variable[f]	Variable[f]	Variable[f]
Recommendation[g]	Continue current therapy. Reevaluate in 1–6 months. May step down if well controlled for 3 months.	Step up therapy by at least 1 step.[h] Reevaluate in 2–6 weeks.	Step up therapy by 1–2 steps.[h] Consider short course of oral systemic glucocorticoids. Reevaluate in 2 weeks.
12 Years and Older			
Symptoms	2 d/wk or less	More than 2 d/wk	Several times/day
Nighttime awakenings	2 times/month or less	1–3 times/wk	4 times/wk or more
SABA use[a]	2 d/wk or less	More than 2 d/wk	Several times/day
Effect on activity	None	Some activity limitation	Severe activity limitation
FEV$_1$ percent of predicted	>80%	60%–80%	<60%
FEV$_1$/FVC	N/A	N/A	N/A
Questionnaires	ATAQ: 0	ATAQ: 1–2	ATAQ: 3–4
• ATAQ[b]	ACQ: 0.75 or less	ACQ: 1.5 or less	ACQ: N/A
• ACQ[c]	ACT: 20 or more	ACT: 16–19	ACT: 15 or less
• ACT[d]			
Risk for exacerbations requiring systemic glucocorticoids[e]	0–1 time/year	2 or more times/year	2 or more times/year
Risk for reduction in lung growth or progressive loss of lung function	Long-term follow-up care required for evaluation	Long-term follow-up care required for evaluation	Long-term follow-up care required for evaluation
Risk for adverse effects of treatment[f]	Variable[f]	Variable[f]	Variable[f]
Recommendation[g]	Continue current therapy. Reevaluate in 1–6 months. May step down if well controlled for 3 months.	Step up therapy by 1 step.[h] Reevaluate in 2–6 weeks.	Step up therapy by 1–2 steps.[h] Consider short course of oral systemic glucocorticoids. Reevaluate in 2 weeks.

[a]Use for control of symptoms, not prophylaxis for exercise-induced bronchospasm

[b]The ATAQ is available at https://getasthmahelp.org/documents/2007Guidelines_ValidatedQuestionnaires.pdf

[c]Access to the ACQ is available at http://www.qoltech.co.uk/obtaining.html

[d]The ACT is available at http://www.pamf.org/asthma/education/handouts/adults/ACT_Eng.pdf

[e]Estimation of risk should take into consideration the intensity of exacerbations and the time between occurrences

[f]Adverse medication effects are highly variable and may not correlate well with certain levels of control; however, general consideration in included in risk assessment

[g]Steps of asthma management are detailed in Table 62.12

[h]Prior to stepping up therapy, review medication adherence, inhaler technique, and environmental factors contributing to asthma. If an alternative treatment was used, switch to preferred treatment for that step. If adverse effects are problematic, consider switching to alternative treatment options.

ACQ, Asthma Control Questionnaire; *ACT*, Asthma Control TestTM; *ATAQ*, Asthma Therapy Assessment Questionnaire; *FEV$_1$*, forced expiratory volume in 1 second; *FVC*, forced vital capacity; *N/A*, not applicable; *SABA*, short-acting β$_2$ agonist

From National Heart, Lung, and Blood Institute. Asthma Care Quick Reference: Diagnosing and managing asthma; 2012. Available at https://www.nhlbi.nih.gov/files/docs/guidelines/asthma_qrg.pdf.

latter is accomplished by preventing COPD progression and by preventing and managing exacerbations.

Treatment goals are based on the overall level of COPD severity. The GOLD Report classifies COPD severity from A to D based on consideration of the patient's symptoms, their airflow limitation severity (see earlier discussion), their risk level for COPD exacerbations, and any comorbid conditions they may have. Symptoms are quantified using instruments such as the COPD Assessment Test and the COPD Control Questionnaire. Both items are available in the GOLD Report available at http://goldcopd.org/gold-reports.

- Group A (few symptoms; low risk): mild/moderate airflow limitation + low symptom scores +1 or fewer exacerbations per year
- Group B (increased symptoms; low risk): mild/moderate airflow limitation + low symptom scores +1 or fewer exacerbations per year
- Group C (few symptoms; high risk): severe/very severe airflow limitation + high symptom scores +2 or more exacerbations per year
- Group D (increased symptoms; high risk): severe/very severe airflow limitation + high symptom scores +2 or more exacerbations per year

Management is often challenging because patients with COPD commonly have comorbidities that complicate management choices.

These four categories are often used to initiate therapy and provide a starting point from which COPD management can then be individualized (Table 62.14).

Management of Stable Chronic Obstructive Pulmonary Disease

Pharmacologic management of stable COPD relies primarily on bronchodilators, glucocorticoids, and PDE4 inhibitors. The GOLD Report offers recommendations to guide selection of each class.

Bronchodilators

Inhaled long-acting formulations of either β_2 agonists or anticholinergics are preferred for bronchodilation. Theophylline is reserved for use only when other bronchodilators are not available.

Glucocorticoids

Long-term inhaled glucocorticoids are recommended when symptoms are severe or when long-acting bronchodilators are inadequate for management of exacerbations. When given for COPD, glucocorticoids should be given in combination with a LABA; glucocorticoid monotherapy is not recommended for long-term therapy because of decreased efficacy when used alone.

Phosphodiesterase-4 Inhibitors

In patients with severe, chronic COPD, the risk for exacerbations may be reduced with roflumilast should be used in combination with a LAMA, a LABA, or an inhaled glucocorticoid.

Management of Chronic Obstructive Pulmonary Disease Exacerbations

Although some of the same drugs used for management of stable COPD are also used for management of COPD exacerbations but are used in combinations. LAMAs have demonstrated better outcomes for exacerbations than LABAs in clinical trials. Systemic glucocorticoids greatly improve outcomes when used in management of COPD exacerbations. Other agents that may be used to control and shorten exacerbations include antibiotics for patients who have signs and symptoms of infection and supplemental oxygen to maintain an oxygen saturation of 88% to 92%.

TABLE 62.13 Classification of COPD Airflow Limitation Severity Post-Bronchodilator Spirometry Determinations

FEV$_1$/FVC <0.7	
Severity	Predicted FEV$_1$
Mild	≥80%
Moderate	50%–79%
Severe	30%–49%
Very Severe	<30%

COPD, Chronic obstructive pulmonary disease; FEV$_1$, forced expiratory volume in 1 second; FVC, Forced vital capacity.

TABLE 62.14 Initiation of COPD Pharmacologic Management

COPD Category	Symptom Control	First-Choice Recommendation	Management of Persistent Symptoms or Further Exacerbations
A (Few symptoms, low risk)	SABA	Consider LAMA or LABA	–
B (Increased symptoms, low risk)	SABA	LAMA or LABA	Combination LAMA/LABA
C (Few symptoms, high risk)	SABA	LAMA	Combination LAMA/LABA (preferred) or LABA/IGC
D (Increased symptoms, low risk)	SABA	LAMA or LAMA/LABA or IGC/LABA	Combination LAMA/LABA/IGC If exacerbations continue, consider adding: Roflumilast Azithromycin

IGC, Inhaled glucocorticoid; LABA, long-acting β_2 agonist; LAMA, long-acting muscarinic antagonist; SABA, short-acting β_2 agonist.

From Global Initiative for Chronic Obstructive Lung Disease. Global strategy for prevention, diagnosis and management of COPD; 2019. Available at https://goldcopd.org/gold-reports.

63

Drugs for Allergic Rhinitis, Cough, and Colds

The drugs addressed in this chapter are prescribed to alleviate symptoms of common upper respiratory disorders. Most are discussed in more depth in other chapters. Our principal focus here is on the symptoms of allergic rhinitis and the common cold.

DRUGS FOR ALLERGIC RHINITIS

Allergic rhinitis is an inflammatory disorder that affects the upper airway. Major symptoms are sneezing, rhinorrhea, pruritus, and nasal congestion caused by dilation and increased permeability of nasal blood vessels. In addition, some patients experience associated conjunctivitis, sinusitis, and even asthma. Symptoms are triggered by airborne allergens, which bind to immunoglobulin E (IgE) antibodies on mast cells and lead to the release of inflammatory mediators, including histamine, leukotrienes, and prostaglandins. Allergic rhinitis is the most common allergic disorder, affecting almost one out of every six people living in the United States.

Allergic rhinitis has two major forms: seasonal and perennial. Seasonal rhinitis, also known as *hay fever*, occurs in the spring and fall in reaction to outdoor allergens such as fungi and pollens from weeds, grasses, and trees. Perennial (nonseasonal) rhinitis is triggered by indoor allergens, especially the house dust mite and pet dander.

Several classes of drugs are used for allergic rhinitis (Table 63.1). Principal among these are (1) glucocorticoids (intranasal), (2) antihistamines (oral and intranasal), and (3) sympathomimetics (oral and intranasal).

The American Academy of Otolaryngology's (AAO) *Clinical Practice Guideline: Allergic Rhinitis* (2015) provides guidance by individualizing drug choice for symptom control. An algorithm for management of allergic rhinitis, developed by the AAO, is shown in Fig. 63.1.

Intranasal Glucocorticoids

The basic pharmacology of the glucocorticoids is discussed in Chapter 58. Consideration here is limited to their use in allergic rhinitis.

Actions and Uses

Intranasal glucocorticoids are the most effective drugs for prevention and treatment of seasonal and perennial rhinitis. Because of their antiinflammatory actions, these drugs can prevent or suppress the major symptoms of allergic rhinitis: congestion, rhinorrhea, sneezing, nasal itching, and erythema in 90% of patients who use them properly. Eight intranasal glucocorticoids are available (Table 63.2). Three of these—budesonide (Rhinocort Aqua), fluticasone propionate (Flonase), and triamcinolone (Nasacort Allergy 24 hours)—are available in the United States without a prescription. All appear equally effective.

Adverse Effects

Adverse effects of intranasal glucocorticoids are generally mild. The most common are *drying of the nasal mucosa* and a *burning or itching sensation. Sore throat, epistaxis,* and *headache* may also occur.

Systemic effects are possible but are rare at recommended doses. The major concerns are adrenal suppression and slowing of linear growth in children (whether final adult height is reduced is unknown). Systemic effects are least likely with ciclesonide, fluticasone, and mometasone, which have very low bioavailability (see Table 63.2).

Preparations, Dosage, and Administration

Intranasal glucocorticoids are administered using a metered-dose spray device. Benefits are greatest when dosing is done daily rather than irregularly. Full doses are given initially (see Table 63.2). After symptoms are under control, the dosage should be reduced to the lowest effective amount. For patients with seasonal allergic rhinitis, maximal effects may require a week or more to develop. However, an initial response can be seen within hours. For patients with perennial rhinitis, maximal responses may take 2 to 3 weeks to develop. If nasal congestion is present, a topical decongestant given before glucocorticoid administration will improve the response.

Antihistamines

The antihistamines are discussed in Chapter 56. Consideration here is limited to their use in allergic rhinitis.

Oral Antihistamines

Oral antihistamines (histamine-1 [H_1] receptor antagonists) are first-line drugs for mild to moderate allergic rhinitis. For therapy of allergic rhinitis, antihistamines are most effective when taken *prophylactically* and less helpful when taken after symptoms appear.

Actions and uses. These drugs can relieve sneezing, rhinorrhea, and nasal itching; however, they do not reduce nasal congestion. Because histamine is only one of several mediators of allergic rhinitis, antihistamines are less effective than glucocorticoids. Antihistamines should be administered on a regular basis throughout the allergy season, even when symptoms are absent, to prevent an initial histamine receptor activation.

Because histamine does not contribute to symptoms of infectious rhinitis, antihistamines are of no value against the common cold. Some patients take first-generation antihistamines for their drying effect; however, this may complicate treatment of colds by increasing the viscosity of secretions.

Adverse effects. Adverse effects are usually mild. The most common complaint is *sedation,* which occurs frequently with the first-generation antihistamines (e.g., diphenhydramine) and much less often with the second-generation agents (e.g., fexofenadine). Accordingly, second-generation agents are clearly preferred for students who need to remain alert in class and for patients who do work that requires alertness. *Anticholinergic effects* (e.g., drying of nasal secretions, dry mouth, constipation, and urinary hesitancy) are common with first-generation agents and relatively rare with the second-generation agents.

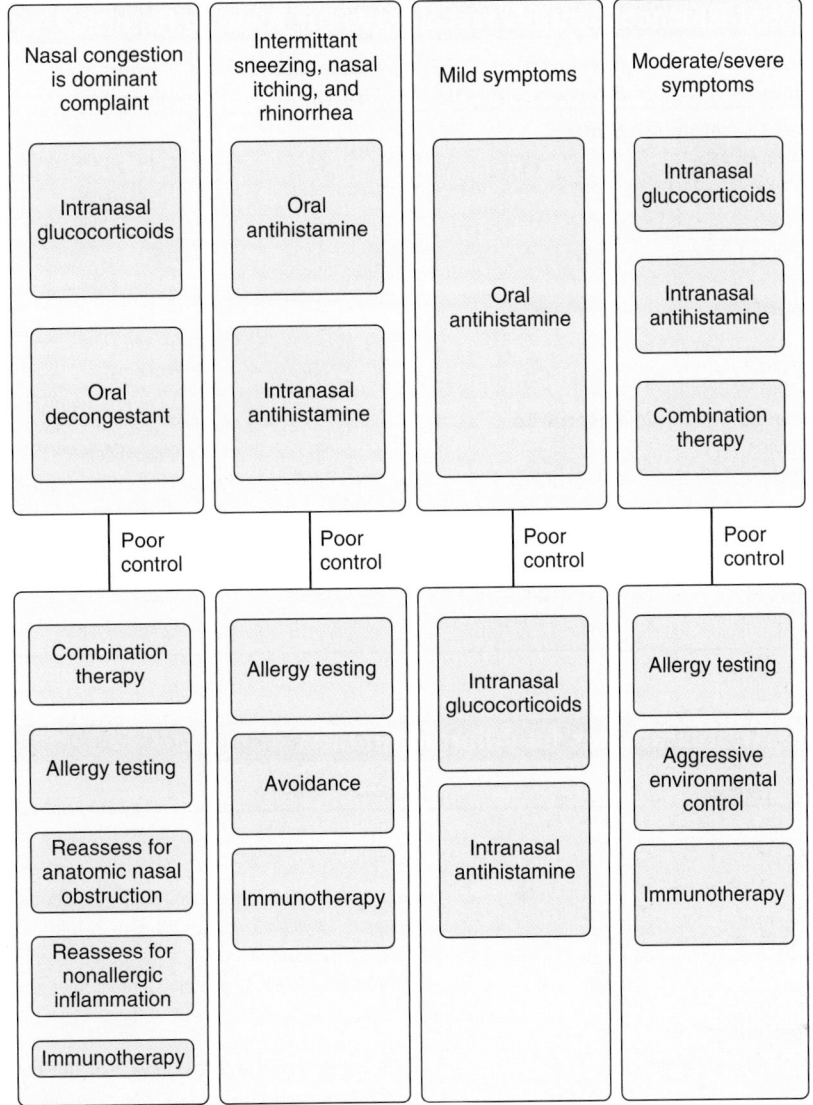

Fig. 63.1 Pharmacologic Management of Allergic Rhinitis. *INS,* Intranasal steroids. (From American Academy of Otolaryngology. Clinical practice guideline: allergic rhinitis; 2015. http://www.entnet.org/content/clinical-practice-guideline-allergic-rhinitis.)

TABLE 63.1 Overview of Drugs for Allergic Rhinitis

Drug or Class	Route	Actions	Adverse Effects
Glucocorticoids	Nasal	Prevent inflammatory response to allergens and thus reduce all symptoms.	Nasal irritation; possible slowing of linear growth in children
Antihistamines	Oral/nasal	Block histamine-1 receptors and thus decrease itching, sneezing, and rhinorrhea; do *not* reduce congestion.	*Oral:* Sedation and anticholinergic effects (mostly with first-generation agents) *Nasal:* Bitter taste
Cromolyn	Nasal	Prevents release of inflammatory mediators from mast cells and thus can decrease all symptoms. However, benefits are modest.	None
Sympathomimetics	Oral/nasal	Activate vascular α_1 receptors and cause vasoconstriction, which reduces nasal congestion; do *not* decrease sneezing, itching, or rhinorrhea.	*Oral:* Restlessness, insomnia, and increased blood pressure *Nasal:* Rebound nasal congestion
Anticholinergics	Nasal	Block nasal cholinergic receptors and hence reduce secretions; do *not* decrease sneezing, nasal congestion, or postnasal drip.	Nasal drying and irritation
Antileukotrienes	Oral	Block leukotriene receptors and thus reduce nasal congestion.	Rare neuropsychiatric effects

TABLE 63.2   Selected Glucocorticoid Nasal Sprays for Allergic Rhinitis

Drug	Trade Name	Intranasal Bioavailability (%)	Dose/Spray (mcg)	Patient Age (Years)	Initial Dosage (Sprays/Nostril)
First Generation: Increased Systemic Absorption					
Beclomethasone	Beconase AQ	44	42	6–11	1 twice daily
				12 and older	1 or 2 twice daily
	Qnasl	—	80	12 and older	2 once daily
Budesonide	Rhinocort Aqua	34	32	6–11	1 or 2 once daily
				12 and older	1–4 once daily
Flunisolide	Generic only	49	25	6–13	2 twice daily or 1 thrice daily
				14 and older	2 twice or thrice daily
Triamcinolone	Nasacort AQ	46	55	6 and older	1 or 2 once daily
Second Generation: Decreased Systemic Absorption					
Ciclesonide	Omnaris	—	50	6 and older	2 once daily
Fluticasone propionate	Flonase	0.5–2	50	4–11	1 once daily
				12 and older	2 once daily
Fluticasone furoate	Veramyst	—	27.5	2–11	1 once daily
				12 and older	2 once daily
Mometasone	Nasonex	0.1	50	2–11	1 once daily
				12 and older	2 once daily

TABLE 63.3   Some Antihistamines for Allergic Rhinitis

Generic Name	Trade Name	Dosage
Oral Antihistamines		
First Generation (Sedating)		
Chlorpheniramine	Chlor-Trimeton Allergy, Chlor-Tripolon ♦ and others	*Adults and children 12 years and older:* 4 mg every 4–6 h *Children 6–11 years:* 2 mg every 4–6 h
Diphenhydramine	Benadryl and others	*Adults:* 25–50 mg every 4–6 h *Children under 10 kg:* 12.5–25 mg three or four times/day
Second Generation (Nonsedating)		
Cetirizine[a]	Zyrtec and Reactine ♦	*Adults and children 6 years and older:* 5 or 10 mg once daily
Levocetirizine	Xyzal	*Adults and children 12 years and older:* 5 mg once daily *Children 6–11 years:* 2.5 mg once daily
Fexofenadine	Allegra	*Adults and children 12 years and older:* 60 mg twice daily or 180 mg once daily
Loratadine	Claritin and Alavert	*Adults and children 6 years and older:* 10 mg once daily
Desloratadine	Clarinex and Aerius ♦	*Adults and children 12 years and older:* 5 mg once daily
Intranasal Antihistamines		
Second Generation (Nonsedating)		
Azelastine[a]	Astelin and Astepro	*Adults and children 12 years and older:* 2 sprays/nostril twice daily *Children 5–11 years:* 1 spray/nostril twice daily[b]
Olopatadine	Patanase	*Adults and children 12 years and older:* 2 sprays/nostril twice daily (665 mcg/spray)

[a]May cause some sedation at recommended doses.
[b]Astelin only. Astepro is not approved for children below the age of 12 years.

Preparations, dosage, and administration. Dosages for some popular H_1 antagonists are presented in Table 63.3. A more complete list appears in Chapter 56.

Intranasal Antihistamines

Two antihistamines—*azelastine* (Astelin and Astepro) and *olopatadine* (Patanase)—are available for intranasal administration. Both drugs are indicated for allergic rhinitis in adults and children older than 12 years. Both drugs are supplied in metered-spray devices.

The usual dosage is two sprays in each nostril twice daily. With both drugs, systemic absorption can cause somnolence. Additionally, some patients experience nosebleeds and headaches with both azelastine and olopatadine. These drugs can also cause an unpleasant taste.

Intranasal Cromolyn Sodium

The basic pharmacology of cromolyn sodium is discussed in Chapter 62. Consideration here is limited to its use in allergic rhinitis.

Actions and Uses

For treatment of allergic rhinitis, intranasal cromolyn (Nasalcrom) is extremely safe but only moderately effective. Benefits are much less than those of intranasal glucocorticoids. Cromolyn reduces symptoms by suppressing the release of histamine and other inflammatory mediators from mast cells. Accordingly, the drug is best suited for prophylaxis and hence should be given before symptoms start. Responses may take a week or two to develop; patients should be informed of this delay. Adverse reactions are minimal—less than with any other drug for allergic rhinitis.

Preparations, Dosage, and Administration

For treatment of allergic rhinitis, cromolyn sodium is available in a metered-dose spray device that delivers 5.2 mg/actuation. The usual dosage for adults and children above the age of 2 years is one spray (5.2 mg) per nostril four to six times a day. If nasal congestion is present, a topical decongestant should be used before cromolyn. Like the antihistamines and glucocorticoids, cromolyn should be dosed on a regular schedule throughout the allergy season.

Sympathomimetics (Decongestants)
Actions and Uses

Sympathomimetics reduce nasal congestion by activating α_1-adrenergic receptors on nasal blood vessels. This causes vasoconstriction, which, in turn, causes shrinkage of swollen membranes followed by nasal drainage. With *topical* administration, vasoconstriction is both rapid and intense. With *oral* administration, responses are delayed, moderate, and prolonged.

In patients with allergic rhinitis, sympathomimetics only relieve congestion. They do not reduce rhinorrhea, sneezing, or itching. In addition to their use in allergic rhinitis, sympathomimetics can reduce congestion associated with sinusitis and colds. Routes and dosages are shown in Table 63.4.

Adverse Effects

Rebound congestion. Rebound congestion develops when *topical* agents are used more than a few days. With prolonged use, as the effects of each application wear off, congestion becomes progressively worse. To overcome this rebound congestion, the patient must use progressively larger and more frequent doses. Once established, rebound congestion can lead to a cycle of escalating congestion and increased drug use. The cycle can be broken by abrupt decongestant withdrawal; however, this tactic can be extremely uncomfortable. A less drastic option is to discontinue the drug in one nostril at a time. An even better option is to use an intranasal glucocorticoid (in both nostrils) for 2 to 6 weeks, starting 1 week before discontinuing the decongestant. Development of rebound congestion can be minimized by limiting topical application to 3 to 5 days. Accordingly, topical sympathomimetics are not appropriate for individuals with chronic rhinitis.

Central nervous system stimulation. Central nervous system (CNS) excitation is the most common adverse effect of the *oral* sympathomimetics. Symptoms include restlessness, irritability, anxiety, and insomnia. These responses are uncommon with topical agents when used as recommended.

Cardiovascular effects. By activating α_1-adrenergic receptors on systemic blood vessels, sympathomimetics can cause widespread vasoconstriction. Generalized vasoconstriction is most likely with *oral* agents. However, if used in excess, even the topical agents can cause significant systemic vasoconstriction. For most patients, effects on systemic vessels are inconsequential. However, for individuals with cardiovascular disorders—hypertension, coronary artery disease, cardiac arrhythmias, and cerebrovascular disease—widespread vasoconstriction can be hazardous.

Abuse. *Pseudoephedrine* is associated with abuse. By causing CNS stimulation, this sympathomimetic can produce subjective effects similar to those of amphetamine. Also, it can be readily converted to methamphetamine, a widely used drug of abuse. To reduce the availability of pseudoephedrine for methamphetamine production, Congress passed the *Combat Methamphetamine Epidemic Act of 2005*, which requires that all products containing pseudoephedrine be placed behind the counter (even though it can still be purchased without a prescription in some states). Furthermore, purchasers must present identification and sign a log. Also, individuals can purchase no more than 9 g per month or 3.6 g on any day. Because of these constraints, many products are being reformulated to contain phenylephrine rather than ephedrine and pseudoephedrine. Unfortunately, although pseudoephedrine is an excellent decongestant, when taken orally, phenylephrine is not very effective. Some randomized controlled trials have demonstrated that phenylephrine is little better than a placebo.

Factors in Topical Administration

General considerations. Because of the risk for rebound congestion, topical sympathomimetics should be used for no more than 3 to 5 consecutive days. To avoid systemic effects, doses should not exceed those recommended by the manufacturer. The applicator should be cleansed after each use to prevent contamination.

Drops. Drops should be administered with the patient in a lateral, head-low position. This causes the drops to spread slowly over the nasal mucosa, thereby promoting beneficial effects while reducing the amount that is swallowed. Because the number of drops can be precisely controlled, drops allow better control of dosage when compared with sprays. Accordingly, because young children are particularly susceptible to toxicity, drops are preferred for them.

Sprays. Sprays deliver the decongestant in a fine mist. Although convenient, sprays are less effective than an equal volume of properly instilled drops.

Contrasts Between Oral and Topical Agents

Oral and topical sympathomimetics differ in several important respects. First, topical agents act faster than the oral agents and are usually more effective. Second, oral agents act longer than topical preparations. Third,

TABLE 63.4   Sympathomimetics Used for Nasal Decongestion

Decongestant	Mode of Use	Dosing Interval	Dosage Size[a]
Phenylephrine (Neo-Synephrine and others)	Drops	Every 4 h or more	*6 years and older:* 2–3 drops (0.25%–1%) *2–6 years:* 2–3 drops (0.125%)
	Spray	Every 4 h or more	*12 years and older:* 2–3 sprays (0.25%–1%) *6–12 years:* 2–3 sprays (0.25%) *2–6 years:* Not recommended
	Oral	Every 4 h	*12 years and older:* 10 mg *6–11 years:* 5 mg *4–5 years:* 2.5 mg *Younger than 4 years:* not recommended
Pseudoephedrine (Sudafed and others)	Oral	Every 4–6 h	*12 years and older:* 60 mg *6–12 years:* 30 mg *Younger than 6 years:* 15 mg
	Oral SR	Every 12 h	*12 years and older:* 120 mg *Younger than 12 years:* not recommended
	Oral CR	Every 24 h	*12 years and older:* 240 mg *Younger than 12 years:* not recommended
Naphazoline (Privine)	Drops	Every 6 h or more	*12 years and older:* 1 or 2 drops (0.05%) *Younger than 12 years:* Not recommended
	Spray	Every 6 h or more	*12 years and older:* 1 or 2 sprays (0.05%) *Younger than 12 years:* Not recommended
Oxymetazoline (Afrin 12-Hour, Neo-Synephrine 12-Hour, Dristan 12-Hour, and others)	Spray	Every 10–12 h	*6 years and older:* 2–3 sprays (0.05%) *Younger than 6 years:* not recommended
Tetrahydrozoline (Tyzine)	Drops	Every 3 h or more	*6 years and older:* 2–4 drops (0.1%) *2–6 years:* 2–3 drops (0.05%)
	Spray	Every 3 h or more	*6 years and older:* 3–4 sprays (0.1%) *Younger than 6 years:* not recommended
Xylometazoline (Otrivin)	Drops	Every 8–10 h	*12 years and older:* 2–3 drops (0.1%) *2–12 years:* 2–3 drops (0.05%)
	Spray	Every 8–10 h	*12 years and older:* 1–3 sprays (0.1%) *2–12 years:* 1 spray (0.05%)

[a]For drops and sprays, dosage listed is applied to *each* nostril; numbers in parentheses indicate concentration of solution employed. *CR,* Controlled release; *SR,* sustained release.

systemic effects (vasoconstriction and CNS stimulation) occur primarily with oral agents; topical agents usually elicit these responses only when dosage is higher than recommended. Fourth, rebound congestion is common with prolonged use of topical agents but is rare with oral agents.

Comparison of Phenylephrine and Pseudoephedrine

Phenylephrine is one of the most widely used nasal decongestants. The drug is administered topically as a single agent and orally as a component of combination preparations. When administered topically, phenylephrine is both fast and effective. When taken orally, the drug is not very effective, in large part because of extensive first-pass metabolism. Although it might seem logical to simply increase the dosage, this is not advisable because, even though absorption is poor, phenylephrine can still cause adverse cardiovascular and CNS effects.

Pseudoephedrine is available for oral administration. Compared with oral phenylephrine, pseudoephedrine is better absorbed, has a longer half-life, and is much more effective.

Antihistamine/Sympathomimetic and Antihistamine/Glucocorticoid Combinations

Some patients require combined therapy with a sympathomimetic or glucocorticoid in addition to an antihistamine. Although antihistamines alone are a first-line treatment, they do not relieve nasal congestion and may be inadequate for some patients. For these patients, addition of a sympathomimetic or glucocorticoid may be indicated. This can be accomplished in one of two ways: by giving the drugs separately or by using a combination product. Some popular combination products are listed in Table 63.5.

Ipratropium, an Anticholinergic Agent

Ipratropium bromide (Atrovent) is an anticholinergic agent. The drug is indicated for allergic rhinitis, asthma, and the common cold. To treat allergic rhinitis, ipratropium is administered as a nasal spray (0.03% and 0.06%). Blockade of cholinergic receptors inhibits secretions from the serous and seromucous glands lining the nasal mucosa and decreases rhinorrhea. The drug does not decrease sneezing, nasal congestion, or postnasal drip. At the doses used for allergic rhinitis, side effects are minimal. The most common side effects are nasal drying and irritation. Ipratropium does not readily cross membranes because it is a quaternary ammonium compound; hence systemic effects are absent. Dosages for allergic rhinitis in patients above the age of 12 years range from two sprays of 0.03% ipratropium (42 mcg total) per nostril two to three times a day to two sprays of 0.06% ipratropium (84 mcg total) per nostril four times a day. The use of ipratropium for asthma is discussed in Chapter 62.

Montelukast, a Leukotriene Antagonist

Montelukast (Singulair), originally approved for asthma, is now approved for seasonal and perennial allergic rhinitis as well. Benefits derive from

TABLE 63.5   Some Antihistamine Combination Products

	Trade Name	Dosage
Antihistamine/Sympathomimetic		
Acrivastine/ pseudoephedrine	Semprex-D Capsules	8 mg/60 mg four times daily
Chlorpheniramine/ pseudoephedrine	Allerest Maximum Strength Tablets	4 mg/60 mg every 4–6 h
Fexofenadine/ pseudoephedrine	Allegra-D 12-Hour Tablets	60 mg/120 mg twice daily
Loratadine/ pseudoephedrine	Claritin-D 12-Hour Tablets	5 mg/120 mg every 12 h
Desloratadine/ pseudoephedrine	Clarinex-D 12-Hour Tablets	2.5 mg/120 mg every 12 h
Triprolidine/ pseudoephedrine	Actifed Cold and Allergy Tablets	2.5 mg/60 mg every 4–6 h
Antihistamine/Glucocorticoid		
Azelastine/ fluticasone propionate	Dymista	*Adults and children 12 years and older:* 1 spray/nostril twice daily

blocking binding of leukotrienes to their receptors. In people with allergic rhinitis, leukotrienes act primarily to cause nasal congestion (by promoting vasodilation and by increasing vascular permeability). Hence, by blocking leukotriene receptors, montelukast relieves nasal congestion, although it has little effect on sneezing or itching. When used alone or in combination with an antihistamine, montelukast is less effective than intranasal glucocorticoids. Although montelukast is generally well tolerated, it can cause rare but serious neuropsychiatric effects including agitation, aggression, hallucinations, depression, insomnia, restlessness, and suicidal thinking and behavior. Because of these adverse effects, along with limited beneficial effects, it is probably best to reserve montelukast for patients who do not respond to or cannot tolerate intranasal glucocorticoids, antihistamines, or both. Administration is oral. Dosage, which varies with age, is the same as that used for asthma.

Omalizumab, a Monoclonal Antibody

Omalizumab (Xolair) is a monoclonal antibody directed against IgE, an immunoglobulin (antibody) that plays a central role in the allergic release of inflammatory mediators from mast cells and basophils. Omalizumab is approved only for allergy-mediated asthma; however, several studies have demonstrated significant improvement of allergic symptoms. Because patients with ragweed-induced seasonal allergic rhinitis have achieved symptom relief with omalizumab when other drugs have been ineffective, this drug is sometimes prescribed off-label for management while clinical trials continue. Monoclonal antibodies and other biologics are discussed in Chapter 84.

DRUGS FOR COUGH

Cough is a complex reflex involving the CNS, the peripheral nervous system, and the muscles of respiration. The cough reflex can be initiated by irritation of the bronchial mucosa as well as by stimuli arising at sites distant from the respiratory tract. Cough is often beneficial, serving to remove foreign matter and excess secretions from the bronchial tree. For example, the productive cough that is characteristic

of chronic lung disease (e.g., emphysema, asthma, and bronchitis) should not be suppressed. Not all cough, however, is useful. When cough is nonproductive, creates discomfort, or deprives patients of comfort or sleep, cough suppressant medication is appropriate. The most common use of cough medicines is suppression of nonproductive cough associated with the common cold and other upper respiratory infections.

Antitussives

Antitussives are drugs that suppress cough. Some agents act within the CNS; others act peripherally. The antitussives fall into two major groups: (1) opioid antitussives and (2) nonopioid antitussives. Interestingly, although the major antitussives—codeine, dextromethorphan, and diphenhydramine—are clearly effective against chronic nonproductive cough and experimentally induced cough, there is no good evidence that these drugs can suppress cough associated with the common cold.

Opioid Antitussives

All the opioid analgesics have the ability to suppress cough. The two opioids used most often for cough suppression are *codeine* and *hydrocodone*. Both drugs act in the CNS to elevate cough threshold. Hydrocodone is somewhat more potent than codeine and carries a greater liability for abuse. The basic pharmacology of the opioids is discussed in Chapter 24.

Codeine is the most effective cough suppressant available. The drug is active orally and can decrease both the frequency and intensity of cough. Doses are low; about $\frac{1}{10}$ of the dose needed to relieve pain. At these doses, when taken as directed and only when needed, the risk for physical dependence is small.

Like all other opioids, codeine can suppress respiration. Accordingly, the drug should be employed with caution in patients with reduced respiratory reserve. In the event of overdose, respiratory depression may prove fatal. An opioid antagonist (e.g., naloxone) should be used to reverse toxicity.

When dispensed by itself, codeine has a significant potential for abuse and therefore is classified under Schedule II of the Controlled Substances Act. However, the abuse potential of the antitussive mixtures that contain codeine is low. Accordingly, these mixtures are classified under Schedule V.

For treatment of cough, the adult dosage is 10 to 20 mg orally, four to six times a day. Codeine is rarely recommended for children.

Nonopioid Antitussives

Dextromethorphan. Dextromethorphan is the most effective over-the-counter (OTC) nonopioid cough medicine and the most widely used of all cough medicines. Like the opioids, dextromethorphan acts in the CNS. Dextromethorphan is a derivative of the opioids; however, it does not produce typical opioid-like euphoria or physical dependence. Nonetheless, when taken in high doses, dextromethorphan can cause euphoria and is sometimes abused for this effect (see Chapter 35). Depending on the dose, subjective effects can range from mild inebriation to a state of mind-body dissociation, much like that caused by phencyclidine (PCP). At therapeutic doses, dextromethorphan does not depress respiration. Adverse effects are mild and rare. Dextromethorphan is the active ingredient in more than 140 nonprescription cough medicines. The usual adult dosage is 10 to 30 mg every 4 to 8 hours.

In the past, dextromethorphan was considered devoid of analgesic actions; however, it now appears the drug *can* reduce pain. The mechanism is blockade of receptors for *N*-methyl-D-aspartate (NMDA) in the brain and spinal cord. In contrast, opioids relieve pain primarily through activation of mu receptors. Although dextromethorphan has minimal analgesic effects when used alone, it can enhance analgesic effects of the opioids. For example, we can double the analgesic response to 30 mg of morphine by combining the morphine with 30 mg of dextromethorphan.

Other nonopioid antitussives. *Diphenhydramine* is an antihistamine with the ability to suppress cough. The mechanism is unclear. Like other antihistamines, diphenhydramine has sedative and anticholinergic properties. Cough suppression is achieved only at doses that produce prominent sedation. The usual adult dosage is 25 mg every 4 hours.

Benzonatate (Tessalon and Zonatuss) is a structural analog of two local anesthetics: tetracaine and procaine. The drug suppresses cough by decreasing the sensitivity of respiratory tract stretch receptors (components of the cough-reflex pathway). Adverse effects are usually mild (e.g., sedation, dizziness, and constipation). Nonetheless, severe effects can occur in children and adults. In children below 2 years of age, accidental ingestion of just one or two capsules has been fatal. In older children and adults, overdose can cause seizures, dysrhythmia, and death. Smaller doses can cause confusion, chest numbness, visual hallucinations, and a burning sensation in the eyes. If the capsules are sucked or chewed, rather than swallowed, the drug can cause laryngospasm, bronchospasm, and circulatory collapse. Accordingly, benzonatate capsules should be swallowed intact. The usual adult dosage is 100 mg three times a day. Safety and efficacy have not been established in children below the age of 10 years.

Expectorants and Mucolytics
Expectorants
An expectorant is a drug that renders cough more productive by stimulating the flow of respiratory tract secretions. A variety of compounds (e.g., ammonium chloride and iodide products) have been promoted for their supposed expectorant actions. However, in almost all cases, efficacy is questionable. One agent—guaifenesin (Mucinex, Humibid, and others]—may be an exception. However, for this drug to be effective, doses higher than those normally employed may be needed.

Mucolytics
A mucolytic is a drug that reacts directly with mucus to make it more watery. This action should help make cough more productive. Two preparations—hypertonic saline and acetylcysteine—are employed for their mucolytic actions. Both are administered by inhalation. Unfortunately, both can trigger bronchospasm. Because of its sulfur content, acetylcysteine has the additional drawback of smelling like rotten eggs.

COLD REMEDIES: COMBINATION PREPARATIONS
Basic Considerations
The common cold is an acute *upper* respiratory infection of viral origin. Between 50% and 80% of colds are caused by the human rhinovirus, which can also cause serious infection of the *lower* respiratory tract. Characteristic symptoms of the common cold are rhinorrhea, nasal congestion, cough, sneezing, sore throat, hoarseness, headache, malaise, and myalgia; fever is common in children but rare in adults. Colds are self-limited and usually benign. Persistence or worsening of symptoms suggests development of a secondary bacterial infection. In the United States, the economic burden of the cold is estimated at more than $60 billion a year.

There is no cure for the cold, so treatment is purely symptomatic. Because colds are caused by viruses, there is no justification for the routine use of antibiotics. These agents are appropriate only if a bacterial coinfection arises. There is also no evidence that vitamin C or zinc can prevent or cure colds.

Because no single drug can relieve all symptoms of a cold, the pharmaceutical industry has formulated a vast number of cold remedies that contain a mixture of ingredients. These combination cold remedies should be reserved for patients with multiple symptoms. In addition, the combination chosen should contain only those agents that are appropriate for the symptoms at hand. Patients who require relief from just a single symptom (e.g., rhinitis, cough, or headache) are best treated with single-drug preparations.

Combination cold remedies frequently contain two or more of the following: (1) a nasal decongestant, (2) an antitussive, (3) an analgesic, (4) an antihistamine, and (5) caffeine. The purpose of the first three agents is self-evident. In contrast, the roles of antihistamines and caffeine require explanation. Because histamine has nothing to do with the symptoms of a cold, the purpose of including antihistamines is not to block histamine receptors. Rather, because of their anticholinergic actions, antihistamines are sometimes included to suppress mucus secretion. (This action can potentially worsen upper respiratory infections by thickening secretions, making them more difficult to drain. This may create an environment conducive to bacterial proliferation, which may lead to secondary bacterial infections such as sinusitis.) Caffeine is added to some preparations to offset the sedative effects of the antihistamine. They may also have an effect on an associated headache.

Although they can be convenient, combination cold remedies do have disadvantages. As with all fixed-dose combinations, there is the chance that a dosage (e.g., 1 capsule or 1 tablet) that produces therapeutic levels of one ingredient may produce levels of other ingredients that are either excessive or subtherapeutic. In addition, the combination may contain ingredients that the patient does not need. Furthermore, under the US Food and Drug Administration (FDA) regulations, a brand-name product can be reformulated and then sold under the same name. Hence, without carefully reading the label, the consumer has no assurance that the brand-name product purchased contains the same amounts of the same drugs that were present in a previous version of that combination product.

Use in Young Children
Many experts believe that OTC cold remedies should not be used by young children. There is no proof of efficacy or safety in pediatric patients—and there *is* proof of the potential for serious harm. According to the Centers for Disease Control and Prevention, thousands of children have been taken to emergency departments for management of adverse effects related to cough or cold products. Presenting symptoms have included convulsions, tachycardia, hallucinations, and impaired consciousness. Some children died. In early 2008, the FDA recommended that OTC cold remedies no longer be given to children below the age of 2 years, owing to the risk for potentially life-threatening events. The FDA is still reviewing the safety of these drugs in children aged 2 to 11 years. In the meantime, citing inadequate effectiveness, significant adverse effects, and common misuse, the American Academy of Pediatrics recommended restricting the use of cough and cold medicines to children above the age of 6 years. Manufacturers voluntarily revised the labels of children's cold and cough preparations to indicate they should not be used in children below the age of 4 years. In addition, for products that contain antihistamine, manufacturers added a warning against using these drugs to sedate children.

After these interventions, emergency visits related to cold and cough medications decreased significantly for children below the age of 4 years. To reduce harm to pediatric patients, parents should do the following:
- Avoid OTC cold remedies in children aged below 4 to 6 years.
- Only use products labeled for pediatric use.

- Consult a health care professional before giving these drugs to a child.
- Read all product safety information before dosing.
- Use the measuring device provided with the product.
- Discontinue the medicine and seek professional care if the child's condition worsens or fails to improve.
- Avoid using antihistamine-containing products to sedate children.

PATIENT EDUCATION

Managing the Common Cold in Children

With so few choices available for managing the common cold in children, parents are often left feeling helpless. In 2018, the American Academy of Pediatrics posted recommendations for parents on its Healthy Children website. The suggestions include:

- Use a nasal bulb to remove nasal secretions in children aged below 6 months.
- Use saline nose drops or nasal spray to decrease nasal stuffiness.
- Use a cool-mist humidifier to thin nasal secretions.
- For children older than 1 year, honey may be given to relieve cough.
- For children older than 2 years, mentholated chest rubs can relieve cough.
- Acetaminophen or ibuprofen can relieve discomfort.

See https://www.healthychildren.org/English/safety-prevention/at-home/medication-safety/Pages/How-to-Manage-Colds-and-Flu.aspx for additional information.

64

Drugs for Peptic Ulcer Disease

Peptic ulcer disease (PUD) refers to a group of upper gastrointestinal (GI) disorders characterized by varying degrees of erosion of the esophagus, stomach, and small intestine. Severe ulcers can be complicated by hemorrhage and perforation. Although peptic ulcers can develop in any region exposed to acid and pepsin, ulceration is most common in the lesser curvature of the stomach and the duodenum. PUD is a common disorder that affects about 10% of Americans at some time in their lives. About 6 million Americans get ulcers each year. Before the mid-1990s, PUD was considered a chronic, relapsing disorder of unknown cause and with no known cure; therapy promoted healing but did not prevent ulcer recurrence. Today, thanks to the pioneering work of two Australians—Barry J. Marshall and J. Robin Warren—we know that most cases of PUD are caused by infection with *Helicobacter pylori* and that eradication of this bacterium not only promotes healing but also greatly reduces the chance of recurrence.

PATHOGENESIS OF PEPTIC ULCERS

Peptic ulcers develop when there is an imbalance between mucosal defensive factors and aggressive factors (Fig. 64.1). The major defensive factors are mucus and bicarbonate. The major aggressive factors are *H. pylori*, nonsteroidal antiinflammatory drugs (NSAIDs), gastric acid, and pepsin.

Defensive Factors

Defensive factors serve the physiologic role of protecting the stomach and duodenum from self-digestion. When defenses are intact, ulcers are unlikely. Conversely, when defenses are compromised, aggressive factors can cause injury. Two important agents that can weaken defenses are *H. pylori* and NSAIDs.

Mucus

Mucus is secreted continuously by cells of the GI mucosa, forming a barrier that protects underlying cells from attack by acid and pepsin.

Bicarbonate

Bicarbonate is secreted by epithelial cells of the stomach and duodenum. Most bicarbonate remains trapped in the mucus layer, where it serves to neutralize any hydrogen ions that penetrate the mucus. Bicarbonate produced by the pancreas is secreted into the lumen of the duodenum, where it neutralizes acid delivered from the stomach.

Blood Flow

Adequate blood flow to cells of the GI mucosa is essential for maintaining mucosal integrity. If submucosal blood flow is reduced, the resultant local ischemia can lead to cell injury, thereby increasing vulnerability to attack by acid and pepsin.

Prostaglandins

Prostaglandins play an important role in maintaining defenses. These compounds stimulate secretion of mucus and bicarbonate, and they promote vasodilation, which helps maintain submucosal blood flow. They provide additional protection by suppressing secretion of gastric acid.

Aggressive Factors

Helicobacter pylori

H. pylori is a gram-negative bacillus that can colonize the stomach and duodenum. By taking up residence in the space between epithelial cells and the mucus barrier that protects these cells, the bacterium manages to escape destruction by acid and pepsin. When established, *H. pylori* can remain in the GI tract for decades. Although about half of the world's population is infected with *H. pylori*, most infected people never develop symptomatic PUD.

Why do we think *H. pylori* causes PUD? First, between 60% and 75% of patients with PUD have *H. pylori* infection. Second, duodenal ulcers are much more common among people with *H. pylori* infection than among people who are not infected. Third, eradication of the bacterium promotes ulcer healing. Fourth, eradication of the bacterium minimizes ulcer recurrence. (One-year recurrence rates approach 80% when *H. pylori* remains present, compared with only 10% when the organism is gone.)

Although the mechanism by which *H. pylori* promotes ulcers has not been firmly established, likely possibilities are enzymatic degradation of the protective mucus layer, elaboration of a cytotoxin that injures mucosal cells, and infiltration of neutrophils and other inflammatory cells in response to the bacterium's presence. Also, *H. pylori* produces *urease*, an enzyme that forms carbon dioxide and ammonia (from urea in gastric juice); both compounds are potentially toxic to the gastric mucosa.

In addition to its role in PUD, *H. pylori* appears to promote gastric cancer. In fact, the bacterium has been declared a type 1 carcinogen by the International Agency for Research on Cancer. There is a strong association between *H. pylori* infection and the presence of gastric mucosa-associated lymphoid tissue (MALT) lymphomas. Furthermore, among patients with localized MALT lymphoma, eradicating *H. pylori* produces tumor regression in 60% to 90% of cases. In one long-term study, treatment of *H. pylori* reduced the risk for gastric adenocarcinoma by 40% after 15 years.

Fig. 64.1 The Relationship of Mucosal Defenses and Aggressive Factors to Health and Peptic Ulcer Sisease. When aggressive factors outweigh mucosal defenses, gastritis and peptic ulcers result. *NSAID,* Nonsteroidal antiinflammatory drug.

Nonsteroidal Antiinflammatory Drugs

NSAIDs are the underlying cause of many gastric ulcers and some duodenal ulcers. As discussed in Chapter 57, aspirin and other NSAIDs inhibit the biosynthesis of prostaglandins. By doing so they can decrease submucosal blood flow, suppress secretion of mucus and bicarbonate, and promote secretion of gastric acid. Furthermore, NSAIDs can irritate the mucosa directly. NSAID-induced ulcers are most likely with long-term, high-dose therapy.

Gastric Acid

Gastric acid is an absolute requirement for peptic ulcer generation: in the absence of acid, no ulcer will form. Acid causes ulcers directly by injuring cells of the GI mucosa and indirectly by activating pepsin, a proteolytic enzyme. In most cases, acid hypersecretion by itself is insufficient to cause ulcers. In fact, in most patients with gastric ulcers, acid secretion is normal or reduced, and among patients with duodenal ulcers, only one-third produce excessive amounts of acid. From these observations we can conclude that, in most patients with peptic ulcers, factors in addition to acid must be involved.

Zollinger-Ellison syndrome is the primary disorder in which hypersecretion of acid alone causes ulcers. The syndrome is caused by a tumor that secretes gastrin, a hormone that stimulates gastric acid production. The amount of acid produced is so large that it overwhelms mucosal defenses. Zollinger-Ellison syndrome is a rare disorder that accounts for only 0.1% of duodenal ulcers.

Pepsin

Pepsin is a proteolytic enzyme present in gastric juice. Like gastric acid, pepsin can injure unprotected cells of the gastric and duodenal mucosa.

Smoking

Smoking delays ulcer healing and increases the risk for recurrence. Possible mechanisms include reduction of the beneficial effects of antiulcer medications, reduced secretion of bicarbonate, and accelerated gastric emptying, which would deliver more acid to the duodenum.

Summary

Infection with *H. pylori* is the most common cause of gastric and duodenal ulcers. However, among people whose PUD can be ascribed to *H. pylori*, additional factors must be involved, because more than

50% of the population harbors *H. pylori* but only 10% develop ulcers. Factors that may increase the risk for PUD in people infected with *H. pylori* include smoking, increased acid secretion, and reduced bicarbonate production. The second most common cause of gastric ulcers is NSAIDs. Hypersecretion of acid underlies a few cases of PUD that are not caused by *H. pylori* or NSAIDs.

OVERVIEW OF TREATMENT

Drug Therapy

The goals of drug therapy are to (1) alleviate symptoms, (2) promote healing, (3) prevent complications (hemorrhage, perforation, and obstruction), and (4) prevent recurrence. Except for antibiotics, the drugs employed do not alter the disease process. Rather, they simply create conditions conducive to healing. Because nonantibiotic therapies do not cure ulcers, the relapse rate after their discontinuation is high. In contrast, the relapse rate after antibiotic therapy is low.

Classes of Antiulcer Drugs

As shown in Table 64.1, the antiulcer drugs fall into five major groups:
- Antibiotics
- Antisecretory agents (proton pump inhibitors [PPIs] and histamine-2 [H$_2$] receptor antagonists)
- Mucosal protectants
- Antisecretory agents that enhance mucosal defenses
- Antacids

From this classification we can see that drugs act in three basic ways to promote ulcer healing. Specifically, they can (1) eradicate *H. pylori* (antibiotics do this), (2) reduce gastric acidity (antisecretory agents, misoprostol, and antacids do this), and (3) enhance mucosal defenses (sucralfate and misoprostol do this).

Drug Selection

Helicobacter pylori–*associated ulcers.* All patients with gastric or duodenal ulcers and documented *H. pylori* infection should be treated with antibiotics. This recommendation applies to patients with newly diagnosed PUD, recurrent PUD, and PUD in which use of NSAIDs is a contributing factor. To hasten healing and relieve symptoms, an antisecretory agent should be given along with the antibiotics. By eliminating *H. pylori*, antibiotics can cure PUD and prevent recurrence. Diagnosis of *H. pylori* infection and specific antibiotic regimens are discussed later under "Antibacterial Drugs."

NSAID-induced ulcers

Prophylaxis. For patients with risk factors for ulcer development (e.g., older than 60 years, history of ulcers, high-dose NSAID therapy), prophylactic therapy is indicated. PPIs (e.g., omeprazole) are preferred. Misoprostol is also effective but can cause diarrhea. Antacids, sucralfate, and H$_2$ receptor blockers are not recommended.

Treatment. NSAID-induced ulcers can be treated with any ulcer medication. However, H$_2$ receptor blockers and PPIs are preferred. If possible, the offending NSAID should be discontinued to accelerate healing. If the NSAID cannot be discontinued, a PPI is the best choice to promote healing.

Evaluation

We can evaluate ulcer healing by monitoring for relief of pain and by radiologic or endoscopic examination of the ulcer site. Unfortunately, evaluation is seldom straightforward because cessation of pain and disappearance of the ulcer rarely coincide—in most cases, pain subsides before complete healing. However, the converse may also be true—pain may persist even though endoscopic or radiologic examination reveals healing is complete.

TABLE 64.1   Classification of Antiulcer Drugs

Class	Drugs	Availability	Usual Daily Adult Dosing	Mechanism of Action
Antibiotics	Amoxicillin (generic only)	250- and 500-mg capsules 500- and 875-mg tablets 775-mg extended-release tablet 125- and 250-mg chewable tablets 125-mg/5 mL, 200-mg/5 mL, 250-mg/5 mL, and 400-mg/5 mL suspension	2000 mg	Eradicate *Helicobacter pylori*
	Bismuth (Pepto-Bismol)	262.4-mg tablets	3000 mg	
	Clarithromycin (Biaxin)	250-, 500-mg tablets 500-mg Extended release tablet 125-mg/5 mL and 250-mg/5 mL solution	1000 mg	
	Metronidazole (Flagyl)	375-mg capsules 250-, 500-mg tablets	1000 mg	
	Tetracycline (generic only)	250- and 500-mg capsules	1500 mg	
	Tinidazole (Tindamax)	250- and 500-mg tablets	1000 mg	
Antisecretory Agents				
H₂ receptor antagonists	Cimetidine (Tagamet)	200-, 300-, 400-, and 800-mg tablets 300-mg/5 mL solution	800 mg Lower dose with renal impairment	Suppress acid secretion by blocking H_2 receptors on parietal cells
	Famotidine (Pepcid)	10-, 20-, and 40-mg tablets 40-mg/5 mL solution	Ulcer treatment 40 mg GERD 20–40 mg	
	Nizatidine (Axid)	150- and 300-mg capsules 15-mg/mL solution	300 mg	
	Ranitidine (Zantac)	75-, 150-, and 300-mg tablets 150-, 300-mg capsules 15-mg/mL syrup	300 mg	
Proton pump inhibitors	Dexlansoprazole (Dexilant)	30- and 60-mg capsules 30-mg orally disintegrating delayed-release tablets	Initial erosive esophagitis: 60 mg Maintenance: 30 mg	Suppress acid secretion by inhibiting H^+,K^+-ATPase, the enzyme that makes gastric acid
	Esomeprazole (Nexium)	20- and 40-mg delayed-release capsules 2.5-, 5-, 10-, 20-, 40-mg enteric-coated granules	20 mg	
	Lansoprazole (Prevacid)	15- and 30-mg delayed-release capsules 15- and 30-mg orally disintegrating delayed-release tablets	30 mg	
	Omeprazole (Prilosec and Losec ♦)	10-, 20-, and 40-mg delayed-release capsules 20-mg delayed-release tablets 2.5- and 10-mg suspension 20-, 40-mg powder for reconstitution	20 mg	
	Pantoprazole (Protonix and Pantoloc ♦)	20- and 40-mg delayed-release tablets 40-mg enteric-coated granules	40 mg	
	Rabeprazole (Aciphex and Pariet ♦)	20-mg delayed-release tablets 5- and 10-mg delayed-release capsules	20 mg	
Mucosal protectant	Sucralfate (Carafate and Sulcrate ♦)	1-mg tablets 1-g/10-mL oral suspension	4 g	Forms a barrier over the ulcer crater that protects against acid and pepsin
Antisecretory agent that enhances mucosal defenses	Misoprostol (Cytotec)	100- and 200-mcg tablets	800 mcg	Protects against NSAID-induced ulcers by stimulating secretion of mucus and bicarbonate, maintaining submucosal blood flow, and suppressing secretion of gastric acid
Antacids	Aluminum hydroxide	Many forms	—	React with gastric acid to form neutral salts
	Calcium carbonate	Many forms	—	
	Magnesium hydroxide	Many forms	—	

GERD, Gastroesophageal reflux disease; *NSAID*, nonsteroidal antiinflammatory drug.

Eradication of *H. pylori* can be determined with several methods, including breath tests, serologic tests, stool tests, and microscopic observation of a stained biopsy sample.

Nondrug Therapy

Optimal antiulcer therapy requires implementation of nondrug measures in addition to drug therapy.

Diet

Despite commonly held beliefs, diet plays a minor role in ulcer management. The traditional "ulcer diet," consisting of bland foods together with milk or cream does not accelerate healing. Furthermore, there is no convincing evidence that caffeine-containing beverages (coffee, tea, and colas) promote ulcer formation or interfere with recovery. A change in *eating pattern* may be beneficial: consumption of five or six small meals a day, rather than three larger ones, can reduce fluctuations in intragastric pH and may facilitate recovery.

Other Nondrug Measures

Smoking is associated with an increased incidence of ulcers and delays recovery. Accordingly, cigarettes should be avoided. Because of their ulcerogenic actions, *aspirin and other NSAIDs* should be avoided by patients with PUD. The exception to this rule is the use of aspirin to prevent cardiovascular disease; in the low doses employed, aspirin is only a small factor in PUD. There are no hard data indicating that *alcohol* contributes to PUD. However, if the patient notes a temporal relationship between alcohol consumption and exacerbation of symptoms, then alcohol consumption should stop. Many people feel that reduction of *stress and anxiety* may encourage ulcer healing; however, there is no good evidence that this is true.

ANTIBACTERIAL DRUGS

Antibacterial drugs should be given to all patients with gastric or duodenal ulcers and confirmed infection with *H. pylori*. Antibiotics are not recommended for asymptomatic individuals who test positive for *H. pylori*.

Antibiotics Employed

The antibiotics employed most often are clarithromycin, amoxicillin, bismuth, metronidazole, and tetracycline. None is effective alone. Furthermore, if these drugs *are* used alone, there is increased risk for developing resistance.

Clarithromycin

Clarithromycin (Biaxin) suppresses growth of *H. pylori* by inhibiting protein synthesis. In the absence of resistance, treatment is highly effective. Unfortunately, the rate of resistance is rising, exceeding 20% in some areas. The most common side effects are nausea, diarrhea, and distortion of taste. The basic pharmacology of clarithromycin is presented in Chapter 73.

Amoxicillin

H. pylori is highly sensitive to amoxicillin. The rate of resistance is low: only about 3%. Amoxicillin kills bacteria by disrupting the cell wall. Antibacterial activity is the highest at neutral pH and hence can be enhanced by reducing gastric acidity with an antisecretory agent (e.g., omeprazole). The most common side effect is diarrhea. The basic pharmacology of amoxicillin is discussed in Chapter 71.

Bismuth

Bismuth compounds—bismuth subsalicylate and bismuth subcitrate—act topically to disrupt the cell wall of *H. pylori*, thereby causing lysis and death. Bismuth may also inhibit urease activity and prevent *H. pylori* from adhering to the gastric surface.

Bismuth can impart a harmless black coloration to the tongue and stool. Patients should be forewarned. Stool discoloration may confound interpretation of gastric bleeding. Long-term therapy may carry a risk for neurologic injury.

Tetracycline

Tetracycline, an inhibitor of bacterial protein synthesis, is highly active against *H. pylori*. Resistance is rare (<1%). Because tetracycline can stain developing teeth, it should not be used by pregnant women or young children. The pharmacology of tetracycline is discussed in Chapter 73.

Metronidazole

Metronidazole (Flagyl) is very effective against sensitive strains of *H. pylori*. Unfortunately, more than 40% of strains are now resistant. The most common side effects are nausea and headache. A disulfiram-like reaction can occur if metronidazole is used with alcohol; hence alcohol must be avoided. Metronidazole should not be taken during pregnancy. The basic pharmacology of metronidazole is discussed in Chapter 83.

Tinidazole

Tinidazole (Tindamax) is very similar to metronidazole and shares that drug's adverse effects and interactions. Like metronidazole, tinidazole can cause a disulfiram-like reaction; hence it must not be combined with alcohol. The basic pharmacology of tinidazole is discussed in Chapter 83.

Antibiotic Regimens

In 2017, the American College of Gastroenterology (ACG) issued updated guidelines for managing *H. pylori* infection. To minimize emergence of resistance, the guidelines recommend using at least two antibiotics, and preferably three. An antisecretory agent—PPI or histamine-2 receptor antagonist (H_2RA)—should be included as well. Eradication rates are good with a 10-day course and slightly better with a 14-day course.

Table 64.2 presents four ACG-recommended regimens. In regions where resistance to clarithromycin is low (below 20%), the preferred treatment is *clarithromycin-based triple therapy*, consisting of clarithromycin plus amoxicillin plus a PPI. For patients with penicillin allergy, metronidazole can be substituted for amoxicillin. In regions where resistance to clarithromycin is high (above 20%), the preferred regimen is *bismuth-based quadruple therapy*, consisting of bismuth subsalicylate plus metronidazole plus tetracycline, all three combined with a PPI or an H_2RA. For patients who can't use triple or quadruple therapy, *sequential therapy* is an option. This regimen consists of taking a PPI plus amoxicillin for 5 days, followed by a PPI plus clarithromycin plus tinidazole for 5 days. At this time, the efficacy of sequential therapy in North America has not been established.

For several reasons, compliance with antibiotic therapy can be difficult. First, antibiotic regimens are complex, requiring the patient to ingest as many as 12 pills a day. Second, side effects—especially nausea and diarrhea—are common. Third, a course of treatment is somewhat expensive. However, it costs much less to eradicate *H. pylori* with antibiotics than it does to treat ulcers repeatedly with traditional antiulcer drugs, which merely promote healing without eliminating the cause.

Combination Packs

Three combination packs—Omeclamox-Pak, Pylera, and Prevpac—are available for treating *H. pylori*-associated ulcers. The purpose of these packs is to simplify the purchase and administration of drugs for triple and quadruple therapy of PUD.

TABLE 64.2   First-Line Regimens for Eradicating *Helicobacter pylori*

Drugs	Duration (Days)	Eradication Rate (%)	Comments
Clarithromycin-Based Triple Therapy 1 Standard-dose PPI[a] Clarithromycin (500 mg twice daily) Amoxicillin (1 g twice daily)	10–14	70–85	Consider in non-penicillin-allergic patients who have not previously received clarithromycin or another macrolide
Clarithromycin-Based Triple Therapy 2 Standard-dose PPI[a] Clarithromycin (500 mg twice daily) Metronidazole (500 mg three times daily)	10–14	70–85	Consider in penicillin-allergic patients who have not previously received a macrolide or are unable to tolerate bismuth quadruple therapy
Bismuth-Based Quadruple Therapy Bismuth subsalicylate (525 mg four times daily) Metronidazole (250 mg four times daily) Tetracycline (500 mg four times daily) Standard-dose PPI[a] or ranitidine (150 mg twice daily)	10–14	75–90	Consider in penicillin-allergic patients and in patients with clarithromycin-resistant *H. pylori*
Sequential Therapy Standard-dose PPI[a] + amoxicillin (1 g twice daily) for 5 days, followed by: Standard-dose PPI[a] + clarithromycin (500 mg once daily) + tinidazole (500 mg twice daily) for 5 days	10	>90	Efficacy in North America requires validation

[a]Standard doses for PPIs are as follows: dexlansoprazole, 30–60 mg once daily; esomeprazole, 40 mg once daily; lansoprazole, 30 mg twice daily; omeprazole, 20 mg twice daily; pantoprazole, 40 mg twice daily; and rabeprazole, 20 mg twice daily.
Modified from American College of Gastroenterology. Treatment of *Helicobacter pylori* infection. *Am J Gastroenterol.* 2017;112:212–238.

HISTAMINE-2 RECEPTOR ANTAGONISTS

The H2RAs are effective drugs for treating gastric and duodenal ulcers. These agents promote ulcer healing by suppressing secretion of gastric acid. Four H2RAs are available: cimetidine, ranitidine, famotidine, and nizatidine. All four are equally effective. Serious side effects are uncommon. We will discuss the prototype, cimetidine, next. Information regarding the other three is in Table 64.1.

Cimetidine

Cimetidine (Tagamet) was the first H2RA available and will serve as our prototype for the group. At one time, cimetidine was the most frequently prescribed drug in the United States.

PROTOTYPE DRUGS

Drugs for Peptic Ulcer Disease

Antibiotic (for *Helicobacter pylori*)
Amoxicillin/clarithromycin/omeprazole

Histamine-2 Receptor Antagonist
Cimetidine

Proton Pump Inhibitor
Omeprazole

Mucosal Protectant
Sucralfate

Antacid
Aluminum hydroxide/magnesium hydroxide

Mechanism of Action

Histamine acts through two types of receptors, named H_1 and H_2. Activation of H_1 receptors produces symptoms of allergy. Activation of H_2 receptors, which are located on parietal cells of the stomach (Fig. 64.2), promotes secretion of gastric acid. By blocking H_2 receptors, cimetidine reduces both the volume of gastric juice and its hydrogen ion concentration. Cimetidine suppresses basal acid secretion and secretion stimulated by gastrin and acetylcholine. Because cimetidine produces selective blockade of H_2 receptors, the drug cannot suppress symptoms of allergy.

Pharmacokinetics

Cimetidine may be administered by the oral, intramuscular (IM), or intravenous (IV) route. Comparable blood levels are achieved with all three routes. When the drug is taken orally, food decreases the rate of absorption but not the extent. Hence, if cimetidine is taken with meals, absorption will be slowed and beneficial effects prolonged. Cimetidine crosses the blood–brain barrier—albeit with difficulty—and side effects associated with central nervous system (CNS) can occur. Although some hepatic metabolism takes place, most of each dose is eliminated intact in the urine. The half-life is relatively short (about 2 hours) but increases in patients with renal impairment. Accordingly, dosage should be reduced in these patients.

Therapeutic Uses

Gastric and duodenal ulcers. Cimetidine promotes healing of gastric and duodenal ulcers. To heal duodenal ulcers, 4 to 6 weeks of therapy are generally required. To heal gastric ulcers, 8 to 12 weeks may be needed. Long-term therapy with low doses may be given as prophylaxis against recurrence of gastric and duodenal ulcers.

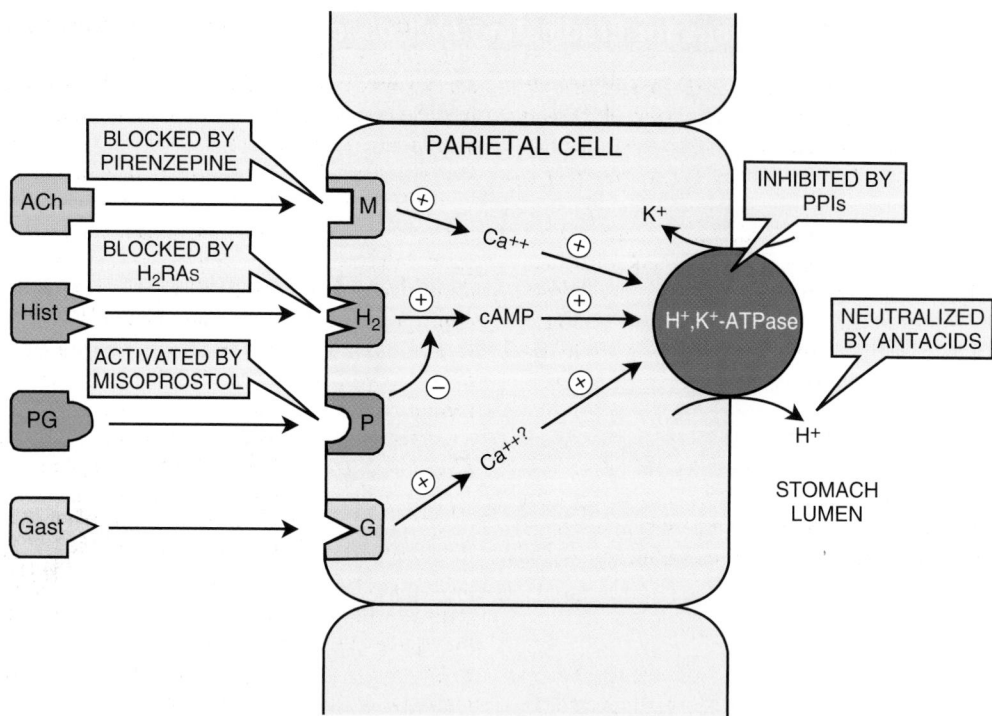

Fig. 64.2 A Model of the Regulation of Gastric Acid Secretion Showing the Actions of Antisecretory Drugs and Antacids. Production of gastric acid is stimulated by three endogenous compounds: (1) acetylcholine *(ACh)* acting at muscarinic *(M)* receptors; (2) histamine *(Hist)* acting at histamine-2 *(H₂)* receptors; and (3) gastrin *(Gast)* acting at gastrin *(G)* receptors. As indicated, all three compounds act through intracellular messengers—either calcium *(Ca²⁺)* or cyclic adenosine monophosphate *(cAMP)*—to increase the activity of H⁺,K⁺-ATPase, the enzyme that actually produces gastric acid. Prostaglandins *(PG)* decrease acid production, perhaps by suppressing production of intracellular cAMP. The actions of H₂ receptor antagonists *(H₂RAs)*, proton pump inhibitors *(PPIs)*, and other drugs are indicated. *P,* Prostaglandin receptor.

Gastroesophageal reflux disease (GERD). Reflux esophagitis is an inflammatory condition caused by reflux of gastric contents back into the esophagus. Cimetidine is a drug of choice for relieving symptoms. However, cimetidine does little to hasten healing.

Zollinger-ellison syndrome. This syndrome is characterized by hypersecretion of gastric acid and development of peptic ulcers. The underlying cause is secretion of gastrin from a gastrin-producing tumor. Cimetidine can promote healing of ulcers in patients with Zollinger-Ellison syndrome, but only if high doses are employed. At these doses, significant adverse effects can occur.

Heartburn, acid indigestion, and sour stomach. Cimetidine is available over the counter to treat these common acid-related symptoms.

Adverse Effects

The incidence of side effects is low, and those that do occur are usually benign.

Antiandrogenic effects. Cimetidine binds to androgen receptors, producing receptor blockade. As a result, the drug can cause gynecomastia, reduced libido, and impotence—all of which reverse when dosing stops.

CNS effects. Effects on the CNS are most likely in older adults who have renal or hepatic impairment. Because of its anticholinergic activity, it can cause confusion, hallucinations, CNS depression, and CNS excitation.

Pneumonia. Elevation of gastric pH with an antisecretory agent increases the risk for pneumonia because when gastric acidity is reduced, bacterial colonization of the stomach increases, resulting in a secondary increase in colonization xf the respiratory tract. Among people using an H₂RA, the *relative* risk for acquiring pneumonia is doubled. However,

the *absolute* risk is still low (about 1 extra case for every 500 people using the drug).

Drug Interactions

Interactions related to inhibition of drug metabolism. Cimetidine inhibits hepatic drug-metabolizing enzymes, thereby increasing the levels of many other drugs. Drugs of particular concern are *warfarin, phenytoin, theophylline,* and *lidocaine,* all of which have a narrow margin of safety. If these drugs are used with cimetidine, their dosages should be reduced.

Antacids. Antacids can decrease absorption of cimetidine. Accordingly, cimetidine and antacids should be administered at least 1 hour apart.

📄 SUMMARY OF KEY PRESCRIBING CONSIDERATIONS

H₂ Receptor Antagonists

Therapeutic Goal: To relieve pain, promote healing, prevent ulcer recurrence, and prevent complications of PUD.

Baseline Data: Consider testing for *H. pylori.*

Monitoring: Consider monitoring of gastric pH (should increase to 5 or above).

Identifying High-Risk Patients: Use with caution in patients with renal or hepatic dysfunction.

Evaluating Therapeutic Effects: Monitor for relief of pain. Eradication of *H. pylori* infection.

Minimizing Adverse Effects: Inform patients to report lethargy, somnolence, restlessness, confusion, or hallucinations.

PROTON PUMP INHIBITORS

The PPIs are the most effective drugs we have for suppressing gastric acid secretion. Indications include gastric and duodenal ulcers and GERD. Similarities among the PPIs are more profound than the differences. Therefore selecting among them is based largely on cost and prescriber preference.

Although PPIs are generally well tolerated, they *can* increase the risk for serious adverse events, including fractures, pneumonia, acid rebound, and, possibly, intestinal infection with *Clostridium difficile*. To ensure that the benefits of treatment outweigh the risks, treatment should be limited to appropriate candidates, who should take the lowest dose needed for the shortest time possible.

Omeprazole

Omeprazole (Prilosec, Prilosec OTC, Zegerid, Zegerid OTC, and Losec ♣) was the first PPI available and will serve as our prototype for the group. Acid suppression is more effective with H_2RAs. Side effects from short-term therapy are minimal. Information on the other PPIs is in Table 64.1.

Mechanism of Action

Omeprazole is a prodrug that undergoes conversion to its active form within parietal cells of the stomach. The active form then causes irreversible inhibition of H^+,K^+-ATPase (proton pump), the enzyme that generates gastric acid (see Fig. 64.2). Because it blocks the final common pathway of gastric acid production, omeprazole can inhibit basal and stimulated acid release. A single 30-mg oral dose reduces acid production by 90% to 97% within 2 hours. Because inhibition of the ATPase is not reversible, effects persist until new enzyme is synthesized. Partial recovery occurs 3 to 5 days after stopping treatment. Full recovery may take weeks.

Pharmacokinetics

After oral dosing, about 50% of the drug reaches the systemic circulation. Omeprazole undergoes hepatic metabolism followed by renal excretion. The plasma half-life is short—about 1 hour. However, because omeprazole acts by irreversible enzyme inhibition, effects persist long after the drug has left the body.

Omeprazole is acid labile and hence must be protected from stomach acid. To accomplish this, the drug is formulated in a capsule that contains protective enteric-coated granules. The capsule dissolves in the stomach, but the granules remain intact until they reach the relatively alkaline environment of the duodenum.

Therapeutic Use

Omeprazole is approved for short-term therapy of duodenal ulcers, gastric ulcers, erosive esophagitis, and GERD and for long-term therapy of hypersecretory conditions (e.g., Zollinger-Ellison syndrome). Except for therapy of hypersecretory states, treatment should be limited to 4 to 8 weeks.

In hospitals, omeprazole and other PPIs are widely used to prevent stress ulcers. However, about two-thirds of patients who receive PPIs don't really need them. Ulcer prophylaxis is indicated only for patients in intensive care units and only if they have an additional risk factor, such as multiple trauma, spinal cord injury, or prolonged mechanical ventilation (more than 48 hours). General medical and surgical patients are at low risk for stress ulcers and should not receive PPIs for prophylaxis.

How does omeprazole compare with H_2RAs? Omeprazole and other PPIs reduce 24-hour acid secretion by 90%, compared with 65% for H_2RAs. Also, PPIs act faster than H_2RAs to reduce gastric acidity and relieve ulcer symptoms. Patients who fail to respond to H_2RAs can often benefit from a PPI.

GERD is a common disorder characterized by heartburn and acid regurgitation. The disease is formally defined by the presence of troublesome symptoms or complications caused by passage of gastric contents into the esophagus. Among American adults, heartburn develops in 44% at least once a month, in 14% at least once a week, and in up to 7% every day. GERD is also common among children.

GERD is associated with a wide range of symptoms and complications. Based on endoscopic examination, patients fall into two major groups: those with *erosive esophagitis* and those with *nonerosive reflux disease* (NERD). Erosive esophagitis is characterized by breaks in the esophageal mucosa. In contrast, mucosal breaks are absent in people with NERD. Less than 50% of patients with GERD have the erosive form. Complications of erosive GERD include difficulty swallowing, painful swallowing, esophageal stricture, ulcers, GI bleeding, anemia, and persistent vomiting. Erosive GERD can also lead to esophageal adenocarcinoma and Barrett esophagus, a premalignant condition that can evolve into adenocarcinoma.

PPIs are considered the drugs of choice. For patients with NERD, PPIs may be taken PRN (when necessary). For patients with erosive GERD, PPIs should be taken continuously until symptoms resolve (typically 4 to 8 weeks). Unfortunately, when PPIs are discontinued, the relapse rate is high, occurring in 80% to 90% of patients within 6 to 12 months. Accordingly, for patients with severe GERD, long-term maintenance therapy is recommended.

Adverse Effects

Pneumonia. Omeprazole and other PPIs increase the risk for community-acquired and hospital-acquired pneumonia. Possible causes include alteration of upper GI flora (owing to reduced gastric acidity) and impairment of white blood cell function. Of note, the time frame for increased risk is limited to the first few days of PPI use. After that, risk is no higher than in nonusers.

Fractures. Long-term therapy, especially in high doses, increases the risk for osteoporosis and fractures by reducing acid secretion, which may decrease absorption of calcium. However, the risk appears to be low. For example, only one extra hip fracture would be expected for every 1200 patients. To minimize fracture risk, treatment should use the lowest dose needed for the shortest duration possible. Also, patients should be encouraged to maintain adequate intake of calcium and vitamin D.

Rebound acid hypersecretion. When patients stop taking PPIs, they often experience dyspepsia brought on by rebound hypersecretion of gastric acid. Acid rebound can be minimized by using PPIs in the lowest effective dose for the shortest time needed and by tapering the dose when stopping treatment. Dyspepsia can be managed with an antacid and perhaps with an H_2RA. Acid rebound can persist for several months after the PPI is discontinued.

Hypomagnesemia. With long-term use, PPIs can lower magnesium levels, perhaps by reducing intestinal magnesium absorption. In severe cases, serum magnesium may drop below 1 mg/dL. The risk for hypomagnesemia is increased by other drugs that lower magnesium, especially thiazide and loop diuretics. If magnesium levels remain low after replacement, the patient can be switched to an H_2 blocker. After PPI withdrawal, magnesium levels usually normalize within 2 weeks. For long-term PPI therapy, consider measuring magnesium at baseline and periodically thereafter.

Diarrhea. In retrospective, observational studies, omeprazole and other PPIs have been associated with a dose-related increase in the risk for infection with *C. difficile*, a bacterium that can cause severe diarrhea. Patients experiencing diarrhea while taking omeprazole or other PPIs should report immediately to their health care provider for testing.

Drug Interactions

By elevating gastric pH, omeprazole and other PPIs can significantly reduce absorption of *atazanavir* (Reyataz), *delavirdine* (Rescriptor), and *nelfinavir* (Viracept), all used to treat HIV/AIDS. These drugs should not be combined with a PPI. Reducing gastric pH can also decrease the absorption of two antifungal drugs: *ketoconazole* and *itraconazole*.

Clopidogrel. Omeprazole and other PPIs can reduce the *adverse* effects of clopidogrel (Plavix) but may also reduce its *beneficial* effects. Clopidogrel is an antiplatelet drug used to decrease thrombotic events. Unfortunately, by suppressing platelet aggregation, the drug can promote gastric bleeding. To reduce the risk for GI bleeding, clopidogrel is often combined with a PPI. Unfortunately, in addition to protecting against GI bleeding, the PPI may reduce the beneficial effects of clopidogrel because PPIs inhibit CYP2C19, the isoenzyme of cytochrome P450 that converts clopidogrel to its active form. Hence the dilemma: if clopidogrel is used alone, there is a significant risk for GI bleeding; however, if clopidogrel is combined with a PPI, the risk for GI bleeding will be reduced, but antiplatelet effects may be reduced as well. After considering the available evidence, three organizations—the American College of Cardiology, the American Heart Association, and the ACG—issued a consensus document on the problem. This document concludes that, although PPIs may reduce the antiplatelet effects of clopidogrel, there is no evidence that the reduction is large enough to be clinically relevant. Accordingly, *for patients with risk factors for GI bleeding* (e.g., advanced age and use of NSAIDs or anticoagulants), the benefits of combining a PPI with clopidogrel probably outweigh any risk from reduced antiplatelet effects; hence combining a PPI with clopidogrel is probably okay. Conversely, *for patients who lack risk factors for GI bleeding,* combined use of clopidogrel with a PPI may reduce the antiplatelet effects of clopidogrel without offering any real benefit, so combining a PPI with clopidogrel in these patients should generally be avoided.

> ## 📄 SUMMARY OF KEY PRESCRIBING CONSIDERATIONS
>
> ### *Proton Pump Inhibitors*
>
> **Therapeutic Goal:** Relieve pain, promote healing, prevent ulcer recurrence, and prevent complications in PUD.
> **Baseline Data:** Magnesium level. Consider testing for *H. pylori.*
> **Monitoring:** Follow magnesium levels periodically.
> **Identifying High-Risk Patients:** These drugs are generally safe.
> **Evaluating Therapeutic Effects:** Monitor for relief of pain. Eradication of *H. pylori* infection.
> **Minimizing Adverse Effects:** When used long term, the risk for osteoporosis and fractures increases. Encourage patients to maintain adequate intake of calcium and vitamin D. Inform patients about symptoms of hypomagnesemia, including muscle cramps, palpitations, and tremors.

OTHER ANTIULCER DRUGS

Sucralfate

Sucralfate (Carafate and Sulcrate) is an effective antiulcer medication notable for minimal side effects and lack of significant drug interactions. The drug promotes ulcer healing by creating a protective barrier against acid and pepsin. Sucralfate has no acid-neutralizing capacity and does not decrease acid secretion.

Mechanism of Antiulcer Action

Sucralfate is a complex substance composed of sulfated sucrose and aluminum hydroxide. Under mildly acidic conditions (pH < 4), sucralfate undergoes polymerization and cross-linking reactions. The resultant product is a viscid and very sticky gel that adheres to the ulcer crater, creating a barrier to back-diffusion of hydrogen ions, pepsin, and bile salts. Attachment to the ulcer appears to last up to 6 hours.

Pharmacokinetics

Sucralfate is administered orally, and systemic absorption is minimal (3% to 5%). About 90% of each dose is eliminated in the feces.

Therapeutic Uses

Sucralfate is approved for acute therapy and maintenance therapy of duodenal ulcers. Rates of healing are comparable to those achieved with cimetidine. Controlled trials indicate that sucralfate can also promote healing of gastric ulcers.

Adverse Effects

Sucralfate has no known serious adverse effects. The most significant side effect is constipation, which occurs in 2% of patients. Because sucralfate is minimally absorbed, systemic effects are absent.

Drug Interactions

Interactions with other drugs are minimal. By raising gastric pH above 4, antacids may interfere with sucralfate's effects. This interaction can be minimized by administering these drugs at least 30 minutes apart.

Sucralfate may impede the absorption of some drugs, including phenytoin, theophylline, digoxin, warfarin, and fluoroquinolone antibiotics (e.g., ciprofloxacin). These interactions can be minimized by administering sucralfate at least 2 hours apart from these other drugs.

Misoprostol
Therapeutic Use

Misoprostol (Cytotec) is an analog of prostaglandin E_1. In the United States, the drug's only approved GI indication is prevention of gastric ulcers caused by long-term therapy with NSAIDs. In other countries, misoprostol is also used to treat peptic ulcers unrelated to NSAIDs. In addition to its use in PUD, misoprostol is used to promote cervical ripening.

> ## 👥 PATIENT-CENTERED CARE ACROSS THE LIFE SPAN
>
> ### *Peptic Ulcer Disease*
>
> | Life Stage | Patient Care Concerns |
> |---|---|
> | Infants | Both PPIs and H_2 receptor antagonists are used safely in infants as young as 1 month to treat GERD and duodenal ulcers. |
> | Children/ adolescents | PPIs and H_2 receptor antagonists can be used safely in children, just in smaller doses. Side-effect profiles resemble those of adults. |
> | Pregnant women | Misoprostol must be avoided at all costs. Some PPIs (esomeprazole) and H_2 receptor antagonists (ranitidine) are safe for use in pregnancy. |
> | Breastfeeding women | Use of drugs such as omeprazole, esomeprazole, and ranitidine is not predicted to cause any adverse effects in breastfed infants. |
> | Older adults | PPIs are associated with increased risk for fractures from osteoporosis. PPIs can also cause medication interactions and vitamin or mineral deficiencies. There should be a clear indication for prescribing these medications in this older population. |

Mechanism of Action

In normal individuals, prostaglandins help protect the stomach by suppressing secretion of gastric acid, promoting secretion of bicarbonate and cytoprotective mucus and maintaining submucosal blood flow (by promoting vasodilation). As discussed in Chapter 57, aspirin and other NSAIDs cause gastric ulcers in part by inhibiting prostaglandin biosynthesis. Misoprostol prevents NSAID-induced ulcers by serving as a replacement for endogenous prostaglandins.

Adverse Effects

The most common reactions are dose-related diarrhea (13% to 40%) and abdominal pain (7% to 20%). Some women experience spotting and dysmenorrhea.

 BLACK BOX WARNING

Misoprostol in Pregnancy

> Misoprostol is contraindicated during pregnancy. Because prostaglandins stimulate uterine contractions, the use of misoprostol during pregnancy has caused partial or complete expulsion of the developing fetus.

Misoprostol is contraindicated in pregnancy. If women of childbearing age are to use misoprostol, they must (1) be able to comply with birth control measures, (2) be given oral and written warnings about the dangers of misoprostol, (3) have a negative serum pregnancy test result within 2 weeks before beginning therapy, and (4) begin therapy only on the second or third day of the next normal menstrual cycle.

Antacids

Antacids are alkaline compounds that neutralize stomach acid. Their principal indications are PUD and GERD.

Beneficial Actions

Antacids react with gastric acid to produce neutral salts or salts of low acidity. By neutralizing acid, these drugs decrease destruction of the gut wall. In addition, if treatment raises gastric pH above 5, these drugs will reduce pepsin activity as well. Antacids may also enhance mucosal protection by stimulating production of prostaglandins. These drugs do not coat the ulcer crater to protect it from acid and pepsin. Except for sodium bicarbonate, antacids are poorly absorbed and therefore do not alter systemic pH.

Therapeutic Uses

Peptic ulcer disease. The primary indication for antacids is PUD. Rates of healing are equivalent to those achieved with H$_2$RAs. In the past, antacids were the mainstay of antiulcer therapy. However, these drugs have been largely replaced by newer options (H$_2$RAs, PPIs, and sucralfate) that are equally effective and more convenient to administer and cause fewer side effects.

Adverse Effects

Constipation and diarrhea. Most antacids affect the bowel. Some (e.g., aluminum hydroxide) promote constipation, whereas others (e.g., magnesium hydroxide) promote diarrhea. Effects on the bowel can be minimized by combining an antacid that promotes constipation with one that promotes diarrhea. Patients should be taught to adjust the dosage of one agent or the other to normalize bowel function.

Sodium loading. Some antacid preparations contain substantial amounts of sodium. Because sodium excess can exacerbate hypertension and heart failure, patients with these disorders should avoid preparations that have high sodium content.

Drug Interactions

By raising gastric pH, antacids can influence the dissolution and absorption of many other drugs, including cimetidine and ranitidine. These interactions can be minimized by providing a gap of 1 hour between taking antacids and these other drugs.

Antacids can interfere with the actions of sucralfate. To minimize this interaction, administer these drugs at least 1 hour apart.

If absorbed in substantial amounts, antacids can alkalinize the urine. Elevation of urinary pH can accelerate excretion of acidic drugs and delay excretion of basic drugs.

Antacid Families

There are four major groups of antacids: (1) aluminum compounds, (2) magnesium compounds, (3) calcium compounds, and (4) sodium compounds. Individual agents that belong to each group are shown in Table 64.3.

Representative Antacids

Antacids differ from one another in terms of onset and duration of action, effects on the bowel, systemic effects, and special applications. These include the two most commonly used antacids—magnesium hydroxide and aluminum hydroxide—and two less commonly used drugs—calcium carbonate and sodium bicarbonate. The distinguishing properties of these agents are shown in Table 64.4.

TABLE 64.3 Classification of Antacids

Aluminum compounds	Aluminum hydroxide
Magnesium compounds	Magnesium hydroxide (milk of magnesia)
	Magnesium oxide
Calcium compounds	Calcium carbonate
Sodium compounds	Sodium bicarbonate
Other	Magaldrate (a complex of magnesium and aluminum compounds)

TABLE 64.4 Representative Antacids: Distinguishing Properties

Antacid	EFFECT ON THE BOWEL		Effect on Systemic pH	Comments
	Constipation	Diarrhea		
Aluminum hydroxide	Yes	No	None	Can cause hypophosphatemia; can treat hyperphosphatemia
Magnesium hydroxide	No	Yes	None	Can cause magnesium toxicity (central nervous system depression) in patients with renal impairment
Calcium carbonate	Yes	No	None	May cause acid rebound or milk-alkali syndrome; releases CO$_2$
Sodium bicarbonate	No	No	Increase	Not used routinely for ulcers; used to treat acidosis and alkalinize urine; high risk for sodium loading; releases CO$_2$

65

Laxatives

Laxatives are used to ease or stimulate defecation. These agents can soften the stool, increase stool volume, hasten fecal passage through the intestine, and facilitate evacuation from the rectum. When properly employed, laxatives are valuable medications. However, these agents are also subject to abuse. Misuse of laxatives is largely the result of misconceptions about what constitutes normal bowel function.

Before we talk about laxatives, we must distinguish between two terms: *laxative effect* and *catharsis*. The term *laxative effect* refers to production of a soft, formed stool over a period of 1 or more days. In contrast, the term *catharsis* refers to a prompt, fluid evacuation of the bowel. Hence a laxative effect is slower and relatively mild, whereas catharsis is relatively fast and intense.

GENERAL CONSIDERATIONS

Function of the Colon

The principal function of the colon is to absorb water and electrolytes. Absorption of nutrients is minimal. Normally about 1500 mL of fluid enters the colon each day and approximately 90% gets absorbed. When the colon is working correctly, the extent of fluid absorption is such that the resulting stool is soft (but formed) and capable of elimination without strain. However, when fluid absorption is excessive, as can happen when transport through the intestine is delayed, the resultant stool is dehydrated and hard. Conversely, if insufficient fluid is absorbed, watery stools result.

The frequency of bowel evacuation varies widely among individuals. For some people, bowel movements occur two or three times a day. For others, elimination may occur only twice a week. Because of this wide individual variation, we can't define a normal frequency for bowel movements. Put another way, although a daily bowel movement may be normal for many people, it may be abnormal for many others.

Constipation

Constipation is one of the most common gastrointestinal (GI) disorders. In the United States, people seek medical help for constipation at least 2.5 million times a year and spend hundreds of millions of dollars on laxatives.

Constipation is defined in terms of symptoms, which include hard stools, infrequent stools, excessive straining, prolonged effort, a sense of incomplete evacuation, and unsuccessful defecation. Scientists who do research on constipation usually define it using the Rome IV criteria (Table 65.1). Constipation is determined more by stool *consistency* (degree of hardness) than by *how often* bowel movements occur. Hence if the interval between bowel movements becomes prolonged but the stool remains soft and hydrated, a diagnosis of constipation would be improper. Conversely, if bowel movements occur with regularity but the feces are hard and dry, constipation can be diagnosed—despite the regular and frequent passage of stool.

A common cause of constipation is poor diet—specifically, a diet deficient in fiber and fluid. Other causes include dysfunction of the pelvic floor and anal sphincter, slow intestinal transit, and use of certain drugs (e.g., opioids, anticholinergics, and some antacids).

In most cases constipation can be readily corrected. Stools will become softer and more easily passed within days of increasing fiber and fluid in the diet. Mild exercise, especially after meals, also helps improve bowel function. If necessary, a laxative may be employed—but only briefly and only as an adjunct to improved diet and exercise.

PATIENT-CENTERED CARE ACROSS THE LIFE SPAN

Laxatives

Life Stage	Patient Care Concerns
Infants	Docusate, lactulose, and glycerin suppositories have been used to treat constipation safely in infants.
Children/ adolescents	Milk of magnesia, mineral oil, senna, docusate, and bisacodyl can be used to treat constipation in children and adolescents.
Pregnant women	Laxatives should be used cautiously in pregnancy because gastrointestinal stimulation can induce labor.
Breastfeeding women	Senna is safe for use during breastfeeding. Data are lacking regarding the use of polyethylene glycol and bisacodyl (Dulcolax); caution is advised.
Older adults	All laxatives discussed in this chapter can be used in the older-adult population. The older adult should be monitored closely for dehydration.

Indications for Laxative Use

Laxatives can be highly beneficial when employed for valid indications. By softening the stool, laxatives can reduce the painful elimination that can be associated with episiotomy and with hemorrhoids and other anorectal lesions. In patients with cardiovascular diseases (e.g., aneurysm, myocardial infarction, disease of the cerebral, or cardiac vasculature), softening the stool decreases the amount of strain needed to defecate, avoiding dangerous elevation of blood pressure. In older adult patients, laxatives can help compensate for loss of tone in abdominal and perineal muscles. As an adjunct to anthelmintic therapy, laxatives can be used for (1) obtaining a fresh stool sample for diagnosis, (2) emptying the bowel before treatment (to increase parasitic exposure to anthelmintic medication), and (3) facilitating the export of dead parasites after anthelmintic use. Additional applications include (1) emptying of the bowel before surgery and diagnostic procedures (e.g., radiologic examination and colonoscopy), (2) modifying the effluent from an ileostomy or colostomy, (3) preventing fecal impaction in bedridden patients, (4) removing ingested poisons, and (5) correcting constipation associated with pregnancy and certain drugs, especially opioid analgesics.

TABLE 65.1 Rome IV Criteria for Constipation

Adults
Two or more of the following for the past 3 months with symptom onset at least 6 months before diagnosis:
- Straining during at least 25% of bowel movements
- Lumpy or hard stools in at least 25% of bowel movements
- Sensation of incomplete evacuation for at least 25% of bowel movements
- Sensation of anorectal blockage for at least 25% of bowel movements
- Manual maneuvers (e.g., digital evacuation; support of the pelvic floor) to facilitate at least 25% of bowel movements
- Fewer than three bowel movements per week
- Loose stools rarely present without the use of laxatives and insufficient criteria to permit diagnosis of irritable bowel syndrome

Infants and Children
Must include 1 month of at least two of the following in infants and children up to the age of 4 years:
- Two or fewer defecations per week
- History of excessive stool retention
- History of painful or hard bowel movements
- History of large-diameter stools that may obstruct the toilet
- At least one episode per week of incontinence after the acquisition of toileting skills

Precautions and Contraindications to Laxative Use

Laxatives are contraindicated for individuals with certain disorders of the bowel. Specifically, laxatives must be avoided by individuals experiencing abdominal pain, nausea, cramps, or other symptoms of appendicitis, regional enteritis, diverticulitis, and ulcerative colitis. Laxatives are also contraindicated for patients with acute surgical abdomen. In addition, laxatives should not be used in patients with fecal impaction or obstruction of the bowel, because increased peristalsis could cause bowel perforation. Last, laxatives should not be employed habitually to manage constipation. Reasons for this are discussed under the section on "Laxative Abuse."

Laxatives should be used with caution during pregnancy (because GI stimulation might induce labor) and during lactation (because the laxative may be excreted in breast milk).

Laxative Classification Schemes

Traditionally, laxatives have been classified according to general *mechanism of action*. This scheme has four major categories: (1) bulk-forming laxatives, (2) surfactant laxatives, (3) stimulant laxatives, and (4) osmotic laxatives. Representative drugs are shown in Table 65.2. An additional class of drugs selective mu opioid antagonists, used specifically for opioid induced constipation, are discussed in Chapter 24.

From a clinical perspective, it can be useful to classify laxatives according to *therapeutic effect* (time of onset and effect on stool consistency). When these properties are considered, most laxatives fall into one of three groups, labeled I, II, and III in this chapter. Group I agents act rapidly (within 2–6 hours) and give a watery consistency to the

TABLE 65.2 Classification of Laxatives by Pharmacologic Category

Class and Agent	Site of Action	Mechanism of Action
Bulk-Forming Laxatives		
Methylcellulose	Small intestine and colon	Absorb water, thereby softening and enlarging the fecal mass; fecal swelling promotes peristalsis
Psyllium		
Polycarbophil		
Surfactant Laxatives		
Docusate sodium	Small intestine and colon	Surfactant action softens stool by facilitating penetration of water and also cause secretion of water and electrolytes into intestine
Docusate calcium		
Stimulant Laxatives		
Bisacodyl	Colon	(1) Stimulate peristalsis and (2) soften feces by increasing secretion of water and electrolytes into the intestine and decreasing water and electrolyte absorption
Senna	Colon	
Castor oil	Small intestine	
Osmotic Laxatives		
Magnesium hydroxide	Small intestine and colon	Osmotic action retains water and, hence, softens the feces; fecal swelling promotes peristalsis
Magnesium sulfate		
Magnesium citrate		
Sodium phosphate		
Polyethylene glycol		
Lactulose		
Miscellaneous Laxatives		
Lubiprostone	Small intestine and colon	Opens chloride channels in the intestinal epithelium and, thus, increases intestinal motility and secretion of fluid into the lumen
Plecanatide	Small intestine and colon	Assists in the regulation of intestinal fluid secretion and motility by indirectly increasing chloride and bicarbonate in the lumen
Polyethylene glycol–electrolyte solution	Small intestine and colon	Similar to osmotic laxatives
Sodium picosulfate/magnesium oxide/anhydrous citric acid	Colon	Stimulates colonic peristalsis and draws water into the GI tract

stool. Laxatives in group I are especially useful when the bowel is being prepared for diagnostic procedures or surgery. Group II agents have an intermediate latency (6–12 hours) and produce a stool that is semifluid. Group II agents are the ones most frequently abused by the general public. Group III laxatives act slowly (in 1–3 days) to produce a soft but formed stool. Uses for this group include treating chronic constipation and preventing straining during bowel movements. Representative members of groups I, II, and III are shown in Table 65.3.

BASIC PHARMACOLOGY OF LAXATIVES

Bulk-Forming Laxatives

The bulk-forming laxatives (e.g., methylcellulose, psyllium, and polycarbophil) have actions and effects much like those of dietary fiber. These agents consist of natural or semisynthetic polysaccharides and celluloses derived from grains and other plant material. The bulk-forming agents belong to therapeutic group III, producing a soft, formed stool after 1 to 3 days of use.

Mechanism of Action

Bulk-forming agents have the same effect on bowel function as dietary fiber. After ingestion, these agents, which are nondigestible and nonabsorbable, swell in water to form a viscous solution or gel, thereby softening the fecal mass and increasing its bulk. Fecal volume may be further enlarged by the growth of colonic bacteria, which can utilize these materials as nutrients. Transit through the intestine is hastened because swelling of the fecal mass stretches the intestinal wall, thereby stimulating peristalsis.

Indications

Bulk-forming laxatives are preferred agents for the temporary treatment of constipation. Also, they are widely used in patients with diverticulosis and irritable bowel syndrome. In addition, by altering fecal consistency, they can provide symptomatic relief of diarrhea and can reduce discomfort and inconvenience for patients with an ileostomy or colostomy.

Adverse Effects

Untoward effects are minimal. Because the bulk-forming agents are not absorbed, systemic reactions are rare. *Esophageal obstruction* can occur if they are swallowed in the absence of sufficient fluid. Accordingly, bulk-forming laxatives should be administered with a full glass of water or juice. If their passage through the intestine is impeded, they may produce *intestinal obstruction* or *impaction*. Accordingly, they should be avoided if there is narrowing of the intestinal lumen.

Preparations, Dosage, and Administration

Psyllium (prepared from *Plantago* seed), *methylcellulose*, and *polycarbophil* are the principal bulk-forming laxatives. All three preparations should be administered with a full glass of water or juice. Dosages and trade names are shown in Table 65.4.

Surfactant Laxatives
Actions

The surfactants (e.g., docusate sodium) are group III laxatives; they produce a soft stool several days after the onset of treatment. Surfactants alter stool consistency by lowering surface tension, which facilitates the penetration of water into the feces. The surfactants may also act on the intestinal wall to (1) inhibit fluid absorption and (2) stimulate secretion of water and electrolytes into the intestinal lumen. In this respect, surfactants resemble the stimulant laxatives (see later).

Preparations, Dosage, and Administration

The surfactant family consists of two *docusate salts:* docusate sodium and docusate calcium. The dosage for docusate sodium (Colace), the

---

PROTOTYPE DRUGS

Laxatives

Bulk-Forming Agent
Methylcellulose

Surfactant
Docusate sodium

Stimulant Laxative
Bisacodyl

Osmotic Laxative
Magnesium hydroxide

Chloride Channel Activator
Lubiprostone

Guanylate Cyclase-C (GC-C) Agonist
Plecanatide

TABLE 65.3   Classification of Laxatives by Therapeutic Response

Group I: Produce Watery Stool in 2–6 Hours	Group II: Produce Semifluid Stool in 6–12 Hours	Group III: Produce Soft Stool in 1–3 Days
Osmotic Laxatives (in High Doses)	Osmotic Laxatives (in Low Doses)	Bulk-Forming Laxatives
Magnesium salts	Magnesium salts	Methylcellulose
Sodium salts	Sodium salts	Psyllium
Polyethylene glycol	Polyethylene glycol	Polycarbophil
Others	Stimulant Laxatives (Except Castor Oil)	Surfactant Laxatives
Castor oil	Bisacodyl, oral[a]	Docusate sodium
Polyethylene glycol electrolyte solution	Senna	Docusate calcium
		Others
		Lactulose
		Lubiprostone
		Plecanatide

[a]Bisacodyl *suppositories* act in 15 minutes.

TABLE 65.4 Representative Laxatives: Trade Names, Dosage Forms, and Dosages

Drug Class and Generic Name	Trade Names	Dosage Forms	Dosage and Administration
Bulk-Forming			
Methylcellulose	Citrucel	Powder	*Powder:* One heaping tbsp in 8 oz of cold water 1–3 times a day
Psyllium	Metamucil, others	Powder, wafer	*Adults:* One rounded tsp (or one packet) mixed with water or other fluid, taken 1–3 times daily *Children older than 6 years:* 1/3–1/2 adult dose
Polycarbophil	FiberCon, others	Tablets	*Adults:* 1250 mg 1–4 times daily *Children 6–12 years:* 625 mg 1–4 times daily
Surfactant			
Docusate sodium	Colace, others	Capsules, tablets, syrup, liquid	*Adults and children older than 12 years:* 50–500 mg/day *Children 6–12 years:* 40–120 mg/day (All doses taken with a full glass of water)
Stimulant			
Bisacodyl	Correctol, Dulcolax, Fleet Laxative, others	Tablets, suppositories	*Adults:* 10–15 mg (tablets) or 10-mg suppository once daily *Children:* 5-mg tablet or 5-mg suppository once daily
Senna	Senokot, Ex-Lax, others	Tablets	*Adults:* two tablets once or twice daily *Children 6–12 years:* one tablet once or twice daily
Osmotic			
Polyethylene glycol	GlycoLax, MiraLax, Peglax ♣	Powder	*Adults:* 17 g (dissolved in 8 oz of water) once daily
Lactulose	Cephulac, Cholac, others	Liquid	*Children:* 1 mL/kg PO once or twice daily
Magnesium hydroxide (milk of magnesia)	Phillips' Milk of Magnesia, others	Liquid	*Adults:* 15–30 mL daily, increased to 60 mL if needed *Children 6 months–1 year:* 40 mg/kg PO daily *Children 2–5 years:* 400–1200 mg PO daily *Children 6–11 years:* 1200–2400 mg PO daily *Children >12 years:* 2400–4800 mg PO daily
Other			
Lubiprostone	Amitiza	Capsule	*Adults:* 24 µg twice daily with food
Plecanatide	Trulance	Tablet	*Adults:* 3 mg daily

prototype surfactant, is shown in Table 65.4. Administration should be accompanied by a full glass of water.

Stimulant Laxatives

The stimulant laxatives (e.g., bisacodyl, senna, and castor oil) have two effects on the bowel. First, they stimulate intestinal motility—hence their name. Second, they increase the amount of water and electrolytes within the intestinal lumen by increasing secretion of water and ions into the intestine and reducing water and electrolyte absorption. Most stimulant laxatives are group II agents: they act on the colon to produce a semifluid stool within 6 to 12 hours.

Stimulant laxatives are widely used—and abused—by the general public and are of concern for this reason. They have few legitimate applications. Two applications that *are* legitimate are (1) treatment of opioid-induced constipation and (2) treatment of constipation resulting from slow intestinal transit. Properties of individual agents are discussed next.

Bisacodyl

Bisacodyl (Correctol, Dulcolax) is unique among the stimulant laxatives, in that it can be administered by rectal suppository as well as by mouth. *Oral* bisacodyl acts within 6 to 12 hours. Hence tablets may be given

at bedtime to produce a response the following morning. Bisacodyl *suppositories* act rapidly (in 15–60 minutes). Dosages for bisacodyl are shown in Table 65.4.

Bisacodyl tablets are enteric-coated to prevent gastric irritation. Accordingly, patients should be advised to swallow them intact, without chewing or crushing. Because milk and antacids accelerate dissolution of the enteric coating, the tablets should be administered no sooner than 1 hour after ingesting these substances.

Bisacodyl suppositories may cause a burning sensation and, with continued use, proctitis may develop. Accordingly, long-term use should be discouraged.

Senna

Senna (Senokot, Ex-Lax) is a plant-derived laxative that contains *anthraquinones* as active ingredients. The actions and applications of senna are similar to those of bisacodyl. Anthraquinones act on the colon to produce a soft or semifluid stool in 6 to 12 hours. Systemic absorption followed by renal secretion may impart a harmless yellow-brown or pink color to the urine. Dosages are presented in Table 65.4.

Castor Oil

Castor oil is the only stimulant laxative that acts on the *small intestine*. As a result, the drug acts quickly (in 2–6 hours) to produce a watery stool. Hence, unlike other stimulant laxatives, which are all group II agents, castor oil belongs to group I. The use of castor oil is limited to situations in which rapid and thorough evacuation of the bowel is desired (e.g., preparation for radiologic procedures). The drug is far too powerful for the routine treatment of constipation. Because of its relatively prompt action, castor oil should not be administered at bedtime. The drug has an unpleasant taste that can be improved by chilling and mixing with fruit juice.

Osmotic Laxatives
Laxative Salts
Actions and uses. The laxative salts (e.g., sodium phosphate and magnesium hydroxide) are poorly absorbed salts whose osmotic action draws water into the intestinal lumen. Accumulation of water causes the fecal mass to soften and swell, thereby stretching the intestinal wall and stimulating peristalsis. When administered in low doses, the osmotic laxatives produce a soft or semifluid stool in 6 to 12 hours. In high doses, these agents act rapidly (in 2–6 hours) to cause a fluid evacuation of the bowel. High-dose therapy is employed to empty the bowel in preparation for diagnostic and surgical procedures. High doses are also employed to purge the bowel of ingested poisons and evacuate dead parasites after anthelmintic therapy.

Preparations. There are two groups of laxative salts: (1) *magnesium salts* (magnesium hydroxide, magnesium citrate, and magnesium sulfate) and (2) one *sodium salt* (sodium phosphate). Dosages for magnesium hydroxide solution (also known as milk of magnesia) and sodium phosphate are shown in Table 65.4.

Adverse effects. Osmotic laxatives can cause substantial *loss of water.* To avoid dehydration, patients should increase fluid intake. Although the osmotic laxatives are poorly and slowly absorbed, some absorption does take place. In patients with renal impairment, *magnesium can accumulate to toxic levels.* Accordingly, magnesium salts are contraindicated in patients with kidney disease. Sodium absorption (from sodium phosphate) can cause *fluid retention,* which, in turn, can exacerbate heart failure, hypertension, and edema. Accordingly, sodium phosphate is contraindicated for patients with these disorders. Sodium phosphate can also cause *acute renal failure* in vulnerable patients, especially those with kidney disease and those taking drugs that alter renal function (e.g., diuretics, angiotensin-converting enzyme inhibitors [ACEIs] and angiotensin receptor blockers [ARBs]). The mechanism involves dehydration and precipitation of calcium and phosphate in renal tubules. Accordingly, sodium phosphate should be avoided in this vulnerable group.

Polyethylene Glycol
Polyethylene glycol (PEG; MiraLax, GlycoLax, Peglax ✦) is an osmotic laxative used widely for chronic constipation. Like the laxative salts, PEG is a nonabsorbable compound that retains water in the intestinal lumen, causing the fecal mass to soften and swell. The most common adverse effects are nausea, abdominal bloating, cramping, and flatulence. High doses may cause diarrhea. For management of chronic constipation, PEG is superior to lactulose with regard to relief of abdominal pain and improvements in stool consistency and frequency per week, although side effects are similar. The recommended dosage is 17 g once daily dissolved in 4 to 8 oz of water, juice, soda, coffee, or tea. Bowel movement may not occur for another 2 to 4 days. As discussed later, products that contain PEG plus electrolytes can be used to cleanse the bowel before colonoscopy and other procedures.

Lactulose
Lactulose (Constulose, Enulose) is a semisynthetic disaccharide composed of galactose and fructose. Lactulose is poorly absorbed and cannot be digested by intestinal enzymes. In the colon, resident bacteria metabolize lactulose to lactic acid, formic acid, and acetic acid. These acids exert a mild osmotic action, producing a soft, formed stool in 1 to 3 days. Although lactulose can relieve constipation, this agent is more expensive than equivalent drugs (bulk-forming laxatives) and causes more unpleasant side effects (flatulence and cramping are common). Accordingly, lactulose should be reserved for patients who do not respond adequately to a bulk-forming agent.

In addition to its laxative action, lactulose can enhance the intestinal excretion of ammonia. This property has been used to lower blood ammonia content in patients with portal hypertension and hepatic encephalopathy secondary to chronic liver disease.

Other Laxatives
Lubiprostone
Lubiprostone (Amitiza) is the first representative of a new class of drugs: the selective *chloride channel activators.* By activating (opening) chloride channels in epithelial cells lining the intestine, lubiprostone (1) promotes secretion of chloride-rich fluid into the intestine and (2) enhances motility in the small intestine and colon. The result is spontaneous evacuation of a semisoft stool, usually within 24 hours. Lubiprostone has three indications: (1) chronic idiopathic constipation in adults, (2) irritable bowel syndrome with constipation (IBS-C) in women at least 18 years old, and (3) treatment of opioid-induced constipation in chronic noncancer pain. In clinical trials, the drug reduced constipation severity, abdominal bloating, and discomfort.

Lubiprostone is taken orally and very little is absorbed. Nausea is the most common side effect and can be reduced by taking lubiprostone with food and water. Other GI effects include diarrhea, abdominal distention, abdominal pain, gas, vomiting, and loose stools. Headache is the major non-GI effect. A small percentage of patients experience difficulty breathing in association with a sense of tightness in the chest, starting 30 to 60 minutes after the first dose and resolving in a few hours. Lubiprostone should be used in pregnant women only if benefits are deemed to outweigh potential risks to the fetus. (In animal studies, lubiprostone was not teratogenic. However, when given to guinea pigs in doses more than 100 times the human dose, lubiprostone did cause fetal loss.) Interactions with other drugs have not been studied but seem unlikely because lubiprostone is poorly absorbed and does not alter the activity of cytochrome P450 drug-metabolizing enzymes.

Lubiprostone is available in 8- and 24-μg soft-gelatin capsules that should be taken with food and water. The recommended dosage is 24 μg twice daily for constipation and 8 μg twice daily for IBS-C.

Plecanatide
Plecanatide (Trulance) is an oral tablet approved for the treatment of chronic idiopathic constipation. Plecanatide is related to the human hormone uroguanylin and assists in regulation of intestinal fluid secretion and motility by acting as a guanylate cyclase-C (GC-C) agonist. Activation of GC-C indirectly stimulates secretion of chloride and bicarbonate into the intestinal lumen. This results in increased intestinal fluid. Plecanatide is taken once daily with or without food.

Bowel Cleansing Products for Colonoscopy
Colonoscopy is the most effective method for early detection of colorectal cancer, the second leading cause of cancer deaths in the United States. Before the procedure, the bowel must be cleansed to permit good visualization. Three kinds of bowel cleansers are used: (1) sodium phosphate; (2) a combination of sodium picosulfate, magnesium oxide, and citric acid; and (3) PEG plus electrolytes (ELS). The PEG-ELS products are isotonic with body fluids and hence do not alter water or electrolyte status. In contrast, the sodium phosphate and combination

TABLE 65.5 Oral Bowel Cleansing Products for Colonoscopy

Product Type and Brand Name	Adult Dosage	TOTAL VOLUME TO SWALLOW	
		Bowel Cleanser	Clear Liquid
Sodium Phosphate Tablets			
Visicol	20 tablets with clear liquid in the evening *plus* 12 tablets with clear liquid the next day		3.4 L
OsmoPrep	20 tablets with clear liquid in the evening *plus* 20 tablets with clear liquid the next day		1.9 L
Polyethylene Glycol Plus Electrolytes			
GoLYTELY, NuLytely, CoLyte, TriLyte	240 mL every 10 min until 4 L is ingested or until rectal effluent is clear	4 L	
GaviLyte-H and bisacodyl	240 mL every 10 min until 2 L is ingested[a]	2 L	
MoviPrep[b]	240 mL every 15 min unti1 1 L is ingested, then repeat 1.5 h later, then drink 1 L of clear liquid[c]	2 L	1 L
Combination Product			
Prepopik	One package (16.1 g) mixed in 5 oz of water the evening before the colonoscopy and one package mixed in 5 oz of water the morning of the colonoscopy.[d]		2.5 L

[a]Before drinking the solution, patients should take four bisacodyl delayed-release tablets and wait for a bowel movement or for 6 hours, whichever comes first.
[b]Formulated with ascorbic acid, which allows use of a smaller volume than traditional polyethylene glycol-electrolyte products.
[c]Dosage can be split by ingesting 1 L of the prep plus 0.5 L clear liquid in the evening, followed by 1 L of the prep plus 0.5 L clear liquid the next day.
[d]Dose should be followed by 40 oz of clear liquid the evening before the colonoscopy and 32 oz of clear liquid in the morning of the procedure.

products are hypertonic and can cause dehydration and electrolyte disturbances. In addition, the sodium phosphate products can cause kidney damage. However, despite their greater potential for harm, the sodium phosphate products have better patient acceptance because the PEG-ELS products require ingestion of a large volume of liquid, whereas the sodium phosphate products do not. Nonetheless, sodium phosphate products should be avoided by patients at risk, including those with electrolyte abnormalities, renal impairment, and hypovolemia. Representative bowel cleansers are shown in Table 65.5.

Polyethylene Glycol–Electrolyte Solutions

These bowel-cleansing solutions (CoLyte, GoLYTELY, and others) contain PEG, a nonabsorbable osmotic agent, together with ELS (usually potassium chloride, sodium chloride, sodium sulfate, and sodium bicarbonate). The mixture is isosmotic with body fluids; hence water and electrolytes are neither absorbed from nor secreted into the intestinal lumen. As a result, dehydration does not occur and electrolyte balance is preserved. Because effects on water and electrolytes are minimal, PEG-ELS solutions can be used safely by patients who are dehydrated and by those who are especially sensitive to alteration of electrolyte levels (e.g., patients with renal impairment or cardiovascular disease).

PEG-ELS products are generally well tolerated. The most common adverse effects are nausea, bloating, and abdominal discomfort. These effects are less intense with the reduced-volume formulations. Because PEG-ELS products don't alter water and electrolyte status, they are safer than sodium phosphate products for patients with electrolyte imbalances, heart failure, kidney disease, or advanced liver disease.

Sodium Phosphate Products

As discussed previously, sodium phosphate is an osmotic laxative that draws water into the intestinal lumen, which then softens and swells the fecal mass and then stretches the intestinal wall to stimulate peristalsis. Dosing consists of swallowing tablets along with a large volume of

water or some other clear liquid. Because the clear liquid is more palatable than the PEG-ELS solutions, patients find the sodium phosphate regimens more appealing.

Like the PEG-ELS products, the sodium phosphate products can cause nausea, bloating, and abdominal discomfort. In addition, the sodium phosphate products can cause adverse effects unlike PEG-ELS products, especially dehydration, electrolyte disturbances, and kidney damage. By drawing a large volume of fluid into the intestinal lumen, sodium phosphate can cause dehydration. To prevent dehydration, patients must drink a large volume of clear fluid before, during, and after dosing.

Rarely, phosphate is absorbed in amounts sufficient to cause hyperphosphatemia, which can cause *acute, reversible renal damage, and possibly chronic, irreversible renal damage*. Risk factors for hyperphosphatemia and kidney damage include hypovolemia, advanced age, delayed bowel transit, active colitis, preexisting kidney disease, and use of drugs that can alter kidney function, including diuretics, ACEIs, ARBs, and nonsteroidal anti-inflammatory drugs. Patients who have these risk factors should probably use a PEG-ELS product rather than sodium phosphate.

Combination Products

One combination product—magnesium oxide/anhydrous citric acid/sodium picosulfate (Prepopik)—is approved for preparation for colonoscopy in adults. Sodium picosulfate is a stimulant laxative, and magnesium oxide and citric acid combine to form magnesium citrate, an osmotic laxative. When this product was given in a split-dose regimen, results were superior to colon preparation with PEG-ELS.

As with sodium phosphate products, Prepopik can cause electrolyte and fluid imbalances, renal impairment, seizures, and dysrhythmia secondary to electrolyte abnormalities. Caution must be employed in patients with reduced renal function. The most common adverse reactions are nausea, headache, and vomiting.

LAXATIVE ABUSE

Causes

Many people believe that a daily bowel movement is a requisite of good health and that any deviation from this pattern merits correction. Such misconceptions are reinforced by aggressive marketing of over-the-counter laxative preparations. Not infrequently, the combination of tradition supported by advertising has led to habitual self-prescribing of laxatives by people who don't need them.

Laxatives can help perpetuate their own use. Strong laxatives can purge the entire bowel. When this occurs, spontaneous evacuation is impossible until bowel content has been replenished, which can take 2 to 5 days. During this time, the laxative user, having experienced no movement of the bowel, often becomes convinced that constipation has returned. In response, he or she takes yet another dose, which purges the bowel once more and therefore sets the stage for a repeating cycle of laxative use and purging.

Consequences

Chronic exposure to laxatives can diminish defecatory reflexes, leading to further reliance on laxatives. Laxative abuse may also cause more serious pathologic changes, including electrolyte imbalance, dehydration, and colitis.

Treatment

The first step in breaking the laxative habit is abrupt cessation of laxative use. After drug withdrawal, bowel movements will be absent for several days; the patient should be informed of this fact. Any misconceptions that the patient has regarding bowel function should be corrected: the patient should be taught that a once-daily bowel movement may not be normal for him or her and that stool *quality* is more important than frequency or quantity. Instruction on bowel training (heeding the defecatory reflex and establishing a consistent time for bowel movements) should be provided. Increased consumption of fiber (bran, fruits, and vegetables) and fluid should be stressed. The patient should be encouraged to exercise daily, especially after meals. Finally, the patient should be advised that, if a laxative must be used, it should be used briefly and in the smallest effective dose. Agents that produce catharsis must be avoided.

 SUMMARY OF KEY PRESCRIBING CONSIDERATIONS

Laxatives

Therapeutic Goal: Reduce painful elimination, decrease the amount of strain needed to defecate, and empty the bowel prior to diagnostic procedures or surgery.

Baseline Data: Normal patterns of bowel function

Monitoring: None needed

Identifying High-Risk Patients: Laxatives are contraindicated in patients with symptoms of appendicitis, enteritis, diverticulitis, ulcerative colitis, acute surgical abdomen, fecal impaction, or bowel obstruction. Magnesium salts and sodium phosphate are contraindicated in patients with renal dysfunction.

Minimizing Adverse Effects: Adequate water intake should be encouraged. Laxatives should be used only when clearly necessary, and then only briefly in the lowest effective dosage.

66

Other Gastrointestinal Drugs

In this chapter we discuss an assortment of gastrointestinal (GI) drugs with indications ranging from emesis to colitis to hemorrhoids. Four groups are emphasized: (1) antiemetics, (2) antidiarrheals, (3) drugs for irritable bowel syndrome (IBS), and (4) drugs for inflammatory bowel disease (IBD).

ANTIEMETICS

The chapter begins by reviewing the emetic response. Next the major antiemetic classes are discussed. Finally, the most important application of these drugs—management of chemotherapy-induced nausea and vomiting (CINV)—is considered.

The Emetic Response

Emesis is a complex reflex brought about by activating the vomiting center, a nucleus of neurons located in the medulla oblongata. Some stimuli activate the vomiting center directly; others act indirectly (Fig. 66.1). Direct-acting stimuli include signals from the cerebral cortex (anticipation or fear), signals from sensory organs (upsetting sights, noxious odors, or pain), and signals from the vestibular apparatus of the inner ear. Indirect-acting stimuli first activate the chemoreceptor trigger zone (CTZ), which, in turn, activates the vomiting center. Activation of the CTZ occurs in two ways: (1) by signals from the stomach and small intestine (traveling along vagal afferents) and (2) by the direct action of emetogenic compounds (e.g., anticancer drugs, opioids, and ipecac) that are carried to the CTZ in the blood. When activated, the vomiting center signals the stomach, diaphragm, and abdominal muscles; the resulting coordinated response expels gastric contents.

Several types of receptors are involved in the emetic response. Important among these are receptors for serotonin, glucocorticoids, substance P, neurokinin-1, dopamine, acetylcholine, and histamine. Many antiemetics, including ondansetron (Zofran), dexamethasone, aprepitant (Emend), prochlorperazine, and dimenhydrinate, act by blocking (or activating) one or more of these receptors.

Antiemetic Drugs

Several types of antiemetics are available. Their classes, trade names, and dosages are shown in Table 66.1. Uses and mechanisms are shown in Table 66.2. Properties of the principal classes are discussed next.

Serotonin Receptor Antagonists

Serotonin receptor antagonists are the most effective drugs available for suppressing nausea and vomiting caused by cisplatin and other highly emetogenic anticancer drugs. These drugs are also highly effective against nausea and vomiting associated with radiation therapy, anesthesia, viral gastritis, and pregnancy. Four serotonin antagonists are available for treating emesis: ondansetron, granisetron, dolasetron, and palonosetron. Further information may be found in Table 66.1.

Ondansetron. Ondansetron (Zofran, Zofran ODT, Zuplenz) was the first serotonin receptor antagonist approved for CINV. The drug is

PROTOTYPE DRUGS
Gastrointestinal Drugs

Serotonin Antagonist
Ondansetron

Glucocorticoids
Dexamethasone

Substance P/Neurokinin-1 Antagonist
Aprepitant

Dopamine Antagonist
Prochlorperazine

Cannabinoid
Dronabinol

Benzodiazepine
Lorazepam

Drug for Constipation-Predominant IBS
Lubiprostone

Drug for Diarrhea-Predominant IBS
Alosetron

5-Aminosalicylate
Sulfasalazine

Glucocorticoid
Budesonide

Immunomodulators/Immunosuppressants
Mercaptopurine
Infliximab

IBS, Irritable bowel syndrome.

also used to prevent nausea and vomiting associated with radiotherapy and anesthesia. In addition, the drug is used off label to treat nausea and vomiting from other causes, including childhood viral gastritis and morning sickness of pregnancy. In all cases, benefits derive from the blockade of type 3 serotonin receptors (5-HT$_3$ receptors[a]) located in the CTZ and on afferent vagal neurons in the upper GI tract. The drug is very effective by itself and even more effective when combined with dexamethasone. Administration may be oral or parenteral. The most common side effects are headache, diarrhea, and dizziness. Of much greater concern, ondansetron prolongs the QT interval and hence poses

[a]Serotonin is also known as 5-hydroxytryptamine (5-HT), so type 3 serotonin receptors are abbreviated as 5-HT$_3$.

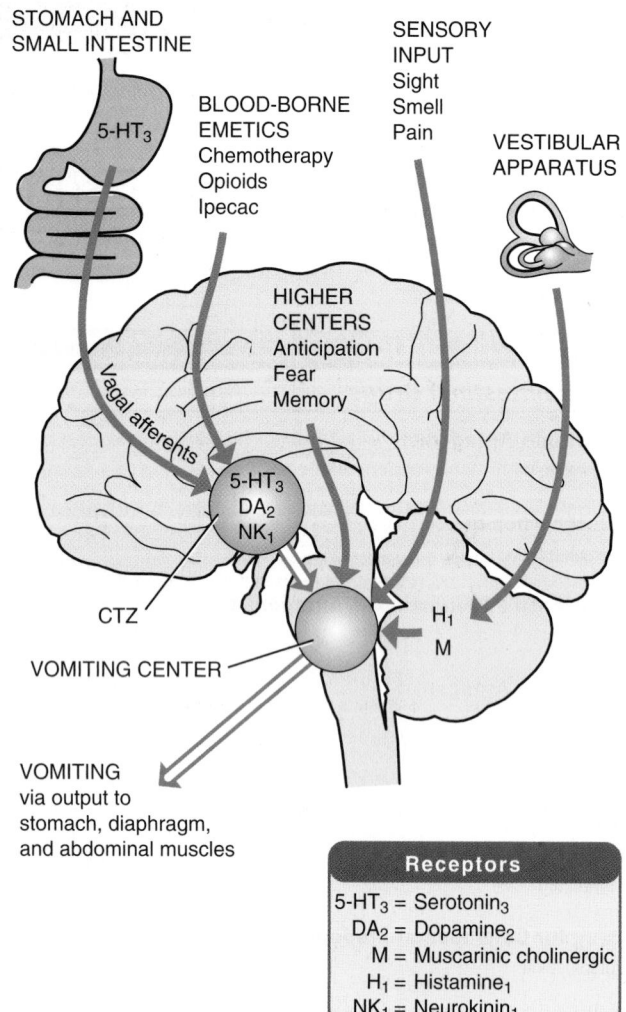

Fig. 66.1 **The Emetic Response: Stimuli, Pathways, and Receptors.** *CTZ,* chemoreceptor trigger zone.

Receptors

5-HT$_3$ = Serotonin$_3$
DA$_2$ = Dopamine$_2$
M = Muscarinic cholinergic
H$_1$ = Histamine$_1$
NK$_1$ = Neurokinin$_1$

a risk for torsades de pointes, a potentially life-threatening dysrhythmia. Accordingly, the drug should not be given to patients with long QT syndrome and should be used with caution in patients with electrolyte abnormalities, heart failure, or bradydysrhythmias and in those taking other QT drugs. Because ondansetron does not block dopamine receptors, it does not cause the extrapyramidal effects (e.g., akathisia and acute dystonia) seen with antiemetic phenothiazines.

Glucocorticoids

Two glucocorticoids—*methylprednisolone* (Solu-Medrol) and *dexamethasone* (Decadron)—are commonly used to suppress CINV, even though they are not approved by the US Food and Drug Administration (FDA) for this application. Glucocorticoids are effective alone and in combination with other antiemetics. The mechanism by which glucocorticoids suppress emesis is unknown. Both dexamethasone and methylprednisolone are administered by the intravenous route. Because antiemetic use is intermittent and short term, serious side effects are absent. The pharmacology of the glucocorticoids is discussed in Chapter 58.

Substance P/Neurokinin-1 Antagonists

Four substance P/neurokinin-1 antagonists are currently available: aprepitant, rolapitant, netupitant, and fosaprepitant, a prodrug that

undergoes conversion to aprepitant in the body. Their principal application is prevention of CINV.

Aprepitant

Actions and use. Aprepitant (Emend) is an important antiemetic. The drug is approved for preventing postoperative nausea and vomiting and CINV. Owing to its unique mechanism of action (blockade of neurokinin-1–type receptors [for substance P] in the CTZ), aprepitant can enhance responses when it is combined with other antiemetic drugs. Aprepitant has a prolonged duration of action and, hence, can prevent *delayed* CINV as well as *acute* CINV. Aprepitant can be used *alone* for managing postoperative nausea and vomiting. However, because the drug is only moderately effective, it must be combined with other antiemetic drugs—specifically, a glucocorticoid (e.g., dexamethasone) and a serotonin antagonist (e.g., ondansetron)—for managing CINV.

Pharmacokinetics. Oral aprepitant is well absorbed both in the presence and absence of food. Plasma levels peak 4 hours after dosing. The drug undergoes extensive hepatic metabolism—primarily by CYP3A4 (the 3A4 isoenzyme of cytochrome P450)—followed by excretion in the urine and feces. The plasma half-life is 9 to 13 hours.

Adverse effects. Aprepitant is generally well tolerated. Compared with patients receiving ondansetron and dexamethasone, those receiving aprepitant plus ondansetron and dexamethasone experience more fatigue and asthenia (17.8% vs 11.8%), hiccups (10.8% vs 5.6%), dizziness (6.6% vs 4.4%), and diarrhea (10.3% vs 7.5%). Aprepitant may also cause a mild, transient elevation of circulating aminotransferases, indicating possible liver injury.

Drug interactions. The potential for drug interactions is complex because aprepitant is a substrate for, inhibitor of, and inducer of CYP3A4, a major drug-metabolizing enzyme. Inhibitors of CYP3A4 (e.g., itraconazole, ritonavir) can raise levels of aprepitant. Conversely, inducers of CYP3A4 (e.g., rifampin and phenytoin) can decrease levels of aprepitant. By inhibiting CYP3A4, aprepitant can raise levels of CYP3A4 substrates, including many drugs used for cancer chemotherapy. Among these are docetaxel, paclitaxel, etoposide, irinotecan, ifosfamide, imatinib, vinorelbine, vinblastine, and vincristine. Also, aprepitant can raise levels of glucocorticoids used to prevent CINV. Accordingly, doses of these drugs (dexamethasone and methylprednisolone) should be reduced.

In addition to affecting CYP3A4, aprepitant can induce CYP2D6, another drug-metabolizing enzyme. As a result, aprepitant can decrease levels of CYP2D6 substrates, including warfarin (an anticoagulant) and ethinyl estradiol (found in oral contraceptives). Patients receiving warfarin should be monitored closely. Patients using oral contraceptives may

TABLE 66.1 Antiemetic Drugs: Classes, Trade Names, and Dosages

Class and Generic Name	Trade Name	Adult Dosage
Serotonin Antagonists		
Ondansetron	Zofran and Zuplenz	CINV: 0.15 mg/kg IV starting 30 min before chemotherapy Radiation therapy: 8 mg PO tid PONV prevention: 16 mg PO 1 h before induction of anesthesia
Granisetron	Kytril ✦ and Sancuso	CINV: either (1) 10 µg/kg IV starting 30 min before chemotherapy or (2) a single transdermal patch applied 24–48 h before chemotherapy and removed 24 h after chemotherapy is completed Radiation therapy: 2 mg given 1 h before chemotherapy PONV prevention: 1 mg IV either before induction of anesthesia or just before reversing anesthesia
Dolasetron	Anzemet	CINV: 100 mg PO 1 h before chemotherapy PONV prevention: 100 mg PO 2 h before anesthesia or 12.5 mg IV 15 min before anesthesia is stopped
Palonosetron	Aloxi	CINV: 250 µg IV 30 min before chemotherapy PONV prevention: 75 µg IV immediately before induction of anesthesia
Glucocorticoids		
Dexamethasone	Decadron	10–20 mg IV before chemotherapy, then 4–8 mg
Methylprednisolone	Solu-Medrol	Two doses of 125–500 mg IV 6 h apart before chemotherapy
Substance P/Neurokinin-1 Antagonists		
Aprepitant	Emend	125 mg PO on day 1, then 80 mg PO on days 2 and 3
Netupitant/Palonosetron	Akynzeo	300/0.5 mg PO 1 h before chemotherapy
Fosaprepitant	Emend	115 mg IV used in place of the first (125-mg) dose of aprepitant in the preceding Emend regimen
Rolapitant	Varubi	180 mg PO 1–2 h before the start of chemotherapy
Benzodiazepine		
Lorazepam	Ativan	1–1.5 mg IV before chemotherapy
Dopamine Antagonists		
Phenothiazines		
Chlorpromazine	Generic only	10–25 mg (PO, IM, and IV) q4–6h PRN
Perphenazine	Generic only	8–16 mg/day in divided doses (PO, IM, and IV)
Prochlorperazine	Generic only	5–10 mg (PO, IM, and IV) 3–4 qid PRN
Promethazine[a]	Phenergan	12.5–25 mg (PO, IM, and IV) q4–6h
Butyrophenones		
Haloperidol[b]	Haldol	1–5 mg (PO, IM, and IV) q12h PRN
Droperidol	Inapsine	0.625–2.5 mg (IM and IV) q4–6h PRN
Others		
Metoclopramide[c]	Reglan	CINV: 1–2 mg/kg IV starting 30 min before chemotherapy PONV prevention: 10 mg IV given prior to cessation of anesthesia
Cannabinoids		
Dronabinol	Marinol	5 mg/m^2 PO q2–4h PRN
Nabilone	Cesamet	1–2 mg PO bid
Anticholinergics		
Antihistamines		
Cyclizine	Cyclivert	50 mg PO q4–6h PRN
Dimenhydrinate	Dramamine	50–100 mg (PO, IM, and IV) q4–6h PRN
Diphenhydramine	Benadryl	10–50 mg (PO, IM, and IV) q4–6h PRN
Hydroxyzine	Vistaril	25–100 mg IM q6h PRN
Meclizine	Bonine and Antivert	25–50 mg PO q24h PRN
Others		
Scopolamine	Transderm Scōp	0.5 mg transdermal q72h PRN

[a]Promethazine is contraindicated for children below 2 years of age owing to a risk for fatal respiratory depression.
[b]Off-label use.
[c]Also blocks serotonin receptors.
CINV, Chemotherapy-induced nausea and vomiting; *IM*, intramuscular; *IV*, intravenous; *PONV*, postoperative nausea and vomiting.

TABLE 66.2   Antiemetic Drugs: Uses and Mechanism of Action

Class	Prototype	Antiemetic Use	Mechanism of Antiemetic Action
Serotonin antagonists	Ondansetron (Zofran and Zuplenz)	Chemotherapy, radiation, postoperative	Block serotonin receptors on vagal afferents and in the CTZ
Glucocorticoids	Dexamethasone (Decadron)	Chemotherapy	Unknown
Substance P/neurokinin-1 antagonists	Aprepitant (Emend)	Chemotherapy	Block receptors for substance P/neurokinin-1 in the brain
Dopamine antagonists	Prochlorperazine (generic only)	Chemotherapy, postoperative, general	Block dopamine receptors in the CTZ
Cannabinoids	Dronabinol (Marinol)	Chemotherapy	Unknown, but probably activate cannabinoid receptors associated with the vomiting center
Anticholinergics	Scopolamine (Transderm Scōp)	Motion sickness	Block muscarinic receptors in the pathway from the inner ear to the vomiting center
Antihistamines	Dimenhydrinate (generic only)	Motion sickness	Block histamine-1 receptors and muscarinic receptors in the pathway from the inner ear to the vomiting center

CTZ, Chemoreceptor trigger zone.

need an alternative form of birth control. Further information may be found in Table 66.1.

Benzodiazepines

Lorazepam (Ativan) is used in combination regimens to suppress CINV. The drug has three principal benefits: sedation, suppression of anticipatory emesis, and production of anterograde amnesia. In addition, lorazepam may help control extrapyramidal reactions caused by phenothiazine antiemetics. The basic pharmacology of lorazepam and other benzodiazepines is discussed in Chapter 30.

Dopamine Antagonists

Phenothiazines. The phenothiazines (e.g., prochlorperazine) suppress emesis by blocking dopamine-2 receptors in the CTZ. These drugs can reduce emesis associated with surgery, cancer chemotherapy, and toxins. Side effects include extrapyramidal reactions, anticholinergic effects, hypotension, and sedation. The basic pharmacology of the phenothiazines is discussed in Chapter 26.

One phenothiazine—*promethazine* (Phenergan)—requires comment. Promethazine is the most widely used antiemetic in young children despite its adverse side effects (respiratory depression and local tissue injury) and despite the availability of potentially safer alternatives (e.g., ondansetron).

⏩ BLACK BOX WARNING

Promethazine

Respiratory depression from promethazine can be severe. Deaths have occurred. Because of this risk, promethazine is contraindicated in children below 2 years of age and should be used with caution in children above that age.

Tissue injury can result in several ways. For example, extravasation of intravenous promethazine can cause abscess formation, tissue necrosis, and gangrene requiring amputation. Severe injury can also occur with inadvertent perivascular or intra-arterial administration or with administration into or near a nerve. Risk for local injury is lower with intramuscular than with intravenous dosing.

Butyrophenones. Two butyrophenones—*haloperidol* (Haldol) and *droperidol*—are used as antiemetics. Similarly to the phenothiazines, the butyrophenones suppress emesis by blocking dopamine-2 receptors in

the CTZ. Butyrophenones are effective against postoperative nausea and vomiting and against emesis caused by cancer chemotherapy, radiation therapy, and toxins. Potential side effects are similar to those of the phenothiazines: extrapyramidal reactions, sedation, and hypotension. The pharmacology of the butyrophenones is discussed in Chapter 26.

⏩ BLACK BOX WARNING

Droperidol

Droperidol may pose a risk for fatal dysrhythmias owing to prolongation of the QT interval. Accordingly, patients receiving the drug should undergo an electrocardiographic evaluation before administration.

Metoclopramide. Metoclopramide (Reglan) suppresses emesis through the blockade of dopamine receptors in the CTZ. The drug can suppress postoperative nausea and vomiting as well as emesis caused by anticancer drugs, opioids, toxins, and radiation therapy. The pharmacology of metoclopramide is discussed under "Prokinetic Agents."

Cannabinoids

Two cannabinoids—*dronabinol* (Marinol) and *nabilone* (Cesamet)—are approved for medical use in the United States. Both drugs are related to marijuana (*Cannabis sativa*). Dronabinol (delta-9-tetrahydrocannabinol; THC) is the principal psychoactive agent in *C. sativa.* Nabilone is a synthetic derivative of dronabinol. A third cannabinoid preparation, sold as *Sativex* (a combination of THC and cannabidiol), is available in Canada (for treating neuropathic pain and intractable cancer pain) but is not FDA-approved in the United States. The basic pharmacology of THC and other cannabinoids is discussed in Chapter 35.

Therapeutic uses. Both dronabinol and nabilone are approved for suppressing CINV. The mechanism underlying their benefits is unknown but most likely results from activating cannabinoid receptors in and around the vomiting center. Because of their psychotomimetic effects and abuse potential (see later), the cannabinoids are considered second-line drugs for CINV and hence should be reserved for patients who are unresponsive to or intolerant of preferred agents.

In addition to its use in suppressing CINV, dronabinol (but not nabilone) is approved for stimulating appetite in patients with AIDS. The goal is to reduce AIDS-induced anorexia and prevent or reverse weight loss.

Adverse effects and drug interactions. In theory, the cannabinoids used medically can produce subjective effects identical to those caused by smoking marijuana. Potential unpleasant effects include temporal disintegration, dissociation, depersonalization, and dysphoria. Because of these effects, cannabinoids are contraindicated for patients with psychiatric disorders. In addition to their subjective effects, cannabinoids can cause tachycardia and hypotension; therefore they must be used with caution in patients with cardiovascular diseases. The cannabinoids can cause drowsiness and hence should not be combined with alcohol, sedatives, or central nervous system (CNS) depressants.

Abuse potential. Because they can mimic the subjective effects of marijuana, cannabinoids have some potential for abuse. When they were first approved for medical use, both drugs were classified under Schedule II of the Controlled Substances Act (CSA). However, in 1998, the manufacturer of dronabinol petitioned the Drug Enforcement Agency (DEA) to reclassify the drug under Schedule III. Two arguments for the reduced classification were offered: (1) because of its slow onset, dronabinol does not produce the same "high" produced by smoking marijuana, and (2) there is little or no interest in dronabinol on the street. Apparently, the DEA agreed: dronabinol is now classified under Schedule III. Nabilone remains under Schedule II, although its abuse potential seems no greater than that of dronabinol.

Chemotherapy-Induced Nausea and Vomiting

Chemotherapy is associated with three types of emesis: (1) anticipatory, (2) acute, and (3) delayed. *Anticipatory emesis* occurs before anticancer drugs are actually given; it is triggered by the memory of severe nausea and vomiting from a previous round of chemotherapy. *Acute emesis* begins within minutes to a few hours after receiving chemotherapy and often resolves within 24 hours. In contrast, *delayed emesis* develops a day or more after drug administration. For example, with cisplatin, emesis is maximum 48 to 72 hours after dosing and can persist for 6 to 7 days.

Antiemetics are more effective at *preventing* CINV than at *suppressing* CINV that has already begun. Accordingly, antiemetics should be administered *before* chemotherapy. For prevention, antiemetics may be given orally or parenterally. Both routes are equally effective (although dosage may differ). In general, oral therapy is preferred. However, if emesis is ongoing, oral therapy won't work; hence parenteral therapy is required.

The antiemetic regimen for a particular patient is based on the emetogenic potential of the chemotherapy drugs being used. For drugs with a low risk for causing emesis, a single antiemetic (dexamethasone) may be adequate. For drugs with a moderate or high risk for causing emesis, a combination of antiemetics is needed. The current regimen of choice for patients taking highly emetogenic drugs consists of three agents: aprepitant plus dexamethasone plus a 5-HT₃ antagonist (e.g., ondansetron and palonosetron). Lorazepam may be added to reduce anxiety and anticipatory emesis and provide amnesia. The superior efficacy of combination therapy suggests that anticancer drugs may induce emesis by multiple mechanisms.

Nausea and Vomiting of Pregnancy

Nausea and vomiting of pregnancy (NVP) is extremely common, especially during the first trimester. About 50% of women experience nausea *plus* vomiting, and another 25% experience nausea alone. A few women experience *hyperemesis gravidarum,* a severe form of NVP characterized by dehydration, ketonuria, hypokalemia, and loss of 5% or more of body weight. Fortunately, most cases of NVP abate early in pregnancy: about 60% resolve within 13 weeks, and 90% resolve by the end of 20 weeks. Although NVP is commonly called *morning sickness,* it can occur at any time of the day.

NVP can be managed with drugs and with nondrug measures. Nondrug measures include (1) eating small portions of food throughout the day; (2) avoiding odors, foods, and supplements that can trigger NVP (e.g., fatty foods, spicy foods, and iron tablets); and (3) use of alternative treatments, such as acupuncture and ginger. Despite the use of these nondrug measures, about 10% of women require drug therapy.

PATIENT-CENTERED CARE ACROSS THE LIFE SPAN

Other Gastrointestinal Drugs

Life Stage	Patient Care Concerns
Children/adolescents	Promethazine is a commonly used antiemetic in children but it is contraindicated in children below 2 years of age. Other antiemetics, including dronabinol, are approved for nausea and vomiting in children. Side effects are similar to those that occur in adults.
Pregnant women	First-line therapy in nausea and vomiting of pregnancy includes doxylamine and vitamin B₆ in addition to diet changes. Other alternatives include prochlorperazine, metoclopramide, and ondansetron. The use of chenodiol is contraindicated during pregnancy.
Breastfeeding women	Prochlorperazine and promethazine appear safe for short-term use in breastfeeding women; their infants should be observed for sedation. Metoclopramide, dronabinol, and droperidol should be avoided while breastfeeding.
Older adults	Benzodiazepines, scopolamine, and metoclopramide should be avoided in older adults.

First-line therapy consists of a two-drug combination: *doxylamine* plus *vitamin B₆ (pyridoxine).* In randomized, controlled trials, the combination reduced NVP by 70% and showed no evidence of adverse fetal outcomes. Doxylamine and vitamin B₆ are available in a fixed-dose combination sold as *Diclectin* ♣ and *Diclegis.* Diclegis is sold in delayed-release tablets containing 10 mg each of doxylamine and pyridoxine. Dosing starts with two tablets at bedtime. If doxylamine and vitamin B₆ fail to suppress NVP, alternatives include prochlorperazine, metoclopramide, and ondansetron. Methylprednisolone may be tried as a last resort, but only after 10 weeks of gestation (earlier use greatly increases the risk for cleft lip with or without cleft palate).

DRUGS FOR MOTION SICKNESS

Motion sickness can be caused by sea, air, automobile, and space travel. Symptoms are nausea, vomiting, pallor, and cold sweats. Drug therapy is most effective when given prophylactically rather than after symptoms begin.

Scopolamine

Scopolamine, a muscarinic antagonist, is the most effective drug for prevention and treatment of motion sickness. Benefits derive from suppressing nerve traffic in the neuronal pathway that connects the vestibular apparatus of the inner ear to the vomiting center (see Fig. 66.1). The most common side effects are dry mouth, blurred vision, and drowsiness. More severe but less common effects are urinary retention, constipation, and disorientation.

Scopolamine is available for oral, subcutaneous, and transdermal dosing. The transdermal system (Transderm Scōp), an adhesive patch that contains scopolamine, is applied behind the ear. Anticholinergic side effects with transdermal administration may be less intense than with oral or subcutaneous dosing.

Antihistamines

The antihistamines used most often for motion sickness are *dimenhydrinate* (Dramamine), *meclizine* (Antivert, others), and *cyclizine* (Cyclivert). Because these drugs block receptors for acetylcholine in addition to receptors for histamine, they appear in Table 66.1 as a subclass under "Anticholinergics." Suppression of motion sickness appears to result from blocking histaminergic (histamine-1, or H_1) and muscarinic cholinergic receptors in the neuronal pathway that connects the inner ear to the vomiting center (see Fig. 66.1). The most prominent side effect—sedation—results from blocking H_1 receptors. Other side effects—dry mouth, blurred vision, urinary retention, and constipation—result from blocking muscarinic receptors. Antihistamines are less effective than scopolamine for treating motion sickness, and sedation further limits their utility. In general, they should be avoided in older adults because their anticholinergic properties may precipitate delirium.

ANTIDIARRHEAL AGENTS

Diarrhea is characterized by stools of excessive volume and fluidity and by increased frequency of defecation. Diarrhea is a symptom of GI disease and not a disease per se. Causes include infection, maldigestion, inflammation, and functional disorders of the bowel (e.g., IBS). The most serious complications of diarrhea are dehydration and electrolyte depletion. Management is directed at (1) diagnosis and treatment of the underlying disease, (2) replacement of lost water and salts, (3) relief of cramping, and (4) reducing passage of unformed stools.

Antidiarrheal drugs fall into two major groups: (1) specific antidiarrheal drugs and (2) nonspecific antidiarrheal drugs. The specific agents are drugs that treat the underlying cause of diarrhea. Included in this group are anti-infective drugs and drugs used to correct malabsorption syndromes. Nonspecific antidiarrheals are agents that act on or within the bowel to provide symptomatic relief; these drugs do not influence the underlying cause.

Nonspecific Antidiarrheal Agents
Opioids

Opioids are the most effective antidiarrheal agents. By activating opioid receptors in the GI tract, these drugs decrease intestinal motility and thus slow down intestinal transit, which allows more time for absorption of fluid and electrolytes. In addition, activation of opioid receptors decreases secretion of fluid into the small intestine and increases absorption of fluid and salt. The net effect is to present the large intestine with less water. As a result, the fluidity and volume of stools are reduced, as is the frequency of defecation.

At the doses employed to relieve diarrhea, subjective effects and dependence do not occur. However, excessive doses *can* elicit typical morphine-like subjective effects. If severe overdose occurs, it should be treated with an opioid antagonist (e.g., naloxone). In patients with IBD, opioids may cause toxic megacolon.

Several opioid preparations—diphenoxylate, difenoxin, loperamide, paregoric, and opium tincture—are approved for diarrhea. Of these, diphenoxylate (Lomotil, others) and loperamide (Imodium, others) are the most frequently employed. Pharmacologic properties of these agents are discussed later. Dosages for diarrhea are shown in Table 66.3.

Diphenoxylate. Diphenoxylate is an opioid used only for diarrhea. The drug is insoluble in water and hence cannot be abused by parenteral routes. When taken orally in antidiarrheal doses, diphenoxylate has no significant effect on the CNS. However, if taken in high doses, it can elicit typical morphine-like subjective effects.

Diphenoxylate is formulated in combination with atropine. The combination, best known as *Lomotil*, is available in tablets and as an oral liquid. Each tablet or 5 mL of liquid contains 2.5 mg of diphenoxylate and 0.025 mg of atropine sulfate. The atropine is present to discourage diphenoxylate abuse: doses of the combination that are sufficiently high to produce euphoria from the diphenoxylate would produce unpleasant side effects from the correspondingly high dose of atropine. Accordingly, the combination has a very low potential for abuse and is classified under Schedule V of the CSA.

Loperamide. Loperamide (Imodium, others) is a structural analog of meperidine. The drug is employed to treat diarrhea and reduce the volume of discharge from ileostomies. Benefits derive from suppressing bowel motility and from suppressing fluid secretion into the intestinal lumen. The drug is poorly absorbed and does not readily cross the blood–brain barrier. Very large oral doses do not elicit morphine-like subjective effects. Loperamide has little or no potential for abuse and is not regulated under the CSA. The drug is supplied in 2-mg capsules, in 2-mg tablets, and in two liquid formulations (1 mg/5 mL and 1 mg/7.5 mL).

TABLE 66.3 Opioids Used to Treat Diarrhea

Generic Name	Trade Name	CSA Schedule	Antidiarrheal Dosage
Diphenoxylate (plus atropine)[a]	Lomotil	V	*Adults:* 5 mg, qid *Children (initial dosage):*[b] Ages 2–5 years: 1 mg qid Ages 5–12 years: 1–2 mg qid
Difenoxin (plus atropine)[a]	Motofen	IV	*Adults:* 2 mg initially, then 1 mg after each loose stool
Loperamide	Imodium, Pepto Diarrhea Control, and others	NR	*Adults* (initial dose): 4 mg *Children (initial dosage):* Ages 2–5 years: 1 mg tid Ages 5–8 years: 2 mg, bid Ages 8–12 years: 2 mg tid
Paregoric (camphorated tincture of opium; contains 0.4 mg morphine/mL)		III	*Adults:* 5–10 mL bid–qid *Children:* 0.25–0.5 mL/kg bid–qid
Opium tincture (opioid content equivalent to 10 mg morphine/mL)		II	0.6 mL qid

[a]Diphenoxylate and difenoxin are available only in combination with atropine. The atropine dose is subtherapeutic and is present to discourage abuse.
[b]Only the liquid product is recommended in children less than 13 years of age.
CSA, Controlled Substances Act; *NR,* not regulated under the CSA.

Management of Infectious Diarrhea
General Considerations

Infectious diarrhea may be produced by enteric infection with a variety of bacteria and protozoa. These infections are usually self-limited. Mild diarrhea can be managed with nonspecific antidiarrheals. In many cases no treatment is required. Antibiotics should be administered only when clearly indicated. Indiscriminate use of antibiotics is undesirable in that it (1) can promote emergence of antibiotic resistance and (2) can produce an asymptomatic carrier state by killing most of the infectious agents. Conditions that *do* merit antibiotic treatment include severe infections with *Salmonella*, *Shigella*, *Campylobacter*, or *Clostridium* species.

Traveler's Diarrhea

Tourists are often plagued by infectious diarrhea. In most cases, the causative organism is *Escherichia coli*. As a rule, treatment is unnecessary: infection with *E. coli* is self-limited and will run its course in a few days. However, if symptoms are especially severe, treatment with a fluoroquinolone antibiotic—*ciprofloxacin* (500 mg bid)—is indicated. *Azithromycin* (Zithromax) is preferred for children (10 mg/kg on day 1 and 5 mg/kg on days 2 and 3) and for pregnant women (1000 mg once or 500 mg once daily for 3 days). *Rifaximin* (Xifaxan) (200 mg tid for 3 days) may also be used provided the patient is not pregnant or febrile and that stools are not bloody. For patients with mild symptoms, relief can be achieved with *loperamide*, a nonspecific antidiarrheal. However, by slowing peristalsis, loperamide may delay export of the offending organism, thereby prolonging the infection.

Several measures can reduce acquisition of traveler's diarrhea. Two measures—avoiding local drinking water and carefully washing foods—are highly effective. Certain drugs—*fluoroquinolones*—can be taken for prophylaxis. However, because these drugs can cause serious side effects, prophylaxis is not generally recommended. Last, travelers can be vaccinated against some pathogens. Oral vaccination with *Dukoral* ♦ protects against diarrhea caused by *E. coli* and *Vibrio cholerae*.

Clostridium difficile–Associated Diarrhea

Clostridium difficile is a gram-positive anaerobic bacillus that infects the bowel. Injury results from release of bacterial toxins. Symptoms range from relatively mild (abdominal discomfort, nausea, fever, and diarrhea) to very severe (toxic megacolon, pseudomembranous colitis, colon perforation, sepsis, and death). *C. difficile* infection and its treatment are discussed in Chapter 72.

DRUGS FOR IRRITABLE BOWEL SYNDROME

IBS is the most common disorder of the GI tract, affecting an estimated 10% to 15% of Americans—about 45 million people. The incidence in women is three times that in men. IBS is responsible for 12% of all visits to primary care physicians and 20% to 40% of all visits to gastroenterologists. The direct medical costs are estimated at $8 billion a year; the indirect costs are much higher—about $21 billion a year. IBS is second only to the common cold as the leading cause of days missed from work.

IBS is a GI disorder characterized by crampy abdominal pain—sometimes severe—occurring in association with diarrhea, constipation, or both. Formally, IBS is defined by the Rome IV criteria as the presence, for at least 12 weeks in the previous year, of abdominal pain or discomfort that cannot be explained by structural or chemical abnormalities and that has at least two of the following features:
- Pain related to defecation.
- Onset associated with a change in frequency of stool.
- Onset of pain associated with a change in stool consistency (from normal to loose, watery, or pellet-like).

IBS has four major forms, characterized as follows:
- Abdominal pain in association with diarrhea (diarrhea-predominant IBS; IBS-D)
- Abdominal pain in association with constipation (constipation-predominant IBS; IBS-C)
- Abdominal pain in association with alternating episodes of diarrhea and constipation (mixed IBS; IBS-M)
- Abdominal pain in association with episodes of diarrhea and/or constipation that do not fit well into the other categories and thus unclassified (IBS-U)

No one knows what causes IBS. Despite extensive research, no underlying pathophysiologic mechanism has been identified. What we do know is that the bowel appears hypersensitive and hyperresponsive. As a result, mild stimuli that would have no effect on most people can trigger an intense response. In addition, we know that symptoms can be triggered by stress, depression, and dietary factors, including caffeine, alcohol, fried foods, high-fat foods, gas-generating vegetables (beans, broccoli, cabbage), and too much sorbitol, a sweetener found in chewing gum and some diet products. Overproduction of gastric acid and excessive bacterial colonization of the small intestine have also been implicated.

Fortunately, many people achieve significant relief with treatment. Nondrug measures and drug therapy are employed. Patients should keep a log to identify foods and stressors that trigger symptoms. Because large meals stretch and stimulate the bowel, switching to smaller, more frequent meals may help. Increasing dietary fluid and fiber may reduce constipation.

Two groups of drugs are used for treatment: nonspecific drugs and drugs specific for IBS. Both groups are discussed next.

Nonspecific Drugs

Four groups of drugs—*antispasmodics* (e.g., hyoscyamine and dicyclomine), *bulk-forming agents* (e.g., psyllium and polycarbophil), *antidiarrheals* (e.g., loperamide), and *tricyclic antidepressants* (TCAs)—have been employed for years to provide symptomatic relief. However, a report from the American College of Gastroenterology (ACG) concluded that, for most of these agents, there is no good proof of clinical benefits. Specifically, after reviewing available data, the authors concluded that loperamide and the bulk-forming agents are no better than placebo at relieving global symptoms of IBS. In contrast, they concluded that there is good evidence that TCAs can reduce abdominal pain and that this benefit is unrelated to relief of depression. Regarding antispasmodic agents, they concluded that the available data are insufficient to make a recommendation for or against use.

Studies suggest that, for some patients, symptoms can be relieved with *antibiotics* or an *acid suppressant*. For example, studies reveal that a large percentage of patients with IBS also suffer from Small Intestine Bacterial Overgrowth (SIBO). When patients with concomitant IBS and SIBO were treated with antibiotics, bacterial colonization was reduced—and so were symptoms of IBS. In a more recent study, treatment with oral rifaximin (a poorly absorbed, broad-spectrum antibiotic) reduced symptoms in some patients with IBS. Meta-analyses of controlled clinical trials report that use of one probiotic, Bifidobacterium infantis, can improve symptoms. Use of the probiotic can address alterations in gut flora that hypothetically lead to inflammation, gas production, abdominal distention, and visceral sensitivity. Further study is needed to identify efficacy. Another study evaluated the effects of drugs that suppress production of stomach acid in patients who routinely experienced exacerbation of symptoms after eating. Two kinds of acid suppressants were used: proton pump inhibitors (lansoprazole or

TABLE 66.4   Drugs for Irritable Bowel Syndrome

Drug	Indication	Mechanism of Action	Preparation	Usual Adult Dose
Alosetron (Lotronex)	IBS-D in women	Selective blockade of 5-HT receptors	0.5-mg, 1-mg tablets	Start 0.5 mg twice daily × 4 weeks. Maxiumum: 2 mg daily.
Eluxadoline (Viberzi)	IBS-D	Mu- and kappa- opioid receptor antagonist	75-mg, 100-mg tablets	100 mg twice daily
Lubiprostone (Amitiza)	IBS-C in women	Selective activation of chloride channels of the intestine	8-μg, 24-μg capsules	8 μg twice daily
Linaclotide (Linzess)	IBS-C	Guanylate Cyclase Agonist- Increases intestinal fluid secretion and motility	72-μg, 145-μg, 290-μg capsules	290 μg daily

IBS-C, Irritable bowel syndrome-Constipation predominant; *IBS-D,* Irritable bowel syndrome-Diarrhea predominant; *5-HT,* Serotonin.

omeprazole) and histamine-2 receptor blockers (famotidine or raniti-dine). In all cases, patients experienced a significant reduction of postprandial urgency and other symptoms. Benefits developed quickly (within days) and reversed when the drugs were stopped.

Inflammatory Bowel Syndrome–Specific Drugs

In this section a drug approved for IBS, alosetron, is discussed. Information regarding the other three approved medications may be found in Table 66.4. These are eluxadoline (approved for IBS-D) and lubiprostone and linaclotide (approved for IBS-C). Although a fifth drug, tegaserod, exists, it is used only in emergency situations owing to a risk for serious cardiovascular events.

Alosetron

Alosetron (Lotronex) is a potentially hazardous drug approved for IBS-D in women. (Safety and efficacy in men have not been demonstrated.) As there have been reports of severe GI toxicity and several deaths, prescribers, patients, and pharmacists must adhere to a strict risk management program (see later).

Indications. Alosetron is approved only for treating women with severe IBS-D that has lasted for 6 months or more and has not responded to conventional treatment. IBS-D is considered severe if the patient experiences one or more of the following: (1) frequent and severe abdominal pain or discomfort, (2) frequent bowel urgency or fecal incontinence, and (3) disability or restriction of daily activities because of IBS. Less than 5% of IBS cases qualify as severe.

Mechanism of action and clinical effects. Alosetron causes selective blockade of 5-HT$_3$ receptors, which are found primarily on neurons that innervate the viscera. In patients with IBS-D, alosetron can decrease abdominal pain, increase colonic transit time, reduce intestinal secretions, and increase absorption of water and sodium. As a result, the drug can increase stool firmness and decrease both fecal urgency and frequency. Presumably, all of these effects result from 5-HT$_3$ blockade. Symptoms decline 1 to 4 weeks after starting the drug and resume 1 week after stopping the drug.

Pharmacokinetics. Administration is oral and absorption is rapid but incomplete (50% to 60%). Bioavailability is decreased by food. Plasma levels peak about 1 hour after dosing. Alosetron undergoes extensive metabolism by hepatic cytochrome P450 enzymes, followed by excretion primarily in the urine. The half-life is 1.5 hours.

Drug interactions. Alosetron does not interact with theophylline, oral contraceptives, cisapride, ibuprofen, alprazolam, amitriptyline, fluoxetine, or hydrocodone combined with acetaminophen. Because alosetron is metabolized by cytochrome P450 enzymes, drugs that interfere with these enzymes (e.g., carbamazepine, phenobarbital, cimetidine, quinolone antibiotics, ketoconazole, clarithromycin, vori-conazole, and protease inhibitors) may alter alosetron levels.

Adverse effects and contraindications. Although alosetron is generally well tolerated, it *can* cause severe adverse effects. Deaths have occurred. The most common problem is constipation (29%), which can be complicated by impaction, bowel obstruction, and perforation.

 BLACK BOX WARNING

Alosetron

Alosetron can cause *ischemic colitis* (intestinal damage secondary to reduced blood flow). Ischemic colitis and complications of constipation have led to hospitalization, blood transfusion, surgery, and death. Owing to its potential for GI toxicity, alosetron is *contraindicated* for patients with ongoing constipation or a history of any of the following:

- Chronic constipation, severe constipation, or sequelae from constipation
- Intestinal obstruction or stricture, toxic megacolon, or GI perforation or adhesions
- Ischemic colitis, impaired intestinal circulation, thrombophlebitis, or hypercoagulable state
- Crohn disease or ulcerative colitis
- Diverticulitis

Risk management program. To ensure the best possible benefit-to-risk ratio, the manufacturer and the FDA have established a risk management program that involves active participation of the patient, prescriber, and pharmacist. Details of this program can be found at lotronexppl.com.

SUMMARY OF KEY PRESCRIBING CONSIDERATIONS

IBS-Specific Drugs

Therapeutic Goal: Decrease in IBS symptoms, including diarrhea, constipation, and abdominal pain.

Baseline Data: Baseline symptoms, including duration and prior treatments as well as defecation patterns.

Monitoring: Laboratory monitoring not needed.

Identifying High-Risk Patients: Women taking alosetron must enroll in a risk-management program for treatment.

Evaluating Therapeutic Effects: Evaluate for decrease in abdominal pain, increase in bowel movements in patients with IBS-C, and decrease in amount or increase in quality of bowel movements in patients with IBS-D.

Minimizing Adverse Effects: Patients who develop constipation or signs of ischemic colitis (rectal bleeding, bloody diarrhea, and new or worsening abdominal pain) should immediately inform the prescriber.

DRUGS FOR INFLAMMATORY BOWEL DISEASE

IBD has two forms: *Crohn disease* and *ulcerative colitis*. Crohn disease is characterized by transmural inflammation and usually affects the terminal ileum but can also affect all other parts of the GI tract. Ulcerative colitis is characterized by inflammation of the mucosa and submucosa of the colon and rectum. Both diseases produce abdominal cramps and diarrhea. Ulcerative colitis may cause rectal bleeding as well. About 15% of patients with ulcerative colitis eventually have an attack severe enough to require hospitalization for intravenous glucocorticoid therapy, which produces remission in 80% of patients; the remaining 20% usually require total colectomy. In the United States IBD afflicts about 3 million people.

There is general agreement that IBD results from an exaggerated immune response directed against normal bowel flora—but only in genetically predisposed people.

Drug therapy of IBD is shown in Table 66.5. Five types of drugs are employed: *5-aminosalicylates* (e.g., sulfasalazine), *glucocorticoids* (e.g., hydrocortisone), *immunosuppressants* (e.g., azathioprine), *immuno-modulators* (e.g., infliximab), and *antibiotics* (e.g., metronidazole). None of these drugs are curative; at best, drugs may control the disease process. Patients frequently require therapy with more than one agent.

TABLE 66.5   Therapeutic Options for Inflammatory Bowel Disease

Disease Intensity	DISEASE FORM	
	Ulcerative Colitis	**Crohn Disease**
Mild	5-Aminosalicylate: PO or rectal	Mesalamine: PO Metronidazole: PO Budesonide: PO Ciprofloxacin: PO
Moderate	5-Aminosalicylate: PO or rectal Infliximab: IV Vedolizumab: IV	Glucocorticoid: PO Azathioprine: PO Mercaptopurine: PO Natalizumab: IV Ustekinumab: IV Vedolizumab: IV
Severe	Glucocorticoid: PO or IV Cyclosporine: IV Infliximab: IV Vedolizumab: IV	Glucocorticoid: PO or IV Methotrexate: IV or subQ Infliximab: IV Certolizumab: subQ Adalimumab: subQ Natalizumab: IV Ustekinumab: IV Vedolizumab: IV
Refractory	Glucocorticoid: PO or IV Azathioprine: PO Mercaptopurine: PO Vedolizumab: IV	Infliximab: IV Certolizumab: subQ Adalimumab: subQ Natalizumab: IV Ustekinumab: IV
Remission	5-Aminosalicylate: PO Azathioprine: PO Mercaptopurine: PO	Mesalamine: PO Azathioprine: PO Metronidazole: PO Mercaptopurine: PO Infliximab: IV Certolizumab: subQ Adalimumab: subQ Natalizumab: IV

IV, Intravenous; *PO*, oral; *subQ*, subcutaneous.

5-Aminosalicylates

The 5-aminosalicylates are used to treat mild or moderate ulcerative colitis and Crohn disease and to maintain remission after symptoms have subsided. Four aminosalicylates are available; sulfasalazine, the prototype, is discussed next.

Sulfasalazine

Sulfasalazine (Azulfidine) belongs to the same chemical family as the sulfonamide antibiotics. However, although similar to the sulfonamides, sulfasalazine is not employed to treat infections. Its only approved indications are IBD and rheumatoid arthritis (see Chapter 59).

Actions. Sulfasalazine is metabolized by intestinal bacteria into two compounds: 5-aminosalicylic acid (5-ASA) and sulfapyridine. 5-ASA is the component responsible for reducing inflammation; sulfapyridine is responsible for adverse effects. Possible mechanisms by which 5-ASA reduces inflammation include suppression of prostaglandin synthesis as well as of the migration of inflammatory cells into the affected region.

Therapeutic uses. Sulfasalazine is most effective against acute episodes of mild to moderate ulcerative colitis. Responses are less satisfactory when symptoms are severe. Sulfasalazine can also benefit patients with Crohn disease.

Adverse effects. Nausea, fever, rash, and arthralgia are common. Hematologic disorders (e.g., agranulocytosis, hemolytic anemia, and macrocytic anemia) may also occur. Accordingly, complete blood counts should be obtained periodically. Sulfasalazine appears safe during pregnancy and lactation.

Glucocorticoids

The basic pharmacology of the glucocorticoids is presented in Chapter 58; discussion here is limited to their use in IBD. Glucocorticoids (e.g., dexamethasone and budesonide) can relieve symptoms of ulcerative colitis and Crohn disease. Benefits derive from antiinflammatory actions. Prolonged use of glucocorticoids can cause severe adverse effects, including adrenal suppression, osteoporosis, increased susceptibility to infection, and a Cushing syndrome.

Glucocorticoids are indicated primarily for the induction of remission—not for long-term maintenance. Administration is either intravenous or by mouth.

Oral *budesonide* (Entocort EC) is approved for mild to moderate Crohn disease that involves the ileum and ascending colon. Entocort EC capsules are formulated to release budesonide when they reach the ileum and ascending colon. As a result, high local concentrations are produced. Systemic effects are lower when compared with other glucocorticoids because absorbed budesonide undergoes extensive first-pass metabolism.

Immunosuppressants

Immunosuppressants are used for long-term therapy in selected patients with ulcerative colitis and Crohn disease. Clinical experience is greatest with azathioprine and mercaptopurine.

Thiopurines: Azathioprine and Mercaptopurine

These drugs are discussed together because one is the active form of the other. (Mercaptopurine is the active drug; azathioprine is a prodrug that undergoes conversion to mercaptopurine in the body.)

Although not approved for IBD, azathioprine (Imuran) and mercaptopurine (Purixan) have been employed with success to induce and maintain remission in both ulcerative colitis and Crohn disease. Because onset of effects may be delayed for up to 6 months, these agents cannot be used for acute monotherapy. Furthermore, because these drugs are potentially more toxic than aminosalicylates or glucocorticoids, they are generally reserved for patients who have not responded to traditional therapy. Major adverse effects are pancreatitis and neutropenia (secondary to bone marrow suppression). At the doses used for IBD, these drugs are neither carcinogenic nor teratogenic.

Cyclosporine

Cyclosporine (Sandimmune, Neoral, and Gengraf) is a stronger immunosuppressant than azathioprine or mercaptopurine—and it acts faster, too. When used for IBD, the drug is generally reserved for patients with acute, severe ulcerative colitis or Crohn disease that has not responded to glucocorticoids. For these patients, continuous intravenous infusion can rapidly induce remission. In addition to intravenous administration, the drug has been administered orally in low doses to maintain remission, but results have been inconsistent. Cyclosporine is a potentially toxic compound that can cause renal impairment, neurotoxicity, and generalized suppression of the immune system.

Methotrexate

In patients with Crohn disease, methotrexate can promote short-term remission and hence reduce the need for glucocorticoids. Because the doses employed are low (25 mg once a week), the toxicity associated with high-dose therapy in cancer patients is lessened.

Immunomodulators

The drugs discussed in this section are monoclonal antibody products that modulate immune responses. Monoclonal antibodies are discussed further in Chapter 84. Three of these drugs—infliximab, certolizumab, and adalimumab—are inhibitors of *tumor necrosis factor-α* (TNF-α). Only infliximab, the prototype, is discussed here. The fourth and fifth drugs—natalizumab and vedolizumab—interfere with α_4 integrin. Finally, ustekinumab, a new drug, blocks the activity of interleukins 12 and 23. These drugs are generally considered second-line agents. However, some authorities now recommend their use early in treatment with the hope of inducing remission quickly and maintaining remission longer.

Infliximab

Infliximab (Remicade) is a monoclonal antibody designed to neutralize TNF-α, a key immunoinflammatory modulator. The drug is indicated for moderate to severe Crohn disease and ulcerative colitis. In clinical trials, infliximab reduced symptoms in 65% of patients with moderate to severe Crohn disease and produced clinical remission in 33%. Good responses are also seen in ulcerative colitis. As discussed in Chapter 59, infliximab is also used for rheumatoid arthritis.

During clinical trials, 5% of patients dropped out because of serious adverse effects. Infections and infusion reactions are most common. Tuberculosis and opportunistic infections are of particular concern. Infusion reactions include fever, chills, pruritus, urticaria, and cardiopulmonary reactions (chest pain, hypotension, hypertension, and dyspnea). Infliximab may also increase the risk for lymphoma, especially among patients with highly active disease or those on long-term immunosuppressive therapy.

For patients with Crohn disease or ulcerative colitis, treatment consists of an induction regimen (5 mg/kg infused at 0, 2, and 6 weeks) followed by maintenance infusions of 5 mg/kg every 8 weeks thereafter.

The basic pharmacology of infliximab is discussed in Chapter 59.

PROKINETIC AGENTS

Prokinetic drugs increase the tone and motility of the GI tract. Indications include gastroesophageal reflux disease (GERD), CINV, and diabetic gastroparesis.

Metoclopramide
Actions

Metoclopramide (Reglan) has two beneficial actions: (1) it suppresses emesis (by blocking receptors for dopamine and serotonin in the CTZ), and (2) it increases upper GI motility (by enhancing the actions of acetylcholine).

Therapeutic Uses

Indications depend on the route (oral or intravenous). *Oral* metoclopramide has two approved uses: diabetic gastroparesis and suppression of gastroesophageal reflux. *Intravenous* metoclopramide has four approved uses: suppression of postoperative nausea and vomiting, suppression of CINV, facilitation of small bowel intubation, and facilitation of radiologic examination of the GI tract. Off-label uses include the treatment of hiccups and nausea and vomiting of early pregnancy.

Adverse Effects

With high-dose therapy, sedation and diarrhea are common. Long-term high-dose therapy can cause irreversible *tardive dyskinesia,* characterized by repetitive, involuntary movements of the arms, legs, and facial muscles. Older adults are especially vulnerable and can develop involuntary movement disorders after a single dose. To reduce the risk for tardive dyskinesia, treatment should be as brief as possible using the lowest effective dose. Owing to its ability to increase gastric and intestinal motility, metoclopramide is contraindicated in patients with GI obstruction, perforation, or hemorrhage. Of note, exposure to metoclopramide during the first trimester of pregnancy is not associated with an excess risk for congenital malformations.

PANCREATIC ENZYMES

The pancreas produces three types of digestive enzymes: lipases, amylases, and proteases. These enzymes are secreted into the duodenum, where they help digest fats, carbohydrates, and proteins. To protect the enzymes from stomach acid and pepsin, the pancreas secretes bicarbonate. The bicarbonate neutralizes acid in the duodenum, and the resulting elevation in pH inactivates pepsin.

Deficiency of pancreatic enzymes can compromise digestion, especially digestion of fats. Fatty stools are characteristic of the deficiency. When secretion of pancreatic enzymes is reduced, replacement therapy is needed. Causes of deficiency include cystic fibrosis, pancreatectomy, pancreatitis, and obstruction of the pancreatic duct.

Pancreatic enzymes for clinical use are available as pancrelipase, a mixture of lipases, amylases, and proteases prepared from hog pancreas. Trade names are Creon, Pancreaze, Pertzye, Viokace, and Zenpep.

ANORECTAL PREPARATIONS
Nitroglycerin for Anal Fissures

Rectiv is a 0.4% nitroglycerin ointment used for relief of moderate to severe pain caused by chronic anal fissures (small tears in the skin that lines the anus). These fissures often cause unrelenting and debilitating pain. Topical nitroglycerin relieves pain and promotes healing by relaxing the internal anal sphincter. Nitroglycerin ointment has been used in other countries for years and is considered by many experts to be a first-line therapy.

Other Anorectal Preparations

Various preparations can help relieve discomfort from hemorrhoids and other anorectal disorders. Local anesthetics (e.g., benzocaine and dibucaine) and hydrocortisone (a glucocorticoid) are common ingredients. Hydrocortisone suppresses inflammation, itching, and swelling. Local anesthetics reduce itching and pain. Anorectal preparations may also contain emollients (e.g., mineral oil and lanolin), whose lubricant properties reduce irritation, and astringents (e.g., bismuth subgallate, witch hazel, and zinc oxide), which reduce irritation and inflammation. Anorectal preparations are available in multiple formulations: suppositories, creams, ointments, lotions, foams, tissues, and pads. Trade names include Preparation H, Rectagene, and Anusol.

67

Vitamins

Vitamins have the following defining characteristics: (1) they are *organic compounds*, (2) they are required in *minute amounts* for growth and maintenance of health, and (3) they do not serve as a source of energy (in contrast to fats, carbohydrates, and proteins) but rather are *essential for energy transformation and regulation of metabolic processes.* Several vitamins are inactive in their native form and must be converted to active compounds in the body.

BASIC CONSIDERATIONS

Dietary Reference Intakes

Reference values on dietary vitamin intake, as set by the Food and Nutrition Board of the National Academy of Medicine (NAM), formerly the Institute of Medicine (IOM), were established to provide a standard for good nutrition. In their report—*Dietary Reference Intakes: The Essential Guide to Nutrient Requirements*—the Food and Nutrition Board defined five reference values: *Recommended Dietary Allowance* (RDA), *Adequate Intake* (AI), *Tolerable Upper Intake Level* (UL), *Estimated Average Requirement* (EAR), and *Acceptable Macronutrient Distribution Range* (AMDR). Collectively, these five values are referred to as *Dietary Reference Intakes* (DRIs). Of these, the RDA, AI, UL, and EAR apply to vitamins. The AMDR is used for macronutrients such as fats and carbohydrates.

Recommended Dietary Allowance

The RDA is the average daily dietary intake sufficient to meet the nutrient requirements of nearly all (97% to 98%) healthy individuals. These figures are not absolutes. RDAs change as people grow older. In addition, they often differ for males and females, and typically increase for women who are pregnant or breastfeeding. Furthermore, RDAs apply only to individuals in good health. Vitamin requirements can be increased by illness; therefore published RDA values may not be appropriate for sick people. RDAs, which are based on extensive experimental data, are revised periodically as new information becomes available. Current values are available at https://www.nal.usda.gov/fnic/dietary-reference-intakes. (See Table 67.1.)

Adequate Intake

The AI is an *estimate* of the average daily intake required to meet nutritional needs. AIs are employed when experimental evidence is not strong enough to establish an RDA. AIs are set with the expectation that they will meet the needs of all individuals. However, because AIs are only estimates, there is no guarantee that they are adequate.

Tolerable Upper Intake Level

The UL is the highest average daily intake that can be consumed by nearly everyone without a significant risk for adverse effects. Note that the UL is not a *recommended* upper limit for intake. It is simply an index of safety.

Estimated Average Requirement

The EAR is the level of intake that will meet nutrition requirements for 50% of the healthy individuals in any life-stage or gender group. By definition, the EAR may be insufficient for the other 50%. The EAR for a vitamin is based on extensive experimental data and serves as the basis for establishing an RDA. If there is not enough information to establish an EAR, no RDA can be set. Instead, an AI is assigned, using the limited data available.

Acceptable Macronutrient Distribution Range

The AMDR is a range for macronutrients (e.g., proteins, carbohydrates, and fats) associated with optimal health. Intake of a nutrient below the established range for that nutrient increases the risk for malnourishment. Intake of a nutrient above the established range for that nutrient increases the risk for chronic diseases.

Classification of Vitamins

The vitamins are divided into two major groups: *fat-soluble* and *water-soluble.* In the fat-soluble group are vitamins A, D, E, and K. The water-soluble group comprises vitamin C and members of the vitamin B complex (thiamine, riboflavin, niacin, pyridoxine, pantothenic acid, biotin, folic acid, and cyanocobalamin). Except for vitamin B_{12}, water-soluble vitamins undergo minimal storage in the body; hence frequent ingestion is needed to replenish supplies. In contrast, fat-soluble vitamins can be stored in massive amounts, which is good news and bad news. The good news is that extensive storage minimizes the risk for deficiency. The bad news is that extensive storage greatly increases the potential for toxicity if intake is excessive.

Should We Take Multivitamin Supplements?

In the United States we spend billions each year on multivitamin and multimineral supplements. Is the money well spent? Maybe, maybe not. An expert panel—convened by the Office of Dietary Supplements at the National Institutes of Health—reports that there is insufficient evidence to recommend either for or against the use of multivitamins by Americans to prevent chronic disease. Exceptions include those who have malabsorption disorders, those who have undergone weight-loss

TABLE 67.1 Recommended Vitamin Intakes for Individuals

Life-Stage Group	RECOMMENDED VITAMIN INTAKE PER DAY												
	Vitamin A (µg)[a]	Vitamin C (mg)	Vitamin D (IU)[b,c]	Vitamin E (mg)[d]	Vitamin K (µg)	Thiamine (mg)	Riboflavin (mg)	Niacin (mg)[e]	Vitamin B_6 (mg)	Folate (µg)[f]	Vitamin B_{12} (µg)	Pantothenic Acid (mg)	Biotin (µg)
Infants													
0–6 months	400*	40*	400*	4*	2*	0.2*	0.3*	2*	0.1*	65*	0.4*	1.7*	5*
7–12 months	500*	50*	400*	5*	2.5*	0.3*	0.4*	4*	0.3*	80*	0.5*	1.8*	6*
Children													
1–3 years	300	15	600	6	30*	0.5	0.5	6	0.5	150	0.9	2*	8*
4–8 years	400	25	600	7	55*	0.6	0.6	8	0.6	200	1.2	3*	12*
Males													
9–13 years	600	45	600	11	60*	0.9	0.9	12	1	300	1.8	4*	20*
14–18 years	900	75	600	15	75*	1.2	1.3	16	1.3	400	2.4	5*	25*
19–30 years	900	90	600	15	120*	1.2	1.3	16	1.3	400	2.4	5*	30*
31–50 years	900	90	600	15	120*	1.2	1.3	16	1.3	400	2.4	5*	30*
51–70 years	900	90	600	15	120*	1.2	1.3	16	1.7	400	2.4[g]	5*	30*
>70 years	900	90	800	15	120*	1.2	1.3	16	1.7	400	2.4[g]	5*	30*
Females													
9–13 years	600	45	600	11	60*	0.9	0.9	12	1	300	1.8	4*	20*
14–18 years	700	65	600	15	75*	1	1	14	1.2	400[h]	2.4	5*	25*
19–30 years	700	75	600	15	90*	1.1	1.1	14	1.3	400[h]	2.4	5*	30*
31–50 years	700	75	600	15	90*	1.1	1.1	14	1.3	400[h]	2.4	5*	30*
51–70 years	700	75	600	15	90*	1.1	1.1	14	1.5	400	2.4[g]	5*	30*
>70 years	700	75	800	15	90*	1.1	1.1	14	1.5	400	2.4[g]	5*	30*
During Pregnancy													
≤18 years	750	80	600	15	75*	1.4	1.4	18	1.9	600[i]	2.6	6*	30*
19–30 years	770	85	600	15	90*	1.4	1.4	18	1.9	600[i]	2.6	6*	30*
31–50 years	770	85	600	15	90*	1.4	1.4	18	1.9	600[i]	2.6	6*	30*
During Lactation													
≤18 years	1200	115	600	19	75*	1.4	1.6	17	2	500	2.8	7*	35*
19–30 years	1300	120	600	19	90*	1.4	1.6	17	2	500	2.8	7*	35*
31–50 years	1300	120	600	19	90*	1.4	1.6	17	2	500	2.8	7*	35*

NOTE: This table presents recommended dietary allowances (RDAs) in **bold type** and Adequate Intakes (AIs) in ordinary type followed by an asterisk (*). RDAs and AIs may both be used as goals for individual intake. RDAs are set to meet the needs of almost all (97% to 98%) individuals in a group. For healthy breastfed infants, the AI is the mean intake. The AI for other life-stage and gender groups is believed to cover needs of all individuals in the group, but lack of data or uncertainty in the data prevents being able to specify with confidence the percentage of individuals covered by this intake.

[a]As retinol activity equivalents (RAEs): 1 RAE = 1 µg retinol, 12 µg β-carotene, 24 µg α-carotene, or 24 µg β-cryptoxanthin. To calculate RAEs from retinol equivalents (REs) of provitamin A carotenoids in foods, divide the REs by 2. For preformed vitamin A in foods or supplements and for provitamin A carotenoids in supplements, 1 RE = 1 RAE.

[b]These new RDAs and AIs were issued by the National Academy of Medicine on November 30, 2010.

[c]In the absence of adequate exposure to sunlight.

[d]As α-tocopherol. α-tocopherol includes RRR-α-tocopherol, the only form of α-tocopherol that occurs naturally in foods, and the 2R-stereoisomeric forms of α-tocopherol (RRR-, RSR-, RRS-, and RSS-α-tocopherol) that occur in fortified foods and supplements. It does not include the 2S-stereoisomeric forms of α-tocopherol (SRR-, SSR-, SRS-, and SSS-α-tocopherol), also found in fortified foods and supplements.

[e]As niacin equivalents (NE): 1 mg of niacin = 60 mg of tryptophan; 0 to 6 months = preformed niacin (not NE).

[f]As dietary folate equivalents (DFEs): 1 DFE = 1 µg food folate = 0.6 µg of folic acid from fortified food or as a supplement consumed with food = 0.5 µg of a supplement taken on an empty stomach.

[g]Because 10% to 30% of older people may absorb food-bound B_{12} poorly, it is advisable for those older than 50 years to meet their RDA mainly by consuming foods fortified with B_{12} or by consuming a supplement containing B_{12}.

[h]In view of evidence linking folate deficiency with neural tube defects in the fetus, the USPSTF recommends that all women capable of becoming pregnant consume 400 to 800 µg from supplements in addition to intake of food folate from a varied diet.

[i]It is assumed that women will continue consuming 400 µg from supplements or fortified food until their pregnancy is confirmed and they enter prenatal care, which ordinarily occurs after the end of the periconceptional period—the critical time for formation of the neural tube.

surgery, and those on restrictive diets (e.g., vegans). (See Table 67.2 for conditions that increase the risk for specific vitamin deficiencies.)

For people who *do* take a multivitamin supplement, the dosage should be moderate, because excessive doses can cause harm. For example, too much vitamin A increases the risk for osteoporosis in postmenopausal women and can cause birth defects when the vitamin is taken early in pregnancy. In older people with chronic health problems, too much vitamin E increases the risk for death. Because of these and other concerns, high-dose multivitamin supplements should be avoided. Instead, supplements that supply 100% or *less* of the RDA should be used.

Although research supporting the use of *multi*vitamin supplements is inconclusive, we do have solid data supporting the use of three *individual* vitamins—vitamin B_{12}, folic acid, and vitamin D. Who should take these vitamins? Nutrition experts recommend vitamin B_{12} for all people above the age of 50 years, folic acid for all women of childbearing age, and vitamin D (plus calcium) for postmenopausal women and other people at risk for fractures.

TABLE 67.2   Conditions That Increase Risk for Vitamin Deficiencies

Vitamin A	Prematurity, breastfed infants of women with vitamin A deficiency, and malabsorption disorders[a]
Vitamin B_1 (thiamine)	Alcohol dependence, older age, HIV/AIDs, diabetes mellitus, and bariatric surgery
Vitamin B_2 (riboflavin)	Pregnant and lactating women and their infants, vegan diet, and infantile Brown-Vialetto-Van Laere syndrome (a rare neurologic disorder)
Vitamin B_3 (niacin)	Alcohol dependence, prolonged treatment with isoniazid, and malabsorption disorders[a]
Vitamin B_5 (pantothenic acid)	Pantothenate kinase–associated neurodegeneration 2 mutation (a rare genetic condition)
Vitamin B_6 (pyridoxine)	Impaired renal function, autoimmune disorders, isoniazid therapy, and alcohol dependence malabsorption disorders[a]
Vitamin B_7 (biotin)	Biotinidase deficiency (a rare inherited disorder), alcohol dependence, and pregnant and breastfeeding women
Vitamin B_9 (folate)	Alcohol dependence, pregnancy, and malabsorption disorders[a]
Vitamin B_{12} (cobalamin)	Older age, strict vegetarian and vegan diets, breastfed infants of women on strict vegetarian or vegan diets, treatment with proton pump inhibitors, H_2 receptor antagonists or metformin, pernicious anemia, gastric disorders or surgery, and other malabsorption disorders[a]
Vitamin C	Smoking (including exposure to passive smoke), use of evaporated or cow's milk (especially if boiled) for infants, inadequate food sources, severe intestinal malabsorption, cancer, and end-stage renal disease with hemodialysis
Vitamin D	Breastfed infants, older age, limited sun exposure, and malabsorption disorders[a]
Vitamin E	Inborn deficiency of α-TTP and malabsorption disorders[a]
Vitamin K	Newborns not receiving vitamin K at birth and malabsorption disorders[a]

[a]Malabsorption disorders encompass a variety of conditions that reduce the ability to absorb dietary fats. Examples include cystic fibrosis, celiac disease, inflammatory bowel disease (e.g., Crohn disease and ulcerative colitis), bariatric surgery, small intestine or colon resections, and some liver diseases. α-*TTP*, Alpha-tocopherol transfer protein.

 PATIENT-CENTERED CARE ACROSS THE LIFE SPAN

Vitamins

Life Stage	Considerations or Concerns
Children	The AAP does not recommend vitamin supplements for healthy children who have a well-balanced diet. Those on vegan diets may require vitamin A, B_{12}, D, and riboflavin. It recommends 400 IU of vitamin D for breastfed infants rather than foregoing sunscreen. (This vitamin is provided in infant formulas.)
Pregnant women	For most vitamins, needs are increased during pregnancy. Prenatal vitamins can be prescribed to ensure adequate vitamin intake.
	Excess vitamin A is associated with multiple congenital abnormalities. Doses greater than the RDA are contraindicated.
	Women of childbearing age should receive folic acid supplementation prior to becoming pregnant and during the pregnancy to prevent neural tube defects.
Breastfeeding women	Vitamin requirements are increased during breastfeeding; however, doses higher than the RDA for breastfeeding women are not recommended.
Older adults	Vitamin D (plus calcium) may be beneficial for adults aged 65 years and older; it is also recommended for postmenopausal women and those at risk for fractures. The NAM recommends vitamin B_{12} for people over 50 years of age.

AAP, American Academy of Pediatrics; *NAM*, National Academy of Medicine; *RDA*, recommended dietary allowance.

What About Protective Antioxidant Effects?

Dietary antioxidants are defined as substances present in food that can significantly decrease cellular and tissue injury caused by highly reactive forms of oxygen and nitrogen, known as *free radicals*. These free radicals, which are normal byproducts of metabolism, readily react with other molecules. The result is tissue injury known as *oxidative stress*. Antioxidants help reduce oxidative stress by neutralizing free radicals before they can cause harm.

Although high doses of antioxidant supplements have been touted for their ability to prevent chronic diseases such as cardiovascular disease and cancer, much of this is information carried over from assumptions made a quarter-century ago. Despite plausible theories and observational studies that provided support for protective effects of antioxidant supplements, more recent and rigorous trials have failed to show protection against heart disease, cancer, or any other long-term illness. The National Center for Complementary and Alternative Medicine examined well-designed experimental studies that included more than 100,000 subjects and concluded that most studies failed to demonstrate a role for antioxidant-related reduction in disease development. Further, they identified that high doses of certain antioxidants might actually increase the risk for disease. For example, high doses of β-carotene were associated with an increase of lung cancer in people who smoked, and high doses of vitamin E were associated with an increase in prostate cancer and stroke. Additionally, some antioxidant supplements were responsible for significant drug interactions.

What's the bottom line? The National Academy of Sciences recommends limiting intake of antioxidant supplements to amounts that will prevent nutritional deficiency and avoiding doses that are potentially harmful. Of course, people should continue to obtain antioxidants as part of a healthy diet.

FAT-SOLUBLE VITAMINS

Vitamin A (Retinol)

Actions

Vitamin A, also known as retinol, has multiple functions. In the eye, vitamin A plays an important role in adaptation to dim light. The vitamin also has a role in embryogenesis, spermatogenesis, immunity, growth, and maintaining the structural and functional integrity of the skin and mucous membranes.

Therapeutic Uses

The only indication for vitamin A is prevention or correction of vitamin A deficiency. Contrary to earlier hopes, it is now clear that vitamin A, in the form of β-carotene supplements, does not decrease the risk for cancer or cardiovascular disease. In fact, in a study comparing placebo with dietary supplements (β-carotene plus vitamin A), subjects taking the supplements had a significantly *increased* risk for lung cancer and overall mortality. As discussed in Chapter 88, certain derivatives of vitamin A (e.g., isotretinoin and etretinate) are used to treat acne and other dermatologic disorders.

Sources

Requirements for vitamin A can be met by (1) consuming foods that contain preformed vitamin A (retinol) and (2) consuming foods that contain provitamin A carotenoids (β-carotene, α-carotene, and β-cryptoxanthin), which are converted to retinol by cells of the intestinal mucosa. Preformed vitamin A is present only in foods of animal origin. Good sources are dairy products, meat, fish oil, and fish. Provitamin A carotenoids are found in dark-colored carotene-rich fruits and vegetables. Especially rich sources are carrots, cantaloupe, mangoes, spinach, tomatoes, pumpkin, and sweet potatoes.

Units

The unit employed to measure vitamin A activity is called the retinol activity equivalent (RAE). By definition, 1 RAE equals 1 μg of retinol, 12 μg of β-carotene, 24 μg of α-carotene, or 24 μg of β-cryptoxanthin. Why are the RAEs for the provitamin A carotenoids 12 to 24 times higher than the RAE for retinol? Because dietary carotenoids are poorly absorbed and incompletely converted into retinol. Hence, to produce the nutritional equivalent of retinol, we must ingest much higher amounts of the carotenoids. In the past, vitamin A activity was measured in international units (IU). This IU designation is still commonly used on product labels. (The Joint Commission recommends spelling out international units rather than using the abbreviation IU if this designation is used when writing prescriptions.)

Requirements

RDA requirements for vitamin A and other vitamins are provided in Table 67.1.

Pharmacokinetics

Under normal conditions, dietary vitamin A is readily absorbed and then stored in the liver. As a rule, liver reserves of vitamin A are large and will last for months if intake of retinol ceases. In the absence of vitamin A intake, levels are maintained through mobilization of liver reserves. As liver stores approach depletion, plasma levels begin to decline. Signs and symptoms of deficiency appear when plasma levels fall below 20 μg/dL.

Additional information on pharmacokinetics of vitamin A and other vitamins is provided in Table 67.3. As it shows, the "usual" pharmacokinetic information for vitamins is limited as compared with most drugs.

Deficiency

Because vitamin A is needed for dark adaptation, night blindness is often the first indication of deficiency. With time, vitamin A deficiency

TABLE 67.3 Pharmacokinetics: Vitamins

Vitamins	Peak	Protein Binding	Metabolism	Half-Life	Elimination
Vitamin A	NA	NA	Converted to retinol in small intestine	NA	Feces Urine
Vitamin B₁ (thiamine)	NA	NA	Hepatic	NA	Urine
Vitamin B₂ (riboflavin)	NA	NA	Hepatic	66–84 min	Urine
Vitamin B₃ (niacin)	IR: 0.5–1 h ER: 4–5 h	Less than 20%	After conjugation with glycine, converted to metabolites	20–48 min	Urine
Vitamin B₅ (pantothenic acid)	NA	NA	Hydrolyzed to coenzyme A in intestine	NA	Urine
Vitamin B₆ (pyridoxine)	NA	NA	Hepatic conversion to active metabolites	NA	Urine
Vitamin B₇ (biotin)	NA	NA	NA	15 h	NA
Vitamin B₉ (folate/folic acid)	1 h	NA	Hepatic	NA	Urine
Vitamin B₁₂ (cobalamin)	0.5–2 h	NA	Converted to active coenzymes in tissues	NA	Urine
Vitamin C	NA	NA	Oxidized to dehydroascorbic acid Degraded in the intestine	10 h	Urine
Vitamin D	NA	50%–80%	Hepatic	NA	NA
Vitamin E	NA	NA	Hepatic	NA	Feces
Vitamin K	12–24 h	NA	Hepatic	NA	Feces Urine

ER, Extended release; *h*, hour(s); *IR*, immediate release; *min*, minutes; *NA*, not available.

may lead to *xerophthalmia* (a dry, thickened conjunctiva) and *keratomalacia* (degeneration of the cornea with keratinization of the corneal epithelium). When vitamin A deficiency is severe, blindness may occur. In addition to effects on the eye, deficiency can produce skin lesions and dysfunction of mucous membranes.

Toxicity

In high doses, vitamin A can cause birth defects, liver injury, and bone-related disorders. To reduce risk, the Food and Nutrition Board has set the UL for vitamin A at 3000 μg/day.

Vitamin A is highly teratogenic. Excessive intake during pregnancy can cause malformation of the fetal heart, skull, and other structures of cranial–neural crest origin. Pregnant women should definitely not exceed the UL for vitamin A and should probably not exceed the RDA.

Excessive doses can cause a toxic state referred to as *hypervitaminosis A*. Chronic intoxication affects multiple organ systems, especially the liver. Symptoms are diverse and may include vomiting, jaundice, hepatosplenomegaly, skin changes, hypomenorrhea, and elevation of intracranial pressure. Most symptoms disappear after vitamin A withdrawal.

Vitamin A excess can damage bone. In infants and young children, vitamin A can cause bulging of the skull at sites where bone has not yet formed. In adult females, too much vitamin A can increase the risk for hip fracture—apparently by blocking the ability of vitamin D to enhance calcium absorption.

Vitamin A supplements were once thought to decrease cancer risk; however, this has not been effectively demonstrated in randomized clinical trials (RCTs). In two large RCTs, vitamin A supplements were given to men deemed at risk for lung cancer as a result of smoking or asbestos exposure. In both trials, the incidence of lung cancer increased among men who received supplements. Another trial identified increased prostate cancer incidence and mortality among men receiving vitamin A supplements.

Preparations

Vitamin A (retinol) is available in drops, tablets, and capsules for oral dosing and in solution for intramuscular (IM) injection. Oral dosing is generally preferred.

Vitamin D

Vitamin D plays a critical role in calcium metabolism and maintenance of bone health. The classic effects of deficiency are *rickets* (in children) and *osteomalacia* (in adults). Recent studies have identified a relationship between vitamin D deficiency and obesity. Does vitamin D offer health benefits beyond bone health? Possibly. Studies suggest that vitamin D may protect against arthritis, diabetes, heart disease, autoimmune disorders, and cancers of the colon, breast, and prostate. However, in the NAM Food and Nutrition Board report titled *Dietary Reference Intakes for Calcium and Vitamin D*, an expert panel concluded that, although such claims might eventually prove true, the current evidence does not prove any benefits beyond bone health. The pharmacology and physiology of vitamin D are discussed in Chapter 61. Values for RDAs and AI are shown in Table 67.1.

Vitamin E (α-Tocopherol)
Actions

Vitamin E (α-tocopherol) is essential to the health of many animal species, but has no clearly established role in human nutrition. Unlike other vitamins, vitamin E has no known role in metabolism.

Vitamin E is an antioxidant. Specifically, the vitamin helps protect against peroxidation of lipids. It also inhibits oxidation of vitamins A and C.

Therapeutic Uses

Observational studies of the past suggested that vitamin E protected against cardiovascular disease, dementia, and cancer. However, more rigorous studies have failed to show any such benefits. There is evidence that 400 IU daily (in combination with vitamin C, β-carotene, zinc, and copper) may delay progression of age-related macular degeneration. The higher dose associated with halting macular degeneration carries substantial risk, as noted earlier, so the *potential* benefit hardly seems worth the risk.

There are some uses for vitamin E. Vitamin E has a role in protecting blood cells from hemolysis. This can be beneficial for premature infants in whom hemolytic anemia occurs in association with vitamin E deficiency. Also, a meta-analysis of available evidence indicated a role in preventing progression of tardive dyskinesia; however, it did not reverse symptoms. Considering that vitamin E deficiency is rare and that, for supplements, there are few benefits and several risks, it is not surprising that many experts recommend against taking vitamin E supplements.

Sources

Most dietary vitamin E comes from vegetable oils (e.g., corn oil, olive oil, cottonseed oil, safflower oil, and canola oil). The vitamin is also found in nuts, wheat germ, whole-grain products, and mustard greens.

Deficiency

Vitamin E deficiency is rare. In the United States, deficiency is limited primarily to people with an inborn deficiency of α tocopherol transfer protein (α-TTP) and to those who have fat malabsorption syndromes and, hence, cannot absorb fat-soluble vitamins. Symptoms of deficiency include ataxia, sensory neuropathy, areflexia, and muscle hypertrophy.

Toxicity

High-dose vitamin E appears to increase the risk for hemorrhagic stroke by inhibiting platelet aggregation. According to one report, for every 10,000 people taking more than 200 IU of vitamin E daily for 1 year, there would be 8 additional cases of hemorrhagic stroke.

Some studies have demonstrated a relationship between high doses of vitamin E (400 IU daily) and increased cancer risk or poor cancer outcomes. These results are consistent with the theory that high doses of antioxidants may cause cancer or accelerate cancer progression.

High-dose vitamin E (in combination with vitamin C) can blunt the beneficial effects of exercise on insulin sensitivity. Under normal conditions, exercising enhances cellular responses to insulin. However, among subjects who took vitamin E (400 IU/day) plus vitamin C (500 mg bid), exercising failed to yield this benefit.

Studies have also linked *high-dose* vitamin E therapy with an increased risk for death, especially in older people. Others have demonstrated higher mortality with *long-term* vitamin E therapy at doses higher than 400 IU (266 mg).

Preparations

Vitamin E is available as tablets, capsules, and solutions for oral administration. It is also added to some over-the-counter skin lotions and crèmes.

Vitamin K
Actions

Vitamin K is required for synthesis of prothrombin and clotting factors VII, IX, and X. All of these vitamin K–dependent factors are needed for coagulation of blood.

Therapeutic Uses

Vitamin K has two major applications: (1) correction or prevention of hypoprothrombinemia and bleeding caused by vitamin K deficiency, and (2) control of hemorrhage caused by warfarin.

Vitamin K deficiency can result from impaired absorption and insufficient synthesis of vitamin K by intestinal flora. Rarely, deficiency results from inadequate diet. For children and adults, the usual dosage for correction of vitamin K deficiency ranges between 5 and 15 mg/day.

As noted, infants are born with vitamin K deficiency. To prevent hemorrhagic disease in neonates, it is recommended that all newborns be given an injection of phytonadione (0.5 to 1 mg) immediately after delivery.

Vitamin K reverses hypoprothrombinemia and bleeding caused by excessive dosing with warfarin, an oral anticoagulant. Bleeding is controlled within 12 to 14 hours of intravenous (IV) vitamin K administration and within 24 to 48 hours of oral administration.

Sources

Vitamin K occurs in nature in two forms: (1) vitamin K_1, or phytonadione (phylloquinone), and (2) vitamin K_2. Phytonadione is present in a wide variety of foods. Vitamin K_2 is synthesized by the normal flora of the gut. Two other forms—vitamin K_4 (menadiol) and vitamin K_3 (menadione)—are produced synthetically.

For most individuals, vitamin K requirements are readily met through dietary sources and vitamin K synthesized by intestinal bacteria. Because bacterial colonization of the gut is not complete until several days after birth, levels of vitamin K may be low in newborns.

Deficiency

Vitamin K deficiency produces bleeding tendencies. If the deficiency is severe, spontaneous hemorrhage may occur. In newborns, intracranial hemorrhage is of particular concern.

An important cause of deficiency is reduced absorption. Because the natural forms of vitamin K require bile salts for their uptake, any condition that decreases availability of these salts (e.g., obstructive jaundice) can lead to deficiency. Malabsorption syndromes (sprue, celiac disease, and cystic fibrosis of the pancreas) can also decrease vitamin K uptake. Other potential causes of impaired absorption are ulcerative colitis, regional enteritis, and surgical resection of the intestine.

Disruption of intestinal flora may result in deficiency by eliminating vitamin K–synthesizing bacteria. Hence deficiency may occur secondary to use of antibiotics. In infants, diarrhea may cause bacterial losses sufficient to result in deficiency.

The normal infant is born vitamin K–deficient. Consequently, to rapidly elevate prothrombin levels and reduce the risk for neonatal hemorrhage, the American Academy of Pediatrics and the Centers for Disease Control and Prevention recommend that all infants receive a single injection of phytonadione (vitamin K_1) immediately after delivery. This previously routine prophylactic intervention has recently been challenged by parents who believe that the risks outweigh benefits. Subsequent to increases in parents declining prophylaxis, there has been an increase in life-threatening vitamin K–deficiency bleeding in recent years.

As discussed in Chapter 46, the anticoagulant warfarin acts as an antagonist of vitamin K and, hence, decreases synthesis of vitamin K–dependent clotting factors. As a result, warfarin produces a state that is functionally equivalent to vitamin K deficiency. If the dosage of warfarin is excessive, hemorrhage can occur secondary to lack of prothrombin.

Toxicity

Vitamin K toxicity can cause hyperbilirubinemia, hemolytic anemia, and jaundice in newborns. This risk is higher with menadione and menadiol, so these are no longer recommended. The oral form of vitamin K_1 is not toxic in adults.

IV phytonadione can cause serious reactions (shock, respiratory arrest, and cardiac arrest) that resemble anaphylaxis or hypersensitivity reactions. Death has occurred. Consequently, phytonadione should not be administered by the IV route unless other routes are not feasible, and then only if the potential benefits clearly outweigh the risks.

Preparations

Phytonadione (vitamin K_1) is available in tablets and in parenteral formulations. Parenteral phytonadione may be administered through IM, subcutaneous (subQ), and IV route. However, because IV administration is dangerous, this route should be used only when other routes are not feasible and only if the perceived benefits outweigh the substantial risks. For example, this might be indicated in management of life-threatening bleeding due to vitamin K antagonists (e.g., poisoning by coumarins in rodenticides).

WATER-SOLUBLE VITAMINS

The group of water-soluble vitamins consists of vitamin C and members of the vitamin B complex. The B vitamins differ widely from one another in structure and function. They are grouped together because they were first isolated from the same sources (yeast and liver). Vitamin C is not found in the same foods as the B vitamins and, hence, is classified by itself.

The B vitamins are known both by their numbers and their names; however, the literature uses one or the other preferentially. As a general rule, for vitamin B6 (pyridoxine) and vitamin B12 (cyanocobalamin), the vitamin numbers are used most often. For the remainder, the names are most often preferred. They are thiamine (vitamin B_1), riboflavin (vitamin B_2), niacin (vitamin B_3), pantothenic acid (vitamin B_5), biotin (vitamin B_7), and folic acid (vitamin B_9).

Two compounds—*pangamic acid* and *laetrile*—have been falsely promoted as B vitamins. Pangamic acid has been marketed as "vitamin B_{15}" and laetrile as "vitamin B_{17}." There is no proof that these compounds act as vitamins or have any other role in human nutrition.

Vitamin C (Ascorbic Acid)
Actions

Vitamin C participates in multiple biochemical reactions. Among these are synthesis of adrenal steroids, conversion of folic acid to folinic acid, and regulation of the respiratory cycle in mitochondria. At the tissue level, vitamin C is required for production of collagen and other compounds that comprise the intercellular matrix, which binds cells together. In addition, vitamin C facilitates absorption of dietary iron.

Therapeutic Use

The only *established* indication for vitamin C is prevention and treatment of scurvy. For severe, acute deficiency, parenteral administration is recommended.

Vitamin C has been advocated for therapy of many conditions unrelated to deficiency, including cancers, asthma, osteoporosis, and the common cold. Claims of efficacy for several of these conditions have been definitively disproved. Other claims remain unproved. Studies have shown that large doses of vitamin C do not reduce the incidence of colds, although the intensity or duration of illness may be decreased slightly. Research has failed to show any benefit of vitamin C therapy for patients with advanced cancer, atherosclerosis, or schizophrenia. Vitamin C does not promote healing of wounds unless severe deficiency has occurred.

Sources

The main dietary sources of ascorbic acid are citrus fruits and juices, tomatoes, potatoes, strawberries, melons, spinach, and broccoli. Orange juice and lemon juice are especially rich sources.

Deficiency

Deficiency of vitamin C can lead to *scurvy*, a disease rarely seen in the United States. Symptoms include faulty bone and tooth development, loosening of the teeth, gingivitis, bleeding gums, poor wound healing, hemorrhage into muscles and joints, and ecchymoses (skin discoloration caused by leakage of blood into subcutaneous tissues). Many of these symptoms result from disruption of the intercellular matrix of capillaries and other tissues.

Though not a common cause of deficiency, smoking creates an increased need for vitamin C. For those who smoke, the RDA is increased by 35 mg/day.

Toxicity

Excessive doses can cause *nausea*, *abdominal cramps*, and *diarrhea*. The mechanism is direct irritation of the intestinal mucosa. To protect against gastrointestinal (GI) disturbances, the Food and Nutrition Board has set 2 g/day as the adult UL for vitamin C.

Preparations

Vitamin C is available in formulations for oral and parenteral administration. Oral products include tablets, timed-release capsules, and syrups, as well as granules, crystals, powders, effervescent powders, and wafers. Vitamin C may be administered parenterally by the subQ, IM, or IV route.

Vitamin B₃ (Niacin)

Niacin (nicotinic acid) has a role as both a vitamin and a medicine. In its medicinal role, niacin is used to reduce cholesterol levels, although it has fallen from favor in recent years. The doses required are much higher than those used to correct or prevent nutritional deficiency. Discussion in this chapter focuses on niacin as a vitamin. Use of nicotinic acid to reduce cholesterol levels is discussed in Chapter 44.

Actions

Before it can exert physiologic effects, niacin must first be converted into nicotinamide adenine dinucleotide (NAD) or nicotinamide adenine dinucleotide phosphate (NADP). NAD and NADP then act as coenzymes in oxidation-reduction reactions essential for cellular respiration.

Therapeutic Uses

In its capacity *as a vitamin*, nicotinic acid is indicated only for the prevention or treatment of niacin deficiency. It is used off-label for the treatment of pellagra.

Sources

Nicotinic acid (or its nutritional equivalent, nicotinamide) is present in many foods of plant and animal origin. Particularly rich sources are liver, poultry, fish, potatoes, peanuts, cereal bran, and cereal germ.

In humans, the amino acid tryptophan can be converted to nicotinic acid. Hence proteins can be a source of the vitamin. About 60 mg of dietary tryptophan is required to produce 1 mg of nicotinic acid.

Deficiency

The syndrome caused by niacin deficiency is called *pellagra*, a term that is a condensation of the Italian words *pelle agra*, meaning "rough skin." As suggested by this name, a prominent symptom of pellagra is dermatitis, characterized by scaling and cracking of the skin in areas exposed to the sun. Other symptoms involve the GI tract (abdominal pain, diarrhea, and soreness of the tongue and mouth) and central nervous system (irritability, insomnia, memory loss, anxiety, and dementia). All symptoms are reversed with niacin replacement therapy.

Toxicity

Nicotinic acid has very low toxicity, and small doses are devoid of adverse effects. When taken in large doses, nicotinic acid can cause vasodilation, with resultant *flushing*, *dizziness*, and *nausea*. Using flushing as an index of excess niacin consumption, the Food and Nutrition Board has set 50 mg as the adult UL.

Nicotinamide, a compound that can substitute for nicotinic acid in the treatment of pellagra, is not a vasodilator and does not produce the adverse effects associated with large doses of nicotinic acid. Accordingly, nicotinamide is often preferred to nicotinic acid for treating pellagra.

Preparations

Niacin is administered orally only. It is available in both immediate release and extended release formulations. A powder is also available.

Vitamin B₂ (Riboflavin)
Actions

Riboflavin participates in numerous enzymatic reactions. However, to do so, the vitamin must first be converted into one of two active forms: flavin adenine dinucleotide (FAD) or flavin mononucleotide (FMN). In the form of FAD or FMN, riboflavin acts as a coenzyme for multiple oxidative reactions.

Therapeutic Uses

Riboflavin is indicated only for prevention and correction of riboflavin deficiency, which usually occurs in conjunction with deficiency of other B vitamins. In its early state, riboflavin deficiency manifests as sore throat and angular stomatitis (cracks in the skin at the corners of the mouth). Later symptoms include cheilosis (painful cracks in the lips), glossitis (inflammation of the tongue), vascularization of the cornea, and itchy dermatitis of the scrotum or vulva. Oral riboflavin is used for treatment.

Sources

In the United States, most dietary riboflavin comes from milk, yogurt, cheese, bread products, and fortified cereals. Organ meats are also rich sources.

Toxicity

Riboflavin appears devoid of toxicity to humans. When large doses are administered, the excess is rapidly excreted in the urine. Because large doses are harmless, no UL has been set.

Riboflavin can help prevent migraine headaches; however, prophylactic effects do not develop until after 3 months of treatment. The daily dosage is 400 mg—much higher than the dosage for riboflavin deficiency.

Preparations

Riboflavin is administered orally. It is available in both capsules and tablets.

Vitamin B₁ (Thiamine)
Actions

The active form of thiamine (thiamine pyrophosphate) is an essential coenzyme for carbohydrate metabolism. Thiamine requirements are related to caloric intake and are greatest when carbohydrates are the primary source of calories.

Therapeutic Use

The only indication for thiamine is treatment and prevention of thiamine deficiency.

Sources

In the United States, the principal dietary sources of thiamine are enriched, fortified, or whole-grain products, especially breads and ready-to-eat cereals. The richest sources of the natural vitamin are fish (especially tuna, salmon, and anchovies) and liver. Chicken, pork, beef, and lamb are also good sources.

Deficiency

Severe thiamine deficiency produces *beriberi*, a disorder having two distinct forms: *wet beriberi* and *dry beriberi*. *Wet beriberi* is so named because its primary symptom is fluid accumulation in the legs. Cardiovascular complications (palpitations, electrocardiogram abnormalities, and high-output heart failure) are common and may progress rapidly to circulatory collapse and death. *Dry beriberi* is characterized by neurologic and motor deficits (e.g., anesthesia of the feet, ataxic gait, footdrop, and wristdrop); edema and cardiovascular symptoms are absent. Wet beriberi responds rapidly and dramatically to replacement therapy. In contrast, recovery from dry beriberi can be very slow.

In the United States, thiamine deficiency occurs most commonly among people with chronic alcohol consumption. In this population, deficiency manifests as *Wernicke-Korsakoff syndrome* rather than frank beriberi. This syndrome is a serious disorder of the central nervous system, having neurologic and psychologic manifestations. Symptoms include nystagmus, diplopia, ataxia, and an inability to remember the recent past. Failure to correct the deficit may result in irreversible brain damage. Accordingly, if Wernicke-Korsakoff syndrome is suspected, parenteral thiamine should be administered immediately.

Toxicity

When taken orally, thiamine is devoid of adverse effects. Accordingly, no UL for the vitamin has been established.

Preparations

Thiamine is available in standard tablets for oral administration and in solution for IM or IV administration. For mild deficiency, oral thiamine is preferred. Parenteral administration is reserved for severe deficiency states (wet or dry beriberi and Wernicke-Korsakoff syndrome).

Vitamin B_6 (Pyridoxine)
Actions

Pyridoxine functions as a coenzyme in the metabolism of amino acids and proteins. However, before it can do so, pyridoxine must first be converted to its active form: pyridoxal phosphate.

Therapeutic Uses

Pyridoxine is indicated for prevention and treatment of all states of vitamin B_6 deficiency. These include dietary deficiency, isoniazid-induced deficiency, and pyridoxine dependency syndrome.

Sources

In the United States, the principal dietary sources of pyridoxine are fortified, ready-to-eat cereals; meat, fish, and poultry; white potatoes and other starchy vegetables; and noncitrus fruits. Especially rich sources are organ meats (e.g., beef liver) and highly fortified cereals or soy-based products.

Deficiency

Pyridoxine deficiency may result from poor diet, isoniazid therapy for tuberculosis, and inborn errors of metabolism. Symptoms include seborrheic dermatitis, anemia, peripheral neuritis, convulsions, depression, and confusion.

In the United States, dietary deficiency of vitamin B_6 is rare except among people who abuse alcohol on a long-term basis. Within this population, vitamin B_6 deficiency is estimated at 20% to 30% and occurs in combination with deficiency of other B vitamins.

Isoniazid (a drug for tuberculosis) prevents conversion of vitamin B_6 to its active form and may induce symptoms of deficiency (peripheral neuritis). Patients who are predisposed to this neuropathy (e.g., people with diabetes or alcoholism) should receive daily pyridoxine supplements.

Inborn errors of metabolism can prevent efficient utilization of vitamin B_6, resulting in greatly increased pyridoxine requirements. Among infants, symptoms include irritability, convulsions, and anemia. Unless treatment with vitamin B_6 is initiated early, permanent cognitive deficits may result.

Toxicity

At low doses, pyridoxine is devoid of adverse effects. However, if extremely large doses are taken, neurologic injury may result. Symptoms include ataxia and numbness of the feet and hands. To minimize risk, adults should not consume more than 100 mg/day, the UL for this vitamin.

Drug Interactions

Vitamin B_6 interferes with the utilization of levodopa, a drug for Parkinson disease. Accordingly, patients receiving levodopa should be advised against taking the vitamin.

Preparations

Pyridoxine is available in solution, standard tablets, extended-release tablets, and capsules for oral use. It is available in solution for IM or IV administration.

Vitamin B_{12} (Cyanocobalamin)

Vitamin B_{12} has several forms. Endogenous B_{12} presents primarily as cobalamin. Vitamin B_{12} supplements are available as cyanocobalamin and hydroxocobalamin. Cyanocobalamin is the primary preparation used in the United States.

Actions

Vitamin B_{12} is involved in carbohydrate and fat metabolism. It is also involved in protein synthesis and is a factor in the synthesis of DNA and in the formation of blood cells.

Therapeutic Uses

Vitamin B_{12} is indicated for treatment of deficiency due to all causes. It is also used to prevent deficiency in patients with increased vitamin B_{12} requirements (e.g., in pregnancy or with hemorrhage or liver disease).

Sources

The greatest sources of vitamin B_{12} are clams and liver. Other sources are meat, fish, poultry, eggs, milk, and other animal products. It is also a component of fortified foods such as processed cereals. It is not available from plants.

Deficiency

Vitamin B_{12} deficiency results in megaloblastic anemia, a macrocytic (large cell) anemia. A deficiency in vitamin B_{12} interferes with mitosis, thus leading to continued cell growth without division. Pernicious anemia is an example of megaloblastic anemia. This autoimmune disorder results in loss of gastric parietal cells that produce intrinsic factor, a substance that promotes absorption of vitamin B_{12}. Conditions other than pernicious anemia (e.g., bariatric surgery, strict vegan diets, and age-associated gastric atrophy) can also result in vitamin B_{12} deficiency sufficient to cause megaloblastic anemia.

Vitamin B_{12} deficiency also causes neurologic damage. This most commonly presents as mental status changes (impaired cognition, mood alterations, and psychosis) and peripheral sensory deficits with weakness, which may progress to ataxia and extrapyramidal symptoms.

Because vitamin B_{12} deficiency interferes with cellular replication, GI effects may occur. Glossitis is the most common presenting symptom.

Toxicity

Vitamin B_{12} has a low potential for toxicity. Two trials using high-dose supplementation—one lasting 40 months and another lasting 5 years—found no serious adverse effects.

Preparations

Most vitamin B_{12} supplements are available for oral administration. This meets most needs for supplementation but is usually inadequate for those with inadequate intrinsic factor due to autoimmune disease, surgery, or other contributing factors. Recent studies, however, suggest that very high doses may be effective for these patients.

Vitamin B_{12} is also available as both an IM injection and an intranasal spray or gel. These have the added advantage of bypassing the GI tract for absorption.

Vitamin B_9 (Folic Acid)

Vitamin B_9 occurs in two forms: folate and folic acid. Many use these terms interchangeably; however, there are differences. Folate is the naturally occurring form of the vitamin; folic acid is the synthetic form. Folic acid is more stable than folate. In the presence of food, the bioavailability of synthetic folic acid is at least 85%. In contrast, bioavailability of folate is less than 50%.

Actions

Folate functions as a coenzyme in the synthesis of nucleic acids (DNA and RNA). It also has a role in the metabolism of amino acids.

Therapeutic Uses

Folic acid supplements are used to prevent neural tube defects (NTDs) in the developing fetus. They are also used to treat megaloblastic anemia due to folate deficiency. Folic acid is used off-label to decrease toxicity due to antifolate chemotherapy.

Sources

Beef liver is the highest source of folate. Other good sources include spinach, black-eyed peas, asparagus, and green leafy vegetables.

To increase folic acid in the American diet, the US Food and Drug Administration (FDA) requires that all enriched grain products (e.g., enriched bread, pasta, flour, breakfast cereal, grits, and rice) must be fortified with folic acid. As a result of grain fortification, the incidence of folic acid deficiency in the United States has declined dramatically. Unfortunately, the incidence of birth defects from folate deficiency (discussed later) has dropped by only 32%.

Deficiency

Folic acid deficiency as a single vitamin deficiency is rare in the United States. When it occurs, it is usually in the form of one of several nutritional deficiencies. Folic acid deficiency, like that of cyanocobalamin, increases the risk for both neurologic damage and megaloblastic anemia.

Deficiency of folic acid during pregnancy can impair development of the central nervous system, resulting in *neural tube defects* and manifesting as *anencephaly* or *spina bifida*. Anencephaly (failure of the brain to develop) is uniformly fatal. Spina bifida, a condition characterized by defective development of the bony encasement of the spinal cord, can result in nerve damage, paralysis, and other complications. The time of vulnerability for NTDs is days 21 through 28 after conception. As a result, damage can occur before a woman recognizes that she is pregnant. Because NTDs occur very early in pregnancy, it is essential that adequate levels of folic acid be present *when pregnancy begins*; women cannot wait until pregnancy is confirmed before establishing AI. To ensure sufficient folate at the onset of pregnancy, the US Preventive Services Task Force (USPSTF) now recommends that *all women who are capable of becoming pregnant consume 400 to 800 μg of supplemental folic acid each day—in addition to the folate they get from food.*

Toxicity

As noted, deficiencies in either folic acid or vitamin B_{12} can result in megaloblastic anemia and neurologic damage. These often occur in concert (i.e., a deficiency in both occurs). In instances where both are responsible, high doses of folate can reverse the anemia, but they cannot reverse the neurologic damage that occurs secondary to vitamin B_{12} deficiency.

In the past, there was a belief that folic acid supplementation could decrease cancer risk. Current research has shown mixed findings, but most suggest that high doses of folic acid may accelerate progression of precancerous lesions. A couple of trials also found an increase in prostate cancer among older men who took high-dose folic acid supplements.

Preparations

Folic acid is available in tablets and capsules for oral administration. It is also available as a solution for SubQ, IM, or IV injection.

Vitamin B_5 (Pantothenic Acid)
Actions

Pantothenic acid is an essential component of two biologically important molecules: coenzyme A and acyl carrier protein. Coenzyme A is an essential factor in multiple biochemical processes, including gluconeogenesis, intermediary metabolism of carbohydrates, and biosynthesis of steroid hormones, porphyrins, and acetylcholine. Acyl carrier protein is required for synthesis of fatty acids.

Therapeutic Uses

Over-the-counter pantothenic acid is taken as a supplement; however, there is no therapeutic use for this supplement. Because deficiency does not occur, no supplement is needed.

Sources

Pantothenic acid is present in virtually all foods. As a result, spontaneous deficiency has not been reported.

Deficiency

The only known cause for pantothenic acid deficiency is pantothenate kinase–associated neurodegeneration 2 mutation, a rare genetic condition. Pantothenic acid kinase is a main enzyme in the metabolic pathway responsible for CoA synthesis.

Toxicity

There are no reports of toxicity from pantothenic acid. Accordingly, no UL has been set.

Preparations

Pantothenic acid is available in single-ingredient tablets and in multivitamin preparations.

Vitamin B$_7$ (Biotin)

Actions

Biotin is an essential cofactor for several reactions involved in the metabolism of carbohydrates and fats.

Therapeutic Uses

The primary reason people take over-the-counter biotin supplements is to treat hair loss and improve skin condition. Biotin is prescribed to treat biotinidase deficiency, a rare inherited disorder.

Sources

The vitamin is found in a wide variety of foods, although the exact amount in most foods has not been determined. In addition to being available in foods, biotin is synthesized by intestinal bacteria.

Deficiency

Biotin deficiency is extremely rare. In fact, to determine the effects of deficiency, scientists had to induce it experimentally. When this was done, subjects experienced dermatitis, conjunctivitis, hair loss, muscle pain, peripheral paresthesias, and psychologic effects (lethargy, hallucinations, and depression).

Toxicity

Biotin appears to be devoid of toxicity: subjects given large doses experienced no adverse effects. Accordingly, no UL has been set.

Although biotin does not cause adverse effects, if taken in excess, it may alter the results of some laboratory findings where testing methods use biotin technology. This can result in indirect adverse effects due to the mismanagement of medical conditions. At least one known death has occurred. In 2017, the FDA issued a safety alert regarding this concern. (See https://www.fda.gov/MedicalDevices/Safety/AlertsandNotices/ucm586505.htm.)

Preparations

Biotin is available in tablet and capsule form for oral dosing.

PATIENT EDUCATION

Vitamin Supplements

Most healthy people who eat a well-balanced diet do not need to take vitamin supplements.

If you decide to take vitamin supplements, do not exceed the RDA unless instructed otherwise by your provider. High doses of most vitamin supplements have been associated with adverse effects.

The National Institutes of Health, Office of Dietary Supplements, offers many fact sheets that include important information on vitamin supplements. Their website is at https://ods.od.nih.gov and their fact sheets for vitamins are located at https://ods.od.nih.gov/factsheets/list-VitaminsMinerals/.

68

Drugs for Weight Loss

In the United States, 70.7% of adults are overweight. Of these, 39.8% are obese. Excessive body fat may be associated with increased risk for morbidity from hypertension, coronary heart disease, ischemic stroke, type 2 diabetes mellitus (DM), gallbladder disease, liver disease, kidney stones, osteoarthritis, sleep apnea, dementia, and certain cancers. Among women, obesity may increase the risk for menstrual irregularities, amenorrhea, and polycystic ovary syndrome. During pregnancy, obesity may increase the risk for morbidity and mortality for both mother and child. In young men, obesity may reduce the quality and quantity of sperm. The National Institutes of Health (NIH) estimates that 300,000 Americans die each year from obesity-associated illnesses.

Pediatric obesity is a special concern. Despite recent declines in obesity prevalence, almost one-third of American children and adolescents are overweight or obese. This increases the risk for hypertension, heart disease, and asthma. In addition, type 2 DM, formerly seen almost exclusively in adults, has increased 10-fold among children and teens, and gallbladder disease has tripled.

Obesity is now viewed as a chronic disease, much like hypertension and DM. Despite intensive research, the underlying cause remains incompletely understood. Contributing factors include genetics, metabolism, and appetite regulation, along with environmental, psychosocial, and cultural factors. Although obese people can lose weight, the tendency to regain weight cannot be eliminated. Put another way, obesity cannot yet be cured. Accordingly, for most patients, lifelong management is indicated.

ASSESSMENT OF WEIGHT-RELATED HEALTH RISK

Health risk is determined by (1) the degree of obesity (as reflected in the body mass index), (2) the pattern of fat distribution (as reflected in the waist circumference measurement), and (3) the presence of obesity-related diseases or cardiovascular risk factors. Accordingly, all three factors must be assessed when a treatment plan is being established.

Body Mass Index

The body mass index (BMI), which is derived from the patient's weight and height, is a simple way to estimate body fat content. Studies indicate a close correlation between BMI and total body fat. These can be calculated manually (Fig. 68.1) or by using an application such as the online CDC resource at http://www.cdc.gov/healthyweight/assessing/bmi/adult_bmi/english_bmi_calculator/bmi_calculator.html. Tables that assign BMI according to height and weight are also available (Fig. 68.2).

According to the federal guidelines, a BMI of 30 or higher indicates obesity. Individuals with a BMI of 25 to 29.9 are considered overweight but not obese. There is evidence that the risk for cardiovascular disease and other disorders rises when the BMI exceeds 25. These associations between BMI and health risk do not apply to older adults, growing children, or women who are pregnant or lactating. Nor do they apply to competitive athletes or bodybuilders, who are heavy because of muscle mass rather than excess fat.

Waist Circumference

Waist circumference (WC) is an indicator of *abdominal* fat content, an independent risk factor for obesity-related diseases. Accumulation of fat in the upper body, and especially within the abdominal cavity, poses a greater risk to health than does accumulation of fat in the lower body (hips and thighs). People with too much abdominal fat are at increased risk for insulin resistance, DM, hypertension, coronary atherosclerosis, ischemic stroke, and dementia. Fat distribution can be estimated simply by looking in the mirror: an apple shape indicates too much abdominal fat, whereas a pear shape indicates fat on the hips and thighs. Measurement of WC provides a quantitative estimate of abdominal fat. A WC exceeding 40 in (102 cm) in men or 35 in (88 cm) in women signifies an increased health risk—but only for people with a BMI between 25 and 34.9.

Risk Status

Overall weight-related health risk is determined by BMI, WC, and the presence of weight-related diseases and cardiovascular risk factors. Certain weight-related diseases—established coronary heart disease, other atherosclerotic diseases, type 2 DM, and sleep apnea—confer a risk for complications and mortality. Other weight-related diseases—gynecologic abnormalities, osteoarthritis, gallstones, and stress incontinence—confer less risk. Cardiovascular risk factors—smoking, hypertension, high levels of low-density lipoprotein (LDL) cholesterol, low levels of high-density lipoprotein (HDL) cholesterol, high fasting glucose, family history of premature coronary heart disease, physical inactivity, and advancing age—confer a high risk when three or more of these factors are present.

Health risk rises as BMI gets larger. In addition, the risk is increased by the presence of an excessive WC. The risk is further increased by weight-related diseases and cardiovascular risk factors. In the absence of an excessive WC and other risk factors, health risk is minimal with a BMI below 25 and relatively low with a BMI below 30. Conversely, a BMI of 30 or more indicates significant risk. In the presence of an excessive WC, health risk is high for all individuals with a BMI above 25.

Several cardiovascular risk calculators are available; two of the most recently developed are provided below. The Multi-Ethnic Study of Atherosclerosis (MESA) Calculator is one of the few that incorporates race and ethnicity in the calculations.

- The American College of Cardiology/American Heart Association (ACC/AHA) pooled cohort hard CVD risk calculator is available at http://www.cvriskcalculator.com.
- The MESA 10-Year CHD Risk Calculator is available at https://www.mesa-nhlbi.org/MESACHDRisk/MesaRiskScore/RiskScore.aspx.

PATHOPHYSIOLOGY

Pathophysiology of Obesity

When we think of weight gain, we tend to focus on the common causes, such as increased food intake and sedentary lifestyles. We may also

$$BMI = \frac{weight\ in\ pounds \times 703}{(height\ in\ inches)^2}$$

OR

$$BMI = \frac{weight\ in\ kilograms}{(height\ in\ metres)^2}$$

BMI	Weight status
Less than 18.5	Underweight
18.5–24.9	Normal weight
25–29.9	Overweight
30–39.9	Obese
40 and greater	Morbidly obese

Fig. 68.1 Calculation of Body Mass Index.

BMI	19	20	21	22	23	24	25	26	27	28	29	30	31	32	33	34	35	36	37	38	39	40	41	42	43	44	45	46	47	48
Height													Weight in Pounds																	
4'10"	91	96	100	105	110	115	119	124	129	134	138	143	148	153	158	162	167	172	177	181	186	191	196	201	205	210	215	220	224	229
4'11"	94	99	104	109	114	119	124	128	133	138	143	148	153	158	163	168	173	178	183	188	193	198	203	208	212	217	222	227	232	237
5'	97	102	107	112	118	123	128	133	138	143	148	153	158	163	168	174	179	184	189	194	199	204	209	215	220	225	230	235	240	245
5'1"	100	106	111	116	122	127	132	137	143	148	153	158	164	169	174	180	185	190	195	201	206	211	217	222	227	232	238	243	248	254
5'2"	104	109	115	120	126	131	136	142	147	153	158	164	169	175	180	186	191	196	202	207	213	218	224	229	235	240	246	251	256	262
5'3"	107	113	118	124	130	135	141	146	152	158	163	169	175	180	186	191	197	203	208	214	220	225	231	237	242	248	254	259	265	270
5'4"	110	116	122	128	134	140	145	151	157	163	169	174	180	186	192	197	204	209	215	221	227	232	238	244	250	256	262	267	273	279
5'5"	114	120	126	132	138	144	150	156	162	168	174	180	186	192	198	204	210	216	222	228	234	240	246	252	258	264	270	276	282	288
5'6"	118	124	130	136	142	148	155	161	167	173	179	186	192	198	204	210	216	223	229	235	241	247	253	260	266	272	278	284	291	297
5'7"	121	127	134	140	146	153	159	166	172	178	185	191	198	204	211	217	223	230	236	242	249	255	261	268	274	280	287	293	299	306
5'8"	125	131	138	144	151	158	164	171	177	184	190	197	203	210	216	223	230	236	243	249	256	262	269	276	282	289	295	302	308	315
5'9"	128	135	142	149	155	162	169	176	182	189	196	203	209	216	223	230	236	243	250	257	263	270	277	284	291	297	304	311	318	324
5'10"	132	139	146	153	160	167	174	181	188	195	202	209	216	222	229	236	243	250	257	264	271	278	285	292	299	306	313	320	327	334
5'11"	136	143	150	157	165	172	179	186	193	200	208	215	222	229	236	243	250	257	265	272	279	286	293	301	308	315	322	329	338	343
6'	140	147	154	162	169	177	184	191	199	206	213	221	228	235	242	250	258	265	272	279	287	294	302	309	316	324	331	338	346	353
6'1"	144	151	159	166	174	182	189	197	204	212	219	227	235	242	250	257	265	272	280	288	295	302	310	318	325	333	340	348	355	363
6'2"	148	155	163	171	179	186	194	202	210	218	225	233	241	249	256	264	272	280	287	295	303	311	319	326	334	342	350	358	365	373
6'3"	152	160	168	176	184	192	200	208	216	224	232	240	248	256	264	272	279	287	295	303	311	319	327	335	343	351	359	367	375	383
6'4"	156	164	172	180	189	197	205	213	221	230	238	246	254	263	271	279	287	295	304	312	320	328	336	344	353	361	369	377	385	394

☐ = Healthy weight: BMI 18.5 to 24.9
▨ = Overweight: BMI 25 to 29.9
▥ = Obese: BMI 30 to 39.9
▩ = Severely obese: BMI 40 and higher

Fig. 68.2 Adult Weight Classification Based on Body Mass Index. (Adapted from National Heart, Lung, and Blood Institute Body Mass Index Table, 2012. Complete table available online at http://www.nhlbi.nih.gov/health/educational/lose_wt/BMI/bmi_tbl.pdf.)

consider economic concerns such as the low cost of ramen noodles compared with fresh vegetables, or we may look to social concerns such as the existence of regional food deserts or unsafe neighborhoods that create barriers for physical activity. Certainly these play a significant role in the rise of obesity, but to fully understand the obesity epidemic, it is also important to recognize pathophysiologic contributors.

Research has determined that weight is controlled by a complex neuroendocrine system in combination with other factors such as genetic contributors. Even the gut microbiome, which metabolizes carbohydrates (thus promoting sugar absorption), can play a role in an individual's tendency to gain weight. A full explanation of these mechanisms is beyond the scope of this text, but a few of the most critical components are examined here.

Several genes contributing to weight gain have been identified. The most significant of these is the fat- and obesity-associated gene, more commonly called the FTO gene for the enzyme that is encoded by the gene. FTO gene variants are thought to cause up to 15% to 20% of obesity cases. These variations can disrupt systems in several ways, but one crucial mechanism is fat cell alteration, resulting in increased fat storage relative to expenditure.

Alterations in neurologic coordination can also promote weight gain. The hypothalamus contains neurons that produce neuropeptides that orchestrate nutrient utilization and storage among pancreatic, hepatic, and muscle tissues. A decrease in these neurons or in their neuropeptide production can result in weight gain even when intake is reasonable. Additionally, these alterations can stimulate appetite and decrease appetite suppression. For example, when dysregulation leads to hyperinsulinemia, appetite is stimulated. Recent research has also identified that neurologic aberrancies can alter the conversion of white fat (fat that stores energy) to brown fat (fat that releases energy). Brown fat stores energy in a smaller space, thus this conversion allows for increased fat storage. Although we may one day be able to exploit the thermogenic ability of brown fat to promote weight loss, for now, its presence appears only as a mechanism by which even more fat is accumulated.

Dysregulation of hormones that stimulate and suppress appetite can also promote weight gain. Two of particular importance are ghrelin, an appetite stimulant, and leptin, an appetite suppressant. Ghrelin is predominantly produced in the stomach and is regulated by food intake and meal schedules. Ghrelin levels typically decrease after eating and create hunger as they rise again before mealtime or after a period of fasting. Leptin, produced by fat cells, has a role in the ongoing control of intake. Because leptin is an appetite suppressant, it would seem logical that overweight people would have less desire to eat because more fat cells create more leptin. Unfortunately many overweight people develop leptin resistance, a condition in which the brain does not respond appropriately to increases in circulating leptin. As a result of this alteration, these people do not experience satiety despite their high levels of leptin.

Pathophysiology of Obesity Maintenance

Why do most overweight and obese people find it so difficult to lose weight? And why do an estimated 80% to 90% (or more) of those who lose weight regain it? Research shows that, in addition to any emotional relationship to food (e.g., feelings of comfort or decreased stress), physiologic adaptive mechanisms work to maintain an overweight or obese state once it occurs.

The same factors that promote weight gain remain in effect following weight loss. Ghrelin and particularly leptin have predominant roles in obesity maintenance because dieting promotes dysregulation. As discussed earlier, elevated leptin levels promote earlier satiety in most people. As people lose weight, leptin levels *drop*; therefore satiety is lessened. Accordingly, people who lose weight find that they are not satisfied with recommended intake. In addition, ghrelin levels *rise* after dieting, thus stimulating hunger.

OVERVIEW OF OBESITY TREATMENT

As is clear from the previous discussion, the best way to manage obesity is to prevent it in the first place. This should begin in childhood before systems become "hard wired" to prevent weight loss.

The foundation of a weight-loss program is lifestyle therapy (Box 68.1). Drugs and surgical therapy are employed as needed based on clinical practice guidelines.

BOX 68.1 Components of Lifestyle Therapy

Food Intake
- Healthy intake at 500- to 750-kcal deficit daily.
- Individualize intake according to personal and cultural preferences.
- Preferred meal plans[a] include the DASH diet; Mediterranean diet; low-carbohydrate, low-fat, high-protein diet; vegetarian diet; and volumetric diet.
- Optional meal plans include meal replacements and very low calorie diets (under supervision).

Physical Activity
- Reduce sedentary activity.
- Individualize activity according to personal preferences and physical ability.
- At least 150 minutes of aerobic activity 3–5 days a week.
- Resistance exercises 2–3 times a week.

Behavior
- Self-monitor intake, weight, and activity.
- Set goals.
- Become educated using reliable resources.
- Obtain counseling and treatment if needed.
- Make use of social support.

[a]Information on preferred meal plans is provided in the 2015–2020 Dietary Guidelines available at https://health.gov/dietaryguidelines/2015/resources/2015-2020_Dietary_Guidelines.pdf.

Who Should Be Treated?

In 2016, the American Association of Clinical Endocrinologists (AACE) and the American College of Endocrinology (ACE) released updated clinical practice guidelines for the care of obese patients (see http://journals.aace.com/doi/pdf/10.4158/EP161365.GL). These more progressive guidelines recommend the following interventions (Fig. 68.3):
- Stage 0: A BMI of 25 or more with no complications
  - Lifestyle therapy (see Box 68.1)
  - Drug therapy to be considered if lifestyle therapy alone is ineffective
- Stage 1: A BMI of 25 or more in the presence of one or more mild to moderate complications amenable to moderate weight loss
  - Lifestyle therapy
  - Drug therapy to be considered if lifestyle therapy alone is ineffective or if BMI is 27 or more
- Stage 2: A BMI of 25 or more at least one complication requiring significant weight loss
  - Lifestyle therapy
  - Drug therapy to be considered for BMI of 25 to 26
  - Drug therapy to be initiated for BMI of 27 or more
  - Bariatric surgery to be considered for BMI of 35 or more

Treatment Goal

Although a goal to attain a normal BMI is desirable, it is rarely achieved in obese individuals, even with drug therapy. A more realistic goal is to target a percentage of body weight at which risk is decreased and comorbidities are prevented. A weight loss of 10% to 15% is typical for those who diligently adhere to medication and lifestyle therapy, whereas a loss greater than 15% is exceptional.

If weight loss plateaus and no additional loss seem imminent, the patients should be evaluated for improvement of weight-associated complications. If the complications have not been improved, weight-loss efforts should be intensified or interventions targeting the weight loss should be employed. If weight loss goals are achieved, it is important to set a goal to prevent lost weight from returning. Patients must recognize that this will be a lifelong effort.

Treatment Modalities

All weight-loss regimens have lifestyle therapy as their foundation (see Box 68.1). Weight loss can be accomplished with five treatment modalities: caloric restriction, physical activity, behavioral therapy, drug therapy, and surgery.

Caloric Restriction

A reduced-calorie diet is central to any weight-loss program. A balanced portion-controlled diet consisting primarily of vegetables, fruits, legumes, and grains is preferable; however, research supports a greater variety of diets than in the past. Success is likely increased by collaborating with the patient to select a safe diet that the patient is most likely to follow (see Box 68.1).

Exercise

Physical activity should be a component of all weight-loss and weight-maintenance programs. Exercise makes a modest contribution to weight loss by increasing energy expenditure. In addition, exercise can help reduce abdominal fat, increase cardiorespiratory fitness, and maintain weight once loss has occurred. According to the American College of Sports Medicine, people trying to *lose* weight should exercise at least 150 minutes per week (and preferably more), and those trying to *maintain* weight loss should exercise 200 to 300 minutes per week.

Algorithm: Guidance for Initiating Weight Loss Therapy

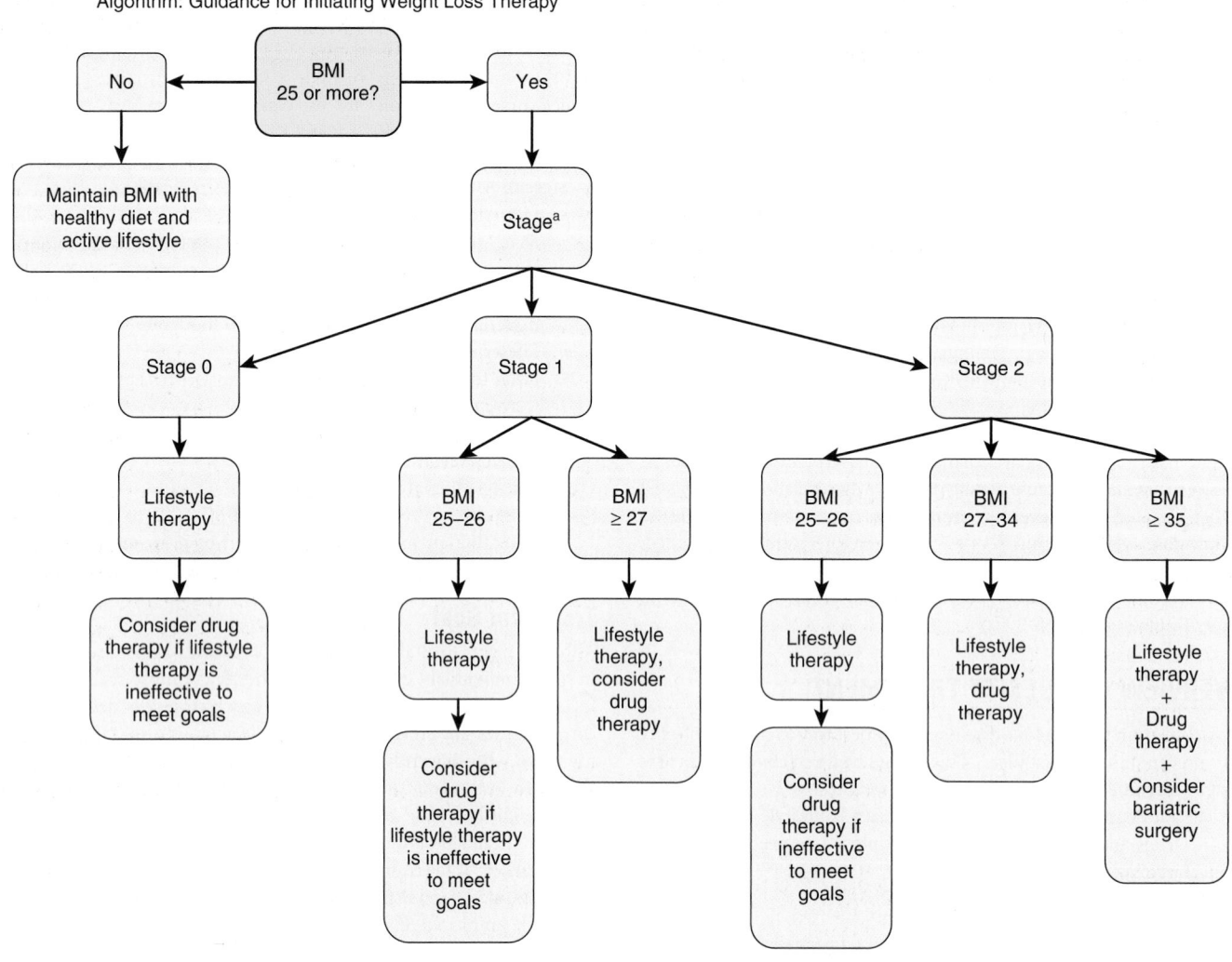

[a]Stage 0 = BMI ≥ 25 with no complications; Stage 1 = BMI ≥ 25 with one or more mild to moderate complications or may be treated effectively with moderate weight loss; Stage 2 = BMI ≥ 25 with at least one severe complication or requires significant weight loss for effective treatment.

Fig. 68.3 Algorithm for weight loss. (Algorithm based on guidance from the American Association of Clinical Endocrinologists [AACE] and American College of Endocrinology [ACE]. Comprehensive Clinical Practice Guidelines for Medical Care of Patients with Obesity available at http://journals.aace.com/doi/pdf/10.4158/EP161365.GL?code=aace-site.)

Behavior Modification

Behavioral therapy is directed at modifying eating and exercise habits; hence it can strengthen a program of diet and exercise. Self-monitoring of eating and exercise habits is essential for most obese patients. Fortunately numerous tools are available to support the patient in this endeavor. Free online resources such as Choose My Plate (www.choosemyplate.gov) are particularly helpful. Social media and face-to-face meetings offer social support, which has been shown to improve adherence.

Drug Therapy

Research demonstrates that the addition of weight loss drugs to obesity management promotes greater success than lifestyle management alone. New drugs for obesity management have provided more options for people who are trying to lose weight. The benefits of drug therapy are usually modest. Weight loss attributable to drugs generally ranges between 4.4 and 22 lb, although some people lose significantly more. As a rule, most weight loss occurs during the first 6 months of treatment.

Duration of therapy varies depending on the drug selected. Today, long-term treatment is recommended more often than in the past because we now know that, when drugs are discontinued, most patients regain lost weight. Accordingly, when treatment has been effective and well tolerated, it may have to continue indefinitely. Unfortunately not all drugs are approved for long-term use.

Not everyone responds to drugs, so regular assessment is required. Patients should lose at least 4 lb during the first 4 weeks of drug treatment. If this initial response is absent, patient adherence to the plan should be evaluated and the appropriateness of drug selection considered. For patients who *do* respond, ongoing assessment must show that (1) the drug is effective at *maintaining* weight loss and (2) serious adverse effects are absent. Otherwise drug therapy should cease.

Bariatric Surgery

Surgical procedures can produce significant weight loss by reducing food intake. The two most widely used procedures are *gastric bypass surgery* (Roux-en-Y procedure) and laparoscopic implantation of an adjustable gastric band, which reduces the effective volume of the upper part of the stomach. Surgery is effective. In 6 months to a year, patients can lose between 110 and 220 pounds. Unfortunately surgery can also carry significant risk: in one study, mortality rates at 30 days, 90 days, and 1 year after gastric surgery were 2%, 2.8%, and 4.6%, respectively.

WEIGHT-LOSS DRUGS

As previously mentioned, weight-loss drugs vary in their ability to promote weight loss. The combination drug topiramate/phentermine is associated with the greatest amount of weight loss (approximately 10% of body weight). Orlistat provides the least weight loss (2% to 3% of body weight). The individual classes of weight loss drugs are discussed next. Pharmacokinetics is presented in Table 68.1. Drug preparations and dosages are summarized in Table 68.2.

Lipase Inhibitor: Orlistat
Actions and Use
Orlistat (Alli, Xenical) is a novel drug approved for promoting and maintaining weight loss in obese patients aged 12 years and older. Unlike most other weight-loss drugs, which act in the brain to curb appetite, orlistat acts in the gastrointestinal (GI) tract to reduce the absorption of fat. Specifically, the drug acts in the stomach and small intestine to cause irreversible inhibition of gastric and pancreatic lipases, enzymes that break down triglycerides into monoglycerides, and free fatty acids. If triglycerides are not broken down, they cannot be absorbed. In patients taking orlistat, absorption of dietary fat is reduced by about 30%. Patients must adopt a reduced-calorie diet in which 30% of calories come from fat.

In clinical trials, orlistat produced modest benefits. Patients treated for 2 years lost an average of 19 lb, compared with 12 lb for those taking placebo. In addition, treatment reduced total and low-density lipoprotein (LDL) cholesterol, raised high-density lipoprotein (HDL) cholesterol, reduced fasting blood glucose, and lowered systolic and diastolic blood pressure.

Adverse Effects
Gastrointestinal effects. Orlistat undergoes less than 1% absorption; hence systemic effects are absent. In contrast, GI effects are common. Approximately 20% to 30% of patients experience oily rectal leakage, flatulence with discharge, fecal urgency, and fatty or oily stools. Another 10% experience increased defecation and fecal incontinence. All of these are the result of reduced fat absorption, and all can be minimized by reducing fat intake. Dosing with psyllium (Metamucil and others), a bulk-forming laxative, can greatly reduce GI effects. The underlying mechanism is adsorption of dietary fat by psyllium.

Possible liver damage. Orlistat has been associated with rare cases of *severe liver damage.* Signs and symptoms include itching, vomiting, jaundice, anorexia, fatigue, dark urine, and light-colored stools. *Patients who experience these signs and symptoms should report them immediately.* Orlistat should be discontinued until liver injury has been ruled out.

Other adverse effects. Rarely, orlistat has been associated with *acute pancreatitis* and *kidney stones,* although a causal relationship has not been established. Cholelithiasis may occur if weight loss is substantial.

Contraindications. Orlistat is contraindicated for patients with malabsorption syndrome or cholestasis.

Drug and Nutrient Interactions
Reduced absorption of vitamins. By reducing fat absorption, orlistat can reduce absorption of fat-soluble vitamins (vitamins A, D, E, and K). Vitamin K deficiency can intensify the effects of *warfarin,* an

TABLE 68.1	**Weight Loss Drugs: Pharmacokinetics**					
Drug Class and Drug	**Peak**	**Protein Binding**	**Metabolism**	**Half-Life**	**Elimination**
Glucagon-Like Peptide-1 Agonist					
Liraglutide (Saxenda)	8–12 h	98%	Metabolism by DPP-IV and endopeptidases	13 h	Urine Feces
Lipase Inhibitor					
Orlistat (Alli and Xenical)	8 h	99%	Metabolized to inactive metabolites within the GI tract	1–2 h	Feces
Serotonin Receptor Agonist					
Lorcaserin (Belviq and Belviq XR)	IR: 1.5–2 h ER: 10 h	70%	Hepatic via multiple pathways	IR: 11 h ER: 12 h	Urine (92%) Feces
Sympathomimetic Amines					
Diethylpropion (generic)	2 h	UK	N-dealkylation and reduction	4–6 h	Urine
Phentermine (Adipex-P and Lomaira)	3–4.4 h	17%–18%	Hepatic primarily by CYP3A4	20 h	Urine
Combination Products					
Phentermine and topiramate (Qsymia)[a]	UK	15%–41%	Hepatic via hydroxylation, hydrolysis, and glucuronidation	65 h	Urine
Naltrexone/bupropion[b] (Contrave)	1 h 2 h	21% 84%	Hepatic (not by CYP450 enzymes) Hepatic primarily by CYP2B6 with minor roles for CYP1A2, CYP2A6, CYP2C9, CYP2D6, CYP2E1, and CYP3A4	4 h Wide range; avg 21 h	Urine Urine (87%) Feces

[a]Topiramate component provided (phentermine pharmacokinetics in prior row).
[b]Naltrexone component provided in the top half of this row; buproprion component in lower half.
avg, Average; *DPP-IV,* dipeptidyl peptidase IV; *ER,* extended release; *h,* hour(s); *IR,* immediate release; *UK,* unknown.

TABLE 68.2   Weight-Loss Drugs: Preparations and Dosages

Drug Class and Drug	Preparation	Dosage
Lipase Inhibitor		
Orlistat (Alli, Xenical)	Alli: 60-mg tablet (over the counter) Xenical: 120-mg tablet	Alli: 60 mg tid with meals Xenical: 120 mg tid with meals
Serotonin 5-HT2C Receptor Agonist		
Lorcaserin (Belviq, Belviq XR)	10-mg tablet	10 mg bid
Sympathomimetic Amines		
Diethylpropion (generic)	25-mg immediate-release tablet 75-mg extended-release tablet	Immediate release: 25 mg tid Extended release: 75 mg qd
Phentermine (Adipex-P and Lomaira)	Adipex-P: 37.5-mg tablet; 37.5-mg capsule Lomaira: 8 mg	Adipex-P: Usual dosage is 37.5 mg qd. Alternate dosing schedules are ½ tablet (18.75 mg) qd or ½ tablet bid. Lowest effective dose is recommended. Lomaira: Usual starting dose is 1 table tid. Individualize to the lowest effective dose.
Glucagon-Like Peptide-1 Agonist		
Liraglutide (Saxenda)	Prefilled multidose pens hold 3 mL of a 6 mg/mL solution. Pen contains a dose selector that allows delivery of specific doses at 0.6-, 1.2-, 1.8-, 2.4-, and 3-mg doses	Week 1: 0.6 mg qd Week 2: 1.2 mg qd Week 3: 1.8 mg qd Week 4: 2.4 mg qd Week 5 and thereafter: 3 mg qd
Combination Products		
Phentermine/topiramate (Qsymia)	24-hour extended-release tablet in four strengths 3.75/23 (Phentermine 3.75 mg/topiramate 23 mg) 7.5/46 (Phentermine 7.5 mg/topiramate 46 mg) 11.25/69 (Phentermine 11.25 mg/topiramate 69 mg) 15/92 (Phentermine 15 mg/topiramate 92 mg)	Weeks 1 and 2: One 3.75/23 tablet qd, followed by one 7.5/46 tablet qd for 12 weeks Evaluate weight loss. If 3% of baseline body weight has not occurred, discontinue or increase to one 11.25/69 tablet once qd for 2 weeks followed by one 15/92 tablet for 12 weeks. Evaluate weight loss. If 5% of baseline weight has not been lost, taper off therapy.
Naltrexone/bupropion (Contrave)	12-h extended-release tablet containing naltrexone 8 mg/bupropion 90 mg	Week 1: one tablet in the morning Week 2: one tablet in the morning; one tablet in the evening Week 3: two tablets in the morning; one tablet in the evening Week 4 and thereafter: two tablets in the morning; two tablets in the evening

anticoagulant. In patients taking warfarin, anticoagulant effects should be monitored closely. To avoid deficiency, patients should take a daily multivitamin supplement. Administration should be done 2 hours before or 2 hours after taking orlistat.

Drug Interactions

Orlistat may cause hypothyroidism in patients taking levothyroxine by decreasing the absorption of thyroid hormone. To minimize this effect, levothyroxine and orlistat should be administered at least 4 hours apart. Orlistat can also reduce absorption of cyclosporine. At least 3 hours is recommended between doses of these two drugs.

Serotonin Receptor Agonist: Lorcaserin
Actions and Use

Lorcaserin (Belviq, Belviq XR) is a selective type 2C serotonin (5-hydroxytryptamine [5-HT2C]) agonist with indications for chronic weight loss. It suppresses appetite and creates a sense of satiety by activating hypothalamic and mesolimbic pathways that control appetite. Studies have demonstrated an average loss of 5.8% of baseline weight

after 1 year, compared with 2.2% in patients taking placebo. In addition, lorcaserin reduces waist circumference, fasting glucose, insulin, total cholesterol, LDL cholesterol, and triglycerides.

Adverse Effects

Ten percent or more of patients will experience headaches, back pain, a decrease in lymphocytes, and upper respiratory infections. About 30% of patients with DM will experience an increase in hypoglycemic episodes.

Less common but serious adverse effects include blood dyscrasias, cognitive impairment, psychiatric disorders, priapism (prolonged penile erection), pulmonary hypertension, and valvular heart disease. Accordingly, this drug should not be given to patients at risk for these conditions.

Lorcaserin has potential for abuse. It is classified as a Schedule IV drug under the Controlled Substances Act (CSA).

Contraindications

Most of the contraindications for lorcaserin are associated with different aspects of the life span.

PATIENT-CENTERED CARE ACROSS THE LIFE SPAN

Weight Loss

Life Stage	Considerations or Concerns
Children	Liraglutide, lorcaserin, and the combination drugs phentermine/topiramate and naltrexone/bupropion are not approved for children. Orlistat is not approved for children younger than 12 years. Diethylpropion and phentermine are not recommended for children younger than 16 years.
Pregnant women	Weight loss is not advisable for pregnant women. All drugs mentioned in this chapter are contraindicated during pregnancy with the exception of diethylpropion. Diethylpropion is not a teratogen; however, neonates born to women who take this drug may experience withdrawal symptoms.
Breastfeeding women	For all drugs listed, breastfeeding is not recommended.
Older adults	For patients with moderate renal impairment, naltrexone/bupropion should be limited to one tablet daily. If the creatinine clearance is less than 50, phentermine/topiramate should be limited to one 7.5/46 capsule daily. If the creatinine clearance is less than 30, lorcaserin should not be given. For patients with hepatic impairment, both naltrexone/bupropion and phentermine/topiramate should be limited to one tablet daily. Phentermine/topiramate should not be prescribed for patients with severe hepatic impairment. The manufacturer of liraglutide recommends caution when prescribing for patients with renal or hepatic impairment. Dosage adjustments are not indicated for orlistat, diethylpropion, and phentermine.

Drug Interactions

Lorcaserin is an inhibitor of the CYP2D6 isoenzyme of cytochrome P450. When given with CYP2D6 substrates (i.e., drugs metabolized by CYP2D6 isoenzymes), the serum levels of the substrates can be increased. To decrease the risk for toxicity when both drugs are prescribed, the substrate may have to be prescribed at a lower dose.

Risk for serotonin syndrome is associated with serotonergic drugs. When serotonergic drugs such as lorcaserin are given with other serotonergic drugs, this risk increases. There are not enough studies yet to evaluate the effects of prescribing lorcaserin with specific serotonergic drugs; therefore caution and close monitoring are advised when administering this drug along with bupropion, dextromethorphan, monoamine oxidase (MAO) inhibitors, serotonin-norepinephrine reuptake inhibitors, selective serotonin reuptake inhibitors, St. John's wort, and triptans.

Sympathomimetic Amines: Diethylpropion and Phentermine

The sympathomimetics fall into two groups: amphetamines and nonamphetamines. The amphetamines are not FDA-approved for weight loss because they have a high abuse potential, so they are not addressed here.

Four noradrenergic drugs are approved for weight loss. However, only two—diethylpropion (generic) and phentermine (Adipex-P, Lomaira)—should be used. The other two—benzphetamine and phendimetrazine—have a higher potential for abuse.

Actions and Use

Diethylpropion and phentermine promote weight loss by decreasing appetite. They are central nervous system (CNS) stimulants that suppress appetite by increasing the availability of norepinephrine at receptors in the brain. This same mechanism underlies their stimulant effects and potential for abuse. Weight loss is usually modest: about 5 to 8 lb. These drugs should be used only in the short term (for 3 months or less).

Adverse Effects

Like the amphetamines, diethylpropion and phentermine can increase alertness, decrease fatigue, and induce nervousness and insomnia. Because they can interfere with sleep, these drugs should be administered no later than 4:00 PM. After drug withdrawal, fatigue and depression may replace CNS stimulation.

Diethylpropion and phentermine have effects in the periphery as well as in the CNS. Peripheral effects of greatest concern are tachycardia, anginal pain, and hypertension. Accordingly, these drugs should be used with caution in patients with cardiovascular disease.

Although the risk for abuse is lower than with the amphetamines, abuse can still occur. Both diethylpropion and phentermine are regulated under Schedule IV of the CSA (benzphetamine and phendimetrazine are regulated under Schedule III). Tolerance is common and may be seen in 6 to 12 weeks. If tolerance develops, the appropriate response is to discontinue the drug rather than to increase the dosage.

Contraindications

Significant life-span contraindications are associated with these drugs. (See box titled Patient-Centered Care Across the Life Span.)

Glucagon-Like Peptide-1 Agonist: Liraglutide
Actions and Use

Liraglutide (Saxenda) is a glucagon-like peptide-1 (GLP-1) agonist that is approved for chronic weight management in adults. It acts by slowing gastric emptying, which increases a feeling of fullness, which leads to decreased food intake. GLP-1 agonists are also used in management of type 2 DM (see Chapter 48) to enhance glycemic control. In this regard, it also increases insulin secretion and decreases glucagon secretion.

Adverse Effects

More than one-third of patients taking liraglutide experience an increase in heart rate of 10 to 20 beats/min from baseline. Approximately 1 in 20 will develop tachycardia. Other common adverse effects include nausea, vomiting, and either constipation or diarrhea. Hypoglycemia is a concern if liraglutide is taken by patients with DM who are taking antidiabetic drugs; however, this is a rare occurrence in patients who do not have DM. Headache may occur, as may generalized fatigue and weakness, although the latter symptoms are less common. Because of the effects on gastric emptying, dyspepsia and abdominal discomfort may occur. Liraglutide is administered subcutaneously; as with any injection, local site reactions such as redness or pruritus may occur.

Several uncommon effects warranting special precautions occur in less than 1% of patients taking liraglutide. These include acute pancreatitis, renal impairment (likely associated with dehydration secondary to nausea, vomiting, and diarrhea) and acute gallbladder disease (typically associated with significant or rapid weight loss regardless of medication).

Contraindications

Liraglutide is known to cause thyroid cancer in rodents, so cautious use is warranted until the effects on humans are known. Liraglutide is contraindicated in patients who have multiple endocrine neoplasia syndrome type 2 (MEN 2) or who have a personal or family history of medullary thyroid carcinoma (MTC).

▶▶ BLACK BOX WARNING

Liraglutide (Saxenda)

Liraglutide is associated with a risk for thyroid C-cell tumors based on studies in rodents. It is contraindicated in patients who have multiple neoplasia syndrome type 2 (MEN 2) or a personal or family history of medullary thyroid carcinoma (MTC).

Life span–associated contraindications are provided the box titled Patient-Centered Care Across the Life Span.

Drug Interactions

Liraglutide may potentiate the hypoglycemic effect of drugs given for glycemic control in DM. Additionally, it will enhance the glucose-lowering side effects of other drugs with this feature, including androgens, fluoroquinolone antibiotics, MAO inhibitors, and selective serotonin reuptake inhibitors (SSRIs).

Combination Products

Currently two combination products are approved for weight loss. Each combination is unique, with different mechanisms of action and different side effect profiles.

Phentermine/Topiramate

Actions and use. The combination product phentermine/topiramate (Qsymia) is a Schedule IV drug indicated for chronic weight-loss therapy. Phentermine, as mentioned previously, is a sympathomimetic amine already approved for the short-term management of obesity. Topiramate is currently approved for seizure disorders (see Chapter 21) and the prophylaxis of migraine (see Chapter 25). Phentermine suppresses appetite and topiramate induces a sense of satiety. Possible mechanisms for topiramate include antagonism of glutamate (an excitatory neurotransmitter), modulation of receptors for γ-aminobutyric acid, and inhibition of carbonic anhydrase. In a 56-week trial, phentermine/topiramate produced a 10% reduction in weight and a significant decrease in systolic blood pressure.

Adverse effects. The most common adverse effects are dry mouth, constipation, altered taste, nausea, blurred vision, dizziness, insomnia, and numbness and tingling in the limbs. The most serious effects are memory impairment, difficulty concentrating, hypertension and tachycardia, birth defects, acute myopia with angle-closure glaucoma, and acidosis. In addition, patients who take insulin or insulin secretagogues face an increased risk for hypoglycemia beyond that of antidiabetic drugs alone.

Contraindications. Phentermine/topiramate is contraindicated for patients with glaucoma or hyperthyroidism. There are also life span–associated contraindications with this drug. (See box titled Patient-Centered Care Across the Life Span.)

Drug interactions. Phentermine/topiramate should not be given with MAO inhibitors. In fact, at least 2 weeks should pass after taking an MAO inhibitor before phentermine/topiramate is begun. Similarly, at least 2 weeks should pass after ending phentermine/topiramate before an MAO inhibitor is begun. Phentermine/topiramate can potentiate CNS depressants. When given with the antiepileptic drugs carbamazepine or phenytoin, levels of topiramate (which is also an antiepileptic drug) may be increased. Administration with carbonic anhydrase inhibitors increases the risk for metabolic acidosis, whereas administration with diuretics that are not potassium-sparing increases the risk for hypokalemia. Finally, studies show that concomitant administration with oral contraceptives increases the estrogen level while decreasing the progestin level.

Naltrexone/Bupropion

Actions and use. The anorexiant naltrexone/bupropion (Contrave) combines the effects of a dopamine and norepinephrine-reuptake inhibitor with an opioid antagonist. The mechanism of action by which this drug combination promotes weight loss is unknown, but it has been hypothesized that it acts on the regulation of appetite in the hypothalamus and on the mesolimbic dopamine system, which is the key reward pathway in the brain. The individual drugs are discussed separately. (See Chapter 24 for naltrexone and Chapter 27 for bupropion.)

Adverse effects. The most common adverse reactions (experienced by more than 10% of those taking naltrexone with bupropion) are nausea, vomiting, constipation, headache, dizziness, and insomnia. Approximately 5% of patients experience an increase in blood pressure, dry mouth, diarrhea, abdominal discomfort, anxiety, and fatigue. There is also a suicide risk associated with this drug.

▶▶ BLACK BOX WARNING

Naltrexone and Bupropion (Contrave)

The naltrexone/bupropion combination is associated with an increased risk for suicidal ideation and suicide attempts in children, adolescents, and young adults.

Contraindications. This product is contraindicated for patients taking other products containing bupropion. Because naltrexone is an opioid antagonist, it will decrease the ability of opioid analgesics to relieve pain. It should not be taken within 2 weeks of MAO inhibitors.

▶▶ BLACK BOX WARNING

Naltrexone and Bupropion (Contrave)

When the naltrexone/bupropion combination is given to patients who are taking or discontinuing bupropion (Aplenzin, Budeprion, Bupropion, Wellbutrin, and Zyban), severe neuropsychiatric reactions, including depression, mania, psychosis, and homicidal ideation, have occurred.

Naltrexone-bupropion is also contraindicated for people with selected conditions. It should not be used for weight loss in patients with uncontrolled hypertension, seizure disorders, or eating disorders such as anorexia or bulimia. Patients who are undergoing alcohol, barbiturate, or benzodiazepine withdrawal should not take this drug. Life span–associated contraindications are listed in the box titled Patient-Centered Care Across the Life Span.

Drug interactions. Drug interactions are numerous and reflect interactions of the individual agents (see Chapter 24 for naltrexone and Chapter 27 for bupropion). Dangerous interactions occur with MAO inhibitors and opioid antagonists.

The bupropion component of naltrexone/bupropion is a minor substrate of numerous hepatic enzyme families and a major substrate of CYP2B6 enzymes. Inhibitors of these enzymes can increase naltrexone/bupropion levels, requiring a lowered dosage. When CYP2B6 inducers are given with this drug, it may result in subtherapeutic doses. Naltrexone/bupropion is also a strong inhibitor of CYP2D6 enzymes. Accordingly, when given with CYP2D6 substrates, naltrexone/bupropion can increase their drug levels.

TABLE 68.3 Prescribing Considerations: Drugs for Weight Loss

Drug	Drug Action	Special Monitoring Needs[a]	High-Risk Patient Conditions	Most Common Adverse Effects	Approximate Cost for 1 Month Supply[b]	Typical Weight Loss at 12 Months	Controlled Drug?
Liraglutide (Saxenda[c])	Promotes satiety Slows gastric emptying promoting a sense of fullness	• Baseline HbA1c, lipids, renal function • Baseline assessment of ability of patient or family to administer injections • HbA1c, every 6 months if stable; more often as needed • Periodic monitoring of triglycerides, if indicated • Assess for s/s of cholecystitis, pancreatitis, depression, and suicidal thoughts	• Pregnancy • Personal or family history of medullary thyroid cancer or multiple endocrine neoplasia 2A or 2B • Patients with or having a history of pancreatitis, renal impairment, or cholecystitis	• Nausea/vomiting • Diarrhea • Elevated heart rate • Hypoglycemia (in patients with DM)	$1100	12 pounds	No
Orlistat (Alli and Xenical)	Decreases fat absorption Inhibits gastric and pancreatic lipases resulting in decreased absorption of dietary fats	• Assess for s/s of deficiency in fat soluble vitamins (Vitamins A, D, E, and K)	• Pregnancy • Malabsorption • Cholestasis • Cholelithiasis • Hepatitis or other liver disorder	• Abdominal cramps • Flatus • Oily rectal leakage • Fecal incontinence	$45	7 pounds or approximately 2%–3% of baseline	No
Lorcaserin (Belviq, Belviq XR)	Promotes satiety Activation of serotonin 5-HT2C receptors stimulates neurons in the hypothalamic and mesolimbic pathways that control appetite	• Baseline assessment to rule out valvular disorders and pulmonary hypertension • Ongoing monitoring for cognitive changes • CBC with differential for s/s of blood dyscrasias	• Pregnancy • Renal failure • Patients taking serotonergic drugs • Patients with (or at risk for) valvular disorders, pulmonary hypertension, blood dyscrasias, or history of priapism	• Headache • Decrease in lymphocytes • Upper respiratory infections • Back pain • Hypoglycemia (patients with DM)	$200	8 pounds or approximately 5.8% of baseline	Yes; Schedule IV
Diethylpropion (generic)	Decreases appetite in response to CNS stimulation with release of norepinephrine in brain	• Baseline cardiac assessment • Baseline renal function in older patients • Ongoing assessment of cardiac status	• Hypertension, angina, or other cardiovascular disease • Hyperthyroidism • Glaucoma • History of drug abuse • Within 14 days of taking MAO inhibitors	• Elevated heart rate • Elevated blood pressure • CNS stimulation (e.g., nervousness and insomnia) • Dry mouth • Constipation	$30	UK	Yes; Schedule IV
Phentermine (Adipex-P, Lomaira)	Decreases appetite in response to CNS stimulation with release of norepinephrine in brain	• Baseline cardiac assessment • Ongoing assessment of cardiac status	• Hypertension, angina, or other cardiovascular disease • Hyperthyroidism • Glaucoma • History of drug abuse • Within 14 days of taking MAO inhibitors	• Elevated heart rate • Elevated blood pressure • CNS stimulation (e.g., nervousness, insomnia) • Dry mouth • Constipation	$30	8 pounds	Yes; Schedule IV

Continued

TABLE 68.3 Prescribing Considerations: Drugs for Weight Loss—cont'd

Drug	Drug Action	Special Monitoring Needs[a]	High-Risk Patient Conditions	Most Common Adverse Effects	Approximate Cost for 1 Month Supply[b]	Typical Weight Loss at 12 Months	Controlled Drug?
Phentermine/topiramate (Qsymia)	Suppresses appetite and promotes satiety. Phentermine produces effects through CNS stimulation Topiramate enhances GABA activity, antagonizes glutamate receptors, and weakly inhibits carbonic anhydrase	• Baseline chemistry panel • Periodic monitoring for electrolyte, serum creatine, s/s acidosis, s/s depression	• Pregnancy • Hypertension, angina, or other cardiovascular disease • Hyperthyroidism • Glaucoma • History of drug abuse • Within 14 days of taking MAO inhibitors	• Elevated heart rate • Elevated blood pressure • CNS stimulation (e.g., nervousness, insomnia) • Blurred vision • Dry mouth • Altered taste • Constipation Anxiety/depression • Paresthesias • Hypoglycemia (patients with DM)	$200	19 pounds or approximately 10% of baseline	Yes; Schedule IV
Bupropion/naltrexone (Contrave)	Unknown; hypothesized to decrease appetite by inhibiting reward system in mesolimbic dopamine circuit and by regulating appetite in the hypothalamus	• Baseline blood glucose, liver function, renal function, and mental status • Periodic assessment for blood glucose, liver and renal function, s/s depression, anxiety or panic attacks, suicidal ideation, and mania	• Pregnancy • Uncontrolled hypertension • Chronic opioid use • Within 14 days of taking a MAO inhibitor	• Nausea/vomiting • Headache • Insomnia • Dizziness • Dry mouth • Constipation • Abdominal discomfort • Fatigue	$200	9 pounds	No

[a]Drug-specific monitoring in addition to that provided in Summary of Key Prescribing Considerations; that is, general health history (including typical intake, eating triggers, past attempts at dieting, activity level, and other associated factors), general physical assessment with cardiovascular emphasis, and pertinent labs based on findings (including thyroid panel), BMI, waist circumference, and cardiovascular risk assessment.

[b]2018 pricing

[c]Liraglutide is available under the brand name Victoza for the management of diabetes mellitus.

5-HT2C, 5-hydroxytryptamine; CBC, compete blood count; CNS, central nervous system; DM, diabetes mellitus; GABA, γ-aminobutyric acid; MAO, monoamine oxidase; s/s, signs or symptoms; UK, unknown.

SUMMARY OF KEY PRESCRIBING CONSIDERATIONS

Drugs for Weight Loss

Therapeutic Goal: To support weight loss as part of a program that includes lifestyle therapy and behavioral interventions

Baseline Data: General health history (including typical intake, eating triggers, past attempts at dieting, activity level, and other associated factors), general physical assessment with cardiovascular emphasis, and pertinent labs based on findings (including thyroid panel), BMI, waist circumference, and cardiovascular risk assessment.

Monitoring: BMI should be evaluated and considered in terms of trend at each clinic visit and adherence to lifestyle therapy should be assessed.

Identifying High-Risk Patients: Patients who are not committed to the process of losing weight and who are not willing to commit to maintaining weight loss are not good candidates for drug therapy because research shows that "yo-yo" dieting (where weight is frequently lost then regained) typically results in physiologic adaptations that support increased weight gain over time.

Prescribing considerations for individual drugs are summarized in the comparison table titled Prescribing Considerations: Drugs for Weight Loss (Table 68.3).

A NOTE REGARDING DRUGS FOR WEIGHT LOSS

Weight-loss drugs share a disturbing history: they receive regulatory approval, undergo widespread use, and then are withdrawn owing to the discovery of serious adverse effects. It is quite likely that new drugs may have been approved by the time this chapter is read. It is also possible that drugs discussed in this chapter, especially those most recently approved, will have been taken off the market by then.

69

Complementary and Alternative Therapy

The National Center for Complementary and Integrative Health (NCCIH) defines a *complementary* health approach as "a nonmainstream practice used together with conventional medicine" and an *alternative* health approach as "a nonmainstream practice that is used in place of conventional medicine." Examples include both products (e.g., herbs, probiotics, and vitamins) and practices (e.g., meditation, acupuncture, and therapeutic touch). According to the National Health Statistics Reports published in 2015, some 32.3% of adults in the United States have used some form of complementary and alternative medicine (CAM).

Dietary supplements are the most common form of CAM. Such a supplement is defined by the US Food and Drug Administration (FDA) as "a product intended for ingestion that contains a 'dietary ingredient' intended to add further nutritional value to (supplement) the diet. A 'dietary ingredient' may be one, or any combination, of the following substances: a vitamin, a mineral, an herb or other botanical, an amino acid, a dietary substance for use by people to supplement the diet by increasing the total dietary intake, a concentrate, metabolite, constituent, or extract."

The popularity of supplements may be explained by several factors (Box 69.1). Some people like the sense of empowerment that comes from self-diagnosis and self-prescribing. Others may turn to supplements out of anger or frustration with their health care providers. Still others may distrust conventional medicine or may feel that it has failed them. In addition, supplements may be a way of saving money: because these products are available without prescription, they can be purchased without the cost of visiting a prescriber. In fact, according to the National Health Interview Survey (NHIS), there is a clear relationship between concern about the costs of conventional care and the likelihood of turning to CAM. However, perhaps the strongest force driving the demand for nutritional supplements is aggressive marketing.

Our understanding of CAM is far from adequate. To advance our knowledge, the National Institutes of Health (NIH) created the National Center for Complementary and Alternative Medicine (NCCAM) in the late 1990s. This organization (renamed the National Center for Complementary and Integrative Health [NCCIH] in 2014) is charged with promoting and funding basic research and clinical trials designed to address open questions on the safety and efficacy of CAM. The NCCIH website, which provides a wealth of information on CAM, is available at https://nccih.nih.gov.

REGULATION OF DIETARY SUPPLEMENTS

Dietary Supplement Health and Education Act of 1994

Core Provisions

In 1994, after intensive lobbying efforts from the multibillion-dollar dietary supplement industry aimed at minimizing FDA oversight, Congress passed the Dietary Supplement Health and Education Act of 1994 (DSHEA). The Food, Drug, and Cosmetic Act requires that conventional drugs—both prescription and over-the-counter agents—undergo rigorous evaluation of safety and efficacy before receiving FDA approval for marketing. The DSHEA categorizes botanical products (herbal supplements), vitamins, and minerals as dietary (food) supplements rather than as drugs. By classifying products as dietary supplements, the DSHEA exempts them from undergoing FDA scrutiny and approval before marketing. In fact, dietary supplements can be manufactured and marketed without giving the FDA any proof that they are safe or effective. All manufacturers must notify the FDA of efficacy claims. If a product eventually proves harmful or turns out to have made false claims, the FDA does have the authority to intervene—but only *after* the product had been released for marketing. Furthermore, to challenge a claim of efficacy, the FDA must file suit in court; the challenge cannot be made through a simple administrative procedure.

Package Labeling

The DSHEA does impose some restrictions on labeling. All herbal products must be labeled as dietary supplements. In addition, the label must not claim that the product can be used to diagnose, prevent, treat, or cure a disease. In fact, it must state the opposite: *this product is not intended to diagnose, treat, cure, or prevent any disease.* However, the label *is* allowed to make claims about the product's ability to favorably influence *body structure or function.* Put another way, the label can insinuate specific benefits but cannot make overt claims. By way of illustration, labels *can* bear statements such as these:

- Helps promote urinary tract health
- Helps maintain cardiovascular function
- Energizes and rejuvenates
- Reduces stress and frustration
- Improves absentmindedness
- Supports the immune system
  But labels *cannot* bear statements or terms such as these:
- Protects against cancer
- Reduces pain and stiffness of arthritis
- Lowers cholesterol
- Supports the body's antiviral capabilities
- Improves symptoms of Alzheimer disease
- Relieves menopausal hot flashes
- "Antibiotic," "antiseptic," "antidepressant," "laxative," or "diuretic"

If all of this sounds like semantic hair splitting—it largely is. Furthermore, regardless of what the label says, common sense assumes that people *will* take herbal products with the intent to prevent or treat disease.

Under the provisions of the DSHEA, there is no assurance that a product actually contains what the label proclaims: the package may contain ingredients that are *not* listed, or it may *lack* ingredients that *are* listed. These shortcomings and others have been addressed by the Current Good Manufacturing Practices (CGMP) ruling, issued by the FDA in 2007.

Adverse Effects

With dietary supplements as with conventional drugs, the manufacturer is responsible for safety. However, the similarity ends there. Under the

DSHEA, a product is presumed safe until proved hazardous. Furthermore, the burden for proving danger lies with the consumer and the FDA. With conventional drugs, the opposite logic and regulations apply: drugs are presumed dangerous until rigorous testing by the manufacturer reveals an absence of serious adverse effects. Because of this system, the number of dangerous drugs that reach the market is kept to a minimum. Ask yourself, "Which product would I be more comfortable using—one that has been tested for adverse effects *before* I take it or one that is evaluated for adverse effects only *after* it caused me harm?"

Impurities, Adulterants, and Variability

The DSHEA does not address the issues of impurities, adulterants, or variability. As a result, dangerous products have been allowed to reach consumers. A few examples illustrate the problem:

* A combination product used to "cleanse the bowel" caused life-threatening heart block. Analysis revealed contamination with *Digitalis lanata*, a plant with powerful effects on the heart.
* Among 125 ephedra products analyzed by the FDA, ephedrine content per dose ranged from undetectable to 110 mg. Also, some products had 6 to 20 additional ingredients.
* Testing of 10 brands of ginseng products revealed a 20-fold variation in ginsenoside content.
* When the California Department of Health Sciences analyzed 243 patent Asian medicines, they found 24 containing lead, 35 containing mercury, and 36 containing arsenic—all at levels above those permitted in drugs. Of these products, 7% were adulterated with undeclared pharmaceuticals, including ephedrine, chlorpheniramine, methyltestosterone, and phenacetin.

As discussed next, the CGMP ruling, issued by the FDA in 2007, should prevent the sale of such products.

Current Good Manufacturing Practices Ruling

In June 2007, the FDA issued a set of standards to regulate the manufacturing and labeling of dietary supplements. These standards, referred to as CGMP, are designed to ensure that dietary supplements be devoid of adulterants, contaminants, and impurities and that package labels accurately reflect the identity, purity, quality, and strength of what is inside. In addition, the label should indicate not only active ingredients but also inactive ingredients. The CGMP also mandates that manufacturers establish quality-control procedures, with the objective of preventing mislabeled, underfilled, or overfilled formulations; variations in tablet size, color, or potency; and contamination with drugs, bacteria, pesticides, glass, lead, and other potential contaminants. Unfortunately, even with standards and rules, there is still no assurance that dietary supplements will be either safe or effective; but at least we do have improved confidence regarding package contents.

Dietary Supplement and Nonprescription Drug Consumer Protection Act

The Dietary Supplement and Nonprescription Drug Consumer Protection Act, passed in 2006, mandates the reporting of serious adverse events for nonprescription drugs and dietary supplements. The following events should be reported: deaths, hospitalizations, life-threatening experiences, persistent or significant disabilities, and birth defects. Manufacturers and distributors must report these to the FDA within 15 days. Reports can be filed by telephone, by mail, or through the MEDWATCH program at http://www.fda.gov/Safety/MedWatch.

A Comment on the Regulatory Status of Dietary Supplements

Although herbal products and other dietary supplements are not regulated for either safety or efficacy, many of these products have components that can produce profound beneficial and adverse pharmacologic effects. Nonetheless, reliable information on clinical effects is largely lacking. Many of those working in the fields of pharmacy, medicine, and nursing are concerned that the exceptions made for dietary supplements are both irrational and dangerous.

PRIVATE QUALITY CERTIFICATION PROGRAMS

Four *private* organizations—the US Pharmacopeia (USP), ConsumerLab, the Natural Products Association, and NSF International (formerly known as the National Sanitation Foundation)—test dietary supplements for quality. A "seal of approval" is given to products that meet their standards, which are very similar to the CGMP described previously. The USP standards are enforceable by the FDA. All four organizations require manufacturers to pay for the tests, and all four report on the following:

* CGMP
* Purity
* Identity
* Potency
* Dissolution
* Accuracy of labeling

In addition, two organizations—the USP and ConsumerLab—report on postapproval surveillance.

STANDARDIZATION OF HERBAL PRODUCTS

With herbal products, there is often uncertainty about the amounts of active ingredients. The concentration of active ingredients in herbal crops can vary from year to year and place to place. Reasons include differences in the amounts of sunshine, rainfall, temperature, and soil nutrients. As a result, the potency of herbal products can vary widely.

Variability can be reduced through standardization, a three-step process in which the manufacturer (1) prepares an *extract* of plant parts, (2) analyzes the extract for one or two known active ingredients, and (3) dilutes or concentrates the extract such that the final product contains a predetermined amount of the active ingredients. The objective is to achieve therapeutic equivalence from batch to batch made by the same manufacturer and among batches made by different manufacturers. Table 69.1 lists the concentrations of active ingredients in some standardized preparations.

Standardization has two important benefits. First, it permits accurate dosing. Second, it permits extrapolation of data obtained in clinical trials to the public in general.

Unfortunately, standardization also has drawbacks. The extraction process might destroy active compounds. Furthermore, the process may fail to extract as-yet unidentified active agents; hence the extract may have a different spectrum of effects than the intact plant. To the extent

TABLE 69.1 Concentrations of Active Agents in Some Standardized Herbal Preparations	
Herb	**Amount of Active Agent**
Black cohosh	2.5% Triterpene glycosides
Echinacea	4% Phenolic compounds
Feverfew	0.2% Parthenolide
Ginkgo biloba	24% Ginkgo flavonoids, 6% terpenoids
St. John's wort	0.3% Hypericin
Valerian root	1% Valerianic acid

that this is true, historical data obtained with whole plants will lose some value as a basis for clarifying clinical responses to the standardized extract.

ADVERSE INTERACTIONS WITH CONVENTIONAL DRUGS

Herbal products and other dietary supplements can interact with conventional drugs, sometimes with significant harmful results. The principal concerns are increased toxicity and decreased therapeutic effects. Clinicians and consumers should be alert to these possibilities. Unfortunately, with many supplements, reliable information on adverse interactions is lacking—in large part because potential interactions have not been systematically studied. Hence, if a patient is taking a conventional medication and a dietary supplement and therapeutic effects are lost or toxicity appears, it may be impossible to say for sure that the supplement was (or was not) responsible.

A few important interactions *have* been identified, including the following:

- St. John's wort can induce CYP3A4 (the 3A4 isoenzyme of cytochrome P450) and can, thereby, accelerate the metabolism of many drugs, causing a loss of therapeutic effects.
- Several herbal products—including *Ginkgo biloba,* feverfew, and garlic—suppress platelet aggregation and, hence, can increase the risk for bleeding in patients receiving antiplatelet drugs (e.g., aspirin) or anticoagulants (e.g., warfarin and heparin).
- Ma huang (ephedra) contains ephedrine, a compound that can elevate blood pressure and stimulate the heart and central nervous system (CNS). Accordingly, ephedra can intensify the effects of pressor agents, cardiac stimulants, and CNS stimulants to counteract the beneficial effects of antihypertensive drugs and CNS depressants.

These interactions, at least, can be avoided—provided that the prescriber is aware of them and that the patient informs the prescriber about supplement use. Unfortunately, up to 70% of patients neglect to do so.

SOME COMMONLY USED DIETARY SUPPLEMENTS

Black Cohosh

Uses

Black cohosh has a long history of use in America. The herb was used by Native Americans and later by American colonists. Between 1820 and 1926, it was listed as an official drug in the USP.

Black cohosh (*Cimicifuga racemosa*) is used for treating symptoms of menopause, including hot flashes, vaginal dryness, palpitations, depression, irritability, and sleep disturbance. The preparation should *not* be used to reduce hot flashes caused by tamoxifen and other selective estrogen receptor modulators (SERMs).

Actions

How black cohosh works is unknown. At one time, we believed that it suppressed the release of luteinizing hormone (LH). However, clinical studies have failed to show an effect on female hormones, including LH, estradiol, prolactin, and follicle-stimulating hormone. In laboratory studies, black cohosh does not interact with estrogen receptors: it does not bind to these receptors, upregulate estrogen-dependent genes, or promote growth of estrogen-dependent tumors (at least in animals).

Effectiveness

Early studies carried out in Germany supported the ability of black cohosh to effectively relieve menopausal symptoms. In 2012, however, a Cochrane meta-analysis of 16 randomized controlled trials involving more than 2000 women concluded that there was insufficient evidence to support black cohosh for the management of menopausal symptoms. After a review of the evidence, the NCCIH concluded, "[T]here is overall insufficient evidence to support the use of black cohosh for menopausal symptoms." These conclusions were echoed by the American College of Obstetricians and Gynecologists (ACOG) when they updated their clinical guidelines for the management of menopausal symptoms in 2014. The following year, the North American Menopause Society withdrew its recommendation for use of black cohosh at this time (pending additional research) and removed it from among the natural remedies listed on its website.

Adverse Effects

Some women taking black cohosh have developed liver inflammation, which, in some instances, has led to liver failure. The association is tenuous, however, because the occurrence has been rare, and other possible causes of liver injury have not been ruled out. Until more is known, it may be wise to check baseline liver function with periodic rechecks.

Less serious and more common adverse effects include rash, headache, dizziness, and abdominal discomfort. Safety in pregnancy and breastfeeding has not been established; however, for those taking black cohosh for menopausal benefit, this would only be a concern in rare circumstances. One caveat acknowledged almost universally is the need to limit the use of black cohosh to 6 months because long-term studies have not been conducted.

Interactions With Conventional Drugs

Black cohosh may potentiate the hypotensive effects of antihypertensive drugs as well as the hypoglycemic effects of insulin and other drugs for diabetes. Black cohosh may potentiate the effects of estrogens used for hormone therapy. Because it may cause liver inflammation, black cohosh may increase the risk for liver damage when taken with other drugs that may harm the liver.

Comments

Users must not confuse black cohosh with blue cohosh (Caulophyllumthalic-troides). Although blue cohosh has legitimate uses, including promotion of menstruation and labor, it is very different from black cohosh and potentially more dangerous. Blue cohosh can elevate blood pressure, increase intestinal motility, and accelerate respiration. It can also induce uterine contractions and, hence, should be avoided during pregnancy. Some commercial products contain both black cohosh and blue cohosh. Women who want only black cohosh should avoid these products.

Butterbur

Butterbur (*Petasiteshybridus*) is a bush that grows in marshy areas across North America. Products are made from itsrhizomes and roots as well as its stems.

Uses

Butterbur is most commonly taken for migraine headaches, allergies, and asthma. It is one of the few botanicals recommended as a drug of first choice based on outcomes of randomized controlled trials.

Actions

Butterbur has antiinflammatory, antispasmodic, and vasodilatory effects. As with many herbal products, the exact mechanism of action is unknown. Some believe that butterbur works as a calcium channel blocker. Laboratory studies point to inhibition of lipoxygenase, an enzyme that contributes to the synthesis of leukotrienes and other proinflammatory substances.

Effectiveness

Although evidence remains lacking for the efficacy of butterbur in the treatment of skin allergies and asthma, substantial evidence supports other uses. According to the NCCIH:

- A sponsored literature review found that butterbur is just as effective as an antihistamine for allergy symptoms.
- Butterbur appears to relieve nasal allergy symptoms.
- Research findings indicate that butterbur can be effective in treating migraine headache.

The American Academy of Neurology (AAN) and the American Headache Society (AHA) also noted the effects of butterbur on preventing migraine headache. In 2012 they published a joint report in which they not only pronounced that butterbur was effective in decreasing migraine headache frequency but also gave it the highest (Level A) rating. Their conclusion? "Petasites (butterbur) is effective for migraine prevention and should be offered to patients with migraine to reduce the frequency and severity of migraine attacks." For this purpose, the AAN recommends 50 to 75 mg twice a day. (See https://www.aan.com/siteassets/home-page/policy-and-guidelines/quality/quality-measures/14headachemeasureset_pg.pdf.)

Adverse Effects

Long-term safety has not been established; however, butterbur appears to be safe for short-term use of less than 4 months' duration when taken at recommended doses. The most common adverse effects are eructation (belching), headache, and fatigue. Those who have allergies to ragweed, daisies, marigolds, and chrysanthemums may have allergic reactions to butterbur.

With the increasing use of butterbur, concern has arisen regarding new reports of liver injury. According to the NCCIH, this can be the result of pyrrolizidine alkaloids (PAs) found in many butterbur preparations. The NCCIH recommends using products in which PAs have been removed or are certified as being PA-free. Whether this type of product was taken by those who developed liver injury is unknown.

Interactions With Conventional Drugs

Interactions can occur if butterbur is given with drugs that induce CYP3A4 isoenzymes. Examples include not only drugs such as carbamazepine, phenobarbital, and phenytoin but also dietary supplements such as echinacea, garlic, and St. John's wort. The greatest concern comes when a non–PA-free form of butterbur is used, because PAs are substrates of CYP3A4 isoenzymes; metabolism converts these to their toxic metabolites.

Coenzyme Q-10

Coenzyme Q-10 (ubiquinone, CoQ-10) is an antioxidant that serves a vital role in cellular energy production. As we age, CoQ-10 levels decrease. This has led to increased interest in the use of CoQ-10 in the treatment of conditions associated with aging and with cellular energy production.

Uses

CoQ-10 is used to treat heart failure, muscle injury caused by HMG-CoA reductase inhibitors (statins), and mitochondrial encephalomyopathies (i.e., muscle and nervous system injury caused by deranged mitochondrial metabolism).

Actions

CoQ-10 is a potent antioxidant. It participates in many metabolic pathways, most notably production of adenosine triphosphate (ATP).

Effectiveness

In patients with documented CoQ-10 deficiency, replacement therapy with CoQ-10 offers clear benefits. Although some study findings have been mixed, the NCCIH reports several positive outcomes associated with the use of CoQ-10.

- Patients with heart failure who took CoQ-10 had improved cardiac function.
- Patients who took CoQ-10 after cardiac surgery had faster recovery.
- CoQ-10 may improve sperm count and semen quality; however, further studies are needed to identify an improvement in conception.

That being said, a 2016 Cochrane systematic review concluded that CoQ-10 did not cause a significant decrease in systolic or diastolic blood pressure. An attempt to perform a substantive review on the primary prevention of cardiovascular disease was hindered by the fact that only six small studies met the criteria for inclusion. Of the five trials that examined the effect of CoQ-10 on hypercholesterolemia, four did not find a significant alteration in lipid levels.

Research studies that examined the effect of CoQ-10 on statin-associated muscle injury and on cancer prevention and treatment were inconclusive.

Adverse Effects

CoQ-10 is well tolerated. High doses may produce gastrointestinal (GI) disturbances, including gastritis, reduced appetite, nausea, and diarrhea. Liver enzymes may increase, although no reports of actual liver injury have been made. Women who are pregnant or breastfeeding should not take CoQ-10 because its safety has not been established.

Interactions With Conventional Drugs

CoQ-10 is structurally similar to vitamin K_2 and, hence, may antagonize the effects of warfarin.

The biosynthesis of CoQ-10 shares a common pathway with cholesterol. As a result, drugs such as the statins, which inhibit the synthesis of cholesterol, can also inhibit the synthesis of CoQ-10, causing levels of endogenous CoQ-10 to decline. (Statin-induced reductions in CoQ-10 may explain why statins cause muscle injury.)

Cranberry Juice

Uses

Cranberry juice is used to prevent urinary tract infections (UTIs) and to decrease urine odor in patients with urinary incontinence.

Actions

Benefits derive from the presence of proanthocyanidins, a group of compounds that prevent bacteria from adhering to the urinary tract wall. Bacteria that have already attached themselves are not affected. Cranberry juice does not acidify the urine, as previously thought.

Effectiveness

Daily consumption of cranberry juice can *prevent* recurrent UTIs, but this has been demonstrated only in certain age groups. Specifically, it appears to benefit older adult women and women in their teens or 20s but not middle-aged adults or young girls. Furthermore, although cranberry juice can prevent UTIs, it is not effective as treatment for an established infection. In patients with urinary incontinence, cranberry juice can reduce unpleasant odor. Little is known about the efficacy of cranberry-extract capsules. Therefore cranberry juice itself is the preferred formulation.

Adverse Effects

Drinking more than 1 L/day may increase the risk for GI upset and the formation of kidney stones.

Interactions With Conventional Drugs

There is some evidence that cranberry juice may increase the risk for bleeding in patients taking warfarin. Therefore, these patients should be monitored closely.

Echinacea

Echinacea is the scientific name of the coneflower plant, which is native to the United States and parts of Canada. Echinacea was listed in the National Formulary from 1916 to 1950 but fell from favor owing to the development of antibiotics and a lack of scientific data to support its use.

Uses

Echinacea (*Echinacea angustifolia, E. purpurea, and E. pallida*) is administered orally and topically. Oral echinacea is taken to stimulate immune function, suppress inflammation, and treat viral infections, including influenza and the common cold. Topical echinacea is used to treat wounds, burns, eczema, psoriasis, and herpes simplex infections.

Actions

Active ingredients in echinacea preparations include cichoric acid, polysaccharides, flavonoids, and essential oils. These ingredients have been thought to produce antiviral, antiinflammatory, and immunostimulant effects through a combination of actions, including mobilization of phagocytes, stimulation of T-lymphocyte proliferation, stimulation of interferon and tumor necrosis factor production, and inhibition of hyaluronidase, a proinflammatory enzyme.

Effectiveness

Research regarding echinacea has yielded mixed results. A 2014 Cochrane review examined the evidence to determine the effectiveness and safety of echinacea in the prevention of common colds. The results identified a very small 10% to 20% risk reduction for those who took echinacea compared with those taking a placebo.

Adverse Effects

Very few adverse effects have been reported. The most common complaint is unpleasant taste. Fever, nausea, and vomiting occur infrequently.

Rarely, echinacea causes allergic reactions, including acute asthma, urticaria, angioedema, and anaphylaxis. Echinacea belongs to the daisy family of plants, whose members include ragweed, asters, chamomile, and chrysanthemums. People allergic to any of these plants are at increased risk for reacting to echinacea. Individuals with atopy (a genetic tendency toward allergic conditions) appear at increased risk for reacting to echinacea.

Until echinacea's effects on the immune system are fully known, it would be prudent to avoid the drug in patients with autoimmune diseases such as lupus erythematosus or rheumatoid arthritis. Although short-term exposure to echinacea *may* stimulate immune function, there is concern that long-term exposure can *suppress* immune function. Research findings published in the *Journal of Medicinal Chemistry* identified a substance in echinacea that blocked CD28 signaling pathway in T-cells creating

an immunosuppressive effect. Hence long-term therapy should be avoided in immunocompromised patients, including those with HIV infection. In addition, prolonged therapy should be avoided in people with tuberculosis and other chronic infections that require optimal immune function for cure.

Interactions With Conventional Drugs

By stimulating the immune system, echinacea can oppose the effects of immunosuppressant drugs. Conversely, by suppressing immune function (in response to long-term use), echinacea can compromise drug therapy of tuberculosis, cancer, and HIV infection.

Feverfew

Feverfew (*Tanacetum parthenium*) is a bushy plaint with small daisy-like flowers that grows throughout North and South America and Europe. Supplements are made from the dried leaves, although sometimes the flowers and stems are included.

Uses

Feverfew is used primarily for the prophylaxis of migraine. It is also taken for a number of conditions associated with hypersensitivity and altered immune responses, such as allergies, asthma, rheumatoid arthritis, and psoriasis.

Actions

The principal active agent in feverfew is *parthenolide*, a compound found in feverfew leaves. How parthenolide suppresses migraine is poorly understood. Possibilities include inhibition of vasoconstriction in the brain, suppression of serotonin release from platelets and leukocytes, and suppression of inflammation secondary to inhibition of arachidonic acid release.

Effectiveness

Clinical studies on feverfew's effect on migraine headaches have had mixed results. Some findings suggest that, when taken prophylactically, the herb can reduce the frequency of attacks and severity of symptoms (nausea, photophobia, phonophobia, and pain). However, feverfew was found less effective when taken to abort an ongoing attack. Furthermore, the doses required are much higher than those used for prophylaxis.

In 2012, the AAN and the AHS published a joint report on the evidence for CAM on the prophylaxis of episodic migraine. Their conclusion was that feverfew was probably effective for this purpose. (See earlier section "Butterbur.") The AAN recommends dosing at 50 to 300 mg twice daily for migraine prophylaxis.

What about the other purposes for which people use feverfew? Unfortunately, there is no reliable evidence that feverfew can benefit patients with rheumatoid arthritis or other inflammatory conditions.

Adverse Effects

Feverfew is very well tolerated. No serious adverse effects have been reported, although long-term studies of safety are lacking. Mild reactions include abdominal pain, indigestion, diarrhea, flatulence, nausea, and vomiting. Chewing feverfew leaves, a rare practice today, can cause oral ulceration, tongue irritation, and swollen lips. Some patients develop *postfeverfew syndrome*, characterized by nervousness, fatigue, insomnia, tension headache, and joint pain or stiffness.

Feverfew belongs to the same plant family as echinacea. Thus individuals allergic to ragweed, chrysanthemums, daisies, and marigolds may also be allergic to feverfew. By suppressing release of arachidonic acid in platelets, feverfew can decrease platelet aggregation and may, therefore, pose a risk for bleeding. Accordingly, the product should be discontinued 2 weeks before elective surgery.

Some reports suggest that feverfew may cause uterine contractions. Therefore women who are pregnant should not take this drug. Safety regarding breastfeeding has not been established.

Interactions With Conventional Drugs

By suppressing platelet aggregation, feverfew can increase the risk for bleeding in patients taking antiplatelet drugs (e.g., aspirin) or anticoagulants (e.g., warfarin and heparin).

Comments

There is great variability in feverfew products. Some contain little or no active ingredient.

Flaxseed

Flaxseeds are small seeds of the flax plant that grows in the northwestern United States and Canada. They may be processed in various products or added whole to cereals and other food products.

Uses

Flaxseed powders are used to treat constipation and dyslipidemias. Because it is a phytoestrogen, some women take it to combat hot flashes associated with menopause. Flaxseed also represents a vegetarian source of omega-3 fatty acids.

Actions

Ground flaxseed provides soluble plant fiber and α-linolenic acid. Like other high-fiber products, flaxseed can reduce serum cholesterol.

Flaxseed is an important food source of phytoestrogens called lignans. In the colon, bacteria convert these lignans into enterolactone and enterodiol, compounds that have both mild estrogenic and antiestrogenic actions. The antiestrogenic actions can decrease cellular proliferation in breast tissue.

Effectiveness

Like other fiber products, flaxseed has the potential to decrease plasma levels of total cholesterol and low-density lipoprotein (LDL) cholesterol but does not affect high-density lipoprotein (HDL) cholesterol or triglycerides. These effects occur predominantly among people with high cholesterol levels and in women who are postmenopausal. In contrast, *defatted* flaxseed may *increase* triglyceride levels, so it should be avoided by patients with hypertriglyceridemia.

Owing to its soluble fiber content, flaxseed acts like a bulk-forming laxative to relieve constipation. As with any bulk-forming laxative, adequate fluid intake is an important component of therapy.

Other than for management of hypercholesterolemia, current studies do not support the use of flaxseed for cardiovascular disease. They also do not support its use for relief of menopausal symptoms or the prevention of cancer. However, NCCIH funding of flaxseed research is ongoing.

Adverse Effects

Similar to other sources of dietary fiber, flaxseed can cause adverse GI effects. These include bloating, flatulence, and abdominal discomfort.

Interactions With Conventional Drugs

Flaxseed may reduce the absorption of conventional medications. Therefore it should be taken 1 hour before or 2 hours after these drugs.

Garlic

Garlic *(Allium sativum)* is a common plant known for its edible bulb. It has been used throughout history for a myriad of purposes and remains one of the most popular dietary supplements in use today.

Uses

Garlic is used primarily for effects on the cardiovascular system. The herb is taken to reduce levels of triglycerides and LDL cholesterol and to raise levels of HDL cholesterol. Garlic is also employed to reduce blood pressure, suppress platelet aggregation, increase arterial elasticity, and decrease the formation of atherosclerotic plaque. In addition, garlic has been used for antimicrobial and anticancer effects.

Actions

Garlic's beneficial effects are presumed to result from the actions of sulfides in garlic oil. Intact garlic cells contain *alliin,* an odorless amino acid. When garlic cells are crushed, they release alliinase, an enzyme that converts alliin into *allicin.* Allicin is the major active agent in garlic oil and the compound that gives garlic its distinctive aroma. In addition to allicin, garlic oil contains *ajoenes* (pronounced AH-ho-weens), biologically active compounds that contribute to beneficial effects.

Garlic is thought to reduce cholesterol levels by interfering with cholesterol synthesis in the liver. There is conflicting evidence regarding inhibition of HMG-CoA reductase, the rate-limiting enzyme in cholesterol synthesis and the enzyme that "statin" drugs inhibit.

Antiplatelet effects, which are well documented, result in part from inhibiting thromboxane synthesis. Methylallyltrisulfide is the chemical in garlic believed responsible. In addition, garlic may suppress platelet aggregation by disrupting calcium-dependent processes. Coagulation is also affected by the ajoenes, which have antithrombotic actions and may also stimulate fibrinolysis.

Lowering of blood pressure may be explained by garlic's ability to increase the activity of nitric oxide synthase, the enzyme in blood vessels that makes nitric oxide. Nitric oxide, also known as endothelium-derived relaxant factor, is a powerful vasodilator.

Effectiveness

As with many dietary supplements, research findings regarding garlic have been mixed. Outcomes of small trials in the 1990s demonstrated that garlic can produce favorable effects on plasma lipids. More recent and larger studies, however, have cast doubt on those findings.

After reviewing the scientific research, the NCCIH has concluded the following for now:

- Garlic does not appear to lower LDL cholesterol.
- Garlic *may* lower blood pressure, but any benefit appears modest at best.
- Garlic *may* decrease the rate of atherosclerosis development.

Regarding the effect of garlic on cancer prevention, at this time the National Cancer Institute recognizes that garlic *may* have a role in cancer prevention but, in the absence of adequate reliable data, does not recommend it. A 2014 Cochrane review found insufficient evidence to determine if garlic has a role in preventing the common cold. Insufficient evidence has also been found regarding garlic's use as an antimicrobial agent. It has been shown to have antibacterial and antifungal properties in vitro but limited to no efficacy in vivo.

Adverse Effects

Garlic is generally well tolerated. The most common side effects are bad breath and body odor. (This occurs because a product of garlic metabolism is allyl methyl sulfide, a sulfur compound that is excreted through respiration and skin pores.) Rarely, garlic causes heartburn, flatulence, nausea, vomiting, diarrhea, and a burning sensation in the mouth. These effects are most pronounced with raw garlic and in people who do not eat garlic often. Patients suffering from infectious or inflammatory GI disorders should avoid garlic owing to its potential for GI irritation.

Interactions With Conventional Drugs

Garlic has significant antiplatelet effects. Thus it can increase the risk for bleeding in patients taking antiplatelet drugs (e.g., aspirin) or anticoagulants (e.g., warfarin and heparin). Garlic can reduce levels of at least two drugs: cyclosporine (an immunosuppressant) and saquinavir (a protease inhibitor used to treat HIV infection).

Ginger Root

Ginger grows primarily in the tropics. Its root, actually a rhizome, is the source of the ginger root used in CAM.

Uses

Ginger root (*Zingiberofficinale*) is used primarily to treat vertigo and to suppress nausea and vomiting associated with motion sickness, morning sickness, seasickness, and general anesthesia. In addition, ginger has antiinflammatory and analgesic properties that may help people with arthritis and other chronic inflammatory conditions. Some practitioners use ginger for URIs, although proof of efficacy is lacking.

Actions

The mechanism by which ginger suppresses nausea and vomiting is unclear. A good possibility is blockade of serotonin (5-hydroxytryptamine$_3$, or 5-HT$_3$) receptors located in the chemoreceptor trigger zone of the medulla and on afferent vagal neurons in the GI tract. Activation of these receptors triggers emesis. Conversely, blockade of these receptors suppresses emesis. In fact, drugs that block 5-HT$_3$ receptors (e.g., ondansetron [Zofran]) are the most effective antiemetics available. Galanolactone, a major constituent of ginger, can block 5-HT$_3$ receptors in vitro, suggesting that receptor blockade may underlie antiemetic effects. Other actions that may contribute to beneficial effects include stimulation of intestinal motility, salivation, gastric mucus production, and suppression of GI spasm secondary to anticholinergic and antihistaminic actions.

The antiinflammatory effects of ginger have been attributed to its ability to inhibit the synthesis of prostaglandins and leukotrienes, which are powerful inflammatory mediators.

How ginger may reduce vertigo is unknown.

Effectiveness

There is good evidence supporting the benefits of ginger root for the prevention and treatment of morning sickness. A 2014 meta-analysis of the evidence demonstrated a decrease in nausea but not in episodes of vomiting. Unfortunately, studies focused on nausea due to motion sickness and postoperative nausea and vomiting (in the absence of opioids) have had conflicting results.

In patients with rheumatoid arthritis, ginger root *appears* to reduce pain, improve joint mobility, and decrease swelling and morning stiffness. However, these studies are inconclusive and further research is ongoing.

Adverse Effects

Ginger is very well tolerated. Severe toxicity has not been reported—although excessive doses (above 5g/d) have the potential to cause CNS depression and cardiac dysrhythmias. Excessive doses may also cause GI disturbances.

Although ginger is effective in relieving nausea due to morning sickness, it should be used with caution during pregnancy because its safety in pregnancy has not been proved. High-dose ginger is believed to stimulate the uterus and, thus, may theoretically cause spontaneous abortion, although there are no reports of this having happened. A 2012 population study of women in Norway included data on 1020 women who used ginger during pregnancy. Research findings showed no increased risk for malformations, spontaneous abortion, or other complications compared with women who did not take ginger.

Interactions With Conventional Drugs

Ginger can inhibit production of thromboxane by platelets and can, hence, suppress platelet aggregation. Accordingly, ginger can increase the risk for bleeding in patients receiving antiplatelet drugs (e.g., aspirin) or anticoagulants (e.g., warfarin and heparin) or other drugs that inhibit clotting such as the direct thrombin and factor xa inhibitors. Ginger can lower blood sugar and, hence, may potentiate the hypoglycemic effects of insulin and other drugs for diabetes.

Ginkgo Biloba

Medicinal ginkgo is prepared by acetone extraction from leaves of the *Ginkgo biloba* tree. These leaves contain two classes of active compounds: *flavonoids* (ginkgo flavone glycosides) and *terpenoids* (ginkgolides and bilobalide). *Ginkgo biloba extracts* (GBEs) are standardized to contain 24% flavonoids and 6% terpenoids. Daily oral doses of standardized GBE range from 60 to 240 mg.

Uses

Ginkgo (*Ginkgo biloba*) is used primarily to improve memory, halt progression of dementia, and decrease intermittent claudication. Less common uses include treatment of erectile dysfunction and other conditions associated with decreased perfusion.

Actions

Any benefits are believed to derive from improved blood flow secondary to ginkgo-induced vasodilation. GBEs also suppress production of platelet-activating factor (PAF), a mediator of platelet aggregation, bronchospasm, and other processes. Reduced PAF production may help protect against thrombosis as well as bronchospasm and other allergic disorders.

Effectiveness

Gingko is one of the most studied herbal products. As with many others, early studies showed promising findings that conflict with more recent and rigorous clinical trials.

Studies that examined the effects of gingko on intermittent claudication have had mixed results. Most have not demonstrated a significant benefit. In those in which improvement was noted, the degree of improvement was small.

What about benefits in dementia? In a large placebo-controlled trial—the Ginkgo Evaluation of Memory (GEM) study, sponsored by the NIH, GBE failed to prevent dementia of any sort, including Alzheimer disease. This study enrolled more than 3000 participants aged 75 years or older. Half received a GBE formulation (120 mg bid), and the other half received a placebo. The result? After 6 years of treatment, the incidence of dementia was nearly identical in both groups.

The NCCIH is currently studying ginkgo's effects in multiple sclerosis, sexual dysfunction caused by antidepressants, insulin resistance, and memory loss due to electroconvulsive therapy. Additional studies continue for intermittent claudication and dementia.

Adverse Effects

Ginkgo is generally well tolerated. In some patients it causes stomach upset, headache, dizziness, or vertigo, all of which can be minimized by avoiding rapid increases in dosage. There have been case reports of spontaneous bleeding, although no bleeding was observed in the GEM study.

There have been reports of people eating raw or roasted ginkgo seeds. Unlike ginkgo leaves, the seeds contain significant amounts of toxins and can cause seizures and fatalities.

Interactions With Conventional Drugs

Ginkgo may suppress coagulation. Therefore it should be used with caution in patients taking antiplatelet drugs (e.g., aspirin) or anticoagulants (e.g., warfarin and heparin).

There is a concern that ginkgo may promote seizures. Hence the herb should be avoided by patients at risk for seizures, including those taking drugs that can lower the seizure threshold as well as some antipsychotics, antidepressants, cholinesterase inhibitors, decongestants, first-generation antihistamines, and systemic glucocorticoids.

Glucosamine and Chondroitin

Glucosamine and chondroitin are individual products that are usually administered together. Both are innate substances in the body that serve as essential components of cartilage. Products containing these substances can come from natural sources (e.g., animal cartilage) or may be manufactured in a laboratory.

Uses

Glucosamine and chondroitin are used widely to treat osteoarthritis. Osteoarthritis primarily affects the knee, hip, and wrist joints.

Actions

Glucosamine is employed by the body in the synthesis of cartilage and synovial fluid. Chondroitin helps keep cartilage hydrated. When given to people with osteoarthritis, glucosamine may help in several ways. First, it can act as a substrate for making cartilage and synovial fluid. Second, it can stimulate the activity of chondrocytes, the cells in joints that make cartilage and synovial fluid. And third, it can suppress production of cytokines that mediate joint inflammation and cartilage degradation. Chondroitin has a role in maintaining cartilage integrity.

Effectiveness

Studies on the efficacy of glucosamine and chondroitin in osteoarthritis have yielded mixed results. Most studies do not show improvement in pain relief; however, some studies have demonstrated a modest improvement in joint structure.

In 2012, the American College of Rheumatology updated their recommendations for the management for osteoarthritis. After an examination of the evidence, the expert panel advised providers *not* to use glucosamine and chondroitin for osteoarthritis management.

Adverse Effects

The most common side effects are GI disturbances, such as nausea and heartburn. Because commercial glucosamine is produced from the exoskeletons of shellfish (shrimp), glucosamine should be used with caution in patients with shellfish allergy. In theory, glucosamine can raise blood levels of glucose, but this has not been observed in clinical trials.

Interactions With Conventional Drugs

Several case reports suggest that glucosamine may increase the risk for bleeding. Therefore patients taking antiplatelet drugs (e.g., aspirin) or anticoagulants (e.g., warfarin and heparin) should probably avoid this product.

Green Tea

Green tea is produced from the *Camellia sinensis* plant. This is the same plant used to produce black tea and oolong tea. The differences lie in the methods of production.

Uses

Green tea and green tea extracts have been used to lose weight, improve mental clarity, and prevent and treat cancers of the stomach, skin, bladder, and breast.

Actions

The mechanism underlying beneficial effects is poorly understood and probably multifactorial. Polyphenols in green tea may underlie antiinflammatory, chemoprotective, and antioxidant effects. Chemoprotection may also stem from epigallocatechin-3-gallate (EGCG), a compound in green tea extracts. The caffeine in green tea may be responsible for weight loss and improved mental clarity.

Effectiveness

Data on the efficacy of green tea are limited. There is evidence that drinking green tea throughout the day can improve mental clarity and may help with weight loss. In both cases, any benefits are probably due to caffeine and not a substance unique to green tea.

Studies done in animals and cultured cancer cells have shown that green tea and EGCG may prevent or slow the growth of certain cancers. Also, there is a small body of evidence indicating that drinking green tea may help prevent recurrence after treatment of early-stage breast cancer. These studies have shown mixed results; however, research is ongoing.

Adverse Effects

Moderate consumption appears to be safe. As with other caffeine-containing products, overconsumption may result in headache, nausea, anxiety, insomnia, increased heart rate, and increased urination. Hepatotoxicity has been reported, primarily in people using concentrated green tea extracts. The mechanism of the hepatotoxicity remains unknown.

Interactions With Conventional Drugs

There is a long list of potential drug interactions. Green tea should be consumed with caution by patients taking vasodilators, stimulants and other psychoactive medications, and medications with a known risk for liver damage. Green tea contains a small amount of vitamin K, which may decrease the anticoagulant effects of warfarin. A small study of subjects taking nadolol and drinking green tea identified a significant decrease in nadolol absorption.

Peppermint

Peppermint (*Mentha piperita*) is a common herb in North America as well as Europe and the Middle East. It is often found near streams, especially in partially shaded areas.

Uses

Peppermint is best known as a culinary flavoring. Peppermint tea is a popular drink in some regions. It is commonly used to decrease nausea. When used as a medicinal preparation, peppermint oil is the form most commonly used. It is available over-the-counter in gel tablets or capsules.

Randomized controlled trials (RCTs) have demonstrated a beneficial effect of peppermint oil for management of irritable bowel syndrome (IBS). In their 2014 monograph on the management of irritable bowel syndrome and chronic idiopathic constipation (available at http://gi.org/wp-content/uploads/2014/08/IBS_CIC_Monograph_AJG_Aug_2014.pdf), the American College of Gastroenterology included peppermint oil among its recommendations for IBS management.

Peppermint oil is also gaining recognition as therapy for small intestinal bacterial overgrowth (SIBO). SIBO is a condition that has become increasingly common as a result of the increasing use of over-the-counter proton pump inhibitor as well as following certain bariatric surgeries such as the Roux-en-Y gastric bypass. As bacteria break down carbohydrates and other substances, excessive gas forms. This results in severe abdominal cramps and low-volume diarrhea. SIBO is typically treated with antibiotics; therefore the antibiotic properties of peppermint oil are beneficial in this regard.

Peppermint water (obtained from distillation of peppermint oil) has been used in many countries to prevent nipple cracking and pain related to breastfeeding. A 2018 report of a randomized clinical trial of 80 breastfeeding women identified a significant decrease of nipple pain, soreness, and trauma in subjects who followed a peppermint water regimen. Small studies have also supported the use of peppermint oil to manage esophageal spasms in adults and functional abdominal pain in children. Numerous anecdotal reports suggest that the topical use of peppermint oil applied to the temples may help ease tension headaches. This is supported by two small trials comparing peppermint oil to a placebo and peppermint oil to acetaminophen. In these trials, peppermint oil was significantly more effective than the placebo and equal in effectiveness compared to acetaminophen.

Actions

Peppermint oil inhibits smooth muscle activity in the gastrointestinal tract. The exact mechanism is unclear; however, animal studies have indicated a possible relationship to blocking of calcium channels in the GI system.

The antibacterial properties of peppermint may come in part from menthol and other volatile oils. Research has demonstrated that peppermint oil has a bacteriostatic effect against 22 strains of both gram-positive and gram-negative bacteria and bactericidal activity against *Escherichia coli*, *Helicobacter pylori*, and *Salmonella enteritidis*.

It has been theorized that peppermint activates opioid receptors. Recent studies point to a different mechanism for pain relief: stimulation of transient receptor potential ion channel melastatin subtype 8 (TRPM8) in gastrointestinal pathways. TRPM8 receptors are activated by cold temperatures and by cooling agents such as menthol, which is a component of peppermint,

Effectiveness

Numerous studies demonstrate that peppermint oil is significantly superior to a placebo for management of IBS. Smaller studies support its use for SIBO, functional abdominal pain, and tension headache.

Adverse Effects

Peppermint can lower esophageal sphincter pressure leading to gastroesophageal reflux. This is more likely to occur with peppermint teas. Peppermint gels do not usually cause such problems because their enteric coating allows them to pass through the stomach intact.

Allergic reactions have been reported. Perianal burning has been reported following high doses. Excessive doses have also been tied to renal problems. At standard doses, peppermint oil appears to be devoid of serious adverse effects.

Interactions With Conventional Drugs

Over a decade ago, questions were raised regarding CYP1A2 inhibition by peppermint oil; however, this has not been demonstrated in humans. Peppermint oil may have an additive effect when administered with antispasmodics.

Probiotics

Probiotics are dietary supplements composed of potentially beneficial bacteria or yeasts. These preparations typically contain two types of bacteria—lactobacilli and bifidobacteria—as well as *Saccharomyces boulardii*, a specific strain of yeast. All of these microorganisms are normal components of our gut flora.

Uses

The *bacteria* in probiotics may help treat IBS, ulcerative colitis, *Clostridium difficile*–associated diarrhea (CDAD), and, in children, rotavirus diarrhea. Products containing *S. boulardii* are used for CDAD.

Actions

Normal intestinal and colonic bacteria play several important roles: they help metabolize foods and some drugs; they promote nutrient absorption; and they reduce colonization of the gut by pathogenic bacteria. *Lactobacillus* and *Bifidobacterium* species adhere to the intestinal wall and, hence, prevent attachment of bacterial pathogens. They also control bacterial overgrowth by producing lactic acid and to some degree by producing hydrogen peroxide. Benefits may also derive from increasing nonspecific cellular and humeral immunity. The yeast *S. boulardii* produces proteases that can degrade toxins produced by *C. difficile*. Benefits of *S. boulardii* in Crohn disease derive in part from increasing intestinal secretion of immunoglobulin A.

Effectiveness

According to information available at NCCIH (https://nccih.nih.gov/health/probiotics), studies on probiotics have yielded conflicting results. There is some evidence that *Lactobacillus* species may reduce the duration of diarrhea in patients with rotavirus infection and other GI conditions. Effectiveness appears to vary among *Lactobacillus* species. VSL#3, a product composed of lactobacilli, bifidobacteria, *Streptococcus thermophilus*, and other bacteria, appears to have a role in inducing remission of ulcerative colitis, perhaps in as many as 50% of patients. In patients with IBS, VSL#3 may reduce bloating and abdominal pain. However, the product does not improve the frequency or consistency of bowel movements.

Fortunately, the number of studies focusing on probiotics has increased in recent years, making this one of the most researched agents in the CAM field. The vast foci (e.g., diarrhea, eczema, ulcerative colitis, candidiasis, bacterial vaginosis, and allergies, to name a few) should yield a rich source of knowledge in the future.

Adverse Effects

Probiotics are generally well tolerated. Flatulence and bloating are the most common adverse effects. Infection of the blood with lactobacilli and fungi has been reported after ingestion of yogurt, but only in severely ill, immunocompromised patients taking broad-spectrum antibiotics long term. Fungemia has occurred most often when packets of *S. boulardii* (Florastor) have been opened at the bedside in the intensive care unit. Florastor is contraindicated in patients who have central lines.

Interactions With Conventional Drugs

Antibacterial and antifungal drugs can kill the bacteria and yeasts in probiotic products. Thus to help preserve probiotic activity, these preparations should be administered no sooner than 2 hours after dosing with antibacterial or antifungal drugs.

Resveratrol

Resveratrol is a chemical found in grapes (mainly the skin), red wine, purple grape juice, blueberries, cranberries, and peanuts. Resveratrol content of dietary supplements ranges from 16 to 600 mg per tablet or capsule. The amount in red wine is quite low, only 0.3 to 1.9 mg per 150-mL serving.

Uses

Resveratrol is an antioxidant promoted for antiaging effects and protection against chronic diseases. Owing to the presence of resveratrol in red wine, researchers thought it might explain the *French paradox*: how it is possible that French people have a relatively low incidence of coronary heart disease despite having a diet relatively high in saturated fats. However, the amount of resveratrol in red wine seems much too low to cause significant cardioprotectant effects.

Recent research findings have opened the door to the potential for resveratrol to improve outcomes in a number of conditions. Research is ongoing to determine resveratrol's role in the management of heart disease, diabetes, obesity, and Alzheimer disease.

Actions

In 2012, a breakthrough NIH study of resveratrol identified the mechanism of action, heretofore believed to result from its direct interaction with sirtuin enzymes. Resveratrol inhibits phosphodiesterases (PDEs). This, in turn, increases levels of cyclic adenosine monophosphate (AMP) and activation of AMP-dependent kinase. This is important because PDEs play a role in many chronic conditions (e.g., heart disease, diabetes, and chronic obstructive pulmonary disease), and PDE inhibitors are proving to be important drugs in managing these.

Effectiveness

Resveratrol has produced clear benefits in animal studies. In middle-aged mice on a high-calorie diet, resveratrol increased insulin sensitivity and reduced mortality. In normal-weight mice, resveratrol failed to reduce mortality but did improve cardiovascular function, bone density, and motor coordination; it also delayed the formation of cataracts. In rodent models of human cancers, resveratrol suppressed tumor growth, including tumors of the lung, skin, breast, and prostate. In diabetic rats, resveratrol lowered blood glucose, and in human cells grown in culture, resveratrol increased glucose uptake. In one human study, resveratrol suppressed production of tumor necrosis factor and free radicals; both actions could reduce blood vessel inflammation and subsequent atherosclerosis.

Although studies done in cell cultures and animals have been encouraging, very little is known about the long-term benefits of resveratrol in humans. In fact, we have no data at all showing that resveratrol either slows aging or reduces the incidence or severity of any disease. A 2013 meta-analysis of the available evidence on the effects of resveratrol on plasma lipids revealed no significant effect of resveratrol compared with placebo.

Adverse Effects and Interactions With Conventional Drugs

Information on adverse effects is limited. We do know that resveratrol has antiplatelet actions, which might intensify the effects of anticoagulants and antiplatelet drugs. Also, resveratrol can mimic the effects of estrogen and, hence, is not recommended for women with estrogen-dependent breast cancer, uterine cancer, ovarian cancer, endometriosis, and uterine fibroids. In addition, resveratrol may increase insulin sensitivity and, hence, should be used with caution by patients taking antidiabetes agents.

Saw Palmetto

The American saw palmetto (*Serenoarepens and Sabal serrulata*) is a small palm tree that grows in the eastern United States. The product employed clinically is an extract made from its berries.

Uses

Saw palmetto is taken to relieve urinary symptoms associated with benign prostatic hyperplasia (BPH). It has also been promoted for treatment of androgenic alopecia.

Actions

How does saw palmetto affect prostate function? Some have postulated that it causes blockade of testosterone receptors, blockade of alpha-adrenergic receptors, and suppression of inflammation. Contrary to prior belief, the preparation does not seem to inhibit 5-α-reductase, the enzyme that converts testosterone into dihydrotestosterone (DHT)—the active form of testosterone in the prostate. Saw palmetto does not reduce prostate size or serum levels of testosterone, DHT, or prostate-specific antigen (PSA).

Effectiveness

At this time, there is insufficient evidence to support using saw palmetto for BPH or any other condition. Although early studies suggested that saw palmetto might reduce symptoms of BPH, these results have not been confirmed by more rigorous studies. Two clinical trials funded by the NIH showed that saw palmetto extract is no more effective than placebo at reducing symptoms of BPH. A 2012 Cochrane review of 32 RCTs involving 5666 men found no significant difference between saw palmetto and placebo. It continues to be widely used, however, and is promoted in nonprofessional magazines and other resources.

Adverse Effects

Saw palmetto is very well tolerated. Significant adverse effects have not been reported. Rarely, saw palmetto causes nausea or headache. Although antiandrogenic effects (e.g., gynecomastia) have not been reported, it may be wise to monitor for them. Saw palmetto may have antiplatelet actions, but increased bleeding has not been reported.

Because of its antiandrogenic effects, saw palmetto represents a danger to the developing fetus. Pregnant women should not ingest this herb.

Interactions With Conventional Drugs

Because of its antiplatelet effects, saw palmetto should be used with caution in patients taking antiplatelet drugs (e.g., aspirin) or anticoagulants (e.g., warfarin and heparin).

Soy

Soy is a member of the pea (legume) family. Although it is processed in tablets and capsules for CAM, it has become a common staple in American diets both in its original form (edamame) and in processed foods such as soy sauce and tofu.

Uses

Soy protein and soy isoflavones have several uses, including prevention of breast cancer and, in postmenopausal women, treatment of vasomotor symptoms (e.g., hot flashes) and prevention of osteoporosis.

Actions

Soy's major active components are phytoestrogens (isoflavones and lignans) and phytosterols (betasitosterol). Two isoflavones—genistein and daidzein—undergo enzymatic conversion to equol, a compound with estrogenic actions. Soy isoflavones are structurally similar to estradiol (the major endogenous estrogen) and can bind with estrogen receptors. However, like the SERMs, isoflavones exert mixed estrogenic and antiestrogenic actions. In women with normal estrogen levels, soy isoflavones appear to *antagonize* endogenous estrogen. By contrast, in postmenopausal women, soy isoflavones act as estrogen agonists.

Effectiveness

Clinical trials using soy-derived phytoestrogens to relieve menopausal hot flashes have yielded mixed results. Overall, the studies lean toward a reduction in hot flashes.

Several epidemiologic studies imply that soy consumption may reduce the risk for developing breast cancer. In particular, population studies have documented that Asian women who eat a diet high in soy are at reduced risk. However, clinical trials confirming this benefit are lacking and there is little evidence of efficacy in Western women.

Several early studies suggested that isoflavones either increase bone mineral density or slow the progression of osteoporosis in perimenopausal and postmenopausal women. However, with one exception, several meta-analyses of studies published between 2010 and 2015 do not demonstrate significant improvement in bone mineral density. The exception? A meta-analysis on the effects of phytoestrogens on osteoporosis in ovariectomized rats.

Adverse Effects

Soy and soy extracts are very well tolerated. Gastrointestinal effects—bloating, nausea, constipation, or diarrhea—are most common. Rarely, soy can cause migraine, probably because of its estrogenic effects. Large amounts of soy products may increase the risk for oxalate kidney stones. There have been several cases of goiter and hypothyroidism in infants who drank soy-based formula. Concerns that soy formulas might cause feminization of male infants were dispelled by a 2008 review from the American Academy of Pediatrics.

Interactions With Conventional Drugs

Soy should not be combined with tamoxifen and other drugs that can block estrogen receptors. By killing intestinal flora, antibiotics may reduce conversion of isoflavones to their active form, thus decreasing any potential positive effects of soy. Because fermented products like soy sauce contain tyramine, they should not be combined with MAO inhibitors.

St. John's Wort

St. John's wort (*Hypericum perforatum*) is a plant that grows wild in the western United States and parts of Canada. Its yellow flowers are used in the preparation of extracts and other preparations.

Uses

St. John's wort is used primarily for oral therapy of mild to moderate depression. The herb has also been used topically to manage local infection and orally to relieve pain and inflammation.

Actions

Benefits of St. John's wort appear to derive from two compounds—hyperforin and hypericin—that are extracted from flowers of the plant. These compounds can decrease reuptake of three neurotransmitters: serotonin, norepinephrine (NE), and dopamine. Blockade of serotonin and NE uptake mimics the actions of some conventional antidepressants. Early research attributed antidepressant effects to inhibition of monoamine oxidase (MAO). However, we now know that the degree of MAO inhibition is too small to explain clinical effects.

Effectiveness

How effective is St. John's wort? At this time, it's hard to say. Although numerous studies have been conducted, evidence for efficacy is mixed, owing to poor study design, heterogeneous study populations, and variable hypericin content of the preparations used, as well as other confounding factors. The bottom line? For patients with *mild to moderate* major depression, St. John's wort appears superior to placebo and equal to tricyclic antidepressants. For patients with *severe* depression, there is no convincing proof of efficacy.

Adverse Effects

St. John's wort is generally well tolerated. Allergic skin reactions may occur, especially in people allergic to ragweed and daisies. In addition, the herb may cause CNS effects (e.g., insomnia, vivid dreams, restlessness, anxiety, agitation, and irritability), as well as GI discomfort, fatigue, dry mouth, and headache. High-dose therapy may pose a risk for phototoxicity. To reduce this risk, patients should minimize exposure to sunlight, wear protective clothing, and apply a sunscreen to exposed skin.

Interactions With Conventional Drugs

St. John's wort is known to interact adversely with many drugs—and the list continues to grow. Three mechanisms are involved: induction

of cytochrome P450 enzymes, induction of P-glycoprotein, and intensification of serotonin effects. Considered one by one, the following may be said:

- *Induction of 3A4 isoenzymes of cytochrome P450* can accelerate the metabolism of many drugs, thereby decreasing their effects. This mechanism appears to be responsible for breakthrough bleeding and unintended pregnancy in women taking oral contraceptives, transplant rejection in patients taking cyclosporine (an immunosuppressant), reduced anticoagulation in patients taking warfarin, and reduced antiretroviral effects in patients taking protease inhibitors or nonnucleoside reverse transcriptase inhibitors.
- *P-glycoprotein* is a transport protein found in cells that line the intestine and renal tubules. In the intestine, P-glycoprotein transports drugs *out* of cells into the intestinal lumen; in renal tubules, P-glycoprotein transports drugs *out* of tubular cells into the urine. Hence, by increasing P-glycoprotein synthesis, St. John's wort can accelerate elimination of drugs and, hence, reduce their effects. This is the mechanism by which St. John's wort greatly reduces levels of *digoxin,* a drug for heart failure. Other drugs whose levels can probably be reduced by this mechanism include calcium channel blockers, steroid hormones, protease inhibitors, and certain anticancer drugs (e.g., etoposide, paclitaxel, vinblastine, and vincristine).
- Combining St. John's wort with certain drugs can intensify serotonergic transmission to a degree sufficient to cause potentially fatal *serotonin syndrome.* Although St. John's wort can enhance serotonergic transmission by itself, its effect is relatively weak. Hence, when used alone, the herb poses little risk. However, if St. John's wort is combined with other serotonin-enhancing agents, the risk is greatly increased; therefore St. John's wort should not be combined with such drugs. Among these are amphetamine, cocaine, and many antidepressants, including MAO inhibitors, selective serotonin reuptake inhibitors, certain tricyclic agents (e.g., amitriptyline and clomipramine), and duloxetine, nefazodone, and venlafaxine.

Because St. John's wort has a variety of known adverse interactions and is likely to have more that are as yet unknown, caution is clearly advised. St. John's wort is not recommended for treating depression in patients taking other medications.

Valerian

Valerian (*Valeriana officinalis*), also known as garden heliotrope, is a common plant in Europe and Asia, although it is grown in some areas of North America. The plant's rhizomes and roots are used in the preparation of medicinal products.

Uses

Valerian root is a sedative preparation used primarily to promote sleep. In addition, some people take it to reduce anxiety-associated restlessness.

Actions

Valerian may work by increasing the availability of γ-aminobutyric acid (GABA, an inhibitory neurotransmitter) at synapses in the CNS. (Benzodiazepines and benzodiazepine-like drugs, which are the major conventional hypnotics, act by potentiating the actions of GABA.) In addition, valerian may act as a direct GABA agonist. The active ingredients in valerian have not been identified.

Effectiveness

Although valerian has been used for centuries in Europe, China, and other countries, objective evidence of its efficacy is lacking. According to the NCCIH at https://nccih.nih.gov/health/providers/digest/sleep-disorders-science, "Various herbs such as valerian, chamomile, and kava, and homeopathic medicines sometimes used as sleep aids have not been shown to be effective for insomnia." Even so, some suggest it may still have mild sedative effects that may be useful for anxiety.

Adverse Effects

Valerian is generally very well tolerated. The FDA has given valerian a Generally Recognized as Safe (GRAS) rating when the product is consumed in amounts commonly used in food. Possible side effects include daytime drowsiness, dizziness, depression, dyspepsia, and pruritus. Prolonged use may cause headache, nervousness, or cardiac abnormalities. Because valerian can reduce alertness, users should exercise caution when performing dangerous activities, such as driving or operating dangerous machinery. In addition, valerian should be used with caution by people with psychiatric illnesses (e.g., depression and dementia). As with benzodiazepines, there may be a risk for paradoxical excitation and physical dependence. We do not know if valerian enters breast milk or harms the developing fetus. Until more is known, valerian should be avoided by women who are pregnant or breastfeeding.

Interactions With Conventional Drugs

In theory, valerian can potentiate the actions of other drugs with CNS-depressant actions. Among these are alcohol, benzodiazepines, barbiturates, opioids, antihistamines, and centrally acting skeletal muscle relaxants. These combinations should be used with caution.

HARMFUL SUPPLEMENTS TO AVOID

To help protect the public from dangerous botanical products, the FDA and the Federal Trade Commission are monitoring adverse event data and issuing warnings to consumers and manufacturers. Three potentially harmful products—comfrey, kava, and Ma huang—are discussed here.

Comfrey

Comfrey (*Symphytum officinale*) is an herbal supplement used topically and orally. Topical use appears safe for short term use but is contraindicated for use on open skin lesions. Oral use is not safe because comfrey contains PAs, which can cause venoocclusive disease (VOD) in animals and hepatic VOD in humans. Hepatic VOD can result in severe liver damage. In addition to causing VOD, PAs may also be carcinogenic. Accordingly, in July of 2001, the FDA issued a letter to dietary supplement manufacturers advising them to remove comfrey from the market. They urged manufacturers to discontinue production, pull existing product off the shelves, and warn consumers of the possible dangers; however, comfrey remains widely available for sale on the internet and elsewhere.

Kava

Kava (*Piper methysticum*), also known as *kava-kava* or *awa*, is used to relieve anxiety, promote sleep, and relax muscles. In the United States,

the herb has been promoted as a natural alternative to benzodiazepines (e.g., diazepam [Valium]) for treating anxiety and stress. Unfortunately, kava can cause severe liver injury, leading the FDA to issue a public warning in March 2002. Later that year, the Centers for Disease Control and Prevention issued a report on kava-related hepatotoxicity. In the report, they discussed 11 cases of hepatotoxicity from the United States and Europe in which the victims required a liver transplant owing to severe liver failure. Because of concerns over hepatotoxicity, kava sales have been restricted in some countries but not yet in the United States.

Ma Huang (Ephedra)

Ma huang (ephedra) contains ephedrine, a compound that can elevate blood pressure and stimulate the heart and CNS. High-dose ephedra has been associated with stroke, myocardial infarction, and death. To date, more than 17 000 adverse events have been reported, and at least 155 users have died. In 2004 the FDA banned US sales of all ephedra products, marking the first time that a dietary supplement has been ordered off the market. The ban was challenged by an ephedra producer and, in 2005, was partially reversed: a federal court upheld the ban for ephedra products that contain more than 10 mg per dose but reversed the ban for products that contain 10 mg or less, arguing that there are insufficient data to prove that low doses pose a "significant or unreasonable risk." In 2006, a federal appeals court upheld the FDA ban of ephedra. This ban was challenged again in 2007, but the US Court of Appeals denied the petition for a rehearing. At this time the FDA ban does not apply to ephedra in traditional Asian medicines or in herbal teas, which are not marketed as dietary supplements.

PATIENT EDUCATION
Dietary Supplements

Make certain that your patients understand the following concerns regarding any dietary supplement.
- Over-the-counter dietary supplements are not necessarily safe. All agents have risks as well as benefits.
- Dietary supplements may interact with medications that patients are taking. In some instances, these interactions can be dangerous. In other instances, they may prevent prescribed medications from being effective.
- It is important for patients to report the use of all drugs, including supplements, at each clinic visit.
- Patients need to know that a lot of inaccurate information may be found on television, online, in magazines, and in other media sources. Be certain to give them an authoritative source for reliable information, such as the National Center for Complementary and Integrative Health website at https://nccih.nih.gov. This is also a good source for patient handouts; the NCCIH's supplement information sheets are in the public domain and duplication is encouraged.

Basic Principles of Antimicrobial Therapy

Modern antimicrobial agents had their debut in the 1930s and 1940s and have greatly reduced morbidity and mortality from infection. As newer drugs are introduced, our ability to fight infections increases even more. However, despite impressive advances, continued progress is needed. There remain organisms that respond poorly to available drugs; there are effective drugs whose use is limited by toxicity; and there is, because of evolving microbial resistance, the constant threat that currently effective antibiotics will be rendered useless.

Here we focus on two principal themes. The first is microbial susceptibility to drugs, with special emphasis on resistance. The second is clinical use of antimicrobials. Topics addressed include criteria for drug selection, host factors that modify drug use, use of antimicrobial combinations, and use of antimicrobial agents for prophylaxis.

Before going further, we need to consider two terms: *antibiotic* and *antimicrobial drug.* In common practice, the terms *antibiotic* and *antimicrobial drug* are used interchangeably, as they are in this book. However, be aware that the formal definitions of these words are not identical. Strictly speaking, an *antibiotic* is a chemical that is produced by one microbe and has the ability to harm other microbes. Under this definition, only those compounds that are actually made by microorganisms qualify as antibiotics. Drugs such as the sulfonamides, which are produced in the laboratory, would not be considered antibiotics under the strict definition. In contrast, an *antimicrobial drug* is defined as any agent, natural or synthetic, that has the ability to kill or suppress microorganisms. Under this definition, no distinction is made between compounds produced by microbes and those made by chemists. From the perspective of therapeutics, there is no benefit to distinguishing between drugs made by microorganisms and drugs made by chemists. Hence the current practice is to use the terms *antibiotic* and *antimicrobial drug* interchangeably.

SELECTIVE TOXICITY

Selective toxicity is defined as the ability of a drug to injure a target cell or target organism without injuring other cells or organisms that are in intimate contact with the target. As applied to antimicrobial drugs, selective toxicity indicates the ability of an antibiotic to kill or suppress microbial pathogens without causing injury to the host. Selective toxicity is the property that makes antibiotics valuable. If it were not for selective toxicity—that is, if antibiotics were as harmful to the host as they are to infecting organisms—these drugs would have no therapeutic utility.

Achieving Selective Toxicity

How can a drug be highly toxic to microbes but harmless to the host? The answer lies with differences in the cellular chemistry of mammals

and microbes. There are biochemical processes critical to microbial well-being that do not take place in mammalian cells. Hence drugs that selectively interfere with these unique microbial processes can cause serious injury to microorganisms while leaving mammalian cells intact. Three examples of how we achieve selective toxicity are discussed here.

Disruption of the Bacterial Cell Wall

Unlike mammalian cells, bacteria are encased in a rigid cell wall. The protoplasm within this wall has a high concentration of solutes, making osmotic pressure within the bacterium high. If it were not for the cell wall, bacteria would absorb water, swell, and then burst. Several families of drugs (e.g., penicillins and cephalosporins) weaken the cell wall and, hence, promote bacterial lysis. Because mammalian cells have no cell wall, drugs directed at this structure do not affect humans.

Inhibition of an Enzyme Unique to Bacteria

The sulfonamides represent antibiotics that are selectively toxic because they inhibit an enzyme critical to bacterial survival but not to our survival. Specifically, sulfonamides inhibit an enzyme needed to make folic acid, a compound required by all cells, both mammalian and bacterial. Because we can use folic acid from dietary sources, sulfonamides are safe for human consumption. In contrast, bacteria must synthesize folic acid themselves (because, unlike us, they cannot take up folic acid from the environment). Hence, to meet their needs, bacteria first take up *para*-aminobenzoic acid (PABA), a precursor of folic acid, and then convert the PABA into folic acid. Sulfonamides block this conversion. Because mammalian cells do not make their own folic acid, sulfonamide toxicity is limited to microbes.

Disruption of Bacterial Protein Synthesis

In bacteria, as in mammalian cells, protein synthesis is completed by ribosomes. However, bacterial and mammalian ribosomes are not identical, and hence we can make drugs that disrupt function of one but not the other. As a result, we can impair protein synthesis in bacteria while leaving mammalian protein synthesis untouched.

CLASSIFICATION OF ANTIMICROBIAL DRUGS

Various schemes are used to classify antimicrobial drugs. The two schemes most suited to our objectives are considered here.

Classification by Susceptible Organism

Antibiotics differ widely in their antimicrobial activity. Some agents, called *narrow-spectrum antibiotics,* are active against only a few species of microorganisms. In contrast, *broad-spectrum antibiotics* are active against a wide variety of microbes. As discussed later, *narrow-spectrum drugs are generally preferred to broad-spectrum drugs.*

Table 70.1 classifies the major antimicrobial drugs according to susceptible organisms. The table shows three major groups: *antibacterial drugs, antifungal drugs,* and *antiviral drugs.* In addition, the table subdivides the antibacterial drugs into narrow-spectrum and broad-spectrum agents, and indicates the principal classes of bacteria against which they are active.

Classification by Mechanism of Action

The antimicrobial drugs fall into seven major groups based on mechanism of action. This classification is shown in Table 70.2. Properties of the seven major classes are discussed briefly here.

- *Drugs that inhibit bacterial cell wall synthesis or activate enzymes that disrupt the cell wall.* These drugs (e.g., penicillins and cephalosporins) weaken the cell wall and, hence, promote bacterial lysis and death.
- *Drugs that increase cell membrane permeability.* Drugs in this group (e.g., amphotericin B) increase the permeability of cell membranes, causing leakage of intracellular material.
- *Drugs that cause lethal inhibition of bacterial protein synthesis.* The aminoglycosides (e.g., gentamicin) are the only drugs in this group. We do not know why inhibition of protein synthesis by these agents results in cell death.
- *Drugs that cause nonlethal inhibition of protein synthesis.* Like the aminoglycosides, these drugs (e.g., tetracyclines) inhibit bacterial protein synthesis. However, in contrast to the aminoglycosides, these agents only slow microbial growth; they do not kill bacteria at clinically achievable concentrations.
- *Drugs that inhibit bacterial synthesis of DNA and RNA or disrupt DNA function.* These drugs inhibit synthesis of DNA or RNA by binding directly to nucleic acids or by interacting with enzymes required for nucleic acid synthesis. They may also bind with DNA and disrupt its function. Members of this group include rifampin, metronidazole, and the fluoroquinolones (e.g., ciprofloxacin).
- *Antimetabolites.* These drugs disrupt specific biochemical reactions. The result is either a decrease in the synthesis of essential cell

TABLE 70.1 Classification of Antimicrobial Drugs by Susceptible Organisms

Antibacterial Drugs
Narrow Spectrum

Gram-positive cocci and gram-positive bacilli	Penicillin G and V
	Penicillinase-resistant penicillins: oxacillin and nafcillin
	Vancomycin
	Erythromycin
	Clindamycin
Gram-negative aerobes	Aminoglycosides: gentamicin and others
	Cephalosporins (first and second generations)
Mycobacterium tuberculosis	Isoniazid
	Rifampin
	Ethambutol
	Pyrazinamide

Broad Spectrum

Gram-positive cocci and gram-negative bacilli	Broad-spectrum penicillins: ampicillin and others
	Extended-spectrum penicillins: piperacillin and others
	Cephalosporins (third generation)
	Tetracyclines: tetracycline and others
	Carbapenems: imipenem and others
	Trimethoprim
	Sulfonamides: sulfisoxazole and others
	Fluoroquinolones: ciprofloxacin and others

Antiviral Drugs

Drugs for HIV infection	Reverse transcriptase inhibitors: zidovudine and others
	Protease inhibitors: ritonavir and others
	Fusion inhibitors: enfuvirtide
	Integrase inhibitors: raltegravir
	CCR5 antagonists: maraviroc
Drugs for influenza	Adamantanes: amantadine and others
	Neuraminidase inhibitors: oseltamivir and others
Other antiviral drugs	Acyclovir
	Ribavirin
	Interferon-α
Antifungal Drugs	Polyene antibiotics: amphotericin B and others
	Azoles: itraconazole and others
	Echinocandins: caspofungin and others

TABLE 70.2 Classification of Antimicrobial Drugs by Mechanism of Action

Drug Class	Representative Antibiotics
Inhibitors of cell wall synthesis	Penicillins
	Cephalosporins
	Imipenem
	Vancomycin
	Caspofungin
Drugs that disrupt the cell membrane	Amphotericin B
	Daptomycin
	Itraconazole
Bactericidal inhibitors of protein synthesis	Aminoglycosides
Bacteriostatic inhibitors of protein synthesis	Clindamycin
	Erythromycin
	Linezolid
	Tetracyclines
Drugs that interfere with synthesis or integrity of bacterial DNA and RNA	Fluoroquinolones
	Metronidazole
	Rifampin
Antimetabolites	Flucytosine
	Sulfonamides
	Trimethoprim
Drugs that suppress viral replication	
Viral DNA polymerase inhibitors	Acyclovir
	Ganciclovir
HIV reverse transcriptase inhibitors	Zidovudine
	Lamivudine
HIV protease inhibitors	Ritonavir
	Saquinavir
HIV fusion inhibitors	Enfuvirtide
HIV integrase inhibitors	Raltegravir
HIV CCR5 antagonists	Maraviroc
Influenza neuraminidase inhibitors	Oseltamivir
	Zanamivir

constituents or synthesis of nonfunctional analogs of normal metabolites. Examples of antimetabolites include trimethoprim and the sulfonamides.

• *Drugs that suppress viral replication.* Most of these drugs inhibit specific enzymes—DNA polymerase, reverse transcriptase, protease, integrase, or neuraminidase—required for viral replication and infectivity.

When considering the *antibacterial* drugs, it is useful to distinguish between agents that are *bactericidal* and agents that are *bacteriostatic*. Bactericidal drugs are directly lethal to bacteria at clinically achievable concentrations. In contrast, *bacteriostatic* drugs can slow bacterial growth but do not cause cell death. When a bacteriostatic drug is used, elimination of bacteria must ultimately be accomplished by host defenses (i.e., the immune system working in concert with phagocytic cells).

ACQUIRED RESISTANCE TO ANTIMICROBIAL DRUGS

In this section, we discuss bacterial resistance to antibiotics, which may be *innate* (natural and inborn) or *acquired* over time. Discussion here is limited to acquired resistance, which is a much greater clinical concern than innate resistance.

Over time, an organism that had once been highly sensitive to an antibiotic may become less susceptible, or it may lose drug sensitivity entirely. In some cases, resistance develops to several drugs. Acquired

resistance is of great concern in that it can render currently effective drugs useless, thereby creating a clinical crisis and a constant need for new antimicrobial agents. As a rule, antibiotic resistance is associated with extended hospitalization, significant morbidity, and excess mortality. Organisms for which drug resistance is currently a serious problem include *Enterococcus faecium, Staphylococcus aureus, Enterobacter* species, *Pseudomonas aeruginosa, Acinetobacter baumannii, Klebsiella* species, and *Clostridiodies difficile* (Table 70.3). Two of these resistant bacteria—methicillin-resistant *S. aureus* and *C. difficile*—are discussed in Chapters 71 and 72, respectively.

In the discussion that follows, we examine the mechanisms by which microbial drug resistance is acquired and the measures by which emergence of resistance can be delayed. As you read this section, keep in mind that it is the *microbe* that becomes drug resistant, *not the patient*.

Microbial Mechanisms of Drug Resistance

Microbes have four basic mechanisms for resisting drugs. They can (1) decrease the concentration of a drug at its site of action, (2) alter the structure of drug target molecules, (3) produce a drug antagonist, and (4) cause drug inactivation.

Reduction of Drug Concentration at Its Site of Action

For most antimicrobial drugs, the site of action is intracellular. Accordingly, if a "bug" can reduce the intracellular concentration of a drug,

TABLE 70.3 Drugs for Highly Resistant Bacteria

Bacterium	Resistance	Resistance Mechanism	Alternative Treatments
Enterococcus faecium	Ampicillin	Mutation and overexpression of PBP5	Quinupristin/dalfopristin, daptomycin, tigecycline, and linezolid
	Linezolid	Production of altered 23S ribosomes	Quinupristin/dalfopristin, daptomycin, and tigecycline
	Daptomycin	Unknown	Quinupristin/dalfopristin
	Quinupristin/dalfopristin	Production of enzymes that inactivate quinupristin/dalfopristin and alter drug target	Daptomycin, tigecycline, and linezolid
	Aminoglycosides	Production of aminoglycoside-modifying enzymes and ribosomal mutations	May attempt to test for streptomycin sensitivity
Staphylococcus aureus[a]	Vancomycin	Thickening of cell wall and altered structure of cell wall precursor molecules	Quinupristin/dalfopristin, daptomycin, tigecycline, linezolid, and telavancin
	Daptomycin	Altered structure of cell wall and cell membrane	Quinupristin/dalfopristin, tigecycline, linezolid, and telavancin
	Linezolid	Production of altered 23S ribosomes	Quinupristin/dalfopristin, daptomycin, tigecycline, telavancin, ceftobiprole, and ceftaroline
Enterobacter species	Ceftriaxone, cefotaxime, ceftazidime, and cefepime	Production of extended-spectrum β-lactamases	Carbapenems, tigecycline
	Carbapenems	Production of carbapenemases and decreased permeability	Polymyxins and tigecycline
Klebsiella species	Ceftriaxone, cefotaxime, ceftazidime, cefepime	Production of extended-spectrum β-lactamases	Carbapenems and tigecycline
	Carbapenems	Production of carbapenemases and decreased permeability	Polymyxins and tigecycline
Pseudomonas aeruginosa	Carbapenems	Decreased permeability, increased drug efflux, and production of carbapenemases	Polymyxins
Acinetobacter baumannii	Carbapenems	Decreased permeability, increased drug efflux, and production of carbapenemases	Polymyxins
Clostridiodies difficile[b]	Metronidazole	Reduced drug activation, increased drug efflux, and increased repair of drug-induced DNA damage	Vancomycin and rifaximin

[a]Methicillin-resistant *Staphylococcus aureus* is discussed in Chapter 71.
[b]*Clostridiodies difficile* infection is discussed in Chapter 72.
PBP5, Penicillin-binding protein 5.

it can resist harm. Two basic mechanisms are involved. First, microbes can *cease active uptake* of certain drugs—tetracyclines and gentamicin, for example. Second, microbes can *increase active export* of certain drugs—tetracyclines, fluoroquinolones, and macrolides, for example.

Alteration of Drug Target Molecules

Most antibiotics, like most other drugs, must interact with target molecules (receptors) to produce their effects. Hence, if the structure of the target molecule is altered, resistance can result. For example, some bacteria are currently resistant to streptomycin because of structural changes in bacterial ribosomes, the sites at which streptomycin acts to inhibit protein synthesis.

Antagonist Production

In rare cases a microbe can synthesize a compound that antagonizes drug actions. For example, by acquiring the ability to synthesize increased quantities of PABA, some bacteria have developed resistance to sulfonamides.

Drug Inactivation

Microbes can resist harm by producing drug-metabolizing enzymes. For example, many bacteria are resistant to penicillin G because of increased production of penicillinase, an enzyme that inactivates penicillin. In addition to penicillins, bacterial enzymes can inactivate other antibiotics, including cephalosporins, carbapenems, and fluoroquinolones.

New Delhi metallo-β-lactamase 1 (NDM-1) gene. Extensive drug resistance is conferred by the *NDM-1* gene, which codes for a powerful form of β-lactamase. As discussed in Chapters 71 and 72, β-lactamases are enzymes that can inactivate drugs that have a β-lactam ring. The form of β-lactamase encoded by *NDM-1* is both unusual and troubling in that it can inactivate essentially all β-lactam antibiotics, a group that includes penicillins, cephalosporins, and carbapenems. Because the *NDM-1* gene is resistant to carbapenems, it is also classified as a type of carbapenem-resistant Enterobacteriaceae (CRE). Worse yet, the DNA segment that contains the *NDM-1* gene also contains genes that code for additional resistance determinants, including drug efflux pumps, and enzymes that can inactivate other important antibiotics, including erythromycin, rifampin, chloramphenicol, and fluoroquinolones. Furthermore, all of these genes are present on a plasmid, a piece of DNA that can be easily transferred from one bacterium to another (see later). Of note, bacteria that have the *NDM-1* gene are resistant to nearly all antibiotics, except for tigecycline and colistin. Since its discovery in *Klebsiella pneumoniae* in 2008, *NDM-1* has been found in other common enteric bacteria, including *Escherichia coli, Enterobacter* and *Salmonella* species, *Citrobacter freundii, Providencia rettgeri,* and *Morganella morganii.*

Mechanisms by Which Resistance Is Acquired

Ultimately, all of the alterations in structure and function discussed previously result from changes in the microbial genome. These genetic changes may result either from spontaneous mutation or from acquisition of DNA from an external source. One important mechanism of DNA acquisition is conjugation with other bacteria.

Spontaneous Mutation

Spontaneous mutations produce random changes in a microbe's DNA. The result is a gradual increase in resistance. Low-level resistance develops first. With additional mutations, resistance becomes greater. As a rule, spontaneous mutations confer resistance *to only one drug.*

Conjugation

Conjugation is a process by which extrachromosomal DNA is transferred from one bacterium to another. To transfer resistance by conjugation,

the donor organism must possess two unique DNA segments, one that codes for the mechanisms of drug resistance and one that codes for the "sexual" apparatus required for DNA transfer. Together, these two DNA segments constitute an *R factor* (resistance factor).

Conjugation takes place primarily among *gram-negative* bacteria. Genetic material may be transferred between members of the same species or between members of different species. Because transfer of R factors is not species specific, it is possible for pathogenic bacteria to acquire R factors from the normal flora of the body. Because R factors are becoming common in normal flora, the possibility of transferring resistance from normal flora to pathogens is a significant clinical concern.

In contrast to spontaneous mutation, conjugation frequently confers *multiple-drug resistance.* This can be achieved, for example, by transferring DNA that codes for several different drug-metabolizing enzymes. Hence, in a single event, a drug-sensitive bacterium can become highly drug resistant.

Relationships Between Antibiotic Use and Emergence of Drug-Resistant Microbes

Use of antibiotics promotes the emergence of drug-resistant microbes. However, please note that although antibiotics promote drug resistance, they are not mutagenic and do not directly cause the genetic changes that underlie reduced drug sensitivity. Spontaneous mutation and conjugation are random events whose incidence is independent of drug use. Drugs simply make conditions favorable for overgrowth of microbes that have acquired mechanisms for resistance.

How Do Antibiotics Promote Resistance?

To answer this question, we need to recall two aspects of microbial ecology: (1) microbes secrete compounds that are toxic to other microbes, and (2) microbes within a given ecologic location (e.g., large intestine, urogenital tract, and skin) compete with each other for available nutrients. Under drug-free conditions, the various microbes in a given region keep each other in check. Furthermore, if none of these organisms is drug resistant, introduction of antibiotics will be equally detrimental to all members of the population and, therefore, will not promote the growth of any individual microbe. However, *if a drug-resistant organism is present, antibiotics will create selection pressure favoring its growth* by killing off sensitive organisms. In doing so, the drug will eliminate the toxins they produce and will, hence, facilitate survival of the microbe that is drug resistant. In addition, elimination of sensitive organisms will remove competition for available nutrients, thereby making conditions even more favorable for the resistant microbe to flourish. Hence, although drug resistance is of no benefit to an organism when there are no antibiotics present, when antibiotics are introduced, they create selection pressure favoring overgrowth of microbes that are resistant.

Which Antibiotics Promote Resistance?

All antimicrobial drugs promote the emergence of drug-resistant organisms. However, some agents are more likely to promote resistance than others. Because broad-spectrum antibiotics kill more competing organisms than do narrow-spectrum drugs, broad-spectrum agents do the most to facilitate emergence of resistance.

Influence of Increased Antibiotic Use on the Emergence of Resistance

The more those antibiotics are used, the faster drug-resistant organisms will emerge. Not only do antibiotics promote emergence of resistant pathogens, they also promote overgrowth of normal flora that possess mechanisms for resistance. Because drug use can increase resistance in normal flora and because normal flora can transfer resistance to pathogens by conjugation, every effort should be made to avoid use of antibiotics by individuals who do not actually need them (i.e., individuals who do not have a bacterial infection). Because all antibiotic use will further lead to the the the emergence of resistance, there can be no excuse for casual or indiscriminate dispensing of these drugs.

Health Care–Associated Infections

Because hospitals are sites of intensive antibiotic use, resident organisms can be extremely drug resistant. As a result, *health care–associated infections (HAIs)* are among the most difficult to treat. According to the Centers for Disease Control and Prevention (CDC), 1 of every 20 patients will fall victim to an HAI. Measures to delay emergence of resistant organisms in hospitals are discussed later.

Superinfection

A superinfection is defined as a *new* infection that appears during the course of treatment for a primary infection.

New infections develop when antibiotics eliminate the inhibitory influence of normal flora, thereby allowing a second infectious agent to flourish. A common example of superinfection is the development of a vaginal *Candida* infection in a female treated with a broad spectrum antibiotic for a urinary tract infection.

Because broad-spectrum antibiotics kill more normal flora than do narrow-spectrum drugs, superinfections are more likely in patients receiving broad-spectrum agents.

Antimicrobial Stewardship

Many organizations have begun to address the issue of antibiotic resistance in health care. In 2012, the Infectious Diseases Society of America (IDSA), in conjunction with the Society for Healthcare Epidemiology of America (SHEA) and the Pediatric Infectious Diseases Society (PIDS), released its first *Statement on Antimicrobial Stewardship.* The statement included five recommendations, with suggestions for monitoring, education, and research to assist in the prevention of antibiotic resistance. The statement can be found online at http://www.jstor.org/stable/10.1086/665010.

The American Board of Internal Medicine (ABIM) Foundation also created the *Choosing Wisely* Campaign in 2012 to decrease the amount of wasteful practice in health care. More than 70 specialty organizations have contributed guidelines to promote evidence-based practice. Many of these guidelines address the appropriate use of antimicrobial therapy. *Choosing Wisely* can be located at http://www.choosingwisely.org. The *Get Smart for Healthcare* Campaign initiated by the CDC provides information on proper use of antibiotics in humans and animals. The campaign has three objectives: to promote adherence to appropriate prescribing guidelines, to decrease demand for antibiotics among healthy adults and parents of young children, and to increase adherence to prescribed antibiotics. Target audiences include patients and providers. More information is available at www.cdc.gov/drugresistance.

In addition to the CDC Campaign, in 2014, the Interagency Task Force on Antimicrobial Resistance published an update to its original publication, *A Public Health Action Plan to Combat Antimicrobial Resistance.* This updated action plan discusses four focus areas developed to decrease resistance to antibiotics:

• *Focus Area I: Surveillance, Prevention, and Control of Antimicrobial Resistant Infections.* Goals include improving the detection, monitoring, and characterization of drug-resistant infections in humans and animals, as well as improving the definition, characterization, and measurement of the impact of antimicrobial drug use.
• *Focus Area II: Research.* Goals include facilitation of basic research on antimicrobial resistance, as well as translation of basic research

into practice. Support for epidemiologic studies to identify key drivers of the emergence and spread of antimicrobial resistance is of great importance.
• *Focus Area III: Regulatory Pathways for New Products.* Aims for product development include provision of information on the status of antibacterial drug product development and encouraging development of rapid diagnostic tests and vaccines.
• *Focus Area IV: Product Development.* Goals include providing a systematic assessment of current and future needs for antimicrobial resistance products and promoting the development of drugs targeted to address areas where unmet needs exist.

SELECTION OF ANTIBIOTICS

When treating infection, the therapeutic objective is to produce maximal antimicrobial effects while causing minimal harm to the host. To achieve this goal, we must select the most appropriate antibiotic for the individual patient. When choosing an antibiotic, three principal factors must be considered: (1) the identity of the infecting organism (Table 70.4), (2) drug sensitivity of the infecting organism, and (3) host factors, such as the site of infection and the status of host defenses.

For any given infection, several drugs may be effective. However, for most infections, there is usually one drug that is superior to the alternatives (Table 70.5). This drug of first choice may be preferred for several reasons, such as greater efficacy, lower toxicity, or more narrow spectrum. Whenever possible, the drug of first choice should be used. Alternative agents should be used only when the first-choice drug is inappropriate. Conditions that might rule out a first-choice agent include (1) allergy to the drug of choice, (2) inability of the drug of choice to penetrate to the site of infection, and (3) heightened susceptibility of the patient to toxicity of the first-choice drug.

Empiric Therapy Before Completion of Laboratory Tests

Optimal antimicrobial therapy requires identification of the infecting organism and determination of its drug sensitivity. However, when the patient has a severe infection, we may have to initiate treatment before test results are available. Under these conditions, drug selection must be based on clinical evaluation and knowledge of which microbes are most likely to cause infection at a particular site. If necessary, a broad-spectrum agent can be used for initial treatment. After the identity and drug sensitivity

TABLE 70.4 Common Infections Caused by Common "Bugs"

Infection	Bacteria
Bacterial meningitis	*Streptococcus pneumoniae* and *Neisseria meningitides*
Acute sinusitis	*S. pneumoniae* and *Haemophilus influenzae*
Pharyngitis	*Streptococcus pyogenes*
Community-acquired pneumonia	*S. pneumoniae, Mycoplasma* spp., *H. influenzae,* and *Staphylococcus aureus*
Hospital-acquired pneumonia	*Pseudomonas* spp., *Klebsiella* spp., and *S. aureus*
Endocarditis	*Streptococcus viridans,* coagulase-negative *Staphylococcus* spp., and *S. aureus*
Cholangitis	Enterobacteriaceae and anaerobes
Urinary tract infection, pyelonephritis	*Escherichia coli* and Enterobacteriaceae
Osteomyelitis	*S. aureus*
Cellulitis	*S. aureus* and *Streptococcus* spp.

TABLE 70.5   Antibacterial Drugs of Choice

Organism	Drug of First Choice	Some Alternative Drugs
Gram-Positive Cocci		
Enterococcus[a]		
Endocarditis and other severe infections	Penicillin G *or* ampicillin *with either* gentamicin or streptomycin	Vancomycin *with either* gentamicin or streptomycin, quinupristin/dalfopristin, linezolid, and daptomycin
Uncomplicated urinary tract infection	Amoxicillin	Nitrofurantoin and a fluoroquinolone; fosfomycin
Staphylococcus aureus or *epidermidis*[a]		
Penicillinase producing	A penicillinase-resistant penicillin	A cephalosporin, vancomycin, imipenem, linezolid, clindamycin, daptomycin, and a fluoroquinolone
Methicillin resistant	Vancomycin or daptomycin	Linezolid, quinupristin/dalfopristin, tigecycline, doxycycline, ceftaroline, and trimethoprim/sulfamethoxazole
Streptococcus pyogenes (group A) and groups C and G	Penicillin G, with clindamycin penicillin	Vancomycin, erythromycin, clarithromycin, azithromycin, daptomycin, linezolid, and a cephalosporin
Streptococcus, group B	Penicillin G or ampicillin	A cephalosporin, vancomycin, erythromycin, and daptomycin
Streptococcus viridans group	Penicillin G or ampicillin	A cephalosporin and vancomycin
Streptococcus bovis	Penicillin G or ampicillin	A cephalosporin and vancomycin
Streptococcus, anaerobic	Cephalosporin	Clindamycin and vancomycin
Streptococcus pneumoniae (pneumococcus)	Penicillin G, penicillin V, and amoxicillin in susceptible strains Resistant strains: a cephalosporin, ampicillin	Erythromycin, azithromycin, clarithromycin, levofloxacin, gemifloxacin, moxifloxacin, meropenem, imipenem, ertapenem, trimethoprim/sulfamethoxazole, clindamycin, a tetracycline, and vancomycin
Gram-Negative Cocci		
Neisseria gonorrhoeae (gonococcus)	See Chapter 82	
Neisseria meningitides (meningococcus)	Third-generation cephalosporin	Penicillin G, chloramphenicol, a sulfonamide, and a fluoroquinolone
Gram-Positive Bacilli		
Bacillus anthracis (anthrax)	Ciprofloxacin	Doxycycline, Amoxicillin
Clostridiodies difficile	See Chapter 72	
Clostridium perfringens	Penicillin G and clindamycin	Metronidazole, chloramphenicol, imipenem, meropenem, and ertapenem
Clostridium tetani	Metronidazole	Penicillin G and doxycycline
Corynebacterium diphtheriae	Erythromycin	Penicillin G
Listeria monocytogenes	Ampicillin or penicillin G with or without gentamicin	Trimethoprim/sulfamethoxazole
Enteric Gram-Negative Bacilli		
Campylobacter jejuni	Fluoroquinolones and azithromycin	Gentamicin and a tetracycline
Escherichia coli	Cefotaxime, ceftazidime, cefepime, and ceftriaxone	Ampicillin *with or without* gentamicin, ticarcillin/clavulanic acid, trimethoprim/sulfamethoxazole, imipenem, meropenem, and others
Enterobacter[a]	Imipenem, meropenem, and cefepime	Trimethoprim/sulfamethoxazole, gentamicin, tobramycin, amikacin, ciprofloxacin, cefotaxime, ticarcillin/clavulanic acid, piperacillin/tazobactam, aztreonam, ceftazidime, and tigecycline
Klebsiella pneumoniae[a]	Cefotaxime, ceftriaxone, cefepime, and ceftazidime	Imipenem, meropenem, ertapenem, gentamicin, tobramycin, amikacin, and others
Proteus, indole positive (including *Providencia rettgeri* and *Morganella morganii*)	Cefotaxime, ceftriaxone, cefepime, and ceftazidime	Imipenem, meropenem, ertapenem, gentamicin, a fluoroquinolone, trimethoprim/sulfamethoxazole, and others
Proteus mirabilis	Ampicillin	A cephalosporin, ticarcillin, trimethoprim/sulfamethoxazole, imipenem, meropenem, ertapenem, gentamicin, and others
Salmonella typhi	Ceftriaxone and a fluoroquinolone	Trimethoprim/sulfamethoxazole, ampicillin, amoxicillin, chloramphenicol, and azithromycin
Other *Salmonella*	Ceftriaxone, cefotaxime, and a fluoroquinolone	Trimethoprim/sulfamethoxazole, chloramphenicol, ampicillin, and amoxicillin

TABLE 70.5 Antibacterial Drugs of Choice—cont'd

Organism	Drug of First Choice	Some Alternative Drugs
Serratia	Imipenem and meropenem	Gentamicin, amikacin, cefotaxime, a fluoroquinolone, trimethoprim/sulfamethoxazole, aztreonam, and others
Shigella	A fluoroquinolone	Trimethoprim/sulfamethoxazole, ampicillin, ceftriaxone, and azithromycin
Yersinia enterocolitica	Trimethoprim/sulfamethoxazole	A fluoroquinolone, gentamicin, tobramycin, amikacin, and cefotaxime
Other Gram-Negative Bacilli		
Acinetobacter[a]	Imipenem and meropenem	An aminoglycoside, trimethoprim/sulfamethoxazole, doxycycline, ciprofloxacin, ceftazidime, ticarcillin/clavulanic acid, and piperacillin/tazobactam
Bacteroides	Metronidazole	Imipenem, ertapenem, meropenem, amoxicillin/clavulanic acid, ticarcillin/clavulanic acid, piperacillin/tazobactam, ampicillin/sulbactam, and chloramphenicol
Bordetella pertussis (whooping cough)	Azithromycin, clarithromycin, and erythromycin	Trimethoprim/sulfamethoxazole
Brucella (brucellosis)	A tetracycline plus rifampin	A tetracycline plus either gentamicin or streptomycin, trimethoprim/sulfamethoxazole with or without gentamicin, chloramphenicol with or without streptomycin, and ciprofloxacin plus rifampin
Klebsiella (formerly Calymmatobacterium) granulomatis	Azithromycin	Doxycycline, trimethoprim/sulfamethoxazole, or ciprofloxacin
Francisella tularensis (tularemia)	Streptomycin	Gentamycin, doxycycline, and ciprofloxacin
Gardnerella vaginalis	Metronidazole (PO)	Topical clindamycin or metronidazole and clindamycin (PO)
Haemophilus ducreyi (chancroid)	Azithromycin and ceftriaxone	Ciprofloxacin, erythromycin
Haemophilus influenzae		
Meningitis, epiglottitis, arthritis, and other serious infections	Cefotaxime and ceftriaxone	Cefuroxime, chloramphenicol, and meropenem
Upper respiratory infection and bronchitis	Trimethoprim/sulfamethoxazole	Cefuroxime, amoxicillin/clavulanic acid, a fluoroquinolone, and others
Helicobacter pylori	Clarithromycin plus amoxicillin plus esomeprazole (a proton pump inhibitor)	Tetracycline plus metronidazole plus bismuth subsalicylate plus esomeprazole (a proton pump inhibitor)
Legionella spp.	Azithromycin and clarithromycin	Doxycycline, trimethoprim/sulfamethoxazole, erythromycin, and fluoroquinolone
Pasteurella multocida	Penicillin G	Doxycycline, a second- or third-generation cephalosporin, amoxicillin/clavulanic acid, and ampicillin/sulbactam
Pseudomonas aeruginosa[a]		
Urinary tract infection	Ciprofloxacin	Levofloxacin, piperacillin/tazobactam, ceftazidime, cefepime, imipenem, meropenem, gentamicin, tobramycin, amikacin, and aztreonam
Other infections	Piperacillin/tazobactam (or ticarcillin/clavulanic acid) with or without tobramycin, gentamicin, or amikacin	Ceftazidime, ciprofloxacin, imipenem, meropenem, aztreonam, or cefepime, any one with or without tobramycin, gentamicin, or amikacin
Spirillum minus (rat-bite fever)	Penicillin G and ceftriaxone	Doxycycline and streptomycin
Streptobacillus moniliformis (rat-bite fever)	Penicillin G and ceftriaxone	Doxycycline and streptomycin
Vibrio cholerae (cholera)	A tetracycline	Trimethoprim/sulfamethoxazole and a fluoroquinolone
Yersinia pestis (plague)	Streptomycin with Gentamycin	Doxycycline, ciprofloxacin, and chloramphenicol
Mycobacteria		
Mycobacterium tuberculosis	See Chapter 77	
Mycobacterium leprae (leprosy)	See Chapter 77	
Mycobacterium avium complex	See Chapter 77	
Actinomycetes		
Actinomycetes israelii	Penicillin G	Doxycycline, erythromycin, and clindamycin
Nocardia	Trimethoprim/sulfamethoxazole	Sulfisoxazole, imipenem, meropenem, amikacin, a tetracycline, linezolid, ceftriaxone, and cycloserine

Continued

TABLE 70.5	Antibacterial Drugs of Choice—cont'd	
Organism	**Drug of First Choice**	**Some Alternative Drugs**
Chlamydiae		
Chlamydia psittaci	Doxycycline	Chloramphenicol
Chlamydia trachomatis	See Chapter 82	
Mycoplasma		
Mycoplasma pneumoniae	Erythromycin, clarithromycin, azithromycin, and a tetracycline	A fluoroquinolone
Ureaplasma urealyticum	Azithromycin	A tetracycline, clarithromycin, erythromycin, and ofloxacin
Rickettsia		
Rocky Mountain spotted fever, endemic typhus (murine), trench fever, typhus, scrub typhus, Q fever	Doxycycline	Chloramphenicol and a fluoroquinolone
Spirochetes		
Borrelia burgdorferi (Lyme disease)	Doxycycline, amoxicillin, and cefuroxime	Ceftriaxone, cefotaxime, penicillin G, azithromycin, and clarithromycin
Borrelia recurrentis (relapsing fever)	A tetracycline and penicillin G	Erythromycin
Leptospira	Penicillin G	Doxycycline and ceftriaxone
Treponema pallidum (syphilis)	Penicillin G	Doxycycline and ceftriaxone
Treponema pertenue (yaws)	Penicillin G	Doxycycline

[a]Many of these drugs have resistant strains that must be treated with alternative antibiotics.
PO, Per os.

of the infecting organism have been determined, we can switch to a more selective antibiotic. When conditions demand that we start therapy in the absence of laboratory data, it is essential that samples of exudates and body fluids be obtained for culture *before initiation of treatment;* if antibiotics are present at the time of sampling, they can suppress microbial growth in culture and can thereby confound identification.

Identifying the Infecting Organism

The first rule of antimicrobial therapy is to *match the drug with the bug.* Hence, whenever possible, the infecting organism should be identified before starting treatment. If treatment is begun in the absence of a definitive diagnosis, positive identification should be established as soon as possible to permit adjustment of the regimen to better conform with the drug sensitivity of the infecting organism.

The quickest, simplest, and most versatile technique for identifying microorganisms is microscopic examination of a *Gram-stained preparation.* Samples for examination can be obtained from exudate, sputum, urine, blood, and other body fluids. The most useful samples are direct aspirates from the site of infection.

In some cases, only a small number of infecting organisms will be present. Under these conditions, positive identification may require that the microbes be grown out in culture. As stressed previously, material for culture should be obtained before initiating treatment. Furthermore, the samples should be taken in a fashion that minimizes contamination with normal body flora. In addition, the samples should not be exposed to low temperature, antiseptics, or oxygen.

A relatively new method, known as the *polymerase chain reaction (PCR) test* or *nucleic acid amplification test,* can detect very low titers of bacteria and viruses. Testing is done by using an enzyme—either DNA polymerase or RNA polymerase—to generate thousands of copies of DNA or RNA unique to the infecting microbe. As a result of this nucleic acid amplification, there is enough material for detection. Microbes that we can identify with a PCR test include important bacterial

pathogens (e.g., *C. difficile, S. aureus, Mycobacterium tuberculosis, Neisseria gonorrhoeae, Chlamydia trachomatis,* and *Helicobacter pylori*) and important viral pathogens (e.g., human immunodeficiency virus [HIV] and influenza virus). Compared with Gram staining, PCR tests are both more specific and more sensitive.

Determining Drug Susceptibility

Owing to the emergence of drug-resistant microbes, testing for drug sensitivity is common. However, sensitivity testing is not always needed. Rather, testing is indicated only when the infecting organism is one in which resistance is likely. Hence, for microbes such as the group A streptococci, which have remained highly susceptible to penicillin G, sensitivity testing is unnecessary. In contrast, when resistance *is* common, as it is with *S. aureus* and the gram-negative bacilli, tests for drug sensitivity should be performed. Most tests currently used are based on one of three methods: disk diffusion, serial dilution, or gradient diffusion.

Before sensitivity testing can be done, we must first identify the microbe so that we can test for sensitivity to the appropriate drugs. For example, if the infection is caused by *C. difficile,* we might test for sensitivity to metronidazole or vancomycin. We would not test for sensitivity to aminoglycosides or cephalosporins—because we already know these drugs will not work.

HOST FACTORS THAT MODIFY DRUG CHOICE, ROUTE OF ADMINISTRATION, OR DOSAGE

In addition to matching the drug with the bug and determining the drug sensitivity of an infecting organism, we must consider host factors when prescribing an antimicrobial drug. Two host factors—host defenses and infection site—are unique to the selection of antibiotics. Other host factors, such as age, pregnancy, and previous drug reactions, are the same factors that must be considered when choosing any other drug.

Host Defenses

Host defenses consist primarily of the immune system and phagocytic cells (macrophages and neutrophils). Without the contribution of these defenses, successful antimicrobial therapy would be rare. In most cases, the drugs we use do not cure infection on their own. Rather, they work in concert with host defense systems to subdue infection. Accordingly, the usual objective of antibiotic treatment is not outright killing of infecting organisms. Rather, the goal is to suppress microbial growth to the point at which the balance is tipped in favor of the host. Underscoring the critical role of host defenses is the grim fact that people whose defenses are impaired, such as those with acquired immunodeficiency syndrome (AIDS) and those undergoing cancer chemotherapy, frequently die of infections that drugs alone are unable to control. When treating the immunocompromised host, our only hope lies with drugs that are rapidly bactericidal, and even these may prove inadequate.

Site of Infection

To be effective, an antibiotic must be present at the site of infection in a concentration greater than the minimal inhibitory concentration (MIC). At some sites, drug penetration may be hampered, making it difficult to achieve the MIC. For example, drug access can be impeded in meningitis (because of the blood-brain barrier), endocarditis (because bacterial vegetations in the heart are difficult to penetrate), and infected abscesses (because of poor vascularity and the presence of purulent material). When treating meningitis, two approaches may be used: (1) we can select a drug that readily crosses the blood-brain barrier, and (2) we can inject an antibiotic directly into the subarachnoid space. When exudate and other fluids hinder drug access, surgical drainage is indicated.

Foreign materials (e.g., cardiac pacemakers, prosthetic joints and heart valves, and synthetic vascular shunts) present a special local problem. Phagocytes react to these objects and attempt to destroy them. Because of this behavior, the phagocytes are less able to attack bacteria, thereby allowing microbes to flourish. Treatment of these infections often results in failure or relapse. In many cases the infection can be eliminated only by removing the foreign material.

Other Host Factors
Previous Allergic Reaction

Severe allergic reactions are more common with the penicillins than with any other family of drugs. As a rule, patients with a history of severe allergy to the penicillins should not receive them again. The exception is treatment of a life-threatening infection for which no suitable alternative is available. In addition to the penicillins, other antibiotics (sulfonamides, trimethoprim, and erythromycin) are associated with a high incidence of allergic responses. However, severe reactions to these agents are rare. It should also be noted that many reported penicillin allergies are not true allergies. Skin testing is available to distinguish true penicillin allergy from other reactions.

Genetic Factors

As with other drugs, responses to antibiotics can be influenced by the patient's genetic heritage. For example, some antibiotics (e.g., sulfonamides) can cause hemolysis in patients who, because of their genetic makeup, have red blood cells that are deficient in glucose-6-phosphate dehydrogenase (G6PD). People with this deficiency should not be given antibiotics that are likely to induce red cell lysis. G6PD deficiency is discussed further in Chapter 5.

Genetic factors can also affect rates of metabolism. For example, hepatic inactivation of isoniazid is rapid in some people and slow in

others. If the dosage is not adjusted accordingly, isoniazid may accumulate to toxic levels in the slow metabolizers and may fail to achieve therapeutic levels in the rapid metabolizers.

PATIENT-CENTERED CARE ACROSS THE LIFE SPAN
Antimicrobials

Life Stage	Patient Care Concerns
Infants	Infants are highly vulnerable to drug toxicity. Because of poorly developed kidney and liver function, neonates eliminate drugs slowly. Use of sulfonamides in newborns can produce kernicterus, a severe neurologic disorder caused by displacement of bilirubin from plasma proteins (see Chapter 75).
Children/ adolescents	The tetracyclines provide another example of toxicity unique to the young: these antibiotics bind to developing teeth, causing discoloration.
Pregnant women	Antimicrobial drugs can cross the placenta, posing a risk to the developing fetus. For example, when gentamicin is used during pregnancy, irreversible hearing loss in the infant may result. Antibiotic use during pregnancy may also pose a risk to the expectant mother.
Breastfeeding women	Antibiotics can enter breast milk, possibly affecting the nursing infant. For example, sulfonamides can reach levels in milk that are sufficient to cause kernicterus in nursing newborns. As a general guideline, antibiotics and all other drugs should be avoided by women who are breastfeeding. If antimicrobial therapy is considered, the benefits should outweigh the risks.
Older adults	In the older adult, heightened drug sensitivity is due in large part to reduced rates of drug metabolism and drug excretion, which can result in accumulation of antibiotics to toxic levels.

DOSAGE AND DURATION OF TREATMENT

Success requires that the antibiotic be present at the site of infection in an effective concentration for a sufficient time. Dosages should be adjusted to produce drug concentrations that are equal to or greater than the MIC for the infection being treated. Drug levels 4 to 8 times the MIC are often desirable.

Duration of therapy depends on a number of variables, including the status of host defenses, the site of the infection, and the identity of the infecting organism.

PATIENT EDUCATION
Finishing the Prescribed Course

It is imperative that antibiotics not be discontinued prematurely. Accordingly, patients should be instructed to take their medication for the entire prescribed course, even though symptoms may subside before the full course has been completed. Early discontinuation is a common cause of recurrent infection, and the organisms responsible for relapse are likely to be more drug resistant than those present when treatment began.

THERAPY WITH ANTIBIOTIC COMBINATIONS

Therapy with a combination of antimicrobial agents is indicated only in specific situations. Under these well-defined conditions, use of multiple drugs may be lifesaving. However, it should be stressed that, although antibiotic combinations do have a valuable therapeutic role, routine use of two or more antibiotics should be discouraged. When an infection is caused by a single, identified microbe, treatment with just one drug is usually most appropriate.

Antimicrobial Effects of Antibiotic Combinations

When two antibiotics are used together, the result may be *additive, potentiative,* or, in certain cases, *antagonistic.* An *additive* response is one in which the antimicrobial effect of the combination is equal to the sum of the effects of the two drugs alone. A *potentiative* interaction (also called a *synergistic* interaction) is one in which the effect of the combination is greater than the sum of the effects of the individual agents. A classic example of potentiation is produced by trimethoprim plus sulfamethoxazole, drugs that inhibit sequential steps in the synthesis of tetrahydrofolic acid (see Chapter 75).

In certain cases a combination of two antibiotics may be *less* effective than one of the agents by itself, indicating *antagonism* between the drugs. Antagonism is most likely when a *bacteriostatic* agent (e.g., tetracycline) is combined with a *bactericidal* drug (e.g., penicillin). Antagonism occurs because bactericidal drugs are usually effective only against organisms that are actively growing. Hence, when bacterial growth has been suppressed by a bacteriostatic drug, the effects of a bactericidal agent can be reduced. If host defenses are intact, antagonism between two antibiotics may have little significance. However, if host defenses are compromised, the consequences can be dire.

Indications for Antibiotic Combinations
Initial Therapy of Severe Infection
The most common indication for using multiple antibiotics is initial therapy of severe infection of unknown etiology, especially in the neutropenic host. Until the infecting organism has been identified, wide antimicrobial coverage is appropriate. Just how broad the coverage should be depends on the clinician's skill in narrowing the field of potential pathogens. After the identity of the infecting microbe is known, drug selection can be adjusted accordingly. As discussed earlier, samples for culture should be obtained before drug therapy starts.

Mixed Infections
An infection may be caused by more than one microbial species. Multiple infectious organisms are common in brain abscesses, pelvic infections, and infections resulting from perforation of abdominal organs. When the infectious microbes differ from one another in drug susceptibility, treatment with more than one antibiotic is required.

Preventing Resistance
Although use of multiple antibiotics is usually associated with *promoting* drug resistance, there is one infectious disease—tuberculosis—in which drug combinations are used for the specific purpose of *suppressing* the emergence of resistant bacteria. Why tuberculosis differs from other infections in this regard is discussed in Chapter 77.

Decreased Toxicity
In some situations, an antibiotic combination can reduce toxicity to the host. For example, by combining flucytosine with amphotericin B in the treatment of fungal meningitis, the dosage of amphotericin B can be reduced, thereby decreasing the risk for amphotericin-induced damage to the kidneys.

Enhanced Antibacterial Action
In specific infections, a combination of antibiotics can have greater antibacterial action than a single agent. This is true of the combined use of penicillin plus an aminoglycoside in the treatment of enterococcal endocarditis. Penicillin acts to weaken the bacterial cell wall; the aminoglycoside acts to suppress protein synthesis. The combination has enhanced antibacterial action because, by weakening the cell wall, penicillin facilitates penetration of the aminoglycoside to its intracellular site of action.

Disadvantages of Antibiotic Combinations

Use of multiple antibiotics has several drawbacks, including (1) increased risk for toxic and allergic reactions, (2) possible antagonism of antimicrobial effects, (3) increased risk for superinfection, (4) selection of drug-resistant bacteria, and (5) increased cost. Accordingly, antimicrobial combinations should be used only when clearly indicated.

PROPHYLACTIC USE OF ANTIMICROBIAL DRUGS

Estimates indicate that between 30% and 50% of the antibiotics used in the United States are administered for prophylaxis. That is, these agents are given to prevent an infection rather than to treat an established infection. Much of this prophylactic use is uncalled for. However, in certain situations, antimicrobial prophylaxis is both appropriate and effective. Whenever prophylaxis is proposed, the benefits must be weighed against the risks for toxicity, allergic reactions, superinfection, and selection of drug-resistant organisms. Generally approved indications for prophylaxis are discussed next.

Surgery

Prophylactic use of antibiotics can decrease the incidence of infection in certain kinds of surgery. Procedures in which prophylactic efficacy has been documented include cardiac surgery, peripheral vascular surgery, orthopedic surgery, and surgery on the gastrointestinal (GI) tract (stomach, duodenum, colon, rectum, and appendix). Prophylaxis is also beneficial for women undergoing a hysterectomy or an emergency cesarean section. In contaminated surgery (operations performed on perforated abdominal organs, compound fractures, or lacerations from animal bites), the risk for infection is nearly 100%. Hence, for these operations, use of antibiotics is considered *treatment,* not prophylaxis. When antibiotics are given for prophylaxis, they should be given before the surgery. If the procedure is unusually long, dosing again during surgery may be indicated. As a rule, postoperative antibiotics are unnecessary. For most operations, a first-generation cephalosporin (e.g., cefazolin) will suffice.

Bacterial Endocarditis

Individuals with congenital or valvular heart disease and those with prosthetic heart valves are unusually susceptible to bacterial endocarditis. For these people, endocarditis can develop after certain dental and medical procedures that dislodge bacteria into the bloodstream. Thus, before undergoing such procedures, these patients may need prophylactic antimicrobial medication. However, according to guidelines released by the American Heart Association, antibiotic prophylaxis is less necessary than previously believed and hence should be done much less often than in the past.

Neutropenia

Severe neutropenia puts individuals at high risk for infection. There is some evidence that the incidence of bacterial infection may be reduced through antibiotic prophylaxis. However, prophylaxis may increase the risk for infection with fungi: by killing normal flora, whose presence helps suppress fungal growth, antibiotics can encourage fungal invasion.

Other Indications for Antimicrobial Prophylaxis

For young women with recurrent urinary tract infection, prophylaxis with trimethoprim/sulfamethoxazole may be helpful. Oseltamivir (an antiviral agent) may be used for prophylaxis against influenza. For individuals who have had severe rheumatic endocarditis, lifelong prophylaxis may be needed. Antimicrobial prophylaxis is indicated after exposure to organisms responsible for sexually transmitted diseases (e.g., syphilis and gonorrhea).

MISUSES OF ANTIMICROBIAL DRUGS

Misuse of antibiotics is common. According to the CDC, one in every three outpatient antibiotic prescriptions is either inappropriate or entirely unnecessary. Ways that we misuse antibiotics are discussed next.

Attempted Treatment of Viral Infection

Most viral infections—including mumps, chickenpox, and the common cold—do not respond to currently available drugs. Hence, when drug therapy of these disorders is attempted, patients are exposed to all the risks of drugs but have no chance of receiving benefits.

Acute upper respiratory tract infections, including the common cold, are a particular concern. When these infections are treated with antibiotics, only 1 patient out of 4000 is likely to benefit. However, the risks remain high: 1 in 4 patients will get diarrhea, 1 in 50 will get a rash, and 1 in 1000 will need to visit an emergency department, usually because of a severe allergic reaction.

Treatment of Fever of Unknown Origin

Although fever can be a sign of infection, it can also signify other diseases, including hepatitis, arthritis, and cancer. Unless the cause of a fever is a proven infection, antibiotics should not be used. If the fever is *not* due to an infection, antibiotics would not only be inappropriate, they would also expose the patient to unnecessary toxicity and delay correct diagnosis of the fever's cause. If the fever *is* caused by infection, antibiotics could hamper later attempts to identify the infecting organism.

The only situation in which fever, by itself, constitutes a legitimate indication for antibiotic use is when fever occurs in the severely immunocompromised host. Because fever may indicate infection and because infection can be lethal to the immunocompromised patient, these patients should be given antibiotics when fever occurs—even if fever is the only indication that an infection may be present.

Improper Dosage

Like all other medications, antibiotics must be used in the right dosage. If the dosage is too low, the patient will be exposed to a risk for adverse effects without the benefit of antibacterial effects. If the dosage is too high, the risks for superinfection and adverse effects become unnecessarily high.

Treatment in the Absence of Adequate Bacteriologic Information

As stressed earlier, proper antimicrobial therapy requires information on the identity and drug sensitivity of the infecting organism. Except in life-threatening situations, therapy should not be undertaken in the absence of bacteriologic information. This important guideline is often ignored.

Omission of Surgical Drainage

Antibiotics may have limited efficacy in the presence of foreign material, necrotic tissue, or exudate. Hence, when appropriate, surgical drainage and cleansing should be performed to promote antimicrobial effects.

MONITORING ANTIMICROBIAL THERAPY

Antimicrobial therapy is assessed by monitoring clinical responses and laboratory results. The frequency of monitoring is directly proportional to the severity of infection. Important clinical indicators of success are reduction of fever and resolution of signs and symptoms related to the affected organ system (e.g., improvement of breath sounds in patients with pneumonia).

Various laboratory tests are used to monitor treatment. Serum drug levels may be monitored for two reasons: to ensure that levels are sufficient for antimicrobial effects and to avoid toxicity from excessive levels. Success of therapy is indicated by the disappearance of infectious organisms from posttreatment cultures. Cultures may become sterile within hours of the onset of treatment (as may happen with urinary tract infections), or they may not become sterile for weeks (as may happen with tuberculosis).

71

Drugs That Weaken the Bacterial Cell Wall I: Penicillins

INTRODUCTION TO THE PENICILLINS

The penicillins are practically ideal antibiotics because they are active against a variety of bacteria and their direct toxicity is low. Allergic reactions are the principal adverse effects. Owing to their safety and efficacy, the penicillins are widely prescribed.

Because they have a β-lactam ring in their structure, the penicillins are known as *β-lactam antibiotics*. The β-lactam family also includes the cephalosporins, carbapenems, and aztreonam (see Chapter 72). All of the β-lactam antibiotics share the same mechanism of action: disruption of the bacterial cell wall.

Mechanism of Action

To understand the actions of the penicillins, we must first understand the structure and function of the bacterial cell wall—a rigid, permeable, mesh-like structure that lies outside the cytoplasmic membrane. Inside the cytoplasmic membrane, osmotic pressure is very high. Hence, were it not for the rigid cell wall, which prevents expansion, bacteria would take up water, swell, and then burst.

Penicillins weaken the cell wall, causing bacteria to take up excessive amounts of water and rupture. As a result, penicillins are generally *bactericidal*.

Penicillins weaken the cell wall by two actions: (1) *inhibition of transpeptidases* and (2) *disinhibition (activation) of autolysins*. Transpeptidases are enzymes critical to cell wall synthesis. Specifically, they catalyze the formation of cross-bridges between the peptidoglycan polymer strands that form the cell wall and, thus, give the cell wall its strength (Fig. 71.1). Autolysins are bacterial enzymes that cleave bonds in the cell wall. Bacteria use these enzymes to break down segments of the cell wall to permit growth and division. By simultaneously inhibiting transpeptidases and activating autolysins, the penicillins (1) disrupt synthesis of the cell wall and (2) promote its active destruction. These combined actions result in cell lysis and death. However, it is important to note that penicillins are active only against bacteria that are undergoing growth and division (see later).

The molecular targets of the penicillins (transpeptidases, autolysins, and other bacterial enzymes) are collectively known as *penicillin-binding proteins* (PBPs). These molecules are so named because penicillins must bind to them to produce antibacterial effects. As indicated in Fig. 71.2, PBPs are located on the outer surface of the cytoplasmic membrane. More than eight different PBPs have been identified. Of these, PBP1 and PBP3 are most critical to penicillin's antibacterial effects. Bacteria express PBPs only during growth and division. Accordingly, because PBPs must be present for penicillins to work, these drugs work only when bacteria are growing.

Because mammalian cells lack a cell wall and because penicillins act specifically on enzymes that affect cell wall integrity, the penicillins have virtually no *direct* effects on cells of the host. As a result, the penicillins are among our safest antibiotics.

Mechanisms of Bacterial Resistance

Bacterial resistance to penicillins is determined primarily by three factors: (1) inability of penicillins to reach their targets (PBPs), (2) inactivation of penicillins by bacterial enzymes, and (3) production of PBPs that have a low affinity for penicillins.

Gram-Negative Cell Envelope

All bacteria are surrounded by a cell envelope. However, the cell envelope of gram-negative organisms differs from that of gram-positive organisms. Because of this difference, some penicillins are ineffective against gram-negative bacteria.

The cell envelope of *gram-positive* bacteria has only two layers: the cytoplasmic membrane and a relatively thick cell wall. Despite its thickness, the cell wall can be readily penetrated by penicillins, giving them easy access to PBPs on the cytoplasmic membrane. As a result, penicillins are generally very active against gram-positive organisms.

The *gram-negative* cell envelope has three layers: the cytoplasmic membrane, a relatively thin cell wall, and an additional *outer membrane* (see Fig. 71.2). Like the gram-positive cell wall, the gram-negative cell wall can be easily penetrated by penicillins. However, the outer membrane is difficult to penetrate. As a result, only certain penicillins (e.g., ampicillin) are able to cross it and, thus, reach PBPs on the cytoplasmic membrane.

Penicillinases (β-Lactamases)

β-Lactamases are enzymes that cleave the β-lactam ring and, therefore, render penicillins and other β-lactam antibiotics inactive. Bacteria produce a large variety of β-lactamases; some are specific for penicillins, some are specific for other β-lactam antibiotics (e.g., cephalosporins), and some act on several kinds of β-lactam antibiotics. β-Lactamases that act selectively on penicillins are known as *penicillinases*.

Penicillinases are synthesized by gram-positive and gram-negative bacteria. Gram-positive organisms produce large amounts of these enzymes and then export them into the surrounding medium. In contrast, gram-negative bacteria produce penicillinases in relatively small amounts and, rather than exporting them to the environment, secrete them into the periplasmic space (see Fig. 71.2).

The genes that code for β-lactamases are located on chromosomes and on plasmids (extrachromosomal DNA). The genes on plasmids may be transferred from one bacterium to another, thereby promoting the spread of penicillin resistance.

Transfer of resistance is of special importance with *Staphylococcus aureus*. When penicillin was first introduced in the early 1940s, all strains of *S. aureus* were sensitive. However, by 1960, as many as 80% of *S. aureus* isolates in hospitals were penicillin resistant. Fortunately, a penicillin derivative (methicillin) that has resistance to the actions of β-lactamases was introduced at this time. To date, no known strains of *S. aureus* produce β-lactamases capable of inactivating methicillin or related penicillinase-resistant penicillins (although some strains are resistant to these drugs for other reasons).

Altered Penicillin-Binding Proteins

Certain bacterial strains, known collectively as methicillin-resistant *S. aureus* (MRSA), have a unique mechanism of resistance: production of PBPs with a low affinity for penicillins and all other β-lactam antibiotics. MRSA developed this ability by acquiring genes that code for low-affinity PBPs from other bacteria.

Methicillin-Resistant *Staphylococcus Aureus*

S. aureus is a gram-positive bacterium that often colonizes the skin and nostrils of healthy people. Infection usually involves the skin and soft tissues, causing abscesses, boils, cellulitis, and impetigo. However, more

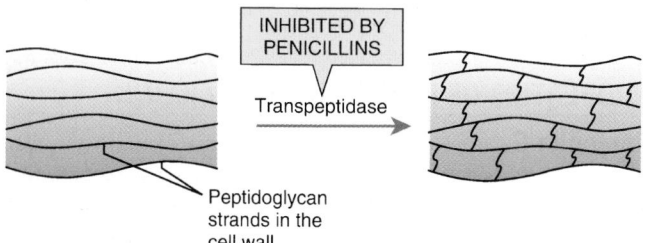

Fig. 71.1 Inhibition of Transpeptidase by Penicillins. The bacterial cell wall is composed of long strands of a peptidoglycan polymer. As depicted, transpeptidase enzymes create cross-bridges between the peptidoglycan strands, giving the cell wall added strength. By inhibiting transpeptidases, penicillins prevent cross-bridge synthesis and, hence, weaken the cell wall.

serious infections can also develop, including infections of the lungs and bloodstream, which can be fatal.

Like other pathogens, *S. aureus* has developed resistance over the years. When penicillins were introduced in the 1940s, all strains of *S. aureus* were susceptible. However, penicillin-resistant strains quickly emerged, owing to bacterial production of penicillinases. In 1959 this resistance was overcome with methicillin, the first penicillinase-resistant penicillin. Unfortunately, by 1968, strains resistant to methicillin had emerged. These highly resistant bacteria, known as *MRSA*, are resistant not only to methicillin (now obsolete), but also to all penicillins and most cephalosporins as well. The basis of MRSA resistance is acquisition of genes that code for PBPs that have very low affinity for penicillins and cephalosporins. Resistant strains were initially limited to health care facilities but are currently found in the community as well.

There are two distinct types of MRSA, referred to as *health care–associated MRSA* (HCA-MRSA) and *community-associated MRSA* (CA-MRSA). Of the two, HCA-MRSA is more prevalent (80% vs. 20%) and emerged earlier (1968 vs. 1981). In addition, HCA-MRSA infection is generally more serious and harder to treat. Molecular typing indicates that HCA-MRSA and CA-MRSA are genetically distinct strains, known as USA100 and USA300, respectively.

Health Care–Associated MRSA

Transmission of HCA-MRSA is usually through person-to-person contact, very often between health care workers and patients. Risk factors for acquiring HCA-MRSA include advanced age, recent surgery or hospitalization, dialysis, treatment in an intensive care unit, prolonged antibiotic therapy, an indwelling catheter, and residence in a long-term care facility.

Fig. 71.2 The Bacterial Cell Envelope. Note that the gram-negative cell envelope has an outer membrane, whereas the gram-positive envelope does not. The outer membrane of the gram-negative cell envelope prevents certain penicillins from reaching their target molecules. *PBP*, Penicillin-binding protein.

The treatment of HCA-MRSA infection is addressed at length in a guideline—Clinical Practice Guidelines by the Infectious Diseases Society of America for the Treatment of Methicillin-Resistant *Staphylococcus aureus* Infections in Adults and Children. The guideline stresses the importance of selecting drugs based on the site of the infection, age of the patient, and drug sensitivity of the pathogen. For complicated skin and soft tissue infections in adults, the preferred drugs are intravenous (IV) vancomycin, linezolid (Zyvox), daptomycin (Cubicin), telavancin (Vibativ), clindamycin, and ceftaroline (Teflaro). IV vancomycin is the preferred drug for children. For bacteremia or endocarditis in adults or children, IV vancomycin and daptomycin are drugs of choice. Preferred drugs for pneumonia in adults and children are IV vancomycin, linezolid, and clindamycin. Because most strains of MRSA are multidrug resistant, many other antibiotics are ineffective, including tetracyclines, clindamycin, trimethoprim/sulfamethoxazole, and β-lactam agents (except ceftaroline).

Community-Associated Methicillin-Resistant *Staphylococcus aureus*

Infection with CA-MRSA, first reported in 1981, is caused by staphylococcal strains that are genetically distinct from HCA-MRSA. For example, most strains of CA-MRSA carry a gene for Panton-Valentine leukocidin (a cytotoxin that causes necrosis), whereas HCA-MRSA strains do not. Many people are currently asymptomatic carriers of CA-MRSA. In fact, between 20% and 30% of the population is colonized, typically on the skin and in the nostrils.

Infection with CA-MRSA is generally less dangerous than with HCA-MRSA but is more dangerous than with methicillin-sensitive *S. aureus*. In most cases, CA-MRSA causes mild infections of the skin and soft tissues, manifesting as boils, impetigo, and so forth. However, CA-MRSA can also cause more serious infections, including necrotizing fasciitis, severe necrotizing pneumonia, and severe sepsis. Fortunately, these invasive infections are relatively rare. On the other hand, infections of the skin and soft tissues are currently common, with CA-MRSA accounting for more than 50% of the *S. aureus* isolates from these sites.

CA-MRSA transmission is by skin-to-skin contact and by contact with contaminated objects, including frequently touched surfaces, sports equipment, and personal items (e.g., razors). In contrast to HCA-MRSA infection, CA-MRSA infection is seen primarily in young, healthy people with no recent exposure to health care facilities. Individuals at risk include athletes in contact sports (e.g., wrestling), men who have sex with men, and people who live in close quarters, such as family members, child care clients, prison inmates, military personnel, and college students.

Several measures can reduce the risk for CA-MRSA transmission. Topping the list is good hand hygiene—washing with soap and water or applying an alcohol-based sanitizer. Other measures include showering after contact sports, cleaning frequently touched surfaces, keeping infected sites covered, and not sharing towels and personal items.

Treatment depends on infection severity. For boils, small abscesses, and other superficial infections, surgical drainage may be all that is needed. For more serious infections, drugs may be indicated. Preferred agents are trimethoprim/sulfamethoxazole, minocycline, doxycycline, and clindamycin. Alternative drugs—vancomycin, daptomycin, and linezolid—should be reserved for severe infections and treatment failures. To eradicate the carrier state, intranasal application of a topical antibiotic—mupirocin or retapamulin—can be effective. Like HCA-MRSA, CA-MRSA does not respond to β-lactam antibiotics, except ceftaroline, a fifth generation cephalosporin.

Chemistry

All of the penicillins are derived from a common nucleus: 6-aminopenicillanic acid. This nucleus contains a β-lactam ring joined to a second ring. The β-lactam ring is essential for antibacterial actions. Properties of individual penicillins are determined by additions made to the basic nucleus. These modifications determine (1) affinity for PBPs, (2) resistance to penicillinases, (3) ability to penetrate the gram-negative cell envelope, (4) resistance to stomach acid, and (5) pharmacokinetic properties.

Classification

The most useful classification of penicillins is based on antimicrobial spectrum. When classified this way, the penicillins fall into four major groups: (1) narrow-spectrum penicillins that are penicillinase sensitive, (2) narrow-spectrum penicillins that are penicillinase resistant (antistaphylococcal penicillins), (3) broad-spectrum penicillins (aminopenicillins), and (4) extended-spectrum penicillins (antipseudomonal penicillins). Table 71.1 lists the members of each group and their principal target organisms.

PROPERTIES OF INDIVIDUAL PENICILLINS

Penicillin G

Penicillin G (benzylpenicillin) was the first penicillin available and will serve as our prototype for the penicillin family. This drug is often referred to simply as *penicillin*. Penicillin G is bactericidal to a number of gram-positive bacteria as well as to some gram-negative bacteria. Despite the introduction of newer antibiotics, penicillin G remains a drug of choice for many infections.

Antimicrobial Spectrum

Penicillin G is active against most *gram-positive bacteria* (except penicillinase-producing staphylococci), gram-negative cocci (*Neisseria meningitidis* and non–penicillinase-producing strains of *Neisseria gonorrhoeae*), anaerobic bacteria, and spirochetes (including *Treponema pallidum*). With few exceptions, gram-negative bacilli are resistant. Although many organisms respond to penicillin G, the drug is considered a narrow-spectrum agent compared with other members of the penicillin family.

TABLE 71.1   Classification of the Penicillins

Penicillin Class	Drug	Clinically Useful Antimicrobial Spectrum
Narrow-spectrum penicillins: penicillinase sensitive	Penicillin G Penicillin V	*Streptococcus* spp., *Neisseria* spp., many anaerobes, spirochetes, and others
Narrow-spectrum penicillins: penicillinase resistant (antistaphylococcal penicillins)	Nafcillin Oxacillin Dicloxacillin	*Staphylococcus aureus*
Broad-spectrum penicillins (aminopenicillins)	Ampicillin Amoxicillin	*Haemophilus influenzae*, *Escherichia coli*, *Proteus mirabilis*, enterococci, and *Neisseria gonorrhoeae*
Extended-spectrum penicillin (antipseudomonal penicillin)	Piperacillin	Same as broad-spectrum penicillins plus *Pseudomonas aeruginosa*, *Enterobacter* spp., *Proteus* (indole positive), *Bacteroides fragilis*, and many *Klebsiella* spp.

Pharmacokinetics

Absorption. Penicillin G is available as four salts: (1) *potassium* penicillin G, (2) *procaine* penicillin G, (3) *benzathine* penicillin G, and (4) *sodium* penicillin G. These salts differ with respect to route of administration and time course of action. With all forms, the salt dissociates to release penicillin G, the active component.

Intramuscular. All forms of penicillin may be administered by the intramuscular (IM) route. However, it is important to note that the different salts are absorbed at very different rates. As indicated in Fig. 71.3, absorption of *potassium* and *sodium* penicillin G is rapid; blood levels peak approximately 15 minutes after injection. In contrast, the *procaine* and *benzathine* salts are absorbed slowly and, hence, are considered *repository* preparations. When benzathine penicillin is administered by IM injection, penicillin G is absorbed for weeks, producing blood levels that are persistent but very low. Consequently, this preparation is useful only against highly sensitive organisms (e.g., *T. pallidum*, the bacterium that causes syphilis).

Distribution. Penicillin distributes well to most tissues and body fluids. In the absence of inflammation, penetration of the meninges into fluids of joints and the eyes is poor. By contrast, in the presence of inflammation, entry into cerebrospinal fluid, joints, and the eyes is enhanced, permitting treatment of infections caused by susceptible organisms.

Metabolism and excretion. Penicillin undergoes minimal metabolism and is eliminated by the kidneys, primarily as the unchanged drug. Renal excretion is accomplished mainly (90%) by active tubular secretion; the remaining 10% results from glomerular filtration. In older children and adults, the half-life is very short (approximately 30 minutes). Renal impairment causes the half-life to increase dramatically and may necessitate a reduction in dosage. In patients at high risk for toxicity (those with renal impairment, the acutely ill, the very young, and older adults), kidney function should be monitored.

Side Effects and Toxicities

Penicillin G is the least toxic of all antibiotics and is among the safest of all medications. Allergic reactions, the principal concern with penicillin, are discussed separately later. Other reactions include *pain at sites of IM injection,* prolonged (but reversible) *sensory and motor dysfunction* after accidental injection into a peripheral nerve, and *neurotoxicity* (seizures, confusion, and hallucinations) if blood levels are too high. Inadvertent *intra-arterial* injection can produce severe reactions—gangrene, necrosis, and sloughing of tissue—and must be avoided.

Certain adverse effects may be caused by compounds coadministered with penicillin. For example, the procaine component of procaine penicillin G may cause bizarre behavioral effects when procaine penicillin is given in large doses. When large IV doses of potassium penicillin G are administered rapidly, hyperkalemia can result, possibly causing dysrhythmias and even cardiac arrest. Similarly, the use of IV sodium penicillin G may lead to electrolyte imbalance. Sodium penicillin G should be used with caution in patients on sodium-restricted diets.

Penicillin Allergy

General considerations. Penicillins are the most common cause of drug allergy. Between 0.4% and 7% of patients who receive penicillins experience an allergic reaction. Severity can range from a minor rash to life-threatening anaphylaxis.

As with most allergic reactions, there is no direct relationship between the size of the dose and the intensity of the response. Although prior exposure to penicillins is required for an allergic reaction, responses may occur in the absence of prior penicillin use because patients may have been exposed to penicillins produced by fungi or to penicillins present in foods of animal origin.

Because of cross sensitivity, patients allergic to one penicillin should be considered allergic to all other penicillins. In addition, a few patients (approximately 1%) display cross sensitivity to *cephalosporins.* If at all possible, patients with penicillin allergy should not be treated with any member of the penicillin family. The use of cephalosporins depends on the intensity of allergic response: if the penicillin allergy is mild, the use of cephalosporins is probably safe; however, if the allergy is severe, cephalosporins should be avoided.

Fig. 71.3 Blood Levels of Penicillin G Following Intramuscular Injection of Four Different Penicillin G Salts.

Individuals allergic to penicillin should be encouraged to wear a medical identification bracelet to alert health care personnel to their condition.

Types of allergic reactions. Penicillin reactions are classified as *immediate, accelerated,* and *delayed.* Immediate reactions occur 2 to 30 minutes after drug administration; accelerated reactions occur within 1 to 72 hours; and delayed reactions occur within days to weeks. Immediate and accelerated reactions are mediated by immunoglobulin E (IgE) antibodies.

Anaphylaxis is an immediate hypersensitivity reaction. Anaphylactic reactions occur more frequently with penicillins than with any other drugs. However, even with penicillins, the incidence of anaphylaxis is extremely low (the estimated incidence is between 0.004% and 0.04%). Nonetheless, when these reactions do occur, the risk for mortality is high (approximately 10%). The primary treatment is *epinephrine* (subcutaneous [subQ], IM, or IV) and respiratory support. To ensure prompt treatment if anaphylaxis should develop, patients should be observed for at least 30 minutes after drug injection (i.e., until the risk for an anaphylactic reaction has passed).

Development of penicillin allergy. Before discussing penicillin allergy further, we need to review development of allergy to small molecules as a class. Small molecules, such as penicillin and most other drugs, are unable to induce antibody formation directly. Therefore, to promote antibody formation, the small molecule must first bond covalently to a larger molecule, usually a protein. In these combinations, the small molecule is referred to as a *hapten.* The hapten-protein combination constitutes the complete *antigen* that stimulates antibody formation.

The hapten that stimulates production of penicillin antibodies is rarely intact penicillin itself. Rather, compounds formed from the degradation of penicillin are the actual cause. As a result, most "penicillin antibodies" are not directed at penicillin itself. Rather, they are directed at various penicillin degradation products.

Skin tests for penicillin allergy. Allergy to penicillin can decrease over time. Hence an intense allergic reaction in the past does not necessarily mean that an intense reaction will occur again. In patients with a history of penicillin allergy, skin tests can be used to assess current risk. These tests are performed by injecting a tiny amount of allergen intradermally and observing for a local allergic response. A positive test indicates the presence of IgE antibodies, which can mediate severe penicillin allergy. Accordingly, if skin testing is negative, anaphylaxis is unlikely.

It is important to note that skin testing can be dangerous: in patients with severe penicillin allergy, the skin test itself can precipitate an anaphylactic reaction. Accordingly, the test should be performed only if epinephrine and facilities for respiratory support are immediately available.

Current guidelines recommend skin testing with two reagents, which test for the major and minor determinants of penicillin allergy. The minor determinants, although less common, mediate most severe penicillin reactions.

Management of patients with a history of penicillin allergy. All patients who are candidates for penicillin therapy should be asked if they have penicillin allergy and what the reaction is. For patients who answer "yes," the general rule is to avoid penicillins. If the allergy is mild, a *cephalosporin* is often an appropriate alternative. However, if there is a history of anaphylaxis or some other severe allergic reaction, it is prudent to avoid cephalosporins as well (because there is an approximately 1% risk for cross sensitivity to cephalosporins). When a cephalosporin is indicated, an oral cephalosporin is preferred (because the risk for a severe reaction is lower than with parenteral therapy). For many infections, *vancomycin, erythromycin,* and *clindamycin* are effective and safe alternatives for patients with penicillin allergy.

Rarely, a patient with a history of anaphylaxis may have a life-threatening infection (e.g., enterococcal endocarditis) for which alternatives to penicillins are ineffective. In these cases the potential benefits of penicillin therapy outweigh the risks, and treatment should be instituted. To minimize the chances of an anaphylactic reaction, penicillin should be administered according to a desensitization schedule. In this procedure, an initial small dose is followed at 60-minute intervals by progressively larger doses until the full therapeutic dose has been achieved. It should be noted that the desensitization procedure is not without risk. Accordingly, epinephrine and facilities for respiratory support should be immediately available.

PATIENT-CENTERED CARE ACROSS THE LIFE SPAN

Penicillins

Life Stage	Patient Care Concerns
Infants	Penicillins are used safely in infants with bacterial infections, including syphilis, meningitis, and group A streptococcus.
Children/adolescents	Penicillins are a common drug used to treat bacterial infections in children.
Pregnant women	Although there are no well-controlled studies in pregnant women, evidence we do have suggests there is no second or third trimester fetal risk.
Breastfeeding women	Amoxicillin is safe for use in breastfeeding mothers. Data are lacking regarding transmission of some other penicillins from mother to infant through breast milk.
Older adults	Doses should be adjusted in older adults with renal dysfunction.

Penicillin V

Penicillin V, also known as penicillin VK, is similar to penicillin G in most respects. The principal difference is acid stability: Penicillin V is stable in stomach acid, whereas penicillin G is not. Because of its acid stability, penicillin V has replaced penicillin G for oral therapy. Penicillin V may be taken with meals.

Penicillinase-Resistant Penicillins (Antistaphylococcal Penicillins)

By altering the penicillin side chain, pharmaceutical chemists have created a group of penicillins that are highly resistant to inactivation by β-lactamases. In the United States, three such drugs are available: *nafcillin, oxacillin,* and *dicloxacillin.* These agents have a very narrow antimicrobial spectrum and are used only against penicillinase-producing strains of staphylococci (*S. aureus* and *S. epidermidis*). Because most strains of staphylococci produce penicillinase, the penicillinase-resistant penicillins are drugs of choice for most staphylococcal infections. It should be noted that these agents should not be used against infections caused by non–penicillinase-producing staphylococci because they are less active than penicillin G against these bacteria.

An increasing clinical problem is the emergence of staphylococcal strains referred to as *MRSA,* a term used to indicate lack of susceptibility to methicillin (an obsolete penicillinase-resistant penicillin) and all other penicillinase-resistant penicillins. Resistance appears to result from production of PBPs to which the penicillinase-resistant penicillins cannot bind. Vancomycin is the treatment of choice.

Broad-Spectrum Penicillins (Aminopenicillins)

Only two broad-spectrum penicillins are available: *ampicillin* and *amoxicillin*. Both have the same antimicrobial spectrum as penicillin G, *plus* increased activity against certain gram-negative bacilli, including *Haemophilus influenzae, Escherichia coli,* and *Salmonella* and *Shigella* species. This broadened spectrum is mainly due to an increased ability to penetrate the gram-negative cell envelope. Both drugs are readily inactivated by β-lactamases and, hence, are ineffective against most infections caused by *S. aureus*.

Ampicillin

Ampicillin was the first broad-spectrum penicillin in clinical use. The drug is useful against infections caused by *Enterococcus fecalis, Proteus mirabilis, E. coli, Salmonella* and *Shigella* species, and *H. influenzae.* The most common side effects are rash and diarrhea, both of which occur more frequently with ampicillin than with any other penicillin. If rash occurs, the provider should evaluate to differentiate between non-allergic rash and rash related to a hypersensitivity reaction. Use of ampicillin can produce non-allergic rash in 5% to 10% of children. Rash generally appears 3 to 10 days after initiation of ampicillin therapy. Administration may be oral or IV. It should be noted that for oral therapy, amoxicillin is preferred (see later). Dosages for patients with normal kidney function are shown in Table 71.2. For patients with renal impairment, dosage should be reduced.

As discussed later, ampicillin is also available in a fixed-dose combination with sulbactam, an inhibitor of bacterial β-lactamase. The combination is sold as *Unasyn*.

Amoxicillin

Amoxicillin (Moxatag) is similar to ampicillin in structure and actions. The drugs differ primarily in acid stability, amoxicillin being the more acid stable. Hence, when the two are administered orally in equivalent doses, blood levels of amoxicillin are greater. Accordingly, when oral therapy is indicated, amoxicillin is preferred. Amoxicillin causes milder diarrhea when compared with ampicillin, perhaps because less amoxicillin remains unabsorbed in the intestine.

As discussed later, amoxicillin is also available in a fixed-dose combination with clavulanic acid, an inhibitor of bacterial β-lactamases. The combination is marketed as *Augmentin*. Amoxicillin, by itself, is one of our most frequently prescribed antibiotics.

Extended-Spectrum Penicillins (Antipseudomonal Penicillins)

Only one extended-spectrum penicillin is available: *piperacillin* antimicrobial spectrum of piperacillin includes organisms that are susceptible to the aminopenicillins plus *Pseudomonas aeruginosa, Enterobacter* species, *Proteus* species (indole positive), *Bacteroides fragilis,* and many *Klebsiella* species. This extended-spectrum penicillin is susceptible to β-lactamases and, hence, is ineffective against most strains of *S. aureus*.

TABLE 71.2 Dosages for Penicillins

Generic Name	Trade Name	Usual Routes	Dosing Interval (h)	TOTAL DAILY DOSAGE[a] Adults	Children
Narrow-Spectrum Penicillins: Penicillinase Sensitive					
Penicillin G	Bicillin C-R, Bicillin LA, and Pfizerpen	IM, IV	4	4–24 million units[b]	100 000–400 000 units/kg[b]
Penicillin V	Generic only	PO	4–6	0.5–2 g	25–75 mg/kg
Narrow-Spectrum Penicillins: Penicillinase-Resistant (Antistaphylococcal Penicillins)					
Nafcillin		IV	4–6	2–12 g	100–200 mg/kg
Oxacillin		IV	4–6	1–12 g	100–200 mg/kg
Dicloxacillin		PO	6	0.5–4 g	12.5–25 mg/kg
Broad-Spectrum Penicillins (Aminopenicillins)					
Ampicillin	Generic only	PO	6–8	2–4 g	50–100 mg/kg
		IV	6–8	4–12 g	50–400 mg/kg
Ampicillin/sulbactam	Unasyn	IV	6	4–8 g[c]	150–600 mg/kg[c]
Amoxicillin	Generic only	PO	8	750–1750 mg	20–90 mg/kg
Amoxicillin, ER	Moxatag	PO	24	775 mg	775 mg
Amoxicillin/clavulanate	Augmentin, Clavulin 🍁	PO	8–12	250–1750 mg[d]	20–90 mg/kg[d]
	Augmentin ES-600	PO	12	—	90 mg/kg
	Augmentin XR	PO	12	4000 mg	—
Extended-Spectrum Penicillin (Antipseudomonal Penicillin)					
Piperacillin/tazobactam	Zosyn, Tazocin 🍁	IV	4–6	12–18 g[e]	80–100 mg/kg[e]

[a]Doses vary widely, depending on the type and severity of infection; doses and dosing intervals presented here may not be appropriate for all patients.
[b]10 000 units = 6 mg.
[c]Dose based on ampicillin content.
[d]Dose based on amoxicillin content.
[e]Dose based on piperacillin content.
ER, Extended release; *IM*, intramuscular; *IV*, intravenous; *PO*, oral.

Piperacillin is used primarily for infections with *P. aeruginosa*. These infections often occur in the immunocompromised host and can be very difficult to eradicate. To increase killing of *Pseudomonas,* an antipseudomonal aminoglycoside (gentamicin, tobramycin, amikacin, and netilmicin) may be added to the regimen. When these combinations are used, the penicillin and the aminoglycoside should not be mixed in the same IV solution because high concentrations of penicillins can inactivate aminoglycosides.

Piperacillin

Piperacillin has a broad antimicrobial spectrum; however, the drug is penicillinase sensitive. Piperacillin is highly active against *P. aeruginosa,* its principal target. Piperacillin can cause bleeding secondary to disrupting platelet function. The drug is acid labile and, hence, must be administered parenterally, usually by the IV route. Dosages for patients with normal kidney function are shown in Table 71.2. Dosage should be reduced in patients with renal impairment. As discussed later, piperacillin is also available in a fixed-dose combination with tazobactam, a β-lactamase inhibitor. The combination is marketed as *Zosyn.*

Penicillins Combined With a β-Lactamase Inhibitor

As their name indicates, β-lactamase inhibitors are drugs that inhibit bacterial β-lactamases. By combining a β-lactamase inhibitor with a penicillinase-sensitive penicillin, we can extend the antimicrobial spectrum of the penicillin. In the United States, three β-lactamase inhibitors are used: *sulbactam, tazobactam,* and *clavulanic acid* (clavulanate). These drugs are not available alone. Rather, they are available only in fixed-dose combinations with a penicillin. Five such combination products are available:

- Ampicillin/sulbactam (Unasyn)
- Amoxicillin/clavulanate (Augmentin and Clavulin)
- Piperacillin/tazobactam (Zosyn and Tazocin)

Because β-lactamase inhibitors have minimal toxicity, any adverse effects that occur with the combination products are due to the penicillin.

📄 SUMMARY OF KEY PRESCRIBING CONSIDERATIONS

Penicillins

Therapeutic Goal: Treatment of infections caused by sensitive bacteria

Baseline Data: Samples for microbiologic culture to identify the infecting organism

Monitoring: Renal impairment can cause penicillins to accumulate to toxic levels. Monitor function in patients with renal disease.

Identifying High-Risk Patients: Penicillins should be used with extreme caution in patients with a history of severe allergic reactions to penicillins, cephalosporins, or carbapenems.

Evaluating Therapeutic Effects: Monitor for indications of antimicrobial effects—reduction in fever, edema, pain, and inflammation.

Minimizing Adverse Effects: For patients with prior allergic responses, a skin test may be ordered to assess current allergy status.

72

Drugs That Weaken the Bacterial Cell Wall II: Other Drugs

Like the penicillins, the drugs discussed here are inhibitors of cell wall synthesis. By disrupting the cell wall, these drugs produce bacterial lysis and death. Much of the chapter focuses on the cephalosporins, our most widely used antibacterial drugs. With only three exceptions—vancomycin, telavancin, and fosfomycin—the agents addressed here are β-lactam drugs.

CEPHALOSPORINS

The cephalosporins are β-lactam antibiotics similar in structure and actions to the penicillins. These drugs are bactericidal, often resistant to β-lactamases, and active against a broad spectrum of pathogens. Their toxicity is low. Because of these attributes, the cephalosporins are popular therapeutic agents and constitute our most widely used group of antibiotics.

Chemistry

All cephalosporins are derived from the same nucleus. This nucleus contains a *β-lactam ring* fused to a second ring. The β-lactam ring is required for antibacterial activity.

Mechanism of Action

The cephalosporins are bactericidal drugs with a mechanism similar to that of the penicillins. These agents bind to penicillin-binding proteins (PBPs) and, hence, (1) disrupt cell wall synthesis and (2) activate autolysins (enzymes that cleave bonds in the cell wall). The resultant damage to the cell wall causes death by lysis. As in the case of the penicillins, cephalosporins are most effective against cells undergoing active growth and division.

Resistance

The principal cause of cephalosporin resistance is production of β-lactamases, enzymes that cleave the β-lactam ring and, thus, render these drugs inactive. β-lactamases that act on cephalosporins are sometimes referred to as *cephalosporinases*. Some of the β-lactamases that act on cephalosporins can also cleave the β-lactam ring of penicillins.

Not all cephalosporins are equally susceptible to β-lactamases. Most *first-generation* cephalosporins are destroyed by β-lactamases; *second-generation* cephalosporins are less sensitive to destruction; and *third-, fourth-, and fifth-generation* cephalosporins are highly resistant.

In some cases, bacterial resistance results from producing altered PBPs that have a low affinity for cephalosporins. Methicillin-resistant staphylococci produce these unusual PBPs and are resistant to most cephalosporins as a result. Ceftaroline, a fifth-generation cephalosporin, has demonstrated activity against methicillin-resistant *Staphylococcus aureus* (MRSA).

Classification and Antimicrobial Spectra

The cephalosporins can be grouped into five "generations" based on the order of their introduction to clinical use. The generations differ significantly with respect to antimicrobial spectrum and susceptibility to β-lactamases (Table 72.1). In general, *as we progress from first-generation*

agents to fifth-generation agents, there is (1) increasing activity against gram-negative bacteria and anaerobes, (2) increasing resistance to destruction by β-lactamases, and (3) increasing ability to reach the cerebrospinal fluid (CSF).

Pharmacokinetics
Absorption

Because of poor absorption from the gastrointestinal (GI) tract, *many cephalosporins must be administered parenterally* (by the intramuscular [IM] or intravenous [IV] route). Of the cephalosporins used in the United States, only 10 can be administered by mouth (Table 72.2). Of these, only one—*cefuroxime*—can be administered orally *and* by injection.

Distribution

Cephalosporins distribute well to most body fluids and tissues. Therapeutic concentrations are achieved in pleural, pericardial, and peritoneal fluids. However, concentrations in ocular fluids are generally low. Penetration to the CSF by first- and second-generation drugs is unreliable; hence these drugs should not be used for bacterial meningitis. In contrast, CSF levels achieved with third-, fourth-, and fifth-generation drugs are generally sufficient for bactericidal effects.

Elimination

Practically all cephalosporins are eliminated by the *kidneys;* excretion is by a combination of glomerular filtration and active tubular secretion. Probenecid can decrease tubular secretion of some cephalosporins, thereby prolonging their effects. In patients with renal insufficiency, dosages of most cephalosporins must be reduced (to prevent accumulation to toxic levels).

One cephalosporin—*ceftriaxone*—is eliminated largely by the liver. Consequently dosage reduction is unnecessary in patients with renal impairment.

Adverse Effects

Cephalosporins are generally well tolerated and constitute one of our safest groups of antimicrobial drugs. Serious adverse effects are rare.

Allergic Reactions

Hypersensitivity reactions are the most frequent adverse events. Maculopapular rash that develops several days after the onset of treatment is most common. Severe, immediate reactions (e.g., bronchospasm and anaphylaxis) are rare. If, during the course of treatment, signs of allergy appear (e.g., urticaria, rash, hypotension, and difficulty in breathing), the cephalosporin should be discontinued immediately. Patients with a history of cephalosporin allergy should not be given these drugs.

Because of structural similarities between penicillins and cephalosporins, a few patients allergic to one type of drug may experience cross-reactivity with the other. In clinical practice, the incidence of cross-reactivity has been low: only 1% of penicillin-allergic patients experience an allergic reaction if given a cephalosporin. For patients with mild penicillin allergy, cephalosporins can be used with minimal concern.

TABLE 72.1   Major Differences Between Cephalosporin Generations

Class	Activity Against Gram-Negative Bacteria	Resistance to β-Lactamases	Distribution to Cerebrospinal Fluid
First generation (e.g., cephalexin)	Low	Low	Poor
Second generation (e.g., cefoxitin)	Higher	Higher	Poor
Third generation (e.g., cefotaxime)	Higher	Higher	Good
Fourth generation (cefepime)	Highest	Highest	Good
Fifth generation (ceftaroline)	High	Highest	Good

TABLE 72.2   Pharmacokinetic Properties of the Cephalosporins

Class	Drug	Routes of Administration	Major Route of Elimination	HALF-LIFE (h) Normal Renal Function	HALF-LIFE (h) Severe Renal Impairment
First generation	Cefadroxil	PO	Renal	1.2–1.3	20–25
	Cefazolin	IM, IV	Renal	1.5–2.2	24–50
	Cephalexin	PO	Renal	0.4–1	10–20
Second generation	Cefaclor	PO	Renal	0.6–0.9	2–3
	Cefotetan	IM, IV	Renal	3–4.5	13–35
	Cefoxitin	IM, IV	Renal	0.7–1	13–22
	Cefprozil	PO	Renal	1.3	5–6
	Cefuroxime	PO, IM, IV	Renal	1–1.9	15–22
Third generation	Cefdinir	PO	Renal	1.7	16
	Cefditoren	PO	Renal	1.6	—
	Cefixime	PO	Renal	3–4	11.5
	Cefotaxime	IM, IV	Renal	0.9–1.4	3–11
	Cefpodoxime	PO	Renal	2–3	9.8
	Ceftazidime	IM, IV	Renal	1.9–2	—
	Ceftibuten	PO	Renal	2	Increased
	Ceftriaxone	IM, IV	Hepatic	5.8–8.7	15.7
Fourth generation	Cefepime	IM, IV	Renal	2	Increased
	Ceftolozane	IV	Renal	2.8–3.1	Increased
Fifth generation	Ceftaroline	IV	Renal	2.6	Increased

However, because of the potential for fatal anaphylaxis, *cephalosporins should not be given to patients with a history of severe reactions to penicillins.*

Drug Interactions

Alcohol

Two cephalosporins—*cefazolin* and *cefotetan*—can induce a state of alcohol intolerance. If a patient taking these drugs were to ingest alcohol, a disulfiram-like reaction could occur. (As discussed in Chapter 33, the disulfiram effect, which can be very dangerous, is brought on by accumulation of acetaldehyde secondary to inhibition of aldehyde dehydrogenase.) Patients using these cephalosporins must not consume alcohol in any form.

Drugs That Promote Bleeding

Cefotetan, cefazolin, and *ceftriaxone* can promote bleeding as they contain a side chain that interferes with Vitamin K metabolism which can inhibit the formation of clotting factors. Caution is needed if these drugs are combined with other agents that promote bleeding (anticoagulants, thrombolytics, nonsteroidal antiinflammatory drugs [NSAIDs], and other antiplatelet agents).

Therapeutic Uses

The therapeutic role of the cephalosporins is continually evolving as new agents are introduced and more experience is gained with older ones. Only general recommendations are considered here.

The cephalosporins are broad-spectrum, bactericidal drugs with a high therapeutic index. They have been employed widely and successfully against a variety of infections. Cephalosporins can be useful alternatives for patients with mild penicillin allergy.

The five generations of cephalosporins differ significantly in their applications. With one important exception—the use of first-generation agents for infections caused by sensitive staphylococci—the *first- and second-generation cephalosporins* are rarely drugs of choice for active infections (Table 72.3). In most cases, equally effective and less expensive alternatives are available. In contrast, the *third-generation agents* have qualities that make them the preferred therapy for several infections. The *fourth- and fifth-generation agents* are effective against resistant organisms. The *fifth-generation* agent is used to treat skin infections, including MRSA, and health care–associated pneumonias.

TABLE 72.3 Therapeutic Uses of Cephalosporin

Generation	Highest Activity	Organism	Preferred Use	Spectrum
First	Gram positive	Staphylococci or streptococci	Use in patients with mild penicillin allergy, surgical prophylaxis	Narrow
Second	Gram positive and gram negative	*Haemophilus influenzae, Klebsiella,* pneumococci, and staphylococci	Otitis, sinusitis, and respiratory tract infections	More broad than first generation
Third	Gram negative	*Pseudomonas aeruginosa, Neisseria gonorrhoeae,* and *Klebsiella, Serratia*	Meningitis	More broad than first and second generations
Fourth	Gram negative	*Pseudomonas aeruginosa*	Hospital-acquired pneumonia and complicated intra-abdominal and urinary tract infections	Narrow
Fifth	Gram positive	Methicillin-resistant *Staphylococcus aureus*	MRSA[a]-associated infections	Narrow

[a]*MRSA*, Methicillin-resistant *Staphylococcus aureus.*

PROTOTYPE DRUGS

Drugs That Inhibit Cell Wall Synthesis

Cephalosporin
Cephalexin

Carbapenem
Imipenem

Other
Vancomycin

Drug Selection

Nineteen cephalosporins are currently employed in the United States, and selection among them can be a challenge. Within each generation, the similarities among cephalosporins are more pronounced than the differences. Hence, aside from cost, there is frequently no rational basis for choosing one drug over another in the outpatient setting. However, there *are* some differences between cephalosporins, and these may render one agent preferable to another for treating a specific infection in a specific host. The differences that do exist can be grouped into three main categories: (1) antimicrobial spectrum, (2) adverse effects, and (3) pharmacokinetics (e.g., route of administration, penetration to the CSF, time course, and mode of elimination) (see Tables 72.1–72.4).

 SUMMARY OF KEY PRESCRIBING CONSIDERATIONS

Cephalosporins

Therapeutic Goal: Treatment of infections caused by susceptible organisms.
Baseline Data: Take samples for culture to determine the identity and sensitivity of the infecting organism.
Monitoring: No routine laboratory monitoring is suggested.
Identifying High-Risk Patients: Cephalosporins are contraindicated for patients with a history of allergic reactions to cephalosporins or severe reactions to penicillin.
Evaluating Therapeutic Effects: Monitor for indications of antimicrobial effects, including reduction in fever, pain, edema, and inflammation.
Minimizing Adverse Effects: All cephalosporins can promote *Clostridiodies difficile* infection. Instruct patients to report increase in stool frequency.

CARBAPENEMS

Carbapenems are β-lactam antibiotics that have very broad antimicrobial spectra, although none is active against MRSA. Four carbapenems are available: imipenem, meropenem, ertapenem, and doripenem. With all four, administration is parenteral. To delay emergence of resistance, these drugs should be reserved for patients who cannot be treated with a more narrow-spectrum agent.

Imipenem

Imipenem (Primaxin), a β-lactam antibiotic, has an extremely broad antimicrobial spectrum—broader, in fact, than that of nearly all other antimicrobial drugs. As a result, imipenem may be of special use for treating mixed infections in which anaerobes, *S. aureus,* and gram-negative bacilli may all be involved. Imipenem is supplied in fixed-dose combinations with cilastatin, a compound that inhibits destruction of imipenem by renal enzymes.

Mechanism of Action

Imipenem binds to two PBPs (PBP1 and PBP2), causing weakening of the bacterial cell wall with subsequent cell lysis and death. Antimicrobial effects are enhanced by the drug's resistance to practically all β-lactamases and by its ability to penetrate the gram-negative cell envelope.

Antimicrobial Spectrum

Imipenem is active against most bacterial pathogens, including organisms resistant to other antibiotics. The drug is highly active against gram-positive cocci and most gram-negative cocci and bacilli. In addition, imipenem is the most effective β-lactam antibiotic for use against anaerobic bacteria.

Pharmacokinetics

Imipenem is not absorbed from the gastrointestinal (GI) tract and, hence, must be given intravenously. The drug is well distributed to body fluids and tissues. Imipenem penetrates the meninges to produce therapeutic concentrations in the CSF.

Elimination is primarily renal. When employed alone, imipenem is inactivated by dipeptidase, an enzyme present in the kidneys. As a result, drug levels in urine are low. To increase urinary concentrations, imipenem is administered in combination with *cilastatin,* a dipeptidase inhibitor. When the combination is used, about 70% of imipenem is excreted unchanged in the urine. The elimination half-life is about 1 hour.

TABLE 72.4   Cephalosporin Dosages

Drug	Trade Name	Route	Dosing Interval (h)	TOTAL DAILY DOSAGE[a] Adults (g)	TOTAL DAILY DOSAGE[a] Children (mg/kg)
First Generation					
Cefadroxil	Generic only	PO	12, 24	1–2	30
Cefazolin	Generic only	IM, IV	6, 8	2–12	80–160
Cephalexin	Keflex	PO	6	1–4	25–100
Second Generation					
Cefaclor	Raniclor	PO	8	0.75–1.5	20–40
Cefotetan	Generic only	IM, IV	12	1–6	—
Cefoxitin	Mefoxin	IM, IV	4, 8	3–12	80–160
Cefprozil	Generic only	PO	12, 24	0.5–1	15–30
Cefuroxime	Ceftin	PO	12	0.5–1	250–500
	Zinacef	IM, IV	8	1.5–6	50–100
Third Generation					
Cefdinir	Omnicef	PO	12, 24	0.6	14
Cefditoren	Spectracef	PO	12	0.4–0.8	—
Cefixime	Suprax	PO	24	0.4	8
Cefotaxime	Claforan	IM, IV	4, 8	2–12	100–200
Cefpodoxime	Vantin	PO	12	0.2–0.4	10
Ceftazidime	Fortaz, Tazicef	IM, IV	8, 12	0.5–6	60–150
Ceftibuten	Cedax	PO	24	0.4	9
Ceftriaxone	Rocephin	IM, IV	12, 24	1–4	50–100
Fourth Generation					
Cefepime	Maxipime	IM, IV	12	1–6	100–150
Ceftolozane/tazobactam	Zerbaxa	IV	8	4.5	—
Fifth Generation					
Ceftaroline	Teflaro	IV	12	1.2	—

[a]With the exception of ceftriaxone, cephalosporins require a dosage reduction in patients with severe renal impairment.

Adverse Effects

Imipenem is generally well tolerated. GI effects (nausea, vomiting, and diarrhea) are most common. Superinfections with bacteria or fungi develop in about 4% of patients. Rarely, seizures have occurred.

Hypersensitivity reactions (rashes, pruritus, and drug fever) have occurred, and patients allergic to other β-lactam antibiotics may be cross-allergic with imipenem. Fortunately, the incidence of cross sensitivity with penicillins is low—only about 1%.

Interaction With Valproate

Imipenem can reduce blood levels of valproate, a drug used to control seizures (see Chapter 21). Breakthrough seizures have occurred. If possible, combined use of imipenem and valproate should be avoided. If no other antibiotic will suffice, supplemental antiseizure therapy should be considered.

Therapeutic Use

Because of its broad spectrum and low toxicity, imipenem is used widely. The drug is effective for serious infections caused by gram-positive cocci, gram-negative cocci, gram-negative bacilli, and and anaerobic bacteria. This broad antimicrobial spectrum gives imipenem special utility for antimicrobial therapy of mixed infections (e.g., simultaneous infection with aerobic and anaerobic bacteria). When imipenem has been given alone to treat infection with *Pseudomonas aeruginosa*, resistant organisms have emerged. Consequently, imipenem should be combined with another antipseudomonal drug when used against this microbe. Dosing as well as information for the remaining carbapenems is provided in Table 72.5.

📄 SUMMARY OF KEY PRESCRIBING CONSIDERATIONS

Carbapenems

Therapeutic Goal: Treatment of infections caused by susceptible organisms.

Baseline Data: Take samples for culture to determine the identity and sensitivity of the infecting organism.

Monitoring: No routine laboratory monitoring is suggested.

Identifying High-Risk Patients: Patients using valproate to control seizures should not be placed on imipenem.

Evaluating Therapeutic Effects: Monitor for indications of antimicrobial effects, including reduction in fever, pain, edema, and inflammation.

Minimizing Adverse Effects: Dosage should be reduced in patients with renal impairment.

TABLE 72.5 Carbapenem Dosages

Drug	Trade Name	Route	Dosing Interval (h)	Adults (g)	Children (mg/kg)
				TOTAL DAILY DOSAGE IN NORMAL RENAL FUNCTION	
Doripenem	Doribax	IV	8	1.5	—
Ertapenem	Invanz	IM, IV	24	1	30
Imipenem/cilastatin	Primaxin	IV	6	1–2	50–100
Meropenem	Merrem	IV	8	3	60–120
Meropenem/vaborbactam	Vabomere	IV	8	12	——

PATIENT-CENTERED CARE ACROSS THE LIFE SPAN

Cephalosporins, Carbapenems, and Others

Life Stage	Patient Care Concerns
Infants	Third-generation cephalosporins are used to treat bacterial infections in neonates as well as infants.
Children/ adolescents	Cephalosporins are commonly used to treat bacterial infections in children, including otitis media and gonococcal and pneumococcal infections.
Pregnant women	Televancin carries a black box warning for use in pregnancy secondary to risk for adverse developmental outcomes. All cephalosporins appear safe for use in pregnancy.
Breastfeeding women	Cephalosporins are generally not expected to cause adverse effects in breastfed infants.
Older adults	Doses should be adjusted in older adults with decreased renal function.

OTHER INHIBITORS OF CELL WALL SYNTHESIS

Vancomycin

Vancomycin (Vancocin) is the most widely used antibiotic in the US hospitals. Principal indications are *Clostridiodies difficile* infection (CDI), MRSA infection, and treatment of serious infections with susceptible organisms in patients allergic to penicillins. The major toxicity is renal failure. Unlike most other drugs discussed here, vancomycin does not contain a β-lactam ring.

Mechanism of Action

As in the case of the β-lactam antibiotics, vancomycin inhibits cell wall synthesis and, therefore, promotes bacterial lysis and death. However, in contrast to the β-lactams, vancomycin does not interact with PBPs. Instead, it disrupts the cell wall by binding to molecules that serve as precursors for cell wall biosynthesis.

Antimicrobial Spectrum

Vancomycin is active only against gram-positive bacteria. The drug is especially active against *S. aureus* and *Staphylococcus epidermidis*, including strains of both species that are methicillin-resistant. Other susceptible organisms include streptococci, penicillin-resistant pneumococci, and *C. difficile*.

Pharmacokinetics

Absorption from the GI tract is poor. Hence vancomycin is given parenterally for most infections. Oral administration is employed only for infections of the intestine, mainly CDI.

Vancomycin is well distributed to most body fluids and tissues. Although it enters the CSF, levels may be insufficient to treat meningitis. Hence, if meningeal infection fails to respond to IV therapy, concurrent intrathecal dosing may be required.

Vancomycin is eliminated unchanged by the kidneys. In patients with renal impairment, dosage must be reduced.

Therapeutic Use

Vancomycin should be reserved for serious infections. This agent is the drug of choice for infections caused by MRSA or *S. epidermidis;* most strains of these bacteria are still sensitive to vancomycin. Vancomycin is also the drug of choice for severe CDI but not for mild CDI. The drug is also employed as an alternative to penicillins and cephalosporins to treat severe infections (e.g., staphylococcal and streptococcal endocarditis) in patients allergic to β-lactam antibiotics.

Adverse Effects

Renal toxicity remains a major adverse effect. Risk is dose-related and increased by concurrent use of other nephrotoxic drugs (e.g., aminoglycosides, cyclosporine, and NSAIDs). To minimize risk, trough serum levels of vancomycin should be no greater than needed (see later). If significant kidney damage develops, as indicated by a 50% increase in serum creatinine level, vancomycin dosage should be reduced.

Clostridiodies difficile Infection

C. difficile (sometimes called *C. diff.*) is a gram-positive, spore-forming, anaerobic bacillus that infects the bowel. Injury results from the release of two toxins: toxins A and B. Symptoms range from mild (abdominal discomfort, nausea, fever, and diarrhea) to very severe (toxic megacolon, pseudomembranous colitis, colon perforation, sepsis, and death). CDI has become more common and more severe owing to the spread of a more virulent strain—known as NAP1/BI/027—that releases more toxin than older strains. In many hospitals, rates of infection caused by *C. diff.* exceed those caused by MRSA. Fortunately, most cases of CDI can be managed well with antibiotics, usually metronidazole (Flagyl) or vancomycin (Vancocin).

CDI is almost always preceded by the use of antibiotics, which kill off normal gut flora and allow *C. diff.* to flourish. Antibiotics most likely to promote CDI are clindamycin, second- and third-generation cephalosporins, and fluoroquinolones. In fact, intensive use of fluoroquinolones such as ciprofloxacin (Cipro) and levofloxacin (Levaquin) is considered responsible for the rapid spread of the NAP1/BI/027 strain.

CDI is acquired by ingesting *C. diff.* spores, which are shed in the feces. Any object that feces contact—including toilets, bathtubs, and rectal thermometers—can be a source of infection. Within hospitals, spores are transferred to patients primarily through the hands of health care workers who have touched a contaminated person or object. Spores of *C. diff.* are resistant to drying, temperature changes, and alcohol, so viable spores can remain in the environment for weeks.

CDI is defined by (1) the passage of three or more unformed stools in 24 hours or less plus (2) a positive stool test for *C. diff.* or its toxins. Intestinal damage is caused by toxins A and B, which attack the lining of the colon. Symptoms range from watery diarrhea to life-threatening pseudomembranous colitis, characterized by patches of severe inflammation and pus. Complications of severe *C. diff.* colitis include dehydration, electrolyte disturbances, toxic megacolon, bowel perforation, renal failure, sepsis, and death. Among patients successfully treated for CDI, the recurrence rate is 15% to 30%.

The principal risk factor for CDI is treatment with antibiotics. Risk is especially high among older adults who take antibiotics. Other risk factors include GI surgery, serious illness, prolonged hospitalization, and immunosuppression, which may result from cancer chemotherapy, immunosuppressive therapy, or HIV.

Treatment of CDI consists of stopping one antibiotic and starting another, as recommended in a clinical guideline issued by the Infectious Disease Society of America (IDSA). As soon as possible after CDI has been diagnosed, the antibiotic that facilitated *C. diff.* overgrowth must be stopped because doing so (1) will reduce the risk for reinfection after CDI has cleared and (2) in 25% of patients with mild CDI, it will cause the infection to resolve. At the same time, an antibiotic to eradicate *C. diff.* should be started. Drug selection is based on number of previous episodes and infection severity as judged by two laboratory values: white blood cell (WBC) counts and serum creatinine (SCr) values. For initial occurrences of CDI, treatment with oral *vancomycin* or fidaxomicin, a narrow spectrum macrolide, is recommended (Table 72.6). If the infection is diagnosed as fulminant—characterized by the presence of shock, megacolon, or hypotension—oral vancomycin is preferred. For the first recurrence of CDI, a pulsed vancomycin regimen with taper should be attempted. Metronidazole can be used in situations where oral vancomycin or fidaxomicin is not available. Fidaxomicin is discussed further in Chapter 73.

Alternatives and supplements to vancomycin and fidaxomicin are as follows:
- *Rifaximin*, approved for diarrhea caused by *Escherichia coli*, can reduce CDI recurrence following treatment with vancomycin.
- *Monoclonal antibodies* directed against *C. diff.* toxins A and B can reduce CDI recurrence when given concurrently with metronidazole or vancomycin. Bezlotoxumab (Zinplava) was the first monoclonal antibody approved for this indication. The actions of monoclonal antibodies are discussed further in Chapter 84.
- Inoculating the bowel with a *benign strain* of *C. diff.* can protect against developing CDI. Presumably, when the benign strain colonizes the bowel, it occupies the same niche that a virulent strain would occupy and, hence, prevents the virulent strain from becoming established.

How can the spread of CDI be controlled? The IDSA guidelines offer the following recommendations:
- Use antibiotics judiciously, especially those associated with a high risk for CDI (clindamycin, cephalosporins, and fluoroquinolones).
- If possible, isolate patients with CDI in a private room or have them share a room with another patient with CDI.
- Wear gloves and a gown when entering the room of a patient with CDI.
- After contact with a patient with CDI, wash hands with soap and running water. Soap and water will not kill *C. diff.* spores but will flush them off the hands. Alcohol-based hand rubs will not kill spores and will not remove them from the hands.
- Use disposable medical equipment when possible.

TABLE 72.6 Recommended Treatments for *Clostridiodies Difficile* Infection

Clinical Definition	Preferred Drug Therapy	Alternative Drug Therapy
Initial episode: mild or moderate	Vancomycin 125 mg PO qid or fidaxomicin 200 mg PO bid for 10 days	Metronidazole, 500 mg PO tid daily for 10 days
Initial episode: fulminant	Vancomycin 500 mg PO qid	Vancomycin, 500 mg PR qid daily in patients with ileus
Initial episode: severe, complicated	Leukocytosis with a WBC count of 15,000/μL or higher *or* SCr 1.5 times baseline or higher, *either one, plus* hypotension/shock, ileus, and megacolon	Metronidazole 500 mg IV q 8 h *plus* vancomycin, 500 mg PO/NG qid for 10–14 days If complete ileus is present, consider adding vancomycin retention enema
First recurrence	Vancomycin as a tapered and pulsed regimen or fidaxomicin for 10 days	Vancomycin standard dose for 10 days if metronidazole was used in the first episode
Second recurrence	Vancomycin PO in a tapered regimen, for example: 125 mg qid for 10–14 days, then 125 mg bid for 7 days, then 125 mg qd for 7 days, then 125 mg q 2–3 d for 2–8 weeks	Addition of rifaximin after vancomycin

μL, nicroliter; *NG*, by nasogastric tube; *PO*, by mouth; *SCr*, serum creatinine; *WBC*, white blood cell.
Adapted from IDSA/SHEA (2018). *Clinical practice guidelines for Clostridiodies difficile infection in adults and children: 2017 update.*

- In areas associated with increased rates of CDI, decontaminate surfaces with a chlorine-containing cleaning agent (or any other agent that can kill *C. diff.* spores).

SUMMARY OF KEY PRESCRIBING CONSIDERATIONS

Vancomycin

- **Therapeutic Goal:** Treatment of serious infections, including *C. diff.* infection, infection with methicillin-resistant *S. aureus*, and serious infections caused by susceptible organisms in patients allergic to penicillin.
- **Baseline Data:** Take samples for culture to determine the identity and sensitivity of the infecting organism.
- **Monitoring:** Vancomycin drug levels should be monitored during IV administration.
- **Identifying High-Risk Patients:** Use with caution in patients with renal impairment.
- **Evaluating Therapeutic Effects:** Monitor for indications of antimicrobial effects, including reduction in fever, pain, edema, and inflammation.

Minimizing Adverse Effects

Monitor patients with renal impairment and avoid concomitant use of additional nephrotoxic medications (NSAIDs, cyclosporine, and aminoglycosides).

Telavancin

Actions and Uses

Telavancin (Vibativ) is the first representative of a new class of agents, the lipoglycoproteins, synthetic derivatives of vancomycin. Like vancomycin, telavancin is active only against gram-positive bacteria. Cell kill results from two mechanisms. First, similar to vancomycin, telavancin inhibits bacterial cell wall synthesis. Second, telavancin binds to the bacterial cell membrane and, thus, disrupts membrane function. Telavancin is approved only for IV therapy of complicated skin and skin structure infections caused by susceptible strains of the following gram-positive organisms: *S. aureus* (including methicillin-sensitive and methicillin-resistant strains), *Streptococcus pyogenes, Streptococcus agalactiae, Streptococcus anginosus* group, and *Enterococcus fecalis* (but only vancomycin-sensitive strains). To delay development of resistance, telavancin should be reserved for treating vancomycin-resistant infections or for use as an alternative to linezolid (Zyvox), daptomycin (Cubicin), or tigecycline (Tygacil) in patients who cannot take these drugs.

Adverse Effects

Telavancin can cause multiple adverse effects. The most common are taste disturbance, nausea, vomiting, and foamy urine. As with vancomycin, rapid infusion can cause "red man syndrome," characterized by flushing, rash, pruritus, urticaria, tachycardia, and hypotension.

 ## BLACK BOX WARNING

Telavancin

> Telavancin, when used to treat hospital-acquired or ventilator-associated bacterial pneumonia in patients with a creatinine clearance of less than 50 mL/min, has been associated with increased mortality compared with vancomycin.

Telavancin can prolong the QT interval. However, serious dysrhythmias have not been reported. Nonetheless, telavancin should not be given to patients at high risk, including those with congenital long-QT syndrome, uncompensated heart failure, or severe left ventricular hypertrophy and those using other QT drugs.

Drug Interactions

Telavancin should be used with caution in patients taking other drugs that can damage the kidneys (e.g., NSAIDs, angiotensin-converting enzyme inhibitors, and aminoglycosides) and in patients taking drugs that prolong the QT interval (e.g., clarithromycin and ketoconazole). Clinically significant interactions involving cytochrome P450 enzymes have not been observed.

Aztreonam

Chemistry

Aztreonam (Azactam and Cayston) belongs to a class of β-lactam antibiotics known as monobactams. These agents contain a β-lactam ring, but the ring is not fused with a second ring.

Mechanism of Action

Aztreonam binds to PBP3. Therefore, as with most β-lactam antibiotics, the drug inhibits bacterial cell wall synthesis and, thus, promotes cell lysis and death. The drug does not bind to PBPs produced by anaerobes or gram-positive bacteria.

Antimicrobial Spectrum and Therapeutic Use

Aztreonam has a narrow antimicrobial spectrum, being active only against gram-negative aerobic bacteria. Susceptible organisms include *Neisseria* species, *H. influenzae, P. aeruginosa,* and Enterobacteriaceae (e.g., *E. coli, Klebsiella, Proteus, Serratia, Salmonella, and Shigella*). Aztreonam is highly resistant to β-lactamases and, therefore, is active against many gram-negative aerobes that produce them. The drug is not active against gram-positive bacteria and anaerobes.

Adverse Effect

Aztreonam is generally well tolerated. Adverse effects are like those of other β-lactam antibiotics. The most common effects are pain and thrombophlebitis at the site of injection. Because aztreonam differs greatly in structure from penicillins and cephalosporins, there is little cross-allergenicity with them. Hence aztreonam appears safe for patients with allergies to other β-lactam antibiotics.

Fosfomycin

Fosfomycin (Monurol) is a unique antibiotic approved for single-dose therapy in women with uncomplicated urinary tract infections (i.e., acute cystitis) caused by *E. coli* or *E. faecalis.* The drug kills bacteria by disrupting synthesis of the peptidoglycan polymer strands that compose the cell wall. (As discussed in Chapter 71, penicillins kill bacteria in part by preventing cross-linking of peptidoglycan strands.)

The most common adverse effects are diarrhea, headache, vaginitis, and nausea. Fosfomycin may also cause abdominal pain, rhinitis, drowsiness, dizziness, and rash.

Fosfomycin dosing may be done with or without food. Symptoms of cystitis should improve in 2 to 3 days. If symptoms fail to improve, additional doses will not help but will increase the risk for side effects.

73

Bacteriostatic Inhibitors of Protein Synthesis

All the drugs discussed in this chapter inhibit bacterial protein synthesis. However, unlike the aminoglycosides, which are bactericidal, the drugs considered here are largely bacteriostatic. That is, they suppress bacterial growth and replication but do not produce outright kill. In general, the drugs presented here are second-line agents, used primarily for infections resistant to first-line agents.

TETRACYCLINES

The tetracyclines are *broad-spectrum* antibiotics. In the United States, seven tetracyclines are available for systemic therapy. All seven—tetracycline, demeclocycline, doxycycline, eravacycline, omadacycline, sarecycline, and minocycline—are similar in structure, antimicrobial actions, and adverse effects. Principal differences among them are pharmacokinetic. Because the similarities among these drugs are more pronounced than their differences, the tetracyclines are discussed as a group rather than in terms of a prototype. Unique properties of individual tetracyclines are indicated as appropriate.

Mechanism of Action

The tetracyclines suppress bacterial growth by inhibiting protein synthesis. These drugs bind to the 30S ribosomal subunit and thereby inhibit binding of transfer RNA to the messenger RNA–ribosome complex. As a result, addition of amino acids to the growing peptide chain is prevented. At the concentrations achieved clinically, the tetracyclines are bacteriostatic.

Selective toxicity of the tetracyclines results from their poor ability to cross mammalian cell membranes. To influence protein synthesis, tetracyclines must first gain access to the cell interior. These drugs enter bacteria by way of an energy-dependent transport system. Mammalian cells lack this transport system and hence do not actively accumulate the drug. Consequently, although tetracyclines are inherently capable of inhibiting protein synthesis in mammalian cells, their levels within host cells remain too low to be harmful.

Antimicrobial Spectrum

The tetracyclines are broad-spectrum antibiotics, active against a wide variety of gram-positive and gram-negative bacteria. Sensitive organisms include *Rickettsia*, spirochetes, *Brucella*, *Chlamydia*, *Mycoplasma*, *Helicobacter pylori*, *Borrelia burgdorferi*, *Bacillus anthracis*, and *Vibrio cholerae*.

Therapeutic Uses
Treatment of Infectious Diseases

Extensive use of tetracyclines has resulted in increasing bacterial resistance. Because of resistance and because antibiotics with greater selectivity and less toxicity are now available, use of tetracyclines has declined. Today tetracyclines are rarely drugs of first choice. Disorders for which they *are* first-line drugs include (1) rickettsial diseases (e.g., Rocky Mountain spotted fever, typhus fever, Q fever); (2) infections caused by *Chlamydia trachomatis* (trachoma, lymphogranuloma

venereum, urethritis, cervicitis); (3) brucellosis; (4) cholera; (5) pneumonia caused by *Mycoplasma pneumoniae;* (6) Lyme disease; (7) anthrax; and (8) gastric infection with *H. pylori*.

Treatment of Acne

Tetracyclines are used topically and orally for severe acne vulgaris. Beneficial effects derive from suppressing the growth and metabolic activity of *Propionibacterium acnes*, an organism that secretes inflammatory chemicals. Oral doses for acne are relatively low. As a result, adverse effects are minimal. Acne is discussed in Chapter 88.

Peptic Ulcer Disease

H. pylori, a bacterium that lives in the stomach, is a major contributing factor to peptic ulcer disease. Tetracyclines, in combination with metronidazole and bismuth subsalicylate, are a treatment of choice for eradicating this bug. The role of *H. pylori* in ulcer formation is discussed in Chapter 64.

Periodontal Disease

Two tetracyclines—*doxycycline* and *minocycline*—are used for periodontal disease. Doxycycline is used orally *and* topically whereas minocycline is used only topically.

Oral therapy. Benefits of oral doxycycline result from inhibiting collagenase, an enzyme that destroys connective tissue in the gums. The small doses employed—20 mg twice daily—are too low to harm bacteria.

Topical therapy. Topical minocycline and doxycycline are employed as adjuncts to scaling and root planing. The objective is to reduce pocket depth and bleeding in adults with periodontitis. Benefits derive from suppressing bacterial growth. Both products are applied directly to the site of periodontal disease.

Pharmacokinetics

Individual tetracyclines differ significantly in their pharmacokinetic properties. Of particular significance are differences in half-life and route of elimination. Also important is the degree to which food decreases absorption. The pharmacokinetic properties of individual tetracyclines are shown in Table 73.1.

PATIENT EDUCATION
Drug Interactions With Tetracyclines

Tetracyclines should not be administered together with (1) *calcium supplements*, (2) *milk products* (because they contain calcium), (3) *iron supplements*, (4) *magnesium-containing laxatives*, and (5) *most antacids* (because they contain magnesium, aluminum, or both).

Distribution

Tetracyclines are widely distributed to most tissues and body fluids. However, penetration to the cerebrospinal fluid (CSF) is poor; hence levels in the CSF are too low to treat meningeal infections. Tetracyclines readily cross the placenta and enter the fetal circulation.

TABLE 73.1   Pharmacokinetic Properties of the Tetracyclines

Class	Drug	Lipid Solubility	Oral Dose Absorbed (%)[a]	Effect of Food on Absorption	Route of Elimination	HALF-LIFE Normal (h)	HALF-LIFE Anuric (h)
Short-acting	Tetracycline	Low	60–80	Large decrease	Urine	8	57–108[b]
Intermediate-acting	Demeclocycline	Moderate	60–80	Large decrease	Urine	12	40–60[b]
Long- acting	Doxycycline	High	90–100	Small decrease	GI (feces), urine	18	18–22
	Eravacycline	High	n/a (IV only)	n/a	GI (feces), renal	20	20–22
	Minocycline	High	90–100	No change	Urine, GI (feces)	16	11–23
	Omadacycline	High	35%	Large decrease	Renal and GI (feces)	16	16
	Sarecycline	Moderate	60%–70%	Large decrease	GI (feces), urine	21	n/a

[a]Percentage absorbed when taken on an empty stomach.
[b]Do not use in patients with renal impairment because the drug could accumulate to toxic levels.
GI, Gastrointestinal.

Adverse Effects

Gastrointestinal Irritation

Tetracyclines irritate the gastrointestinal (GI) tract. As a result, oral therapy is frequently associated with epigastric burning, cramps, nausea, vomiting, and diarrhea. These reactions can be reduced by giving tetracyclines with meals, although food may decrease absorption. Occasionally tetracyclines cause esophageal ulceration. The risk for this can be minimized by avoiding dosing at bedtime. Because diarrhea may result from superinfection of the bowel (in addition to nonspecific irritation), it is important that the cause of diarrhea be determined.

Effects on Bones and Teeth

Tetracyclines bind to calcium in developing teeth, resulting in yellow or brown discoloration; hypoplasia of the enamel may also occur. The intensity of tooth discoloration is related to the total cumulative dose: staining is darker with prolonged and repeated treatment. When taken by a pregnant woman after the fourth month of gestation, tetracyclines can cause staining of *deciduous* teeth of the infant. However, use during pregnancy will not affect *permanent* teeth. Discoloration of permanent teeth occurs when tetracyclines are taken by patients aged 4 months to 8 years, the interval during which tooth enamel is being formed. Accordingly, these drugs should be avoided by children younger than 8 years. The risk for tooth discoloration with *doxycycline* may be less than with other tetracyclines.

Tetracyclines taken by a pregnant woman can suppress the growth of long bones in premature infants. This effect is reversible on discontinuation of treatment.

Superinfection

A superinfection is an overgrowth with drug-resistant microbes, which occurs secondary to suppression of drug-sensitive organisms. Because the tetracyclines are broad-spectrum agents and therefore can decrease viability of a wide variety of microbes, the risk for superinfection is greater than that with antibiotics having a narrower spectrum.

Superinfection of the bowel with staphylococci or with *Clostridium difficile* produces severe diarrhea and can be life-threatening. The infection caused by *C. difficile* is known as *C. difficile*–associated diarrhea (CDAD), also known as *antibiotic-associated pseudomembranous colitis*. Patients should notify the prescriber if significant diarrhea occurs so that the possibility of bacterial superinfection can be evaluated. If a diagnosis of superinfection with staphylococci or *C. difficile* is made, tetracyclines should be discontinued immediately. Treatment of CDAD consists of oral *vancomycin* or *metronidazole* plus vigorous fluid and electrolyte replacement (see Chapter 66).

Overgrowth with fungi (commonly *Candida albicans*) may occur in the mouth, pharynx, vagina, and bowel. Symptoms include vaginal or anal itching; inflammatory lesions of the anogenital region; and a black, furry appearance of the tongue. Superinfection with *Candida* can be managed by discontinuing tetracyclines. When this is not possible, antifungal therapy is indicated.

Hepatotoxicity

Tetracyclines can cause fatty infiltration of the liver. Hepatotoxicity manifests clinically as lethargy and jaundice. Rarely, the condition progresses to massive liver failure. Liver damage is most likely when tetracyclines are administered intravenously in high doses (greater than 2 g/d). Pregnant and postpartum women with kidney disease are at especially high risk.

Renal Toxicity

Tetracyclines may exacerbate renal impairment in patients with preexisting kidney disease. Because *tetracycline* and *demeclocycline* are eliminated by the kidneys, these agents should not be given to patients with renal impairment. If a patient with renal impairment requires a tetracycline, either *doxycycline* or *minocycline* should be used because these drugs are eliminated primarily by the liver.

PATIENT EDUCATION

Sun Exposure Risk With Tetracyclines

All tetracyclines can increase the sensitivity of the skin to ultraviolet light. The most common result is exaggerated sunburn. Advise patients to avoid prolonged exposure to sunlight, to wear protective clothing, and to apply a sunscreen to exposed skin.

Drug and Food Interactions

As noted, tetracyclines can form nonabsorbable chelates with certain metal ions (calcium, iron, magnesium, aluminum, zinc). Substances that contain these ions include *milk products, calcium supplements, iron supplements, magnesium-containing laxatives,* and *most antacids.* If a tetracycline is administered with these agents, its absorption will be decreased. To minimize interference with absorption, tetracyclines should be *administered at least 1 hour before or 2 hours after ingestion of chelating agents.* Usual dosing is located in Table 73.2.

Tetracyclines can also increase digoxin levels through increasing absorption in the GI tract and increase international normalized ratio (INR) levels by altering the vitamin K–producing flora in the gut. Patients on digoxin or warfarin should undergo careful drug level monitoring.

TABLE 73.2 Tetracyclines: Routes of Administration, Dosing Interval, and Dosage

Class	Drug	Trade Names	Route	Usual Dosing Interval (h)	TOTAL DAILY DOSE Adult (mg)	TOTAL DAILY DOSE Pediatric (mg/kg)[a]
Short-acting	Tetracycline	Generic only	PO	6	1000–2000	25–50
Intermediate- acting	Demeclocycline	Generic only	PO	12	600	7–13
Long-acting	Doxycycline	Vibramycin, others	PO	24	100–200	2.2[b]
			IV	24	100–200[c]	2.2–4.4[d]
	Eravacycline	Xerava	IV	12	1 mg/kg	n/a
	Minocycline	Minocin, others	PO	12	200[e]	4[f]
			IV	12	200[e]	4[f]
	Omadacycline	Nuzyra	PO, IV	24	300–450	n/a
	Sarecycline	Seysara	PO	24	60–150	60–150

[a]Doses presented are for children older than 8 years. Use in children younger than this age may cause permanent staining of teeth.
[b]First-day regimen is 2.2 mg/kg initially, followed by 2.2 mg/kg 12 h later.
[c]First-day regimen is 200 mg in one or two slow infusions (1–4 h).
[d]First-day regimen is 4.4 mg/kg in one or two slow infusions (1–4 h).
[e]First-day regimen is 200 mg initially, followed by 100 mg 12 h later.
[f]First-day regimen is 4 mg/kg initially, followed by 2 mg/kg 12 h later.

PATIENT-CENTERED CARE ACROSS THE LIFE SPAN

Tetracyclines

Life Stage	Patient Care Concerns
Children/ adolescents	Tetracyclines should not be used in children younger than 8 years because they may cause permanent discoloration of the teeth..
Pregnant women	Animal studies reveal that tetracyclines can cause fetal harm in pregnancy. Thus this class of drugs should be avoided in pregnant women.
Breastfeeding women	Use of tetracyclines during tooth development can cause permanent staining. Tetracyclines should be avoided by breastfeeding women.
Older adults	Tetracyclines can interact with drugs, including digoxin. In the older adult who takes many medications, check for interactions.

Major Precautions

Two tetracyclines—*tetracycline* and *demeclocycline*—are eliminated primarily in the urine and hence will accumulate to toxic levels in patients with kidney disease. Accordingly, patients with kidney disease should not use these drugs.

Tetracyclines can cause discoloration of deciduous and permanent teeth. Tooth discoloration can be avoided by withholding these drugs from pregnant women and from children younger than 8 years of age.

Diarrhea may indicate a potentially life-threatening superinfection of the bowel. Advise patients to notify the prescriber if diarrhea occurs.

High-dose intravenous therapy has been associated with severe liver damage, particularly in pregnant and postpartum women with kidney disease. As a rule, these women should not receive tetracyclines.

MACROLIDES

The macrolides are broad-spectrum antibiotics that inhibit bacterial protein synthesis. They are called macrolides because they are big. Erythromycin is the oldest member of the family. The newer macrolides—azithromycin and clarithromycin—are derivatives of erythromycin (Table 73.3).

SUMMARY OF KEY PRESCRIBING CONSIDERATIONS

Tetracyclines

Therapeutic Goal: Treatment of tetracycline-sensitive infections, acne, and periodontal disease.
Baseline Data: None required.
Monitoring: None recommended.
Identifying High-Risk Patients: Contraindicated in pregnant women and in children younger than 8 years.
Evaluating Therapeutic Effects: Monitor for indications of antimicrobial effects—reduction in fever, pain, or inflammation.
Minimizing Adverse Effects: GI distress can be reduced by taking tetracyclines with meals. Advise patients to avoid prolonged exposure to sunlight.

Erythromycin

Erythromycin has a relatively broad antimicrobial spectrum and is a preferred or alternative treatment for a number of infections. The drug is one of our safer antibiotics and will serve as prototype for the macrolide family.

PROTOTYPE DRUGS

Bacteriostatic Inhibitors of Protein Synthesis

Tetracycline
Tetracycline

Macrolide
Erythromycin

Oxazolidinone
Linezolid

Glycylcycline
Tigecycline

Other
Clindamycin

TABLE 73.3 Macrolides: Routes of Administration, Dosing Interval, and Dosage

Drug	Trade Names	Route	Usual Dosing Interval (h)	Total Daily Dose Adult (mg)	Total Daily Dose Pediatric (mg/kg)
Azithromycin	Zithromax	PO	24	250–500[b]	5–12[a]
		IV	24	500	5–10[a]
Clarithromycin	Biaxin Biaxin XL	PO	12–24	500–1000	15
Erythromycin	Ery-Tab	PO	6	1000–2000	30–50
	E.E.S.	IV	24	1000–4000	15–50

[a]10 mg/kg on days 1–2 and 5 mg/kg on days 3–5.
[b]500 mg on day 1 and 250 mg on days 2–4.

Mechanism of Action

Antibacterial effects result from the inhibition of protein synthesis: erythromycin binds to the 50S ribosomal subunit and thereby blocks the addition of new amino acids to the growing peptide chain. The drug is usually bacteriostatic but can be bactericidal against highly susceptible organisms or when present in high concentration. Erythromycin is selectively toxic to bacteria because ribosomes in the cytoplasm of mammalian cells do not bind the drug. Also, in contrast to chloramphenicol (see later), erythromycin cannot cross the mitochondrial membrane and therefore does not inhibit protein synthesis in host mitochondria.

Antimicrobial Spectrum

Erythromycin has an antibacterial spectrum similar to that of penicillin. The drug is active against most gram-positive bacteria as well as some gram-negative bacteria. Bacterial sensitivity is determined in large part by the ability of erythromycin to gain access to the cell interior.

Therapeutic Uses

Erythromycin is a commonly used antibiotic. *The drug is a treatment of first choice for* Corynebacterium diphtheriae *and may be used as an alternative to penicillin G in patients with penicillin allergy.* Accordingly, erythromycin is the treatment of choice for *acute diphtheria* and for eliminating the diphtheria carrier state.

Several infections respond equally well to macrolides and tetracyclines. Both are drugs of first choice for certain chlamydial infections (urethritis, cervicitis) and for pneumonia caused by *Mycobacterium pneumoniae*.

Pharmacokinetics

Absorption and bioavailability. Erythromycin for oral administration is available in three forms: *erythromycin base* and two derivatives of the base, *erythromycin stearate* and *erythromycin ethylsuccinate*. The base is unstable in stomach acid and its absorption can be variable; the derivatives were synthesized to improve bioavailability. Bioavailability has also been enhanced by formulating tablets with an acid-resistant coating, which protects erythromycin while in the stomach and then dissolves in the duodenum, permitting absorption from the small intestine. As a rule, *food decreases the absorption of erythromycin base and erythromycin stearate,* whereas absorption of erythromycin ethylsuccinate is not affected. Only erythromycin base is biologically active; the derivatives must be converted to the base (either in the intestine or after absorption) in order to work. When used properly (i.e., when dosage is correct and the effects of food are accounted for), all of the oral erythromycins produce equivalent responses.

In addition to its oral forms, erythromycin is available as *erythromycin lactobionate* for intravenous use. Intravenous dosing produces drug levels higher than those achieved with oral dosing (see Table 73.3).

Distribution. Erythromycin readily distributes to most tissues and body fluids. Penetration to the CSF, however, is poor. Erythromycin crosses the placenta, but adverse effects on the fetus have not been observed.

Elimination. Erythromycin is eliminated primarily by hepatic mechanisms, including metabolism by CYP3A4 (the 3A4 isoenzyme of cytochrome P450). Erythromycin is concentrated in the liver and then excreted in the bile. A small amount (10% to 15%) is excreted unchanged in the urine.

Adverse Effects

Erythromycin is generally free of serious toxicity and is considered one of the safest antibiotics. However, the drug does carry a very small risk for sudden cardiac death from QT prolongation.

Gastrointestinal effects. Gastrointestinal disturbances (epigastric pain, nausea, vomiting, diarrhea) are the most common side effects. These can be reduced by administering erythromycin with meals. However, this should be done only with erythromycin products whose absorption is unaffected by food (erythromycin ethylsuccinate, certain enteric-coated formulations of erythromycin base). Patients who experience persistent or severe GI reactions should notify the prescriber.

QT prolongation and sudden cardiac death. When present in high concentrations, erythromycin can prolong the QT interval, thereby posing a risk for torsades de pointes, a potentially fatal ventricular dysrhythmia. Sudden death can result. When erythromycin is combined with a CYP3A4 inhibitor, there is a fivefold increase in the risk for sudden cardiac death—or 6 extra deaths for every 100,000 patients using the drug. To minimize risk, erythromycin should be avoided by patients with congenital QT prolongation and by those taking class IA or III antidysrhythmic drugs. Also, the drug should be avoided by patients taking CYP3A4 inhibitors, including certain calcium channel blockers (verapamil and diltiazem), azole antifungal drugs (e.g., ketoconazole, itraconazole), HIV protease inhibitors (e.g., ritonavir, saquinavir), and nefazodone (an antidepressant).

Drug Interactions

Erythromycin can increase the plasma levels and half-lives of several drugs, thereby posing a risk for toxicity. The mechanism is inhibition of hepatic cytochrome P450 drug-metabolizing enzymes. Elevated levels are a concern with *theophylline* (used for asthma), *carbamazepine* (used for seizures and bipolar disorder), and *warfarin* (an anticoagulant).

Accordingly, when these agents are combined with erythromycin, the patient should be monitored closely for signs of toxicity.

Erythromycin prevents binding of *chloramphenicol* and *clindamycin* to bacterial ribosomes, thereby antagonizing their antibacterial effects. Accordingly, concurrent use of erythromycin with these two drugs is not recommended.

As noted, erythromycin should not be combined with drugs that can inhibit erythromycin metabolism. Among these are verapamil, diltiazem, HIV protease inhibitors, and azole antifungal drugs.

 ## SUMMARY OF KEY PRESCRIBING CONSIDERATIONS

Macrolides

Therapeutic Goal: Treatment of respiratory infections, infections caused by *H. pylori*, disseminated *Mycobacterium*, and as alternatives to penicillin in patients with penicillin allergy.

Baseline Data: None indicated.

Monitoring: None recommended.

Identifying High-Risk Patients: Use with caution in patients with QT prolongation.

Evaluating Therapeutic Effects: Monitor for indications of antimicrobial effects—reduction in fever, pain, or inflammation.

Minimizing Adverse Effects: Avoid use in patients with QT prolongation. GI disturbances can be reduced by administering with meals.

OTHER BACTERIOSTATIC INHIBITORS OF PROTEIN SYNTHESIS

Clindamycin

Clindamycin (Cleocin, Dalacin C ✦) can promote severe CDAD, a condition that can be fatal. Because of the risk for CDAD, indications for clindamycin are limited. Currently, systemic use is indicated only for certain anaerobic infections located outside the central nervous system (CNS).

Mechanism of Action

Clindamycin binds to the 50S subunit of bacterial ribosomes and thereby inhibits protein synthesis. The site at which clindamycin binds overlaps the binding sites for erythromycin and chloramphenicol. As a result, these agents may antagonize each other's effects. Accordingly, there are no indications for concurrent use of clindamycin with these other antibiotics.

Antimicrobial Spectrum

Clindamycin is active against most anaerobic bacteria (gram-positive and gram-negative) and most gram-positive aerobes. Gram-negative aerobes are generally resistant. Susceptible anaerobes include *Bacteroides fragilis*, *Fusobacterium* species, *Clostridium perfringens*, and anaerobic streptococci. Clindamycin is usually bacteriostatic. However, it can be bactericidal if the target organism is especially sensitive. Resistance can be a significant problem with *B. fragilis*.

Therapeutic Use

Because of its efficacy against gram-positive cocci, clindamycin has been used widely as an alternative to penicillin. The drug is employed primarily for anaerobic infections outside the CNS (it does not cross the blood–brain barrier). Clindamycin is the drug of choice for severe group A streptococcal infection and for gas gangrene (an infection caused by *C. perfringens*), owing to its ability to rapidly suppress synthesis of bacterial toxins. (Table 73.4).

Adverse Effects

Clostridium difficile–associated diarrhea. CDAD, formerly known as *antibiotic-associated pseudomembranous colitis*, is the most severe toxicity of clindamycin. The cause is superinfection of the bowel with *C. difficile*, an anaerobic gram-positive bacillus. CDAD is characterized by profuse, watery diarrhea (10 to 20 watery stools per day), abdominal pain, fever, and leukocytosis. Stools often contain mucus and blood. Symptoms usually begin during the first week of treatment but may develop as long as 4 to 6 weeks after clindamycin withdrawal. Left untreated, the condition can be fatal. CDAD occurs with parenteral and oral therapy. Because of the risk for CDAD, patients should be instructed to report significant diarrhea (more than five watery stools per day). If superinfection with *C. difficile* is diagnosed, clindamycin should be discontinued and the patient given oral vancomycin or metronidazole, which are drugs of choice for eliminating *C. difficile* from the bowel. Diarrhea usually ceases 3 to 5 days after starting vancomycin. Vigorous replacement therapy with fluids and electrolytes is usually indicated. Drugs that decrease bowel motility (e.g., opioids, anticholinergics) may worsen symptoms and should not be used. CDAD is discussed further in Chapter 66.

 ## BLACK BOX WARNING

Clindamycin

> Clindamycin can cause potentially fatal *Clostridium difficile* diarrhea. Patients should promptly report any diarrhea to their health care provider.

Linezolid

Linezolid (Zyvox) is a first-in-class *oxazolidinone* antibiotic. The drug is important because it has activity against multidrug-resistant gram-positive pathogens, including vancomycin-resistant enterococci (VRE) and methicillin-resistant *Staphylococcus aureus* (MRSA). For treatment of MRSA, the drug is at least as effective as vancomycin. To delay the emergence of resistance, linezolid should generally be reserved for infections caused by VRE or MRSA, even though it has additional approved uses.

Mechanism, Resistance, and Antimicrobial Spectrum

Linezolid is a bacteriostatic inhibitor of protein synthesis. The drug binds to the 23S portion of the 50S ribosomal subunit and thereby blocks formation of the initiation complex. As a result, cross-resistance with other agents is unlikely. In clinical trials, development of resistance to linezolid was rare and occurred only in association with prolonged treatment of VRE infections and the presence of a prosthetic implant or undrained abscess. In actual practice, resistance has been reported in association with extensive linezolid use.

Linezolid is active primarily against aerobic and facultative gram-positive bacteria. Susceptible pathogens include *Enterococcus faecium* (vancomycin-sensitive and vancomycin-resistant strains), *Enterococcus faecalis* (vancomycin-resistant strains), *S. aureus* (methicillin-sensitive and methicillin-resistant strains), *Staphylococcus epidermidis* (including methicillin-resistant strains), and *Streptococcus pneumoniae* (penicillin-sensitive and penicillin-resistant strains). Linezolid is not active against gram-negative bacteria, which readily export the drug.

Therapeutic Use

Linezolid has five approved indications:
- Infections caused by VRE
- Hospital-acquired pneumonia caused by *S. aureus* (methicillin-susceptible and methicillin-resistant strains) or *S. pneumoniae* (penicillin-susceptible strains only)

TABLE 73.4 Other Bacteriostatic Inhibitors

Drug	Class and Mechanism of Action	Therapeutic Use	Pharmacokinetics	Adverse Effects	Drug Interactions
Clindamycin (Cleocin)	Lincosamide antibiotic Binds to 50S subunit of bacterial ribosomes	Anaerobic infections outside the CNS *Clostrodium perfringes* Group A streptococcus	Metabolism: hepatic Elimination: renal Poor CSF distribution	CDAD	May decrease oral contraceptive activity.
Linezolid (Zyvox)	Oxazolidinone antibiotic Binds to 23S portion of the 50S ribosomal subunit	Aerobic and facilitative gram-positive bacteria *Enterococcus* *Staphylococcus*	Metabolism: hepatic, elimination: renal	Diarrhea, nausea, headache. Myelosuppression	MAO inhibitors, SSRIs.
Tedizolid (Sivextro)	Oxazolidinone antibiotic Binds to 23S portion of the 50S ribosomal subunit	Skin and soft tissue infections caused by MRSA, *Streptococcus*, and *Enterococcus*	Metabolism: hepatic Elimination: GI (feces)	Diarrhea, nausea, headache, myelosuppression	MAO inhibitors, SSRIs.
Dalfopristin/ quinupristin (Synercid)	Streptogramin antibiotics Separately bacteriostatic; in combination, bactericidal	*Enterococcus*, specifically resistant to vancomycin MRSA, drug-resistant *Streptococcus pneumoniae*	Metabolism: hepatic Elimination: GI (feces)	Hepatotoxicity	Drugs metabolized through CYP3A4, including cyclosporine and tacrolimus.
Chloramphenicol (generic only)	Binds to the 50S subunit of bacterial ribosomes	Broad-spectrum aerobic and anaerobic bacteria Life-threatening infections for which safer drugs are ineffective or contraindicated	Metabolism: hepatic Elimination: hepatic and renal Highly penetrable to CSF	Aplastic anemia, Gray syndrome	Phenytoin and warfarin.
Tigecycline (Tygacil)	Glycylcycline antibiotic Binds to the 50S ribosomal subunit	Broad-spectrum with gram-positive and gram-negative bacteria Approved only for intra-abdominal infections, CAP, and complicated skin infections.	Metabolism: very little metabolized Elimination: GI (bile) and renal	Nausea and vomiting, CDAD, acute pancreatitis	Warfarin.
Mupirocin (Bactroban)	Binds with bacterial isoleucyl transfer RNA synthetase	Topical antibiotic for impetigo caused by *Staphylococcus* or *Streptococcus* and elimination of nasal colonization by MRSA	Metabolism: minimal absorption with rapid conversion to inactive products Elimination: urine	Local skin irritation, headache, rhinitis	None.

CAP, Community-acquired pneumonia; *CDAD*, *Clostridium difficile*–associated diarrhea; *CNS*, central nervous system; *CSF*, cerebrospinal fluid; *GI*, gastrointestinal; *MAO*, monoamine oxidase; *MRSA*, methicillin-resistant *Staphylococcus aureus*; *MSSA*, methicillin-sensitive *Staphylococcus aureus*; *SSRI*, selective serotonin reuptake inhibitor.

- Community-associated pneumonia (CAP) caused by *S. pneumoniae* (penicillin-susceptible strains only)
- Complicated skin and skin structure infections caused by *S. aureus* (methicillin-susceptible and methicillin-resistant strains), *Streptococcus pyogenes*, or *Streptococcus agalactiae*
- Uncomplicated skin and skin structure infections caused by *S. aureus* (methicillin-susceptible strains only) or *S. pyogenes*

As noted previously, to delay the emergence of resistance, linezolid should generally be reserved for infections caused by VRE or MRSA, even though it has other approved uses (see Table 73.4).

Adverse Effects

Linezolid is generally well tolerated. The most common side effects are diarrhea, nausea, and headache. Linezolid oral suspension contains phenylalanine and hence must not be used by patients with phenylketonuria.

Linezolid can cause reversible *myelosuppression*, manifesting as anemia, leukopenia, thrombocytopenia, or even pancytopenia. Risk is related to duration of use. Complete blood counts should be done weekly. Special caution is needed in patients with preexisting myelosuppression,

those taking other myelosuppressive drugs, and those receiving linezolid for more than 2 weeks. If existing myelosuppression worsens or new myelosuppression develops, discontinuing linezolid should be considered.

Rarely, prolonged therapy has been associated with *neuropathy*. Patients taking the drug for more than 5 months have developed reversible optic neuropathy and irreversible peripheral neuropathy.

Drug Interactions

Linezolid is a weak inhibitor of monoamine oxidase (MAO) and hence poses a risk for hypertensive crisis. As discussed in Chapter 27, MAO inhibitors can cause severe hypertension if combined with *indirect-acting sympathomimetics* (e.g., ephedrine, pseudoephedrine, methylphenidate, cocaine) or with foods that contain large amounts of *tyramine*. Accordingly, patients using linezolid should be warned to avoid these agents.

Combining linezolid with a *selective serotonin reuptake inhibitor* (SSRI) can increase the risk for serotonin syndrome (because inhibition of MAO increases the serotonin content of CNS neurons). Deaths have been reported. Patients using SSRIs (e.g., paroxetine [Paxil, Pexeva], duloxetine [Cymbalta]) should not take linezolid.

Tedizolid

Tedizolid (Sivextro) was the second *oxazolidinone* antibiotic approved after linezolid. Like linezolid, tedizolid is effective in the treatment of MRSA as well as other bacterial skin and soft tissue infections caused by sensitive *Staphylococcus* and *Streptococcus* species.

Therapeutic Use

Tedizolid is used in the treatment of skin and soft tissue infections caused by MRSA, methicillin-sensitive *S. aureus* (MSSA), *S. pyogenes*, *S. agalactiae*, *Streptococcus anginosus* group (including *Streptococcus anginosus, Streptococcus intermedius,* and *Streptococcus constellatus)*, and *E. fecalis* (see Table 73.4).

Adverse Effects

The most common side effects associated with tedizolid are diarrhea, nausea, vomiting, dizziness, and headache. More serious adverse effects such as neuropathy and myelosuppression were seen with tedizolid as with linezolid.

Drug Interactions

Tedizolid interacts with few drugs. Of note, both tedizolid and linezolid are weak inhibitors of MAO and hence pose a risk for hypertensive crisis. Accordingly, patients using tedizolid should be warned to avoid these agents. The same principle applies to the SSRIs as well.

74

Aminoglycosides: Bactericidal Inhibitors of Protein Synthesis

The aminoglycosides are narrow-spectrum antibiotics used primarily against aerobic gram-negative bacilli. These drugs disrupt protein synthesis, resulting in rapid bacterial death. The aminoglycosides can cause serious injury to the inner ears and kidneys. Because of these toxicities, indications for these drugs are limited. All of the aminoglycosides carry multiple positive charges. As a result, they are not absorbed from the gastrointestinal (GI) tract and must be administered parenterally to treat systemic infections. In the United States, seven aminoglycosides are approved for clinical use. The agents employed most commonly are gentamicin, tobramycin, and amikacin.

BASIC PHARMACOLOGY OF THE AMINOGLYCOSIDES

Chemistry

The aminoglycosides are composed of two or more amino sugars connected by a glycoside linkage. At physiologic pH, these drugs are highly polar polycations (i.e., they carry several positive charges) and therefore cannot readily cross membranes. As a result, aminoglycosides are not absorbed from the GI tract, do not enter the cerebrospinal fluid, and are rapidly excreted by the kidneys.

Mechanism of Action

The aminoglycosides disrupt bacterial protein synthesis. As indicated in Fig. 74.1, these drugs bind to the 30S ribosomal subunit, causing (1) inhibition of protein synthesis, (2) premature termination of protein synthesis, and (3) production of abnormal proteins (secondary to misreading of the genetic code).

The aminoglycosides are *bactericidal*. Cell kill is *concentration dependent*. Hence the higher the concentration, the more rapidly the infection will clear. Of note, bactericidal activity persists for several hours *after* serum levels have dropped below the minimal bactericidal concentration, a phenomenon known as the *postantibiotic effect.*

Bacterial kill appears to result from the production of abnormal proteins rather than from simple inhibition of protein synthesis. Studies suggest that abnormal proteins become inserted in the bacterial cell membrane, causing it to leak. The resultant loss of cell contents causes death. Inhibition of protein synthesis per se does not seem the likely cause of bacterial death because complete blockade of protein synthesis by other antibiotics (e.g., tetracyclines, chloramphenicol) is usually bacteriostatic, not bactericidal.

Microbial Resistance

The principal cause for bacterial resistance is the production of enzymes that can inactivate aminoglycosides. Among gram-negative bacteria, the genetic information needed to synthesize these enzymes is acquired through the transfer of R factors. To date, more than 20 different aminoglycoside-inactivating enzymes have been identified. Because each of the aminoglycosides can be modified by more than one of these enzymes and each enzyme can act on more than one aminoglycoside, patterns of bacterial resistance can be complex.

Of all the aminoglycosides, *amikacin* is least susceptible to inactivation by bacterial enzymes. As a result, resistance to amikacin is uncommon. To minimize the emergence of resistant bacteria, amikacin should be reserved for infections that are unresponsive to other aminoglycosides.

Antimicrobial Spectrum

Bactericidal effects of the aminoglycosides are limited almost exclusively to aerobic *gram-negative bacilli*. Sensitive organisms include *Escherichia coli, Klebsiella pneumoniae, Serratia marcescens, Proteus mirabilis*, and *Pseudomonas aeruginosa*. Aminoglycosides are inactive against most gram-positive bacteria.

Aminoglycosides *cannot kill anaerobes*. To produce antibacterial effects, aminoglycosides must be transported across the bacterial cell membrane, a process that is oxygen dependent. Because by definition anaerobic organisms live in the absence of oxygen, these microbes cannot take up aminoglycosides and hence are resistant. For the same reason, aminoglycosides are inactive against facultative bacteria when these organisms are living under anaerobic conditions.

Therapeutic Use
Parenteral Therapy

The principal use for parenteral aminoglycosides is treatment of *serious infections due to aerobic gram-negative bacilli*. Primary target organisms are *P. aeruginosa* and the Enterobacteriaceae (e.g., *E. coli, Klebsiella* and *Serratia* species, *P. mirabilis*).

One aminoglycoside—gentamicin—is used in combination with either vancomycin or a beta-lactam antibiotic to treat *serious infections with certain gram-positive cocci*, specifically *Enterococcus* species, some streptococci, and *Staphylococcus aureus.*

The aminoglycosides used most commonly for parenteral therapy are gentamicin, tobramycin, and amikacin. Selection among the three depends in large part on patterns of resistance in a given community or hospital. In settings where resistance to aminoglycosides is uncommon, either gentamicin or tobramycin is usually preferred. Of the two, gentamicin is less expensive and may be selected on this basis. Organisms resistant to both gentamicin and tobramycin are usually sensitive to amikacin. Accordingly, in settings where resistance to gentamicin and tobramycin is common, amikacin may be preferred for initial therapy.

Topical Therapy

Aminoglycosides are also used topically to treat infection. Gentamicin and tobramycin can treat eye infections (see Chapter 87), while neomycin can treat infections of the ear and eye (see Chapters 87 and 89).

Pharmacokinetics

All of the aminoglycosides have similar pharmacokinetic profiles. Pharmacokinetic properties of the principal aminoglycosides are shown in Table 74.1.

Normal Protein Synthesis

Effects of Aminoglycosides

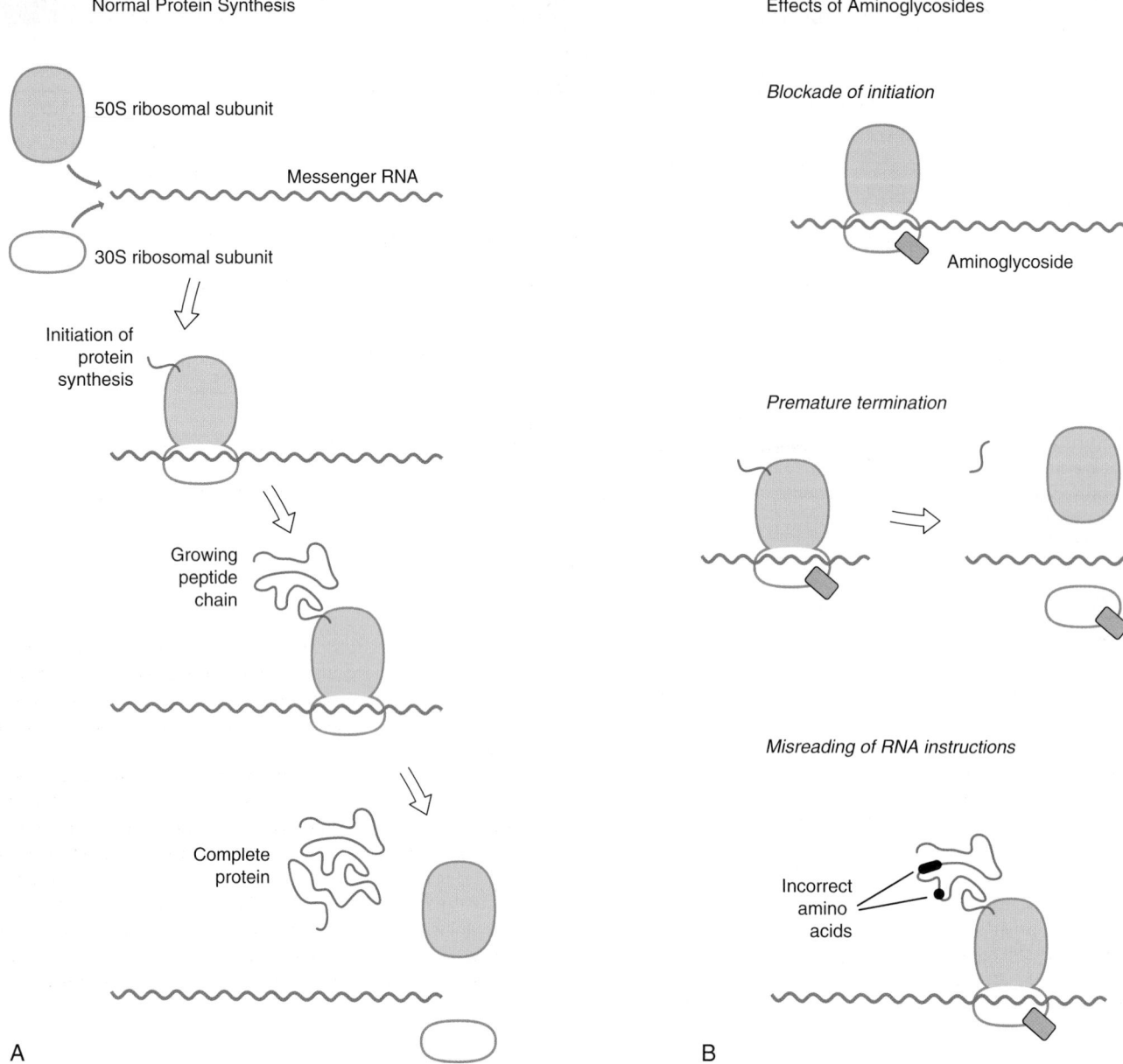

Fig. 74.1 Mechanism of Action of Aminoglycosides. (A) Protein synthesis begins with binding of the 50S and 30S ribosomal subunits to messenger RNA (mRNA), followed by attachment of the first amino acid of the new protein to the 50S subunit. As the ribosome moves down the mRNA strand, additional amino acids are added to the growing peptide chain. When the new protein is complete, it separates from the ribosome and the ribosomal subunits separate from the mRNA. (B) Aminoglycosides bind to the 30S ribosomal subunit and can (1) block initiation, (2) terminate synthesis before the new protein is complete, and (3) cause misreading of the genetic code, which leads to the synthesis of faulty proteins.

Absorption

Because they are polycations, the aminoglycosides cross membranes poorly. As a result, very little (about 1%) of an oral dose is absorbed. Hence for treatment of systemic infections, aminoglycosides must be given parenterally (by intramuscular (IM) or intravenous (IV) administration). Absorption after application to the intact skin is minimal. However, when used for wound irrigation, aminoglycosides may be absorbed in amounts sufficient to produce systemic toxicity.

Distribution

Distribution of aminoglycosides is limited largely to extracellular fluid. Entry into the cerebrospinal fluid is insufficient to treat meningitis in adults. Aminoglycosides bind tightly to renal tissue, achieving levels in the kidneys up to 50 times higher than levels in serum. These high levels are responsible for nephrotoxicity (see later). Aminoglycosides penetrate readily to the perilymph and endolymph of the inner ears and can thereby cause ototoxicity (see later). Aminoglycosides can cross the placenta and may be toxic to the fetus.

Elimination

The aminoglycosides are eliminated primarily by the kidneys. These drugs are not metabolized. In patients with normal renal function, half-lives of the aminoglycosides range from 2 to 3 hours. However, because elimination is almost exclusively renal, half-lives increase

TABLE 74.1 Dosages and Pharmacokinetics of Systemic Aminoglycosides

Generic Name	Trade Name	TOTAL DAILY DOSE (mg/kg)[a,b]		HALF-LIFE IN ADULTS (h)		Therapeutic (Peak) Level[c,d] (µg/mL)	Recommended Trough Level[e,f] (µg/mL)
		Adults	Children	Normal	Anuric		
Amikacin	Generic only	15	15	2–3	24–60	15–30	Less than 5–10
Gentamicin	Generic only	3–5[g]	6–7.5[g]	2	24–60	4–10[h]	Less than 1–2[i]
Tobramycin	Generic only	3–6	6–7.5	2–2.5	24–60	4–10	Less than 1–2[i]

[a]The total daily dose may be administered as one large dose each day or as two or three divided doses given at equally spaced intervals around the clock.

[b]Because of interpatient variability, standard doses cannot be relied on to produce appropriate serum drug levels; hence dosage should be adjusted on the basis of serum drug measurements.

[c]Measured 30 minutes after intramuscular injection or after completing a 30-minute intravenous infusion.

[d]The peak values presented refer to levels obtained when the total daily dosage is given in *divided* doses rather than as a single large daily dose.

[e]Measured just before the next dose.

[f]To minimize ototoxicity and nephrotoxicity, drug levels should drop *below* the listed values between doses.

[g]When gentamicin is combined with either vancomycin or a β-lactam antibiotic to treat certain gram-positive infections, the total daily dose is much lower (e.g., about 1 mg/kg for adults).

[h]These peak values apply when gentamicin is used to treat gram-negative infections, not when gentamicin is combined with vancomycin or a β-lactam antibiotic to treat gram-positive infections.

[i]For severe infections, the trough may be higher (e.g., less than 2–4 µg/mL).

PATIENT-CENTERED CARE ACROSS THE LIFE SPAN

Aminoglycosides

Life Stage	Patient Care Concerns
Infants	Aminoglycosides are approved to treat bacterial infections in infants younger than 8 days. Dosing is based on weight and length of gestation.
Children/adolescents	Aminoglycosides are safe for use against bacterial infections in children and adolescents.
Pregnant women	There is evidence that use of aminoglycosides in pregnancy can harm the fetus.
Breastfeeding women	Gentamicin is probably safe to use during lactation. There is limited information regarding its use in this way.
Older adults	Caution must be used regarding decreased renal function in the older adult.

dramatically in patients with renal impairment. *Accordingly, to avoid serious toxicity, we must reduce dosage size or increase the dosing interval in patients with kidney disease.*

Interpatient Variation

Different patients receiving the same aminoglycoside dosage (in milligrams per kilogram of body weight) can achieve widely different serum levels of drug. This interpatient variation is caused by several factors, including age, percent body fat, and pathophysiology (e.g., renal impairment, fever, edema, dehydration). Because of the variability among patients, aminoglycoside dosage must be individualized. As dramatic evidence of this need, in one clinical study it was observed that, to produce equivalent serum drug levels, the doses required ranged from as little as 0.5 mg/kg in one patient to a high of 25.8 mg/kg in another—a difference of more than 50-fold.

Adverse Effects

The aminoglycosides can produce serious toxicity, especially to the inner ears and kidneys. These structures are vulnerable because aminoglycosides become concentrated within their cells.

Ototoxicity

All aminoglycosides can accumulate within the inner ears, causing cellular injury that can impair both hearing and balance. *Hearing impairment* is caused by damage to sensory hair cells in the *cochlea*. *Disruption of balance* is caused by damage to sensory hair cells of the *vestibular apparatus*.

The risk for ototoxicity is related primarily to excessive *trough levels* of drug rather than to excessive *peak* levels. When trough levels remain persistently elevated, aminoglycosides are unable to diffuse out of inner ear cells; hence the cells are exposed to the drug continuously for an extended time. It is this prolonged exposure, rather than brief exposure to high levels, that underlies cellular injury. In addition to high trough levels, the risk for ototoxicity is increased by (1) renal impairment (which can cause accumulation of aminoglycosides), (2) concurrent use of loop diuretics, and (3) administering aminoglycosides in excessive doses or for more than 10 days.

BLACK BOX WARNING

Aminoglycoside Neurotoxicity/Ototoxicity

Use of aminoglycosides is associated with irreversible ototoxicity. Neurotoxic symptoms may also include numbness, tingling, muscle twitching, and seizures. This risk increases in patients on high doses or with prolonged use and in patients with preexisting renal impairment.

Patients on aminoglycoside therapy should be monitored for ototoxicity. The first sign of impending *cochlear* damage is high-pitched tinnitus. Ototoxicity is largely *irreversible*. Accordingly, if permanent injury is to be avoided, aminoglycosides should be withdrawn at the first sign of damage (i.e., tinnitus, persistent headache, or both).

As injury to cochlear hair cells proceeds, hearing in the high-frequency range begins to decline. Loss of low-frequency hearing develops with continued drug use. Because the initial decline in high-frequency hearing is subtle, audiometric testing is needed to detect it. The first sign of impending *vestibular* damage is headache, which may last for 1 or 2 days. After that, nausea, unsteadiness, dizziness, and vertigo begin to appear. Patients should be informed about the symptoms of vestibular and cochlear damage and instructed to report them.

 BLACK BOX WARNING

Aminoglycoside Nephrotoxicity

> Use of aminoglycosides is associated with nephrotoxicity. This risk increases in patients using high doses, with prolonged use, and in patients with preexisting renal impairment.

Nephrotoxicity

Aminoglycosides can injure cells of the proximal renal tubules. These drugs are taken up by tubular cells and achieve high intracellular concentrations. As with ototoxicity, nephrotoxicity correlates with (1) the *total cumulative dose* of aminoglycosides and (2) *high trough levels.* High *peak levels* do not seem to increase toxicity. Aminoglycoside-induced nephrotoxicity usually manifests as acute tubular necrosis. Prominent symptoms are proteinuria, casts in the urine, production of dilute urine, and elevations in serum creatinine and blood urea nitrogen (BUN). Serum creatinine and BUN should be monitored. The risk for nephrotoxicity is especially high in older adults, in patients with preexisting kidney disease, and in patients receiving other nephrotoxic drugs (e.g., amphotericin B, cyclosporine). Fortunately, cells of the proximal tubule readily regenerate. As a result, injury to the kidneys usually reverses after aminoglycoside use.[a] The most significant consequence of renal damage is accumulation of aminoglycosides themselves, which can lead to ototoxicity and even more kidney damage.

 BLACK BOX WARNING

Aminoglycoside-Induced Neuromuscular Blockade

> Aminoglycosides can inhibit neuromuscular transmission, causing flaccid paralysis and potentially fatal respiratory depression. Most episodes of neuromuscular blockade have occurred after intraperitoneal or intrapleural instillation of aminoglycosides.

Beneficial Drug Interactions
Penicillins

Penicillins and aminoglycosides are frequently employed in combination to enhance bacterial kill. The combination is effective because penicillins disrupt the cell wall and thereby facilitate access of aminoglycosides to their site of action.

Cephalosporins and Vancomycin

Like the penicillins, cephalosporins and vancomycin weaken the bacterial cell wall and can thereby act in concert with aminoglycosides to enhance bacterial kill.

Adverse Drug Interactions
Ototoxic Drugs

The risk for injury to the inner ears is increased by concurrent use of loop diuretics—these combinations should be avoided.

---

[a]If interstitial fibrosis or renal tubular necrosis develops, damage to the kidneys may be permanent.

Nephrotoxic Drugs

The risk for renal damage is increased by concurrent therapy with other nephrotoxic agents. Additive or potentiative nephrotoxicity can occur with *amphotericin B, cephalosporins, polymyxins, vancomycin,* and *cyclosporine* as well as with *aspirin* and *other nonsteroidal antiinflammatory drugs (NSAIDs).*

Dosing Schedules

Systemic aminoglycosides may be administered as a single large dose each day or as two or three smaller doses. Traditionally, these drugs have been administered in divided doses, given at equally spaced intervals around the clock (e.g., every 8 hours). Today, however, it is common to administer the total daily dose all at once rather than dividing it up. Several studies have shown that once-daily doses are just as effective as divided doses and probably safer. Because once-daily dosing is both safe and effective and it's easier and cheaper than giving divided doses, once-daily dosing has become the preferred schedule. However, this schedule is not appropriate for some patients, including neonates, patients who are pregnant, patients undergoing dialysis, and patients with ascites.

Monitoring Serum Drug Levels

Monitoring serum drug levels provides the best basis for adjusting aminoglycoside dosage. To produce bacterial kill, peak levels must be sufficiently high. To minimize ototoxicity and nephrotoxicity, trough levels must be sufficiently low.

How monitoring is done depends on the dosing schedule employed (i.e., once-daily dosing or use of divided doses). When once-daily dosing is employed, only trough levels need to be measured. As a rule, there is no need to measure peak levels because, when the entire daily dose is given at once, high peak levels are guaranteed. (They are typically three to four times those achieved with divided doses.) In contrast, when divided doses are employed, we need to measure both the peak and the trough.

When blood samples for aminoglycoside levels are being drawn, timing is important. Samples for *peak* levels should be taken 30 minutes after giving an IM injection or after completing an IV infusion. Sampling for *trough* levels depends on the dosing schedule. For patients receiving *divided doses,* trough samples should be taken just before the next dose. For patients receiving *once-daily doses,* a single sample can be drawn 1 hour before the next dose. The value should be very low, preferably close to zero.

PROPERTIES OF INDIVIDUAL AMINOGLYCOSIDES
Gentamicin
Therapeutic Use

Gentamicin is used primarily to treat serious infections caused by aerobic gram-negative bacilli. Primary targets are *P. aeruginosa* and the Enterobacteriaceae (e.g., *E. coli, Klebsiella* and *Serratia* species, *P. mirabilis*). In hospitals where resistance is not a problem, gentamicin is often the preferred aminoglycoside for use against these bacteria because it is cheaper than the alternatives (tobramycin and amikacin). Unfortunately, resistance to gentamicin is increasing, and cross-resistance to tobramycin is common. For infections that are resistant to gentamicin and tobramycin, amikacin is usually effective.

In addition to its use against gram-negative bacilli, gentamicin can be combined with vancomycin, a cephalosporin, or a penicillin to treat serious infections caused by certain gram-positive cocci, namely *Enterococcus* species, some streptococci, and *S. aureus* (Table 74.2).

Adverse Effects and Interactions

As in the case of all other aminoglycosides, gentamicin is toxic to the kidneys and inner ears. Caution must be exercised when gentamicin is

TABLE 74.2	**Aminoglycosides**		
Drug	**Therapeutic Use**	**Preparations**	**Usual Adult Dosage**
Gentamicin	Bacterial infections caused by aerobic gram-negative bacilli: *Pseudomonas aeruginosa* Enterobacteriaceae	Injection (IV/IM, intrathecal)	1–1.7 mg/kg q 8 h
Tobramycin	Bacterial infections caused by aerobic gram-negative bacilli: *Pseudomonas aeruginosa* Enterobacteriaceae	Injection (IV/IM) Nebulizer solution 300 mg/5 mL	1–1.7 mg/kg q 8 h 300 mg q 12 h
Amikacin	Bacterial infections caused by gram-negative bacilli	Injection (IV/IM)	15 mg/kg/d divided q 8–12 h
Neomycin	Topical infection Prevention in minor cuts Ocular bacterial infections	Topical cream Topical ointment	Apply 1–3 times daily Apply q 3–4 h
Kanamycin	Bacterial infections caused by gram-negative bacilli—not to be used for *Serratia* and *Pseudomonas*, as these bacteria are now resistant	Injection (IV/IM)	7.5 mg/kg q 12 h
Streptomycin	Used in combination with other drugs to treat tuberculosis; also used to treat tularemia and plague	Injection (IV/IM)	1–2 g/d divided q 6–12 h
Paromycin	Treatment of intestinal amebiasis	250-mg capsules	25–35 mg/kg per day divided q 8 h
Plazomicin (Zemdri)	Complicated UTI caused by Enterobacteriaceae	Injection (IV)	15 mg/kg q 24 h

UTI, Urinary tract infection.

combined with other nephrotoxic or ototoxic drugs. Gentamicin is inactivated by direct chemical interaction with penicillins; hence these drugs should not be mixed in the same parenteral solution.

Tobramycin
Uses, Adverse Effects, and Interactions
Tobramycin is similar to gentamicin with respect to uses, adverse effects, and interactions. The drug is more active than gentamicin against *P. aeruginosa* but less active against enterococci and *Serratia* species (see Table 74.2). Tobramycin is used for patients with cystic fibrosis. Like all other aminoglycosides, tobramycin can injure the inner ears and kidneys. If possible, concurrent therapy with other ototoxic or nephrotoxic drugs should be avoided. Tobramycin may also cause *C. difficile*–associated diarrhea.

Amikacin
Uses, Adverse Effects, and Interactions
Amikacin has two outstanding features. Of all the aminoglycosides, (1) amikacin is active against the broadest spectrum of gram-negative bacilli, and (2) it is the least vulnerable to inactivation by bacterial enzymes. Because most aminoglycoside-inactivating enzymes do not affect amikacin, the incidence of bacterial resistance to this agent is lower than that with other major aminoglycosides (gentamicin and tobramycin). In hospitals where resistance to gentamicin and tobramycin is common, amikacin is the preferred agent for initial treatment of infections caused by aerobic gram-negative bacilli (see Table 74.2). However, in settings

where resistance to the other aminoglycosides is infrequent, amikacin should be reserved for infections of proven aminoglycoside resistance because this practice will delay the emergence of organisms resistant to amikacin. Similarly to all other aminoglycosides, amikacin is toxic to the kidneys and inner ears. Caution should be exercised if amikacin is used in combination with other ototoxic or nephrotoxic drugs.

SUMMARY OF KEY PRESCRIBING CONSIDERATIONS

Aminoglycosides

Therapeutic Goal: Treatment of serious infections caused by gram-negative aerobic bacilli.

Baseline Data: Blood and/or urine cultures.

Monitoring: Aminoglycoside levels (peaks and troughs) and renal function must be monitored.

Identifying High-Risk Patients: Aminoglycosides should be used with caution in patients with renal impairment, preexisting hearing impairment, and those receiving ototoxic and nephrotoxic drugs.

Evaluating Therapeutic Effects: Patients must be monitored for indications of antimicrobial effects, including reduction in fever, pain, or inflammation.

Minimizing Adverse Effects: Caution must be exercised when aminoglycosides are used in combination with other nephrotoxic or ototoxic drugs. Patients must be instructed to report symptoms of ototoxicity.

75

Sulfonamide Antibiotics and Trimethoprim

The sulfonamides and trimethoprim are broad-spectrum antimicrobials that have closely related mechanisms. In approaching these drugs, the sulfonamides are discussed first, followed by trimethoprim, and then by trimethoprim/sulfamethoxazole, an important fixed-dose combination.

SULFONAMIDES

Sulfonamides were the first drugs available for the systemic treatment of bacterial infections. After their introduction in the 1930s, their use produced a sharp decline in morbidity and mortality from susceptible infections. With the advent of penicillin and newer antimicrobial drugs, use of sulfonamides has greatly declined. Nonetheless, the sulfonamides still have important uses, primarily against urinary tract infections (UTIs). With the introduction of trimethoprim/sulfamethoxazole in the 1970s, indications for the sulfonamides expanded.

Sulfonamides are usually bacteriostatic. Accordingly, adequate host defenses are essential for elimination of infection.

The similarities among the sulfonamides are more striking than the differences. Accordingly, the sulfonamides are discussed as a group as opposed to focusing on a representative prototype.

Mechanism of Action

The general structural formula for the sulfonamides is shown in Fig. 75.1. Sulfonamides are structural analogs of para-aminobenzoic acid (PABA), a component of folate. The antimicrobial actions of sulfonamides are based on this similarity.

Sulfonamides suppress bacterial growth by inhibiting the synthesis of tetrahydrofolate, a derivative of folate. In the absence of tetrahydrofolate bacteria are unable to synthesize DNA, RNA, and proteins.

If all cells require folate, why don't sulfonamides harm us? The answer lies in how bacteria and mammalian cells acquire folate. Bacteria are unable to take up folate from their environment, so they must synthesize it from precursors. In contrast to bacteria, mammalian cells do not manufacture their own folate. Rather, they simply take up folate from the diet, using a specialized transport system for uptake. Because mammalian cells use preformed folate rather than synthesizing it, sulfonamides are harmless to us.

Antimicrobial Spectrum

The sulfonamides are active against a broad spectrum of microbes comprising gram-positive cocci (including methicillin-resistant *Staphylococcus aureus*), gram-negative bacilli, *Listeria monocytogenes*, actinomycetes (e.g., *Nocardia*), chlamydiae (e.g., *Chlamydia trachomatis*), some protozoa (e.g., *Toxoplasma* species, plasmodia, *Isospora belli*), and two fungi: *Pneumocystis jirovecii* (formerly thought to be *Pneumocystis carinii*) and *Paracoccidioides brasiliensis*.

Microbial Resistance

Many bacterial species have developed resistance to sulfonamides. Resistance is especially high among gonococci, meningococci, streptococci, and shigellae. Resistance may be acquired by spontaneous mutation or by transfer of plasmids that code for antibiotic resistance (R factors). Principal resistance mechanisms are (1) reduced sulfonamide uptake, (2) synthesis of PABA in amounts sufficient to overcome sulfonamide-mediated inhibition of dihydropteroate synthetase (Fig. 75.2), and (3) alteration in the structure of dihydropteroate synthetase such that binding and inhibition by sulfonamides is reduced.

Therapeutic Uses

Although the sulfonamides were once employed widely, their applications are now limited due to the introduction of bactericidal antibiotics that are less toxic than the sulfonamides; and the development of sulfonamide resistance. Today, UTI is the principal indication for these drugs.

Urinary Tract Infections

Sulfonamides are often preferred drugs for acute UTIs. About 90% of these infections are due to *Escherichia coli*, a bacterium that is usually sulfonamide sensitive. Of the sulfonamides available, *sulfamethoxazole* (in combination with trimethoprim) is generally favored. Sulfamethoxazole has good solubility in urine and achieves effective concentrations within the urinary tract. UTIs are discussed in Chapter 76.

Other Uses

Sulfonamides are useful drugs for nocardiosis (infection with *Nocardia asteroides*), *Listeria* species infection, and infection with *P. jirovecii*. In addition, sulfonamides are alternatives to doxycycline and erythromycin for infections caused by *C. trachomatis* (trachoma, inclusion conjunctivitis, urethritis, lymphogranuloma venereum). Sulfonamides are used in conjunction with pyrimethamine to treat two protozoal infections: toxoplasmosis and malaria caused by chloroquine-resistant *Plasmodium falciparum*. Topical sulfonamides are used to treat superficial infections of the eyes and to suppress bacterial colonization in burn patients.

One sulfonamide—sulfasalazine—is used to treat ulcerative colitis. However, benefits in this disorder do not result from inhibiting microbial growth. Ulcerative colitis is discussed in Chapter 66.

Pharmacokinetics

Sulfonamides are well absorbed after oral administration. When applied topically to the skin or mucous membranes, these drugs may be absorbed in amounts sufficient to cause systemic effects.

Sulfonamides are well distributed to all tissues. Concentrations in pleural, peritoneal, ocular, and similar body fluids may be as much as 80% of the concentration in blood. Sulfonamides readily cross the placenta, and levels achieved in the fetus are sufficient to produce antimicrobial effects and toxicity. See Table 75.1 for additional information on pharmacokinetics for sulfonamides and trimethoprim. Typical dosages are provided in Table 75.2.

Adverse Effects

Sulfonamides can cause multiple adverse effects. Prominent among these are hypersensitivity reactions, blood dyscrasias, and kernicterus, which occurs in newborns.

Hypersensitivity Reactions

Sulfonamides can induce a variety of hypersensitivity reactions, which are seen in about 3% of patients. Mild reactions—rash, drug fever, photosensitivity—are relatively common. To minimize photosensitivity reactions, patients should avoid prolonged exposure to sunlight, wear protective clothing, and apply sunscreen to exposed skin.

PATIENT EDUCATION

Sulfonamides

- Instruct patients to complete the prescribed course of treatment even though symptoms may abate before the full course is over.
- Patients taking oral sulfonamides should drink at least 8 to 10 glasses of water or other noncaffeinated fluids per day to decrease the risk for crystalluria. (Caffeine may be taken in addition to the other fluids.)
- To prevent photosensitivity reactions, advise patients to avoid prolonged exposure to sunlight, to wear protective clothing, and to apply sunscreen to exposed skin. Tanning beds are to be avoided.
- Patients should be instructed to observe for alterations that may indicate hypersensitivity (e.g., rash) and to report these promptly if they occur.

Hypersensitivity reactions are especially frequent with *topical* sulfonamides. As a result, these preparations are no longer employed routinely. Rather, they are usually reserved for ophthalmic infections, burns, and bacterial vaginosis caused by *Gardnerella vaginalis* and a mixed population of anaerobic bacteria.

The most severe hypersensitivity response to sulfonamides is *Stevens-Johnson syndrome,* a rare reaction with a mortality rate of about 25%. Symptoms include widespread lesions of the skin and mucous membranes combined with fever, malaise, and toxemia. The reaction is most likely to occur with long-acting sulfonamides, which are now banned in the United States. Short-acting sulfonamides may also induce the syndrome, but the incidence is low. To minimize the risk for severe reactions, sulfonamides should be discontinued immediately if skin rash of any sort is observed. In addition, sulfonamides should not be given to patients with a history of severe hypersensitivity to chemically related drugs (See Box 75.1)—although the risk for cross-reactivity with these agents is probably low (see later section titled "Drug Interactions").

Hematologic Effects

Sulfonamides can cause *hemolytic anemia* in patients with glucose-6-phosphate dehydrogenase (G6PD) deficiency. This inherited trait is most common among blacks and people of Mediterranean origin. Rarely, hemolysis occurs in the absence of G6PD deficiency. Red cell lysis can produce fever, pallor, and jaundice; patients should be observed for these signs. In addition to hemolytic anemia, sulfonamides can cause agranulocytosis, leukopenia, thrombocytopenia, and, very rarely, aplastic anemia. When sulfonamides are used for a long time, periodic blood tests should be obtained.

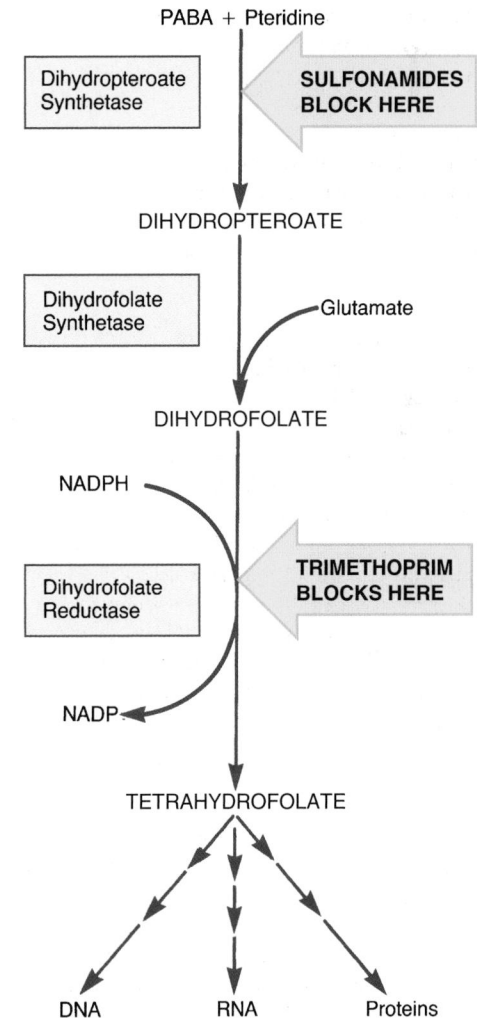

Fig. 75.2 Sites of Action of Sulfonamides and Trimethoprim. Sulfonamides and trimethoprim inhibit sequential steps in the synthesis of tetrahydrofolate (FAH_4). In the absence of FAH_4, bacteria are unable to synthesize DNA, RNA, and proteins.

Fig. 75.1 Structural relationships among sulfonamides, para-aminobenzoic acid *(PABA)*, and folate.

TABLE 75.1 Pharmacokinetics: Sulfonamide Antibiotics and Trimethoprim

Drug Class and Drugs	Peak	Protein Binding	Metabolism	Half-Life	Elimination
Sulfonamide Antibiotics					
Sulfadiazine (generic)	3–6 h	38%–48%	Acetylation	10 h	Urine
Trimethoprim					
Trimethoprim (Primsol)	1–4 h	44%	Demethylation, oxidation, and hydroxylation	8–10 h	Urine Feces
Combination Product					
Sulfamethoxazole + Trimethoprim (Bactrim, Bactrim DS, Protrin, Trisulfa)	1–4 h	SMX: 70% TMP: 44%	SMX: Hepatic (CYP2C9) TMP: trimethoprim: Demethylation, oxidation, and hydroxylation	SMX: 9–12 TMP: 8–10	Urine

SMX, Sulfamethoxazole; *TMP,* trimethoprim.

TABLE 75.2 Dosages[a] and Administration Sulfonamide Antibiotics and Trimethoprim

Generic Name	Trade Name	Typical Dosage	Administration
Oral Sulfonamides			
Sulfadiazine	Generic only	Adults: 2–4 g initially, followed by 2–4 g q 24 h given as three to six divided doses. Children >2 months: *Initial:* 75 mg/kg per day divided into 4–6 doses *Maintenance:* 150 mg/kg (or 4 g/m^2) per day (6 g max) given as 4–6 divided doses	Giving with vitamin C or acidifying drinks such as cranberry juice may increase the risk for crystalluria.
Sulfamethoxazole (+ trimethoprim)	Bactrim, Bactrim DS, Protrin, Trisulfa ♦	Adults: 800 mg SMZ/160 mg TMP tablets q 12–24 h. Children >2 months (based on trimethoprim [TMP]): 4 mg TMP/kg every 12 hours. May be increased to 20 mg TMP/kg per day	Should be taken with a full glass of water.
Topical Sulfonamides			
Silver sulfadiazine	Silvadene, Thermazene, Flamazine ♦	Apply a thin layer to affected skin 1–2 times per day	Do not use on the face; may cause a blue-green or gray discoloration.
Mafenide	Sulfamylon	Apply a thin layer to affected skin 1–2 times per day	Cream should cover the burned area at all times. If dressings are used, only a thin, nonocclusive dressing should be used.
Sulfacetamide ophthalmic	Bleph-10, Diosulf ♦, Sodium Sulamyd ♦	Solution: 1–2 drops q 2–3 h. Ointment: ½ in q 3–4 h	When tapering off, increase time interval between doses.
Trimethoprim			
Trimethoprim	Primsol	Adults: 100 mg q 12 h or 200 mg q 24 h. Children >2 months: 4–12 mg/kg per day divided into two 12-h doses	Administer with food or milk.

[a]Dosing is for most infections. Dosing for specific conditions (e.g., shigellosis) and for prophylaxis of *Pneumocystis jirovecii* pneumonia in patients with AIDS varies. Length of treatment is controversial, especially for UTIs, and may range from 3 to 14 days.
SMZ, Sulfamethoxazole; *TMP,* trimethoprim

Kernicterus

Kernicterus is a disorder in newborns caused by deposition of bilirubin in the brain. Bilirubin is neurotoxic and can cause severe neurologic deficits and even death. Under normal conditions, infants are not vulnerable to kernicterus. Any bilirubin present in their blood is tightly bound to plasma proteins and therefore is not free to enter the central nervous system (CNS). Sulfonamides promote kernicterus by displacing bilirubin from plasma proteins. Because the blood–brain barrier of infants is poorly developed, the newly freed bilirubin has easy access to sites within the brain. *Because of the risk for kernicterus, sulfonamides should not be administered to infants younger than 2 months. In addition, sulfonamides should not be given to pregnant patients after 32 weeks of gestation or to those who are breastfeeding.*

Renal Damage

Because of their low solubility, older sulfonamides tended to come out of solution in the urine, forming crystalline aggregates in the kidneys, ureters, and bladder. These aggregates cause irritation and obstruction, sometimes resulting in anuria and even death. Renal damage is uncommon with today's sulfonamides owing to their increased water solubility;

BOX 75.1 Other Sulfonamide Drugs

Alpha₁ Blocker
- Tamsulosin (Flomax)

Anticonvulsant
- Topiramate (Topamax)
- Zonisamide (Zonegran)

Antidiabetic, Sulfonylureas
- Chlorpropamide (generic)
- Glimepiride (Amaryl)
- Glipizide (Glucotrol)
- Glyburide (Glynase)
- Tolbutamide (generic)
- Tolazamide (generic)

Antidysrhythmic Drugs
- Ibutilide (Corvert)
- Sotalol (Betapace)

Antimigraine, Serotonin Receptor Agonists
- Naratriptan (Amerge)
- Sumatriptan (Imitrex)

Diuretics, Carbonic Anhydrase Inhibitors
- Acetazolamide (generic)
- Brinzolamide (Azopt)

- Dorzolamide (Trusopt)
- Methazolamide (generic)

Diuretics, Loop
- Bumetanide (Bumex, Burinex)
- Furosemide (Lasix)
- Torsemide (Demadex)

Diuretics, Thiazide and Thiazide-Related
- Chlorothiazide (Diuril)
- Chlorthalidone (generic)
- Hydrochlorothiazide (Microzide, Urozide)
- Indapamide (generic)
- Metolazone (Zaroxolyn)

Protease Inhibitors
- Darunavir (Prezista)
- Fosamprenavir (Lexiva, Telzir)
- Simeprevir (Olysio)
- Tipranavir (Aptivus)

Nonsteroidal Antiinflammatory Drugs
- Celecoxib (Celebrex)

Urocosuric Drug
- Probenecid (generic)

PATIENT-CENTERED CARE ACROSS THE LIFE SPAN

Sulfonamides and Trimethoprim

Life Stage	Patient Care Concerns
Infants	Use of sulfonamides in infants younger than 2 months can cause kernicterus, a potentially fatal condition.
Pregnant women	Systemic sulfonamides may cause birth defects, especially if taken during the first semester. If taken near term, the infant may develop kernicterus.
Breastfeeding women	Sulfonamides are secreted in breast milk. Breastfeeding women on sulfonamides should be warned that breastfeeding an infant younger than 2 months can cause kernicterus.
Older adults	Older patients are more likely to experience adverse effects, and when experienced, the effects are more likely to be severe. Life-threatening effects—including neutropenia, Stevens-Johnson syndrome, and toxic epidermal necrolysis—occur more frequently in older adults.

however, there is still a risk. To minimize the risk for renal damage, adults should maintain a daily urine output of at least 1200 mL. This can be accomplished by consuming 8 to 10 glasses of water each day.

Sulfonamides are contraindicated for patients with severe renal disease. For patients with a creatinine clearance (CrCl) of 15 to 30 mL/minute, providers should prescribe 50% of the typical recommended dose.

Drug Interactions
Metabolism-Related Interactions
Sulfonamides can intensify the effects of warfarin, phenytoin, and sulfonylurea-type oral hypoglycemics (e.g., glipizide, glyburide). The principal mechanism is inhibition of hepatic metabolism. When they are combined with sulfonamides, these drugs may require a reduction in dosage to prevent toxicity.

Cross-Hypersensitivity
There is theoretical concern that people who are hypersensitive to sulfonamide antibiotics may be cross-hypersensitive to other drugs that contain a sulfonamide moiety (see Box 75.1). Current evidence demonstrates only a shared sensitivity among sulfonamide antibiotics but not a cross-sensitivity to nonantibiotic sulfonamides. The exception is sulfasalazine (Azulfidine, Salazopyrin), an antiinflammatory drug that breaks down into sulfaypridine, an antibiotic no longer available for prescription. Does that mean that this is no longer a concern? Probably, but experts still recommend precaution for severe hypersensitivity reactions to sulfonamide antibiotics, and product labeling includes warnings and precautions for these drugs. As with all prescribing situations, a thoughtful consideration of benefits versus risks is needed.

Sulfonamide Preparations
Sulfonamide antibiotics fall into two major categories: (1) systemic sulfonamides and (2) topical sulfonamides. The systemic agents are used more often.

Systemic Sulfonamides
There are two groups of systemic sulfonamides—short acting and intermediate acting. These differ primarily with regard to dosing interval, which is much shorter for the short-acting drugs.

Sulfamethoxazole. Sulfamethoxazole is the only *intermediate-acting* sulfonamide available. The risk for renal damage from crystalluria can be reduced by maintaining adequate hydration. Sulfamethoxazole is not available for use by itself but *is* available in combination with trimethoprim.

Sulfadiazine. Sulfadiazine is a short-acting sulfonamide. It is more likely to cause crystalluria than sulfamethoxazole. Accordingly, if renal damage is to be avoided, high urine flow must be maintained.

Topical Sulfonamides

Topical sulfonamides have been associated with a high incidence of hypersensitivity and are not used routinely. The preparations discussed here have proven utility and a relatively low incidence of hypersensitivity.

Sulfacetamide. Sulfacetamide (Bleph-10) is widely used for superficial infections of the eyes (e.g., conjunctivitis, corneal ulcer). The drug may cause blurred vision, sensitivity to bright light, headache, brow ache, and local irritation. Hypersensitivity is rare but severe reactions have occurred. Accordingly, sulfacetamide should not be used by patients with a history of severe hypersensitivity to sulfonamides, sulfonylureas, or thiazide or loop diuretics. Sulfacetamide is available in a 10% solution for application to the eyes.

In addition to its ophthalmologic use, topical sulfacetamide is used for dermatologic disorders. The drug is available as a 10% solution in lotions, gels, washes, and shampoos for treating seborrheic dermatitis, acne vulgaris, and bacterial infections of the skin.

Silver sulfadiazine and mafenide. These sulfonamides are employed to suppress bacterial colonization in patients with second- and third-degree burns. Mafenide (Sulfamylon) acts by the same mechanism as other sulfonamides. In contrast, the antibacterial effects of silver sulfadiazine are due primarily to the release of free silver—not to the sulfonamide portion of the molecule. Local application of mafenide is frequently painful, but application of silver sulfadiazine is usually pain-free. After application, both agents can be absorbed in amounts sufficient to produce systemic effects. Mafenide, but not silver sulfadiazine, is metabolized to a compound that can suppress renal excretion of acid, causing acidosis. Accordingly, patients receiving mafenide should be monitored for acid–base status. If acidosis becomes severe, mafenide should be discontinued for 1 to 2 days. Silver sulfadiazine (Silvadene, SSD Cream, Flamazine ❧) can cause a blue-green or gray skin discoloration, so facial application should be avoided. A Cochrane review questioned the ability of silver sulfadiazine to promote healing but noted that good-quality research studies were lacking.

TRIMETHOPRIM

Like the sulfonamides, trimethoprim (generic) suppresses the synthesis of tetrahydrofolate. Trimethoprim is active against a broad spectrum of microbes.

Mechanism of Action

Trimethoprim *inhibits dihydrofolate reductase,* the enzyme that converts dihydrofolate to its active form: tetrahydrofolate. Thus, like the sulfonamides, trimethoprim suppresses the bacterial synthesis of DNA, RNA, and proteins. Depending on conditions at the site of infection, trimethoprim may be bactericidal or bacteriostatic.

Although mammalian cells also contain dihydrofolate reductase, trimethoprim is selectively toxic to bacteria because bacterial dihydrofolate reductase differs in structure from mammalian dihydrofolate reductase. As a result, trimethoprim inhibits the bacterial enzyme at concentrations about 40,000 times lower than those required to inhibit the mammalian enzyme. This allows it to suppress bacterial growth with doses that have essentially no effect on the host.

Antimicrobial Spectrum

Trimethoprim is active against most enteric gram-negative bacilli of clinical importance, including *E. coli, Klebsiella pneumoniae, Proteus mirabilis, Serratia marcescens,* and *Salmonella* and *Shigella* species. The drug is also active against some gram-positive bacilli (e.g., *Corynebacterium diphtheriae, L. monocytogenes*) as well as some pathogenic protozoa (e.g., *Toxoplasma gondii)* and one fungus (*P. jirovecii*).

Microbial Resistance

Bacteria acquire resistance to trimethoprim in three ways: (1) synthesizing increased amounts of dihydrofolate reductase, (2) producing an altered dihydrofolate reductase that has a low affinity for trimethoprim, and (3) reducing cellular permeability to trimethoprim. Resistance has resulted from spontaneous mutation and from the transfer of R factors. Bacterial resistance is uncommon in the United States.

Therapeutic Uses

Trimethoprim is approved only for the initial therapy of acute, uncomplicated UTIs due to susceptible organisms (e.g., *E. coli, P. mirabilis, K. pneumoniae, Enterobacter* species, and coagulase-negative *Staphylococcus* species, including *S. saprophyticus*). Combined with sulfamethoxazole, trimethoprim has considerably more applications, as discussed later.

PATIENT EDUCATION

Trimethoprim

- Inform patients about early signs of blood dyscrasias (e.g., sore throat, fever, pallor) and instruct them to report these promptly if they occur.

Adverse Effects

Trimethoprim is generally well tolerated. The most frequent adverse effects are itching and rash. GI reactions (e.g., epigastric distress, nausea, vomiting, glossitis, stomatitis) occur occasionally.

Hematologic Effects

Because mammalian dihydrofolate reductase is relatively insensitive to trimethoprim, toxicities related to impaired tetrahydrofolate production are rare. These rare effects—*megaloblastic anemia, thrombocytopenia,* and *neutropenia*—occur only in individuals with preexisting folic acid deficiency. Therefore caution is needed when trimethoprim is being administered to patients in whom folate deficiency might be likely (e.g., patients with excessive alcohol intake, pregnant women, debilitated patients). If early signs of bone marrow suppression occur (e.g., sore throat, fever, pallor), complete blood counts should be performed. If a significant reduction in blood cell counts is observed, trimethoprim should be discontinued. Administration of leucovorin, a reduced form of folic acid, will restore normal hematopoiesis.

Hyperkalemia

Trimethoprim suppresses renal excretion of potassium and can thereby promote hyperkalemia. Patients at greatest risk are those taking high doses, those with renal impairment, and those taking other drugs that can elevate potassium, including angiotensin-converting enzyme inhibitors (ACEIs), angiotensin receptor blockers (ARBs), potassium-sparing diuretics, aldosterone antagonists, and potassium supplements. Patients older than 65 years who are taking an ACEI or ARB are at especially high risk. Risk can be reduced by checking serum potassium, preferably 4 days after starting treatment (hyperkalemia typically develops within 5 days of starting treatment).

Effects in Pregnancy and Lactation

Large doses of trimethoprim have caused fetal malformations in animals. To date, developmental abnormalities have not been observed in humans.

Nonetheless, because trimethoprim readily crosses the placenta, prudence dictates avoiding its routine use during pregnancy. The risk for exacerbating pregnancy-related folate deficiency is an additional reason to avoid the drug.

Trimethoprim is excreted in breast milk and may interfere with folic acid utilization by the nursing infant. It should be administered with caution to women who are breastfeeding.

TRIMETHOPRIM/SULFAMETHOXAZOLE

Trimethoprim (TMP) and sulfamethoxazole (SMZ) are marketed together in a fixed-dose combination product. This combination (TMP/SMZ or one of the variations: TMP/SMX, SMZ/TMP, SMX/TMP) is a powerful antimicrobial preparation whose components act in concert to inhibit sequential steps in tetrahydrofolate synthesis. Trade names for TMP/SMZ are *Bactrim*, *Protrin*, Septra ♣, and *Trisulfa*.

Mechanism of Action

The antimicrobial effects of TMP/SMZ result from inhibiting consecutive steps in the synthesis of tetrahydrofolate: SMZ acts first to inhibit incorporation of PABA into folate; TMP then inhibits dihydrofolate reductase, the enzyme that converts dihydrofolate into tetrahydrofolate (see Fig. 75.2). As a result, the ability of the target organism to make nucleic acids and proteins is greatly suppressed. By inhibiting two reactions required for synthesis of tetrahydrofolate, TMP and SMZ potentiate each other's effects. That is, the antimicrobial effect of the combination is more powerful than the sum of the effects of TMP alone plus SMZ alone. TMP/SMZ is selectively toxic to microbes because (1) mammalian cells use preformed folic acid and therefore are not affected by SMZ and (2) dihydrofolate reductases of mammalian cells are relatively insensitive to inhibition by TMP.

Antimicrobial Spectrum

TMP/SMZ is active against a wide range of gram-positive and gram-negative bacteria. This should be no surprise in that TMP and SMZ by themselves are broad-spectrum antimicrobial drugs. About 80% of urinary tract pathogens are susceptible. Specific bacteria against which TMP/SMZ is consistently effective include *E. coli*, *P. mirabilis*, *L. monocytogenes*, *S. aureus* (including methicillin-resistant isolates), *C. trachomatis*, *Salmonella typhi*, *Shigella* species, *Vibrio cholerae*, *Haemophilus influenzae*, and *Yersinia pestis*. TMP/SMZ is also active against *Nocardia* species, certain protozoa (e.g., *T. gondii*), and two fungi (*P. jirovecii* and *P. brasiliensis*).

Microbial Resistance

Resistance to TMP/SMZ is less than that to either drug alone. This is logical in that the chances of an organism acquiring resistance to both drugs are less than its chances of developing resistance to just one or the other.

Therapeutic Uses

TMP/SMZ is a preferred or alternative medication for a variety of infectious diseases. The combination is especially valuable for UTIs, otitis media, bronchitis, shigellosis, and pneumonia caused by *P. jirovecii*.

Urinary Tract Infections

TMP/SMZ is indicated for the treatment of uncomplicated UTIs caused by susceptible strains of *E. coli*, *Klebsiella* and *Enterobacter* species, *P. mirabilis*, *Proteus vulgaris*, and *Morganella morganii*. The combination is particularly useful for treating chronic and recurrent infections.

Pneumocystis jirovecii Pneumonia

TMP/SMZ is the treatment of choice for infections caused by *P. jirovecii*, an opportunistic fungus that thrives in immunocompromised hosts (e.g., cancer patients, organ transplant recipients, individuals with AIDS). Unfortunately, when given to patients with AIDS, TMP/SMZ produces a high incidence of adverse effects, which often limits its use in this group.

Gastrointestinal Infections

TMP/SMZ is a drug of choice for infections caused by several gram-negative bacilli, including *Yersinia enterocolitica* and *Aeromonas* species. In addition, the combination is a preferred treatment for shigellosis caused by susceptible strains of *Shigella flexneri* and *S. sonnei*.

Other Infections

TMP/SMZ can be used for the treatment of otitis media and acute exacerbations of chronic bronchitis when these infections are due to susceptible strains of *H. influenzae* or *Streptococcus pneumoniae*. The preparation is also useful against urethritis and pharyngeal infection caused by penicillinase-producing *Neisseria gonorrhoeae*. Other infections that can be treated with TMP/SMZ include whooping cough, nocardiosis, brucellosis, melioidosis, listeriosis, and chancroid.

Pharmacokinetics

TMP/SMZ may be administered orally or by intravenous infusion. Both components of TMP/SMZ are well distributed throughout the body. Therapeutic concentrations are achieved in tissues and body fluids (e.g., vaginal secretions, cerebrospinal fluid, pleural effusions, bile, aqueous humor). Both TMP and SMZ readily cross the placenta and both enter breast milk.

Optimal antibacterial effects are produced when the ratio of TMP to SMZ is 1:20. To achieve this ratio in plasma, TMP and SMZ must be administered in a ratio of 1:5. Hence standard tablets contain 80 mg of TMP and 400 mg of SMZ. Because the plasma half-lives of TMP and SMZ are similar (10 hours for TMP and 11 hours for SMZ), levels of both drugs decline in parallel, and the 1:20 ratio is maintained as the drugs are eliminated. See Table 75.1 for additional information on pharmacokinetics.

Adverse Effects

TMP/SMZ is generally well tolerated; toxicity from routine use is rare. The most common adverse effects are nausea, vomiting, and rash. However, although infrequent, all of the serious toxicities associated with sulfonamides alone and trimethoprim alone can occur with TMP/SMZ.

Like sulfonamides, the combination can cause the following:
- Hypersensitivity reactions (including Stevens-Johnson syndrome)
- Blood dyscrasias (hemolytic anemia, agranulocytosis, leukopenia, thrombocytopenia, aplastic anemia)
- Kernicterus in neonates
- Renal damage

Like trimethoprim, the combination can cause the following:
- Megaloblastic anemia (but only in patients who are folate deficient)
- Hyperkalemia (especially in patients on high doses, in those with renal impairment, and in those taking other drugs that can raise potassium levels)
- Birth defects (especially during the first trimester)

TMP/SMZ may also cause adverse CNS effects (headache, depression, hallucinations). Patients suffering from AIDS are unusually susceptible to TMP/SMZ toxicity. In this group, the incidence of adverse effects (rash, recurrent fever, leukopenia) is about 55%.

Several measures can reduce the incidence and severity of adverse effects. Crystalluria can be avoided by maintaining adequate hydration. Periodic blood tests permit early detection of hematologic disorders. To avoid kernicterus, TMP/SMZ should be withheld from pregnant patients near term, nursing mothers, and infants younger than 2 months. To avoid possible birth defects, TMP/SMZ should be withheld during the first trimester. The risk for megaloblastic anemia can be reduced by withholding sulfonamides from individuals likely to be folate deficient (e.g., debilitated patients, pregnant patients, patients with excessive alcohol intake). Hypersensitivity reactions can be minimized by avoiding TMP/SMZ in patients with a history of hypersensitivity to sulfonamides or to chemically related drugs, including thiazide diuretics, loop diuretics, and sulfonylurea-type oral hypoglycemics. Injury from hyperkalemia can be reduced by checking serum potassium and exercising caution in patients taking other drugs that can elevate potassium.

Drug Interactions

Interactions of TMP/SMZ with other drugs are due primarily to the presence of SMZ. Consequently, like sulfonamides used alone, SMZ in the combination can intensify the effects of warfarin, phenytoin, and sulfonylurea-type oral hypoglycemics (e.g., glipizide). Accordingly, when these drugs are combined with TMP/SMZ, a reduction in their dosage may be needed. TMP/SMZ may also intensify bone marrow suppression in patients receiving methotrexate. As noted, drugs that raise potassium levels can increase the risk for hyperkalemia from TMP.

📄 SUMMARY OF KEY PRESCRIBING CONSIDERATIONS

Trimethoprim/Sulfamethoxazole

Therapeutic Goal: Absence of infection

Baseline Data: Establish infection: Urinalysis (if UTI is suspected) with culture and sensitivity as indicated. (Collect urine sample before starting therapy but don't wait for results before prescribing treatment; treat empirically until results are available.) Obtain complete blood count (CBC) with white cell differential if indicated or if treatment will be prolonged. Renal function should be checked if there is concern that it may be compromised.

Monitoring: CBC should be monitored if the patient develops signs or symptoms of blood disorders, as should CD4+ count for patients with HIV infection. Signs and symptoms of hypersensitivity reactions and of resolution of infection should also be assessed. If hyperkalemia is suspected due to use of trimethoprim, potassium must be checked 4 days after starting treatment.

Identifying High-Risk Patients: Sulfonamides are contraindicated for nursing mothers, pregnant women in the first trimester and also those near term, and infants younger than 2 months. An alternative antibiotic must be chosen for patients with G6PD deficiency.

It is important to *exercise caution* in prescribing sulfonamides for patients with renal impairment.

In patients with renal impairment (creatinine clearance of 15–30 mL/min), dosage should be decreased by 50%. If creatinine clearance falls below 15 mL/min, drug use must be discontinued.

Trimethoprim is *contraindicated* in patients with folate deficiency (manifested as megaloblastic anemia). When possible, trimethoprim should be avoided during pregnancy and lactation.

Patients with renal dysfunction require a reduced dosage.

Trimethoprim should be avoided when folate deficiency is likely (e.g., in patients with alcoholism or debilitation and in women who are pregnant).

Evaluating Therapeutic Effects: Absence of evidence of infection (negative urinalysis, white cell differential returns to normal, signs and symptoms resolve).

76

Drug Therapy of Urinary Tract Infections

Urinary tract infections (UTIs) are the second most common infections encountered today. In the United States, UTIs account for nearly 10 million visits to health care providers each year. It is estimated that 50% to 80% of women will have a UTI in their lifetimes. Among older women in nursing homes, between 30% and 50% have bacteriuria at any given time. UTIs occur much less frequently in males but are more likely to be associated with complications (e.g., septicemia, pyelonephritis).

Infections may be limited to bacterial colonization of the urine, or bacteria may invade tissues of the urinary tract. When bacteria invade tissues, characteristic inflammatory syndromes result: *urethritis, cystitis, pyelonephritis,* and *prostatitis.*

UTIs can be classified according to their location, in either the lower urinary tract (bladder and urethra) or upper urinary tract (kidney). Within this classification scheme, *cystitis* and *urethritis* are considered *lower tract infections,* whereas *pyelonephritis* is considered an *upper tract infection.*

UTIs are referred to as *complicated* or *uncomplicated. Complicated* UTIs occur in both males and females and are associated with some predisposing factor, such as calculi, prostatic hypertrophy, an indwelling catheter, or an impediment to the flow of urine (e.g., physical obstruction). *Uncomplicated* UTIs occur primarily in women of childbearing age and are not associated with any particular predisposing factor.

Several classes of antibiotics are used to treat UTIs. Among these are sulfonamides, trimethoprim, penicillins, aminoglycosides, carbapenems, cephalosporins, fluoroquinolones, and two urinary tract antiseptics: nitrofurantoin and methenamine. With the exception of the urinary tract antiseptics, these drugs are discussed in other chapters. The basic pharmacology of the urinary tract antiseptics is introduced here.

ORGANISMS THAT CAUSE URINARY TRACT INFECTIONS

The bacteria that cause UTIs differ between community-associated infections and hospital-associated infections. Most (more than 80%) uncomplicated, community-associated UTIs are caused by *Escherichia coli.* Rarely, other gram-negative bacilli—*Klebsiella pneumoniae* and *Enterobacter, Proteus, Providencia,* and *Pseudomonas* species—are the cause. Gram-positive cocci, especially *Staphylococcus saprophyticus,* account for 10% to 15% of community-associated infections. Hospital-associated UTIs are frequently caused by *Klebsiella, Proteus, Enterobacter* and *Pseudomonas* species, staphylococci, and enterococci; *E. coli* is responsible for less than 50% of these infections. Although most UTIs involve only one organism, infection with multiple organisms may occur, especially in patients with an indwelling catheter, renal stones, or chronic renal abscesses.

SPECIFIC URINARY TRACT INFECTIONS AND THEIR TREATMENT

This section covers the characteristics and treatment of the major UTIs: acute cystitis, acute urethral syndrome, acute pyelonephritis, acute

bacterial prostatitis, and recurrent UTIs. Most of these can be treated with oral therapy at home. The principal exception is severe pyelonephritis, which requires intravenous therapy in a hospital. A treatment algorithm for outpatient therapy in nonpregnant women is shown in Fig. 76.1.

Acute Cystitis

Acute cystitis is a lower UTI that occurs most often in women of childbearing age. Clinical manifestations are dysuria, urinary urgency, urinary frequency, suprapubic discomfort, pyuria, and bacteriuria (more than 100,000 bacteria per milliliter of urine). It is important to note that many women (30% or more) with symptoms of acute cystitis also have asymptomatic upper UTI (subclinical pyelonephritis). In uncomplicated, community-associated cystitis, the principal causative organisms are *E. coli* (80%), *S. saprophyticus* (11%), and *Enterococcus faecalis.*

For community-associated infections, three types of oral therapy can be employed: (1) single-dose therapy, (2) short-course therapy (3 days), and (3) conventional therapy (7 days). *Single-dose* therapy and *short-course* therapy are recommended only for uncomplicated, community-associated infections in women who are not pregnant and whose symptoms began less than 7 days before starting treatment. As a rule, short-course therapy is more effective than single-dose therapy and hence is generally preferred. Advantages of short-course therapy over conventional therapy are lower cost, greater adherence, fewer side effects, and less potential for promoting the emergence of bacterial resistance. *Conventional* therapy is indicated for all patients who do not meet the criteria for short-course therapy. Among these are males, children, pregnant women, and women with suspected upper tract involvement.

Several drugs can be used for treatment (see Fig. 76.1). For uncomplicated cystitis, trimethoprim/sulfamethoxazole and nitrofurantoin are the drugs of first choice. In communities where resistance to these drugs exceeds 20%, the fluoroquinolones (e.g., ciprofloxacin) are good alternatives. When adherence is a concern, fosfomycin, which requires just one dose, is a good choice.

Acute Uncomplicated Pyelonephritis

Acute uncomplicated pyelonephritis is an infection of the kidneys. The disorder is common in young children, older adults, and women of childbearing age. Clinical manifestations include fever, chills, severe flank pain, dysuria, urinary frequency, urinary urgency, pyuria, and usually bacteriuria (more than 100,000 bacteria per milliliter of urine). *E. coli* is the causative organism in 90% of initial community-associated infections.

Mild to moderate infection can be treated at home with oral antibiotics. Preferred options are fluroquinolones or trimethoprim/sulfamethoxazole. Treatment should last 7 to 14 days (Table 76.1).

Severe pyelonephritis requires hospitalization and intravenous antibiotics. Options include ciprofloxacin, ceftriaxone, ceftazidime, ampicillin plus gentamicin, and ampicillin/sulbactam. After the infection has been controlled with intravenous antibiotics, a switch to oral antibiotics should be made, usually within 24 to 48 hours.

Fig. 76.1 Treatment of Uncomplicated Acute Cystitis.

Complicated Urinary Tract Infections

Complicated UTIs occur in males and females who have a structural or functional abnormality of the urinary tract that predisposes them to developing infection. Such predisposing factors include prostatic hypertrophy, renal calculi, nephrocalcinosis, renal or bladder tumors, ureteric stricture, or an indwelling urethral catheter. Symptoms of complicated UTIs can range from mild to severe. Some patients even develop systemic illness, manifesting as fever, bacteremia, and septic shock.

The microbiology of complicated UTIs is less predictable than that of uncomplicated UTIs. Although *E. coli* is a common pathogen, it is by no means the only one. Other possibilities include *Klebsiella, Proteus, Pseudomonas, Enterobacter, Serratia,* and even *Candida* species, as well as *Staphylococcus aureus.* Accordingly, if treatment is to succeed, the identity and drug sensitivity of the causative organism must be determined. To do so, urine for microbiologic testing should be obtained *before* giving any antibiotics. If symptoms are relatively mild, treatment should wait until test results are available. However, if symptoms are severe, immediate treatment with a broad-spectrum antibiotic can be instituted. After test results are known, a drug specific to the pathogen can be substituted. Duration of treatment ranges from 7 days (for cystitis) to 14 days (for pyelonephritis or when there is systemic involvement).

Recurrent Urinary Tract Infection

Recurrent UTIs result from *relapse* or from *reinfection. Relapse* is caused by recolonization with the same organism responsible for the initial infection. In contrast, *reinfection* is caused by colonization with a new organism.

Reinfection

More than 80% of recurrent UTIs in females are due to reinfection. These usually involve the lower urinary tract and may be related to sexual intercourse or use of a contraceptive diaphragm. If reinfections are *infrequent* (only one or two a year), each episode should be treated as a separate infection. Single-dose or short-course therapy can be used.

When reinfections are *frequent* (three or more a year), long-term prophylaxis may be indicated. Prophylaxis can be achieved with low daily doses of several agents, including trimethoprim (100 mg), nitrofurantoin (50 or 100 mg), or trimethoprim/sulfamethoxazole (40 mg/200 mg). Prophylaxis should continue for at least 6 months. During this time, periodic urine cultures should be obtained. If a symptomatic episode occurs, standard therapy for acute cystitis should be given. If reinfection is associated with sexual intercourse, the risk can be decreased by voiding after intercourse and by single-dose prophylaxis (e.g., trimethoprim/sulfamethoxazole [80 mg/400 mg] taken after intercourse).

Relapse

Recolonization with the original infecting organism accounts for 20% of recurrent UTIs. Symptoms that reappear shortly after completion of a course of therapy suggest either a structural abnormality of the urinary tract, involvement of the kidneys, or chronic bacterial prostatitis, the most common cause of recurrent UTI in males. If obstruction of the urinary tract is present, it should be corrected surgically. If renal calculi are the cause, they should be removed.

Drug therapy is progressive. When relapse occurs in women after short-course therapy, a 2-week course of therapy should be tried. If this fails, an additional 4 to 6 weeks of therapy should be tried. If this, too, is unsuccessful, long-term therapy (6 months) may be indicated. Drugs employed for long-term therapy of relapse include fluroquinolones or trimethoprim/sulfamethoxazole.

Acute Bacterial Prostatitis

Acute bacterial prostatitis is defined as inflammation of the prostate caused by local bacterial infection. Clinical manifestations include high

TABLE 76.1 Regimens for Oral Therapy of Complicated Urinary Tract Infections in Nonpregnant Women

Drug	Dose	Duration
Acute Cystitis		
First-Line Drugs		
Trimethoprim/sulfamethoxazole	160/800 mg bid	3 days
Nitrofurantoin (monohydrate/ macrocrystals)	100 mg bid	5 days
Fosfomycin	3 g once	1 day
Second-Line Drugs		
Ciprofloxacin	250 mg bid	3 days
Levofloxacin	250 mg bid	3 days
Complicated Urinary Tract Infections and Acute Uncomplicated Pyelonephritis		
First-Line Drugs		
Trimethoprim/sulfamethoxazole[a]	160/800 mg bid	14 days
Ciprofloxacin	500 mg bid	5–7 days
Levofloxacin	750 mg qd	5–7 days
Second-Line Drugs		
Amoxicillin (with clavulanic acid)	875 mg bid	10–14 days
Cefadroxil	1 g bid	10–14 days
Cefdinir	300 mg bid	10–14 days
Cefpodoxime	200 mg bid	10–14 days
Complicated Urinary Tract Infections		
Trimethoprim/sulfamethoxazole	160/800 mg bid	7–14 days
Ciprofloxacin	500 mg bid	5–14 days
Levofloxacin	750 mg qd	5–14 days
Amoxicillin (with clavulanic acid)	500 mg tid	7–14 days
Cephalexin	500 mg tid	7–14 days
Prophylaxis of Recurrent Infections		
Trimethoprim/sulfamethoxazole	40/200 mg[b] hs 3 times a week	6 months
Trimethoprim	100 mg hs	6 months
Nitrofurantoin	50–100 mg hs	6 months

[a]Use only if bacterial sensitivity is known.
[b]Using half of a single-strength tablet.

fever, chills, malaise, myalgia, localized pain, and various urinary tract symptoms (dysuria, nocturia, urinary urgency, urinary frequency, urinary retention). In most cases (80%), *E. coli* is the causative organism. Infection is frequently associated with an indwelling urethral catheter, urethral instrumentation, or transurethral prostatic resection. However, in many patients, the infection has no obvious cause.

Bacterial prostatitis responds well to antimicrobial therapy. Because of local inflammation, antibiotics can readily penetrate to the site of infection. (In the absence of inflammation, penetration of the prostate is difficult.) Drug selection and route depend on the causative organism and infection severity. For severe infection with *E. coli,* treatment starts with an intravenous agent (a fluoroquinolone [e.g., ciprofloxacin]), followed by 2 to 4 weeks with an oral agent (either doxycycline or a fluoroquinolone). For severe infection with vancomycin-sensitive *E. faecalis,* treatment starts with intravenous ampicillin/sulbactam,

followed by 2 to 4 weeks with oral (PO) amoxicillin, levofloxacin, or doxycycline.

URINARY TRACT ANTISEPTICS

Two urinary tract antiseptics are available: nitrofurantoin and methenamine. Both are used only for UTIs. These drugs become concentrated in the urine and are active against the common urinary tract pathogens. Neither drug achieves effective antibacterial concentrations in blood or tissues. Nitrofurantoin is a first-choice drug for uncomplicated cystitis.

Nitrofurantoin
Mechanism of Action
Nitrofurantoin (Furadantin, Macrodantin, Macrobid) is a broad-spectrum antibacterial drug, producing bacteriostatic effects at low concentrations and bactericidal effects at high concentrations. Therapeutic levels are achieved only in urine. Nitrofurantoin can cause serious adverse effects.

Nitrofurantoin injures bacteria by damaging DNA. However, to damage DNA, the drug must first undergo enzymatic conversion to a reactive form. Nitrofurantoin is selectively toxic to bacteria because, unlike mammalian cells, bacteria possess relatively high levels of the enzyme needed for drug activation.

Antimicrobial Spectrum
Nitrofurantoin is active against a large number of gram-positive and gram-negative bacteria. Susceptible organisms include staphylococci, streptococci, *Neisseria* and *Bacteroides* species, and most strains of *E. coli.* These sensitive bacteria rarely acquire resistance. Organisms that are frequently resistant include *Proteus, Pseudomonas, Enterobacter,* and *Klebsiella* species.

Therapeutic Use
Nitrofurantoin is indicated for acute infections of the lower urinary tract caused by susceptible organisms (Table 76.2). In addition, the drug can be used for prophylaxis of recurrent lower UTI. Nitrofurantoin is not recommended for infections of the upper urinary tract.

Adverse Effects
Gastrointestinal effects. The most frequent adverse reactions are GI disturbances (e.g., anorexia, nausea, vomiting, diarrhea). These can be minimized by administering nitrofurantoin with milk or with meals, by reducing the dosage, and by using the macrocrystalline formulations.

Pulmonary reactions. Nitrofurantoin can induce two kinds of pulmonary reactions: acute and subacute. Acute reactions, which are most common, manifest as dyspnea, chest pain, chills, fever, cough, and alveolar infiltrates. These symptoms resolve 2 to 4 days after discontinuing the drug. Acute pulmonary responses are thought to be hypersensitivity reactions. Patients with a history of these responses should not receive nitrofurantoin again. Subacute reactions are rare and occur during prolonged treatment. Symptoms (e.g., dyspnea, cough, malaise) usually regress over weeks to months after nitrofurantoin withdrawal. However, in some patients, permanent lung damage may occur.

Hematologic effects. Nitrofurantoin can cause a variety of hematologic reactions, including agranulocytosis, leukopenia, thrombocytopenia, and megaloblastic anemia. In addition, hemolytic anemia may occur in infants and in patients whose red blood cells have an inherited deficiency in glucose-6-phosphate dehydrogenase. Because of the potential for hemolytic anemia in newborns, nitrofurantoin is contraindicated for pregnant women near term and for infants younger than 1 month.

Peripheral neuropathy. Damage to sensory and motor nerves is a serious concern. Demyelinization and nerve degeneration can occur and may be irreversible. Early symptoms include muscle weakness,

TABLE 76.2   Antibiotics Specific for the Treatment of Urinary Tract Infection

Drug	Name	Availability	Usual Dose	Use	Absorption and Distribution	Metabolism and Excretion
Nitrofurantoin microcrystals	Furadantin	5 mg/mL oral suspension	50–100 mg qid 50–100 mg hs	Treatment of UTI UTI prophylaxis	Absorbed faster than the macrocrystals Distributed to tissues in very small amounts	Primarily hepatic metabolism. One-third excreted intact in the urine.
Nitrofurantoin macrocrystals	Macrodantin	25-, 50-, 100-mg capsules	50–100 mg qid 50–100 mg hs	Treatment of UTI UTI prophylaxis	Absorbed relatively slowly Produce less GI distress than the microcrystals Distributed to tissues in very small amounts	
Nitrofurantoin monohydrate/ macrocrystals	Macrobid	100-mg extended-release capsules	100 mg bid	Treatment of UTI		
Methenamine hippurate	Hiprex, Urex	1-g tablets	1 g bid	UTI prophylaxis/ suppression	Approximately 30% may be converted to ammonia and formaldehyde in the stomach Distributed throughout total body water	Excreted by the kidneys. Within the urinary tract, 20% decomposes to form formaldehyde.
Methenamine mandelate	Generic only	0.5-, 1-g tablets	1 g qid	UTI prophylaxis/ suppression		

tingling sensations, and numbness. Patients should be informed about these symptoms and instructed to report them immediately. Neuropathy is most likely in patients with renal impairment and in those taking nitrofurantoin chronically.

Hepatotoxicity. Rarely, nitrofurantoin has caused severe liver injury, manifesting as hepatitis, cholestatic jaundice, and hepatic necrosis. Deaths have occurred. To reduce risk, patients should undergo periodic tests of liver function. Those who develop liver injury should discontinue nitrofurantoin immediately and never use it again.

Birth defects. Data are conflicted about the use of nitrofurantoin in pregnancy. Results of the *National Birth Defects Prevention Study,* published in 2009, showed an association between nitrofurantoin and four types of birth defects: anophthalmia (the absence of one or both eyes), hypoplastic left heart syndrome (marked hypoplasia of the left ventricle and ascending aorta), atrial septal defects, and cleft lip with cleft palate. However, an additional study completed in Norway in 2013 did not find an increased incidence of these birth defects in babies delivered by mothers who had taken nitrofurantoin. However, this study did reveal an increased incidence of neonatal jaundice in neonates exposed to nitrofurantoin in the last 30 days of gestation. Because of the possibility of hemolytic anemia, the drug is contraindicated in pregnant patients at term (38–42 weeks of gestation). Until more is known, it seems prudent to use alternate antibiotics when needed during any gestational age.

Methenamine
Mechanism of Action
Methenamine (Hiprex, Urex) is a prodrug that, under acidic conditions, breaks down into ammonia and formaldehyde. The formaldehyde denatures bacterial proteins, causing cell death. For formaldehyde to be released, the urine must be acidic (pH 5.5 or less). Because formaldehyde is not formed at physiologic systemic pH, methenamine is devoid of systemic toxicity.

Antimicrobial Spectrum
Virtually all bacteria are susceptible to formaldehyde; there is no resistance. Certain bacteria (e.g., *Proteus* species) can elevate urinary pH (by splitting urea to form ammonia). Because formaldehyde is not released under alkaline conditions, infections with urea-splitting organisms are often unresponsive.

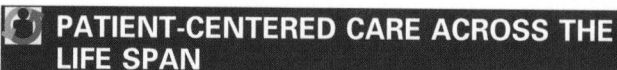

PATIENT-CENTERED CARE ACROSS THE LIFE SPAN

Drugs for Urinary Tract Infection

Life Stage	Patient Care Concerns
Infants	Ampicillin and gentamycin are recommended to treat infants with UTI. Nitrofurantoin is contraindicated in infants less than one month of age. Often the UTI coincides with other infections or urinary tract abnormalities. The source should be sought immediately. Trimethoprim/sulfamethoxazole should also be avoided in the early stages of infancy.
Children/ adolescents	Methenamine hippurate is approved for use in children between 6 and 12 years of age. Methanamine mandelate can be used in children less than 6 years of age.
Pregnant women	UTIs in pregnancy must be treated as complicated infections. Nitrofurantoin is contraindicated in the third trimester of pregnancy. Fluoroquinolones should also be avoided in pregnancy.
Breastfeeding women	Fluoroquinolones have been detected in breast milk at low doses. Short-term use during breastfeeding is acceptable. For greatest safety, breastfeeding should be avoided between 4 and 6 hours after a dose.
Older adults	Nitrofurantoin should be avoided in older adults with decreased renal function.

Therapeutic Uses
Methenamine is used for chronic infection of the lower urinary tract. However, trimethoprim/sulfamethoxazole is preferred. Methenamine is not active against upper tract infections because there is insufficient time for formaldehyde to form as the drug passes through. Methenamine does not prevent UTIs associated with catheters.

Adverse Effects and Precautions
Chronic high-dose therapy can cause bladder irritation, manifested as dysuria, frequent voiding, urinary urgency, proteinuria, and hematuria.

Because decomposition of methenamine generates ammonia (in addition to formaldehyde), the drug is contraindicated for patients with liver dysfunction. Methenamine salts (methenamine mandelate, methenamine hippurate) should not be used by patients with renal impairment because crystalluria may be caused by precipitating the mandelate or hippurate moiety.

Drug Interactions

Urinary alkalinizers. Drugs that elevate urinary pH (e.g., acetazolamide, sodium bicarbonate) inhibit formaldehyde production and can thereby reduce the antibacterial effects. Patients taking methenamine should not receive alkalinizing agents.

Sulfonamides. Methenamine should not be combined with sulfonamides because formaldehyde forms an insoluble complex with sulfonamides, thereby posing a risk for urinary tract injury from crystalluria.

SUMMARY OF KEY PRESCRIBING CONSIDERATIONS

Urinary Tract Antiseptics

Therapeutic Goal: Resolution of infection with improvement in urinary symptoms

Baseline Data: Renal function, urinalysis with culture

Monitoring: Monitoring not recommended

Identifying High-Risk Patients: Pregnant patients should be treated for complicated infections, and fluroquinolones and nitrofurantoin should be avoided in this population. Patients with decreased renal impairment should not be treated with nitrofurantoin.

Evaluating Therapeutic Effects: Inquire about resolution of symptoms

Minimizing Adverse Effects: Drugs that elevated urinary pH should be avoided in combination with methenamine.

77

Drug Therapy for Tuberculosis

Tuberculosis (TB) is a leading cause of death worldwide. According to the World Health Organization, in 2016 there were 10.4 million new TB cases worldwide. Also in 2016, some 1.7 million people died of TB worldwide. More than 95% of these deaths occurred in developing countries.

In the United States we are more fortunate. TB trends have declined over recent decades (down from 20,673 in 1992 to 9272 in 2016). Approximately 70% of these cases occur in people born outside of the United States.

PATHOGENESIS OF TUBERCULOSIS

Tuberculosis is caused by *Mycobacterium tuberculosis*, a slow-growing organism also known as the tubercle bacillus. Infections may be limited to the lungs or may become disseminated. In most cases the bacteria are quiescent and the infected individual has no symptoms. However, when the disease is active, morbidity can be significant.

Primary Infection

Infection with *M. tuberculosis* is transmitted from person to person by inhaling infected sputum that has been aerosolized, usually by coughing or sneezing. As a result, initial infection occurs in the lungs. In the lungs, tubercle bacilli are taken up by the phagocytic macrophages and neutrophils. At first, the bacilli are resistant to the destructive activity of phagocytes and multiply freely within them. Infection can spread from the lungs to other organs through the lymphatic and circulatory systems.

In most cases, immunity to *M. tuberculosis* develops within a few weeks, and the infection is brought under complete control. The immune system facilitates control by increasing the ability of phagocytes to suppress multiplication of tubercle bacilli. Because of this rapid response by the immune system, approximately 90% of individuals with primary infection never develop clinical or radiologic evidence of disease. This condition is defined as latent infection. Even though symptoms are absent and the progression of infection is halted, the infected individual is likely to harbor tubercle bacilli lifelong unless drugs are given to eliminate quiescent bacilli. In 5% to 10% of individuals, reactivation, a renewed multiplication of tubercle bacilli, can occur after a period of dormancy. Hence, in the absence of treatment, there is always some risk that latent infection may become active.

If the immune system fails to control the primary infection, clinical disease (tuberculosis) develops. The result is necrosis and cavitation of lung tissue. Lung tissue may also become caseous (cheese-like in appearance). In the absence of treatment, tissue destruction progresses, and death may result.

OVERVIEW OF TREATMENT

The goals of treatment are to eliminate infection and prevent relapse while also preventing the development of drug-resistant organisms. To accomplish this, treatment must kill tubercle bacilli that are actively dividing as well as those that are dormant.

Drug Resistance

Drug resistance is a major impediment to successful therapy. The emergence of *multi-drug–resistant TB* (MDR-TB) and *extensively drug-resistant TB* (XDR-TB) is a recent and ominous development. MDR-TB is defined as TB that is resistant to both isoniazid and rifampin, our two most effective antituberculosis (anti-TB) drugs. XDR-TB, a severe form of MDR-TB, is defined as TB that is resistant not only to isoniazid and rifampin but also to all fluoroquinolones (e.g., moxifloxacin) and at least one of the injectable second-line anti-TB drugs (amikacin, or capreomycin). Infection with multi-drug–resistant organisms greatly increases the risk for death, especially among patients with AIDS. In addition, multi-drug resistance is expensive. In 2017 the average cost of treating one case of TB was about $18,000, whereas the average costs of treating one case of MDR-TB or XDR-TB were $294,000 or $694,000, respectively.

Infection with a resistant organism may be acquired in two ways: (1) through contact with someone who harbors resistant bacteria and (2) through repeated ineffectual courses of therapy. Common causes of ineffectual therapy are treatment that is too short; dosages that are too low; erratic patient adherence; and, perhaps most important, a regimen that contains too few drugs.

The Prime Directive: Tuberculosis Must Always Be Treated With Two or More Drugs

Antituberculosis regimens must always contain two or more drugs to which the infecting organism is sensitive. Because treatment is prolonged, there is a high risk that drug-resistant bacilli will emerge if only one anti-TB agent is employed. Because the chances of a bacterium developing resistance to two drugs is lower, treatment with two or more drugs minimizes the risk for drug resistance.

Not only do drug combinations decrease the risk for resistance, they can also reduce the incidence of relapse. Because some drugs are especially effective against actively dividing bacilli whereas other drugs are most active against intracellular (quiescent) bacilli, the chances of killing all tubercle bacilli present, whether they are actively multiplying or dormant, is increased when proper combinations of anti-TB agents are used.

In Chapter 70, we noted that treatment with multiple antibiotics broadens the spectrum of antimicrobial coverage, thereby increasing the risk for superinfection. This is not the case with multi-drug therapy of TB. The major drugs used against *M. tuberculosis* are *selective* for this organism. As a result, these drugs, even when used in combination, do not kill off beneficial microorganisms and therefore do not create the conditions that lead to superinfection.

Determining Drug Sensitivity

Because resistance to one or more anti-TB drugs is common and many patterns of resistance are possible, it is essential that we determine drug sensitivity in isolates from each patient at treatment onset. The traditional method is to culture sputum samples in the presence of antimycobacterial drugs. Unfortunately the process is slow, usually taking 6 to 16 weeks to complete. (Although rapid tests for drug sensitivity have been developed in recent years, these can be very expensive. For this reason their use is often restricted.)

Initial drug selection is empiric, based on (1) patterns of drug resistance in the community and (2) the immunocompetence of the patient. After test results have become available, the regimen should be adjusted accordingly. In the event of treatment failure, sensitivity tests should be repeated.

Treatment of Active Tuberculosis

In 2016, the American Thoracic Society, Centers for Disease Control and Prevention, and Infectious Diseases Society of America published new clinical practice guidelines (*ATS/CDC/IDSA Guidelines*) for the treatment of drug-susceptible tuberculosis. (See http://cid.oxfordjournals.org/content/63/7/e147.full.pdf.) These updates, along with current CDC guidelines for other types of TB, inform TB treatment indications in this chapter.

Several regimens may be employed for active TB. Drug selection is based largely on the susceptibility of the infecting organism and the immunocompetence of the host. Life-span considerations are also a factor.

PATIENT-CENTERED CARE ACROSS THE LIFE SPAN

First-Line Drugs for Tuberculosis

Life Stage	Considerations or Concerns
Children	First-line antitubercular drugs with the exception of rifapentine are approved for children; rifapentine is approved for children 12 years of age and older. Ethambutol is usually reserved for children older than 8 years.
Pregnant women	Rifabutin is deemed the safest during pregnancy. The CDC reports that the benefit justifies the risk for isoniazid, rifampin, and pyrazinamide. The CDC does not recommend rifapentine due to insufficient data in pregnant women. Ethambutol has caused teratogenesis in animal studies and there have been reports of eye abnormalities in children; therefore ethambutol should be given only if the benefits are judged to be greater than the risks.
Breastfeeding women	According to the CDC, mothers taking isoniazid and rifampin should be encouraged to breastfeed. For other drugs, it is important to weigh the benefits of breastfeeding against any possible risks to the infant. The amounts of drugs excreted in milk are not sufficient for neonatal treatment against TB.
Older adults	No contraindications are identified for older patients. Dosing may need to be adjusted for patients with decreased renal function.

Four drugs—isoniazid, rifampin, pyrazinamide, and ethambutol—are first-line drugs for TB treatment and are used in most treatment regimens. The rifamycin antibiotics rifapentine and rifabutin are also considered first-line drugs. For latent TB infection, rifapentine is commonly used

instead of rifampin. For patients taking multiple drugs, rifabutin may be used to replace rifampin and reduce drug interactions, but rifampin or rifapentine should be used over rifabutin when possible.

The *ATS/CDC/ISDA Guidelines* identify the following as second-line drugs for TB treatment: cycloserine, ethionamide, capreomycin, *para*-aminosalicylic acid (PAS), the aminoglycosides streptomycin and amikacin, and the quinolones levofloxacin and moxifloxacin. Additional antibiotics are sometimes employed when necessary due to severe adverse effects or other complications in therapy.

Therapy is usually initiated with a *four-drug* regimen. In the event of suspected or proved resistance, more drugs are added; the total may be as high as seven. A sample drug regimen is shown in Table 77.1 and discussed next.

Treatment of Drug-Sensitive Tuberculosis

If the infecting organisms are not resistant to isoniazid or rifampin, therapy is relatively simple. Treatment is divided into two phases. The goal of the initial (intensive) phase is to eliminate actively dividing extracellular tubercle bacilli and thereby render the sputum noninfectious. The goal of the second (continuation) phase is to eliminate persistent intracellular organisms.

The intensive phase, which lasts 8 weeks, consists of four drugs: *isoniazid, rifampin, pyrazinamide,* and *ethambutol*. The continuation phase, which lasts 18 weeks, consists of two drugs—*isoniazid* and *rifampin* (see Fig. 77.1).

Isoniazid- or rifampin-resistant tuberculosis. Infections that are resistant to a single drug—isoniazid or rifampin—usually respond well. Isoniazid-resistant TB can be treated for 6 months with three drugs: rifampin, ethambutol, and pyrazinamide. Rifampin-resistant TB can also be treated with three drugs—isoniazid, ethambutol, and pyrazinamide—but the duration is longer: 18 to 24 months rather than 6 months.

Multi-drug-resistant tuberculosis and extensively drug-resistant tuberculosis. MDR-TB and XDR-TB are much harder to manage than drug-sensitive TB. Treatment is prolonged (to at least 24 months) and must use second- and third-line drugs, which are less effective than the first-line drugs (e.g., isoniazid and rifampin) and are generally more toxic. Initial therapy may consist of five, six, or even seven drugs. Hence an initial regimen might include (1) isoniazid; (2) rifampin; (3) pyrazinamide;

TABLE 77.1 Recommended Treatment Regimen for Drug-Sensitive Active Tuberculosis[a]

Phase of Treatment	Drug Combination	Treatment Intervals	Minimal Length of Treatment
Intensive	Isoniazid Rifampin Pyrazinamide Ethambutol	7 days/week for 56 doses or 5 days/week for 40 doses	8 weeks 8 weeks
Continuation	Isoniazid Rifampin	7 days/week for 126 doses or 5 days/week for 90 doses	18 weeks 18 weeks

[a]Recommendation of the 2016 ATS/CDC/IDSA Clinical Practice Guidelines for Drug-Susceptible TB. Additional regimens are available online at http://www.cdc.gov/tb/publications/guidelines/pdf/clin-infect-dis.-2016-nahid-cid_ciw376.pdf.

Fig. 77.1 Algorithm Indicating the Preferred Empiric Treatment for Adults With Drug-Susceptible Tuberculosis. Although daily administration is preferred, administration 5 days a week under direct observation is an acceptable alternative for preferred care. (Developed from the 2016 ATS/CDC/ISDA Clinical Practice Guidelines: Treatment of Drug-Susceptible Tuberculosis. Alternative choices and recommendations for special situations are available in the report at http://cid.oxfordjournals.org/content/63/7/e147.full.pdf.)

(4) ethambutol; (5) amikacin or capreomycin; (6) levofloxacin; and (7) cycloserine, ethionamide, or PAS. As a last resort, infected tissue may be removed by surgery. Even with all of these measures, the prognosis is often poor: of patients with XDR-TB, between 40% and 60% die. Factors that determine outcome include the extent of drug resistance, infection severity, and the immunocompetence of the host.

Patients With Tuberculosis Plus HIV Infection

Between 2% and 20% of patients with HIV infection develop active TB. Because of their reduced ability to fight infection, these patients require therapy that is more aggressive than that in immunocompetent patients and should last several months longer. In some instances, treatment has lasted 30 months or more.

Interactions among drugs for TB infection and those used for HIV infection are a common problem, especially for patients taking *rifampin*. Rifampin, a cornerstone of TB therapy, can accelerate the metabolism of most protease inhibitors and most nonnucleoside reverse transcriptase inhibitors (NNRTIs) prescribed to treat HIV, and this can decrease the effects of the latter. Accordingly, it is best to avoid combining rifampin with these agents. Unfortunately, this means that patients will be denied optimal treatment for one of their infections. That is, if they take rifampin to treat TB, they will be unable to take most protease inhibitors or NNRTIs for HIV. Conversely, if they take protease inhibitors and NNRTIs to treat HIV, they will be unable to take rifampin for TB. This dilemma does not have an easy solution.

Like rifampin, *rifabutin* can accelerate the metabolism of antiretroviral drugs. However, the degree of acceleration is much less. As a result, many of the antiretroviral drugs that must be avoided in patients taking rifampin can still be used in patients taking rifabutin.

Promoting Adherence: Directly Observed Therapy With Intermittent Dosing

Patient nonadherence is the most common cause of treatment failure, relapse, and increased drug resistance. Because patients with TB must take multiple drugs for 6 months or more, adherence can be a very real problem.

Directly observed therapy (DOT) is now considered the standard of care for TB. In DOT, administration of each dose is done in the presence of an observer, usually a representative of the health department. DOT, combined with intermittent dosing (2 to 3 times a week), helps ensure adherence.

Additionally, DOT facilitates the ongoing evaluation of the clinical response and adverse drug effects.

Evaluating Treatment

Three primary modes are employed to evaluate therapy: bacteriologic evaluation of sputum, chest radiographs, and clinical evaluation.

In patients with positive pretreatment sputum tests, sputum should be evaluated monthly until two consecutive specimens are negative. With proper drug selection and good adherence, sputum cultures become negative in more than 90% of patients after 3 months of treatment.

In patients with negative pretreatment sputum tests, treatment is monitored by chest radiographs and clinical evaluation. The chest radiograph should be repeated at 2 months after initiating therapy, at which time it should show improvement.

Clinical manifestations (e.g., fever, malaise, anorexia, cough) must be evaluated at every clinic visit. These should decrease markedly within 2 weeks.

Treatment failures should be evaluated for drug resistance and patient adherence. In the absence of demonstrated drug resistance, treatment with the same regimen should continue, using DOT to ensure that medication is being taken as prescribed. In patients with drug-resistant TB, *two* effective drugs should be added to the regimen.

End-of-treatment sputum cultures and radiographs are optional if negative results were obtained with monitoring during treatment. If negative results were not obtained during treatment, and positive results are obtained following treatment, patients should continue therapy for another 31 weeks.

TREATMENT OF LATENT TUBERCULOSIS

In the United States, an estimated 13 million people have latent TB infection (LTBI). In the absence of treatment, 5% to 10% of these people will develop active TB. Because LTBI can become active, the condition poses a threat to the infected individual and to the community as well.

Before starting treatment for LTBI, active TB must be ruled out. This is important because if it is treated with just one or two drugs and active TB is present, treatment would promote the emergence of resistant bacilli. To exclude active disease, the patient should receive a physical examination and chest radiograph; if indicated, bacteriologic studies may also be ordered.

The CDC recommends four different treatments for LTBI, using either *isoniazid alone, rifampin alone, or isoniazid plus rifapentine* (Table 77.2). Because dosing with isoniazid plus rifapentine is so simple—just 12 doses instead of up to 270—the chances that a patient will complete the full course are greater than with isoniazid alone.

Treatment decisions are based in part on patient status. Three of the regimens contain isoniazid. Rifampin alone is the obvious choice for patients who cannot take isoniazid or who are presumed to be infected with isoniazid-resistant *M. tuberculosis*. Isoniazid plus rifapentine is recommended for individuals 12 years of age and older, including

TABLE 77.2 Recommended Treatment Regimens for Drug-Sensitive Latent Tuberculosis[a]

Treatment Options	Treatment Intervals	Minimal Length of Treatment	Treatment Considerations
Isoniazid	Daily or twice weekly	9 months	A 9-month regimen of isoniazid is recommended for pregnant women, children age 2–11 years, and patients with HIV. Children and patients with HIV should receive medication daily. Pregnant women should receive pyridoxine supplements.
Isoniazid	Daily or twice weekly	6 months	This option may be used for non-pregnant patients without HIV/AIDS and without chest x-ray findings suggestive of previous TB disease.
Rifampin	Daily	4 months	Rifampin alone is an alternative for patients who are unable to take isoniazid due to resistant organisms or patient status.
Isoniazid plus rifapentine	Once weekly	3 months	Isoniazid plus rifapentine should *not* be used for women who are pregnant or who plan to become pregnant while receiving treatment. It also should not be used for patients younger than 2 years, patients taking antiretroviral treatment for HIV/AIDS, or patients with isoniazid or rifamycin-resistant *M. tuberculosis*. Must be administered under direct observation.

[a]Recommendation of the Centers for Disease Control and Prevention (2017). Retrieved from https://www.cdc.gov/tb/topic/treatment/.htm.

those with HIV infection who are not taking antiretroviral drugs. Other selection criteria are provided in Table 77.2.

VACCINATION AGAINST TUBERCULOSIS

Protection against TB can be conferred by vaccination with bacillus Calmette-Guérin (BCG), a freeze-dried preparation of attenuated *Mycobacterium bovis*. In countries where TB is endemic, the World Health Organization recommends BCG vaccination in infancy in order to protect children against severe, life-threatening TB infection (i.e., miliary TB and tuberculous meningitis). In the United States, routine vaccination is not done because there is a low risk for infection with *M. tuberculosis* and protection against pulmonary TB in adulthood is variable.

PHARMACOLOGY OF INDIVIDUAL ANTITUBERCULOSIS DRUGS

As mentioned earlier, the anti-TB drugs are divided into two groups: first-line drugs and second-line drugs. The first-line drugs are *isoniazid*, *rifampin*, *pyrazinamide*, and *ethambutol* (with rifapentine or rifabutin sometimes substituting for rifampin). Of these, isoniazid and rifampin are the most important. The second-line drugs are generally less effective, more toxic, and more expensive than the primary drugs. Second-line agents are used in combination with the primary drugs to treat disseminated TB and TB caused by organisms resistant to first-line drugs. The major adverse effects of the anti-TB drugs are shown in Table 77.3.

PROTOTYPE DRUGS

Drugs for Tuberculosis

Isoniazid
Rifampin
Pyrazinamide
Ethambutol

Isoniazid

Isoniazid (generic in United States; in Canada, Isotamine ♣) is the primary agent for treatment and prophylaxis of TB. This drug has early bactericidal activity and is superior to alternative drugs with regard to efficacy, toxicity, ease of use, patient acceptance, and affordability. With the exception of patients who cannot tolerate the drug, isoniazid should

TABLE 77.3 Antituberculosis Drugs: Major Adverse Effects

Drug	Major Adverse Effects
First-Line Drugs	
Isoniazid	Hepatotoxicity, peripheral neuritis
Rifampin	Hepatotoxicity
Rifapentine	Hepatotoxicity
Rifabutin	Hepatotoxicity
Pyrazinamide	Hepatotoxicity, polyarthritis
Ethambutol	Optic neuritis
Second-Line Drugs	
Fluoroquinolones	
Levofloxacin	GI intolerance
Moxifloxacin	GI intolerance
Injectable Drugs	
Capreomycin	Eighth cranial nerve damage, nephrotoxicity
Amikacin	Eighth cranial nerve damage, nephrotoxicity
Streptomycin	Eighth cranial nerve damage, nephrotoxicity
Others	
Para-aminosalicylic acid	GI intolerance
Ethionamide	GI intolerance, hepatotoxicity
Cycloserine	Psychoses, seizure, rash

be taken by all individuals infected with isoniazid-sensitive strains of *M. tuberculosis*.

Antimicrobial Activity and Therapeutic Use

Isoniazid is highly selective for *M. tuberculosis*. The drug can kill tubercle bacilli at concentrations 10,000 times lower than those needed to affect gram-positive and gram-negative bacteria. Isoniazid is bactericidal to mycobacteria that are actively dividing but is only bacteriostatic to dormant organisms.

Isoniazid is indicated only for treating active and LTBI. When used for active TB, it must be taken in combination with at least one other agent (e.g., rifampin). For patient convenience, isoniazid is available in fixed-dose combinations: (1) capsules, sold as Isonarif and Rifamate, containing 150 mg of isoniazid and 300 mg of rifampin; and (2) tablets, sold as Rifater, containing 50 mg of isoniazid, 120 mg of rifampin, and 300 mg of pyrazinamide.

Mechanism of Action

Isoniazid suppresses bacterial growth by inhibiting the synthesis of mycolic acid, a component of the mycobacterial cell wall. Because mycolic acid is not produced by other bacteria or by cells of the host, this mechanism would explain why isoniazid is so selective for tubercle bacilli.

Dosing

Although best-practice recommendations for dosing are daily or 5 days a week, providers may select other options after discussing options with patients and their families. Dosing for isoniazid and other drugs is provided in Table 77.4.

Pharmacokinetics

Pharmacokinetics for isoniazid and other drugs used for the treatment of tuberculosis are provided in Table 77.5.

Adverse Effects

Hepatotoxicity. Isoniazid can cause hepatocellular injury and multilobular necrosis. Consequently the US Food and Drug Administration (FDA) has issued a black box warning. Deaths have occurred. Liver injury is thought to result from the production of a toxic isoniazid metabolite. The greatest risk factor for liver damage is advancing age: the incidence is extremely low in patients younger than 20 years. It is 1.2% in those aged 35 to 49 years, 2.3% in those aged 50 to 64 years, and 8% in those older than 65 years. Patients should be informed about signs and symptoms of hepatitis and instructed to notify the provider immediately if these develop. Patients should also undergo monthly evaluation for these signs. Some clinicians perform monthly determinations of serum aspartate aminotransferase (AST) activity because elevation of AST activity is indicative of liver injury. However, because AST levels may rise and then return to normal despite continued isoniazid use, increases in AST may not be predictive of clinical hepatitis. It is recommended that isoniazid be withdrawn if signs of hepatitis develop or if AST activity exceeds three to five times the pretreatment baseline. Caution should be exercised when isoniazid is given to individuals who consume large amounts of alcohol or who have preexisting liver disorders.

TABLE 77.4   Preparations and Dosages[a] of Drugs for Tuberculosis

Drug	Preparation	Daily	Three Times a Week	Twice a Week	Weekly
Isoniazid (generic)	Tablets: 50, 100, 300 mg Oral syrup: 10 mg/mL Solution for injection: 100 mg/mL	Adults: 5 mg/kg/day (usual dose 300 mg) Children: 10–15 mg/kg/day	Adults: 15 mg/kg (usual dose 900 mg) Children: no recommendation	Adults: 15 mg/kg (usual dose 900 mg) Children: 20–30 mg/kg	Adults: 15 mg/kg (usual dose 900 mg) Children: no recommendation
Rifampin (Rifadin, Rofact)	Capsules: 150 mg, 300 mg IV: 600 mg for reconstitution	Adults: 10 mg/kg (usual dose 600 mg) Children: 10–20 mg/kg	Adults: 10 mg/kg (usual dose 600 mg) Children: no recommendation	Adults: 10 mg/kg (usual dose 600 mg) Children: 10–20 mg/kg	Adults: no recommendation Children: no recommendation
Rifapentine (Priftin)	Tablets: 150 mg	Adults: only given weekly in continuation phase Children: not approved for children < 12 years	Adults: only given weekly Children: not approved	Adults: only given weekly Children: not approved	Adults: 20 mg/kg Children: not approved
Rifabutin (Mycobutin)	Capsules: 150 mg	Adults: 5 mg/kg (usual dose 300 mg) Children: 5 mg/kg (suggested)[b]	Adults: no recommendation Children: no recommendation	Adults: no recommendation Children: no recommendation	Adults: no recommendation Children: no recommendation
Pyrazinamide (Tebrazid ✦)	Tablet: 500 mg	Adults: Weight 40–55 kg = 1000/mg per kilogram; Weight 56–75 kg = 1500 mg/kg; Weight 76–90 kg = 2000 mg/kg Children: 30–40 mg/kg	Adults: Weight 40–55 kg = 1500/mg per kilogram; Weight 56–75 kg = 2500 mg/kg; Weight 76–90 kg = 3000 mg/kg Children: no recommendation	Adults: Weight 40–55 kg = 2000 mg/kg; Weight 56–75 kg = 3000 mg/kg; Weight 76–90 kg = 4000 mg/kg Children: 50 mg/kg	Adults: no recommendation Children: no recommendation
Ethambutol (Myambutol, Etibi)	Tablets: 100 mg, 400 mg	Adults: Weight 40–55 kg = 800 mg/kg; Weight 56–75 kg = 1200 mg/kg; Weight 76–90 kg = 1600 mg/kg Children: 15–25 mg/kg	Adults: Weight 40–55 kg = 1200/mg/kg; Weight 56–75 kg = 2000 mg/kg; Weight 76–90 kg = 2400 mg/kg Children: no recommendation	Adults: Weight 40–55 kg = 2000 mg/kg; Weight 56–75 kg = 2800 mg/kg; Weight 76–90 kg = 4000 mg/kg Children: 50 mg/kg	Adults: no recommendation Children: no recommendation
Para-aminosalicylate (Paser Granules)	Packets: 4-g delayed-release granules	Adults: 4000 mg 2–3 times per day (usual dose 8–12 g/d) Children: 100 mg/kg given bid or tid (usual total dose 200–300 mg/kg per day)	Adults: no recommendation Children: no recommendation	Adults: no recommendation Children: no recommendation	Adults: no recommendation Children: no recommendation

TABLE 77.4 Preparations and Dosages[a] of Drugs for Tuberculosis—cont'd

Drug	Preparation	Daily	Three Times a Week	Twice a Week	Weekly
Ethionamide (Trecator)	Tablets: 250 mg	Adults: 15–20 mg/kg per day (usual dose 250–500 mg qd or bid) Children: 15–20 mg/kg per day total in 1–2 doses	Adults: no recommendation Children: no recommendation	Adults: no recommendation Children: no recommendation	Adults: no recommendation Children: no recommendation
Cycloserine (generic)	Capsules: 250 mg	Adults: 10–15 mg/kg per day (usual dose 250–500 mg qd or bid) Children: 15–20 mg/kg per day in 1–2 doses	Adults: no recommendation Children: no recommendation	Adults: no recommendation Children: no recommendation	Adults: no recommendation Children: no recommendation
Capreomycin (Capastat)	Solution for injection: 1-g vial	Adults: 15 mg/kg Children: 15–20 mg/kg	Adults: 25 mg/kg Children: no recommendation	Adults: no recommendation Children: 25–30 mg/kg	Adults: no recommendation Children: no recommendation
Streptomycin (generic)	Solution for injection: 1-g vial	Adults: 15 mg/kg Children: 15–20 mg/kg	Adults: 25 mg/kg Children: no recommendation	Adults: no recommendation Children: 25–30 mg/kg	Adults: no recommendation Children: no recommendation
Amikacin (generic)	Solution for injection: 500 mg/2mL	Adults: 15 mg/kg Children: 15–20 mg/kg	Adults: 25 mg/kg Children: no recommendation	Adults: no recommendation Children: 25–30 mg/kg	Adults: no recommendation Children: no recommendation
Levofloxacin (Levaquin)	Tablets: 250-, 500-, 750-mg Solution for injection: 500-mg vial	Adults: 500–1000 mg Children: ±15–20 mg/kg (suggested)[b]	Adults: no recommendation Children: no recommendation	Adults: no recommendation Children: no recommendation	Adults: no recommendation Children: no recommendation
Moxifloxacin (Avelox, Avelox ABC Pack)	Tablets: 400 mg Solution for injection: 400 mg/250 mL	Adults: 400 mg Children: ±10 mg/kg (suggested)[b]	Adults: no recommendation Children: no recommendation	Adults: no recommendation Children: no recommendation	Adults: no recommendation Children: no recommendation

[a]Alternate dosing is often used, as treatment regimens are commonly individualized.
[b]Optimal dosing unknown; dosing is suggested by experts in the field.
IM, Intramuscular; *IV*, intravenous; *PAS, para*-aminosalicylic acid; *TB*, tuberculosis.

TABLE 77.5 Pharmacokinetics of First-Line Antituberculosis Drugs

Drug	Peak	Protein Binding	Distribution	Metabolism	Half-Life	Elimination
Isoniazid	1–2 h	10%–15%	Widely distributed; crosses blood-brain barrier	Hepatic	0.5–1 h (fast acetylators) 2–5 h (slow acetylators)	Urine
Rifampin	2–4 h	80%	Widely distributed; crosses blood-brain barrier	Hepatic	3–4 h	Feces (approximately 65%; undergoes enterohepatic recirculation); urine
Rifapentine	3–10 h	98%	Widely distributed; crosses blood-brain barrier	Hepatic by esterases	17–24 h	Feces (70%); urine
Rifabutin	2–4 h	85%	Widely distributed; crosses blood-brain barrier	Hepatic	45 h (range 16–69 h)	Urine (53%); feces
Pyrazinamide	<2 h	50%	Widely distributed; crosses blood-brain barrier	Hepatic	9–10 h	Urine
Ethambutol	2–4 h	20%–30%	Widely distributed, crosses blood-brain barrier in presence of inflammation	Hepatic	2.5–3.6 h	Urine; feces

BLACK BOX WARNING

Isoniazid (Generic)

Isoniazid therapy may cause severe hepatitis. Fatalities have been reported.

Peripheral neuropathy. Dose-related peripheral neuropathy is the most common adverse event. Principal symptoms are symmetric paresthesias of the hands and feet. Clumsiness, unsteadiness, and muscle ache may develop. Peripheral neuropathy results from isoniazid-induced deficiency in pyridoxine (vitamin B$_6$).

Other adverse effects. Because isoniazid crosses the blood–brain barrier, a variety of central nervous system (CNS) effects can occur, including optic neuritis, seizures, dizziness, ataxia, and psychologic disturbances (depression, agitation, impairment of memory, hallucinations, toxic psychosis). GI distress, and hematologic reactions (decreases in blood cell production, hemolytic anemia) occur on occasion. There is also an increased risk for pancreatitis; however, this is rare. Allergy to isoniazid can produce fever and rashes. Antinuclear antibodies develop in 20% of patients taking this drug.

Drug Interactions

Isoniazid is a strong inhibitor of three cytochrome P450 isoenzymes: CYP2C9, CYP2C19, and CYP2E1. By inhibiting these isoenzymes, isoniazid can raise levels of drugs that are metabolized by these isoenzymes, including phenytoin, carbamazepine, diazepam, and triazolam. Phenytoin is of particular concern. Plasma levels of phenytoin should be monitored, and phenytoin dosage should be reduced as appropriate. Dosage of isoniazid should not be changed.

Rifampin

Rifampin (Rifadin, Rofact) equals isoniazid in importance as an anti-TB drug. Before the appearance of resistant tubercle bacilli, the combination of rifampin plus isoniazid was the most frequently prescribed regimen for uncomplicated pulmonary TB.

Antimicrobial Activity and Therapeutic Use

Rifampin is one of our most effective anti-TB drugs. This agent is bactericidal to M. tuberculosis at extracellular and intracellular sites. It is a drug of choice for treating pulmonary TB and disseminated disease. Because resistance can develop rapidly when rifampin is employed alone, the drug is always given in combination with at least one other anti-TB agent. Despite the capacity of rifampin to produce a variety of adverse effects, toxicity rarely requires discontinuing treatment.

Rifampin is also used to treat infections other than TB. This broad spectrum drug is active against most gram-positive bacteria as well as many gram-negative bacteria. Rifampin is bactericidal to *M. leprae* and has become an important agent for treating Hansen disease (leprosy), a rare condition in North America. Rifampin is highly active against *Neisseria meningitidis* and is indicated for short-term therapy to eliminate this bacterium from the nasopharynx of asymptomatic carriers. (Because resistant organisms emerge rapidly, rifampin should not be used against active meningococcal disease.) Other bacteria that are highly sensitive include *N. meningitidis, Haemophilus influenzae, Staphylococcus aureus,* and *Legionella* species.

Mechanism of Action

Rifampin inhibits bacterial DNA-dependent RNA polymerase and thereby suppresses RNA synthesis and, consequently, protein synthesis. The results are bactericidal. The drug is lipid soluble and hence has ready access to intracellular bacteria. Because mammalian RNA polymerases are not affected, rifampin is selectively toxic to microbes.

SUMMARY OF KEY PRESCRIBING CONSIDERATIONS

Isoniazid

Therapeutic Goal: Cure the disease, decrease its transmission, and prevent development of antimicrobial resistance.

Baseline Data: See Table 77.6 for a summary of baseline recommendations. Specific baseline data for isoniazid: Obtain sputum smear and culture; drug susceptibility testing for isoniazid: chest radiograph (and other imaging as appropriate if there is extrapulmonary TB), liver function (AST, ALT, bilirubin, alkaline phosphate), and complete a clinical assessment.

Monitoring: See Table 77.6 for general monitoring for all patients treated for TB. Additional considerations for isoniazid: Monitor for signs and symptoms of hepatotoxicity and peripheral neuropathy at each clinic visit.

Identifying High-Risk Patients: Isoniazid is *contraindicated* for patients with acute liver disease or a history of isoniazid-induced hepatotoxicity. Use with *caution* in patients with high alcohol intake, patients with diabetes, patients with vitamin B$_6$ deficiency, patients older than 50 years, and patients who are taking phenytoin, rifampin, rifabutin, rifapentine, or pyrazinamide.

Evaluating Therapeutic Effects: Success is indicated by (1) reductions in fever, malaise, anorexia, cough, and other clinical manifestations of TB; (2) radiographic evidence of improvement; and (3) an absence of *M. tuberculosis* in sputum. Improvement in other presenting signs and symptoms (e.g., evidence of extrapulmonary TB) are also expected.

Minimizing Adverse Effects: Prophylactic use of pyridoxine at 25 to 50 mg/day can decrease the risk of acquiring peripheral neuropathy. Preventive supplementation is especially important for at-risk people with diabetes or with high alcohol intake. If peripheral neuropathy develops, it can be reversed by administering pyridoxine, however, higher than prophylactic doses are required (typically 100 mg daily).

TABLE 77.6 Monitoring Recommendations

Providers should assess the following prior to beginning treatment with first-line drugs for TB. Follow-up recommendations should be obtained periodically as indicated.

Assessment	Timing
Sputum smears and culture	Baseline, then monthly until two consecutive specimens are negative
Drug susceptibility	Baseline, then repeat at 3 months if sputum cultures remain positive
Chest radiograph	Baseline, then repeat at 2 months if baseline sputum cultures were negative
Weight	Baseline, then monthly
Symptom assessment	Baseline, then monthly
Adherence to treatment	Baseline, then monthly
Visual acuity and color discrimination	Baseline, then monthly if taking ethambutol
AST, ALT, bilirubin, alkaline phosphate	Baseline, then monthly if baseline abnormal, if signs or symptoms of liver injury develop, or for patients at high risk of liver injury (e.g., high alcohol intake, HIV infection, taking drugs associated with liver injury)
Creatinine	Baseline, then as indicated
Platelet count	Baseline, then monthly if abnormal
HIV	Baseline, then, if HIV positive, obtain CD4 lymphocyte count and HIV RNA load
Hepatitis B and C screen	Baseline for patients with risk factors
Diabetes screen	Baseline for patients with risk factors

ALT, Alanine aminotransferase; *AST,* aspartate aminotransferase

Adverse Effects

Rifampin is generally well tolerated. When employed at recommended dosages, the drug rarely causes significant toxicity.

Hepatotoxicity. Rifampin can cause hepatotoxicity, posing a risk for jaundice and even hepatitis. Asymptomatic elevation of liver enzymes occurs in about 14% of patients; however, the incidence of overt hepatitis is less than 1%. Hepatotoxicity is most likely in people with heavy alcohol intake and patients with preexisting liver disease. These individuals should be monitored closely for signs of liver dysfunction. Patients should be informed about symptoms of hepatitis and instructed to notify the prescriber if they develop.

Discoloration of body fluids. Rifampin frequently imparts a red-orange color to urine, sweat, saliva, and tears. Patients should be informed of this harmless effect. Permanent staining of soft contact lenses has occurred on occasion.

Other adverse effects. Gastrointestinal (GI) disturbances (anorexia, nausea, abdominal discomfort) and cutaneous reactions (flushing, itching, rash) occur occasionally. Rarely, intermittent high-dose therapy has produced a flu-like syndrome, characterized by fever, chills, muscle aches, headache, and dizziness. This reaction appears to have an immunologic basis. In some patients, high-dose therapy has been associated with shortness of breath, thrombocytopenia, hemolytic anemia, shock, and acute renal failure.

Drug Interactions

Rifampin is a powerful inducer of CYP1A2, CYP2A6, CYP2B6, CYP2C19, CYP2C8, CYP2C9, and CYP3A4 cytochrome P450 isoenzymes. It can hasten the metabolism of many drugs, thereby reducing their effects. This interaction is of special concern with oral contraceptives, warfarin, and certain protease inhibitors and NNRTIs used for HIV infection.

Rifampin can also increase the risk for hepatotoxicity when given with other drugs that are hepatotoxic. For example, rifampin, isoniazid, and pyrazinamide are all hepatotoxic. Hence when these drugs are used in combination, as they often are, the risk for liver injury is greater than when they are used alone.

Rifapentine

Rifapentine (Priftin) is a long-acting analog of rifampin. Both drugs have the same mechanism of action, adverse effects, and drug interactions.

Actions and Uses

Rifapentine is indicated only for pulmonary TB. At therapeutic doses, the drug is lethal to *M. tuberculosis*. The mechanism underlying cell kill is inhibition of DNA-dependent RNA polymerase.

Adverse Effects

Rifapentine is well tolerated at recommended doses. Similarly to rifampin, the drug imparts a red-orange color to urine, sweat, saliva, and tears. Permanent staining of contact lenses can occur.

Hepatotoxicity is the principal concern. In clinical trials, serum transaminase levels increased in 5% of patients. However, overt hepatitis occurred in only one patient. Because of the risk for hepatotoxicity, liver function tests should be performed at baseline and monthly thereafter. Patients should be informed about symptoms of hepatitis and instructed to notify the prescriber if these develop.

Drug Interactions

Similarly to rifampin, rifapentine is a powerful inducer of cytochrome P450 drug-metabolizing enzymes. As a result, it can decrease the levels of other drugs. Important among these are protease inhibitors and NNRTIs (used for HIV infection), oral contraceptives, and warfarin.

SUMMARY OF KEY PRESCRIBING CONSIDERATIONS

Rifampin and Other Rifamycins

Therapeutic Goal: Cure the disease, decrease its transmission, and prevent development of antimicrobial resistance.

Baseline Data: See Table 77.6 for a summary of baseline recommendations. Specific baseline data for rifampin: Obtain sputum smear and culture; drug susceptibility testing for rifampin: chest radiograph (and other imaging as appropriate if there is extrapulmonary TB), liver function (AST, ALT, bilirubin, alkaline phosphate), and complete a clinical assessment. A pregnancy test should be conducted.

Monitoring: See Table 77.6 for general monitoring for all patients treated for TB. Additional considerations for rifamycins: Monitor for signs and symptoms of hepatotoxicity, GI problems, rashes, and potential immunologic reaction at each clinic visit.

Identifying High-Risk Patients: Rifampin is *contraindicated* for patients taking delavirdine (an NNRTI) and most protease inhibitors.

Use with *caution* in people with high alcohol intake, patients with liver disease, and patients taking warfarin.

Evaluating Therapeutic Effects: Success is indicated by (1) reductions in fever, malaise, anorexia, cough, and other clinical manifestations of TB; (2) radiographic evidence of improvement; and (3) an absence of *M. tuberculosis* in sputum. Improvement in other presenting signs and symptoms (e.g., evidence of extrapulmonary TB) are also expected.

Minimizing Adverse Effects: If a patient wears soft contact lenses, he or she should be informed that these drugs may impart a harmless red-orange color to body secretions; therefore permanent staining of contact lenses may occur.

For patients taking warfarin, PT/INR must be monitored closely. Warfarin dosage must then be adjusted as needed.

Alternative nonhormonal birth control measures should be recommended for women of childbearing age.

Rifabutin

Actions and Uses

Rifabutin (Mycobutin) is a close chemical relative of rifampin. Similarly to rifampin, rifabutin inhibits mycobacterial DNA-dependent RNA polymerase and thereby suppresses protein synthesis. The drug is approved for prevention of disseminated *M. avium* complex (MAC) disease in patients with advanced HIV infection (CD4 lymphocyte counts below 200/mm³). In addition to this approved indication, rifabutin is used off label as an alternative to rifampin to treat TB in patients with HIV infection. Rifabutin is preferred to rifampin in HIV patients because it has less effect on the metabolism of protease inhibitors and NNRTIs.

Adverse Effects

Rifabutin is generally well tolerated. The most common side effects (affecting less than 5% of patients) are rash, GI disturbances, and neutropenia. Similarly to rifampin, rifabutin can impart a harmless red-orange color to urine, sweat, saliva, and tears; soft contact lenses may be permanently stained. Rifabutin poses a risk for uveitis and hence should be discontinued if ocular pain or blurred vision develops. Other adverse effects include myositis, hepatitis, arthralgia, chest pain with dyspnea, and a flu-like syndrome.

Drug Interactions

Similarly to rifampin, rifabutin induces cytochrome P450 isoenzymes, although less strongly than rifampin does. By increasing enzyme activity, rifabutin can decrease blood levels of other drugs, especially oral contraceptives and delavirdine, an NNRTI (see Chapter 81). Women using oral contraceptives should be advised to use a nonhormonal method of birth control.

Pyrazinamide
Antimicrobial Activity and Therapeutic Use

Pyrazinamide is bactericidal to *M. tuberculosis*, particularly those that are dormant. Currently, the combination of pyrazinamide with rifampin, isoniazid, and ethambutol is a preferred regimen for initial therapy of active disease caused by drug-sensitive *M. tuberculosis*.

Mechanism of Action

In the body, pyrazinamide is metabolized to pyrazinoic acid, which lowers the pH and increases its activity. It is also thought to inhibit fatty acid synthetase I, a *M. tuberculosis* enzyme.

Adverse Effects and Drug Interactions

Hepatotoxicity. Pyrazinamide is the most hepatotoxic of all the first-line drugs. High-dose therapy has caused hepatitis and, rarely, fatal hepatic necrosis.

The risk for liver injury is increased by concurrent therapy with isoniazid or rifampin, both of which are hepatotoxic. Pyrazinamide plus rifampin is contraindicated for patients with active liver disease or a history of isoniazid-induced liver injury and should be used with caution in patients who are taking hepatotoxic drugs or who drink alcohol in excess.

Other adverse effects. Polyarthralgias develop in 40% of patients. Pyrazinamide and its metabolites can inhibit renal excretion of uric acid, causing hyperuricemia. Although this drug does not usually produce symptoms, pyrazinamide-induced hyperuricemia has (rarely) resulted in gouty arthritis. Additional adverse effects include GI disturbances (nausea, vomiting, diarrhea), rash, and photosensitivity with associated dermatitis.

ETHAMBUTOL
Antimicrobial Activity and Therapeutic Use

Ethambutol (Myambutol, Etibi ♦) is active only against mycobacteria; nearly all strains of *M. tuberculosis* are sensitive. In most cases, ethambutol is active against tubercle bacilli that are resistant to isoniazid and rifampin.

Ethambutol is employed for initial treatment of TB and for treating patients who have received therapy previously. Like other drugs for TB, ethambutol is always employed as part of a multi-drug regimen.

Mechanism of Action

Ethambutol is bacteriostatic, not bactericidal. It inhibits the enzyme arabinosyl transferase; this impairs mycobacterial cell wall synthesis.

Adverse Effects

Ethambutol is generally well tolerated. The most significant adverse effect is optic neuritis.

Optic Neuritis

Ethambutol can produce dose-related optic neuritis, resulting in blurred vision, constriction of the visual field, and disturbance of color discrimination. The mechanism underlying these effects is unknown. Symptoms usually resolve on discontinuation of treatment. Fortunately, this adverse effect is uncommon; however, for some patients, visual disturbance may persist. Because visual changes can be difficult to monitor in pediatric patients, ethambutol is not usually recommended for children younger than 8 years.

SUMMARY OF KEY PRESCRIBING CONSIDERATIONS
Pyrazinamide

Therapeutic Goal: Cure the disease, decrease its transmission, and prevent development of antimicrobial resistance

Baseline Data: See Table 77.6 for a summary of baseline recommendations. Specific baseline data for rifampin: Obtain sputum smear and culture; drug susceptibility testing for pyrazinamide: chest radiograph (and other imaging as appropriate if there is extrapulmonary TB), liver function tests (AST, ALT, bilirubin, alkaline phosphate), and complete a thorough clinical assessment.

Monitoring: See Table 77.6 for general monitoring for all patients treated for TB. Additional considerations for pyrazinamide: Monitor for signs and symptoms of hepatotoxicity at each clinic visit. Assess for joint pain, GI disturbances and rashes. If symptoms of gout occur, check uric acid levels.

Identifying High-Risk Patients: Pyrazinamide is *contraindicated* for patients with severe liver dysfunction or acute gout. Use with *caution* in patients with high alcohol intake.

Evaluating Therapeutic Effects: Success is indicated by (1) reductions in fever, malaise, anorexia, cough, and other clinical manifestations of TB; (2) radiographic evidence of improvement; and (3) an absence of *M. tuberculosis* in sputum. Improvements in other presenting signs and symptoms (e.g., evidence of extrapulmonary TB) are also expected.

Minimizing Adverse Effects: Pain due to polyarthralgias can usually be managed with a nonsteroidal antiinflammatory drug (NSAID), such as aspirin or ibuprofen. A few patients may need to reduce the dosage of pyrazinamide or discontinue treatment.

Other Adverse Effects

Ethambutol can produce allergic reactions (dermatitis, pruritus), GI upset, and confusion. The drug inhibits renal excretion of uric acid, causing asymptomatic hyperuricemia in about 50% of patients; occasionally elevation of uric acid levels results in acute gouty arthritis. Rare adverse effects include peripheral neuropathy, renal damage, and thrombocytopenia.

SUMMARY OF KEY PRESCRIBING CONSIDERATIONS
Ethambutol

Therapeutic Goal: Cure the disease, decrease its transmission, and prevent development of antimicrobial resistance

Baseline Data: See Table 77.6 for a summary of baseline recommendations. Specific baseline data for ethambutol: Obtain sputum smear and culture; drug susceptibility testing for pyrazinamide: chest radiograph (and other imaging as appropriate if there is extrapulmonary TB), and complete a thorough clinical assessment. Tests for visual acuity and color discrimination should be included.

Monitoring: See Table 77.6 for general monitoring for all patients treated for TB. Additional considerations for ethambutol: Monitor color discrimination monthly. Ask about changes in vision or presence of eye pain at each visit. Assess for rashes, GI upset, and changes in mental status. If signs and symptoms of gout occur, check a uric acid level.

Identifying High-Risk Patients: Ethambutol is *contraindicated* for patients with optic neuritis.

Evaluating Therapeutic Effects: Success is indicated by (1) reductions in fever, malaise, anorexia, cough, and other clinical manifestations of TB; (2) radiographic evidence of improvement; and (3) an absence of *M. tuberculosis* in sputum. Improvements in other presenting signs and symptoms (e.g., evidence of extrapulmonary TB) are also expected.

Minimizing Adverse Effects: Withdraw ethambutol immediately if signs or symptoms of optic neuritis develop.

SECOND-LINE ANTITUBERCULOSIS DRUGS

The group of second-line anti-TB drugs consists of two fluoroquinolones (levofloxacin and moxifloxacin), three injectable drugs (capreomycin, amikacin, streptomycin), and three other drugs (PAS, ethionamide, and cycloserine). In general, these drugs are less effective, more toxic, and more expensive than the first-line drugs. As a result, their principal indication is TB caused by organisms that have proved resistant to first-line agents. In addition, second-line drugs are used to treat severe pulmonary TB as well as disseminated (extrapulmonary) infection. The second-line drugs are always employed in conjunction with a first-line anti-TB drug.

Fluoroquinolones

Levofloxacin (Levaquin) and moxifloxacin (Avelox) are fluoroquinolone antibiotics indicated for a wide variety of bacterial infections (see Chapter 78). Both drugs have good activity against *M. tuberculosis*. As therapy for TB, these drugs are reserved for infection caused by multi-drug–resistant organisms. Both drugs are generally well tolerated, although GI disturbances are relatively common. Tendon rupture occurs rarely but may result in permanent damage, especially in patients more than 60 years old. The FDA has issued a black box warning to address this concern. These drugs are not recommended for children.

 BLACK BOX WARNING

Fluoroquinolones

Systemic fluoroquinolones (e.g., levofloxacin and moxifloxacin) may cause tendinitis, tendon rupture, and permanent and disabling adverse effects of the tendons, muscles, joints, nerves, and CNS.

Fluoroquinolones may worsen myasthenia gravis–associated muscle weakness.

Injectable Drugs

Capreomycin

Capreomycin (Capastat Sulfate) is an antibiotic derived from a species of *Streptomyces*. Antibacterial effects probably result from inhibiting protein synthesis. The drug is bacteriostatic to *M. tuberculosis*. Capreomycin is used only for TB that is resistant to primary agents. The principal toxicity is renal damage; hence the drug should not be taken by patients with kidney disease. Capreomycin may also cause damage to the eighth cranial nerve, resulting in hearing loss, tinnitus, and disturbed balance (see the accompanying black box warning). Administration is by deep intramuscular injection (the drug is not absorbed from the GI tract and therefore cannot be administered orally).

 BLACK BOX WARNING

Capreomycin

Capreomycin is nephrotoxic and ototoxic and can cause renal impairment and cranial nerve VIII impairment. It should not be given to patients with renal insufficiency or auditory impairment. It also should not be given with aminoglycosides or other drugs having similar nephrotoxic and ototoxic effects.

Amikacin and Streptomycin

Amikacin (Amikin), kanamycin (generic only), and streptomycin (generic only) are aminoglycoside antibiotics with good activity against *M. tuberculosis*. Similarly to other aminoglycosides, these drugs are nephrotoxic and may also damage the eighth cranial nerve. The FDA issued a black box warning regarding this concern. These drugs are not absorbed from the GI tract; hence administration is parenteral (intramuscular or intravenous). The pharmacology of these and other aminoglycosides is discussed in Chapter 74.

 BLACK BOX WARNING

Aminoglycosides

Aminoglycosides (e.g., streptomycin and amikacin) are ototoxic and can cause permanent hearing loss. Vertigo may occur as a result of vestibular injury. Aminoglycosides are nephrotoxic and may cause renal impairment.

Para-Aminosalicylic Acid

Actions and uses. PAS (Paser Granules) is similar in structure and actions to the sulfonamides. Similarly to the sulfonamides, PAS exerts its antibacterial effects by inhibiting synthesis of folic acid. However, in contrast to the sulfonamides, which are broad-spectrum antibiotics, PAS is active only against mycobacteria. In the United States, PAS has been employed primarily as a substitute for ethambutol in pediatric patients. The drug is always used in combination with other anti-TB agents.

Adverse effects. PAS is poorly tolerated by adults; children accept the drug somewhat better. The most frequent adverse effects are GI disturbances (nausea, vomiting, diarrhea). Because PAS is administered in large doses as a sodium salt, substantial sodium loading may occur. Additional adverse effects are allergic reactions, hepatotoxicity, and goiter.

Storage. PAS loses its effectiveness if exposed to heat. Packets should be stored in a cool location (below 59°F).

Ethionamide

Actions and uses. Ethionamide (Trecator), a relative of isoniazid, is active against mycobacteria, but less so than isoniazid itself. Ethionamide is administered with other anti-TB drugs to treat TB that is resistant to first-line agents. GI disturbances limit patient acceptance. Ethionamide is the least well tolerated of all anti-TB agents and hence should be used only when there is no alternative.

Adverse effects. GI effects (anorexia, nausea, vomiting, diarrhea, metallic taste) occur often; intolerance of these effects frequently leads to discontinuation. Ethionamide is toxic to the liver. Hepatotoxicity is assessed by measuring serum transaminases (AST, ALT) before treatment and periodically thereafter. Additional adverse effects include peripheral neuropathy, CNS effects (convulsions, mental disturbance), and allergic reactions. Hypoglycemia has occurred; patients with diabetes need close monitoring and possible dosage adjustment of medications used to manage diabetes.

Cycloserine

Actions and uses. Cycloserine (generic) is an antibiotic produced by a species of *Streptomyces*. The drug is bacteriostatic and acts by inhibiting cell wall synthesis. Cycloserine is used against TB that is resistant to first-line drugs.

Adverse effects. CNS effects occur frequently and can be severe. Possible reactions include anxiety, depression, confusion, hallucinations, paranoia, hyperreflexia, and seizures. Psychotic episodes occur in approximately 10% of patients; symptoms usually subside within 2 weeks after drug withdrawal. Pyridoxine may prevent neurotoxic effects. Other adverse effects include peripheral neuropathy, hepatotoxicity, and folate deficiency. To minimize the risk for adverse effects, serum concentrations of cycloserine should be measured periodically; peak concentrations, measured 2 hours after dosing, should be 25 to 35 µg/mL.

Alternative Drug

Bedaquiline

When the FDA granted accelerated approval of bedaquiline (Sirturo) in December 2012, it was heralded as the first unique drug in the anti-TB arsenal to emerge in more than 40 years. The drug appears to work faster and better than all other anti-TB drugs. In addition, bedaquiline does not accelerate the metabolism of other drugs and hence can be used in patients taking drugs for HIV. Nevertheless, it is not among those drugs recommended as first- or second-line drugs in the *ATS/CDC/IDSA Guidelines* pending results of additional clinical trials. It also has some serious adverse effects and costs approximately $36,000 for 100 tablets.

▶▶ BLACK BOX WARNING

Bedaquiline (Sirturo)

Subjects in a bedaquiline clinical trial had an increased mortality rate: 11.4% died compared with 2.5% in the group taking a placebo.

Bedaquiline can cause QT prolongation. The drug must be discontinued if QT prolongation exceeds 500 msec.

Actions and uses. Bedaquiline has a unique mechanism of action: bacterial kill results from inhibiting adenosine triphosphate (ATP) synthase, an enzyme required by *M. tuberculosis* to make ATP. Few drugs share this mechanism, which explains why there's no cross-resistance between bedaquiline and conventional drugs. Because humans make ATP by a different pathway, bedaquiline does not interfere with ATP synthesis in humans.

Bedaquiline is approved for multi-drug–resistant pulmonary TB in patients at least 18 years of age. It is not approved for treatment of latent, nonpulmonary, or drug-sensitive tuberculosis (i.e., TB that is effectively treated by other drugs). It also should not be used for mycobacterial infections other than TB.

Although resistance to bedaquiline is uncommon, it does occur: about 1 in 200 million tubercle bacilli make a form of ATP synthase that is not inhibited by the drug. Accordingly, to prevent overgrowth with these resistant microbes, the regimen should always contain other anti-TB drugs.

Adverse effects. Bedaquiline labeling includes a black box warning related to the risk for prolonged QT interval and risk for hepatotoxicity.

There was an increased risk for death in clinical trials; therefore labeling recommends that bedaquiline be used only if there is no other effective treatment. Beyond the adverse effects listed in the black box warning, bedaquiline has few adverse effects. Approximately 10% to 40% of patients may experience nausea, arthralgia, headache, chest pain, and hemoptysis. Fewer than 10% experience rash and anorexia. It may be taken during pregnancy.

Drug interactions. In a clinical trial, rifampin significantly reduced blood levels of bedaquiline. This interaction with rifampin occurs because rifampin induces the activity of CYP3A4, the isoenzyme of cytochrome P450 that metabolizes bedaquiline.

PATIENT EDUCATION

Drugs for Tuberculosis

To promote adherence, educate the patient about the rationale for multi-drug therapy and the need for long-term treatment. Encourage patients to take their medication exactly as prescribed and to continue treatment until the infection has resolved.

All first-line drugs except ethambutol carry a risk of hepatotoxicity; therefore the combination of drugs for TB increases the risk for liver damage. Inform patients to be alert to the occurrence of jaundice, anorexia, malaise, fatigue, and nausea and instruct them to report any of these symptoms if they develop. Urge patients who drink alcohol to minimize or eliminate alcohol consumption so as to avoid increasing the risk for liver damage. Also, instruct patients to avoid acetaminophen and other drugs that can cause liver damage.

Inform patients taking isoniazid about symptoms of tingling, numbness, burning, or pain in the hands or feet that can signal onset of peripheral neuropathy and instruct them to report such symptoms if they occur. Explain the importance of taking vitamin B6, if prescribed, to prevent this.

Inform patients taking rifampin that it may impart a harmless red-orange color to urine, sweat, saliva, and tears. Warn patients that soft contact lenses may undergo permanent staining. Advise them to consult their eye care specialist about continued use of the lenses.

When rifampin is being prescribed, advise women taking oral contraceptives to use a nonhormonal form of birth control.

Advise patients taking pyrazinamide who develop polyarthralgias to take an NSAID (e.g., aspirin, ibuprofen) to relieve pain.

Instruct patients taking ethambutol to report any alteration in vision such as blurring of vision or reduced color discrimination.

78

Miscellaneous Antibacterial Drugs

FLUOROQUINOLONES

The fluoroquinolones are fluorinated analogs of nalidixic acid, a narrow-spectrum quinolone antibiotic used only for urinary tract infections (UTIs). However, unlike nalidixic acid, the fluoroquinolones are broad-spectrum agents that have multiple applications. Benefits derive from disrupting DNA replication and cell division. Fluoroquinolones do not disrupt synthesis of proteins or the cell wall. All of the systemic fluoroquinolones can be administered orally. As a result, these drugs are attractive alternatives for people who might otherwise require intravenous antibacterial therapy. Although side effects are generally mild, all fluoroquinolones can cause tendinitis and tendon rupture, usually of the Achilles tendon. Fortunately the risk is low. Bacterial resistance develops slowly but has become common in *Neisseria gonorrhoeae*; hence these drugs are no longer recommended for this infection. Six fluoroquinolones are currently available for systemic therapy (Table 78.1). Fluoroquinolones used solely for topical treatment of the eyes are discussed in Chapter 87.

Ciprofloxacin

Ciprofloxacin (Cipro) was among the first fluoroquinolones available and can serve as the prototype for the group. The drug is active against a broad spectrum of bacterial pathogens and may be administered by the oral or intravenous route. Oral ciprofloxacin has been used as an alternative to parenteral antibiotics for treatment of several serious infections. Because it can be administered by mouth, patients receiving ciprofloxacin can be treated at home rather than going to the hospital for intravenous antibacterial therapy.

PROTOTYPE DRUGS

Miscellaneous Antibacterial Drugs

Fluoroquinolone
Ciprofloxacin

Nitroimidazole
Metronidazole

Cyclic Lipopeptide
Daptomycin

Mechanism of Action

Ciprofloxacin inhibits two bacterial enzymes: *DNA gyrase* and *topoisomerase IV*. Both are needed for DNA replication and cell division. DNA gyrase converts closed circular DNA into a supercoiled configuration. In the absence of supercoiling, DNA replication cannot take place. Topoisomerase IV helps separate daughter DNA strands during cell division. Because the mammalian equivalents of DNA gyrase and topoisomerase IV are largely insensitive to fluoroquinolones, cells of the host are spared. Ciprofloxacin is rapidly bactericidal.

Antimicrobial Spectrum

Ciprofloxacin is active against a broad spectrum of bacteria, including most aerobic gram-negative bacteria and some gram-positive bacteria. Most urinary tract pathogens, including *Escherichia coli* and *Klebsiella* species, are sensitive. The drug is also highly active against most bacteria that cause enteritis (e.g., *Salmonella* and *Shigella* species, *Campylobacter jejuni, E. coli*). Other sensitive organisms include *Bacillus anthracis, Pseudomonas aeruginosa, Haemophilus influenzae*, meningococci, and many streptococci. Activity against anaerobes is fair to poor. *Clostridium difficile* is resistant.

Pharmacokinetics

Ciprofloxacin may be given by the oral or intravenous route. After oral dosing, the drug is absorbed rapidly but incompletely. High concentrations are achieved in urine, stool, bile, saliva, bone, and prostate tissue. Drug levels in cerebrospinal fluid remain low. Ciprofloxacin has a plasma half-life of about 4 hours. Elimination is by hepatic metabolism and renal excretion.

Therapeutic Uses

Ciprofloxacin is approved for a wide variety of infections. Among these are infections of the respiratory tract, urinary tract, gastrointestinal (GI) tract, bones, joints, skin, and soft tissues. Also, ciprofloxacin is a preferred drug for preventing anthrax in people who have inhaled anthrax spores. Because ciprofloxacin is active against a variety of pathogens and can be given orally, the drug represents an alternative to parenteral treatment for many serious infections. Owing to high rates of resistance, ciprofloxacin is a poor choice for staphylococcal infections. The drug is not useful against infections caused by anaerobes.

Because of concerns about tendon injury (see later), *systemic* ciprofloxacin is generally avoided in individuals younger than 18 years. Nonetheless, the drug does have two approved pediatric uses: (1) treatment of complicated urinary tract and kidney infections caused by *E. coli*, and (2) postexposure prophylaxis and treatment of anthrax.

Adverse Effects

Ciprofloxacin can induce a variety of mild adverse effects, including GI reactions (nausea, vomiting, diarrhea, abdominal pain) and central nervous system (CNS) effects (dizziness, headache, restlessness, confusion). *Candida* infections of the pharynx and vagina may develop during treatment. Very rarely, seizures have occurred. In older adults, ciprofloxacin poses a significant risk for confusion, somnolence, psychosis, and visual disturbances.

Fluoroquinolones damage tendons by disrupting the extracellular matrix of cartilage in immature animals. A similar mechanism may underlie tendon rupture in humans. Because tendon injury is reversible if diagnosed early, fluoroquinolones should be discontinued at the first sign of tendon pain, swelling, or inflammation. In addition, patients should refrain from exercise until tendinitis has been ruled out. Although there are no controlled studies on the use of ciprofloxacin during

711

TABLE 78.1 Systemic Fluoroquinolones

Drug	Therapeutic Uses	Pharmacokinetics	Adverse Effects	Drug Interactions
Ciprofloxacin (Cipro)	Infections of the respiratory tract, urinary tract, GI tract, bones, joints, skin and soft tissues; Inhalational anthrax	Metabolism: hepatic; Excretion: renal; Poor CSF absorption	Tendonitis and tendon rupture; Exacerbation of muscle weakness in MG	Antacids; Calcium supplements; Milk and dairy products; Iron salts; Zinc salts; Sucralfate
Levofloxacin (Levaquin)	Infections of the respiratory tract, urinary tract, GI tract, skin and soft tissues; Inhalational anthrax	Metabolism: minimal hepatic; Elimination: renal	Peripheral neuropathy; Phototoxicity	Warfarin
Ofloxacin	Infections of the respiratory tract, urinary tract, GI tract, skin and soft tissues	Metabolism: minimal hepatic; Elimination: renal primary		Antacids; Calcium supplements; Milk and dairy products; Iron salts; Zinc salts; Sucralfate
Moxifloxacin (Avelox)	Infections of the respiratory tract, intra-abdominal infections, skin and skin structures	Metabolism: hepatic; Elimination: renal	Prolonged QT interval; Tendonitis and tendon rupture; Exacerbation of muscle weakness in MG	Drugs that prolong the QT interval; Antacids; Calcium supplements; Milk and dairy products; Iron salts; Zinc salts; Sucralfate
Gemifloxacin (Factive)	Respiratory tract infections (1) CAP (2) Acute bacterial exacerbation of chronic bronchitis	Metabolism: minimal hepatic; Elimination: GI tract (feces) primary, renal	Peripheral neuropathy; Phototoxicity	
Delafloxacin (Baxdela)	Infections of the skin or skin structures	Metabolism: hepatic; Excretion: renal primary, GI tract (feces)	Tendonitis and tendon rupture; Exacerbation of muscle weakness in MG; Peripheral neuropathy; Phototoxicity	Antacids; Calcium supplements; Milk and dairy products; Iron salts; Zinc salts; Sucralfate

CSF, Cerebrospinal fluid; *CAP*, community-acquired pneumonia; *GI*, gastrointestinal; *MG*, myasthenia gravis.

PATIENT-CENTERED CARE ACROSS THE LIFE SPAN

Antibacterial Drugs

Life Stage	Patient Care Concerns
Children/ adolescents	Ciprofloxacin and levofloxacin are the only fluoroquinolones approved for use in children. Because of concerns regarding tendon injury, fluoroquinolones are generally avoided in this population.
Pregnant women	Although data reveal little potential for fluoroquinolone toxicity in the fetus, these data are limited. Risks and benefits must be considered for administration during pregnancy.
Breastfeeding women	Effects of fluoroquinolones on the nursing infant are largely unknown. Other medications should be considered if possible.
Older adults	Fluoroquinolones are generally well tolerated in older adults. For safe dosing, creatinine clearance should be calculated.

BLACK BOX WARNING

Fluoroquinolones and Tendon Rupture

Rarely, ciprofloxacin and other fluoroquinolones have caused tendon rupture, usually of the Achilles tendon. The incidence is 1 in 10,000 or less. People at highest risk are those 60 years of age and older, those taking glucocorticoids, and those who have undergone heart, lung, or kidney transplantation.

pregnancy or lactation, limited data indicate that such use poses little or no risk for tendon damage to either the fetus or nursing infant. Because of the relative lack of data, alternative drugs should be given if possible.

Ciprofloxacin and other fluoroquinolones pose a risk for *phototoxicity* (severe sunburn), characterized by burning, erythema, exudation, vesicles, blistering, and edema. This can occur after exposure to direct sunlight, indirect sunlight, and sunlamps—even if a sunscreen has been applied. Patients should be warned about phototoxicity and advised to avoid sunlight and sunlamps. People who must go outdoors should wear protective clothing and apply a sunscreen. Ciprofloxacin should be withdrawn at the first sign of a phototoxic reaction (e.g., burning sensation, redness, rash).

Ciprofloxacin and other fluoroquinolones increase the risk for developing *C. difficile* infection (CDI), a potentially severe infection of the bowel. CDI results from killing off intestinal bacteria that normally keep *C. difficile* in check.

BLACK BOX WARNING

Ciprofloxacin and Myasthenia Gravis

Ciprofloxacin and other fluoroquinolones can exacerbate muscle weakness in patients with myasthenia gravis. Accordingly, patients with a history of myasthenia gravis should not receive these drugs.

Drug and Food Interactions

Cationic compounds. Absorption of ciprofloxacin can be reduced by compounds that contain cations. Among these are (1) aluminum- or magnesium-containing antacids, (2) iron salts, (3) zinc salts, (4) sucralfate,

(5) calcium supplements, and (6) milk and other dairy products, all of which contain calcium ions. These cationic agents should be administered at least 6 hours before ciprofloxacin or 2 hours after.

Elevation of drug levels. Ciprofloxacin can increase plasma levels of several drugs, including *theophylline* (used for asthma), *warfarin* (an anticoagulant), and *tinidazole* (an antifungal drug). Toxicity could result. For patients taking theophylline, drug levels should be monitored and the dosage adjusted accordingly. For patients taking warfarin, prothrombin time should be monitored and the dosage of warfarin reduced as appropriate.

SUMMARY OF KEY PRESCRIBING CONSIDERATIONS

Fluoroquinolones

Therapeutic Goal: Treatment of fluoroquinolone-sensitive infections

Baseline Data: None indicated

Monitoring: None recommended

Identifying High-Risk Patients: Fluoroquinolones are contraindicated in patients with a history of myasthenia gravis. They should be used with caution in patients with renal impairment, patients over 60 years of age, and patients taking glucocorticoids.

Evaluating Therapeutic Effects: Patients should be monitored for indications of antimicrobial effects such as reduction in fever, pain, or inflammation.

Minimizing Adverse Effects: Patients must be instructed to report early signs of tendon injury and to avoid prolonged sun exposure.

ADDITIONAL ANTIBACTERIAL DRUGS

Metronidazole

Metronidazole (Flagyl) is used to treat protozoal infections and infections caused by obligate anaerobic bacteria. The basic pharmacology of metronidazole is discussed in Chapter 83, as is the drug's use against protozoal infections. Consideration here is limited to antibacterial applications.

Mechanism of Antibacterial Action

Metronidazole is lethal to anaerobic organisms only. To exert bactericidal effects, metronidazole must first be taken up by cells and then converted into its active form; only anaerobes can perform the conversion. The active form interacts with DNA to cause strand breakage and loss of helical structure, effects that result in inhibition of nucleic acid synthesis and, ultimately, cell death. Because aerobic bacteria are unable to activate metronidazole, they are insensitive to the drug.

Antibacterial Spectrum

Metronidazole is active against obligate anaerobes only. Sensitive bacterial pathogens include *Bacteroides fragilis* (and other *Bacteroides* species),

C. difficile (and other *Clostridium* species), *Fusobacterium* species, *Gardnerella vaginalis*, *Peptococcus* species, and *Peptostreptococcus* species.

Therapeutic Uses

Metronidazole is active against a variety of anaerobic bacterial infections, including infections of the CNS, abdominal organs, bones and joints, skin and soft tissues, and genitourinary tract. Frequently these infections also involve aerobic bacteria; hence therapy must include a drug active against them. Metronidazole is used for treatment of *C. difficile* infection, as discussed in Chapter 72. In addition, the drug is employed for prophylaxis in surgical procedures associated with a high risk for infection by anaerobes (e.g., colorectal surgery, abdominal surgery, gynecologic surgery). Metronidazole is also used in combination with a tetracycline and bismuth subsalicylate to eradicate *Helicobacter pylori* in people with peptic ulcer disease.

⯈⯈ BLACK BOX WARNING

Metronidazole

Metronidazole has been associated with increased carcinogenic risk in mice and rats. Unnecessary use is to be avoided.

Daptomycin

Daptomycin (Cubicin) is the first representative of a class of antibiotics known as the *cyclic lipopeptides* (Table 78.2). The drug has a unique mechanism and can rapidly kill virtually all clinically relevant gram-positive bacteria, including methicillin-resistant *Staphylococcus aureus.* Daptomycin is devoid of significant drug interactions, and the only notable side effect is possible muscle injury. The drug is given once daily by intravenous infusion, and there is no need to monitor its plasma level.

Mechanism of Action

Daptomycin has a novel mechanism of action. The drug inserts itself into the bacterial cell membrane and thereby forms channels that permit efflux of intracellular potassium (and possibly other cytoplasmic ions). Loss of intracellular ions has two effects. First, it depolarizes the cell membrane; second, it inhibits the synthesis of DNA, RNA, and proteins, thereby causing cell death.

Antibacterial Spectrum

Daptomycin is active only against gram-positive bacteria. The drug cannot penetrate the outer membrane of gram-negative bacteria and hence cannot harm them. Daptomycin is rapidly bactericidal to staphylococci (including methicillin- and vancomycin-resistant *S. aureus* and

TABLE 78.2 Cyclic Lipopeptides and Glycopeptides				
Drug	**Therapeutic Uses**	**Pharmacokinetics**	**Severe Adverse Effects**	**Drug Interactions**
Daptomycin (Cubicin)	(1) Bloodstream infection (2) Endocarditis (3) Skin and skin structure infections	Metabolism: Minimal hepatic Excretion: Renal	Myopathy	Statins
Dalbavancin (Dalvance)	Skin and skin structure infections	Metabolism: Minimal hepatic. Excretion: Renal primary, GI tract (feces)	CDAD Hypersensitivity reactions	None Known
Oritavancin (Orbactiv)		Metabolism: Not metabolized. Excretion: Minimal renal and GI tract (feces)		Warfarin Phenytoin

CDAD, Clostridium difficile associated diarrhea.

methicillin-resistant *Staphylococcus epidermidis*), enterococci (including vancomycin-resistant *Enterococcus faecium and Enterococcus faecalis*), streptococci (including penicillin-resistant *Streptococcus pneumoniae*), and most other aerobic and anaerobic gram-positive bacteria. As a rule, daptomycin is more rapidly bactericidal than either vancomycin, linezolid, or quinupristin/dalfopristin.

Therapeutic Use

Daptomycin has two approved indications: (1) bloodstream infection (including endocarditis) with *S. aureus*; and (2) complicated skin and skin structure infections caused by susceptible strains of the following gram-positive bacteria: *S. aureus* (including methicillin-resistant strains), *Streptococcus pyogenes*, *Streptococcus agalactiae*, *Streptococcus dysgalactiae* subspecies *equisimilis*, and *E. faecalis* (vancomycin-susceptible strains only). Daptomycin should not be used to treat community-acquired pneumonia (CAP). Clinical trials have shown that in CAP patients receiving daptomycin, the rate of death and serious cardiorespiratory events is higher than that in patients receiving equally effective alternatives.

Pharmacokinetics

Daptomycin is administered by intravenous infusion, and a significant fraction (92%) becomes bound to plasma proteins. The drug undergoes minimal metabolism. Most of each dose is excreted unchanged in the urine. In patients with normal renal function, the half-life is 9 hours. However, in those with severe renal impairment (creatinine clearance less than 30 mL/min) and those on hemodialysis or continuous ambulatory peritoneal dialysis, the half-life increases threefold. As a result, if the dosage is not reduced, plasma drug levels can rise dangerously high.

Adverse Effects

Daptomycin is generally well tolerated. The most common adverse effects are constipation, nausea, diarrhea, injection-site reactions, headache, insomnia, and rash.

Daptomycin may pose a small risk for myopathy (muscle injury). In clinical trials with doses that were larger and more frequent than those used now, patients often experienced muscle pain and weakness in association with increased levels of creatine phosphokinase (CPK), a marker for muscle injury. However, with currently approved doses, elevation of CPK is rare.

PATIENT EDUCATION
Daptomycin

Patients should be warned about possible muscle injury, and told to report any muscle pain or weakness.

In addition, CPK levels should be measured weekly. If the level rises markedly (to more than 10 times the upper limit of normal), daptomycin should be discontinued. Daptomycin should also be discontinued in patients who report muscle pain or weakness in conjunction with a more moderate rise in CPK.

Drug Interactions

Daptomycin appears to be devoid of significant drug interactions. It does not induce or inhibit cytochrome P450 and should not affect drugs that are metabolized by this enzyme system. In clinical studies, daptomycin did not affect the kinetics of warfarin, simvastatin, or aztreonam. Concurrent use of daptomycin plus tobramycin caused a moderate increase in daptomycin levels and a moderate decrease in tobramycin levels. Accordingly, caution is needed when these drugs are combined.

Like daptomycin, the HMG-CoA reductase inhibitors (e.g., simvastatin [Zocor]) can cause myopathy. However, in clinical trials, no patient receiving simvastatin plus daptomycin developed signs of muscle injury. Nonetheless, given our limited experience with daptomycin, it may be prudent to suspend HMG-CoA reductase inhibitors while daptomycin is being used.

79

Antifungal Agents

The antifungal agents fall into two major groups: drugs for *systemic mycoses* (i.e., systemic fungal infections) and drugs for *superficial mycoses*. A few drugs are used for both. Systemic infections occur much less frequently than superficial infections but are much more serious. Accordingly, therapy of systemic mycoses is our main focus.

DRUGS FOR SYSTEMIC MYCOSES

Systemic mycoses can be subdivided into two categories: opportunistic infections and nonopportunistic infections. The opportunistic mycoses—*candidiasis, aspergillosis, cryptococcosis,* and *mucormycosis*—are seen primarily in debilitated or immunocompromised hosts. In contrast, nonopportunistic infections can occur in any host. These latter mycoses, which are relatively uncommon, include *sporotrichosis, blastomycosis, histoplasmosis,* and *coccidioidomycosis.* Treating systemic mycoses can be difficult: these infections often resist treatment and hence may require prolonged therapy with drugs that frequently prove toxic. Drugs of choice for systemic mycoses are shown in Table 79.1.

The systemic antifungal drugs fall into four classes: polyene antibiotics, azoles, echinocandins, and pyrimidine analogs. Class members and mechanisms of action are shown in Table 79.2.

Amphotericin B, a Polyene Antibiotic

Amphotericin B [Abelcet, Amphotec, AmBisome, Fungizone ✤] belongs to a drug class known as *polyene antibiotics,* so named because their structures contain a series of conjugated double bonds. Nystatin, another antifungal drug, is in the same family.

Amphotericin B is active against a broad spectrum of pathogenic fungi and is a drug of choice for most systemic mycoses. Unfortunately, amphotericin B is highly toxic: infusion reactions and renal damage occur in many patients. Because of its potential for harm, amphotericin B should be employed only against infections that are progressive and potentially fatal.

Amphotericin B is available in four formulations: a conventional formulation (amphotericin B deoxycholate) and three lipid-based formulations. The lipid-based formulations are as effective as the conventional formulation and cause less toxicity—but are much more expensive. For treatment of systemic mycoses, all formulations are administered by intravenous (IV) infusion. Infusions are given daily or every other day for several months.

Mechanism of Action

Amphotericin B binds to components of the fungal cell membrane, increasing permeability. The resultant leakage of intracellular cations (especially potassium) reduces viability. Depending on the concentration of amphotericin B and the susceptibility of the fungus, the drug may be fungistatic or fungicidal.

The component of the fungal membrane to which amphotericin B binds is *ergosterol,* a member of the *sterol* family of compounds. Hence, for a cell to be susceptible, its cytoplasmic membrane must contain sterols. Because bacterial membranes lack sterols, bacteria are not affected.

Much of the toxicity of amphotericin is attributable to the presence of sterols (principally cholesterol) in mammalian cell membranes. When amphotericin binds with cholesterol in mammalian membranes, the effect is similar to that seen in fungi. However, there *is* some degree of selectivity: amphotericin binds more strongly to ergosterol than it does to cholesterol, so fungi are affected more than we are.

Microbial Susceptibility and Resistance

Amphotericin B is active against a broad spectrum of fungi. Some protozoa (e.g., *Leishmania braziliensis*) are also susceptible. As noted, bacteria are resistant.

Emergence of resistant fungi is extremely rare and occurs only with long-term amphotericin use. In all cases of resistance, the fungal membranes had reduced amounts of ergosterol or none at all.

Therapeutic Uses

Amphotericin B is a drug of choice for most systemic mycoses. Before this drug became available, systemic fungal infections usually proved fatal. Treatment is prolonged; 6 to 8 weeks is common. In some cases, treatment may last for 3 or 4 months. In addition to its antifungal applications, amphotericin B is a drug of choice for leishmaniasis.

Pharmacokinetics

Absorption and distribution. Amphotericin is poorly absorbed from the gastrointestinal (GI) tract, and hence oral therapy cannot be used for systemic infection. Rather, amphotericin must be administered intravenously. When the drug leaves the vascular system, it undergoes extensive binding to sterol-containing membranes of tissues. Levels about half those in plasma are achieved in aqueous humor and in peritoneal, pleural, and joint fluids. Amphotericin B does not readily penetrate to the cerebrospinal fluid (CSF).

Metabolism and excretion. Little is known about the elimination of amphotericin B. We do not know if the drug is metabolized or if it is ultimately removed from the body. Renal excretion of unchanged amphotericin is minimal. However, dose or frequency reduction may be considered in patients with preexisting renal impairment. Complete elimination of amphotericin takes a long time; the drug has been detected in tissues more than a year after cessation of treatment.

Adverse Effects

Amphotericin can cause a variety of serious adverse effects. Patients should be under close supervision, preferably in a hospital.

▶▶ **BLACK BOX WARNING**
Amphotericin Toxicity

Because of its toxicity, amphotericin should be used only in the setting of a potentially life-threatening infection.

TABLE 79.1 Drugs of Choice for Systemic Mycoses

Infection	Causative Organism	Drugs of Choice	Alternative Drugs
Aspergillosis	*Aspergillus* spp.	Voriconazole	Amphotericin B, isavuconazonium, itraconazole, posaconazole, caspofungin, micafungin
Blastomycosis	*Blastomyces dermatitidis*	Amphotericin B *or* itraconazole	No alternative recommended
Candidiasis	*Candida* spp.	Amphotericin B *or* fluconazole, either one ± flucytosine	Itraconazole, voriconazole, caspofungin
Coccidioidomycosis	*Coccidioides immitis*	Amphotericin B *or* fluconazole	Itraconazole, ketoconazole
Cryptococcosis	*Cryptococcus neoformans*	Amphotericin B ± flucytosine	Itraconazole
Chronic suppression		Fluconazole	Amphotericin B
Histoplasmosis	*Histoplasma capsulatum*	Amphotericin B *or* itraconazole	Fluconazole, ketoconazole
Chronic suppression		Itraconazole	Amphotericin B
Mucormycosis	*Mucor*	Amphotericin B	Isavuconazonium
Paracoccidioidomycosis	*Paracoccidioides brasiliensis*	Amphotericin B *or* itraconazole	Ketoconazole
Sporotrichosis	*Sporothrix schenckii*	Amphotericin B *or* itraconazole	Fluconazole

TABLE 79.2 Classes of Systemic Antifungal Drugs

Drug Class	Mechanism of Action	Class Members
Polyene antibiotics	Bind to ergosterol and disrupt the fungal cell membrane	Amphotericin B
Azoles	Inhibit synthesis of ergosterol and disrupt the fungal cell membrane	Fluconazole Isavuconazonium Itraconazole Ketoconazole Posaconazole Voriconazole
Echinocandins	Inhibit synthesis of β-1,3-d-glucan and disrupt the fungal cell wall	Anidulafungin Caspofungin Micafungin
Pyrimidine analogs	Disrupt synthesis of RNA and DNA	Flucytosine

Infusion reactions. Intravenous amphotericin frequently produces fever, chills, rigors, nausea, and headache. These reactions are caused by release of proinflammatory cytokines (tumor necrosis factor, interleukin-1, interleukin-6) from monocytes and macrophages. Symptoms begin 1 to 3 hours after starting the infusion and persist about an hour. Mild reactions can be reduced by pretreatment with diphenhydramine plus acetaminophen. If other measures fail, hydrocortisone can be used to decrease fever and chills. However, because glucocorticoids can reduce the patient's ability to fight infection, routine use of hydrocortisone should be avoided. Infusion reactions are less intense with lipid-based amphotericin formulations than with the conventional formulation.

Amphotericin infusion produces a high incidence of phlebitis. This can be minimized by changing peripheral venous sites often, administering amphotericin through a large central vein, and pretreatment with heparin.

Nephrotoxicity. Amphotericin is toxic to cells of the kidneys. Renal impairment occurs in practically all patients. The extent of kidney damage is related to the total dose administered over the full course of treatment. In most cases, renal function normalizes after amphotericin use stops. However, if the total dose exceeds 4 g, residual impairment is likely. Kidney damage can be minimized by infusing 1 L of saline on the days amphotericin is given. Other nephrotoxic drugs should be avoided. To evaluate renal injury, tests of kidney function should be performed every 3 to 4 days, and intake and output should be monitored. If plasma creatinine content rises above 3.5 mg/dL, amphotericin dosage should be reduced. As noted, the degree of renal damage is less with lipid-based amphotericin than with the conventional formulation.

Hematologic effects. Amphotericin can cause bone marrow suppression, resulting in normocytic, normochromic anemia. Hematocrit determinations should be conducted to monitor red blood cell status.

Drug Interactions

Nephrotoxic drugs. Use of amphotericin with other nephrotoxic drugs (e.g., aminoglycosides, cyclosporine, nonsteroidal antiinflammatory drugs [NSAIDs]) increases the risk for kidney damage. Accordingly, these combinations should be avoided if possible.

Azoles

Like amphotericin B, the azoles are broad-spectrum antifungal drugs. As a result, azoles represent an alternative to amphotericin B for most systemic fungal infections. In contrast to amphotericin, which is highly toxic and must be given intravenously, the azoles have lower toxicity and can be given by mouth. However, azoles do have one disadvantage: they inhibit hepatic cytochrome P450 drug-metabolizing enzymes and can increase the levels of many other drugs. Of the azoles in current use, only six—itraconazole, ketoconazole, fluconazole, voriconazole, posaconazole, and isavuconazonium—are indicated for systemic mycoses (Table 79.3). Azoles used for superficial mycoses are discussed separately later.

Itraconazole

Itraconazole [Sporanox] is an alternative to amphotericin B for several systemic mycoses and will serve as our prototype for the azole family. The drug is safer than amphotericin B and has the added advantage of oral dosing. Principal adverse effects are cardiosuppression and liver injury. Like other azoles, itraconazole can inhibit drug-metabolizing enzymes and raise levels of other drugs.

Mechanism of action. Itraconazole inhibits the synthesis of *ergosterol*, an essential component of the fungal cytoplasmic membrane. The result is increased membrane permeability and leakage of cellular components. Accumulation of ergosterol precursors may also contribute to antifungal actions. Itraconazole suppresses ergosterol synthesis by inhibiting fungal cytochrome P450–dependent enzymes.

Therapeutic use. Itraconazole is active against a broad spectrum of fungal pathogens. At this time, it is a drug of choice for *blastomycosis*,

TABLE 79.3 The Azole Drugs

Drug	Therapeutic Uses	Availability	Usual Adult Dose	Pharmacokinetics	Adverse Effects
Itraconazole [Sporanox]	Blastomycosis, histoplasmosis, paracoccidioidomycosis	100-mg capsules 10-mg/mL solution	200 mg 1–2 times daily	Metabolism: hepatic Elimination: urine	Cardiac suppression, liver injury
Fluconazole [Diflucan]	Blastomycosis, Candidiasis, histoplasmosis	50-, 100-, 150-, 200-mg tablets 10-mg and 40-mg/mL suspension Solution for IV injection	Oropharyngeal candidiasis, 100–200 mg PO/IV daily Esophageal candidiasis, 200–400 mg PO/IV daily Vulvovaginal candidiasis, uncomplicated, 150 mg PO once Cryptococcal meningitis, 400 mg once, then 200 mg PO/IV daily	Metabolism: hepatic Elimination: urine	Nausea, headache, Stevens-Johnson syndrome
Voriconazole [Vfend]	Aspergillosis, Candidiasis, Histoplasmosis	50-, 200-mg tablets 40-mg/mL suspension Solution for IV injection	Aspergillosis: 6 mg/kg on day 1, followed by 4 mg/kg IV twice daily × 7 days, then 100 mg PO every 12 h	Metabolism: hepatic Elimination: urine	Hepatotoxicity, visual disturbances, hypersensitivity reactions
Ketoconazole (generic only)	Systemic mycoses in patients not tolerant of amphotericin B	200-mg tablets	200–400 mg PO daily	Metabolism: hepatic Elimination: hepatic	Nausea, vomiting, hepatic necrosis (potentially fatal)
Posaconazole [Noxafil]	Aspergillosis, Candidiasis	100-mg delayed-release tablets 40-mg/mL suspension Solution for IV injection	Oropharyngeal candidiasis, 100 mg PO daily Invasive fungal infections in immunocompromised patients, 300 mg IV daily	Metabolism: hepatic Elimination: fecal	Nausea, vomiting, headache, QT prolongation
Isavuconazonium [Cresemba]	Aspergillosis, mucormycosis	186-mg capsules Solution for IV injection	372 mg PO/IV 3 times daily × 6 doses, then 372 mg PO/IV daily	Metabolism: hepatic Elimination: feces, urine	Hepatotoxicity, Stevens-Johnson syndrome, nausea, vomiting

PROTOTYPE DRUGS

Antifungal Agents

Polyene Macrolide
Amphotericin B

Azole
Itraconazole

Echinocandin
Caspofungin

histoplasmosis, *paracoccidioidomycosis*, and *sporotrichosis* and is an alternative to amphotericin B for *aspergillosis*, *candidiasis*, and *coccidioidomycosis*. Itraconazole may also be used for superficial mycoses.

Pharmacokinetics. Itraconazole is administered orally, in capsules or suspension. Food increases absorption of capsules but decreases absorption of suspension. Interestingly, administration with cola enhances absorption. When absorbed, the drug is widely distributed to lipophilic tissues. Concentrations in aqueous fluids (e.g., saliva, CSF) are negligible. The drug undergoes extensive hepatic metabolism. About 40% of each dose is excreted in the urine as inactive metabolites.

Adverse effects. Itraconazole is well tolerated in usual doses. Gastrointestinal reactions (nausea, vomiting, diarrhea) are most common. Other reactions include rash, headache, abdominal pain, and edema. Itraconazole may also cause two potentially serious effects: cardiac suppression and liver injury.

Cardiac suppression. Itraconazole has negative inotropic actions that can cause a transient decrease in ventricular ejection fraction. Cardiac function returns to normal by 12 hours after dosing. The drug may still be used to treat serious fungal infections in patients with heart failure but only with careful monitoring and only if the benefits clearly outweigh the risks. If signs and symptoms of heart failure worsen, itraconazole should be stopped.

▶ BLACK BOX WARNING
Negative Inotropic Actions With Itraconazole

Because of its negative inotropic actions, itraconazole should not be used for superficial fungal infections (dermatomycoses, onychomycosis) in patients with heart failure, a history of heart failure, or other indications of ventricular dysfunction.

Liver injury. Itraconazole has been associated with rare cases of liver failure, some of which were fatal. Although a causal link has not been established, caution is nonetheless advised. Patients should be informed about signs of liver impairment and, if they appear, should seek medical attention immediately.

Drug interactions

Inhibition of hepatic drug metabolizing enzymes. Itraconazole inhibits CYP3A4 (the 3A4 isoenzyme of cytochrome P450) and thus can increase levels of many other drugs (see Table 79.3). The most important are cisapride, pimozide, dofetilide, and quinidine. When present at high levels, these drugs can cause potentially fatal ventricular dysrhythmias. Accordingly, concurrent use with itraconazole is contraindicated. Other drugs of concern include cyclosporine, digoxin, warfarin, and sulfonylurea-type oral hypoglycemics. In patients taking cyclosporine or digoxin, levels of these drugs should be monitored; in patients taking warfarin, prothrombin time should be monitored; and in patients taking sulfonylureas, blood glucose levels should be monitored.

Drugs that raise gastric pH. Drugs that decrease gastric acidity—antacids, histamine-2 (H₂) antagonists, and proton pump inhibitors—can greatly reduce absorption of oral itraconazole. Accordingly, these agents should be administered at least 1 hour before itraconazole or 2 hours after. (Because proton pump inhibitors have a prolonged duration of action, patients using these drugs may have insufficient stomach acid for itraconazole absorption, regardless of when the proton pump inhibitor is given.)

SUMMARY OF KEY PRESCRIBING CONSIDERATIONS

Azoles

Therapeutic Goal: Treatment of systemic and superficial mycoses.
Baseline Data: Baseline tests of liver function.
Monitoring: No recommended monitoring.
Identifying High-Risk Patients: Use with great caution in patient with liver disease.
Evaluating Therapeutic Effects: Monitor for indications of antifungal effects—reduction in fever, pain, or inflammation.
Minimizing Adverse Effects: Instruct patients to report signs of liver dysfunction. Avoid use with drugs metabolized by CYP3A4 (warfarin, cyclosporine, digoxin, quinidine).

PATIENT-CENTERED CARE ACROSS THE LIFE SPAN

Antifungal Agents

Life Stage	Patient Care Concerns
Infants	Nystatin is used to treat oral candidiasis in premature and full-term infants. Fluconazole is also used safely to treat systemic candidiasis in newborn infants.
Children/adolescents	Many antifungal agents are used safely in children, in lower doses. Side-effect profiles are similar to those of adults.
Pregnant women	Risks and benefits must be considered for administration during pregnancy.
Breastfeeding women	Data are lacking regarding most antifungals and breastfeeding. Most antifungals are considered safe in lower doses. The exception to this is ketoconazole. Because it has high potential for hepatotoxicity, it should be avoided in breastfeeding women.
Older adults	Older adults have a higher risk for achlorhydria than do younger individuals and may not predictably absorb some antifungal agents. In addition, common drugs prescribed to older adults, including warfarin, phenytoin, and oral hypoglycemic agents, are increased by azoles.

Echinocandins

The echinocandins are the newest class of antifungal drugs. In contrast to amphotericin B and the azoles, which disrupt the fungal cell membrane, the echinocandins disrupt the fungal cell wall. Echinocandins cannot be dosed orally, and their antifungal spectrum is narrow, being limited mainly to *Aspergillus* and *Candida* species. Three echinocandins are available: caspofungin, micafungin, and anidulafungin (Table 79.4). When dosage is appropriate, all three appear therapeutically equivalent.

Caspofungin

Actions and uses. Caspofungin [Cancidas] was the first echinocandin available. Antifungal effects result from inhibiting the biosynthesis of β-1,3-d-glucan, an essential component of the cell wall of some fungi, including *Candida* and *Aspergillus*. Caspofungin is approved for IV therapy of (1) invasive aspergillosis in patients unresponsive to or intolerant of traditional agents (e.g., amphotericin B, itraconazole) and (2) systemic *Candida* infections, including candidemia and *Candida*-related esophagitis, peritonitis, pleural space infections, and intra-abdominal abscesses. The drug is better tolerated than amphotericin B and appears just as effective.

Pharmacokinetics. Caspofungin is not absorbed from the GI tract and hence must be given parenterally (by IV infusion). In the blood, 97% of the drug is protein bound. Caspofungin is cleared from the blood with a half-life of 9 to 11 hours. The principal mechanism of plasma clearance is redistribution to tissues, not metabolism or excretion. Over time, the drug undergoes gradual metabolism followed by excretion in the urine and feces.

Adverse effects. Caspofungin is generally well tolerated. The most common adverse effects are fever and phlebitis at the injection site. Less common reactions include headache, rash, nausea, and vomiting. In addition, caspofungin can cause effects that appear to be mediated by histamine release. Among these are rash, facial flushing, pruritus, and a sense of warmth. One case of anaphylaxis has been reported.

Drug interactions. Drugs that induce cytochrome P450 may decrease levels of caspofungin. Powerful inducers include efavirenz, nelfinavir, rifampin, carbamazepine, dexamethasone, and phenytoin. Patients taking these drugs may need to increase caspofungin dosage.

Caspofungin can decrease levels of tacrolimus [Prograf], an immunosuppressant. If these drugs are taken concurrently, levels of tacrolimus should be monitored and dosage increased as needed.

Combining caspofungin with cyclosporine [Sandimmune, others] increases the risk for liver injury, as evidenced by a transient elevation in plasma levels of liver enzyme. Accordingly, the combination should generally be avoided.

SUMMARY OF KEY PRESCRIBING CONSIDERATIONS

Echinocandins

Therapeutic Goal: Treatment of aspergillus and candida species.
Baseline Data: Liver function tests
Monitoring: None recommended
Identifying High-Risk Patients: Echinocandins should be avoided in pregnancy. Patients with underlying liver dysfunction should be monitored closely.
Evaluating Therapeutic Effects: Monitor for indications of antifungal effects: reduction in fever, pain, or inflammation.
Minimizing Adverse Effects: Instruct patients to report signs of liver dysfunction. Caspofungin can decrease levels of tacrolimus.

Flucytosine, a Pyrimidine Analog

Flucytosine [Ancobon], a pyrimidine analog, is employed for serious infections caused by susceptible strains of *Candida* and *Cryptococcus neoformans*. Because development of resistance is common, flucytosine is almost always used in combination with amphotericin B. Extreme caution is needed in patients with renal impairment and hematologic disorders.

Mechanism of Action

Flucytosine is taken up by fungal cells, which then convert it to 5-fluorouracil (5-FU), a powerful antimetabolite. The ultimate effect

TABLE 79.4 The Echinocandins

Drug	Therapeutic Uses	Availability	Usual Adult Dosing	Pharmacokinetics	Adverse Effects
Caspofungin [Cancidas]	Aspergillosis, *Candida*	Solution for IV injection	70 mg IV × 1 then 50 mg daily	Metabolism: minimal; redistributes to tissues Elimination: urine, feces	Fever, phlebitis at injection site
Micafungin [Mycamine]	Candida	Solution for IV injection	100 mg IV daily	Metabolism: hepatic Elimination: feces	Headache, nausea, vomiting, phlebitis at injection site
Anidulafungin [Eraxis]	Candida	Solution for IV injection	100–200 mg IV daily	Metabolism: chemical degradation Elimination: feces	Diarrhea, hypokalemia, histamine-mediated infusion reactions

is disruption of fungal DNA and RNA synthesis. Flucytosine is relatively harmless to us because mammalian cells lack cytosine deaminase, the enzyme that converts flucytosine to 5-FU.

Antifungal Spectrum and Therapeutic Uses

Flucytosine has a narrow antifungal spectrum. Fungicidal activity is highest against *Candida* species and *C. neoformans*. Most other fungi are resistant. Because of this narrow spectrum, flucytosine is indicated only for candidiasis and cryptococcosis. For treatment of serious infections (e.g., cryptococcal meningitis, systemic candidiasis), flucytosine should be combined with amphotericin B. This combination offers two advantages over flucytosine alone: (1) antifungal activity is enhanced and (2) emergence of resistant fungi is reduced.

Pharmacokinetics

Flucytosine is readily absorbed from the GI tract and is well distributed throughout the body. The drug has good access to the central nervous system; levels in the CSF are about 80% of those in plasma. Flucytosine is eliminated by the kidneys, principally as unchanged drug. The half-life is about 4 hours in patients with normal renal function. However, in patients with renal insufficiency, the half-life is greatly prolonged, and hence dosage must be reduced.

Adverse Effects

Hematologic effects. Bone marrow suppression is the most serious complication of treatment. Marrow suppression usually manifests as reversible neutropenia or thrombocytopenia. Rarely, fatal agranulocytosis develops. Platelet and leukocyte counts should be determined weekly. Adverse hematologic effects are most likely when plasma levels of flucytosine exceed 100 mcg/mL. Accordingly, the dosage should be adjusted to keep drug levels below this value. Flucytosine should be used with caution in patients with preexisting bone marrow suppression.

Hepatotoxicity. Mild and reversible liver dysfunction occurs frequently, but severe hepatic injury is rare. Liver function should be monitored (by making weekly determinations of serum transaminase and alkaline phosphatase levels).

▶▶ BLACK BOX WARNING

Flucytosine and Renal Impairment

Flucytosine should be used with extreme caution in patients with renal impairment.

Drug Interactions

Flucytosine is often combined with amphotericin B. This combination offers several advantages. However, the combination can also be detrimental. Because amphotericin B is nephrotoxic, and because flucytosine

is eliminated by the kidneys, amphotericin B–induced kidney damage may suppress flucytosine excretion, promoting flucytosine toxicity. Therefore it is important to monitor renal function and flucytosine levels when amphotericin B and flucytosine are combined.

Like itraconazole, flucytosine inhibits hepatic drug-metabolizing enzymes and can raise levels of several other drugs. With at least four drugs—cisapride, pimozide, dofetilide, and quinidine—elevated levels can lead to potentially fatal dysrhythmias. Accordingly, flucytosine must not be combined with these drugs.

DRUGS FOR SUPERFICIAL MYCOSES

The superficial mycoses are caused by two groups of organisms: (1) *Candida* species and (2) dermatophytes (species of *Epidermophyton*, *Trichophyton*, and *Microsporum*). *Candida* infections usually occur in mucous membranes and moist skin; chronic infections may involve the scalp, skin, and nails. Dermatophytoses are generally confined to the skin, hair, and nails. Superficial infections with dermatophytes are more common than superficial infections with *Candida*.

Overview of Drug Therapy

Superficial mycoses can be treated with a variety of topical and oral drugs. For mild to moderate infections, topical agents are generally preferred. Specific indications for the drugs used against superficial mycoses are shown in Table 79.5. Some of these drugs are also used for systemic mycoses.

Dermatophytic Infections (Ringworm)

Dermatophytic infections are commonly referred to as *ringworm*. There are four principal dermatophytic infections, defined by their location: *tinea pedis* (ringworm of the foot, or "athlete's foot"), *tinea corporis* (ringworm of the body), *tinea cruris* (ringworm of the groin), and *tinea capitis* (ringworm of the scalp).

Tinea pedis. Tinea pedis, the most common fungal infection, generally responds well to topical therapy. Patients should be advised to wear absorbent cotton socks, change their shoes often, and dry their feet after bathing.

Tinea corporis. Tinea corporis usually responds to a topical azole or allylamine. Treatment should continue for at least 1 week after symptoms have cleared. Severe infection may require a systemic antifungal agent (e.g., griseofulvin).

Tinea cruris. Tinea cruris responds well to topical therapy. Treatment should continue for at least 1 week after symptoms have cleared. If the infection is severely inflamed, a systemic antifungal drug (e.g., clotrimazole) may be needed; topical or systemic glucocorticoids may be needed as well.

Tinea capitis. Tinea capitis is difficult to treat. Topical drugs are not likely to work. Oral griseofulvin, taken for 6 to 8 weeks, is considered

TABLE 79.5 Drugs for Superficial Fungal Infections

Drug	Route	Availability	Ringworm[a]	CANDIDA INFECTION Skin	Mouth	Vulvovaginal	Onychomycosis[b]
Azoles							
Butoconazole [Gynazole-1]	Topical	2% vaginal cream				✔	
Clotrimazole [Desenex, Lotrimin, Gyne-Lotrimin]	Topical	1% cream 2% powder 100-, 200-mg vaginal tablets 2% vaginal cream	✔	✔	✔	✔	
Econazole [Ecoza]	Topical	1% foam 1% cream	✔	✔			
Fluconazole [Diflucan]	Oral	50-, 100-, 150-, 200-mg tablets 10 mg/mL and 40 mg/mL suspension	✔		✔	✔	✔
Itraconazole [Sporanox]	Oral	100-mg capsules	✔				✔
Ketoconazole [Nizoral, Xolgel, Extina]	Oral Topical	200-mg tablets 2% shampoo 2% gel 2% foam	✔ ✔	✔	✔		✔
Miconazole [Monistat 1, Monistat 3, Monistat 7, Micatin]	Topical	200-, 1200-mg vaginal ovules 100-mg vaginal cream 2% topical skin cream	✔	✔		✔	
Oxiconazole [Oxistat]	Topical	1% cream 1% lotion	✔				
Sertaconazole [Ertaczo]	Topical	2% cream	✔				
Sulconazole [Exelderm]	Topical	1% cream 1% solution	✔				
Terconazole [Terazol 3, Terazol 7]	Topical	80-mg vaginal suppository 0.4% and 0.8% vaginal cream				✔	
Tioconazole [Monistat 1]	Topical	6.5% vaginal ointment				✔	
Allylamines							
Butenafine [Lotrimin Ultra Cream]	Topical	1% cream	✔				
Naftifine [Naftin]	Topical	1% and 2% cream 2% gel	✔				
Terbinafine [Lamisil, LamisilAT]	Oral Topical	250-mg tablets 1% spray 1% gel 1% powder 1% cream	✔ ✔				✔
Others							
Ciclopirox [Loprox, Penlac Nail Lacquer]	Topical	1% shampoo 0.77% cream, gel, suspension	✔	✔			✔
Griseofulvin [Gris-PEG]	Oral	125- and 250-mg ultra-microcrystalline tablets 500-mg microcrystalline tablets 125 mg/5 mL solution	✔				✔
Nystatin [Mycostatin]	Topical	100,000 units/gm cream, powder, and ointment 100,000-unit vaginal tablets		✔	✔	✔	
Tolnaftate [Tinactin]	Topical	1% spray, cream, powder, solution	✔				
Undecylenate [Fungi-Nail]	Topical	25% solution	✔				

[a]*Ringworm* is a popular term for dermatophytic infections, including tinea pedis, tinea cruris, tinea corporis, and tinea capitis.
[b]*Onychomycosis* is a clinical term for fungal infection of the toenails and fingernails.

standard therapy. However, oral terbinafine, taken for only 2 to 4 weeks, may be more effective.

Candidiasis

Vulvovaginal candidiasis. Vulvovaginal candidiasis is very common, occurring in 75% of women at least once in their life. Most cases are caused by *Candida albicans*, and many of the rest are caused by *Candida glabrata*, especially in patients with HIV/AIDS. Factors that predispose to *Candida* infection include pregnancy, obesity, diabetes, debilitation, HIV infection, and use of certain drugs, including oral contraceptives, systemic glucocorticoids, anticancer agents, immunosuppressants, and systemic antibiotics. With current drugs, just 1 or 3 days of *topical* therapy can be curative. In addition, *oral* therapy may be used: a single 150-mg dose of fluconazole can be curative—but it causes more side effects (headache, rash, GI disturbance) than topical agents. For women with recurrent vulvovaginal candidiasis, weekly prophylaxis with oral fluconazole is highly effective—but relapse is common when treatment is stopped. Major drugs for uncomplicated vulvovaginal candidiasis are shown in Table 79.5. All appear equally effective, so drug selection is based largely on patient preference. Longer regimens have no demonstrated advantage over shorter ones.

Oral candidiasis. Oral candidiasis, also known as *thrush*, is seen often. Topical agents—*nystatin*, *clotrimazole*, and *miconazole*—are generally effective. In the immunocompromised host, oral therapy with *fluconazole* or *ketoconazole* is usually required.

Onychomycosis

Onychomycosis is difficult to eradicate and requires prolonged treatment. Infections may be caused by dermatophytes or *Candida* species. Because onychomycosis is largely a cosmetic concern, treatment is usually optional.

Onychomycosis may be treated with oral antifungal drugs or with topical ciclopirox. Success rates with oral therapy are quite low, and rates with topical therapy are even lower.

Oral therapy. The drugs used most often are *terbinafine* [Lamisil] and *itraconazole* [Sporanox]. Both are active against *Candida* species and dermatophytes. When in the body, these drugs become incorporated into keratin as the nails grow. Drug may also diffuse into the nails from the tissue below. Side effects include headache, GI disturbances (e.g., nausea, vomiting, abdominal pain), and skin reactions (e.g., itching, rash). Treatment generally lasts 3 to 6 months. Unfortunately, even with this prolonged therapy, the cure rate is relatively low (about 50%).

Topical therapy

Ciclopirox. *Ciclopirox* [Penlac Nail Lacquer] is one of three topical agents for onychomycosis available in the United States. In contrast to oral terbinafine or itraconazole, which are active against *Candida* species and several dermatophytes, topical ciclopirox is active against only one dermatophyte—*Trichophyton rubrum*—and has no activity against *Candida*. Ciclopirox is applied once a day to the nails and immediately adjacent skin. New coats are applied over old ones. Once a week, all coats are removed with alcohol. Side effects are minimal and localized. Unfortunately, despite prolonged use (up to 48 weeks), ciclopirox confers only modest benefits: complete cure occurs in less than 12% of patients, and even when complete cure *does* occur, the recurrence rate is high—about 40%. Compared with oral therapy, topical ciclopirox is safer and cheaper but is much less effective.

Use of ciclopirox for superficial fungal infections of the *skin* is discussed later.

Tavaborole. Tavaborole [Kerydin] is an oxaborole antifungal medication that treats onychomycosis from the dermatophytes *T. rubrum* and *Trichophyton mentagrophytes*. An oxaborole antifungal contains Boron, which is thought to decrease fungal protein synthesis. Tavaborole is available in a 5% solution for topical application. Patients should apply tavaborole to the entire nail surface and under the tip of affected toenails once daily for 48 weeks.

Efinaconazole. Efinaconazole [Jublia] belongs to the azole family of antifungal medications. Efinaconazole is available as a 10% gel. Patients cover the entire nail, including the folds, bed, and undersurface of the toenail plate, with the brush applicator supplied with the medication. Like tavaborole, the dosing is one application to affected nails daily for 48 weeks.

Azoles

Twelve members of the azole family are used for superficial mycoses (see Table 79.5). The usual route is topical. Three of the 12—itraconazole,

fluconazole, and ketoconazole—are also used for systemic mycoses (see earlier).

The azoles are active against a broad spectrum of pathogenic fungi, including dermatophytes and *Candida* species. Antifungal effects result from inhibiting the biosynthesis of ergosterol, an essential component of the fungal cytoplasmic membrane.

Griseofulvin

Griseofulvin [Gris-PEG] is administered orally to treat superficial mycoses. The drug is inactive against organisms that cause systemic mycoses.

Mechanism of Action

After absorption, griseofulvin is deposited in the keratin precursor cells of skin, hair, and nails. Because griseofulvin is present, newly formed keratin is resistant to fungal invasion. Hence as infected keratin is shed, it is replaced by fungus-free tissue.

Griseofulvin kills fungi by inhibiting fungal mitosis by binding to components of microtubules, the structures that form the mitotic spindle. Because griseofulvin acts by disrupting mitosis, the drug only affects fungi that are actively growing.

Pharmacokinetics

Administration is oral, and absorption can be enhanced by dosing with a fatty meal. As noted, griseofulvin is deposited in the keratin precursor cells of skin, hair, and nails. Elimination is by hepatic metabolism and renal excretion.

Therapeutic Uses

Griseofulvin is employed orally to treat dermatophytic infections of the skin, hair, and nails. The drug is not active against *Candida* species, nor is it useful against systemic mycoses. Dermatophytic infections of the skin respond relatively quickly (in 3 to 8 weeks). However, infections of the palms may require 2 to 3 months of treatment, and a year or more may be needed to eliminate infections of the toenails.

Polyene Antibiotics
Nystatin

Actions, uses, and adverse effects. Nystatin [Mycostatin ♣] is a polyene antibiotic used only for candidiasis. Nystatin is the drug of choice for intestinal candidiasis and is also employed to treat candidal infections of the skin, mouth, esophagus, and vagina. Nystatin can be administered orally and topically. There is no significant absorption from either route. Oral nystatin occasionally causes GI disturbance (nausea, vomiting, diarrhea). Topical application may produce local irritation.

Allylamines
Naftifine

Naftifine [Naftin] was the first allylamine available. Although approved only for topical treatment of dermatophytic infections, naftifine is active against a broad spectrum of pathogenic fungi. The drug works by inhibiting squalene epoxidase, thus inhibiting synthesis of ergosterol, a key component of the fungal cell membrane. The most common adverse effects are burning and stinging. Absorption after topical administration is relatively low (about 6%). Systemic effects have not been reported. Naftifine is supplied in two formulations: 1% and 2% cream and 1% gel. The cream is applied once daily, the gel twice daily. Treatment usually lasts 2 to 4 weeks.

Terbinafine

Terbinafine [Lamisil] belongs to the same chemical family as naftifine and has the same mechanism of action: inhibition of squalene epoxidase with resultant inhibition of ergosterol synthesis. The drug is highly active against dermatophytes and less active against *Candida* species. Terbinafine is available in topical and oral formulations. Topical therapy is used for ringworm infections (e.g., tinea corporis, tinea cruris, tinea pedis). Oral therapy is used for ringworm and onychomycosis (fungal infection of the nails).

Butenafine

Butenafine [Lotrimin Ultra Cream, Mentax] is chemically similar to naftifine and terbinafine, although butenafine is not a true allylamine. However, it does have the same mechanism of action: inhibition of squalene epoxidase with resultant inhibition of ergosterol synthesis. Butenafine is indicated for topical therapy of tinea pedis, tinea corporis, tinea cruris, and tinea versicolor. Absorption is minimum, and systemic side effects have not been reported. Local reactions include burning, stinging, erythema, irritation, and itching. Butenafine 1% cream is applied once daily for 2 to 4 weeks.

Other Drugs for Superficial Mycoses

Tolnaftate

Tolnaftate [Tinactin, others] is employed topically to treat a variety of superficial mycoses. The drug is active against dermatophytes, but not against *Candida* species. The mechanism of antifungal action is unknown. Adverse effects (sensitization, irritation) are extremely rare. Tolnaftate is available in several formulations. Creams, powders, and solutions are most effective; powders are used adjunctively. The drug is applied twice daily for 2 to 4 weeks.

Undecylenic Acid

Undecylenic acid [Fungi-Nail, others] is a topical agent used to treat superficial mycoses. The drug is active against dermatophytes but not *Candida* species. Its major indication is tinea pedis (athlete's foot). However, other drugs (tolnaftate, the azoles) are more effective.

Ciclopirox

When applied to the skin, ciclopirox is active against dermatophytes and *Candida* species. The drug is effective against superficial candidiasis and tinea pedis, tinea cruris, and tinea corporis. Ciclopirox penetrates the epidermis to the dermis, but systemic absorption is minimum, and hence no significant systemic accumulation occurs. There is no toxicity from local application. For treatment of skin infections, ciclopirox is available as a 1% shampoo and as a 0.77% cream, gel, and suspension. The shampoo is used twice weekly for 4 weeks. The cream, gel, and suspension are applied twice daily for 2 to 4 weeks.

80

Antiviral Agents I: Drugs for Non-HIV Viral Infections

Antiviral drugs are discussed in this chapter and Chapter 81. Here we consider drugs used to treat infections caused by viruses other than human immunodeficiency virus (HIV). In Chapter 81, we consider drugs used against HIV infection. Drugs for non-HIV infections are shown in Table 80.1.

Unlike antibiotics, which may be used to treat a variety of bacterial infections, antiviral agents are more specific. For this reason, we present these agents based on associated viral infections.

DRUGS FOR INFECTION WITH HERPES SIMPLEX VIRUSES AND VARICELLA ZOSTER VIRUS

Herpes simplex virus (HSV) and *varicella zoster virus* (VZV) are members of the herpesvirus group. HSV causes infection of the genitalia, mouth, face, and other sites. VZV is the cause of *varicella* (chickenpox) and *herpes zoster* (shingles), a painful condition resulting from reactivation of VZV that has been dormant within sensory nerve roots. Both conditions are discussed in Chapter 55, along with the vaccine used to prevent chickenpox. Genital herpes is discussed in Chapter 82.

Acyclovir

Acyclovir (Zovirax) is the agent of first choice for most infections caused by HSV and VZV. The drug can be administered topically, orally, and intravenously. Serious side effects are uncommon.

Antiviral Spectrum

Acyclovir is active only against members of the herpesvirus family, a group that includes *herpes simplex viruses, varicella zoster virus,* and *cytomegalovirus* (CMV). Of these, HSVs are most sensitive, VZV is moderately sensitive, and most strains of CMV are resistant.

Mechanism of Action

Acyclovir inhibits viral replication by suppressing the synthesis of viral DNA. To exert antiviral effects, acyclovir must first undergo activation. The critical step in activation is conversion of acyclovir to acyclo-guanosine monophosphate (GMP) by *thymidine kinase*. When formed, acyclo-GMP is converted to acyclo-guanosine triphosphate (GTP), the compound directly responsible for inhibiting DNA synthesis. Acyclo-GTP suppresses DNA synthesis by (1) inhibiting viral DNA polymerase and (2) becoming incorporated into the growing strand of viral DNA, which blocks further strand growth.

The selectivity of acyclovir is based in large part on the ability of certain viruses to activate the drug. HSVs are especially sensitive to acyclovir because the drug is a much better substrate for thymidine kinase produced by HSVs than it is for mammalian thymidine kinase. Hence formation of acyclo-GMP, the limiting step in the activation of acyclovir, occurs almost exclusively in cells infected with HSV. CMV is inherently resistant to the drug because acyclovir is a poor substrate for the form of thymidine kinase produced by this virus.

Resistance

Herpesviruses develop resistance to acyclovir by three mechanisms: (1) decreased production of thymidine kinase, (2) alteration of thymidine kinase such that it no longer converts acyclovir to acyclo-GMP, and (3) alteration of viral DNA polymerase such that it is less sensitive to inhibition. Of these mechanisms, thymidine kinase deficiency is the most common. Resistance is rare in immunocompetent patients, but many cases have been reported in transplant recipients and patients with AIDS. Lesions caused by resistant HSVs can be extensive and severe, progressing despite continued acyclovir therapy. Acyclovir-resistant HSVs and VZV usually respond to intravenous foscarnet or cidofovir, which are primarily used for treatment of CMV infection (see later discussion).

Therapeutic Uses

Mucocutaneous herpes simplex infections. Herpes infections of the face and oropharynx are usually caused by HSV type 2 (HSV-2). For immunocompetent patients, *oral* acyclovir can be used to treat primary infections of the gums and mouth. Oral acyclovir can also be taken *prophylactically* to prevent episodes of *recurrent* herpes labialis (cold sores). However, there is no truly effective treatment for active herpes labialis. Mucocutaneous herpes infections can be especially severe in immunocompromised patients. For these people, *intravenous* acyclovir is the treatment of choice.

Varicella Zoster infections. High doses of *oral* acyclovir are effective for herpes zoster (shingles) in older adults. Oral therapy is also effective for varicella (chickenpox) in children, adolescents, and adults provided that dosing is begun early (within 24 hours of rash onset). *Intravenous* acyclovir is the treatment of choice for VZV infection in the immunocompromised host.

Herpes simplex genitalis. The characteristics and treatment of genital HSV infection are discussed in Chapter 82.

Pharmacokinetics

Acyclovir may be administered topically, orally, and intravenously. Oral bioavailability is low, ranging from 15% to 30%. No significant absorption occurs with topical use. It is important to note that, with normal kidney function, acyclovir has a half-life of 2.5 hours; however, the half-life is prolonged by renal impairment, reaching 20 hours in anuric patients. (This very prolonged half-life is true for other agents in this category, as well.) Accordingly, dosages should be reduced in patients with kidney disease. Additional information on pharmacokinetics for acyclovir and other drugs used to treat HSV and VZV are provided in Table 80.2.

Adverse Effects

Oral. Acyclovir is devoid of serious adverse effects. Renal impairment has not been reported. The most common reactions are nausea, vomiting, diarrhea, headache, and vertigo. Topical acyclovir frequently causes transient local burning or stinging; systemic reactions do not occur.

TABLE 80.1 Major Drugs for Non-HIV Viral Infections

Drug	Antiviral Spectrum
Drugs for HSV and VZV Infections	
Systemic Drugs	
Acyclovir	HSV, VZV
Famciclovir	HSV, VZV
Foscarnet	HSV, VZV
Valacyclovir	HSV, VZV
Topical Drugs	
Penciclovir	HSV
Trifluridine	HSV keratitis
Docosanol	HSV keratitis
Ganciclovir	HSV keratitis
Drugs for Hepatitis	
Protease Inhibitors	
Glecaprevir	HCV
Grazoprevir	HCV
Paritaprevir	HCV
Simeprevir	HCV
Voxilaprevir	HCV
NS5A Inhibitors	
Daclatasvir	HCV
Elbasvir	HCV
Ledipasvir	HCV
Ombitasvir	HCV
Pibrentasvir	HCV
Velpatasvir	HCV
NS5B Nucleoside Polymerase Inhibitors	
Sofosbuvir	HCV
NS5B Nonnucleoside Polymerase Inhibitors	
Dasabuvir	HCV
Alfa Interferons	
Interferon alfa-2b	HCV[a], HBV
Peginterferon alfa-2a	HCV[a], HBV
Nucleoside Analogs	
Ribavirin (oral)	HCV
Adefovir	HBV[b]
Entecavir	HBV[b]
Lamivudine	HBV[b]
Telbivudine	HBV
Tenofovir	HBV[b]
Drugs for Cytomegalovirus Infection	
Ganciclovir	CMV
Valganciclovir	CMV
Cidofovir	CMV
Foscarnet	CMV
Drugs for Influenza	
Oseltamivir	Influenza A and B
Zanamivir	Influenza A and B

[a]FDA approved for HCV but is not recommended in current clinical guidelines.
[b]Also active against HIV.
CMV, Cytomegalovirus; *HBV*, hepatitis B virus; *HCV*, hepatitis C virus; *HSV*, herpes simplex virus; *VZV*, varicella zoster virus.

Oral acyclovir is safe during pregnancy, so it can be used to suppress recurrent genital herpes near term.

Intravenous. Unlike oral formulations of alcyclovir, intravenous (IV) acyclovir can cause renal failure. Patients with preexisting renal disease and dehydration are at increased risk.

PATIENT EDUCATION
Acyclovir

Inform patients that acyclovir only decreases symptoms; it does not eliminate the virus and does not produce cure.

Advise patients to apply topical acyclovir with a finger cot or rubber glove to avoid viral transfer to other body sites or other people. Explain that some transient local burning or stinging may occur and that this does not indicate a reaction.

Preparations and Dosage

Preparations and dosages for acyclovir and other antiviral drugs for HSV and VZV infections are presented in Table 80.3.

PATIENT-CENTERED CARE ACROSS THE LIFE SPAN
Systemic Drugs for Herpesvirus and Varicella Zoster Virus Infections

Life Stage	Considerations or Concerns
Children	Acyclovir is approved for children as young as 3 months of age. Valacyclovir is approved for children 2 years of age. The safety and efficacy of foscarnet have not been established for children. The efficacy of famciclovir in children has not been established.
Pregnant women	Epidemiologic reviews of the use of acyclovir, famciclovir, and valacyclovir in pregnant women did not find a significant increase in abnormal outcomes compared with the general population. Foscarnet, which is deposited in bone and teeth, has caused abnormal development of tooth enamel in animal students and therefore is not recommended during pregnancy.
Breastfeeding women	Sufficient acyclovir is present in breast milk to give the nursing infant a dose of 0.3 mg/kg per day. For those taking valacyclovir, the amount of acyclovir in breast milk is higher, resulting in a dose of 0.6 mg/kg per day. In animal studies of famciclovir, the active metabolite penciclovir was excreted in breast milk at amounts higher than plasma levels. For these reasons and because serious adverse events could occur in infants exposed to these drugs, It is therefore recommended that women who are taking systemic drugs for HSV and VZV should avoid breastfeeding.
Older adults	There are no contraindications for this age group; however, those with renal impairment should be started on lower doses, with dosage adjustments made cautiously. Older adults taking acyclovir and valacyclovir are at greater risk for adverse CNS effects.

Valacyclovir
Actions and Uses

Valacyclovir (Valtrex), is a prodrug form of acyclovir. When acyclovir is given orally, its bioavailability is only 15% to 30%. In contrast, when valacyclovir is given orally, the effective bioavailability of acyclovir is

TABLE 80.2 Pharmacokinetics: Drugs for the Treatment of Herpes Simplex Virus and Varicella Zoster Virus Infections[a]

Drug Class and Drugs	Peak	Protein Binding	Metabolism	Half-Life	Elimination
Acyclovir (Sitavig, Zovirax)	NA	9%–33%	Cellular enzymes	2.5 h[b]	Urine
Valacyclovir (Valtrex)	1.5 h	14%–18%	Hepatic conversion to acyclovir, then cellular enzymes	2.5–3.3 h[b]	Urine
Famciclovir (Famvir ♦)	1 h	20%	Deacetylated and oxidized to penciclovir	2–4 h[c]	Urine (73%) Feces (25%)
Foscarnet (Foscavir)	NA	14%–17%	None	3–4 h	Urine

[a]Topical preparations omitted because formulations for these antiviral agents have negligible absorption.
[b]Half-life may be extended to 20 hours in patients with renal failure.
[c]Half-life may be extended to 13 hours in patients with renal failure.
NA, Not available.

PROTOTYPE DRUGS

Drugs for Non-HIV Viral Infections

Drugs for Herpes Simplex Virus Infection
Acyclovir

Drug for Cytomegalovirus Infection
Ganciclovir

Drugs for Hepatitis
Lamivudine (nucleoside analog)
Simeprevir (protease inhibitor)
Daclatasvir (NS5A inhibitor)
Sofosbuvir (NS5B inhibitor)
Peginterferon alfa-2a (an interferon)

Drugs for Influenza
Influenza vaccine
Oseltamivir (neuraminidase inhibitor)
Baloxavir marboxil (endonuclease inhibitor)

Drugs for Prophylaxis of Respiratory Syncytial Virus Infection
Palivizumab (monoclonal antibody)

greatly increased to about 55%. Therefore valacyclovir represents a more efficient way of getting acyclovir into the body.

Valacyclovir is approved for the management of four conditions: (1) herpes labialis, (2) varicella (chickenpox), (3) herpes zoster infection (shingles), and (4) herpes simplex genitalis (genital herpes). Genital herpes is discussed in Chapter 82.

Valacyclovir is sometimes used off label for prophylaxis of HSV, VZV, and CMV infections in patients with cancer. It is also sometimes used to treat cancer-related HSV and VZV.

Adverse Effects

In the course of clinical research regarding the use of valacyclovir in immunocompromised patients, a syndrome known as thrombotic thrombocytopenic purpura/hemolytic uremic syndrome (TTP/HUS) has occurred. This syndrome, which can be fatal, has not occurred in immunocompetent patients. For this reason, the US Food and Drug Administration (FDA) has not approved the use of valacyclovir in immunocompromised patients with the exception of chronic suppressive therapy for recurrent genital herpes in patients with HIV infection.

That being said, we are seeing more recommendations in the literature for its use in patients with immunosuppression. Because TTP/HUS occurred in clinical trials where immunocompromised patients were receiving 8 g/day of valacyclovir; therefore daily doses should be lower than 8 g.

Aside from causing TTP/HUS among immunocompromised patients, valacyclovir is generally well tolerated, producing the same side effects seen with oral acyclovir (e.g., nausea, vomiting, diarrhea, headache, vertigo).

Famciclovir
Actions and Uses

Famciclovir is a prodrug of penciclovir. Famciclovir undergoes enzymatic conversion to penciclovir, its active form. Penciclovir then undergoes intracellular conversion to penciclovir triphosphate, a compound that inhibits viral DNA polymerase and thereby prevents replication of viral DNA. Under clinical conditions, formation of penciclovir triphosphate requires viral thymidine kinase. As a result, inhibition of DNA synthesis is limited to cells that are infected, leaving most host cells unharmed. In vitro, penciclovir is active against HSV type 1 (HSV-1), HSV-2, and VZV.

Famciclovir is approved for the treatment of acute herpes zoster and herpes simplex genitalis. In patients with herpes zoster, the drug can decrease the time to full crusting from 7 days down to 5 days. Famciclovir does not decrease the incidence of postherpetic neuralgia but can decrease its duration (from 112 days down to 61 days).

Adverse Effects

Famciclovir is very well tolerated. In clinical trials, only headache and nausea were reported by more than 10% of the subjects. If famciclovir is given in higher than recommended doses, acute renal failure can occur.

Topical Drugs for Herpes Labialis

There are three topical drugs for the treatment of recurrent herpes labialis. Two of these drugs—penciclovir and docosanol—are discussed next. The third drug—acyclovir—was discussed earlier.

Penciclovir Cream

Penciclovir (Denavir) is a topical drug indicated for recurrent herpes labialis, an infection caused by HSV-1 and HSV-2. The drug suppresses viral replication by inhibiting DNA polymerase, the enzyme that makes DNA. Penciclovir is supplied as a 1% cream to be applied every 2 hours (except when sleeping) for 4 days. In clinical trials, benefits were modest: the average time to healing and duration of pain were decreased by

TABLE 80.3   Preparations, Dosages, and Considerations of Drugs for the Acute Treatment of Herpes Simplex Virus and Varicella Zoster Virus Infections

Drug	Preparations	Dosage	Considerations
Acyclovir (Zovirax), oral	Capsule: 200 mg Tablet: 400 and 800 mg Suspension: 200 mg/5 mL	*Orolabial HSV:* 200 mg five times daily *or* 400 mg tid for 7–10 days *Orolabial HSV in ICH:* 400 mg tid for 5–10 days or until lesions have healed *Varicella, children under 40 kg:* 20 mg/kg per dose four times daily for 5 days *Varicella, children over 40 kg and adults:* 800 mg four times daily for 5 days *Herpes zoster:* 800 mg five times daily for 7–10 days	Decrease dosing in patients with impaired renal function.
Acyclovir (Sitavig, Zovirax), topical	Topical cream (Zovirax): 5% Topical ointment (Zovirax): 5% Buccal tablet (Sitavig): 50 mg	*Orolabial HSV:* Apply cream five times daily for 4 days *Orolabial HSV:* Apply buccal tablet to upper gum above cuspid (canine) tooth *Mucocutaneous HSV in ICH:* Apply a $\frac{1}{2}$ -in ribbon of ointment for each 4-in² affected area q 3 h (up to six times daily) for 7 days	Begin therapy for orolabial HSV at the first onset of symptoms (e.g., tingling or burning) when possible.
Acyclovir (Zovirax), IV	IV solution: 50 mg/mL	*Orolabial HSV in ICH:* 5 mg/kg IV q 8 h (Change to oral therapy when lesions begin to regress and then continue therapy until lesions have healed.) *Mucocutaneous HSV in ICH:* 5 mg/kg IV q 8 h for 7–10 days *Neonatal HSV:* 10 mg/kg IV q 8 h for 14–21 days *HSV encephalitis:* 10 mg/kg q 8 h for 14–21 days *Varicella:* 800 mg IV qid for 5 days *Varicella in ICH:* 10 mg/kg IV q 8 h for 7–10 days or until all lesions have crusted *Herpes zoster in ICH:* 10–15 mg/kg IV q 8 h until there are no new lesions, then change to oral therapy	To decrease the risk for renal injury and neurologic toxicity, ensure adequate hydration before beginning IV therapy with acyclovir. Begin therapy for orolabial HSV at the first onset of symptoms when possible.
Valacyclovir (Valtrex),[a] oral	Tablet: 500 mg, 1 g	*Orolabial HSV:* 2 g bid for one day *Mucocutaneous HSV:* 1 g bid for 7–10 days or until lesions have healed *Varicella:* 1 g tid for 5–7 days or until lesions have crusted *HZV:* 1 g tid for 7 days	Decrease dosing in patients with impaired renal function. For HSV, varicella, and VZV, treatment should begin with first onset of symptoms when possible.
Famciclovir (Famvir 🍁) (generic in the United States)	Tablet: 125, 250, and 500 mg	*Orolabial HSV:* 1500 mg once *Orolabial HSV in ICH:* 500 mg bid for 5–10 days *HZV[b]:* 500 mg tid for 7 days	
Foscarnet (Foscavir)[c]	IV solution, 24 mg/mL	*Acyclovir-resistant HSV:* 40 mg/kg q 8–12 h for 14–21 days	High risk for renal injury. Ensure adequate hydration before beginning therapy.
Penciclovir (Denavir)	Topical cream, 1%	*Orolabial HSV:* 1% cream q 2 h while awake for 4 days	When possible, begin therapy at the first sign of a cold sore. Not indicated for application to mucous membranes.
Docosanol (Abreva)	Topical cream, 10%	*Orolabial HSV:* 10% cream five times a day for 4 days or until lesions have healed	Available over the counter. When possible, begin therapy at the first sign of a cold sore.
Ganciclovir, ophthalmic (Zirgan)	Topical gel 0.15%	*Keratoconjunctivitis:* 1 drop in affected eye five times a day until symptoms abate, then 1 drop three times a day for 7 days	Instruct patients to apply drops directly to the affected eye and to avoid contact lenses until lesions heal.
Trifluridine (Viroptic)	Ophthalmic solution, 1%	*Keratoconjunctivitis:* Place 1 drop on cornea q 2 h while awake (maximum 9 drops daily); after reepithelialization of the cornea, decrease to 1 drop q 4 h while awake for an additional 7 days	Limit treatment to 21 days. If no improvement after 1–2 weeks, switch to another drug.

[a]Valacyclovir is not currently approved for the acute treatment of HSV and VZV infections in immunocompromised patients. This could change in the near future as more is learned from off-label prescribing for this population.
[b]HZV in ICH should be treated with intravenous acyclovir.
[c]Foscarnet should be reserved for acyclovir-resistant infection.
ICH, Immunocompromised host; *IV,* intravenous.

just half a day, from 5 days down to 4.5 days. The only common adverse effect is mild local erythema.

Docosanol Cream

Docosanol (Abreva) is a topical preparation indicated for recurrent herpes labialis. The drug is available over the counter as a 10% cream. Application is done five times a day, beginning at the first sign of recurrence. Benefits are modest. In one trial, treatment reduced the time to healing from 4.8 days down to 4.1 days—about the same response seen with penciclovir. Docosanol cream appears to be devoid of adverse effects.

Docosanol has a broad antiviral spectrum and a unique mechanism of action. Unlike penciclovir, which inhibits viral DNA synthesis (and thereby suppresses replication), docosanol blocks viral entry into host cells. The drug does not kill viruses and does not prevent them from binding to cells. As a result, viable virions can remain attached to the cell surface for a long time. Because docosanol does not affect processes of replication, it is unlikely to promote resistance.

Topical Drugs for Ocular Herpes Infections
Trifluridine Ophthalmic Solution

Trifluridine (Viroptic) is indicated only for topical treatment of ocular infections caused by HSV-1 and HSV-2. The drug is given to treat acute keratoconjunctivitis and recurrent epithelial keratitis. Antiviral actions result from the inhibition of DNA synthesis. The most common side effects are localized burning and stinging. Edema of the eyelid occurs in about 3% of patients. Systemic absorption is minimal after topical administration, so the drug is devoid of systemic toxicity.

Ganciclovir Gel

Ganciclovir 0.15% ophthalmic gel (Zirgan) is indicated for acute herpetic keratitis (inflammation and ulceration of the cornea caused by infection with a herpes simplex virus). As discussed later (see Ganciclovir), benefits derive from suppressing viral replication. Principal adverse effects are blurred vision, eye irritation, and red eyes. Systemic effects are absent.

DRUGS FOR CYTOMEGALOVIRUS INFECTION

Cytomegalovirus is a member of the herpesvirus group, which includes HSV-1 and HSV-2, VZV (the cause of chickenpox), and Epstein-Barr virus (the cause of infectious mononucleosis). Transmission of CMV occurs person to person—through direct contact with saliva, urine, blood, tears, breast milk, semen, and other body fluids. Infection can also be acquired by way of blood transfusion or organ transplantation. Infection with CMV is very common: between 50% and 85% of Americans 40 years of age and older harbor the virus. After the initial infection, which causes minimal symptoms in healthy people, the virus remains dormant within cells for life without causing detectable injury or clinical illness. Hence for most healthy people, CMV infection is of little concern. By contrast, people who are immunocompromised—owing to HIV infection, cancer chemotherapy, or the use of immunosuppressive drugs—are at high risk for serious morbidity and even death, both from initial CMV infection and from reactivation of dormant CMV. Common sites for infection are the lungs, eyes, and gastrointestinal (GI) tract. Among people with AIDS, CMV retinitis is the principal reason for loss of vision (see Chapter 81). The four drugs used against CMV are discussed next. A fifth drug, letermovir (Prevymis), approved in 2017, is approved only for prophylaxis.

Ganciclovir

Ganciclovir (Cytovene, Zirgan) is a synthetic antiviral agent with activity against herpesviruses, including CMV. Because the drug can cause serious adverse effects, especially granulocytopenia and thrombocytopenia, it

SUMMARY OF KEY PRESCRIBING CONSIDERATIONS

Systemic Drugs for Herpes Simplex Virus and Varicella Zoster Virus Infections

Therapeutic Goal: To alleviate signs and symptoms associated with HSV and VZV outbreaks

Baseline Data: Serum creatinine, blood urea nitrogen (BUN), urinalysis, CBC with WBC differential.

Additional Drug-Specific Baseline Data:
- Acyclovir: liver enzymes
- Valacyclovir: liver enzymes
- Foscarnet: Electrolytes, 24-hour creatinine clearance, and electrocardiogram (ECG)

Monitoring: Serum creatinine (with BUN if clinically indicated), CBC
- Acyclovir: Urinalysis (check specific gravity for evidence of dehydration), urine output, liver enzymes
- Valacyclovir: Urinalysis, liver enzymes
- Foscarnet: Electrolytes, calcium, ionized calcium, magnesium, and phosphorus

Identifying High-Risk Patients: Impaired renal function

Additional Drug-Specific High-Risk Patients:
- Foscarnet: Patients with QT prolongation; hypocalcemia, hyper/hypophosphatemia, hypomagnesemia, or hypokalemia; heart failure (due to high sodium content of drug)

Evaluating Therapeutic Effects: Signs and symptoms of acute infection abate and infection is held in check.

should be used only for the prevention and treatment of CMV infection in the immunocompromised host.

Mechanism of Action

Ganciclovir is converted to its active form, ganciclovir triphosphate, inside infected cells. As ganciclovir triphosphate, it suppresses the replication of viral DNA by (1) inhibiting viral DNA polymerase and (2) undergoing incorporation into the growing DNA chain, which causes premature chain termination.

Therapeutic Use

Ganciclovir is approved only to prevent and treat CMV infection in immunocompromised patients, including transplant recipients, those with HIV infection, and those receiving immunosuppressive drugs.

In patients with AIDS, CMV retinitis has an incidence of 15% to 40%. Although most AIDS patients respond initially, the relapse rate is high. Accordingly, maintenance therapy should continue indefinitely for most patients. The risk for relapse is higher with oral ganciclovir than with intravenous ganciclovir. Because viral resistance can develop during treatment, this possibility should be considered if the patient responds poorly.

PATIENT EDUCATION
Ganciclovir

Advise patients against becoming pregnant. Inform male patients about possible sterility.

Teach patients to report symptoms of bone marrow suppression (anemia, leukocytopenia, and thrombocytopenia) such as pallor, weakness, fever, chills, increased bruising, or petechiae.

When topical ophthalmic gel drops are prescribed, teach proper methods of administration and instruct patients to avoid the use of contact lenses.

Pharmacokinetics

The pharmacokinetics of ganciclovir and other antiviral drugs for CVM infection is provided in Table 80.4.

Adverse Effects

Granulocytopenia and thrombocytopenia. The adverse effect of greatest concern is bone marrow suppression, which can result in granulocytopenia and thrombocytopenia. These effects, which are usually reversible, are more likely with intravenous therapy than with oral therapy. These hematologic responses can be exacerbated by concurrent therapy with zidovudine. Conversely, granulocytopenia can be reduced with granulocyte colony-stimulating factors. Because of the risk for adverse hematologic effects, blood cell counts must be monitored. Treatment should be interrupted if the absolute neutrophil count falls below 500/mm³ or if the platelet count falls below 25,000/mm³. Cell counts usually begin to recover within 3 to 5 days. Ganciclovir should be used with caution in patients with preexisting cytopenias, in those with a history of cytopenic reactions to other drugs, and in those taking other bone marrow suppressants (e.g., zidovudine).

BLACK BOX WARNING

Ganciclovir and Its Prodrug Valganciclovir

> Ganciclovir may cause anemia, granulocytopenia, and thrombocytopenia. In animal studies, ganciclovir was associated with teratogenic effects, carcinogenic effects, and inhibited sperm formation.

Reproductive toxicity. Ganciclovir is teratogenic and embryotoxic in laboratory animals and probably also in humans. Women should be advised to avoid pregnancy during therapy and for 90 days after ending treatment. At doses equivalent to those used therapeutically, ganciclovir inhibits spermatogenesis in mice; sterility is reversible with low doses and irreversible with high doses. Female infertility may also occur. Patients should be forewarned of these effects.

Other adverse effects. Incidental effects include nausea, fever, rash, anemia, liver dysfunction, and confusion and other central nervous system (CNS) symptoms.

Preparations and Dosages

Preparations and dosages for ganciclovir and other drugs for CMV infections are provided in Table 80.5.

Valganciclovir

Mechanism of Action

Valganciclovir (Valcyte) is a prodrug version of ganciclovir but has the advantage of greater oral bioavailability (60% vs 9%) over ganciclovir. After absorption from the GI tract, valganciclovir is rapidly metabolized to ganciclovir, its active form. It eventually undergoes excretion as unchanged ganciclovir in the urine.

Therapeutic Use

Indications are CMV retinitis and prevention of CMV disease in high-risk organ transplant recipients. In patients with active CMV retinitis, oral

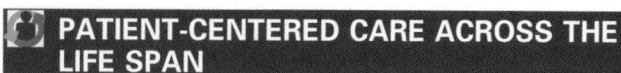
PATIENT-CENTERED CARE ACROSS THE LIFE SPAN

Drugs for Cytomegalovirus Infection

Life Stage	Considerations or Concerns
Children	Ganciclovir and valganciclovir are approved for infants, children, and adolescents. The safety and effectiveness of cidofovir and foscavir have not been established for children. Additionally, foscavir is deposited in bones and teeth and, in animal studies, resulted in abnormal development of tooth enamel.
Pregnant women	Ganciclovir, valganciclovir, and cidofovir were teratogenic in animal studies and thus should be avoided during pregnancy. Effects of foscarnet on pregnancy outcomes are unknown; however, due to deposition in bones and tooth enamel, it may create problems in young children born to patients who took foscarnet during pregnancy.
Breastfeeding women	Breastfeeding is not recommended for these drugs due to the potential for serious adverse effects
Older adults	Risk for renal impairment is increased in older adults. Monitor closely.

valganciclovir is just as effective as intravenous ganciclovir and much more convenient.

Adverse Effects

Adverse effects are the same as with ganciclovir. The principal concern is blood dyscrasias—granulocytopenia, anemia, and thrombocytopenia—secondary to bone marrow suppression. In addition, any of the following adverse effects will typically occur in 20% to 40% of patients: diarrhea, nausea, vomiting, fever, and headache. Valganciclovir is presumed to pose the same risks for mutagenesis, aspermatogenesis, and carcinogenesis as ganciclovir.

Cidofovir

Cidofovir (Vistide) is an intravenous drug with just one indication: CMV retinitis in patients with AIDS who have failed to respond to ganciclovir or foscarnet. Cidofovir is always administered with probenecid, a drug that competes with cidofovir for renal tubular secretion and thereby delays elimination. As a result, cidofovir has a prolonged intracellular half-life (17 to 65 hours), and a long interval (2 weeks) can separate doses. Compared with intravenous foscarnet or intravenous ganciclovir, cidofovir has the distinct advantage of needing fewer infusions: Whereas foscarnet and ganciclovir must be infused daily, cidofovir is infused just once a week or every other week.

Mechanism of Action

Inside cells, cidofovir is converted to cidofovir diphosphate, its active form. As the diphosphate, cidofovir causes selective inhibition of viral DNA polymerase and thereby inhibits viral DNA synthesis. Intracellular concentrations of cidofovir diphosphate are too low to inhibit human DNA polymerases; thus host cells are spared.

TABLE 80.4 Pharmacokinetics: Drugs for Cytomegalovirus Infection

Drug Class and Drugs	Peak	Protein Binding	Metabolism	Half-Life	Elimination
Ganciclovir (Cytovene)	NA	1%–2%	Little to none	2.4–5 h	Urine
Valganciclovir (Valcyte)	1.7–3 h	1%–2%	Minimal	2.8–6 h	Urine
Cidofovir (Vistide) (with probenecid)	NA	Less than 6%	Minimal	2.6 h	Urine
Foscarnet (Foscavir)	NA	14%–17%	None	3–4 h	Urine

NA, Not available.

TABLE 80.5   Preparations, Dosages, and Considerations for Drugs to Treat Cytomegalovirus Infections

Drug	Preparations	Dosage	Considerations
Ganciclovir (Cytovene)	IV solution, 500 mg/250 mL Reconstituted IV solution: 500 mg each Capsule: 250 and 500 mg	CMV retinitis, acute therapy, and CMV prophylaxis in ICH, initial therapy: 5 mg/kg IV q 12 h for 14–21 days CMV retinitis, maintenance therapy or CMV prophylaxis in ICH: 5 mg/kg IV qd for 7 days or 6 mg/kg qd for 5 days CMV prevention in transplant recipients and patients with advanced HIV infection: 500 mg six times daily or 1 g tid	Administer over 1 h or more to decrease risk for toxicity Oral ganciclovir should be taken with food.
Valganciclovir (Valcyte)	Oral Solution: 50 mg/mL Tablet: 450 mg	CMV retinitis, acute therapy: 900 mg bid for 21 days CMV retinitis, maintenance therapy: 900 mg qd	Administration with a high-fat meal increase absorption by 30%
Cidofovir (generic)	75 mg/mL	CMV retinitis, acute therapy: 5 mg/kg once weekly for 2 weeks with probenecid 2 g 3 h before cidofovir dosing CMV retinitis, maintenance therapy: 5 mg/kg once every 2 weeks (with probenecid)	Administer with probenecid as follows: • 2 g 3 h prior to cidofovir • 1 g 2 h after beginning cidofovir • 1 g 8 h after cidofovir infusion • Hydrate with IV NS as follows: • 1 L over 1–2 h prior to infusion • 1 L over 1–3 h with, or immediately following cidofovir infusion, as tolerated
Foscarnet (Foscavir)	IV Solution, 24 mg/mL	CMV retinitis, acute therapy: 60 mg/kg q 8 h for 14–21 days or 90 mg/kg q 12 h for 14–21 days CMV retinitis, maintenance therapy: 90–120 mg/kg daily	High risk for renal injury. Ensure adequate hydration before beginning therapy. Reduce dosage for impaired renal function. Do not prescribe for CrCl less than 0.4

CrCl, Creatinine clearance; *ICH*, immunocompromised host; *NS*, normal saline.

▶ BLACK BOX WARNING

Cidofovir (Vistide)

Cidofovir has been associated with severe renal impairment. Dialysis has been required after only one or two doses.

Cidofovir can cause neutropenia.

In animal studies, cidofovir was associated with teratogenic effects, carcinogenic effects, and inhibited sperm formation.

Therapeutic Use

Cidofovir is active against herpesviruses, including CMV, HSV-1, HSV-2, and VZV. However, the drug is approved only for CMV retinitis in patients with AIDS. Whether cidofovir is active against CMV infections in other patients or at other sites (e.g., GI tract, lungs) is unknown. In clinical trials in patients with AIDS and established CMV retinitis, cidofovir significantly delayed the progression of retinitis.

Adverse Effects

The principal adverse effect is dose-dependent nephrotoxicity, manifesting as decreased renal function and symptoms of a Fanconi-like syndrome manifesting as proteinuria, glucosuria, and bicarbonate wasting. The bicarbonate wasting may be sufficient to cause metabolic acidosis.

To reduce the risk for renal injury, all patients must receive probenecid and intravenous hydration therapy with each infusion (see Table 80.5). Also, serum creatinine and urine protein should be checked within 48 hours before each dose; if these values indicate kidney damage, cidofovir should be withheld or the dosage reduced. Cidofovir is contraindicated for patients taking other drugs that can injure the kidney and for patients with proteinuria (2+ or greater) or baseline serum creatinine greater than 1.5 mg/dL.

Neutropenia develops in about 20% of patients, so neutrophil counts should be monitored. Ocular disorders—iritis, uveitis, or ocular hypotony (low intraocular pressure)—can also occur. In animal studies, cidofovir

was carcinogenic and teratogenic and caused hypospermia. Adverse effects are more likely in patients taking antiretroviral drugs (i.e., drugs for HIV).

Foscarnet

Foscarnet is an intravenous drug active against all known herpesviruses, including CMV, HSV-1, HSV-2, and VZV. Compared with ganciclovir, foscarnet is more difficult to administer, less well tolerated, and much more expensive. The major adverse effect is renal injury.

Mechanism of Action

Foscarnet, an analog of pyrophosphate, inhibits viral DNA polymerases and reverse transcriptases and thereby inhibits the synthesis of viral nucleic acids. At the concentrations achieved clinically, the drug does not inhibit host DNA replication. Unlike many other antiviral drugs, which must undergo conversion to an active form, foscarnet is active as administered.

Therapeutic Use

Foscarnet has two approved indications: (1) CMV retinitis in patients with AIDS and (2) acyclovir-resistant mucocutaneous HSV and VZV infection in the immunocompromised host. CMV retinitis resistant to ganciclovir may respond to foscarnet.

Adverse Effects and Interactions

In general, foscarnet is less well tolerated than ganciclovir. Serious concerns include nephrotoxicity, electrolyte and mineral imbalances, seizures, blood disorders (specifically, anemia and granulocytopenia), and QT prolongation and associated dysrhythmias.

Renal injury, as evidenced by a rise in serum creatinine, is the most common dose-limiting toxicity. Most patients develop some degree of renal impairment. Renal injury occurs most often during the second week of therapy. The risk for nephrotoxicity is increased by concurrent use of other nephrotoxic drugs, including amphotericin B, aminoglycosides (e.g., gentamicin), and pentamidine. Prehydration with intravenous saline may reduce the risk for renal injury. Renal function (creatinine clearance) should be monitored closely, and the dosage should be reduced if renal impairment develops.

▶▶ BLACK BOX WARNING
Foscarnet (Foscavir)

Renal impairment due to foscarnet has occurred. Seizures have occurred in relation to alterations in electrolytes and mineral composition in plasma.

Foscarnet frequently causes hypocalcemia, hypokalemia, hypomagnesemia, and hypo/hyperphosphatemia. Ionized serum calcium may be reduced despite normal levels of total serum calcium. Patients should be informed about symptoms of low ionized calcium (e.g., paresthesias, numbness in the extremities, perioral tingling) and instructed to report these. Severe hypocalcemia can result in dysrhythmias, tetany, and seizures. Serum levels of calcium, magnesium, potassium, and phosphorus should be measured frequently. Special caution is required in patients with preexisting electrolyte, cardiac, or neurologic abnormalities. The risk for hypocalcemia is increased by the concurrent use of pentamidine.

Common reactions (seen in 25% to 50% of patients) include fever, nausea, anemia, diarrhea, vomiting, and headache. In addition to those conditions previously mentioned, foscarnet can cause fatigue, tremor, irritability, and elevated liver enzymes.

SUMMARY OF KEY PRESCRIBING CONSIDERATIONS
Drugs for Cytomegalovirus Infections

Therapeutic Goal: To control viral progression and associated signs and symptoms of cytomegalovirus infection.
Baseline Data: Nucleic acid testing (NAT) using the polymerase chain reaction (PCR) to detect CMV DNA. Thorough ophthalmic examination, including visual acuity and intraocular pressure. Pregnancy test in women capable of becoming pregnant. CBC with differential, serum creatinine.
Additional Drug-Specific Baseline Data:
- Foscarnet: Electrolytes, 24-hour creatinine clearance, and ECG.
Monitoring: Eye exam at each clinic visit. PCR each week to monitor treatment response. Serum creatinine and CBC each week and adjust dosage or hold administration as indicated by product labeling.
Additional Drug-Specific Monitoring:
- Ganciclovir and valganciclovir: Monitor platelet count twice weekly during therapy.
- Cidofovir: Check urinalysis for protein before each dose. Monitor for signs and symptoms of metabolic acidosis.
- Foscarnet: Serum creatinine, electrolytes, calcium, ionized calcium, magnesium, and phosphorus twice weekly during acute therapy and once weekly during maintenance therapy. Repeat 24-hour creatinine clearance and ECG whenever clinically indicated. Assess hydration with each treatment.
Identifying High-Risk Patients: Renal impairment, blood disorders
Additional Drug-Specific High-Risk Patients:
- Foscarnet: Patients with QT prolongation; hypocalcemia, hyperphosphatemia/hypophosphatemia, hypomagnesemia, or hypokalemia; heart failure (due to high sodium content of drug)
Evaluating Therapeutic Effects: Signs and symptoms of acute infection abate and infection is held in check.

Viral Hepatitis

Viral hepatitis is the most common liver disorder, affecting millions of Americans. The disease can be caused by six different hepatitis viruses labeled A, B, C, D, E, and G. All six can cause *acute* hepatitis, but only B, C, and D also cause *chronic* hepatitis.

Acute hepatitis lasts for 6 months or less and is characterized by liver inflammation, jaundice, and elevation of serum alanine aminotransferase (ALT) activity. In most cases, acute hepatitis resolves spontaneously, so intervention is generally unnecessary. In contrast, chronic hepatitis can lead to cirrhosis, hepatocellular carcinoma, and life-threatening liver failure; hence treatment should be considered.

Most cases (90%) of chronic hepatitis are caused by either hepatitis B virus (HBV) or hepatitis C virus (HCV). Accordingly, this discussion focuses on hepatitis B and hepatitis C. About 1.5% of Americans are infected with HBV or HCV, which is five times more than the number infected with HIV. Vaccines for hepatitis A and B are discussed in Chapter 55. Drugs for hepatitis B and C are discussed here.

DRUGS FOR HEPATITIS C

According to the Centers for Disease Control and Prevention (CDC), more people in the United States die from hepatitis C than from any other infectious disease, including HIV infection. Transmission occurs primarily through exchange of blood, with injection drug use being the most common means. Transmission may also occur as the result of sexual intercourse with an HCV-infected partner, although this occurs far less frequently. Pregnant women who are infected can transfer the virus to their offspring.

Among people who acquire HCV, 75% to 85% develop active infection manifested by jaundice, nausea, abdominal pain, myalgias and arthralgias. However, most people with chronic hepatitis C have no symptoms and are unaware that they are infected, although they can transmit HCV to others. Chronic HCV infection undergoes slow progression and, in some people, eventually causes liver failure, cancer, and death.

It is important to note that not all hepatitis C viruses are the same. There are six genotypes of HCV and more than 50 subtypes. In the United States 75% of HCV infections are caused by HCV genotype 1, which, unfortunately, is less responsive to treatment than other HCV genotypes.

The options for hepatitis C management have increased dramatically over the past decade. The expanse in knowledge and understanding of the HCV genome led to the development of direct-acting antiviral (DAA) drugs.

DAAs are drugs that target specific steps in the process of HCV replication. There are currently four categories of DAAs: NS3/4A protease inhibitors (PIs), NS5A inhibitors, NS5B nucleoside polymerase inhibitors (NPIs), and NS5B nonnucleoside polymerase inhibitors (NNPIs). To decrease the development of viral resistance and to increase the likelihood of successful outcomes, all of these drugs are used in combination therapy.

In 2015, when the European Association for the Study of the Liver (EASL) released its groundbreaking recommendations for the treatment of HCV infection; the first sentence following the introduction was astounding: "The primary goal of HCV therapy is to cure the infection." For the patients, their families, and the health care providers who had accepted the long-held belief that there is no cure, hope had truly arrived.

In 2018, joint guidelines by the American Association for the Study of Liver Diseases (AASLD) and the Infectious Diseases Society of America (IDSA) were released (see http://www.hcvguidelines.org). These guidelines complement those of the EASL. As with the EASL guidelines, they focus on genotype-specific treatment that considers liver status (i.e., presence or absence of cirrhosis) and treatment history (i.e., treatment-naive and previous treatment failure) to optimize therapy (Fig. 80.1).

With the rapid advance of knowledge and development of new drugs, it is quite likely that, by the time this chapter is published, there will be new updates on the treatment of HCV infection. The most current recommendations are maintained at the AASLD/IDSA website at http://www.hcvguidelines.org.

Treatment of HCV infection is typically managed in specialty practices. Rather than give detailed information about drugs that nonspecialist providers may never prescribe or encounter, the goal here is to provide a summary of information that will benefit health care providers who see these patients in their practice for other conditions.

Protease Inhibitors

In 2011, the FDA approved two PIs—boceprevir and telaprevir—for treatment of chronic hepatitis C, making them the first new drugs for hepatitis C in 20 years. These were the first of the direct-acting antivirals that would revolutionize hepatitis C treatment. (Telaprevir was

subsequently withdrawn from the market in 2014 by the manufacturer, who cited dwindling sales of this first-generation DAA among increased competition from new products, including DAAs with fewer interactions and fewer adverse effects. Boceprevir is no longer available in the United States.)

PIs inhibit viral protease, an enzyme required for HCV replication. There are currently five "second-wave" PIs approved in the United States: glecaprevir, grazoprevir, paritaprevir, simeprevir, and voxilaprevir. Of these, only simeprevir is available as a single agent (with indications to use it only in combination with other drugs). The other PIs are available only in fixed combination with other drugs.

In the present discussion, the second-wave PI simeprevir is examined. Properties of the combination drugs are presented in Table 80.6.

Simeprevir

Action and use. Simeprevir (Olysio, Galexos ♣) is a second-wave protease inhibitor and DAA against HVC. Simeprevir is approved for the treatment of chronic hepatitis C for HCV genotype 1 or 4. It must always be used in combination with other anti-HCV drugs.

Fig. 80.1 Drug selection for initial treatment of hepatitis C virus (HCV) infection by genotype in the patient without cirrhosis. Treatment is often complicated by comorbidities, life-span considerations, and other factors affecting drug choice. Consult evidence-based practice guidelines at https://www.hcvguidelines.org for additional information. Drugs are listed by highest level of evidence. When the level of evidence is the same, drugs are listed alphabetically. [a]Length of dosing may be decreased to 8 weeks for patients who are not black, are not coinfected with HIV, and have an HCV RNA level lower than 6 million IU/mL. (Based on joint recommendations of the American Association for the Study of Liver Diseases [AASLD] and Infectious Diseases Society of America [IDSA]. Initial treatment of HCV infection, 2018. https://www.hcvguidelines.org/treatment-naive.)

TABLE 80.6 Properties of Anti-HCV Direct-Acting Antiviral Drug Combinations

Drug Combinations	Elbasvir/ Grazoprevir (Zepatier)	Elbasvir-Grazoprevir (Zepatier)	Ledipasvir/ Sofosbuvir (Harvoni)	Ombitasvir/ Paritaprevir/ Ritonavir[a] (Technivie)	Ombitasvir/ Paritaprevir/ Ritonavir[a] With Dasabuvir (Viekira Pak. Viekira XR, Holkira Pak ♦)	Sofosbuvir-velpatasvir (Epclusa)	Sofosbuvir-velpalasvir-voxilaprevir (Vosevi)
Classification	NS5A inhibitor + PI	NS5A Inhibitors + PI	NS5A inhibitor + NPI	NS5A inhibitor + PI + CYP3A inhibitor	NS5A inhibitor + PI + CYP3A inhibitor + NNPI	NS5A inhibitor + NS5B inhibitor	NS5A inhibitor + PI + NS5B inhibitor
HCV genotype treated	1a, 1b, & 4	1a, 1b (4 off label)	1a, 1b, 4, 5, 6	4	1a, 1b	1a, 1b, 2, 3, 4, 5, 6	1a, 1b, 2, 3, 4, 5, 6
Adverse effects	Significant ALT elevations have occurred. The most common adverse reactions are headache, nausea, and fatigue. About 5% develop anemia	Fatigue, headache, and nausea. ALT elevation occurs in up to 10% of patients	Common adverse effects are headache, fatigue, and weakness	ALT elevations up to five times normal have occurred. Patients with cirrhosis may develop hepatic failure. Common adverse reactions are nausea, fatigue, insomnia, weakness	Significant ALT elevations have occurred. Hepatic failure has occurred, primary in patients with advanced cirrhosis. Common adverse reactions include nausea, fatigue, insomnia, weakness, pruritus, and skin reactions	Significant creatine phosphokinase elevations up to 10 times normal in 1–2%. Headache, fatigue	Fatigue, headache, nausea, and diarrhea. Bilirubin elevation occurs in up to 13% of patients
Administration	Administer with or without food	Administer with or without food	Administer with or without food	Administer with meals (increases absorption)	Administer with meals (increases absorption)	Administer with or without food	Administer with food

[a]Ritonavir is an HIV protease inhibitor with no inherent anti-HCV activity. It boosts the HCV antiviral drugs through its CYP3A inhibitor activity.
ALT, Alanine aminotransferase; *CBC,* complete blood count; *HCV,* hepatitis C virus; *NNPI,* nonnucleoside polymerase inhibitor; *NPI,* nucleoside polymerase inhibitor; *PI,* protease inhibitor.

Adverse effects. FDA labeling warns of the potential for hepatic injury, significant photosensitivity, and severe rashes. The most common adverse effects experienced are headache, nausea, and fatigue.

 BLACK BOX WARNING

Simeprevir (Olysio, Galexos ♦) and Other Protease Inhibitors

> HBV reactivation has occurred in patients undergoing or previously treated for HBV. Hepatic failure and death have occurred. Patient should be prescreened for HBV infection.

Pharmacokinetics. Taking simeprevir with food will enhance its absorption to 62% bioavailability. Its half-life is 10 to 13 hours in healthy individuals, In HCV-infected patients, however, the half-life may be as long as 41 hours. Additional pharmacokinetics for simeprevir and other drugs used to treat HCV are provided in Table 80.7. Preparations and dosages are provided in Table 80.8.

Contraindications. There are no absolute contraindications to the use of simeprevir. Although not contraindicated, simeprevir is not recommended for patients with severe liver impairment and should not be administered with peginterferon and ribavirin if the patient has decompensated cirrhosis. Also, simeprevir contains a component of sulfonamide, so caution is advised for patients who have had previous reactions to sulfonamides.

Drug interactions. Simeprevir exerts mild inhibition of CYP1A2 isoenzyme activity, but it is unlikely to have a significant effect. On the other hand, it is a substrate of CYP3A4 isoenzymes; therefore drugs that are CYP3A4 inducers may lower simeprevir levels, whereas CYP3A4 inhibitors may raise levels. Significant adverse effects may occur when simeprevir is given with amiodarone (i.e., serious symptomatic bradycardia). It may elevate levels of HMG-CoA reductase inhibitors, so lower doses of statin drugs may be necessary. It may also raise levels of sedative anxiolytics such as midazolam and triazolam, which both have a narrow therapeutic index. Labeling warns against coadministration of a number of drugs. As with any drug, it is important to consult drug interaction software before prescribing a new drug to patients taking anti-HCV therapy.

NS5A Inhibitors

NS5A inhibitors target a nonstructural protein, NS5A, that is necessary for HCV RNA replication and assembly. In so doing, these drugs prevent the replication and construction of HCV. Unfortunately, resistance to these agents can build easily. Hence, as with other HCV regimens, they should never be given alone.

Currently six NS5A inhibitors are approved for use in the United States. Daclatasvir is approved as a single agent to be added to other anti-HCV regimens. Elbasvir, ledipasvir, ombitasvir, pibrentasvir, and velpatasvir are combined in fixed dosages with other antiviral drugs. As with our previous classification, those in combinations are summarized in Tables 80.6 and 80.8.

Daclatasvir

Action and use. Daclatasvir (Daklinza) is an NS5A inhibitor antiviral drug approved for treatment of chronic hepatitis C infection with HCV genotype 1 or 3. It should be used with sofosbuvir, with or without the addition of ribavirin.

TABLE 80.7 Pharmacokinetics: Drugs for Hepatitis C

Drugs and Class	Peak	Protein Binding	Metabolism	Half-Life	Elimination
Protease Inhibitors					
Glecaprevir	5 h	97.5	CYP3A	6 h	Feces (92.1%)
Grazoprevir	2 h	98.8%	CYP3A	31 h	Feces (90%)
Paritaprevir	4–5 h	97%–98.6%	CYP3A4 (primarily) and CYP3A5	5.5 h	Feces (88%)
Ritonavir	2 h (fasting) 4 h (not fasting)	98%–99%	CYP3A4 and 2D6	2–5 h	Feces (86%)
Simeprevir	4–6 h	99.9%	CYP3A4 (primarily)	41 h[a]	Feces (91%)
NS5A Inhibitors					
Daclatasvir	2 h	99%	CYP3A4	12–15 h	Feces (88%)
Elbasvir	3–6 h	99.9%	CYP3A	24 h	Feces (90%)
Ledipasvir	4–4.5 h	99.8%	Oxidative metabolism	47 h	Feces (86%)
Ombitasvir	5 h	99.9%	Amide hydrolysis and oxidative metabolism	21–25 h	Feces (90%)
Pibrentasvir	5 h	99.9%	NA	13 h	Feces (96.6%)
Velpatasvir	3 h	99.5%	Hepatic, multiple mechanisms	15 h	Feces (94%)
NS5B Nucleoside Polymerase Inhibitors					
Sofosbuvir (Sovaldi)	0.5–2 h	61%–65%	Hepatic (non-CYP450) and phosphorylation	0.5 h	Urine (80%)
NS5B Nonnucleoside Polymerase Inhibitors					
Dasabuvir	IR: 4 h ER: 8 h	99.5%	CYP2C8 (primary) and CYP3A	5.5–6 h	Feces (94.4%)
Alfa Interferons					
Interferon alfa-2b (Intron A)	IM, SubQ: 3–12 h IV: less than 30 min	NA	Renal	SubQ: 2–3 h IV: 2 h	Urine
Peginterferon alfa-2a (Pegasys, Pegasys ProClick)	72–96 h	NA	Hepatic and renal	50–160 h	Urine
Nucleoside Analogs					
Ribavirin (systemic)	2–3 h	None	Intracellular and hepatic	Capsule: 24–48 h Tablet: 120–170 h	Urine (61%) Feces (12%)

[a]Half-life is for patients with HCV infection. Patients without HCV infection have a half-life of 10–13 h.
ER, Extended release; *IR*, immediate release; *NA*, not available.

PATIENT-CENTERED CARE ACROSS THE LIFE SPAN

Drugs for Hepatitis C

Life Stage	Considerations or Concerns
Children	Direct-acting antivirals are recommended for children older than 3 years. Preferred regimens are ledipasvir-sofosbuvir for genotypes 1, 4, 5, and 6 and sofosbuvir plus ribavirin for genotypes 2 and 3. Interferons are not recommended (see https://www.hcvguidelines.org/unique-populations/children).
Pregnant women	Current evidence recommends against HCV treatment during pregnancy (see https://www.hcvguidelines.org/unique-populations/pregnancy). Women considering pregnancy should be tested for HCV and, when possible, treated before conception.
Breastfeeding women	HCV infection is not a contraindication for breastfeeding as long as the nipples are healthy and without cracks or bleeding. Manufacturers recommend carefully weighing benefits versus risks, because adverse effects of drugs for HCV are not fully known.
Older adults	Because older patients are more likely than other age groups to have decreased renal and hepatic function, they are at increased risk for toxicity and adverse events. In particular, older patients taking ribavirin are at an increased risk for the development of anemia, especially if renal function is compromised. Older patients are also more likely to be susceptible to interferon alfa–associated neuropsychiatric disorders, infections, and ischemia. When possible, interferon alfa and ribavirin combinations are best avoided in older patients.

TABLE 80.8   Preparations and Dosages: Drugs for Hepatitis C

Drugs and Drug Class	Preparations	Usual Dosage
Protease Inhibitors Available as a Single Drug		
Simeprevir (Olysio, Galexos ♣)	Capsule: 150 mg	1 capsule qd with sofosbuvir (with or without ribavirin)
NS5A Inhibitors Available as a Single Drug		
Daclatasvir (Daklinza)	Tablet: 30, 60, and 90 mg	60 mg qd
NS5B Nucleoside Polymerase Inhibitors Available as a Single Drug		
Sofosbuvir (Sovaldi)	Tablet: 400 mg	400 mg qd
Nucleoside Analogs		
Ribavirin (systemic)	Solution (oral): 40 mg/mL Capsule: 200 mg Tablet: 200, 400, and 600 mg	Varies
Alfa Interferons		
Interferon alfa-2b (Intron A)	Solution: 6 million U/mL and 1 million U/mL Solution: reconstituted: 10,000,000 units; 18,000,000 units; 50,000,000 units	IM or subQ: 3 million units three times weekly[a]
Peginterferon alfa-2a (Pegasys, Pegasys ProClick)	Pegasys: 180 µg/0.5 mL, 180 µg/1 mL Pegasys ProClick: 135 µg/0.5 mL, 180 µg/0.5 mL	SubQ: 180 µg once weekly, subQ[a]
Combination Products		
Elbasvir-grazoprevir (Zepatier)	Tablet: Elbasvir 50 mg + grazoprevir 100 mg	1 tablet qd
Glecaprevir-pibrentasvir (Mavyret, Maviret ♣)	Tablet: Glecaprevir 100 mg + pibrentasvir 40 mg	1 tablet tid
Ledipasvir-sofosbuvir (Harvoni)	Tablet: Ledipasvir 90 mg + sofosbuvir 400 mg	1 tablet qd
Ombitasvir-paritaprevir-ritonavir (Technivie)	Tablet: Ombitasvir 12.5 mg + paritaprevir 75 mg + ritonavir 50 mg	2 tablets qd
Ombitasvir-paritaprevir-ritonavir-dasabuvir (Viekira Pak, Viekira XR, Holkira Pak ♣)	Viekira Pak: IR tablets: Ombitasvir 12.5 mg + paritaprevir 75 mg + ritonavir 50 mg with IR tablet: Dasabuvir 250 mg Viekira XR: ER tablet: Ombitasvir 8.33 mg + paritaprevir 50 mg + ritonavir 33.33 mg + dasabuvir 200 mg	IR tablets: 2 tablets ombitasvir-paritaprevir-ritonavir every morning and 1 tablet dasabuvir bid ER tablet: 3 tablets qd
Sofosbuvir-velpatasvir (Epclusa)	Tablet: Sofosbuvir 400 mg + velpatasvir 100 mg	1 tablet qd
Sofosbuvir-velpalasvir-voxilaprevir (Vosevi)	Tablet: Sofosbuvir 400 mg + velpatasvir 100 mg + voxilaprevir 100 mg	1 tablet qd

[a]The FDA has approved interferon for treatment of hepatitis C; however, it is not recommended in the current guidelines for hepatitis C virus treatment.
ER, Extended release; *IR*, immediate release.

Adverse effects. The most common adverse reactions are headache and fatigue (in combination with sofosbuvir). With the addition of ribavirin, nausea and anemia also occurred in at least 10% of those taking the triple therapy.

Contraindications. There are no absolute contraindications. However, product labeling includes drug interactions with strong CYP3A inducers and amiodarone (see Drug Interactions, next).

Drug interactions. Because daclatasvir is a CYP3A substrate, strong CYP3A inducers can significantly lower levels of daclatasvir. Examples of strong inducers include the antiepileptic drugs carbamazepine and phenytoin and the herbal supplement St. John's wort. Similarly, CYP3A inhibitors can raise levels of daclatasvir. Both situations may require dosage adjustments of daclatasvir. Although not a contraindication per se, there is a strong warning and recommendation against adding the daclatasvir/sofosbuvir combination to amiodarone because dangerous symptomatic bradycardia may occur. In addition to the interactions mentioned as contraindications, a large number of others can occur.

Most notably, substances that induce or inhibit CYP3A isoenzymes may affect levels of daclatasvir. Others, when given together, include elevations of HMG-CoA reductase inhibitors (statins) and of digoxin. Use of drug interaction software is needed to screen potential interactions when new drugs are being prescribed to patients taking daclatasvir.

NS5B Inhibitors

NS5B is a nonstructural HCV protein that, like NS5A, is vital for HCV RNA replication. There are two classes of drugs that target this protein: NS5B NPIs and NS5B NNPIs. Beyond structural composition, they differ primarily in respect to properties of resistance and genotype. NPIs have a low likelihood of development of viral resistance, whereas the likelihood of viral resistance is high for NNPIs. In contrast, NPIs have high efficacy for all genotypes, whereas the NNPIs have lower efficacy and are effective for fewer genotypes.

The only NPI currently approved is sofosbuvir (Sovaldi). The only NNPI is dasabuvir, which is available only in a fixed-dose combination with ombitasvir, paritaprevir, and ritonavir. As before, sofosbuvir is examined here as an individual drug whereas dasabuvir is examined in the combined form. It is important to note that ritonavir has an associated black box warning.

 BLACK BOX WARNING

Ritonavir

> Life-threatening adverse effects can occur when ritonavir is administered with sedative hypnotics, antidysrhythmics, and ergot preparations.

Sofosbuvir

Action and use. Sofosbuvir (Sovaldi) is an NS5B NPI. It is activated by metabolism, after which it incorporates into the HCV RNA through NS5B polymerase. It is approved as a component of antiviral treatment for chronic hepatitis C of HCV genotype 1, 2, 3, or 4.

Adverse effects. Headaches and fatigue affect about 20% of patients when sofosbuvir given in combination with ribavirin. When interferon alfa is added to the combination, nausea, anemia, and insomnia may also occur.

Contraindications. There are no contraindications for sofosbuvir. Those mentioned in product labeling apply only to drugs with which sofosbuvir may be combined.

Drug interactions. If sofosbuvir is administered with amiodarone, dangerous symptomatic bradycardia may occur. Sofosbuvir is a substrate of P-glycoprotein (P-gp), a drug transporter with a role in determining the amount of drug that is absorbed and distributed. If administered with P-gp inducers such as St. John's wort, the level of sofosbuvir may decrease.

Interferon Alfa and Ribavirin

Long the cornerstone of HCV treatment, interferon alfa and ribavirin are not included among the recommendations for treatment in the 2018 evidence-based practice guidelines (see https://www.hcvguidelines.org). Because they are still commonly prescribed, we include them briefly here.

Effects in Chronic Hepatitis C

In patients with chronic hepatitis C, serum ALT normalizes in 40% to 50% of patients, and serum levels of HCV-RNA become undetectable in 30% to 40% of patients after 12 months of treatment. Unfortunately about half of these people relapse when treatment is stopped; sustained responses are maintained in only 5% to 15% of patients. Combining interferon alfa with other agents can improve response rates. Ribavirin is the drug most commonly used for this purpose. Ribavirin is discussed next. Additional information on interferon alfa is provided under the heading Drugs for Hepatitis B, further on.

Ribavirin

Actions and use. For decades, oral ribavirin (Copegus, Moderiba Rebetol, Ribasphere) was combined with interferon alfa as the treatment of choice for HCV infection. When used alone against HCV, ribavirin is not effective: treatment produces a transient normalization of serum ALT but does not reduce serum HCV-RNA. The purpose of combining ribavirin with interferon alfa was to greatly improve response rates. Ribavirin is a nucleoside analog with a broad spectrum of antiviral activity, but its mechanism of action remains unclear.

In addition to its use against HCV, ribavirin is available as an aerosol for treating children infected with respiratory syncytial virus.

Adverse effects. Although ribavirin and interferon alfa are generally well tolerated, both drugs can cause significant adverse effects. The principal concerns with ribavirin are *hemolytic anemia* and *fetal injury.*

 BLACK BOX WARNING

Ribavirin

> Ribavirin may cause hemolytic anemia and cardiac decompensation secondary to hemolytic anemia.

Hemolytic anemia, characterized by a hemoglobin (Hb) level below 10 g/dL, develops in 10% to 13% of patients receiving dual therapy with ribavirin/interferon alfa. Onset is typically 1 to 2 weeks after starting treatment. Hemolytic anemia can worsen heart disease and may lead to nonfatal or fatal myocardial infarction.

Ribavirin is both embryolethal and teratogenic. In laboratory animals, the drug has caused fetal death as well as malformations of the skull, palate, eyes, jaw, limbs, GI tract, and skeleton—all at doses as low as 5% of those used to treat humans. Of note, among men being treated, ribavirin can be present in sperm. It is not known whether ribavirin-containing sperm will be teratogenic on fertilizing an ovum.

Contraindications. Ribavirin should not be prescribed for pregnant women or women who want to become pregnant. It should also not be prescribed for men with female partners who are or want to become pregnant.

Because ribavirin increases the risk for hemolytic anemia, careful consideration should be given before prescribing this drug for patients with a history of blood disorders or cardiac disease. Patients with renal dysfunction are also at an increased risk for anemia.

Drug interactions. Ribavirin is commonly prescribed with alfa interferons. Numerous adverse effects are associated with this drug combination. These include an increased risk for autoimmune disorders, infections, and hypersensitivity reactions. Bone marrow suppression has occurred, resulting in low levels of circulating blood cells. Periodontal problems, ophthalmologic disorders, and severe skin reactions have occurred. Pancreatitis and diabetes have developed in some patients. Others have experienced pulmonary complications and psychiatric disorders.

PATIENT EDUCATION

Ribavirin

> Instruct patients to report signs and symptoms of anemia such as pallor or fatigue.
>
> Counsel both female and male patients to avoid pregnancy. Couples should use two reliable forms of birth control during treatment and for 6 months after stopping. Furthermore, if ribavirin is used in conjunction with a protease inhibitor, hormonal contraceptives may not work, and hence two barrier contraceptives should be used.

DRUGS FOR HEPATITIS B

In the United States about 1.2 million people have chronic hepatitis B. Unlike hepatitis C, hepatitis B has been on a decreasing trend since 2013. Transmission is primarily through the exchange of blood or semen. Between 45% and 60% of exposed adults develop acute hepatitis. In adults, acute infection usually leads to viral clearance by the immune

SUMMARY OF KEY PRESCRIBING CONSIDERATIONS

Drugs for Hepatitis C

Therapeutic Goal: A sustained virologic response (SVR), which represents elimination of HCV RNA. The SVR occurs if there is no detectable HCV RNA at 12 weeks (SVR12) after therapy.

Baseline Data: Complete history and physical exam, HCV RNA (i.e., HCV viral load), HCV genotype and subtype, liver function panel (see components listed earlier for HBV), liver ultrasound or computed tomography (CT) if indicated, complete blood count (CBC), international normalized ratio (INR), serum creatinine, and glomerular filtration rate (GFR). Pregnancy test.

Additional Drug-Specific Baseline Data:

- Daclatasvir: Hepatitis B surface antigen (HBsAg) and hepatitis B core antibody (anti-HBc). For patients taking or recently discontinuing amiodarone, therapy should be initiated on an inpatient basis under continuous cardiac monitoring for the first 48 hours.
- Ribavirin: Focused cardiac examination.
- Simeprevir: HBsAg and anti-HBc.
- Elbasvir-grazoprevir: HBsAg and anti-HBc.
- Glecaprevir-pibrentasvir: HBsAg and anti-HBc.
- Ledipasvir-sofosbuvir: HBsAg and anti-HBc. For patients taking or recently discontinuing amiodarone, initiate therapy on an inpatient basis under continuous cardiac monitoring for the first 48 hours.
- Ombitasvir-paritaprevir-ritonavir (with or without dasabuvir): HBsAg and anti-HBc.
- Sofosbuvir-velpatasvir: HBsAg and anti-HBc. For patients taking or recently discontinuing amiodarone, initiate therapy as an inpatient under continuous cardiac monitoring for the first 48 hours.

Monitoring: HCV RNA at week 4 after starting therapy (should be undetectable) and, if positive, again at week 6, then HCV RNA at 12 weeks after therapy. Every 4 weeks check CBC, creatinine, GFR, ALT, AST, bilirubin, and pregnancy test.

Additional Drug-Specific Monitoring:

- Daclatasvir: For patients taking or recently discontinuing amiodarone, have patient monitor heart rate and rhythm for first 2 weeks of treatment.

- Elbasvir-grazoprevir: ALT/AST may increase to more than five times normal limits. If this occurs, check other tests of liver function (e.g., total and direct bilirubin, alkaline phosphatase, albumin) and assess for physical evidence of liver problems. If other evidence of liver problems, discontinue drug. If no other evidence of liver problems but ALT/AST continues to increase to 10 times normal limits, discontinue drug even if there are no other signs or symptoms of liver injury.
- Interferon and peginterferon: Thyroid-stimulating hormone (TSH) every 3 months.
- Ribavirin: In addition to routine scheduling for all HCV drugs (see earlier), recheck CBC 2 weeks after beginning therapy and for any signs or symptoms of anemia during treatment. Check a pregnancy test every month during treatment and for 6 months after treatment.
- Sofosbuvir: For patients taking or recently discontinuing amiodarone, have patient monitor heart rate and rhythm for first 2 weeks of treatment.

Identifying High-Risk Patients:

- Daclatasvir: May reactivate HBV.
- Elbasvir-grazoprevir: May reactivate HBV. Contraindicated for patients with moderate to severe hepatic impairment.
- Glecaprevir-pibrentasvir: May reactivate HBV. Contraindicated for patients with severe hepatic impairment.
- Ledipasvir-sofosbuvir: May reactivate HBV.
- Ombitasvir-paritaprevir-ritonavir (with or without dasabuvir): May reactivate HBV. Contraindicated for patients with moderate to severe hepatic impairment.
- Sofosbuvir-velpatasvir: May reactivate HBV.
- Ribavirin: Avoid for patients with significant heart disease and in those with hemoglobinopathies, including sickle cell anemia and thalassemia major.

---

system. As a result, only 3% to 5% of infected adults develop chronic infection. However, when chronic infection does develop, it can lead to cirrhosis, hepatic failure, hepatocellular carcinoma, and death. The best strategy against HBV is prevention: all children should receive HBV vaccine before entering school (see Chapter 55).

Six drugs are used to treat chronic HBV. Two are alfa interferons—*interferon alfa-2b* (Intron A) and *peginterferon alfa-2a* (Pegasys), and four are nucleoside analogs—*lamivudine* (Epivir HBV, Heptovir ✤), *adefovir* (Hepsera), *entecavir* (Baraclude), and *tenofovir* (Viread). (A fifth nucleoside, *telbivudine* (Sebivo ✤), is currently unavailable in the United States but is available in Canada.) The alfa interferons are administered subcutaneously; the nucleoside analogs are administered orally. The interferons are more effective than the nucleoside analogs but are also more expensive and less well tolerated. Development of resistance is common with lamivudine and relatively rare with the other drugs. Four agents—lamivudine, adefovir, entecavir, and tenofovir—are also active against HIV and hence may promote the emergence of resistant HIV in people coinfected with that virus.

With all six drugs—and especially the nucleoside analogs—the rate of relapse after cessation of treatment is high. As a result, treatment is usually prolonged, thereby amplifying concerns about adverse effects and drug cost. To decrease unnecessary drug exposure and expense, current guidelines recommend treatment only for patients at highest risk, indicated by elevated aminotransferase levels, or those with histologic evidence of moderate or severe hepatic inflammation or advanced

fibrosis. Given that relapse is common, patients should be followed closely if these drugs are withdrawn. Comparisons among the six drugs are shown in Table 80.9.

Interferon Alfa

Human interferons are naturally occurring compounds with complex antiviral, immunomodulatory, and antineoplastic actions. The interferon family has three major classes designated alpha, beta, and gamma. All of the interferons used to treat hepatitis belong to the alpha class.

Mechanism of Action

Interferon alfa has multiple effects on the viral replication cycle. After binding to receptors on host cell membranes, the drug blocks viral entry into cells, synthesis of viral messenger RNA and viral proteins, and viral assembly and release. The pharmacokinetics for interferon alfa and other drugs for hepatitis B is provided in Table 80.10.

Conventional Versus Long-Acting Interferons

The alfa interferons can be divided into two groups—conventional and long acting—based on their time course of action. The conventional preparation (interferon alfa-2b) has a short half-life, so it must be administered three times a week. In contrast, the long-acting preparation (peginterferon alfa-2a) is administered just once a week. Preparations and dosages for the alfa interferons and other drugs for hepatitis B are provided in Table 80.11.

TABLE 80.9   Drugs for Chronic Hepatitis B

Drug	Route	Relapse Rate[a]	Adverse Effects	Resistance Rate	Active Against HIV
Interferon Alfa Preparations					
Interferon alfa-2b (Intron A)	SubQ	Moderate	Flu-like symptoms, fatigue, neutropenia, depression	Zero	No
Peginterferon alfa-2a (Pegasys)	SubQ	Moderate	Same as interferon alfa-2b	Zero	No
Nucleoside Analogs					
Lamivudine (Epivir HBV, Heptovir ♦)	PO	High	Well tolerated; lactic acidosis and hepatomegaly are possible	15%–30% in year 1; 70% by year 5	Yes
Adefovir (Hepsera)	PO	High	Nephrotoxic at high doses; lactic acidosis and hepatomegaly are possible	Zero in year 1; 29% by year 5	Yes
Entecavir (Baraclude)	PO	High	Well tolerated; lactic acidosis and hepatomegaly are possible	Zero in year 1; 1% or less by year 3	Yes
Tenofovir (Viread)	PO	High	Weakness, headache, gastrointestinal reactions; lactic acidosis and hepatomegaly are possible	—	Yes
Telbivudine (Sebivo ♦) (no longer available in U.S.	PO	Moderate	Myopathy, lactic acidosis, hepatomegaly are possible	6%–12% in year 1; 9%–22% by year 2	No

[a]After discontinuation of treatment.

TABLE 80.10   Pharmacokinetics: Drugs for Hepatitis B

Drugs and Class	Peak	Protein Binding	Metabolism	Half-Life	Elimination
Interferon Alfa Preparations					
Interferon alfa-2b (Intron A)	IM, SubQ: 3–12 h IV: less than 30 min	NA	Renal	SubQ: 2–3 h IV: 2 h	Urine
Peginterferon alfa-2a (Pegasys)	72–96 h	NA	Hepatic and renal	50–160 h	Urine
Nucleoside Analogs					
Lamivudine (Epivir HBV, Heptovir ♦)	0.5–1 h (fasting) 3.2 h (not fasting)	36% or less	Minor	10–15 h	Urine
Adefovir (Hepsera)	1–4 h	4% or less	Intestinal	7.5 h	Urine
Entecavir (Baraclude)	0.5–1.5 h	13%	Minor	24 h	Urine
Tenofovir (Viread)	0.5–1.25 h (fasting) 1.5–2.5 h (not fasting)	7% or less	Hydrolysis and phosphorylation	17 h	Urine

Adverse Effects

All formulations of interferon alfa produce the same spectrum of adverse effects, some of which can be life threatening. The incidence is higher with the long-acting preparations.

▶ BLACK BOX WARNING

Interferon Alfa (Intron A, Pegasys)

Alfa interferons may cause or worsen life-threatening disorders, including autoimmune, infectious, and ischemic conditions. Serious neuropsychiatric conditions have also occurred.

The most common side effect is a *flu-like syndrome* characterized by fever, fatigue, myalgia, headache, and chills. The incidence is about 50%. Fortunately, symptoms tend to diminish with continued therapy. Some symptoms (fever, headache, myalgia) can be reduced with acetaminophen.

Interferon alfa frequently causes *neuropsychiatric effects*—especially *depression*. Suicidal ideation and suicide have occurred. The risk for depression is increased by large doses and prolonged treatment. The mechanism underlying depression is unknown. In many patients, depression responds to antidepressant drugs (e.g., paroxetine). If depression persists, a reduction in dosage or cessation of treatment is indicated.

Prolonged or high-dose therapy can cause fatigue, thyroid dysfunction, heart damage, and bone marrow suppression, manifesting as neutropenia and thrombocytopenia.

Other adverse effects include alopecia and GI effects: nausea, diarrhea, anorexia, and vomiting. Injection-site reactions (inflammation, bruising, itching, irritation) are common, especially with long-acting formulations. Also, interferon may induce or exacerbate autoimmune diseases, such as thyroiditis and autoimmune chronic hepatitis.

Only two forms of interferon alfa—interferon alfa-2b (Intron A) and peginterferon alfa-2a (Pegasys)—are approved for the treatment of chronic hepatitis B. In clinical trials, treatment for 4 months reduced

TABLE 80.11   Preparations and Dosages: Drugs for Hepatitis B

Drugs and Drug Class	Preparations	Usual Dosage
Interferon Alfa Preparations		
Interferon alfa-2b (Intron A)	Solution: 6 million U//mL, 1 million U/mL Solution reconstituted: 10 million U; 18 million U; 50 million U	IM or SubQ: 5 million U qd for 16 weeks *or* 10 million U three times weekly for 16 weeks
Peginterferon alfa-2a (Pegasys)	Pegasys: 180 μg/0.5 mL, 180 μg/1 mL Pegasys ProClick: 135 μg/0.5 mL, 180 μg/0.5 mL	IM, SubQ: 180 μg once weekly for 48 weeks
Nucleoside Analogs		
Lamivudine (Epivir HBV, Heptovir ✦)	Oral solution: 5 mg/mL, 10 mg/mL Tablet: 100, 150, and 300 mg	100 mg qd[a]
Adefovir (Hepsera)	Tablet: 10 mg	10 mg qd[a]
Entecavir (Baraclude)	Oral solution: 0.05/mL Tablet: 0.5 and 1 mg	0.5 mg qd[a]
Tenofovir (Viread)	Powder: 40 mg/g Tablet: 150, 200, 250, and 300 mg	300 mg qd[a]

[a]Lower dosing for decreased creatinine clearance.

serum ALT and improved liver histology in about 40% of recipients. Remissions have been prolonged in some patients, and resistance has not been reported. Unfortunately, although alfa interferons are effective, they are also expensive, and adverse effects—flu-like syndrome, depression, fatigue, and leukopenia—are common.

Nucleoside Analogs

Lamivudine

Therapeutic use. Lamivudine (Epivir HBV, Heptovir ✦) is a nucleoside analog approved for infections caused by HBV or HIV. The drug was originally developed for HIV infection and later approved for HBV. Formulations and dosages for treating HIV and HBV infections differ, so they must not be considered interchangeable. Discussion here is limited to the treatment of HBV.

Mechanism of action. Lamivudine suppresses HBV replication by inhibiting viral DNA synthesis. The process begins with intracellular conversion of lamivudine to lamivudine triphosphate, the drug's active form. As the triphosphate, lamivudine undergoes incorporation into the growing DNA chain and thereby causes premature chain termination.

Lamivudine offers at least some benefit to most patients. In one trial, 52 weeks of daily lamivudine normalized serum ALT in 72% of patients and reduced liver inflammation and fibrosis in 56%. Unfortunately, the rate of relapse is high when treatment stops. Also, emergence of resistance is a concern: resistant isolates appear in 24% of patients after 1 year of continuous treatment, 42% after 2 years, 53% after 3 years, and 70% after 4 years.

Adverse effects. At the dosage employed to treat hepatitis B, side effects are minimal. In clinical trials, the incidence of most side effects was no greater than that with placebo. *Lactic acidosis, pancreatitis,* and *severe hepatomegaly* are rare but dangerous complications. If one of these conditions develops, lamivudine should be discontinued.

PATIENT-CENTERED CARE ACROSS THE LIFE SPAN

Drugs for Hepatitis B

Life Stage	Considerations or Concerns
Children	The AASLD recommends interferon alfa-2b but not peg-interferon alfa 2a if prescribed for children. For treatment of HBV infection, lamivudine and entecavir are approved for children aged 2 years and older; adefovir and tenofovir are approved for children aged 12 years and older.
Pregnant women	Lamivudine and tenofovir are considered safest for treatment of HBV in pregnant women. Teratogenesis has occurred in animal studies with both adefovir and entecavir.
Breastfeeding women	The AASLD treatment guidelines for chronic hepatitis B do not identify antiviral therapy as a contraindication to breastfeeding; however, manufacturers recommend weighing benefits vs. risk, citing a possibility for dangerous adverse reactions in the nursing infant.
Older adults	Because older patients are more likely than other age groups to have decreased renal and hepatic function, they are at increased risk for toxicity and adverse events. Older patients are also more likely to be susceptible to interferon alfa–associated neuropsychiatric disorders, infections, and ischemia.

AASLD, American Association for the Study of Liver Diseases; *HBV*, hepatitis B virus.

Precautions. Because lamivudine is also used against HIV, if a patient is infected with HIV, giving lamivudine in the low doses employed against HBV may allow emergence of HIV viruses resistant to nucleoside analogs. Accordingly, HIV infection should be ruled out before lamivudine is used.

Patients with a history of autoimmune disorders may experience immune reconstitution inflammatory syndrome (IRIS). This is a worsening or reemergence of inflammatory conditions. It is usually temporary but can be debilitating.

Adefovir

Therapeutic use. Adefovir (Hepsera) is indicated for oral therapy of chronic hepatitis B. The drug was originally developed to fight HIV infection but was not approved owing to a high incidence of nephrotoxicity at the doses required. The doses used for hepatitis B are much lower, and thus the risk for renal injury is lower too.

Mechanism of action. Adefovir is a nucleoside analog with a mechanism similar to that of acyclovir. Both drugs inhibit viral DNA synthesis, and both must be converted to their active form within the body. Activation of adefovir is mediated by cellular kinases—enzymes that convert the drug into adefovir diphosphate, a compound with two actions: (1) it directly inhibits viral DNA polymerase (by competing with deoxyadenosine triphosphate, a natural substrate for the enzyme) and (2) it undergoes incorporation into the growing strand of viral DNA and thereby causes premature strand termination. Host cells are spared because adefovir diphosphate is a poor inhibitor of human DNA polymerase.

Adverse effects and precautions. Nephrotoxicity is the principal concern. Increased serum creatinine was seen in 4% of patients who received 48 weeks of therapy and in 9% of patients who received 96 weeks of therapy. To reduce risk, kidney function should be assessed at baseline and periodically thereafter, paying special attention to patients at high risk (i.e., patients with preexisting renal impairment and those taking nephrotoxic drugs [e.g., cyclosporine, tacrolimus, aminoglycosides, vancomycin, aspirin, and other nonsteroidal antiinflammatory drugs]).

When adefovir is discontinued, patients may experience acute exacerbation of hepatitis B. In clinical trials, serum ALT levels rose dramatically in 25% of patients when treatment was stopped. Liver function should be assessed periodically after adefovir withdrawal.

Because adefovir is related to the nucleoside analogs used against HIV, there is a concern that giving adefovir in the low doses used to treat HBV may allow emergence of HIV viruses resistant to nucleoside analogs.

The nucleoside analogs used to treat HIV infection can cause lactic acidosis and severe hepatomegaly. There is concern that adefovir can cause these effects, too. If the patient develops clinical or laboratory findings that suggest lactic acidosis or pronounced hepatotoxicity, adefovir should be withdrawn.

Entecavir

Therapeutic use. Entecavir (Baraclude) is indicated for oral therapy of chronic hepatitis B. Candidates for treatment should have evidence of active viral replication along with persistently elevated serum aminotransferases or histologic evidence of active disease. In clinical trials, entecavir was more effective than lamivudine. In patients with lamivudine-resistant HBV, responses to entecavir were somewhat reduced, but were still better than responses to lamivudine. Recent evidence indicates that, with long-term use (3 years), entecavir can reverse fibrosis and cirrhosis.

Mechanism of action. Entecavir is a nucleoside analog that undergoes conversion to entecavir triphosphate (its active form) within the body. As entecavir triphosphate, the drug inhibits HBV DNA polymerase and thereby prevents viral replication. Entecavir triphosphate is a weak inhibitor of human DNA polymerases, both nuclear and mitochondrial: hence host cells are spared. As with lamivudine and adefovir, entecavir may impede HIV replication, so it may promote emergence of resistant HIV.

Adverse effects and precautions. Entecavir is very well tolerated. The most common adverse effects are dizziness, headache, fatigue, and nausea—and even these occur in less than 5% of patients.

Patients treated with other nucleoside analogs have developed lactic acidosis and severe hepatomegaly, and hence there is concern that entecavir may cause these effects, too. If the patient develops clinical or laboratory findings that suggest lactic acidosis or pronounced hepatotoxicity, entecavir should be withdrawn.

Acute severe exacerbations of hepatitis B have developed after discontinuation of entecavir and other drugs for hepatitis B. Accordingly, if entecavir is discontinued, liver function should be monitored closely for several months.

Tenofovir

As with lamivudine and adefovir, tenofovir (Viread) was originally approved for HIV infection, and then later approved for HBV in adults. When it was compared directly with adefovir in patients with HBV, tenofovir was considerably more effective. However, as with other nucleoside analogs, discontinuation of treatment is followed by exacerbation of hepatitis. Adverse effects include weakness, headache, lactic acidosis with hepatomegaly, and GI reactions: diarrhea, vomiting, and flatulence. Similarly to some other nucleoside analogs, tenofovir can impede HIV replication and hence may promote the emergence of resistant HIV.

DRUGS FOR INFLUENZA

Influenza is a serious respiratory tract infection that constitutes a major cause of morbidity and mortality worldwide. Complications of influenza (e.g., bronchitis, pneumonia) cause up to 300,000 American

---

 SUMMARY OF KEY PRESCRIBING CONSIDERATIONS

Drugs for Hepatitis B

Therapeutic Goal: Suppression of HBV DNA. Absence of HBsAG and, for those previously HBeAG-positive, absence of HBeAg.

Baseline Data: Complete history and physical exam, HBV DNA, hepatitis Be antigen (HBeAg), antibody to HBeAg (anti-HBe), liver function panel (alanine aminotransferase [ALT] and aspartate aminotransferase [AST], total and direct bilirubin, alkaline phosphatase, albumin), CBC, INR, serum creatinine and estimated GFR.

Additional Drug-Specific Baseline Testing:
- Adefovir: HIV status: Bone density if osteopenia or osteoporosis suspected
- Entecavir: HIV status
- Lamivudine: HIV status
- Tenofovir: HIV status; bone density if osteopenia or osteoporosis suspected

Monitoring: HBV DNA every 3 months until undetectable on two consecutive 3-month tests, then decrease HBV DNA testing to twice yearly. Also, every 3 months, ALT, AST until HBV DNA undetectable then every 6 months. For patients who were HbeAg-positive, HBeAg and antibody to HBeAg every 6 months. HBsAg yearly.

Additional Drug-Specific Monitoring:
- Adefovir: Lactic acidosis, if suspected; for patients at risk for renal impairment, obtain annual creatinine clearance, serum phosphate, urine glucose, and urine protein
- Entecavir: Lactic acidosis for patients with decompensated cirrhosis (if suspected)
- Lamivudine: Lactic acidosis, if suspected; amylase for symptoms of pancreatitis
- Telbivudine: Lactic acidosis, if suspected; creatine kinase for symptoms of myopathy
- Tenofovir: Lactic acidosis, if suspected; annual creatinine, serum phosphate, urine glucose, and urine protein
- Interferon alfa and Peginterferon alfa: Thyroid stimulating hormone (TSH) every 3 months

Identifying High-Risk Patients:
- Adefovir: Renal impairment (requires lowered dosage)
- Entecavir: Renal impairment (requires lowered dosage)
- Lamivudine: Renal impairment (requires lowered dosage), auto-immune disorders, pancreatitis
- Tenofovir: Renal impairment (requires lowered dosage plus comparative increased risk for renal toxicity), auto-immune disorders, decreased bone mineral density
- Interferon alfa and Peginterferon alfa: blood disorders, periodontal and dental disorders, hypertriglyceridemia, psychiatric disorders, eye disorders, pulmonary disorders

Evaluating Therapeutic Effects: See Therapeutic Goal.

---

hospitalizations a year. Annual deaths vary widely, depending on the strain of flu in circulation. During the influenza epidemic of 2017–18, there were 185 deaths in children due to influenza. Of those who died, 80% had not been vaccinated. Adult deaths due to influenza are not notifiable as they are for children; however, there were an estimated 710,000 hospitalizations for influenza during this period. Approximately 58% of those were patients age 65 years and older. The cost of influenza is huge: direct costs are estimated to be greater than $10 billion a year and indirect costs related to lost income are greater than $16 billion annually.

Influenza is caused by influenza viruses, of which there are two major types: *influenza A* and *influenza B*. Type A influenza viruses cause far more infections than type B influenza viruses (about 96% vs. 4%).

The influenza A viruses are further subclassified on the basis of two types of surface antigens: hemagglutinin (H) and neuraminidase (N). The predominant subgroups of seasonal influenza A viruses in circulation today are known as H1N1 and H3N2, because of the specific types of hemagglutinin and neuraminidase that they carry. Keep in mind, however, that viral strains undergo constant evolution. As a result, the strains of H1N1 and H3N2 in circulation this year are likely to differ from the strains of H1N1 and H3N2 in circulation next year.

Influenza is a highly contagious infection spread by aerosolized droplets produced by coughing or sneezing. The virus enters the body through mucous membranes of the nose, mouth, or eyes. Viral replication takes place in the respiratory tract. Symptoms begin 2 to 4 days after exposure and last 5 to 6 days. Influenza is characterized by fever, cough, chills, sore throat, headache, and myalgia (muscle pain). For typical patients, infection results in 5 to 6 days of restricted activity or 3 to 4 days of bed disability and 3 days of absence from work or school.

Influenza is managed by vaccination and with drugs. Vaccination is the primary management strategy; drug therapy is secondary. For very current information on influenza vaccines and drugs, see www.cdc.gov/flu, a comprehensive website maintained by the CDC.

Influenza Vaccines

Annual vaccination is the best protection against influenza. Because influenza viruses are constantly evolving, influenza vaccines must continuously change too. Each year, manufacturers produce a new vaccine directed against the three (trivalent) or four (quadrivalent) strains of influenza virus deemed most likely to cause disease during the upcoming flu season. Identification of the strains is done jointly by the CDC, FDA, and World Health Organization.

Types of Influenza Vaccines

Three basic kinds of influenza vaccine are available: (1) inactivated influenza vaccine (IIV); (2) recombinant hemagglutinin vaccine (RIV); and (3) live, attenuated influenza vaccine (LAIV). IIV and RIV are administered by intramuscular injection with one exception, Fluzone Intradermal, which is administered by intradermal injection. (The intradermal injection was not an option for the 2018–19 season; whether it will return for future seasons will be announced on the CDC site.) The LAIV is administered by intranasal spray. Information on individual vaccines is provided in Table 80.12.

The vaccination recommendations differ regarding the age groups for which they are approved. Most vaccine recipients get just one dose a year; however, there are exceptions. Children age 2 through 8 years who have not been vaccinated before require two doses administered at least 1 month apart. Protection begins 1 to 2 weeks after vaccination. Immunity generally lasts 6 months or longer; however, among older vaccine recipients, protection may be lost in 4 months or even less. (A high-dose vaccine and a vaccine with an adjuvant to improve efficacy are developed especially for patients age 65 and older.) Because antibody titers can decline fairly quickly, annual *revaccination* is recommended for some people even if the vaccine formulation does *not* change.

Efficacy

Each year the CDC conducts vaccine effectiveness (VE) studies. The study findings determine the vaccines that will be offered. For example, in the years from 2013 to 2016, VE study data demonstrated a decline in LAIV efficacy. Subsequently, the CDC's Advisory Committee on Immunization Practices (ACIP) advised against the use of LAIV for the 2016–17 influenza season (see https://www.cdc.gov/mmwr/volumes/65/rr/rr6505a1.htm). For the 2018–19 influenza season, however,

it was reintroduced as a recommended option after the manufacturer assured "improved replicative fitness" over the earlier LAIV.

Adverse Effects

Adverse effects differ for the inactivated vaccine versus the LAIV. However, with all vaccines, significant adverse effects are rare.

Inactivated influenza vaccine. Adverse effects are uncommon except for possible soreness at the site of intramuscular or intradermal injection. People who have not been vaccinated previously may experience fever, myalgia, and malaise lasting 1 or 2 days.

Influenza vaccination may carry a very small risk for *Guillain-Barré syndrome* (GBS), a severe paralytic illness. In 1976 swine flu vaccine was associated with GBS. However, there has been no clear link between GBS and influenza vaccines used since then. If there *is* a risk, it is very small, estimated by the CDC to be only about one or two cases per million vaccine recipients—much smaller than the risk posed by severe influenza.

Live attenuated influenza vaccine. LAIV has been given to millions of people since it was first approved in 2003, and reports of serious adverse events have been relatively rare. The most common side effects for all ages are nasal congestion with rhinorrhea, lethargy, headache, sore throat, and decreased appetite.

Precautions and Contraindications

People with an acute febrile illness should defer vaccination until symptoms abate. Minor illnesses (e.g., the common cold), with or without fever, do not preclude vaccination.

Previously, there was great concern for people with hypersensitivity to eggs. The rationale was that vaccines are produced from viruses grown in eggs and hence may contain trace amounts of egg proteins. Although FDA labeling continues to warn against giving such vaccines to people with severe egg allergies, recommendations published in the *Morbidity and Mortality Weekly Report* in August, 2018, state that "persons with a history of egg allergy *of any severity* may receive *any licensed, recommended, and age-appropriate influenza vaccine* (IIV, RIV4, or LAIV4)" (see https://www.cdc.gov/mmwr/volumes/67/rr/rr6703a1.htm). These recommendations come following extensive reviews of vaccine usage by people with reported egg allergies demonstrating that this practice is not as risky as once believed.

Who Should Be Vaccinated?

The ACIP recommends annual vaccination for *all people 6 months of age and older.* Although an annual flu shot is recommended for everyone, an annual shot is especially important for persons at high risk for flu complications and for those who live with or care for persons at high risk. Persons at high risk include the following:

- Children younger than 5 years of age, especially children younger than 2 years
- Children 18 years of age or younger receiving long-term aspirin therapy
- Pregnant women
- People 65 years of age and older
- People who are morbidly obese
- People who live in nursing homes and other long-term care facilities
- Native Americans/Alaskan Natives
- People who are immunosuppressed (e.g., owing to HIV infection or the use of immunosuppressant drugs)
- People with certain chronic medical conditions, including spinal cord injury; asthma; anemia; diabetes; heart, kidney, or lung disease; also those with neurologic disorders, such as epilepsy or cerebral palsy, that can lead to breathing or swallowing problems

TABLE 80.12 Influenza Vaccines

Type of Vaccine	Trade Name	Formulation(s)	Source	Mercury Content[a] (µg/0.5-mL Dose)	Route	Approved Age Group
Inactivated Influenza Vaccine, Quadrivalent (IIV4)	Afluria Quadrivalent	0.5-mL single-dose prefilled syringe	Egg-grown virus	None	IM	3 years and older
		5.0-mL multi-dose vial	Egg-grown virus	24.5	IM	6 months[b] and older (traditional syringe) 18–64 years (jet injector)
	Fluarix Quadrivalent	0.5-mL single-dose prefilled syringe	Egg-grown virus	None	IM	6 months and older
	Flucelvax Quadrivalent	0.5-mL single-dose prefilled syringe	Cell culture–grown virus[c]	None	IM	4 years and older
		5.0-mL multi-dose vial	Cell culture–grown virus[c]	25		
	FluLaval Quadrivalent	0.5-mL single-dose prefilled syringe	Egg-grown virus	None	IM	6 months and older
		5.0-mL multi-dose vial	Egg-grown virus	< 25		
	Fluzone Quadrivalent	0.25-mL single-dose prefilled syringe	Egg-grown virus	None	IM	6–35 months
		0.5-mL single-dose prefilled syringe	Egg-grown virus	None	IM	3 years and older
		0.5-mL single-dose vial	Egg-grown virus	None		
		5.0-mL multi-dose vial	Egg-grown virus	25	IM	6 months and older
	Fluzone Intradermal Quadrivalent[a]	0.1-mL single-dose prefilled microinjection system	Egg-grown virus	None	ID	18–64 years
Inactivated Influenza Vaccine, Trivalent (IIV3)	Afluria	0.5-mL single-dose prefilled syringe	Egg-grown virus	None	IM	3 years and older
		5.0-mL multi-dose vial	Egg-grown virus	24.5	IM	6 months[b] and older (traditional syringe) 18–64 years (jet injector)
	Fluad	0.5-mL single-dose prefilled syringe	Egg-grown virus	None	IM	65 years and older
	Fluzone High-Dose	0.5-mL single-dose prefilled syringe	Egg-grown virus	None	IM	65 years and older
Recombinant Influenza Vaccine, quadrivalent (RIV4)[d]	Flublok Quadrivalent	0.5-mL prefilled syringe	Recombinant hemagglutinin	None	IM	18 years and older
Live Attenuated Influenza Vaccine, quadrivalent (LAIV4)[d]	FluMist Quadrivalent	0.2-mL single-dose prefilled intranasal sprayer	Egg-grown virus	None	INS	2–49 years

[a]Mercury, in the form of thimerosal, is used as a preservative in multi-dose vials of vaccines.
[b]Although Afluria is approved for children as young as 6 months, ACIP recommends avoiding Afluria in children younger than 9 years owing to a possible risk for fever and febrile seizures in younger children.
[c]Flucelvax is grown in dog kidney cells; however, some viruses provided to the manufacturer are grown in eggs, so the CDC does not consider this to be truly egg-free.
[d]Not available in the United States for the 2018–19 influenza season.
ID, Intradermal; *IM*, intramuscular; *INS*, intranasal spray
Adapted from Centers for Disease Control and Prevention. (2018). *Influenza vaccines—United States, 2018–19 influenza season.* https://www.cdc.gov/flu/protect/vaccine/vaccines.htm.

Important note: These people at high risk should receive only the *inactivated* influenza vaccine. They should not receive the live influenza vaccine. Why? Because the safety of the live vaccine has not been adequately evaluated in these populations.

Who Should NOT Be Vaccinated?

As noted earlier, people at high risk for flu complications, including pregnant women, should not receive the *live* influenza vaccine. Instead, they should receive the *inactivated* vaccine. Current recommendations have one contraindication, namely, a severe allergic reaction to influenza vaccine or a vaccine component. Previously, GBS occurring within 6 weeks following vaccine administration was a contraindication for further vaccinations, but the most current guidelines have given this precautionary status. The other precaution is the presence of a moderate to severe acute illness at the time of planned vaccination.

When Should Vaccination Be Administered?

In the United States the influenza "season" begins in November and extends through March or April, but it can also start earlier and last later. It usually peaks in January or February but this may also vary. To ensure full protection, the best time to vaccinate is October or November. However, for people who missed the best time, vaccinating as late as April may be of benefit. Influenza vaccine may be given at the same time as other vaccines, including pneumococcal vaccine.

Antiviral Drugs for Influenza

Antiviral drugs are available for the prevention and treatment of influenza. Three classes are available: adamantanes, neuraminidase inhibitors, and an endonuclease inhibitor.

Adamantanes

The adamantanes—amantadine (Symmetrel) and rimantadine (Flumadine)—were the first influenza drugs available. Although they remain on the market and are approved for influenza infection, most current strains of influenza A are resistant. Because all strains of influenza B are resistant, the CDC recommends against using these drugs for any influenza patients, whether infected with influenza A or influenza B. For this reason these vaccines are not discussed further here.

Neuraminidase Inhibitors

The neuraminidase inhibitors are active against influenza A and influenza B. At this time, three neuraminidase inhibitors are available: oseltamivir, peramivir, and zanamivir. Peramivir (Rapivab) is available only for intravenous delivery. For this reason, most providers do not routinely offer it in nonacute settings. Therefore the following discussion focuses on oseltamivir and zanamivir.

Both oseltamivir and zanamivir are approved for influenza prophylaxis and treatment. Although approved for prophylaxis, these drugs are not as adequate as vaccination and should not be considered as a substitute for annual vaccination against influenza. However, because it takes about 2 weeks after vaccination for antibodies to develop against the influenza virus, oseltamivir can provide some protection for unvaccinated people during a community outbreak. It may also be given to vaccinated people when there are community outbreaks despite widespread vaccination, as can happen when viruses other than those used in vaccine development are responsible for outbreaks.

When used for treatment, dosing must begin early—ideally no later than 2 days after symptom onset and preferably much sooner, because benefits decline greatly when treatment is delayed. When treatment is started within 12 hours of symptom onset, symptom duration is reduced by more than 3 days; when started within 24 hours, symptom duration is reduced by less than 2 days; and when started within 36 hours, symptom duration is reduced by only 29 hours. Unfortunately, in the real world, patients may be unable to obtain and fill a prescription soon enough for the drug to be of significant benefit.

Oseltamivir

Actions and uses. Oseltamivir (Tamiflu) is an oral drug approved for the prevention and treatment of influenza in patients 1 year of age and older. In addition to reducing symptom duration, oseltamivir can reduce symptom severity and the incidence of complications (sinusitis, bronchitis). Because of the harmful effects of influenza on the developing embryo and fetus, the American College of Obstetricians and Gynecologists (ACOG) recommends oseltamivir for both prophylaxis and treatment in pregnant women (see https://www.cdc.gov/flu/professionals/antivirals/avrec_ob.htm).

Antiviral effects derive from inhibiting *neuraminidase,* a viral enzyme required for replication. As a result of neuraminidase inhibition, newly formed viral particles are unable to bud off from the cytoplasmic membrane of infected host cells. Hence viral spread is stopped. Oseltamivir is active against most strains of influenza A and influenza B. Emergence of resistance over the course of treatment is rare.

The pharmacokinetics for oseltamivir and the other antiviral drugs for influenza is presented in Table 80.13. Preparations and dosages are presented in Table 80.14.

Adverse effects and interactions. Oseltamivir has few adverse effects. The most common, occurring in fewer than 10% of people taking the drug, are headache, nausea, and vomiting. Nausea can be reduced by giving oseltamivir with food.

In theory, oseltamivir can blunt responses to LAIV. Accordingly, oseltamivir should be discontinued at least 2 days before giving LAIV. After dosing with LAIV, at least 2 weeks should elapse before starting oseltamivir.

Indications for prophylactic therapy. Candidates for prophylactic therapy include family members of someone with flu and residents of nursing homes. To protect family members, dosing should begin within 48 hours of exposure and should continue for 10 days. To protect residents of nursing homes or high-risk members of the community at large, dosing can be done continuously for up to 42 days.

Zanamivir

Actions and uses. Zanamivir (Relenza), administered by oral inhalation, is approved for treatment of acute uncomplicated influenza in patients at least 7 years of age and for prophylaxis of influenza in patients at least 5 years of age. As with oseltamivir, benefits derive from inhibiting viral neuraminidase, an enzyme required for viral replication. Like oseltamivir, zanamivir is well tolerated except in patients with underlying airway disease. Indications for prophylactic therapy are the same as for oseltamivir. The ACOG recommends zanamivir for pregnant women; however, if there is an option to give oseltamivir, it is preferred (see https://www.cdc.gov/flu/professionals/antivirals/avrec_ob.htm).

Adverse effects and interactions. In patients with healthy lung function, serious adverse effects are uncommon. Because zanamivir is administered as an inhaled powder, patients may experience cough or throat irritation. Also, as with oseltamivir, there have been rare reports of severe allergic reactions and neuropsychiatric effects.

In patients with preexisting lung disorders (e.g., asthma, chronic obstructive pulmonary disease), zanamivir may cause severe bronchospasm and respiratory decline. Some patients have required immediate treatment or hospitalization. Deaths have occurred. However, given the effect of flu itself on lung function, it is not clear that zanamivir was

TABLE 80.13 Pharmacokinetics: Antiviral Drugs for Influenza and Respiratory Syncytial Virus Infection

Drugs	Peak	Protein Binding	Metabolism	Half-Life	Elimination
Drugs for Influenza Treatment and Prophylaxis					
Oseltamivir (Tamiflu)	Unavailable	42% Active metabolite: 3%	Hepatic	1–3 h Active metabolite: 6–10 h	Urine
Zanamivir (Zanamivir)	1–2 h	<10%	None	2.5–5 h	Urine
Baloxavir marboxil (Xofluza)	4 h	93%–94%	Hepatic	79 h	Feces Feces (80%) Urine
Drugs for Respiratory Syncytial Virus Infection Prophylaxis					
Palivizumab (Synagis)ᵃ	Unavailable	Unavailable	Unavailable	20 days	Unavailable

ᵃFDA labeling and other sources have limited information on pharmacokinetics on this newly approved drug.

TABLE 80.14 Preparation, Dosage, and Considerations for Antiviral Drugs for Influenza and Respiratory Syncytial Virus Infection

Drug Class and Drugs	Preparation	Dosage	Considerations
Neuraminidase Inhibitors			
Oseltamivir (Tamiflu)	Oral suspension: 6 mg/mL Capsule: 30 mg, 45 mg, 75 mg	Treatment: 75 mg twice daily Prophylaxis: 75 mg once daily for length of exposure	Treatment: Should be taken within 48 h of symptom onset.
Zanamivir (Relenza)	Diskhaler: 5 mg each	Treatment: Two inhalations twice daily Prophylaxis: Two inhalations once daily	Treatment: Should be taken within 48 h of symptom onset. Inhalations should be every 12 h except for initiation of treatment when they should be given about 2 h apart. Prophylaxis: Duration of treatment should continue until 7 days after last exposure (home use) or last illness identified (institutional outbreak)
Endonuclease Inhibitor			
Baloxavir marboxil (Xofluza)	20 mg, 40 mg	40–79 kg: one dose of 40 mg 80 kg and above: one dose of 80 mg	Should be taken within 48 h of symptom onset
Monoclonal Antibody			
Palivizumab (Synagis)	Solution for IM injection: 50 mg/mL, 100 mg/mL	15 mg/kg once monthly	Dosing should commence before the RSV season and continue until the season ends.

the cause. Nonetheless, owing to the potential risk, zanamivir is not recommended for patients with underlying airway disease.

Zanamivir appears to be devoid of drug interactions. However, like oseltamivir, zanamivir may blunt responses to LAIV and hence should be stopped 2 days before giving LAIV; it should not be started for 2 weeks after giving LAIV.

Endonuclease Inhibitor
Baloxavir Marboxil

Actions and uses. Baloxavir marboxil (Xofluza), the newest antiviral drug against influenza, received FDA approval for the treatment of influenza in 2018. It may be used in patients 12 years of age and older when symptoms have been present for 2 days or less. It is active against both influenza A and influenza B viruses. In clinical trials, symptoms were relieved within 54 hours for those taking the drug compared to 80 hours for those taking a placebo.

Baloxavir marboxil is a prodrug. After administration, it is converted to its active metabolite, baloxavir, which inhibits the activity of a protein required for viral gene transcription. By inhibiting transcription, it prevents viral replication

Adverse effects and interactions. Adverse effects are uncommon. Only five symptoms were noted in clinical trials: diarrhea (3%), bronchitis (2%), nausea, nasopharyngitis, and headache (all 1%). Of note, those taking the placebo experienced these in higher percentages for diarrhea (5%), bronchitis (4%), and headache (2%).

Baloxavir marboxil should not be administered with salts (e.g., calcium salts, iron salts, magnesium salts). Administration with LAIV may decrease the effectiveness of the vaccination. Though not yet tested with inactivated vaccines, similar results may be anticipated. At this time we there are not enough data to adequately determine safety during pregnancy, breastfeeding, use in children younger than 12 years of age, or use in adults above 65 years of age.

Drugs for the Prophylaxis of Respiratory Syncytial Virus

Respiratory syncytial virus (RSV) infection is a major cause of lower respiratory tract disease. Symptomatic infection with RSV is most likely in the very young, older adults, and persons with disorders involving the respiratory tract, heart, or immune system. In the United States, RSV infection is the most common cause of lower respiratory tract disease in infants and young children, leading to between 132,000 and 172,000 hospitalizations each year. Among children 5 years of age and younger, RSV is a leading cause of viral death. Like influenza, infection with RSV is seasonal, with most cases occurring during the winter months. Only one drug, palivizumab (Synagis) is currently approved for RSV prophylaxis in the United States.

Palivizumab

Actions and uses. Palivizumab (Synagis) is a monoclonal antibody indicated for preventing RSV infection in premature infants and in young children with chronic lung disease. The antibody binds to a surface protein on RSV and thereby prevents replication. In clinical trials, the rate of hospitalization was 1.8% for premature infants treated with palivizumab compared with 8.1% for those receiving placebo. In young children with chronic lung disease, the hospitalization rate was 7.9% for those receiving the antibody versus 12.8% for those receiving placebo. Additional information on monoclonal antibodies is available in Chapter 84.

Dosing should commence before the RSV season (December through March in the United States) and continue until the season ends. The cost for a full season of treatment is about $7000. However, although this seems high, it could save more than $50,000 by avoiding hospitalization.

Adverse effects. Except for hypersensitivity reactions, which are rare, palivizumab appears to be devoid of significant adverse effects. Acute hypersensitivity reactions have occurred with initial drug use and with subsequent use. Very rarely (less than 1 in 100,000 cases), palivizumab has caused anaphylaxis, but only with reexposure, not with the initial dose. If a mild hypersensitivity reaction occurs, cautious use of palivizumab can continue. However, if a severe reaction occurs, the drug should be stopped and never used again. Severe reactions are managed with parenteral epinephrine and supportive care.

81

Antiviral Agents II: Drugs for HIV Infection

In this chapter we discuss drug therapy of infection with the *human immunodeficiency virus* (HIV), the microbe that causes *acquired immunodeficiency syndrome* (AIDS). HIV specialists typically carry out pharmacologic management of HIV/AIDS. Still, because a vast number of people have HIV/AIDS, it is important that all providers be familiar with these drugs and their effects on patients. Because it is unlikely that most reading this chapter will be prescribing these drugs, our focus will be on providing generalized information with a representative prototype for each antiviral classification.

HIV promotes immunodeficiency by killing CD4 T lymphocytes (CD4 T-cells), which are key components of the immune system (see Chapter 54). As a result of HIV-induced immunodeficiency, patients are at risk for opportunistic infections and certain neoplasms.

It is important to appreciate that HIV infection is not synonymous with AIDS, which develops years after HIV infection is acquired. The definition of AIDS, established by the Centers for Disease Control and Prevention (CDC), is a syndrome in which the individual is HIV positive and has either (1) CD4 T-cell counts below 200 cells/mL or (2) an AIDS-defining illness. Included in the CDC's long list of AIDS-defining illnesses are *Pneumocystis* pneumonia, cytomegalovirus retinitis, disseminated histoplasmosis, tuberculosis, and Kaposi sarcoma.

Since being identified as a new disease in 1981, AIDS has become a global epidemic. According to the HIV Surveillance Report published in 2018, in the United States approximately 1.1 million people are now infected and about 50,000 more become infected each year. More than 658,000 have died since the epidemic began. The World Health Organization (WHO) reports that, worldwide, an estimated 36.9 million people are now infected, and approximately 34 million have died; however, there is good news. According to the CDC, in the 6 years between 2008 and 2014, new HIV infections declined by 18% in the United States. Also, according to a United Nations report released in 2014, the number of new HIV infections has declined by 35%, and AIDS-related deaths declined by 42% in the previous decade, owing in large part to more widespread use of HIV drugs.

Therapy of HIV infection has made dramatic advances. Today, standard *antiretroviral therapy* (ART) consists of three or four drugs. These combinations, often referred to as *HAART* (for *highly active antiretroviral therapy*), can decrease plasma HIV to levels that are undetectable with current technology and can therefore delay or reverse loss of immune function, decrease certain AIDS-related complications, preserve health, prolong life, and decrease HIV transmission; however, these benefits have not come without a price: ART is expensive, poses a risk for long-term side effects and serious drug interactions, and must continue lifelong. Accordingly, if treatment is to succeed, patients must be highly motivated and well informed about all aspects of the treatment program. A strong support network is extremely valuable, too.

ART cannot cure HIV infection. Although treatment *can* greatly reduce HIV levels—often rendering the virus undetectable—discontinuation

has consistently been followed by a rebound in HIV replication. Because ART does not eliminate HIV, patients continue to be infectious and must be warned to avoid behaviors that can transmit the virus to others.

Understanding this chapter requires a basic understanding of the immune system. Accordingly, you may find it helpful to read Chapter 54 before proceeding.

PATHOPHYSIOLOGY OF HUMAN IMMUNODEFICIENCY VIRUS INFECTION

Characteristics of Human Immunodeficiency Virus

HIV is a *retrovirus*. Like all other viruses, retroviruses lack the machinery needed for self-replication and are therefore obligate intracellular parasites; however, in contrast to other viruses, retroviruses have positive-sense, single-stranded RNA as their genetic material. Accordingly, to replicate, retroviruses must first transcribe their RNA into DNA. The enzyme employed for this process is viral *RNA-dependent DNA polymerase*, commonly known as *reverse transcriptase*. (The enzyme is called reverse transcriptase to distinguish it from DNA-dependent RNA polymerase, the host enzyme that transcribes DNA into RNA, which is the usual ["forward"] transcription process.) The name *retrovirus* is derived from the first two letters of *reverse* and *transcriptase*.

There are two types of HIV, referred to as HIV-1 and HIV-2. HIV-1 is found worldwide, whereas HIV-2 is found mainly in West Africa. Although HIV-1 and HIV-2 differ with respect to genetic makeup and antigenicity, they both cause similar disease syndromes. Not all drugs that are effective against HIV-1 are also effective against HIV-2.

Target Cells

The principal cells attacked by HIV are *CD4 T-cells* (helper T lymphocytes). As discussed in Chapter 54, these cells are essential components of the immune system. They are required for production of antibodies by B lymphocytes and for activation of cytolytic T lymphocytes. Accordingly, as HIV kills CD4 T-cells, the immune system undergoes progressive decline. As a result, infected individuals become increasingly vulnerable to opportunistic infections, a major cause of death among people with AIDS. HIV targets CD4 T-cells because the CD4 proteins on the surface of these cells provide points of attachment for HIV (see later). Without such a receptor, HIV would be unable to connect with and penetrate these cells. After HIV has infected a CD4 T-cell, the cell dies in approximately 1.25 days. It is important to appreciate that only a few percent of CD4 T-cells circulate in the blood; most reside in lymph nodes and other lymphoid tissues.

In addition to infecting CD4 T-cells, HIV infects *macrophages* and *microglial cells* (the central nervous system [CNS] counterparts of macrophages), both of which carry CD4 proteins. Because macrophages and microglial cells are resistant to destruction by HIV, they can survive

744

despite being infected. As a result, they serve as a reservoir of HIV during chronic infection.

Structure of Human Immunodeficiency Virus

The structure of HIV is very simple. As shown in Fig. 81.1, the HIV *virion* (i.e., the entire virus particle) consists of *nucleic acid* (RNA) surrounded by *core proteins*, which, in turn, are surrounded by a *capsid* (protein shell), which, in turn, is surrounded by a *lipid bilayer envelope* (derived from the membrane of the host cell).

The central core contains two separate but identical single strands of RNA, each with its own molecule of *reverse transcriptase* attached. The RNA serves as the template for DNA synthesis.

The outer envelope of HIV contains *glycoproteins* that are needed for attachment to host cells. Each glycoprotein (gp) consists of two subunits, known as *gp41* and *gp120*. The smaller protein (gp41) is embedded in the lipid bilayer of the viral envelope; the larger protein (gp120) is connected firmly to gp41. (The numbers 41 and 120 simply indicate the mass of these glycoproteins in thousands of daltons.)

Replication Cycle of Human Immunodeficiency Virus

The replication cycle of HIV is shown in Fig. 81.2. The numbered steps listed here correspond to the numbers in the figure.

- *Step 1*—The cycle begins with attachment of HIV to the host cell. The primary connection takes place between *gp120* on the HIV envelope and a *CD4* protein on the host cell membrane. Other host proteins, known as coreceptors, act in concert with CD4 to tighten the bond with HIV. Two of these coreceptors—known as chemokine receptor 5 (CCR5) and CXCR4—are of particular importance. (One drug—maraviroc—blocks HIV entry by binding CCR5.)

- *Step 2*—The lipid bilayer envelope of HIV fuses with the lipid bilayer of the host cell membrane. Fusion is followed by release of HIV RNA into the host cell. (One drug—enfuvirtide—works by blocking the fusion process.)

- *Step 3*—HIV RNA is transcribed into single-stranded DNA by HIV *reverse transcriptase.*

- *Step 4*—Reverse transcriptase converts the single strand of HIV DNA into double-stranded HIV DNA.

- *Step 5*—Double-stranded HIV DNA becomes integrated into the host's DNA, under the direction of a viral enzyme known (aptly) as *integrase.* (The integrase strand transfer inhibitors inhibit this enzyme.)

- *Step 6*—HIV DNA undergoes transcription into RNA. Some of the resulting RNA becomes the genome for daughter HIV virions (step 6a). The rest of the RNA is messenger RNA that codes for HIV proteins (step 6b).

- *Step 7*—Messenger RNA is translated into HIV glycoproteins (step 7a) and HIV enzymes and structural proteins (step 7b).

- *Step 8*—The components of HIV migrate to the cell surface and assemble into a new virus. Before assembly, HIV glycoproteins become incorporated into the host cell membrane (step 8a). In steps 8b and 8c, the other components of the virion migrate to the cell surface, where they undergo assembly into the new virus.

- *Step 9*—The newly formed virus buds off from the host cell. As indicated, the outer envelope of the virion is derived from the cell membrane of the host.

- *Step 10*—In this step, which occurs either during or immediately after budding off, HIV undergoes final maturation under the influence of *protease*, an enzyme that cleaves certain large polyproteins into

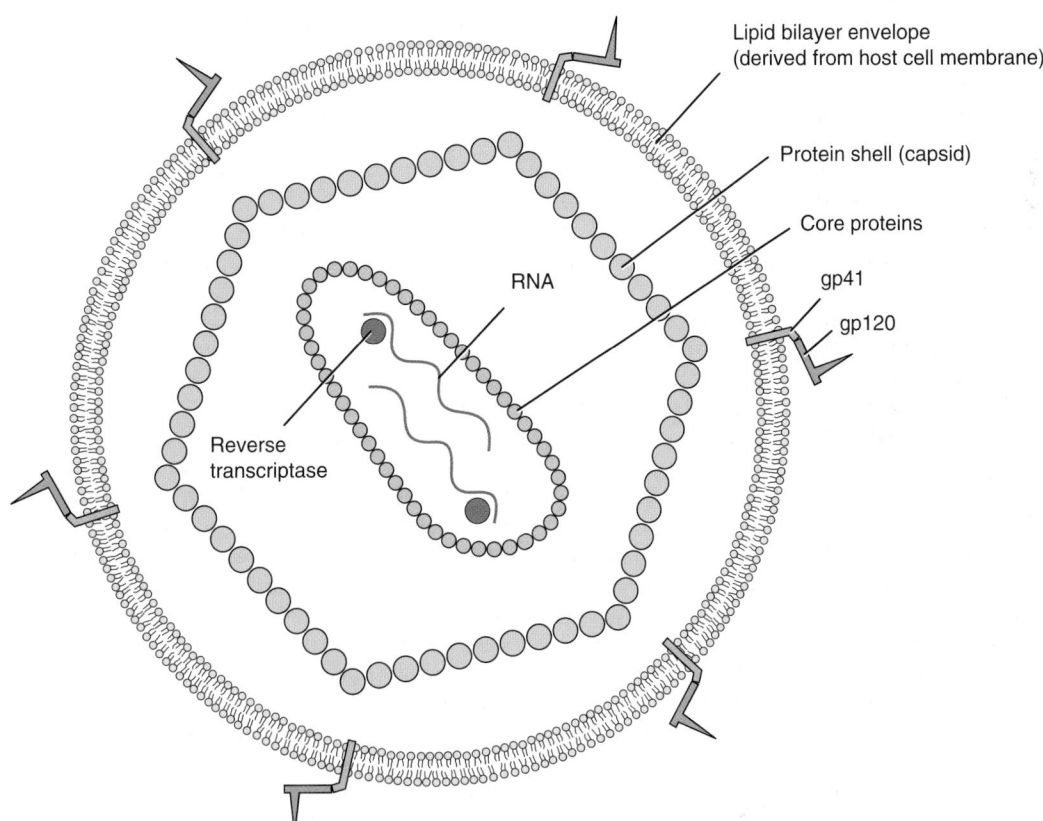

Fig. 81.1 Structure of the Human Immunodeficiency Virus. Note that human immunodeficiency virus has two single strands of RNA and that each strand is associated with a molecule of reverse transcriptase. *gp41,* Glycoprotein 41; *gp120,* glycoprotein 120.

Fig. 81.2 Replication Cycle of the Human Immunodeficiency Virus. See text for description of events. *CCR5*, Chemokine receptor 5 coreceptor; *CD4*, CD4 receptor; *CXCR4*, CXCR4 coreceptor; *dsDNA*, double-stranded DNA; *gp120*, glycoprotein 120; *mRNA*, messenger RNA; *ssDNA*, single-stranded DNA; *ssRNA*, single-stranded RNA.

their smaller, functional forms. If protease fails to cleave these proteins, HIV will remain immature and noninfectious. HIV protease is the target of several important drugs.

Replication Rate

HIV replicates rapidly during *all* stages of the infection. During the initial phase of infection, replication is massive. Why? Because (1) the population of CD4 cells is still large, thereby providing a large viral breeding ground, and (2) the host has not yet mounted an immune response against HIV, so replication can proceed unopposed. As a result of massive replication, plasma levels of HIV can exceed 10 million virions/mL. During this stage of high viral load, patients often experience an *acute retroviral syndrome* (discussed later).

Over the next few months, as the immune system begins to attack HIV, plasma levels of HIV undergo a sharp decline and then level off. A typical steady-state level is between 1000 and 100,000 virions/mL. Please note, however, that steady-state numbers can be deceptive. The plasma half-life of HIV is only 6 hours; that is, every 6 hours, half of the HIV virions in plasma are lost. Accordingly, to maintain the steady-state levels typically seen during chronic HIV infection, the actual

rate of *replication* is between 1 and 10 *billion* virions/day. Despite this high rate of ongoing replication, infected persons typically remain asymptomatic for approximately 10 years, after which symptoms of advanced HIV disease appear.

Mutation and Drug Resistance

HIV mutates rapidly because HIV reverse transcriptase is an error-prone enzyme. Therefore whenever it transcribes HIV RNA into single-stranded DNA and then into double-stranded DNA, there is a high probability of introducing base-pair errors. In fact, according to one estimate, up to 10 incorrect bases may be incorporated into HIV DNA during each round of replication. Because of these errors, HIV can rapidly mutate from a drug-sensitive form into a drug-resistant form. The probability of developing resistance in the individual patient is directly related to the total viral load; hence the more virions the patient harbors, the greater the likelihood that some will become resistant. To minimize the emergence of resistance, patients must be treated with a combination of antiretroviral drugs. This is the same strategy we employ to prevent emergence of resistance when treating tuberculosis (see Chapter 77).

Transmission of Human Immunodeficiency Virus

HIV is transmitted by body fluids from an infected person. This transmission can occur by sexual contact, transfusion, sharing intravenous (IV) needles, and accidental needle sticks. In addition, HIV can be transmitted to the fetus by an infected mother, usually during the perinatal period.

Clinical Course of Human Immunodeficiency Virus Infection

HIV infection follows a triphasic clinical course. During the initial phase, HIV undergoes massive replication, causing blood levels of HIV to rise very high. As a result, between 50% and 90% of patients experience a flu-like *acute retroviral syndrome.* Signs and symptoms include fever, lymphadenopathy, pharyngitis, rash, myalgia, and headache (Box 81.1). Soon, however, the immune system mounts a counterattack, causing HIV levels to fall. As a result, symptoms of the acute syndrome fade. Very often, the acute retroviral syndrome is perceived as influenza, so it goes unrecognized for what it really is.

The middle phase of HIV infection is characterized by prolonged *clinical latency* lasting approximately 10 years. During this time, blood levels of HIV remain relatively low, and most patients are asymptomatic. HIV continues to replicate, however, and CD4 T-cells undergo progressive decline.

During the late phase of HIV infection, CD4 T-cells drop below a critical level (200 cells/mL), rendering the patient highly vulnerable to opportunistic infections and certain neoplasms (e.g., Kaposi sarcoma). The late phase is when AIDS occurs.

Many patients with HIV infection experience neurologic complications. Both the peripheral and CNSs may be involved. *Peripheral neuropathies* affect 20% to 40% of patients and may develop at any time over the course of HIV infection. In contrast, *CNS complications* usually occur late in the disease. Symptoms of CNS injury include decreased cognition, reduced concentration, memory loss, mental slowness, and motor complaints (e.g., ataxia, tremors). Neuronal injury may be the direct result of HIV infection or may develop secondary to an opportunistic infection in the CNS.

ANTIRETROVIRAL DRUGS

Drug Interactions

Before we begin our discussion of the different classes of antiretroviral drugs, it will be wise to explore a topic of great concern. Drug interactions are common and significant with these drugs. Many are inducers or inhibitors of one or more (and sometimes many) CYP450 isoenzymes and many are also substrates of one or more of these. As a result, interactions are common. Some drugs have the same adverse effect; therefore giving them together can intensify an effect so that it becomes dangerous. Moreover, patients with HIV infection, especially those with advanced infection and AIDS, often take drugs for multiple other illnesses and infections. When we consider all the various combinations of these drugs plus drugs taken for other conditions and illnesses that the patient may have, the possibility of dangerous drug interactions increases dramatically. Although we provide the most common or concerning drug interactions, we recognize that simple lists of common drug interactions are inadequate to address this issue.

Every provider needs access to reliable drug interaction software that is capable of simultaneously checking for interactions among multiple drugs. These are widely available online and as downloads for mobile devices.

Classification of Antiretroviral Drugs

At this time, we have five classes of antiretroviral drugs. Three types—*reverse transcriptase inhibitors, integrase strand transfer inhibitors* (INSTIs), and *protease inhibitors* (PIs)—inhibit enzymes required for HIV replication. The other two types—*fusion inhibitors* and *CCR5 antagonists*—block viral entry into cells. As discussed later, the reverse transcriptase inhibitors are subdivided into two groups: *nucleoside/ nucleotide reverse transcriptase inhibitors* (NRTIs), which are structural analogs of nucleosides or nucleotides; and (2) *nonnucleoside reverse transcriptase inhibitors* (NNRTIs). Drugs that belong to these groups are shown in Table 81.1.

BOX 81.1   Acute Retroviral Syndrome: Associated Signs and Symptoms

- Fever (96%)
- Lymphadenopathy (74%)
- Pharyngitis (70%)
- Rash and mucocutaneous ulceration (70%)
- Erythematous maculopapular rash with lesions on face and trunk and sometimes extremities, including palms and soles
- Mucocutaneous ulceration involving mouth, esophagus, or genitals
- Myalgia or arthralgia (54%)
- Diarrhea (32%)
- Headache (32%)
- Nausea and vomiting (27%)
- Hepatosplenomegaly (14%)
- Weight loss (13%)
- Thrush (12%)
- Neurologic symptoms (12%)
- Meningoencephalitis or aseptic meningitis
- Peripheral neuropathy or radiculopathy
- Facial palsy
- Guillain-Barré neuritis
- Brachial neuritis
- Cognitive impairment or psychosis

PROTOTYPE DRUGS

Drugs for HIV Infection

Nucleoside/Nucleotide Reverse Transcriptase Inhibitors
Abacavir

Nonnucleoside Reverse Transcriptase Inhibitors
Efavirenz

Protease Inhibitors
Darunavir

Integrase Strand Transfer Inhibitors
Raletgravir

HIV Fusion Inhibitors
Enfuvirtide

Chemokine Receptor 5 Antagonists
Maraviroc

TABLE 81.1 Classification of Antiretroviral Drugs

Generic Name	Trade Name	Abbreviation
DRUGS THAT INHIBIT HIV ENZYMES		
Nucleoside/Nucleotide Reverse Transcriptase Inhibitors (NRTIs)		
Single-Drug Products		
Abacavir	Ziagen	ABC
Didanosine	Videx	ddI
Emtricitabine	Emtriva	FTC
Lamivudine	Epivir	3TC
Stavudine	Zerit	d4T
Tenofovir	Viread	TDF
Zidovudine	Retrovir	ZDV
Nonnucleoside Reverse Transcriptase Inhibitors (NNRTIs)		
Delavirdine	Rescriptor	DLV
Doravirine	Pifeltro	DOR
Efavirenz	Sustiva	EFV
Etravirine	Intelence	ETR
Nevirapine	Viramune	NVP
Rilpivirine	Edurant	RPV
Protease Inhibitors		
Atazanavir	Reyataz	ATV
Darunavir	Prezista	DRV
Fosamprenavir	Lexiva, Telzir ✦	FPV
Indinavir	Crixivan	IDV
Nelfinavir	Viracept	NFV
Ritonavir	Norvir	RTV
Saquinavir	Invirase	SQV
Tipranavir	Aptivus	TPV
Lopinavir/ritonavir	Kaletra	LPV/r
Integrase Strand Transfer Inhibitor		
Raltegravir	Isentress	RAL
Dolutegravir	Tivicay	DTG
DRUGS THAT BLOCK HIV ENTRY INTO CELLS		
Fusion Inhibitor		
Enfuvirtide	Fuzeon	T-20
CCR5 Antagonist		
Maraviroc	Selzentry, Celsentri ✦	MVC

Generic Name	Trade Name	Abbreviation
FIXED-DOSE COMBINATIONS		
Abacavir 600 mg Lamivudine 300 mg	Epzicom	ABC/3TC
Abacavir 600 mg Dolutegravir 50 mg Lamivudine 300 mg	Triumeq	ABC/DTG/3TC
Abacavir 300 mg Lamivudine 150 mg Zidovudine 300 mg	Trizivir	ABC/3TC/ZDV
Atazanavir 300 mg Cobicistat[a] 150 mg	Evotaz	ATV/COBI
Bictegravir 50 mg Emtricitabine 200 mg Tenofovir alafenamide 25 mg	Biktarvy	(BIC/TAF/FTC)
Darunavir 800 mg Cobicistat[a] 150 mg	Prezcobix	DRV/COBI
Efavirenz 600 mg Emtricitabine 200 mg Tenofovir DF 300 mg	Atripla	EFV/FTC/TDF
Elvitegravir 150 mg Cobicistat[a] 150 mg Emtricitabine 200 mg Tenofovir AF 10 mg	Genvoya	EVG/COBI/FTC/TAF
Elvitegravir 150 mg Cobicistat[a] 150 mg Emtricitabine 200 mg Tenofovir DF 300 mg	Stribild	EVG/COBI/FTC/TDF
Emtricitabine 200 mg Rilpivirine 25 mg Tenofovir AF 25 mg	Odefsey	FTC/RPV/TAF
Emtricitabine 200 mg Rilpivirine 25 mg Tenofovir DF 300 mg	Complera	FTC/RPV/TDF
Emtricitabine 200 mg Tenofovir AF 25 mg	Descovy	FTC/TAF
Emtricitabine 200 mg Tenofovir DF 300 mg	Truvada	FTC/TDF
Lamivudine 150 mg Zidovudine 300 mg	Combivir	ZDV/3TC
Lopinavir 200 mg Ritonavir 50 mg	Kaletra[b]	LPV/r₁LPV[c]/RTV)

[a]Cobicistat is a CYP3A inhibitor.
[b]Oral solution contains lopinavir 80 mg/ritonavir 20 mg per mL.
[c]Ritonavir-boosted lopinavir.

Nucleoside/Nucleotide Reverse Transcriptase Inhibitors

The NRTIs were the first drugs used against HIV infection. As their name suggests, the NRTIs are chemical relatives of naturally occurring nucleosides or nucleotides, the building blocks of DNA.

The NRTIs are effective against both HIV-1 and HIV-2; however, their activity is greater for HIV-1. The NRTIs are ineffective as monotherapy because resistance develops rapidly. First-line antiretroviral regimens include two NRTIs and one other drug and the availability of combination antiretroviral products has simplified treatment. The fixed-dose combinations are shown in Table 81.1.

Mechanism of Action

All NRTIs are prodrugs that inhibit HIV replication by suppressing synthesis of viral DNA. To do this, they must first undergo intracellular conversion to their active (phosphate) form. In their active form, they act as substrates for reverse transcriptase; however, after they become incorporated into the growing DNA strand, they prevent reverse transcriptase from adding more bases. As a result, all further growth of the DNA strand is blocked. In addition to causing premature strand termination, the activated NRTI competes with natural nucleoside triphosphates for binding to the active site of reverse transcriptase.

Adverse Effects

The NRTIs share a core of adverse effects associated with mitochondrial toxicity. Recall that mitochondria are cellular organelles that take in nutrients and convert them into adenosine triphosphate (ATP) for energy. NRTIs can disrupt synthesis of mitochondrial DNA and can thereby impair mitochondrial function.

Lactic acidosis. A major consequence of mitochondrial impairment is lactic acidosis. Lactic acid accumulates because dysfunctional mitochondria cannot break down lactic acid. Symptoms include nausea, malaise, fatigue, anorexia, and hyperventilation (blowing off carbon dioxide can reduce acidosis). Left untreated, the syndrome can be fatal. Diagnosis is based on lactic acid measurement in arterial blood.

The United States Food and Drug Administration (FDA) requires all NRTIs to carry black box warnings about this possibility, even though it is rare for most. Those for which this is most likely to occur are didanosine and stavudine.

Hepatic steatosis. Hepatic steatosis (fatty degeneration of the liver) and hepatomegaly are also adverse effects of NRTIs. This is also associated with mitochondrial impairment because there is decreased breakdown of fatty acids by mitochondria leading to fatty deposits in the liver.

Other adverse effects. NRTIs may also cause pancreatitis and myopathies, which are likely tied to lactic acidosis. Adverse effects of individual NRTIs are discussed separately.

Drug Interactions

NRTIs have fewer drug interactions than most antiretroviral drugs, in part because most are not metabolized by the P450 enzymes. Interactions of individual drugs are discussed separately.

Individual Nucleoside/Nucleotide Reverse Transcriptase Inhibitors

At this time, seven NRTIs are available: abacavir [Ziagen], didanosine [Videx], emtricitabine [Emtriva], lamivudine [Epivir], stavudine [Zerit], tenofovir [Viread], and zidovudine [Retrovir]. They are commonly identified by assigned abbreviations: abacavir (ABC), didanosine (ddI), emtricitabine (FTC), lamivudine (3TC), stavudine (d4T), tenofovir (TDF), and zidovudine (ZDV).

Pharmacokinetic properties of NRTIs are shown in Table 81.2. Preparation, dosage, and administration are provided in Table 81.3. Significant adverse effects are provided in Table 81.4.

Abacavir

Abacavir [Ziagen] will serve as our prototype for the NRTIs. Abacavir is an analog of guanine, a naturally occurring pyrimidine. It is one of the most commonly used antiretrovirals, especially in combination with lamivudine, another NRTI.

Actions and use. Abacavir is taken up by host cells and then undergoes conversion to its active form, carbovir triphosphate. Carbovir triphosphate then suppresses HIV replication by (1) causing premature termination of the growing DNA strand and (2) competing with natural nucleoside triphosphates for binding to reverse transcriptase. When employed in combination with other antiretroviral drugs, abacavir can decrease viral load, increase CD4 T-cell counts, delay onset of disease symptoms, and reduce symptom severity.

Adverse effects

Lactic acidosis and hepatomegaly with steatosis. There is a relatively small risk for the lactic acidosis and hepatomegaly with steatosis that is associated with all NRTIs. Still, it is important to be alert to this possibility.

Hypersensitivity reactions. Hypersensitivity reactions occur in 5% to 8% of patients treated with abacavir. These reactions, which usually develop during the first 6 weeks of treatment, can cause multiorgan failure and anaphylaxis, and they are sometimes fatal. Symptoms include fever, rash, myalgia, arthralgia, and gastrointestinal (GI) disturbances (nausea, vomiting, diarrhea, abdominal pain). Abacavir hypersensitivity

TABLE 81.2 Pharmacokinetic Properties of Nucleoside/Nucleotide Reverse Transcriptase Inhibitors

Drug Name	Route	Peak	Serum Half-Life	Intracellular Half-Life	Metabolism	Excretion
Abacavir (ABC) [Ziagen]	PO	0.7–1.7 h	1.5 h	12–26 h	Metabolized intracellularly to active form, then hepatic (non-P450)	Urine (primary), feces
Didanosine (ddI) [Videx]	PO	Suspension: 0.25–15 h Capsules: 2 h	1.5 h	> 20 h	Metabolized intracellularly to active form. Further metabolism not studied in humans	Urine
Emtricitabine (FTC) [Emtriva]	PO	1–2 h	10 h	> 20 h	Metabolized intracellularly to active form, then oxidation and glucuronidation	Urine (primary), feces
Lamivudine (3TC) [Epivir]	PO	Taken on empty stomach: ±1 h Taken with food: 3.2 h	5–7 h	18–22 h	Metabolized intracellularly to active form	Urine
Stavudine (d4T) [Zerit]	PO	1 h	1 h	7.5 h	Metabolized intracellularly	Urine
Tenofovir (TDF) [Viread]	PO	On empty stomach: 36–84 min; With high-fat food: 96 to 144 min	17 h	>60 h	Metabolized intracellularly	Urine
Zidovudine (ZDV) [Retrovir]	PO IV	PO: 0.5–1.5 hr	1.1 h	7 h	Metabolized intracellularly to active form, then hepatic by glucuronidation	Urine

hr, Hour(s); *IM*, intramuscular; *IV*, intravenous; *min*, minute(s); *PO*, oral.

TABLE 81.3 Preparation, Dosage, and Administration of Nucleoside/Nucleotide Reverse Transcriptase Inhibitors

Drug Name	Preparation	Typical Adult Dosage[a]	Administration
Abacavir (ABC) [Ziagen]	Tablets: 300 mg Oral solution: 20 mg/mL	300 mg twice daily	Administer with or without food
Didanosine (ddI) [Videx]	ER capsules: 125 mg, 200 mg, 250 mg, 400 mg Oral suspension: 2 g/100 mL, 4 g/200 mL	Capsules: <60 kg: 250 mg once daily >60 kg: 400 mg once daily Solution: <60 kg: 125 mg twice daily >60 kg: 200 mg twice daily	Administer on empty stomach.[b] Swallow capsule whole; do not crush or chew.
Emtricitabine (FTC) [Emtriva]	Oral solution: 10 mg/mL Capsule: 200 mg	Solution: 240 mg once daily Capsule: 200 mg once daily	Administer with or without food.
Lamivudine (3TC) [Epivir]	Oral solution: 5 mg/mL, 10 mg/mL Tablets: 100 mg, 150 mg, 300 mg	150 mg twice daily or 300 mg once daily	Administer with or without food.
Stavudine (d4T) [Zerit]	Oral solution: 1 mg/mL Capsules: 15 mg, 20 mg, 30 mg, 40 mg	<60 kg: 30 mg every 12 h ≥60 kg: 40 mg every 12 h	Administer with or without food. Capsule can be opened and contents sprinkled in water.
Tenofovir (TDF) [Viread]	Powder: 40 mg/g Tablets: 150 mg, 200 mg, 250 mg, 300 mg	300 mg once daily	Administer with or without food. Powder may be mixed with food but it is bitter. Will not dissolve in water.
Zidovudine (ZDV) [Retrovir]	Oral syrup: 50 mg/5 mL Tablets: 300 mg Capsules: 100 mg IV solution: 10 mg/mL	PO: 300 mg every 12 h IV: 1 mg/kg administered every 4 h	Oral: Administer with or without food IV: Infuse over 1 h

[a]These are representative manufacturer recommendations for HIV treatment (not prophylaxis). In practice, dosage is individualized.
[b]Food decreases serum levels by 55%.
ER, Extended release.

reactions can also manifest initially as respiratory symptoms (e.g., pharyngitis, dyspnea, cough).

A specific genetic variation, known as HLA-B*5701, is strongly associated with abacavir hypersensitivity; therefore all candidates for abacavir should be screened for this variation before starting therapy. Those who test negative are less likely to experience hypersensitivity but should be counseled about the symptoms of the reaction.

Myocardial infarction. There has been some controversy regarding an association between abacavir and myocardial infarction (MI). After analyzing 26 randomized controlled trials, the FDA found no statistically significant association between MI and abacavir-containing regimens. (See https://www.fda.gov/Drugs/DrugSafety/ucm245164.htm) Still, others have expressed a need for more rigorous research. Therefore if a patient has a history of coronary artery disease, some experts recommend using another drug.

Other adverse effects. Approximately 10% of patients experience fatigue and headache. Lipodystrophy with redistribution of adipose tissue may occur. The outcome is a Cushingoid appearance with truncal obesity, thin extremities, and a fat pad at the base of the neck.

Contraindications. Patients who test positive for HLA-B*5701 should never receive abavacir. This should also be noted on their allergy list.

Drug interactions. Alcohol can compete with abacavir for metabolism by alcohol dehydrogenase. This can thereby increase abacavir levels substantially.

Nonnucleoside Reverse Transcriptase Inhibitors

The NNRTIs differ from the NRTIs in structure and mechanism of action. As their name suggests, the NNRTIs have no structural relationship with naturally occurring nucleosides. Also, unlike NRTIs, the NNRTIs are only active against HIV-1. In practice, they are usually combined with an NRTI.

PATIENT-CENTERED CARE ACROSS THE LIFE SPAN

Nucleoside Reverse Transcriptase Inhibitors

Life Stage	Considerations or Concerns
Children	Both stavudine and zidovudine are approved for neonates. Abacavir and lamivudine are approved for infants as young as 3 months. Tenofovir is approved for children age 2 and older. Didanosine is approved for children 6 years and older weighing at least 20 kg.
Pregnant women	Antiretroviral therapy is recommended for all HIV-infected pregnant women to lower the viral load and decrease the risk of perinatal transmission. The choice of antiretroviral drug for the pregnant woman must consider not only the risk for harm to the fetus from the drug but also the risk for harm to the fetus from the adverse effects tied to the drug. Didanosine, emtricitabine, and tenofovir are associated with less risk than lamivudine, stavudine, and zidovudine. Less is known about abacavir, but there are currently no known long-term adverse effects to the fetus despite a high level of placental transfer. Combined NRTIs during pregnancy increase the risk for lactic acidosis, which can be life threatening.
Breastfeeding women	Breastfeeding should be avoided by women with HIV because there is a danger of transmitting the virus.
Older adults	Older patients taking didanosine have a higher risk for developing pancreatitis than younger patients. Peripheral neuropathy may be increased for older patients taking stavudine.

TABLE 81.4 Significant Adverse Effects of Nucleoside/Nucleotide Reverse Transcriptase Inhibitors

Drug	Adverse Effect
Abacavir (ABC) [Ziagen]	Lactic acidosis,[a] severe hepatomegaly with steatosis,[a] severe hypersensitivity reactions,[a] headache, nausea, vomiting, fatigue, malaise, sleep disorders
Didanosine (ddI) [Videx]	Lactic acidosis,[a] severe hepatomegaly with steatosis,[a] severe pancreatitis,[a] hepatotoxicity,[b] noncirrhotic portal hypertension,[b] immune reconstitution syndrome,[b] redistribution of adipose tissue,[b] peripheral neuropathy,[b] retinal disorders and/or optic neuritis,[b] headache, nausea, vomiting, rash
Emtricitabine (FTC) [Emtriva]	Lactic acidosis,[a] severe hepatomegaly with steatosis,[a] hepatitis B exacerbations,[a] immune reconstitution syndrome,[b] redistribution of adipose tissue,[b] headache, nausea, fatigue, malaise, weakness, sleep disorders, depression, rash, dermal hyperpigmentation, rhinitis, cough, abdominal discomfort, diarrhea
Lamivudine (3TC) [Epivir]	Lactic acidosis,[a] severe hepatomegaly with steatosis,[a] hepatitis B exacerbations,[a] risk for HIV-1 resistance if used in a patient with untreated HIV-1 infection,[a] ENT infections, sore throat, diarrhea
Stavudine (d4T) [Zerit]	Lactic acidosis,[a] severe hepatomegaly with steatosis,[a] severe pancreatitis,[a] hepatotoxicity,[b] immune reconstitution syndrome,[b] redistribution of adipose tissue,[b] neurologic symptoms (e.g., motor weakness, peripheral neuropathy),[b] headache, nausea, vomiting, rash, diarrhea
Tenofovir (TDF) [Viread]	Lactic acidosis,[a] severe hepatomegaly with steatosis,[a] hepatitis B exacerbations,[a] immune reconstitution syndrome,[b] redistribution of adipose tissue,[b] renal impairment,[b] decreased bone mineral density,[b] headache, nausea, weakness, depression, rash, diarrhea
Zidovudine (ZDV) [Retrovir]	Lactic acidosis,[a] severe hepatomegaly with steatosis,[a] severe anemia and neutropenia,[a] serious myopathy and myositis,[a] immune reconstitution syndrome,[b] redistribution of adipose tissue,[b] headache, nausea, vomiting, anorexia, malaise, fever, cough

[a]Black box warnings issued.
[b]Warnings issued.
Note: *Immune reconstitution syndrome* describes the paradoxical inflammatory response to and exacerbation of preexisting infections after initiation of antiretroviral therapy. *Redistribution of adipose tissue* results in increased fat deposits in the trunk, abdomen, and dorsocervical region and decreased body fat in the extremities and face.

Mechanism of Action

In contrast to the NRTIs, the NNRTIs bind to the active center of reverse transcriptase enzyme. At this location, the NNRTI causes stereochemical (i.e., changes in the spatial arrangement of atoms forming the structure of molecules). This hampers the ability of nucleosides to bind, which inhibits DNA replication and promotes premature termination of the growing DNA strand.

Adverse Effects

Unlike NRTIs, there are no adverse effects shared by all NNRTIs; however, two of the NNRTIs, efavirenz and rilpivirine, can both cause CNS effects. Table 81.5 provides the significant adverse effects of individual NNRTIs.

PATIENT EDUCATION

Nucleoside/Nucleotide Reverse Transcriptase Inhibitors

Instruct patients to adhere closely to the prescribed dosing schedule. Emphasize the need to avoid taking any over-the-counter drugs or supplements without first checking with the provider to verify safety. Teach patients how to access and use drug interaction checkers.

All NRTIs, except didanosine, may be taken without regard to meals.

Patients taking NRTIs are at risk of lactic acidosis and hepatic steatosis. Inform patients about symptoms—nausea, vomiting, abdominal pain, malaise, fatigue, anorexia, and hyperventilation—and instruct them to report these immediately.

Inform patients that, even when HIV RNA is undetectable, they are still infectious and hence should avoid behaviors that can transmit HIV.

Abacavir

Inform patients of hypersensitivity reactions that are possible with abacavir. Teach them common symptoms—fever, rash, myalgia, arthralgia, nausea, vomiting, diarrhea, abdominal pain, pharyngitis, dyspnea, and cough—and instruct them to report these immediately.

Didanosine

Instruct patients to take didanosine 30 min before meals or 2 h after. Instruct patients taking powdered didanosine to pour the contents of one packet into 4 ounces of water (not fruit juice or any other acid-containing beverage), stir the mixture until the drug dissolves (about 2–3 min), and then drink the solution immediately. Also, inform patients about early signs of neuropathy (numbness, tingling, or pain in hands and feet) and instruct them to report these immediately.

Zidovudine

Instruct patients to report new or worsening symptoms of anemia (e.g., pallor, weakness) or neutropenia (evidence of infection). To prevent exposure to illness, patients should be cautioned to avoid contact with people who are ill and to avoid areas where people may congregate in large numbers.

Drug Interactions

The NNRTIs have multiple drug interactions with commonly used drugs across many drug classes. These vary according to the individual NNRTI in question.

Individual Nonnucleoside Reverse Transcriptase Inhibitors

At this time, six NNRTIs are available: efavirenz [Sustiva], delavirdine [Rescriptor], doravirine [Pifeltro], etravirine [Intelence], nevirapine [Viramune], and rilpivirine [Edurant]. Their assigned abbreviations are efavirenz (EFV), delavirdine (DLV), doravirine (DOR), etravirine (ETR), nevirapine (NVP), and rilpivirine (RPV). Pharmacokinetic properties of the NNRTIs are shown in Table 81.6. Preparation, dosage, and administration are displayed in Table 81.7.

Our discussion continues with an examination of efavirenz. Efavirenz will serve as the prototype for the NNRTIs.

Efavirenz

Efavirenz [Sustiva] is the only NNRTI deemed a preferred agent for treating HIV and so it will serve as the prototype for the NNRTIs. The drug is effective and, because of its long half-life, can be administered once a day. Its principal drawbacks are teratogenicity and transient adverse CNS effects.

Mechanism of action. Efavirenz binds directly to HIV reverse transcriptase and thereby disrupts the active center of the enzyme. As a result, replication is suppressed.

Therapeutic use. Efavirenz is the only NNRTI recommended as first-line therapy for HIV-1 infection. In clinical trials, the combination of efavirenz plus two NRTIs (zidovudine and lamivudine) was at least as effective as indinavir (a PI) combined with the same two NRTIs. Furthermore, the efavirenz-based regimen was better tolerated. Because efavirenz crosses the blood-brain barrier, it can reduce HIV levels in the CNS, making it particularly useful in patients with CNS complications.

Adverse effects

CNS effects. *CNS symptoms* occur in more than 50% of patients. The most common are dizziness, insomnia, impaired consciousness, drowsiness, vivid dreams, and nightmares. Delusions, hallucinations, and severe acute depression may also occur, primarily in patients with a history of mental illness or drug abuse. Patients who experience these severe reactions should discontinue the drug. CNS symptoms are prominent at the onset of treatment but generally resolve within 2 to 4 weeks, despite continuous drug use.

Rash. *Rash*, which can be severe, occurs often. In clinical trials, rash developed in 27% of adults and 40% of children. The median time to rash onset was 11 days, and the median duration was 14 days. Rash can range in severity from mild (erythema, pruritus) to moderate (diffuse maculopapular rash, dry desquamation) to severe (vesiculation, moist desquamation, ulceration). Very rarely, rash evolves into potentially fatal Stevens-Johnson syndrome, erythema multiforme, or toxic epidermal necrolysis. Accordingly, if severe rash occurs, efavirenz should be withdrawn immediately. Mild rash may respond to antihistamines and topical glucocorticoids.

Teratogenicity. Efavirenz is teratogenic. In monkeys, doses equivalent to those used in humans produced a high incidence of fetal malformation. Women using the drug must avoid getting pregnant, so two methods of birth control, such as a barrier method (e.g., condom) in conjunction with a hormonal method (e.g., oral contraceptive), should be used. Pregnancy must be ruled out before efavirenz is used.

Other adverse effects. Efavirenz may pose a risk of *liver damage.* Liver enzymes should be monitored, especially in patients with hepatitis B or C.

Hyperlipidemia may occur. Interestingly, drug screens of people taking efavirenz may show a false positive result for cannabinoids and benzodiazepines.

Drug interactions. Efavirenz is a substrate, inhibitor, and inducer of several cytochrome P450 enzymes. Because of this role, it has many drug interactions.

Efavirenz is metabolized by CYP2B6 (primarily), CYP3A4, and CYP2A6. Accordingly, drugs that are inducers of these enzyme systems may decrease efavirenz levels and drugs that are inhibitors of these enzyme systems may increase efavirenz levels.

Efavirenz *induces* CYP3A4 and CYP2B6 enzymes. It can thereby accelerate its own metabolism as well as the metabolism of drugs that are CYP3A4 substrates. Increased metabolism of two PIs—saquinavir and indinavir—is of particular concern. If efavirenz is combined with indinavir, the dosage of indinavir should be increased. Combined use with saquinavir, a drug with low bioavailability, should be avoided.

By inducing these P450 enzymes, efavirenz can decrease the effects of *hormonal contraceptives*, including oral contraceptives and the contraceptive implants. Contraceptive failure can result. Since efavirenz is teratogenic, it is essential that women of child-bearing potential use a barrier contraceptive in addition to any hormonal contraceptive.

TABLE 81.5 Significant Adverse Effects of Nonnucleoside Reverse Transcriptase Inhibitors

Delavirdine (DLV) [Rescriptor]	Rash ranging from erythema and pruritus (16.7%) to desquamation and ulceration (4.4%), headache, nausea, vomiting, fatigue, weakness, diarrhea
Doravirine (DOR) [Pifeltro]	Immune reconstitution syndrome,[a] fatigue, headache, nausea, abdominal pain, diarrhea
Efavirenz (EFV) [Sustiva]	Rash,[a] hepatotoxicity,[a] severe depression with/without suicidal ideation,[a] nervous system symptoms,[a] convulsions,[a] immune reconstitution syndrome,[a] redistribution of adipose tissue,[a] hyperlipidemia,[a] headache, nausea, vomiting, fatigue, dizziness, impaired concentration, sleep disorders
Etravirine (ETR) [Intelence]	Severe rashes, including Stevens–Johnson syndrome and toxic epidermal necrolysis,[a] peripheral neuropathy
Nevirapine [Viramune] (NVP)	Life-threatening skin reactions,[b] hepatotoxicity,[b] immune reconstitution syndrome,[a] redistribution of adipose tissue[a]
Rilpivirine [Edurant] (RPV)	Rash,[a] hypersensitivity reactions,[a] hepatotoxicity,[a] immune reconstitution syndrome,[a] redistribution of adipose tissue,[a] depression,[a] headache, sleep disorders

[a]Warnings issued.
[b]Black box warnings issued.
Note: *Immune reconstitution syndrome* describes the paradoxical inflammatory response to and exacerbation of preexisting infections after initiation of antiretroviral therapy. *Redistribution of adipose tissue* results in increased fat deposits in the trunk, abdomen, and dorsocervical region and decreased body fat in the extremities and face.

TABLE 81.6 Pharmacokinetic Properties of Nonnucleoside Reverse Transcriptase Inhibitors

Drug Name	Route	Peak	Serum Half-Life	Metabolism	Excretion
Delavirdine (DLV) [Rescriptor]	PO	IR: 4 h ER: 24 h	5.8 h	Hepatic by CYP3A and possibly CYP2D6	Urine (primary), feces
Doravirine (DOR) [Pifeltro]	PO	2 h	15 h	Hepatic by CYP3A	Urine (primary), feces
Efavirenz (EFV) [Sustiva]	PO	3–5 h	40–55 h	Hepatic by CYP3A4 and CYP2B6	Feces (primary), urine
Etravirine (ETR) [Intelence]	PO	2.5–4 h	41 h	Hepatic by CYP3A4, CYP2C9, and CYP2C19	Feces (primary, 93.7%), urine
Nevirapine (NVP) [Viramune]	PO	IR: 4 h ER: 24 h	25–30 h	Hepatic by CYP3A4 and CYP2B6	Urine (primary, 80%), feces (10%)
Rilpivirine (RPV) [Edurant]	PO	4–5 h	50 h	Hepatic by CYP3A4	Feces (primary, 85%), urine (6.1%)

ER, Extended release; *hr,* hour(s); *IR,* immediate release; *PO,* oral.

TABLE 81.7   Preparation, Dosage, and Administration of Nonnucleoside Reverse Transcriptase Inhibitors

Drug Name	Preparation	Typical Adult Dosage[a]	Administration
Delavirdine (DLV) [Rescriptor]	Tablets: 100 mg, 200 mg	400 mg 3 times daily	Take with or without food. Swallow 200 mg tablets intact. Can mix 4 × 100 mg tablets in 3 or more ounces of water to produce a slurry
Doravirine (DOR) [Pifeltro]	Tablets: 100 mg	100 mg once daily	Take with or without food
Efavirenz (EFV) [Sustiva]	Capsules: 50 mg, 200 mg Tablets: 600 mg	600 mg once daily, preferably at bedtime	Take on an empty stomach.[b]
Etravirine (ETR) [Intelence]	Tablets: 100 mg, 200 mg	200 mg twice daily	Take following a meal.
Nevirapine (NVP) [Viramune]	Tablets, IR: 200 mg Tablets, ER: 400 mg PO suspension: 100 mg/10 mL	200 mg once daily for 14 days, then either 200 mg twice daily (with IR tablets or oral suspension) or 400 mg once daily (with ER tablets)	Take with or without food.
Rilpivirine (RPV) [Edurant]	Tablets: 25 mg	25 mg once daily	Take with food.

[a]These are representative manufacturer recommendations for HIV treatment (not prophylaxis). In practice, dosage is individualized.
[b]High-fat meals increase plasma levels by 39% with capsules and by 79% with tablets.
ER, Extended release; *IR,* immediate release.

Combining efavirenz with ritonavir (a PI that inhibits CYP3A4) can increase levels of efavirenz. Toxicity may result.

At this point, we have only mentioned efavirenz's activities as a P450 inducer. It is also a CYP2C9 and CYP2C19 *inhibitor.* Drugs that are substrates for these enzymes may have increased serum levels, and increased adverse effects, if dosage adjustments are not made.

Protease Inhibitors

PIs are active against both HIV-1 and HIV-2. They are among the most effective antiretroviral drugs available. When used in combination with NRTIs, they can reduce viral load to a level that is undetectable with current assays.

As with other antiretroviral drugs, HIV resistance can be a significant problem. Mutant strains of HIV that are resistant to one PI are likely to be cross-resistant to other PIs. In contrast, because PIs do not share the same mechanism as other antiretroviral drugs, cross-resistance between PIs and these drugs does not occur. To reduce the risk for resistance, PIs should never be used alone; rather, they should always be combined with at least one reverse transcriptase inhibitor, and preferably two.

Mechanism of Action

Maturation is necessary for HIV to infect CD4 cells; immature forms are noninfectious. PIs prevent HIV maturation by blocking the HIV enzyme protease.

It may help to look at the process of HIV maturation. When the various enzymes and structural proteins of HIV are synthesized, they are not produced as separate entities; rather, they are strung together in large polyproteins. Protease catalyzes the cleavage of bonds in the polyproteins, thereby freeing the individual enzymes and structural proteins. Once these components have been freed, HIV uses them to complete its maturation. PIs bind to the active site of HIV protease and prevent the enzyme from cleaving HIV polyproteins. As a result, the structural proteins and enzymes of HIV are unable to function, and hence the virus remains immature and noninfectious.

Adverse Effects

There are several adverse effects that all PIs have in common. These include hyperglycemia and the development of diabetes, lipodystrophy (fat redistribution), elevation of serum transaminases, and decreased cardiac conduction velocity. They can also increase bleeding in patients with hemophilia.

Hyperglycemia/diabetes. PIs have been associated with hyperglycemia, new-onset diabetes, abrupt exacerbation of existing diabetes, and diabetic ketoacidosis. Onset typically occurs after 2 months of drug use, but can also develop much earlier. Hyperglycemia can be managed

PATIENT-CENTERED CARE ACROSS THE LIFE SPAN

Nonnucleoside Reverse Transcriptase Inhibitors

Life Stage	Considerations or Concerns
Children	Nevirapine may be given to infants as young as 15 days. Efavirenz is approved for children older than 3 months and weighing at least 3.5 kg. Etravirine may be given to children who are 3 years and older. Safety and efficacy have not been established for rilpivirine and, for delavirdine, safety has not been established for patients younger than 16 years.
Pregnant women	Antiretroviral therapy is recommended for all HIV-infected pregnant women to lower the viral load and decrease the risk of perinatal transmission. Etravirine, nevirapine, and rilpivirine are among the safest drugs in this category. Delavirdine carries a slightly higher risk for complications. Efavirenz is teratogenic. Pregnancy must be ruled out before efavirenz is used. For women capable of becoming pregnant, two forms of contraception are recommended during treatment and for 3 months after treatment is discontinued.
Breastfeeding women	Breastfeeding should be avoided by women with HIV because there is a danger of transmitting the virus.
Older adults	Each drug in this category identified insufficient numbers of older adults in clinical trials. Consider individual patient status regarding cardiac, hepatic, and renal status or comorbidities that may necessitate alternate regimens.

Nonnucleoside Reverse Transcriptase Inhibitors

Explain the need to adhere closely to the prescribed dosing schedule.

Inform patients about signs and symptoms of an evolving hypersensitivity reaction—severe rash, or rash accompanied by fever, malaise, fatigue, blisters, oral lesions, conjunctivitis, facial edema, hepatitis, muscle aches, or joint aches—and instruct them to report these immediately.

Explain to patients that, even when HIV RNA is undetectable, they are still infectious and hence should avoid behaviors that can transmit HIV.

Delavirdine

Inform patients that delavirdine may be taken with or without food. Inform patients who cannot swallow delavirdine tablets whole that they can mix the 100-mg tablets (but not the 200-mg tablets) with 3 or more ounces of water. Advise patients with achlorhydria to take delavirdine with an acidic beverage, such as orange or cranberry juice.

Efavirenz

Inform patients that CNS symptoms typically resolve in 2 to 4 weeks, despite ongoing efavirenz use, and that taking efavirenz at bedtime can minimize CNS effects. Also, inform women about the potential for fetal harm, and instruct them to use effective contraception, preferably a barrier method of birth control (e.g., condom) in conjunction with a hormonal method (e.g., oral contraceptive) unless contraindicated.

Rilpivirine

Instruct patients to contact their provider immediately if they start feeling sad, hopeless, or suicidal.

---

with insulin and oral antidiabetic agents (e.g., metformin). Owing to the possible risk for diabetes, patients should be instructed to report signs of the disease, such as polydipsia (increased fluid intake), polyphagia (increased food intake), and polyuria (frequent urination). In patients with existing diabetes, blood glucose should be monitored closely. In others, blood glucose should be measured at baseline every 3 to 4 months during the first year of treatment, and less frequently thereafter. Although withdrawing PIs may restore normal glucose metabolism, discontinuation is not recommended.

Lipodystrophy. Use of PIs has been associated with redistribution of body fat, sometimes referred to as *lipodystrophy syndrome* or *pseudo-Cushing syndrome (Cushingoid appearance).* Fat accumulates in the abdomen, in the breasts of men and women, and between the shoulder blades at the base of the neck. Fat is lost from the face, arms, buttocks, and legs. The underlying mechanism has not been determined. Although these fat changes resemble those of Cushing syndrome, which is caused by excessive cortisol, elevated cortisol has not been observed. Health risks of the syndrome are unknown, although it can be psychologically distressing. Drug withdrawal may cause symptoms to resolve but is not recommended.

Hyperlipidemia. All PIs can elevate plasma levels of cholesterol and triglycerides. These effects may occur with or without redistribution of fat. Elevation of cholesterol can lead to atherosclerosis and associated cardiovascular events. Elevation of triglycerides can lead to pancreatitis. Changes in plasma lipids can be detected by monitoring lipid levels every 3 to 4 months. Potential interventions for hyperlipidemia include diet, exercise, and lipid-lowering drugs; however, benefits of these interventions have not been established. If lipid-lowering drugs are employed, lovastatin and simvastatin should be avoided because cytochrome P450 inhibition by PIs can cause lovastatin and simvastatin to accumulate to dangerous levels.

Increased bleeding in people with hemophilia. PIs may increase the risk for bleeding in patients with hemophilia. Bleeding typically occurs in the joints and soft tissues, where danger is lower; however, serious bleeds in the brain and GI tract have also occurred. The mean time to increased bleeding is 22 days after the onset of treatment. Patients may need to increase their dosage of coagulation factors.

Elevation of serum transaminases. PIs can increase serum levels of transaminases, indicating injury to the liver. Exercise caution in patients with chronic liver disease (e.g., hepatitis B or C, cirrhosis). Serum transaminases should be measured at baseline and periodically thereafter.

Decreased cardiac conduction velocity. PIs can decrease the speed of cardiac conduction. The most common effect is prolongation of the PR interval; however, studies have shown that this may also lead to bundle branch blocks. This effect may be worsened if patients are taking other drugs that promote this effect, such as β blockers.

Drug Interactions

All PIs are metabolized by cytochrome P450 enzymes, and all PIs can inhibit selected cytochrome P450 enzymes. Typically, they will also induce other enzymes. As a result, PIs can interact with drugs that inhibit or induce P450 enzymes, and with drugs that are substrates for P450 enzymes.

Not all interactions are harmful, of course. By inhibiting selected P450 enzymes, one PI can increase the level of another PI and can therefore intensify therapeutic effects. One PI—*ritonavir* [Norvir]—is routinely combined with other PIs with the specific purpose of increasing the therapeutic effects of the other PI. In this technique, known as *ritonavir boosting,* the dose of ritonavir is low: 100 to 400 mg/day. This dosage is too low to contribute significant antiviral effects but still high enough to inhibit P450 metabolism. Unfortunately, most interactions with PIs are not beneficial.

Individual Protease Inhibitors

Nine PIs are available: atazanavir [Reyataz], darunavir [Prezista], fosamprenavir [Lexiva, Telzir], indinavir [Crixivan], lopinavir with ritonavir [Kaletra], nelfinavir [Viracept], ritonavir [Norvir], saquinavir [Invirase], and tipranavir [Aptivus]. Abbreviations for these are atazanavir (ATV), darunavir (DRV), fosamprenavir (FPV), indinavir (IDV), lopinavir with ritonavir (LPV/r), nelfinavir (NFV), ritonavir (RTV), saquinavir (SQV), and tipranavir (TPV). Pharmacokinetic properties of PIs are shown in Table 81.8. Preparations, dosages, and administration are provided in Table 81.9. Significant adverse effects are provided in Table 81.10.

Darunavir

Darunavir [Prezista] is a second-generation PI with activity against HIV strains that are resistant to other PIs. It will serve as our prototype for this class.

Actions and use. As mentioned, darunavir has more activity against HIV strains that develop resistance to other PIs. Strains resistant to darunavir are generally cross-resistant with all other PIs, except possibly tipranavir. Darunavir is typically boosted with ritonavir and combined with other antiretroviral drugs. The combination can be especially useful in treatment-experienced patients infected with PI-resistant HIV strains.

Adverse effects. Darunavir causes the same adverse effects shared with other PIs (see earlier discussion). Of particular importance for darunavir is hyperlipidemia. As many as 23% to 25% experience elevated cholesterol levels with associated increases in low-density lipoprotein cholesterol and triglycerides. On the other hand, the hyperglycemia that occurs with all PIs occurs less often with darunavir.

TABLE 81.8 Pharmacokinetic Properties of Protease Inhibitors

Drug Name	Route	Peak	Serum Half-Life	Metabolism	Excretion
Atazanavir (ATV) [Reyataz]	PO	2–3 h	7 h	Hepatic, primarily by CYP3A	Feces (primary), urine
Darunavir (DRV) [Prezista]	PO	2.5–4 h	15 h (with ritonavir)	Hepatic by CYP3A	Feces (primary), urine
Fosamprenavir (FPV) [Lexiva, Telzir]	PO	1.5–4 h	7.7 h	GI metabolism to amprenavir; hepatic metabolism primarily by CYP3A4	Feces (primary), urine
Indinavir (IDV) [Crixivan]	PO	0.5–1.1 h	1.5–2 h	Hepatic by CYP3A4	Feces (primary), urine
Lopinavir/Ritonavir (LPV/r) [Kaletra]	PO	4 h	5–6 h	Hepatic by CYP3A4	Feces (primary), urine
Nelfinavir (NFV) [Viracept]	PO	2–4 h	3.5–5 h	Hepatic by CYP2C19 and CYP3A4	Feces (primary), urine
Ritonavir (RTV) [Norvir]	PO	2 h (taken on empty stomach) 4 h (taken with food)	3–5 h	Hepatic by CYP3A4 and CYP2D6	Feces (primary), urine
Saquinavir (SQV) [Invirase]	PO	NA[a]	1–2 h	Hepatic by CYP3A4	Feces (primary), urine
Tipranavir (TPV) [Aptivus]	PO	3 h	6 h	Hepatic by CYP3A4	Feces (primary), urine

[a]Information not provided in product labeling.
ER, Extended release; *hr*, hour(s); *IM*, intramuscular; *IR*, immediate release; *IV*, intravenous; *min*, minute(s); *NA*, not available; *PO*, oral.

TABLE 81.9 Preparation, Dosage, and Administration of Protease Inhibitors

Drug Name	Preparation	Typical Adult Dosage[a]	Administration
Atazanavir (ATV) [Reyataz]	PO powder packet: 50 mg Capsules: 150 mg, 200 mg, 300 mg	300 mg once daily (with other drugs)	Administer with food. Mix powder with food or liquid. Swallow capsules whole.
Darunavir (DRV) [Prezista]	PO Suspension: 100 mg/mL Tablets: 75 mg, 150 mg, 600 mg, 800 mg	600 mg twice daily (with other drugs) 800 mg once daily (with other drugs)	Administer with food and ritonavir.
Fosamprenavir (FPV) [Lexiva, Telzir]	PO suspension: 50 mg/mL (225 mL) Tablets: 700 mg	1400 mg once daily (with other drugs) 700 twice daily (with other drugs)	Administer with food and ritonavir (recommended); otherwise, administer on empty stomach
Indinavir (IDV) [Crixivan]	Capsules: 200 mg, 400 mg	800 mg every 8 h	Administer on empty stomach or light meal. Administer with food if taken with ritonavir
Lopinavir/Ritonavir (LPV/r) [Kaletra]	PO solution: Lopinavir 80 mg/ ritonavir 20 mg/mL Tablets: Lopinavir 100 mg/ritonavir 25 mg Lopinavir 200 mg/ritonavir 50 mg	400 mg/100 mg twice daily 800 mg/200 mg once daily	Solution: Administer with food. Tablets: Administer with or without food. Swallow whole.
Nelfinavir (NFV) [Viracept]	Tablets: 250 mg, 625 mg	750 mg 3 times daily 1250 mg twice daily (with other drugs)	Administer with foods. Tablets may be crushed and added to soft food or dissolved in liquids.
Ritonavir (RTV) [Norvir]	PO solution: 80 mg/mL EC Tablets: 100 mg Capsules: 100 mg	600 mg twice daily	Administer with food. Swallow tablets whole.
Saquinavir (SQV) [Invirase]	Tablets: 500 mg Capsules: 200 mg	1000 mg twice daily (with other drugs)	Administer 2 h after meals with ritonavir. Capsules may be opened and mixed with food. (Manufacturer recommends syrup or jam.)
Tipranavir (TPV) [Aptivus]	PO solution: 100 mg/mL Capsules: 250 mg	200 mg twice daily 500 mg twice daily	Administer with food and ritonavir.

[a]These are a sampling of representative manufacturer recommendations for HIV treatment (not prophylaxis). In practice, dosage is individualized.
EC, Enteric-coated; *ER*, extended release; *IR*, immediate release; *PO*, oral.

Approximately 10% of patients taking this drug develop a rash. Darunavir has a sulfonamide component that may be a contributing factor; however, other factors are likely also involved.

Other common adverse effects include nausea, diarrhea, and headache. When administered with cobicistat, increases in serum creatinine have occurred.

Drug interactions. Darunavir is both a CYP3A4 substrate and inhibitor. It is also a CYP2C9 inducer. Because these two enzyme systems are responsible for the metabolism of so many drugs, the number of drug interactions is *extensive*. For patients with HIV infection, the following drugs included in product labeling present special concerns.

Darunavir can increase serum levels of several antiretroviral drugs, including maraviroc and indinavir. Darunavir can decrease serum levels of the antiretroviral drug abacavir.

Darunavir levels may also be affected by co-administration of antiretroviral drugs. Indinavir increases darunavir levels; lopinavir/ritonavir and saquinavir decrease darunavir levels.

Darunavir has interactions with two drugs used to treat hepatitis C infection. Co-administration with boceprevir decreases levels of both

TABLE 81.10	Significant Adverse Effects of Protease Inhibitors
Drug	**Adverse Effects**
Atazanavir (ATV) [Reyataz]	Dangerous drug interactions,[a] severe skin reactions,[a] PR interval prolongation,[a] hepatotoxicity,[a] hyperbilirubinemia,[a] kidney stones and gallstones,[a] diabetes (new onset or exacerbation),[a] immune reconstitution syndrome,[a] redistribution of adipose tissue,[a] renewed bleeding in patients with hemophilia,[a] headache, dizziness, nausea, vomiting, abdominal discomfort, fever, rash, peripheral neurologic symptoms, depression, sleep disorders
Darunavir (DRV) [Prezista]	Dangerous drug interactions,[a] severe skin reactions, including SJS and TEN, hepatitis, diabetes (new onset or exacerbation),[b] immune reconstitution syndrome,[b] redistribution of adipose tissue,[b] renewed bleeding in patients with hemophilia,[b] headache, nausea, vomiting, abdominal discomfort, diarrhea, rash
Fosamprenavir (FPV) [Lexiva]	Dangerous drug interactions,[b] severe skin reactions, including SJS and TEN, transaminase elevations (especially in patients with hepatitis B or C),[a] diabetes (new onset or exacerbation),[a] immune reconstitution syndrome,[a] redistribution of adipose tissue,[a] hyperlipidemia,[a] hemolytic anemia,[a] renewed bleeding in patients with hemophilia,[a] kidney stones,[a] headache, nausea, vomiting, diarrhea, rash
Indinavir (IDV) [Crixivan]	Dangerous drug interactions,[a] hepatitis, including reports of liver failure,[a] hyperglycemia or diabetes (new onset or exacerbation),[a] hemolytic anemia,[a] renewed bleeding in patients with hemophilia,[a] kidney stones,[a] hyperbilirubinemia, headache, nausea, vomiting, abdominal pain, back pain
Lopinavir with ritonavir (LPV/r) [Kaletra]	Dangerous drug interactions,[a] hepatotoxicity,[a] pancreatitis,[a] PR interval prolongation,[a] QT interval prolongation,[a] hyperglycemia or diabetes (new onset or exacerbation),[a] immune reconstitution syndrome,[a] redistribution of adipose tissue,[a] hyperlipidemia,[a] renewed bleeding in patients with hemophilia,[a] headache, nausea, vomiting, abdominal discomfort, indigestion, weakness
Nelfinavir (NFV) [Viracept]	Dangerous drug interactions,[a] diabetes (new onset or exacerbation),[a] diarrhea
Ritonavir (RTV) [Norvir]	Dangerous drug interactions,[b] hepatotoxicity,[a] pancreatitis,[a] severe hypersensitivity reactions,[a] PR interval prolongation,[a] hyperlipidemia,[a] diabetes (new onset or exacerbation),[a] immune reconstitution syndrome,[a] redistribution of adipose tissue,[a] renewed bleeding in patients with hemophilia,[a] nausea, vomiting, abdominal discomfort, diarrhea, fatigue, weakness, paresthesias, rash
Saquinavir (SQV) [Invirase]	Dangerous drug interactions (including danger with ritonavir),[a] PR interval prolongation,[a] QT interval prolongation,[a] diabetes (new onset or exacerbation),[a] immune reconstitution syndrome,[a] redistribution of adipose tissue,[a] renewed bleeding in patients with hemophilia,[a] exacerbation of comorbid hepatic disease,[a] hyperlipidemia,[a] nausea, vomiting, abdominal pain, diarrhea, fatigue
Tipranavir (TPV) [Aptivus]	Hepatotoxicity,[b] intracranial hemorrhage,[b] dangerous drug interactions,[a] renewed bleeding in patients with hemophilia,[a] serious rash,[a] hyperglycemia and diabetes (new onset or exacerbation),[a] immune reconstitution syndrome,[a] redistribution of adipose tissue,[a] renewed bleeding in patients with hemophilia,[a] increased bleeding risk in the absence of hemophilia,[a] hyperlipidemia,[a] headache, nausea, vomiting, indigestion, diarrhea

[a]Warnings issued.
[b]Black box warnings issued.
Note: Immune reconstitution syndrome describes the paradoxical inflammatory response to and exacerbation of preexisting infections after initiation of antiretroviral therapy. *Redistribution of adipose tissue* results in increased fat deposits in the trunk, abdomen, and dorsocervical region and decreased body fat in the extremities and face.
SJS, Stevens–Johnson syndrome; *TEN,* toxic epidermal necrolysis.

boceprevir and darunavir. Coadministration with simeprevir increases levels of both drugs.

Darunavir increases levels of β blockers, calcium channel blockers, amiodarone, lidocaine, disopyramide, flecainide, mexiletine, propafenone, and quinidine. This is significant because this can further worsen the decreased conduction velocity that can be an adverse effect of darunavir.

Integrase Strand Transfer Inhibitors
Actions and Use

HIV INSTIs, or simply *integrase inhibitors,* target HIV by terminating the integration of HIV into DNA. Integrase is one of three viral enzymes needed for HIV replication. As its name implies, integrase inserts HIV genetic material into the DNA of CD4 cells. By inhibiting integrase, these drugs prevent insertion of HIV DNA and thereby stop HIV replication. Integrase inhibitors are combined with other antiretroviral agents to treat adults infected with HIV-1.

Adverse Effects

INSTIs have few adverse effects, the most common being dizziness and insomnia. Rarely, and primarily among patients with a history of psychiatric problems, depression and suicidal ideation have occurred.

Rhabdomyolysis and other skeletal muscle complications have occurred and are reflected in elevated creatine phosphokinase levels.

Individual Integrase Strand Transfer Inhibitors

We currently have four approved INSTIs: raltegravir [Isentress], dolutegravir [Tivicay], bictegravir, and elvitegravir. They are often referenced by their abbreviations: raltegravir (RAL), dolutegravir (DTG), bictegravir (BIC), and elvitegravir (EVG). Bictegravir and elvitegravir are only available in combination with other drugs. Pharmacokinetic properties for INSTIs, as well as for the representative drugs in the two categories that follow, are provided in Table 81.11. Preparations, dosages, and administration are available in Table 81.12. Significant adverse reactions are detailed in Table 81.13.

Raltegravir

Actions and use. Raltegravir [Isentress] was the first HIV INSTI to be developed. Raltegravir stops HIV replication by preventing insertion of HIV DNA. Raltegravir is active against HIV strains resistant to some of the other drugs.

Raltegravir was originally approved only for treatment-experienced patients but is now approved for treatment-naïve patients as well. In

PATIENT-CENTERED CARE ACROSS THE LIFE SPAN

Protease Inhibitors

Life Stage	Considerations or Concerns
Children	Lopinavir/ritonavir[a] may be given to infants as young as 14 days. Atazanavir is approved for infants as young as 3 months who weigh at least 5 kg. Fosamprenavir and ritonavir are approved for those older than 4 weeks. Nelfinavir and tipranavir are approved for children aged 2 years. Darunavir may be given to children aged at least 3 years and weighing at least 10 kg. Safety and effectiveness have not been established for use of indinavir to treat children. For saquinavir, safety and effectiveness have not been established for those younger than 16 years.
Pregnant women	Antiretroviral therapy is recommended for all HIV-infected pregnant women to lower the viral load and decrease the risk of perinatal transmission. Nelfinavir, ritonavir, and saquinavir are the safest drugs in this class. Darunavir, fosamprenavir, indinavir, lopinavir/ritonavir, and tipranavir have slightly higher risk profiles. Less is known about atazanavir, but updated labeling reports that there is no evidence that atazanavir causes major birth defects. Labeling emphasizes that atazanavir should be accompanied by ritonavir when prescribed for pregnant women.
Breastfeeding women	Breastfeeding should be avoided by women with HIV because there is a danger of transmitting the virus.
Older adults	Clinical trials did not enroll sufficient numbers of patients 65 years and older to adequately determine comparative responses to younger subjects. Consider hepatic, renal, or cardiac function and comorbidity in monitoring.

[a]Lopinavir/ritonavir oral solution should not be given to preterm infants until 14 days after their *predicted due date*. The solution contains 42% alcohol and 15% propylene glycol, which can accumulate to toxic levels causing potentially fatal cardiac, renal, and respiratory problems.

current guidelines, raltegravir (in combination with tenofovir plus either emtricitabine or lamivudine) is considered a first-choice drug for HIV treatment. In clinical trials, raltegravir demonstrated increased viral suppression when compared to PIs and the NNRTI efavirenz. Unfortunately, HIV resistance was also more likely to develop.

PATIENT EDUCATION

Protease Inhibitors

All PIs can cause hyperglycemia and diabetes. Instruct patients on signs and symptoms.

Forewarn patients that all PIs may cause accumulation of fat on the waist, stomach, breasts, and back of the neck, and loss of fat from the face, arms, buttocks, and legs.

To reduce risk of bone loss, encourage patients to ensure adequate intake of calcium and vitamin D.

Teach patients how to access and use drug interaction checkers. Explain importance of considering interactions for both over-the-counter and herbal supplements. St. John's wort induces P450 and can reduce levels of PIs. Warn patients not to use St. John's wort.

Inform patients that even when HIV RNA is undetectable, they are still infectious and hence should avoid behaviors that can transmit HIV.

Indinavir and fosamprenavir: Inform patients that these drugs may cause kidney stones. Instruct patients to report symptoms: pain in the abdomen, groin, testicles, or side of the back. To decrease the risk for nephrolithiasis, instruct patients to consume at least 48 ounces (1.5 L) of water daily.

Adverse effects. Raltegravir is generally well tolerated by most. The most common adverse effect is an elevation in liver enzymes that occurs in approximately 10% of those taking the drug. Approximately 4% to 5% will have elevations in serum amylase and lipase.

Symptomatic adverse effects occur infrequently; in fact, the most common adverse effects, insomnia and headache, occur in only 2% to 4% of those taking this drug. In clinical trials, a few patients experienced myopathy and rhabdomyolysis, but a causal relationship has not been established.

Rarely, patients have developed *severe hypersensitivity reactions*. Skin reactions include Stevens–Johnson syndrome and toxic epidermal necrolysis, which can be fatal. Organ dysfunction, including liver failure, may also develop. Patients who develop signs of a hypersensitivity reaction (e.g., severe rash, or rash associated with blisters, fever, malaise, fatigue, oral lesions, facial edema, hepatitis, angioedema, muscle or joint aches) should discontinue raltegravir immediately.

Contraindications. There are no contraindications to taking raltegravir. Those with pre-existing hepatic impairment may be at risk for worsening of this condition. Caution should be maintained when taken by patients with a history of rhabdomyolysis or by those taking other drugs that have this adverse effect.

TABLE 81.11 Pharmacokinetic Properties of Integrase Strand Transfer Inhibitors, Human Immunodeficiency Virus Fusion Inhibitors, and Chemokine Receptor 5 Antagonists

Drug Category	Drug Name	Route	Peak	Serum Half-Life	Metabolism	Excretion
Integrase Strand Transfer Inhibitors	Raltegravir (RAL) [Isentress]	PO	3 h	9 h	Hepatic glucuronidation mediated by UGT1A1	Feces (primary), urine
	Dolutegravir (DTG) [Tivicay]	PO	2–3 h	14 h	Metabolism by UGT1A1 (primary) and CYP3A enzymes	Feces (primary), urine
HIV Fusion Inhibitors	Enfuvirtide (ENF) [Fuzeon]	SubQ	3–13 h	3.2–4.4 h	Hepatic and renal by peptidases and proteinases	NA[a]
CCR5 Antagonists	Maraviroc (MVC) [Selzentry, Celsentri ✦]	PO	0.5–4 h	14–18 h	Hepatic by CYP3A enzymes	Feces (primary), urine

[a]Product labeling reports studies to identify elimination route have not been carried out in humans.
ER, Extended release; *hr*, hour(s); *IM*, intramuscular; *IR*, immediate release; *IV*, intravenous; *min*, minute(s); *NA*, not available; *PO*, oral; *SubQ*, subcutaneous.

TABLE 81.12 Preparation, Dosage, and Administration of Integrase Strand Transfer Inhibitors, Human Immunodeficiency Virus Fusion Inhibitors, and Chemokine Receptor 5 Antagonists

Drug Category	Drug Name	Preparation	Typical Adult Dosage[a]	Administration
Integrase Strand Transfer Inhibitors[b]	Raltegravir (RAL) [Isentress]	Packet for PO suspension: 100 mg Chewable tablets: 25 mg, 100 mg EC tablet: 400 mg	400 mg twice daily	Mix packet with 5 mL water to make a suspension. Chewable tablets may be chewed, divided, or swallowed whole. EC tablet must be swallowed whole.
	Dolutegravir (DTG) [Tivicay]	Tablets: 10 mg, 25 mg, 50 mg	50–100 mg once daily (with other drugs)	Administer with or without food.
HIV Fusion Inhibitors	Enfuvirtide (ENF) [Fuzeon]	Solution for injection: 90 mg	90 mg twice daily	Administer subcutaneously. Rotate sites.
CCR5 Antagonists	Maraviroc (MVC) [Selzentry, Celsentri ✦]	Tablets: 25 mg, 75 mg, 150 mg, 300 mg	300 mg twice daily	Administer with or without food.

[a]These are a sampling of representative manufacturer recommendations for HIV treatment (not prophylaxis). Dosage is individualized in practice.
[b]Elvitegravir is omitted because it is no longer available as a single product; it is only available in fixed combination products.
IR, Immediate release; *ER,* extended release; *PO,* oral; *EC,* enteric-coated.

TABLE 81.13 Significant Adverse Effects of Integrase Strand Transfer Inhibitors, Human Immunodeficiency Virus Fusion Inhibitors, and Chemokine Receptor 5 Antagonists

Integrase Strand Transfer Inhibitors

Raltegravir (RAL) [Isentress]	Immune reconstitution syndrome,[a] headache, nausea, insomnia, fatigue, weakness, CK elevation.
Dolutegravir (DTG) [Tivicay]	Neural tube birth defects,[b] immune reconstitution syndrome,[a] hypersensitivity,[a] hepatotoxicity,[a] hyperglycemia, insomnia, CK elevation.

HIV Fusion Inhibitors

Enfuvirtide (T-20) [Fuzeon]	Injection site reactions (98%),[a] hypersensitivity,[a] postinjection bleeding,[a] immune reconstitution syndrome,[a] pneumonia, nausea, diarrhea, fatigue.

CCR5 Antagonists

Maraviroc (MVC) [Selzentry, Celsentri ✦]	Hepatotoxicity,[b] myocardial ischemia or infarction,[a] orthostatic hypotension (in patients with impaired renal function),[a] immune reconstitution syndrome,[a] increased risk for infection,[a] potential risk for malignancy,[a] fever, upper respiratory infections, cough, rash, dizziness.

[a]Warnings issued.
[b]Black box warnings issued.
Note: *Immune reconstitution syndrome* describes the paradoxical inflammatory response to and exacerbation of preexisting infections after initiation of antiretroviral therapy.
CK, Creatine kinase.

Drug interactions. Because raltegravir is metabolized by glucuronidation, it does not have as many drug interactions as those with roles in P450 enzyme systems. Atazanavir and other inhibitors of uridine glucuronyl transferases (UGT) can increase levels of raltegravir. Conversely, inducers of UGT (e.g., efavirenz, fosamprenavir, rifabutin, tipranavir) can lower raltegravir levels.

Human Immunodeficiency Virus Fusion Inhibitors

Unlike most other drugs for HIV, which inhibit essential viral enzymes (i.e., reverse transcriptase, integrase, protease), HIV fusion inhibitors block entry of HIV into CD4 T-cells. Earlier in the chapter, we discussed the replication cycle of HIV. Recall that in step 2, the lipid bilayer envelope of HIV fuses with the lipid bilayer of the host cell membrane. HIV fusion inhibitors block this fusion process.

Enfuvirtide

Enfuvirtide [Fuzeon], widely known as T-20, is the first and only HIV fusion inhibitor approved by the FDA. Unfortunately, although enfuvirtide is effective, it is also inconvenient (treatment requires twice-daily subQ injections) and very expensive (treatment costs approximately $52,000 a year). Furthermore, injection-site reactions (ISRs) occur in nearly all patients.

Mechanism of action. Enfuvirtide prevents the HIV envelope from fusing with the cell membrane of CD4 cells (see Fig. 81.2, step 2) and thereby blocks viral entry and replication. Fusion inhibition results from binding of enfuvirtide to gp41, a subunit of the glycoproteins embedded in the HIV envelope (see Fig. 81.1). As a result of enfuvirtide binding, the glycoprotein becomes rigid and hence cannot undergo the configurational change needed to permit fusion of HIV with the cell membrane.

Resistance. Resistance to enfuvirtide has developed in cultured cells and in patients. The cause is a structural change in gp41. In clinical trials, reductions in drug susceptibility have ranged from 4- to 422-fold. Fortunately, the HIV mutations that confer resistance to enfuvirtide do not confer cross-resistance to NRTIs, NNRTIs, PIs, INSTIs, or CCR5 antagonists. Conversely, resistance to NRTIs, NNRTIs, PIs, INSTIs, or CCR5 antagonists does not confer cross-resistance to enfuvirtide.

The rate at which resistance develops depends on the efficacy of the drugs used concurrently. When the patient's other antiretroviral drugs

PATIENT-CENTERED CARE ACROSS THE LIFE SPAN

Integrase Strand Inhibitors, Human Immunodeficiency Virus Fusion Inhibitors, and Chemokine Receptor 5 Antagonists

Life Stage	Considerations or Concerns
Children	*ISTIs:* Raltegravir is approved for use in infants aged 4 months and older. Dolutegravir is approved for children 12 years and older weighing at least 30 kg. Safety of elvitegravir has not been adequately evaluated for patients under 12 years old. *Fusion inhibitor:* Enfuvirtide is approved for children age 6 and older. *CCR5 Antagonist:* Maraviroc is not indicated for children younger than 16 years because safety and efficacy have not been established.
Pregnant women	Antiretroviral therapy is recommended for all HIV-infected pregnant women to lower the viral load and decrease the risk of perinatal transmission. Dolutegravir, elvitegravir, enfuvirtide, and maraviroc are considered among the safest in these classes. Raltegravir has a slightly higher risk profile.
Breastfeeding women	Breastfeeding should be avoided by women with HIV because there is a danger of transmitting the virus.
Older adults	Clinical trials did not enroll sufficient numbers of patients 65 years and older to adequately determine comparative responses to younger subjects. Consider hepatic, renal, or cardiac function and comorbidity in considering therapy.

PATIENT EDUCATION

Integrase Strand Inhibitors: Raltegravir

Inform patients about signs of a hypersensitivity reaction (e.g., severe rash, or rash associated with blisters, fever, malaise, fatigue, oral lesions, facial edema, hepatitis, angioedema, or muscle or joint aches) and instruct them to discontinue raltegravir immediately and report their occurrence.

are still effective, resistance to enfuvirtide develops relatively slowly; however, when there is significant resistance to the other drugs, resistance to enfuvirtide develops rapidly.

Therapeutic use. Enfuvirtide is reserved for treating HIV-1 infection that has become resistant to other antiretroviral agents. Specifically, the drug is indicated for HIV-1 infection in patients who are treatment experienced and have evidence of HIV replication despite ongoing ART. To delay emergence of resistance, enfuvirtide should always be combined with other antiretroviral drugs.

Adverse effects

Injection-site reactions. In clinical trials, ISRs developed in 98% of patients, usually within the first week of treatment. Principal manifestations are pain and tenderness, erythema and induration, nodules or cysts, pruritus, and ecchymosis (small hemorrhagic spots). Although generally mild to moderate, symptoms can also be severe. In 17% of patients, individual ISRs persisted more than 7 days. Because ISRs are

both common and long lasting, 23% of patients had six or more ongoing ISRs at any given time. The intensity of ISRs can be reduced by rotating the injection site, avoiding sites with an active ISR, and avoiding unnecessarily deep injections. If a severe ISR occurs, or if local infection develops, patients should seek immediate medical attention.

Pneumonia. Enfuvirtide appears to increase the risk for bacterial pneumonia. Patients should be informed about signs of pneumonia (cough, fever, breathing difficulties), and instructed to report them immediately. Enfuvirtide should be used with caution in patients who have pneumonia risk factors: low initial CD4 cell counts, high initial viral load, IV drug use, smoking, and a history of lung disease.

Hypersensitivity reactions. Because enfuvirtide is a foreign peptide, it can trigger hypersensitivity reactions. Typical symptoms, which may occur individually and in combination, are rash, fever, nausea, vomiting, chills, rigors, hypotension, and elevated serum transaminases. Enfuvirtide has also been associated with respiratory distress, glomerulonephritis, Guillain-Barré syndrome, and primary immune complex reaction, all of which may be immune mediated. If a systemic hypersensitivity reaction occurs, enfuvirtide should be discontinued immediately and never used again.

Drug interactions. Enfuvirtide appears devoid of significant drug interactions. There are no interactions with other antiretroviral drugs that would require a dosage adjustment for either enfuvirtide or the other agent.

PATIENT EDUCATION

Human Immunodeficiency Virus Fusion Inhibitors: Enfuvirtide

Inform patients about manifestations of ISRs—pain, tenderness, erythema, induration, nodules, cysts, pruritus, and ecchymosis—and forewarn them that these occur in nearly everyone. Inform patients that they can reduce the risk for a severe ISR by rotating the injection site, avoiding sites with an active ISR, and avoiding unnecessarily deep injections. Instruct patients to promptly report a severe ISR or localized infection.

Explain that the risk for bacterial pneumonia is increased. Inform patients about signs of pneumonia—cough, fever, and breathing difficulties—and instruct them to report these immediately.

Inform patients about signs of hypersensitivity and advise them to report them immediately.

Chemokine Receptor 5 Antagonists

The *CCR5* antagonists, like the fusion inhibitors, block entry of HIV into CD4 T-cells; however, the mechanism by which this is accomplished differs.

Maraviroc

Maraviroc [Selzentry, Celsentri ✦] is the first and, currently, only representative of the CCR5 antagonists. It often appears as its abbreviation MVC. Maraviroc isn't usually used for initial treatment of HIV. It appears most effective in treating patients with drug-resistant HIV.

Mechanism of action. As discussed earlier, CCR5 is a coreceptor that some strains of HIV must bind with to enter CD4 cells. Maraviroc binds with CCR5 and thereby blocks viral entry. HIV strains that require CCR5 for entry are referred to as being *CCR5 tropic*. Between 50% and

60% of patients are infected with this type of HIV. Maraviroc and enfuvirtide (a fusion inhibitor) are the only antiretroviral drugs that block HIV entry.

Therapeutic use. Maraviroc is indicated for combined use with other antiretroviral agents to treat patients age 16 years and older who are infected with CCR5-tropic HIV-1 strains. The drug was originally approved only for treatment-experienced patients but is now approved for treatment-naïve patients as well. Before maraviroc is used, a test must be performed to confirm that the infecting HIV strain is CCR5 tropic.

Adverse effects. The most common side effects are cough, dizziness, pyrexia, rash, abdominal pain, musculoskeletal symptoms, and upper respiratory tract infections. Intensity is generally mild to moderate.

Liver injury has been seen in some patients and may be preceded by signs of an allergic reaction (e.g., eosinophilia, pruritic rash, elevated immunoglobulin E). Patients should be informed about signs of an evolving reaction (itchy rash, jaundice, vomiting and/or abdominal pain), and instructed to stop maraviroc and seek medical attention.

During clinical trials, a few patients experienced *cardiovascular events,* including myocardial ischemia and MI. Maraviroc should be used with caution in patients with cardiovascular risk factors.

Drug interactions. Because maraviroc is metabolized by CYP3A4, drugs that inhibit or induce this enzyme will affect maraviroc levels. Levels will be raised by strong CYP3A4 inhibitors, including PIs (except tipranavir/ritonavir) and delavirdine; conversely, maraviroc levels will be lowered by strong CYP3A4 inducers, including etravirine and efavirenz. As always, it is important to check for interactions via a comprehensive database before administering drugs such as this one.

PATIENT EDUCATION

Chemokine Receptor 5 *Antagonist: Maraviroc*

Teach patients how to access and use drug interaction checkers. Explain the importance of drug-drug interactions and that this includes herbal supplements.

Advise patients that if they forget to take a dose, they should take the missed dose as soon as possible and take the next scheduled dose at its regular time. If the time to the next dose is less than 6 h, the patient should skip the missed dose and take the next dose as scheduled.

Inform patients about signs of an evolving reaction (pruritic rash, jaundice, dark urine, and vomiting and/or abdominal pain) and instruct them to stop maraviroc and seek medical attention.

MANAGEMENT OF HUMAN IMMUNODEFICIENCY VIRUS INFECTION

Thanks to the drugs we have today, HIV infection has been transformed from a near-certain death sentence to a manageable chronic disease. Most patients take several antiretroviral drugs—typically two NRTIs combined with either a PI or NNRTI. These highly effective regimens can reduce plasma HIV to undetectable levels, causing CD4 T-cell counts to return toward normal and thereby restoring some immune function; however, despite these advances, treatment cannot cure HIV. In all cases, discontinuation of antiretroviral drugs has led to a rebound in plasma HIV.

Therapy of HIV disease is often complex. Patients take a combination of drugs for HIV itself, and may take additional drugs to manage treatment side effects (e.g., hyperlipidemia, lipodystrophy, depression) along with drugs to prevent or treat opportunistic infections. As a result, the potential for adverse effects and drug interactions is large. Also, among the drugs used for HIV, emergence of resistance is common. Furthermore, adverse effects and pill burden make adherence difficult. Owing to these complexities, management is best done by a specialist who has extensive experience in treating HIV.

Much of the discussion that follows is based on *Guidelines for the Use of Antiretroviral Agents in Adults and Adolescents Living with HIV,* available online at https://aidsinfo.nih.gov/guidelines. The guidelines were developed by the Panel on Clinical Practices for Treatment of HIV Infection, convened by the U.S. Department of Health and Human Services (DHHS), and undergo periodic updates (the one used here was updated in October 2018). The website also contains guidelines for pediatric patients, pregnant patients, and HIV pre-exposure and post-exposure prophylaxis. We encourage you to examine these guidelines for additional information because much of it is beyond the scope of a pharmacology textbook.

Laboratory Tests

The principal laboratory tests employed to monitor and guide therapy are *CD4 T-cell counts* and *plasma HIV RNA* (viral load) *assays.* Measurement of viral load indicates the magnitude of HIV replication and predicts the rate of CD4 T cell destruction. In contrast, CD4 T-cell counts indicate how much damage the immune system has already suffered. In addition to these tests, evaluation of *HIV drug resistance* is now done routinely. Some patients will also need tests for *HLA-B*5701* (a genetic variant linked to abacavir hypersensitivity) and for *HIV CCR5 tropism* (a determinant of responsiveness to maraviroc). Additionally, it is important to monitor labs that reflect adverse effects (e.g., liver function) and general status (e.g., chemistry panel and complete blood count with differential). A summary of common laboratory testing recommendations is provided in Box 81.2. Additional information with rationales for testing is available in the document *Guidelines for the Use of Antiretroviral Agents in Adults and Adolescents Living with HIV* (2018) available at https://aidsinfo.nih.gov/contentfiles/lvguidelines/adultandadolescentgl.pdf

HUMAN IMMUNODEFICIENCY VIRUS INFECTION PROPHYLAXIS

Although nonspecialists are less likely to manage HIV infection, they may be commonly involved in treating patients prophylactically. The following section focuses on prevention of HIV infection.

Preexposure Prophylaxis

The term *preexposure prophylaxis* (PrEP) refers to the use of antiretroviral drugs to *prevent* HIV infection, rather than treat it. In this section, we consider the ability of antiretroviral drugs to reduce HIV *acquisition* when given to an HIV-*negative* person.

In 2010, results of the *Pre-Exposure Prophylaxis Initiative* study, a study of HIV-negative men, demonstrated that tenofovir/emtricitabine [Truvada] could reduce infection risk by 44% to 73%. These results led the CDC to recommend use of tenofovir/emtricitabine for PrEP for people at high risk for HIV acquisition. The CDC identifies high-risk people as those who (1) have sexual partners with known HIV-1 infection *or* are sexually active with people who belong to social networks with high HIV-1 prevalence *and* (2) have one or more of the following risk factors:

- Do not regularly use condoms.
- Have sexually transmitted infections.
- Engage in sex for money, drugs, or other supplies.
- Use recreational drugs or are dependent on alcohol.
- Are imprisoned.

Preexposure guidelines were updated in 2017. (The guidelines, *Pre-Exposure Prophylaxis for the Prevention of HIV Infection in the United States,* are available at https://www.cdc.gov/hiv/pdf/risk/prep/cdc-hiv-prep-guidelines-2017.pdf.) Interestingly, years after the first clinical trials, the drug combination tenofovir/emtricitabine [Truvada] remains the only FDA-approved drug for PrEP. (Tenofovir without emtricitabine

BOX 81.2 Laboratory Testing Recommendations for Patients Receiving Human Immunodeficiency Virus Therapy

HIV Serology
- Entry into care (for confirmation of HIV diagnosis)

CD4 Count
- Entry into care
- ART modification
- Every 3–6 months during the first 2 years
- Every 12 months after 2 years on ART with suppressed viral load
- Treatment failure
- When clinically indicated

HIV Viral Load
- Entry into care
- ART modification
- 2–8 weeks after ART initiation or modification
- Every 3–6 months
- Treatment failure
- When clinically indicated

Resistance Testing
- Entry into care
- ART modification
- Treatment failure
- When clinically indicated

Hepatitis B Serology (HBsAb, HBsAg, HBcAb total)
- Entry into care
- ART modification (if indicated, for nonimmune patients without HBV infection)
- Every 12 months (if indicated, for nonimmune patients without HBV infection)
- Prior to starting HCV direct-acting antiviral drugs for patients with HCV/HIV coinfection

Hepatitis C Screening (HCV Antibody or HCV RNA)
- Entry into care
- Every 12 months for patients at risk for HCV
- Prior to starting HCV direct-acting antiviral drugs for patients with HCV/HIV coinfection
- When clinically indicated

Basic Chemistry Panel (Serum Na, K, HCO$_3$, Cl, BUN, Creatinine, Fasting Glucose, and Creatinine-Based Estimated Glomerular Filtration Rate. Serum Phosphorus for Patients With Chronic Kidney Disease Who Are on TAF- or TDF-Containing Regimens)
- Entry into care
- ART modification

- 2–8 weeks after ART initiation or modification
- Every 3–6 months
- When clinically indicated

Liver Function (ALT, AST, Total Bilirubin)
- Entry into care
- ART modification
- 2–8 weeks after ART initiation or modification
- Every 3–6 months
- When clinically indicated

CBC With WBC Differential
- Entry into care
- ART modification
- 2–8 weeks after ART initiation or modification if on ZDV
- Every 6 months (every 3–6 months if on ZDV)
- When clinically indicated

Fasting Lipid Profile
- Entry into care
- ART modification
- Every 6 months if last profile abnormal
- Every 12 months if last profile normal
- When clinically indicated

Fasting Glucose or Hemoglobin A1C
- Entry into care
- ART modification
- Every 3–6 months if last test abnormal
- Every 12 months if last test normal
- When clinically indicated

Urinalysis
- Entry into care
- ART modification
- Every 12 months (every 6 months if on TAF or TDF)
- When clinically indicated

Pregnancy Test
- Entry into care
- ART modification
- When clinically indicated

ALT, Alanine aminotransferase; *ART*, antiretroviral therapy; *AST*, aspartate aminotransferase; *BUN*, blood urea nitrogen; *CBC*, complete blood count; *HBV*, hepatitis B virus; *HCV*, hepatitis C virus; *HIV*, human immunodeficiency virus; *TAF*, tenofovir AF; *TDF*, tenofovir DF; *WBC*, white blood count; *ZDV*, zidovudine.

has been given alone with success in some groups but has been less effective among men who have sex with men.)

How is PrEP prescribed? It should be taken once daily for as long as the risk for acquiring HIV is present. The PrEP guidelines recommend prescribing a 90-day supply, and requiring HIV testing as an incentive for a refill increases the chances that at-risk patients will return for monitoring.

Postexposure Prophylaxis

One-time exposure to HIV carries a small, but nonetheless real, risk for infection. Sources of exposure include unprotected vaginal or anal intercourse, receptive oral intercourse, shared needles for drug injection, accidental needle sticks, and blood and other body fluid splashes. Risk is especially high after exposure to a large quantity of infected blood or blood with a high virus titer, and after deep percutaneous penetration with a needle recently removed from the vein of an infected person.

The risk for developing HIV disease after a single exposure can be reduced—but not eliminated—with prophylactic antiretroviral drugs. Presumably, protection results from preventing initial cellular infection and local propagation of HIV, thereby allowing host immune defenses to eliminate the virus before it can become established. To be effective, postexposure prophylaxis (PEP) should be initiated as soon as possible after HIV exposure—preferably within 1 or 2 hours, and no later than 72 hours—and should continue for 28 days. All patients should undergo testing for antibodies against HIV, preferably at the time of exposure, and then 6 weeks, 12 weeks, and 6 months after exposure.

Recommendations for PEP are based on whether the exposure was nonoccupational or occupational, defined as exposure of health care personnel while on the job.

Nonoccupational Postexposure Prophylaxis

For nonoccupational PEP, current guidelines recommend ART regimens much like those employed for initial therapy of established HIV infection. The preferred regimen for healthy adults is tenofovir disoproxil fumarate 300 mg and emtricitabine 200 mg once daily *plus* either raltegravir 400 mg twice daily *or* dolutegravir[a] 50 mg once daily. An alternative option is tenofovir DF 300 mg and emtricitabine (200 mg) once daily *plus* darunavir 800 mg *and* ritonavir 100 mg once daily. Options for children, pregnant women, and patients with impaired renal function, along with detailed information on nonoccupational PEP, is available in a document titled *Updated Guidelines for Antiretroviral Postexposure Prophylaxis After Sexual, Injection Drug Use, or Other Nonoccupational Exposure to HIV—United States, 2016*, which is available online at https://www.cdc.gov/hiv/pdf/programresources/cdc-hiv-npep-guidelines.pdf.

Occupational Postexposure Prophylaxis

Recommendations for occupational PEP are based on the risk for acquiring HIV, which is determined by multiple factors, including (1) the nature of the exposure (skin penetration vs. body fluid splashed onto nonintact skin or mucous membrane); (2) the severity of the exposure (e.g., shallow skin penetration with a solid probe, deep skin penetration with a large-bore hollow needle, surface exposure to small volume of sputum, surface exposure to a large volume of blood); and (3) the HIV status of the exposure source (e.g., asymptomatic with a low viral load, symptomatic with a high viral load).

PEP should begin as early as possible after exposure, should contain at least three antiretroviral drugs, and should be continued for 4 weeks post exposure. The preferred regimen includes tenofovir DF 300 mg and emtricitabine 200 mg once daily plus raltegravir 400 mg twice daily. Close follow-up and counseling should be provided along with monitoring for drug-related side effects.

Please note that our discussion of this important topic is greatly simplified. For detailed information, you can refer to a document titled *Updated U.S. Public Health Service Guidelines for the Management of Occupational Exposures to HIV and Recommendations for Postexposure Prophylaxis* (updated 2015), which is available at https://npin.cdc.gov/publication/updated-us-public-health-service-guidelines-management-occupational-exposures-human.

Another valuable resource for recommendations on managing PEP (occupational, nonoccupational, or perinatal) is a 24-hour National HIV/AIDS Clinicians' Consultative Center through the University of California, San Francisco. Information is available by calling the PEP hotline at 1-888-448-4911. (See http://nccc.ucsf.edu/clinician-consultation/pep-post-exposure-prophylaxis)

KEEPING CURRENT

Drug therapy of HIV infection is continuously evolving. New drugs are being developed, knowledge of existing drugs is expanding, and new drug combinations are being studied. The AIDSinfo website, maintained by the DHHS, has the most current information on treatment guidelines, drugs, vaccines, and clinical trials. There are also links to other HIV/AIDS-related sites there. Content is presented in English and Spanish. You can sign up for e-mail notification of updates.

 SUMMARY OF KEY PRESCRIBING CONSIDERATIONS

Drugs for Human Immunodeficiency Virus Infection

Therapeutic Goal: Treatment has five goals: (1) maximal and long-lasting suppression of viral load, (2) restoration and preservation of immune function, (3) improved quality of life, (4) reduction of HIV-related morbidity and mortality, and (5) prevention of HIV transmission.

Baseline Data: In addition to a complete history and physical exam: CD4 count, HIV viral load, resistance testing, HBsAb, HBsAg, HBcAb total, HCV antibody, serum Na, K, HCO3, Cl, BUN, creatinine, estimated glomerular filtration rate, ALT, AST, total bilirubin, CBC with differential, fasting lipid profile, fasting glucose or hemoglobin A1c, urinalysis, pregnancy test if capable of becoming pregnant, HLA-B*5701 testing if considering abacavir, tropism testing if considering maraviroc, and serum phosphorus if considering tenofovir for patients with chronic kidney disease.

Monitoring: See Box 81.2.

Identifying High-Risk Patients:

- Didanosine's risk for pancreatitis is increased by a history of alcoholism or pancreatitis and by use of IV pentamidine.
- Zidovudine's risk for hematologic toxicity is increased by a low granulocyte count; low levels of hemoglobin, vitamin B_{12}, or folic acid; and concurrent use of drugs that are myelosuppressive, nephrotoxic, or toxic to circulating blood cells.
- Lopinavir/ritonavir oral solution is contraindicated for full-term infants (until 14 days after birth) and preterm infants (until 14 days after their predicted due date).
- Use atazanavir, saquinavir, and lopinavir/ritonavir with caution in patients with structural heart disease, cardiac conduction disturbances, and ischemic heart disease, and in those taking other drugs that prolong the PR interval.
- Avoid lopinavir/ritonavir and saquinavir in patients with congenital long QT syndrome, and in those taking drugs that prolong the QT interval.
- Use enfuvirtide with caution in patients who have pneumonia risk factors: low initial CD4 cell counts, high initial viral load, IV drug use, smoking, and a history of lung disease.
- Patients with elevated liver function and cardiovascular disease who take maraviroc must be monitored carefully.

Evaluating Therapeutic Effects:

HIV RNA

Success is indicated by a reduction in plasma HIV RNA. With ART, plasma HIV RNA should decline to 10% of baseline within 2 to 8 weeks. After 16 to 20 weeks of treatment, plasma HIV RNA should reach its minimum. Ideally, the minimum will be undetectable with sensitive assays.

CD4 T-Cell Counts

As viral load decreases, CD4 T-cell counts may rise, indicating some restoration of immune function.

---

[a]Dolutegravir should not be prescribed for pregnant women or for women who may become pregnant.

82

Drug Therapy for Sexually Transmitted Diseases

Sexually transmitted diseases (STDs), also known as *sexually transmitted infections*, are infectious diseases transmitted primarily through sexual contact. STDs are very common in the United States and constitute a major public health problem. In 2018, the Centers for Disease Control and Prevention (CDC) reported sharp increases in the number of reported STDs. For the top three reportable STDs in 2017 there were 1.7 million new cases of chlamydia (an increase of 22% since 2013), 555,608 new cases of gonorrhea (up 67%), and 30,644 new cases of syphilis (up 76%). Because many STDs are unreported, actual numbers are likely much higher.

Our objective in this chapter is to describe the principal STDs and provide an overview of their treatment (Table 82.1). Because keeping this straight can be challenging at first, we developed a chart that aligns treatment with pharmacological categories (Box 82.1).

The basic pharmacology of these drugs is discussed in other chapters. HIV infection is covered separately in Chapter 81.

In 2015, the CDC updated its *Sexually Transmitted Diseases Treatment Guidelines*. The treatment recommendations presented in this chapter reflect those guidelines, which are available at http://www.cdc.gov/std/tg2015.

CHLAMYDIA TRACHOMATIS INFECTIONS

Characteristics

Chlamydia trachomatis is the most frequently reported bacterial STD (Fig. 82.1). The various strains of *Chlamydia* can cause genital tract infections, proctitis, conjunctivitis, and lymphogranuloma venereum (LGV), as well as ophthalmia and pneumonia in infants. Infection is frequently asymptomatic in women and may also be asymptomatic in men. In women, untreated infection can cause pelvic inflammatory disease (PID), ectopic pregnancy, and infertility. The CDC estimates that chlamydial infections cause sterility in up to 50,000 women each year, primarily from fallopian tube scarring. Because infection is often asymptomatic in women, and because sequelae can be serious, the CDC now recommends annual screening for all sexually active women 25 years or younger. Screening is also recommended for women older than 25 years who have a new sex partner, multiple partners, or a partner with a history of an STD.

Treatment
Adults and Adolescents

For uncomplicated urethral, cervical, or rectal infections in adults or adolescents, treatment with either *azithromycin* [Zithromax] or *doxycycline* [Vibramycin, others] is recommended. Patients who are unable to take these medications may take erythromycin, levofloxacin [Levaquin], or ofloxacin [generic]. Table 82.1 provides a detailed summary of specific dosages of drugs used to treat chlamydia and other STDs.

Infection in Pregnancy

Azithromycin is the preferred treatment for *C. trachomatis* infection. Although doxycycline and other tetracyclines are active against *C.*

trachomatis, these drugs are contraindicated because they can damage fetal teeth and bones. If the patient cannot take azithromycin, the approved alternatives are amoxicillin, erythromycin base, or erythromycin ethylsuccinate [E.E.S., Ery-Tab, Erybid, Erythrocin, others].

Infants

About half the infants born to women with cervical *C. trachomatis* acquire the infection during delivery, putting them at risk for *pneumonia* and *conjunctivitis* (ophthalmia neonatorum). Pneumonia is generally not severe and lasts about 6 weeks. Conjunctivitis does not result in blindness and spontaneously resolves in 6 months. The preferred treatment for both infections is oral *erythromycin base* or *erythromycin ethylsuccinate*. Azithromycin suspension may be given as an alternative. Although topical erythromycin, tetracycline, or silver nitrate may be given to prevent conjunctivitis, these drugs are not completely effective—and they have no effect on neonatal pneumonia caused by *C. trachomatis*.

Preadolescent Children

Although infection in preadolescent children can result from perinatal transmission, sexual abuse is the more likely cause, especially in children older than 2 years. Because of the legal implications, diagnosis must be definitive. Treatment depends on the age and weight of the child. For children who weigh less than 45 kg, the preferred treatment is oral *erythromycin base* or *erythromycin ethylsuccinate*. For children who weigh 45 kg or more, but are younger than 8 years, the preferred treatment is *azithromycin*. For children at least 8 years old, the preferred treatments are *azithromycin* or *doxycycline*.

Lymphogranuloma Venereum

LGV is caused by a unique strain of *C. trachomatis*. Transmission is strictly by sexual contact. LGV is most common in tropical countries but does occur in the United States, especially in the South. Infection begins as a small erosion or papule in the genital region. From this site, the organism migrates to regional lymph nodes, causing swelling, tenderness, and blockage of lymphatic flow. Tremendous enlargement of the genitalia may result. The enlarged nodes, called buboes, may break open and drain.

The treatment of choice for genital, inguinal, and anorectal LGV is *doxycycline*. Erythromycin base serves as an alternative for those who cannot take tetracycline antibiotics.

GONOCOCCAL INFECTIONS

Characteristics

Gonorrhea is caused by *Neisseria gonorrhoeae*, a gram-negative diplococcus, often referred to as the gonococcus. Gonorrhea is second only to chlamydia as our most common STD. Gonorrhea is transmitted almost exclusively by sexual contact.

The intensity of symptoms differs between men and women. In men, the main symptoms are a burning sensation during urination

TABLE 82.1 Drug Therapy Recommendations for Sexually Transmitted Diseases[a]

Disease or Syndrome	Recommended Treatment	Causative Organism(s)
Chlamydia Trachomatis Infections		*Chlamydia trachomatis*
Adults and adolescents	Azithromycin, 1 g PO once *or*	
	Doxycycline, 100 mg PO 2 times/day × 7 days	
Children		
<45 kg	Erythromycin base/ethylsuccinate, 12.5 mg/kg PO 4 times/day × 14 days	
≥45 kg but <8 year old	Azithromycin, 1 g PO once	
≥8 year old	Azithromycin, 1 g PO once *or*	
	Doxycycline, 100 mg PO 2 times/day × 7 days	
Pregnant women	Azithromycin, 1 g PO once	
Newborns: ophthalmia or pneumonia	Erythromycin base/ethylsuccinate, 12.5 mg/kg PO 4 times/day × 14 days	
Lymphogranuloma venereum	Doxycycline, 100 mg PO 2 times/day × 21 days	
Gonococcal Infections (Gonorrhea)		*Neisseria gonorrhoeae*
Urethritis, cervicitis, proctitis	Ceftriaxone, 250 mg IM once, *plus* azithromycin, 1 g PO once	
Pharyngitis	Ceftriaxone, 250 mg IM once, *plus* azithromycin, 1 g PO once	
Disseminated gonococcal infection (DGI) in adults	Ceftriaxone, 1 g IM or IV every 24 h, *plus* azithromycin, 1 g PO once	
DGI with meningitis	Ceftriaxone, 1–2 g IV every 12 h × 10–14 days, *plus* azithromycin, 1 g PO once	
DGI with endocarditis	Ceftriaxone, 1–2 g IV every 12 h × 28 days or more, *plus* azithromycin, 1 g PO once	
Conjunctivitis	Ceftriaxone, 1 g IM once, *plus* azithromycin 1 g PO once	
Newborns		
Ophthalmia neonatorum prophylaxis	Erythromycin 0.5% ophthalmic ointment in each eye at birth	
Ophthalmia neonatorum	Ceftriaxone 25–50 mg/kg (not to exceed 125 mg) IM or IV once	
Disseminated infection or scalp abscess	Ceftriaxone, 25–50 mg/kg IM or IV once daily × 7 days *or*	
	Cefotaxime, 25 mg/kg IM or IV every 12 h × 7 days	
	(Dosing of both drugs is increased to 10–14 days if meningitis is present.)	
Children		
Arthritis, bacteremia	If 45 kg or less, ceftriaxone, 50 mg/kg IM or IV once daily × 7 days, not to exceed 1 g	
	If more than 45 kg, ceftriaxone 1 g IM or IV once daily × 7 days	
Vulvovaginitis, cervicitis, proctitis, pharyngitis, urethritis	If 45 kg or less, ceftriaxone 25–50 mg/kg (not to exceed 125 mg) IM or IV once	
	If more than 45 kg, same as adult	
Nongonococcal Urethritis		*Chlamydia trachomatis, Ureaplasma urealyticum, Trichomonas vaginalis, Mycoplasma genitalium*
Acute infection	Azithromycin, 1 g PO once *or*	
	Doxycycline, 100 mg PO 2 times/day × 7 days	
Recurrent/persistent	Azithromycin, 1 g PO once if original treatment was with doxycycline	
	Moxifloxacin 400 mg PO daily × 7 days if original treatment was azithromycin	
	Metronidazole (2 g PO once) or tinidazole (2 g PO once) in areas where *Trichomonas* outbreaks are common	
Pelvic Inflammatory Disease		*Neisseria gonorrhoeae, Chlamydia trachomatis,* others
Inpatients	Doxycycline (100 mg IV or PO every 12 h), *plus* either cefoxitin (2 g IV every 6 h) or cefotetan (2 g IV every 12 h); or clindamycin (900 mg IV every 8 h), *plus* gentamicin (3–5 mg/kg IM or IV once or 2 mg/kg IM or IV once then 1.5 mg/kg every 8 h)	
Outpatients	Doxycycline (100 mg PO 2 times/day × 14 days), *plus* either cefoxitin (2 g IM once, boosted with probenecid 1 g PO once) or ceftriaxone (250 mg IM once), *with or without* metronidazole (500 mg PO 2 times/day × 14 days)	

TABLE 82.1 Drug Therapy Recommendations for Sexually Transmitted Diseases—cont'd

Disease or Syndrome	Recommended Treatment	Causative Organism(s)
Sexually Acquired Epididymitis		Chlamydia trachomatis, Neisseria gonorrhoeae, enteric organisms
Sexually acquired epididymitis without history of insertive anal sex	Ceftriaxone (250 mg IM once) plus doxycycline (100 mg PO 2 times/day × 10 days)	
Sexually acquired epididymitis with history of insertive anal sex	Ceftriaxone (250 mg IM once) plus either levofloxacin (500 mg PO daily × 10 days) or ofloxacin (300 mg PO 2 times/day × 10 days)	
Syphilis		Treponema pallidum
Primary syphilis, secondary syphilis, and early latent syphilis	Adults: Benzathine penicillin G, 2.4 million units IM once Children: Benzathine penicillin G, 50,000 units/kg IM once (up to a max. of 2.4 million units)	
Late latent syphilis or latent syphilis of unknown duration	Adults: Benzathine penicillin G, 2.4 million units IM once/week for 3 weeks Children: Benzathine penicillin G, 50,000 units/kg IM once/week for 3 weeks (up to a max. of 7.2 million units over the course of treatment)	
Tertiary syphilis	Benzathine penicillin G, 2.4 million units IM once/week for 3 weeks (must rule out CNS involvement)	
Neurosyphilis	Aqueous crystalline penicillin G, 18–24 million units IV daily for 10–14 days, administered by continuous infusion or in separate doses of 3–4 million units each every 4 h	
Congenital syphilis	Aqueous crystalline penicillin G, 50,000 units/kg IV every 12 h for the first 7 days of life, followed by 50,000 units/kg every 8 h for the next 3 days or Procaine penicillin G, 50,000 units/kg IM once daily for 10 days	
Acquired immunodeficiency syndrome (AIDS)	See Chapter 81	Human immunodeficiency virus (HIV)
Bacterial Vaginosis		Gardnerella vaginalis, Mycoplasma hominis, various anaerobes
	Metronidazole, 500 mg PO 2 times/day × 7 days or Metronidazole gel (0.75%), 1 full applicator (5 g) intravaginally once/day × 5 days or Clindamycin cream (2%), 1 full applicator (5 g) intravaginally at bedtime × 7 days	
Trichomoniasis	Metronidazole, 2 g PO once or Tinidazole, 2 g PO once	Trichomonas vaginalis
Chancroid	Azithromycin, 1 g PO once or Ceftriaxone, 250 mg IM once or Ciprofloxacin, 500 mg PO 2 times/day × 3 days or Erythromycin base, 500 mg PO 3 times/day × 7 days	Haemophilus ducreyi
Genital Herpes Simplex Virus Infections		Herpes simplex virus
First episode, genital herpes	Acyclovir, 400 mg PO 3 times/day × 7–10 days (or longer) or Acyclovir, 200 mg PO 5 times/day × 7–10 days (or longer) or Famciclovir, 250 mg PO 3 times/day × 7–10 days (or longer) or Valacyclovir, 1 g PO 2 times/day × 7–10 days (or longer)	
Severe infection	Acyclovir, 5–10 mg/kg IV every 8 h for 2–7 days or until clinical improvement, then PO acyclovir to complete at least 10 days	
Recurrent episodes	Acyclovir, 800 mg PO 2 times/day × 5 days or Acyclovir, 800 mg PO 3 times/day × 2 days or Acyclovir, 400 mg PO 3 times/day × 5 days or Famciclovir, 125 mg PO 2 times/day × 5 days or Famciclovir, 1 g 2 times/day × 1 day or Famciclovir, 500 mg once, followed by 200 mg 2 times/day for 2 days or Valacyclovir, 500 mg PO 2 times/day × 3 days or Valacyclovir, 1 g PO once/day × 5 days	

Continued

TABLE 82.1	Drug Therapy Recommendations for Sexually Transmitted Diseases—cont'd	
Disease or Syndrome	**Recommended Treatment**	**Causative Organism(s)**
Daily suppressive therapy	Acyclovir, 400 mg PO 2 times/day *or* Famciclovir, 250 mg PO 2 times/day *or* Valacyclovir, 500 mg PO once/day *or* Valacyclovir, 1 g PO once/day	
Neonatal herpes	Acyclovir, 20 mg/kg IV every 8 h × 14 days (for skin or mucous membrane infection) or × 21 days (for disseminated or CNS infection)	
Proctitis	Ceftriaxone (250 mg IM once) *plus* doxycycline (100 mg PO 2 times/day × 7 days)	*Chlamydia trachomatis, Neisseria gonorrhoeae, Treponema pallidum,* herpes simplex virus
Venereal warts	*See* Chapter 88	Human papillomavirus

aRecommendations from Centers for Disease Control and Prevention. Sexually transmitted diseases treatment guidelines, 2015. *MMWR Morb Mortal Wkly Rep* 2016;64:1–137. Dosing for alternative regimens is available at http://www.cdc.gov/std/tg2015/tg-2015-print.pdf. *CNS,* Central nervous system.

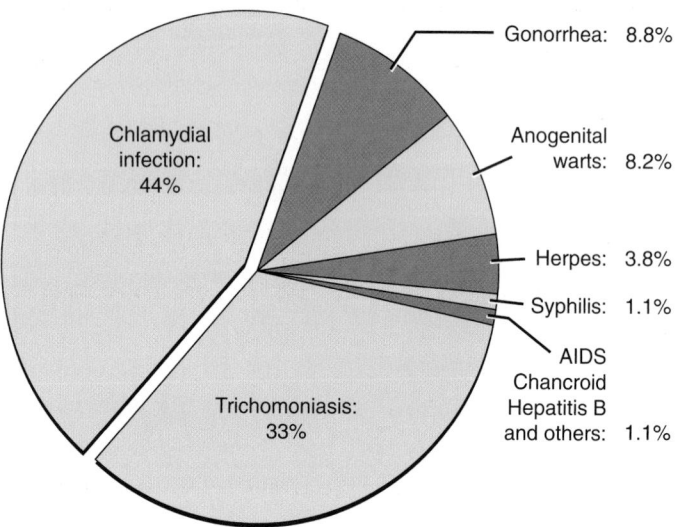

Fig. 82.1 Prevalence of Sexually Transmitted Diseases.

Gonorrhea: 8.8%
Chlamydial infection: 44%
Anogenital warts: 8.2%
Herpes: 3.8%
Syphilis: 1.1%
AIDS Chancroid Hepatitis B and others: 1.1%
Trichomoniasis: 33%

and a purulent discharge from the penis. In contrast, gonorrhea in women is often asymptomatic or may present as mild cervicitis. However, serious infection of female reproductive structures (vagina, urethra, cervix, ovaries, fallopian tubes) can occur, ultimately resulting in sterility. Among people who engage in oral sex, the mouth and throat can become infected, causing sore throat and tonsillitis. Among people who engage in receptive anal sex, the rectum can become infected, causing a purulent discharge and tenesmus. Bacteremia can develop in males and females, causing cutaneous lesions, arthritis, and, rarely, meningitis and endocarditis.

Treatment

Owing to antibiotic resistance, treatment of gonorrhea has changed over the years. In the 1930s, virtually all strains of the gonococcus were sensitive to sulfonamides. However, within a decade, sulfonamide resistance had become common. Fortunately, by that time penicillin had become available, and the drug was active against all gonococcal strains. However, in 1976, organisms resistant to penicillin began to emerge. More recently, resistance to fluoroquinolones has become common. As a result, in 2007, *the CDC recommended against using fluoroquinolones for gonorrhea*, leaving cephalosporins as the preferred

treatments. This recommendation was changed yet again in 2012, also triggered by antimicrobial resistance—this time to oral cephalosporins.

Urethral, Cervical, and Rectal Infection

Because of increasing resistance to cephalosporins, preferred treatment now consists of a combination of two drugs: *ceftriaxone* intramuscular (IM) plus *azithromycin* oral (PO). If a patient refuses IM therapy, PO cefixime [Suprax] can be substituted for IM ceftriaxone; however, the CDC recommends not routinely substituting this drug, because resistance to cefixime has been documented and is anticipated to increase.

If a patient is allergic to azithromycin, a 7-day course of doxycycline may be substituted. For patients with cephalosporin allergies, the options are not as clear. Although prescribing double the azithromycin dose as monotherapy will cure gonorrhea in most cases, the CDC does not recommend this because of treatment failures and rapid development of resistance. Although acknowledging a lack of data for recommendation, the CDC suggests substituting gemifloxacin [Factive] for the cephalosporin component, despite having recommended against using quinolones to treat gonorrhea. Spectinomycin, an aminoglycoside, has also been suggested; however, it is not currently available in the United States. For additional information on this dilemma, see http://www.cdc.gov/std/tg2015/gonorrhea.htm.

Pharyngeal Infection

Gonococcal infection of the pharynx is more difficult to treat than infection of the urethra, cervix, or rectum; therefore parenteral therapy is recommended for all patients. The preferred treatment is *ceftriaxone* combined with *azithromycin*. Azithromycin is preferred over doxycycline because patients are more likely to adhere to a single-dose regimen of azithromycin than the full-week regimen of doxycycline taken twice a day.

Conjunctivitis

Gonococcal conjunctivitis can be reliably eradicated with *ceftriaxone* plus azithromycin. Treatment also includes washing the infected eye with saline solution once.

Disseminated Gonococcal Infection

Disseminated gonococcal infection (DGI) occurs secondary to gonococcal bacteremia. Symptoms include petechial or pustular skin lesions, arthritis, arthralgia, and tenosynovitis. Endocarditis and meningitis occur rarely.

BOX 82.1 Drug Categories Used in Treatment of Sexually Transmitted Infections

Amebicide, Antiprotozoal, Miscellaneous Antibiotic
Metronidazole
- Pelvic inflammatory disease, outpatient (with other drugs)
- Bacterial vaginosis
- Trichomoniasis
- Nongonococcal urethritis, resistant/persistent (in areas where *Trichomonas* outbreaks are common)

Tindazole
- Nongonococcal urethritis, recurrent/persistent
- Trichomoniasis

Aminoglycoside
Gentamicin
- Pelvic inflammatory disease, inpatient (with other drugs)

Antivirals
Acyclovir
- Genital herpes, first episode, severe, recurrent, suppressive
- Neonatal herpes

Famicyclovir
- Genital herpes, first episode, recurrent, suppressive

Valacyclovir
- Genital herpes, first episode, recurrent, suppressive

Cephalosporins
Cefotetan
- Pelvic inflammatory disease, inpatient (with other drugs)

Cefoxitin
- Pelvic inflammatory disease, inpatient (with other drugs)
- Pelvic inflammatory disease, outpatient (with other drugs)

Ceftriaxone
- Gonorrhea in men: gonococcal urethritis, proctitis (with azithromycin)
- Gonorrhea in women: vulvovaginitis, cervicitis, urethritis (with azithromycin)
- Gonococcal pharyngitis (with azithromycin)
- Gonococcal conjunctivitis (with azithromycin)
- Disseminated gonococcal infection, all types (with azithromycin)
- Disseminated gonococcal infection or scalp abscess in neonates
- Ophthalmia neonatorum
- Gonococcal arthritis, bacteremia in children
- Pelvic inflammatory disease, outpatient (with other drugs)
- Sexually acquired epididymitis (with other drugs)
- Chancroid
- Proctitis

Cefotaxime
- Disseminated gonococcal infection or scalp abscess in neonates

Lincosamide
Clindamycin
- Pelvic Inflammatory disease, inpatient (with other drugs)
- Bacterial vaginosis

Macrolides
Azithromycin
- Chlamydia (except for children weighing less than 45 kg)
- Chlamydia in pregnant women
- Gonorrhea in men: gonococcal urethritis, proctitis (with ceftriaxone)
- Gonorrhea in women: vulvovaginitis, cervicitis, urethritis (with ceftriaxone)
- Gonococcal pharyngitis (with ceftriaxone)
- Gonococcal conjunctivitis (with ceftriaxone)
- Disseminated gonococcal infection, all types (with ceftriaxone)
- Nongonococcal urethritis, acute
- Nongonococcal urethritis, recurrent/persistent (if original treatment was doxycycline)
- Chancroid

Erythromycin
- Chlamydia in children weighing less than 45 kg (erythromycin base/ethylsuccinate)
- Newborn ophthalmia or pneumonia caused by *C. trachomatis* (erythromycin base/ethylsuccinate)
- Prophylaxis for newborn ophthalmia caused by *N. gonorrhoeae* (Erythromycin 0.5% ophthalmic ointment)
- Chancroid (erythromycin base)

Penicillins
Penicillin G
- Syphilis, primary, secondary, tertiary, latent (benzathine penicillin G)
- Neurosyphilis (aqueous crystalline penicillin G)
- Congenital syphilis (aqueous crystalline penicillin G or procaine penicillin G)

Quinolone
Ciprofloxacin
- Chancroid

Moxifloxacin
- Nongonococcal urethritis, recurrent/persistent (if original treatment was azithromycin)

Levofloxacin
- Sexually acquired epididymitis with insertive anal sex (with ceftriaxone)

Ofloxacin
- Sexually acquired epididymitis with insertive anal sex (with ceftriaxone)

Tetracycline
Doxycycline
- *C. trachomatis* infections in non-pregnant adults and children 8 years and older
- Lymphogranuloma venereum
- Nongonococcal urethritis, acute
- Pelvic inflammatory disease, inpatient and outpatient (with other drugs)
- Sexually acquired epididymitis without insertive anal sex (with ceftriaxone)
- Proctitis (with ceftriaxone)

Strains of *N. gonorrhoeae* that cause DGI are uncommon in the United States. In the absence of endocarditis or meningitis, treatment consists of IM or intravenous (IV) *ceftriaxone* plus azithromycin. For patients with endocarditis or meningitis, the preferred treatment is IV *ceftriaxone* plus PO azithromycin.

Neonatal Infection

Neonatal gonococcal infection is acquired through contact with infected cervical exudates during delivery. Infection can be limited to the eyes or it may be disseminated.

Gonococcal *neonatal ophthalmia* is a serious infection. The initial symptom is conjunctivitis. Over time, other structures of the eye become involved. Blindness can result. The recommended therapy is a single dose of *ceftriaxone* given by either IM injection or IV infusion.

To protect against neonatal ophthalmia, a topical antibiotic should be instilled into both eyes immediately postpartum—as required by law in most states. According to the 2015 CDC guidelines, the only approved topical agent is *0.5% erythromycin* ophthalmic ointment. If this antimicrobial is not available, parenteral therapy with ceftriaxone is to be used.

In neonates, *DGI* is rare. Possible manifestations include sepsis, arthritis, meningitis, and scalp abscesses. There are two recommended treatments: *ceftriaxone and cefotaxime*.

Preadolescent Children

Among preadolescent children, the most common cause of gonococcal infection is sexual abuse. Vaginal, anorectal, and pharyngeal infections are most common. Because of legal implications, diagnosis must be definitive. Growing a specimen in culture is the preferred technique.

Treatment depends on the type of infection and the weight of the child. For children who have localized infection (vulvovaginitis, cervicitis, urethritis, pharyngitis, proctitis) and who weigh 45 kg or less, the preferred treatment is a single dose of IM or IV *ceftriaxone*. For children with localized infection who weigh more than 45 kg, treatment is the same as for adults. For children of any weight who have systemic infection (bacteremia, arthritis), the preferred treatment is IM or IV *ceftriaxone*, once daily for 7 days. Specific dosing is provided in Table 82.1.

NONGONOCOCCAL URETHRITIS

Characteristics

Nongonococcal urethritis (NGU) is defined as urethritis caused by any organism other than *N. gonorrhoeae*, the gonococcus. The most common infectious agent is *C. trachomatis*. Other likely agents are *Ureaplasma urealyticum*, *Trichomonas vaginalis*, and *Mycoplasma genitalium*. NGU is diagnosed by the presence of polymorphonuclear leukocytes and a negative culture for *N. gonorrhoeae*. The infection is especially prevalent among sexually active adolescent girls.

Treatment

The recommended treatment is either *azithromycin* or *doxycycline*. Alternative regimens are erythromycin base, erythromycin ethylsuccinate, levofloxacin, or ofloxacin. For persistent or recurrent NGU, one of two drugs, *metronidazole* [Flagyl] or *tinidazole* [Tindamax], is recommended if *T. vaginalis* transmission is a suspected cause. *Azithromycin* should be added to the regimen if it had not been used during initial therapy. If the infection still fails to respond, the cause may be *M. genitalium*. Unfortunately, we have no easy tests for this bacterium, and hence definitive diagnosis may not be possible. Nonetheless, when *M. genitalium* is suspected, a trial with *moxifloxacin* [Avelox] may be warranted.

ⓘ PAITENT-CENTERED CARE ACROSS THE LIFE SPAN

Drugs for STDs

Life Stage	Considerations or Concerns
Children	Some drugs used to treat sexually transmitted diseases (STDs), such as doxycycline, are contraindicated for children. It is important to use regimens specifically indicated for children.
Pregnant Women	Some drugs used to treat STDs (doxycycline, tinidazole, gentamicin) may cause congenital anomalies. Macrolides, penicillins, and cephalosporins are generally safe. It is important to use alternative regimens specifically designated for pregnant women when indicated (see Table 82.1).
Breast-Feeding Women	Tinidazole is contraindicated in breast-feeding women. When taken, breast-feeding should be withheld during treatment and for 3 days after treatment is completed. For women taking metronidazole, some providers advise avoidance of breast-feeding for 12 to 24 hours after treatment. Breastfeeding while taking doxycycline carries a theoretical risk for tooth discoloration; however, the WHO reports that a single dose will not be a risk. Macrolides (e.g., erythromycin, azithromycin) and cephalosporins (e.g., ceftriaxone, cefotetan) and penicillins are considered safe for lactating women; however, the infants may develop diarrhea, modified bowel flora, and other side effects of the drugs.
Older Adults	For many antimicrobials, adverse effects in older adults may be more severe and recovery from infection may be slower or complicated.

PELVIC INFLAMMATORY DISEASE

Characteristics

Acute pelvic inflammatory disease (PID) is a syndrome that includes endometritis, pelvic peritonitis, tuboovarian abscess, and inflammation of the fallopian tubes. Infertility can result. Prominent symptoms are abdominal pain, vaginal discharge, and fever. Most frequently, PID is caused by *N. gonorrhoeae*, *C. trachomatis*, or both. However, *Mycoplasma hominis*, as well as assorted anaerobic and facultative bacteria, may also be present. In recent years, the United States has experienced an almost 40% decrease in PID despite the increase in diseases that cause this condition. This may be attributable to intensified patient education efforts, increased and improved screening practices, or improved adherence to single-dose treatment.

Treatment

Because multiple organisms are likely to be involved, drug therapy must provide broad coverage. Because no single drug can do this, combination therapy is required. For the *hospitalized patient*, treatment can be initiated with either *cefoxitin* (generic) or *cefotetan* [Cefotan], combined with *doxycycline*. After symptoms resolve, IV therapy can be discontinued—but must be followed by oral *doxycycline* to complete a 14-day course of treatment. An alternative recommended regimen consists of IV *clindamycin* [Cleocin] plus IV or IM *gentamicin* (generic).

Outpatients can be treated with either *ceftriaxone* or *cefoxitin*. Treatment should also include *doxycycline*, with or without *metronidazole*. Because PID can be difficult to treat, and because the consequences of failure can be severe (e.g., sterility), many experts recommend that *all* patients receive IV antibiotics in a hospital.

ACUTE EPIDIDYMITIS

Characteristics

Epididymitis may be acquired by sexual contact or nonsexually. Sexually acquired epididymitis is usually caused by *N. gonorrhoeae*, *C. trachomatis*, or both. The syndrome occurs primarily in young adults (under 35 years old) and may be associated with urethritis. Primary symptoms are fever accompanied by pain in the back of the testicles that develops over the course of several hours.

Treatment

For patients with gonococcal or chlamydial infection, the recommended treatment is *ceftriaxone* plus *doxycycline*. For patients who engage in insertive anal sex, the addition of levofloxacin or ofloxacin is recommended to target enteric bacteria. Testicular pain can be managed with analgesics, bed rest, and ice packs.

Non–sexually transmitted epididymitis generally occurs in older men and in men who have had urinary tract instrumentation. Causative organisms are gram-negative enteric bacilli and *Pseudomonas* species. Ofloxacin can be used for treatment.

SYPHILIS

Syphilis is caused by the spirochete *Treponema pallidum*. In the United States, the incidence of syphilis has risen steadily since 2000. Fortunately, *T. pallidum* has remained highly responsive to penicillin, the treatment of choice.

Characteristics

Syphilis develops in three stages, termed *primary*, *secondary*, and *tertiary*. *T. pallidum* enters the body by penetrating the mucous membranes of the mouth, vagina, or urethra of the penis. After an incubation period of 1 to 4 weeks, a primary lesion, called a chancre, develops at the site of entry. The chancre is a hard, red, protruding, painless sore. Nearby lymph nodes may become swollen. Within a few weeks the chancre heals spontaneously, although *T. pallidum* is still present. In clinical practice, chancres are rarely seen, especially in females.

Two to 6 weeks after the chancre heals, secondary syphilis develops. Symptoms result from spread of *T. pallidum* through the bloodstream. Skin lesions and flu-like symptoms (fever, headache, reduced appetite, general malaise) are typical. Enlarged lymph nodes and joint pain may also be present. The symptoms of secondary syphilis resolve in 4 to 8 weeks—but may recur episodically over the next 3 to 4 years.

Tertiary syphilis develops 5 to 40 years after the initial infection. Almost any organ can be involved. Infection of the brain—neurosyphilis—is common and can cause senility, paralysis, and severe psychiatric symptoms. The heart valves and aorta can be damaged. Lesions can also occur in the skin, bones, joints, and eyes. The risk for neurosyphilis is increased in individuals with HIV infection.

Infants exposed to *T. pallidum* in utero can be born with syphilis. Early signs of congenital syphilis include sores, rhinitis, and severe tenderness over bones.

Treatment

Penicillin G is the drug of choice for all stages of syphilis. The form and dosage of penicillin G depend on the disease stage. *Early syphilis* (primary, secondary, or latent syphilis of less than 1 year's duration) is treated with a single IM dose of benzathine penicillin G. *Late latent syphilis* (more than 1 year's duration) and tertiary syphilis are also treated with IM benzathine penicillin G. However, instead of receiving a single dose, adults and children receive three doses 1 week apart. *Neurosyphilis* requires more aggressive therapy. The recommended treatment is IV penicillin G daily for 10 to 14 days, administered either by continuous infusion or in separate doses every 4 hours. For *congenital syphilis*, treatment options are either IV penicillin G or IM procaine penicillin. *Syphilis in pregnancy* should be treated with penicillin G, using a dosage appropriate to the stage of the disease.

How should patients with *penicillin allergy* be treated? For *nonpregnant* patients with early or late syphilis, either *doxycycline* or *tetracycline* may be used. For patients with *neurosyphilis*, ceftriaxone can be effective, but possible cross-reactivity with penicillin is a concern. If the patient is a child or a pregnant woman, the CDC recommends a penicillin-allergy desensitization protocol to permit penicillin use, rather than substituting another drug for penicillin.

BACTERIAL VAGINOSIS

Characteristics

Bacterial vaginosis (BV) is a common vaginal infection in women of childbearing age. The condition results from an alteration in vaginal microflora. Organisms responsible for the syndrome include *Gardnerella vaginalis* (also known as *Haemophilus vaginalis*), *M. hominis*, and various anaerobes. The syndrome occurs most commonly in sexually active women, although it may be transmitted in other ways. BV is characterized by a malodorous vaginal discharge, elevation of vaginal pH (above 4.5), and generation of a fishy odor when vaginal secretions are mixed with 10% potassium hydroxide. Clue cells (epithelial cells whose borders are obscured by bacteria) are typically found on microscopic examination of vaginal secretions.

Treatment

The recommended therapy for BV is either oral or vaginal *metronidazole* or vaginal clindamycin cream. Clindamycin cream is available as a *short-acting 2% clindamycin cream* [Cleocin] and a *long-acting 2% clindamycin cream* [Clindesse]. Clindesse cream is formulated to adhere to the vaginal mucosa for several days and hence can clear BV with just one application. Approved alternative regimens are tinidazole [Tindamax], oral clindamycin, or clindamycin ovules (intravaginal suppositories). Unlike the other drugs approved for BV, tinidazole should not be prescribed for pregnant women.

TRICHOMONIASIS

Characteristics

Trichomoniasis, caused by *T. vaginalis*, is the most common nonviral STD in the United States. In men, infection is usually asymptomatic. In women, infection may be asymptomatic or may cause a diffuse, malodorous, yellow-green vaginal discharge, along with burning and itching. The rapid movement of *T. vaginalis* protozoa are notable on microscopic examination of vaginal secretions.

Treatment

Most infections can be eliminated with a single oral dose of either *metronidazole* or *tinidazole*. Dosing can be repeated in the event of treatment failure. Male partners of infected women should always be treated, even if free of symptoms. Although some clinicians remain concerned about giving metronidazole during pregnancy, there is no evidence that the drug causes birth defects in humans. Tinidazole, on the other hand, should not be prescribed for pregnant women.

CHANCROID

Characteristics

Chancroid, also known as soft chancre, is one of the few STDs for which prevalence has declined both in the United States and worldwide. It is caused by *Haemophilus ducreyi*. Transmission is primarily by sexual contact. The infection is characterized by a painful, ragged ulcer at the site of inoculation, usually the external genitalia. Regional lymph nodes may be swollen. Multiple secondary lesions may develop.

Treatment

Four antibiotics are recommended for treatment. These are (1) *azithromycin*, (2) *ceftriaxone*, (3) *ciprofloxacin* [Cipro], and (4) *erythromycin base*.

HERPES SIMPLEX VIRUS INFECTIONS

Characteristics

Most genital herpes infections are caused by herpes simplex virus type 2 (HSV-2). However, an increasing number of anogenital infections are caused by HSV-1, the herpes virus that causes cold sores. In the United States, the infection has reached epidemic proportions: more than 50 million people are affected.

Symptoms of primary infection develop 6 to 8 days after contact. Some people with HSV infection are asymptomatic or have relatively mild symptoms; however, for others there is a common presentation. In females, blisters or vesicles can appear on the perianal skin, labia, vagina, cervix, and foreskin of the clitoris. In males, vesicles develop on the penis and occasionally on the testicles. Painful urination and a watery discharge can occur in both sexes. Also, the patient may experience systemic symptoms: fever, headache, myalgia, and tender, swollen lymph nodes in the affected region. Within days, the original blisters can evolve into large, painful, ulcer-like sores. Over the next 2 to 3 weeks, all symptoms resolve spontaneously. However, this does not indicate cure. The virus remains present in a latent state and can cause recurrence. Because available drugs cannot eliminate the virus, there is no cure. Symptoms may recur for life; however, for some patients, subsequent episodes become progressively shorter and less severe, and in rare cases they may cease entirely.

Neonatal Infection

Genital herpes in pregnant women can be transmitted to the infant. Transmission can occur in utero, which is very rare, or during delivery. Infection acquired in utero can result in spontaneous abortion or fetal malformation. Infection acquired during delivery can cause blindness, severe neurologic damage, and even death. To protect the infant during delivery, birth should be accomplished by cesarean delivery if the mother has an active infection. Infants who acquire the infection should be treated with acyclovir.

Treatment

Genital herpes can be treated with three drugs: *acyclovir* [Zovirax], *famciclovir* [Famvir], and *valacyclovir* [Valtrex] at dosage regimens recommended in Table 82.1. These agents cannot eliminate the virus, but they can reduce symptoms and shorten the duration of pain and viral shedding. Patients with recurrent infections may take these drugs every day (suppressive therapy) or just when symptoms appear (episodic therapy). Continuous daily administration reduces the frequency and intensity of episodes, whereas episodic treatment reduces symptom intensity after an episode has begun.

Reduction of Transmission

Transmission of HSV can occur when symptoms are absent as well as when symptoms are present. *Valacyclovir* (500 mg once daily) can decrease transmission of genital herpes by almost 50%. No other drug has been shown to reduce transmission of this STD, or any other STD, for that matter. Valacyclovir only *reduces* transmission; it does not stop it entirely. Accordingly, patients must continue to use condoms for insertive sexual activity and dental dams for oral sexual activity. Because viral shedding is increased when the infection is active, it is advisable to abstain from sexual activity during breakouts.

PROCTITIS

Characteristics

Sexually acquired proctitis (inflammation of the rectum) results primarily from receptive anal intercourse. Symptoms include anorectal pain, tenesmus, and rectal discharge. Usual causative organisms are *N. gonorrhoeae*, *C. trachomatis*, *T. pallidum*, and HSV.

Treatment

Empiric treatment is *ceftriaxone* plus *doxycycline*. If perianal ulcers are present, treatment for HSV should also be included.

ANOGENITAL WARTS

Genital and perianal warts are caused by human papillomaviruses (HPVs). Characteristics of these warts and their treatment are presented in Chapter 88. As discussed in Chapter 55, an HPV vaccine, sold as Gardasil 9, can protect against both venereal warts and cervical cancer.

83

Anthelmintics

Helminths are parasitic worms, and *anthelmintics* are the drugs used against them. Helminthiasis (worm infestation) is the most common affliction of humans, affecting more than 2 billion people worldwide. The intestine is a frequent site of infestation. Other sites include the liver, lymphatic system, and blood vessels. Infestation is frequently asymptomatic. However, infestation with some parasites can cause severe complications. Helminthiasis is most prevalent where sanitation is poor. Cleanliness greatly reduces infestation risk.

Treatment of helminthiasis is not always indicated. Most parasitic worms do not reproduce in the human body. Therefore in the absence of reinfestation, many infections simply subside as adult worms die. Accordingly, treatment may be optional. In countries where providers and medication are readily available, drug therapy is definitely indicated. However, in less fortunate locales, several factors—cost of medication, limited medical facilities, and high probability of reinfestation—may render individual treatment impractical. In these places, preventative measures, such as improved hygiene and elimination of carriers, may be the most valuable interventions.

In approaching the anthelmintic drugs, we begin by reviewing classification of the parasitic worms. Next we briefly discuss the characteristics of the more common helminthic infestations. After this, we discuss preferred drugs for treatment.

CLASSIFICATION OF PARASITIC WORMS

The most common parasitic worms belong to three classes: Nematoda (roundworms), Cestoda (tapeworms), and Trematoda (flukes). Nematodes belong to the phylum Nemathelminthes. Cestodes and trematodes belong to the phylum Platyhelminthes (flat worms).

Nematodes (Roundworms)

Parasitic nematodes can be subdivided into two groups: (1) those that infest the intestinal lumen and (2) those that inhabit tissues. There are five major species of intestinal nematodes. Their common names are giant roundworm, pinworm, hookworm, whipworm, and threadworm. Official names (e.g., Ascaris lumbricoides) are shown in Table 83.1. Two types of nematodes invade tissues: (1) pork roundworms (responsible for trichinosis) and (2) filariae. The three species of filariae encountered most commonly are also found in Table 83.1.

Cestodes (Tapeworms)

Three species of cestodes infest humans. Common names for these parasites are beef tapeworm, pork tapeworm, and fish tapeworm. Their official names appear in Table 83.1.

Trematodes (Flukes)

Five species of trematodes infest humans. These organisms fall into four groups having the following common names: blood fluke, liver fluke, intestinal fluke, and lung fluke. Official names of the five species belonging to these groups are given in Table 83.1.

HELMINTHIC INFESTATIONS

This section describes the major characteristics of infestation by specific helminths. These infestations can differ with respect to anatomic site and danger to the host. Infestations also differ with respect to the drugs employed for treatment.

The name applied to an infestation is based on the official name of the invading organism. For example, infestation with the giant round-worm, whose official name is *Ascaris lumbricoides*, is referred to as ascariasis.

In the following discussion, the helminthic infestations are grouped in four categories: (1) nematode infestations of the intestine, (2) nematode infestations of extraintestinal sites, (3) cestode infestations, and (4) trematode infestations.

Nematode Infestations (Intestinal)
Ascariasis (Giant Roundworm Infestation)

Ascariasis is the most prevalent helminthic infestation. Worldwide, one of every three people is affected. In the United States, the condition is isolated to rural areas without adequate sanitation. Worms in feces from humans or pigs enter the soil and are taken up by human hosts who consume food grown in the soil. Adult worms inhabit the small intestine. Ascariasis is usually asymptomatic. However, serious complications can result if worms migrate into the pancreatic duct, bile duct, gallbladder, or liver. In addition, if infestation is extremely heavy, intestinal blockage may occur. Because of these potential hazards, ascariasis should always be treated. Drugs of choice are albendazole, mebendazole, and ivermectin.

Enterobiasis (Pinworm Infestation)

Enterobiasis is the most common helminthic infestation in the United States. Adult pinworms inhabit the ileum and large intestine. Their life span is approximately 2 months. Although usually asymptomatic, some patients experience intense perianal itching. Itching leads to the most common mode of transmission. Pinworm eggs deposited in the perianal are transferred to scratching fingers. If hands are not washed well immediately, the eggs can be transferred to everything the person touches. Drugs of choice are albendazole, mebendazole, and pyrantel pamoate. Because enterobiasis is readily transmitted, all family members of an infected individual should be treated simultaneously.

Ancylostomiasis and Necatoriasis (Hookworm Infestation)

Hookworm infestation was once thought to be eliminated in the United States, and it remains so for most of the country. Regional outbreaks occur primarily in rural areas where inhabitants do not have adequate sewer or septic systems and walk barefoot. Worms from feces enter the soil and then enter their human host by attaching to their feet as they walk over the infested soil. Adult hookworms attach to the wall of the small intestine and suck blood. As a result, infestation is associated with chronic blood loss and progressive anemia. Symptomatic anemia is most likely in menstruating women and undernourished individuals. Nausea, vomiting, and abdominal pain may accompany the infestation.

TABLE 83.1 Drugs of Choice for Parasitic Worms

Worm Class	PARASITIC ORGANISM		Drugs of Choice
	Common Name	Official Name	
Nematodes (roundworms): intestinal	Giant roundworm	*Ascaris lumbricoides*	Albendazole *or* mebendazole *or* ivermectin
	Pinworm	*Enterobius vermicularis*	Albendazole *or* mebendazole *or* pyrantel pamoate
	Hookworm	*Ancylostoma duodenale, Necator americanus*	
	Whipworm	*Trichuris trichiura*	Albendazole
	Threadworm	*Strongyloides stercoralis*	Ivermectin
Nematodes (roundworms): extraintestinal	Pork roundworm	*Trichinella spiralis*	Albendazole[a]
	Filariae	*Brugia malayi, Loa loa, Wuchereria bancrofti*	Diethylcarbamazine[b]
		Onchocerca volvulus	Ivermectin
			Moxidectin
Cestodes (tapeworms)	Beef tapeworm	*Taenia saginata*	Praziquantel[a]
	Pork tapeworm	*Taenia solum*	
	Fish tapeworm	*Diphyllobothrium latum*	
Trematodes (flukes)	Blood fluke	*Schistosoma* species	Praziquantel
	Intestinal fluke	*Fasciolopsis buski*	
	Lung fluke	*Paragonimus westermani*	
	Liver flukes	*Fasciola hepatica* (sheep liver fluke)	Triclabendazole[c]
		Clonorchis sinensis (Chinese liver fluke)	Praziquantel *or* albendazole[a]

[a]Not approved by the U.S. Food and Drug Administration for this indication.
[b]Available from the Centers for Disease Control and Prevention.
[c]Not available in the United States.

Albendazole, mebendazole, and pyrantel pamoate are treatments of choice.

Trichuriasis (Whipworm Infestation)

Trichuriasis are most commonly found in rural areas in Southeast United States. Like roundworms and hookworms, they infest the soil by way of feces. They enter the human host as they eat food grown in infested soil. Larvae and adult worms inhabit the large intestine. Mature worms may live for 10 years or more. The disease is usually devoid of symptoms; however, it may cause abdominal pain and gastrointestinal bleeding. When the worm burden is very large, rectal prolapse may occur. In children, infestation can cause iron deficiency anemia and impaired cognitive development. Patients with severe infestation require therapy. Albendazole is the treatment of choice.

Strongyloidiasis (Threadworm Infestation)

Strongyloidiasis is common in the southern United States. Larval and adult threadworms inhabit the small intestine. The disease can be very dangerous, although symptoms are usually absent. Mild infestation may cause abdominal pain and occasional diarrhea. Severe infestation can cause vomiting, massive diarrhea, dehydration, electrolyte imbalance, secondary bacteremia, and sometimes death. Affected individuals should always be treated; ivermectin is the treatment of choice.

Nematode Infestations (Extraintestinal)
Trichinosis (Pork Roundworm Infestation)

Trichinosis, also called trichinellosis, is acquired by eating undercooked pork that contains encysted larvae of *Trichinella spiralis*. Adult worms reside in the intestine, whereas larvae migrate to skeletal muscle and become encysted. Some encysted larvae live for years; others die and calcify within months. Symptoms of trichinosis include gastrointestinal (GI) upset, fever, muscle pain, and sore throat. Potentially lethal complications (heart failure, meningitis, and neuritis) arise in some patients. Albendazole is the drug of choice for killing adult worms and migrating larvae. However, this agent may not be active against larvae that have become encysted. Prednisone (a glucocorticoid) is given to reduce inflammation during larval migration.

Wuchereriasis and Brugiasis (Lymphatic Filarial Infestation)

Wuchereria bancrofti and *Brugia malayi* are filarial nematodes that are spread by mosquito bites. The nematodes subsequently invade the lymphatic system. Infestation with either organism can cause severe complications. When infestation is heavy, lymphatic obstruction occurs, resulting in elephantiasis (usually of the scrotum or legs). In addition, "filarial fever" may develop. Symptoms include chills, fever, headache, nausea, vomiting, constipation, and lymphadenitis. The drug of choice for killing both filarial species is diethylcarbamazine. They have been no cases of this infestation originating in the North America since the 20th century, but those who care for immigrants and refuges need to be alert to these conditions. This drug is not marketed in the United States but is available from the CDC as part of an Investigational New Drug policy.

Onchocerciasis (River Blindness)

Onchocerca volvulus is a filarial nematode found in streams and rivers of Mexico, Guatemala, northern South America, and equatorial Africa. The parasite is transmitted to humans by the bite of certain flies. Heavy infestation with *O. volvulus* causes dermatologic and ophthalmic symptoms. Dermatologic manifestations include subcutaneous nodules (filled with adult worms) and persistent pruritic dermatitis. Ocular lesions, caused by the infiltration and death of microfilariae within the eye, result in optic neuritis, optic atrophy, and then blindness. The drug of choice for treating onchocerciasis is ivermectin.

Cestode Infestations
Taeniasis (Beef and Pork Tapeworm Infestation)

Taeniasis is acquired by eating undercooked beef or pork that contains tapeworm larvae. Adult tapeworms live attached to the wall of the small intestine. Infestation is usually asymptomatic. Taeniasis is treated with praziquantel.

Diphyllobothriasis (Fish Tapeworm Infestation)

Diphyllobothriasis is acquired by ingestion of undercooked fish that is infested with tapeworm larvae. Adult worms inhabit the ileum. Infestation is usually devoid of symptoms. Worms can be killed with praziquantel.

Trematode Infestations
Schistosomiasis (Blood Fluke Infestations)
The term *schistosomiasis* refers to infestation with blood flukes of any species (e.g., *Schistosoma mansoni, Schistosoma japonicum*). Specific snails serve as intermediate hosts for these flukes. Schistosomiasis cannot be acquired in the continental United States because the appropriate snails are not indigenous.

Schistosomiasis has an acute and a chronic phase. The acute phase subsides in 3 to 4 months. Symptoms during this phase include lymphadenopathy, fever, anorexia, malaise, muscle pain, and rash. During the chronic phase, schistosomes take up residence in the vascular system, primarily in veins of the intestines and liver. This late infestation can produce intestinal polyposis, hepatosplenomegaly, and portal hypertension. For either the acute or the chronic stage, praziquantel is the treatment of choice.

Fascioliasis (Liver Fluke Infestation)
Fascioliasis is caused by two liver flukes: *Fasciola hepatica* (sheep liver fluke) and *Clonorchis sinensis* (Chinese liver fluke). Both parasites inhabit the biliary tract. Symptoms (anorexia, mild fever, fatigue, and aching in the region of the liver) are delayed for 1 to 3 months.

Liver flukes differ in drug sensitivity. The preferred drug for use against *F. hepatica* is triclabendazole (a veterinary anthelmintic). It is not approved by the U.S. Food and Drug Administration (FDA), but it is available through the Centers for Disease Control and Prevention (CDC) under an investigational drug protocol. The preferred drugs for use against *C. sinensis* are praziquantel and albendazole.

Fasciolopsiasis (Intestinal Fluke Infestation)
Fasciolopsiasis is most common in Southeast Asia. Adult worms inhabit the small intestine. The disease is usually asymptomatic. However, some people experience ulcer-like pain; some develop constipation or diarrhea; and, in the presence of massive infestation, bowel obstruction may occur, requiring surgery for clearance. Praziquantel is the treatment of choice.

DRUGS OF CHOICE FOR HELMINTHIASIS

The major anthelmintic drugs are considered next. These agents differ in antiparasitic spectra: some are active against several worms and others are more selective. Because of these differences, it is important to identify the invading organism so that the most appropriate drug can be chosen. Table 83.2 lists the major anthelmintic drugs and indicates the parasites against which each is most effective. Although the discussion that follows is limited to drugs of choice, be aware that additional anthelmintics are available.

Mebendazole
Target Organisms
Mebendazole (Emverm and Vermox) is a drug of choice for most intestinal roundworms. This agent clears infestation with pinworms, hookworms, and giant roundworms. Because of its relatively broad spectrum of action, mebendazole is especially useful for treatment of mixed infestations.

Mechanism of Action
Mebendazole prevents uptake of glucose by susceptible intestinal worms. Glucose deprivation results in immobilization followed by slow death. Because the worms die slowly, up to 3 days may elapse between treatment onset and complete clearance of parasites. Mebendazole does not influence glucose uptake or utilization by humans.

TABLE 83.2   First-Choice Anthelmintic Drugs: Target Organisms and Dosages

Generic Name (Trade Name)	Target Organism	Adult and Pediatric Dosages
Mebendazole (Vermox)	Roundworm	100 mg 2 times/day for 3 days *or* 500 mg once
	Hookworm	500 mg once
	Pinworm	100 mg; repeat in 2 weeks
Albendazole (Albenza)	Giant roundworm	400 mg once
	Hookworm	
	Whipworm	400 mg/day for 3 days
	Pork roundworm	400 mg 2 times/day for 8–14 days
	Pinworm	400 mg; repeat in 2 weeks
	Chinese liver fluke	10 mg/kg/day for 7 days
Triclabendazole[a]	Sheep liver fluke	10 mg/kg once or twice
Pyrantel pamoate (Reese's Pinworm Medicine, Combantrin)	Hookworm	11 mg/kg (max. 1 g) for 3 days
	Pinworm	11 mg/kg (max. 1 g); repeat in 2 weeks
Praziquantel (Biltricide)	Beef tapeworm[b]	5–10 mg/kg once
	Pork tapeworm[b]	
	Fish tapeworm[b]	
	Blood flukes (*Schistosoma*)	20 mg/kg 3 doses 4–6 hours apart
	S. japonicum, S. mekongi	20 mg/kg 3 times/day for 1 day
	S. mansoni, S. haematobium	20 mg/kg 2 times/day for 1 day
	Intestinal fluke	25 mg/kg 3 times/day for 1 day
	Chinese liver fluke Lung fluke	25 mg/kg 3 times/day for 2 days
Diethylcarbamazine[c]	*Wuchereria bancrofti* *Brugia malayi*	Day 1: 50 mg Day 2: 50 mg 3 times/day Day 3: 100 mg 3 times/day Days 4–21: 6 mg/kg/day in 3 divided doses
	Loa loa	Day 1: 50 mg Day 2: 50 mg 3 times/day Day 3: 100 mg 3 times/day Days 4–21: 9 mg/kg/day in 3 divided doses
Ivermectin (Stromectol)	Threadworm	200 mcg/kg/day for 2 days
	Giant roundworm	150–200 mcg/kg once
	Onchocerca volvulus	150 mcg/kg every 6–12 months until asymptomatic
Moxidectin (Moxidectin)	*Onchocerca volvulus*	8 mg once

[a]Not available in the United States.
[b]Treatment of adult (intestinal) stage.
[c]Available from the Centers for Disease Control and Prevention.

Pharmacokinetics
Pharmacokinetic information for mebendazole and other anthelmintics is provided in Table 83.3.

Adverse Effects
Systemic effects are rare at usual doses, perhaps because the drug is so poorly absorbed. The most concerning are bone marrow

TABLE 83.3　Pharmacokinetics of Anthelmintics

Generic Name [Trade Name]	Route	Peak	Half Life	Metabolism	Excretion
Mebendazole[a] (Emverm and Vermox)	PO	0.5–6 h	3–6 h	Hepatic	Feces
Albendazole (Albenza)	PO	2–5 h	8–12 h	Hepatic	Urine
Triclabendazole[b]	PO	—	—	—	—
Pyrantel pamoate (Reese's Pinworm Medicine, Combantrin)[a]	PO	1–2 h	2.5–5.5 h	Hepatic	Feces (primary) and urine
Praziquantel (Biltricide)	PO	1–3 h	1–1.5 h	Hepatic	Urine
Diethylcarbamazine[b]	PO	1–2 h	10–12 h	Hepatic	Urine (primary) and feces
Ivermectin (Stromectol)	PO	4 h	16–18 h	Hepatic	Feces (primary) and urine
Moxidectin	PO	4 h	23 days	Minimal	Feces

[a]Absorption is poor, so plasma levels are low.
[b]Not available in the United States. Limited data is available.

suppression and liver impairment; however, these are typically only a problem with high doses or prolonged treatment. In patients with massive parasitic infestations, transient abdominal pain and diarrhea may occur.

Relatively low doses are embryotoxic and teratogenic in some animal reproduction studies. See Lifespan Considerations for Anthelmintics for mebendazole and other drugs in this chapter.

Albendazole

Target Organisms

Albendazole (Albenza) is active against many cestode and nematode parasites, including larval forms of *Taenia solium* and *Echinococcus granulosus*. In the United States, the drug is approved only for (1) parenchymal neurocysticercosis caused by larval forms of the pork tapeworm, *T. solium*; and (2) cystic hydatid disease of the liver, lung, and peritoneum caused by larval forms of the dog tapeworm, *E. granulosus*. However, despite lack of FDA approval, albendazole is considered a drug of choice for infestation with hookworms, pinworms, whipworms, Chinese liver flukes, giant roundworms, and pork roundworms, the cause of trichinosis.

Mechanism of Action

Albendazole inhibits polymerization of tubulin and hence prevents the formation of cytoplasmic microtubules. As a result, microtubule-dependent uptake of glucose is prevented.

Adverse Effects

Albendazole is generally well tolerated. Mild to moderate liver impairment has occurred in 16% of patients, as indicated by elevation of liver transaminases in plasma. Liver function should be assessed before each cycle of treatment and 14 days later.

Albendazole suppresses bone marrow function and can, hence, cause granulocytopenia, agranulocytosis, and even pancytopenia. Liver impairment may increase risk. Blood cell counts should be obtained before each cycle of treatment and 14 days later. In post-marketing studies, some patients developed renal failure. This occurred rarely and the association with albendazole has not been established.

Albendazole is teratogenic in animals and hence should not be used during pregnancy. If pregnancy occurs, the drug should be discontinued immediately.

Pyrantel Pamoate

Target Organisms

Pyrantel pamoate (Reese's Pinworm Medicine, Combantrin) is active against intestinal nematodes. The drug is an alternative to mebendazole or albendazole for infestations with hookworms or pinworms.

PATIENT-CENETERED CARE ACROSS THE LIFE SPAN

Anthelmintics[a]

Life Stage	Considerations or Concerns
Children	There are inadequate studies in children taking most of these drugs. Pyrantel pamoate formulations containing benzyl alcohol or its derivatives should not be prescribed for neonates. As with all drugs the benefits of treatment must be weighed against the risk of adverse effects.
Pregnant Women	Praziquantel appears to be the safest of the anthelmintics. No abnormalities occurred in animal studies. Moxidectin has also demonstrated apparent safety; however, it was only approved in June 2018 and post-marketing studies are unavailable. Animal reproduction studies have demonstrated abnormalities for mebendazole, albendazole, and ivermectin; however, the risk to humans has not been established. The World Health Organization (WHO) allows use of mebendazole, albendazole, and pyrantel pamoate in the second and third trimesters, but not the first trimester, and does not recommend the use of ivermectin and diethylcarbamazine as treatment for women who are pregnant.
Breast-Feeding Women	The WHO advises women taking mebendazole and pyrantel pamoate to continue breastfeeding but advises caution with albendazole and ivermectin. The manufacturer of pyrantel pamoate, however, does not recommend breastfeeding when taking this drug. The manufacturer of praziquantel notes that significant amounts of the drug are excreted into breast milk and advises that women not nurse on the day of praziquantel treatment and during the subsequent 72 hours. Data are lacking for moxidectin.
Older Adults	There are no current contraindications for older adults taking these drugs; however, because there are relatively few studies on the effects of these drugs on older adults, insufficient data are available to determine safety.

[a]Life span information is limited for triclabendazole and diethylcarbamazine, which are not available in the United States.

Mechanism of Action

Pyrantel is a depolarizing neuromuscular blocking agent that causes spastic paralysis of intestinal parasites. The paralyzed worms are cleared in the feces.

Adverse Effects

Neonates given formulations with benzyl alcohol or its derivatives had developed a potentially fatal "gasping syndrome" with complications that include respiratory distress, cardiovascular collapse, seizures, and metabolic acidosis. Otherwise, serious reactions are rare. The most common effects are GI reactions (nausea, vomiting, diarrhea, stomach pain, and cramps). Possible central nervous system effects include dizziness, drowsiness, headache, and insomnia.

Praziquantel
Target Organisms

Praziquantel (Biltricide) is very active against flukes and cestodes (tapeworms), and is the drug of choice for tapeworms, schistosomiasis, and other fluke infestations.

Mechanism of Action

Praziquantel is readily absorbed by helminths. At low therapeutic concentrations, the drug produces spastic paralysis, causing detachment of worms from body tissues. At high therapeutic concentrations, praziquantel disrupts the integument of the worms, rendering the parasites vulnerable to lethal attack by host defenses.

Adverse Effects

Praziquantel is relatively free of toxicity. Transient headache and abdominal discomfort are the most frequent reactions. Drowsiness may occur, and hence patients should avoid driving and other hazardous activities. Post-marketing studies identified an uncommon (less than 1%) occurrence of bradycardia, atrioventricular heart block, and dysrhythmias and elevated liver enzymes.

Ivermectin
Target Organisms

Ivermectin (Stromectol) is active against many nematodes. Currently, the drug has two approved indications: onchocerciasis (a major cause of blindness worldwide) and intestinal strongyloidiasis. Ivermectin is active against the tissue microfilariae of *O. volvulus* (the cause of onchocerciasis), but not against the adult form. However, because adults are unable to produce microfilariae that remain viable, they are not replaced. Ivermectin can also be used to kill mites and lice, although these parasites are not approved targets. In addition to its use in humans, ivermectin is used widely in veterinary medicine.

Mechanism of Action

Ivermectin disrupts nerve traffic and muscle function in target parasites by opening chloride channels on the cell surface, which allows chloride ions to rush into nerve and muscle cells. The resultant hyperpolarization of these cells causes paralysis followed by death. Host cells are not affected, because ivermectin is selective for chloride channels in parasites.

Adverse Effects

Patients treated for onchocerciasis commonly develop pruritus, rash, fever, lymph node tenderness, and bone and joint pain. This reaction, known as a Mazotti reaction, is an allergic and inflammatory response to the death of *O. volvulus* rather than a reaction to the drug. (Mazotti-type reactions do not occur in patients treated for strongyloidiasis.) Abdominal pain and headache are seen in less than 5% of patients. Hypotension develops rarely.

Ivermectin is teratogenic in mice, rats, and rabbits. Cleft palate is the most common effect. There are no adequate data on teratogenesis in humans. Until more is known, ivermectin should be avoided during pregnancy.

Moxidectin
Target Organisms

Moxidectin (Moxidectin) received the FDA approval for treatment of onchocerciasis due to *O. volvulus* in 2018. Activity against other helminths is unknown at this time.

Mechanism of Action

The exact mechanism of moxidectin is unknown, but the end result, like ivermectin, is increased cellular permeability followed by influx of calcium. Also, like ivermectin, the resultant hyperpolarization leads to paralysis.

Adverse Effects

Patients typically experience the flu-like symptoms of the Mazotti-response associated with death of the microfilariae during the first week. Adverse effects mirror those of ivermectin. Early studies suggest that a major advantage over ivermectin is moxidectin's apparent decreased risk for teratogenesis. In animal studies with rats (at 15 times the human dose) and rabbits (at 24 times the human dose), there were no significant effects on the embryo or fetus. Human studies are lacking, though, and we do not yet know what post-marketing studies may reveal.

 SUMMARY OF KEY PRESCRIBING CONSIDERATIONS

Anthelmintic Drugs[a]

Therapeutic Goal: To eradicate parasitic worm infestation
Baseline Data: Confirmation of infestation. Pregnancy test. Drugs requiring additional baseline data are albendazole (liver function and complete blood count [CBC] with differential); mebendazole (liver function, CBC with differential, and renal function); praziquantel (liver function); and ivermectin and moxidectin (ophthalmologic exam for evidence of eye infestation).
Monitoring: Drugs requiring monitoring (other than confirmation of a cure, if needed) are: albendazole (liver function and CBC with differential); mebendazole (liver function, CBC with differential, and renal function); praziquantel (liver function); and ivermectin and moxidectin (ophthalmologic exam if abnormal at baseline).
Identifying High-Risk Patients:
- Albendazole – Because bone marrow suppression, impaired liver function, and possibly renal function may occur, patients with liver or kidney disease, anemia, bleeding disorders, and infections are at increased risk.
- Mebendazole – Because bone marrow suppression and liver impairment may occur, patients with liver disease, anemia, bleeding disorders, and infections are at increased risk.
- Pyrantel pamoate – Patients with liver impairment are at a higher risk for adverse effects. Neonates should not be prescribed formulations containing benzyl alcohol or its derivatives.
- Praziquantel – Patients with cardiac disease, liver impairment, or seizure disorders are at increased risk for complications.
- Ivermectin and Moxidectin – Patients with hypotension or taking antihypertensive drugs may be at risk for increased hypotension and falls.

Evaluating Therapeutic Effects: Follow-up testing confirms cure.
Minimizing Adverse Effects: For most of these drugs, adverse reactions do not require special treatment. Mazotti reactions can be treated with antihistamines and NSAIDs. Rarely, glucocorticoids are needed. Ensuring adequate hydration is important.

[a]Only those available in the United States without restriction are included.

Introduction to Immunomodulators

With the developments in genetics and pharmacogenomics, providers are able to deliver more targeted drug therapy to patients. Although some of these types of drugs entered the market decades ago, it is only with new research that the U.S. Food and Drug Administration (FDA) recently approved increasing numbers of these new drugs. As you will see, many of these drugs treat diseases of the immune system or oncologic disease. In fact, many of these drugs are mislabeled as chemotherapy when they are not chemotherapy, but immunotherapy. In the text that follows, we will discuss both the novel and more common drugs used. Many of these are mentioned in further depth in other chapters of this text. As the classifications of drugs are rapidly increasing, the most commonly used—monoclonal antibodies (mAbs), tyrosine kinase inhibitors (nibs), and proteasome inhibitors (mibs)—are included here.

MONOCLONAL ANTIBODIES "MABS"

Definition and Creation

Something important to notice in the classification of immunotherapy drugs is the ending of the drug name. mAbs contain the three letters *mab* attached to the end of each medication. A mAb is a protein (antibody) derived from a human, a mouse or similar rodent, or a combination of the two. An antigen is introduced into a host, and the host makes antibodies to the antigen. These cells with antibodies are then combined with tumor cells to form *hybridomas* that divide without restriction. Once these cells divide to make enough copies, the antibodies are isolated to make a drug (Fig. 84.1). mAbs work at the site of cell membrane receptors and target specific antigens (Table 84.1). Just like antibodies, mAbs activate the body's natural immune response. Review Chapter 54 for discussion of how antibodies and antigens interact.

MAbs have many uses, including treatment of cancer, asthma, and hemophilia and prevention of migraine headache. The drugs specifically discussed in this chapter include the newer drugs for the treatment of asthma and *Clostridium difficile* and prevention of migraine headache (Table 84.2). mAbs for the treatment of cancer and rheumatoid arthritis are discussed in Chapters 85 and 59.

MONOCLONAL ANTIBODIES FOR ASTHMA

Omalizumab

Omalizumab (Xolair), as discussed in Chapter 62, was the first mAb approved for the treatment of allergy-related asthma. Omalizumab works by combining with free immunoglobulin E (IgE), therefore reducing the available IgE to bind to receptors on the surface of mast cells. By decreasing mast cell activation, airway bronchospasm and airway inflammation are also decreased.

Interleukin Antagonists
Mepolizumab, Benralziumab, and Reslizumab

Mepolizumab (Nucala), benralziumab (Fasenra), and reslizumab (Cinqair) are approved for the treatment of eosinophilic asthma. These drugs bind to interleukin-5 (IL-5), which is responsible for the functioning and survival of eosinophils. As discussed in Chapter 62, eosinophil activation promotes airway inflammation and bronchial hyperreactivity. When these drugs bind to IL-5, it is unable to react with receptors on the surface of eosinophils, therefore decreasing their production and survival.

Dupilumab (Dupixent)

Like the aforementioned drugs, dupilumab is approved for the treatment of eosinophilic asthma. However, dupilimab differs in the specific IL targets. Dupilimab focuses on binding with IL-4 type I and II receptors on mast cells and eosinophils. IL-13 also binds to these type II receptors. IL-4 plays a role in allergic inflammation through many means. Its inhibition of eosinophil apoptosis and induction of eosinophil chemotaxis is hindered with the administration of dupilumab.

MONOCLONAL ANTIBODIES FOR INFECTIOUS DISEASE—*CLOSTRIDIUM DIFFICILE*

Bezlotoxumab

Bezlotoxumab (Zinplava) is used in patients currently undergoing antimicrobial treatment for *C. difficile* who are at high risk for recurrence. This human-derived antibody binds to *C. difficile* toxin B and reduces recurrence in adults. As bezlotoxumab lacks antimicrobial properties, it must be used with another agent in treatment of *C. difficile*. Bezlotoxumab is administered as a single-dose intravenous infusion over 60 minutes.

MONOCLONAL ANTIBODIES FOR MIGRAINE PREVENTION

Erenumab

Erenumab (Aimovig) was the first FDA-approved mAb for the prevention of migraine headaches. As discussed in Chapter 25, it is thought that calcitonin gene–related peptide (CGRP) plays a role in the promotion of migraine headache by promoting vasodilation and release of

Fig. 84.1 Schematic Representation of the Production of Monoclonal Antibodies. (From Andronescu E, Grumezescu MA. *Nanostructures for Drug Delivery.* St. Louis: Elsevier; 2017.)

TABLE 84.1   Differences in Immunotherapy

Type of Immunotherapy	Site of Action	Type of Action	Formulation	Drug Examples	Common Uses
Monoclonal Antibodies (mAbs)	Outside cell at the receptor sites	Increase body's own immune system	Parenteral	Adalimumab, bevacizumab, infliximab, anibizumab, rituximab	Asthma, rheumatoid arthritis, psoriasis, psoriatic arthritis, breast cancer
Tyrosine Kinase Inhibitors (Nibs)	Inside the cell	Block tyrosine kinases that signal cell growth	Oral	Alectinib, cobimetinib, lenvatinib, osimertinib	Hepatocellular carcinoma, renal cell carcinoma, melanoma
Proteasome Inhibitors (Mibs)	Inside the cell	Block proteasomes that breakdown unwanted proteins	Oral Parenteral	Bortezomib, carfilzomib	Multiple myeloma, mantle cell lymphoma

TABLE 84.2   Monoclonal Antibodies

Drug	Trade Name	Target
Asthma		
Omalizumab	Xolair	Free IgE
Mepolizumab	Nucala	IL-5
Benralziumab	Fasenra	IL-5
Reslizumab	Cinqair	IL-5
Duplilumab	Dupixent	IL-4 and IL-13
Infectious Disease—*Clostridium difficile*		
Bezlotoxumab	Zinplava	*C. difficile* toxin B
Prevention of Migraine Headache		
Erenumab (Aimovig)	Aimovig	CGRP
Galcanezumab	Emgality	CGRP
Fremanezmab	Ajovy	CGRP

CGRP, Calcitonin gene–related peptide; *IgE*, immunoglobulin E; *IL*, Interleukin

inflammatory neuropeptides. Plasma levels of CGRP rise during a migraine attack. Erenumab blocks the receptors for CGRP.

Erenumab is produced with Chinese hamster ovary cells. It is administered by the patient as a 70-mg subcutaneous injection given monthly. In clinical trials, erenumab was shown to be effective in the reduction of both episodic and chronic migraine. Soon after the approval of erenumab, galcanezumab (Emgality) and fremanezmab (Ajovy) were also approved for the same indication in late 2018.

COMMON ADVERSE REACTIONS TO MONOCLONAL ANTIBODIES

Immunogenicity

Because immunomodulators boost the patient immune system, immunogenicity, the development of adverse immune reactions, can occur. These reactions occur secondary to the production of antidrug-antibodies (ADAs) that cause inactivation of the drug and can cause dangerous effects for patients, including anaphylaxis.

Characteristics that may increase immunogenicity include prior exposure to a similar protein-derived drug, route of administration, dose, and frequency of administration. Intravenous administration has been associated with decreased risk of sensitization. If the drug is developed from a nonhuman (foreign) source, higher immune responses are likely.

Anaphylaxis

Production of ADAs can lead to anaphylaxis when a specific immunomodulator is administered, although presence of these antibodies does not necessarily indicate anaphylaxis will occur.

Cytokine Release Syndrome

Cytokine release syndrome (CRS) occurs when proinflammatory cytokines are released from leukocytes after the administration of an immunomodulator. Key cytokines involved in the mediation of CRS include primarily IL-6 and can also include IL-1 and IL-2. Common symptoms associated with CRS include fever, nausea, vomiting, diarrhea, and rash. If serious, CRS can present with hypotension, tachycardia, tachypnea, delirium, and seizure. Management of CRS is largely supportive. If severe, tocilizumab, a mAb against IL-6, can be administered.

Nonacute Reactions

Nonacute reactions include delayed hypersensitivity reactions. These reactions generally occur a period of time after administration of the immunomodulator. Reactions are often consistent with serum sickness and can include fever, rash, hemolytic anemia, hematuria, myalgias, and arthralgias. As with CRS, treatment is supportive. Corticosteroids are considered in severe cases.

Toxicity

Certain mAbs are associated with organ toxicity, specifically avelumab, durvalumab, ipilimumab, nivolumab, and pembrolizumab. Signs and symptoms may occur during or up to several months after completion of treatment. Although immunomodulators can affect any organ system, the most common systems are discussed here.

Dermatologic

Many of the mAbs target epidermal growth factor receptor (EGFR). As evident by its name, EGFR is expressed in skin epithelial cells and regulates the differentiation and migration of keratinocytes to the skin surface. Blockade of EGFR has led to skin fissures, acneiform rash, pruritis, and xerosis. Although these may seem minor, patients can become infected with herpes simplex or *Staphylococcus aureus* through loss of integrity due to itchy, dry skin. It is recommended that all patients use sun protectant to help prevent excessive exposure. If dermatologic toxicity occurs, treatment includes topical or systemic corticosteroids, topical or oral antibiotics, or retinoids.

Gastrointestinal

Although many mAbs cause gastrointestinal (GI) toxicity, ipilimumab- and pertuzumab-related diarrhea appears to be very common, occurring in approximately 30% to 50% of patients. The incidence also increases with increases in dose. Severe colitis is seen in 5% to 8% of patients. Treatment includes cessation of the drug and administration of glucocorticoids.

Hepatic

Hepatotoxicity has been witnessed with the administration of mAbs, usually occurring approximately 6 weeks after therapy. Drug-induced liver damage occurs as a result of immune-mediated hepatocyte necrosis and damage to the biliary tree. Elevations in liver enzymes can reach up to 5 times that of normal. This is often of higher concern if there is a concomitant rise in bilirubin levels. Resolution often occurs with cessation of the drug. Severe liver injury is uncommon, although deaths have occurred.

TYROSINE KINASE INHIBITORS "NIBS"

Tyrosine kinase inhibitors contain the letters "nib" at the end of their name. Nibs work intracellularly by blocking tyrosine kinases that send growth signals (see Table 84.1). If the cell cannot send growth signals,

it cannot grow or divide. This is especially helpful in stopping the spread of cancer. Nibs are synthetically created in laboratories and available in oral forms for ingestion. Currently, tyrosine kinase inhibitors are used to treat hepatocellular carcinoma, differentiated thyroid cancer, renal cell carcinoma, metastatic melanoma, and other malignancies. More than 30 tyrosine kinase inhibitors currently exist, as listed in Chapter 85.

Common Tyrosine Kinase Inhibitor Toxicities
Dermatologic

Many of the tyrosine kinase inhibitors target EGFR. Therefore the mechanism for dermatologic toxicity is the same as mentioned previously with the MAbs. Erlotinib appears to produce higher grades (3 to 4) of rash. It has been demonstrated that degree of skin toxicity correlates positively to therapy response to the tyrosine kinase inhibitor.

Gastrointestinal

EGFR is also highly expressed in the epithelial cells of the GI tract. The mechanism of toxicity is likely related to excess chloride secretion, motility dysfunction, and inflammation that occurs with blockade of EGFR. The most common side effect is diarrhea. Also commonly seen is stomatitis, resulting from mucosal inflammation. Incidence of GI toxicity appears higher in patients receiving chemotherapy. Treatment is largely supportive, including administration of loperamide, rehydration, and potentially the use of antibiotics if the patient presents with fever.

PROTEASOME INHIBITORS "MIBS"

Much like the tyrosine kinase inhibitors, proteasome inhibitors work intracellularly (see Table 84.1). Proteasomes break down unused or unwanted proteins existing within a cell. By blocking proteasomes, these unwanted proteins build up, eventually causing cell death. Mibs are used to cause the death of cancer cells. Proteasome inhibitors are used in the treatment of multiple myeloma and mantle cell lymphoma (see Chapter 85). It should be noted that Mibs are substrates of cytochrome P450 enzymes and therefore may cause more medication interactions that other immunotherapies.

Common Proteasome Inhibitor Toxicities
Cardiologic

Although rare, serious adverse cardiac events have been associated with the use of proteasome inhibitors. Most commonly noted include heart failure and arrhythmias. The mechanism for cardiotoxicity is not yet clearly understood, although it is thought to be related to endothelial dysfunction and inflammation. Assessment of cardiac risk factors should be assessed prior to administration. It is not currently recommended to provide routine screening with transthoracic echocardiogram prior to initiation of therapy. It has been demonstrated that higher rates of heart failure are associated with the use of carfilzomib.

Gastrointestinal

GI side effects are commonly reported with the use of proteasome inhibitors. Frequently reported symptoms include nausea, vomiting, diarrhea, and constipation. More severe instances of toxicity, including colitis and colonic ulceration, have occurred. The mechanism behind these side effects is not fully understood but is potentially related to proinflammatory cytokine secretion. Risk factors for development of GI toxicity include increased age, concurrent administration of chemotherapy, history of colitis/diverticulitis/irritable bowel syndrome, or receipt of radiation therapy. It appears that patients experience similar amounts of GI toxicity whether using carfilzomib or bortezomib.

IMMUNOTHERAPY OF THE FUTURE

The rapid and explosive growth of pharmacogenomics continues to produce new and improved targeted drug therapy for patients. We have seen the scope of treatment expand from specific cancers and rheumatoid arthritis to prevention of migraine headaches and asthma exacerbations.

Areas of current and future research include immunotherapy for aging, advanced solid tumors, IgA nephropathy, and Parkinson disease. Undoubtedly, as research on the human genome advances, so will the pharmacologic options for therapy. As practitioners, it is important to maintain current knowledge of emerging treatments.

85

Anticancer Drugs for the Nonspecialist

THE ROLE OF THE NONSPECIALIST

Oncologists and affiliated specialists oversee cancer treatment. The nonspecialist provider does not typically have an active role in deciding how to treat cancer; however, as part of the interdisciplinary team caring for the patient, it remains essential for them to provide preventive care and promote optimal well-being for those patients who receive treatment. Hence it is important to have a basic understanding of cancer, the drugs used to treat cancer, and the effects that anticancer drugs have on patients.

WHAT IS CANCER?

In the discussion that follows, we consider properties shared by neoplastic cells as a group. However, although this discussion addresses cancers in general, the term *cancer* refers to a large group of disorders and not to a single disease. There are more than 100 different types of cancer, most of which have multiple subtypes. These various forms of cancer differ in clinical presentation, aggressiveness, drug sensitivity, and prognosis. Because of this diversity, treatment is individualized on the basis of the specific biology of the cells involved.

Characteristics of Neoplastic Cells
Persistent Proliferation

Cancer cells are genetically altered cells. Unlike normal cells, whose proliferation is carefully controlled, cancer cells undergo unrestrained growth and division. This capacity for persistent proliferation is the most distinguishing property of malignant cells. In the absence of intervention, cancerous tissues will continue to grow until they cause death.

It was once believed that cancer cells divided more rapidly than normal cells and that this excessive rate of division was responsible for the abnormal growth patterns of cancerous tissues. We now know that this concept is not correct. The correct explanation for the relentless growth of tumors is that *malignant cells are unresponsive to the feedback mechanisms that regulate cellular proliferation in healthy tissue.* As a result, cancer cells can continue multiplying under conditions that would suppress further growth and division of normal cells. In other words, instead of dividing more rapidly, they divide more frequently than normal cells.

Invasive Growth

In the absence of malignancy, various types of cells that compose a tissue remain segregated from one another; cells of one type do not invade territory that belongs to cells of a different type. In contrast, malignant cells are free of the constraints that inhibit invasive growth. As a result, cells of a solid tumor can penetrate adjacent tissues, thereby allowing the cancer to spread.

Formation of Metastases

Metastases are secondary tumors that appear at sites distant from the primary tumor. Metastases result from the unique ability of malignant cells to break away from their site of origin, migrate to other parts of the body (through the lymphatic and circulatory systems), and then reimplant to form a new tumor.

Immortality

Unlike normal cells, which are programmed to differentiate and eventually die, cancer cells can undergo endless divisions. The underlying cause for this difference is *telomerase,* an enzyme that is active in most cancers and expressed only rarely in normal cells. Telomerase permits repeated division by preserving *telomeres*—the DNA–protein "caps" found on the ends of all chromosomes. As normal cells divide and differentiate, their telomeres become progressively shorter. Once telomeres lose a critical portion of their length, the cells are unable to keep on dividing. In cancer cells, telomerase continually adds back lost pieces of the telomere and hence preserves or extends telomere length. As a result, cancer cells can divide indefinitely.

Etiology of Cancer

The abnormal behavior of cancer cells results from alterations in their DNA. Specifically, malignant transformation results from a combination of activating *oncogenes* (cancer-causing genes) and inactivating *tumor suppressor genes* (genes that prevent the replication of cells that have become cancerous). These genetic alterations are caused by chemical carcinogens, viruses, and radiation (x-rays, ultraviolet light, and radioisotopes). Malignant transformation occurs in three major stages, namely initiation, promotion, and progression. These stages suggest that DNA in cancer cells undergoes a series of small modifications rather than a single large change. This accumulated genetic damage leads to the dysregulation of cell division and protection against cell death.

It is important to appreciate that the changes in cellular function caused by malignant transformation are primarily *quantitative* rather than *qualitative.* That is, malignant transformation simply results in the over- or underexpression of the same gene products made by normal cells. As a result, cancer cells employ the same metabolic machinery as normal cells, use the same signaling pathways as normal cells, and express the same surface antigens as normal cells. Nonetheless, even though these changes in cellular function are only quantitative, they are still sufficient to allow unrestrained growth and avoidance of cell death.

Epidemiology

The American Cancer Society estimated that 609,640 Americans died from cancer in 2018. Cancer is one of the leading causes of death among all age groups, including children aged 1 to 18 years, in whom it is the leading nonaccidental cause of death. Among women, the most common cancers are breast, lung, and colorectal cancer. Among men, the most common cancers are prostate, lung, and colorectal cancer. (See Table 85.1 for current cancer statistics.)

Although these statistics are grim, the death rate from cancer has been steadily declining for the past two decades. For patients with some

TABLE 85.1   Estimated New Cancer Cases and Deaths, United States, 2018

Type of Cancer	New Cases	Percent of All New Cancer Cases	Deaths	Percent of All Cancer Deaths	5-Year Survival (%)
All types	1,735,350		609,640		66.9
Brain and other CNS	23,880	1.4	16,830	2.8	33.2
Bone and Joint	3,450	0.2	1,590	0.3	66.9
Breast	266,120	15.3	40,920	6.7	89.7
Cervix	13,240	0.8	4,170	0.7	66.2
Colon and rectum	140,250	8.1	50,630	8.3	64.5
Esophagus	17,290	1.0	15,850	2.6	19.2
Kidney and renal pelvis	65,340	3.	14,970	2.5	74.5
Larynx	13,150	0.8	3,710	0.6	60.9
Liver and intrahepatic bile duct	42,220	2.4	30,200	5.0	17.7
Leukemia	60,300	3.5	24,370	4.0	61.4
Lung and bronchus	234,030	13.5	154,050	25.3	18.6
Lymphoma, Hodgkin	8,500	0.5	1,050	0.2	86.6
Lymphoma, Non-Hodgkin	74,680	4.3	19,910	3.3	71.4
Melanoma of skin	91,270	5.3	9,320	1.5	91.8
Myeloma	30,770	1.8	12,770	2.	50.7
Oral cavity and pharynx	51,540	3.0	10,030	1.6	64.8
Ovary	22,240	1.3	14,070	2.3	47.4
Pancreas	55,440	3.2	44,330	7.3	8.5
Prostate	164,690	9.5	29,430	4.8	98.2
Small intestine	10,470	0.6	1,450	0.2	67.6
Soft tissue (including heart)	13,040	0.8	5,150	0.8	64.5
Stomach	26,240	1.5	10,800	1.8	31.0
Testis	9,310	0.5	400	0.1	95.3
Thyroid	53,990	3.1	2,060	0.3	98.1
Urinary bladder	81,190	4.7	17,240	2.8	76.8
Uterus	63,230	3.6	11,350	1.9	81.1
Vulva	6,190	0.4	1,200	0.2	71.0

CNS, Central nervous system
National Cancer Institute. (2018). Surveillance, Epidemiology, and End Results Program. Available at https://seer.cancer.gov/statfacts.
American Cancer Society. (2018). Cancer Statistics 2018. Available at https://www.cancer.org/content/dam/cancer-org/research/cancer-facts-and-statistics/annual-cancer-facts-and-figures/2018/cancer-statistics-presentation-2018.pptx.

forms of cancer, drugs can often be curative. Cancers with a high cure rate include Hodgkin disease, testicular cancer, and acute lymphocytic leukemia. For many patients whose cancer is not yet curable, anticancer therapy can still be of value, offering realistic hopes of palliation and a prolonged life. However, although progress in chemotherapy has been encouraging, the ability to cure most cancers with drugs alone remains elusive.

TREATMENT OF CANCER

There are four major modalities for treating cancer: *surgery, radiation therapy, drug therapy,* and *immunotherapy.* Surgery is the most common treatment for *solid* cancers. In contrast, drug therapy is the treatment of choice for *disseminated* cancers (leukemias, disseminated lymphomas, and metastases) along with several localized cancers (e.g., choriocarcinoma and testicular carcinoma). Drug therapy also plays an important role as an adjunct to surgery and irradiation by suppressing or killing malignant cells that surgery and irradiation leave behind; adjuvant drug therapy can reduce recurrence and improve survival. Immunotherapy is a newer but promising intervention that uses the body's natural defense system to target and kill cancerous cells. It is expected to revolutionize cancer treatment in the future but is still in its early stages. (See Chapter 84.)

Anticancer drugs fall into four major classes: *cytotoxic agents* (i.e., drugs that kill cells directly), *hormones and hormone antagonists, biologic response modifiers* (e.g., immunomodulating agents), and *targeted drugs* (i.e., drugs that bind with specific molecules [targets] that promote cancer growth). Of the four classes, the cytotoxic agents are used most often. Importantly, the term *cancer chemotherapy* applies *only to the cytotoxic drugs*—it does not apply to the use of hormones, biologic response modifiers, or targeted drugs.

INTRODUCTION TO THE CYTOTOXIC ANTICANCER DRUGS

The cytotoxic agents constitute the largest class of anticancer drugs. As their name implies, these agents act directly on cancer cells to cause their death. The cytotoxic drugs can be subdivided into eight major groups: (1) alkylating agents, (2) platinum compounds, (3) antimetabolites, (4) hypomethylating agents, (5) antitumor antibiotics, (6) mitotic inhibitors, (7) topoisomerase inhibitors, and (8) miscellaneous cytotoxic drugs. Individual cytotoxic agents are shown in Table 85.2.

Mechanisms of Cytotoxic Action

Most cytotoxic agents disrupt processes related to the synthesis of DNA or its precursors. In addition, some agents (e.g., vinblastine and

TABLE 85.2 Cytotoxic Anticancer Drugs

Generic Name	Trade Name	Cell-Cycle Phase Specificity	Route	Dose-Limiting Toxicity
Alkylating Agents				
Nitrogen Mustards				
Bendamustine	Treanda	Phase nonspecific	IV	Bone marrow suppression and infusion reactions
Chlorambucil	Leukeran	Phase nonspecific	PO	Bone marrow suppression
Cyclophosphamide	Generic only	Phase nonspecific	PO, IV	Bone marrow suppression
Ifosfamide	Ifex	Phase nonspecific	IV	Bone marrow suppression and hemorrhagic cystitis
Mechlorethamine	Mustargen	Phase nonspecific	IV, IC, IP	Bone marrow suppression
Melphalan	Alkeran	Phase nonspecific	PO, IV	Bone marrow suppression
Nitrosoureas				
Carmustine	BiCNU, Gliadel	Phase nonspecific	IV, CNS implant	Bone marrow suppression
Lomustine	CeeNU	Phase nonspecific	PO	Bone marrow suppression
Streptozocin	Zanosar	Phase nonspecific	IV	Nephrotoxicity
Others				
Busulfan	Myleran, Busulfex	Phase nonspecific	PO, IV	Bone marrow suppression and pulmonary fibrosis
Temozolomide	Temodar and Temodal ♣	Phase nonspecific	PO	Bone marrow suppression
Platinum Compounds				
Carboplatin	Generic only	Phase nonspecific	IV	Bone marrow suppression
Cisplatin	Generic only	Phase nonspecific	IV	Nephrotoxicity
Oxaliplatin	Eloxatin	Phase nonspecific	IV	Peripheral neuropathy
Antimetabolites				
Folic Acid Analogs				
Methotrexate	Rheumatrex and Trexall	S phase–specific	IV, IM, PO, IT	Bone marrow suppression and mucositis
Pemetrexed	Alimta	S phase–specific	IV	Bone marrow suppression
Pralatrexate	Folotyn	S phase–specific	IV	Bone marrow suppression and mucositis
Pyrimidine Analogs				
Capecitabine	Xeloda	Kills dividing cells only, mainly in S phase	PO	Bone marrow suppression, diarrhea, and hand-and-foot syndrome
Cytarabine	DepoCyt and Tarabine PFS ♣	S phase–specific	IV, subQ, and IT	Bone marrow suppression
Floxuridine	FUDR	Kills dividing cells only, mainly in S phase	IA	Bone marrow suppression, oral and GI ulceration
Fluorouracil	Adrucil	Kills dividing cells only, mainly in S phase	IV	Bone marrow suppression and oral and GI ulceration
Gemcitabine	Gemzar	S phase–specific	IV	Bone marrow suppression
Purine Analogs				
Cladribine	Generic only	Kills dividing cells only, mainly in S phase	IV	Bone marrow suppression
Clofarabine	Clolar	S phase–specific	IV	Bone marrow suppression
Fludarabine	Fludara	S phase–specific	IV	Bone marrow suppression
Mercaptopurine	Purinethol	S phase–specific	PO	Bone marrow suppression
Nelarabine	Arranon and Atriance ♣	S phase–specific	IV	Neurotoxicity
Pentostatin	Nipent	S phase–specific	IV	Bone marrow suppression
Thioguanine	Tabloid and Lanvis ♣	S phase–specific	PO, IV	Bone marrow suppression
Hypomethylating Agents				
Azacitidine	Vidaza	S phase–specific	SubQ	Bone marrow suppression
Decitabine	Dacogen	S phase–specific	IV	Bone marrow suppression
Antitumor Antibiotics				
Anthracyclines				
Daunorubicin (conventional)	Cerubidine	Phase nonspecific	IV	Bone marrow suppression and cardiotoxicity

Continued

TABLE 85.2   Cytotoxic Anticancer Drugs—cont'd

Generic Name	Trade Name	Cell-Cycle Phase Specificity	Route	Dose-Limiting Toxicity
Daunorubicin (liposomal)	DaunoXome	Phase nonspecific	IV	Bone marrow suppression and cardiotoxicity
Doxorubicin (conventional)	Adriamycin	Phase nonspecific	IV	Bone marrow suppression, cardiotoxicity
Doxorubicin (liposomal)	Doxil, Caelyx ♣	Phase nonspecific	IV	Bone marrow suppression and heart failure
Epirubicin	Ellence	Phase nonspecific, but S and G_2 most sensitive	IV	Bone marrow suppression and cardiotoxicity
Idarubicin	Idamycin	Phase nonspecific, but S most sensitive	IV	Bone marrow suppression and cardiotoxicity
Valrubicin	Valstar	G_2 phase–specific	Intravesical	Dysuria inadequately controlled by phenazopyridine and hematuria lasting more than 2 days
Mitoxantrone[a]	Novantrone	Phase nonspecific	IV	Bone marrow suppression and cardiotoxicity
Nonanthracyclines				
Bleomycin	Generic only	G_2 phase–specific	IV, IM, subQ, IP	Pneumonitis and pulmonary fibrosis
Dactinomycin	Cosmegen	Phase nonspecific	IV	Bone marrow suppression and mucositis
Mitomycin	Generic only in United States, Mutamycin ♣	Phase nonspecific, but G_1 and S most sensitive	IV	Bone marrow suppression
Mitotic Inhibitors				
Vinca Alkaloids				
Vinblastine	Velban	M phase–specific	IV	Bone marrow suppression
Vincristine (conventional)	Oncovin and Vincasar PFS	M phase–specific	IV	Peripheral neuropathy
Vincristine (liposomal)	Marqibo	M phase–specific	IV	Peripheral neuropathy
Vinorelbine	Navelbine	M phase–specific	IV	Bone marrow suppression
Taxanes				
Cabazitaxel	Jevtana	G_2/M phase–specific	IV	Bone marrow suppression and diarrhea
Docetaxel	Docefrez and Taxotere	G_2/M phase–specific	IV	Bone marrow suppression
Paclitaxel	Abraxane, Onxol, and Taxol ♣	G_2/M phase–specific	IV	Bone marrow suppression
Others				
Eribulin	Halaven	G_2/M phase–specific	IV	Bone marrow suppression and peripheral neuropathy
Estramustine	Emcyt	M phase–specific	PO	Nausea and vomiting
Ixabepilone	Ixempra	G_2/M phase–specific	IV	Bone marrow suppression and neurotoxicity
Topoisomerase Inhibitors				
Etoposide	Toposar	S and G_2 most sensitive	IV, PO	Bone marrow suppression
Irinotecan	Camptosar	S phase–specific	IV	Bone marrow suppression and late diarrhea
Teniposide	Vumon	S and G_2 most sensitive	IV	Bone marrow suppression
Topotecan	Hycamtin	S phase–specific	IV	Bone marrow suppression
Miscellaneous				
Altretamine	Hexalen	Specificity unknown	PO	Bone marrow suppression
Asparaginase	Elspar, Erwinase ♣, and Kidrolase ♣	G_1 phase–specific	IV, IM	None
Dacarbazine	DTIC-Dome	Phase nonspecific	IV	Bone marrow suppression
Hydroxyurea	Hydrea	S phase–specific	PO	Bone marrow suppression
Mitotane	Lysodren	Phase nonspecific	PO	CNS depression
Pegaspargase	Oncaspar	G_1 phase–specific	IV, IM	None
Procarbazine	Matulane	Phase nonspecific	PO	Bone marrow suppression

[a]Mitoxantrone is classified chemically as an anthracenedione, which is very similar to an anthracycline.
CNS, Central nervous system; *GI*, gastrointestinal; *IA*, intra-arterial; *IC*, intracavitary; *IM*, intramuscular; *IP*, intrapleural; *IT*, intrathecal; *IV*, intravenous; *PO*, oral; *subQ*, subcutaneous.

vincristine) act specifically to block mitosis, and one drug—asparaginase—disrupts the synthesis of proteins. Note that, with the exception of asparaginase, all of the cytotoxic drugs disrupt processes carried out exclusively by cells that are undergoing replication. As a result, these drugs are most toxic to tissues that have a high growth fraction (i.e., a high proportion of proliferating cells).

Cell-Cycle Phase Specificity

Some anticancer agents, known as *cell-cycle phase–specific drugs*, are effective only during a specific phase of the cell cycle (Box 85.1). Other anticancer agents, known as cell-cycle phase–nonspecific drugs, can affect cells during any phase of the cell cycle. About half of the cytotoxic anticancer drugs are phase-specific and the other half are phase-nonspecific. The cell-cycle phase specificity of individual cytotoxic agents is shown in Table 85.2.

Cell-Cycle Phase–Specific Drugs

Phase-specific agents are toxic only to cells during replication as they pass through a particular phase of the cell cycle (Fig. 85.1). Vincristine, for example, acts by causing mitotic arrest and hence is effective only during M phase. Other agents act by disrupting DNA synthesis and hence are effective only during S phase. Because of their phase specificity, these drugs are toxic only to cells that are active participants in the cell cycle; cells that are "resting" in G_0 are not harmed. Obviously if these drugs are to be effective, they must be present as neoplastic cells cycle through the specific phase in which they act. Accordingly, these drugs must be present for an extended time. To accomplish this, phase-specific drugs are often administered by prolonged infusion. Alternatively, they can be given in multiple doses at short intervals over an extended time. Because the dosing schedule is so critical to the therapeutic response, phase-specific drugs are also known as *schedule-dependent drugs*.

Cell-Cycle Phase–Nonspecific Drugs

The phase-nonspecific drugs can act during any phase of the cell cycle, including G_0. Among the phase-nonspecific drugs are the alkylating agents and most antitumor antibiotics. Because phase-nonspecific drugs can injure cells throughout the cell cycle whereas phase-specific drugs cannot, phase-nonspecific drugs can increase cell kill when combined with phase-specific drugs.

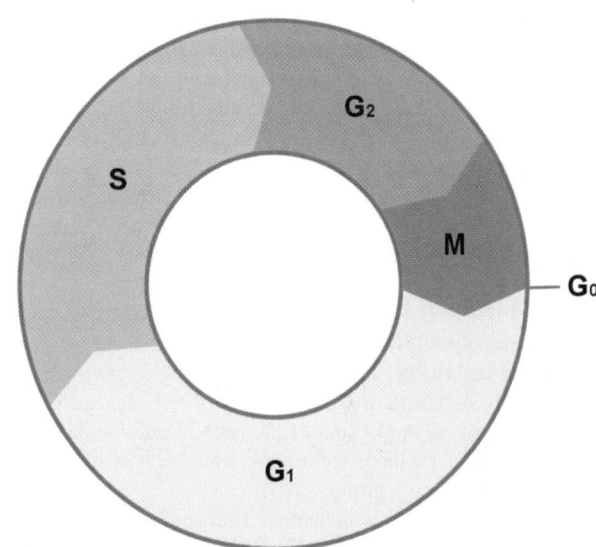

Fig. 85.1 The Cell Cycle. G_0 – Cell in resting phase; G^1 – Synthesis of components needed for DNA synthesis; S – Synthesis of DNA; G_2 – Synthesis of components needed for mitosis; M – Mitosis (cell division).

BOX 85.1 The Growth Fraction and Its Relationship to Chemotherapy

The growth fraction of a tissue is a major determinant of its responsiveness to chemotherapy. Consequently, before we discuss the anticancer drugs, we must first understand the growth fraction. To define the growth fraction, we must review the cell cycle.

The Cell Cycle

The cell cycle is the sequence of events that a cell goes through from one mitotic division to the next. As shown in Fig. 85.1, the cell cycle consists of four major phases, namely G_1, S, G_2, and M. (The length of the *arrows* in the figure is proportional to the time spent in each phase.) For our purpose, we can imagine the cycle as beginning with G_1, the phase in which the cell prepares to make DNA. After G_1, the cell enters S phase, the phase in which DNA synthesis actually takes place. After synthesis of DNA is complete, the cell enters G_2 and prepares for mitosis (cell division). Mitosis occurs next during M phase. On completing mitosis, the resulting daughter cells have two options: they can enter G_1 and repeat the cycle or they can enter the phase known as G_0. Cells that enter G_0 become mitotically dormant; they do not replicate and are not active participants in the cycle. Cells may remain in G_0 for days, weeks, or even years. Under appropriate conditions, resting cells may leave G_0 and resume active participation in the cycle.

The Growth Fraction

In any tissue, some cells are going through the cell cycle whereas others are "resting" in G_0. The ratio of proliferating cells to G_0 cells is called the *growth fraction*. A tissue with a large percentage of proliferating cells and few cells in G_0 has a *high* growth fraction. Conversely, a tissue composed mostly of G_0 cells has a *low* growth fraction.

Impact of Tissue Growth Fraction on Responsiveness to Chemotherapy

As a rule, *chemotherapeutic drugs are much more toxic to tissues that have a high growth fraction than to tissues that have a low growth fraction*. Why? Because most cytotoxic agents are more active against proliferating cells than against cells in G_0. Proliferating cells are especially sensitive to chemotherapy because cytotoxic drugs usually act by disrupting either DNA synthesis or mitosis—activities that only proliferating cells carry out. Unfortunately the toxicity of anticancer drugs is not restricted to cancers: These drugs are also toxic to normal tissues that have a high growth fraction (e.g., bone marrow, GI epithelium, hair follicles, and sperm-forming cells).

Having established the relationship between growth fraction and drug sensitivity, we can apply this knowledge to predict how specific cancers will respond to chemotherapy. As a rule, *the most common cancers*—solid tumors of the breast, lung, prostate, colon, and rectum—have a *low* growth fraction, so they respond *poorly to cytotoxic drugs*. In contrast, only some rarer cancers—such as acute lymphocytic leukemia, Hodgkin disease, and certain testicular cancers—have a *high* growth fraction, so they tend to respond *well to cytotoxic drugs*. In practical terms, this means that the most common cancers, which don't respond well to drugs, must be managed primarily with surgery. Only a few cancers can be managed primarily with drugs.

Although the phase-nonspecific drugs can cause biochemical lesions at any time during the cell cycle, *as a rule these drugs are more toxic to proliferating cells than to cells in G_0.* There are two reasons why this is so. First, cells in G_0 have time to repair drug-induced damage before it can result in significant harm. In contrast, proliferating cells often lack time for repair. Second, toxicity may not become manifest until the cells attempt to proliferate. For example, many alkylating agents act by producing cross-links between DNA strands. Although these biochemical lesions can be made at any time, they are largely without effect until cells attempt to replicate DNA. This is much similar to putting a flat tire on an automobile: the tire can deflate at any time; however, loss of air is consequential only if the car is moving. Carrying the analogy further, if the flat occurs while the car is stopped and is repaired before travel is attempted, the flat will have no functional effect at all.

It should be noted that some dividing cells are more vulnerable than others. Specifically, cells that divide frequently are harmed more readily than cells that divide infrequently because the cytotoxic drugs have more opportunities to act.

Toxicity to Normal Cells

Toxicity to normal cells is a major barrier to successful chemotherapy. Injury to normal cells occurs primarily in tissues where the growth fraction is high: bone marrow, gastrointestinal (GI) epithelium, hair follicles, and germinal epithelium of the testes. Drug-induced injury to each of these tissues is discussed in detail later. For now, let's consider injury to normal cells as a group.

Toxicity to normal cells is dose-limiting. That is, dosage cannot exceed an amount that produces the maximally tolerated injury to normal cells. Although very large doses of cytotoxic drugs might be able to produce cure, these doses cannot be given because they are likely to kill the patient.

Why are cytotoxic anticancer drugs so harmful to normal tissues? Because these drugs lack selective toxicity. That is, they cannot kill target cells without also killing other cells with which the target cells are in intimate contact. We encountered this concept in Chapter 70. As noted there, successful antimicrobial therapy is possible because antimicrobial drugs are highly selective in their toxicity. Penicillin, for example, can readily kill invading bacteria while being virtually harmless to cells of the host. This high degree of selective toxicity stands in sharp contrast to the lack of selectivity displayed by cytotoxic anticancer drugs.

Why have we been unable to develop drugs that selectively kill neoplastic cells? Because neoplastic cells and normal cells are very similar; differences between them are quantitative rather than qualitative. To make a cytotoxic drug that is truly selective, the target cell must have a biochemical feature that normal cells lack. Unfortunately, we have yet to identify unique biochemical features that would render cancer cells vulnerable to selective attack. Nevertheless, there is reason for hope: our expanding knowledge of cancer biology is revealing potential new targets for anticancer drugs. Exploiting these targets may lead to anticancer drugs that are more selective than the drugs we have now.

Major Toxicities of Cytotoxic Drugs

The agents used for cancer chemotherapy constitute our most toxic group of medicines. In the discussion that follows, we consider the more common toxicities of the *cytotoxic* anticancer drugs along with steps that can be taken to minimize harm and discomfort.

Bone Marrow Suppression

Chemotherapeutic drugs are highly toxic to the bone marrow, a tissue with a high proportion of proliferating cells. Myelosuppression reduces the number of circulating neutrophils, platelets, and erythrocytes. Loss of these cells has three major consequences: (1) infection (from loss of

neutrophils), (2) bleeding (from loss of platelets), and (3) anemia (from loss of erythrocytes).

Neutropenia. Neutrophils (neutrophilic granulocytes) are white blood cells that play a critical role in fighting infection. In patients with neutropenia (a reduction in circulating neutrophils), both the incidence and severity of infection are increased. Infections that are normally benign (e.g., candidiasis) can become life-threatening. Infection secondary to neutropenia is one of the most serious complications of chemotherapy.

With most anticancer drugs, onset of neutropenia is rapid and recovery develops relatively quickly. Neutropenia begins to develop a few days after dosing, and the lowest neutrophil count, called the *nadir,* occurs between days 10 and 14. Neutrophil counts then recover a week or so later. Patients are at highest risk during the nadir. Accordingly, special care should be taken at this time to prevent infection.

With some anticancer drugs, neutropenia is *delayed.* Neutrophil counts begin to fall in 1 to 2 weeks and reach their nadir between weeks 3 and 4. Full recovery may not occur until after week 7.

Neutrophil counts must be monitored. Normal cell counts range from 2500 to 7000/mm^3. If neutropenia is substantial (absolute neutrophil count below 500/mm^3), chemotherapy should be withheld until neutrophil counts return toward normal. Fortunately normal cells such as neutrophils repopulate faster than malignant cells (Fig. 85.2).

Lack of neutrophils confounds the diagnosis of infection because the usual signs of infection (e.g., purulent drainage, abscesses, and infiltrates on the chest radiograph) depend on neutrophils being present. In the absence of neutrophils, *fever* is the principal early sign of infection.

Patients must be their own first line of defense against infection. They should be made aware of their elevated risk for infection and taught how to minimize contagion. They should be informed that fever may be the only indication of infection and instructed to report immediately if fever develops. Because infection is commonly acquired through contact with other people, hospitalized patients should be instructed to refuse direct contact with anyone who has not washed his or her hands in the patient's presence. This rule applies not only to visiting friends and relatives but also to nurses, providers, and all other hospital staff. The normal flora of the body is a major source of infection;

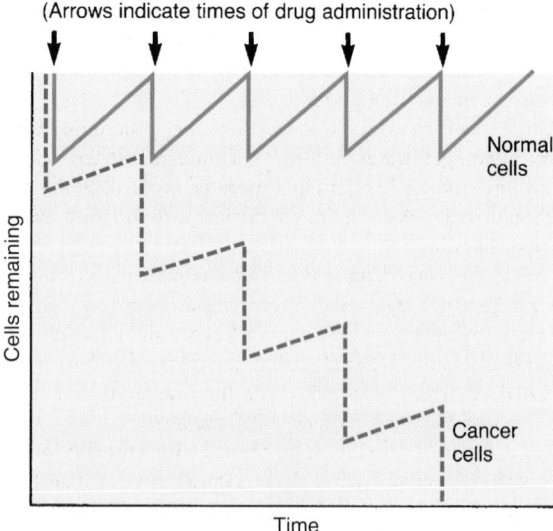

(Arrows indicate times of drug administration)

Fig. 85.2 Recovery of Critical Normal Cells. Cancer cells and normal cells (e.g., cells of the bone marrow) are killed each time cytotoxic drugs are given. In the interval between doses, both types of cells proliferate. Because normal cells repopulate faster than cancer cells, normal cells are able to recover in higher numbers between doses, whereas regrowth of the cancer cells is slower.

the risk for acquiring an infection with these microbes can be reduced by daily examination and cleansing of the skin and oral cavity.

Hospitalization of the infection-free neutropenic patient is controversial. Some providers feel that hospitalization *increases* the risk for acquiring a serious infection because hospitals harbor drug-resistant microbes, which can make hospital-acquired (nosocomial) infections especially difficult to treat. Accordingly, these providers recommend that neutropenic patients stay at home as long as they remain infection-free.

If neutropenic patients *are* hospitalized, every precaution must be taken to prevent nosocomial infection. Patients should be given an isolation room and monitored frequently for fever. Certain foods (e.g., lettuce) abound in pathogenic bacteria and must be avoided.

When a neutropenic patient develops an infection, immediate and vigorous intervention is required. Specimens for culture should be taken to determine the identity and drug sensitivity of the infecting organism. While awaiting reports on the cultures, empiric therapy with intravenous antibiotics should be instituted. Therapy is usually initiated with a single drug active against *Pseudomonas* species and other gram-negative bacteria. Options include ceftazidime, imipenem, and doripenem. If the patient develops sepsis, an aminoglycoside (e.g., tobramycin and amikacin) is added. If the patient remains febrile, vancomycin is added (for gram-positive coverage).

Colony-stimulating factors can minimize neutropenia. Three preparations are available: *granulocyte colony-stimulating factor* (filgrastim), long-acting granulocyte colony-stimulating factor (pegfilgrastim), and *granulocyte-macrophage colony-stimulating factor* (GM-CSF) (sargramostim). All three drugs act on the bone marrow to enhance granulocyte (neutrophil) production. Colony-stimulating factors can decrease the incidence, magnitude, and duration of neutropenia. As a result, they can decrease the incidence and severity of infection as well as the need for intravenous antibiotics and hospitalization.

Thrombocytopenia. Bone marrow suppression can cause thrombocytopenia (a reduction in circulating platelets), thereby increasing the risk for serious bleeding. Bleeding from the nose and gums is relatively common. Bleeding from the gums can be reduced by avoiding vigorous tooth brushing. Drugs that promote bleeding (e.g., aspirin and anticoagulants) should not be used. When a mild analgesic is required, acetaminophen, which does not promote bleeding, is preferred to aspirin. For patients with severe thrombocytopenia, platelet infusions are the mainstay of treatment. Platelet production can be stimulated with *oprelvekin* (Neumega). However, owing to limited efficacy and flu-like reactions, oprelvekin is not often used.

Caution should be exercised when performing procedures that might promote bleeding. Intravenous needles should be inserted with special care and intramuscular injections should be avoided. Blood pressure cuffs should be applied cautiously because overinflation may cause bruising or bleeding.

Anemia. Anemia is defined as a reduction in the number of circulating erythrocytes (red blood cells). Although anticancer drugs can suppress erythrocyte production, anemia is much less common than neutropenia or thrombocytopenia because circulating erythrocytes have a long life span (120 days), which usually allows erythrocyte production to recover before levels of existing erythrocytes fall too low.

If anemia does develop, it can be treated with a transfusion or with erythropoietin (*epoetin α* or *darbepoetin α*), a hormone that stimulates production of red blood cells. Because transfusions require the patient to make arrangements for treatment at an outpatient facility whereas epoetin can be administered at home, epoetin therapy can spare the patient inconvenience. However, erythropoietin has two huge drawbacks. First, it cannot be used in patients with leukemias and other myeloid malignancies (because it can stimulate proliferation of these cancers). Second, it *shortens* survival in all cancer patients and hence is indicated only when the treatment goal is *palliation.* Clearly erythropoietin should not be used when the goal is cure or prolongation of life. Erythropoietin is discussed in Chapter 46.

Digestive Tract Injury

The epithelial lining of the GI tract has a very high growth fraction, so it is exquisitely sensitive to cytotoxic drugs. Stomatitis and diarrhea are common. Severe GI injury can be life-threatening.

Stomatitis. Stomatitis (inflammation of the oral mucosa) often develops a few days after the onset of chemotherapy and may persist for 2 or more weeks after treatment has ceased. Inflammation can progress to denudation and ulceration and is often complicated by infection. Pain can be severe, inhibiting eating, speaking, and swallowing. Management includes good oral hygiene and a bland diet. Topical antifungal drugs may be needed to control infection with *Candida albicans*. For patients with mild stomatitis, pain can be managed with a mouthwash containing a topical anesthetic (e.g., lidocaine) plus an antihistamine (e.g., diphenhydramine). For patients with severe stomatitis, a systemic opioid is needed for pain. In some cases, stomatitis is so severe that chemotherapy has to be interrupted. For patients being treated for hematologic malignancies, *palifermin* (Kepivance), a chemoprotective agent and keratinocyte growth factor, can decrease the severity of stomatitis.

Diarrhea. By injuring the epithelial lining of the intestine, anticancer drugs can impair absorption of fluids and other nutrients, thereby causing diarrhea. Diarrhea can be reduced with oral loperamide, a nonabsorbable opioid that slows gut motility by activating local opioid receptors.

Nausea and vomiting. Chemotherapy-induced nausea and vomiting (CINV) are common sequelae of cancer chemotherapy. These responses, which result in part from direct stimulation of the chemoreceptor trigger zone, can be both immediate and dramatic and may persist for hours or even days. In some cases, discomfort is so great as to prompt refusal of further treatment.

It should be noted that nausea and vomiting associated with chemotherapy are much more severe than with other medications. Although these reactions are generally unremarkable with most drugs, they must be considered major and characteristic toxicities of cytotoxic drugs. The emetogenic potential of several intravenous agents is shown in Table 85.3.

Nausea and vomiting can be reduced by premedication with antiemetics. These drugs offer three benefits: (1) reduction of anticipatory nausea and vomiting, (2) prevention of dehydration and malnutrition secondary to frequent nausea and vomiting, and (3) promotion of compliance with chemotherapy by reducing discomfort. Combinations of antiemetics are more effective than single-drug therapy. The regimen of choice for patients taking highly emetogenic drugs consists of a neurokinin-1 receptor antagonists (e.g., aprepitant [Emend] or its prodrug fosaprepitant [Emend IV]), a glucocorticoid (e.g., dexamethasone), and a serotonin antagonist (e.g., ondansetron [Zofran]) or atypical antipsychotic (e.g., olanzapine [Zyprexa]). These drugs are typically administered prior to chemotherapy and continued for up to 4 days. Other antiemetics may also be used to supplement or replace one or more of these drugs if their use is contraindicated. The use of antiemetics for CINV is discussed in Chapter 66.

Many patients have reported relief from smoking marijuana. There have been relatively few studies on botanical marijuana. However, whether because of the drug or a placebo effect, anecdotal reports by patients who perceive relief and report vomiting less are plentiful. In states where it is legal to prescribe cannabinoids, the determination of results has been more promising. A review of CINV management with cannabinoids, published in *Cancer Chemotherapy and Pharmacology* (2017),

TABLE 85.3 Emetogenic Potential of Selected Intravenous Anticancer Drugs

Severe	Carmustine
	Cisplatin
	Cyclophosphamide (high dose)
	Dacarbazine
	Dactinomycin
	Mechlorethamine
	Streptozocin
Moderate	Carboplatin
	Cyclophosphamide (low dose)
	Daunorubicin
	Doxorubicin
	Epirubicin
	Idarubicin
	Ifosfamide
	Irinotecan
	Oxaliplatin
Low	Cytarabine
	Docetaxel
	Etoposide
	Fluorouracil
	Gemcitabine
	Methotrexate (high dose)
	Mitomycin
	Mitoxantrone
	Paclitaxel
	Pemetrexed
	Topotecan
	Trastuzumab
Minimal	Bevacizumab
	Bleomycin
	Busulfan
	Cetuximab
	Fludarabine
	Pralatrexate
	Rituximab
	Vinblastine
	Vincristine
	Vinorelbine

demonstrated improved outcomes for patients taking these drugs in a large majority of cases. A series of meta-analyses comparing cannabinoids with other antiemetics found that cannabinoids were not only more effective than a placebo but also more effective than commonly used antiemetics such as chlorpromazine, haloperidol, metoclopramide, or prochlorperazine.

It should be noted that the degree of relief from cannabinoids does not approach that of the recommended first-line agents for CINV, but perhaps their best use is as an add-on drug. The reason for this is their unique mechanism of action—the binding of cannabinoid receptors—which offers a benefit that other antiemetics do not have.

Other Important Toxicities

Alopecia. Reversible alopecia (hair loss) results from injury to hair follicles. Alopecia can occur with most cytotoxic anticancer drugs. Hair loss begins 7 to 10 days after the onset of treatment and reaches maximal loss in 1 to 2 months. Regeneration begins 1 to 2 months after the last course of treatment.

Although alopecia is not dangerous, it is still very upsetting. In fact, for many cancer patients, alopecia is second only to vomiting as their greatest treatment-related fear. If drugs are expected to cause hair loss, the patient should be forewarned. For patients who choose to wear a hairpiece or wig, one should be selected before hair loss occurs. Hairpieces are tax-deductible as medical expenses and are covered by some insurance plans.

To some degree, hair loss can be prevented by cooling the scalp while chemotherapy is being administered. Cooling causes vasoconstriction and therefore reduces drug delivery to hair follicles. Unfortunately, scalp cooling is uncomfortable, causes headache, and creates a small risk for cancer recurrence in the scalp (because drug delivery is reduced).

Reproductive toxicity. The developing fetus and the germinal epithelium of the testes have high growth fractions. As a result, both are highly susceptible to injury by cytotoxic drugs, especially the alkylating agents. These drugs can interfere with embryogenesis, causing death of the early embryo. They may also cause fetal malformation. Risk is the highest during the first trimester; hence chemotherapy should generally be avoided during this time. However, after 18 weeks of gestation, risk appears to be very low: according to a report in *Lancet*, exposure during this time does not cause neurologic, cardiac, or any other fetal abnormalities. Drug effects on the ovaries may result in amenorrhea, menopausal symptoms, and atrophy of the vaginal epithelium.

Cytotoxic drugs can cause irreversible sterility in males. Men should be forewarned and counseled about sperm banking.

Hyperuricemia. Hyperuricemia is defined as an excessive level of uric acid in the blood. Uric acid, a compound with low solubility, is formed by the breakdown of DNA after cell death. Hyperuricemia is especially common after treatment for leukemias and lymphomas (because therapy results in massive cell kill). The major concern with hyperuricemia is injury to the kidneys secondary to deposition of uric acid crystals in renal tubules. The risk for crystal formation can be reduced by increasing fluid intake. In patients with leukemias and lymphomas, in whom hyperuricemia is likely, prophylaxis with *allopurinol* is the standard of care. (As discussed in Chapter 60, allopurinol prevents hyperuricemia by inhibiting xanthine oxidase, an enzyme involved in converting nucleic acids to uric acid. If hyperuricemia develops despite the use of allopurinol, it can be managed with *rasburicase,* an enzyme that catalyzes uric acid degradation).

Local Injury from Extravasation of Vesicants

Certain anticancer drugs, known as *vesicants,* are highly chemically reactive. These drugs can cause severe local injury if they make direct contact with tissues. Vesicants are administered intravenously, usually into a central line because rapid dilution in venous blood minimizes the risk for injury. When a peripheral line is used, administration is by intravenous push into a freely flowing intravenous line. Sites of previous irradiation should be avoided. Extreme care must be exercised to prevent extravasation because leakage can produce high local concentrations, resulting in prolonged pain, infection, and loss of mobility. Severe injury can lead to necrosis and sloughing, requiring surgical débridement and skin grafting. If extravasation occurs, the infusion should be stopped immediately. Because of the potential for severe tissue damage, vesicants should be administered only by clinicians specially trained to handle them safely.

Unique Toxicities

In addition to the toxicities discussed previously, which generally apply to the cytotoxic drugs as a group, some agents produce unique toxicities. For example, a number of drugs can cause peripheral sensory neuropathy, manifesting as numbness or tingling in the fingers and toes and around the mouth and throat. Neuropathy may impede activities of daily living, such as buttoning clothing, writing, or just holding things. Anthracyclines such as daunorubicin and doxorubicin can cause serious injury to the heart. Ifosfamide, a nitrogen mustard, can cause severe hemorrhagic cystitis.

Carcinogenesis

Along with their other adverse actions, anticancer drugs have one final and ironic toxicity: these drugs, which are used to treat cancer, have caused cancer in some patients. Such cancer results from drug-induced damage to DNA and is most likely to occur with alkylating agents. Cancers caused by anticancer drugs may take many years to appear and are hard to treat.

Making the Decision to Treat With Cytotoxic Drugs

From the preceding discussion of toxicities, it is clear that cytotoxic anticancer drugs can cause great harm. Given the known dangers of these drugs, we must ask why such toxic substances are given to sick people at all. The answer lies with the primary rule of therapeutics, which states that the benefits of treatment must outweigh the risks. For most patients undergoing chemotherapy, the conditions of this rule are met. That is, although the toxicities of the anticancer drugs can be significant, the potential benefits (cure, prolonged life, and palliation) justify the risks. However, the desirability of treating cancer with drugs is not always obvious. There are patients whose chances of being helped by chemotherapy are remote, whereas the risk for serious toxicity is high. Because the potential benefits for some patients are small and the risks are large, the decision to institute chemotherapy must be made with care.

Before a decision to treat can be made, the patient must be given some idea of the benefits the proposed therapy might offer. Three basic benefits are possible: cure, prolongation of life, and palliation. For treatment to be justified, there should be reason to believe that at least one of these benefits will be forthcoming. If a patient cannot be offered some reasonable hope of cure, prolonged life, or palliation, it would be difficult to justify treatment.

The most important factors for predicting the outcome of chemo- therapy are (1) the general health of the patient and (2) the responsiveness of the type of cancer the patient has. General health status is assessed by measuring performance status, frequently using the Karnofsky Performance Scale (Table 85.4). A Karnofsky score of less than 40 indicates the patient is debilitated and not likely to tolerate the additional stress of chemotherapy. Accordingly, patients with a low Karnofsky rating should not receive anticancer drugs unless their cancer is known to be especially responsive. Similar rating scales have been developed by the Eastern Cooperative Oncology Group (ECOG) available at http:// www.npcrc.org/files/news/ECOG_performance_status.pdf and the Palliative Performance Scale (PPSv2) available at http://www.npcrc.org/ files/news/palliative_performance_scale_PPSv2.pdf).

The responsiveness of specific cancers is not highly predictable: some patients with a specific type of cancer may respond well, but others may not. Nonetheless, we should still try to assess whether treatment is likely to produce cure, palliation, or prolonged life. If a positive outcome is deemed likely, the patient should almost always be treated, even if his or her Karnofsky score is low. In contrast, if a positive outcome is deemed highly unlikely, the patient should be treated only after careful consideration so as to avoid the discomforts of a course of treatment that has little to offer.

An important requirement for deciding in favor of chemotherapy is that the effect of treatment be measurable. That is, there must be some objective means of determining the cancer's response to drugs. For solid tumors, we should be able to measure a decrease in tumor size (or at least inhibition of further growth). For hematologic cancers, we should be able to measure a decrease in neoplastic cells in blood

TABLE 85.4   Karnofsky Performance Scale

Definition	Percentage	Criteria
Able to carry on normal activity and work; no special care needed	100	Normal; no complaints; no evidence of disease
	90	Able to carry on normal activity; minor signs or symptoms of disease
	80	Normal activity with effort; some signs or symptoms of disease
Unable to work; able to live at home and care for most personal needs; a varying amount of assistance needed	70	Cares for self; unable to carry on normal activity or do active work
	60	Requires occasional assistance; able to care for most needs
	50	Requires considerable assistance and frequent medical care
Unable to care for self; requires equivalent of institutional or hospital care; disease may be progressing rapidly	40	Disabled; requires special care and assistance
	30	Severely disabled; hospitalization is indicated although death not imminent
	20	Very sick, hospitalization necessary; active supportive treatment necessary
	10	Moribund; fatal processes progressing rapidly
	0	Dead

and bone marrow. If we have no way to measure the response of a cancer, then we have no way of knowing if treatment has done any good. If we cannot determine that drugs are doing something beneficial, there is little justification for giving them.

Clearly not all patients are candidates for chemotherapy. The decision to institute treatment must be individualized. Patients should be informed as accurately as possible about the potential risks and benefits of the proposed therapy. When the decision to treat is made, it should be the result of collaboration between the patient, family, and physician and should reflect a conviction on the part of the patient that, within his or her set of values, the potential benefits outweigh the inherent risks.

CYTOTOXIC AGENTS

Alkylating Agents

The family of alkylating agents consists of nitrogen mustards, nitro- soureas, and other compounds. The alkylating agents are shown in Table 85.2.

Shared Properties

Mechanism of action. The alkylating agents are highly reactive compounds that can transfer an alkyl group to various cell constituents. Cell kill results primarily from alkylation of DNA. As a rule, alkylating agents interact with DNA by forming a covalent bond with a specific nitrogen atom in guanine.

Some alkylating agents have two reactive sites whereas others have only one. Alkylating agents with two reactive sites (*bifunctional* agents) are able to bind DNA in two places to form *crosslinks*. These bridges may be formed within a single DNA strand or between parallel DNA

Fig. 85.3 Crosslinking of DNA by an Alkylating Agent. (A) Reactions leading to cross-linkage between guanine moieties in DNA. (B) Schematic representation of interstrand crosslinking within the DNA double helix. *A,* Adenine; *C,* cytosine; *G,* guanine; *T,* thymine.

strands. Fig. 85.3 shows the production of interstrand crosslinks by nitrogen mustard. Alkylating agents with only one reactive site (*monofunctional* agents) lack the ability to form crosslinks but can still bind to a single guanine in DNA.

The consequences of guanine alkylation are miscoding, scission of DNA strands, and, if crosslinks have been formed, inhibition of DNA replication. Because crosslinking of DNA is especially injurious, cell death is more likely with bifunctional agents than with monofunctional agents.

Because alkylation reactions can take place at any time during the cell cycle, alkylating agents are considered *cell-cycle phase–nonspecific.* However, *most of these drugs are more toxic to dividing cells—especially cells that divide more frequently—than they are to cells in G$_0$.* The reason for this toxicity to dividing cells is because (1) alkylation of DNA produces its most detrimental effects when cells attempt to replicate DNA and (2) quiescent cells are often able to repair damage to DNA before it can affect cell function.

Toxicities. Alkylating agents are toxic to tissues that have a high growth fraction. Accordingly, these drugs may injure cells of the bone marrow, hair follicles, GI mucosa, and germinal epithelium. Blood dyscrasias—neutropenia, thrombocytopenia, and anemia—caused by bone marrow suppression are of greatest concern. Nausea and vomiting occur with all alkylating agents. Also, several of these drugs are vesicants and hence must be administered through a free-flowing intravenous line. The major dose-limiting toxicities of individual drugs are provided in Table 85.2.

Nitrosoureas

The nitrosoureas are bifunctional alkylating agents and are active against a broad spectrum of neoplastic diseases. Cell kill results from crosslinking DNA. Unlike many anticancer drugs, the nitrosoureas are highly lipophilic and hence can readily penetrate the blood-brain barrier. As a result, these drugs are especially useful against *cancers of the CNS.* The major dose-limiting toxicity is *delayed bone marrow suppression.*

Platinum Compounds

The platinum-containing anticancer drugs—cisplatin, carboplatin, and oxaliplatin—are similar to the alkylating agents and are often classified as such. Similar to the bifunctional alkylating agents, the platinum compounds produce crosslinks in DNA and hence are cell-cycle phase–nonspecific.

Antimetabolites

Antimetabolites are structural analogs of important natural metabolites. Because they resemble natural metabolites, these drugs can disrupt critical metabolic processes. Some antimetabolites inhibit enzymes that synthesize essential cellular constituents. Others undergo incorporation into DNA and therefore disrupt DNA replication and function.

Antimetabolites are effective only against cells that are active participants in the cell cycle. Most antimetabolites are S phase–specific, although some can act during any phase of the cycle except G_0. To be effective, agents that are S phase–specific must be present for an extended time.

There are three classes of antimetabolites: (1) folic acid analogs, (2) pyrimidine analogs, and (3) purine analogs. Members of each class, along with their dose-limiting toxicities, are shown in Table 85.2.

Folic Acid Analogs

Folic acid in its active form is needed for several essential biochemical reactions. The folic acid analogs block the conversion of folic acid to its active form. At this time, three analogs of folic acid are used against cancer: methotrexate, pemetrexed, and pralatrexate. Other folate analogs are used to treat bacterial infections (trimethoprim), malaria (pyrimethamine), and *Pneumocystis jirovecii* pneumonia (trimetrexate).

Pyrimidine Analogs

The pyrimidine analogs are cytarabine, fluorouracil, capecitabine, floxuridine, and gemcitabine.

Pyrimidines—cytosine, thymine, and uracil—are bases employed in the biosynthesis of DNA and RNA. The pyrimidine analogs, because of their structural similarity to naturally occurring pyrimidines, can act in several ways: (1) they can inhibit biosynthesis of pyrimidines, (2) they can inhibit biosynthesis of DNA and RNA, and (3) they can undergo incorporation into DNA and RNA and hence disrupt nucleic acid function. All pyrimidine analogs are prodrugs that must be converted to their active forms in the body.

Purine Analogs

The purine analogs are cladribine, clofarabine, fludarabine, mercaptopurine, nelarabine, pentostatin, and thioguanine. Similar to the pyrimidines, the purines—adenine, guanine, and hypoxanthine—are bases employed for biosynthesis of nucleic acids. Purine analogs discussed in other chapters are used for immunosuppression, antiviral therapy, and gout.

Hypomethylating Agents

Hypomethylating agents are so-called because they inhibit DNA methyltransferase, an enzyme that puts methyl groups onto DNA components. Drugs in this category include azacitidine and decitabine. Both are analogs of cytidine, a component of RNA.

Antitumor Antibiotics

The antitumor antibiotics are cytotoxic drugs originally isolated from cultures of *Streptomyces* species. They fall into two major groups: anthracyclines and nonanthracyclines. These drugs injure cells through direct interaction with DNA. Antitumor antibiotics are used only to treat cancer; they are not used to treat infections.

Anthracyclines

Five of the antitumor antibiotics are derivatives of anthracycline: doxorubicin (conventional and liposomal), daunorubicin (conventional and liposomal), epirubicin, idarubicin, and valrubicin. A sixth drug, mitoxantrone, is often categorized as an anthracycline because of its close similarity to drugs in this category. All can cause severe bone marrow suppression and heart damage. In some patients, cardiotoxicity has led to fatal heart failure.

Nonanthracyclines

There are three nonanthracycline antitumor antibiotics: dactinomycin, bleomycin, and mitomycin. In contrast to anthracyclines, nonanthracyclines do not injure the heart. However, these drugs do have serious toxicities of their own. Table 85.2 details dose-limiting toxicities of each drug.

Mitotic Inhibitors

Mitotic inhibitors are drugs that act during M phase to prevent cell division. There are two major groups of these drugs—vinca alkaloids and taxanes—as well as three other drugs that belong to neither group. Of these, vincristine is unique in that it spares the bone marrow and thus causes very little damage with regard to hematopoiesis.

Topoisomerase Inhibitors

Topoisomerases are nuclear enzymes that alter the shape (topology) of supercoiled DNA. Without the actions of topoisomerases, the double helix would be too tangled to permit DNA replication, RNA synthesis, or DNA repair. How do topoisomerases alter DNA configuration? They make a cut in the DNA strand—which permits the strand to relax in the vicinity of the cut—and then later they reseal the cut. There are two types of topoisomerase, known as topoisomerase I and topoisomerase II. Topoisomerase I makes single-strand cuts, and topoisomerase II makes double-strand cuts. Of the four topoisomerase inhibitors in current use, two—topotecan and irinotecan—inhibit topoisomerase I, and the other two—etoposide and teniposide—inhibit topoisomerase II. The actions of these drugs are partly similar to those of the antitumor antibiotics discussed previously, which inhibit topoisomerase II and intercalate DNA.

Miscellaneous Cytotoxic Drugs

Some cytotoxic drugs are in categories of their own. A few examples follow.

Asparaginase

Asparaginase (Elspar, Erwinase ♣, and ♣) is an enzyme that converts asparagine, an essential amino acid, into aspartic acid. By converting asparagine to aspartic acid, the drug deprives cells of the asparagine needed to synthesize proteins. However, not all cells are affected. In fact, toxicity from asparaginase is limited almost exclusively to leukemic lymphoblasts because these cells are unable to manufacture their own asparagine, as normal cells can. Therefore normal cells can replace the asparagine that asparaginase took away, but leukemic lymphoblasts can't. Asparaginase appears to act selectively during G_1.

Hydroxyurea

Hydroxyurea (Hydrea and Droxia) inhibits DNA replication by suppressing synthesis of DNA precursors. Specifically, the drug inhibits ribonucleoside diphosphate reductase, the enzyme that converts ribonucleotides into their corresponding deoxyribonucleotides. In the absence of deoxyribonucleotides, DNA cannot be made. Hydroxyurea is S phase–specific.

Mitotane

Mitotane (Lysodren) is a structural analog of two insecticides: DDD and DDT. For reasons that are not understood, the drug is selectively toxic to cells of the adrenal cortex, both normal and neoplastic. The only indication for mitotane is palliative therapy of inoperable adrenocortical carcinoma.

HORMONAL AGENTS, TARGETED DRUGS, AND OTHER NONCYTOTOXIC ANTICANCER DRUGS

As we continue our discussion of anticancer agents, we will focus on two large groups of drugs: hormonal agents and targeted drugs. Unlike the cytotoxic agents discussed previously, many of which are cell-cycle phase–specific, the drugs addressed here lack phase specificity. In addition, many of these drugs lack the serious toxicities associated with cytotoxic agents, including bone marrow suppression, stomatitis, alopecia, and severe nausea and vomiting. Nonetheless, most of these have severe toxicities of their own.

The hormonal agents mimic or suppress the actions of endogenous hormones. Because hormonal agents are used primarily for breast cancer and prostate cancer, we will discuss hormonal agents within the context of treatment for these conditions. The so-called targeted drugs bind with specific molecular targets on cancer cells and hence suppress tumor growth and promote cell death.

Drugs for Breast Cancer

Principal modalities for breast cancer treatment are surgery, radiation, cytotoxic drugs (chemotherapy), and hormonal drugs. Surgery and radiation are considered primary therapy; chemotherapy and hormonal therapy are used as adjuvants. For a woman with early breast cancer, treatment typically consists of surgery (using total mastectomy or partial mastectomy [lumpectomy]) followed by local radiation. After that, chemotherapy is used to kill cells left behind after surgery and radiation and to kill cells that may have metastasized to other sites. Finally, hormonal agents are taken for several years to reduce recurrence. Increasingly, chemotherapy is used before surgery—so-called neoadjuvant therapy—to shrink large tumors and hence permit lumpectomy in women who would otherwise require mastectomy. Drugs for adjuvant therapy are shown in Table 85.5.

Hormonal agents for breast cancer fall into two major groups: antiestrogens (e.g., tamoxifen]Nolvadex]) and aromatase inhibitors (e.g., anastrozole [Arimidex]). Antiestrogens block receptors for estrogen, whereas aromatase inhibitors block estrogen biosynthesis. In both cases, tumor cells are deprived of the estrogen they need for growth. However, there is a caveat: for these drugs to work, tumor cells must have estrogen receptors (ERs). Fortunately most breast cancers are ER-positive.

In addition to chemotherapy and hormonal therapy, four other drugs—trastuzumab (Herceptin), ado-trastuzumab emtansine (Kadcyla), pertuzumab (Perjeta), and lapatinib (Tykerb)—can be used for adjuvant treatment. Trastuzumab, pertuzumab, and ado-trastuzumab emtansine block receptors such as as human epidermal growth factor receptor type 2 (HER2). In addition, when ado-trastuzumab emtansine binds with HER2 receptors, it releases cytotoxic catabolites that cause cell apoptosis (programmed cell death). Lapatinib inhibits two enzymes, known as HER2 tyrosine kinase and epidermal growth factor receptor (EGFR) tyrosine kinase. These drugs are indicated only for cancers that are HER2-positive. Last, patients may take denosumab (Xgeva) or zoledronate (Zometa) to minimize hypercalcemia (caused by bone metastases) and fractures (caused by bone metastases as well as hormonal therapy).

What about breast cancer prevention? Currently, two drugs are approved for preventing breast cancer in women at high risk. Both are selective estrogen receptor modulators, or SERMS. One of the drugs—raloxifene (Evista)—is approved only for postmenopausal women. The other drug—tamoxifen (Nolvadex)—is approved for premenopausal and postmenopausal women. Raloxifene is discussed in Chapter 61. Tamoxifen is discussed in the next section. Another drug—exemestane (Aromasin)—can also prevent breast cancer, but currently it is approved only for breast cancer treatment.

Antiestrogens

Antiestrogens are drugs that block ERs and, hence, work only against cells that are ER-positive. Benefits derive from depriving tumor cells of the growth-promoting influence of estrogen. Three antiestrogens—tamoxifen, toremifene, and fulvestrant—are approved for adjuvant treatment. Of these, tamoxifen is by far the most widely used.

Tamoxifen. Tamoxifen (Nolvadex) is considered the gold standard for endocrine treatment of breast cancer. The drug is approved for treating established disease and for primary prevention in women at risk.

Mechanism of action in breast cancer. Tamoxifen is a prodrug that undergoes hepatic conversion to active metabolites. These metabolites then block ERs on breast cancer cells and, hence, prevent receptor activation by estradiol, the principal endogenous estrogen. Estrogen acts on tumor cells to stimulate growth and proliferation; hence, in the absence of the influence of estradiol, the rate of tumor cell proliferation declines. Tumors regress in size as the rate of cell death outpaces new cell production. Obviously, if treatment is to be effective, target cells must be ER-positive.

Use for treatment of breast cancer. Tamoxifen has two treatment applications: (1) as adjuvant therapy to suppress growth of residual cancer cells after surgery and (2) as treatment of metastatic disease. Tamoxifen can be used in both premenopausal and postmenopausal women.

Use for prevention of breast cancer. Tamoxifen is approved for reducing the development of breast cancer in healthy women at high risk. Unfortunately, tamoxifen increases the incidence of endometrial cancer, pulmonary embolism, and deep venous thrombosis. Hence women considering tamoxifen for chemoprevention must carefully weigh the benefits of treatment (reduced risk for breast cancer) against the risks (increased risk for endometrial cancer and thromboembolic events). According to current guidelines issued by the US Preventive Services Task Force (USPSTF), tamoxifen chemoprevention is appropriate only for women at increased risk for breast cancer and at low risk for tamoxifen adverse effects.

To help determine who is at high risk for breast cancer, the National Cancer Institute has created an internet-based Breast Cancer Risk Assessment Tool. You can access the tool at www.cancer.gov/bcrisktool.

In the liver, CYP2D6 (the 2D6 isoenzyme of cytochrome P450) converts tamoxifen to two active metabolites: 4-hydroxy-N-desmethyltamoxifen (endoxifen) and 4-hydroxytamoxifen.

Not surprisingly, benefits of tamoxifen are greatly reduced in women with an inherited deficiency in the gene that codes for CYP2D6. Cancer recurrence rates in poor metabolizers may be higher than in good metabolizers. Between 8% and 10% of women of European descent have gene variants that prevent them from converting tamoxifen to its active metabolites. However, at this time, the US Food and Drug Administration (FDA) neither requires nor recommends testing for variants in the CYP2D6 gene, although a test kit is available.

Adverse effects. The most common adverse effects are hot flashes, fluid retention, vaginal discharge, nausea, vomiting, and menstrual irregularities. In women with bone metastases, tamoxifen may cause transient hypercalcemia and a flare in bone pain. Because of its estrogen agonist actions, tamoxifen poses a small risk for thromboembolic events, including deep venous thrombosis, pulmonary embolism, and stroke.

TABLE 85.5   Drugs for Adjuvant Therapy of Breast Cancer

Generic Name	Trade Name	Route	Mechanism	Indications	Major Adverse Effects
Hormonal Therapies					
Antiestrogens					
Tamoxifen	Nolvadex	PO	Blockade of estrogen receptors	ER-positive breast cancer in premenopausal and postmenopausal women	Increased risk for endometrial cancer and thrombosis
Toremifene	Fareston	PO	Blockade of estrogen receptors	ER-positive breast cancer in postmenopausal women only	Hot flashes, fluid retention, vaginal discharge, nausea, vomiting, and menstrual irregularities
Fulvestrant	Faslodex	IM	Blockade of estrogen receptors	ER-positive breast cancer in postmenopausal women only	
Aromatase Inhibitors					
Anastrozole	Arimidex	PO	Inhibition of estrogen synthesis	ER-positive breast cancer in postmenopausal women only	Musculoskeletal pain, osteoporosis, and related fractures
Letrozole	Femara	PO			
Exemestane	Aromasin	PO			
Other Drugs for Breast Cancer					
Anti-HER2 Antibodies					
Trastuzumab	Herceptin	IV	Blockade of HER2 receptors	HER2-positive breast cancer in premenopausal and postmenopausal women	Cardiotoxicity and hypersensitivity reactions
Ado-trastuzumab	Kadcyla	IV	Blockade of HER2 receptors	HER2-positive breast cancer	Hepatotoxicity, cardiotoxicity, and neurotoxicity
Pertuzumab	Perjeta	IV	Blockade of HER2 receptors	HER2-positive breast cancer	Cardiotoxicity and hypersensitivity reactions
Kinase Inhibitor					
Lapatinib	Tykerb	PO	Inhibits HER2 tyrosine kinase and EGFR tyrosine kinase	HER2-positive breast cancer in premenopausal and postmenopausal women	Diarrhea, hepatotoxicity, cardiotoxicity, and interstitial lung disease
Cytotoxic Drugs (Representative Agents)					
Doxorubicin *plus* cyclophosphamide	Adriamycin; Cytoxan, Neosar	IV	Direct cell kill by DNA intercalation, topoisomerase II inhibition, and DNA alkylation	Breast cancer in all women, regardless of ER, HER2, or menopausal status	Together, these drugs can cause cardiotoxicity, bone marrow suppression, alopecia, oral and GI ulceration, and hemorrhagic cystitis
Paclitaxel	Taxol ♣, Onxol, and Abraxane	IV	Direct cell kill by mitotic arrest	Breast cancer in all women, regardless of ER, HER2, or menopausal status	Bone marrow suppression, peripheral neuropathy, alopecia, cardiotoxicity, and muscle and joint pain. Severe hypersensitivity reactions with Taxol ♣ and Onxol, but not Abraxane
Eribulin	Halaven	IV	Direct cell kill by mitotic arrest	Breast cancer in all women, regardless of ER, HER2, or menopausal status	Bone marrow suppression and peripheral neuropathy
Drugs to Delay Skeletal Events					
Zoledronate	Zometa[a]	IV	Inhibits osteoclast function	Hypercalcemia of malignancy, prevention of malignancy-related skeletal events	Kidney damage, osteonecrosis of the jaw, and rare atrial fibrillation
Denosumab	Xgeva[b]	SubQ	Inhibits osteoclast function and production	Hypercalcemia of malignancy, prevention of malignancy-related skeletal events	Hypocalcemia, serious infections, skin reactions, osteonecrosis of the jaw

[a]Zoledronate is also available as *Reclast* for treating osteoporosis and Paget disease.
[b]Denosumab is also available as *Prolia* for treating postmenopausal osteoporosis.
EGFR, Epidermal growth factor receptor; *ER,* estrogen receptor; *GI,* gastrointestinal; *HER2,* human epidermal growth factor receptor 2; *IM,* intramuscular; *IV,* intravenous; *PO,* oral; *subQ,* subcutaneous.

Perhaps the biggest concern is *endometrial cancer.* Tamoxifen acts as an estrogen agonist at receptors in the uterus, causing proliferation of endometrial tissue. Proliferation initially results in endometrial hyperplasia and may eventually lead to endometrial cancer. In women taking tamoxifen to *treat* breast cancer, the benefits likely outweigh this risk. However, in women taking the drug to *prevent* breast cancer, the risk/benefit balance is less obvious. In postmenopausal women, endometrial cancer is usually caught early, owing to abnormal menstrual bleeding.

Tamoxifen can harm the developing fetus. Accordingly, women using the drug should avoid getting pregnant.

Interaction with CYP2D6 inhibitors. Inhibitors of CYP2D6 can prevent activation of tamoxifen and, hence, negate the benefits of treatment. Put another way, when tamoxifen is combined with a CYP2D6 inhibitor, the risk for breast cancer recurrence is greater than when tamoxifen is used alone. Accordingly, women using tamoxifen should avoid strong CYP2D6 inhibitors. Important among these are *fluoxetine* (Prozac), *paroxetine* (Paxil and Pexeva), and *sertraline* (Zoloft)—selective serotonin reuptake inhibitors (SSRIs) taken by many women to suppress tamoxifen-induced hot flashes. Fortunately alternatives with less effect on CYP2D6 are available. Among these are *escitalopram* (Lexapro and Cipralex, an SSRI) and *venlafaxine* (Effexor, a serotonin/norepinephrine reuptake inhibitor).

Toremifene

Actions and use. Toremifene (Fareston) is an antiestrogen indicated for metastatic breast cancer in postmenopausal women with ER-positive tumors or tumors for which the ER status is unknown. The drug is a structural analog of tamoxifen and shares most of that drug's properties. Similar to tamoxifen, toremifene is a SERM with antiestrogenic actions in some tissues and estrogenic actions in others. In women with breast cancer, toremifene blocks ERs on tumor cells, thereby depriving them of estrogen's growth-promoting effects.

Adverse effects and drug interactions. Adverse effects are similar to those of tamoxifen. Hot flashes are most common. Other common reactions are sweating, nausea, and vaginal discharge. Patients may also experience dizziness, vomiting, and vaginal bleeding. Hypercalcemia may occur in women with bone metastases. There is a small risk for thromboembolic events. Cataracts and elevation of liver enzymes have been reported.

Toremifene prolongs the QT interval and, hence, poses a risk for potentially fatal dysrhythmias. To reduce risk, toremifene should be avoided in patients with hypokalemia, hypomagnesemia, or preexisting QT prolongation and in those taking other QT drugs.

Similar to tamoxifen, toremifene activates ERs in the uterus. As a result, the drug can promote uterine hyperplasia and uterine cancer.

Drugs that induce CYP3A4 will reduce toremifene levels. Drugs that inhibit the enzyme will raise toremifene levels.

Fulvestrant

Actions and use. Fulvestrant (Faslodex) is an antiestrogen indicated for metastatic ER-positive breast cancer in postmenopausal women. Unlike tamoxifen and toremifene, which block some ERs and activate others, fulvestrant is a pure estrogen receptor antagonist—the first one available. As with other antiestrogens, benefits derive from depriving breast cancer cells of required hormonal stimulation.

Adverse effects and drug interactions. Fulvestrant is generally well tolerated. The most common adverse effects are GI disturbances, hot flashes, headache, pharyngitis, and bone and back pain. Thromboembolism can occur but is uncommon. In contrast to tamoxifen, fulvestrant poses no risk for endometrial cancer. Fulvestrant has no known drug interactions.

Aromatase Inhibitors

The aromatase inhibitors are used to treat ER-positive breast cancer in *postmenopausal* women. These drugs block the production of estrogen

from androgenic precursors and, hence, deprive breast cancer cells of the estrogen they need for growth. Aromatase inhibitors do not block production of estrogen by the ovaries and hence are of little benefit in premenopausal women. In fact, aromatase inhibitors may cause a compensatory rise in estradiol in premenopausal patients. Aromatase inhibitors are more effective than tamoxifen and have a different toxicity profile. Unlike tamoxifen, aromatase inhibitors pose no risk for endometrial cancer and only rarely cause thromboembolism. However, they *can* increase the risk for fractures and have been associated with moderate to severe myalgias.

Anastrozole

Actions and use. Anastrozole (Arimidex) is approved for first-line oral therapy of *postmenopausal* women with early or advanced *ER-positive breast cancer.* The drug works by depriving breast cancer cells of estrogen. In postmenopausal women, the major source of estrogen is adrenal androgens, which are converted into estrogen by the enzyme *aromatase* in peripheral tissues. Anastrozole inhibits aromatase and therefore reduces estrogen production. With regular use, the drug lowers estrogen to undetectable levels. In women with estrogen-dependent cancer, estrogen deprivation can arrest tumor growth and may cause outright cell death. Anastrozole may be used as initial therapy or as a follow-up to therapy with tamoxifen.

Adverse effects. Anastrozole is generally well tolerated. At a daily dose of 1 mg, the most common adverse effects are musculoskeletal pain, asthenia, headache, and menopausal symptoms, including hot flashes, vaginal dryness, and GI disturbances. Other reactions include anorexia, vomiting, diarrhea, constipation, dyspnea, peripheral edema, vaginal hemorrhage, and hypertension.

Up to 50% of women experience *musculoskeletal pain.* The cause may be estrogen deprivation. Persistent or severe pain drives about 5% of users to discontinue treatment. For women who choose to continue anastrozole, pain can often be managed with a mild analgesic (e.g., acetaminophen and ibuprofen). High-dose vitamin D may help.

Estrogen depletion increases the risk for *osteoporosis and related fractures.* To reduce bone loss, women should ensure adequate intake of calcium and vitamin D. Women at high risk should take a bisphosphonate (e.g., zoledronate [Zometa] or denosumab [Prolia]).

Comparison with tamoxifen. Anastrozole is more effective than tamoxifen. Anastrozole is less likely to cause hot flashes, weight gain, or vaginal bleeding, although it may cause more nausea and irritability. In contrast to tamoxifen, anastrozole is devoid of all estrogenic activity and, hence, does not promote endometrial cancer or thromboembolic events, although it does increase the risk for fractures. Because of their superior efficacy and tolerability, aromatase inhibitors have replaced tamoxifen as the drugs of first choice for treating ER-positive breast cancer in postmenopausal women.

Letrozole.
Letrozole (Femara), a selective aromatase inhibitor, is indicated for (1) first-line therapy of early and advanced ER-positive breast cancer in postmenopausal women and (2) extended adjuvant therapy of early breast cancer after 5 years of adjuvant therapy with tamoxifen. Similar to anastrozole, letrozole blocks conversion of androgens into estrogens and therefore deprives breast cancer cells of estrogen's growth-promoting influence. Letrozole's most common adverse effects are musculoskeletal pain and nausea. Other reactions include headache, arthralgia, fatigue, constipation, dyspnea, cough, vomiting, diarrhea, and hot flashes. Extremely low doses are embryotoxic and fetotoxic in animals. Similar to anastrozole and unlike tamoxifen, letrozole poses no risk for endometrial cancer. However, it can cause osteoporosis and fractures and, rarely, thromboembolism. Osteoporosis can be managed with denosumab (Prolia) or a bisphosphonate (e.g., zoledronate [Zometa]). No significant drug interactions have been reported.

Exemestane. Exemestane (Aromasin) is indicated for oral therapy of (1) advanced ER-positive breast cancer in postmenopausal women whose disease has progressed despite treatment with tamoxifen and (2) early ER-positive breast cancer in postmenopausal women who have received 2 to 3 years of tamoxifen therapy and then are switched to adjuvant exemestane to complete a 5-year course of treatment. Similar to anastrozole, exemestane inhibits aromatase and therefore reduces estrogen levels.

Exemestane is generally well tolerated. The most common adverse effects are fatigue, nausea, hot flashes, depression, and weight gain. Similar to anastrozole and letrozole, exemestane often causes musculoskeletal pain. Increased risk for osteoporosis and fractures is a concern. Women at high risk for osteoporosis can be treated with denosumab (Prolia) or a bisphosphonate (e.g., zoledronate [Zometa]).

Drugs that induce CYP3A4 (e.g., phenytoin, phenobarbital, rifampin, and St. John's wort) can cause a significant drop in exemestane levels. Accordingly, if these drugs are combined, exemestane dosage may have to be increased.

Monoclonal Antibodies

Monoclonal antibodies mimic the body's natural immune system. They are designed to target antigens that present on cancer cells. This class of drugs is discussed in depth in Chapter 84.

Trastuzumab

Actions and use. Trastuzumab (Herceptin) is a monoclonal antibody originally approved for *HER2-positive metastatic breast cancer* and for *adjuvant therapy of HER2-positive breast cancer.* Trastuzumab is also approved for treatment of *HER2-positive metastatic gastric cancer.* Discussion here is limited to breast cancer.

Trastuzumab is effective only against tumors that overexpress *HER2,* a transmembrane receptor that helps regulate cell growth. Trastuzumab binds with HER2 and, hence, (1) inhibits cell proliferation and (2) promotes antibody-dependent cell death. Between 25% and 30% of metastatic breast cancers produce excessive HER2. High numbers of HER2 receptors are associated with unusually aggressive tumor growth. For treatment of breast cancer, trastuzumab may be used (1) alone in women who failed to respond to prior chemotherapy; (2) in combination with paclitaxel as first-line therapy; and (3) for adjuvant treatment as part of a regimen containing doxorubicin, cyclophosphamide, and paclitaxel.

Adverse effects. The principal concern with trastuzumab is *cardiotoxicity,* manifesting as ventricular dysfunction and congestive heart failure. Because of cardiotoxicity, trastuzumab should be used with caution in women with preexisting heart disease. Concurrent use with other drugs that can cause cardiotoxicity, such as doxorubicin and other anthracyclines, should generally be avoided. In contrast to the cytotoxic anticancer drugs, trastuzumab does not cause bone marrow suppression or alopecia.

Many patients experience a *flu-like syndrome,* which also occurs with other monoclonal antibodies. Symptoms include chills, fever, pain, weakness, nausea, vomiting, and headache. The syndrome develops in 40% of patients receiving their first infusion and then diminishes with subsequent infusions.

Ado-trastuzumab emtansine

Actions and use. Ado-trastuzumab emtansine (Kadcyla) is a monoclonal antibody approved for *HER2-positive metastatic breast cancer* in patients previously treated with trastuzumab and/or a taxane.

Like trastuzumab, ado-trastuzumab emtansine is effective only against tumors that overexpress *HER2.* Ado-trastuzumab emtansine binds with HER2 and releases cytotoxic catabolites, thereby (1) inhibiting the cell cycle and (2) promoting cell death. In addition, ado-trastuzumab emtansine inhibits HER2 receptor signaling and shedding of HER2 in breast cancer cells.

Adverse effects. Ado-trastuzumab emtansine can cause hepatotoxicity, cardiotoxicity, and neurotoxicity. Serious hepatotoxicity, including liver failure and death, has been reported. Liver function tests should be obtained before each dose. Left ventricular dysfunction was seen in 1.8% of patients. Ejection fraction should be monitored at regular intervals. The incidence of neurotoxicity, expressed as peripheral neuropathy, was 2.2%.

Ado-trastuzumab emtansine can also cause toxicity in the embryo or fetus. Because exposure can result in birth defects or death of the fetus, ado-trastuzumab emtansine should be avoided by pregnant women and nursing mothers.

The most common reactions include nausea, fatigue, musculoskeletal pain, headache, and constipation. Other common but more serious reactions include thrombocytopenia, increases in liver function test results, anemia, and hypokalemia.

Like trastuzumab, ado-trastuzumab emtansine can cause potentially fatal *hypersensitivity reactions, infusion reactions,* and *pulmonary events.* If a patient experienced trastuzumab-related infusion reactions in the past, ado-trastuzumab emtansine should be avoided.

Pertuzumab. Pertuzumab (Perjeta) is used in combination with trastuzumab and docetaxel for the treatment of women with *HER2-positive metastatic breast cancer* who have not received prior therapy for metastatic disease. Similar to trastuzumab, pertuzumab is an antibody that blocks HER2 receptors, resulting in cell growth arrest and cell death.

Adverse effects include infusion-related reactions. Patients should be closely monitored for 60 minutes after the first infusion and for 30 minutes after subsequent infusions. Other adverse effects include cardiotoxicity, diarrhea, leukopenia, and neuropathy. Oligohydramnios has been reported in pregnancy; therefore pregnant women should avoid use of pertuzumab.

Lapatinib

Actions and use. Lapatinib (Tykerb) is an oral inhibitor of two enzymes—HER2 tyrosine kinase and EGFR tyrosine kinase—that are involved in cell signal transduction. Enzyme inhibition results in apoptosis and suppression of tumor cell growth. Lapatinib is approved for treating advanced HER2-positive breast cancer, but only in combination with either (1) capecitabine (in patients who have received prior therapy with multiple drugs, including an anthracycline, a taxane, and trastuzumab) or (2) letrozole (in postmenopausal women for whom estrogen deprivation therapy is indicated). EGFR tyrosine kinase is discussed further in the later section titled "EGFR Tyrosine Kinase Inhibitors."

Adverse effects. The most common adverse effects of lapatinib plus capecitabine are GI disturbances (diarrhea, nausea, and vomiting), fatigue, rash, and palmar-plantar erythrodysesthesia (swelling and numbness of the hands and feet). The most common adverse effects of lapatinib plus letrozole are diarrhea, rash, nausea, and fatigue. Diarrhea occurs in 65% of patients and is the most common reason for stopping treatment. Similar to other HER2 inhibitors, lapatinib may pose a risk for cardiotoxicity. Accordingly, the drug should be used with caution in patients with existing cardiac impairment. Rarely, letrozole has been associated with severe liver injury. Liver function tests should be performed at baseline and periodically throughout treatment. When used alone and together with other drugs, letrozole has been associated with interstitial lung disease and pneumonitis. In laboratory animals, giving letrozole during pregnancy resulted in death of the pups a few days after birth. Women using the drug should avoid getting pregnant.

Drug interactions. Lapatinib is metabolized by CYP3A4, and hence CYP3A4 inducers (e.g., phenytoin, carbamazepine, rifampin, rifabutin, phenobarbital, and St. John's wort) can lower lapatinib levels, and CYP3A4 inhibitors (e.g., ketoconazole, itraconazole, erythromycin, indinavir, and nelfinavir) can raise lapatinib levels. If possible, CYP3A4 inducers and inhibitors should be avoided.

Cytotoxic Drugs (Chemotherapy)

Cytotoxic drugs may be used before or after breast surgery. When used before surgery, chemotherapy can shrink large tumors, thereby permitting lumpectomy in women who would otherwise require a mastectomy. When used after surgery, chemotherapy can kill cancer cells that remain in the breast as well as cells that may have metastasized to distant sites. A common regimen for breast cancer consists of doxorubicin (an anthracycline-type anticancer antibiotic) plus cyclophosphamide (an alkylating agent) followed by paclitaxel (a mitotic inhibitor).

Management of Skeletal-Related Events

Women with breast cancer are at risk for skeletal-related events (SREs), especially hypercalcemia and fractures. There are two causes: the cancer itself and the drugs used for treatment. In breast cancer, most metastases occur in bone. These metastases promote hypercalcemia by increasing the activity of osteoclasts, the cells that promote bone resorption. Resorption not only promotes hypercalcemia but also weakens bone and therefore increases the risk for fractures. Fracture risk is further increased by the use of antiestrogens and aromatase inhibitors. As discussed in Chapter 50, estrogens promote bone health by inhibiting bone resorption and promoting bone deposition. Hence, by removing the influence of estrogen, the antiestrogens and aromatase inhibitors accelerate bone resorption and reduce bone deposition. Both actions weaken bone and therefore increase the risk for fractures. To reduce the risk for SREs, we can treat patients with denosumab or a bisphosphonate (usually zoledronate).

Bisphosphonates. In women with breast cancer, bisphosphonates can help preserve bone integrity and therefore decrease the risk for hypercalcemia and fractures. Benefits derive from inhibiting the activity of osteoclasts. At this time, two bisphosphonates—*zoledronate* (Zometa) and *pamidronate* (Aredia)—are approved for treating hypercalcemia of malignancy, and one of them—pamidronate—is also approved for managing osteolytic bone metastases. However, although zoledronate is not *approved* for osteolytic bone metastases, it is just as effective as pamidronate. Furthermore, compared with pamidronate, zoledronate has three advantages: its onset is faster, its duration is longer, and the infusion time is shorter (15 minutes vs. 2 to 4 hours). Accordingly, zoledronate is generally preferred to pamidronate. Principal adverse effects of the bisphosphonates are kidney damage and osteonecrosis of the jaw.

In addition to reducing fractures and hypercalcemia, bisphosphonates may actually prevent metastases and prolong life. How do bisphosphonates suppress metastases? When cancer cells spread to bone, they stimulate the activity of osteoclasts, the cells responsible for bone resorption. In turn, osteoclasts release growth factors that stimulate the cancer cells, thereby setting up a self-reinforcing cycle. Bisphosphonates interrupt the cycle by inhibiting osteoclast function and blocking tumor adhesion to bone. The basic pharmacology of the bisphosphonates is discussed in Chapter 61.

Denosumab. Denosumab, marketed as *Xgeva*, is indicated for preventing (delaying) SREs in patients with breast cancer and other solid tumors that have metastasized to bone. Benefits derive from inhibiting the formation and function of osteoclasts. Principal adverse effects of denosumab are hypocalcemia, serious infections, skin reactions, and osteonecrosis of the jaw. The pharmacology of denosumab is presented in Chapter 61.

Drugs for Prostate Cancer

Cancer of the prostate is the most common cancer among men in the United States. In 2018, an estimated 164,690 new cases were diagnosed, and 29,430 were fatal. For men with *localized* prostate cancer, the preferred treatments are surgery and radiation, with or without

adjunctive use of drugs. For men with *metastatic* prostate cancer, drug therapy and castration are the only options. Among the drugs employed, agents for *androgen deprivation therapy* (ADT) comprise the largest and most widely used group. Other choices are cytotoxic drugs and a new immunotherapy known as sipuleucel-T (Provenge). As with breast cancer, most metastases (65% to 75%) go to bone. To minimize hypercalcemia and fractures caused by bone metastases, men may take *zoledronate* (Zometa) or *denosumab* (Xgeva) (see previous discussion of breast cancer). The drugs used to treat prostate cancer are shown in Table 85.6.

The term *androgen deprivation therapy* refers to the use of castration, drugs, or both to deprive prostate cancers of the androgens they need for growth. By implementing ADT, we can slow disease progression and increase comfort. Initially, ADT was reserved for patients with metastatic disease. However, ADT is now used as an adjuvant in earlier-stage disease. Unfortunately, the benefits of ADT are time-limited: after 18 to 24 months of treatment, disease progression often resumes. Side effects of ADT include hot flashes, reduced libido, erectile dysfunction, gynecomastia, decreased muscle mass, and decreased bone mass with associated increased risk for fractures.

Where do androgens come from, and how can we reduce their influence? About 90% of circulating androgens are produced by the testes. The remaining 10% are produced by the adrenal glands and the prostate cancer itself. Accordingly, we can reduce the influence of androgens in three ways. Specifically we can block testosterone receptors with drugs, lower testosterone production with drugs, and lower testosterone production by castration. Drug therapy is more effective than castration because castration eliminates only testicular androgens, leaving androgen synthesis by the adrenal glands and cancer cells intact. In contrast, by using drugs to block testosterone receptors and testosterone synthesis, we can reduce the influence of testosterone from all sources (testes, adrenal glands, and prostate cancer).

Four classes of drugs are used for androgen deprivation therapy. These classes—gonadotropin-releasing hormone agonists, gonadotropin-releasing hormone antagonists, androgen receptor blockers, and a CYP17 inhibitor—are discussed next.

Gonadotropin-Releasing Hormone Agonists

The gonadotropin-releasing hormone (GnRH) agonists suppress production of androgens by the testes—but not by the adrenal glands and prostate cancer cells. Currently, four GnRH agonists are available: leuprolide, triptorelin, goserelin, and histrelin. All four are indicated for the treatment of cancer of the prostate. In addition, leuprolide is used to treat endometriosis.

Leuprolide

Use. Leuprolide (Eligard, Lupro ✦, Lupron Depot, and Viadur) is a synthetic analog of GnRH, also known as *luteinizing hormone–releasing hormone* (LHRH). Leuprolide is indicated for *advanced carcinoma of the prostate*. Palliation is the primary benefit. For patients with prostate cancer, leuprolide represents an alternative to orchiectomy (surgical castration).

Cells of the prostate, both normal and neoplastic, are androgen-dependent. Leuprolide provides palliation by suppressing androgen production in the *testes*. During the initial phase of treatment, leuprolide *mimics* GnRH. That is, the drug acts on the pituitary to *stimulate* release of interstitial cell–stimulating hormone (ICSH), which acts on the testes to *increase* production of testosterone. As a result, there may be a transient "flare" in prostate cancer symptoms. However, with continuous exposure to leuprolide, GnRH receptors in the pituitary become desensitized. As a result, release of ICSH declines, causing testosterone production to decline too. After several weeks of treatment, testosterone levels are equivalent to those seen after surgical castration. Because leuprolide

TABLE 85.6 Drugs for Prostate Cancer

Generic Name	Trade Name	Route	Major Adverse Effects
Drugs for Androgen Deprivation Therapy			
GnRH Agonists[a]			
Leuprolide	Lupron 🍁, Lupron Depot	IM	Hot flashes, erectile dysfunction, decreased libido, decreased muscle mass, gynecomastia, and osteoporosis
	Eligard	SubQ	
	Viadur	SubQ implant	
Triptorelin	Trelstar	IM	
Goserelin	Zoladex	SubQ	
Histrelin	Vantas	SubQ implant	
GnRH Antagonist			
Degarelix	Firmagon	SubQ	Same as the GnRH agonists *plus* hepatotoxicity
Androgen Receptor Blockers			
Flutamide	Generic only	PO	Same as the GnRH agonists *plus* hepatotoxicity
Bicalutamide	Casodex	PO	Same as the GnRH agonists *plus* hepatotoxicity
Nilutamide	Nilandron, Anandron 🍁	PO	Same as the GnRH agonists *plus* hepatotoxicity and interstitial pneumonitis
CYP17 Inhibitor			
Abiraterone	Zytiga	PO	Same as the GnRH agonists *plus* hepatotoxicity, edema, hypertension, hypokalemia, and glucocorticoid insufficiency
Other Drugs for Prostate Cancer			
Immunotherapy			
Sipuleucel-T	Provenge	IV	Infusion reactions, fatigue, and fever
Cytotoxic Drugs			
Cabazitaxel	Jevtana	IV	Neutropenia, hypersensitivity reactions, and diarrhea
Docetaxel	Taxotere	IV	Neutropenia, anemia, hypersensitivity reactions, and fluid retention
Estramustine	Emcyt	PO	Gynecomastia and thrombosis
Drugs to Delay Skeletal Events			
Zoledronate	Zometa[b]	IV	Kidney damage, osteonecrosis of the jaw, and rare atrial fibrillation
Denosumab	Xgeva[c]	SubQ	Hypocalcemia, serious infections, skin reactions, and osteonecrosis of the jaw

[a]Gonadotropin-releasing hormone agonists, also known as luteinizing hormone–releasing hormone (LHRH) agonists.
[b]Zoledronate is also available as *Reclast* for treating osteoporosis and Paget disease.
[c]Denosumab is also available as *Prolia* for treating postmenopausal osteoporosis.
IM, Intramuscular; *IV*, intravenous; *PO*, oral; *subQ*, subcutaneous.

therapy mimics the effects of orchiectomy, treatment is often referred to as *chemical castration.*

It is important to note that leuprolide does *not* decrease production of androgens made by the adrenal glands or by the prostate cancer itself. As noted, these nontesticular sources account for about 10% of the androgens in circulation. Hence even though production of testicular androgens is essentially eliminated, adrenal and prostatic androgens can still provide some support for prostate cancer cells.

Cotreatment with an androgen receptor blocker. In patients receiving leuprolide, an androgen receptor blocker can help in two ways. Specifically (1) it can prevent cancer cells from undergoing increased stimulation during the initial phase of GnRH therapy, when androgen production is increased, and (2) it can block the effects of adrenal and prostatic androgens, whose production is not reduced by GnRH agonists. The current trend is to use an androgen receptor blocker during the first weeks of leuprolide therapy (to prevent leuprolide-induced tumor flare), after which the drug is discontinued unless there is tumor progression despite continued leuprolide treatment.

Adverse effects. Leuprolide is generally well tolerated. Hot flashes are the most common adverse effect, but these usually decline as treatment continues. Reduced testosterone may also lead to erectile dysfunction, loss of libido, gynecomastia, reduced muscle mass, new-onset diabetes, myocardial infarction, and stroke. During the initial weeks of treatment, elevation of testosterone levels may aggravate bone pain and urinary obstruction caused by prostate cancer. As a result, patients with vertebral metastases or preexisting obstruction of the urinary tract may find treatment intolerable. As noted, concurrent treatment with an androgen receptor blocker can minimize these problems.

By suppressing testosterone production, leuprolide may increase the risk for osteoporosis and related fractures. Bone loss can be minimized by consuming adequate calcium and vitamin D and performing regular weight-bearing exercise. In addition, a bisphosphonate (e.g., zoledronate [Zometa] or denosumab [Xgeva]) can be used to preserve bone and reduce fracture risk (see earlier discussion of breast cancer).

Triptorelin, goserelin, and histrelin. Triptorelin, goserelin, and histrelin are GnRH analogs indicated for palliative treatment of advanced prostate cancer. All three have the same mechanism and adverse effects as leuprolide, our prototype GnRH agonist.

Gonadotropin-Releasing Hormone Antagonists

Like the GnRH agonists, the GnRH *antagonists* suppress production of androgens by the testes. However, in contrast to the GnRH agonists, the GnRH antagonists do not produce an initial tumor flare. Currently, only one GnRH antagonist—degarelix—is available.

Degarelix. Degarelix (Firmagon) is a synthetic decapeptide GnRH antagonist indicated for palliative therapy of *advanced prostate cancer* in men who are not candidates for a GnRH agonist and who do not want surgical castration. Benefits derive from suppressing testosterone production by the testes. The underlying mechanism is blockade of GnRH receptors in the anterior pituitary, which decreases release of luteinizing hormone and follicle-stimulating hormone, which in turn deprives the testes of the stimulus they need for testosterone production. Because degarelix works through direct blockade of GnRH receptors, the drug does not cause the initial surge in testosterone production seen with GnRH agonists; hence there is no early tumor flare.

As with other drugs for ADT, major side effects are hot flashes, reduced libido, erectile dysfunction, gynecomastia, decreased muscle mass, and decreased bone mass with associated increased risk for fractures. In addition, degarelix often causes injection-site reactions (pain, erythema, and swelling), weight gain, and elevation of liver transaminases. After a year of treatment, about 10% of patients develop antibodies against degarelix. However, the antibodies do not reduce the effectiveness of treatment.

Androgen Receptor Blockers

Androgen receptor blockers, or simply *antiandrogens,* are indicated only for advanced androgen-sensitive prostate cancer, and only in combination with surgical castration or chemical castration using a GnRH agonist. Currently three androgen receptor blockers are available: flutamide, bicalutamide, and nilutamide.

Flutamide. Flutamide is indicated for *prostate cancer* only. Benefits derive from the blockade of androgen receptors in tumor cells, thereby depriving them of needed androgenic support. In patients taking a GnRH agonist, flutamide can serve two purposes: (1) it can prevent tumor flare when GnRH therapy is started, and (2) it can block the effects of adrenal and prostatic androgens. As a rule, the combination of an androgen antagonist plus a GnRH agonist—so-called complete androgen blockade—is reserved for suppressing the initial flare and suppressing the tumor after it has stopped responding to a GnRH agonist alone. The combination is not used continuously because it does not increase survival; however, it does increase toxicity.

Flutamide is administered orally and undergoes rapid and complete absorption. Most of each dose is converted to an active metabolite on the first pass through the liver. Parent drug and metabolites are excreted in the urine.

As with other drugs for ADT, prominent side effects are hot flashes, reduced libido, erectile dysfunction, gynecomastia, decreased muscle mass, and decreased bone mass with associated increased risk for fractures. Nausea, vomiting, and diarrhea are also common. Rarely, potentially fatal liver toxicity has occurred. To reduce the risk for serious harm, liver function should be assessed at baseline, monthly during the first 4 months of treatment, and periodically thereafter.

Flutamide may cause fetal harm. There are no current indications for use of in women. Accordingly, the drug should not be used during pregnancy.

Bicalutamide. Like flutamide, bicalutamide (Casodex) is an androgen receptor blocker used for advanced androgen-sensitive prostate cancer in men undergoing therapy with a GnRH agonist (e.g., leuprolide).

Bicalutamide is just as effective as flutamide and dosing is more convenient. As a result, bicalutamide is often preferred. The rationale for the combination of androgen receptor blocker and GnRH agonist is explained in the discussion of flutamide. When bicalutamide is used alone, the most common side effects are breast pain and gynecomastia. When the drug is combined with leuprolide, the most common side effect is hot flashes. Similar to all other drugs used for ADT, bicalutamide can also cause reduced libido, erectile dysfunction, decreased muscle mass, and decreased bone mass with associated increased risk for fractures. Also, similar to flutamide, bicalutamide poses a small risk for liver injury; hence liver function should be monitored. Bicalutamide poses a significant risk for fetal harm; therefore it should not be taken by pregnant women. Because it is indicated only for prostate cancer, this should not be an issue of concern.

Nilutamide. Nilutamide (Nilandron and Anandron ✦) is another androgen receptor blocker. The drug is approved for metastatic prostate cancer in men who have undergone surgical castration. Benefits derive from blocking the actions of adrenal androgens, which are not reduced by castration.

Although nilutamide is structurally similar to flutamide, it is not as well tolerated. The most common adverse effects are hot flashes, delayed adaptation to darkness, nausea, constipation, insomnia, and gynecomastia. In addition, nilutamide can cause reduced libido, erectile dysfunction, decreased muscle mass, and decreased bone mass with associated increased risk for fractures. Other reactions occur less frequently but are more dangerous. About 2% of patients experience dyspnea secondary to interstitial pneumonitis. If this develops, nilutamide should be withdrawn. About 1% of patients develop hepatitis. To ensure early diagnosis, liver function should be monitored.

Cytochrome P450 Enzyme 17 Inhibitor

Actions and use. Abiraterone (Zytiga) is indicated for combined use with prednisone to treat *metastatic castration-resistant prostate cancer* in men previously treated with docetaxel. Benefits derive from inhibiting the production of androgens by the adrenal gland and by the prostate cancer itself. (If castration has not been done, abiraterone can also inhibit androgen production by the testes.) In all cases, the underlying mechanism is inhibition of the cytochrome P450 enzyme 17 (CYP17), an enzyme needed by the adrenals, testes, and prostate tumors for androgen synthesis. When tested in men with metastatic castration-resistant prostate cancer, the combination of abiraterone plus prednisone increased overall survival by nearly 4 months and progression-free survival by 2 months.

Adverse effects. The most common adverse effects are hypokalemia, edema, joint swelling and discomfort, muscle discomfort, hot flashes, diarrhea, urinary tract infection, cough, and hypertension. Similar to all other drugs for ADT, abiraterone can also decrease libido, muscle mass, and bone mass and can cause erectile dysfunction and gynecomastia.

Inhibition of CYP17 in the adrenals can lead to overproduction of mineralocorticoids and underproduction of glucocorticoids. High levels of mineralocorticoids can cause retention of sodium and loss of potassium, leading to fluid retention, edema, hypertension, and hypokalemia. Low levels of glucocorticoids can increase the risk for death from traumatic events. Cotreatment with prednisone (a glucocorticoid) helps compensate for reduced production of glucocorticoids by the adrenal glands, and, by suppressing release of adrenocorticotropic hormone from the pituitary, prednisone can reduce excessive production of mineralocorticoids.

Hepatotoxicity, manifesting as a marked elevation of liver transaminases—alanine aminotransferase (ALT) and aspartate aminotransferase (AST)—develops in about 30% of patients. To monitor liver status, ALT and AST should be measured at baseline, every 2 weeks for the first 3 months of treatment, and once a month thereafter. If these tests indicate significant liver injury, abiraterone should be discontinued or the dosage reduced.

Abiraterone can harm the developing fetus. Accordingly, the drug should be avoided by women who are pregnant.

Drug interactions. Abiraterone is a substrate for CYP3A4; hence its levels can be raised by CYP3A4 inhibitors (e.g., ketoconazole, clarithromycin, and ritonavir) and lowered by CYP3A4 inducers (e.g., phenytoin, carbamazepine, and rifampin). Abiraterone inhibits hepatic CYP2D6 and, hence, can raise levels of CYP2D6 substrates (e.g., dextromethorphan and thioridazine).

Ketoconazole

Ketoconazole (Nizoral), used primarily for fungal infections (see Chapter 79), can be used off label for prostate cancer. As with abiraterone, benefits derive from inhibiting testicular, adrenal, and prostatic production of androgens. Ketoconazole is employed as secondary therapy in men who have rising prostate-specific antigen levels despite treatment with a GnRH agonist plus an antiandrogen. Dosages are higher than those used for antifungal therapy; hence side effects are common. Among these are nausea, vomiting, fatigue, skin changes, liver damage, and gynecomastia. Because high-dose ketoconazole can suppress adrenal production of glucocorticoids, the drug is usually combined with hydrocortisone (to avoid adrenal insufficiency).

Other Drugs for Prostate Cancer

Sipuleucel-T. Sipuleucel-T (Provenge) is the name of a patient-specific form of immunotherapy designed to stimulate an immune attack against prostate cancer cells. Each dose is custom made from the patient's own immune cells and hence cannot be used by any other patient. Unfortunately, sipuleucel-T is very expensive and only moderately effective. Nonetheless, sipuleucel-T is of great interest in that it represents an entirely new approach to cancer treatment.

Therapeutic use. Sipuleucel-T is indicated for treatment of asymptomatic or minimally symptomatic metastatic castration-resistant (hormone-refractory) prostate cancer. Treatment consists of three infusions given 2 weeks apart. Of note, although sipuleucel-T improves survival, it does not cause measurable tumor regression, nor does it delay the time to tumor progression—suggesting that the mechanism underlying prolonged survival may be something other than immune-mediated injury to cancer cells.

Production. Sipuleucel-T is produced in two steps: collection of circulating immune cells (macrophages) from the patient, followed by modification of those cells in the laboratory. This process—cell collection plus modification—takes about 2 days and must be done for *each dose.*

Macrophage collection is done by *leukapheresis,* a process in which venous blood is circulated from the patient, through a machine, and then back into the patient. The machine separates out macrophages (along with some platelets and other blood cells) and then returns the remaining cells and serum to the patient. The whole procedure takes 3 to 4 hours.

In the laboratory, the macrophages—also known as *antigen-presenting cells,* or *APCs*—are modified by incubation with a recombinant human protein consisting of prostatic acid phosphatase (PAP) linked with GM-CSF. PAP is a protein that is highly expressed by more than 95% of prostate cancer cells. GM-CSF is a blood growth factor that stimulates the production and function of macrophages and some other blood cells. During incubation, the APCs engulf the PAP–GM-CSF, break it into small peptides, and then express those peptides on the APC surface. The modified APCs can now activate cytolytic T cells (killer T cells), causing them to attack prostate cancer cells by recognizing the PAP molecules on their surface.

Adverse effects. Sipuleucel-T can cause multiple adverse effects. The most common are chills, fatigue, fever, back pain, nausea, joint ache, and headache. Other common reactions include paresthesias, vomiting, anemia, constipation, dizziness, weakness, and extremity pain.

Acute infusion reactions develop in more than 70% of patients. Symptoms include fever, chills, nausea, vomiting, fatigue, hypertension, tachycardia, and respiratory reactions (dyspnea, hypoxia, and bronchospasm). Severe reactions may require hospitalization. Infusion reactions can be reduced by premedication with acetaminophen plus an antihistamine, such as diphenhydramine (Benadryl).

Cytotoxic drugs

Docetaxel and cabazitaxel. Docetaxel (Taxotere) and cabazitaxel (Jevtana) are cytotoxic anticancer drugs indicated for hormone-refractory prostate cancer (i.e., prostate cancer that no longer responds to ADT). Either drug, in combination with prednisone, can prolong overall survival as well as progression-free survival. At this time, docetaxel is considered a first-line drug for hormone-refractory prostate cancer. Cabazitaxel is reserved for patients who have already been treated with docetaxel. The major adverse effects of docetaxel are neutropenia, hypersensitivity reactions, and fluid retention. The major adverse effects of cabazitaxel are neutropenia, hypersensitivity reactions, anemia, and diarrhea. With both drugs, benefits derive from causing mitotic arrest.

Estramustine. Estramustine (Emcyt) is a hybrid molecule composed of estradiol (an estrogen) coupled to nitrogen mustard (an alkylating agent). The only indication for the drug is palliative therapy of advanced prostate cancer. Estramustine is administered orally and becomes concentrated in prostate cells, apparently through the actions of a unique "estramustine-binding protein." Injury to prostate cells appears to result from three mechanisms. First, estramustine acts as a weak alkylating agent. Second, hydrolysis of estramustine releases free estradiol, which suppresses ICSH release by the pituitary, thereby depriving prostate cells of hormonal support. Third and most important, the drug binds to microtubules of mitotic spindles and, hence, disrupts mitosis. As a result, estramustine has M-phase specificity.

Adverse effects are caused primarily by free estradiol. Gynecomastia is common. The most serious effect is thrombosis, with resultant myocardial infarction and stroke. Other adverse effects include fluid retention, nausea, vomiting, diarrhea, and hypercalcemia.

Targeted Anticancer Drugs

Targeted anticancer drugs are designed to bind with specific molecules (targets) with the goal of suppressing tumor growth. The hope is that these drugs will be more selective than hormones and cytotoxic anticancer drugs and, hence, will be able to destroy cancer cells while leaving normal cells untouched. A few targeted drugs, such as imatinib (Gleevec), have been remarkably successful, producing complete responses with relatively mild adverse effects. Unfortunately, responses have been less impressive with many other targeted drugs, whereas adverse effects have been more severe. Nonetheless the concept of targeted therapy has great appeal, and intensive research is under way to make it more of a reality.

How do targeted drugs work? Many of these drugs are *antibodies* that bind with specific antigens on tumor cells; others are *small molecules* that inhibit intracellular enzymes. Some antibodies mark cancer cells for immune attack, some block cell surface receptors, some deliver toxic drugs or radioactivity, and some inhibit angiogenesis and therefore deprive tumor cells of their blood supply. Most of the small molecules inhibit specific tyrosine kinases and, hence, disrupt intracellular signaling pathways. Properties of the targeted drugs are shown in Table 85.7.

Kinase Inhibitors

A kinase is an enzyme that catalyzes the transfer of a phosphate group from a nucleoside triphosphate donor (e.g., adenosine triphosphate

TABLE 85.7   Targeted Anticancer Drugs

Drug	Molecular Target	Drug Structure	Indications	Major Toxicities
Kinase Inhibitors				
EGFR Tyrosine Kinase Inhibitors				
Cetuximab (Erbitux)	Inhibits EGFR	Antibody	EGFR-positive colorectal cancer and head and neck cancer	Rash, infusion reactions, interstitial and lung disease
Panitumumab (Vectibix)	Inhibits EGFR	Antibody	EGFR-positive colorectal cancer	Rare infusion reactions, rash, and rare interstitial pneumonitis
Gefitinib (Iressa)	Inhibits EGFR tyrosine kinase	Small molecule	Non–small cell lung cancer	Rash, diarrhea, and interstitial lung disease
Erlotinib (Tarceva)	Inhibits EGFR tyrosine kinase	Small molecule	Non–small cell lung cancer	Blistering, GI perforation, interstitial lung disease, and corneal ulceration/perforation
Afatinib (Gilotrif)	Inhibits EGFR tyrosine kinase and HER2 and HER4 tyrosine kinase	Small molecule	Metastatic non–small cell lung cancer	Diarrhea, cutaneous reactions, and keratitis
Lapatinib (Tykerb)	Inhibits EGFR tyrosine kinase and HER2 tyrosine kinase	Small molecule	HER2-positive breast cancer	Diarrhea, hepatotoxicity, cardiotoxicity, and interstitial lung disease
BCR-ABL Tyrosine Kinase Inhibitors				
Imatinib (Gleevec)	Inhibits BCR-ABL tyrosine kinase	Small molecule	Chronic myeloid leukemia and GI stromal tumors	Nausea, diarrhea, myalgia, edema, and liver injury
Dasatinib (Sprycel)	Inhibits BCR-ABL tyrosine kinase	Small molecule	Chronic myeloid leukemia	Myelosuppression, QT prolongation, fluid retention, and pulmonary arterial hypertension
Nilotinib (Tasigna)	Inhibits BCR-ABL tyrosine kinase	Small molecule	Chronic myeloid leukemia	Myelosuppression, QT prolongation
Bosutinib (Bosulif)	Inhibits BCR-ABL tyrosine kinase	Small molecule	Philadelphia chromosome–positive chronic myelogenous leukemia	Myelosuppression, hepatotoxicity, and anaphylactic shock
Ponatinib (Iclusig)	Inhibits BCR-ABL tyrosine kinase	Small molecule	Chronic myeloid leukemia or Philadelphia chromosome–positive lymphoblastic leukemia	Venous thromboembolism, cardiotoxicity, pancreatitis, and cardiac dysrhythmias
Multi–Tyrosine Kinase Inhibitors				
Sorafenib (Nexavar)	Inhibits multiple cell-surface and intracellular tyrosine kinases	Small molecule	Renal cell carcinoma, hepatocellular carcinoma	Rash, diarrhea, hand-and-foot syndrome, bleeding, QT prolongation, and hypertension
Sunitinib (Sutent)	Inhibits multiple tyrosine kinases	Small molecule	Renal cell carcinoma, GI stromal tumors, and pancreatic neuroendocrine tumors	Hepatotoxicity, heart failure, QT prolongation, hypertension, and hemorrhage
Pazopanib (Votrient)	Inhibits multiple tyrosine kinases	Small molecule	Renal cell carcinoma	Bone marrow suppression and hepatotoxicity
Vandetanib (Caprelsa)	Inhibits multiple tyrosine kinases	Small molecule	Medullary thyroid cancer	QT prolongation, rash, and diarrhea/colitis
Axitinib (Inlyta)	Inhibits multiple tyrosine kinases	Small molecule	Advanced renal cell carcinoma	Hypertensive crisis, venous thromboembolism, and hypothyroidism
Cabozantinib (Cometriq)	Inhibits multiple tyrosine kinases	Small molecule	Metastatic medullary thyroid cancer	Thromboembolism, GI perforation, and posterior leukoencephalopathy
Regorafenib (Stivarga)	Inhibits multiple tyrosine kinases	Small molecule	Metastatic colon cancer and metastatic GI stromal cancer	Hepatotoxicity, toxic cutaneous reactions, and cardiotoxicity

TABLE 85.7 Targeted Anticancer Drugs—cont'd

Drug	Molecular Target	Drug Structure	Indications	Major Toxicities
mTOR Kinase Inhibitors				
Temsirolimus (Torisel)	Inhibits mTOR kinase	Small molecule	Renal cell carcinoma	Mucositis, bone marrow suppression, and metabolic abnormalities
Everolimus (Afinitor)	Inhibits mTOR kinase	Small molecule	Renal cell carcinoma	Oral ulceration, bone marrow suppression, and metabolic abnormalities
BRAF V600E Kinase Inhibitors				
Vemurafenib (Zelboraf)	Inhibits BRAF V600E kinase	Small molecule	BRAF V600E–positive melanoma	Cutaneous squamous cell carcinoma, arthralgia, QT prolongation, severe skin reactions, and photosensitivity
Dabrafenib (Tafinlar)	Inhibits BRAF V600E kinase	Small molecule	BRAF V600E–positive melanoma	Retinal vein occlusion and cutaneous malignancies
Trametinib (Mekinist)	Inhibits BRAF V600E pathway through inhibition of MEK1 and MEK2	Small molecule	BRAF V600E–positive melanoma	Cutaneous malignancies, hemorrhage, thromboembolism, and retinal vein occlusion
Anaplastic Lymphoma Kinase (ALK) Inhibitor				
Crizotinib (Xalkori)	Inhibits ALK	Small molecule	ALK-positive non–small cell lung cancer	Pneumonitis, hepatotoxicity, and QT prolongation
Other Targeted Drugs				
CD20-Directed Antibodies				
Rituximab (Rituxan)	Binds CD20 antigen, causing apoptosis and immune attack	Antibody	B-cell chronic lymphocytic leukemia and B-cell non-Hodgkin lymphoma	Severe infusion reactions, severe mucocutaneous reactions, tumor lysis syndrome, and PML
Ofatumumab (Arzerra)	Binds CD20 antigen, causing apoptosis and immune attack	Antibody	B-cell chronic lymphocytic leukemia	Severe infusion reactions, cytopenias, and PML
Ibritumomab tiuxetan/yttrium-90 (Zevalin)	Binds CD20 antigen, causing radiation injury	Antibody/yttrium-90 hybrid	B-cell non-Hodgkin lymphoma	Bone marrow suppression and infusion reactions
Antibody-Drug Conjugate				
Brentuximab vedotin (Adcetris)	Binds CD30 antigen, to deliver a toxin that causes mitotic arrest	Antibody/drug hybrid	Hodgkin lymphoma and anaplastic large cell lymphoma	Peripheral neuropathy and neutropenia
Angiogenesis Inhibitor				
Bevacizumab (Avastin)	Binds VEGF and thereby inhibits angiogenesis	Antibody	Colorectal cancer, non–small cell lung cancer, glioblastoma, and renal cell carcinoma	Hypertension, GI perforation, impaired wound healing, hemorrhage, thromboembolism, and nephrotic syndrome
Proteasome Inhibitors				
Bortezomib (Velcade)	Inhibits proteasome activity	Small molecule	Multiple myeloma	Bone marrow suppression, GI disturbances, peripheral neuropathy, and weakness
Carfilzomib (Kyprolis)	Inhibits proteasome activity	Small molecule	Multiple myeloma	Cardiac arrest, cardiotoxicity, and infusion reactions
Histone Deacetylase (HDAC) Inhibitors				
Vorinostat (Zolinza)	Inhibits HDAC	Small molecule	Cutaneous T-cell lymphoma	Pulmonary embolism, bone marrow suppression, fatigue, nausea, diarrhea

Continued

TABLE 85.7   Targeted Anticancer Drugs—cont'd

Drug	Molecular Target	Drug Structure	Indications	Major Toxicities
Romidepsin (Istodax)	Inhibits HDAC	Small molecule	Cutaneous T-cell lymphoma	Bone marrow suppression, infection, and QT prolongation
Additional Targeted Anticancer Drugs				
Ipilimumab (Yervoy)	Binds CTLA-4 to unleash an immune attack	Antibody	Melanoma	Severe immune-mediated enterocolitis, hepatitis, dermatitis, neuropathies, and endocrinopathies
Alemtuzumab (Campath)	Binds CD52 antigen	Antibody	B-cell chronic lymphocytic leukemia	Bone marrow suppression, infusion reactions, and infection

CTLA-4, Cytotoxic T lymphocyte–associated antigen-4; *EGFR*, epidermal growth factor receptor, which is coupled with tyrosine kinase; *GI*, gastrointestinal; *HER2*, human epidermal growth factor receptor 2; *MEK*, MAP (mitogen-activated protein)/ERK (extracellular signal–regulated) kinase; *mTOR*, mammalian target of rapamycin; *PML*, progressive multifocal leukoencephalopathy; *VEGF*, vascular endothelial growth factor.

[ATP]) to an acceptor molecule, often a protein involved in regulation of cell behavior. This process, known as phosphorylation, alters the structure of the acceptor protein and thus increases or decreases its activity. Put another way, the result of phosphorylation is similar to flipping a switch, turning it on or turning it off. Of interest to us are the protein "switches" that help promote cancer growth. For example, certain regulatory proteins, when phosphorylated, activate signaling pathways that increase cell proliferation and cell survival. Accordingly, if we prevent phosphorylation with a kinase inhibitor, we can shut down the signaling pathway and thus inhibit proliferation and promote apoptosis.

Most of the drugs discussed next inhibit *tyrosine kinases* of one type or another. What's a tyrosine kinase? It's simply a kinase that transfers a phosphate group specifically to tyrosine, one of the amino acid components of the protein undergoing phosphorylation. Other kinases phosphorylate different amino acids, often serine or threonine.

Epidermal growth factor receptor tyrosine kinase inhibitors. The *epidermal growth factor receptor* (EGFR) is a transmembrane regulatory molecule that works through activation of intracellular tyrosine kinase. The receptor portion of EGFR, which is found on the outer surface of the cell membrane, is coupled with tyrosine kinase on the inner surface of the cell membrane. Binding of an agonist to EGFR activates tyrosine kinase, which in turn activates signaling pathways that regulate cell proliferation and survival. EGFRs are expressed constitutively in many normal epithelial tissues (e.g., skin and hair follicles) and are overexpressed in several cancers, including cancers of the lung, breast, prostate, bladder, ovary, colon, and rectum. Overexpression is associated with unregulated cell growth and poor prognosis. Drugs that inhibit EGFR suppress cell proliferation and promote apoptosis. At present there are six EGFR tyrosine kinase inhibitors. Two of these drugs—cetuximab and panitumumab—are monoclonal antibodies that bind with the receptor portion of EGFR tyrosine kinase and thus prevent its activation by agonists. The other four drugs—erlotinib, gefitinib, afatinib, and lapatinib—are small molecules that work inside the cell to inhibit tyrosine kinase directly. It should be noted that EGFRs belong to the same receptor family as HER2, the target through which trastuzumab (Herceptin) works.

Cetuximab. Cetuximab (Erbitux) is a monoclonal antibody that blocks EGFRs. The drug is approved for refractory colorectal cancer and for carcinoma of the head and neck. Infusion reactions, acneiform rash, low magnesium, and GI symptoms are common.

Cetuximab acts as a competitive antagonist at EGFRs. As noted, these receptors, which help regulate cell growth, are overexpressed in certain cancers, including those of the colon and rectum. EGFR blockade inhibits cell growth and promotes apoptosis. In animal studies, cetuximab decreased the growth and survival of cancer cells that overexpressed EGFR but had no effect on cancer cells that lacked EGFR.

Cetuximab is approved for metastatic, EGFR-positive colorectal cancer. The drug may be added to an irinotecan-based regimen (if the cancer has progressed despite irinotecan treatment), or it may be used alone (in patients who cannot tolerate irinotecan). Treatment improves quality of life and can improve survival rate at 3 years.

Cetuximab, in combination with radiation, is approved for initial treatment of locally or regionally advanced squamous cell carcinoma of the head and neck. In addition, the drug can be used for recurrent or metastatic cancers that have progressed despite treatment with a platinum-based regimen.

Cetuximab causes adverse effects in most patients. The effects of greatest concern are severe infusion reactions, severe rash, and interstitial lung disease (ILD). Interstitial lung disease begins with acute-onset dyspnea, sometimes with cough or fever. Rapid deterioration may ensue.

Cetuximab causes severe *infusion reactions* in 2% to 5% of patients. Manifestations include rapid-onset airway obstruction, hypotension, shock, loss of consciousness, myocardial infarction, and cardiopulmonary arrest. Severe reactions can happen with any infusion, but most (90%) occur with the first infusion. If a severe reaction develops, cetuximab should be discontinued immediately and never used again. Agents for medical management—epinephrine, glucocorticoids, intravenously administered antihistamines, bronchodilators, and oxygen—should always be on hand. To reduce the risk for a severe reaction, premedication with an intravenous antihistamine (e.g., 50 mg diphenhydramine) is recommended.

Acne-like rash, mainly on the face and upper torso, develops in 88% of patients and is severe in 12%. Severe rash has led to *Staphylococcus aureus* sepsis and abscesses that require incision and drainage. Sunlight can exacerbate dermatologic reactions; hence patients should limit sun exposure, use a sunblock, and wear protective clothing.

Very rarely, cetuximab has been associated with *interstitial lung disease,* characterized by inflammation, scarring, and hardening of the lungs. One case of fatal interstitial pneumonitis with pulmonary edema has been reported. Whether cetuximab is truly the cause of these lung disorders has not been established.

The combination of cetuximab and irinotecan often causes *GI toxicity,* manifesting as diarrhea, nausea, abdominal pain, vomiting, anorexia, and constipation.

Hypomagnesemia is common. Magnesium supplements are often required.

Cetuximab can cross the placenta, but whether it causes fetal harm has not been studied in humans. Animal studies do show adverse fetal effects. Until more is known, prudence dictates avoiding cetuximab during pregnancy.

Panitumumab. Panitumumab (Vectibix) is a monoclonal antibody similar to cetuximab with respect to mechanism, indications, and adverse effects. The principal difference between the drugs is that panitumumab is a fully human antibody whereas cetuximab is not. Similar to cetuximab, panitumumab blocks EGFRs, causing inhibition of tyrosine kinase and, ultimately, apoptosis. At this time, the drug has only one indication: treatment of EGFR-expressing metastatic colorectal cancer in patients who have already received chemotherapy.

The most common adverse effect is acne-like rash. Other adverse effects include fatigue, nausea, diarrhea, and hypomagnesemia. Because panitumumab is a fully human antibody, severe infusion reactions are less frequent than with cetuximab (1% vs 3%).

Gefitinib. Gefitinib (Iressa) is approved for oral therapy of advanced non–small cell lung cancer (NSCLC) that has been refractory to first-line treatment (platinum- or docetaxel-based therapy). Unfortunately, postmarketing studies have failed to show any survival benefit. As a result, gefitinib is restricted to patients enrolled in a medical trial in the United States. NSCLC is the most common form of lung cancer, and cells of this cancer often overexpress EGFRs.

Like cetuximab, gefitinib disrupts cellular processes regulated by EGFRs. However, unlike cetuximab, which acts on the cell surface to block EGFRs, gefitinib acts within the cell to inhibit tyrosine kinase that is linked to EGFR. Under normal conditions, activation of EGFR leads to activation of tyrosine kinase, which in turn activates signaling pathways that regulate cell proliferation and survival. By inhibiting EGFR-linked tyrosine kinase, gefitinib has the same effect as EGFR blockade: suppression of cell proliferation and promotion of apoptosis.

A mutation in the EGFR tyrosine kinase gene predicts who will respond to gefitinib. This mutation is more likely in women, Asians, and patients with the adenocarcinoma subtype of NSCLC. People in these populations are more likely to respond.

Gefitinib is generally well tolerated. As with cetuximab, the most frequent reactions are diarrhea and acne-like rash. Other fairly common reactions are dry skin, nausea, and vomiting. Ocular effects—amblyopia, conjunctivitis, eye pain, and corneal erosion or ulceration—occur infrequently. Asymptomatic elevation of liver transaminases has been reported.

Interstitial lung disease is the most serious adverse effect. The overall incidence is about 1%, with one-third of cases being fatal. If respiratory symptoms develop, gefitinib should be interrupted and the patient evaluated. If ILD is diagnosed, gefitinib should not be used again. The risk for ILD is highest among patients with prior radiation or chemotherapy.

Drugs that inhibit CYP3A4 (e.g., itraconazole and ketoconazole) can decrease gefitinib metabolism and may in turn increase its plasma level. Conversely, agents that induce CYP3A4 (e.g., rifampin, phenytoin, carbamazepine, and St. John's wort) can accelerate gefitinib metabolism and may, in turn, reduce its level. (For patients taking a potent inducer of CYP3A4, dosage may be increased.) Furthermore, drugs that lower gastric pH (e.g., histamine-2 antagonists, proton pump inhibitors, and antacids) can decrease gefitinib absorption and may in turn lower its level.

Gefitinib can harm the developing fetus and hence should not be used by pregnant women. In laboratory animals, the drug decreased the number of live births, increased neonatal mortality, and reduced fetal weight. We don't know if gefitinib is safe during breastfeeding.

Erlotinib. Erlotinib (Tarceva) has three indications: (1) advanced NSCLC after previous chemotherapy has failed; (2) maintenance therapy of advanced NSCLC when the disease has remained stable after four cycles of platinum-based first-line therapy, and (3) first-line treatment of inoperable pancreatic cancer in combination with gemcitabine.

Like gefitinib, erlotinib inhibits tyrosine kinase coupled with EGFR and thus suppresses cell proliferation and promotes apoptosis. However, in contrast to gefitinib, erlotinib has been shown to prolong survival. Survival was longest among patients who had never smoked and those with high levels of EGFR.

As with gefitinib, a mutation in the EGFR tyrosine kinase gene predicts who will respond to erlotinib. As noted, this mutation is more likely in women, Asians, and patients with the adenocarcinoma subtype of NSCLC; hence people in these populations are more likely to respond.

Although erlotinib is generally well tolerated, adverse effects often occur. The most common are rash, diarrhea, nausea, and vomiting. Diarrhea can usually be managed with loperamide. Rarely, patients develop ILD. Hepatotoxicity, manifesting as asymptomatic elevation of liver transaminases, occurs in some patients. Rarely, erlotinib causes GI perforation or severe skin reactions, both of which can be fatal. The drug can also cause ocular disorders, including corneal perforation, corneal ulceration, and abnormal eyelash growth. In animal studies, erlotinib caused fetal death and abortion; hence it should not be used during pregnancy.

Strong inhibitors of CYP3A4 (e.g., itraconazole, clarithromycin, and ritonavir) can decrease metabolism of erlotinib, causing its level to rise. Conversely, inducers of CYP3A4 (e.g., rifampin and carbamazepine) can accelerate metabolism of erlotinib, causing its level to fall, sometimes dramatically. Erlotinib may increase the risk for bleeding in patients taking warfarin; close monitoring of prothrombin time or the international normalized ratio (INR) is recommended.

Afatinib. Afatinib (Gilotrif) is approved for treatment of metastatic NSCLC in patients whose tumors have EGFR deletions or other mutations as detected by an FDA-approved test.

Like gefitinib and erlotinib, afatinib inhibits tyrosine kinase coupled with EGFR and, hence, suppresses cell proliferation and promotes apoptosis. In addition, afatinib also inhibits tyrosine kinase coupled with HER2 and HER4.

Afatinib has caused severe diarrhea leading to dehydration and death. Diarrhea can usually be managed with loperamide. Skin and eye reactions have also occurred. These are characterized by blistering or exfoliating lesions as well as keratitis of the eye. Afatinib should be withheld in these cases. Liver test abnormalities have been seen. Periodic liver testing should be completed to monitor this adverse effect. Afatinib may cause fetal harm and should be avoided in pregnancy.

As with erlotinib, strong inhibitors of CYP3A4 (e.g., itraconazole, clarithromycin, and ritonavir) can decrease metabolism of afatinib, causing its level to rise. Conversely, inducers of CYP3A4 (e.g., rifampin and carbamazepine) can accelerate metabolism of afatinib, causing its level to fall, sometimes dramatically.

Lapatinib. Lapatinib (Tykerb) is a small-molecule inhibitor of EGFR tyrosine kinase and HER2 tyrosine kinase. Lapatinib and its use in breast cancer were discussed earlier.

BCR-ABL tyrosine kinase inhibitors. The BCR-ABL tyrosine kinase inhibitors are the preferred agents for treating *chronic myeloid leukemia* (CML). Five of these drugs are available: imatinib, dasatinib, bosutinib, ponatinib, and nilotinib. Imatinib is the "gold standard" for CML therapy. Unfortunately, relapse can occur, owing to evolution of subclones that have imatinib-resistant BCR-ABL mutations. The other drugs—dasatinib, bosutinib, ponatinib, and nilotinib—are active against all but one of these resistant subclones and hence can be effective even in patients who no longer respond to imatinib.

Imatinib. Imatinib (Gleevec) was approved for oral therapy of CML, but only after treatment with interferon α had failed. Because of clear superiority, imatinib had displaced interferon α as the initial treatment of choice. Imatinib may be continued as long as there is no evidence of disease progression and as long as side effects remain tolerable.

Imatinib is also approved for *myelodysplastic/myeloproliferative diseases, aggressive systemic mastocytosis, acute lymphoblastic leukemia, dermatofibrosarcoma protuberans, hypereosinophilic syndrome, chronic eosinophilic leukemia,* and unresectable or metastatic malignant *gastrointestinal stromal tumor,* a rare form of stomach and intestinal cancer. These applications are not discussed further.

CML is a cancer in which myeloid cells undergo massive clonal expansion. The disease begins with a chronic phase, progresses through an accelerated phase, and ends with the blast crisis phase. The underlying cause is a genetic abnormality known as the *Philadelphia chromosome,* which is produced by translocation of genetic material between chromosomes 9 and 22. Because of this genetic change, CML cells make an abnormal, continuously active enzyme, called *BCR-ABL tyrosine kinase.* This enzyme phosphorylates and, hence, activates as yet unidentified regulatory proteins, which in turn inhibit apoptosis and stimulate cell proliferation. Major treatment options are the BCR-ABL tyrosine kinase inhibitors, interferon-based regimens, and stem cell transplantation (the only potentially curative treatment).

Imatinib is a highly specific competitive inhibitor of BCR-ABL tyrosine kinase. By inhibiting this enzyme, imatinib prevents the phosphorylation and resultant activation of regulatory proteins and, hence, suppresses proliferation of CML cells and promotes apoptosis. Imatinib is selective for cells that express BCR-ABL tyrosine kinase; normal cells are not affected. When tested during the chronic phase of CML, imatinib was superior to the combination of interferon α plus cytarabine. After 18 months, disease progression was stopped in 92% of imatinib users, compared with 74% of those getting interferon. Furthermore, imatinib was better tolerated. Long-term follow-up is needed to determine how long responses to imatinib will last and whether imatinib prolongs survival.

Over time, resistance to imatinib may develop because the genes that code for BCR-ABL can mutate, causing production of imatinib-resistant forms of the enzyme.

Imatinib causes adverse effects in most patients. The incidence and severity of adverse effects is lowest during the chronic phase of CML, higher during the accelerated phase, and highest during blast crisis. Common reactions include nausea, vomiting, diarrhea, rash, headache, fatigue, fever, and musculoskeletal complaints, including muscle cramps, muscle pain, and arthralgia. Fluid retention occurs in 52% to 68% of patients and may lead to pleural effusion, pericardial effusion, pulmonary edema, or ascites. Neutropenia and thrombocytopenia develop often, posing a risk for infection and bleeding. Accordingly, complete blood counts should be obtained weekly during the first month of treatment, biweekly during the second month, and periodically thereafter. Hepatotoxicity, indicated by severe elevations of transaminases or bilirubin, develops in 1.1% to 3.5% of patients. Other reported effects include severe congestive heart failure, serious skin reactions (e.g., erythema multiforme and Stevens-Johnson syndrome), and hypothyroidism in thyroidectomy patients receiving thyroid hormone replacement therapy.

In animal studies, dosages equivalent to those used clinically have caused major fetal malformations. Accordingly, imatinib should be avoided during pregnancy. Women of childbearing age should use adequate contraception.

Imatinib achieves high concentrations in breast milk and poses a risk to the breastfed infant. The manufacturer recommends against breastfeeding while taking the drug.

Imatinib is a substrate for and competitive inhibitor of CYP3A4, CYP2C9, and CYP2D6. By inhibiting these CYP isoenzymes, imatinib can raise levels of warfarin and other drugs that are metabolized by them.

Drugs that inhibit CYP3A4 (e.g., ketoconazole and erythromycin) can raise levels of imatinib. Conversely, drugs that induce CYP3A4 (e.g., carbamazepine, rifampin, and St. John's wort) can reduce levels of imatinib.

Dasatinib. Dasatinib (Sprycel) is indicated for all three phases of CML: chronic, accelerated, and blast crisis. Initially, the drug was approved only for patients who were unresponsive to or intolerant of imatinib. Soon after, the FDA approved dasatinib as first-line therapy.

Dasatinib inhibits BCR-ABL tyrosine kinase more effectively than imatinib. First, dasatinib binds to both the active and inactive conformations of BCR-ABL tyrosine kinase, whereas imatinib binds only to the inactive conformation. Second, dasatinib binds the enzyme with greater affinity than imatinib. Third, dasatinib binds a wider variety of protein kinases. As a result of these differences, dasatinib is active against nearly all imatinib-resistant mutant clones. In fact, the only exception is the T315I mutation, which is resistant to all available drugs.

Adverse effects of dasatinib are much similar to those of imatinib, with one important exception: dasatinib produces more myelosuppression and therefore poses a risk for severe neutropenia, thrombocytopenia, and anemia. Fluid retention is seen in about 35% of patients. Severe cases can cause pulmonary edema. Rarely, dasatinib has been associated with pulmonary arterial hypertension, although a causal relationship has not been established. Dasatinib has the potential to prolong the QT interval, but the clinical significance of this is unclear.

Levels of dasatinib can be affected by other drugs. Dasatinib is a substrate for CYP3A4; therefore drugs that induce CYP3A4 can lower dasatinib levels, and drugs that inhibit CYP3A4 can raise dasatinib levels. Solubility of dasatinib is pH dependent, so drugs that raise gastric pH (antacids, proton pump inhibitors, and histamine-2 receptor blockers) can reduce dasatinib absorption.

Nilotinib. Nilotinib (Tasigna) is indicated for (1) accelerated-phase CML in patients resistant to or intolerant of imatinib and (2) chronic-phase CML in treatment-naive patients as well as patients previously treated with imatinib. Both imatinib and nilotinib bind to the inactive form of BCR-ABL. However, nilotinib's binding affinity is much greater. Both drugs are also active against all imatinib-resistant clones, except those with the T315I mutation.

In general, patients tolerate nilotinib better than imatinib. The most common adverse effects are thrombocytopenia, neutropenia, rash, pruritus, nausea, fatigue, headache, and constipation. Of much greater concern, nilotinib prolongs the QT interval, posing a risk for severe dysrhythmias and sudden cardiac death. Accordingly, the drug should not be used in patients with hypokalemia, hypomagnesemia, or long QT syndrome. Also, it should not be combined with other QT drugs or with strong inhibitors of CYP3A4 (e.g., ketoconazole, clarithromycin, and ritonavir).

Similar to dasatinib, nilotinib is a substrate for CYP3A4; therefore drugs that induce CYP3A4 can lower nilotinib levels, and drugs that inhibit CYP3A4 can raise nilotinib levels.

Bosutinib. Bosutinib (Bosulif) has one indication: treatment of adults with Philadelphia chromosome–positive CML resistant to prior therapy. Bosutinib inhibits the tyrosine kinase that promotes CML.

Myelosuppression has occurred in patients taking bosutinib. A complete blood count should be performed weekly during the first month and then monthly thereafter. Because of the potential for hepatotoxicity, liver function tests should be obtained monthly for the first 3 months. Bosutinib can result in fetal harm and should be avoided in pregnancy.

As bosutinib is metabolized by the CYP3A system, drugs that affect this system may alter the metabolism of bosutinib. Taking CYP3A inhibitors (clarithromycin, grapefruit juice, ketoconazole, and ritonavir) and CYP3A inducers (carbamazepine, phenytoin, and rifampin) in conjunction with bosutinib may increase adverse reactions.

Ponatinib. Ponatinib (Iclusig) is indicated for treatment of (1) adults with CML that is resistant to or intolerant of prior therapy and (2) those with Philadelphia chromosome–positive lymphoblastic leukemia resistant to prior therapy with tyrosine kinase inhibitors.

Ponatinib, similar to dasatinib, inhibits multiple tyrosine kinases and is therefore used as an alternative treatment after use of other tyrosine kinase inhibitors such as imatinib.

Venous thromboembolic events have been reported in patients taking ponatinib. Reduction or cessation of the drug should be considered in patients who develop serious thromboembolism. Other adverse effects include pancreatitis, hypertension, cardiotoxicity, heart dysrhythmias, GI perforation, and myelosuppression. Blood pressure, complete blood counts, and ejection fraction should be closely followed during treatment with ponatinib.

Like bosutinib, ponatinib is metabolized by the CYP3A system. Drugs that affect this system may alter the metabolism of ponatinib.

Ponatinib is available in 15- and 45-mg tablets. Dosing is 45 mg daily. Treatment should be continued until the disease progresses or unacceptable toxicity is experienced.

Multi–tyrosine kinase inhibitors. In contrast to the EGFR tyrosine kinase inhibitors and the BCR-ABL tyrosine kinase inhibitors, which inhibit just one type of tyrosine kinase, the drugs in this section inhibit several types of tyrosine kinase. However, despite their diverse actions, the multi–tyrosine kinase inhibitors have limited indications: four of the available agents—sorafenib, sunitinib, axitinib, and pazopanib—are approved for advanced renal cell carcinoma. In addition, sorafenib is approved for hepatocellular carcinoma, and sunitinib is approved for GI stromal tumor and pancreatic neuroendocrine tumor (PNET). Two additional drugs—vandetanib and cabozantinib—are approved for medullary thyroid cancer. A seventh drug—regorafenib—is approved for metastatic colon cancer and metastatic GI stromal tumor.

Sorafenib. Sorafenib (Nexavar) is an oral multi–tyrosine kinase inhibitor approved for advanced renal cell carcinoma, recurrent thyroid carcinoma refractory to iodine treatment, and unresectable hepatocellular carcinoma. The drug inhibits multiple cell-surface and intracellular kinases that are associated with angiogenesis, apoptosis, and cell proliferation.

The most common adverse effects are diarrhea, rash, fatigue, and hand-and-foot syndrome. Hypertension is developed in between 15% and 20% of patients. Nausea and vomiting are usually mild. Sorafenib prolongs the QT interval and therefore poses a risk for serious dysrhythmias. In addition, the drug doubles the risk for bleeding (by inhibiting vascular endothelial growth factor [VEGF] tyrosine kinase). Myocardial ischemia and GI perforation occur rarely. Sorafenib (in low doses) is teratogenic and embryolethal in animals and hence should be avoided during pregnancy.

Sunitinib. Sunitinib (Sutent) is an oral multi–tyrosine kinase inhibitor with three indications: advanced renal cell carcinoma, PNET, and GI stromal tumor in patients unresponsive to or intolerant of imatinib. The drug inhibits multiple tyrosine kinases and, hence, disrupts angiogenesis, cellular growth, and tumor metastasis.

Adverse effects are very common. Twenty percent or more of patients experience fatigue, weakness, anorexia, altered taste, fever, dyspnea, cough, GI disturbances (nausea, vomiting, diarrhea, dyspepsia, and abdominal pain), pain (headache, back pain, arthralgia, and extremity pain), and skin reactions (rash, dryness, hand-and-foot syndrome, and discolored skin and hair). Of much greater concern, sunitinib can cause heart damage, liver damage, and hemorrhage. About 15% of patients develop irreversible heart failure, hence cardiac function should be monitored closely. Both sorafenib and sunitinib prolong the QT interval and, hence, can cause severe dysrhythmias. Sunitinib can cause potentially fatal liver injury. Accordingly, liver function tests should be conducted

at baseline and periodically throughout the treatment period. By suppressing platelet production, sunitinib can cause hemorrhage. To reduce risk, serial blood counts should be conducted. About 25% of patients develop mild to moderate hypertension, which responds to standard antihypertensive drugs. Other serious effects include impairment of wound healing, adrenal function, and thyroid function. In animal studies, sunitinib has been teratogenic and fetotoxic.

Sunitinib is a substrate for CYP3A4, so medications that inhibit CYP3A4 (e.g., ketoconazole and erythromycin) can raise levels of sunitinib and increase toxicity. Conversely, drugs that induce CYP3A4 (e.g., carbamazepine, rifampin, and St. John's wort) can reduce levels and therefore decrease efficacy.

Pazopanib. Pazopanib (Votrient) is an oral multi–tyrosine kinase inhibitor indicated only for advanced renal cell carcinoma. Similar to sunitinib and sorafenib, pazopanib disrupts tumor growth and angiogenesis by inhibiting multiple forms of tyrosine kinase.

Adverse effects are common and sometimes severe. Effects seen often include hepatotoxicity, diarrhea, hypertension, hyperglycemia, change in hair color, leukopenia, and thrombocytopenia, sometimes associated with hemorrhage. Rarely, pazopanib has caused fatal GI perforation, fatal thrombotic events, and potentially fatal torsades de pointes secondary to prolonging the QT interval. In pregnant animals, pazopanib has been teratogenic, embryolethal, and abortifacient.

Both sunitinib and pazopanib are metabolized by CYP3A4; hence medications that inhibit CYP3A4 can raise levels of pazopanib (thus increasing toxicity) and medications that induce CYP3A4 can reduce levels of pazopanib (thus decreasing efficacy).

Vandetanib. Vandetanib (Caprelsa) is indicated for advanced medullary thyroid cancer, a rare disease that accounts for just 3% to 5% of all thyroid cancers. In the United States this translates to about 1300 to 2200 cases a year. Benefits of vandetanib appear to result from inhibiting multiple tyrosine kinases, including EGFR tyrosine kinase.

The most common adverse effects are diarrhea/colitis, rash, acne, nausea, hypertension, headache, fatigue, decreased appetite, and abdominal pain. More important, vandetanib poses a significant risk for QT prolongation, which can lead to potentially fatal dysrhythmias. Furthermore, because vandetanib has a long half-life (19 days), this risk can persist long after dosing is stopped. To monitor QT effects, an electrocardiogram should be obtained at baseline, between weeks 2 and 4, between weeks 8 and 12, and every 3 months thereafter. Other drugs that prolong the QT interval should be avoided. In laboratory animals, low-dose vandetanib is fetotoxic and teratogenic. Accordingly, the drug should be avoided by women who are pregnant.

Axitinib. Axitinib (Inlyta) is approved for the treatment of advanced renal cell carcinoma after failure of one prior systemic therapy. Axitinib inhibits VEGF receptors, resulting in the inhibition of cell proliferation, survival, and tumor growth.

Hypertension and hypertensive crises have been reported with the use of axitinib. Blood pressure should be monitored closely, and dosage should be reduced if persistent hypertension occurs. As there is potential for hepatotoxicity, liver function should also be monitored periodically.

Cabozantinib. Cabozantinib (Cometriq), similar to pazopanib, is an oral multi–tyrosine kinase inhibitor. Cabozantinib is indicated for the treatment of metastatic medullary thyroid cancer.

Common adverse effects include diarrhea, stomatitis, nausea, and fatigue. More concerning adverse effects include posterior leukoencephalopathy syndrome. Patients present with seizures, headache, confusion, or visual disturbances. Osteonecrosis of the jaw has also been reported with cabozantinib use. If these adverse effects are present, treatment should cease. Fetal harm has been reported with cabozantinib, so it should be avoided in pregnant women. As with other kinase inhibitors, cabozantinib interacts with strong inducers and inhibitors of CYP3A4.

Regorafenib. Regorafenib (Stivarga) is a multi–tyrosine kinase inhibitor approved for the treatment of metastatic colorectal cancer previously treated with chemotherapy. Regorafenib is also indicated for the treatment of unresectable GI stromal tumor previously treated with imatinib and sunitinib.

Severe and sometimes fatal hepatotoxicity has occurred with regorafenib. Liver function tests should be monitored every 2 weeks for the first 2 months of therapy, then monthly thereafter. Severe skin reactions, including Stevens-Johnson syndrome, have been reported. As with the other kinase inhibitors, regorafenib should be avoided in combination with CYP3A4 inhibitors or inducers. Patients on warfarin should also have frequent INR monitoring.

Mammalian target of rapamycin kinase inhibitors

Temsirolimus. Temsirolimus (Torisel) is indicated for intravenous therapy of advanced renal cell carcinoma. After conversion to its active form—sirolimus—the drug inhibits mammalian target of rapamycin (mTOR), a protein kinase that helps regulate cell growth, proliferation, and survival. Inhibition of mTOR leads to G_1 arrest and apoptosis. Adverse effects, which are common, include weakness, rash, mucositis, nausea, edema, anorexia, dyspnea, pain, and fever. Common laboratory abnormalities include anemia, neutropenia, hyperglycemia, and increases in cholesterol, triglycerides, and alkaline phosphatase. Sirolimus (the active metabolite of temsirolimus) is metabolized by CYP3A4; hence levels of sirolimus can be altered by drugs that induce or inhibit CYP3A4.

Everolimus. Everolimus (Afinitor) has four anticancer indications: (1) advanced renal cell carcinoma after failure with sorafenib or sunitinib; (2) subependymal giant cell astrocytoma (SEGA) in patients who are not candidates for curative surgical resection; (3) advanced hormone receptor–positive, HER2-negative breast cancer in postmenopausal women; and (4) PNETs that are unresectable, locally advanced, or metastatic. As with temsirolimus, benefits derive from inhibiting mTOR kinase. In addition to its use in cancer, everolimus, sold as Zortress, is used to prevent organ rejection in transplant recipients.

Everolimus causes multiple adverse effects, including weakness, fatigue, diarrhea, nausea, cough, dyspnea, rash, and peripheral edema. Hematologic effects include reduced hemoglobin levels, reduced lymphocyte counts, and reduced platelet counts. Neutropenia predisposes to infections. Metabolic abnormalities include elevations of cholesterol, triglycerides, and glucose. About 44% of patients develop oral mucositis, stomatitis, or mouth and tongue ulcers. Everolimus is toxic to the developing fetus.

BRAF V600E kinase inhibitors

Vemurafenib. Vemurafenib (Zelboraf) is a kinase inhibitor indicated for patients with unresectable or metastatic *melanoma* that expresses *BRAF V600E kinase*, a variant form of BRAF kinase that is found in 30% to 60% of melanoma cells. In healthy cells, BRAF kinase (a cell-membrane protein) stimulates cell proliferation, but only when activated by specific growth factors. BRAF V600E differs from normal BRAF kinase in that BRAF V600E is highly active in the *absence* of stimulation by growth factors. As a result, cells with the BRAF V600E mutation undergo excessive proliferation and metastasis. Vemurafenib is a small molecule that inhibits BRAF V600E kinase activity and thus suppresses tumor growth. Before vemurafenib is used, the BRAF V600E mutation must be confirmed using an FDA-approved assay, such as the *cobas 4800 BRAF V600 mutation test.*

Vemurafenib can cause serious adverse effects. *Cutaneous squamous cell carcinoma,* seen in 24% of patients, is of greatest concern. Other serious effects include hepatotoxicity, severe hypersensitivity reactions (e.g., anaphylaxis), severe skin reactions (e.g., Stevens-Johnson syndrome and toxic epidermal necrolysis), serious ophthalmic reactions (e.g.,

uveitis, iritis, and retinal vein occlusion), and QT prolongation, which poses a risk for severe dysrhythmias. Less serious effects include arthralgia, hair loss, fatigue, rash, photosensitivity reactions, itching, nausea, and diarrhea. Because of its mechanism, vemurafenib is likely to cause fetal harm. Accordingly, women using the drug should avoid getting pregnant.

Vemurafenib is subject to multiple drug interactions, which could be hard to predict. Vemurafenib is a substrate for CYP3A4 and P-glycoprotein (a transporter that pumps drugs out of cells); hence levels of vemurafenib can be altered by drugs that induce or inhibit these pathways. Also, vemurafenib itself is an inhibitor of P-glycoproteins as well as several CYP isoenzymes; hence vemurafenib can increase levels of drugs that employ these pathways. Last, vemurafenib can induce CYP3A4 and thus can reduce levels of CYP3A4 substrates.

Dabrafenib. Dabrafenib (Tafinlar) is used as a single agent or in combination with trametinib for the treatment of unresectable metastatic *melanoma* with BRAF V600E mutation. Dabrafenib acts as a kinase inhibitor that inhibits melanoma cell growth.

In addition to fatigue, rash, diarrhea, and nausea, dabrafenib is associated with retinal vein occlusion and venous thromboembolism. Providers should assess for changes in vision. Also of concern is the potential development of new cutaneous malignancies. Dermatologic evaluations should be performed at the beginning and throughout therapy. Cardiomyopathy may also occur with dabrafenib use. Ejection fraction should be assessed before initiation as well as periodically during treatment. Dabrafenib should be avoided during pregnancy and breastfeeding. As in the case of vemurafenib, the metabolism of dabrafenib is altered when combined with drugs that inhibit the cytochrome systems.

Trametinib. Trametinib (Mekinist) is an inhibitor of the MAP (mitogen-activated protein)/ERK (extracellular signal–regulated) kinases 1 and 2 (MEK1 and MEK2). Because MEK1 and MEK2 are part of the BRAF pathway, trametinib is an indirect inhibitor of the BRAF V600E kinase. Trametinib is used to treat unresectable or metastatic *melanoma* with BRAF V600E or V600K mutations.

Adverse effects are similar to those of dabrafenib, including thromboembolism, new cutaneous malignancies, and retinal vein occlusion. Increased toxicity has been reported when trametinib is used in conjunction with other kinase inhibitors and cytotoxic agents. Trametinib should not be used in pregnancy.

Crizotinib, an anaplastic lymphoma kinase inhibitor. Crizotinib (Xalkori) is indicated for advanced non–small cell lung cancer that is anaplastic lymphoma kinase (ALK)–positive. Benefits derive from inhibiting ALK, a tyrosine kinase found in normal and cancerous cells. However, the form of ALK found in normal cells differs from the form found in cancer cells. Because of this difference, ALK activity in normal cells is low, whereas ALK activity in certain cancer cells is high—so high, in fact, that it drives proliferation and prolongs survival. Hence, by inhibiting ALK, crizotinib can suppress tumor growth. Because crizotinib is approved only for NSCLC that is ALK positive, the cancer must be tested for ALK before treatment. Among patients with NSCLC, about 2% to 10% have the ALK-positive type.

Crizotinib is generally well tolerated. The most common adverse effects are nausea, diarrhea, vomiting, constipation, edema, fatigue, dizziness, and neuropathies. Elevation of liver enzymes is seen in 4% to 7% of patients. Crizotinib prolongs the QT interval and hence poses a risk for serious dysrhythmias. The most serious adverse effect—potentially fatal pneumonitis—develops in 1.6% of patients. If pneumonitis is diagnosed, crizotinib should be stopped and never used again. In laboratory animals, crizotinib was fetotoxic at doses close to those used clinically. Accordingly, women using the drug should avoid pregnancy.

Crizotinib is a substrate for and inhibitor of CYP3A4. Accordingly, crizotinib levels can be increased by CYP3A4 inhibitors (e.g., ketoconazole, clarithromycin, and ritonavir) and can be decreased by CYP3A4 inducers (e.g., carbamazepine, phenytoin, and St. John's wort). By inhibiting CYP3A4, crizotinib can raise levels of CYP3A4 substrates, including cyclosporine, fentanyl, and alfentanil.

Other Targeted Drugs

CD20-Directed Antibodies

Antibodies directed against CD20 are used to treat B-cell non-Hodgkin lymphoma and B-cell chronic lymphocytic leukemia. CD20 is a molecule found on the cell membrane surface of B lymphocytes (B cells). When antibodies bind with CD20, they trigger an immune attack against the B cell itself. Because most other cells do not have CD20, injury is limited to normal and malignant B lymphocytes.

At present, three products containing anti-CD20 antibodies are available. One of these products—ibritumomab (Zevalin)—consist of a monoclonal antibody that has been linked with a radioactive isotope. With these drugs, cell kill results largely from radiation damage rather than from immune attack. The other two drugs—rituximab (Rituxan) and ofatumumab (Arzerra)—have no radioactivity; thus cell kill results from immune attack promoted by the antibody.

Rituximab

Actions and use. Rituximab (Rituxan) is a monoclonal antibody indicated for IV therapy of *B-cell non-Hodgkin lymphoma* and *B-cell chronic lymphocytic leukemia*. The antibody is directed against the CD20 antigen, which is found on the surface of most normal and malignant B cells. Binding of rituximab recruits components of the immune system, which then cause cell lysis.

In addition to its use in cancer, rituximab is used to treat rheumatoid arthritis (see Chapter 59) and two inflammatory disorders of blood vessels: microscopic polyangiitis and Wegener granulomatosis.

Adverse effects. Rituximab can cause severe infusion-related hypersensitivity reactions. Prominent symptoms are hypotension, bronchospasm, and angioedema. Deaths have occurred. Management includes slowing or discontinuing the infusion and injecting epinephrine.

Rapid and massive death of tumor cells can lead to tumor lysis syndrome (TLS), characterized by acute renal failure, hyperkalemia, hypocalcemia, hyperuricemia, or hyperphosphatemia. Rarely, the syndrome proves fatal. TLS begins within 12 to 24 hours of the first rituximab infusion. The risk for TLS is increased by a high tumor burden. Management includes dialysis and correction of fluid and electrolyte abnormalities.

Rituximab has been associated with severe mucocutaneous reactions, including Stevens-Johnson syndrome, lichenoid dermatitis, vesiculobullous dermatitis, and toxic epidermal necrolysis. Deaths have occurred. Reaction onset is typically 1 to 3 weeks after rituximab exposure. Patients who experience these reactions should seek immediate medical attention and should not receive rituximab again.

There have been reports of hepatitis B virus (HBV) reactivation, leading to fulminant hepatitis, hepatic failure, and death. Patients at high risk for HBV should be screened before getting rituximab. Asymptomatic carriers should be closely monitored for clinical and laboratory signs of active HBV infection while taking rituximab and for several months after stopping.

Rituximab has been associated with rare cases of progressive multifocal leukoencephalopathy (PML), a severe infection of the CNS caused by reactivation of the JC virus, an opportunistic pathogen resistant to all available drugs.

Similar to other monoclonal antibodies, rituximab can cause a flu-like syndrome, especially during the initial infusion. Symptoms include fever, chills, nausea, vomiting, and myalgia. Rituximab causes transient neutropenia, but this does not appear to increase the risk for infection.

Ofatumumab

Actions and use. Ofatumumab (Arzerra) is a monoclonal antibody directed against the CD20 antigen on B lymphocytes. The drug was approved as second-line therapy for B-cell chronic lymphocytic leukemia in patients refractory to fludarabine (Fludara) and alemtuzumab (Campath). Both rituximab and ofatumumab bind with CD20 antigens on B cells and hence promote immune-mediated cell lysis. In patients refractory to fludarabine and alemtuzumab, the overall response rate to ofatumumab is 42%, with a median response duration of 6.5 months.

Adverse effects. Ofatumumab can cause severe adverse effects. Similar to rituximab, the drug can cause infusion reactions, PML, and reactivation of HBV. In addition, ofatumumab can cause severe neutropenia and thrombocytopenia, increasing the risk for infections and bleeding. Intestinal obstruction may also occur. Common but less serious effects include fever, cough, dyspnea, diarrhea, fatigue, rash, and nausea.

Zevalin (Ibritumomab Tiuxetan Linked With Yttrium-90)

Actions and use. Ibritumomab tiuxetan (IT), marketed as Zevalin, is a compound molecule composed of ibritumomab (a monoclonal antibody) that has been covalently bound with tiuxetan. Both rituximab and IT bind selectively with the CD20 antigen present on most normal and malignant B cells. However, unlike rituximab, which is used by itself to treat cancer, IT is first linked with yttrium-90 (Y90), a β particle–emitting radioisotope. When the IT-Y90 complex binds with cellular CD20 antigens, cell kill results from radiation-induced injury rather than from injury caused by ibritumomab itself. Because β particles have a relatively short path length (about 5 mm), injury is restricted to CD20-containing cells and neighboring cells within a 5-mm radius. The radioactive drug poses no danger to people in proximity. IT-Y90 was the first anticancer treatment to employ an antibody complexed with a radioactive compound. IT-Y90 was originally approved for low-grade, B-cell non-Hodgkin lymphoma and then was later approved for follicular non-Hodgkin lymphoma.

Before patients receive IT-Y90, they are given two small doses of rituximab, 7 to 9 days apart. The contribution of rituximab is twofold. First, it binds with circulating B cells and thus greatly reduces their numbers. Second, it occupies nonspecific binding sites that could otherwise attract IT-Y90 and hence would reduce the amount of IT-Y90 available to bind with target cells. For the purpose of diagnostic imaging, the first dose of rituximab is accompanied by a small dose of IT that has been linked to radioactive indium-111.

Adverse effects. Adverse effects of treatment are due to IT-Y90 itself and to the rituximab given before it. As noted earlier, rituximab can cause severe infusion reactions. With IT-Y90, hematologic toxicity is the major concern: severe, prolonged cytopenias develop in more than 50% of patients. Counts of neutrophils and platelets reach their nadir 7 to 9 weeks after treatment and take 3 to 7 weeks to recover. Infection risk is high. Deaths have occurred. Because of its hematologic toxicity, IT-Y90 is contraindicated for patients with (1) lymphoma bone marrow involvement of 25% or more or (2) limited bone marrow reserve (e.g., platelet count below 100,000/mm^3 or neutrophil count below 1500/mm^3; history of prior myeloablative therapy).

Brentuximab Vedotin, an Antibody-Drug Conjugate

Brentuximab vedotin (Adcetris) is an antibody-drug conjugate (ADC), composed of brentuximab coupled with monomethyl auristatin E (MMAE). Brentuximab is a monoclonal antibody that selectively binds with CD30, an antigen expressed on the surface of certain cancer cells. MMAE is a toxic compound that binds with intracellular tubulin. Cell kill results as follows: after binding with CD30 on the cell surface, the entire ADC is rapidly internalized and then cleaved to release free MMAE, which then binds with tubulin to cause mitotic arrest.

Brentuximab vedotin has two indications: *Hodgkin lymphoma* after failure of autologous stem cell transplantation or after failure of at least two multidrug chemotherapy regimens and (2) systemic *anaplastic large cell lymphoma* after failure of at least one multidrug chemotherapy regimen. In clinical trials, the drug demonstrated response rates that were higher than those produced with any available chemotherapy regimen.

Adverse effects are generally "manageable." The most common are peripheral sensory neuropathy, neutropenia, anemia, fatigue, nausea, diarrhea, and fever. Of these, neuropathy and neutropenia are the greatest concerns. If neuropathy or neutropenia develops, dosage should be reduced or the dosing interval increased.

In laboratory animals, low-dose brentuximab vedotin was teratogenic and fetotoxic. Accordingly, the drug should be avoided in women who are pregnant.

Angiogenesis Inhibitors

Cancer cells, similar to other cells, need oxygen and nutrients to survive and multiply. To meet this need, cancer cells produce growth factors such as VEGF to promote the formation of new blood vessels. This process is called angiogenesis.

Angiogenesis inhibitors suppress formation of new blood vessels and, hence, deprive solid tumors of the expanding blood supply they need for continued growth. It is important to note, however, that although tumor growth is suppressed, angiogenesis inhibitors, by themselves, cannot kill tumor cells that already exist.

Since the first angiogenesis inhibitor was approved in 2004, there has been a boon in the approval of drugs for this purpose. Currently, thirteen angiogenesis inhibitors have received FDA approval (see Table 85.8). Angiogenesis is usually not the only attribute of these agents, as

TABLE 85.8 Angiogenesis Inhibitors

Generic Name	Trade Name	Targeted Cancers
Axitinib	Inlyta	Renal cell carcinoma
Bevacizumab	Avastin	Cervical cancer, colorectal cancer, glioblastoma, non-small cell lung cancer, ovarian cancer, and renal cell carcinoma
Cabozantinib	Cabometyx, Cometriq	Renal cell carcinoma and medullary thyroid cancer
Everolimus	Afinitor	Breast cancer, neuroendocrine tumors, and renal cell carcinoma
Lenalidomide	Revlimid	Mantle cell lymphoma[a] and multiple myeloma
Pazopanib	Votrient	Renal cell carcinoma and soft tissue sarcoma
Ramucirumab	Cyramza	Colorectal cancer, gastric cancer, and non-small cell lung cancer
Regorafenib	Stivarga	Colorectal cancer, gastrointestinal stromal tumors, and hepatocellular carcinoma
Sorafenib	Nexavar	Hepatocellular cancer, renal cell cancer, and thyroid cancer
Sunitinib	Sutent	Gastrointestinal stromal tumor, pancreatic neuroendocrine tumors, and renal cell carcinoma
Thalidomide	Thalomid	Multiple myeloma
Vandetanib	Caprelsa	Medullary thyroid cancer
Ziv-aflibercept	Zaltrap	Colorectal cancer

[a]A type of non-Hodgkin lymphoma

evidenced by the fact that we have covered most of these drugs earlier in this chapter.

Bevacizumab

Bevacizumab (Avastin) became the first angiogenesis inhibitor approved for clinical use. In patients with metastatic colorectal cancer or non-squamous NSCLC, the drug can delay tumor progression and prolong life. Unfortunately, bevacizumab can also cause life-threatening side effects, including GI perforation, hemorrhage, and thromboembolism.

Mechanism of action. Bevacizumab is a monoclonal antibody that binds with VEGF, an endogenous compound that stimulates blood vessel growth. Binding with bevacizumab prevents VEGF from binding with its receptors on vascular endothelial cells, preventing VEGF from promoting new vessel formation. As a result, further tumor growth is suppressed.

Therapeutic use. Bevacizumab has five approved uses:
- Persistent, recurrent, or metastatic *cervical cancer*, in combination with paclitaxel and either cisplatin or topotecan
- Metastatic *cancer of the colon or rectum,* in combination with a regimen based on IV 5-fluorouracil (5-FU)
- *Nonsquamous non–small cell lung cancer,* in combination with carboplatin and paclitaxel
- Metastatic *renal cell carcinoma,* in combination with interferon α
- *Glioblastoma,* as a single agent after prior therapy

In addition to its use in cancer, bevacizumab is used off label to treat the neovascular form of *age-related macular degeneration.*

Adverse effects. The most serious adverse effects are GI perforation, hemorrhage, thromboembolism, nephrotic syndrome, disruption of wound healing, and hypertensive crisis. Less serious effects include diarrhea, rhinitis, proteinuria, taste alteration, dry skin, headache, and back pain.

Some cases of GI perforation have been fatal. Primary symptoms are abdominal pain in association with constipation and vomiting. If GI perforation occurs, bevacizumab should be stopped and never used again.

Bevacizumab greatly increases the risk for *severe or fatal hemorrhage.* Patients have experienced GI bleeding, intracranial bleeding, vaginal bleeding, and nosebleeds. In addition, patients with NSCLC have experienced life-threatening *pulmonary hemorrhage.* The risk for a life-threatening or fatal lung bleed is very high (31%) in patients with squamous cell histology and much lower (4%) in those with non–squamous cell histology. Onset of pulmonary bleeding is sudden and presents as major or massive hemoptysis (expectoration of blood). Bevacizumab should be avoided in patients with recent hemoptysis or serious hemorrhage.

When added to a regimen based on 5-FU, bevacizumab doubles the risk for *arterial thromboembolic events,* including ischemic stroke, myocardial infarction, and transient ischemic attacks. Deaths have occurred. Patients who experience a thromboembolic event should stop bevacizumab and never use it again.

Bevacizumab *impairs wound healing* and can induce wound dehiscence (splitting open). Because of these effects, if bevacizumab is initiated too soon after surgery, or if it is not discontinued soon enough before surgery, impaired wound healing can result. To minimize healing complications, guidelines suggest waiting at least 28 days after surgery before using the drug and stopping the drug at least 28 days before elective surgery.

Bevacizumab can cause *severe hypertension* that may persist for months after the drug is withdrawn. Some patients have experienced hypertensive encephalopathy and subarachnoid hemorrhage. Blood pressure should be monitored in all patients. If severe hypertension develops, bevacizumab should be permanently discontinued.

Nephrotic syndrome may develop. Patients should be monitored for development or worsening of proteinuria, a sign of kidney injury. If moderate to severe proteinuria occurs, bevacizumab should be withdrawn.

Effect in pregnancy. Angiogenesis is critical to fetal development, and hence angiogenesis inhibition is likely to cause fetal harm. Although human data are lacking, animal studies indicate that bevacizumab decreases fetal weight, increases fetal resorption, and can promote gross malformations. Bevacizumab should be used only if the benefits to the mother are judged to outweigh the risks to the fetus.

Proteasome Inhibitors

Proteasomes are intracellular multienzyme complexes that degrade proteins. Their physiologic role is to rid cells of proteins that are not needed, including proteins that regulate transcription, cell adhesion, apoptosis, and progression through the cell cycle. Proteasome inhibitors can cause these proteins to accumulate and can thus disrupt various aspects of cell physiology. In cancer cells, these drugs appear to promote accumulation of proteins that promote apoptosis. Three proteasome inhibitors are currently approved by the FDA: bortezomib (Velcade), carfilzomib (Kyprolis), and ixazomib (Ninlaro).

Bortezomib

Mechanism of actions. Bortezomib (Velcade) was the first proteasome inhibitor available for general use. The drug inhibits a specific proteasome, known as the 26S proteasome, and, hence, alters the concentration of proteins that regulate cell growth and division. The result is reduced cell viability, increased apoptosis, and increased sensitivity to the lethal effects of radiation and cytotoxic anticancer drugs. Does bortezomib hurt normal cells too? Yes. However, in vitro studies suggest that normal cells are less vulnerable than cancer cells.

Therapeutic use. Bortezomib is approved for (1) multiple myeloma, both as first-line therapy and for patients who have not responded adequately to other therapies and (2) mantle cell lymphoma (a type of non-Hodgkin lymphoma) in patients with at least 1 prior year of therapy.

Adverse effects. Adverse effects are common and often serious. Approximately half of patients develop fatigue, peripheral neuropathy, nausea, diarrhea and thrombocytopenia. In addition to thrombocytopenia, anemia and leukopenia develop in 20% to 25% of patients. Other adverse effects occurring in 20% to 25% of patients are headaches, neuralgia, paresthesia, dizziness rash, constipation, vomiting, and fever. Hypotension occurs in approximately 10% of patients.

Bortezomib has demonstrated fetotoxicity in animal reproduction studies. Accordingly, pregnancy should be avoided.

Drug interactions. St. John's wort may decrease the levels of bortezomib, so this combination should be avoided. Both hypoglycemia and hyperglycemia were reported in patients taking oral antidiabetic agents in conjunction with bortezomib. Blood glucose levels should be monitored closely. Bortezomib is metabolized in the liver by CYP isoenzymes. Accordingly, inhibitors or inducers of these isoenzymes might be expected to alter bortezomib levels.

Carfilzomib

Carfilzomib (Kyprolis) works like bortezomib by binding to the active sites of the core particle within the 26S proteasome. It is approved for treatment of patients with multiple myeloma who have received at least two prior therapies.

Adverse effects are common. In some studies, more than 50% of patients experienced dyspnea, fever, thrombocytopenia, fatigue and nausea. Approximately 20% to 40% developed hypertension, peripheral edema, chest pain, headache, cough, insomnia, dizziness, vomiting, diarrhea, anorexia, leukopenia, back pain, muscle spasm, and elevated serum creatinine.

A serious adverse effect of carfilzomib is cardiac arrest. This can occur within 1 day of administration. Cardiac function should be monitored closely during treatment with carfilzomib. Other infusion reactions have also occurred, including shortness of breath, chest tightness, fever, and chills. Dexamethasone can be administered before treatment in an attempt to reduce infusion-associated incidences. Similar to bortezomib, carfilzomib should be avoided in pregnancy.

Carfilzomib can potentiate the immunosuppressant effects of drugs prescribed for immunosuppression. It is important to monitor these closely.

Ixazomib

Ixazomib (Ninlaro) induces cell-cycle arrest and apoptosis by inhibiting activity of the β 5 subunit of the 20S proteasome. It is approved for treatment of multiple myeloma.

Adverse effects are common among large numbers of patients. Thrombocytopenia develops in 78% of patients and neutropenia develops in 67%. Over 40% develop diarrhea. Approximately one-quarter to one-third of patients develop peripheral edema, peripheral neuropathy, nausea, vomiting, constipation, and eye problems. About 20% develop a rash, back pain, and upper respiratory infections. Ixazomib should be avoided in pregnancy.

Ixazomib is a substrate of hepatic CYP3A4 isoenzymes. Drugs that are strong inhibitors or inducers of these isoenzymes can cause significant drug interactions. Ixazomib will also increase immunosuppressive effects of other immunosuppressants.

Histone Deacetylase Inhibitors

The histone deacetylase (HDAC) inhibitors are a relatively new class of targeted anticancer drugs. Vorinostat and romidepsin were the first approved drugs in this class. Both drugs are indicated only for cutaneous T-cell lymphoma (CTCL), a rare form of cancer with only 1500 new cases a year in the United States. As their name implies, these drugs inhibit HDAC and, hence, increase the acetylation of histones, regulatory proteins in the cell nucleus that help control DNA transcription. When histones are in their acetylated state, they turn on gene transcription. In tumor cells, increased transcription leads to cell-cycle arrest and apoptosis.

Vorinostat

Vorinostat (Zolinza), the first HDAC inhibitor available, is indicated for oral therapy of CTCL that has progressed or returned after treatment with two systemic therapies. Unfortunately, benefits of vorinostat are modest. The most common adverse effects are fatigue, diarrhea, nausea, altered taste, anorexia, weight loss, thrombocytopenia, and anemia. Pulmonary embolism is the most common serious effect. When used with warfarin, prolonged levels of prothrombin time and INR have been noted. These levels must be monitored closely. Severe thrombocytopenia has also occurred when vorinostat is combined with valproic acid. Platelet levels should be checked every 2 weeks for the first 2 months.

Romidepsin

Romidepsin (Istodax) is indicated for intravenous therapy of CTCL and peripheral T-cell lymphoma that has progressed or returned despite treatment with at least one systemic agent. As with vorinostat, benefits are modest.

Romidepsin can cause multiple adverse effects. The most common are nausea, vomiting, fatigue, anorexia, taste disturbance, and hematologic deficits: anemia, leukopenia, and thrombocytopenia. Because of leukopenia, patients are at increased risk for serious infections. Primary cardiac effects are electrocardiographic T-wave changes and QT prolongation. Romidepsin can harm the developing fetus and hence should not be used during pregnancy. In contrast to vorinostat, romidepsin has not been associated with pulmonary embolism.

Romidepsin undergoes extensive metabolism by CYP3A4 and, hence, strong inhibitors (e.g., clarithromycin) and inducers (e.g., carbamazepine) should be avoided. Romidepsin binds with receptors for estrogen and can in turn reduce the effects of estrogen-containing contraceptives.

Ipilimumab

Ipilimumab (Yervoy) is indicated for unresectable or metastatic melanoma. Benefits derive from unleashing an immune attack on cancer cells. Here's how it works. Ipilimumab is a monoclonal antibody directed against cytotoxic T-lymphocyte–associated antigen 4 (CTLA-4), a regulatory molecule that puts a brake on T-cell function. When ipilimumab binds with CTLA-4, it releases the brake, thereby allowing T cells to attack and kill cancer cells.

By promoting T-cell activation and proliferation, ipilimumab can cause severe or fatal immune-mediated effects. Among these are enterocolitis, hepatitis, dermatitis (including toxic epidermal necrolysis), neuropathies (both motor and sensory), and endocrinopathies (e.g., hypopituitarism, hypothyroidism, and adrenal insufficiency). Patients should be closely monitored for signs and symptoms. If a severe immune-mediated reaction is diagnosed, ipilimumab should be immediately and permanently discontinued, and patients should be treated with high-dose systemic glucocorticoids.

Immunostimulants

As their name implies, the immunostimulants enhance the body's immune attack on cancer cells. The following discussion focuses on three agents: interferon α-2b, aldesleukin, and bacillus Calmette-Guérin (BCG) vaccine. Indications and routes are shown in Table 85.9.

Interferon α-2b

Interferons are naturally occurring proteins with complex antiviral, anticancer, and immunomodulatory actions. Release of endogenous interferons is triggered by viral infections and other stimuli. Interferons are active against a variety of solid tumors and hematologic malignancies.

Discussion here is limited to two interferons: interferon α-2b (Intron A) and peginterferon α-2b (Sylatron). (Peginterferon α-2b is simply a long-acting form of interferon α-2b produced by a process known as pegylation, in which a polymer of polyethylene glycol (PEG) is attached

to native interferon α-2b.) Although the active component of interferon α-2b and peginterferon α-2b is the same, these preparations have different indications. Specifically, interferon α-2b is approved for melanoma, hairy cell leukemia, chronic myelogenous leukemia, follicular lymphoma, and AIDS-related Kaposi sarcoma, whereas peginterferon α-2b is approved only for melanoma.

Anticancer effects of interferon α-2b are thought to result from two basic processes: (1) enhancement of host immune responses and (2) direct antiproliferative effects on cancer cells. Both processes are mediated by binding of interferon α-2b to cell surface receptors, with resultant increased expression of certain genes and reduced expression of others. Interferon α-2b can cause G_0 cells to remain dormant, preventing proliferation. In addition, it can cause proliferating cells to differentiate into nonproliferative mature forms.

Interferon α can cause multiple adverse effects. The most common is a flu-like syndrome characterized by fever, fatigue, myalgia, headache, and chills. Symptoms tend to diminish with continued therapy. Some symptoms (fever, headache, and myalgia) can be reduced with acetaminophen. Other common effects include anorexia, weight loss, diarrhea, abdominal pain, dizziness, and cough. Prolonged or high-dose therapy can cause fatigue, cardiotoxicity, thyroid dysfunction, and bone marrow suppression, manifesting as neutropenia and thrombocytopenia. Neuropsychiatric effects—especially depression—are a serious concern, owing to a risk for death by suicide.

Aldesleukin

Interleukin 2 (IL-2) is a type of cytokine signaling molecule that is produced primarily by leukocytes. Aldesleukin (Proleukin), is a type of IL-2 produced in the laboratory. It is an immunostimulant indicated for advanced renal carcinoma and melanoma. Because severe adverse effects occur often, the drug must be administered in a hospital that has an intensive care facility; a specialist in cardiopulmonary or intensive care medicine must be available.

Therapeutic use. Aldesleukin has two approved uses: metastatic renal cell carcinoma and metastatic melanoma. Among patients with renal cell cancer, 4% respond completely and 11% respond partially. The median response duration is 2 years.

Mechanism of action. Aldesleukin is a large glycoprotein nearly identical in structure and actions to human IL-2. The drug is produced by recombinant DNA technology. Similar to IL-2, aldesleukin stimulates immune function. Specific responses include enhanced production and cytotoxicity of lymphocytes; increased production of IL-1, interferon γ, and tumor necrosis factor; and induction of lymphokine-activated killer cell activity. These powerful immunostimulant actions are believed to underlie antitumor effects.

Adverse effects. Practically all patients experience significant toxicity. The fatality rate is high (4%). Effects seen most frequently are fever and chills, nausea and vomiting, hypotension, anemia, diarrhea, altered mental status, sinus tachycardia, impaired renal function, impaired liver function, pulmonary congestion, dyspnea, and pruritus. Depression may also occur.

Capillary leak syndrome (CLS) is of particular concern. This potentially fatal reaction is characterized by hypotension and reduced organ perfusion (secondary to loss of vascular tone and extravasation of plasma proteins and fluid). Symptoms begin to develop immediately after treatment. CLS may be associated with angina pectoris, cardiac dysrhythmias, myocardial infarction, pronounced respiratory insufficiency, renal insufficiency, GI bleeding, and altered mental status. Because of the risk for CLS, aldesleukin must not be given to patients with cardiac, pulmonary, renal, hepatic, or CNS impairment. Careful monitoring is essential.

TABLE 85.9 ■ Immunostimulants

Generic Name	Trade Name	Route	Indications
Interferon α-2b	Intron A	SubQ, IM, IV	Melanoma, hairy cell leukemia, chronic myelogenous leukemia, follicular lymphoma, and AIDS-related Kaposi sarcoma
Peginterferon α-2b	Sylatron[a]	SubQ	Melanoma
Aldesleukin (interleukin-2)	Proleukin	IV	Metastatic renal cell cancer and metastatic melanoma
BCG vaccine	TheraCys, TICE BCG	Intravesical	In situ bladder cancer

[a]Peginterferon α-2b is also marketed as *PegIntron* for treatment of hepatitis.
BCG, Bacillus Calmette-Guérin; *IM,* intramuscular; *IV,* intravenous; *subQ,* subcutaneous.

Bacillus Calmette-Guérin Vaccine

Therapeutic use. BCG vaccine (TheraCys and TICE BCG) is a freeze-dried preparation of live, attenuated *Mycobacterium bovis*. It is approved for primary and relapsed carcinoma in situ of the bladder in both the presence and absence of associated papillary tumors. To treat bladder cancers, BCG vaccine is administered intravesically (i.e., directly into the bladder through a urethral catheter). In addition to its use in cancer therapy, BCG vaccine is used to protect against tuberculosis (see Chapter 77).

Mechanism of action. BCG vaccine is a nonspecific immunostimulant. Instillation in the bladder produces a local inflammatory response that, by an unknown mechanism, promotes regression of tumors in the urothelial lining.

Adverse effects. The most common adverse effects, which result from bladder irritation, are dysuria, urinary frequency, urinary urgency, and hematuria. Urinary status should be monitored closely. The most common systemic reactions are malaise, fatigue, fever, and chills.

Because BCG vaccine consists of live *M. bovis*, the therapy carries a risk for systemic infection, including fatal septic shock. Accordingly, the vaccine is contraindicated for (1) immunocompromised patients (e.g., those taking immunosuppressant drugs and those with symptomatic or asymptomatic HIV infection); (2) patients with fever of unknown origin (because it may signify infection); and (3) patients with urinary tract infections (because there is an increased risk for systemic absorption of BCG vaccine).

Because BCG vaccine is infectious, it must be handled using aseptic technique. All materials employed during administration should be disposed of in plastic bags labeled "Infectious Waste." Urine voided within 6 hours of BCG instillation should be disinfected with an equal volume of 5% hypochlorite before flushing.

Other Noncytotoxic Anticancer Drugs
Glucocorticoids

The basic pharmacology of the glucocorticoids is discussed in Chapter 58. Discussion here is limited to their use in cancer. To benefit patients with cancer, dosages must be high; hence adverse effects with long-term use are a concern.

Glucocorticoids (e.g., prednisone and dexamethasone) are used in combination with other agents to treat cancers arising from lymphoid tissue. Specific indications are *acute and chronic lymphocytic leukemias, Hodgkin disease, non-Hodgkin lymphomas,* and *multiple myeloma.* Glucocorticoids are beneficial in these cancers because they are directly toxic to lymphoid tissues: high-dose therapy causes suppression of mitosis, dissolution of lymphocytes, regression of lymphatic tissue, and cell death. When glucocorticoids are used acutely, toxicity is limited and manageable. However, with prolonged treatment, multiple serious toxicities can occur, including osteoporosis, adrenal insufficiency, increased susceptibility to infection, GI ulcers, fluid and electrolyte disturbances, myopathy, growth delay in children, cutaneous atrophy, and diabetes. Unlike the short-term toxicities, these long-term toxicities are hard to manage.

In addition to their use against lymphoid-derived cancers, glucocorticoids are used to manage complications of cancer and cancer therapy. Specific benefits include suppression of CINV, reduction of cerebral edema (caused by brain metastasis and irradiation to the brain), reduction of pain (caused by nerve compression or edema), and suppression of hypercalcemia in patients with steroid-responsive tumors. In addition, glucocorticoids can improve appetite and promote weight gain.

Retinoids

Retinoids are derivatives of retinol (vitamin A) that bind to and activate retinoid receptors. In their active state, retinoid receptors regulate the proliferation and differentiation of cells, both normal and neoplastic. In patients with cancer, retinoids inhibit cancer cell growth.

Alitretinoin. Alitretinoin (Panretin), an analog of retinol, is indicated for topical therapy of cutaneous lesions in patients with AIDS-related Kaposi sarcoma. When alitretinoin is added to Kaposi sarcoma cells in culture, it inhibits their growth.

The drug should be applied only to cutaneous Kaposi sarcoma lesions, not to normal skin. After application, the area should be allowed to dry for 3 to 5 minutes before putting clothing over it. Occlusive dressings should be avoided.

Adverse effects are limited to the site of application. Local reactions—erythema, scaling, irritation, rash, and dermatitis—occur in 25% to 77% of patients. The incidence of severe reactions is 10%. Other retinoids are known to cause photosensitivity reactions. Although photosensitivity has not been reported with alitretinoin, exposing the treated area to sunlight or sunlamps should nonetheless be minimized. Retinoids are highly teratogenic. Accordingly, women using alitretinoin should avoid getting pregnant (even though systemic absorption of alitretinoin appears to be minimal).

Bexarotene

Actions and use. Bexarotene (Targretin) is indicated for oral therapy of cutaneous T-cell lymphoma in patients who have been refractory to prior systemic therapy. Similar to alitretinoin, bexarotene is an analog of vitamin A (retinol) and can activate retinoid receptors. The result is altered regulation of cellular proliferation and differentiation. In vitro, bexarotene can inhibit growth of some tumor cell lines.

Adverse effects. Major lipid abnormalities are common. Plasma triglycerides rise to a level 2.5 times above the upper limit of the normal range in 70% of patients. Sixty percent of patients have significant elevations in total cholesterol and low-density lipoprotein cholesterol. Levels of high-density lipoprotein cholesterol (good cholesterol) are reduced.

Bexarotene frequently causes headache, asthenia, leukopenia, anemia, infection, rash, and photosensitivity. The incidence of clinically significant hypothyroidism is 30%. Fatal pancreatitis and fatal cholestasis have been reported.

Bexarotene and other retinoids are powerful teratogens. Accordingly, bexarotene is absolutely contraindicated for use during pregnancy. Women taking the drug must ensure that pregnancy does not occur.

Drug interactions. Drugs that inhibit CYP3A4 can increase bexarotene levels, and drugs that induce CYP3A4 can reduce its levels. Combining vitamin A with bexarotene could result in increased toxicity.

Tretinoin. Tretinoin (Vesanoid), also known as all-trans retinoic acid (ATRA), is approved for induction of remission in patients with acute promyelocytic leukemia (APL). Rates of complete remission are high. Unfortunately, although tretinoin can be very effective, it can also cause severe toxicity, and hence the benefits of treatment must be carefully weighed against the risks. The mechanism underlying beneficial effects is not well established.

The most common adverse effects are rash, dry skin, and CNS toxicity, manifesting as headache, depression, confusion, and anxiety. The most serious effect, seen in 25% of patients, is retinoic acid–APL syndrome, characterized by fever, pleural and pericardial effusions, and hypoxia. In its most severe form, the syndrome can lead to respiratory failure and death. Milder reactions generally respond to high-dose intravenous glucocorticoids without interruption of tretinoin. In severe cases, tretinoin should be withdrawn.

Tretinoin is a substrate for hepatic CYP enzymes, and hence CYP inducers (e.g., rifampin, phenytoin, and St. John's wort) and inhibitors (e.g., erythromycin, azole antifungals, and diltiazem) should be avoided.

The use of tretinoin for dermatologic disorders is discussed in Chapter 88.

Arsenic Trioxide

Arsenic trioxide (Trisenox) is approved for the treatment of acute promyelocytic leukemia (APL), a rare subtype of acute myelogenous leukemia in which myeloid cells are blocked from undergoing normal differentiation and apoptosis. In patients who have relapsed after standard therapy for APL, arsenic trioxide has produced a high rate of complete remission. The drug works by fragmenting DNA and causing structural changes that lead to apoptosis.

Toxicity occurs in most patients. Common side effects include nausea, vomiting, diarrhea, fatigue, edema, hyperglycemia, dyspnea, cough, rash, headache, and dizziness. Leukocytosis (elevation of white blood cell counts) occurs in 50% of patients. Of greater concern, about 23% experience a potentially fatal condition known as APL differentiation syndrome, characterized by fever, weight gain, pulmonary infiltrates, dyspnea, musculoskeletal pain, and pleural and pericardial effusions. Symptoms can be reduced by immediate therapy with high-dose glucocorticoids. Prolongation of the QT interval is common and can lead to life-threatening dysrhythmias. An electrocardiogram should be obtained before treatment and at least weekly thereafter. If possible, drugs known to cause QT prolongation should be withdrawn. Among these are class I and class III antidysrhythmics, clarithromycin, daunorubicin, mesoridazine, and thioridazine. Arsenic trioxide has the potential to cause fetal harm. In contrast to cytotoxic anticancer drugs, arsenic trioxide does not cause alopecia or mucositis.

Denileukin Diftitox

Therapeutic use. Denileukin diftitox (Ontak) is an intravenously administered drug approved for the treatment of cutaneous T-cell lymphoma. Unfortunately, adverse events are very common and sometimes severe. Denileukin can cause life-threatening hypersensitivity reactions and, hence, must be administered in a facility equipped for cardiopulmonary resuscitation.

Mechanism of action. Denileukin is a hybrid molecule consisting of IL-2 coupled to diphtheria toxin. The IL-2 portion of the molecule enables it to bind with CTCL cells that have IL-2 receptors. After the drug is bound, the diphtheria toxin moiety inhibits protein synthesis, causing cell death within hours. Denileukin is produced by recombinant DNA technology.

Adverse effects. Acute hypersensitivity reactions occur in 69% of patients. Prominent symptoms are hypotension, back pain, dyspnea, vasodilation, rash, chest pain, and tachycardia. Management consists of stopping the infusion and, if necessary, administering IV epinephrine, antihistamines, and glucocorticoids.

Denileukin can cause potentially fatal capillary leak syndrome, characterized by hypoalbuminemia, edema, and hypotension. Onset usually occurs during the first or second week of treatment. Because of vascular leak, hypoalbuminemia occurs in 83% of patients. Serum albumin should be monitored, and, if it falls below 3 g/dL, the next round of treatment should be postponed.

A flu-like syndrome occurs in 91% of patients. Symptoms include fever or chills, asthenia, nausea and vomiting, myalgia, and arthralgia. Diarrhea occurs in 29% of patients and leads to dehydration in 9%.

Denileukin can cause eye damage, manifesting as a decrease in color vision and vision acuity. For a few patients, these effects are irreversible. However, most report persistent impairment.

Thalidomide

Thalidomide (Thalomid) is a drug with complex pharmacologic actions, including the ability to cause severe birth defects. In the United States, thalidomide has two approved indications: (1) erythema nodosum leprosum, a complication of leprosy, and (2) multiple myeloma, a cancer of the bone marrow. Promising results have also been seen with other cancers, including plasma cell leukemia and various solid tumors, including renal cell carcinoma, AIDS-related Kaposi sarcoma, and cancers of the brain, breast, ovary, prostate, and colon. Anticancer effects are thought to derive from (1) effects on the immune system and (2) inhibition of angiogenesis. Compared with cytotoxic anticancer drugs, thalidomide is relatively well tolerated but can cause clinically important neuropathy, sedation, and constipation. Neuropathy can be a chronic dose-limiting toxicity. Because thalidomide is a powerful teratogen, patients must comply with a strict set of FDA-mandated safeguards, known as the System for Thalidomide Education and Prescribing Safety (STEPS).

Lenalidomide

Lenalidomide (Revlimid), an analog of thalidomide, is indicated for (1) multiple myeloma, (2) relapsed mantle cell lymphoma after two prior therapies, and (3) raising RBC counts in patients with transfusion-dependent anemia due to myelodysplastic syndrome—but only if their MDS is associated with a specific cytogenetic abnormality known as a 5q deletion, which is seen in up to 30% of MDS patients. In these patients, lenalidomide increases RBC production and greatly reduces the need for RBC transfusions. The mechanism underlying benefits in multiple myeloma and MDS is unclear.

Lenalidomide has serious toxicities, including thrombocytopenia and neutropenia. In patients with multiple myeloma, the drug has caused deep venous thrombosis and pulmonary embolism. Both thalidomide and lenalidomide are teratogenic in primates and thus must not be used during pregnancy. To reduce risk, the drug is available only through a restricted distribution program, known as RevAssist, similar to the STEPS program used for thalidomide.

Progestins

Two progestins can be employed to treat cancer: medroxyprogesterone acetate (Depo-Provera) and megestrol acetate (Megace). Medroxyprogesterone is indicated for advanced endometrial and renal cancer. Megestrol is indicated for advanced endometrial and breast cancer. In women with metastatic endometrial cancer, progestins promote palliation and tumor regression. About 30% of patients have an objective response. Among those who respond, survival time is increased to about 2 years. This compares with survival times of 6 months among nonresponders. Benefits appear to derive from depriving these cancers of estrogen by inducing enzymes that metabolize estradiol, the primary endogenous estrogen. The principal adverse effects of progestins are fluid retention and nonfluid weight gain. Hypercalcemia may occur if bone metastases are present. Progestins may be teratogens and hence should be avoided during pregnancy. The basic pharmacology of the progestins is discussed in Chapter 50.

CHEMOPREVENTION AND CANCER IMMUNOTHERAPY

A substantial portion of this chapter has been devoted to the discussion of drugs to treat cancer. However, this chapter would not be complete without acknowledging the strides made in chemoprevention and cancer immunotherapy.

Chemoprevention

Chemoprevention is one of the exciting buzzwords in the science of cancer treatment. In fact, "cancer treatment" is a misnomer here because drugs used in chemoprevention aren't typically used to treat cancer;

rather, they are used to prevent cancer or at least to lower the risk for developing cancer. Chemoprevention isn't new. Vaccines are one type of chemoprevention. Recombinant human papillomavirus 9-valent vaccine (Gardasil 9) lowers the risk for cervical, anal, and throat cancer by targeting the human papillomavirus. Similarly, the hepatitis B vaccine lowers the risk for hepatic cancer by targeting the hepatitis B virus. Taking drugs to prevent cancer is another type of chemoprevention. For example, the US Preventive Services Task Force recently began recommending daily low-dose aspirin for the prevention of colorectal cancer after evidence demonstrated its benefit. Raloxifene and tamoxifen, mentioned earlier, decrease the risk for developing estrogen receptor–positive breast cancer. Although the field of chemoprevention isn't new, it hasn't seen the growth experienced in some other cancer therapies. With an increased emphasis on research in this area, we can expect increases in chemopreventive agents in the near future.

Cancer Immunotherapy

At the beginning of this chapter we briefly discussed how cancers cells result are capable of unrestricted growth. Our immune system is amazingly effective at identifying bacteria, viruses and other organisms as "foreign" and subsequently exterminating them. Unfortunately, the abnormal mutant cancer cells often aren't recognized as foreign, and so they continue to grow unrestrained.

Cancer immunotherapy is a revolutionary approach to cancer treatment. Unlike cancer drugs that poison cancer cells, along with some normal cells in the process, immunotherapy harnesses the body's own natural defense mechanism, the immune system, to attack cancer cells in the same ferocious manner that it attacks other invasive organisms.

Adverse effects of immunotherapy are relatively minor when compared to the adverse effects associated with some cancer drugs. Injection site reactions are common but usually mild. Some cause fever and chills, myalgias and arthralgias, nausea, vomiting, and weakness. Patients are also at risk for hypersensitivity reactions.

Antibody-Dependent Cell-Mediated Cytotoxicity

One of the challenges of immunotherapy is to overcome the inability of T cells and other immune cells to recognize cancer cells as foreign cells. Cancer cells have several ways to evade detection. For example, genetic changes can result in a decreased expression of tumor antigen. Cancer cells also carry "checkpoint" proteins that allow them to go undetected among healthy cells. Some of these proteins have been identified; two in particular are PD-1/PD-L1 and CTLA-4. Scientists discovered that they could use monoclonal antibodies as "checkpoint inhibitors" to attach to these proteins on cancer cells. Subsequently, the T cells were able to recognize the cancer cells and annihilate them.

Clinical trials centered on antibody-dependent cell-mediated cytotoxicity (ADCC) have demonstrated remarkable success for melanoma. Early reports from other clinical trials show promise for treatment of head and neck cancers, breast cancer, lung cancer, liver cancer, and bladder cancer in particular.

Examples of checkpoint inhibitors are the PD-1 inhibitors pembrolizumab (Keytruda) and nivolumab (Opdivo) and the PD-L1 inhibitors atezolizumab (Tecentriq), avelumab (Bavencio), durvalumab (Imfinzi). Ipilimumab (Yervoy) is a checkpoint inhibitor targeting CTLA-4 proteins.

Adverse effects associated with checkpoint inhibitors include immune mediated reactions involving the digestive, nervous, renal, and endocrine. Outcomes of these include hepatitis, colitis, renal dysfunction, hypothyroidism, and hyperthyroidism. Autoimmune conditions may also result.

Adoptive Cell Therapy

Another type of immunotherapy is adoptive cell therapy or adoptive immunotherapy. There are two types of approaches.

Chimeric antigen receptor T-cell therapy. In chimeric antigen receptor (CAR) T-cell therapy, T cells are removed from the patient's bloodstream and genetically modified to express CAR. CAR is a T-cell receptor protein that allows T cells to effectively recognize, attach to, and destroy cancer cells. These more responsive T cells are then returned to the circulation.

This type of immunotherapy has demonstrated effectiveness in treating leukemia and is in trials for other types of cancer. Tisagenlecleucel (Kymriah) is currently approved for CAR T-cell therapy but is available only through a risk evaluation and mitigation strategy (REMS).

The most significant adverse reaction is cytokine release syndrome. This occurs when immune cells rapidly release a large volume of cytokines into the circulation. The resulting effects include fever, nausea, headache, and tachycardia. Skin reactions and dyspnea may also occur.

Tumor infiltrating lymphocytes. Tumor infiltrating lymphocytes (TILs) are T cells that are able to infiltrate deep inside solid tumors. Researchers determined that there must be some recognition of these cancer cells as foreign based on the TILs location. Despite this, they were not effectively killing the cells, perhaps because of their relatively small number. Scientists remove these TILs, allow them to replicate into large numbers in the laboratory, and then treat them with IL-2. These supercharged TILs are then injected back into the patient's circulation. These are currently being tested in clinical trials, but early reports have been promising.

Capillary leak syndrome is an adverse effect associated with this therapy. In this condition, proteins and fluids leak out of capillaries and into the tissues. This can significantly decrease the blood pressure, leading to shock and multiple organ failure.

Vaccines

Earlier, vaccines were discussed in relation to chemoprevention. A number of vaccines are also being studied for cancer *treatment*. So far, the only one to receive FDA approval is Sipuleucel-T (Provenge). (See earlier discussion.)

86

Pain Management in Patients With Cancer

Our topic—management of cancer pain—is noteworthy for both its good news and its bad news. The good news is that cancer pain can be relieved with simple interventions in 90% of patients. The bad news is that, despite the availability of effective treatments, pain goes unrelieved far too often. Multiple factors contribute to undertreatment (Box 86.1). Important among these are inadequate prescriber training in pain management; unfounded fears of addiction (shared by prescribers, patients, and families); and a health care system that focuses more on treating disease than relieving suffering.

Pain has a profound effect on both the patient and family. Pain undermines quality of life for the patient and puts a heavy burden on the family. Unrelieved pain compromises the patient's ability to work, enjoy leisure activities, and fulfill his or her role in the family and in society at large. Furthermore, pain can impede recovery, hasten death from cancer, and possibly even create a risk for suicide.

Every patient has the right to expect that pain management will be an integral part of treatment throughout the course of his or her disease. The goal is to minimize pain and thereby maintain a reasonable quality of life, including the ability to function at work and at play and within the family and society. In addition, if the cancer is incurable, treatment should permit the patient a relatively painless death when that time comes.

PAIN IN CANCER PATIENTS

Among patients with cancer, pain can be caused by the cancer itself and by therapeutic interventions. Cancer can cause pain through direct invasion of surrounding tissues (e.g., nerves, muscles, and visceral organs) and through metastatic invasion at distant sites. Metastases to bone are very common, causing pain in up to 50% of patients. Cancer can cause neuropathic pain through infiltration of nerves, and visceral pain through infiltration, obstruction, and compression of visceral structures.

The incidence and intensity of cancer-induced pain is a function of cancer type and the stage of disease progression. Among patients with advanced disease, about 75% experience significant pain. Of these, 40% to 50% report moderate to severe pain, and 25% to 30% report very severe pain.

Therapeutic interventions—especially chemotherapy, radiation, and surgery—cause significant pain in at least 25% of patients, and probably more. Chemotherapy can cause painful mucositis, diffuse neuropathies, and aseptic necrosis of joints. Radiation can cause osteonecrosis, chronic visceral pain, and peripheral neuropathy (secondary to causing fibrosis of nerves). Surgery can cause a variety of pain syndromes, including phantom limb syndrome and postmastectomy syndrome.

MANAGEMENT STRATEGY

Management of cancer pain is an ongoing process that involves repeating cycles of assessment, intervention, and reassessment. The goal is to create and implement a flexible treatment plan that can meet the changing needs of the individual patient. Fig. 86.1 shows the steps involved. Management begins with a comprehensive assessment. After the nature of the pain has been determined, a treatment modality is selected. Analgesic drugs are preferred and hence are usually tried first. If drugs are ineffective, other modalities can be implemented. Among these are radiation, surgery, and nerve blocks. After each intervention, pain is reassessed. When relief has been achieved, the effective intervention is continued, accompanied by frequent reassessments. If severe pain returns or new pain develops, a new comprehensive assessment should be performed—followed by appropriate interventions and reassessment. Throughout this process, the health care team should make every effort to ensure active involvement of the patient and his or her family. Without their involvement, maximal benefits cannot be achieved.

ASSESSMENT AND ONGOING EVALUATION

Assessment is the foundation of treatment. In the absence of thorough assessment, effective pain management is impossible. Assessment begins with a comprehensive evaluation and then continues with regular follow-up evaluations. The initial assessment provides the basis for designing the treatment program. Follow-ups let us know how well treatment is working.

Comprehensive Initial Assessment

The initial assessment employs an extensive array of tests. The primary objective is to characterize the pain and identify its cause. This information provides the basis for designing a pain management plan. In addition, by documenting the patient's baseline pain status, the initial assessment provides a basis for evaluating the efficacy of treatment.

Assessment of Pain Intensity and Character: The Patient Self-Report

The patient's description of his or her pain is the cornerstone of pain assessment. The best way to ensure an accurate report is to ask the right questions and listen carefully to the answers. We cannot elicit comprehensive information by asking, "How do you feel?" Rather, we must ask a series of specific questions. The answers should be recorded on a pain inventory form.

Physical and Neurologic Examinations

The physical and neurologic examinations help further characterize the pain, identify its source, and identify any complications related to the underlying pathology. The clinician should examine the site of pain and determine whether palpation or manipulation makes it worse. Nonverbal cues (e.g., protecting the painful area and limited movement in an arm or leg) that may indicate pain should be noted. Common patterns of referred pain should be assessed. For example, if the patient has hip pain, the assessment should determine whether the pain actually originates in the hip or if it is referred pain caused by pathology in the

BOX 86.1 Barriers to Cancer Pain Management

Barriers Related to Health Care Professionals
Inadequate knowledge of pain management
Poor assessment of pain
Concerns stemming from regulations on controlled substances
Fear of patient addiction
Concern about side effects of analgesics
Concern about tolerance to analgesics

Barriers Related to Patients
Reluctance to report pain
Fear of distracting physicians from treating the cancer
Fear that pain means the cancer is worse
Concern about not being a "good" patient
Reluctance to take pain medication
Fear of addiction or being thought of as an addict
Worries about unmanageable side effects
Concern about becoming tolerant to pain medications
Inability to pay for treatment

Barriers Related to the Health Care System
Low priority given to cancer pain management
Inadequate reimbursement: the most appropriate treatment may not be reimbursed
Restrictive regulation of controlled substances
Treatment is unavailable or access is limited

Adapted from Kwon JH. Overcoming barriers in cancer pain management. *J Clin Oncol.* 2014;32:1727–1733.

lumbar spine. Potential neurologic complications should be considered. For example, patients with back pain should be evaluated for impaired motor and sensory function in the limbs and for impaired rectal and urinary sphincter function, which may indicate spinal cord involvement.

Diagnostic Tests

Diagnostic tests are performed to identify the underlying cause of pain (e.g., progression of cancer and tissue injury caused by cancer treatments). The battery of diagnostic tests includes imaging studies (e.g., computed tomography scan and magnetic resonance imaging), neurophysiologic tests, and tests for tumor markers in blood. To ensure that abnormalities identified in the diagnostic tests really do explain the patient's pain, these findings should be correlated with findings from the physical and neurologic examinations.

Psychosocial Assessment

Psychosocial assessment is directed at both the patient and his or her family. The information is used in making pain management decisions. Some important issues to address include the following:
- The effect of significant pain on the patient in the past
- The patient's usual coping responses to pain and stress
- The patient's preferences regarding pain management methods
- The patient's concerns about using opioids and other controlled substances (anxiolytics, stimulants)
- Changes in the patient's mood (anxiety and depression) brought on by cancer and pain
- The effect of cancer and its treatment on the family
- The level of care the family can provide and the potential need for outside help (e.g., hospice)

Ongoing Evaluation

After a treatment plan has been implemented, pain should be reassessed frequently. The objective is to determine the efficacy of treatment and allow early diagnosis and treatment of new pain. Each time an analgesic drug is administered, pain should be evaluated after sufficient time has elapsed for the drug to take effect. Because most patients are treated at home, patients and caregivers should be taught to conduct and document pain evaluations. The prescriber will use the documented record to make adjustments to the pain management plan.

Prescribers, patients, and caregivers should be alert for new pain. In most cases, new pain results from a new cause (e.g., metastasis, infection, and fracture). Accordingly, whenever new pain occurs, a rigorous diagnostic workup is indicated.

DRUG THERAPY

Analgesic drugs are the most powerful weapons we have for overcoming cancer pain. With proper use, these agents can relieve pain in 90% of patients. Because analgesics are so effective, drug therapy is the principal modality for pain treatment. Three types of analgesics are employed:
- Nonopioid analgesics (nonsteroidal antiinflammatory drugs [NSAIDs] and acetaminophen)
- Opioid analgesics (e.g., oxycodone, fentanyl, and morphine)
- Adjuvant analgesics (e.g., amitriptyline, carbamazepine, and dextroamphetamine)

These classes differ in their abilities to relieve pain. With the nonopioid and adjuvant analgesics, there is a ceiling to how much relief we can achieve. In contrast, there is no ceiling to relief with the opioids.

Selection among the analgesics is based on pain intensity and pain type. To help guide drug selection, the World Health Organization (WHO) devised a drug selection ladder (Fig. 86.2). The first step of the ladder—for mild to moderate pain—consists of nonopioid analgesics: NSAIDs and acetaminophen. The second step—for more severe pain—*adds* opioid analgesics of moderate strength (e.g., oxycodone and hydrocodone). The top step—for severe pain—substitutes powerful opioids (e.g., morphine and fentanyl) for the weaker ones. Adjuvant analgesics, which are especially effective against neuropathic pain, can be used on any step of the ladder. Specific drugs to *avoid* are listed in Table 86.1.

Traditionally, patients have been given opioid analgesics only after a trial with nonopioids has failed. Guidelines from the National Comprehensive Cancer Network (NCCN) recommend a different approach, in which initial drug selection is based on pain intensity. Specifically, if the patient reports pain in the 4 to 10 range, then treatment should start directly with an opioid; an initial trial with a nonopioid is considered unnecessary. If the patient reports pain in the 1 to 3 range, then treatment usually begins with a nonopioid, although starting with an opioid remains an alternative.

It is common practice to combine an opioid with a nonopioid because the combination can be more effective than either drug alone. When pain is only moderate, opioids and nonopioids can be given in a fixed-dose combination formulation, thereby simplifying dosing. However, when pain is severe, these drugs must be given separately because, with a fixed-dose combination, side effects of the nonopioid would become intolerable as the dosage grew large and hence would limit how much opioid could be given.

Drug therapy of cancer pain should adhere to the following principles:
- Perform a comprehensive pretreatment assessment to identify pain intensity and the underlying cause.
- Individualize the treatment plan.
- Use the WHO analgesic ladder and NCCN guidelines to guide drug selection.

Fig. 86.1 Flow Chart for Pain Management in Patients With Cancer. *NSAID,* Nonsteroidal antiinflammatory drug. (Adapted from Jacox A, Carr DB, Payne R, et al. *Management of Cancer Pain* [Clinical Practice Guideline No. 9; AHCPR Publication No. 94-0592]. Rockville, MD: Agency for Health Care Policy and Research; 1994.)

- Use oral therapy whenever possible.
- Avoid intramuscular (IM) injections whenever possible.
- For persistent pain, administer analgesics on a fixed schedule around-the-clock (ATC), and provide additional rescue doses of a short-acting agent if breakthrough pain occurs.
- If a particular activity is associated with breakthrough pain (for example bathing, provide an "incident dose" of short-acting medication before the procedure.
- Evaluate the patient frequently for pain relief and drug side effects.

Nonopioid Analgesics

The nonopioid analgesics—NSAIDs and acetaminophen—constitute the first rung of the WHO analgesic ladder. These agents are the initial drugs of choice for patients with mild pain. There is a ceiling to how much pain relief nonopioid drugs can provide, so there is no benefit to exceeding recommended dosages. Acetaminophen is about equal to the NSAIDs in *analgesic* efficacy but lacks *antiinflammatory* actions. Because of this difference and others, acetaminophen is considered

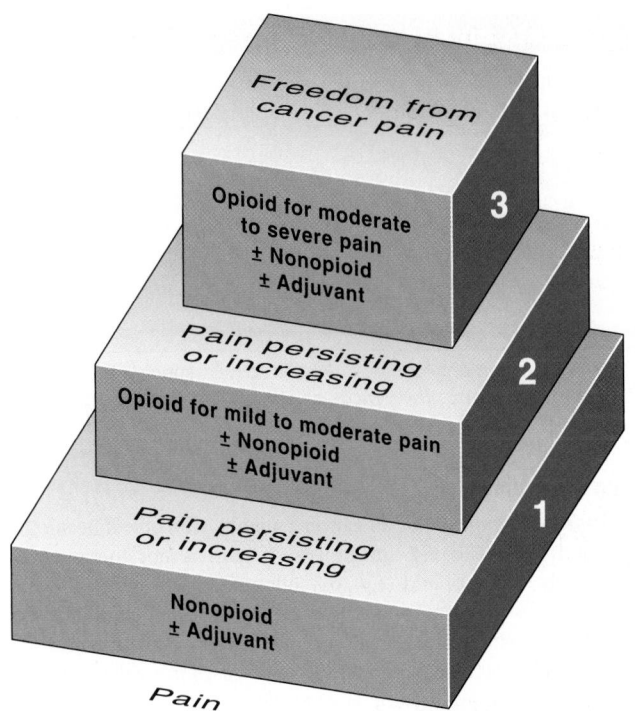

Fig. 86.2 The World Health Organization Analgesic Ladder for Cancer Pain Management. Note that steps represent pain intensity. Accordingly, if a patient has intense pain at the outset, then treatment can be initiated with an opioid (step 2), rather than trying a nonopioid first (step 1). (Adapted from *Cancer Pain Relief*, 2nd ed. Geneva: World Health Organization; 1996.)

TABLE 86.1	Drugs That Are Not Recommended for Treating Cancer Pain	
Drug Class	**Drug**	**Why the Drug Is Not Recommended**
Pure Opioid Agonists	Meperidine	A toxic metabolite accumulates with prolonged use
	Codeine	Maximal pain relief is limited owing to dose-limiting side effects
Opioid Agonist-Antagonists	Buprenorphine Butorphanol Nalbuphine Pentazocine	Ceiling to analgesic effects; can precipitate withdrawal in opioid-dependent patients; cause psychotomimetic reactions
Opioid antagonists	Naloxone Naltrexone	Can precipitate withdrawal in opioid-dependent patients; limit use to reversing life-threatening respiratory depression caused by opioid overdose
Benzodiazepines	Diazepam Lorazepam others	Sedation from benzodiazepines limits opioid dosage; no demonstrated analgesic action
Barbiturates	Amobarbital Secobarbital Others	Sedation from barbiturates limits opioid dosage; no demonstrated analgesic action
Miscellaneous	Marijuana	Side effects (dysphoria, drowsiness, hypotension, and bradycardia) preclude routine use as an analgesic

separately later. The NSAIDs and acetaminophen are discussed in Chapter 56.

Nonsteroidal Antiinflammatory Drugs

NSAIDs (e.g., aspirin and ibuprofen) can produce a variety of effects. Primary beneficial effects are pain relief, suppression of inflammation, and reduction of fever. Primary adverse effects are gastric ulceration, acute renal failure, and bleeding. In addition, all NSAIDs *except aspirin* increase the risk for thrombotic events (e.g., myocardial infarction and stroke). In contrast to opioids, NSAIDs do not cause tolerance, physical dependence, or psychologic dependence.

NSAIDs are effective analgesics that can relieve mild to moderate pain. All of the NSAIDs have essentially equal analgesic efficacy, although individual patients may respond better to one NSAID than to another. NSAIDs relieve pain by a mechanism different from that of the opioids. As a result, combined use of an NSAID with an opioid can produce greater pain relief than either agent alone.

NSAIDs produce their effects—both good and bad—by inhibiting cyclooxygenase (COX), an enzyme that has two forms, known as cyclooxygenase-1 (COX-1) and cyclooxygenase-2 (COX-2). Most NSAIDs inhibit both COX-1 and COX-2, although a few are selective for COX-2. The selective COX-2 inhibitors (e.g., celecoxib [Celebrex]) cause less gastrointestinal (GI) damage than the nonselective inhibitors. Unfortunately, the selective inhibitors pose a greater risk for thrombotic events, and hence long-term use of these drugs is not recommended.

For patients undergoing chemotherapy, inhibition of platelet aggregation by NSAIDs is a serious concern. Many anticancer drugs suppress bone marrow function and thereby decrease platelet production. The resultant thrombocytopenia puts patients at risk for bruising and

bleeding. Obviously, this risk will be increased by drugs that inhibit platelet function. Among the conventional NSAIDs, only one subclass—the nonacetylated salicylates (e.g., magnesium salicylate)—does not inhibit platelet aggregation and hence is safe for patients with thrombocytopenia. All other conventional NSAIDs should be avoided. *Aspirin* should be avoided because it causes *irreversible* inhibition of platelet aggregation. Hence its effects persist for the life of the platelet (about 8 days). Because COX-2 inhibitors do not affect platelets, these drugs are safe for patients with thrombocytopenia.

Acetaminophen

Acetaminophen (Tylenol and others) is similar to the NSAIDs in some respects and different in others. Like the NSAIDs, acetaminophen is an effective analgesic and hence can relieve mild to moderate pain. Benefits derive from inhibiting COX in the central nervous system (CNS), but not in the periphery. Combining acetaminophen with an opioid can produce greater analgesia than either drug alone (because acetaminophen and opioids relieve pain by different mechanisms).

Acetaminophen differs from the NSAIDs in several important ways. Because it does not inhibit COX in the periphery, acetaminophen lacks antiinflammatory actions, does not inhibit platelet aggregation, and does not promote gastric ulceration, renal failure, or thrombotic events. Because acetaminophen does not affect platelets, the drug is safe for patients with thrombocytopenia.

Acetaminophen has important interactions with two other drugs: alcohol and warfarin (an anticoagulant). Combining acetaminophen with alcohol, even in moderate amounts, can result in potentially fatal liver

TABLE 86.2   Equianalgesic Doses of Pure Opioid Agonists and Tramadol

Opioid	Oral Dose (PO)	Parenteral Dose (IV/SC)	Conversion Factor: Parenteral to Oral Opioid	Conversion Factor: Oral Opioid to Oral Morphine
Morphine	30 mg	10 mg	3	1
Oxycodone	20 mg	N/A	N/A	1.5
Hydrocodone	30 mg	N/A	N/A	1
Oxymorphone	10 mg	1 mg	10	3
Hydromorphone	7.5 mg	3 mg	2.5	4
Fentanyl	N/A	120 mcg	N/A	Variable
Methadone	Variable	Variable	0.5	Variable[a]

[a]Methadone should only be initiated and managed by clinicians experienced in pain management. Consider consult to pain specialists if needed. This Equianalgesic Opioid Dose Conversion chart is based on the CDC's recommendations (https://www.cdc.gov/drugoverdose/resources/data.html).

damage. Accordingly, patients taking acetaminophen should minimize alcohol consumption. Acetaminophen also can increase the risk for bleeding in patients taking warfarin. The mechanism appears to be inhibition of warfarin metabolism, which causes warfarin to accumulate to toxic levels. Although evidence regarding use of bleeding with acetaminophen in patient taking warfarin is scarce, it is prudent to increase monitoring of INR in patients taking scheduled acetaminophen.

Opioid Analgesics

Opioids are the most effective analgesics available and hence are the primary drugs for treating moderate to severe cancer pain. With proper dosing, opioids can safely relieve pain in about 90% of cancer patients. Unfortunately, many patients are denied adequate doses, owing largely to unfounded fears of addiction.

Opioids produce a variety of pharmacologic effects. In addition to analgesia, they can cause sedation, euphoria, constipation, respiratory depression, urinary retention, and miosis. With continuous use, tolerance develops to most of these effects, with the notable exceptions of constipation and miosis. Continuous use also results in physical dependence, which must not be equated with addiction.

The opioids are discussed in Chapter 23. Discussion here focuses on their use in patients with cancer.

Mechanism of Action and Classification

Opioid analgesics relieve pain by mimicking the actions of endogenous opioid peptides (enkephalins, dynorphins, and endorphins), primarily at mu receptors and partly at kappa receptors.

Based on their actions at mu and kappa receptors, the opioids fall into two major groups: (1) pure (full) agonists (e.g., morphine) and (2) agonist-antagonists (e.g., butorphanol). The pure agonists can be subdivided into (1) agents for mild to moderate pain and (2) agents for moderate to severe pain. The pure agonists act as agonists at mu receptors and at kappa receptors. In contrast, the agonist-antagonists act as agonists only at kappa receptors; at mu receptors, these drugs act as antagonists. Because their agonist actions are limited to kappa receptors, the agonist-antagonists have a ceiling to their analgesic effects. Furthermore, because of their antagonist actions, the agonist-antagonists can block access of the pure agonists to mu receptors, and can thereby prevent the pure agonists from relieving pain. Accordingly, agonist-antagonists are not recommended for managing cancer pain.

Tolerance and Physical Dependence

Over time, opioids cause tolerance and physical dependence. These phenomena, which are generally inseparable, reflect neuronal adaptations to prolonged opioid exposure. Some degree of tolerance and physical dependence develops after 1 to 2 weeks of opioid use. Tolerance, physical dependence, and addiction are discussed in Chapter 31.

Drug Selection

Preferred opioids. For all cancer patients, pure opioid agonists are preferred to the agonist-antagonists. If pain is not too intense, a moderately strong opioid (e.g., oxycodone) is appropriate. If pain is moderate to severe, a strong opioid (e.g., morphine) should be used. Because morphine is inexpensive, available in multiple dosage forms, and clinically well understood, this opioid is used more than any other. Preferred opioids are listed in Table 86.2.

Opioid rotation. Opioid rotation—switching from one opioid to another—is now an accepted practice. Because opioids have different side-effect profiles, rotation can help minimize adverse effects while maintaining good analgesia. To make the switch, the current opioid is stopped abruptly and immediately replaced with an equianalgesic dose of an alternative opioid.

Opioids to use with special caution. Methadone (Dolophine and Methadose) and levorphanol must be used with caution. Both drugs have prolonged half-lives, which makes dosage titration difficult. If dosing is not done skillfully, these drugs can accumulate to dangerous levels, causing excessive sedation and respiratory depression. Use of methadone should be limited to those with specialty training.

Codeine deserves special comment. Although codeine is capable of producing significant analgesia, side effects limit the dose that can be given. As a result, the degree of pain relief that can be achieved safely is quite low.

Opioids to avoid. Meperidine (Demerol), a pure opioid agonist, may be used for a few days, but no longer. When the drug is taken chronically, a toxic metabolite—normeperidine—can accumulate, thereby posing a risk for adverse CNS effects (dysphoria, agitation, and seizures) especially in older adults.

The agonist-antagonists—buprenorphine, butorphanol, nalbuphine, and pentazocine—should be avoided for several reasons. First, they are less effective than pure opioid agonists, and hence there is little reason to choose them. Second, if given to a patient who is physically dependent on a pure opioid agonist, these drugs can prevent the pure agonist from working and can thereby block analgesia and precipitate withdrawal. Third, the agonist-antagonists can cause adverse psychologic reactions (nightmares, hallucinations, and dysphoria).

Dosage

Dosage must be individualized. The objective is to find a dosage that can relieve pain without causing intolerable side effects. For patients with moderate pain and low opioid tolerance, very low doses (e.g., 2 mg of parenteral morphine every 4 hours) can be sufficient. In contrast, when pain is severe or tolerance is high, much larger doses (e.g., 600 mg of parenteral morphine every few hours) may be required. The upper limit to dosage is determined only by the intensity of side effects. Accordingly, as pain or tolerance increases, dosage should be increased until pain is relieved—unless intolerable side effects (e.g., excessive respiratory depression) occur first.

The dosing schedule is determined by the temporal pattern of the pain. If pain is intermittent and infrequent, as-needed or pro re nata (PRN) dosing can suffice. However, because most patients have persistent pain, PRN dosing is inappropriate. Instead, dosing should be done *on a fixed schedule* around the clock (ATC). A fixed schedule can prevent opioid levels from becoming subtherapeutic and can thereby prevent pain recurrence. As a result, the patient is spared needless suffering, both from the pain itself and from anxiety about its return.

What dose should be used when switching from one opioid to another, or from one route of administration to another? To help make this decision, an equianalgesia table such as Table 86.2 should be consulted. Equianalgesia tables indicate equivalent analgesic doses for different opioids and for the same opioid administered by different routes. Let's assume, for example, that our patient has been getting 10 mg of IV morphine every 4 hours, and we want to switch to oral hydromorphone. Table 86.2 shows that 7.5 mg of oral hydromorphone is about equivalent to 10 mg of parenteral morphine, with both drugs being given every 4 hours. Hence we might begin oral hydromorphone at 7.5 mg. However, there is a caveat: because cross-tolerance among opioids is incomplete, the listed equianalgesic dose may actually produce a *stronger* effect than advertised. Accordingly, when switching drugs, it is safer to use a dose that is somewhat *lower* than the equianalgesic dose, and then titrate up.

Routes of Administration

Because most patients with cancer pain must take analgesics continuously, the route should be as convenient, affordable, and noninvasive as possible. Oral administration meets these criteria best and hence is preferred for most patients. If oral medication cannot be used, the preferred alternative routes are rectal and transdermal: both are relatively convenient, affordable, and noninvasive. If these routes are ineffective or inappropriate, then parenteral administration (intravenous [IV] or subcutaneous [subQ]) is indicated (IM injections should be avoided). For patients who cannot be managed with IV or subQ therapy, more invasive routes—intraspinal or intraventricular—can be tried.

Managing Breakthrough Pain

Many patients whose pain is well controlled most of the day experience transient episodes of moderate to severe pain, known as breakthrough pain. Breakthrough pain develops quickly, reaches peak intensity in minutes, and may persist from minutes to hours (the median duration is 30 minutes). At least 50% of cancer patients experience these episodes, typically 1 to 4 times a day. Breakthrough pain may occur spontaneously, or it may be precipitated by coughing or other movements. In contrast to end-of-dose pain, which occurs because analgesic levels are lowest at that time, breakthrough pain can occur at any time during the dosing interval.

All patients receiving ATC opioids for persistent pain should have access to a rescue medication to manage breakthrough pain. Because breakthrough pain is both severe and self-limited, the best medication is a strong opioid with a rapid onset and short duration. The rapid onset permits speedy relief, and the short duration facilitates dosage titration. For ease of administration, oral, transmucosal, and intranasal formulations are preferred; examples include immediate-release oral morphine, transmucosal fentanyl (Abstral, Actiq, Fentora, and Subsys), and fentanyl nasal spray (Lazanda). The dosage, as recommended by the American Pain Society and the WHO, should be equivalent to one-sixth (17%) of the total daily opioid dose, repeated in 2 hours if needed.

Managing Side Effects

Side effects of the opioids include respiratory depression, constipation, sedation, orthostatic hypotension, miosis, nausea, and vomiting. All can be effectively managed. In many patients, side effects can be reduced

simply by decreasing the dosage (typically by 25%). If dosage reduction causes pain to return, adding a nonopioid analgesic may take care of the problem. Over time, tolerance develops to sedation, respiratory depression, nausea, and vomiting—but not to constipation or miosis.

Adjuvant Analgesics

Adjuvant analgesics are used to *complement* the effects of opioids. Accordingly, these drugs are employed in *combination* with opioids—not as substitutes. Adjuvant analgesics can (1) enhance analgesia from opioids, (2) help manage concurrent symptoms that exacerbate pain, and (3) treat side effects caused by opioids. Several of the adjuvants are especially useful for *neuropathic pain*. The adjuvant analgesics differ from opioids in that pain relief is limited and less predictable and often develops slowly.

Adjuvant agents may be employed at any step on the analgesic ladder. The adjuvants are interesting in that, although they can relieve pain, all of them were developed to treat other conditions (e.g., depression, seizures, and dysrhythmias). Accordingly, it is important to reassure patients that the adjuvant is being used to alleviate pain, and not for its original purpose. Dosages for the adjuvant analgesics are shown in Table 86.3.

Antidepressants

Tricyclic antidepressants. Amitriptyline (Elavil) and other tricyclic antidepressants (TCAs) can reduce pain of *neuropathic* origin. TCAs have analgesic effects of their own, and they enhance the effects of opioids and may thereby allow a reduction in opioid dosage. As a side benefit, TCAs can elevate mood. Important adverse effects are orthostatic hypotension, sedation, anticholinergic effects (dry mouth, urinary retention, constipation), and weight gain (secondary to improved appetite). Dosing at bedtime takes advantage of sedative effects and minimizes hypotension during the day. Effects begin in 1 to 2 weeks and reach their maximum in 4 to 6 weeks. Typically doses used for pain are lower than those used for depression. The TCAs are discussed in Chapter 26.

Other antidepressants. In addition to the tricyclic agents, certain other antidepressants (e.g., bupropion, duloxetine, and venlafaxine) can help with neuropathic pain.

Antiseizure Drugs

Certain antiseizure drugs can help relieve *neuropathic pain*. Acute pain (sharp, darting pain) is especially responsive, although other forms of neuropathic pain (cramping pain, aching pain, and burning pain) also respond. Analgesia is thought to result from suppressing spontaneous neuronal firing. Of the available antiseizure drugs, *carbamazepine* (Tegretol) has been used most widely. Because carbamazepine is myelosuppressive, it must be used with caution in patients receiving anticancer drugs that suppress bone marrow function. As discussed in Chapter 20, caution is also needed in patients of Asian descent, owing to an increased risk for severe dermatologic reactions. Another drug—*gabapentin* (Neurontin)—is also very effective and causes fewer side effects than carbamazepine. Dosage should be low initially (100 mg once a day) and then gradually increased; dosages as high as 1200 mg 3 times a day have been employed. Antiseizure drugs are discussed in Chapter 20.

Topical Anesthetics

Lidocaine (Lidoderm) is considered a second-line agent for *neuropathic pain*. It is supplied in a topical 5% patch that may be applied to the area of pain for up to 12 hours. Lidocaine is discussed in Chapter 22.

Central Nervous System Stimulants

The CNS stimulants, such as *dextroamphetamine* (Dexedrine) and *methylphenidate* (Ritalin), have two beneficial effects: they can enhance opioid-induced analgesia; and they can counteract opioid-induced

TABLE 86.3   Adjuvant Drugs for Cancer Pain

Drug	Usual Adult Dosage	Beneficial Actions
Tricyclic Antidepressants		
Amitriptyline (Elavil)	25–150 mg/day PO	Reduce
Desipramine (Norpramin)[a]	10–150 mg/day PO	neuropathic pain
Doxepin (Sinequan)[a]	25–150 mg/day PO	
Imipramine (Tofranil)	20–100 mg/day PO	
Nortriptyline (Aventyl and Pamelor)[a]	10–150 mg/day PO	
Other Antidepressants		
Duloxetine (Cymbalta)	30–60 mg/day PO	Reduce
Venlafaxine (Effexor)[a]	37.5–225 mg/day PO	neuropathic pain
Antiseizure Drugs		
Carbamazepine (Tegretol)	200–1600 mg/day PO	Reduce
Gabapentin (Neurontin)	300–3600 mg/day PO	neuropathic pain
Lamotrigine (Lamictal)[a]	25–400 mg/day PO	
Phenytoin (Dilantin)[a]	300–500 mg/day PO	
Pregabalin (Lyrica)	100–600 mg/day PO	
Local Anesthetics/Antidysrhythmics		
Lidocaine (Lidoderm)	Apply 5% topical patch for up to 12 hours daily	Reduce neuropathic pain
CNS Stimulants		
Dextroamphetamine (Dexedrine)	5–10 mg/day PO	Enhance analgesia and reduce sedation from opioids
Methylphenidate (Ritalin)	10–15 mg/day PO	
Glucocorticoids		
Dexamethasone (Decadron and others)	16–96 mg/day PO or IV	Reduce pain associated with brain metastases and epidural spinal cord compression
Prednisone	40–100 mg/day PO	
Bisphosphonates		
Pamidronate	60–90 mg IV once	Reduce hypercalcemia and possibly bone pain
Zoledronic acid	4 mg IV once	

[a]Off-label use.

IM, Intramuscular; *IV,* intravenous; *PO,* oral; *subQ,* subcutaneous.

sedation. In addition, they can be used for rapid elevation of mood. Principal adverse effects are weight loss (from appetite suppression) and insomnia (from CNS stimulation). To minimize interference with sleep, dosing late in the day should be avoided. The CNS stimulants are discussed in Chapter 30.

Glucocorticoids

Although glucocorticoids lack direct analgesic actions, they can help manage painful cancer-related conditions. Because glucocorticoids can reduce cerebral and spinal edema, they are essential for the emergency management of elevated intracranial pressure and epidural spinal cord compression. Similarly, glucocorticoids are part of the standard therapy for tumor-induced spinal cord compression. In addition to these benefits, glucocorticoids can improve appetite and impart a general sense of well-being; both actions help in managing anorexia and cachexia associated with terminal illness.

Glucocorticoids are very safe when used short term (even in high doses) and very dangerous when used long term (even in low doses). In particular, long-term therapy can cause adrenal insufficiency, osteoporosis, glucose intolerance (hyperglycemia), increased vulnerability to infection, thinning of the skin, and, possibly, peptic ulcer disease. The risk for osteoporosis can be reduced by giving calcium supplements and vitamin D along with calcitonin or a bisphosphonate (e.g., etidronate). The glucocorticoids are discussed in Chapter 57.

Bisphosphonates

Bisphosphonates, such as *zoledronic acidpamidronate* (Aredia), can reduce cancer-related *bone pain* in some patients. Bone pain is common when cancers metastasize to bone. The cause of pain may be tumor-induced bone resorption, which can also cause hypercalcemia, osteoporosis, and related fractures. Bisphosphonates inhibit bone resorption and are approved for treating hypercalcemia of malignancy and bone metastases in breast cancer—but not bone pain itself. However, when these drugs are given to treat hypercalcemia, many patients report a reduction in bone pain, although others do not. Hence although these drugs appear promising, their use for management of bone pain is still considered investigational. The bisphosphonates are discussed in Chapter 60.

NONDRUG THERAPY

Neurolytic Nerve Block

The goal of this procedure is to destroy neurons that transmit pain from a limited area, thereby providing permanent pain relief. Nerve destruction is accomplished through local injection of a neurolytic (neurotoxic) substance, typically alcohol or phenol. To ensure that the correct nerves are destroyed, reversible nerve block is done first, using a local anesthetic. If the local anesthetic relieves the pain, a neurolytic agent is then applied to the same site. Neurolytic nerve block can eliminate pain in up to 80% of patients. However, even if pain relief is only partial, the procedure can still permit some reduction in opioid dosage and can thereby decrease side effects, such as sedation and constipation. When nerve block is successful and opioids are discontinued, opioid dosage should be tapered gradually to avoid withdrawal. Nerve block is not without risk. Potential complications include hypotension, paresis, paralysis, and disruption of bowel and bladder function (e.g., diarrhea and incontinence). The incidence of complications ranges from 0.5% to 2%.

Radiation Therapy

Radiation therapy relieves pain by causing tumor regression. Palliative treatment can be directed at primary tumors and at metastases anywhere in the body.

Radiation can be delivered in four forms: *brachytherapy* (implanted radioactive pellets), *teletherapy* (external beam radiation therapy), *radiofrequency ablation,* and *IV radiopharmaceuticals.* With brachytherapy, cell kill is limited to the immediate area of the implanted pellets; hence the technique is suited only for localized tumors. With teletherapy, cell kill can be localized or widespread, depending on the size of the beam employed; hence the technique can be used for both localized tumors and metastases. Radiofrequency ablation uses a thin, needle-like probe inserted into a tumor through an incision in the skin. The probe extends electrodes that emit high-frequency electrical current, producing heat to destroy cancer cells; hence the technique is best suited for localized tumors. IV radiopharmaceuticals travel throughout the body and hence are best suited for widespread metastases.

With radiation therapy, as with chemotherapy, damage to normal tissue is dose limiting. Therefore the challenge is to deliver a dose of radiation that is large enough to kill cancer cells but not so large that it causes intolerable damage to healthy tissue.

Some side effects of radiation occur early, and some are late. Early effects develop during or immediately after radiation exposure. Late reactions develop months or years later. The most common early effects are skin inflammation and lesions of the GI mucosa. Fortunately, in the regimens employed for palliation, these acute effects are generally mild. The most common late reaction is fibrosis, which occurs mainly in tissues that have a limited ability to regenerate (e.g., brain, peripheral neurons, and lung).

PATIENT EDUCATION

Patient education is an integral part of cancer pain management. When education is successful, it can help reduce anxiety, dispel hopelessness, facilitate assessment, enhance compliance, decrease complications, provide a sense of control, and enable patients to take an active role in their care. All of these will promote pain relief.

General Issues

Patient education should be accurate, comprehensive, and understandable. To reinforce communication, information should be presented at least twice and in more than one way. Major topics to discuss are (1) the nature and causes of pain, (2) assessment and the importance of honest self-reporting, and (3) plans for drug and nondrug therapy. Patients should be encouraged to express their fears and concerns about cancer, cancer pain, and pain treatment—and they should be reassured that pain can be effectively controlled in most cases. All patients should receive a written pain management plan. To facilitate ongoing education, patients should be invited to contact care providers whenever they feel the need—be it to discuss specific concerns with treatment or simply to acquire new information. Finally, patients should know when and how to contact the prescriber to report treatment failure, serious side effects, or new pain.

Drug Therapy

The goal in teaching patients about analgesic drugs is to maximize pain relief and minimize harm. To help achieve this goal, patients should know the following about each drug they take:
- Drug name and therapeutic category
- Dose size and schedule
- Route and technique of administration
- Expected therapeutic response and when it should develop

- Duration of treatment
- Method of drug storage and disposal
- Symptoms of major adverse effects and measures to minimize discomfort and harm
- Major adverse drug–drug and drug–food interactions
- Whom to contact in the event of therapeutic failure, severe adverse effects, or severe adverse interactions

The dosing schedule should be discussed. Patients should understand that PRN dosing is appropriate only if pain is intermittent. When pain is persistent, as it is for most patients, the objective is to *prevent* pain from returning. Hence dosing should be done on a fixed schedule ATC, not PRN. However, even with ATC dosing, breakthrough pain can occur. Hence patients should be taught what drug and dosage to use for rescue treatment.

Fears based on misconceptions about opioids can impair compliance and can thereby impair pain control. The misconceptions that influence compliance the most relate to tolerance, physical dependence, addiction, and side effects. To correct these misconceptions and, hence, dispel fears and improve compliance, the following topics should be discussed:
- *Tolerance*—Some patients fear that, because of tolerance, taking opioids now will decrease their effectiveness later. Hence to help ensure pain relief in the future, they limit opioid use now and thus suffer needless pain. These patients should be reassured that if tolerance does develop, efficacy can be restored by increasing the dosage; tolerance does not mean that efficacy is lost.
- *Physical dependence and addiction*—Many patients fear opioid addiction and hence are reluctant to take these drugs. This fear is based largely on the misconception that physical dependence (which eventually develops in all patients) equals addiction. Patients should be taught that physical dependence is not the same as addiction and that physical dependence itself is nothing to fear. In addition, they should be taught that the behavior pattern that constitutes addiction rarely develops in people who take opioids in a therapeutic setting.
- *Fear of severe side effects*—Some patients fear that opioids cannot relieve pain without causing severe side effects. These patients should be reassured that, when used correctly, opioids are both safe and effective.

The rationale for using an adjuvant analgesic should be discussed. With all of the adjuvants, the objective is to *complement* the effects of opioid and nonopioid analgesics. Adjuvants are not intended to substitute for these drugs. Furthermore, because the drugs we use as adjuvants were originally developed to treat disorders other than pain, the rationale for prescribing specific adjuvants should be explained. For example, when imipramine is prescribed, the patient should understand that the objective is to relieve neuropathic pain and not depression, the disorder for which this drug was originally developed.

Basic issues related to patient education in drug therapy are discussed in Chapter 3.

87

Drugs for the Eye

The drugs addressed in this chapter are used to diagnose and treat disorders of the eye. The primary focus is on glaucoma. Many of the drugs considered here are discussed in other chapters, so discussion in this chapter is limited to ophthalmologic applications.

GLAUCOMA

Glaucoma refers to a group of diseases characterized by a decrease in peripheral vision secondary to optic nerve damage. The most common forms of glaucoma are primary open-angle glaucoma (POAG) and acute angle-closure glaucoma. These forms differ with respect to underlying pathology and treatment.

Glaucoma is the leading cause of preventable blindness in the United States. Of the 120,000 Americans blinded each year by glaucoma, 90% could have saved their sight with timely treatment. Unfortunately, many afflicted persons are unaware of their condition: of the 4 million Americans with glaucoma, only 50% are diagnosed.

Before we discuss glaucoma, we must review the role of aqueous humor in maintaining intraocular pressure (IOP). As shown in Fig. 87.1, aqueous humor is produced by the ciliary body and secreted into the posterior chamber of the eye. From there it circulates around the iris into the anterior chamber and then exits the anterior chamber through the trabecular meshwork and canal of Schlemm. If outflow from the anterior chamber is impeded, back pressure will develop and IOP will rise. Conversely, if production of aqueous humor falls, IOP will decline.

Pathophysiology of Glaucoma and Treatment Overview
Primary Open-Angle Glaucoma

Characteristics. POAG is the most common form of glaucoma in the United States. About 90% of people with glaucoma have this type. POAG is a leading cause of blindness in the United States.

POAG is characterized by progressive optic nerve damage with eventual impairment of vision. Visual loss develops first in the peripheral visual field. As the disease advances, loss occurs in the central visual field. The pathologic process that leads to optic nerve damage is not understood. IOP is often elevated, but it may also be normal. POAG is a painless, insidious disease in which injury develops over years. Symptoms are absent until extensive optic nerve damage has been produced.

Management. Treatment of POAG is directed at reducing elevated IOP, the only risk factor we can modify. Although POAG has no cure, reduction of IOP can slow or even stop disease progression. Management is usually initiated by specialists; however, primary care providers often play a role in the ongoing monitoring and follow-up of patients taking these medications.

The principal method for reducing IOP is chronic therapy with drugs. Drugs lower IOP by either (1) facilitating aqueous humor outflow or (2) reducing aqueous humor production. As indicated in Table 87.1, the first-line drugs for glaucoma belong to three classes: *β-adrenergic blocking agents* (β blockers), *$α_2$-adrenergic agonists,* and *prostaglandin analogs.* Other options—*cholinergic drugs* and *carbonic anhydrase inhibitors*—are considered second-line choices. All antiglaucoma drugs are available for topical administration, which is the preferred route. For more than 25 years, the β blockers (e.g., timolol) have been considered drugs of first choice. However, the $α_2$ agonists (e.g., brimonidine) and prostaglandin analogs (e.g., latanoprost) are just as effective as the β blockers and have a more desirable side-effect profile. Accordingly, these drugs have joined the β blockers as first-choice agents. Because drugs in different classes lower IOP by different mechanisms, combined therapy can be more effective than monotherapy. These drugs are applied topically; therefore systemic effects are relatively uncommon. Nonetheless, serious systemic reactions *can* occur if sufficient absorption takes place.

If drugs are unable to reduce IOP to an acceptable level, surgical intervention to promote outflow of aqueous humor is indicated. Options include trabeculectomy and laser trabeculoplasty.

Angle-Closure Glaucoma

Angle-closure glaucoma is precipitated by displacement of the iris such that it covers the trabecular meshwork, thereby preventing exit of aqueous humor from the anterior chamber. As a result, IOP increases rapidly and to dangerous levels. This disorder is referred to as *angle-closure* or *narrow-angle* glaucoma because the angle between the cornea and the iris is greatly reduced (Fig. 87.2). Angle-closure glaucoma develops suddenly and is extremely painful. In the absence of treatment, irreversible loss of vision occurs in 1 to 2 days. This disorder is much less common than open-angle glaucoma.

Treatment consists of *drug therapy* (to control the acute attack) followed by *corrective surgery*. A combination of drugs (osmotic agents, short-acting miotics, carbonic anhydrase inhibitors, and topical β-adrenergic blocking agents) is employed to suppress symptoms. After IOP has been reduced with drugs, definitive treatment can be rendered with surgery. Options include *iridectomy* and *laser iridotomy*. Both procedures alter the iris to permit unimpeded outflow of aqueous humor.

Drugs Used to Manage Glaucoma

Before we discuss the drugs used to treat glaucoma, a short word about nonadherence is in order. Nonadherence to medication regimens for glaucoma is high, and various reasons for these high rates have been proposed. They include the asymptomatic nature of the condition, frequent dosing intervals, and age-related issues. The latter may include

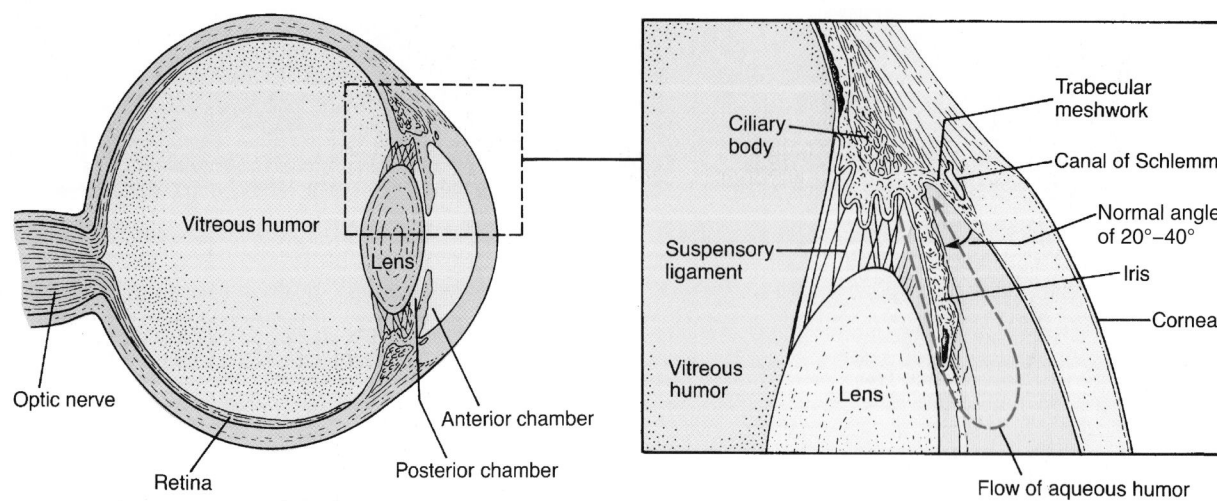

Fig. 87.1 Anatomy of the Normal Eye.

TABLE 87.1   Topical Drugs for Open-Angle Glaucoma

Class	Drugs	Mechanism	Adverse Effects
First-Line Agents			
β blockers		Decreased aqueous humor formation	
Nonselective	Timolol		Heart block, bradycardia, and bronchospasm
	Carteolol		
	Levobunolol		
	Metipranolol		
β₁-selective drugs	Betaxolol		Heart block, bradycardia, and hypotension
Prostaglandin analogs	Latanoprost	Increased aqueous humor outflow	Heightened brown pigmentation of the iris and eyelid
	Latanoprostene bunod		
	Travoprost		
	Bimatoprost		
α₂-adrenergic agonists	Apraclonidine[a]	Decreased aqueous humor formation	Headache, dry mouth, dry nose, altered taste, conjunctivitis, lid reactions, and pruritus
	Brimonidine		
Second-Line Agents			
Cholinergic drugs		Increased aqueous humor outflow	
Muscarinic agonists	Pilocarpine		Miosis and blurred vision
Cholinesterase inhibitors	Echothiophate		Miosis and blurred vision
Carbonic anhydrase inhibitors	Acetazolamide	Decreased aqueous humor formation	Ocular stinging, bitter taste, conjunctivitis, and lid reactions
	Methazolamide		
	Dorzolamide		
	Brinzolamide		
Rho kinase inhibitor	Netarsudil	Increased aqueous humor outflow	Eye discomfort, hyperemic conjunctiva, and conjunctival hemorrhage

[a]Apraclonidine is indicated for short-term use only and therefore is *not* a first-line drug for glaucoma.

forgetfulness associated with dementia or failure of providers to continue medications when patients are admitted to tertiary care facilities. For some drugs, cost is a concern. For these reasons it is essential not to assume that these drugs are being taken as directed. Monitoring to ascertain progress and identify worsening is critical.

β-Adrenergic Blocking Agents

Actions and use in glaucoma. Five β blockers—*betaxolol, carteolol, levobunolol, metipranolol,* and *timolol*—are approved for use in glaucoma. Dosing is topical. These agents cause minimal disturbance of vision and are considered first-line drugs for glaucoma, although prostaglandin analogs are becoming favored. Formulations and dosages of the β blockers are shown in Table 87.2.

The β-adrenergic blockers lower IOP by decreasing production of aqueous humor. Reductions in IOP occur with "nonselective" β blockers (drugs that block β₁ *and* β₂ receptors) as well as with "cardioselective" β blockers (drugs that block β₁ receptors only).

β blockers are used primarily for open-angle glaucoma. They are suitable for initial therapy as well as maintenance therapy. β blockers in combination with other drugs are also employed for emergency management of acute angle-closure glaucoma.

The basic pharmacology of the β blockers is discussed in Chapter 16.

Adverse effects

Local. Local effects are generally minimal, although patients commonly complain of transient ocular stinging. β blockers occasionally cause conjunctivitis, blurred vision, photophobia, and dry eyes.

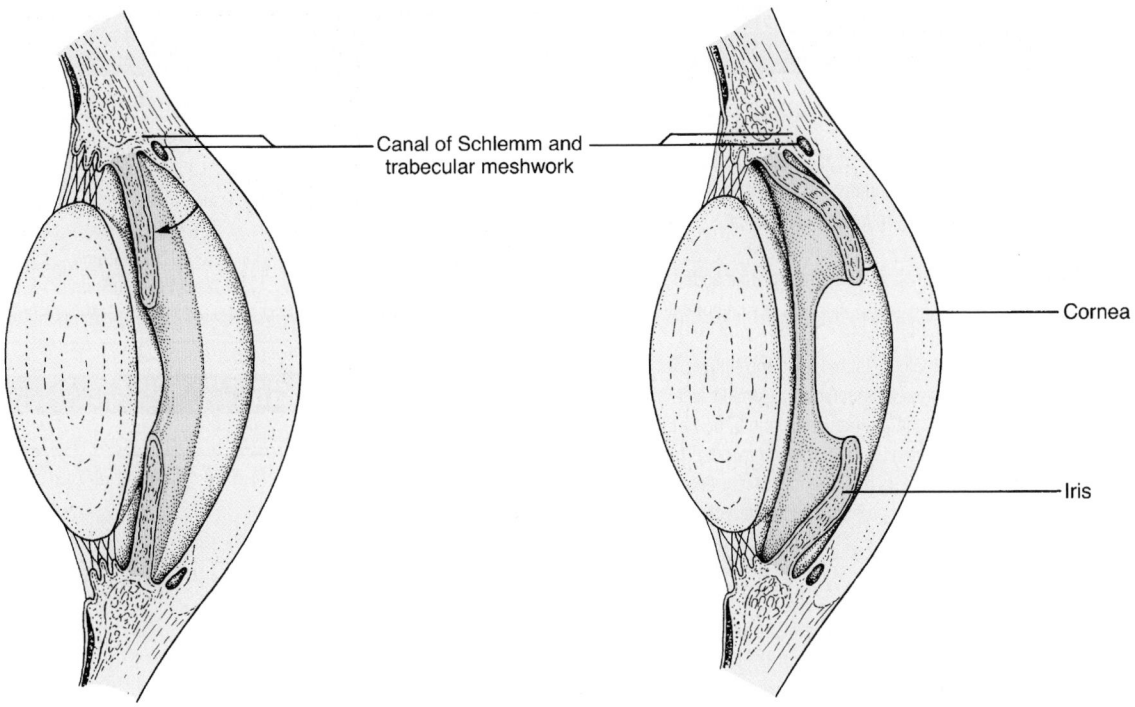

A   Open-angle glaucoma

B   Angle-closure glaucoma

Fig. 87.2 Comparative Anatomy of the Eye in Open-Angle and Angle-Closure Glaucoma. (A) The angle between the iris and cornea is open in open-angle glaucoma, permitting unimpeded outflow of aqueous humor through the canal of Schlemm and trabecular meshwork. (B) The angle between the iris and cornea is constricted in angle-closure glaucoma, thereby blocking outflow of aqueous humor through the canal of Schlemm and trabecular meshwork.

TABLE 87.2   β Blockers Used in Glaucoma

Drug	Receptor Specificity	Formulation	Usual Dosage
Betaxolol (Betoptic S)	β_1	0.25% suspension	1 drop bid
Carteolol	β_1, β_2	1% solution	1 drop bid
Levobunolol (Betagan and AKBeta)	β_1, β_2	0.25% solution	1 drop bid
		0.5% solution	1 drop qd–bid
Metipranolol (OptiPranolol)	β_1, β_2	0.3% solution	1 drop bid
Timolol (Timoptic, Timoptic XE, Betimol, and Istalol)	β_1, β_2	0.25% solution	1 drop qd–bid
		0.5% solution	1 drop qd–bid
		0.25% gel	1 drop qd
		0.5% gel	1 drop qd

Systemic. β blockers can be absorbed in amounts sufficient to cause systemic effects. For example, instilling 1 drop of 0.5% timolol in each eye can produce the same blood level as taking 10 mg of timolol by mouth (the usual starting dose for hypertension). Effects on the heart and lungs are of greatest concern.

Blockade of cardiac β_1 receptors can produce bradycardia and atrioventricular (AV) heart block. Pulse rate should be monitored. Because of their ability to depress cardiac function, β blockers are contraindicated for patients with AV heart block, sinus bradycardia, and cardiogenic shock. In addition, they should be used with caution in patients with heart failure.

Blockade of β_2 receptors in the lung can cause bronchospasm. Constriction of the bronchi can occur with β_1-selective antagonists as well as with "nonselective" β-adrenergic blockers, although the risk is greatest with the nonselective agents. Only one ophthalmic β blocker—betaxolol—is β_1-selective. This drug is preferred to other β blockers for patients with asthma or chronic obstructive pulmonary disease.

Prostaglandin Analogs

Four prostaglandin analogs are approved for topical therapy of glaucoma. These drugs are as effective as the β blockers and cause fewer side effects. Accordingly, they are considered first-line medications for glaucoma. Formulations and dosages are shown in Table 87.3.

Latanoprost. Latanoprost (Xalatan), an analog of prostaglandin F_2 α, was the first prostaglandin approved for glaucoma and can serve as the prototype for the group. The drug is applied topically to lower IOP in patients with open-angle glaucoma and ocular hypertension. Latanoprost lowers IOP by facilitating aqueous humor outflow, in part by relaxing the ciliary muscle. The recommended dosage is 1 drop (0.005% solution) applied once daily in the evening. At this dosage, latanoprost produces the same reduction in IOP as does timolol twice daily.

PAITENT-CENTERED CARE ACROSS THE LIFE SPAN

Drugs for Glaucoma

Life Stage	Considerations or Concerns
Children	Compared with adults, children usually have greater systemic absorption following ophthalmic administration.
	Most drug classes include drugs not recommended for children. These are the β blockers, levobunolol and metipranolol; the α₂ agonist, apraclonidine; the prostaglandin analogs, latanoprost and tafluprost; the carbonic anhydrase inhibitors, brinzolamide and methazolamide; and the rho kinase inhibitor, netarsudil. Additionally, brimonidine is not recommended for children under 2 years old. The manufacturers of travoprost and latanoprostene bunod do not recommend its use for children under 16 years of age because of possible long-term effects involving pigmentary changes.
	The muscarinic agonist pilocarpine may cause paradoxical *increases* in intraocular pressure. It is indicated for the treatment of primary congenital glaucoma but not glaucoma secondary to other conditions.
Pregnant women	The intraocular pressure is usually decreased during pregnancy. This aids in the use of lower drug doses.
	For all β-blocker preparations except betaxolol, adverse events have occurred in animal studies. No animal studies have been conducted for ophthalmic preparations of betaxolol; however, oral betaxolol crosses the placenta.
	Of the α-adrenergic agonists, brimonidine is generally considered safest because no adverse events have been observed in animal studies. Adverse events occurred in animals when apraclonidine was used.
	Both adverse and teratogenic effects were noted in animal reproduction studies with prostaglandin analogs and carbonic anhydrase inhibitors.
	No adverse effects were identified in animal reproduction studies using netarsudil.
	Risk has not been determined for the cholinesterase inhibitor echothiophate and the muscarinic agonist pilocarpine because there are inadequate animal reproduction studies on which to base any conclusion.
Breastfeeding women	For all these drugs, manufacturers recommend considering the possibility of benefits versus drug adverse effects in deciding whether or not to breastfeed. If the patient will be breastfeeding, the lowest effective dose should be used, along with punctual occlusion after administration to decrease absorption.
Older adults	β blockers, even when administered topically, may worsen heart failure in patients with this condition.
	α₂ agonists can cause orthostatic hypotension. This creates a fall risk for older patients.
	Patients with marked renal impairment should not take carbonic anhydrase inhibitors. This applies to topical as well as systemic formulations.
	Cholinesterase inhibitors may cause bradycardia and hypotension leading to a fall risk.

TABLE 87.3   Prostaglandin Analogs Used in Glaucoma

Generic Name	Trade Name	Formulation	Usual Dosage
Latanoprost	Xalatan	0.005% solution	1 drop qd hs
Travoprost	Travatan	0.004% solution	1 drop qd hs
Bimatoprost	Lumigan	0.01% solution	1 drop qd hs
		0.03% solution	1 drop qd hs
Tafluprost	Zioptan	0.0015% solution	1 drop qd hs
Latanoprostene bunod	Vyzulta	0.024% solution	1 drop qd hs

PROTOTYPE DRUGS

Drugs for the Eye

β Blockers
Betaxolol (β₁-selective)
Timolol (blocks β₁ and β₂ receptors)

α-Adrenergic Agonists
Brimonidine

Prostaglandin Analogs
Latanoprost

Angiogenesis Inhibitors
Ranibizumab

Latanoprost is generally well tolerated, and systemic reactions are rare. The most significant side effect is a harmless heightened brown pigmentation of the iris, which is most noticeable in patients whose irides are green-brown, yellow-brown, or blue/gray-brown. The effect is rare in patients whose irides are blue, green, or blue-green. Heightened pigmentation stops progressing when latanoprost is discontinued but does not usually regress. Topical latanoprost may also increase pigmentation of the eyelid and may increase the length, thickness, and pigmentation of the eyelashes. Other side effects include blurred vision, burning, stinging, conjunctival hyperemia, conjunctival edema, and punctate keratopathy. Rarely, latanoprost may cause macular edema.

Other prostaglandin analogs. In addition to latanoprost, three other topical prostaglandins are approved for topical therapy of glaucoma. Like latanoprost, these drugs—travoprost (Travatan), bimatoprost (Lumigan), latanoprostene bunod, and tafluprost (Zioptan)—reduce IOP by increasing aqueous humor outflow. In clinical trials, these agents were at least as effective as timolol, a representative β blocker. Interestingly, one drug—travoprost—was more effective in blacks than in nonblacks. Like latanoprost, these prostaglandins can cause a gradual increase in brown pigmentation of the iris, which may be irreversible. In addition, these drugs can increase pigmentation of the eyelid and growth of the eyelashes. In fact, bimatoprost, marketed as Latisse, is used for the specific purpose of increasing eyelash length, darkness, and thickness. The most common adverse conjunctival effects are blurred vision, eye discomfort, ocular pruritus, allergic conjunctivitis, dry eye syndrome, light intolerance, and tearing. Macular edema has occurred.

α₂-Adrenergic Agonists

Two α₂ agonists are approved for glaucoma. One agent—apraclonidine—is used only for short-term therapy. The other agent—brimonidine—has emerged as a first-line drug for long-term therapy. (Brimonidine also is available over-the-counter as Lumify. This formulation is used for its vasoconstrictor properties as an ocular decongestant.)

Brimonidine. Brimonidine (Alphagan P, Alphagan ♦) is the first and only topical α_2-adrenergic agonist approved for the *long-term* reduction of elevated IOP in patients with open-angle glaucoma or ocular hypertension. Effects on IOP are similar to those achieved with timolol. The drug lowers IOP by reducing the production of aqueous humor and perhaps by increasing outflow. In addition to lowering IOP, brimonidine may delay optic nerve degeneration and protect retinal neurons from death. This possibility arises from the ability of α_2 agonists to protect neurons from injury caused by ischemia. The most common adverse effects are dry mouth, ocular hyperemia, local burning and stinging, headache, blurred vision, foreign body sensation, and itching. In contrast to apraclonidine (see later), brimonidine can cross the blood–brain barrier and hence can cause drowsiness, fatigue, and hypotension. (Recall from Chapter 15 that activation of α_2 receptors in the brain decreases sympathetic outflow to blood vessels, thereby lowering the blood pressure.) Brimonidine can be absorbed onto soft contact lenses. Accordingly, at least 15 minutes should elapse between drug administration and lens installation.

Apraclonidine. Apraclonidine (Iopidine), a topical α_2-adrenergic agonist, lowers IOP by reducing aqueous humor production and possibly by increasing outflow. The drug is indicated only for (1) short-term therapy of open-angle glaucoma in patients who have not responded adequately to maximal doses of other IOP-lowering drugs and (2) preoperative medication before laser trabeculoplasty or iridotomy. Side effects include headache, dry mouth, dry nose, altered taste, conjunctivitis, lid reactions, pruritus, tearing, and blurred vision. Apraclonidine does not cross the blood-brain barrier and thus does not promote hypotension.

α_2 Agonist/β-Blocker Combination

A fixed-dose combination of brimonidine (an α_2 agonist) and timolol (a nonselective β blocker) is available for lowering IOP in patients with glaucoma or ocular hypertension. Benefits and adverse effects are about equal to those seen when the two drugs are applied separately. Formulations and dosages for the α_2 agonist and the α_2 agonist/β blocker combination are shown in Table 87.4.

α_2 Agonist/Carbonic Anhydrase Inhibitor Combination

A fixed-dose combination of the α_2 agonist brimonidine and the carbonic anhydrase inhibitor brinzolamide is available as Simbrinza to lower IOP. Therapeutic and adverse effects are the same as the single agents. Formulations and dosages are provided in Table 87.4.

Pilocarpine, a Direct-Acting Muscarinic Agonist

Pilocarpine is a direct-acting muscarinic agonist (parasympathomimetic agent). Although used widely in the past, pilocarpine is now considered a second-line drug for open-angle glaucoma. Pilocarpine can also be used for emergency treatment of acute angle-closure glaucoma.

Administration is topical. The basic pharmacology of the muscarinic agonists is discussed in Chapter 13. Consideration here is limited to the use of pilocarpine in glaucoma.

By stimulating cholinergic receptors in the eye, pilocarpine produces two direct effects: (1) miosis (constriction of the pupil secondary to contraction of the iris sphincter) and (2) contraction of the ciliary muscle (an action that focuses the lens for near vision). IOP is lowered indirectly. In patients with open-angle glaucoma, IOP is reduced because the tension generated by contracting the ciliary muscle promotes widening of the spaces within the trabecular meshwork, thereby facilitating outflow of aqueous humor. In angle-closure glaucoma, contraction of the iris sphincter pulls the iris away from the pores of the trabecular meshwork, thereby removing the impediment to aqueous humor outflow.

The major side effects of pilocarpine concern the eye. Contraction of the ciliary muscle focuses the lens for near vision; corrective lenses can provide partial compensation for this problem. Occasionally sustained contraction of the ciliary muscle causes retinal detachment. Constriction of the pupil, caused by contraction of the iris sphincter, may decrease visual acuity. Pilocarpine may also produce local irritation, eye pain, and brow ache.

Rarely, pilocarpine is absorbed in amounts sufficient to cause systemic effects. Stimulation of muscarinic receptors throughout the body can produce a variety of responses, including bradycardia, bronchospasm, hypotension, urinary urgency, diarrhea, hypersalivation, and sweating. Caution should be exercised in patients with asthma or bradycardia. Systemic toxicity can be reversed with a muscarinic antagonist (e.g., atropine).

Formulations and dosages are shown in Table 87.5.

Echothiophate, a Cholinesterase Inhibitor

Only one cholinesterase inhibitor—echothiophate (Phospholine Iodide)—is available for glaucoma. Echothiophate is indicated for

TABLE 87.4 α_2 Agonists Used in Glaucoma

Generic Name	Trade Name	Formulation	Usual Dosage
Brimonidine	Alphagan P	0.1% and 0.15% solutions (0.2% solution available in Canada)	1 drop ~q 8 h
Apraclonidine	Iopidine	0.5% solution	1–2 drops ~q 8 h
Brimonidine + timolol (a β blocker)	Combigan	0.2% brimonidine + 0.5% timolol	1 drop ~q 12 h
Brimonidine + brinzolamide (a carbonic anhydrase inhibitor)	Simbrinza	0.2% brimonidine + 1% brinzolamide	1 drop q 8 h

TABLE 87.5 Direct and Indirect Parasympathomimetic Preparations Used in Glaucoma

Generic Name	Trade Name	Formulation	Usual Dosage
Pilocarpine solution	Isopto Carpine, Akarpine ♦, and Diocarpine ♦	0.5%–8% solution	Open-angle maintenance: 1 drop of solution (0.5%–4%) qid. Acute angle-closure: 1 drop q 5–10 min for 3–6 doses, then 1 drop q 1–3 h
Echothiophate	Phospholine Iodide	0.03%–0.25% reconstituted solution	1 drop bid. Maintenance may be once daily, twice daily, or every other day

POAG; however, because of concerns about adverse effects, the drug is not a first-choice agent. Rather, it is reserved for patients who have responded poorly to preferred medications (e.g., β blockers, α₂ agonists, and prostaglandins).

The drug has a long duration of action. The basic pharmacology of cholinesterase inhibitors is discussed in Chapter 13. Consideration here is limited to its use in glaucoma.

Cholinesterase inhibitors inhibit breakdown of acetylcholine by cholinesterase and thereby promote accumulation of acetylcholine at muscarinic receptors. As a result, they can produce the same ocular effects as pilocarpine (i.e., miosis, focusing of the lens for near vision, and reduction of IOP).

Like pilocarpine, echothiophate can cause myopia (secondary to contraction of the ciliary muscle) and excessive pupillary constriction. However, of much greater concern is the association between long-acting cholinesterase inhibitors and development of cataracts. Absorption of echothiophate into the systemic circulation can produce typical parasympathomimetic responses, including bradycardia, bronchospasm, sweating, salivation, urinary urgency, and diarrhea.

Echothiophate iodide is supplied as a powder for reconstitution to solution. Formulations and dosages are shown in Table 87.5.

Carbonic Anhydrase Inhibitors: Topical

Carbonic anhydrase inhibitors tend to be less effective than other drug therapy for glaucoma. They remain useful as adjuncts and as alternatives for treatments that are less well tolerated.

Dorzolamide. Dorzolamide (Trusopt) was the first carbonic anhydrase inhibitor available for topical administration. The drug is used to reduce IOP in patients with open-angle glaucoma and ocular hypertension. Dorzolamide lowers IOP by decreasing production of aqueous humor. Responses are similar to those produced with β blockers.

Dorzolamide is generally well tolerated. The most common side effects are ocular stinging and bitter taste immediately after dosing. Between 10% and 15% of patients experience allergic reactions, primarily conjunctivitis and lid reactions. If these occur, the patient should stop dorzolamide and contact the prescriber. Other reactions include blurred vision, tearing, eye dryness, and photophobia. In contrast to systemic carbonic anhydrase inhibitors, dorzolamide does not produce acidosis or electrolyte imbalance.

Dorzolamide is also available in a fixed-dose combination with timolol, marketed as Cosopt. The combination produces a greater reduction in IOP than either component used alone. Formulations and dosages for these products as well as other carbonic anhydrase inhibitors are shown in Table 87.6.

Brinzolamide. Brinzolamide (Azopt) is approved for topical treatment of elevated IOP in patients with open-angle glaucoma or ocular hypertension. The drug is as effective as dorzolamide and is better tolerated. Like other carbonic anhydrase inhibitors, brinzolamide reduces IOP by slowing production of aqueous humor. The most common adverse effects are bitter aftertaste and transient blurred vision. Brinzolamide causes less ocular stinging and burning than dorzolamide. Both brinzolamide and dorzolamide contain the preservative benzalkonium chloride. This is absorbed by soft contact lenses. Patients wearing these should wait 15 minutes after administration before inserting contact lenses.

Brinzolamide is available in combination with brimonidine, marketed as Simbrinza. With this combination producing a greater reduction in IOP than either component used alone.

Carbonic Anhydrase Inhibitors: Systemic

Oral carbonic anhydrase inhibitors have mostly been replaced by topical drugs. Two carbonic anhydrase inhibitors—acetazolamide and methazolamide—are available for systemic therapy of glaucoma. Of these, acetazolamide is used more often.

Carbonic anhydrase inhibitors lower IOP by decreasing production of aqueous humor. Maximally effective doses reduce aqueous flow by 50%. Administration is oral.

Carbonic anhydrase inhibitors are employed primarily for long-term treatment of open-angle glaucoma. They are not drugs of first choice. Rather, they should be reserved for patients who have been refractory to preferred medications (e.g., β blockers, α₂ agonists, and prostaglandin analogs). Carbonic anhydrase inhibitors may also be given (in combination with other antiglaucoma drugs) to produce rapid lowering of IOP in patients with angle-closure glaucoma.

Systemic carbonic anhydrase inhibitors can produce a variety of adverse effects. Effects on the central nervous system (CNS), which are relatively common, include malaise, anorexia, fatigue, and paresthesias. The sense of malaise causes many patients to discontinue treatment. Reduced appetite, coupled with GI disturbances (nausea, vomiting, and diarrhea), may result in weight loss. Carbonic anhydrase inhibitors are teratogenic in animals and should be avoided during pregnancy, especially the first trimester. Additional concerns are acid–base disturbances, electrolyte imbalance, and nephrolithiasis.

Netarsudil, a Rho Kinase Inhibitor

Netarsudil (Rhopressa), approved in 2017, is the most recent drug to be added to the glaucoma arsenal. Netarsudil decreases IOP by increasing aqueous humor outflow through the trabecular meshwork; however, the exact mechanism by which this is accomplished is unknown. Dosage is 1 drop daily of a 0.02% solution.

Other than eye discomfort, in part from the benzalkonium chloride, there are few known adverse effects. Subconjunctival hemorrhage may occur and, while it is visually disturbing, is not a serious condition. Postmarketing studies are ongoing.

TABLE 87.6   Carbonic Anhydrase Inhibitors Used in Glaucoma

Generic Name	Trade Name	Formulation	Usual Dosage
Dorzolamide	Trusopt	2% solution	1 drop tid
Dorzolamide + timolol (a β-blocker)	Cosopt	2% dorzolamide + 0.5% timolol	1 drop bid
Brinzolamide	Azopt	1% solution	1 drop 3 times/d
Acetazolamide	Diamox, Diamox Sequels, and Acetazolam ✦	125- and 250-mg tablets 500-mg sustained-release capsules	250 mg–1 g qd
Methazolamide	Neptazane	25- and 50-mg tablets	50–100 mg bid–tid

PATIENT EDUCATION

Glaucoma

- It is important to take the prescribed medications according to schedule. If days are skipped or if prescriptions are not refilled, loss of vision may occur.
- Notify the provider immediately if experiencing vision loss, severe eye pain, headache, or nausea and vomiting. These could indicate angle-closure glaucoma.
- If photophobia is a problem outdoors, sunglasses, wide-brimmed hats, visors, or baseball caps may be helpful.
- Check labels of ophthalmic drugs to see if they contain benzalkonium as a preservative. These drugs may be absorbed by soft contact lenses. Allow at least 15 min to elapse between administration and insertion of the lenses.
- Take care not to touch the dropper to the eyes and not to touch the tip with your fingers. Contamination can cause an eye infection.
- To improve topical absorption and minimize systemic absorption, close the eye(s) for 3 minutes after administering the eye drop(s) and lightly press a thumb or finger over the medial canthus (inner corner of the eye).

ALLERGIC CONJUNCTIVITIS

Pathophysiology of Allergic Conjunctivitis

Allergic conjunctivitis (AC) is defined as inflammation of the conjunctiva in response to an allergen. AC may be seasonal or perennial (chronic). Primary symptoms are itching, burning, and a thin, watery discharge. In addition, the conjunctivae are usually red and congested.

Symptoms of AC result from a biphasic immune response. Initially, symptoms are caused by release of inflammatory mediators—histamine, prostaglandins, leukotrienes, and kinins—from mast cells. These mediators stimulate mucus production (hence cause discharge), activate nerve endings (hence cause itching and burning sensations), and promote vasodilation and increase capillary permeability (hence cause redness and congestion). These symptoms peak about 20 minutes after allergen exposure and abate 20 minutes later. After this early response, symptoms typically reappear 6 or more hours later. The late phase is due to recruitment of immune cells—eosinophils, neutrophils, and macrophages—that amplify the inflammatory response.

Drugs Used to Manage Allergic Conjunctivitis

AC can be managed with a variety of topical drugs (Table 87.7). *Mast cell stabilizers* (e.g., cromolyn and lodoxamide) prevent release of inflammatory

📄 SUMMARY OF KEY PRESCRIBING CONSIDERATIONS

Drugs for Glaucoma

Therapeutic Goal: Reduce elevated IOP and prevent loss of vision.

Baseline Data: IOP measurement, fundoscopic exam, visual field testing using automated perimetry. (Assessment of visual fields by confrontation is inadequate, even when performed correctly.) Baseline IOP is typically measured in ophthalmology clinics using specialized equipment.

Monitoring: IOP should be assessed every 1 to 3 months initially and then as indicated. Fundoscopic exams can be carried out in most settings.

Patients taking β blockers must be monitored for hypotension, bradycardia, AV block, and wheezing due to bronchoconstriction. Patients taking the α_2 agonist brimonidine should be assessed for CNS effects (e.g., excessive drowsiness) and hypotension. Assessment of visual acuity can be important for patients taking the parasympathomimetics pilocarpine and echothiophate. If changes are noted, refer to an optometrist because new glasses may be

needed. These patients should also be assessed for cholinergic effects (e.g., wheezing, slowed heart rate, decreased blood pressure, urinary urgency, diarrhea, excessive salivation, and excessive perspiration).

Identifying High-Risk Patients: Patients with a history of medication nonadherence are at risk for permanent visual deficits. Those with a history of heart failure, bradycardia, heart block, asthma, or obstructive pulmonary disease may be poor candidates for β-blocker therapy.

Evaluating Therapeutic Effects: Periodic evaluations compared with baseline data. May refer for specialty evaluation.

Minimizing Adverse Effects: All agents can cause eye discomfort and itching. Artificial tears may be helpful but should not be used within 30 minutes of drug administration. Warm compresses may also be helpful.

TABLE 87.7 Topical Drugs for Allergic Conjunctivitis

Class and Generic Name	Trade Name	Concentration	Usual Daily Dosage
Mast-Cell Stabilizers			
Cromolyn sodium	Crolom, Opticrom	4%	1–2 drops every 4–6 h
Lodoxamide tromethamine	Alomide	0.1%	1–2 drops qid
Nedocromil sodium	Alocril	2%	1–2 drops bid
H₁-Receptor Blocker			
Emedastine difumarate	Emadine	0.05%	1 drop qid
H₁ Blockers With Mast-Cell Stabilizing Properties			
Alcaftadine	Lastacaft	0.25%	1 drop once daily
Azelastine hydrochloride	Optivar	0.05%	1 drop bid
Epinastine	Elestat	0.05%	1 drop bid
Ketotifen fumarate	Zaditor and Alaway	0.025%	1 drop q 8–12 h
Olopatadine hydrochloride	Patanol	0.1%	1 drop bid
	Pataday	0.2%	1 drop qd
Bepotastine besylate	Bepreve	1.5%	1 drop bid

Continued

TABLE 87.7   Topical Drugs for Allergic Conjunctivitis—cont'd

Class and Generic Name	Trade Name	Concentration	Usual Daily Dosage
NSAIDs			
Ketorolac tromethamine	Acular LS	0.4%	1 drop qid
	Acuvail	0.45%	1 drop twice daily
	Acular and Acular PF	0.5%	1 qid
Glucocorticoids			
Loteprednol etabonate	Alrex	0.2%	1 drop qid
	Lotemax	0.5%	1–2 drops qid
Dexamethasone sodium phosphate	Various	0.1%	1 drop q 6–8 h
Fluorometholone	FML (ointment)	0.1%	1/2-in ribbon qd–tid
	Flarex (suspension)	0.1%	1 drop q 4 h for 24–48 h, then 1–2 drops qid
Prednisolone acetate	Various	1%	2 drops every 6–12 h
Prednisolone sodium phosphate	Various	1%	1 drop q 6–8 h
Rimexolone[a]	Vexol	1%	1–2 drops q 1–4 h
Decongestants (Vasoconstrictors)			
Naphazoline	Clear Eyes	0.012%	1–2 drops up to qid
Oxymetazoline	Visine L.R., OcuClear	0.025%	1–2 drops 4 times/d
Phenylephrine	Neo-Synephrine	0.12%	1–2 drops qid
Tetrahydrozoline	Visine Moisturizing	0.05%	1–2 drops qid
Decongestant/H₁ Blocker			
Naphazoline/pheniramine	Naphcon-A	0.025%/0.3%	1–2 drops qd–qid
	Opcon-A	0.27%/0.325%	1–2 drops qd–qid

[a]Off-label use.

NSAIDs, Nonsteroidal antiinflammatory drugs

mediators. Patients should be informed that benefits take several days to develop and 2 or more weeks to become maximally effective. In contrast to mast cell stabilizers, *histamine-1* (H₁)-*receptor antagonists* (antihistamines) can provide immediate symptomatic relief. Some drugs (e.g., azelastine and olopatadine) have both actions: they block H₁ receptors and prevent mediator release from mast cells. Ketorolac, a *nonsteroidal antiinflammatory drug* (NSAID), reduce symptoms by inhibiting cyclooxygenase, an enzyme required for synthesis of prostaglandins.

Like the NSAIDs, *glucocorticoids* (e.g., loteprednol) inhibit production of prostaglandins. In addition, glucocorticoids inhibit production of leukotrienes and thromboxane. As a result, these drugs are highly effective.

The *ocular decongestants* (e.g., naphazoline and phenylephrine) decrease redness and edema by activating α₁-adrenergic receptors on blood vessels, thereby causing vasoconstriction. Benefits are only symptomatic; these drugs do not interrupt any phase of the immune response. Furthermore, with regular use, rebound congestion is likely. For this reason, short-term use for no longer than 2 weeks is recommended. Fortunately that gives time for drugs such as mast cell stabilizers to become effective.

Before making a decision for therapy, it is important to determine the severity of symptoms. This can be used to guide treatment decisions (Fig. 87.3).

- Mild symptoms: mild pruritus that is intermittent or short-lived
- Moderate symptoms: mild to severe pruritus lasting a few days to 2 weeks without eye redness
- Severe symptoms: moderate to severe pruritus that is chronic with eye redness

SUMMARY OF KEY PRESCRIBING CONSIDERATIONS

Topical Drugs for Allergic Conjunctivitis

Therapeutic Goal: Relief of ocular pruritis, watery discharge, and redness. Prevention of associated complications that occur secondary to eye irritation or vigorous eye rubbing.

Baseline Data: Focused history and physical exam.

Monitoring: For patients using topical glucocorticoids, assess for evidence of eye infection.

Identifying High-Risk Patients: Ocular decongestants are contraindicated for patients with a history of angle-closure glaucoma. Glucocorticoids may increase IOP if prescribed long term.

Evaluating Therapeutic Effects: Evaluate extent of symptom control.

Minimizing Adverse Effects: Mast cell stabilizers—Because full efficacy takes days to weeks, acute symptoms must be managed with other medications.

H₁-receptor blockers—Emedastine may cause headache. This can be relieved with over-the-counter (OTC) NSAIDs.

H₁-receptor blockers with mast cell–stabilizing properties—saline drops may help to decrease sensation of dryness or burning.

NSAIDs—If symptoms are not adequately controlled, consider using a topical antihistamine.

Glucocorticoids—Reserve for short-term therapy of severe conditions. Establish that symptoms are caused by allergies and that there is no underlying viral infection.

Decongestants—Reserve for short-term therapy (no longer than 2 weeks) to avoid rebound congestion.

Fig. 87.3 Management of Allergic Conjunctivitis. *OTC,* Over-the-counter. (From Bielory L, Meltzer EO, Nichols KK, et al. An algorithm for the management of allergic conjunctivitis. *Allergy Asthma Proc.* 2013;34:408–420. Copyright © 2013, OceanSide Publications, Inc., USA.)

PATIENT EDUCATION

Allergic Conjunctivitis

- Allergen avoidance can reduce the severity of symptoms; for example, avoid being outside on windy days during pollen season if allergic to pollen.
- Mast-cell stabilizers, if prescribed, should not be abandoned prematurely. They require several days to develop symptom relief and several weeks to achieve maximal benefit.
- If oral antihistamines are taken for allergy symptoms, they will probably cause eye dryness. Artificial tears or other eye lubricants may provide relief from dryness and the associated discomfort.
- Artificial tears will help flush out allergens that are causing symptoms. These are available OTC. Application of cold compresses for 5–10 min at a time may help if discomfort is severe.
  Avoid rubbing eyes and wearing contact lenses, as this may result in worsening of symptoms.
- Notify the provider if symptoms worsen or if there is no relief after 2 weeks of therapy. (This could indicate an underlying problem other than allergic conjunctivitis.)
- Benzalkonium chloride is a common preservative in OTC and prescription eye drops. These drugs may be absorbed by soft contact lenses. Allow at least 15 min to elapse between administration and insertion of the lenses.
- If multiple topical drugs are prescribed, wait at least 5 min between drugs so that the second drug administered doesn't flush out the first drug administered.

ADDITIONAL OPHTHALMIC DRUGS

Drugs for Dry Eyes

Ophthalmic demulcents (artificial tears) are isotonic solutions employed as substitutes for natural tears. Most preparations contain polyvinyl alcohol, cellulose esters, or both. Artificial tears are indicated for relieving dry-eye syndromes and discomfort and dryness caused by irritants, wind, and sun. In addition, demulcents may be used to lubricate artificial eyes. Artificial tears are devoid of adverse effects and hence may be administered as often and as long as desired.

Topical cyclosporine ophthalmic emulsion (Restasis) is prescribed for dry eyes due to inflammation. It suppresses the immune response, thereby promoting resumption of tear production. Despite its mechanism of action, clinical trials and post-marketing reports have not identified an increase of ophthalmic infections in patients using this drug. Adverse effects are eye discomfort (burning, stinging, foreign body sensation), pruritus, conjunctival hyperemia, and blurred vision.

Ocular Decongestants

Ocular decongestants are weak solutions of adrenergic agonists applied topically to constrict dilated conjunctival blood vessels. These preparations are used to reduce redness of the eye caused by minor irritation. The adrenergic agents employed as decongestants are phenylephrine, naphazoline, oxymetazoline, brimonidine, and tetrahydrozoline. When applied to the eye in the low concentrations found in decongestant products, adrenergic agonists rarely cause adverse effects. Local reactions (stinging, burning, and reactive hyperemia) may occur with overuse. The adrenergic agonists are discussed in Chapter 15.

TABLE 87.8   Commonly Prescribed Topical Ophthalmic Antibacterial Agents

Class and Generic Name	Trade Name	Formulation	Typical Dosage[a]
Fluoroquinolones			
Besifloxacin	Besivance	0.6% suspension	Instill 1 drop in affected eye tid administered 4–12 h apart for 7 days
Ciprofloxacin	Ciloxan	0.3% solution, 0.3% ointment	Solution: Instill 1 or 2 drops in affected eye q 2 h while awake for 2 days, then 1 or 2 drops q 4 h while awake for 5 days Ointment: Apply 1/2-in ribbon tid for 2 days, then bid for 5 days
Gatifloxacin	Zymar 🍁 🍁	0.3% solution	Instill 1 drop in affected eye(s) q 2 h while awake for 2 days (maximum 8 times daily), then 1 drop qid while awake for 5 days
	Zymaxid	0.5% solution	Instill 1 drop in affected eye q 2 h while awake (maximum 8 times) the first day then 1 drop bid–qid while awake for 6 days
Levofloxacin	Quixin	0.5% solution	Instill 1–2 drops in affected eye q 2 h while awake for 2 days (maximum 8 times daily) then 1–2 drops q 4 h while awake for 5 days (maximum 4 times daily)
Moxifloxacin	Moxeza and Vigamox	0.5% solution	Moxeza: Instill 1 drop in affected eye bid for 7 days Vigamox: Instill 1 drop in affected eye tid for 7 days
Ofloxacin	Ocuflox	0.3% solution	Instill 1–2 drops in affected eye q 2–4 h for 2 days then instill 1–2 drops qid for 5 days
Macrolides			
Azithromycin	AzaSite	1% solution	Instill 1 drop in affected eye(s) bid for 2 days then 1 drop in affected eye qd for 5 days
Erythromycin	Ilotycin	0.5% ointment	Apply 1 cm in affected eye up to 6 times a day for 7 days
Aminoglycosides			
Gentamicin	Diogent 🍁 and Gentak	0.3% solution, 0.3% ointment	Solution: Instill 1–2 drops in affected eye q 4 h or 2 drops qh for more severe infection Ointment: Apply 1/2 in (1.25 cm) in affected eye bid–tid 3–4 h apart
Tobramycin	Tobrex and Tobrexan 🍁	0.3% solution, 0.3% ointment 0.3% viscous solution (Tobrexan)	Ointment: Apply half-inch in affected eye bid–tid or q 3–4 h if infection is severe Solution: Instill 1–2 drops in affected eye q 4 h for mild to moderate infections or 2 drops qh for severe infections Viscous solution (Tobrexan [Canadian product]): Instill 1 drop in affected eye bid for 7 days for mild to moderate infections or 1 drop qid on the first day then 1 drop bid for 5 days for more severe infections
Sulfonamides			
Sulfacetamide	Bleph-10 and Sodium Sulamyd 🍁	10% solution, 10% ointment	Solution: Instill 1–2 q 2–3 h Ointment: Apply 1/2 in q 3–4 h and hs
Polymyxin B–Containing Mixtures			
Polymyxin B/ bacitracin	AK-Poly-Bac	Ointment	Apply the ointment q 3–4 h for 7–10 days depending on the severity of the infection
Polymyxin B/ bacitracin/ neomycin	Neo-Polycin	Ointment	Apply 0.5 in to affected eye q 3–4 h for acute infections or bid–tid for mild to moderate infections for 7–10 days
Polymyxin B/ gramicidin/ neomycin	Neosporin and Optimyxin 🍁	Solution	Instill 1–2 drops to affected eye q 4 h or 2 drops qh for 7–10 days
Polymyxin B/ trimethoprim	Polytrim	Solution	Instill 2 drops in the affected eye q 3 h (maximum of 6 doses/d) for 7–10 days

[a]Dosage is typical for infections such as bacterial conjunctivitis and does not include treatment of corneal ulcers or prophylaxis of neonatal conjunctivitis secondary to sexually transmitted infections.

Glucocorticoids

Glucocorticoids are used to treat inflammatory disorders of the eye (e.g., uveitis, iritis, and conjunctivitis). Short-term therapy in the absence of infection is generally devoid of adverse effects. In contrast, prolonged therapy may cause cataracts, reduced visual acuity, and glaucoma. In addition, there is an increased risk for infection secondary to glucocorticoid-induced suppression of host defenses. Because eye infections may present with symptoms similar to inflammatory disorders of the eye, prescribing should be done in consult with an ophthalmologist or other specialist with the equipment to verify that symptoms are not caused by an underlying viral or fungal infection. When administered in the presence of these infections, permanent vision loss can occur. The glucocorticoids are discussed in Chapter 58.

Topical Drugs for Eye Infections

Topical drugs are available for treating viral and bacterial infections of the eye. Two antiviral drugs—trifluridine, and ganciclovir—are employed. The pharmacology of antiviral drugs is discussed in Chapter 80. Important antibacterial drugs are shown in Table 87.8. These drugs are used to treat serious ophthalmic infections and prevent infection after ocular surgery. As a rule, anti-infective drugs are not needed for simple conjunctivitis. Patients should be made aware that bacterial and viral infections are contagious. Bacterial infections will remain contagious until they have been treated for 24 to 48 hours. Viral infections may remain contagious until they are completely gone. Patients should not use contact lenses while they have an eye infection and while they are treating the infection with a topical drug.

Dyes for Evaluation of Eye Problems

Fluorescein is a water-soluble dye that produces an intense green color. This agent is applied to the surface of the eye to detect lesions of the corneal epithelium; intact areas of the cornea remain uncolored, whereas abrasions and other defects turn bright green. Intravenous fluorescein is used to facilitate visualization of retinal blood vessels; intravenous fluorescein has been employed to help evaluate diabetic retinopathy and other abnormalities of the retinal vasculature. Fluorescein can also be used topically and intravenously to assess flow of aqueous humor. Adverse effects from systemic administration include nausea, vomiting, paresthesias, and pruritus. Severe reactions (anaphylaxis, pulmonary edema, and cardiac arrest) are rare.

Rose bengal is applied topically to visualize abrasions of the corneal and conjunctival epithelium. Injured tissue appears rose colored when viewed with a slit lamp. The dye is also employed for the diagnosis of dryness of conjunctival tissue; however, this can be painful.

Lissamine green, another topical dye, turns bright green in the presence of conjunctival defects and dryness. Because it is less likely to cause stinging, it is beginning to replace rose bengal as a diagnostic tool.

88

Drugs for the Skin

When one considers the vast number of skin conditions and the even greater number of pharmacologic agents used in their management, it is easy to see that the topic of dermatologic conditions alone could fill a separate textbook. Our objective is to discuss dermatologic drugs used to manage a select group of conditions commonly managed by nonspecialists. Most are dosed topically; some are given systemically.

ANATOMY OF THE SKIN

Before discussing the dermatologic drugs, it will help to review the anatomy of the skin.

The skin is composed of three distinct layers: the epidermis, the dermis, and a layer of subcutaneous fat.

Epidermis

The epidermis is the outermost layer of the skin and is composed almost entirely of closely packed cells. The epidermis itself consists of several layers. The deepest, known as the *basal layer* or *stratum germinativum*, contains the only epidermal cells that are mitotically active. All cells of the epidermis arise from this layer. Production of new cells within the basal layer pushes older cells outward. During their migration, these cells become smaller and flatter. As epidermal cells near the surface of the skin, they die and their cytoplasm is converted to *keratin*, a hard, proteinaceous material. Because of its high content of keratin, the outer layer of the epidermis has a rough, horny texture. Because of its texture, this layer is referred to as the *cornified layer* or *stratum corneum*. The surface of the stratum corneum undergoes continuous exfoliation (shedding). This shedding completes the epidermal growth cycle.

In addition to germinal cells, the basal layer of the epidermis contains *melanocytes*. These cells, which are few in number, produce *melanin*, the pigment that determines skin color. After its synthesis within melanocytes, melanin is transferred to other cells of the epidermis. Melanin protects the skin against ultraviolet (UV) radiation, which is the principal stimulus for melanin production.

Dermis

The dermis underlies the epidermis and is composed largely of connective tissue, primarily collagen. A major function of the dermis is to provide support and nourishment for the epidermis. Structures found in the dermis include blood vessels, nerves, and muscle. The dermis also contains sweat glands, sebaceous glands, and hair follicles. Sebaceous glands secrete an oily composite known as sebum. Almost all sebaceous glands are associated with hair follicles.

Subcutaneous Tissue

Subcutaneous tissue consists largely of fat. This fatty layer provides protection and insulation. In addition, the stored fat constitutes a reserve source of calories.

TOPICAL DRUG FORMULATIONS

Topical drugs are provided by a number of vehicles. The most popular are ointments, creams, lotions, gels, foams, powders, and pastes.

Ointments are thick, greasy preparations with an oil or petroleum jelly base and little if any water. They provide the highest medication absorption of all formulations. Their enhanced penetration makes them especially useful in the management of conditions with thickened skin (e.g., with lichenification secondary to prolonged scratching) or inflamed skin. Because an ointment provides an occlusive film that retains moisture, it is not a good choice for weeping or oozing skin conditions or in areas prone to heavy perspiration. It is often an excellent choice, however, for dry skin conditions.

A cream is an emulsion of oil and water. Some creams contain more oil than water, whereas others contain more water than oil. This affects the thickness of their consistency and how oily or sticky they feel on the skin. They are not as thick as ointments but thicker than lotions. Creams tend to be good for inflamed skin and dry, sensitive skin. They may or may not be useful for oozing lesions depending on the ratio of water to oil. Creams tend to be more appropriate than ointments for intertriginous areas.

Lotions are water based. Some may contain alcohol or acids, which can cause a burning sensation. They have little if any oil; as a result, they have a lighter feel than creams. Lotions are nongreasy, a feature that tends to promote patient satisfaction. Another advantage of lotions is that they are easy to spread, which makes them a good choice for large and/or hairy areas. They are suitable for intertriginous areas. Unlike ointments and creams, they are suitable for oily skin and may even decrease oiliness depending on the ingredients.

Gels are transparent preparations with a water or alcohol base that usually contain cellulose. They liquefy on skin contact and often have a cooling effect as they dry. Because they are nongreasy and tend to have drying effects, gels are good choices for oily skin. They spread easily, so they are good for covering large or hairy areas. Because they dry clear and invisible, they may be more acceptable for facial regions. They may cause burning, but when this occurs, it is often the fault of the inactive ingredients rather than the medication.

Foams are aerated solutions. They spread easily, dry quickly, and leave negligible residue. They tend to be good choices for oily skin and large and/or hairy areas.

Most powders have a talc or cornstarch base. They are dry, with a silky feel that reduces friction between surfaces. This can make them useful between skin folds. The dryness of the vehicle can be helpful when it is applied to regions that tend to perspire, such as the feet or axillae.

Pastes are mixtures of an ointment and a powder. The addition of a powder increases adherence to the skin. Because the powder disrupts the occlusive nature of an ointment, allowing air to reach the covered skin, most pastes can be used safely in areas that are occluded, as in applying a diaper rash paste to the skin under a diaper.

Topical Glucocorticoids

The basic pharmacology of the glucocorticoids is discussed in Chapter 58. Consideration here is limited to their use for skin disorders.

Actions and Uses

Topical glucocorticoids are employed to relieve inflammation and itching associated with a variety of dermatologic conditions (e.g., insect bites, dermatitis, psoriasis, eczema, pemphigus).

The vehicle in which a glucocorticoid is dispersed (e.g., cream, ointment, gel) can enhance the therapeutic response by helping the glucocorticoid penetrate to its site of action. The vehicle may provide additional benefits by acting as a drying agent or an emollient.

Relative Potency

Glucocorticoid preparations vary widely in potency. As indicated in Table 88.1, these drugs can be assigned to groups that range in potency from low to super high. Preparations within each group are equipotent.

It is important to note that the intensity of the response to topical glucocorticoids depends not only on the concentration and inherent activity of the glucocorticoid but also on the vehicle employed and the method of application. Occlusive dressings can enhance percutaneous absorption by as much as 10-fold, thereby greatly increasing pharmacologic effects.

Absorption

Topical glucocorticoids can be absorbed into the systemic circulation. The extent of absorption is proportional to the duration of use and the surface area covered. Absorption is higher from regions where the skin is especially permeable (axilla, face, eyelids, neck, perineum, genitalia) and lower from regions where penetrability is poor (palms, soles). Absorption through intact skin is lower than through inflamed skin. As noted, absorption is influenced by the vehicle and can be greatly increased by an occlusive dressing.

Adverse Effects

Adverse effects may be local or systemic. Factors that increase the risk for adverse effects include use of a high-potency glucocorticoid, use of an occlusive dressing, prolonged therapy, and application over a large area.

Local reactions. Glucocorticoids increase the risk for local infection and may also produce irritation. With prolonged use, glucocorticoids can cause atrophy of the dermis and epidermis, resulting in thinning of the skin, striae, purpura, and telangiectasias. Long-term therapy may induce acne and hypertrichosis (excessive growth of hair, especially on the face).

Systemic toxicity. Topical glucocorticoids can be absorbed in amounts sufficient to produce systemic toxicity. Principal concerns are growth delay (in children) and adrenal suppression (in all age groups). Systemic toxicity is more likely under extreme conditions of use (prolonged therapy in which a large area is treated with big doses of a high-potency agent covered with an occlusive dressing). When these conditions are present, adrenal suppression can occur.

Administration

Topical glucocorticoids should be applied in a thin film and gently rubbed into the skin. Patients should be advised not to use occlusive dressings (bandages, plastic wraps) unless the prescriber tells them to. Tight-fitting diapers and plastic pants can act as occlusive dressings

and should not be worn when glucocorticoids are applied to the diaper region of infants. The same would be true of adults who wear diapers owing to urinary or bowel incontinence.

Keratolytic Agents

Keratolytic agents are drugs that promote shedding of the stratum corneum. They are used to treat conditions where there is an overgrowth or abnormal thickening of the skin. Effects range from peeling to extensive desquamation of the stratum corneum. Two keratolytic compounds—*salicylic acid* and *sulfur*—are considered next. Other keratolytic drugs are discussed later under "Topical Drugs for Acne."

Salicylic Acid

Salicylic acid promotes desquamation by dissolving the intracellular cement that binds scales to the stratum corneum. Keratolytic effects are achieved with concentrations between 3% and 6%. At concentrations above 6%, tissue injury is likely. Low (3% to 6%) concentrations are used to treat dandruff, seborrheic dermatitis, acne, and psoriasis. Higher concentrations (up to 40%) are used to remove warts and corns.

Salicylic acid is readily absorbed through the skin. Though rare, systemic salicylate toxicity (salicylism) can result when large amounts are used for a prolonged period. Symptoms of salicylism include tinnitus, hyperpnea, and psychologic disturbances. Systemic effects can be minimized by avoiding prolonged use of high concentrations over large areas.

Sulfur

Sulfur promotes peeling and drying. Compounds containing sulfur have been used to treat acne, dandruff, psoriasis, and seborrheic dermatitis. Sulfur is available in lotions, gels, and shampoos. It is commonly combined with salicylic acid for additive effects (e.g., Sebex shampoo). Concentrations range from 2% to 10%.

ACNE

Acne is the most common dermatologic disease. About 85% of teenagers develop acne, which often persists into adulthood. Acne accounts for more visits to dermatologists than any other disorder. In the United States the direct costs of acne exceed $1 billion a year, including about $100 million spent on acne products sold over the counter.

PROTOTYPE DRUGS

Drugs for Acne

Topical Drug for Acne
Benzoyl peroxide
Tretinoin

Oral Drugs for Acne
Isotretinoin
Doxycycline

Pathophysiology

Acne is a chronic skin disorder that usually begins during puberty. It is more common and more severe in males. Lesions typically develop on the face, neck, chest, shoulders, and back. In mild acne, *open comedones* (blackheads) are the most common lesion. A comedo forms when sebum combines with keratin to create a plug within a pore (oxidation of the sebum causes the exposed surface of the plug to turn black). *Closed*

TABLE 88.1   Relative Potency of Topical Glucocorticoids

Potency Class and Drug	Formulation	Concentration
Super-High Potency		
Betamethasone dipropionate (Diprolene)	Ointment, lotion, gel	0.05%
Clobetasol propionate (Clobex, Cormax, Temovate)	Cream, ointment, gel, spray, foam, lotion, shampoo	0.05%
Diflorasone diacetate ointment (Psorcon)	Ointment	0.05%
Fluocinonide (Vanos)	Cream	0.1%
Flurandrenolide (Cordran tape)	Tape	4 mcg/m^2
Halobetasol propionate (Ultravate)	Cream, ointment	0.05%
High Potency		
Amcinonide (Cyclocort)	Cream, ointment, lotion	0.1%
Betamethasone dipropionate (Diprolene, Diprolene AF)	Cream, ointment, lotion	0.05%
Desoximetasone (Topicort)	Cream, ointment, gel, spray	0.5%, 0.25%
Diflorasone diacetate cream (ApexiCon, Florone, Maxiflor, Psorcon)	Cream	0.05%
Fluocinonide (Fluonex, Lidex, Vanos)	Cream, ointment, gel, solution	0.05%
Halcinonide (Halog)	Cream, ointment	0.1%
Triamcinolone acetonide	Ointment	0.5%
Medium to High Potency		
Amcinonide cream (Cyclocort)	Cream	0.1%
Betamethasone dipropionate cream (Diprosone)	Cream	0.05%
Diflorasone diacetate (ApexiCon, Psorcon)	Cream, ointment	0.05%
Fluocinonide emollient cream (Lidex E)	Cream	0.05%
Fluticasone propionate ointment (Cutivate)	Ointment	0.005%
Triamcinolone acetonide ointment (Aristocort A)	Ointment	0.01%
Triamcinolone high-potency cream (Aristocort-HP)	Cream	0.05%
Medium Potency		
Betamethasone dipropionate	Lotion	0.05%
Betamethasone valerate (Beta-Val, Luxiq, Valisone)	Cream, ointment, lotion, foam	0.1%, 0.12%
Clocortolone pivalate (Cloderm)	Cream	0.1%
Desoximetasone (Topicort LP)	Cream, ointment, gel, spray	0.05%
Fluocinolone acetonide (Synalar)	Cream, ointment	0.025%, 0.2%
Flurandrenolide (Cordran, Cordran SP)	Cream, lotion	0.05%
Fluticasone propionate (Cutivate)	Cream	0.05%
Hydrocortisone butyrate (Locoid, Locoid Lipocream)	Cream, ointment, lotion, solution	0.1%
Hydrocortisone valerate (Westcort)	Cream, ointment	0.2%
Mometasone furoate (Elocon)	Cream, ointment, lotion, solution	0.1%
Prednicarbate (Dermatop)	Cream, ointment	0.1%
Triamcinolone acetonide (Kenalog)	Cream, lotion	0.1%
	Ointment	0.025%
	Aerosol	0.2%
Low Potency		
Alclometasone dipropionate (Aclovate)	Cream, ointment	0.05%
Desonide (DesOwen, LoKara, Verdeso)	Cream, ointment, gel, lotion, foam	0.05%
Fluocinolone acetonide (Capex, Synalar)	Cream, oil, shampoo, solution	0.01%
Hydrocortisone acetate (Lanacort 10, U-Cort)	Cream, ointment	1%
Hydrocortisone butyrate (Locoid)	Cream, ointment, lotion, solution	0.1%
Triamcinolone acetonide (Kenalog)	Cream, ointment, lotion	0.025%
Least Potency		
Hydrocortisone (Ala-Cort, Anusol-HC, Cortaid, Cortizone-10, Hytone)	Cream, ointment, lotion	1%, 2.5%

comedones (whiteheads) develop when pores become blocked with sebum and scales below the skin surface. In its most severe form, acne is characterized by abscesses and inflammatory cysts. As a rule, acne begins to improve after puberty and, for some, clears entirely during the early 20s. However, with some people, the disease continues for decades.

Onset of acne is initiated by increased production of androgens during adolescence. Under the influence of androgens, sebum production and the turnover of follicular epithelial cells are increased, leading to plugging of pores. Symptoms are intensified by the activity of *Propionibacterium acnes,* a microbe that converts sebum into irritant fatty acids. This bacterium also releases chemotactic factors that promote inflammation. Oily skin and a genetic predisposition also contribute.

Overview of Treatment

Because acne is a chronic disease, treatment is prolonged. Fortunately, almost all patients respond well. Effective treatment will prevent scarring and limit the duration of symptomatic disease, thereby minimizing the psychologic effects of the disorder.

Nonpharmacologic Therapy

Nonpharmacologic measures can help minimize acne lesions, especially in patients with milder acne. Surface oiliness should be reduced by cleansing with a gentle nonirritant soap a couple of times a day. Care should be taken to avoid irritation from vigorous scrubbing or the use of abrasives. Oil-based makeup or moisturizing products should not be used. Additional measures (e.g., comedo extraction, dermabrasion) may be indicated for some individuals. Research has demonstrated that dietary changes provide no benefit.

Drug Therapy

Drugs for acne fall into two major groups: topical and oral. The topical drugs have two principal subgroups: antibiotics and retinoids. Likewise, the oral drugs have two principal subgroups: antibiotics and retinoids. Occasionally other agents, such as keratolytic agents (e.g., salicylic or azelaic acid) or hormonal agents (e.g., oral contraceptives [OCs]), may be used.

Drug selection is based on symptom severity. For patients with relatively mild symptoms, topical therapy can suffice. When symptoms are more severe, oral therapy is required. *Mild* acne can be managed with *topical* antibiotics and topical retinoids. *Moderate* acne can be treated with *oral* antibiotics (e.g., doxycycline, minocycline) and

comedolytics (retinoids and azelaic acid). In addition, hormonal agents—combination oral contraceptives (OCs) and spironolactone—can be used in young women whose acne is unresponsive to other drugs. The principal agent for *severe* acne is isotretinoin.

Topical Drugs for Acne
Antibiotics

Benzoyl peroxide. Benzoyl peroxide, a first-line drug for mild to moderate acne, is both an antibiotic and keratolytic. Improvement can be seen within days of starting treatment. Benefits derive primarily from suppressing the growth of *P. acnes*. The presumed mechanism is release of active oxygen. In addition to suppressing *P. acnes,* benzoyl peroxide can reduce inflammation and promote keratolysis (peeling of the horny layer of the epidermis).

Unlike other topical antimicrobials, benzoyl peroxide does not promote emergence of resistant *P. acnes.*

The pharmacokinetics of benzoyl peroxide and other antiacne drugs is presented in Table 88.2.

Benzoyl peroxide may produce drying and peeling of the skin. If signs of severe local irritation occur (e.g., burning, blistering, scaling, swelling), the frequency of application should be reduced. (See Table 88.3 for preparations and dosages of antiacne drugs.) Benzoyl peroxide has been associated with potentially serious hypersensitivity reactions, especially in patients with asthma. In Canada, 131 instances of severe allergies experienced by patients using benzoyl peroxide and/or salicylic acid prompted a safety review. In December 2015, Health Canada issued a public warning. Revised drug monographs include information on sensitivity testing. (See http://healthycanadians.gc.ca/recall-alert-rappel-avis/hc-sc/2015/56268a-eng.php.)

Clindamycin and erythromycin. Like benzoyl peroxide, topical clindamycin (Cleocin, Clinda-T, others) and erythromycin (Ery, Erygel, Erysol) suppress growth of *P. acnes*. In addition, these drugs can decrease

TABLE 88.2 Pharmacokinetics of Drugs for the Treatment of Acne

Topical Drugs[a] Drug Class and Drug[b]	Absorption	Metabolism	Elimination
Antibiotics			
Benzoyl peroxide (generic only)	Approximately 5%	Skin—conversion to benzoic acid	Unknown
Clindamycin (Cleocin, Clinda-T, others]	0–3 ng/mL	Hepatic	Urine
Dapsone (Aczone)	0%–1%	Unknown	Unknown
Erythromycin (Ery, Erygel, Erysol)	Unknown	Hepatic	Urine
Retinoids			
Adapalene (Differin)	Trace	Unknown	Bile
Tazarotene (Fabior, Tazorac)	Trace	Unknown	Biliary
Tretinoin (Atralin, Avita, Retin-A, Retin-A Micro, Stieva-A)	Trace	Hepatic	Urine, feces
Keratolytics			
Azelaic acid (Azelex, Finacea ✦)	Trace	Negligible	Urine
Salicylic acid (Stridex pads, Acnomel Acne Mask, others)	Minimal for low-strength acne preparations	Unknown	Urine

Oral Drugs[c] Retinoids	Peak	Protein Binding	Metabolism	Half-Life	Elimination
Isotretinoin (Absorica, Amnesteem, Claravis, Myorisan, Zenatane, Accutane, Clarus, Epuris)	3–5 h	99%–100%	Hepatic (CYP2B6, 2C8, 2C9, 3A4)	21 h	Urine, feces

[a]Systemic absorption of topical drugs is very low when applied as directed, thus the pharmacokinetics table is abbreviated.
[b]For combination agents, see individual drugs.
[c]Pharmacokinetics of oral antibiotics are presented in Unit XVI; pharmacokinetics of hormonal agents are presented in Chapter 50 (for oral contraceptives) and Chapter 36 (for spironolactone).

TABLE 88.3 Preparation, Dosage, and Administration Considerations for Drugs for Acne

Drug or Drug Class	Preparation	Dosage	Administration Considerations
Antibiotics			
Benzoyl peroxide (generic only)	10% cream 5.3%, 9.8% foam 6% foaming cloths 2.5%, 2.75%, 5%, 5.25%, 6.5%, 8%, 10% gel 5%, 8%, 10% lotion 2.5%, 5%, 5.25%, 7%, 10% liquid cleansers Variety of kits containing medicated cleansers and lotion	Cream, foam, gels, lotions: Thin film once daily initially; increase to 2–3 times daily as needed. Cleansers: Wash once or twice daily.	If excessive stinging occurs, wash off medication with mild soap and water then resume use the next day.
Clindamycin (Cleocin, Clinda-T, others)	1% foam, gel, lotion, solution, swab	Thin film once or twice daily.	Foam melts on contact to skin; instruct patient to dispense into cap and then apply to face in sections.
Dapsone (Aczone)	5% gel 7.5% gel	Thin film twice daily. Thin film once daily.	Use with benzoyl peroxide can discolor skin yellow-orange. There is a slight risk that patients with glucose 6-phosphate dehydrogenase (G6PD) deficiency will hematologic effects with topical use.
Erythromycin (Ery, Erygel, Erysol)	2% gel, pads, solution	Gel: Thin film once or twice daily. Pads, solution: Thin film twice daily.	Anticipate a wait of 6–8 weeks before improvement is seen.
Retinoids			
Adapalene (Differin)	0.1% cream, gel, lotion 0.3% gel	Thin film of cream or gel or 3–4 pumps of lotion once daily.	Transient warmth and stinging commonly occur after application. These effects decrease after 2–4 weeks.
Isotretinoin (Absorica, Amnesteem, Claravis, Myorisan, Zenatane, Accutane, Clarus, Epuris)	10 mg, 20 mg, 25 mg, 30 mg, 35 mg, 40 mg	0.5–2 mg/kg per day divided into two doses.	All except Absorica must be taken with meals to increase bioavailability.
Tazarotene (Fabior, Tazorac)	0.05%, 0.1% gel and cream	Thin film once daily in the evening.	Dry skin with itching and burning is more common than with other topical retinoids. Prescribe lower initial doses.
Tretinoin (Atralin, Avita, Retin-A, Retin-A Micro, Stieva-A)	0.02%, 0.025%, 0.0375%, 0.05% cream 0.01%, 0.025%, 0.04%, 0.05%, 0.06%, 0.08% gel	Thin film once daily in the evening.	Products containing alcohol, astringents, spices, or lime should not be used in affected areas to avoid excessive stinging and burning.
Keratolytics			
Azelaic acid (Azelex, Finacea ✦)	20% cream[a] 15% gel 15% foam	Thin film to affected area twice daily.	Decrease to once daily for excessive skin irritation. Improvement should occur within 4 weeks.
Salicylic acid (Stridex pads, Acnomel Acne Mask, others)	0.5%–2%[b] cleanser, creams, gels, lotions, pads, mask	Creams, gels, lotions, and pads: Thin film 1–3 times daily. Cleanser products: 1–2 times daily Mask: 1–2 times weekly.	Cleansers and mask should be rinsed off after use. Decrease number of applications for excessive skin dryness, peeling, or irritation.

[a]Only the cream is approved for acne. The foam and gel are approved for treatment of rosacea.
[b]Formulations greater than 2% are used for other purposes such as wart and callus removal.

inflammation. Monotherapy with either drug quickly leads to resistance. To protect against emergence of resistance, these drugs can be combined with benzoyl peroxide. Two fixed-dose combinations are available: clindamycin/benzoyl peroxide (Acanya, BenzaClin, Clindoxyl ✦) and erythromycin/benzoyl peroxide (Benzamycin).

Dapsone. Dapsone (Aczone) has been used for oral therapy of leprosy for decades. In patients with acne, the drug yields a modest decrease in inflammation and number of lesions. The mechanism of action underlying antiacne benefits has not been established. The most common side effects of dapsone gel are oiliness, peeling, dryness, and erythema. These effects are caused primarily by the gel vehicle and not by dapsone. Like oral dapsone, topical dapsone poses a risk for hemolytic anemia in patients with glucose-6-phosphate dehydrogenase (G6PD) deficiency; however, the risk is slight. Unlike oral dapsone, topical dapsone is not known to cause peripheral neuropathy. Combining dapsone with benzoyl peroxide can turn the skin yellow or orange.

Retinoids

The topical retinoids—derivatives of vitamin A (retinol)—are a cornerstone of acne therapy. These drugs can unplug existing comedones and prevent development of new ones. In addition, they can reduce inflammation and improve penetration of other topical agents. Topical retinoids currently approved for acne use are tretinoin, adapalene, and tazarotene. They may be used alone or in combination with other drugs, including topical and oral antimicrobials. In 2016, adapalene became the first topical retinoid approved for over-the-counter treatment of acne in people aged 12 years and older.

Tretinoin. Topical tretinoin, a derivative of vitamin A, is used for acne and to remove fine wrinkles. Formulations for acne are marketed as Atralin, Avita, Retin-A, and Retin-A Micro. The formulation for wrinkles, which is nearly identical to one of the formulations for acne, is marketed as Refissa and Renova. Topical tretinoin should not be confused with isotretinoin, a powerful *oral* antiacne medicine (discussed later in this chapter) or with the oral form of tretinoin, which is approved for remission induction of acute promyelocytic leukemia but not for skin conditions.

Use for acne. Tretinoin is approved for the topical treatment of mild to moderate acne. Benefits derive from normalizing the hyperproliferation of epithelial cells within hair follicles. Tretinoin also causes thinning of the stratum corneum and can thereby facilitate penetration of other drugs. Therapeutic effects can be enhanced by combining tretinoin with benzoyl peroxide, topical antibiotics, and oral antibiotics.

Use for fine wrinkles. Tretinoin is approved for reducing fine wrinkles, tactile roughness, and mottled hyperpigmentation ("liver spots," age spots) in facial skin. Benefits may derive from suppressing genes that code for specific proteases that break down collagen and elastin. In clinical trials, responses to tretinoin were modest. In fact, many patients achieved equivalent effects with a program of comprehensive skin care and sun protection. It is important to appreciate that tretinoin does *not* repair deep, coarse wrinkles and other damage caused by chronic sun exposure. Furthermore, the drug does not reverse photoaging or restore the microscopic structure of skin to a more youthful pattern. Benefits in patients older than 50 years have not been established.

Adverse effects. Tretinoin can cause *localized* reactions, but absorption is insufficient to cause systemic toxicity. In patients with sensitive skin, tretinoin may induce blistering, peeling, crusting, burning, and edema. These effects can be intensified by concurrent use of abrasive soaps and keratolytic agents (e.g., sulfur, resorcinol, benzoyl peroxide, salicylic acid). Accordingly, these preparations should be discontinued before beginning tretinoin therapy. Skin reactions with two formulations—Avita and Retin-A Micro—may be less intense than those caused by Retin-A, an older formulation.

Tretinoin increases susceptibility to sunburn. Patients should be warned to apply a sunscreen with a sun protection factor (SPF) of 15 or greater and to wear protective clothing. Patients with existing sunburn should not apply the drug.

Adapalene. Adapalene (Differin) is a topical antiacne drug similar to tretinoin. Through actions in the cell nucleus, adapalene modulates inflammation, epithelial keratinization, and differentiation of follicular cells. As a result, the drug reduces formation of comedones and inflammatory lesions. Benefits take 8 to 12 weeks to develop. During the early weeks, adapalene may appear to exacerbate acne by affecting previously invisible lesions. In clinical trials, 0.1% adapalene gel was as effective as 0.025% tretinoin gel in reducing the total number of comedones, and it was more effective than tretinoin in reducing the total number of acne lesions and inflammatory lesions.

Tazarotene. Tazarotene (Avage, Fabior, Tazorac) is indicated for topical therapy of acne, wrinkles, and psoriasis. (Avage has approval for treatment of wrinkles, mottled complexions, and and benign facial lentigines, but not for acne.) Like tretinoin and adapalene, tazarotene is a derivative of vitamin A.

Keratolytic Agents

As mentioned earlier, keratolytic agents promote shedding of the outermost layer of the epidermal skin cells. Keratolytic drugs used to treat acne include benzoyl peroxide, the combination antibiotic and keratolytic agent discussed earlier, azelaic acid, and salicylic acid.

Azelaic acid. Azelaic acid (Azelex, Finacea ✤) is a topical keratolytic drug for the treatment of mild to moderate acne. It is also commonly prescribed for rosacea, a condition with some similarities to acne. Azelaic acid appears to work by suppressing the growth of *P. acnes* and decreasing the proliferation of keratinocytes, thereby decreasing the thickness of the stratum corneum. In clinical trials, topical azelaic acid (20% cream) was as effective as 5% benzoyl peroxide, 0.05% tretinoin, or 2% erythromycin. For severe acne, azelaic acid was much less effective than oral isotretinoin. Adverse effects—which are uncommon and less intense than with tretinoin or benzoyl peroxide—include pruritus, burning, stinging, tingling, and erythema. Azelaic acid may reduce pigmentation in patients with dark complexions, so people using this product should be monitored for hypopigmentation.

Salicylic acid. Salicylic acid is another topical keratolytic drug for mild to moderate acne. Adverse effects such as local irritation and peeling are usually mild, but Health Canada has issued safety alerts regarding the association between salicylic acid and severe allergic reactions. Salicylate toxicity is not a problem when it is applied only to the face; however, if acne is extensive and the drug is applied to the trunk, back, and other locations, this could possibly occur. Monitoring for signs and symptoms of salicylism (e.g., hyperpnea, tinnitus, nausea and vomiting, and mental status changes) is indicated.

PATIENT EDUCATION

Topical Drugs for Acne

- Topical anti-acne drugs can increase the risk for sunburn; avoid exposure to sunlight, sunlamps, and tanning beds during treatment.
- Avoid irritant soaps and scrubs.
- Wash and dry skin before applying medication and then wash hands afterward.
- Keep the drug away from the eyes, mouth, and mucous membranes as well as inflamed, denuded, or sunburned skin.
- Some drying, slight burning, and peeling is expected; however, report severe irritation such as blistering, intense burning, or swelling. A dosage adjustment or a different drug may be necessary.
- Dapsone: Do not use with benzoyl peroxide to avoid skin discoloration.
- Tretinoin: Women who may become pregnant must strictly adhere to their birth control regimens.

Oral Drugs for Acne
Antibiotics

Oral antibiotics are used to treat moderate to severe acne. These drugs suppress the growth of *P. acnes* and directly suppress inflammation. Oral antibiotics can be combined with a topical retinoid.

Doxycycline (Vibramycin, others) and minocycline (Minocin, others) are considered agents of choice. Tetracycline (generic) and erythromycin (Ery-Tab, others) are alternatives, but resistance to these drugs, which are discussed in Chapter 73, is common. With all antibiotics, benefits develop slowly, taking 3 to 6 months to become maximal. After symptoms have been controlled with an oral antibiotic, patients should switch to a topical antibiotic for long-term maintenance.

Isotretinoin

Actions and use. Isotretinoin (Accutane, Amnesteem, Claravis, others), a derivative of vitamin A, is used to treat *severe nodulocystic acne vulgaris,* a condition for which this drug is highly effective. For most patients, a single course of therapy can produce complete and prolonged remission. Because isotretinoin can cause serious side effects, its use is restricted to patients with severe, disfiguring acne that has not responded to more conventional agents, including oral antibiotics.

Isotretinoin has several actions that may contribute to antiacne effects. The drug decreases sebum production, sebaceous gland size, inflammation, and keratinization. In addition, by decreasing the availability of sebum, a nutrient for *P. acnes,* isotretinoin lowers the skin population of this microbe.

The pharmacokinetics of this and other drugs for acne is provided in Table 88.2.

 BLACK BOX WARNING

Isotretinoin

> Isotretinoin carries a high risk of severe structural and cognitive defects in the developing fetus. It is also associated with an increased risk for spontaneous abortion.

Adverse effects

Physical effects. The most common reactions are nosebleeds (80%), inflammation of the lips (90%); inflammation of the eyes (40%); and dryness or itching of the skin, nose, and mouth (80%). About 15% of patients experience pain, tenderness, or stiffness in muscles, bones, and joints. Among pediatric patients, nearly 30% experience back pain. Premature epiphyseal closure may also be a problem for those who are still growing. Other reactions include skin rash, headache, hair loss, and peeling of skin from the palms and soles. Reduction in night vision has occurred, sometimes with sudden onset. The skin may become sensitized to UV light, thus increasing the risk for sunburn. Isotretinoin increases the risk for several significant problems including pseudotumor cerebri (benign elevation of intracranial pressure), pancreatitis, hearing impairment (with or without tinnitus), decreased bone mineral density, and mental health changes, including depression with suicidal ideation. A 2017 safety alert from Health Canada noted identification of a possible association between isotretinoin and erectile dysfunction.

Triglyceride levels may become elevated. Alcohol can potentiate hypertriglyceridemia and should be avoided.

Depression. Isotretinoin may pose a risk for depression and suicide, although proof of a causal relationship is lacking. Nonetheless, because the potential consequences of depression are severe, steps should be taken to minimize risk. Accordingly, providers should ask patients to report signs of depression (e.g., depressed mood, loss of interest or pleasure) or thoughts of suicide. If these occur, isotretinoin should be withdrawn and psychiatric evaluation considered.

Drug interactions. Adverse effects of isotretinoin can be increased by *tetracyclines* and *vitamin A.* Tetracyclines increase the risk for pseudotumor cerebri and papilledema. Vitamin A, a close relative of isotretinoin, can produce generalized intensification of isotretinoin toxicity. Because of the potential for increased toxicity, tetracyclines and vitamin A supplements should be discontinued before isotretinoin therapy.

Contraindication: pregnancy. Isotretinoin is teratogenic and must not be used during pregnancy. Major fetal abnormalities that have occurred include hydrocephalus, microcephaly, facial malformation, cleft palate, cardiovascular defects, and abnormal formation of the outer ear.

iPLEDGE program. iPLEDGE is a very strict risk management program designed to ensure that no woman starting isotretinoin *is*

Isotretinoin

- This drug may affect vision in the dark; therefore avoid driving at night if this affects you.
- You may sunburn easily; protect skin from sunlight and avoid sunlamps and tanning beds.
- Your provider will need you to come in periodically for blood tests and other assessments.
- Women who can become pregnant should use two kinds of reliable birth control. Notify your provider if you miss a period.
- You cannot donate blood while taking this drug and for 1 month after you stop.
- Avoid supplements containing vitamin A.
- Avoid alcohol.
- Scarring may occur if you have cosmetic skin procedures while taking this drug and up to 6 months after stopping. Avoid waxing, laser therapy, dermabrasion, or similar procedures.
- It is important to notify your provider of *any* new problems that develop while taking this drug. It is especially important to report the following:
  - Severe headaches, vision changes (other than decreased night vision), vomiting, weakness, or seizures. These may be signs of increased pressure in the brain.
  - Symptoms of depression or thoughts of harming yourself or others.
  - Problems obtaining or maintaining an erection.

pregnant and that no woman taking isotretinoin *becomes* pregnant. Under iPLEDGE, all transactions involving isotretinoin must be processed through a *central automated system,* which tracks and verifies critical elements that control access to the drug. The program has rules that apply to the prescriber, patient, pharmacist, and wholesaler. Details regarding iPLEDGE are available online at www.ipledgeprogram.com.

Requirements for female patients. Each patient must receive oral and written warnings about the high risk for fetal harm if isotretinoin is taken during pregnancy.

Pregnancy must be ruled out before the initial prescription and again before each monthly refill. Before the initial prescription, the patient must undergo *two* pregnancy tests, both of which must be negative. For the monthly refills, only one negative test result is required.

Each patient must use *two* effective forms of birth control, even if one of them is tubal ligation or vasectomy of the male partner. In addition, the patient must review educational material, provided through iPLEDGE, on contraceptive methods, possible reasons for contraceptive failure, and the importance of using effective contraception while taking a teratogenic drug. Birth control measures must be implemented at least 1 month before starting isotretinoin and must continue at least 1 month after stopping. Birth control is not required after hysterectomy or for women who commit to total abstinence from sexual intercourse.

Each patient must sign the Patient Information/Informed Consent document, designed to reinforce the benefits and risks of isotretinoin use.

Each patient must be registered with iPLEDGE by her prescriber and must contact iPLEDGE (through the Internet or by phone) before starting treatment, once a month during treatment, and, finally, 1 month after stopping treatment. At each contact, the patient must answer questions on program requirements and must indicate her two chosen methods of birth control.

Requirements for prescribers. Prescribers must register with iPLEDGE and must agree to follow key points of the iPLEDGE program, as described in the *iPLEDGE Program Guide to Best Practices for Isotretinoin.* Also, the prescriber must register each patient with iPLEDGE, enter the results of each monthly pregnancy test, and indicate what methods of contraception the patient is using. The initial prescription for isotretinoin and each monthly refill must be entered into the iPLEDGE system.

 SUMMARY OF KEY PRESCRIBING CONSIDERATIONS

Isotretinoin

Therapeutic Goal: To control acne, decrease the number of nodular lesions, and decrease or prevent scarring.

Baseline Data: Complete blood count with white cell differential, glucose, lipid panel, liver function tests. Assess vision and mental health status. Check height of patients under 18 years of age.

Monitoring: Check lipids and liver function at least every 2 weeks initially then decrease once stable. For women who can become pregnant, verify adherence to birth control measures at every visit. Ask about changes in vision and hearing, pain, nausea, alterations in mood, or other concerns and follow up with targeted assessment as indicated.

Identifying High-Risk Patients: These include women who can become pregnant and are not capable of or committed to strict adherence to birth control measures, younger patients who have not reached full height, patients with a history of diabetes or hyperlipidemia, and patients with a history of depression or other mental illness.

Evaluating Therapeutic Effects: Assess for decrease of nodular lesions and skin improvement.

Minimizing Adverse Effects: Advise patients to avoid prolonged exposure to sunlight. If vision is decreased in the dark, have them increase ambient light in the home and avoid driving at night. Discontinue if the patient becomes pregnant; develops depression, aggression, or other mood disturbance; develops papilledema or other signs or symptoms of pseudotumor cerebri (and refer to neurologist); develops evidence of hepatitis or has elevated liver enzymes that do not normalize; has significant hyperlipidemia that is uncontrolled with treatment.

Hormonal Agents

Hormonal therapies can be used for acne in young women. Combination OCs and spironolactone are the main agents employed. In both cases, benefits derive from decreasing androgen activity, leading to decreased production of sebum.

Oral contraceptives. Four combination OCs—Estrostep, Ortho Tri-Cyclen, Beyaz, and YAZ—are approved for managing acne in women. Treatment is limited to females at least 15 years of age who want contraception, have reached menarche, and have not responded to topical drugs. Acne may take 6 or more months to improve. Benefits are due primarily to the *estrogen* in combination OCs, not the progestin. Two mechanisms are involved: (1) suppression of ovarian androgen production and (2) increased production of *sex hormone–binding globulin*, a protein that binds androgens and thereby renders them inactive. By decreasing androgen availability, estrogens decrease production of sebum. Although only four OCs are approved for acne, all estrogen-containing OCs should work. Accordingly, selection among them should be based primarily on tolerability.

Spironolactone. Spironolactone (Aldactone) blocks a variety of steroid receptors, including those for aldosterone and sex hormones. Blockade of aldosterone receptors underlies the drug's use as a diuretic (see Chapter 37) as well as its use in heart failure (see Chapter 42). Blockade of androgen receptors underlies benefits in females with acne. As a rule, spironolactone is added to the regimen after an OC has proved inadequate. This sequence makes sense because spironolactone is teratogenic, and hence contraception should be implemented before

taking the drug. Adverse effects include menstrual irregularities, breast tenderness, and hyperkalemia.

In 2016, the American Academy of Dermatology published *Guidelines of Care for the Management of Acne Vulgaris*. Their algorithm for acne management is included in this chapter (Fig. 88.1). The complete guidelines are available online at https://www.aad.org/File%20Library/Main%20navigation/Practice%20tools/Quality%20care%20and%20guidelines/Acne-guideline.pdf.

PATIENT-CENTERED CARE ACROSS THE LIFE SPAN

Antiacne Drugs

Life Stage	Considerations or Concerns
Children	Retinoids are not recommended for children younger than 12 years of age with the exception of Atralin, a brand name tretinoin gel for which labeling specifies use for patients age 10 years and older. Benzoyl peroxide, sulfacetamide, dapsone, azelaic acid, salicylic acid are recommended for age 12 and older. Hormone therapy for acne is not recommended for prepubertal children.
Pregnant women	Benzoyl peroxide and topical salicylic acid are preferred over other agents for pregnant women. Both are available over the counter. Retinoids are teratogens. Absence of pregnancy should be verified prior to use. Both oral and topical dapsone are associated with complications in the neonate, including hyperbilirubinemia, methemoglobinemia, and hemolysis. Animal reproduction studies using azelaic acid identified a potential for adverse effects; however, the amount of systemic absorption is minimal. Hormone therapy should not be prescribed for women who are pregnant.
Breastfeeding women	The amount of retinoids, benzoyl peroxide, dapsone, and salicylic acid excreted in breast milk is unknown. Caution is advised by the manufacturers. The excretion of systemic sulfonamides in breast milk has caused kernicterus in breastfed neonates. Topical sulfacetamide poses a risk for this complication if sufficient amounts are absorbed. Manufacturer labeling for azelaic acid gel and foam discourages breastfeeding by patients using this drug; however, the manufacturer of the cream urges caution. Hormone therapy may decrease milk production and protein content.[a]
Older adults	The safety and efficacy of some of these drugs, especially the retinoids, have not been established in older populations for whom anti-acne medication is not usually indicated. There are no special requirements for benzoyl peroxide, sulfacetamide, dapsone, azelaic acid, and salicylic acid. Hormone therapy for the purpose of acne treatment is not recommended for older adults.

Life-span considerations for common antibiotics is provided in Unit XVI.
[a]According to the American Academy of Pediatrics, use of combination oral contraceptives is compatible with breastfeeding.

Diagnosis of acne			
	Mild	Moderate	Severe
First-line treatment	Benzoyl peroxide (BP) or topical retinoid -or- Topical combination therapy[a] BP + antibiotic or retinoid + BP or retinoid + BP + antibiotic	Topical combination therapy[a] BP + antibiotic or retinoid + BP or retinoid + BP + antibiotic -or- Oral antibiotic + topical retinoid + BP -or- Oral antibiotic + topical retinoid + BP + topical antibiotic	Oral antibiotic + Topical combination therapy[a] BP + antibiotic or retinoid + BP or retinoid + BP + antibiotic -or- Oral isotretinoin
Alternative treatment	Add topical retinoid or BP (if not on already) -or- Consider alternate retinoid -or- Consider topical dapsone	Consider alternate combination therapy -or- Consider change in oral antibiotic -or- Add combined oral contraceptive or oral spironolactone (females) -or- Consider oral isotretinoin	Consider change in oral antibiotic -or- Add combined oral contraceptive or oral spironolactone (females) -or- Consider oral isotretinoin

Fig. 88.1 Treatment of Acne Vulgaris. [a]The drug may be prescribed as a fixed combination product or as separate component. *BP,* Benzoyl peroxide. (From Zaenglein, A. L., Pathy, A. L., Schlosser, B. J., Alikhan, A., Baldwin, H. E., Berson, D. S., et al. (2016) Guidelines of care for the management of acne vulgaris. *Journal of the American Academy of Dermatology, 74,* 945-973. Available at https://www.jaad.org/article/S0190-9622(15)02614-6/pdf.)

SUNSCREENS

Sunlight causes a variety of harmful dermatologic effects. These include sunburns, premature aging of the skin, skin cancer, and immunosuppression. Sun exposure can also induce photosensitivity reactions to drugs. All of these effects are caused by UV radiation, and all can be greatly reduced by using a sunscreen.

Dermatologic Effects of Ultraviolet Radiation

Solar UV radiation that reaches the earth's surface is classified by wavelength into two basic types: ultraviolet B (UVB) and ultraviolet A (UVA). Most (95%) of this UV radiation is UVA.

The dermatologic effects of UVA and UVB differ. UVA penetrates the epidermis and deep into the dermis. In contrast, UVB penetrates into the epidermis but goes no deeper. Tanning and sunburn are caused primarily by UVB. Because UVA penetrates much deeper than UVB, UVA is the primary cause of immunosuppression, photosensitive drug reactions, and photoaging of the skin (wrinkling, thickening, yellowing, breakdown of elastic fibers). Both UVA and UVB promote damage to DNA, hence both can cause premalignant actinic keratoses, basal cell carcinoma, squamous cell carcinoma, and malignant and nonmalignant melanoma.

Benefits of Sunscreens

Sunscreens impede penetration of UV radiation to viable cells of the skin. As a result, sunscreens can protect against many harmful effects of UV radiation.

Compounds Employed as Sunscreens

There are two categories of sunscreens: *organic* screens (also known as *chemical* screens) and *inorganic* screens (also known as *physical* screens). Organic screens *absorb* UV radiation and then dissipate it as heat. Inorganic screens *scatter* UV radiation. At this time, 17 compounds are approved by the U.S. Food and Drug Administration (FDA) for use as sunscreens (Fig. 88.2).

Organic (Chemical) Screens

Most (15) of the approved sunscreens are organic. Almost all of them absorb UVB, but only six absorb UVA. Of these six, five absorb UVA2, and only one—*avobenzone*—absorbs UVA1. Therefore to provide protection against the full range of UV radiation, products must contain a mixture of compounds, one of which must be avobenzone.

Inorganic (Physical) Screens

Physical screens act primarily as barriers to the sun's rays. Hence rather than absorbing solar radiation, they *reflect and scatter* sunlight, thereby preventing penetration to the skin. Only two agents are employed as physical screens: *titanium dioxide* and *zinc oxide.* Preparations containing these compounds are especially useful for protecting limited areas (e.g., nose, lips, tips of ears). In the formulations used today, titanium dioxide and zinc oxide are "micronized." As a result, unlike older formulations, which were white, they are clear when applied to the skin.

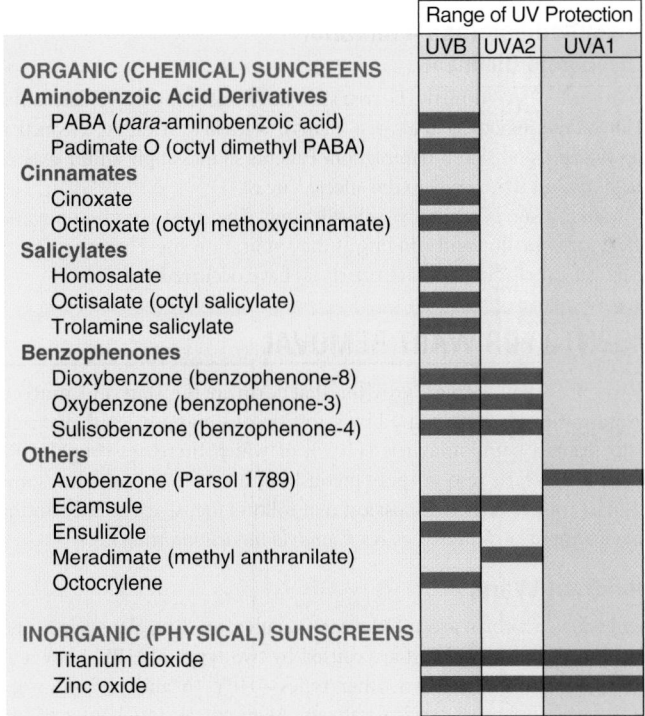

Fig. 88.2 Range of ultraviolet B and ultraviolet A protection conferred by sunscreens that have been approved by the U.S. food and drug administration. *UV*, ultraviolet.

Sun Protection Factor

All sunscreen products are labeled with an SPF. The SPF is an index of protection against UVB. The SPF says nothing about protection against UVA.

The relationship between SPF and protection against sunburn is not linear. That is, an SPF of 30 does not indicate twice as much protection as an SPF of 15. In fact, as the SPF increases, the increment in protection gets progressively smaller. For example, SPF 15 indicates 93% block of UVB, SPF 30 indicates 96.7% block, and SPF 40 indicates 97.5% block. Because SPF values above 30 provide only a small additional benefit, the FDA no longer allows companies to advertise high SPF values (e.g., SPF 80). Instead, products with an SPF greater than 50 can be labeled only as SPF 50+.

Range of Ultraviolet Protection and Sun Protection Factor

All sunscreens protect against UVB radiation, but only some protect against UVA. Products that protect against UVA *and* UVB are labeled with the words *broad spectrum*. Product labeling allows consumers to distinguish between three basic groups of sunscreens:

- *Highly protective*—Broad-spectrum sunscreens with an SPF of 15 or higher. These protect against sunburn, skin cancer, and photoaging.
- *Moderately protective*—Broad-spectrum sunscreens with an SPF of 2 to 14. These protect against sunburn but do not protect against skin cancer and photoaging.
- *Least protective*—Sunscreens with UVB protection only. These protect against sunburn but do not protect against skin cancer and photoaging.

Moderately protective and least protective sunscreens must also carry a warning that they do not protect against skin cancer or photoaging.

Water and Sweat Resistance

Sunscreens can no longer claim to be *waterproof* or *sweatproof*. Rather, they can claim to be *water resistant* or *sweat resistant*. Furthermore, they must indicate how long the resistance lasts, as determined by laboratory testing. Products that retain their SPF after 40 minutes of water exposure will be labeled *Water Resistant 40 Minutes*. Products that retain their water resistance after 80 minutes will be labeled *Water Resistant 80 Minutes*. Regardless of the stated duration of water and sweat resistance, the label must advise reapplication after swimming or sweating.

DRUGS FOR ATOPIC DERMATITIS (ECZEMA)

Atopic dermatitis, also known as eczema, is a chronic inflammatory skin disease. The condition is characterized by dry, scaly skin and intense pruritus that often leads to scratching and rubbing, which in turn can lead to erythema, abrasions, rash, erosions with an exudate, and increased susceptibility to skin infection. Continued scratching will typically result in lichenification of the affected skin. The underlying cause is abnormal activity of T lymphocytes. First-line therapy consists of moisturizers (e.g., Cetaphil Moisturizing Cream, Eucerin Original Cream) and topical glucocorticoids. Unfortunately, the glucocorticoids can cause skin atrophy, hypopigmentation, telangiectasias (permanent focal red lesions), and, in high doses, possible systemic effects, including adrenal suppression. If topical glucocorticoids are insufficient, patients may be treated with a topical immunosuppressant (see later). A sedating antihistamine can help to control itching and facilitate sleeping at night.

Topical Immunosuppressants

Two topical immunosuppressants—tacrolimus and pimecrolimus—are approved for atopic dermatitis. Both drugs are calcineurin inhibitors. Although effective against atopic dermatitis, both drugs may pose a risk for skin cancer and lymphoma. Because of this potential for serious harm, tacrolimus and pimecrolimus are considered second-line drugs for atopic dermatitis and should be reserved for patients who have not responded to glucocorticoids.

Tacrolimus Ointment

Tacrolimus (Protopic) is available as an ointment for moderate to severe atopic dermatitis. The drug relieves symptoms by attenuating local immune responses. Specifically, the drug inhibits calcineurin and thereby suppresses the activity of T cells and decreases the release of inflammatory mediators from cutaneous mast cells and basophils. The result is reduced inflammation.

Systemic absorption of topical tacrolimus is low, and it gets even lower as the skin heals. Absolute bioavailability is less than 0.05%. Blood levels of tacrolimus are usually low.

Tacrolimus ointment is generally well tolerated. The most common side effects are erythema, pruritus, and a burning sensation at the application site. As the skin heals, these local reactions abate. In children, tacrolimus may increase the risk for varicella zoster virus infection. Adverse effects associated with systemic tacrolimus (nephrotoxicity, neurotoxicity, hypertension, diarrhea, nausea) have not occurred with topical therapy. Unlike topical glucocorticoids, tacrolimus does not cause thinning of the skin.

There is concern that tacrolimus may pose a risk for cancer. The drug increases the incidence of skin cancer in laboratory animals exposed to UV light. In mice, tacrolimus increases the incidence of lymphoma. There have been reports of skin cancer and lymphoma in humans, although a causal relationship has not been established. To reduce any risk for skin cancer, patients should protect treated areas from direct sunlight and should avoid sunlamps and tanning beds.

Tacrolimus ointment (Protopic) is available in two concentrations: 0.03% and 0.1%. Adults may use either formulation; children 2 to 16 years of age should use the 0.03% formulation; and children younger than 2 years should not use the drug. All patients should apply a thin layer twice daily. Occlusive dressings should be avoided. Treatment should be intermittent or short term.

Pimecrolimus Cream

Pimecrolimus 1% cream (Elidel) is a topical immunosuppressant approved for mild to moderate atopic dermatitis. The drug is very similar to tacrolimus with regard to mechanism, therapeutic effects, and adverse effects. In clinical trials, twice-daily application for 3 weeks reduced signs and symptoms of eczema by 72%. Initial improvement could be seen in 2 days. Pimecrolimus may be less effective than topical glucocorticoids. Although studies comparing pimecrolimus directly with tacrolimus have not been done, the clinical efficacy of the drugs appears to be similar.

Pimecrolimus is generally well tolerated. The most common adverse effects are erythema, pruritus, and burning sensations at the application site, especially during the first few days of treatment. As with tacrolimus, there have been reports of skin cancer and lymphoma, but a causal relationship has not been established. Like tacrolimus, pimecrolimus sensitizes the skin to UV light; hence patients should use a sunscreen and should limit exposure to natural and artificial sunlight. Systemic absorption of pimecrolimus is minimal; in clinical trials, blood levels were at or below the limit of detection. As with tacrolimus, prolonged treatment should be avoided.

PATIENT-CENTERED CARE ACROSS THE LIFE SPAN

Drugs for Actinic Keratoses and Atopic Dermatis

Life Stage	Considerations or Concerns
Children	Imiquimod is approved for children 12 years of age or older. Tacrolimus, pimecrolimus, and crisaborole are approved for children 2 years of age and older.
Pregnant women	Animal reproduction studies yielded abnormalities for imiquimod and tacrolimus but not for pimecrolimus.
Breastfeeding women	Breastfeeding is not recommended for patients receiving therapy with tacrolimus, and pimecrolimus. Labeling recommends caution for those taking imiquimod.
Older adults	No age-specific precautions were listed for drugs used to treat these conditions.

Phosphodiesterase 4 Inhibitor
Crisaborole Ointment

Crisaborole 2% ointment (Eucrisa) is a novel agent for atopic dermatitis. It inhibits phosphodiesterase type 4 (PDE4), which in turn leads to a reduction in cytokines and skin inflammation. Patients should apply a thin layer of the ointment twice-daily to the affected areas.

Crisaborole is generally well tolerated. The most common adverse effects are burning and stinging at the application site. Hypersensitivity reactions, including contact urticaria, have occurred.

AGENTS FOR WART REMOVAL

Warts are small, benign growths that form in the skin and mucous membranes. They are caused by infection of squamous epithelial cells with human papillomavirus (HPV), of which there are roughly 100 types. Most warts resolve spontaneously within a few months, but some can last for years. The discussion that follows focuses primarily on the management of venereal warts (Condyloma acuminatum).

Venereal Warts

Venereal warts form around the cervix, vulva, urethra, glans penis, and anus and anal canal. Most are caused by two types of HPV, known as HPV-6 and HPV-11. Two other types—HPV-16 and HPV-18—are responsible for most cervical cancers. As discussed in Chapter 55, an HPV vaccine, sold as Gardasil 9, can protect against all four HPV types as well as HPV-31, 33, 45, 52, and 58, and hence can help prevent venereal warts as well as cancer of the cervix.

Infection with HPV can be transmitted by sexual contact. Individuals with anogenital warts should be warned that they can transmit the infection to sexual partners. Partners of infected individuals should be examined for warts. Using a condom can reduce the risk for transmission.

Genital warts can be removed in two basic ways: with topical drugs or with physical measures such as cryotherapy (freezing), electrodesiccation (destruction with an electric current), laser surgery, and conventional surgery. Physical measures are much faster than drugs but also more painful. Neither drugs nor physical measures can eradicate the virus because, even after successful wart removal, the virus remains. Treatments for genital warts are shown in Table 88.4.

The drugs used to remove venereal warts can be divided into two groups: agents that must be administered by a health care provider and agents that can be applied at home. With both groups, application is done repeatedly until the warts disappear. Provider-applied drugs are podophyllin, trichloroacetic acid (TCA), and bichloroacetic acid (BCA). Drugs for home application are podofilox, imiquimod, and kunecatechins (sinecatechins). All of these drugs act slowly, and all cause local irritation. The pharmacology of six topical drugs is discussed later.

Provider-Applied Drugs

Podophyllin. Podophyllin (podophyllum resin) (Podocon-25, Podofilm ♣) is used primarily for perianal and venereal warts. The drug is not very effective against common warts. Podophyllin is a mixture of resins from the May apple or mandrake (Podophyllum peltatum Linne). The active ingredient in the resin is podophyllotoxin, a compound that inhibits DNA synthesis and mitosis. These actions eventually lead to cell death and erosion of warty tissue. Formulations employed to remove warts contain 25% podophyllum resin. These preparations are highly caustic and should be applied only by a trained clinician. To minimize the risk for toxicity from systemic absorption, the resin should be washed off with alcohol or soap and water a few hours after application. Each treatment should be limited to a small surface area and to a small number of warts.

Podophyllin can be absorbed in amounts sufficient to cause systemic toxicity. Potential reactions include central and peripheral neuropathy,

TABLE 88.4   Treatment and Prevention of Venereal Warts

Treatment

External genital	*Patient administered:*
	Podofilox 0.5% solution or gel (topical) *or*
	Imiquimod 3.75% or 5% cream (topical) *or*
	Kunecatechins (sinecatechins) 15% ointment (topical)
	Provider administered:
	Cryotherapy with liquid nitrogen or cryoprobe *or*
	Podophyllin 10%–25% (topical) *or*
	TCA or BCA 80%–90% (topical) *or*
	Surgical excision.
Anal	Cryotherapy with liquid nitrogen *or*
	TCA or BCA (80%–90%) applied to warts *or*
	Surgical excision.
Vaginal	Cryotherapy with liquid nitrogen *or*
	TCA or BCA (80%–90%) applied to warts.
Urethral meatus	Cryotherapy with liquid nitrogen *or*
	Podophyllin resin 10%–25% (topical).

Prevention

All sites	Gardasil 9 vaccine: protects against HPV-6 and HPV-11, which cause 90% of venereal warts, as well as HPV-16 and HPV-18, which cause 70% of cervical cancers.

BCA, Bichloroacetic acid; *HPV*, human papillomavirus; *TCA*, trichloroacetic acid

kidney damage, and blood dyscrasias. These effects are most likely when the drug is applied to large areas in excessive amounts. Podophyllin is teratogenic and must not be used during pregnancy.

Podophyllin is supplied in a 25% solution for topical use. Application should be limited to small areas. The drug should not be applied to moles or birthmarks, nor should it be applied to warts that are bleeding or friable or that have undergone recent biopsy. When used to remove venereal warts, podophyllin should be washed off 1 to 4 hours after application. Treatment may be repeated at weekly intervals for up to 4 weeks.

Bichloroacetic acid and trichloroacetic acid. When applied in high concentration (80% to 90%), BCA and TCA can destroy warts by chemical coagulation. Application is repeated weekly if needed. Solutions of these acids are very watery and hence can easily spread to and thereby injure surrounding tissue. To minimize spread, the solution should be allowed to dry before the patient sits or stands. If pain develops, BCA and TCA can be neutralized with liquid soap or sodium bicarbonate (baking soda). If too much solution is applied, it should be neutralized with soap or sodium bicarbonate or removed by applying talc.

Patient-Applied Drugs

Patient-applied drugs are used for topical therapy of external genital and perianal warts. Like podophyllin, these drugs require a prescription. Because they are applied at home, they are more convenient than the provider-applied drugs.

Imiquimod. Imiquimod cream (Aldara, Zyclara) stimulates production of interferon alpha, tumor necrosis factor (TNF), and several interleukins and thereby intensifies immune responses to HPV, the virus that causes venereal warts. Imiquimod has no direct antiviral effects of its own. Principal adverse effects are erythema, erosion, and flaking at the site of administration. Local itching, burning, and pain may also occur. Imiquimod undergoes minimal absorption, and hence systemic effects are usually absent.

Imiquimod cream is available in two formulations: a 3.75% cream sold as Zyclara and a 5% cream sold as Aldara. Zyclara is applied once a day for up to 8 weeks; Aldara is applied 3 times a week for up to 16 weeks. Both formulations are applied at bedtime and washed off in the morning. Imiquimod use for actinic keratoses was discussed earlier.

Podofilox. As with podophyllin, podofilox (Condylox) inhibits mitosis. Whether this action underlies beneficial effects (erosion of warty tissue) is unknown. Podofilox is supplied as a 0.5% gel or 0.5% solution to be applied twice daily for 3 consecutive days followed by 4 days off. This pattern is repeated four times or until the warts are gone, whichever comes first. Patients should wash their hands before and after applying the drug. However, unlike imiquimod, podofilox need not be washed from the site of application. Treatment frequently causes local inflammation, burning, erosion, pain, itching, and bleeding. These can be minimized by limiting the application area to 10 cm^2, applying no more than 0.5 g/d, and avoiding application to normal skin. Podofilox causes more discomfort than imiquimod but works faster and costs less.

Kunecatechins (sinecatechins) ointment. Kunecatechins (Veregen) is made by extraction from the leaves of *Camellia sinensis* (green tea). The primary active component in this extract is epigallocatechin, a compound in the catechin family. The extract also contains small amounts of gallic acid and three methylxanthines: caffeine, theophylline, and theobromine. Although the mechanism of action has not been determined, possibilities include antioxidative effects, induction of apoptosis (programmed cell death), and inhibition of telomerase (an enzyme cells use to extend the telomere cap on DNA). Kunecatechins is supplied as a 15% ointment to be applied three times daily until all warts clear, or for 16 weeks, whichever comes first. In one trial, treatment for 16 weeks produced complete wart removal in 53.6% of patients, compared with 35.3% in those treated with placebo. Adverse effects, which are common, include erythema (70%), pruritus (69%), burning (67%), pain (56%), erosion or ulceration (49%), edema (45%), induration (35%), and rash (2%). Moderate reactions develop in 37% of patients, and severe reactions in 30%. Kunecatechins is only indicated for external genital and perianal warts. It should not be inserted into the vagina or rectum and should not be applied to open wounds. Patients should avoid sexual contact while the ointment is present. Kunecatechins is not recommended for HIV-infected patients, immunocompromised patients, or patients with genital herpes infection because safety and efficacy in these patients have not been established.

Common Warts

Common warts—also known as verruca vulgaris—manifest as hard, rough, horny papules. These benign lesions may appear anywhere on the body but are most common on the hands and feet. Most common warts are caused by just three types of HPV, known as HPV-1, HPV-2, and HPV-3.

As with venereal warts, common warts may be removed by physical procedures and with topical drugs. The physical methods are cryotherapy, electrodesiccation, curettage (surgical removal with a loop-shaped cutting tool), and laser therapy. Pharmacologic agents include salicylic acid, podophyllin, podofilox, imiquimod, trichloroacetic acid, and topical fluorouracil.

DRUGS FOR MISCELLANEOUS SKIN CONDITIONS

Drugs have been developed to treat a variety of other conditions related to skin and hair. These are discussed next.

Onabotulinumtoxina for Nonsurgical Cosmetic Procedures

OnabotulinumtoxinA (Botox) is an acetylcholine release inhibitor and neuromuscular blocking agent. Botulinum toxin type A is a protein produced by the gram-negative bacterium *Clostridium botulinum*. This is the same powerful toxin that causes botulism, a potentially fatal condition brought on by eating foods contaminated with *C. botulinum*; however, the doses approved for cosmetic use are much too small to produce toxic effects.

In the United States, two licensed Botox products are available: Botox and Botox Cosmetic. Botox Cosmetic is approved only for treating frown lines, whereas plain Botox is approved for treating cervical dystonia, detrusor overactivity, upper limb spasticity, strabismus, blepharospasm, hyperhidrosis, and for migraine headache prophylaxis. However, except for the packaging, both Botox products are identical. The drug is available as a powder in 100-unit vials under the name Botox. Immediately before use, the powder is reconstituted with 2.5 mL of preservative-free normal saline to form a clear, colorless solution. According to the package label, reconstituted botulinum toxin is unstable and hence should be stored cold and used within 4 hours. However, data indicate that if the drug is diluted in normal saline that contains the preservative benzyl alcohol, it retains its potency for 5 weeks and causes less pain when injected.

Actions and Use

OnabotulinumtoxinA is a neurotoxin that acts on cholinergic neurons to block release of acetylcholine. After injection, the drug is taken up by cholinergic nerve terminals, where it inactivates SNAP-25, a protein critical to the function of acetylcholine-containing vesicles. In the absence of SNAP-25, the vesicles are unable to fuse with the terminal membrane and hence cannot release their acetylcholine. Restoration of neuronal function requires sprouting of new terminals, a process that can take several months. Botulinum toxin blocks transmission at neuromuscular junctions and at cholinergic synapses of the autonomic nervous system, including synapses in autonomic ganglia.

The FDA has approved Botox for reducing frown lines, known formally as "glabellar" lines (because they appear on the glabella—the smooth area located between the eyebrows, directly above the nose). Botox is also used to soften lines on the forehead and neck and to diminish "crow's feet" (lines that form near the outer corners of our eyes when we squint).

Administration

Botox is administered by injection. (Pretreatment with a topical anesthetic cream is commonly done to reduce discomfort.) To reduce frown lines, for example, Botox is injected directly into the small muscles that produce a frown when they contract. Five injections are made, each consisting of four units of botulinum toxin in 0.1 mL of fluid. Two injections go into each corrugator muscle and one into the procerus muscle. The whole procedure takes just a few minutes.

Results are neither instantaneous nor permanent. Rather, muscle paralysis develops slowly—over 3 to 10 days—and fades within 3 to 6 months. Botox injections may be repeated to maintain cosmetic benefits. However, at least 3 months should separate treatments. There are no data on long-term effects.

Adverse Effects

The FDA has issued a black box warning related to spread of the toxin from the site of injection to other areas, leading to life-threatening injuries; however, this has not occurred with the small doses used for cosmetic treatment. For cosmetic treatment, the most common side effects are headache, facial pain, swelling, and bruising. Swelling and bruising can be reduced by applying ice to the site and by avoiding alcohol, vitamin E, and aspirin (and related nonsteroidal antiinflammatory drugs, or NSAIDs) for the week before treatment.

Injection into the wrong site or diffusion from the right site into surrounding tissues can weaken muscles that were not intended as targets, causing multiple undesired effects. Ptosis occurs in about 5% of patients and can persist for 3 to 6 months. Injections in the lower face can result in drooling, an asymmetric smile, drooping mouth, and biting of the inside of the cheek. Injections in the neck can make swallowing difficult and can change vocal pitch.

Contraindications and Precautions

The drug should be avoided by women who are pregnant or breastfeeding and by patients who may be allergic to human albumin, a protein in Botox preparations. In addition, Botox should be avoided by people using aminoglycoside antibiotics or any other agent that has neuromuscular blocking properties. The drug should be used with caution in patients with myasthenia gravis and other neuromuscular disorders that can intensify muscle paralysis. Lastly, Botox should be avoided by people above 65 years of age because it is unlikely to help: in older people, the major cause of lines and wrinkles is loss of elasticity in the skin—a phenomenon that cannot be reversed by neuromuscular blockade.

Over time, some patients develop antibodies against botulinum toxin type A. The only consequence is a reduction in Botox benefits. The risk for antibody production may be increased by using high doses and short dosing intervals. If antibodies do develop, patients may still respond to a product known as Myobloc, which consists of botulinum toxin type B (instead of botulinum toxin type A).

Drugs for Seborrheic Dermatitis and Dandruff

Seborrheic dermatitis is a chronic, relapsing condition characterized by inflammation and scaling of the scalp and face. Skin of the underarms, chest, and anogenital region may also be affected. Symptoms result from an inflammatory reaction to infection with *Malassezia* (formerly *Pityrosporum*), a microbe in the yeast family.

Symptoms respond rapidly to topical treatment with ketoconazole, an antifungal drug with activity against yeast (see Chapter 79). For treatment of seborrhea, ketoconazole is available in a 2% cream (Ketoderm ✦), 2% foam (Extina), 2% gel (Xolegel), and 1% and 2% shampoos (Nizoral). The cream and foam formulations are applied twice daily for 4 weeks. The gel is more convenient, being applied just daily and for only 2 weeks. Concurrent use of topical glucocorticoids can accelerate initial responses. After the yeast infection has been controlled, remission can be maintained by periodic use of a shampoo that contains a yeast-suppressing drug, such as ketoconazole (in Nizoral), pyrithione zinc (in Head & Shoulders), or selenium sulfide (in Selsun Blue and Head & Shoulders Intensive Treatment).

Drugs for Hair Loss

Two drugs are approved to promote hair growth: minoxidil and finasteride. Minoxidil is applied topically; finasteride is taken orally. Neither drug was originally developed for baldness: minoxidil was developed for hypertension and finasteride for benign prostatic hyperplasia (BPH). (Dutasteride is sometimes prescribed off label; however, studies supporting its use for hair loss are lacking.)

Topical Minoxidil

Minoxidil is a direct-acting vasodilator used primarily to treat severe hypertension. The drug's basic pharmacology is discussed in Chapter 40. Consideration here is limited to its use against patterned hair loss in men and women.

TABLE 88.5   Preparation and Dosage of Selected Antibiotics for Impetigo

Generic Name	Trade Name	Formulation	DOSAGE Pediatric	Adult
Topical				
Mupirocin	Bactroban	Ointment, cream	Apply tid for 3–5 days	Apply tid for 3–5 days
Retapamulin	Altabax	Ointment	Apply bid for 5 days	Apply bid for 5 days
Oral				
Cephalexin	Keflex	Capsules, suspension	6.25 mg/kg qid	500 mg q 6–12 h
Dicloxacillin	Generic only	Capsules	6.25 mg/kg 4 times a day	250 mg qid
Clindamycin	Cleocin	Capsules, suspension	10–20 mg/kg per day in three doses	300–450 mg tid
Amoxicillin/clavulanate	Augmentin	Tablets, suspension	*3 months and older and under 40 kg:* 20–40 mg/kg per day (amoxicillin component) divided q 8 h *or* 25–45 mg/kg per day (amoxicillin component) divided q 12 h *40 kg and greater:* 500 mg q 12 h *or* 250 mg q 8 h *Severe infections, 40 kg and greater:* 875 mg q 12 h *or* 500 mg q 8 h	875 mg amoxicillin/125 mg clavulanate bid

Minoxidil for baldness is available in three formulations, a 2% solution (generic only), a 5% solution (Rogaine Extra Strength for Men), and a 5% foam (Rogaine Men's Extra Strength). All formulations are approved for men, but only the 2% solution is approved for women. Nonetheless, all formulations are routinely prescribed for women. All formulations are applied to the scalp twice a day.

The mechanism by which minoxidil promotes hair growth is unknown. One possibility is that it causes resting hair follicles to enter a state of active growth. Improved cutaneous blood flow secondary to vasodilation does not seem to be involved.

Minoxidil can delay loss of hair and stimulate hair growth. Benefits take several months to develop. Unfortunately, response rates are somewhat disappointing: only about one-third of patients experience significant restoration of hair to regions of baldness. Hair regrowth is most likely when baldness has developed recently and has been limited to a small area. Responses with the 5% solution are only 50% greater than with the 2% solution. When minoxidil is discontinued, newly gained hair is lost in 3 to 4 months, and the natural progression of hair loss resumes. In some cases, beneficial effects may decline even with uninterrupted treatment.

Topical minoxidil is generally devoid of adverse effects. A few patients have reported pruritus and local allergic responses (e.g., rash, swelling, burning sensation). Absorption is low; hence systemic reactions (e.g., hypotension, headache, flushing) are rare.

Finasteride

Finasteride is an oral drug with two indications: androgenic alopecia (male-pattern baldness) and BPH. For treatment of androgenic alopecia, finasteride is sold in 1-mg tablets under the trade name Propecia. For treatment of BPH, the drug is sold in 5-mg tablets under the trade name Proscar (see Chapter 53).

Male-pattern baldness is caused by dihydrotestosterone (DHT), a powerful androgenic hormone formed from testosterone. In balding men, the scalp has high levels of DHT, which acts on hair follicles to induce shrinkage. Finasteride promotes hair growth by inhibiting the enzyme that converts testosterone into DHT. A 1-mg dose reduces serum levels of DHT by 65% after 24 hours. In the prostate gland, levels of

testosterone increase by sixfold (because conversion of testosterone into DHT has been suppressed).

Regrowth of hair with finasteride is very modest. The drug has been evaluated in men 18 to 41 years old. Only 50% grew any hair. Furthermore, even when hair growth did occur, the amount was small: 1 year of treatment with 1 mg/d increased hair count by only 12% (in a 5.1-cm^2 circle on the scalp, the average hair count rose by 107 hairs, up from a baseline of 867 hairs). In older men taking 5 mg/d to treat BPH, no hair growth has been reported.

At the dosage employed to treat baldness (1 mg/d), adverse effects are few. About 4% of men experience reduced libido, erectile dysfunction, impaired ejaculation, and reduced ejaculate volume. Orthostatic hypotension and dizziness may occur. Finasteride is a teratogen that can cause genitourinary abnormalities in males exposed to the drug in utero. Accordingly, women who are or may become pregnant should not take finasteride, nor should they handle tablets that are crushed or broken.

Eflornithine for Unwanted Facial Hair

Eflornithine (Vaniqa) is an old drug with a new indication and new formulation. It has been available since 1990 for systemic therapy of African trypanosomiasis (sleeping sickness). Today the drug is also available in a 13.9% cream for use by women to remove facial hair. Topical eflornithine acts on cells in hair follicles to inhibit ornithine decarboxylase, an enzyme required for synthesis of polyamines, which in turn are required for cell division and subsequent hair growth.

In clinical trials, eflornithine cream was moderately effective in some women and had no effect in others. All subjects had beards or mustaches that required removal (e.g., by shaving, waxing, tweezing) at least twice a week. Participants were randomized to receive either (1) eflornithine cream twice a week or (2) the vehicle alone (i.e., the cream without eflornithine). Substantial hair reduction occurred in 40% of treated women in one study and 20% of treated women in another, compared with a 10% response in women receiving the vehicle alone. Among the women who did respond, benefits developed slowly—over 4 to 8 weeks or more—and then faded entirely within 8 weeks of stopping treatment. It should be noted that eflornithine does not remove facial hair entirely. Rather, it slows hair growth, causes hair to be finer and lighter, and decreases (but does not eliminate) the need for shaving and other hair removal procedures. Because effects are not permanent, continuous treatment is required.

Very little of topical eflornithine gets absorbed: about 1% of each dose reaches the systemic circulation. Absorbed drug is eliminated intact in the urine. No metabolism occurs.

Eflornithine cream is generally well tolerated—although there is some concern about possible fetal harm. The most common reactions are transient stinging, burning, tingling, or rash at the application site. Although eflornithine absorption is minimal, it may still be sufficient to cause fetal injury. In animal studies, there was no evidence that topical eflornithine is teratogenic or fetotoxic. However, of the 19 pregnancies that occurred during clinical trials, there were four spontaneous abortions and one birth defect (Down syndrome). Until more is known, avoiding pregnancy would seem prudent.

Eflornithine is supplied in 45-g tubes (a 2-month supply). Applications are made twice daily, 8 hours apart. Women should rub the cream in thoroughly and should not wash the treated area for at least 4 hours. Cosmetics and sunscreens can be applied as soon as the cream dries.

Drugs for Impetigo

Impetigo is the most common bacterial infection of the skin. The usual pathogen is *S. aureus*. Most cases are seen in children 2 to 5 years old, although all age groups are susceptible. Impetigo is highly contagious and usually spread by person-to-person contact. Fortunately the infection is superficial and usually is self-limited.

Impetigo has two forms: bullous and nonbullous. Bullous impetigo is caused by a toxin from *S. aureus* and manifests as rapidly spreading papules that may evolve into large, thin-walled vesicles. The usual location is a warm, moist area of the skin. Nonbullous impetigo, also known as crusted impetigo, is caused by *S. aureus* and/or *Streptococcus pyogenes*. This infection typically manifests as a single small macule or papule that evolves into a vesicle that oozes a yellow-brown exudate, which then dries into a honey-colored crust. The usual location is skin of the hands, feet, and legs. Most (70%) impetigo cases are nonbullous.

Impetigo is treated with antibiotics. Mild to moderate infection can be treated with topical agents. More serious infection is treated with oral agents. Dosages for representative antibiotics are shown in Table 88.5.

Local Anesthetics

Local anesthetics (e.g., benzocaine, lidocaine, pramoxine) can be applied topically to relieve pain and itching associated with various skin disorders, including sunburn, plant poisoning, fungal infection, diaper rash, and eczema. Selection of a topical anesthetic is based on duration of action, desired vehicle (cream, ointment, solution, gel), and prior history of hypersensitivity reactions. The pharmacology of the local anesthetics is discussed in Chapter 23.

89

Drugs for the Ear

In this chapter, drugs used to treat disorders of the middle and external ear are discussed. Information on these drugs is provided in Unit XVIII.

OTITIS MEDIA AND ITS MANAGEMENT

Otitis media (OM), defined as an inflammation of the middle ear, is the most prevalent disorder of childhood. The condition affects more than 75% of children by 3 years of age and about 95% by 12 years of age. In the United States, OM is responsible for more than 16 million clinic visits a year.

OM may result from bacterial or viral infection or from noninfectious causes. Only bacterial OM responds to antibiotics. Furthermore, most cases resolve spontaneously, making antibiotics largely unnecessary even when bacteria *are* the cause. Nonetheless, antibiotics have been used routinely. In fact, OM is the most common reason antibiotics are prescribed for children—at an estimated cost of $5 billion a year.

Acute Otitis Media

Characteristics, Pathogenesis, and Microbiology

Acute OM (AOM) is defined by *infection, inflammation,* and *fluid in the middle ear.* Otalgia (ear pain) is characteristic, often causing the young child to tug at or hold the affected ear. Other signs and symptoms accompanying AOM may include fever, vomiting, anorexia, irritability, sleeplessness, and diarrhea.

AOM results from a bacterial or viral infection of the middle ear. It occurs most commonly among children. The middle ear is filled with purulent fluid, which can cause the tympanic membrane (TM) to bulge outward. If the membrane is perforated, purulent otorrhea results.

AOM commonly develops after a viral upper respiratory infection, which can cause inflammation and swelling of the eustachian tube. The swelling can lead to blockage, resulting in negative pressure in the middle ear that, in turn, leads to fluid accumulation in the middle ear. When the eustachian tube opens, causing pressure equalization, bacteria and viruses can be sucked in. If the mucociliary system is sufficiently impaired, it will be unable to transport these pathogens back to the nasopharynx. OM results when bacteria colonize the fluid of the middle ear or when viruses colonize cells of the middle ear mucosa.

Prior to the introduction of pneumococcal conjugate vaccine (PCV), *Streptococcus pneumoniae* was the primary cause of AOM (40% to 50% of cases). A 2015 report revealed that *S. pneumoniae* is now responsible for only 12% of cases. (See Table 89.1 for common pathogens.)

Diagnosis

To diagnose AOM, three elements must be present: (1) acute onset of signs and symptoms; (2) middle ear effusion (MEE) or, if the TM is ruptured, purulent otorrhea; and (3) middle ear inflammation. The presence of MEE is indicated by a bulging TM with limited mobility, or, if the TM is perforated, purulent otorrhea. MEE is the best predictor of AOM. Middle ear inflammation is indicated by either distinct erythema of the TM or distinct otalgia. Because TM erythema can be caused by

TABLE 89.1 Primary Pathogens Found in Fluid From the Middle Ear of Children With Acute Otitis Media

Pathogen	Children With the Pathogen
Haemophilus influenzae	56%
Moraxella catarrhalis	22%
Streptococcus pneumoniae	12%
Others (e.g., *Streptococcus pyogenes, Staphylococcus aureus,* and gram-negative bacilli)	Uncommon
No bacteria found	10%–30%
Both bacteria and viruses	66%
Viruses alone[a]	4%

[a]It is uncommon for viruses to be present in the absence of bacteria.

things other than inflammation (e.g.. crying in a child), it is not always reliable as an indicator for AOM.

It is important to distinguish between AOM and otitis media with effusion (OME). Children with OME have fluid in the middle ear but no signs of local or systemic illness. Prolonged OME is common after resolution of AOM.

Standard Treatment

All children with AOM should receive pain medication, and *some* should receive antibiotics. Prescribing antibiotics for *all* children should be discouraged because most (over 80%) of AOM episodes resolve spontaneously within a week. If antibiotics are prescribed routinely, most recipients will be taking drugs they don't really need. This generates unnecessary expense and, worse yet, puts children at needless risk for adverse drug effects, increases their risk for recurrent AOM, and accelerates the emergence of antibiotic-resistant bacteria.

In 2013, the American Academy of Pediatrics (AAP) released updated guidelines for treating AOM in children (Fig. 89.1). These build on earlier guidelines developed jointly by the AAP and the American Academy of Family Physicians. For many patients, the guidelines include an important option—*observation*—rather than immediate treatment with antibiotics. Observation is defined as management by symptomatic relief alone for 48 to 72 hours, thereby allowing time for AOM to resolve on its own. If symptoms persist or worsen, antibacterial therapy is started. As part of this strategy, parents are informed about (1) the high probability of spontaneous AOM resolution and (2) the drawbacks of giving antibiotics when they are not needed. Observation is considered appropriate only when follow-up can be ensured. The recommendation for observation is based on studies showing the following:

- Most episodes of AOM resolve spontaneously.
- Immediate antibacterial therapy is only marginally superior to observation at causing AOM resolution and is no better at relieving pain or distress.
- Parents find the observation approach acceptable.

- Delaying antibacterial therapy does not significantly increase the risk for mastoiditis, which can occur when bacteria invade the mastoid bone.

Criteria for choosing between observation and initial antibacterial therapy are shown in Table 89.2. As indicated, all children younger than 6 months should receive antibiotics, regardless of diagnostic certainty or symptom severity. Among children 6 months to 2 years old, antibiotics are indicated whenever the diagnosis is certain. For children 2 years and older, antibacterial therapy is indicated only if the diagnosis is certain, and then only if symptoms are severe. In all other cases, observation is the preferred strategy.

When antibacterial drugs *are* indicated, *high-dose amoxicillin* is the treatment of choice (Table 89.3). Benefits of amoxicillin are efficacy, safety, low cost, acceptable taste, and narrow microbiologic spectrum. The duration of treatment ranges from 5 to 10 days, depending on patient age and illness severity.

For patients with penicillin allergy, drug selection depends on allergy severity. If the allergy is *not* severe (type II allergy), a cephalosporin may be used (e.g., cefdinir and cefuroxime). However, if the allergy is *severe* (type I allergy, causing urticaria or anaphylaxis), cephalosporins should be avoided, owing to concerns of cross-reactivity. In this case azithromycin and clarithromycin are recommended.

Regardless of whether antibiotics are prescribed, pain management must be included when AOM is being treated. Analgesics such as acetaminophen or ibuprofen are commonly used to manage mild to moderate pain. For moderate to severe pain, codeine and similar drugs may be needed. For children older than 5 years, the 2013 AAP guidelines also recommend a topical anesthetic such as procaine or lidocaine drops for pain relief. (The 2013 guidelines also recommended benzocaine drops; however, because they lacked US Food and Drug Administration [FDA] approval, the FDA required their removal from the market in 2015.) To relieve pain, the external auditory canal (EAC) is filled with the solution and then a solution-soaked cotton pledget is placed in the EAC to prevent drainage. This must typically be repeated every 1 to 2 hours until the pain is relieved. It is contraindicated if the TM is perforated.

Treatment of Antibiotic-Resistant Acute Otitis Media

Antibiotic resistance is indicated by persistence of symptoms (fever, earache, otorrhea, and a red and bulging TM) for 2 to 3 days despite

TABLE 89.2   Criteria for Choosing Initial Antibacterial Therapy Versus Observation in Children With Acute Otitis Media

Age	MANAGEMENT RECOMMENDATION	
	Certain Diagnosis	Uncertain Diagnosis
Less than 6 months	Antibacterial therapy	Antibacterial therapy
6 months to 2 years	Antibacterial therapy[a]	Antibacterial therapy if illness is severe; observation if illness is not severe[b]
2 years and older	Antibacterial therapy if illness is severe; observation if illness is not severe[b]	Observation, regardless of symptom severity

[a]If AOM is unilateral without otorrhea and with mild symptoms, observation may be appropriate.
[b]Severe illness = moderate to severe otalgia or fever of 39°C (102.2°F) or higher; nonsevere illness = mild otalgia and fever below 39°C in the past 24 hours.

TABLE 89.3   Recommended Antibacterial Drugs for Acute Otitis Media

Patient Group and Illness Severity	RECOMMENDED DRUGS	
	For Most Patients	For Patients With Penicillin Allergy[a]
Patients Receiving Immediate Antibiotic Therapy		
Nonsevere illness	Amoxicillin, 40–45 mg/kg bid	*Non–type I allergy:* Cefdinir, 14 mg/kg per day in one dose or two divided doses, *or* Cefuroxime, 15 mg/kg bid, *or* Cefpodoxime, 5 mg/kg bid *Type I allergy:* Azithromycin, 10 mg/kg on day 1, then 5 mg/kg on days 2, 3, 4, and 5. *or* Clarithromycin, 7.5 mg/kg bid
Severe illness	Amoxicillin, 45 mg/kg bid *plus* clavulanate, 3.2 mg/kg bid[b]	Ceftriaxone, 50 mg/kg IM for 1 or 3 days
Patients With Persistent Symptoms After 48–72 h of Observation (With No Antibiotic Therapy)		
	Same as for patients receiving immediate antibiotic therapy	
Patients With Persistent Symptoms After 48–72 h of Antibiotic Therapy (Indicating Drug Resistance)		
Nonsevere illness	Amoxicillin, 45 mg/kg bid *plus* clavulanate, 3.2 mg/kg bid[b]	*Non–type I allergy:* Ceftriaxone, 50 mg/kg IM or IV for 3 days *Type I allergy:* Clindamycin, 30–40 mg/kg/d in 3 divided doses
Severe illness	Ceftriaxone, 50 mg/kg IM for 3 days	Clindamycin (plus a third-generation cephalosporin if non–type I penicillin allergy) and tympanocentesis

[a]Type I allergy is severe (urticaria or anaphylaxis); type II is less severe.
[b]This ratio of amoxicillin to clavulanate can be achieved with Augmentin ES-600, a fixed-dose combination containing amoxicillin and clavulanic acid.
IM, Intramuscular; *IV*, intravenous.

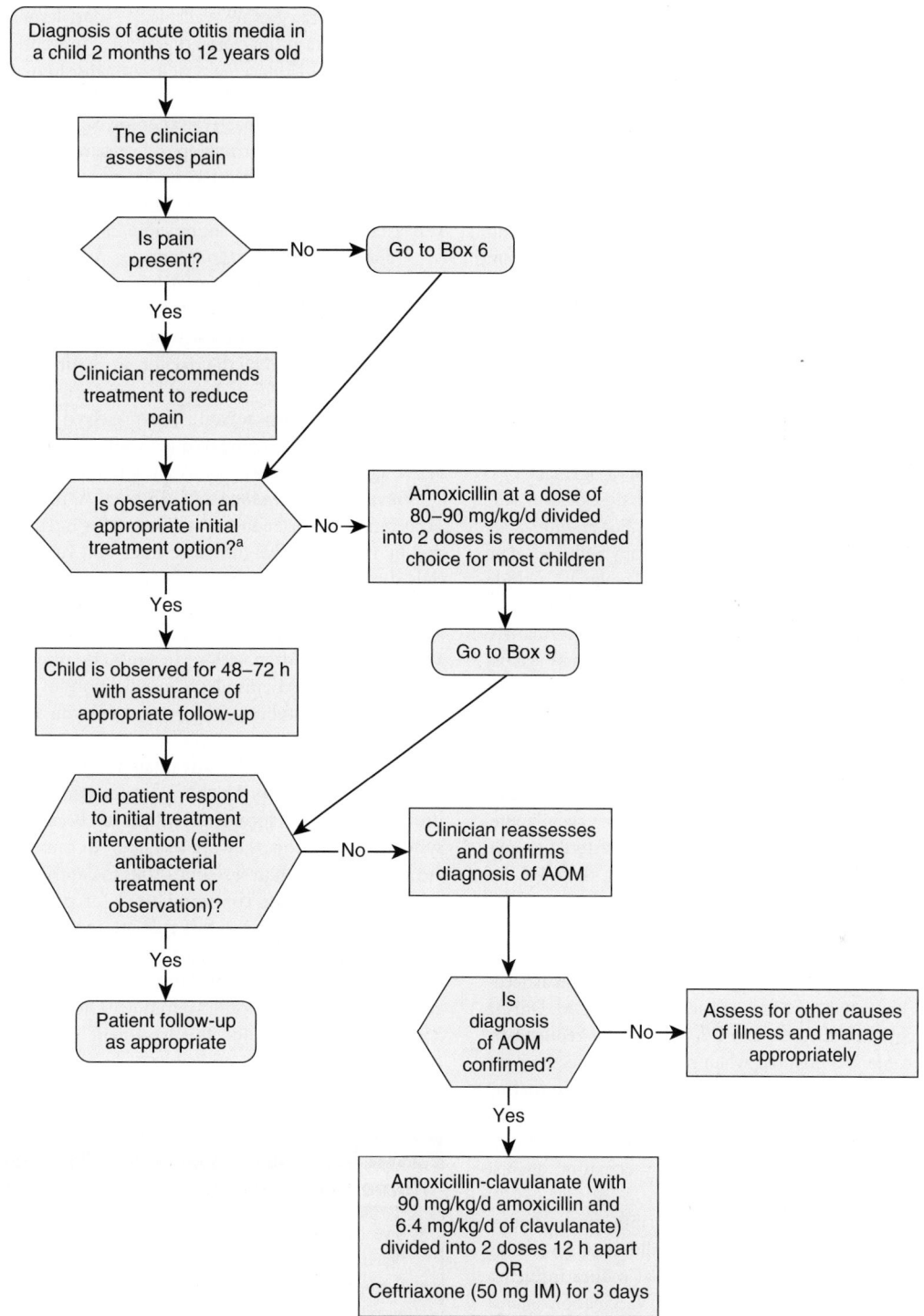

Fig. 89.1 Management of Acute Otitis Media. *AOM,* acute otitis media; *IM,* intramuscular. (Data from http://pediatrics. aappublications.org/content/113/5/1451.figures-only; http://pediatrics.aappublications.org/content/pediatrics/early/ 2013/02/20/peds.2012-3488.full.pdf.)

ª Criteria for antibacterial treatment or observation in children with uncomplicated AOMᵇ

1) <6 months: antibacterial treatment
2) 6 months - 2 years: antibacterial treatment if AOM diagnosis is certain unless AOM is unilateral without otorrhea
3) 2 yr and older: antibacterial treatment if severe pain >48 h, fever ≥39°C (102.2°F) during the preceding 48 h, or if there is a possibility that the caregiver may not reliably arrange for follow-up, if needed. For mild earache of <48 h or if temperature is <39°C, observation is appropriate

ᵇCaregiver is informed and agrees to the option of observation.
Caregiver is able to monitor child and return should condition worsen.
Systems are in place for ready communication with the clinician, evaluation, and obtaining medication if necessary.

ªAppropriate medication alternatives should be used for the child with penicillin allergy.

antibiotic therapy. Major risk factors for developing resistant AOM are the following:

- Day care attendance
- Age younger than 2 years
- Exposure to antibiotics in the prior 1 to 3 months
- Winter and spring seasons

In the United States, the incidence of resistant AOM is on the rise because overuse of antibiotics has favored emergence of resistant pathogens. Resistance among strains of *Haemophilus influenzae* and *Moraxella catarrhalis* is limited to β-lactam antibiotics. The mechanism involves the production of β-lactamase, an enzyme that inactivates amoxicillin and certain other β-lactam antibiotics. In contrast, strains of *S. pneumoniae* are resistant to multiple antibiotics, including erythromycin and trimethoprim/sulfamethoxazole as well as amoxicillin and other β-lactam antibiotics. Interestingly, *S. pneumoniae* resistance to amoxicillin does not result from β-lactamase production. Rather, it results from synthesis of altered penicillin-binding proteins (PBPs), whose affinity for amoxicillin is much lower than that of normal PBPs.

How should resistant AOM be treated? Using a high dose of amoxicillin increases activity against resistant *S. pneumoniae*. For *H. influenzae* and *M. catarrhalis*, the preferred approach is oral therapy with *high-dose amoxicillin/clavulanate*. Alternatives to amoxicillin/clavulanate include *intramuscular or intravenous ceftriaxone* and *oral clindamycin*.

The clavulanate (clavulanic acid) in the amoxicillin/clavulanate combination inhibits beta-lactamase and thereby increases activity against resistant *H. influenzae* and *M. catarrhalis*. Because the clavulanate in the combination can cause diarrhea, the dosage of clavulanate should be low. It is important to be aware that the ratio of amoxicillin to clavulanate is not constant. For example, Augmentin (amoxicillin with clavulanate) is available as tablets containing 250 mg amoxicillin with 125 mg clavulanate and as tablets containing 500 mg amoxicillin with 125 mg clavulanate. If two tablets containing 250 mg amoxicillin are administered to give a patient a 500-mg dose of the amoxicillin component, the excess of clavulanate can result in worsening diarrhea.

Prevention

The risk for acquiring AOM can be decreased in several ways. Breastfeeding for at least 6 months seems to reduce early episodes of AOM. During infancy and early childhood, AOM can be significantly reduced by avoiding child care centers, if possible, when respiratory infections are prevalent. Measures believed to help prevent AOM include eliminating exposure to tobacco smoke, reducing pacifier use in the second 6 months of life, and avoiding supine bottle feeding. Two additional measures are prevention and treatment of influenza and vaccination against pneumococcal infection.

Prevention and treatment of influenza. As noted, influenza and other viral infections of the respiratory tract predispose children to developing bacterial and viral OM. Accordingly, measures that reduce influenza can reduce OM risk. Two methods are available: (1) vaccination against influenza and (2) treatment of active influenza infection. Although both immunization against and treatment of influenza can help during the flu season, they do nothing to alter AOM risk the rest of the year.

Vaccination against Streptococcus pneumoniae. Vaccination with *pneumococcal conjugate vaccine* (PCV) (Prevnar) can reduce the risk for AOM. As mentioned earlier, *S. pneumoniae* was once responsible for 40% to 50% of bacterial AOM. This has decreased significantly since the first PCV was introduced in 2000.

Recurrent Otitis Media

Recurrent AOM can be defined as AOM that occurs three or more times within 6 months or 4 or more times within 12 months. Four management strategies are available: (1) short-term antibacterial therapy, (2) prophylactic antibacterial therapy, (3) prevention and treatment of influenza, and (4) placement of a tympanostomy tube.

Short-term antibacterial therapy. There is disagreement among experts regarding antibacterial therapy. Some authorities recommend antibiotics for each recurrent episode, regardless of presentation. Others recommend reserving antibiotics for episodes in which symptoms are severe. In both cases, high-dose amoxicillin is the treatment of choice. If resistance is suspected, amoxicillin/clavulanate can be used.

Prophylactic antibacterial therapy. Antibacterial prophylaxis is *not* generally recommended. An analysis of several studies indicates that for each year of prophylaxis (with *trimethoprim/sulfamethoxazole* or *amoxicillin*), only 1.3 episodes of AOM are prevented. This small benefit is largely outweighed by the risk for promoting antibiotic resistance. If prophylaxis *is* elected, it should be conducted only during the upper respiratory infection season. The preferred drug for prophylaxis is amoxicillin because, compared with sulfonamides, amoxicillin is more active against multi-drug–resistant strains of *S. pneumoniae*.

Prevention and treatment of influenza. As discussed previously, AOM occurrence can be reduced by vaccinating against the influenza virus and by treating active influenza infection. However, benefits are seen only during the flu season.

Tympanostomy tubes. A tympanostomy tube permits drainage and aeration of the middle ear. Tube insertion is performed under general anesthesia. In children with recurrent AOM, the procedure can significantly reduce AOM episodes. Complications of the procedure include obstruction of the tube, secondary infection with otorrhea, and premature tube extrusion.

Otic preparations have advantages over oral preparations because the can go directly to the source of infection in the middle ear; this provides for high local concentration. Because there is decreased systemic absorption, they are less likely to cause adverse effects. They are also less likely than systemic drugs to contribute to resistance. Most otic preparations are contraindicated for patients who do not have intact TMs. Exceptions to this rule are some of the fluoroquinolones and fluoroquinolone/glucocorticoid combination products. The combination products ciprofloxacin/dexamethasone (Ciprodex) and ciprofloxacin/fluocinolone acetonide (Otovel) are topical solutions approved specifically for the treatment of AOM in patients with tympanostomy tubes.

PATIENT EDUCATION
Home Management of Acute Otitis Media

- Give acetaminophen or ibuprofen for pain. Avoid aspirin in children. Demonstrate administration of otic analgesics if prescribed.
- Symptoms should start to improve within 2 days to 3 days. If this does not occur or if the symptoms increase in severity, return to the clinic.
- If antibiotics are prescribed, take exactly as ordered.

OTITIS MEDIA WITH EFFUSION

OME (previously called secretory or serous otitis media) is more common than AOM. It often occurs with upper respiratory tract infections and may precede or follow an episode of AOM. The condition is characterized by fluid in the middle ear but without evidence of local or systemic illness. OME may cause mild hearing loss while present, but not pain. The condition typically resolves without treatment; however, it may persist for weeks to months after AOM has resolved. Because it is not caused by a bacterial infection, antibiotics have no effect on OME and should not be used.

ACUTE OTITIS EXTERNA

Acute otitis externa (AOE) is an inflammation of the EAC. The usual cause is bacterial infection, which may be limited to the EAC or may spread to adjacent tissues. Most cases of AOE respond to topical drugs.

Characteristics, Pathogenesis, and Microbiology

AOE, also known as "swimmer's ear," is a bacterial infection of the EAC. The most common pathogens are *Pseudomonas aeruginosa* and *Staphylococcus aureus*. Other pathogens include *Staphylococcus epidermidis* and *Microbacterium otitidis*. Patients who have AOE present with one or more of the following: rapid-onset ear pain associated with pruritus, a sensation of ear fullness, tenderness on manipulation of the external ear, or edema or erythema of the EAC. Impaired hearing and purulent discharge may occur.

Susceptibility to AOE is precipitated primarily by two factors: abrasion and excessive moisture. Both facilitate bacterial colonization. Abrasion of the epithelium creates a site for bacterial entry. Most often, abrasion results from cleaning or scratching the EAC with a cotton-tipped swab or some other foreign object (e.g., finger, pencil, and toothpick). Abrasion can also be caused by hearing aids and earplugs. Moisture can wash away the protective layer of cerumen. As a result, keratin debris in the EAC is able to absorb water, thereby creating a nourishing medium for bacterial growth. Moisture in the EAC may come from swimming, perspiration, and even high humidity.

Treatment

AOE is a painful condition, often severe, so analgesics are indicated. The same analgesics used for AOM are appropriate for AOE pain management.

AOE usually responds well to simple treatment. The goal is to eradicate the pathogen and reduce pain. For most patients, cleaning and using topical antimicrobials will suffice. If the infection is extensive, oral antibiotics may be needed. To facilitate healing, the ear should be kept as dry as possible. Most infections begin to improve in 3 days and resolve completely by 10 days.

Topical Medications

The most recent (2014) AOE clinical practice guidelines published by the American Academy of Otolaryngology recommend topical antimicrobials over systemic drugs for uncomplicated AOE (Fig. 89.2). There are two reasons for this recommendation. First, topical agents achieve very high local concentrations (often 100 to 1000 times the concentration achieved with systemic drugs), antibacterial effects are superior, disease persistence is lower, and recurrence is less likely. Second, with topical therapy, systemic side effects are absent. Exceptions are made for patients with diabetes, immune deficiencies, or those who would have difficulty with proper administration of topical drugs. These patients should have systemic therapy. Systemic therapy should also be prescribed if the infection has spread beyond the EAC. In severe cases, both systemic and topical antibiotics are needed.

A variety of topical medications can be used. A *2% solution of acetic acid* is safe, effective, and inexpensive. A solution of *alcohol plus acetic acid* offers the additional benefit of promoting tissue drying. For many patients, acidification and drying are all that is needed.

If the infection is more extensive or cannot be cleared with acetic acid and alcohol, a topical antibiotic should be employed. In the past,

a three-drug combination—*hydrocortisone, neomycin,* and *polymyxin B*—was considered standard therapy. The hydrocortisone reduces inflammation and edema; neomycin and polymyxin kill bacterial pathogens. Unfortunately, although this combination is effective and inexpensive, it has drawbacks. Specifically, the neomycin component is ototoxic and causes local swelling and erythema in about 15% of patients. Today, *quinolones* (e.g., ciprofloxacin) are preferred because these drugs are highly effective, do not cause local reactions, and are not ototoxic. Fluoroquinolone and glucocorticoid combination products have the added benefit of decreasing pain by reducing swelling caused by inflammation. Principal drawbacks of these preparations are expense and the potential to promote resistance to fluoroquinolone antibiotics.

Applying ear drops correctly can improve outcomes and reduce drug-related discomfort. Instillation of cold solutions can cause dizziness; therefore ear drops should be warmed before administration. Wiggling the earlobe, if tolerated, can facilitate transit of solutions down the EAC. If edema results in EAC closure that is sufficient to impede drug penetration, insertion of a wick can help. A wick is like a very tiny elongated tampon. After it is carefully inserted into the edematous EAC, ear drops are applied to the exposed tip. (It will be important to apply enough medication to keep the wick moist.) Drug solutions are absorbed into the wick, which then delivers them to the epithelium of the entire canal. The wick should be replaced at least every 48 hours to allow cleaning and to determine whether further wicking is still needed.

Oral Medications

Oral antibacterials are indicated if the infection extends beyond the EAC to involve the pinna. For adults, *ciprofloxacin* (Cipro) is a good choice; however, because oral quinolones can cause tendon rupture in younger patients, this drug should not be given to patients younger than 18 years of age. For children, *cephalexin* (Keflex) is preferred.

PATIENT EDUCATION
Prevention of Acute Otitis Externa

The best way to prevent bacterial AOE is to keep the natural defenses of the EAC healthy. Ear hygiene can be promoted by following these rules:
- Don't put *anything* in the ear—including cotton swabs, fingers, pencils, toothpicks, liquids, or sprays—all of which can remove cerumen and damage the EAC lining.
- Dry the EAC after swimming and showering by toweling off and promoting water drainage by tipping the head to each side while pulling the auricle in different directions.
- Don't remove cerumen (earwax).
- Don't use earplugs (except when swimming).

Necrotizing Otitis Externa

Necrotizing otitis externa (NOE) is a rare but potentially fatal complication of AOE that develops when bacteria in the EAC invade the mastoid or temporal bone. Spread of infection to the skull base can affect cranial nerves, and spread to the dura mater can cause meningitis and possibly lateral sinus thrombosis. The usual pathogen is *P. aeruginosa*. Patients typically present with progressive severe otic pain, purulent discharge from the ear, and granulation of tissue in the EAC. NOE occurs almost exclusively in two groups of high-risk people, specifically older people with diabetes and people who are immunocompromised, especially people with HIV infection. All patients should receive antipseudomonal ear drops (e.g., ofloxacin solution) along with oral ciprofloxacin. Referral for specialist care should also be considered. Progression to severe disease will likely require intravenous antipseudomonal therapy.

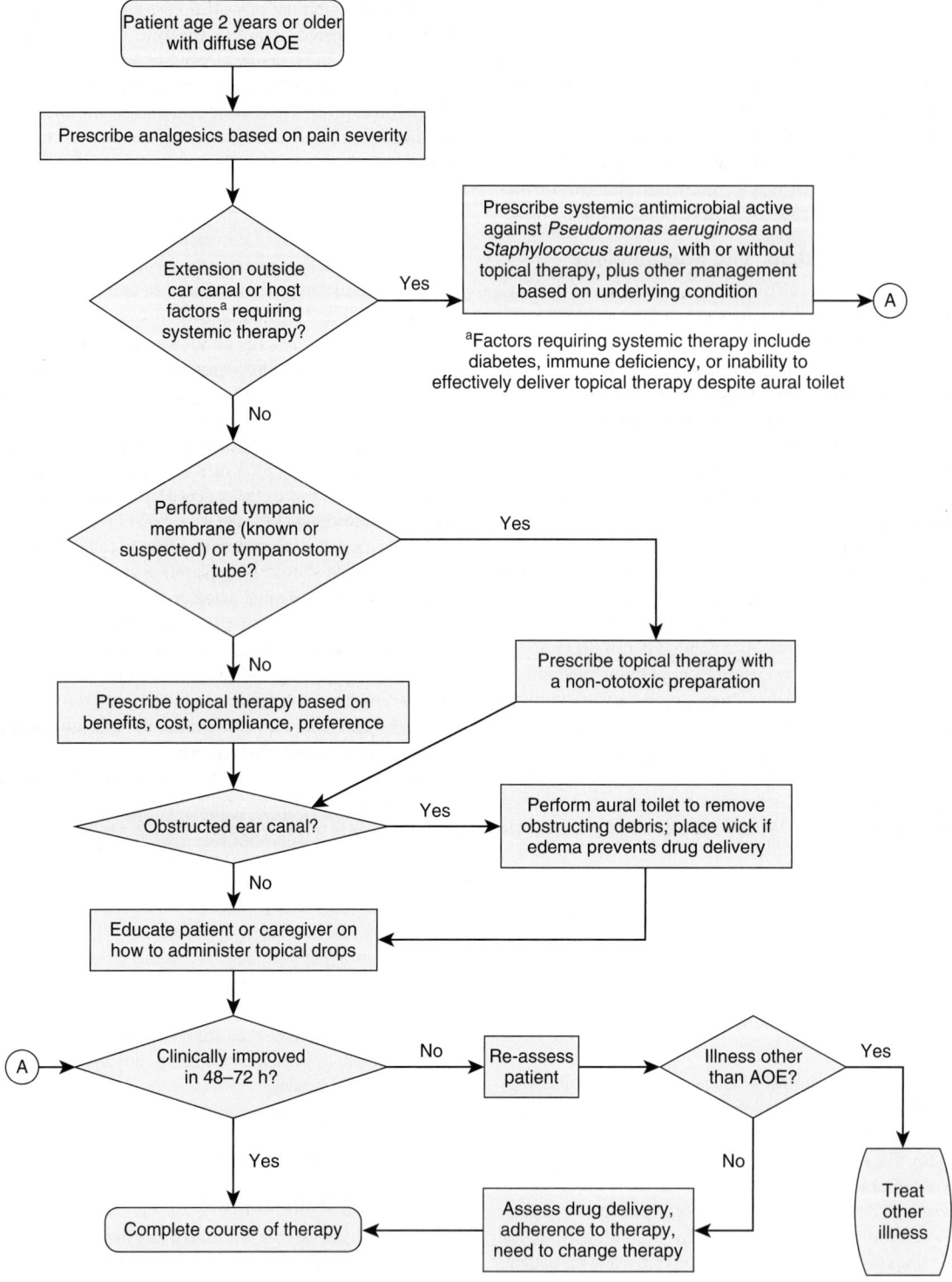

Fig. 89.2 Management of Acute Otitis Externa. *AOE,* Acute otitis externa. (From Rosenfeld RM, Schwartz SR, Cannon CR, et al. Clinical practice guideline: acute otitis externa. *Otolaryngol Head Neck Surg.* 2014;150(1 Suppl):S1–S24. © American Academy Otolaryngology—Head and Neck Surgery Foundation 2014. Reprints and permission: sagepub.com/journalsPermissions.nav.)

Fungal Otitis Externa (Otomycosis)

In about 10% of patients, OE is caused by fungi and not bacteria. The two most common pathogens are *Aspergillus,* which causes 80% to 90% of otomycoses, and *Candida.* Fungal OE typically manifests as intense pruritus and erythema, with or without pain or hearing loss. As a rule, otomycosis can be managed with thorough cleansing and application of acidifying drops (e.g., 2% acetic acid solution must be applied three to four times a day for 7 days). If these measures prove inadequate, a solution that contains an antifungal drug (e.g., *1% clotrimazole* [Lotrimin]) can be applied twice daily for 7 days. If the infection fails to respond, *oral* antifungal therapy may be needed. Options include *itraconazole* (Sporanox) and *fluconazole* (Diflucan).

🖹 SUMMARY OF KEY PRESCRIBING CONSIDERATIONS

Therapeutic Goal: The goals of management of ear infections are to reduce inflammation, eliminate infection, and prevent complications due to AOM and AOE. Complications include development of language problems secondary to hearing deficits and development of drug-resistant bacteria. Rare but serious complications of AOM include mastoiditis and meningitis. As noted, NOE can occur from an extension of AOE.

Baseline Data: Document local and systemic signs and symptoms of infection, inflammation, and pain. Note TM mobility with pneumatic otoscopy or tympanometry. Assess hearing if deficits are a concern.

Identifying High-Risk Patients

- Assess for penicillin allergy before prescribing amoxicillin or amoxicillin/clavulanate. For patients who have experienced a mild reaction to penicillin, guidelines recommend a cephalosporin such as cefdinir, cefuroxime, or cefpodoxime. For a severe reaction such as anaphylaxis, azithromycin or clarithromycin is recommended.
- Determine whether the patient with AOM has taken amoxicillin in the past 30 days. If so, amoxicillin/clavulanate should be prescribed. This should also be prescribed if *H. influenzae* or *M. catarrhalis* is suspected.
- Have there been three or more episodes of AOM in the past 6 months or four episodes in the past year (indicative of recurrent AOM)? If so, consider referral to an otolaryngologist. Tympanostomy tubes may be indicated, especially if hearing loss is a concern.

- Is the TM intact? If not, avoid ototoxic drops such as aminoglycoside preparations. Instead, prescribe a quinolone or quinolone/glucocorticoid combination because these are safe for patients who have perforated TMs.
- For AOE, if the canal is significantly swollen, insert a wick to ensure that the medication reaches all affected tissues.
- Patients with AOE who have diabetes or immune deficiencies should receive systemic therapy or a combination of systemic and topical therapy. Systemic therapy or referral is indicated if the infection has spread beyond the EAC.

Evaluating Therapeutic Effects

- Patients with both AOM and AOE should have improvement in 48–72 h. Before leaving the clinic, they should be instructed to return if they do not have improvement or if their condition worsens.
- Keep in mind that MME will continue long after the AOM has resolved. For this reason, tympanometry and pneumatic otoscopy will not reflect a normal response to pressure changes for several weeks or even months.

Minimizing Adverse Effects

- For young children who have not yet developed language, reassess for resolution of MEE a few months after treatment.
- If young children with recurrent or prolonged AOM experience language problems, consider early referral for intervention.

Agents Affecting the Volume and Ion Content of Body Fluids

The drugs discussed in this chapter are used to correct disturbances in the volume and ionic composition of body fluids. Standard guidelines do not exist for electrolyte and fluid replacement. Most facilities will have their own protocols regarding recommended replacement. Many of these protocols allow for the replacement of electrolytes by the registered nurse. Three groups of agents are considered for replacement: (1) drugs used to correct disorders of fluid volume and osmolality, (2) drugs used to correct disturbances of hydrogen ion concentration (acid–base status), and (3) drugs used to correct electrolyte imbalances.

DISORDERS OF FLUID VOLUME AND OSMOLALITY

Good health requires that both the volume and osmolality of extracellular and intracellular fluids remain within a normal range. If a substantial alteration in either the volume or osmolality of these fluids develops, significant harm can result.

Maintenance of fluid volume and osmolality is primarily the job of the kidneys, and even under adverse conditions, renal mechanisms usually succeed in keeping the volume and composition of body fluids within acceptable limits. However, circumstances can arise in which the regulatory capacity of the kidneys is exceeded. When this occurs, disruption of fluid volume, osmolality, or both can result.

Abnormal states of hydration can be divided into two major categories: volume contraction and volume expansion. *Volume contraction* is defined as a *decrease* in total body water; conversely, *volume expansion* is defined as an *increase* in total body water. States of volume contraction and volume expansion have three subclassifications based on alterations in extracellular osmolality. For volume contraction, the subcategories are *isotonic contraction, hypertonic contraction,* and *hypotonic contraction.* Volume expansion may also be subclassified as *isotonic, hypertonic,* or *hypotonic.* Descriptions and causes of these abnormal states are discussed next.

In the clinical setting, changes in osmolality are described in terms of the sodium content of plasma. Sodium is used as the reference for classification because this ion is the principal extracellular solute. In most cases, the total osmolality of plasma is about twice the osmolality of sodium. That is, total plasma osmolality usually ranges from 280 to 300 mOsm/kg water.

Volume Contraction
Isotonic Contraction
Definition and causes. Isotonic contraction is defined as volume contraction in which *sodium and water are lost in isotonic proportions.* Hence although there is a decrease in the total volume of extracellular fluid, there is no change in osmolality. Causes of isotonic contraction include vomiting, diarrhea, kidney disease, and misuse of diuretics.

Treatment. Lost volume should be replaced with fluids that are isotonic to plasma. This can be accomplished by infusing isotonic (0.9%) sodium chloride in sterile water, a solution in which both sodium and chloride are present at a concentration of 145 mEq/L.

Hypertonic Contraction
Definition and causes. Hypertonic contraction is defined as volume contraction in which *loss of water exceeds loss of sodium.* Hence there is a reduction in extracellular fluid volume coupled with an increase in osmolality. Because of extracellular hypertonicity, water is drawn out of cells, thereby producing intracellular dehydration and partial compensation for lost extracellular volume.

Causes of hypertonic contraction include excessive sweating, osmotic diuresis, and feeding excessively concentrated formula or foods to infants. Hypertonic contraction may also develop secondary to extensive burns or disorders of the central nervous system (CNS) that render the patient unable to experience or report thirst.

Treatment. Volume replacement in hypertonic contraction should be accomplished with hypotonic fluids (e.g., 0.45% sodium chloride) or with fluids that contain no solutes at all. Initial therapy may consist simply of drinking water. Alternatively, 5% dextrose can be infused intravenously. (Because dextrose is rapidly metabolized to carbon dioxide and water, dextrose solutions can be viewed as the osmotic equivalent of water alone.) Volume replenishment should be done in stages. About 50% of the estimated loss should be replaced during the first 24 hours of treatment. The remainder should be replenished over the next 1 to 2 days.

Hypotonic Contraction
Definition and causes. Hypotonic contraction is defined as volume contraction in which *loss of sodium exceeds loss of water.* Hence both the volume and osmolality of extracellular fluid are reduced. Because intracellular osmolality now exceeds extracellular osmolality, extracellular volume becomes diminished further by movement of water into cells.

The principal cause of hypotonic contraction is excessive loss of sodium through the kidneys. This may occur because of diuretic therapy, chronic renal insufficiency, or lack of aldosterone (the adrenocortical hormone that promotes renal retention of sodium).

Treatment. If hyponatremia is mild and if renal function is adequate, hypotonic contraction can be corrected by infusing *isotonic* sodium chloride solution for injection. When this is done, plasma tonicity will be adjusted by the kidneys. However, if the sodium loss is severe, a *hypertonic* (e.g., 3%) solution of sodium chloride should be infused. Administration should continue until plasma sodium concentration has been raised to about 130 mEq/L. Patients should be monitored for signs of fluid overload (distention of neck veins and peripheral or pulmonary edema). When hypotonic contraction is due to aldosterone insufficiency, patients should receive hormone replacement therapy along with intravenous infusion of isotonic sodium chloride.

Volume Expansion

Volume expansion is defined as an *increase in the total volume of body fluid.* As with volume contraction, volume expansion may be *isotonic, hypertonic,* or *hypotonic.* Volume expansion may result from an overdose with therapeutic fluids (e.g., sodium chloride infusion) or may be associated with disease states, such as heart failure, nephrotic syndrome, or cirrhosis of the liver with ascites. The principal drugs employed to correct volume expansion are *diuretics* and the *agents used for heart failure.* These drugs are discussed in Chapters 36 and 41, respectively. An additional class of drugs, the vaptans, is used in the acute care setting for euvolemic and hypervolemic hyponatremia and is discussed in Chapter 91.

ACID–BASE DISTURBANCES

Maintenance of acid–base balance is a complex process, the full discussion of which is beyond the scope of this text. Hence discussion here is condensed.

Acid–base status is regulated by multiple systems. The most important are (1) the bicarbonate–carbonic acid buffer system, (2) the respiratory system, and (3) the kidneys. The respiratory system influences pH through control of CO_2 exhalation. Because CO_2 represents volatile carbonic acid, exhalation of CO_2 tends to elevate pH (reduce acidity), whereas retention of CO_2 (secondary to respiratory slowing) tends to lower pH. The kidneys influence pH by regulating bicarbonate excretion. By *retaining* bicarbonate, the kidneys can raise pH. Conversely, by increasing bicarbonate *excretion,* the kidneys can lower pH and thereby compensate for alkalosis.

There are four principal types of acid–base imbalance: (1) respiratory alkalosis, (2) respiratory acidosis, (3) metabolic alkalosis, and (4) metabolic acidosis. Causes and treatments are discussed next.

Respiratory Alkalosis
Causes

Respiratory alkalosis is produced by hyperventilation. Deep, rapid breathing increases CO_2 loss, which in turn lowers the PCO_2 (partial pressure of carbon dioxide) of blood and increases pH. Mild hyperventilation may result from a number of causes, including hypoxia, pulmonary disease, and drugs (especially aspirin and other salicylates). Severe hyperventilation can be caused by CNS injury and extreme anxiety states.

Treatment

Management of respiratory alkalosis is dictated by the severity of pH elevation. When alkalosis is mild, no specific treatment is indicated. Severe respiratory alkalosis can be treated with a sedative (e.g., diazepam [Valium]), which can help suppress the anxiety.

Respiratory Acidosis
Causes

Respiratory acidosis results from retention of CO_2 secondary to hypoventilation. Reduced CO_2 exhalation raises plasma PCO_2, which in turn causes plasma pH to fall. Primary causes of impaired ventilation are (1) depression of the medullary respiratory center and (2) pathologic changes in the lungs (e.g., status asthmaticus and airway obstruction). Over time, the kidneys compensate for respiratory acidosis by excreting less bicarbonate.

Treatment

Primary treatment of respiratory acidosis is directed at correcting respiratory impairment. The patient may also need oxygen and ventilatory assistance. Infusion of sodium bicarbonate may be indicated if acidosis is severe (pH ≤6.9).

Metabolic Alkalosis
Causes

Metabolic alkalosis is characterized by increases in both the pH and bicarbonate content of plasma. Causes include excessive loss of gastric acid (through vomiting or suctioning) and administration of alkalinizing salts (e.g., sodium bicarbonate). The body compensates for metabolic alkalosis by (1) hypoventilation (which causes retention of CO_2), (2) increased renal excretion of bicarbonate, and (3) accumulation of organic acids.

Treatment

In most cases, metabolic alkalosis can be corrected by targeting the specific cause of the acidosis (e.g., medicating for vomiting or decreasing gastric suction). One may also consider infusing a solution of *sodium chloride plus potassium chloride.* This facilitates renal excretion of bicarbonate and thereby promotes normalization of plasma pH.

Metabolic Acidosis
Causes

Principal causes of metabolic acidosis are chronic renal failure, loss of bicarbonate during severe diarrhea, and metabolic disorders that result in overproduction of lactic acid (lactic acidosis) or ketoacids (ketoacidosis). Metabolic acidosis may also result from poisoning by methanol and certain medications (e.g., aspirin and other salicylates).

Treatment

Treatment consists of correcting the underlying cause of acidosis and, if the acidosis is severe, administering an alkalinizing salt (e.g., sodium bicarbonate, sodium carbonate).

When an alkalinizing salt is indicated, *sodium bicarbonate* is generally preferred. Administration may be oral or intravenous. If acidosis is mild, oral administration is preferred. Intravenous infusion is usually reserved for severe reductions of pH. When sodium bicarbonate is given intravenously to treat acute, severe acidosis, caution must be exercised to avoid excessive elevation of plasma pH because rapid conversion from acidosis to alkalosis can be hazardous. Also, because of the sodium content of sodium bicarbonate, care should be taken to avoid hypernatremia.

Potassium Imbalances
Regulation of Potassium Levels

Serum levels of potassium are regulated primarily by the kidneys. Under steady-state conditions, urinary output of potassium equals intake. Renal excretion of potassium is increased by aldosterone, an adrenal steroid that promotes conservation of sodium while increasing potassium loss. Potassium excretion is also increased by most diuretics. Potassium-sparing diuretics (e.g., spironolactone) are the exception.

Potassium levels are influenced by extracellular pH. In the presence of extracellular *alkalosis,* potassium uptake by cells is *enhanced,* causing a *reduction* in extracellular potassium levels. Conversely, extracellular *acidosis* promotes the exit of potassium from cells, thereby causing extracellular *hyperkalemia.*

Insulin has a profound effect on potassium: in high doses, insulin stimulates potassium uptake by cells. This ability has been used to treat hyperkalemia.

Hypokalemia
Causes and Consequences

The most common cause of hypokalemia is treatment with a thiazide or loop diuretic (see Chapter 36). Other causes include insufficient potassium intake; alkalosis and excessive insulin (both of which decrease extracellular potassium levels by driving potassium into cells); increased renal excretion of potassium (e.g., as caused by aldosterone); and potassium loss associated with vomiting, diarrhea, and abuse of laxatives. Hypokalemia may also occur because of excessive potassium loss in sweat. As a rule, potassium depletion is accompanied by loss of chloride. Insufficiency of both ions produces *hypokalemic alkalosis.* Hypomagnesemia is found in 40% of patients with hypokalemia, and can be a potential cause of hypokalemia. This mechanism is not completely understood, although it is thought to occur through an increase in open potassium channels causing renal excretion of potassium.

Prevention and Treatment

Before treating hypokalemia, it is important to assess magnesium levels. If hypomagnesemia is present, hypokalemia cannot be adequately treated without prior magnesium replacement.

Potassium depletion can be treated with four potassium salts: potassium chloride, potassium phosphate, potassium gluconate, and potassium bicarbonate. These may also be used for prophylaxis against potassium insufficiency. For either treatment or prophylaxis, the preferred salt is *potassium chloride* because chloride deficiency frequently coexists with potassium deficiency.

Potassium chloride may be administered orally or intravenously. Oral therapy is preferred for prophylaxis and for treating mild deficiency. Intravenous therapy is reserved for severe deficiency and for patients who cannot take potassium by mouth.

Oral potassium chloride

Uses, dosage, and preparations. Oral potassium chloride may be used for both prevention and treatment of potassium deficiency. Dosages for prevention range from 16 to 24 mEq/d. Dosages for deficiency range from 40 to 100 mEq/d (Table 90.1). In a perfect world, giving 10 mEq of potassium should raise the serum potassium level by about 0.1 mEq/L.

Adverse effects. Potassium chloride irritates the gastrointestinal (GI) tract, frequently causing abdominal discomfort, nausea, vomiting, and diarrhea. With the exception of the sustained-release tablets, solid formulations can produce high local concentrations of potassium, resulting in severe intestinal injury (ulcerative lesions, bleeding, and perforation); it can also cause death. To minimize GI effects, oral potassium chloride should be taken with meals or a full glass of water. If symptoms of irritation occur, dosing should be discontinued. Rarely, oral potassium chloride produces hyperkalemia. This dangerous development is much more likely with intravenous therapy.

The principal complication is *hyper*kalemia, which can prove fatal. To reduce the risk for hyperkalemia, serum potassium levels should be measured before the infusion and periodically throughout the treatment interval. Also, renal function should be assessed before and during treatment to ensure adequate output of urine. If renal failure develops, the infusion should be stopped immediately. Changes in the electrocardiogram (ECG) can be an early indication that potassium toxicity is developing.

Contraindications to potassium use. Potassium should be avoided under conditions that predispose to hyperkalemia (e.g., severe renal impairment, use of potassium-sparing diuretics, and hypoaldosteronism). Potassium must also be avoided when hyperkalemia already exists.

Hyperkalemia

Causes

Hyperkalemia can result from a number of causes. These include severe tissue trauma, untreated Addison disease, acute acidosis (which draws potassium out of cells), acute renal failure, misuse of potassium-sparing diuretics, and overdose with intravenous potassium.

Consequences

The most serious consequence of hyperkalemia is disruption of the electrical activity of the heart. Because hyperkalemia alters the generation and conduction of cardiac impulses, alterations in the ECG and cardiac rhythm are usually the earliest signs that potassium levels are growing dangerously high. With mild elevation of serum potassium (5 to 7 mEq/L), the T wave heightens and the PR interval becomes prolonged. When serum potassium reaches 8 to 9 mEq/L, cardiac arrest can occur, possibly preceded by ventricular tachycardia or fibrillation.

Effects of hyperkalemia are not limited to the heart. Noncardiac effects include confusion, anxiety, dyspnea, weakness or heaviness of the legs, and numbness or tingling of the hands, feet, and lips.

Treatment

Treatment is begun by withholding any foods that contain potassium and any medicines that promote potassium accumulation (e.g., potassium-sparing diuretics and potassium supplements). After this, management consists of measures that (1) counteract potassium-induced cardiotoxicity and (2) lower extracellular levels of potassium. Specific steps include infusion of a *calcium salt* (e.g., calcium gluconate) to offset effects of hyperkalemia on the heart and infusion of *glucose* and *insulin* to promote uptake of potassium by cells and thereby decrease extracellular potassium levels. If these measures prove inadequate, steps can be taken to remove potassium. These include (1) oral or rectal administration of *sodium polystyrene sulfonate* (Kayexalate and Kionex), an exchange resin that absorbs potassium (Table 90.2), and (2) peritoneal or extracorporeal dialysis.

Additional potassium binders. In 2015, the US Food and Drug Administration approved the first new drug to treat hyperkalemia in many years. Patiromer (Veltassa) is a powder that works by decreasing absorption of potassium by binding potassium within the GI tract. Patiromer is useful in reducing potassium levels in patients with chronic kidney disease or those treated with a drug that affects the renin-angiotensin-aldosterone system. Because of its slower onset, patiromer is not approved for the treatment of acute hyperkalemia.

In 2018, a similar drug, sodium zirconium cyclosillcate (Lokelma), followed suit. Lokelma increases fecal potassium excretion, just as patiromer does, through binding of potassium in the GI tract. As with patiromer, Lokelma is not to be used in the treatment of acute hyperkalemia. It is supplied in a 5- and 10-g powder for oral suspension. The patient empties the foil-lined packet into a glass of water for ingestion.

TABLE 90.1   Potassium Chloride Uses, Dosage, and Preparations

Drug	Forms	Uses	Usual Adult Doses
K-Dur	Tablets	Prevention of hypokalemia	20–40 mEq/d PO in 1–2 divided doses
Micro-K	Powder	Treatment of mild hypokalemia	40–100 mEq/d PO in 2–5 divided doses
Klor-Con	Tablets and powder	Treatment of mild to moderate hypokalemia	40–100 mEq/d PO in 3–4 divided doses
Potassium chloride IV solution		Treatment of moderate to severe hypokalemia	10 mEq/h IV Maximum 24-h dose: 200 mEq

TABLE 90.2	**Potassium Binding Drugs**		
Drug	**Forms**	**Uses**	**Usual Adult Doses**
Sodium Polystyrene Sulfonate (Kayexalate)	15-g/60 mL solution, 15-g powder for suspension	Treatment of hyperkalemia in infants, children, and adults	15 g PO qd–qid
Patiromer (Veltassa)	8.4-g, 16.8-g, 25.2-g powder for oral suspension	Treatment of hyperkalemia in patients taking an ACEI medication or with chronic kidney disease	Start with 8.4-g packet dissolved in water daily. May increase dose by 8.4 g weekly to max of 25.2 g/d
Sodium zirconium cyclosilicate (Lokelma)	5-g and 10-g powder for oral suspension	Treatment of hyperkalemia in adults	Start with 10-g packet dissolved in water tid for 48 h Then 10 g/d if continuing treatment

ACEI, Angiotensin-converting enzyme inhibitor

TABLE 90.3	**Magnesium Uses, Dosage, and Preparations**		
Drug	**Forms**	**Uses**	**Usual Adult Doses**
Magnesium oxide	Tablets	Prevention of hypomagnesemia	400–800 mg/d PO in 1–2 divided doses
Magnesium sulfate	Intravenous solution	Treatment of mild hypomagnesemia	1–2 g IV as indicated by serum magnesium concentrations
		Treatment of moderate hypomagnesemia	2–4 g IV as indicated by serum magnesium concentrations
		Treatment of severe hypomagnesemia	4–8 g IV as indicated by serum magnesium concentrations

MAGNESIUM IMBALANCES

Magnesium is required for the activity of many enzymes and for binding of messenger RNA to ribosomes. In addition, magnesium helps regulate neurochemical transmission and the excitability of muscle. The concentration of magnesium within cells is about 40 mEq/L, much higher than its concentration outside cells (~2 mEq/L).

Hypomagnesemia
Causes and Consequences

Low levels of magnesium may result from a variety of causes, including diarrhea, hemodialysis, kidney disease, and prolonged intravenous feeding with magnesium-free solutions. Hypomagnesemia may also be seen in people with chronic alcoholism, diabetes, or pancreatitis. Frequently, patients with magnesium deficiency also present with hypocalcemia and hypokalemia.

Prominent symptoms of hypomagnesemia involve cardiac and skeletal muscle. In the presence of low levels of magnesium, release of acetylcholine at the neuromuscular junction is enhanced. This can increase muscle excitability to the point of tetany. Hypomagnesemia also increases excitability of neurons in the CNS, causing disorientation, psychosis, and seizures.

Prevention and Treatment

Frank hypomagnesemia is treated with parenteral magnesium sulfate. For prophylaxis against magnesium deficiency, an oral preparation (magnesium oxide) may be used (Table 90.3).

Adverse effects. Excessive levels of magnesium cause *neuromuscular blockade*. Paralysis of the respiratory muscles is of particular concern. By suppressing neuromuscular transmission, magnesium excess can intensify the effects of neuromuscular blocking agents (e.g., succinylcholine and atracurium). Hence caution must be exercised in patients receiving these drugs. The neuromuscular blocking actions of magnesium can be counteracted with calcium. Accordingly, when parenteral magnesium is being employed, an injectable form of calcium (e.g., calcium gluconate) should be immediately available.

In the heart, excessive magnesium can suppress impulse conduction through the atrioventricular (AV) node. Accordingly, magnesium sulfate is contraindicated for patients with AV heart block.

To minimize the risk for toxicity, serum magnesium levels should be monitored. Respiratory paralysis occurs at 12 to 15 mEq/L. When magnesium levels exceed 25 mEq/L, cardiac arrest may set in.

Hypermagnesemia

Toxic elevation of magnesium levels is most common in patients with renal insufficiency, especially when magnesium-containing antacids or cathartics are being used. Symptoms of mild intoxication include muscle weakness (resulting from inhibition of acetylcholine release), hypotension, sedation, and ECG changes. As noted, respiratory paralysis is likely when plasma levels reach 12 to 15 mEq/L. At higher magnesium concentrations, there is a risk for cardiac arrest. Muscle weakness and paralysis can be counteracted with intravenous calcium.

 SUMMARY OF KEY PRESCRIBING CONSIDERATIONS

Electrolytes and Potassium Binders

Therapeutic Goal: To maintain serum potassium and magnesium levels within normal range.

Baseline Data: ECG, magnesium, potassium levels.

Monitoring: ECG, magnesium, potassium levels.

Identifying High-Risk Patients: Potassium and magnesium supplements must be used with caution in patients with renal dysfunction or in those taking angiotensin-converting enzyme inhibitors or potassium sparing diuretics. In patients with ECG changes, cardiac monitoring should be initiated.

Evaluating Therapeutic Effects: Patients must be monitored for ECG changes, change in muscle spasticity or weakness, and changes in sensation. Serum potassium and magnesium levels according to replacement protocols and severity must also be monitored.

Minimizing Adverse Effects: Recommended facility protocols for electrolyte replacement must be followed.

91

Management of ST-Segment Elevation Myocardial Infarction

Myocardial infarction (MI) is defined as necrosis of the myocardium resulting from local ischemia. The underlying cause is partial or complete blockage of a coronary artery. In this chapter, discussion is limited to *ST-segment elevation myocardial infarction* (STEMI). Management of STEMI differs from management of non ST–elevation MI, which occurs when blockage of blood flow is only partial.

PATHOPHYSIOLOGY OF STEMI

Acute MI occurs when blood flow to a region of the myocardium is stopped owing to platelet plugging and thrombus formation in a coronary artery—almost always at the site of a fissured or ruptured atherosclerotic plaque. Myocardial injury is ultimately the result of an imbalance between oxygen demand and oxygen supply.

In response to local ischemia, a dramatic redistribution of ions takes place. Hydrogen ions accumulate in the myocardium, and calcium ions become sequestered in mitochondria. The resultant acidosis and functional calcium deficiency alter the distensibility of cardiac muscle. Sodium ions accumulate in myocardial cells and promote edema. Potassium ions are lost from myocardial cells, setting the stage for dysrhythmias.

Local metabolic changes begin rapidly after coronary artery occlusion. Within seconds, metabolism shifts from aerobic to anaerobic. High-energy stores of adenosine triphosphate (ATP) and creatine phosphate become depleted. As a result, contraction ceases in the affected region.

If blood flow is not restored, cell death begins within 20 minutes. Clear indices of cell death—myocyte disruption, coagulative necrosis, elevation of cardiac proteins in serum—are present by 24 hours. By 4 days, monocyte infiltration and removal of dead myocytes weaken the infarcted area, making it vulnerable to expansion and rupture. Structural integrity is partially restored with deposition of collagen, which begins in 10 to 12 days and ends with dense scar formation by 4 to 6 weeks.

Myocardial injury also triggers ventricular remodeling, a process in which ventricular mass increases and the chambers change in volume and shape. Remodeling is driven in part by local production of angiotensin II. Ventricular remodeling increases the risk for heart failure and death.

The degree of residual cardiac impairment depends on how much of the myocardium was damaged. With infarction of 10% of left ventricular (LV) mass, the ejection fraction is reduced. With 25% LV infarction, cardiac dilation and heart failure occur. With 40% LV infarction, cardiogenic shock and death are likely.

MANAGEMENT OF ST-SEGMENT ELEVATION MYOCARDIAL INFARCTION

The acute phase of management refers to the interval between the onset of symptoms and discharge from the hospital. The goal is to bring cardiac oxygen supply back in balance with oxygen demand. This can be accomplished by reperfusion therapy, which restores blood flow to the myocardium, and by reducing myocardial oxygen demand. The first few hours of treatment are most critical. The major threats to life during acute STEMI are ventricular dysrhythmias, cardiogenic shock, and heart failure.

To aid clinicians in the management of STEMI, the American College of Cardiology Foundation (ACCF), the American Heart Association (AHA), and the Society for Cardiovascular Angiography and Interventions (SCAI) have updated a series of evidence-based guidelines, including the following:

- *2013 ACCF/AHA Guideline for the Management of ST-Elevation Myocardial Infarction: A Report of the American College of Cardiology Foundation/American Heart Association Task Force on Practice Guidelines*
- *2015 ACC/AHA/SCAI Focused Update on Primary Percutaneous Coronary Intervention for Patients with ST-Elevation Myocardial Infarction: An Update of the 2011 ACCF/AHA/SCAI Guideline for Percutaneous Coronary Intervention and the 2013 ACCF/AHA Guideline for the Management of ST-Elevation Myocardial Infarction*

These guidelines are available at www.circ.ahajournals.org. The following discussion reflects recommendations in these documents.

Routine Drug Therapy

When a patient presents with suspected STEMI, several interventions should begin immediately. The objective is to minimize possible myocardial necrosis while waiting for a clear diagnosis. After STEMI has been diagnosed, more definitive therapy—reperfusion—can be implemented (see later).

Oxygen

Supplemental oxygen, administered by nasal cannula, can increase arterial oxygen saturation and hence increase oxygen delivery to the ischemic myocardium. Accordingly, current guidelines recommend giving oxygen to all patients with reduced arterial oxygen saturation (below 90%). However, although oxygen is recommended and using it seems to make sense, the practice is not evidence-based. That is, we have no hard evidence to show that oxygen is beneficial. In fact, there is some evidence that oxygen may actually be harmful, causing mortality to increase rather than decline.

Aspirin

Aspirin suppresses platelet aggregation, producing an immediate antithrombotic effect. In the Second International Study of Infarct Survival (ISIS-2), aspirin caused a substantial reduction in mortality. Moreover, benefits were synergistic with fibrinolytic drugs: mortality was 13.2% with fibrinolytics alone and dropped to 8% with the addition of aspirin. Because of these benefits, virtually all patients with evolving STEMI should get aspirin. Therapy should begin immediately after onset of symptoms and should continue indefinitely. The first dose (162 to 325 mg) should be chewed to allow rapid absorption across the buccal mucosa. Prolonged therapy (with 81 to 162 mg/d) reduces the risk for reinfarction, stroke, and death.

Nonaspirin Nonsteroidal Antiinflammatory Drugs

According to the 2013 guideline updates, routine use of nonsteroidal antiinflammatory drugs (NSAIDs) other than aspirin should be *discontinued*. Unlike aspirin, these agents increase the risk for mortality, reinfarction, hypertension, heart failure, and myocardial rupture.

Morphine

Intravenous morphine is the treatment of choice for STEMI-associated pain. In addition to relieving pain, morphine can improve hemodynamics. By promoting venodilation, the drug reduces cardiac preload. By promoting modest arterial dilation, morphine may cause some reduction in afterload. The combined reductions in preload and afterload lower cardiac oxygen demand, helping preserve the ischemic myocardium.

β Blockers

When given to patients undergoing acute STEMI, cardioselective β blockers reduce cardiac pain, infarct size, and short-term mortality. Recurrent ischemia and reinfarction are also decreased. Reduction in myocardial wall tension may decrease the risk for myocardial rupture. Continued use of an oral β blocker increases long-term survival. Unfortunately, although nearly all patients can benefit from β blockers, many don't get them. Furthermore, among patients who *do* get a β blocker, the dosage is often too low.

Benefits result from several mechanisms. As STEMI evolves, traffic along sympathetic nerves to the heart increases greatly, as does the number of β receptors in the heart. As a result, heart rate and force of contraction rise substantially, increasing cardiac oxygen demand. By preventing β-receptor activation, β blockers reduce heart rate and contractility and, hence, reduce oxygen demand. They reduce oxygen demand even more by lowering blood pressure. By prolonging diastolic filling time, β blockers increase coronary blood flow and myocardial oxygen supply. Additional benefits derive from antidysrhythmic actions.

Beta blockers should be used routinely in the absence of specific contraindications (e.g., bradycardia and significant LV dysfunction). The initial dose may be oral or intravenous; oral dosing is used thereafter. Treatment with an oral β blocker should begin within 24 hours. β blockers are especially good for patients with reflex tachycardia, systolic hypertension, atrial fibrillation, and atrioventricular conduction abnormalities. Contraindications include overt severe heart failure, pronounced bradycardia, persistent hypotension, advanced heart block, and cardiogenic shock. The basic pharmacology of the β blockers is presented in Chapter 15.

Nitroglycerin

In patients with STEMI, nitroglycerin has several beneficial effects: it can (1) reduce preload and thereby reduce oxygen demand, (2) increase collateral blood flow in the ischemic region of the heart, (3) control hypertension caused by STEMI-associated anxiety, and (4) limit infarct size and improve LV function. However, despite these useful effects, nitroglycerin does not reduce mortality. Nonetheless, because the drug is easily administered, offers hemodynamic benefits, and helps relieve ischemic chest pain, it continues to be used. According to the current guidelines, patients with ongoing ischemic discomfort should be given sublingual nitroglycerin (0.4 mg) every 5 minutes for a total of three doses and then be assessed to determine whether intravenous nitroglycerin should be given. Indications for intravenous therapy include persisting ischemic discomfort, hypertension, and pulmonary congestion. Nitroglycerin should be avoided in patients with hypotension (systolic pressure <90 mm Hg), severe bradycardia (heart rate <50 beats/min), marked tachycardia (heart rate >100 beats/min), or suspected right ventricular infarction. In addition, nitroglycerin should be avoided in patients who have taken sildenafil, avanafil, or vardenafil for erectile dysfunction or pulmonary hypertension within the last 24 hours or tadalafil within the last 48 hours.

Reperfusion Therapy

The goal of reperfusion therapy is to restore blood flow through the blocked coronary artery. Reperfusion is the most effective way to preserve myocardial function and limit infarct size. Reperfusion is accomplished with either fibrinolytic drugs or percutaneous coronary intervention (PCI), usually balloon angioplasty coupled with placement of a stent. Both options are very effective. However, PCI is generally preferred. The relative advantages of fibrinolytic therapy and primary PCI are shown in Table 91.1. With either intervention, rapid implementation is essential.

Primary Percutaneous Coronary Intervention

The term *primary PCI* refers to the use of angioplasty rather than fibrinolytic therapy to recanalize an occluded coronary artery. In almost all cases, PCI consists of balloon angioplasty coupled with placement of a drug-eluting stent. Under current guidelines, the institutional goal is to implement PCI within 90 minutes of initial patient contact. As discussed later, all patients undergoing PCI should receive an anticoagulant (intravenous heparin and bivalirudin) combined with antiplatelet drugs: aspirin plus either clopidogrel, ticagrelor, or prasugrel, and perhaps a glycoprotein (GP) IIb/IIIa inhibitor.

The success rate with primary PCI is somewhat higher than with fibrinolytic therapy. Moreover, studies indicate that the benefits of PCI last longer. After 30 days, the rate of death, reinfarction, or disabling stroke after PCI is 8% versus 13.7% after fibrinolytic therapy using tissue plasminogen activator (tPA). After 7.8 years, the rate of all-cause mortality after PCI is 34.88%, versus 41.3% with streptokinase—the difference being due entirely to lower cardiovascular mortality in PCI-treated patients. Benefits of primary PCI over fibrinolytic therapy are greatest in high-risk patients.

Fibrinolytic Therapy

Fibrinolytic drugs dissolve clots by converting plasminogen into plasmin, a proteolytic enzyme that digests the fibrin meshwork that holds clots together. In the United States, three fibrinolytic drugs are available: *alteplase (tPA), reteplase,* and *tenecteplase.* The basic pharmacology of these drugs is discussed in Chapter 91. Discussion here is limited to their use in STEMI.

TABLE 91.1 Comparison of Fibrinolytic Therapy With Primary Percutaneous Coronary Intervention	
Advantages of fibrinolytic therapy	• More universal access • Shorter time to treatment • Results less dependent on physician experience • Lower system cost
Advantages of primary PCI	• Higher initial reperfusion rates • Less residual stenosis • Lower recurrence rates of ischemia/infarction • Does not promote intracranial bleeding • Defines coronary anatomy and LV function • Can be used when fibrinolytic therapy is contraindicated

LV, Left ventricular; *PCI,* percutaneous coronary intervention

Fibrinolytic therapy is most effective when presentation is early. When thrombolytics are given soon enough, the occluded artery can be opened in 80% of patients. Current guidelines suggest a target of 30 minutes or less for the time between entering the emergency department and starting fibrinolysis. Clinical trials have shown that timely therapy improves ventricular function, limits infarct size, and reduces mortality. Restoration of blood flow reduces or eliminates chest pain and often reduces ST elevation. Current guidelines restrict fibrinolytic therapy to patients with ischemic pain that has been present no more than 12 to 24 hours. Patients for whom fibrinolytic therapy is contraindicated are listed in Table 91.2.

Under *typical* conditions, all fibrinolytics are equally beneficial. However, under *ideal* conditions (i.e., treatment within 4 to 6 hours of

pain onset), alteplase is most effective, especially in patients younger than 75 years, as shown in the Global Utilization of Streptokinase and TPA for Occluded Coronary Arteries (GUSTO-I) trial. Unfortunately alteplase is very expensive.

The major complication of fibrinolytic therapy is bleeding, which occurs in 1% to 5% of patients. Intracranial hemorrhage (ICH) is the greatest concern. ICH has an incidence of 0.5% to 1% and is most likely in older adults. Nonetheless, the benefits of fibrinolysis generally outweigh the risks.

As discussed later, all patients undergoing fibrinolytic therapy should receive an anticoagulant (intravenous heparin, bivalirudin, enoxaparin, and fondaparinux) plus antiplatelet drugs (aspirin plus clopidogrel—but not a GP IIb/IIIa inhibitor, such as abciximab).

Adjuncts to Reperfusion Therapy
Anticoagulants
Heparin. Heparin is recommended for all STEMI patients undergoing fibrinolytic therapy or PCI. For those receiving fibrinolytic drugs, treatment should begin before giving the fibrinolytic and should continue for at least 48 to 72 hours after. For patients undergoing PCI, heparin is given once, immediately before the procedure.

Heparin is available as the intact (unfractionated) drug and in low-molecular-weight (LMW) forms. When heparin is used as an adjunct to fibrinolytic therapy, selection of a heparin product depends on duration of use. For treatment lasting less than 48 hours, *unfractionated* heparin can be employed. However, for treatment lasting more than 48 hours, enoxaparin (Lovenox), an *LMW* heparin, should be chosen because prolonged use of unfractionated heparin poses a risk for heparin-induced thrombocytopenia (Table 91.3).

Antiplatelet Drugs
Thienopyridines: clopidogrel, ticagrelor, and prasugrel. Clopidogrel (Plavix), ticagrelor (Brilinta), and prasugrel (Effient) suppress platelet aggregation by blocking receptors for adenosine diphosphate. These drugs are recommended for all MI patients undergoing PCI. In all cases, clopidogrel, ticagrelor, or prasugrel should be *combined* with aspirin. In patients undergoing PCI with stenting, duration of treatment should be at least 12 months unless the risk for bleeding outweighs the benefits of continued drug use. In patients undergoing fibrinolytic therapy, clopidogrel is the only recommended antiplatelet drug. Dosing should continue for at least 14 days up to a period of 1 year. These drugs are discussed in detail in Chapter 45.

Glycoprotein IIb/IIIa inhibitors. The GP IIb/IIIa inhibitors (e.g., abciximab [ReoPro]) are powerful intravenous antiplatelet drugs that inhibit the final step in platelet aggregation. These drugs are recommended for patients undergoing PCI but not for those undergoing fibrinolytic therapy. Of the three GP IIb/IIIa inhibitors available, abciximab is preferred. Treatment should begin as soon as possible before PCI and should continue for 12 hours thereafter. For further information, refer to Chapter 91.

Aspirin. As discussed earlier, *low-dose* aspirin (81 to 162 mg/d) should be taken indefinitely by all people who have had an MI. This should be combined with antiplatelet drugs (clopidogrel, ticagrelor, and prasugrel) for a period of 1 year. The duration of therapy does not change with placement of a drug-eluting stent or bare metal stent.

Angiotensin-Converting Enzyme Inhibitors and Angiotensin II Receptor Blockers
When used after acute STEMI, angiotensin-converting enzyme inhibitors (ACEIs; e.g., captopril and lisinopril) decrease short-term mortality in all patients and long-term mortality in patients with reduced LV function. Benefits derive from reducing preload and afterload, promoting water

TABLE 91.2 Contraindications and Cautions Regarding Use of Fibrinolytics for Myocardial Infarction

Absolute contraindications	• Any prior intracranial hemorrhage • Known structural cerebrovascular lesion • Ischemic stroke within last 3 months *except* ischemic stroke within 4.5 h • Known intracranial neoplasm • Active internal bleeding (other than menses) • Severe uncontrolled hypertension (unresponsive to emergency therapy) • Suspected aortic dissection • For streptokinase, prior treatment within the previous 6 months • Intracranial or intraspinal surgery within 2 months • Significant closed head or facial trauma within 3 months
Relative contraindications and cautions	• Severe, uncontrolled hypertension on presentation (blood pressure above 180/110 mm Hg) • History of chronic, severe, poorly controlled hypertension • History of prior ischemic stroke (>3 months earlier), dementia, or known intracerebral pathology not covered in contraindications • Current use of anticoagulants in therapeutic doses (INR 2–3 or greater); known bleeding diathesis • Traumatic or prolonged (>10 min) CPR or major surgery (<3 weeks ago) • Recent internal bleeding (within 2–4 weeks) • Noncompressible vascular punctures • Pregnancy • Active peptic ulcer • Oral anticoagulant therapy

CPR, Cardiopulmonary resuscitation; *INR*, international normalized ratio.
Adapted from O'Gara PT, Kushner FG, Ascheim DD, et al. 2013 ACCF/AHA guideline for the management of ST-Elevation Myocardial Infarction: a report of the American College of Cardiology Foundation/American Heart Association Task Force on practice guidelines. *J Am Coll Cardiol.* 2013;61:e78–e140.

TABLE 91.3	**Adjuncts to Reperfusion Therapy**			
Drug	**Class**	**Usual Adult Dose**	**Preferred Use**	**Contraindications**
Enoxaparin (Lovenox)	Low-molecular-weight heparin	30-mg IV bolus followed by 1 mg/kg q 12 h subcutaneously Continue until revascularization or for a period of 8 days	Treatment lasting >48 h	Patients >75 years should not receive IV bolus Adjust dose for CrCl <30 mL/min
Fondaparinux (Arixtra)	Factor Xa inhibitor	2.5-mg IV followed by 2.5 mg daily subcutaneously Continue until revascularization or for a period of 8 days	Alternative to therapy with heparin in patients undergoing reperfusion with thrombolytics	Not recommended as sole anticoagulant in PCI Do not use in patients with CrCl <30 mL/min
Bivalirudin (Angiomax)	Direct thrombin inhibitor	0.75-mg/kg bolus IV followed by continued infusion at 1/75 mg/kg per hour	Preferred agent with GP IIb/IIIa inhibitors in patients undergoing PCI Alternative to heparin in patients with heparin-induced thrombocytopenia	Reduce doses for patients with CrCl <3 mL/min

IV, Intravenous; *CrCl,* Creatinine clearance; *PCI,* percutaneous coronary intervention.

loss and favorably altering ventricular remodeling. Because of their benefits, ACEIs are recommended for all STEMI patients in the absence of specific contraindications. Treatment should start within 24 hours of symptom onset. The possibility that long-term therapy may also benefit patients who do not have LV dysfunction is being evaluated in large-scale trials. The major adverse effects of ACEIs are hypotension and cough. Contraindications to ACEIs are hypotension, bilateral renal artery stenosis, renal failure, and a history of ACEI-induced cough or angioedema. The basic pharmacology of the ACEIs is described in Chapter 37.

Therapy with angiotensin receptor blockers (ARBs) in STEMI patients has not been studied as extensively as has therapy with ACEIs. However, one major trial—Valsartan in Acute Myocardial Infarction Trial (VALIANT)—demonstrated that, in patients with post-MI heart failure or LV dysfunction, valsartan (an ARB) was as effective as captopril (an ACEI) at reducing short-term and long-term mortality. In the current guidelines, ARBs are recommended for STEMI patients who are intolerant of ACEIs and have heart failure or reduced LV function.

COMPLICATIONS OF STEMI

MI predisposes the heart and vascular system to serious complications. Among the most severe are ventricular dysrhythmias, cardiogenic shock, and heart failure.

Ventricular Dysrhythmias

These dysrhythmias develop frequently and are the major cause of death after MI. Sudden death from dysrhythmias occurs in 15% of patients during the first hour. Ultimately, ventricular dysrhythmias cause 60% of infarction-related deaths. Acute management of ventricular fibrillation consists of defibrillation followed by intravenous amiodarone for 24 to 48 hours. Programmed ventricular stimulation with guided antidysrhythmic therapy may be lifesaving for some patients.

Cardiogenic Shock

Shock results from greatly reduced tissue perfusion secondary to impaired cardiac function. Shock develops in 7% to 10% of patients in the first few days after MI and has a mortality rate of up to 50% in hospitalized patients. Patients at highest risk are those with large infarcts, a previous infarct, a low ejection fraction (<35%), diabetes, and advanced age. Drug therapy includes inotropic agents (e.g., dopamine and dobutamine) to increase cardiac output and vasodilators (nitroglycerin and

nitroprusside) to improve tissue perfusion and reduce cardiac work and oxygen demand. Unfortunately, although these drugs can improve hemodynamic status, they do not seem to reduce mortality. Restoration of cardiac perfusion with PCI or coronary artery bypass grafting may be of value.

Heart Failure

Heart failure secondary to acute MI can be treated with a combination of drugs. A diuretic (e.g., furosemide) is given to decrease preload and pulmonary congestion. Inotropic agents (e.g., digoxin) increase cardiac output by enhancing contractility. Vasodilators (e.g., nitroglycerin and nitroprusside) improve hemodynamic status by reducing preload, afterload, or both. ACEIs (or ARBs), which reduce both preload and afterload, can be especially helpful. β blockers may also improve outcome. Drug therapy of heart failure is discussed in Chapter 41.

Cardiac Rupture

Weakening of the myocardium predisposes the heart wall to rupture. After rupture, shock and circulatory collapse develop rapidly. Death is often immediate. Fortunately cardiac rupture is relatively rare (less than 2% incidence). Patients at highest risk are those with a large anterior infarction. Cardiac rupture is most likely within the first days after MI. Early treatment with vasodilators and β blockers may reduce the risk for wall rupture.

SECONDARY PREVENTION OF STEMI

As a rule, patients who survive the acute phase of STEMI can be discharged from the hospital as early as 72 hours after admission if they remain free from complications. However, they are still at risk for reinfarction (5% to 15% incidence within the first year) and other complications (e.g., dysrhythmias and heart failure). Outcome can be improved with risk factor reduction, exercise, and long-term therapy with drugs.

Reduction of risk factors for MI can increase long-term survival. Patients who smoke must be encouraged to quit; the goal is total cessation. Patients with high serum cholesterol should be given an appropriate dietary plan and treated with a high-dose statin. Hypertension and diabetes increase the risk for mortality and must be controlled. For patients with hypertension, blood pressure should be decreased to below 130/80 mm Hg. For patients with diabetes, the goal is a level of hemoglobin A_{1c} below 7%.

Exercise training can be valuable for two reasons: it reduces complications associated with prolonged bed rest, and it accelerates return to an optimal level of functioning. The goal is 30 minutes of exercise at least 3 to 4 days a week. Although exercise is safe for most patients, there is a concern regarding cardiac risk and impairment of infarct healing in patients whose infarcts are large.

All post-MI patients should take four drugs: (1) a β blocker; (2) an ACEI or an ARB, either (3a) an antiplatelet drug (aspirin or clopidogrel, ticagrelor, or prasugrel) or (3b) an anticoagulant (warfarin); and (4) a statin. All four should be taken indefinitely.

Estrogen therapy for postmenopausal women is not effective as secondary prevention and should not be initiated.

SUMMARY OF KEY PRESCRIBING CONSIDERATIONS

STEMI Treatment

Therapeutic Goal: Increase oxygen supply to the myocardium while decreasing oxygen demand and preventing complications from STEMI.

Baseline Data: Weight, vital signs, coagulation levels, CBC, CMP, troponins, and ECG.

Monitoring: Continuous cardiac monitoring, repeat ECGs, coagulation levels, physical examination for bleeding, and CBC for platelets and hemoglobin levels.

Identifying High-Risk Patients: Risk factors for MI include history of cardiovascular disease, smoking, hypertension, hyperlipidemia, sedentary lifestyle, and diabetes.

Evaluating Therapeutic Effects: Monitor for chest pain, dysrhythmias, bleeding, and hypotension.

Minimizing Adverse Effects: PCI or fibrolytic therapy should be initiated as soon as possible to minimize myocardial damage.

92

Drugs for Acute Care

Most of the medications discussed throughout this book are available in oral form or are used in primary care settings. There are a few medications that are reserved for the prehospital, emergency department, or inpatient hospital setting. These medications are given to treat acute illness.

ANESTHESIA, NEUROMUSCULAR BLOCKERS, AND ANALGESIA

Intravenous Regional Anesthesia

Intravenous regional anesthesia is employed to anesthetize the extremities—hands, feet, arms, and lower legs (but not the entire leg because too much anesthetic would be needed). Anesthesia is produced by injection into a distal vein of an arm or leg. Before giving the anesthetic, blood is removed from the limb (by gravity or by application of an Esmarch bandage) and a tourniquet is applied to the limb (proximal to the site of anesthetic injection) to prevent anesthetic from entering the systemic circulation. To ensure complete blockade of arterial flow throughout the procedure, a double tourniquet is used. After injection, the anesthetic diffuses out of the vasculature and becomes evenly distributed to all areas of the occluded limb. When the tourniquet is loosened at the end of surgery, about 15% to 30% of administered anesthetic is released into the systemic circulation. Lidocaine is the preferred agent for this type of anesthesia.

Alfentanil and Sufentanil

Alfentanil (Alfenta) and sufentanil are intravenous opioids related to fentanyl. Both drugs are used for the induction of anesthesia, for maintenance of anesthesia (in combination with other agents), and as sole anesthetic agents. Pharmacologic effects are similar to those of morphine. Sufentanil has an especially high milligram potency (about 1000 times that of morphine). Alfentanil is about 10 times more potent than morphine. Both drugs have a rapid onset, and both are schedule II agents.

Remifentanil

Remifentanil (Ultiva) is an intravenous opioid with a rapid onset and brief duration. The brief duration results from rapid metabolism by plasma and tissue esterases and not from hepatic metabolism or renal excretion. Similar to fentanyl, remifentanil is about 100 times more potent than morphine. Remifentanil is approved for analgesia during surgery and during the immediate postoperative period. Administration is by continuous intravenous infusion. Effects begin in minutes and terminate 5 to 10 minutes after the infusion is stopped. Adverse effects during the infusion include respiratory depression, hypotension, bradycardia, and muscle rigidity sufficient to compromise breathing. Postinfusion effects include nausea, vomiting, and headache. Remifentanil is regulated as a schedule II substance.

Dexmedetomidine

Actions and therapeutic use. Dexmedetomidine (Precedex), similar to clonidine, is a selective α_2-adrenergic agonist. The drug acts in the central nervous system (CNS) to cause sedation and analgesia. It has two approved indications: (1) short-term sedation in critically ill patients who are initially intubated and undergoing mechanical ventilation and (2) sedation for nonintubated patients before and/or during surgical and other procedures. However, in addition to these approved uses, dexmedetomidine has a variety of off-label uses, including sedation during awake craniotomy, prevention and treatment of postanesthetic shivering, and enhancement of sedation and analgesia in patients undergoing general anesthesia. In contrast to clonidine, which is administered by epidural infusion, dexmedetomidine is administered by intravenous infusion.

Pharmacokinetics. With intravenous infusion, dexmedetomidine undergoes wide distribution to tissues. In the blood, the drug is 94% protein-bound. Dexmedetomidine undergoes rapid and complete hepatic metabolism, followed by excretion in the urine. The elimination half-life is 2 hours.

Adverse effects. The most common adverse effects are hypotension and bradycardia. The mechanism is activation of α_2-adrenergic receptors in the CNS and periphery, which results in decreased release of norepinephrine from sympathetic neurons innervating the heart and blood vessels. If these cardiovascular effects are too intense, they can be managed in several ways, including (1) decreasing or stopping the infusion, (2) infusing fluid, and (3) elevating the lower extremities. Giving a muscarinic antagonist (e.g., atropine) can increase heart rate.

Additional adverse effects include nausea, dry mouth, and transient hypertension. Importantly, dexmedetomidine does not cause respiratory depression.

Drug interactions. Dexmedetomidine can enhance the actions of anesthetics, sedatives, hypnotics, and opioids. Excessive CNS depression can be managed by reducing the dosage of dexmedetomidine or the other agents.

Etomidate

Etomidate is a potent hypnotic agent used for the induction of anesthesia. Unconsciousness develops rapidly and lasts about 5 minutes. The drugs have no analgesic actions. Adverse effects associated with single injections include transient apnea, venous pain at the injection site, and suppression of plasma cortisol levels for 6 to 8 hours. Repeated administration can cause hypotension, oliguria, and electrolyte disturbances.

Ketamine

Ketamine produces a state known as dissociative anesthesia in which the patient feels dissociated from his or her environment. In addition, the drug causes sedation, immobility, analgesia, and amnesia. Intravenous induction is rapid and emergence begins within 10 to 15 minutes. Ketamine is especially valuable for anesthesia in patients undergoing minor surgical procedures.

Midazolam

Intravenous midazolam may be used for induction of anesthesia and to produce conscious sedation. Unconsciousness develops in 80 seconds. Conscious sedation can be produced by combining midazolam with an opioid analgesic. Midazolam can cause dangerous cardiorespiratory effects, including respiratory depression and respiratory and cardiac arrest.

Benzodiazepine Overdose
Flumazenil

Flumazenil (Romazicon) is a competitive benzodiazepine receptor antagonist. The drug can reverse the sedative effects of benzodiazepines, but may not reverse respiratory depression. Flumazenil is approved for benzodiazepine overdose and for reversing the effects of benzodiazepines after general anesthesia. The principal adverse effect is precipitation of seizures in patients who are physically dependent on benzodiazepines. This is most likely in patients taking benzodiazepines to treat epilepsy and in those who are physically dependent on benzodiazepines. Flumazenil is administered intravenously. Although flumazenil can be used to reverse the effects of benzodizepines, the risks often outweigh the benefits and should be reserved for severe symptoms. Consutation with a toxicologist should be considered.

Epidural Anesthesia

Epidural anesthesia is achieved by injecting a local anesthetic into the epidural space (i.e., within the spinal column but outside the dura mater). A catheter placed in the epidural space allows administration by bolus or by continuous infusion. After administration, diffusion of anesthetic across the dura into the subarachnoid space blocks conduction in nerve roots and in the spinal cord. Diffusion through intervertebral foramina blocks nerves located in the paravertebral region. With epidural administration, anesthetic can reach the systemic circulation in significant amounts. As a result, when the technique is used during delivery, neonatal depression may result. Lidocaine and bupivacaine are popular drugs for epidural anesthesia. Because of the risk for death from cardiac arrest, the concentrated (0.75%) solution of bupivacaine must not be used in obstetric patients.

Spinal (Subarachnoid) Anesthesia
Technique

Spinal anesthesia is produced by injecting local anesthetic into the subarachnoid space. Injection is made in the lumbar region below the termination of the cord. Spread of anesthetic within the subarachnoid space determines the level of anesthesia achieved. Movement of anesthetic within the subarachnoid space is determined by two factors: (1) the density of the anesthetic solution and (2) the position of the patient. Anesthetics employed most commonly are bupivacaine, lidocaine, and tetracaine. All must be free of preservatives.

Analgesia
Acetaminophen

Intravenous acetaminophen (Ofirmev) is indicated for fever and mild to moderate pain (when used alone) and for moderate to severe pain (when combined with an opioid). Dosages are as follows:

- Adults and children 13 years and older who weigh more than 50 kg—1000 mg every 6 hours or 650 mg every 4 hours as needed. The daily maximum is 4000 mg.
- Children 2 to 12 years old, and children 13 years and older who weigh less than 50 kg—15 mg/kg every 6 hours or 12.5 mg/kg every 4 hours as needed. The daily maximum is 75 mg/kg.

Acetaminophen Overdose—Acetylcysteine

For intravenous therapy, acetylcysteine is supplied in solution (200 mg/mL), sold as Acetadote; it should be diluted in 5% dextrose. Three doses are given in sequence. The first dose—150 mg/kg (in 200 mL of 5% dextrose)—is infused over 15 minutes to 1 hour. The second dose—50 mg/kg (in 500 mL of 5% dextrose)—is infused over 4 hours. And the third dose—100 mg/kg (in 1000 mL of 5% dextrose)—is infused over 16 hours. Rarely, intravenous acetylcysteine causes allergic reactions (rash, itching, angioedema, bronchospasm, and hypotension), most often in response to the first dose. Fortunately, these reactions tend to be mild and self-limited and can be minimized by infusing the initial dose slowly (over a 1-hour interval).

Reversal of Opioid Effects

Naloxone. Naloxone may be employed to reverse excessive respiratory and CNS depression caused by opioids. Dosage should be titrated with care; the objective is to achieve adequate ventilation and alertness without reversing opioid actions to the point of unmasking pain. The initial dose is 0.4 mg for adults and 0.1 mg/kg for children. The intravenous route is preferred.

If intravenous administration is not possible, intramuscular, intranasal, or subcutaneous injection may be employed. Dosing is repeated at 2- to 3-minute intervals until a satisfactory response has been achieved. Additional doses may be needed at 1- to 2-hour intervals or more frequently for up to 72 hours, depending on the duration of the offending opioid.

Alvimopan. Alvimopan (Entereg) is a selective, peripherally acting mu opioid antagonist developed to counteract the adverse effects of opioids on bowel function. At therapeutic doses, alvimopan does not reduce opioid-mediated analgesia, in part because of its limited ability to cross the blood-brain barrier. In contrast to methylnaltrexone, which is approved for long-term therapy of constipation in patients taking opioids for chronic pain, alvimopan is approved by the Food and Drug Administration (FDA) only for short-term therapy of opioid-induced ileus after partial small or large bowel resection with primary anastomosis. The goal is to accelerate time to recovery of upper and lower bowel function, which can be impaired by opioids used for analgesia during and after surgery.

When used short term in postoperative patients, alvimopan is very well tolerated. However, when used long term in patients taking opioids for chronic pain, the drug has been associated with an increased incidence of MI, although a causal relationship has not been established. Because MI may be a risk with prolonged dosing, the drug is approved only for short-term (7-day) use, and only for hospitalized patients. Furthermore, hospitals that dispense the drug must enroll in the Entereg Access Support and Education program, designed to minimize risk for MI.

Nonsteroidal Anti-inflammatory Drugs

Ibuprofen. An intravenous formulation of ibuprofen is sold as Caldolor. Caldolor is indicated for fever and pain in adults. The drug may be used alone for mild to moderate pain or combined with an opioid for moderate to severe pain. For patients with pain, the usual dosage is 400 to 800 mg every 6 hours as needed. For patients with fever, treatment consists of an initial 400-mg dose, followed by either (1) 400 mg every 4 to 6 hours or (2) 100 to 200 mg every 4 hours as needed.

Ketorolac. Parenteral therapy with ketorolac can be accomplished with one injection or with several. When a single injection is used, the intramuscular dose is 30 or 60 mg and the intravenous dose is 15 or 30 mg. When multiple injections are given, the dosage (intramuscular or intravenous) is 15 or 30 mg every 6 hours as needed. In all cases, the smaller dosage option is employed for patients older than 65 years, patients with impaired kidney function, and patients who weigh less than 50 kg (110 lb). Intravenous doses should be administered over 15 seconds or longer. Intramuscular injections should be done slowly and deep in the muscle. Treatment should not exceed 5 days.

Neuromuscular Blockers
Competitive (Nonedpolarizing)

All competitive neuromuscular blockers share the same mechanism of action—blockade of acetylcholine binding to nicotinic receptors—and they all have the same indications: production

TABLE 92.1   Properties of Competitive and Depolarizing Neuromuscular Blockers

Drug	Time to Maximum Paralysis (min)	Duration of Effective Paralysis (min)	Time to Nearly Full Spontaneous Recovery	Promotes Histamine Release	Primary Mode of Elimination
Competitive Agents					
Atracurium	2–5	20–35	60–70	Yes	Plasma Cholinesterase
Cisatracurium	2–5	20–35	—	Minimal	Spontaneous degradation
Mivacurium	2–5	15–20	20–35	Yes	Plasma Cholinesterase
Pancuronium	3–4	35–45	60–70	No	Renal
Rocuronium	1–3	20–40	—	No	Hepatic/biliary
Vecuronium	3–5	25–30	45–60	No	Hepatic/biliary
Depolarizing Agent					
Succinylcholine	1	4–6	—	Yes	Plasma Cholinesterase

of muscle relaxation during intubation, general anesthesia, and mechanical ventilation. Differences among the drugs relate primarily to histamine release and mode of elimination (Table 92.1). With all of these agents, respiratory depression secondary to meuromuscular blockade is the major concern.

Depolarizing

Succinylcholine. Succinylcholine, an ultra short–acting drug, is the only depolarizing neuromuscular blocker in clinical use in the United States. This drug differs from the competitive blockers with regard to time course, mechanism of action, mode of elimination, and interaction with cholinesterase inhibitors.

Succinylcholine binds to nicotinic receptors, causing depolarization and transient muscle contractions. It then remains bound to the receptor on the motor end plate, causing a constant state of depolarization and thus paralysis. Succinylcholine is used primarily for muscle relaxation during endotracheal intubation. Due to its rapid onset, providers should be prepared for immediate airway management.

CARDIOLOGY
Anticoagulants and Thrombolytics
Continuous Unfractionated Heparin Intravenous Infusion
Intravenous infusion provides steady levels of heparin and therefore is preferred to intermittent injections. Indications for the use of heparin infusion include treatment of deep venous thrombosis (DVT) or pulmonary embolism (PE); it may also be used in patients with myocardial ischemia or infarction. Dosing may consist of an initial weight-based bolus followed by a weight-based infusion titrated to laboratory results. Whether or not a bolus is indicated depends on the indication for treatment and the facility's policy. During the initial phase of treatment, the activated partial thromboplastin time (aPTT) or anti-Xa level should be measured once every 4 to 6 hours and the infusion rate adjusted accordingly. For additional information on unfractionated heparin, see Chapter 45.

Low-Dose Unfractionated Heparin Therapy
Heparin in low doses is given for prophylaxis against thromboembolism in hospitalized patients. Doses of 5000 U are given subcutaneously every 8 to 12 hours depending on patient weight. During low-dose therapy, monitoring of the aPTT or anti-Xa level is not usually required.

Protamine Sulfate for Heparin Overdose
Protamine sulfate is an antidote to severe heparin overdose. Protamine is a small protein that has multiple positively charged groups. These groups bond ionically with the negative groups on heparin, thereby

forming a heparin-protamine complex that is devoid of anticoagulant activity. Neutralization of heparin occurs immediately and lasts for 2 hours, after which additional protamine may be needed. Protamine is administered by slow intravenous injection. Dosage is based on the fact that 1 mg of protamine will inactivate 100 U of heparin. Hence for each 100 U of heparin in the body, 1 mg of protamine should be injected.

Direct Thrombin Inhibitors
Bivalirudin. Bivalirudin (Angiomax), an intravenous direct thrombin inhibitor, has actions similar to those of dabigatran (see Chapter 45). Bivalirudin is a synthetic drug chemically related to hirudin, an anticoagulant isolated from the saliva of leeches.

Bivalirudin is given in combination with aspirin, clopidogrel, or prasugrel to prevent clot formation in patients undergoing coronary angioplasty. At this time, the standard therapy for these patients is aspirin combined with a platelet glycoprotein (GP) IIb/IIIa inhibitor combined with low-dose unfractionated heparin. Bivalirudin, an alternative to heparin in this regimen, has been studied in combination with aspirin as well as GP IIb/IIIa inhibitors. In one trial—the Hirulog Angioplasty Study—bivalirudin plus aspirin was compared with heparin plus aspirin. Bivalirudin was at least as effective as heparin at preventing ischemic complications (myocardial infarction [MI], abrupt vessel closure, and death) and caused fewer bleeding complications. In a subgroup of patients—those with postinfarction angina—bivalirudin was significantly more effective than heparin.

Adverse effects. The most common side effects are back pain, nausea, hypotension, and headache. Other relatively common effects (incidence >5%) include vomiting, abdominal pain, pelvic pain, anxiety, nervousness, insomnia, bradycardia, and fever.

Bleeding is the effect of greatest concern. However, compared with heparin, bivalirudin causes fewer incidents of major bleeding (3.7% vs 9.3%), and fewer patients require transfusions (2% vs 5.7%). Coadministration of bivalirudin with heparin, warfarin, or thrombolytic drugs increases the risk for bleeding.

Pharmacokinetics. With intravenous dosing, anticoagulation begins immediately. Drug levels are maintained by continuous infusion. Bivalirudin is eliminated primarily by renal excretion and partly by proteolytic cleavage. The half-life is short (25 minutes) in patients with normal renal function but may be longer in patients with renal impairment. Coagulation returns to baseline about 1 hour after stopping the infusion. Anticoagulation can be monitored by measuring activated clotting time.

Argatroban. Similar to bivalirudin, argatroban is an intravenous anticoagulant that works by direct inhibition of thrombin. The drug is indicated for the prophylaxis and treatment of thrombosis in patients with heparin-induced thrombocytopenia (HIT). In clinical trials, argatroban reduced development of new thrombosis and permitted restoration of platelet counts. Similar to other anticoagulants, argatroban poses a risk for hemorrhage. About 12% of patients experience hematuria. Allergic reactions (dyspnea, cough, and rash), which develop in 10% of patients, occur almost exclusively in those receiving either thrombolytic drugs (e.g., alteplase) or contrast media for coronary angioplasty. Argatroban has a short half-life (about 45 minutes) owing to rapid metabolism by the liver. Treatment is monitored by measuring the aPTT. When infusion of argatroban is discontinued, the aPTT returns to baseline in 2 to 4 hours.

Antithrombin

AT is an endogenous compound that suppresses coagulation, primarily by inhibiting thrombin and factor Xa. Clinically, AT is used to prevent thrombosis in patients with inherited AT deficiency. Currently, there are two AT preparations, marketed as ATryn and Thrombate III. Atryn is made by recombinant DNA technology; Thrombate III is made by extraction from human plasma. Nonetheless, the actions of both products are the same: suppression of coagulation mediated by thrombin and factor Xa.

Recombinant human antithrombin

Production. Recombinant human AT (rhAT), sold as ATryn, is produced in goats that have been given the DNA sequence for human AT, along with genetic instructions that cause the AT to be expressed into their milk. The rhAT produced in goats is nearly identical to endogenous AT.

Therapeutic use. rhAT is approved for prevention of perioperative or peripartum thromboembolic events in patients with inherited AT deficiency, a disorder that puts these people at high risk for venous thromboembolism (VTE). In fact, to protect against thromboembolism, these people typically require lifelong therapy with an anticoagulant, usually warfarin. During surgery or childbirth, the risk for thrombosis increases. However, there is also an obvious increase in the risk for serious bleeding. Accordingly, when patients with hereditary AT deficiency are facing childbirth or surgery, anticoagulant therapy is usually discontinued—reducing the risk for bleeding but increasing the risk for thrombosis. To reduce the risk for thrombosis, rhAT is given until anticoagulant therapy can be safely resumed. In clinical trials, rhAT prevented thromboembolism associated with childbirth or surgery in 30 of 31 patients with inherited AT deficiency.

Plasma-derived antithrombin.
Plasma-derived AT (Thrombate III) is made by extraction from the plasma of human volunteers. Thrombate III is similar to rhAT in most regards: Both drugs share the same indication (prevention of thromboembolic events associated with surgery or childbirth in patients with inherited AT deficiency), both pose a risk for hemorrhage, both increase the anticoagulant effects of heparin, and both are given by intravenous infusion. The drugs differ primarily in that plasma-derived AT carries a risk for hepatitis C and other infections, whereas rhAT does not. As with rhAT, dosage is based on AT activity and body weight.

Glycoprotein IIb/IIIa Receptor Antagonists
Group Properties

The GP IIb/IIIa receptor antagonists, sometimes called "super aspirins," are the most effective antiplatelet drugs on the market. Three agents are available: abciximab, tirofiban, and eptifibatide. All three are administered intravenously, usually in combination with aspirin and low-dose heparin.

Actions

The GP IIb/IIIa antagonists cause *reversible* blockade of platelet GP IIb/IIIa receptors and thus inhibit the final step in aggregation. As a result, these drugs can prevent aggregation stimulated by all factors, including collagen, thromboxane A_2 adenosine diphosphate, thrombin, and platelet activating factor.

Therapeutic Use

The GP IIb/IIIa antagonists are used short term to prevent ischemic events in patients with acute coronary syndrome (ACS) and those undergoing PCI.

Acute Coronary Syndromes

ACSs have two major manifestations: unstable angina and non–ST-segment elevation MI (non-STEMI). In both cases, symptoms result from thrombosis triggered by disruption of atherosclerotic plaque. When added to traditional drugs for ACS (heparin and aspirin), GP IIb/IIIa antagonists reduce the risk for ischemic complications.

Percutaneous Coronary Intervention

GP IIb/IIIa antagonists reduce the risk for rapid reocclusion after coronary artery revascularization with percutaneous coronary intervention (PCI; balloon or laser angioplasty or atherectomy using an intra-arterial rotating blade). Reocclusion is common because PCI damages the arterial wall, encouraging platelet aggregation.

Properties of Individual Glycoprotein IIb/IIIa Antagonists

Abciximab. Abciximab (ReoPro) is a purified Fab fragment of a monoclonal antibody. The drug binds to platelets in the vicinity of GP IIb/IIIa receptors and thus prevents the receptors from binding fibrinogen. Abciximab in conjunction with aspirin and heparin is approved for intravenous therapy of ACS and for patients undergoing PCI. In addition, studies indicate that it can accelerate revascularization in patients undergoing thrombolytic therapy for acute MI. Antiplatelet effects persist for 24 to 48 hours after stopping the infusion.

Eptifibatide. Eptifibatide (Integrilin) is a small peptide that causes reversible and highly selective inhibition of GP IIb/IIIa receptors. The drug is approved for patients with ACS and those undergoing PCI. Antiplatelet effects reverse within 4 hours of stopping the infusion. The most important adverse effect is bleeding, which occurs most often at the site of PCI catheter insertion and in the GI and urinary tracts. As with other GP IIb/IIIa inhibitors, the risk for bleeding is increased by concurrent use of other drugs that impede hemostasis.

Tirofiban. Tirofiban (Aggrastat) causes selective and reversible inhibition of GP IIb/IIIa receptors. The drug—neither an antibody nor a peptide—was modeled after a platelet inhibitor isolated from the venom of the saw-scaled viper, a snake indigenous to Africa. Similar to other GP IIb/IIIa inhibitors, tirofiban is used to reduce ischemic events associated with ACS. Platelet function returns to baseline within 4 hours of stopping the infusion. Bleeding is the primary adverse effect. The risk for bleeding can be increased by other drugs that suppress hemostasis.

Thrombolytic (Fibrinolytic) Drugs

As their name implies, thrombolytic drugs are given to remove thrombi that have already formed. This contrasts with the anticoagulants, which are given to prevent thrombus formation. In the United States, three thrombolytic drugs are available: alteplase, reteplase, and tenecteplase. These drugs are employed acutely and only for severe thrombotic disease: acute MI, PE, and ischemic stroke. Principal differences among the drugs concern specific uses, duration of action, and ease of dosing. All thrombolytics pose a risk for serious bleeding and hence should be administered only by clinicians skilled in their use. Because of their mechanism, thrombolytic drugs are also known as *fibrinolytics* (and informally as *clot busters*). Properties of individual agents are shown in Table 92.2.

TABLE 92.2	**Properties of Thrombolytic (Fibrinolytic) Drugs**		
	Alteplase (tPA)	**Tenecteplase**	**Reteplase**
Trade name	Activase, Cathflo Activase	TNKase	Retavase
Description	A compound identical to human tPA	Modified form of tPA with a prolonged half-life	A compound that contains the active sequence of amino acids present in tPA
Source	All three drugs are made using recombinant DNA technology.		
Mechanism	All three drugs promote conversion of plasminogen to plasmin, an enzyme that degrades the fibrin matrix of thrombi.		
Indications:			
Acute MI	Yes	Yes	Yes
Acute ischemic stroke	Yes	No	No
Acute pulmonary embolism	Yes	No	No
Clearing a blocked central venous catheter	Yes	No	No
Adverse effect: bleeding	With all three drugs, bleeding is the primary adverse effect.		
Half-life (min)	5	20–24	13–16
Dosage and administration for acute MI	*Intravenous:* 15-mg bolus, then 50 mg infused over 30 min, then 35 mg infused over 60 min[a]	*Intravenous:* Single bolus based on body weight (see text)	*Intravenous:* 10-unit bolus twice, separated by 30 min

[a]Dosage for patients who weigh more than 67 kg.
MI, Myocardial infarction; *tPA*, tissue plasminogen activator.

Alteplase (Tissue Plasminogen Activator)

Alteplase (Activase and Cathflo Activase)—also known as a *tissue plasminogen activator (tPA)*—is identical to naturally occurring human tPA. The drug is manufactured using recombinant DNA technology.

The drug first binds with *plasminogen* to form an active complex. The alteplase-plasminogen complex then catalyzes the conversion of other plasminogen molecules into *plasmin,* an enzyme that digests the fibrin meshwork of clots. In addition to digesting fibrin, plasmin degrades fibrinogen and other clotting factors. These actions do not contribute to lysis of thrombi, but they do increase the risk for hemorrhage.

Therapeutic uses. Alteplase has three major indications: (1) acute MI, (2) acute ischemic stroke, and (3) acute massive PE. In all three settings, timely intervention is essential: the sooner alteplase is administered, the better the outcome.

The importance of early intervention was first demonstrated in the Global Utilization of Streptokinase and tPA for Occluded Coronary Arteries (GUSTO-I) trial, a huge study that evaluated the benefits of two thrombolytic drugs—alteplase (tPA) and streptokinase—in patients with acute MI. Results for alteplase were as follows: among patients treated within 2 hours of symptom onset, the death rate was only 5.4%; among those treated 2 to 4 hours after symptom onset, the rate increased to 6.6%; and among those treated 4 to 6 hours after symptom onset, the rate jumped to 9.4%. Clearly outcomes are best when thrombolytic therapy is started quickly, preferably within 2 to 4 hours of symptom onset and even earlier if possible. Thrombolytic therapy of acute MI is discussed further in Chapter 90.

In addition to its use for acute thrombotic disease, alteplase can be used to restore patency in a clogged central venous catheter.

Owing to the risk for hemorrhage, alteplase and other thrombolytic drugs must be avoided in patients at high risk for bleeding complications and must be used with great caution in patients at lower risk for bleeding. Absolute and relative contraindications to thrombolytic therapy are shown in Table 92.3.

Tenecteplase

Tenecteplase (TNKase), a variant of human tPA (alteplase), is approved only for acute MI. Except for the substitution of three amino acids, the

TABLE 92.3	**Contraindications and Cautions Regarding the Use of Thrombolytics for Myocardial Infarction**
Absolute contraindications	• Any prior intracranial hemorrhage • Known structural cerebral vascular lesion • Ischemic stroke within last 3 months *except* ischemic stroke within 4.5 h • Known intracranial neoplasm • Active internal bleeding (other than menses) • Suspected aortic dissection
Relative contraindications/ cautions	• Severe, uncontrolled hypertension on presentation (blood pressure above 180/110 mm Hg) • History of chronic, severe, poorly controlled hypertension • History of prior ischemic stroke, dementia, or known intracerebral pathology not covered in absolute contraindications • Current use of anticoagulants in therapeutic doses (INR 2–3 or greater); known bleeding diathesis • Traumatic or prolonged (more than 10 min) CPR or major surgery (less than 3 weeks earlier) • Recent internal bleeding (within 2–4 weeks) • Noncompressible vascular punctures • Pregnancy • Active peptic ulcer

CPR, Cardiopulmonary resuscitation; *INR,* international normalized ratio.

drug is structurally identical to tPA. However, because of this small structural change, the pharmacokinetics of tenecteplase is much different. Specifically, tenecteplase is 80 times more resistant than tPA to circulating inhibitors and has a much longer half-life (20 to 24 minutes vs 5 minutes for tPA). Similar to tPA, tenecteplase acts by converting plasminogen into plasmin, an enzyme that digests fibrin clots. Tenecteplase is just as safe and effective as tPA but much easier to use: whereas tPA must be infused over 90 minutes, tenecteplase is given as a single intravenous bolus. As a result, thrombolysis develops faster and emergency personnel are spared the trouble of monitoring a prolonged infusion. Because tenecteplase is so easy to administer, it has the potential to allow dosing before the patient reaches a hospital.

Tenecteplase was compared with tPA in the second Assessment of the Safety and Efficacy of a New Thrombolytic (ASSENT-2) study, which enrolled 16,949 patients. Tenecteplase was given as a 5-second intravenous bolus; tPA was infused over 90 minutes. The median time between symptom onset and starting treatment was 2.7 hours for tenecteplase and 2.8 hours for tPA. Thirty days after treatment, outcomes were equivalent with respect to mortality (6.2% with each drug), ICH (0.93% with tenecteplase vs 0.94% with tPA), and total stroke (1.78% vs 1.66% with tPA). Of significance, the incidence of major hemorrhage (other than intracranial) was lower with tenecteplase (4.7% vs 5.9%).

Reteplase

Reteplase (Retavase) is a derivative of tPA produced by recombinant DNA technology. Similar to tPA, reteplase converts plasminogen to plasmin, which in turn digests the fibrin matrix of the thrombus. Reteplase has a short half-life (13 to 16 minutes), owing to rapid clearance by the liver and kidneys. As with other thrombolytic drugs, bleeding is the major adverse effect. The risk for bleeding is increased by concurrent use of heparin, aspirin, and other drugs that impair hemostasis.

Antidysrhythmics
Lidocaine

Lidocaine (Xylocaine), an intravenous agent, is used only for ventricular dysrhythmias. In addition to its antidysrhythmic applications, lidocaine is employed as a local anesthetic (see Chapter 22).

Effects on the heart and electrocardiogram. Lidocaine has three significant effects on the heart: (1) similar to other class I drugs, lidocaine blocks cardiac sodium channels and thus *slows conduction* in the atria, ventricles, and His-Purkinje system; (2) the drug *reduces automaticity* in the ventricles and His-Purkinje system by a mechanism that is poorly understood; and (3) lidocaine *accelerates repolarization* (shortens the action potential duration and event-related potential). In contrast to quinidine and procainamide, lidocaine is devoid of anticholinergic properties. Also, lidocaine has no significant effect on the electrocardiogram (ECG): a small reduction in the QT interval may occur, but there is no QRS widening.

Pharmacokinetics. Lidocaine undergoes rapid hepatic metabolism. If the drug were administered orally, most of each dose would be inactivated on its first pass through the liver. For this reason, administration is parenteral, almost always by intravenous infusion.

Because lidocaine is rapidly degraded, plasma drug levels can easily be controlled: if levels climb too high, the infusion can be slowed and the liver will quickly remove excess drug from the circulation. The therapeutic range for lidocaine is 1.5 to 5 µg/mL.

Antidysrhythmic use. Antidysrhythmic use of lidocaine is limited to short-term therapy of *ventricular dysrhythmias* (Table 92.4). Lidocaine is not active against supraventricular dysrhythmias.

Adverse effects. Lidocaine is generally well tolerated. However, adverse CNS effects can occur. High therapeutic doses can cause *drowsiness, confusion,* and *paresthesias.* Toxic doses may produce *seizures* and *respiratory arrest.* Consequently, whenever lidocaine is used, equipment for resuscitation must be available. Seizures can be managed with diazepam.

Procainamide

Procainamide blocks cardiac sodium channels, thereby decreasing conduction velocity in the atria, ventricles, and His-Purkinje system. Also, the drug delays repolarization. In contrast to quinidine, procainamide is only weakly anticholinergic and hence is not likely to increase ventricular rate.

Procainamide is effective against a broad spectrum of atrial and ventricular dysrhythmias. Similar to quinidine, the drug can be used for long-term suppression (see Table 92.3). However, because prolonged therapy is often associated with serious adverse effects, procainamide

TABLE 92.4 Properties of Antidysrhythmic Drugs

Drug	Acute Care Route	Effects on the Electrocardiogram	Major Antidysrhythmic Applications
Class IA			
Procainamide	IV	Widens QRS, prolongs QT	Broad spectrum: similar to quinidine, but toxicity makes it less desirable for long-term use
Class IB			
Lidocaine	IV	No significant change	Ventricular dysrhythmias
Class II			
Esmolol	IV	Prolongs PR, bradycardia	Control of ventricular rate in patients with supraventricular tachydysrhythmias
Class III			
Amiodarone	IV	Prolongs QT and PR and widens QRS	Life-threatening ventricular dysrhythmias and atrial fibrillation[a]
Ibutilide	IV	Prolongs QT	Atrial flutter and atrial fibrillation
Class IV			
Diltiazem	IV	Prolongs PR, bradycardia	Control of ventricular rate in patients with supraventricular tachydysrhythmias
Others			
Adenosine	IV	Prolongs PR	Termination of paroxysmal supraventricular tachycardia

[a]Amiodarone is widely used for atrial fibrillation, but it is not approved for this use.
ECG, Electrocardiogram; *IV,* intravenous.

is less desirable than quinidine for long-term use. In contrast to quinidine, procainamide can be used to terminate ventricular tachycardia and ventricular fibrillation.

Esmolol

Esmolol (Brevibloc) is a cardioselective β blocker with a very short half-life (9 minutes). Administration is by intravenous infusion. The drug is employed for immediate control of ventricular rate in patients with supraventricular tachycardia (SVT), atrial flutter, and atrial fibrillation. The use is short term only (e.g., in patients with dysrhythmias associated with surgery). The most common adverse reaction is hypotension. However, as in the case of other β blockers, esmolol can also cause bradycardia, heart block, HF, and bronchospasm (at higher doses). In addition, pain can occur at the infusion site.

Amiodarone

Intravenous amiodarone is approved only for initial treatment and prophylaxis of recurrent ventricular fibrillation and hemodynamically unstable ventricular tachycardia in patients refractory to safer drugs. For these indications, amiodarone may be lifesaving.

In addition to its approved uses, intravenous amiodarone has been used with success against other dysrhythmias, including atrial fibrillation, atrioventricular (AV) nodal reentrant tachycardia, and shock-resistant ventricular fibrillation.

Effects on the heart and electrocardiogram. In contrast to oral amiodarone (discussed in Chapter 42), which affects multiple aspects of cardiac function, intravenous amiodarone affects primarily the AV node. Specifically, the drug slows AV conduction and prolongs AV refractoriness. Both effects probably result from antiadrenergic actions. The mechanism underlying antidysrhythmic effects is unknown.

Adverse effects. The most common adverse effects are hypotension and bradydysrhythmias. Hypotension develops in 15% to 20% of patients and may require discontinuation of treatment. Bradycardia or AV block occurs in 5% of patients; discontinuation of treatment or insertion of a pacemaker may be needed. Infusions containing more than 2 mg/mL (in 5% dextrose in water) produce a high incidence of phlebitis and therefore should be administered through a central venous line. Torsades de pointes in association with QT prolongation occurs rarely.

Ibutilide

Ibutilide (Corvert) is an intravenous agent used to terminate atrial flutter and atrial fibrillation of recent onset (i.e., that has been present no longer than 90 days). Conversion to sinus rhythm occurs during the infusion or within 90 minutes of its termination. Ibutilide is more effective against atrial flutter (49% to 70% success) than atrial fibrillation (22% to 43% success). Similar to other class III agents, ibutilide blocks potassium channels and hence prolongs the action potential duration and QT interval. Up to 8% of patients develop torsades de pointes, frequently in association with QT prolongation. Oral doses are teratogenic and embryocidal in rats.

Verapamil

The pharmacology of verapamil, a calcium channel blocker, is discussed in Chapter 38. Dosing of verapamil may be intravenous or oral. Intravenous therapy is preferred for initial treatment of dysrhythmia. Oral therapy is used for maintenance of sinus rhythm. Intravenous verapamil can cause serious cardiovascular effects. Accordingly, BP and the ECG should be monitored, and equipment for resuscitation should be immediately available.

Diltiazem

Similar to verapamil, diltiazem is also a calcium channel blocker. Diltiazem may be given by intravenous or oral route and is discussed in

Chapter 38. Intravenous therapy is preferred for initial treatment of dysrhythmia, and oral therapy is used for maintenance of sinus rhythm.

Adenosine

Adenosine (Adenocard), a naturally occurring nucleotide, is a drug of choice for terminating paroxysmal SVT. Adenosine has an extremely short half-life and thus must be administered intravenously. Adverse effects are minimal because adenosine is rapidly cleared from the blood.

Effects on the heart and electrocardiogram. Adenosine decreases automaticity in the sinoatrial (SA) node and greatly slows conduction through the AV node. The most prominent ECG change is prolongation of the PR interval, brought on by delayed AV conduction. Although it is not uncommon to see asystole lasting several seconds immediately following injection. Adenosine works in part by inhibiting cyclic adenosine monophosphate (cAMP)–induced calcium influx, thereby suppressing calcium-dependent action potentials in the SA and AV nodes.

Therapeutic use. Adenosine is approved only for termination of paroxysmal SVT, including Wolff-Parkinson-White syndrome. The drug is not active against atrial fibrillation, atrial flutter, or ventricular dysrhythmias.

Pharmacokinetics. Adenosine has an extremely short half-life (estimated at 1.5 to 10 seconds), owing primarily to rapid uptake by cells and partly to deactivation by circulating adenosine deaminase. Because of its rapid clearance, adenosine must be administered by intravenous bolus as close to the heart as possible.

Adverse effects. Adverse effects are short-lived, lasting less than 1 minute. The most common are sinus bradycardia, dyspnea (from bronchoconstriction), hypotension and facial flushing (from vasodilation), and chest discomfort (perhaps from stimulation of pain receptors in the heart).

Drug interactions. Methylxanthines (aminophylline, theophylline, and caffeine) block receptors for adenosine. Hence asthma patients taking aminophylline or theophylline need larger doses of adenosine; even then, adenosine may not work.

Dipyridamole, an antiplatelet drug, blocks cellular uptake of adenosine and can thus intensify its effects.

Acute Decompensated Heart Failure
Inotropic Agents

In addition to digoxin, there are two other types of inotropic drugs: sympathomimetics and phosphodiesterase (PDE) inhibitors. Unlike digoxin, which can be taken orally, these other inotropics must be given by intravenous infusion. Accordingly, their use is restricted to acute care of hospitalized patients. Because digoxin can be given orally, it is the only inotropic agent suited for long-term therapy.

Sympathomimetic drugs: dopamine and dobutamine. The basic pharmacology of dopamine and dobutamine is presented in Chapter 14. Discussion here is limited to their use in HF. Both drugs are administered by intravenous infusion.

Dopamine. Dopamine is a catecholamine that can activate (1) β₁-adrenergic receptors in the heart, (2) dopamine receptors in the kidney, and (3) at high doses, α₁-adrenergic receptors in blood vessels. Activation of β₁ receptors increases myocardial contractility, thereby improving cardiac performance. β₁ activation also increases heart rate, creating a risk for tachycardia. Activation of dopamine receptors dilates renal blood vessels, thereby increasing renal blood flow and urine output. Activation of α₁ receptors increases vascular resistance (afterload) and can thus reduce cardiac output. Dopamine is administered by continuous infusion. Constant monitoring of blood pressure, the ECG, and urine output is required. Dopamine is employed as a short-term rescue measure for patients with severe acute cardiac failure.

Dobutamine. Dobutamine is a synthetic catecholamine that causes selective activation of β₁-adrenergic receptors. By doing so, the drug can increase myocardial contractility and can thus improve cardiac performance. Similar to dopamine, dobutamine can cause tachycardia and induce myocardial ischemia. In contrast to dopamine, dobutamine does not activate α_1 receptors and therefore does not increase vascular resistance. As a result, the drug is generally preferred to dopamine for short-term treatment of acute HF. Administration is by continuous infusion.

Phosphodiesterase Inhibitors

Milrinone. Milrinone has been called an inodilator because it increases myocardial contractility and promotes vasodilation. Increased contractility results from accumulation of cAMP secondary to inhibition of PDE-3, an enzyme that degrades cAMP. Milrinone is administered by intravenous infusion and is indicated only for short-term therapy of severe HF. The use should be reserved for patients with severe reduction in cardiac output resulting in decreased organ perfusion because ionotropes can induce dysrhythmias and cause myocardial ischemia from increased metabolic demand.

Intravenous Vasodilators

Intravenous nitroglycerin. Intravenous nitroglycerin is indicated for perioperative control of blood pressure, production of controlled hypotension during surgery, and treatment of HF associated with acute MI. In addition, intravenous nitroglycerin is used to treat unstable angina and chronic angina when symptoms cannot be controlled with preferred medications.

Intravenous nitroglycerin is employed only rarely to treat angina pectoris. When used for angina, intravenous nitroglycerin is limited to patients who have failed to respond to other medications. Additional uses of intravenous nitroglycerin include treatment of HF associated with acute MI, treatment of perioperative hypertension, and production of controlled hypotension for surgery.

Nesiritide. Nesiritide (Natrecor) is a synthetic form of human brain natriuretic peptide (BNP) indicated only for short-term intravenous therapy of hospitalized patients with acutely decompensated HF, which is characterized by increased pulmonary capillary wedge pressure (PCWP) and dyspnea at rest. Nesiritide is produced by recombinant DNA technology and has the same amino acid sequence as naturally occurring BNP. The drug was approved after a relatively small trial showed a modest decrease in dyspnea and PCWP. However, after 10 years of use, a much larger trial—the Acute Study of Clinical Effectiveness of Nesiritide in Decompensated Heart Failure (ASCEND-HF)—failed to show any benefit. The incidence of dyspnea, rehospitalization, and 30-day mortality was the same for patients receiving nesiritide as it was for patients receiving placebo. Worse yet, although nesiritide offered no benefit, it nearly doubled the incidence of hypotension. These results led the authors to conclude that "Nesiritide cannot be recommended for routine use in the broad population of patients with heart failure." Nesiritide my be considered for use in patients without hypotension or cardiogenic shock who continue to have severe symptoms despite routine therapy.

Mechanism of action. Nesiritide affects hemodynamics by three mechanisms: suppression of the renin-angiotensin-aldosterone system, suppression of sympathetic outflow from the CNS, and direct dilation of arterioles and veins. In patients with HF, benefits derive primarily from direct vasodilation. To promote vasodilation, nesiritide binds with receptors on vascular smooth muscle (VSM) and thus stimulates production of cyclic guanosine monophosphate (cGMP), a second messenger that causes VSM to relax. This mechanism is similar to that of nitroglycerin, which also stimulates cGMP production. However, whereas nitroglycerin acts primarily on veins, nesiritide dilates arterioles as well. By dilating arterioles and veins, nesiritide reduces both preload and afterload. The net result is a decrease in PCWP and increased cardiac output. Also, by dilating afferent renal arterioles, nesiritide increases glomerular filtration rate and thus increases excretion of sodium and

water. The result is a reduction in blood volume, which further reduces cardiac preload.

Pharmacokinetics. With continuous infusion, nesiritide achieves steady-state levels that are three to six times greater than the level of endogenous BNP present at baseline. Nesiritide is eliminated by three mechanisms: (1) proteolytic cleavage by endopeptidases present on the luminal surface of blood vessels; (2) binding to clearance receptors on the surface of cells, followed by cellular uptake and proteolytic cleavage; and (3) renal filtration. The drug's half-life is short, about 18 minutes.

Adverse effects. The principal adverse effect is symptomatic hypotension. In the ASCEND-HF trial, hypotension developed in 26.6% of patients receiving nesiritide, compared with 15.3% of those receiving placebo. The risk for hypotension is increased by high doses of nesiritide and by concurrent use of angiotensin-converting enzyme inhibitors and other vasodilators. In addition to causing hypotension, nesiritide can cause ventricular tachycardia, headache, back pain, dizziness, and nausea. An analysis of several clinical trials suggested that nesiritide might cause renal damage. However, ASCEND-HF revealed no evidence of renal harm.

Drugs for Hypertensive Emergencies

A hypertensive emergency exists when systolic BP exceeds 180 mm Hg, diastolic BP exceeds 100 mm Hg, and there is evidence of end-organ damage. When excessive BP is associated with papilledema (edema of the retina), intracerebral hemorrhage (ICH), MI, or acute congestive heart failure (CHF), a severe emergency exists—and BP must be lowered rapidly (within 1 hour). If severe hypertension is present but does not yet pose an immediate threat of organ damage, reducing BP more slowly (over 24 to 48 hours) is preferable. This situation is often referred to as hypertensive urgency. Because rapid reductions can cause cerebral ischemia, MI, and renal failure, pressure should be reduced gradually whenever possible.

The major drugs used for hypertensive emergencies are discussed next. All reduce BP by causing vasodilation, and all are given intravenously.

Sodium nitroprusside

When acute, severe hypertension demands a rapid but controlled reduction in BP, intravenous nitroprusside (Nitropress) is usually the drug of first choice. Effects begin in seconds and then fade rapidly when administration ceases.

Cardiovascular effects. Nitroprusside is a direct-acting vasodilator that relaxes smooth muscle of arterioles and veins. Curiously, although nitroprusside is an effective arteriolar dilator, reflex tachycardia is minimal. Nitroprusside can trigger retention of sodium and water; furosemide can help counteract this effect.

Mechanism of action. When in the body, nitroprusside breaks down to release nitric oxide, which then activates guanylate cyclase, an enzyme present in VSM. Guanylate cyclase catalyzes the production of cyclic GMP, which, through a series of reactions, causes vasodilation. This mechanism is similar to that of nitroglycerin.

Metabolism. Nitroprusside contains five *cyanide groups,* which are split free in the first step of nitroprusside metabolism. *Nitric oxide,* the active component, is released next. Both reactions take place in smooth muscle. When freed, the cyanide groups are converted to *thiocyanate* by the liver, using *thiosulfate* as a cofactor. Thiocyanate is eliminated by the kidneys over several days.

Adverse effects.

Excessive hypotension. If administered too rapidly, nitroprusside can cause a precipitous drop in blood pressure, resulting in headache, palpitations, nausea, vomiting, and sweating. Blood pressure should be monitored continuously.

Cyanide poisoning. Rarely, lethal amounts of cyanide have accumulated. Cyanide buildup is most likely in patients with liver disease and in those with low stores of thiosulfate, the cofactor needed for cyanide detoxification. The chances of cyanide poisoning can be minimized by avoiding rapid infusion (faster than 5 µg/kg per minute) and by coadministering thiosulfate. If cyanide toxicity occurs, nitroprusside should be withdrawn.

Thiocyanate toxicity. When nitroprusside is given for several days, thiocyanate may accumulate. Although much less hazardous than cyanide, thiocyanate can also cause adverse effects. These effects, which involve the CNS, include disorientation, psychotic behavior, and delirium. To minimize toxicity, patients receiving nitroprusside for more than 3 days should undergo monitoring of plasma thiocyanate, which must be kept below 0.1 mg/mL.

Fenoldopam

Fenoldopam (Corlopam) is an intravenous drug indicated for short-term management of hypertensive emergencies. Benefits equal those of nitroprusside. Fenoldopam lowers BP by activating dopamine-1 receptors on arterioles to cause vasodilation. In animal models, the drug dilates renal, coronary, mesenteric, and peripheral vessels.

Fenoldopam differs from other antihypertensives in that it helps maintain (or even improve) renal function. Two mechanisms are involved. First, the drug dilates renal blood vessels, increasing renal blood flow (despite reducing arterial pressure). Second, fenoldopam promotes sodium and water excretion through direct effects on renal tubules.

Fenoldopam has a rapid onset and short duration. Effects begin in less than 5 minutes. The drug undergoes rapid hepatic metabolism followed by renal excretion. Its plasma half-life is only 5 minutes.

Fenoldopam is generally well tolerated. The most common side effects are hypotension, headache, flushing, dizziness, and reflex tachycardia—all of which occur secondary to vasodilation. Tachycardia may cause ischemia in patients with angina. Combined use with a β blocker can minimize tachycardia, but may also result in excessive lowering of BP. Fenoldopam can elevate intraocular pressure (IOP) and hence should be used with caution in patients with glaucoma.

Labetalol

Labetalol blocks α- and β-adrenergic receptors. Blood pressure is reduced by arteriolar dilation secondary to α blockade. β blockade prevents reflex tachycardia in response to reduced arterial pressure; hence the drug is probably safe for patients with angina or MI. β blockade can aggravate bronchial asthma, HF, AV block, cardiogenic shock, and bradycardia. Accordingly, labetalol should not be given to patients with these disorders.

Clevidipine

Clevidipine (Cleviprex) is a dihydropyridine calcium channel blocker with an ultrashort half-life (about 1 minute). Administration is by intravenous infusion. As with nitroprusside, effects begin rapidly and then fade rapidly when the infusion is slowed or stopped. As a result, BP can be easily titrated. The most common side effects are headache, nausea, and vomiting. The basic pharmacology of clevidipine is discussed in Chapter 38.

HEMATOLOGY

Drugs for Anemia

Parenteral Iron Preparations

Iron is available in four forms for parenteral therapy. However, only one of these forms—iron dextran—is approved for iron deficiency of all causes. Approval of the other three forms—iron sucrose, sodium–ferric gluconate complex (SFGC), and ferumoxytol—is limited to treating iron deficiency anemia in patients with chronic kidney disease (CKD).

Iron dextran. Iron dextran (INFeD, Dexferrum, Infufer, and Dexiron) is the most frequently used parenteral iron preparation. The drug is a complex consisting of ferric hydroxide and dextrans (polymers of glucose). The rate of response to parenteral iron is equal to that of oral iron.

> ## ⟫ BLACK BOX WARNING
> ### *Iron Dextran*
>
> This preparation should be used for treatment of iron deficiency only in patients in whom oral administration is infeasible or ineffective due to increased risk for anaphylaxis. A test dose is required before administration.

Indications. Iron dextran is reserved for patients with a clear diagnosis of iron deficiency and for whom oral iron is either ineffective or intolerable. Primary candidates for parenteral iron are patients who, because of intestinal disease, are unable to absorb iron taken orally. Iron dextran is also indicated when blood loss is so great (500 to 1000 mL/wk) that oral iron cannot be absorbed fast enough to meet hematopoietic needs. Parenteral iron may also be employed when there is concern that oral iron might exacerbate preexisting disease of the stomach or bowel. Last, parenteral iron can be given to the rare patient for whom the gastrointestinal (GI) effects of oral iron are intolerable.

Adverse effects.

Anaphylactic reactions. Potentially fatal anaphylaxis is the most serious adverse effect. Anaphylactic reactions are triggered by dextran in the product, not by the iron. Although these reactions are rare, their possibility demands that iron dextran be used only when clearly required. Furthermore, whenever iron dextran is administered, injectable epinephrine and facilities for resuscitation should be at hand. To reduce risk, each full dose must be preceded by a small test dose. However, be aware that even the test dose can trigger anaphylactic and other hypersensitivity reactions. In addition, even when the test dose has no adverse effects, patients can still experience anaphylaxis.

Other adverse effects. Hypotension is common in patients receiving parenteral iron. In addition, iron dextran can cause headache, fever, urticaria, and arthralgia. More serious reactions—circulatory failure and cardiac arrest—may also occur. When administered intramuscularly, iron dextran can cause persistent pain and prolonged, localized discoloration. Very rarely, tumors develop at sites of intramuscular injection. Intravenous administration may result in lymphadenopathy and phlebitis.

Sodium–ferric gluconate complex, iron sucrose, and ferumoxytol. SFGC, iron sucrose, and ferumoxytol represent alternatives to iron dextran for parenteral iron therapy. With all three drugs, the risk for anaphylaxis is very low, so there is little or no need for giving test doses. As a result, these drugs are more convenient than iron dextran. Unfortunately, indications for these drugs are limited to treatment of iron deficiency anemia in patients with CKD. They are not approved for iron deficiency from other causes.

Sodium–ferric gluconate complex. SFGC, sold under the trade name Ferrlecit, is a parenteral iron product indicated for iron deficiency anemia in patients with CKD who are undergoing chronic hemodialysis. The drug is always used in conjunction with erythropoietin, an agent that stimulates RBC production.

SFGC can cause transient flushing and hypotension associated with lightheadedness, malaise, fatigue, weakness, and severe pain in the chest, back, flanks, or groin. This reaction can be minimized by infusing the drug slowly. In contrast to iron dextran, SFGC poses little risk for anaphylaxis. SFGC is supplied in 5-mL ampules that contain 62.5 mg of elemental iron. For most patients, a single dose consists of 125 mg. The typical patient requires a cumulative dose of 1 g (eight

125-mg infusions on separate days). Every time the drug is administered, facilities for cardiopulmonary resuscitation should be immediately available.

Iron Sucrose. Similar to SFGC, iron sucrose (Venofer) is a parenteral form of iron indicated for iron deficiency anemia in patients with CKD. However, in contrast to SFGC, whose indications are limited to CKD patients undergoing hemodialysis in conjunction with erythropoietin therapy, iron sucrose is indicated for a broader range of CKD patients, specifically the following:

- Nondialysis-dependent (NDD) patients receiving erythropoietin
- NDD patients *not* receiving erythropoietin
- Hemodialysis-dependent (HDD) patients receiving erythropoietin
- Peritoneal dialysis–dependent (PDD) patients receiving erythropoietin

Ferumoxytol. Ferumoxytol (Feraheme) is a parenteral form of iron indicated for iron deficiency anemia in all patients with CKD, whether or not they are on dialysis or using erythropoietin. Compared with SFGC and iron sucrose, ferumoxytol is much more convenient because it requires only two doses (given over 3 to 8 days), whereas SFGC and iron sucrose require 3 to 10 doses (given over several weeks).

NEPHROLOGY

Diuretics

Furosemide

Furosemide is usually given intravenously for the treatment of pulmonary edema or acute decompensated HF in the hospital setting. Furosemide (discussed further in Chapter 36) is available in solution for intravenous and intramuscular administration. The usual dosage for adults is 20 to 40 mg, repeated in 1 or 2 hours if needed. For high-dose therapy, furosemide can be administered by continuous infusion at a rate of 4 mg/min or slower.

Mannitol, an Osmotic Diuretic

Osmotic diuretics differ from other diuretics with regard to mechanisms and uses. At this time, mannitol is the only osmotic diuretic available in the United States. Mannitol (Osmitrol) is a simple six-carbon sugar that embodies the following four properties of an ideal osmotic diuretic:

- Is freely filtered at the glomerulus
- Undergoes minimal tubular reabsorption
- Undergoes minimal metabolism
- Is pharmacologically inert (i.e., it has no direct effects on the biochemistry or physiology of cells)

After intravenous administration, mannitol is filtered by the glomerulus. However, unlike other solutes, the drug undergoes minimal reabsorption. As a result, most of the filtered drug remains in the nephron, creating an osmotic force that inhibits passive reabsorption of water. Hence urine flow increases. The degree of diuresis produced is directly related to the concentration of mannitol in the filtrate: the more mannitol present, the greater the diuresis. Mannitol has no significant effect on the excretion of potassium and other electrolytes.

Pharmacokinetics. Mannitol does not diffuse across the GI epithelium and cannot be transported by the uptake systems that absorb dietary sugars. Accordingly, to reach the circulation, the drug must be given parenterally. After intravenous injection, mannitol distributes freely to extracellular water. Diuresis begins in 30 to 60 minutes and persists 6 to 8 hours. Most of the drug is excreted intact in the urine.

Therapeutic uses

Prophylaxis of renal failure. Under certain conditions (e.g., dehydration, severe hypotension, and hypovolemic shock), blood flow to the kidney is decreased, causing a great reduction in filtrate volume. When the volume of filtrate is very low, transport mechanisms of the nephron are able to reabsorb virtually all of the sodium and chloride present, causing complete reabsorption of water as well. As a result, urine production ceases and kidney failure ensues. The risk for renal failure can be reduced with mannitol in the following way. Because filtered mannitol is not reabsorbed—even when filtrate volume is small—filtered mannitol will remain in the nephron, drawing water with it. Hence mannitol can preserve urine flow and may thus prevent renal failure. Thiazides and loop diuretics are not as effective for this application because, under conditions of low filtrate production, there is such an excess of reabsorptive capacity (relative to the amount of filtrate) that these drugs are unable to produce sufficient blockade of reabsorption to promote diuresis.

Reduction of intracranial pressure. Intracranial pressure (ICP) that has been elevated by cerebral edema can be reduced with mannitol. The drug lowers ICP because its presence in the blood vessels of the brain creates an osmotic force that draws edematous fluid from the brain into the blood. There is no risk for increasing cerebral edema because mannitol cannot exit the capillary beds of the brain.

Reduction of intraocular pressure. Mannitol and other osmotic agents can lower IOP by rendering the plasma hyperosmotic with respect to intraocular fluids. The hyperosmotic plasma creates an osmotic force that draws ocular fluid into the blood. The use of mannitol to lower IOP is reserved for patients who have not responded to more conventional treatment.

Adverse effects

Edema. Mannitol can leave the vascular system at all capillary beds except those of the brain. When the drug exits capillaries, it draws water along with it, causing edema. Mannitol must be used with extreme caution in patients with heart disease because it may precipitate CHF and pulmonary edema. If signs of pulmonary congestion or CHF develop, the use of the drug must cease immediately. Mannitol must also be discontinued in patients with HF or pulmonary edema who develop renal failure, because the resultant accumulation of mannitol would increase the risk for cardiac or pulmonary injury.

Vasopressin Receptor Antagonists (Vaptans)

The vaptans are vaspression receptor antagonists; that is, they selectively antagonize vasopressin (V2) receptors located in the collecting ducts, thus increasing the excretion of free water by the kidneys. Two drugs compose the vaptan class; tolvaptan (Samsca) and conivaptan (Vaprisol). Conivaptan is used for the inpatient treatment of hyponatremia and tolvaptan (Jynarque) is also approved for the treatment of autosomal dominant polycystic kidney disease.

Therapeutic Uses

Hyponatremia. By decreasing the amount of circulating free water in the body, conivaptan and tolvaptan indirectly increase the serum sodium levels in euvolemic and hypervolemic hyponatremia. Although conivaptan is used for hypervolemic hypernatremia, it has not been used successfully in patients with heart failure. Tolvaptan, on the other hand, is used for patients with hypervolemic hyponatremia related to heart failure. In clinical trials with conivaptan, the average rise in sodium after intravenous administration was greater than 6 mEq/L.

Autosomal dominant polycystic kidney disease. Tolvaptan is also available in an oral formulation sold as *Jynarque*. Oral tolvaptan inhibits in vitro cyst growth and chloride-dependent fluid secretion into cysts, thereby slowing the progression of renal decline in polycystic kidney disease.

Adverse effects

Rapid overcorrection of sodium. The use of the intravenous vaptans for treating hyponatremia is approved only within a hospital setting. Because of the risk of osmotic demyelination syndrome (ODS), frequent monitoring of serum sodium levels and volume status is required.

Canadian Drug Information

CANADIAN DRUG LEGISLATION

Two acts form the basis of the drug laws in Canada: the Food and Drugs Act and the Controlled Drugs and Substance Act. The Health Products and Food Branch within Health Canada is responsible for ensuring that health products and foods approved for sale to Canadians are safe and of high quality. The Therapeutic Products Directorate (TPD) is responsible for regulating pharmaceutical drugs and medical devices. The Biologics & Genetic Therapies Directorate regulates biologic drugs (drugs derived from living sources) and radiopharmaceuticals. Examples of biologic products are insulin analogs, blood products, and vaccines. The Natural and Non-prescription Health Products Directorate is the regulating authority for natural health products for sale in Canada. Natural Health Products (NHPs) are a class of health products that include vitamin and mineral supplements, herbal preparations, traditional and homeopathic medicines, probiotics, and enzymes.

The Food and Drug Act (1927), accompanied by the Food and Drug Regulations (1953, 1954, 1979), reviews the safety and efficacy of drugs before they are marketed, and the legislation determines whether the medicine is classified as having prescription or nonprescription status. The act controls the requirements for good manufacturing practices, labeling, distribution, and sale, including advertising of the drug. It also prescribes the standards of composition, strength, potency, purity, and quality of drugs in Canada.

Prescription Drugs (Schedule F)

All drugs that require a prescription except for narcotics and controlled substances are listed in Schedule F of the Food and Drug Regulations. Prescriptions for Schedule F medications may be written, including facsimiles and electronic prescriptions (depending on the province), or transmitted verbally (i.e., by telephone order directly to the pharmacist) by a duly qualified medical practitioner authorized to issue prescriptions. The symbol Pr must appear on all manufacturing labels. Individual provinces can legislate more restrictive control and require a prescription for a medication classified by the TPD as a nonprescription drug (e.g., digoxin). Provinces cannot legislate less restrictive control on any drug.

The Controlled Drugs and Substances Act (1997) establishes the requirements for the control and sale of opioids, controlled drugs, and substances of abuse in Canada. This act lists eight schedules of controlled substances. Assignment to a schedule is based on potential for abuse and the ease with which illicit substances can be manufactured in illegal laboratories. The degree of control, the conditions of record keeping, and other regulations depend on the specific schedule. For example, Schedule I, which includes the opioid agents, requires written orders only, and no repeat prescriptions are allowed. Some provinces require prescriptions for certain opioids, such as morphine, to be written on a triplicate prescription form with one copy to be sent to the practitioner's regulatory body. The symbol ◇ must appear on the labels of controlled products, and the letter N is printed on the label of all the opioid agents.

Schedules I through VIII are defined in the following list. Benzodiazepines are classified as Targeted Substances, and the symbol must appear on all the labels for these drugs.

- Schedule I: Opium poppy and its derivatives (e.g., morphine, heroin); methadone; coca and its derivatives (e.g., cocaine)
- Schedule II: Cannabis and its derivatives (e.g., marijuana, hashish)[a]
- Schedule III: Amphetamines, methylphenidate, lysergic acid diethylamide (LSD), methaqualone, psilocybin, mescaline
- Schedule IV: Sedative-hypnotic agents (e.g., barbiturates, benzodiazepines); anabolic steroids
- Schedule V: Propylhexedrine and any salt thereof
- Schedule VI: Compounds that can serve as precursors for manufacturing controlled substances
    - *Part 1: Class A Precursors.* Acetic anhydride, N-acetylanthranilic acid, anthranilic acid, ephedrine, ergometrine, ergotamine, isosafrole, lysergic acid, 3,4-methylenedioxyphenyl-2-propanone, norephedrine, 1-phenyl-2-propanone, phenylacetic acid, piperidine, piperonal, potassium permanganate, pseudoephedrine, safrole, gamma-butyrolactone, 1,4-butanediol, red and white phosphorus, hypophosphorous acid, hydriodic acid
    - *Part 2: Class B Precursors.* Acetone, ethyl ether, hydrochloric acid, methyl ethyl ketone, sulphuric acid, toluene
    - *Part 3:* Any preparation or mixture that contains a precursor set out in Part 1 or in Part 2
- Schedule VII: Cannabis resin 3 kg; Cannabis (marijuana) 3 kg
- Schedule VIII: Cannabis resin 1 g; Cannabis (marijuana) 30 g

The Controlled Drugs and Substance Act also provides for the nonprescription sale of certain codeine preparations. The content must not exceed the equivalent of 8 mg codeine phosphate per solid dosage unit or 20 mg/30 mL of a liquid, and the preparation must also contain two additional nonnarcotic medicinal ingredients (usually acetylsalicylic acid or acetaminophen and caffeine). These preparations may not be advertised or displayed and may be sold only by pharmacists. Some provinces choose to restrict the amount that can be sold at any given time. The Royal Canadian Mounted Police (RCMP) is responsible for enforcing the Controlled Drugs and Substances Act and related sections of the *Criminal Code*.

[a]Cannabis: Medical cannabis has been legal in Canada since 2001 and is regulated primarily by the *Cannabis Act*. Patients may obtain medical cannabis with a Medical Document written by any physician from a licensed producer via mail. On October 17, 2018, cannabis was descheduled from the *Controlled Drugs and Substances Act* and became regulated by the federal *Cannabis Act*. Canadians can obtain cannabis products from any provincially licensed retailer. Each province has set a minimum age requirement, similar to restrictions of alcohol use. Currently, only cannabis plants, oil, and seeds can be sold. Additional categories will be announced in October 2019.

Nonprescription Medications—National Drug Schedules

As previously mentioned, individual provinces have enacted their own legislation controlling the sale of both prescription and nonprescription products. As a result, the National Association of Pharmacy Regulatory Authorities (NAPRA) has endorsed a proposal for a national drug scheduling model. This model attempts to align the provincial drug schedules so that the conditions for the sale of drugs will be consistent across the country. The harmonized model includes all classes of medications. Opioids, controlled substances, and prescription medications are listed in Schedule I, whereas nonprescription medications are assigned to one of the three categories described further on. There is general support among the provincial regulatory bodies for the National Drug Schedules, although there are some differences from province to province of the actual list of drugs in each schedule. For a complete drug list proposed by NAPRA, visit their web site at *www.napra.ca*.

- **Schedule I** drugs require a prescription for sale and are provided to the public by the pharmacist following the diagnosis and professional intervention of a practitioner. The sale is controlled in a regulated environment as defined by provincial pharmacy regulation.
- **Schedule II** drugs, though less strictly regulated, do require professional intervention from the pharmacist at the point of sale and possibly referral to a practitioner. Whereas a prescription is not required, the drugs are available only from the pharmacist and must be retained within an area of the pharmacy where there is no public access and no opportunity for patient self-selection.
- **Schedule III** drugs may present risks to certain populations in self-selection. Although available without a prescription, these drugs are to be sold from the self-selection area of the pharmacy, operated under the direct supervision of the pharmacist and subject to any local professional discretionary requirements that may increase the degree of control. Such an environment is accessible to the patient and clearly identified as the "professional services area" of the pharmacy. The pharmacist is available, accessible, and approachable to assist the patient in making an appropriate self-medication selection.
- **Unscheduled** drugs can be sold without professional supervision. Adequate information is available for the patient to make a safe and effective choice and labeling is deemed sufficient to ensure the appropriate use of the drug. These drugs are not included in Schedules I, II, or III and may be sold from any retail outlet.

New Drug Development in Canada

The process for approving a new drug in Canada is very similar if not identical to the process in the United States. The same drug data that are required for approval by the US Food and Drug Administration are required by the TPD in Canada. The principal difference between Canada and the United States is one of nomenclature: Once preclinical testing has been completed, the manufacturer in Canada applies for a Preclinical New Drug Submission versus an Investigational New Drug in the United States. At the end of clinical testing, the manufacturer in Canada seeks a New Drug Submission (NDS), versus a New Drug Application in the United States.

After all the information on a new drug has been submitted—including results of preclinical and clinical testing, method of manufacturing, packaging, labeling, and results of stability testing—the pharmaceutical company receives a Notice of Compliance (NOC) from the TPD, and the drug enters the market.

Although data collection for a new drug is thorough, there is no guarantee that all adverse reactions are known, especially when the drug is used concurrently with other drugs. Also, long-term effects are not fully appreciated. For these reasons postmarketing surveillance plays a major role in monitoring new drugs. The Canada Vigilance Program is Health Canada's postmarketing surveillance program; it collects and assesses reports of suspected adverse reactions to health products marketed in Canada. Postmarketing surveillance enables Health Canada to monitor the safety profile of health products once they have been marketed to ensure that the benefits of the products continue to outweigh the risks. The manufacturer and all health care practitioners must immediately report any new clinical findings, unexpected adverse effects, or therapeutic failures to the TPD. The Canada Vigilance Program also collects information on nonprescription drugs, natural health products, biologics, radiopharmaceuticals, and disinfectants and sanitizers with disinfectant claims.

Patent Laws

In 1969, the Patent Act was changed to include compulsory licensing. This new provision allowed generic drug companies to manufacture and distribute patented drugs in Canada provided that a minimal 4% royalty fee was paid to the patent holder. This system was introduced to help control drug prices. Unfortunately the system caused a decline in revenue to "innovative" pharmaceutical companies, with a resultant decline in research on new drug development. After much debate and retroactive to June 1987, the Patent Act was amended to give patent holders market exclusivity either (1) for 7 to 10 years or (2) until the 17-year patent (from date of filing) expires, whichever comes first. The Patent Act was then further amended to "make Canada's intellectual property legislation more in line with that of the major industrialized countries."

In response to provisions of the North American Free Trade Agreement (NAFTA) and the General Agreement on Tariffs and Trade (GATT), Bill C-91 was introduced in 1993. This bill (1) eliminated compulsory licensing and (2) extended patent protection on brand-name drugs to 20 years, thereby making Canadian patent laws similar to those of the United States and other industrialized nations. Section 14 of Bill C-91 called for a parliamentary review of legislation in 1997. A special committee reviewed the impact of Bill C-91 on such factors as drug prices, drug research and development, and job creation. No changes to the legislation were made.

In order to respond to concerns arising from changes in the Patent Act, a Patented Medicine Prices Review Board (PMPRB) was created. Its mandate is to (1) ensure that prices of patented medicines are not excessive and (2) report on the ratios of research and development expenditures relative to sales for individual patentees and for the pharmaceutical industry as a whole. There is, however, some pressure by the pharmaceutical industry to adopt worldwide patent laws for pharmaceutical products.

An amendment to the Patented Medicines Regulations is currently being proposed to modernize the way the prices of patented drugs are regulated in Canada. The list of countries used for comparison when drug prices are being assessed will be revised and new price regulatory factors added to equip the PMPRB to be a more effective price regulator.

DRUG ADVERTISING

Direct-to-consumer advertising is restricted in Canada to giving names of prescription drugs only, which is different from that in the United States. Advertisements to health professionals are permitted to contain claims for product effectiveness and prescribing information. The Pharmaceutical Advertising Advisory Board (PAAB) and Advertising Standards Canada (ASC) review and clear advertisements according to standards set by the Food and Drugs Act.

Table A.1   Therapeutic Serum Drug Concentrations

Drugs	SI Reference Interval	SI Unit	Conversion Factor	Traditional Reference Interval	Traditional Reference Unit
Acetaminophen	13–40	µmol/L	66.15	0.2–0.6	mg/dL
Acetylsalicylic acid	7.2–21.7	µmol/L	0.0724	100–300	mg/dL
Amikacin[a]	—	—	—	15–25[b]; <8[c]	µg/mL
Amitriptyline	430–9000[d]	mmol/L	3.605	120–250[d]	ng/mL
Carbamazepine	17–42	µmol/L	4.233	4–10	µg/mL
Desipramine	430–750	nmol/L	3.754	115–200	ng/mL
Digoxin	0.6–2.8	nmol/L	1.282	0.5–2.2	ng/mL
Disopyramide	6–18	µmol/L	2.946	2–6	µg/mL
Gentamicin[a]	—	—	—	6–10[b]; <2[c]	µg/mL
Imipramine	640–1070[d]	nmol/L	3.566	180–300[d]	ng/mL
Lidocaine	4.5–21.5	µmol/L	4.267	1–5	µg/mL
Lithium	0.4–1.2	mmol/L	1	0.4–1.2	mEq/L
Netilmicin[a]	—	—	—	6–10[b]; <2[c]	µg/mL
Nortriptyline	190–570	nmol/L	3.797	50–150	ng/mL
Phenobarbital	65–170	µmol/L	4.306	15–40	µg/mL
Phenytoin	40–80	µmol/L	3.964	10–20	µg/mL
Primidone	25–46	µmol/L	4.582	6–10	µg/mL
Procainamide	17–34[d]	µmol/L	4.249	4–8[d]	µg/mL
Quinidine	4.6–9.2	µmol/L	3.082	1.5–3	µg/mL
Theophylline	55–110	µmol/L	5.55	10–20	µg/mL
Tobramycin[a]	—	—	—	6–10[b]; <2[c]	µg/mL
Valproic acid	300–700	µmol/L	6.934	50–100	µg/mL
Vancomycin[a]	—	—	—	25–40[b]; <10[c]	µg/mL

[a]Aminoglycosides (amikacin, gentamicin, netilmicin, tobramycin) and vancomycin are not reported in SI units because of the variability of their molecular weights.
[b]Peak drug level.
[c]Trough drug level.
[d]Drug level reported as the total of the parent drug and its active metabolite.

INTERNATIONAL SYSTEM OF UNITS

In an attempt to standardize the large number of different units used worldwide and thus improve communication, the Système International d'Unités (International System of Units [SI]) was recommended in 1954. In 1971, the mole (mol) was adopted as the standard for designating the amount of substance present, and the liter (L) was adopted as the standard for designating volume. The World Health Organization recommended the adoption of SI units in 1977. However, Canada had already implemented an equivalent system in 1971.

In the area of therapeutics, the major change caused by adopting the SI was to express drug concentrations present in body fluids in molar units (e.g., mmol/L) rather than in mass units (e.g., mg/L). This allows a better comparison between the pharmacologic and pharmacodynamic effects of different drugs, since these properties are relative to the number of molecules (e.g., mmol) of drug present rather than to the number of mass units (e.g., mg).

DRUG SERUM CONCENTRATIONS

Many drugs have known therapeutic or toxic levels that are monitored in patients to ensure safety and efficacy. In Canada, clinical laboratories report these levels in SI units. Levels traditionally reported as milligrams per milliliter (mg/mL) can be converted to millimoles per liter (mmol/L) using the conversion factor (CF) for that specific drug:

$$CF = 1000/\text{molecular weight of the drug}$$

To convert from micrograms per milliliter to SI units, the following equation is used:

$$\mu g/mL \times CF = \mu mol/L$$

To convert from SI units to micrograms per milliliter, the following equation is used:

$$(\mu mol/L)/CF = \mu g/mL$$

Table A.1 shows some important drugs for which therapeutic or toxic levels have been established. For most of these drugs, the levels presented are trough (minimum) values, which are measured in blood samples drawn just prior to the next dose. For the aminoglycosides and vancomycin, two levels are listed: a trough level and a peak (maximum) level. Levels must remain between the peak and trough to ensure efficacy of these drugs and at the same time to minimize toxicity.

REFERENCES

Bachynsky J: Nonprescription drugs in health care. In *Nonprescription Drug Reference for Health Professionals*. Ottawa: Canadian Pharmaceutical Association, 1996.
Canada Vigilance Program web site: http://www.hc-sc.gc.ca/dhp-mps/medeff/vigilance-eng.php
Cannabis Act (S.C. 2018, c. 16)

Controlled Drugs and Substances Act (S.C. 1996, c. 19).

Evans WE, Schentag JJ, Jusko WJ (eds): *Applied Pharmacokinetics: Principles of Therapeutic Drug Monitoring.* Spokane, WA: Applied Therapeutics, Inc., 1992.

Food and Drugs Act (R.S.C., 1985, c. F-27).

Forward Regulatory Plan 2019-2021: Regulations Amending the Patented Medicines Regulations web site: https://www.canada.ca/en/health-canada/corporate/about-health-canada/legislation-guidelines/acts-regulations/forward-regulatory-plan/plan/patented-medicines.html.

Health Protection and Drug Laws. Ottawa: Health and Welfare Canada, Canadian Publishing Center, 1988.

Health Protection Branch: Information Newsletter No. 798, 1991.

Johnson GE, Hannah KJ, Zerr SR: *Pharmacology and the Nursing Process*, 3rd ed. Philadelphia: WB Saunders, 1992.

Mailhot R: The Canadian drug regulatory process. *J Clin Pharmacol* 26:232, 1986.

McLeod DC: SI units in drug therapeutics. *Drug Intell Clin Pharm* 22:990, 1988.

National Association of Pharmacy Regulatory Authorities web site: www.napra.ca.

Subcommittee of Metric Commission Canada, Sector 9.10: SI Manual in Health Care, 2nd ed. Ottawa: Health and Welfare Canada, 1982.

Sullivan P: CMA to support increased patent protection for drugs but will attach strong qualifications. *CMAJ* 147:1669, 1992.

INDEX

Note: Page numbers followed by "f" refer to illustrations; page numbers followed by "t" refer to tables; page numbers followed by "b" refer to boxes.